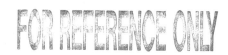

Werner & Ingbar's

THE THYROID

A Fundamental and Clinical Text

Ninth Edition

Werner & Ingbar's

THE THYROID

A Fundamental and Clinical Text

Ninth Edition

Editors

LEWIS E. BRAVERMAN, MD

Professor of Medicine
Boston University School of Medicine
Chief, Section of Endocrinology, Diabetes, and Nutrition
Department of Medicine
Boston Medical Center
Boston, Massachusetts

ROBERT D. UTIGER, MD

Clinical Professor of Medicine
Harvard Medical School
Boston, Massachusetts

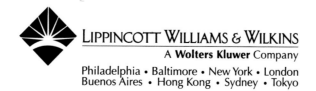

LIPPINCOTT WILLIAMS & WILKINS
A **Wolters Kluwer** Company
Philadelphia • Baltimore • New York • London
Buenos Aires • Hong Kong • Sydney • Tokyo

Acquisitions Editor: Lisa McAllister
Developmental Editor: Jenny Kim
Project Manager: David Murphy
Manufacturing Manager: Benjamin Rivera
Marketing Manager: Angela Panetta
Production Services: Print Matters, Inc.
Compositor: Compset, Inc.
Printer: Courier

© 2005 by LIPPINCOTT WILLIAMS & WILKINS
530 Walnut Street
Philadelphia, PA 19106 USA
LWW.com

Library of Congress Cataloging-in-Publication Data

Werner & Ingbar's the thyroid : a fundamental and clinical text / editors, Lewis E.
    Braverman, Robert D. Utiger.—9th ed.
       p. ; cm.
    Includes bibliographical references and index.
    ISBN 0-7817-5047-4 (HC)
    1. Thyroid gland—Diseases. 2. Thyroid gland—Physiology. I. Title: Werner
and Ingbar's the thyroid. II. Title: Thyroid. III. Werner, Sidney C. IV. Ingbar,
Sidney H. V. Braverman, Lewis E., 1929– VI. Utiger, Robert D.
    [DNLM: 1. Thyroid Diseases. 2. Thyroid Gland—physiology. WK 200
W492 2004]
    RC655.W39 2004
    616.4′4—dc22

                                                                        2004056722

10 9 8 7 6 5 4 3 2

CONTENTS

Section D. Management of Thyrotoxicosis

PART V. THYROID DISEASES: HYPOTHYROIDISM

Section A. Introduction

Section B. Causes of Hypothyroidism

Section C. Organ System Manifestations of Hypothyroidism

PREFACE TO THE NINTH EDITION

The first edition of the *The Thyroid,* published in 1955, was the culmination of the vision of Sidney Werner that there was a need for a comprehensive textbook of thyroidology and of his efforts to meet that need. The continued success of the book has confirmed the wisdom of his vision. As knowledge about the thyroid gland, its physiology, and its diseases has expanded, the scope and size of the book have increased substantially. We like to think that *The Thyroid* has become a standard textbook of the biochemistry and physiology of the thyroid gland and the pathophysiology, clinical manifestations, and treatment of thyroid disease.

Sidney Werner's vision and skill in creating the book and developing its basic organization of multiple chapters, each written by an expert, was undoubtedly responsible for its rapid acceptance. This basic organization has changed little from what he created, although chapters and subchapters about particular topics have been added, and subtracted, in later editions.

Dr. Werner, who died in 1994, not only conceived the book but also guided it through its first two editions. He was joined by Dr. Sidney H. Ingbar as co-editor for the third and fourth editions, after which he stepped down as editor. Dr. Ingbar's role continued through the fifth edition, which was completed 2 years before his untimely death in 1988.

The creation of this book was just one of Dr. Werner's many contributions to thyroidology. Long interested in Graves' disease, he carried out many of the early studies of the therapeutic efficacy and side effects of radioiodine therapy for Graves' thyrotoxicosis, and was one of the first to question whether it was a pituitary disease, as many had thought. He was responsible for the first system for classifying the ocular manifestations of Graves' disease, and he carried out many studies of the pathogenesis and therapy of Graves' ophthalmopathy. He was a long-time member of the American Thyroid Association, a member of its board of directors from 1968 to 1974, and its president in 1973. In short, he was a leader in the field of thyroidology for many years.

Dr. Ingbar was equally accomplished. He was at the forefront of thyroid research for over 40 years, and his studies spanned all of thyroidology. He made seminal contributions to our understanding of the mechanisms of action of thyroid hormone, the physiology of thyroid hormone secretion, the transport and metabolism of thyroid hormones, the mechanisms of action of antithyroid drugs, and the diagnosis and treatment of virtually every thyroid disease. He too was a long-time member of the American Thyroid Association, a member of its Board of Directors from 1971 to 1975, and president in 1976.

In his preface to the first edition, which is reprinted on the following pages, Dr. Werner commented that the book "is intended for those who must deal with the problems of thyroid function and thyroid disease in man." That has been our intention as well. To be more specific, we want the book to be useful to anyone who is interested in any aspect of the thyroid gland and of its products and their actions, in both health and disease. This includes not only clinicians and investigators, but also research and clinical fellows just entering the field, and maybe even younger students at the time of their first exposure to thyroidology.

This ninth edition of *The Thyroid* owes much to its predecessors, but it has been changed, too. Authorship has become more international. There are new chapters, and some old ones are missing, their contents incorporated into related chapters. As in the past, we have tried to minimize overlap among different chapters, but some is inevitable and probably essential. For example, the topics of iodine metabolism and the effects of iodine deficiency and excess on thyroid function are so central to any understanding of the thyroid gland and its diseases, and yet so diverse, that they must be considered in many chapters. The same is true for the actions of thyroid hormone, and to the many different yet related aspects of thyroid autoimmunity.

Research into the thyroid gland and its disorders has flourished in recent years, as a result of application of a wide array of new research methods, from those of molecular biology to those of clinical trials and meta-analysis. We know much more about the mechanisms of action of thyroid hormone and the metabolism of thyroid hormones than just a few years ago. The genes for the transporters and enzymes involved in thyroid iodine metabolism and thyroid hormone production have been cloned. Studies of these and other previously cloned thyroid-related genes (e.g., those of the thyrotropin receptor and thyroglobulin) have provided much new knowledge about both normal and abnormal physiology. With respect to the common thyroid diseases, iodine deficiency is still the most common, and we have the knowledge if not the will to eradicate it. The success of programs for screening newborn infants for hypothyroidism is surely a major triumph, and the continued expansion of these programs has the potential to eliminate the most common treatable cause of mental retardation. We still know little about the pathogenesis of the thyroid autoimmune diseases or thyroid nodular disease, but even in these areas advances are being made with regularity. For example, it is now possible to induce something very similar to Graves' disease in animals, and one cannot help but think that this will lead to much greater understanding of, and hopefully also treatment for, the disease itself.

We wish to thank all the contributors to the book. Their charge was to ensure that their chapters are current and comprehensive, and to provide interpretation and guidance in areas of controversy. We have tried to guide but not dictate to them. We also wish to thank Mr. Brian Brown and Ms. Jenny Kim of Lippincott Williams and Wilkins for their encouragement and assistance in the production of the book.

In this era of ready access to many small packets of information, we think there is a need for comprehensive review and evaluation of what is known and what is not known—in other words, a book, and it has been our goal to provide this review and evaluation. We hope this new edition of *The Thyroid* will match up with the preceding ones, and that it will provide guidance and even inspiration to those who seek to increase understanding of the thyroid gland and to treat or prevent its diseases.

Lewis E. Braverman
Robert D. Utiger

PREFACE TO THE FIRST EDITION

This book is intended for those who must deal with the problems of thyroid function and thyroid disease in man. It is designed for use in the clinic and in the basic science laboratory connected with the clinic. The information made available has been brought together from widely diverse sources, and in some instances is reported here for the first time. Many subjects have been presented both in broad outline and in more comprehensive detail to meet differing requirements. It has been planned to provide sufficient documentation to satisfy most needs and, for more exhaustive requirements, to provide a bibliography adequate enough to initiate a search of the literature.

The introduction of a book into a field of clinical medicine today requires considerable justification. In the thyroid field particularly, there already is a profusion of books including the almost classic works of Means in this country and of Joll in England, recently and capably revised by Rundle. Nevertheless, the recent growth of medical knowledge in general, and about the thyroid in particular, appears to have created need for a new volume constructed on a somewhat different basis from those of previous works.

Barry Wood has compared the growth of medical information to that of bacteria. Bacteria show a lag at the beginning of growth and then multiply at a logarithmic rate. Wood considers the growth of current-day medicine to have reached the logarithmic phase. The accumulation of data about the thyroid provides a good example of this acceleration. One author of a recent review claims to have unearthed 3,000 new references pertaining to the gland and published during the single year before he wrote his article. *The Quarterly Cumulative Index Medicus* offers about 7,800 references to the thyroid in the past decade. More than this, the thyroid field is permeated by contributions from the cardiologist, neurologist, muscle physiologist, and many others, bringing the highly unique techniques of their particular specialties to bear on the subject.

It is evident that the ability of any one individual to follow progress in all directions at once has all but vanished. As a consequence, marked subspecialization of interest has developed and advances have come to depend upon the interchange of information among many specialist, each providing his own orientation. This trend has suggested that the information in a book about the healthy and diseased thyroid should also be subjected to the process of sifting

and appraising through many eyes. The various specialists present material with which they have had direct experience, and the editor functions as the overseer to provide orientation and preserve the inherent orderliness of the entire subject. The total clinical and research experience made available in this way exceeds that of one person alone. Each topic can be subjected to the critique of a man who has worked intensively with the problem. Finally, a book of this sort can be readily kept current, because of the authors' continued contact with investigation and the fact that there are no large sections to be rewritten by any one individual.

Every effort has been made to make available sufficient basic and clinical knowledge to satisfy curiosity about either of these aspects. For example, sections on the fundamental properties of radioiodine that permit the use of the isotope and on the instrumentation that facilitates such use are presented as well as a discussion of the clinical application. Most basic sections are separated from the clinical material, but are incorporated with it where this has seemed reasonable.

The fundamental aspects of thyroid function is man and the mechanisms which control the activity of the gland; the biochemistry of the hormone; and histology and comparative anatomy make up Part I. The mechanisms of action of the antithyroid drugs are included because of the intimate relationship of their effects to the problems of basic physiology.

Part II presents the laboratory methods which supplement the clinical appraisal of thyroid secretory activity. The presentations of the basic principles involved in radioiodine usage and the instrumentation which is employed are included within the laboratory section and are available here for later reference when the therapeutic as well as diagnostic use of the isotope are considered.

The diseases of the thyroid are considered in Part III. The disorders first described are those in which the level of thyroid hormone in the circulation and tissues is within normal limits—euthyroidism. After this come the derangements in which hormone levels are increased—toxic goiter or hyperthyroidism—or decreased—hypothyroidism or myxedema. The effects of hyperthyroidism and of hypothyroidism upon the individual body systems have been subjected to fairly detailed analysis.

The plan to arrange disease by functional categories breaks down in relation to inflammation of the thyroid including the peculiar composite entity, chronic thyroiditis. Inflammations of the thyroid tend to inactivate the gland but chronic thyroiditis is almost as often associated with evidence of hyperthyroidism as with hypothyroidism. The inflammations have been placed under a separate heading on this account.

Before the disease states are presented, several important preliminary subjects are considered in Part III. The normal and abnormal developments of the gland are described, together with the surgical anatomy and a method of physical examination that is an essential procedure because of the accessibility of the thyroid to this approach. The pathology is presented in its entirety in the introductory sections and is not dispersed among the various diseases. A concept of change in thyroid disease emerges in this way which could not otherwise become evident.

A major goal throughout the volume has been to assess the validity of the facts on which current information or procedure is based. Corroborative information is often documented beyond reasonable doubt, but too often is based only on speculation or custom or is wanting altogether. The fact that a critical appraisal has been accomplished is a tribute to the contributors. The world today, as in the past, is threatened by prejudice, of which racial, social, and economic prejudices are but a few. Equally influential, but less well recognized, is the prejudice of "experience," derived from uncritical or uncontrolled observation, from the word of an "authority," or from emotional bias.* Fortunately there are those who are willing to give time and effort to seek out and correct such distortions of the truth.

Considerable aid has come to the editor from several sources. Dr. John Stanbury has been particularly helpful. The members of the Thyroid Clinic at the Presbyterian Hospital need recognition for their influence upon the formulation of many of the views presented herein. Credit must be given to the patience and forbearance of the many contributors who tolerated changes in style and length of manuscript in the interest of creating an integrated volume out of a series of individual essays. The editor's wife has acted as guardian of clarity, upon the thesis that even the layman should be able to read and understand a well-written article. Miss Anne Powell, of the librarian staff at P. & S., was extremely generous with her time. Finally, Mrs. R. Levine and Mrs. K. Sorenson were more than patient with the secretarial details.

Sidney C. Werner
New York City

---

*"Conviction is by no means devoid of emotion but is a disciplined and differentiated emotion, pointed to the removal of a realistic obstacle. By contrast, the emotion behind prejudice is diffused and overgeneralized, saturating unrelated objects."—Gordon W. Allport: *The Nature of Prejudice.*

CONTRIBUTORS

Mubarak Al-Gahtany, MD   Division of Neurosurgery, Department of Surgery, King Khalid University, and Consultant Neurosurgeon, Department of Neurosurgery, Asir Central Hospital, Abha, Saudi Arabia

Mubarak M. Al-Shraim, MD   Department of Laboratory Medicine and Pathobiology, King Khalid University, Abha, Saudi Arabia, and Department of Laboratory Medicine and Pathobiology, St. Michel's Hospital, Toronto, Ontario, Canada

Peter Arvan, MD, PhD   Department of Internal Medicine, University of Michigan, Ann Arbor, MI

Zubair Wahid Baloch, MD, PhD   Department of Pathology and Laboratory Medicine, University of Pennsylvania, and Academic Pathologist, Department of Pathology and Laboratory Medicine, University of Pennsylvania Medical Center, Philadelphia, PA

Michael Bauer, MD, PhD   Department of Psychiatry and Psychotherapy, University Medicine, Charité-University Medicine, Berlin, Germany

Robert M. Beazley, MD   Department of Surgical Oncology, Boston Medical Center, Boston, MA

Paolo Beck-Peccoz, MD   Institute of Endocrine Sciences, University of Milan, and Department of Endocrinology, IRCCS Ospedale Maggiore, Milan, Italy

Geoffrey J. Beckett, BSc, PhD, FRCPath   Department of Clinical Biochemistry, University of Edinburgh, and Consultant Clinical Scientist, Department of Clinical Biochemistry, Edinburgh Royal Infirmary, Edinburgh, United Kingdom

Finn Noe Bennedbaek, MD, PhD   Department of Endocrinology and Metabolism, Odense University Hospital, Odense, Denmark

Salvatore Benvenga, MD   Department of Clinical Experimental Medicine and Pharmacology, University of Messina School of Medicine, and Head, Program of Molecular and Clinical Endocrinology, Azienda Ospedaliera Universitaria, Policlinico Gaetano Martino, Messina, Italy

Antonio C. Bianco, MD, PhD   Department of Medicine, and Director of Research, Thyroid Section, Division of Endocrinology, Diabetes and Hypertension, Harvard Medical School, Boston, MA

Rosalind S. Brown, MD   Division of Endocrinology, Department of Pediatrics, Harvard Medical School, and Children's Hospital, Boston, MA

Albert G. Burger, MD   Thyroid Unit, Hospital Cantonal Universitaire, Geneva, Switzerland

Nancy Carrasco, MD   Department of Molecular Pharmacology, Albert Einstein College of Medicine, Yeshiva University, Bronx, NY

Vivian Cody, PhD   Department of Structural Biology, Hauptman-Woodward Medical Research Institute, Buffalo, NY

Ronald N. Cohen, MD   Division of Endocrinology, Department of Medicine, University of Chicago School of Medicine, Chicago, IL

David S. Cooper, MD   Johns Hopkins School of Medicine, and Director, Division of Endocrinology, Sinai Hospital of Baltimore, Baltimore, MD

Sabine Costagliola, PhD   Institut de Recherche Interdisciplinaire, Free University of Brussels, Brussels, Belgium

Gilbert J. Cote, PhD   Department of Endocrine Neoplasia and Hormonal Disorders, M.D. Anderson Cancer Center, Houston, TX

Sara Danzi, PhD   Division of Endocrinology, North Shore–Long Island Jewish Research Institute, Manhasset, NY

Terry F. Davies, MD   Division of Endocrinology and Metabolism, Department of Medicine, Mount Sinai Medical Center, New York, NY

Jan J.M. de Vijlder, PhD   Department of Pediatric Endocrinology, Academic Medical Center, Amsterdam, The Netherlands

François M. Delange, MD, PhD   International Council for Control of Iodine Deficiency Disorders, University of Brussels, and Honorary Head of Clinics, Department of Pediatrics, Hospital Saint Pierre, Brussels Belgium

A. Jane Dickinson, MB ChB, MRCP, FRCOphth   School of Neurology, Neurobiology, and Psychiatry (Ophthalmology), University of Newcastle upon Tyne, and Consultant Oculoplastic and Orbital Surgeon, Eye Department, Royal Victoria Infirmary, Newcastle upon Tyne, United Kingdom

Bruno Di Jeso, MD   Laboratorio di Patologia Generale, Dipartimento di Fisiche e Naturali, Universit degli Studi di Lecce, Lecce, Italy

Robert G. Dluhy, MD   Department of Medicine, Harvard University, and Associate Director, Division of Endocrinology, Diabetes and Hypertension, Brigham and Women's Hospital, Boston, MA

*John T. Dunn, MD   Department of Health Sciences, University of Virginia, Charlottesville, VA

James A. Fagin, MD   Department of Medicine, University of Cincinnati, and Director, Division of Endocrinology and Metabolism, University Hospital, Cincinnati, OH

Alan P. Farwell, MD   Division of Endocrinology and Metabolism, University of Massachusetts Medical Center, Worcester, MA

Vahab Fatourechi, MD   Department of Diabetes, Metabolism, and Nutrition, Mayo Clinic, Rochester, MN

Stephanie A. Fish, MD   Department of Medicine, University of Pennsylvania, Philadelphia, PA

Delbert A. Fisher, MD   Department of Pediatrics and Medicine, David Geffen School of Medicine at UCLA, Los Angeles, and Vice President of Science and Innovation, Quest Diagnostics, Nichols Institute, San Juan Capistrano, CA

Jayne A. Franklyn, MD, PhD   Department of Medicine, Queen Elizabeth Hospital, Birmingham, United Kingdom

Dagmar Führer, III MD   Department of Medicine, University of Leipzig, Leipzig, Germany

Michael D. Gammage, MD, FRCP   Department of Medicine, Queen Elizabeth Hospital, Birmingham, United Kingdom

Robert F. Gagel, MD   Department of Endocrine Neoplasia and Hormonal Disorders, M.D. Anderson Cancer Center, Houston, TX

David F. Gardner, MD   Department of Medicine, Virginia Commonwealth University School of Medicine, Richmond, VA

Neil J.L. Gittoes, BSc, PhD, FRCP   Department of Medicine, Division of Medical Sciences, University of Birmingham, Birmingham, United Kingdom

Daniel Glinoer, MD, PhD   School of Medicine, Free University of Brussels, and Chief of Endocrinology, Department of Internal Medicine, Hospital Saint Pierre, Brussels, Belgium

Loukas Gourgiotis, MD   Clinical Endocrinology Branch, National Institute of Diabetes, Digestive, and Kidney Diseases, National Institutes of Health, Bethesda, MD

Cheryl E. Hanna, MD   Department of Pediatrics, Oregon Health and Science University, Portland, OR

Laszlo Hegedüs, MD   Department of Endocrinology, Odense University Hospital, Odense, Denmark

James V. Hennessey, MD   Rhode Island Hospital, Brown University, Providence, RI

Ad R. Hermus, MD, PhD   Department of Endocrinology, Radboud University Medical Center, Nijmegen, The Netherlands

Jerome M. Hershman, MD   Endocrinology Division, VA Medical Center–West Los Angeles, Los Angeles, CA

Ana O. Hoff, MD   Department of Endocrine Neoplasia and Hormonal Disorders, University of Texas M.D. Anderson Cancer Center, Houston, TX

Anthony N. Hollenberg, MD   Division of Endocrinology, Department of Medicine, Beth Israel Deaconess Medical Center, Boston, MA

Eva Horvath, PhD   Department of Pathology, St. Michael's Hospital and University of Toronto, Toronto, Ontario, Canada

Stephen A. Huang, MD   Division of Endocrinology, Children's Hospital, Boston, MA

Dyde A. Huysmans, MD, PhD   Department of Endocrinology, Catharina Hospital, Eindhoven, The Netherlands

David H. Ingbar, MD   Director of the Pulmonary Allergy and Critical Care Division, Department of Medicine Physiology and Pediatrics, University of Minnesota, and Medical Director, Medical ICU and

*Deceased.

Respiratory Care, Fairview University Medical Center, Minneapolis, MN

Michael M. Kaplan, MD   Associated Endocrinologists, Bloomfield, MI

Elaine M. Kaptein, MD   Department of Medicine, University of Southern California, Los Angeles, CA

Pat Kendall-Taylor, MD, FRCP   Department of Endocrinology, University of Newcastle, Newcastle-on-Tyne, United Kingdom

Irwin L. Klein, MD   Department of Medicine and Cell Biology, New York University School of Medicine, New York, NY, and Chief, Division of Endocrinology, North Shore University Hospital, Manhasset, NY

Richard T. Kloos, MD   Departments of Medicine and Radiology, Ohio State University, Columbus, OH

Peter Kopp, MD   Division of Endocrinology, Metabolism and Molecular Medicine, Northwestern University, and Northwestern Memorial Hospital, Chicago, IL

Kalman C. Kovacs, MD   Department of Pathology, St. Michael's Hospital, Toronto, Ontario, Canada

Gerasimos E. Krassas, MD   Department of Endocrinology, Diabetes and Metabolism, Panagia General Hospital, Thessaloniki, Greece

Knut Krohn III, MD   Department of Medicine and Interdisciplinary Center for Clinical Research, University of Leipzig, Leipzig, Germany

Paul W. Ladenson, MD   Division of Endocrinology and Metabolism, Johns Hopkins University, and Director, Division of Endocrinology and Metabolism, Johns Hopkins Hospital, Baltimore, MD

Stephen H. LaFranchi, MD   Department of Pediatrics, Oregon Health and Science University, and Staff Physician, Department of Pediatrics, Doernbecher Children's Hospital, Portland, OR

P. Reed Larsen, MD   Thyroid Division, Department of Medicine, Brigham and Women's Hospital, Harvard Institute of Medicine, Boston, MA

John H. Lazarus, MA, MD, FRCP, FACE   Department of Endocrine and Diabetic Sciences, Cardiff University, University Hospital of Wales, and Consultant Physician, Department of Medicine, Llandough Hospital, Cardiff, United Kingdom

Virginia A. LiVolsi, MD   Department of Pathology and Laboratory Medicine, University of Pennsylvania, and Pathologist, Department of Pathology and Laboratory

Medicine, University of Pennsylvania Medical Center, Philadelphia, PA

Susan J. Mandel, MD   Department of Medicine, University of Pennsylvania School of Medicine, and Associate Chief for Clinical Affairs, Division of Endocrinology, Diabetes, and Metabolism, Hospital of the University of Pennsylvania, Philadelphia, PA

Claudio Marcocci, MD   Department of Endocrinology and Metabolism, University of Pisa, Pisa, Italy

Michele Marinò, MD   Department of Endocrinology, University of Pisa, Pisa, Italy

Ellen Marqusee, MD   Thyroid Division, Harvard Medical School, and Associate Physician, Brigham and Women's Hospital, Boston, MA

Enio Martino, MD   Department of Endocrinology and Metabolism, University of Pisa, Pisa, Italy

Ernest L. Mazzaferri, MD   Department of Medicine, University of Florida, and Staff Physician, Department of Medicine/Endocrinology, Shands Hospital, Gainesville, FL

I. Ross McDougall, MD   Division of Nuclear Medicine, Department of Radiology, Stanford University School of Medicine, Stanford, CA

Christoph A. Meier, MD   Laboratory of Molecular Endocrinology, Department of Cellular Physiology and Metabolism, University Medical Center, and Head, Endocrine Unit, Department of Internal Medicine, University Hospital of Geneva, Geneva, Switzerland

Ralf Paschke, MD   Medical Clinic and Poliklinik III, University of Leipzig, Leipzig, Germany

Elizabeth N. Pearce, MD   Department of Medicine, Boston University School of Medicine, and Section of Endocrinology, Diabetes, and Nutrition, Boston Medical Center, Boston, MA

Simon H.S. Pearce, MD   Institute of Human Genetics, Newcastle University, and Honorary Consultant Physician, Endocrine Unit, Royal Victoria Infirmary, Newcastle upon Tyne, United Kingdom

Petros Perros, MD   Endocrine Unit, Freeman Hospital, Newcastle upon Tyne, United Kingdom

Luca Persani, MD, PhD   Institute of Endocrine Sciences, University of Milan, Milan, Italy, and Head, Laboratory of Experimental Endocrinology, IRCCS Istituto Auxologico Italiano, Cusano Milanino, Italy

Aldo Pinchera, MD   Department of Endocrinology, University of Pisa, Pisa, Italy

H. Lester Reed, MD Department of Medicine, University of Auckland, South Auckland Clinical School, and Clinical Director, Centre Clinical Research and Effective Practice, Middlemore Hospital, Auckland, New Zealand

Samuel Refetoff, MD University of Chicago, Chicago, IL

Elaine Ron, PhD Department of Medicine, Radiation Epidemiology Branch, Division of Cancer Epidemiology and Genetics, National Cancer Institute, National Institutes of Health, Bethesda, MD

Douglas S. Ross, MD Harvard Medical School, and Co-Director, Thyroid Associates, Massachusetts General Hospital, Boston, MA

Elio Roti, MD Cattedra Endocrinologia, University of Parma, Parma, Italy

Joshua D. Safer, MD Section of Endocrinology, Department of Medicine, Boston University School of Medicine, Boston, MA

Pilar Santisteban, MD, PhD Department of Molecular Endocrinology, Instituto de Investigaciones Biomédicas "Alberto Sols," Consejo Superior de Investigaciones Científicas, Universidad Autónoma de Madrid, Madrid, Spain.

Nicholas J. Sarlis, MD, PhD Department of Endocrine Neoplasia and Hormonal Disorders, University of Texas–M.D. Anderson Cancer Center, Houston, TX

***Clark T. Sawin, MD** Department of Veterans Affairs, Office of the Medical Inspector, Veterans Administration, Washington, DC

Arthur B. Schneider, MD, PhD Department of Medicine, and Chief, Section of Endocrinology and Metabolism, University of Illinois College of Medicine, Chicago, IL

Joseph H. Sellin, MD Division of Gastroenterology, University of Texas Medical Branch, Galveston, TX

Michael C. Sheppard, MD, PhD Department of Medicine, University of Birmingham School of Medicine, and Consultant Endocrinologist, Department of Medicine, Queen Elizabeth Hospital, Birmingham, United Kingdom

J. Enrique Silva, MD Department of Medicine and Physiology, McGill University Faculty of Medicine, and Chief, Division of Endocrinology and Metabolism, Department of Medicine, Sir Mortimer B. Davis Jewish General Hospital, Montreal, Quebec, Canada

Peter A. Singer, MD Department of Medicine, USC Keck School of Medicine, Los Angeles, CA

Peter J. Snyder, MD Department of Medicine, University of Pennsylvania, Philadelphia, PA

Stephen W. Spaulding, MD VA Medical Center, Buffalo, NY

Carole Ann Spencer, PhD Department of Medicine, University of Southern California, Los Angeles, CA

Anthony D. Toft, BSc, MD Endocrine Clinic, Royal Infirmary, Edinburgh, United Kingdom

Apostolos G. Vagenakis, MD Department of Internal Medicine, University of Patras Medical School, Patras, Greece

Guy Van Vliet, MD Department of Pediatrics, Hôpital Sainte Justine, Montreal, Quebec, Canada

Mark P.J. Vanderpump, MD Department of Endocrinology, Royal Free and University College Medical School, and Consultant Physician, Department of Endocrinology, Royal Free Hapsted NHS Trust, London, United Kingdom

Gilbert Vassart, MD, PhD Institut de Recherche Interdisciplinaire, Free University of Brussels, and Chief, Department of Medical Genetics, Hôpital Erasme, Brussels, Belgium

Rena Vassilopoulou-Sellin, MD Department of Endocrinology, M.D. Anderson Cancer Center, Houston, TX

Thomas Vulsma, MD Department of Pediatric Endocrinology, Academic Medical Center, Amsterdam, The Netherlands

Leonard Wartofsky, MD, MPH Department of Anatomy, Physiology and Genetics, Uniformed Services University of Healthy Sciences, Professor of Medicine, Georgetown University School of Medicine, and Chairman, Department of Medicine, Washington Hospital Center, Washington, DC

Sanjeev M. Wasan, MD Division of Gastroenterology, Department of Medicine, University of Texas Medical School, Houston, TX

Anthony P. Weetman, MD, DSc The Medical School, University of Sheffield, and Honorary Consultant, Department of Endocrinology, Northern General Hospital, Sheffield, United Kingdom

Peter C. Whybrow, MD Neuropsychiatric Institute, Department of Psychiatry and Biobehavioral Sciences, UCLA, and Physician-in-Chief, UCLA Neuropsychiatric Hospital, Los Angeles, CA

---

*Deceased.

Wilmar M. Wiersinga, MD, PhD Department of Internal Medicine, University of Amsterdam, and Chief Department of Endocrinology and Metabolism, Academic Medical Center, Amsterdam, The Netherlands

Kenneth A. Woeber, MD, FRCPE Department of Medicine, University of California at San Francisco, and Clinical Chief, Division of Endocrinology and Metabolism, UCSF Medical Center, San Francisco, CA

Frederic E. Wondisford, MD Section of Endocrinology, Department of Medicine, University of Chicago School of Medicine, Chicago, IL

Paul M. Yen, MD Department of Medicine, Johns Hopkins University School of Medicine, and Endocrine Division, Department of Medicine, Johns Hopkins Bayview Medical Center, Baltimore, MD

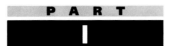

PART I

THE NORMAL THYROID

HISTORY, DEVELOPMENT, ANATOMY

1

THE HERITAGE OF THE THYROID: A BRIEF HISTORY

CLARK T. SAWIN

The occurrence of goiter was no surprise to Europeans 2 millennia ago, especially to those living in the Alps (1). They did not know, however, that goiter was related to the thyroid gland, or that the thyroid gland existed (2). The ancient Greeks called the goitrous swelling in the neck a *bronchocele* ("tracheal outpouch"); the name was still used in the 19th century, despite the fact that the thyroid gland had been discovered and named 200 years earlier (Fig. 1.1).

The thyroid gland had not been identified as a discrete entity until the Renaissance and the expansion of inquiry into the human body. Leonardo da Vinci probably found it by about 1500, and Vesalius definitely knew about it in 1543 (although he used the term *laryngeal glands* for the entire gland we now know as the thyroid gland). By the early 1600s, anatomists definitely identified the thyroid gland in humans and realized that its enlargement caused swelling in the neck, as documented by Fabricius in 1619. The modem name arose in 1656, when Thomas Wharton called it the thyroid gland, after the Greek for "shield-shaped," not by virtue of its own shape, but because of the shape of the nearby thyroid cartilage (3).

Alpine travelers' observations of cretinism, a thyroid-linked disorder, can be traced to the 13th century, but clinically relevant descriptions appeared only in the 16th century, when Paracelsus (c. 1527) and Platter (in 1562) made the connection between goiter and cretinism (4).

This was the extent of our knowledge of thyroid physiology and disease until the 19th century. Until then, medical theories behind disease causation were humorally based. An imbalance of the four humors (blood, phlegm, bile, and black bile) caused illness. Some thought that goiter was caused by an excess of phlegm. Treatment was empiric, however, and not based on the theoretical cause. Numerous remedies for goiter were proposed; some were complex mixtures of seaweed and marine sponge. These aquatic substances were well known in medieval Europe and had been used to treat goiter a thousand years earlier in China (some historians believe that the Europeans may have learned of these substances from the Chinese indirectly via traders).

Courtois discovered iodine in the residue of burnt seaweed in about 1812 as an indirect consequence of the British blockade of French ports during the Napoleonic wars. Subsequently, Coindet, an Edinburgh-trained physician working among goitrous people in Geneva, Switzerland, considered iodine to be the active ingredient of the empiric therapies for goiter. In 1820, he gave iodine, mostly as the potassium salt, to patients with goiter, after which their goiters shrank remarkably (5). To his chagrin, he also saw major toxic effects in some patients (not his own) who took too much of the astonishing remedy, which consequently fell into disfavor. Still, iodine continued to be

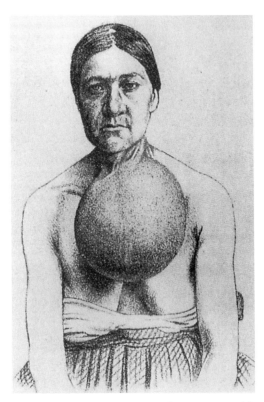

FIGURE 1.1. Large goiter in a woman from an area with a high rate of endemic goiter (Bern, Switzerland). The woman was a patient of the Bern surgeon E. Theodor Kocher, a Nobel laureate. (From Kocher T. Zur Pathologic and Therapie des Kropfes. *Dtsch Z Chir* 1874;4:417, with permission.)

given for other disorders (6), such as scrofula, syphilis, and tuberculosis. Coindet had in fact discovered iodine-induced thyrotoxicosis , the cause of the major toxic effects he had seen; this was the earliest description of any form of thyrotoxicosis, although the true nature of the disorder was not recognized for several decades. Despite the controversy over the use of iodine in Geneva, the therapy represented a shift from an empiric, folk medicine to a rational treatment of a defined illness with a specific substance.

The use of iodine as a drug, even though it was effective at shrinking the goiter in many patients, by no means meant that practitioners knew that they were replacing a deficiency. For most of the 19th century, few accepted the idea that disease could be due to the lack of something. Although the use of iodine to prevent goiter was proposed in 1831—based on observations in Colombia, South America (7), and later in 1850 by Chatin, a Parisian pharmacist, botanist, and physician (8)—these suggestions were not in tune with the times, were not accepted by the practitioners of that era, and were put aside. Most believed that goiter must be due to something in the water—a toxin, a bacterium, or a parasite. The issue was not resolved until the early 20th century, when small amounts of iodine were found to prevent goiter in schoolgirls in Akron, Ohio (9).

Even then, there was no evidence that these girls were iodine deficient to begin with; the existence of iodine deficiency in certain areas of the United States was not proven for another decade or so.

What has happened since the 1920s is curiously reminiscent of the 19th century: iodine replacement never became widespread and was eventually abandoned because it was seen as toxic or irrational. This attitude resulted in continued goiter and the associated, but less common, cretinism. After the Akron experiment, the notion of deficiency was slowly becoming accepted, but iodine replacement would still not become widespread for decades. The lesson that iodine is a useful prophylaxis against, and therapy for, goiter and cretinism has still not been put into practice universally. Today, an international consortium (the International Council for the Control of Iodine Deficiency Disorders) attempts to ensure that all people receive sufficient amounts of iodine.

The thyroid dysfunctions we know as hypothyroidism and thyrotoxicosis were not thought to be thyroid diseases when described in the 19th century. There was instead a slow accumulation of clinical and physiologic evidence that gradually defined these conditions as we know them today.

Coindet was not the only one to describe thyrotoxicosis without realizing it. Parry, who saw spontaneous thyrotoxicosis before Coindet, but whose observations went unpublished until after his death (10) (and then in an obscure book published by one of his sons, rather than in a journal), saw a few patients with rapid heartbeat, goiter, and sometimes exophthalmos (exophthalmos was not described by Coindet). Parry thought that this constellation of signs represented some form of heart disease. A few years later, Graves described in his Meath Hospital lectures three women who seemed alike (they had goiter and palpitations). His published lectures (11) included a fourth patient who also had exophthalmos. This extra patient had been mentioned to him by his student, friend, and colleague Stokes. Both Graves and Stokes believed that the illness was cardiac. Graves' description was not widely known on the European continent, so when Basedow reported somewhat similar patients in 1840 (12), he was thought to be the first to describe the illness. As a result, many Europeans still use the term *Basedow's disease,* rather than *Graves' disease,* for what in fact should probably be called "Parry's disease." Even after Basedow's report, however, the goiter itself was not considered of much importance. The belief that the syndrome was of cardiac origin faded after about 1860, in part because of Charcot's emphasis on the nervousness of most patients (13); a neurologic hypothesis was then dominant for the rest of the 19th century. The disorder was still not thought to be a thyroid disease.

By the 1880s, surgeons were able to remove the goiters, at least partially, in these nervous, overactive patients without killing many of them, a clear change from 20 years before, when this surgery did in fact kill the majority of patients operated upon. Interestingly, the nervousness often disappeared in the survivors. This fact, plus the observation in the 1890s that too much thyroid extract led to similar nervousness and weight loss, brought a shift in thinking toward the thyroid origin of the syndrome. Only in reference to the 1890s and early 1900s can we really speak of thyrotoxicosis, because only then did the concept of an excessive amount of thyroid hormone come into existence as the cause of the syndrome. The concept was applied to both the spontaneous disease and the disease induced by administration of desiccated thyroid. Note that the term *thyrotoxicosis* is based on another idea of the 1890s, namely, that the thyroid gland in this syndrome either secretes or fails to inactivate a toxin (i.e., a deleterious substance not found in a normal person). The word is still in common use, but it does not reflect the actual pathophysiology, one cause of which is hyperthyroidism, an excess synthesis and secretion of thyroid hormone. The success of partial thyroidectomy over 100 years ago helped focus attention on the thyroid gland, eventually leading to the now more commonly used treatments, radioiodine (14,15) and antithyroid drugs (16).

Hypothyroidism as a clinical syndrome was recognized even later than hyperthyroidism, and at first its cause was equally obscure. First defined in London in the 1870s (17), what we call hypothyroidism was named *myxedema* because of the swollen skin *(edema)* and its excess content of mucin *(myx-)* (18). It was considered either a neurologic or a skin disease. There was no cure, and its course was inexorably progressive. There was only palliation with drugs such as pilocarpine, to be given in an attempt to reverse the patient's decreased sweating. At about the same time, in the latter part of the 19th century, it became evident that the same surgical skill that allowed thyrotoxic patients to survive thyroidectomy also permitted survival when a goiter was removed from patients who were not nervous or overactive. The ability to remove the entire thyroid gland, however, led to a peculiar and disastrous outcome: the patient lived but became puffy-faced, slow of mind, and socially nonfunctional (19, 20). Again, no one knew why, and there was no cure.

The Swiss, writing in German or French, and the English, writing in English, did not read each others' reports of this peculiar syndrome or this disastrous outcome, and so neither were aware of the other's work. That situation changed in 1883, when Felix Semon, an immigrant Prussian practicing laryngology in London, noted to others present at a meeting of the Clinical Society of London that the Swiss patients who had undergone total thyroidectomy seemed quite similar to the English ones with myxedema. Scoffed at, Semon persisted. The Society finally named a committee to investigate his observation. The report was not finished until 1888, 5 years later, and is now considered a classic (21).

The Committee found that cretinism, myxedema, and the Swiss postthyroidectomy changes all were the result of loss of the function of the thyroid body (21). Despite this major step in understanding, the report did not offer an ef-

fective therapy. In 1889, however, Brown-Séquard's work in Paris on the supposed rejuvenating effects of testicular extracts of dogs and guinea pigs (22) led to the use of extracts of other tissues as treatments for many disorders. Most extracts eventually proved to be ineffective, but the idea led indirectly to the successful and remarkable cure of myxedema (i.e., Murray's injection of sheep thyroid extract) in 1891 (23). A year later, the treatment was made even easier by simply eating, instead of injecting, ground or fried sheep thyroid, or tablets of dried thyroid tissue. This affirmation that Brown-Séquard's organotherapy was effective in at least one serious illness was the origin of modern endocrinology; this despite the fact that Murray was preceded in his discovery of a successful therapy by two Portuguese, Bettancourt and Serrano, who published, naturally enough, in a local Portuguese journal in Lisbon, but which was completely unknown to Murray. It was another example of simultaneous discovery.

Nevertheless, no one knew just what it was in thyroid extract that made it work, even though the therapy was extended in 1894 to the treatment of goiter (24). [The 15th century Chinese may have used the same therapy for goiter on the basis of "like treating like" (25).] A vigorous search for the "active principle" then took place, but no one found anything helpful until 1895, when Baumann, to his great surprise, found iodine in the thyroid gland (26). Twenty years later, Kendall at the Mayo Clinic, using iodine as a marker for the isolation of the active substance, succeeded in isolating bioactive crystalline material on Christmas Day, 1914 (27). He and his associate, Osterberg, named it *thyroxin* while waiting for a train. The name was a contraction of *thyroxyindole,* and stemmed from Kendall's erroneous belief that the compound had an indole nucleus with three iodine atoms per molecule. He never changed his ideas, despite his repeated failure to synthesize an active molecule based on his presumed structure, and was much disappointed when, in 1926, an Englishman, Harington, not only found the correct structure, but found that it had four (not three) iodine atoms per molecule (28). Harington, to Kendall's greater chagrin, then synthesized it (29). Harington also added an *e* to the name and called it *thyroxine* to fit the convention at the time for naming amino acid derivatives. Kendall agreed with this change.

Kendall's extracted thyroxine was patented and commercially licensed, but was far more expensive and not as effective as desiccated thyroid. (In the 1920s, no one knew that thyroxine as the free acid is not well absorbed.) Even so, Harington's synthetic product was far too costly. Therefore, until the 1960s, the usual therapy for thyroid deficiency and goiter was the administration of desiccated thyroid. The successful synthesis of thyroxine in high yield in 1949 (30) (in the form of sodium L-thyroxine, which, in contrast to thyroxine itself, is quite well absorbed from the gut) made therapy with this form of thyroxine economically sensible. Thyroxine is used now in almost all treatment with thyroid hormone. Although in 1999, based on one report (31), some have added triiodothyronine to the thyroxine; however, several recent studies have not been able to confirm this report (32–34).

Both Kendall and Harington suspected that there might be another thyroid hormone other than thyroxine, but they were never able to find it. Kendall moved on to work with adrenal steroids, which won him a Nobel Prize in 1950, almost 3 decades later. Harington gave up the idea of a second thyroid hormone and became director of London's National Institute for Medical Research. He was much surprised when his associate, Pitt-Rivers, and her postdoctoral fellow, Gross, found and synthesized triiodothyronine and then showed it to be more active than thyroxine in a bioassay (35,36). Harington was elated when, with Gross on a vacation in France, the bioassay was successfully repeated and confirmed the high biologic activity of triiodothyronine. It was found almost simultaneously across the English Channel in Paris by Roche, Lissitsky, and Michel (37,38). There was indeed a second thyroid hormone.

Gaps in our knowledge remain, for example, an identification of the cause of goiter in the absence of iodine deficiency, or an explanation of the initial causes of thyrotoxicosis. The record of the past does suggest a certain optimism; surely some of these gaps will be filled in. Only Kocher, among all those mentioned earlier, won a Nobel Prize for work in the area of thyroid studies, although several others were considered worthy by one or another Nobel committee. No matter; our patients are still the better for it.

REFERENCES

1. Merke F. *History and iconography of endemic goitre and cretinism.* Lancaster, UK: MTP Press Limited, 1984.
2. Sawin CT. Goiter. In: Kiple KF, ed. *Cambridge world history of human disease.* Cambridge: Cambridge University Press, 1993:750.
3. Wharton T. Adenographia: sive glandularum totius corporis descriptio. Noviomagi (now Nijmegen): Andreas ab Hoogenhuyse, 1664. (This endocrine classic has been translated into English. See: Freer 5, translator. *Thomas Wharton's Adenographia.* Oxford: Clarendon Press, 1996.)
4. Cranefield PF. The discovery of cretinism. *Bull Hist Med* 1962;36:489.
5. Coindet J-F. Découverte d'un nouveau remède contre le goitre. *Ann Chim Phys* 1820;15:49 (originally published in the Swiss Biblioteque Universelle, 1820, and reprinted in its entirety in *J Pharmacie* 1820;6:485).
6. Lugol JGA. *Mémoire sur 1 'emploi de 1 'iode dans les maladies scrophuleuses.* Paris: 1829.
7. Boussingault J-B. Recherches sur la cause qui produit le goitre dans les Cordilieres de la Nouvelle-Grenade. *Ann Chim Phys* 1831;48:41.
8. Chatin A. Existence de l'iode dans les plarites d'eau douce: consequences de ce fait pour le géognosie, la physiologie végétale, la thérapeutique et peut-etre pour l'industrie. *Compt Rend Acad Sci* 1850;30:352.
9. Marine D, Kimball OP. Prevention of simple goiter in man. *Arch Intern Med* 1920;25:661.
10. Parry CH. *Collections from the unpublished medical writings.* London: Underwoods, 1825:111.
11. Graves RJ. Clinical lectures delivered by Robert J. Graves, M.D., at the Meath Hospital during the Session of 1834–5. *Lond Med Surg J* 1835;7:516.
12. Basedow CA. Exophthalmos durch hypertrophie des Zeilgewebes in der Augenhohle. *WochenschrHeilkd* 1840;6:197, 220.
13. Charcot JM. Mémoire sur une affection caractérisée par des palpitations du coeur et des arteres, la tumefaction de la glande thyroide et une double exophthalmie. *Compt Rend Soc Biol* 1857; 3(2nd series):43.
14. Hertz S, Roberts A. Radioactive iodine in the study of thyroid physiology. vii. The use of radioactive iodine therapy in hyperthyroidism. *JAMA* 1946;131:81.
15. Chapman E, Evans RD. The treatment of hyperthyroidism with radioactive iodine. *JAMA* 1946;131:86.
16. Astwood EB. Treatment of hyperthyroidism with thiourea and thiouracil. *JAMA* 1943;122:78.
17. Gull WW. On a cretinoid state supervening in adult life in women. *Trans Clin Soc Lond* 1874;7:180.
18. Ord WM. On myxoedema, a term proposed to be applied to an essential condition in the "cretinoid" affection occasionally observed in middle-aged women. *Med Chir Trans* 1878;61:57.
19. Reverdin JL. Accidents consécutifs a l'ablation totale du goitre. *Rev Med Suisse Romande* 1882;2:539.
20. Kocher T. Ueber Kropfexstirpation und ihre Folgen. *Arch Klin Chir* 1883;29:254.
21. Ord WM. Report of a committee of the Clinical Society of London nominated December 14, 1883, to investigate the subject of myxoedema. *Trans Clin Soc Lond* 1888;21[Suppl].
22. Brown-Séquard CE. Des effets produits chez l'homme par les injections sous-cutanées d'un liquide retire des testicules frais de cobaye et de chien. *Compt Rend Soc Biol* 1889;41:415.
23. Murray GR. Note on the treatment of myxoedema by hypodermic injections of an extract of the thyroid gland of a sheep. *BMJ* 1891;2:796.
24. Bruns P. Ueber die Kropfbehandlung mit Schildrusenfutterung. *Dtsch Med Wochenschr* 1894;41:785.
25. Needham J. Proto-endocrinology in medieval China. In: Needham J, Ling W, Gwei-Djen L, Ping-Yu H, eds. *Clerks and craftsmen in China and the West.* Cambridge: Cambridge University Press, 1970:294.
26. Baumann E. Ueber das normale Vorkommen von Jod im Thierkorper. *Hoppe-Seyler's Z Physiol Chem* 1895;21:319.
27. Kendall EC. The isolation in crystalline form of the compound which occurs in the thyroid: its chemical nature and physiologic activity. *JAMA* 1915;64:2042.
28. Harington CR. Chemistry of thyroxine. II. Constitution and synthesis of desiodo-thyroxine. *Biochem J* 1926;20:300.
29. Harington CR, Barger G. Chemistry of thyroxine. III. Constitution and synthesis of thyroxine. *Biochem J* 1927;21:169.
30. Chalmers JR, Dickson GT, Elks J, et al. The synthesis of thyroxine and related substances. Part V. A synthesis of L-thyroxine from L-tyrosine. *J Chem Soc* 1949;3424.
31. Bunevicius R, Kazanavicius G, Zalinkevicius R, et al. Effects of thyroxine as compared with thyroxine plus triiodothyronine in patients with hypothyroidism. *N Engl J Med* 1999;340:424.
32. Sawka AM, Gerstein MJ, Marriott MJ, et al. Does a combination regimen of thyroxine (T$_4$) and 3,5,3'-triiodothyronine improve depressive symptoms better than T$_4$ alone in patients with hypothyroidism? Results of a double-blind, randomized, controlled trial. *J Clin Endocrinol Metab* 2003;88:4551.
33. Walsh JP, Shiels L, Mun Lim EE, et al. Combined thyroxine/liothyronine treatment does not improve well-being, quality of life,

or cognitive function compared to thyroxine alone: a randomized controlled trial in patients with primary hypothyroidism. *J Clin Endocrinol Metab* 2003;88:4543.

34. Clyde PW, Harari AE, Cetka EJ, et al. Combined levothyroxine plus liothyronine compared with levothyroxine alone in primary hypothyroidism: a randomized controlled trial. *JAMA* 2003; 290:2952.

35. Gross J, Pitt-Rivers R. The identification of 3:5:38-L-triiodothyronine in human plasma. *Lancet* 1952;1:439.

36. Gross J, Pitt-Rivers R. Physiological activity of 3:5:38-L-triiodothyronine. *Lancet* 1952;1:593.

37. Roche J, Lissitsky S, Michel R. Sur la triiodothyronine, produit intermédiaire de la transformation de la diiodothyronine en thyroxine. *Compt Rend Acad Sci* 1952;234:997.

38. Roche J, Lissitsky S, Michel R. Sur la presence de triiodothyronine dans la thyroglobuline. *Compt Rend Acad Sci* 1952;234: 1228.

SUGGESTED READINGS

In addition to the references given above, readers will find more historical detail in the following:

Harington CR. *The thyroid gland: its chemistry and physiology.* London: Oxford University Press, 1933.

Pitt-Rivers R, Vanderlaan WP. The therapy of thyroid disease. In: Pamham MJ, Bruinvels J, eds. *Discoveries in pharmacology.* Vol 2. Amsterdam: Elsevier, 1984:391.

Rolleston HD. *The endocrine organs in health and disease with an historical review.* London: Oxford University Press, 1936.

Sawin CT. Defining thyroid hormone: its nature and control. In: McCann SM, ed. *Endocrinology: people and ideas.* Bethesda, MD: American Physiological Society, 1988:149.

2

DEVELOPMENT AND ANATOMY OF THE HYPOTHALAMIC–PITUITARY–THYROID AXIS

PILAR SANTISTEBAN

The thyroid gland is an organ composed primarily of endoderm-derived follicular cells and is responsible for thyroid hormone production in all vertebrates. The main regulator of thyroid function is thyrotropin (thyroid-stimulating hormone, TSH), which is synthesized and secreted from the pituitary gland and is under the control of thyrotropin-releasing hormone (TRH), secreted by the hypothalamus. Thyroid secretion and serum concentrations of thyroxine (T_4) and 3,5,3′-triiodothyronine (T_3) are maintained by a negative feedback loop involving inhibition of TSH and TRH secretion by T_4 and T_3, and by tissue-specific and hormone-regulated expression of the three iodothyronine deiodinase enzymes that metabolize thyroid hormones. Thus, the regulation of thyroid function depends on the normal development of the hypothalamic–pituitary–thyroid axis, which occurs independently but coordinately during embryonic and neonatal life.

This chapter will focus on the development of the thyroid gland, with emphasis on recent studies of the morphogenesis and differentiation of the gland, as well as the hypothalamic–pituitary axis, which is required for normal thyroid function. The recent identification of several transcription factors expressed specifically in the thyroid has helped to define the molecular events responsible for thyroid development. Most of the recent advances in the understanding in the formation of the hypothalamus, pituitary, and thyroid have come from studies in animals, but where possible this information will be integrated with what is known about the anatomy, morphology, and development of the axis in humans.

THE HYPOTHALAMIC–PITUITARY AXIS

The vertebrate embryo relies on complex inductive interactions to orchestrate pattern formation, organogenesis, and ultimately, the development of integrated organ systems. The hypothalamic–pituitary axis is a prime example of such a system. The regulated functions of the hypothalamus and pituitary are intrinsically linked throughout life, and they result from the coordinated development of the two organs. Experimental embryology and molecular genetic studies have yielded evidence that the determination,

development, and differentiation of the pituitary gland and hypothalamus are intimately coupled. How both organs, of different embryonic origin, codevelop introduces a level of complexity still not well understood.

The hypothalamus emerges from the ventral-caudal prosencephalon (diencephalon) during the sixth week of gestation in humans, and between embryonic (E) days E-11 and E-18 in rats. The progenitor of the central and peripheral nervous systems is the neural plate, which is first seen as a thickening of the midline ectoderm that overlies the notochord. Ten days later, this thickened ectoderm forms neural folds that fuse to form the neural tube; some cells in the dorsal region of the neural tube, the neural crest, migrate and give rise to neurons, glia, melanocytes, connective tissue of the head, and numerous endocrine derivatives, such as the parafollicular cells of the thyroid. The rest of the neural tube becomes the central nervous system. The primitive hypothalamic region is initially localized at the most rostral region of the neural tube, and later has a more caudal and ventral position. During development of the hypothalamus, neurosecretory cells are organized into several nuclei, including the paraventricular, supraoptic, and arcuate nuclei. Two different neurosecretory systems are organized in the hypothalamus, one formed of magnocellular neurons, whose axons migrate directly into the posterior lobe of the pituitary gland, and the other formed of parvocellular neurons, which synthesize, among other neuropeptides, TRH for regulating the TSH–thyroid axis (Fig. 2.1).

In the ventral hypothalamus, the infundibulum forms as an evagination that gives rise to multiple structures, including the posterior pituitary gland, the median eminence, and the pituitary stalk, which connects the hypothalamus and the pituitary gland. The median eminence is the site where nerves, whose cell bodies originate in the hypothalamus, release neurosecretory peptides into the hypothalamic–pituitary portal venous system (1). The anterior pituitary is derived from Rathke's pouch, an invagination of an ectodermal layer of cells beneath the diencephalon that, in mice, appears at around day E-8.5 and detaches from the ectoderm by E-12.5 (2–4). Even before the pouch is visible, certain cells are committed to develop into the anterior pituitary. Thus, the pituitary gland originates from two embryonic tissues; the anterior and intermediate lobes (adenohypophysis) are

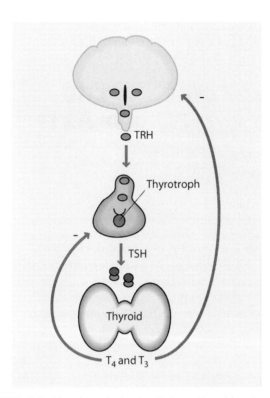

FIGURE 2.1. The hypothalamic–pituitary–thyroid axis. Thyrotropin-releasing hormone (TRH) is synthesized in the hypothalamus and secreted into the hypothalamic–pituitary portal venous system, in which it is carried to the pituitary, where it stimulates the synthesis and secretion of thyrotropin (TSH). TSH binds to its receptor in the thyroid gland, stimulating the synthesis and secretion of thyroxine (T_4) and triiodothyronine (T_3). Precise control of the axis is maintained by the inhibitory actions of T_4 and T_3 on both TRH and TSH secretion.

derived from the oral ectoderm and the posterior lobe (neurohypophysis) from the neural ectoderm (5). During this process there is a direct association between the neuroectoderm of the diencephalon and Rathke's pouch, and it is a unique region in the developing head in which there is no intervening mesoderm between neuroectoderm and ectoderm. The close apposition of these tissues suggests that cell–cell contact and inductive tissue interactions may be important for their determination and differentiation. Many early studies focused on the role of neural contact in the determination and differentiation of the adenohypophysis (6). Recently, it has become clear that several genes expressed in the ventral diencephalon are involved in the formation and development of Rathke's pouch, providing evidence that the infundibulum acts as a key organizing center (7). For example, mice with deletion of the gene for the homeodomain protein, thyroid transcription factor-1 (TTF-1; also called T/EBP or Nkx2.1, see later in this chapter), which is expressed in the ventral diencephalon (but not Rathke's pouch), lack some ventral regions of the brain, including the infundibulum, and have no pituitary gland (8). These data are consistent with the critical role of the infundibular signals in pituitary organogenesis.

The role of the pituitary primordium in the development of the hypothalamus has been less extensively studied, but contact between the two organs is important for proper formation of the ventral hypothalamus and median eminence, and for differentiation and proliferation of the different types of pituitary cells.

Signaling and Transcriptional Mechanisms Involved in Pituitary Organogenesis

The development of the pituitary gland is a model system in which to study the complex processes involved in intercellular signaling, because it contains different cell types that are derived from a common ectodermal primordium and arise in a distinct spatial and temporal fashion in response to intrinsic and extrinsic signals.

Each cell type of the anterior pituitary gland is characterized by the secretion of different trophic hormones that regulate a diverse range of biological processes in response to signals from the hypothalamus and peripheral organs. Two cell types synthesize proopiomelanocortin (POMC), which is cleaved by proteolytic processing to generate melanocyte-stimulating hormone in melanotrophs and corticotropin, or adrenocorticotropic hormone (ACTH), in corticotrophs. The somatotrophs secrete growth hormone, lactotrophs secrete prolactin, thyrotrophs secrete TSH, and gonadotrophs secrete follicle-stimulating hormone and luteinizing hormone. The last three hormones are heterodimeric glycoproteins consisting of a common α subunit and a specific β subunit (see section on chemistry and biosynthesis of thyrotropin in Chapter 10). Recent studies have identified some of the molecules (morphogens) that signal differentiation of these different cells from the common population of progenitor cells (3). These signals have a central role in early organogenesis and are especially important in development of the pituitary gland (see Chapter 3).

Morphogenic Signals Involved in Early Steps of Pituitary Development

The signaling molecules called bone-morphogenic proteins (BMPs) are members of the transforming-growth factor-β superfamily, which play critical roles in patterning and cell-type specification in several species (9). In the case of the pituitary, multiple BMPs play different roles in morphogenesis of the pituitary gland.

BMP-4 is expressed in the ventral diencephalon where the infundibulum makes contact with Rathke's pouch at E-8.5 to E-9.0 in mice, and it is one of the early signals required for the initial commitment of some cells of the oral ectoderm to form the pituitary gland (Fig. 2.2). However, the signals required for the initial invagination of Rathke's pouch are still unclear, although the notochord may have a

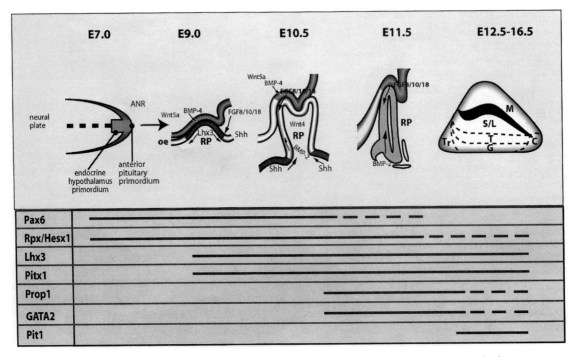

FIGURE 2.2. Schematic diagram of the development of the hypothalamic–pituitary axis showing the main transcription factors involved in pituitary organogenesis in mice. At embryonic day E-7, the anterior neural ridge *(ANR)*, primordial endocrine hypothalamus, and primordial anterior pituitary are present. The signals originating on E-9.0 in the ventral diencephalon include Wnt-5a, bone-morphogenic protein (BMP)-4, and fibroblast growth factors (FGFs)-8 and -10. At E-10.5, the ectoderm provides the ventral signal Shh and the mesenchyme signal BMP-2, both of which signal ventrally to dorsally in Rathke's pouch *(RP)*. All these signals control the expression of specific transcription factors involved in the commitment of cell lineages at E-11.5. Cell types later arise in a temporal and spatial fashion, starting on E-12.5 for corticotrophs *(C)* and rostral thyrotrophs *(Tr)*, and subsequently from E-15.5 to E-17.5 for somatotrophs *(S)*, lactotrophs *(L)*, thyrotrophs *(T)*, gonadotrophs *(G)*, and melanotrophs *(M)*. The temporal expression of the main transcription factors controlling specification of pituitary cell types and organogenesis are shown in the table below the diagram. (From Scully KM, Rosenfeld MG. Pituitary development: regulatory codes in mammalian organogenesis. *Science* 2002;295:2231, modified with permission.)

role in this process. Blockade of the BMP-4 signal results in arrest of pituitary gland development and absence of all pituitary endocrine cell types (10–12).

Several members of the fibroblast growth factor (FGF) family (FGF-8 and FGF-10) are expressed in the infundibulum and control pituitary proliferation and positional-restricted determination of pituitary cell lineage (10,13). The requirement for FGF-8 has been further suggested by studies in mice lacking TTF-1, in which FGF-8 is not expressed in the ventral diencephalon. This absence is linked to the absence of Rathke's pouch-specific transcription factors (Rpx) (14). FGF receptors are also important in the process of pituitary development. In addition to BMP-4 and FGF-8 and -10, signals that originate in the dorsal region of the infundibulum, ventral signals, and intrinsic pouch signals [such as BMP-2 and sonic hedgehog (Shh)], contribute to the establishment of the positional identity of pituitary cells at days E-9.5 through E-10.5 in mice (13). BMP-2 controls the expression of different, ventrally

expressed pituitary transcription factors, and also expression of the gene for the α subunit of the glycoprotein hormones, which is an early marker of cells destined to be thyrotrophs and gonadotrophs. Together, these data suggest that BMP-2 signaling specifies the progenitors that will later give rise to the ventral pituitary cell types.

In vertebrates, the Shh protein is expressed in several organizing centers during embryogenesis, during which it exerts crucial roles in patterning (15). During the early development of the pituitary gland, Shh is expressed in the oral ectoderm, although not in the region that forms Rathke's pouch (16). It may act in a signaling cascade with BMP-2 in the determination of ventral pituitary cell lineages (Fig. 2.2).

Other morphogenic factors have also been implicated in the formation of different cell types within the pituitary. The Wnt proteins are a family of secreted proteins involved in a variety of early embryonic events that function through transcriptional mediators such as β-catenin and T-cell factor lymphoid-enhancing factor (17,18). In the pituitary,

Wnt-4 and Wnt-5 are expressed in the ventral diencephalon and within the cells of Rathke's pouch, respectively. Mice lacking Wnt-4 have a hypocellular pituitary gland with differentiated but incompletely expanded ventral cells (18). In cultured Rathke's pouch cells, Wnt-5 and BMP-4 induce expression of the α subunit gene (2,19,20), suggesting that both signals may act in synergy to expand pituitary cell lineages and induce cell determination. All the morphogens that contribute to pituitary development are important for thyroid development and function, because pituitary TSH is the main regulator of the thyroid gland function.

Transcription Factors Controlling the Early Phases of Pituitary Development

Many transcription factors responsible for the differentiation of pituitary cells have been identified (4,5,21–23), establishing a hierarchy of expression during pituitary development (Fig. 2.2). Thus, multiple members of the LIM homeodomain family of transcription factors are expressed in Rathke's pouch, including Lhx-3, Lhx-4, and Isl-1. Lhx-3 is specifically expressed in Rathke's pouch on E-9.5 in mice, and it plays a decisive role, together with Lhx-4, in the earliest phases of pituitary organogenesis. Lhx-3 knockout mice have a rudimentary Rathke's pouch, but the ectoderm fails to continue to proliferate and all pituitary cell types are absent, with the exception of a few corticotrophs (24). Isl-1 is initially expressed in Rathke's pouch during early pituitary development, but is later (E-10.5) restricted to the ventral cell population. The expression of this gene is regulated by both BMP-4 and BMP-2.

Two pituitary homeobox (*Pitx*) genes (previously referred to as **P-Otx** and **Pitx-1**) are expressed throughout the pituitary, with distinct overlapping patterns of expression. Pitx-1 interacts with the amino-terminal domain of the pituitary-specific POU-domain protein Pit-1 (see later in this chapter), and is expressed, in the earliest stages of pituitary organogenesis, in the anterior region of the neural plate, the oral ectoderm. Targeted disruption of Pitx-1 leads to decreased expression of terminal differentiation markers for the gonadotrophs and thyrotrophs (25). The Pitx-2 gene was identified through positional cloning of the gene responsible for the Rieger's syndrome in humans (26). Both Pitx genes, Pitx-1 and -2, are expressed in most pituitary cell types from early to late pituitary ontogeny, and also in other developing organs. Pitx-2-null mice have many severe developmental defects, including arrest of the early stage of pituitary development after establishment of the contact between the infundibulum and Rathke's pouch, and arrest of the subsequent signaling gradients; the pituitary gland fails to develop after E-10.5, which results in marked hypoplasia of the gland. The similarity of the phenotypes of **Pitx-2**-null and **Lhx-3**-null mice suggests that these two classes of homeodomain factors collaborate to regulate the same pituitary-specific genes. Indeed, both factors act synergistically to activate the expression of the α subunit gene (27). In summary, the induction of Lhx-3 expression in response to infundibular FGF signals is the critical step in the selection of oral ectoderm for development into the pituitary gland, and it acts synergistically with Pitx-2 to direct pituitary-specific gene expression.

The paired homeodomain factors Prop-1 and Rpx are expressed in a sequential overlapping temporal pattern and are required for Rathke's pouch cell types to populate the anterior lobe of the pituitary. By positional cloning in Ames dwarf mice, a gene named Prophet of Pit-1 (Prop-1) was identified. Its expression is coincident with the closure of Rathke's pouch at E-10.5, and it is down-regulated on days E-15.5 through E-16.5, at the time of terminal differentiation of pituitary-specific cells. Prop-1-deficient mice do not express Pit-1, and consequently lack somatotrophs, lactotrophs, and thyrotrophs. Prop-1 is also required for the generation of gonadotrophs and corticotrophs, indicating that it is important for the expansion of all anterior pituitary cell lineages. Mutations in the Prop-1 gene are the cause of combined pituitary hormone deficiency in humans (see Chapter 48) (28–31).

The Rathke's pouch factor Rpx is the homologue of the Hesx-1 gene, a homeodomain protein that contains a conserved repressor domain named eh1. Rpx expression is restricted to the oral ectoderm and pouch. The attenuation of Rpx/Hesx-1 expression by different corepressors coincides with the appearance of terminal differentiation markers for anterior pituitary cell types, suggesting that down-regulation of this gene is required for progression of pituitary development. This gene can dimerize with Prop-1 and inhibit Prop-1 activity, suggesting that Rpx/Hesx-1 acts to antagonize Prop-1 function (32).

Another paired-domain factor important in the early development of Rathke's pouch is *Pax-6*. This gene is transiently expressed in the dorsal part of the pouch, and is down-regulated when cell-type differentiation starts. The pituitary glands of *Pax-6*-null mice have expansion of the ventral cell types that express α subunits, predominantly thyrotrophs, with a corresponding loss of the more dorsal somatotrophs (33,34). Thus, Pax-6 is required for delineating the dorsal/ventral boundaries between the thyrotroph/gonadotroph and the somatotroph/lactotroph progenitor regions of the pituitary gland.

Transcription Factors Controlling Specification of Different Pituitary Cell Types

Pit-1 is a member of the family of POU domain–containing transcription factors, which have a paired DNA-binding domain. The POU domain consists of an amino-terminal POU-specific domain separated by a short linker to a carboxy-terminal POU homeodomain. Both subdomains contain helix-turn-helix motifs that directly associate with two DNA binding-sites (35). Referred to also as GHF-1, Pit-1 was originally identified through analysis of the nuclear proteins regulating the transcription of growth hormone and prolactin (36,37). Later, Pit-1 was found to be required for generation and cell-type specification of three pituitary cell lineages: somatotrophs, lactotrophs, and thyrotrophs (38). Pit-1 binds to the promoter region of the genes for growth hormone, prolactin, the β subunit of TSH, the receptor for growth hormone-releasing hormone, the type-1 somatostatin receptor 1, and the TRH receptor (35), where it interacts with other transcription factors to form functionally active heterodimers. Pit-1 also interacts with various members of the nuclear-receptor family including, thyroid hormone receptors (TRs) and retinoic acid receptors (RARs) (39).

An interaction between Pit-1 and the zinc finger protein GATA-2 is a critical determinant of the development of both thyrotrophs and gonadotrophs. In the thyrotrophs, this interaction leads to synergistic activation of thyrotroph-specific genes such as the gene for the β subunit of TSH. In gonadotrophs, Pit-1 inhibits GATA-2 binding to promoters not containing an adjacent Pit-1 site (40). In Snell dwarf mice, in which the Pit-1 gene is mutated, Pit-1 and GATA-2 do not interact, and the thyrotrophs assume the fate of gonadotrophs.

Taken together, these studies indicate that there are extrinsic and intrinsic signaling mechanisms that govern the early and late aspects of the development of the hypothalamus and the pituitary gland (Fig. 2.2). Coordination between signal molecules and transcription factors is necessary for the early patterning, proliferation, and positional determination of pituitary cell types, including the thyrotrophs.

THE THYROID GLAND

The thyroid, like the anterior pituitary gland, develops from a diverticulum of the pharynx. It consists of two lobes on either side of larynx, in the middle of the neck, connected by an isthmus that normally overlies the second or third cartilaginous rings of the trachea in humans; this gland also includes cells (the parafollicular or C-cells) derived from the ultimobranchial bodies. Its name comes from its topographic relationship to the laryngeal thyroid cartilage, whose shape resembles a Greek shield. Differential growth of the neck structures is fundamental for the development and anatomy of the thyroid gland (41). The thyroid is the largest endocrine gland in humans; it weighs 1 to 2 g at birth and 10 to 20 g in adults.

Morphogenesis

The thyroid gland of vertebrates has a dual embryonic origin, and its several cell types derive from all three germ lay-

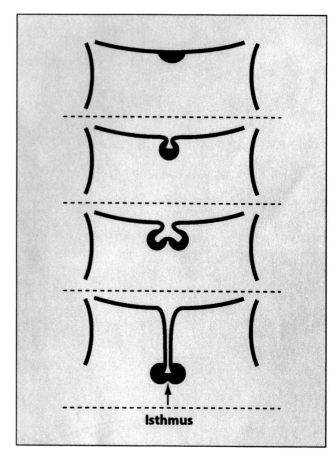

FIGURE 2.3. Frontal view of the stages of development of the median thyroid anlagen. The anlagen first appears as a group of cells located on the floor of the primitive pharynx **(upper panel)**, which then form as a visible bud on embryonic day (E)-16 or E-17 in humans, and E-8.5 or E-9.0 in mice. The bud proliferates ventrally, then expands laterally, forming the characteristic bilobed structure of the thyroid gland. Caudal migration occurs between E-24 to E-32 in humans and E-10.5 to E-14.5 in mice; the thyroid reaches its final position on about E-40 to E-50 in humans and E-15.5 in mice. The association between the medial and lateral (C-cells) thyroid anlagen with an isthmus connecting the two lateral lobes appears on E-50 to E-51 in humans. (From Van Vliet G. Development of the thyroid gland: lessons from congenitally hypothyroid mice and men. *Clin Genetics* 2003; 63:445, modified with permission.)

ers. The most abundant cells, the thyroid follicular cells (thyrocytes), arise from the embryonic endoderm as a thickening in the floor of the primitive pharynx (Fig. 2.3). It is the first endocrine structure that becomes recognizable in humans. This thickening, the so-called median anlagen, is located between the first and second branchial arches and is adjacent to the newly differentiating myocardium (Fig. 2.4A). The anlagen appear as a visible bud on E-16 or E-17 in humans and E-8.5 or E-9.0 in mice. The bud expands ventrally as a diverticulum, with rapid proliferation of the cells at its distal end (Fig. 2.3), but it remains attached to the pharyngeal floor by a tubular stalk called the thyroglossal duct (Fig. 2.4B). The thyrocyte progenitor

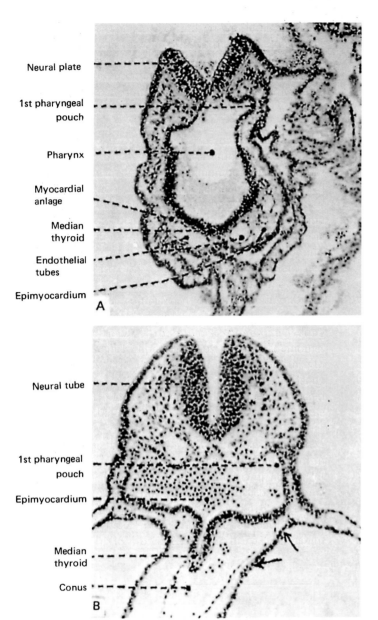

Neural plate

1st pharyngeal pouch

Pharynx

Myocardial anlage

Median thyroid

Endothelial tubes

Epimyocardium

A

Neural tube

1st pharyngeal pouch

Epimyocardium

Median thyroid

Conus

B

FIGURE 2.4. Sections of human embryos showing thyroid development. **A:** Section through a 2-somite embryo (150× magnification). **B:** Section through the thyroid anlagen of a 10-somite embryo (150× magnification).

cells continue to proliferate distally and then begin to proliferate laterally, which leads to the formation of the characterized bilobed structure connected by an isthmus (Fig. 2.3). Because of its close association with the embryonic heart, the thyroid can be viewed as being pulled downward by the heart during its descent. This caudal migration is accompanied by rapid elongation of the thyroglossal duct, which eventually fragments and degenerates. This migration occurs from E-24 to E-32 in humans and E-10.5 to E-14.5 in mice.

The thyroid reaches its final position at about E-40 to E-50 in humans and about E-15.5 in mice. At that time it connects with the two lateral anlagen, the ultimobranchial bodies, resulting in the incorporation of C-cells into the thyroid. These lateral anlagen are derived from the endo-

derm of the fourth pharyngeal pouch and the ectoderm of the abortive fifth pouch (41) (Fig. 2.5). In the mature thyroid gland, the C-cells occur either singly or in small groups, and their contribution to the total thyroid mass is minimal (10%). They are more concentrated in the central parts of the lobes, but can be found throughout the gland (42). The origin of the C-cells is still debated [for more details, see the previous edition of this book (43)].

The association between the medial and lateral thyroid anlagen is complete by about E-50 in humans, at which time the thyroid gland exhibits its definitive external form, with an isthmus connecting the two lateral lobes (Figs. 2.3 and 2.5). The foramen cecum at the base of the tongue is the remnant of the origination of the gland in the floor of the primitive pharynx. The development and migration of

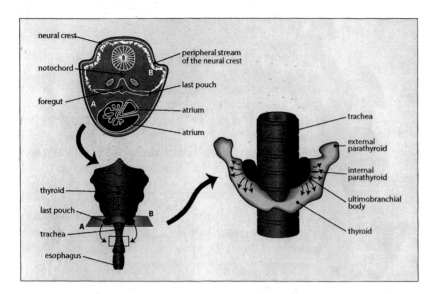

FIGURE 2.5. Schematic diagrams showing the neural crest origin of C-cells and their incorporation into the thyroid gland. Primordial cells arising from the neural crest migrate ventrally during embryonic life to become incorporated in the last (ultimobranchial) pharyngeal pouch. The ultimobranchial body fuses with the primordial thyroid gland, and the C-cells are distributed throughout the thyroid gland. (From Foster GV, Byfield PGH, Gudmundsson TV. Calcitonin. *Clin Endocrinol Metab* 1972;1:93, modified with permission.)

the medial and lateral thyroid anlagen should be viewed in conjunction with the development and migration of other structures of the head and neck, such as the parathyroid glands and thymus (Fig. 2.6).

Most of the critical events in thyroid morphogenesis take place in the first 60 days of gestation in humans or the first 15 days of gestation in mice. For that reason, most developmental thyroid abnormalities result from morphogenetic errors during this period, which lead to displacement of cells derived from the medial anlagen. Ectopic thyroid tissue can result from abnormal thyroid migration that is secondary to abnormal morphogenesis of the heart, or from abnormal interactions between the thyroid primordium and the heart. As a result, ectopic thyroid cells have been found throughout the regions through which the developing thyroid migrates, including sublingual, high cervical, mediastinal, and even intracardiac locations. In the first three cases, interaction between the heart and median anlagen is abrogated earlier in development than normal, whereas in the last, thyroid tissue differentiates within the cardiac endothelium. Finally, the thyroglossal duct may not degenerate, but instead persist as a fistulous tract, which may include some thyroid follicular cells and in which thyroid carcinoma may arise. Recent studies have related mutations in thyroid transcription factors to abnormalities in thyroid development resulting in congenital hypothyroidism (see later in this chapter and Chapter 48; also see section on congenital hypothyroidism in Chapter 75) [reviewed in (44,45)].

Histology and Ultrastructure

The structure of the thyroid is unique among endocrine glands in that it is the only endocrine gland in which the

hormonal products are stored in an extracellular location. It is composed of follicles of varying size that consist of an outer layer of thyroid follicular cells, which enclose a lumen that contains thyroglobulin-rich colloid. The follicular cells are surrounded by a basement membrane. Thyroid folliculogenesis is a complex process that begins with the proliferation of irregularly arranged cell cords derived from the endoderm of the thyroglossal duct. The follicles are formed by proliferation of follicular cells, coalescence of colloid-containing droplets in individual cells, and extrusion of the droplets into the follicular lumen. Studies in rats showed that the volumetric fractions of the different histologic components (follicular cells, C-cells, colloid, and interstitial tissue) change considerably during development (birth to 120 days of age). The fraction of follicular cells decreased from 61% at birth to 37% at 120 days. The fraction of C-cells increased from 3% at birth to 4% at 15 days, with no further change at 120 days. Colloid and stroma together represented 36% of the volume at birth and 59% at 120 days. During this period, the absolute volumes occupied by follicular cells, C-cells, colloid, and stroma increased 13-, 31-, 39-, and 34-fold, respectively (46).

Follicular structure is maintained by the integrity of the cytoskeleton, including microtubules and microfilaments (47), through which TSH and intercellular contact may regulate adhesion of follicular cells to each other and to the extracellular matrix, and also influence thyroid-cell behavior. The extracellular matrix plays a role in the adhesion, proliferation, differentiation, and migration of thyroid follicular cells. Molecules involved in these processes include type I and type IV collagen, fibronectin, laminin (48), and cadherin (49). Type IV collagen and laminin (major components of the basement membrane surrounding each follicle) play an important positive role in the proliferation

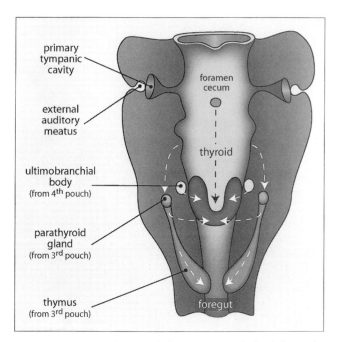

FIGURE 2.6. Frontal view of the structures derived from the pharyngeal organ. The thyroid gland forms from the posterior migration of the thyroid anlagen, which, as shown in Figure 2.3, is derived from the ventral floor of the pharynx. As it migrates downward, it is joined by the ultimobranchial bodies (derived from the fourth branchial pouch), which contains C-cells, to form the mature thyroid gland. The foramen cecum is an opening formed by the evagination of the thyroid anlagen that closes later in development. The parathyroid glands and thymus are derived from the third branchial pouch. The tympanic cavity and external auditory meatus are formed from the first pouch. (From Manley NR, Capecchi MR. The role of Hoxa-3 in mouse thymus and thyroid development. *Development* 1995;121:1989, modified with permission.)

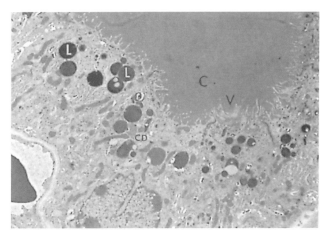

FIGURE 2.7. Electron micrograph of normal thyroid follicular cells with long microvilli (*V*) that extend into the luminal colloid (*C*). Pseudopods from the apical plasma membrane surround a portion of the colloid to form an intracellular colloid droplet (*CD*). Numerous lysosomes (*L*) are present in the apical cytoplasm in proximity to the colloid droplets. An intrafollicular capillary is visible in the lower left.

and differentiation of follicular cells, and E-cadherin plays an important role in the maintenance of the thyroid epithelial cell phenotype throughout organogenesis (50).

Thyroid follicular cells have long profiles of rough endoplasmic reticulum and a large Golgi apparatus in their cytoplasm for synthesis and packaging of thyroglobulin that is then transported into the follicular lumen (see Chapter 5). The cytoplasm also contains numerous electron-dense lysosomal bodies, which are important in the secretion of thyroid hormones. The surface characteristics of the apical (luminal) and the basolateral sides of the cells are different, according to the role of the particular surface in thyroid hormonogenesis (see Chapter 4) (51). The secretory polarity of the cells is directed toward the lumen of the follicles; this polarity is important for iodine uptake. The apical (luminal) surfaces of the follicular cells have numerous microvilli that protrude into the follicular lumen, greatly increasing the surface area in contact with the colloid (Fig. 2.7) (46). The follicular structure seems to be required for normal thyroid hormone synthesis and secretion (52).

An extensive network of interfollicular and intrafollicular capillaries provides the follicular cells with an abundant blood supply. There is also a network of lymphatics in the gland. The stroma also contains nerve fibers, some of which are parasympathetic, but most are sympathetic. These nerves terminate on blood vessels or in apposition to the follicular cells. Growth factors and vasoactive factors are produced in the thyroid. They include fibroblast growth factor and vascular-endothelial growth factor, which are potent angiogenic proteins, and which, in cooperation with TSH, may regulate the growth and function of follicular cells (53). The role of these growth factors in thyroid development during embryonic life has not been explored, but they are likely to be important, by analogy with their effects on other organs derived from endoderm such as the liver (54) and pancreas (55).

The follicular cells vary in height, depending on degree of stimulation by TSH—between low cuboidal and tall columnar (Fig. 2.8). In humans, the cells are more cuboidal, whereas in rats, in which the rates of production and clearance of T_4 and T_3 are more rapid, the cells are more columnar. In the normal human thyroid, the size of the follicles is quite variable, and there is no discernible pattern in the distribution of small and large follicles within the gland. The histologic appearance of the thyroid is dramatically influenced by TSH (56). When TSH secretion increases, the first response is formation of numerous cytoplasmic pseudopods, which result in increased endocytosis of thyroglobulin-rich colloid from the follicular lumen (57). If the increase in secretion of TSH is sustained, thyroid follicular cells become more columnar, and the lumens of the follicles become smaller (even to the

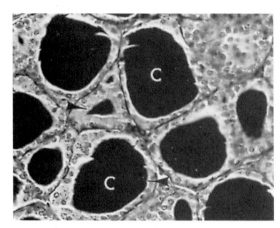

FIGURE 2.8. Microscopic section of the thyroid gland of a normal rat showing colloid-filled (*C*) follicles of varying size (*arrows*) lined by cuboidal follicular cells. An extensive network of capillaries is present between the thyroid follicles (periodic acid–Schiff-stained section).

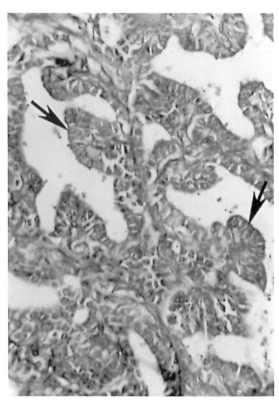

FIGURE 2.9. Microscopic section of thyroid tissue from a rat showing diffuse hyperplasia induced by a chronic increase in thyrotropin secretion. The follicles are small and lined by columnar thyroid follicular cells, and there are projections of the cells (*arrows*) into the follicular lumens. The small size and partial collapse of some follicles are due to increased endocytosis of colloid.

point of collapse) because of the increase in endocytosis of colloid (53,55,56), and numerous periodic acid-Schiff (PAS)–positive colloid droplets are present along the luminal side of the hypertrophied follicular cells. Whether caused by iodine deficiency or goitrogens, a sustained increase in TSH secretion results in thyroid follicular-cell hyperplasia and enlargement of the entire thyroid gland (see section on biological actions of TSH in Chapter 10). The hyperplasia is accompanied by the formation of papillary projections of follicular cells into the lumens of follicles or of multiple layers of cells lining follicles (Fig. 2.9). The opposite changes occur when TSH secretion is inhibited. In this situation, thyroid follicular cells become flat (atrophic), their microvilli disappear, and the follicles become greatly enlarged, due to accumulation of colloid (Fig. 2.10).

Thyroid Follicular Cells

Thus, functional unit of the mature thyroid gland is the thyroid follicle enclosed by a basement membrane. C-cells are found within this basement membrane in contact with follicular cells, but they do not abut the lumen.

During thyroid development, there are three stages of histologic differentiation of the thyroid follicular cells: the precolloid stage (7 to 13 weeks in humans), the beginning colloid stage (13 to 14 weeks), and the follicular stage (> 14 weeks). The three stages are characterized by the appearance and enlargement of canaliculi, which are extensions of the smooth endoplasmic reticulum (Fig. 2.11). The coalescence of the canaliculi, and finally their extrusion through the apical membrane, forms the lumen that is surrounded by the follicular cells. The major component within these canaliculi, and ultimately the colloid, is thyroglobulin.

Multiple proteins are involved in the process of synthesis and secretion of T_4 and T_3 by the thyroid follicles (Fig. 2.12). In addition to thyroglobulin (60), they include the sodium/iodide symporter (NIS), located on the basolateral membrane of the cells, which transports iodide into the cells (see section on thyroid iodine transport in Chapter 4) (61,62). Once within the cells, the iodide is transported through the apical membrane into the follicular lumen by anion transporters, among which is pendrin, an iodide/chloride transporter (63,64). Iodide oxidation and binding to the tyrosine residues of thyroglobulin, as well as the coupling of iodotyrosines to form T_4 and T_3, is catalyzed by thyroid peroxidase (TPO) in the presence of hydrogen peroxide (H_2O_2) (65). The H_2O_2-generating system of the thyroid is a membrane system composed of at least two NADPH thyroid oxidases, THOX-1 and THOX-2, localized in the apical membrane (66). For production of individual molecules of T_4 and T_3, thyroglobulin in the follicular lumen is absorbed across the apical membrane in the form of colloid droplets by endocytosis. These droplets then fuse with lysosomes, and most of the thyroglobulin is hydrolyzed by proteolytic enzymes, forming T_4 and T_3 for release into the circulation. This proteolysis also releases

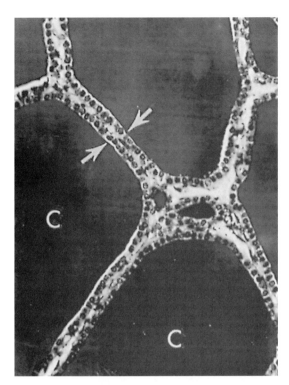

FIGURE 2.10. Microscopic section of thyroid tissue of a rat in which thyrotropin secretion was chronically inhibited. The follicular cells (*arrows*) are low-cuboidal, and the thyroid follicles are distended with dense colloid (*C*).

mono- and diiodotyrosine (MIT and DIT), the precursors of T_4 and T_3, which then are deiodinated by a dehalogenase (67) (see section on thyroid hormone synthesis in Chapter 4).

TSH is the main regulator of thyroid hormone synthesis and secretion; it acts through its thyroid-specific G protein–coupled receptor in the cell surface of thyroid cells (see section on the thyrotropin receptor in Chapter 10) (68,69). The action of TSH is largely mediated by an increase in intracellular cyclic adenosine monophosphate (cAMP), which activates multiple signaling pathways to increase thyroid hormone synthesis and release, and also contributes to thyroid differentiation and proliferation (see section on biological actions of thyrotropin in Chapter 10) (70,71).

The genes encoding these proteins and enzymes are expressed either specifically in thyroid follicular cells, for example, thyroglobulin and TPO, or in a very restricted number of tissues, such as NIS and the TSH receptor (TSHR). Fully differentiated thyroid follicular cells express all these genes; they become expressed in a coordinate way during thyroid morphogenesis. Thyroglobulin has been detected in human thyroid tissue as early as the fifth gestational week, when morphogenesis is still occurring. Iodine uptake and T_4 production occur by the 10th to 14th weeks, during a period that corresponds to the final stages of formation of the lumen of follicles (see Chapter 74). In mice thyroglobulin and TSHR expression occur at E-15, and other markers of thyroid-cell differentiation such as TPO or NIS are detected at E-16 during the process of formation of thyroid follicles (72).

Thyroid-Specific Transcription Factors

The promoter regions of the genes for thyroglobulin, TPO, the TSHR, and NIS are well characterized, and transcription factors that bind to these genes and regulate their activity have been identified (Fig 2.13). Three thyroid-specific transcription factors—TTF-1, TTF-2, and Pax-8—that have decisive roles in thyroid gland morphogenesis have been cloned (73–75).

Thyroid Transcription Factor-1

Thyroid transcription factor-1 (TTF-1, also called T/EBP or Nkx2.1) is a homeodomain transcription factor encoded by the genetic locus named *Titf-1*. Genomic regions and complementary DNAs for TTF-1 have been cloned from various species (76,77). In humans, the *Titf-1* gene, located on chromosome 14q13, contains three exons and two introns of 150 and 850 bp, respectively; its structure is well conserved among mammals. It encodes a 42 kDa protein that binds DNA through its homeodomain sequence of 61 amino acids that consist of three helical regions (I, II, and III) folded in a globular structure (78). Helix I is preceded by an N-terminal arm and separated by a loose loop from helix II, which together with helix III forms a helix-turn-helix motif. Helix III is the recognition helix that binds to DNA. In addition to the DNA-binding domain, TTF-1 contains two transcriptional activation domains in its N- and C-terminal regions (79).

Thyroid Transcription Factor-1 Expression during Development
In mice, TTF-1 is expressed in the endodermal cells of the primitive pharynx, in the thyroid anlagen (8,80), as well as in the fourth branchial pouch and the ultimobranchial body (76,77) between days E-8.5 to E-10. Its expression coincides with the proliferation of cells that give rise to the primitive thyroid bud, before the start of migration of the precursor follicular cells (Fig. 2.14). Consistent with this time of expression, *Titf-1*-null mice have only a rudimentary thyroid gland that is later eliminated by apoptosis (8,81). Therefore, TTF-1 is necessary for survival and proliferation of primitive thyroid cells, but not for initial specification of endodermal cells to give rise to the primitive thyroid cells.

TTF-1 is also expressed in the embryonic ventral forebrain, certain hypothalamic areas, the posterior pituitary, and in the lung. Furthermore, it has been detected in several tissues, including thyroid C-cells and parathyroid cells in adult rats (82). In the brain of mice, TTF-1 is expressed in the median ganglionic eminence that gives rise to the

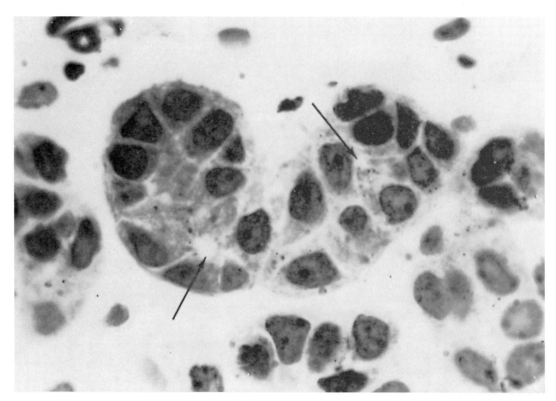

FIGURE 2.11. Photomicrograph of thyroid tissue from a human fetus of 50 mm crown-to-rump length. The *arrows* indicate two intracellular canaliculi (2,400× magnification). (From Shepard TH. Onset of function in the human fetal thyroid: biochemical and radioautographic studies from organ culture. *J Clin Endocrinol Metab* 1967;27:945, with permission.)

pallidal component of the basal ganglia at E-10.5. Consistent with this expression, *Titf-1*-null mice do not form the pallidal structures due to a ventral to dorsal transformation of the pallidal primordium into a striatum-like structure (8,83). The expression of TTF-1 in the early developing diencephalon (E-10.5) is restricted to the hypothalamic areas and to the infundibulum, which gives rise to the posterior lobe of the pituitary gland (see previous section on the hypothalamic–pituitary axis). TTF-1 expression continues during all stages of development of the posterior pituitary, whereas expression has not been detected in Rathke's pouch, which gives rise to the anterior pituitary gland. In *Titf-1*-null mice the pituitary gland is completely missing, both in its epithelial (from Rathke's pouch) and diencephalic (from infundibulum) components (8). A rudimentary Rathke's pouch is initially formed from the diencephalon, but is eliminated by apoptosis before definitive formation of the gland (8,14). Altogether, these data suggest that the presence of TTF-1 in the diencephalon is essential to induce full development of Rathke's pouch, and therefore to form the anterior and intermediate lobes of the pituitary gland. FGF-8 expression is not detectable in the diencephalon of mutant mice, suggesting that this factor is involved in the signaling events.

In the lung, TTF-1 expression is detected at E-9.5 and is restricted to the ventral migrating edge of the lung bud in which the tracheal diverticulum forms. Later, TTF-1 is expressed in all pulmonary epithelial cells. *Titf-1*-null mice die at birth because they have severely hypoplastic lungs, with dilated sac-like structures and only rudimentary bronchial branching (8). These findings suggest that TTF-1 is not required for initial commitment of endodermal cells to originate the lung, but is required for differentiation of lung cells (84).

In conclusion, the phenotypic analysis of *Titf-1*-null mice indicates that TTF-1 is necessary for development of the thyroid, lung, and ventral brain structures, but not for the selection of precursor cells for these structures.

Thyroid Transcription Factor-2

TTF-2 is another transcription factor, also called FOXE-1, due to a recent change in the nomenclature of this family of transcription factors (85). The gene, named *Titf-2/Foxe1*, is located on chromosome 9q22.3 in humans and chromosome 4–4C2 in mice. It encodes a 42-kDa protein that binds DNA through its forkhead domain (fkh), a well-conserved domain described initially in hepatocyte nuclear factor-3, a factor involved in the development of organs derived from the primitive endoderm. The fkh domain is 100 amino acids long with three α-helices in its

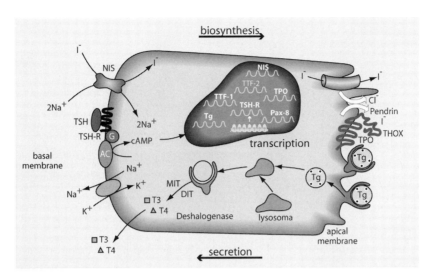

FIGURE 2.12. Schematic diagram of a thyroid follicular cell showing the major intracellular structures and the main proteins and other substances involved in the biosynthesis and secretion of the thyroid hormones thyroxine (T$_4$) and triiodothyronine (T$_3$). Iodide ions (I$^-$) are concentrated by follicular cells from the circulation by the sodium-iodide symporter (NIS) **(left)**, then rapidly transported into the follicular lumen by pendrin and other channels **(right)**. Amino acids (tyrosine and others) and sugars are assembled into thyroglobulin (Tg) in apical vesicles that are released into the follicular lumen. Iodination of tyrosine residues occurs within Tg, after the I$^-$ is oxidized by thyroid peroxidase (TPO), using H$_2$O$_2$ generated by two oxidases, THOX-1 and THOX-2. The iodinated Tg is taken up by endocytosis of colloid, and the colloid droplets fuse with lysosomes, after which Tg is enzymatically cleaved with the release of monoiodotyrosine (MIT), diiodotyrosine (DIT), T$_4$, and T$_3$. The MIT and DIT are deiodinated by a deshalogenase, whereas the T$_4$ and T$_3$ are released into the extracellular fluid. The cell nucleus contains the genes for NIS, TPO, Tg, and TSH receptors, the transcription factors TTF-1 and TTF-2, and Pax-8, which augments the transcription of these and other genes within the thyroid.

N-terminal half, forming a compact structure that presents the third helix to DNA. These proteins bind to DNA as monomers, and are able to bend it; their main property as transcriptional activators is in the remodeling of chromatin structure (86). These factors are expressed early in development, and they appear to alter the chromatin structure in such a way that allow the other specific transcription factors to bind and transactivate the DNA (87).

Thyroid Transcription Factor-2 Expression during Development

In mice, TTF-2 mRNA is detected at E-8.5 in the endoderm lining the foregut, the developing thyroid, and in the

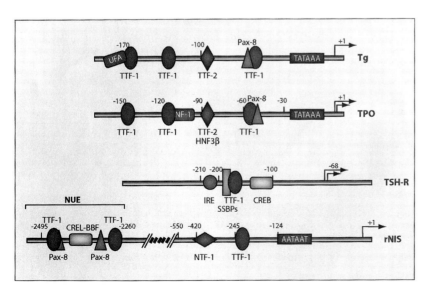

FIGURE 2.13. Schematic diagram showing interactions of multiple transcription factors with the promoter regions of the genes for thyroglobulin (Tg), thyroid peroxidase (TPO), thyrotropin receptors (TSHR), and sodium-iodide symporter (NIS). The structures of the promoter regions of the Tg and TPO genes are similar. *NUE* denotes the NIS upstream enhancer element, which is the main promoter region of the NIS gene.

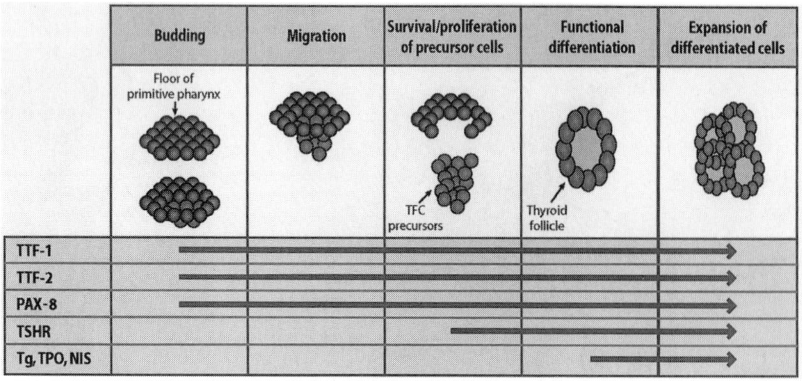

FIGURE 2.14. Schematic representation of the stages of development of the thyroid gland. The *upper boxes* are the names of the different steps of thyroid organogenesis and differentiation. The *middle boxes* show representative diagrams of these steps. The *arrows* in the *lower boxes* show the thyroid transcription factors and their target genes. *TFC* denotes thyroid follicular cells. (From Macchia PE. Recent advances in understanding the molecular basis of primary congenital hypothyroidism. *Mol Med Today* 2000;6:36, modified with permission.)

ectoderm that gives rise to the anterior pituitary (75). In addition, TTF-2 is expressed at E-9 in the palate, nasal choanae, and hair follicles (88). The expression at the beginning of development of the anterior pharynx is restricted to a group of cells in the midline that give rise to the thyroid anlagen, whereas expression is more widespread in the posterior region of the primitive pharynx, where TTF-1 is not expressed. Both TTF-1 and TTF-2 transcripts are detectable in the migrating thyroid anlagen at E-9.5 and thereafter (Fig. 2.14). Hence, both transcription factors seem to be coexpressed in the same cells during a defined temporal window at the time of early thyroid development. The expression pattern of TTF-2 suggests that this factor has only a marginal role in the specification of thyroid follicular-cell precursors. This was confirmed by the thyroid phenotype of *Titf-2*-null mice; at E-8.5 these mice have normal budding of the thyroid anlagen, but at E-9.5 the thyroid precursor cells are unable to migrate downward, and remain contiguous to the pharyngeal endoderm (89). Therefore, the main function of TTF-2 in thyroid development is control of the migration of the thyroid to its position alongside of the trachea. In these mice two phenotypes have been observed. In half, the precursor cells remain in their initial position (thyroid ectopia), and in the other half the cells are not detected (agenesis) (89).

On E-15.5, *Titf-2*-null mice have a small ectopic thyroid that is able to complete the differentiation program because it expresses thyroglobulin, indicating that terminal differentiation of thyroid follicular cells is independent of the position of the cells. In these null mice the shelves of the palate do not fuse with each other, resulting in a cleft palate (89). This anomaly correlates with the expression of TTF-2 in the posterior region of the primitive pharynx (88).

TTF-2 is also expressed in ectodermal cells close to the pharyngeal membrane that give rise to the anterior lobe of the pituitary gland. At E-10.5 in mice, it can be detected in the migrating Rathke's pouch, which is moving upward, but its expression disappears at E-12 to E-12.5, when Rathke's pouch is no longer connected to the oral cavity and the cells of the pouch begin to proliferate. The pattern of expression of TTF-2 in the developing pituitary is similar to that of Rpx. Both factors are down-regulated before the expression of pituitary terminal differentiation markers, suggesting that both could be a repressor of late differentiation events (4). The onset of TTF-2 expression precedes that of the α subunit, and cessation of its expression correlates with the expression of proopiomelanocortin.

Pax-8

This factor is a member of the Pax family of transcription factors defined by a common element, the Paired (Prd) domain, by which they bind to specific DNA sequences (90). Based on the similarity of this domain, these proteins are grouped in several classes, such as Pax-2, Pax-5, and Pax-8. In addition to the Prd domain, these three proteins have a truncated homeodomain, a conserved octapeptide sequence, and sequence homology in the transcriptional activation domain located at the carboxy-terminal end of the molecules. The *Pax-8* gene is located on human chromosome 2q12-q14 and on mouse chromosome 4, and encodes a protein of approximately 46 kDa. The molecular structure of *Pax* genes is known (91). The Prd is 128 amino acids long and consists of two different domains, each containing a helix-turn-helix motif, joined by a linker region. The amino-terminal domain is named PAI and the carboxy terminal domain RED. Because of this independent subdomain structure, each Pax protein binds to different DNA sequences. The binding sites for Pax-8 and TTF-1 in the promoter regions of the thyroglobulin and TPO genes partially overlap (Fig. 2.13), and the two factors therefore compete for binding. In the case of the thyroglobulin promoter, both subdomains of Pax-8 are required for efficient binding (92). In addition, Pax-8 interacts with TTF-1 for full expression of the thyroglobulin promoter (93).

Pax-8 Expression during Development

Pax genes display dynamic patterns of expression during ontogenesis and are involved in pattern formation during organogenesis (94). In mice, the *Pax-8* gene is expressed during development in thyroid, kidney, and neural tissue.

In the thyroid, it is expressed on E-8.5 in the endoderm from the primitive pharynx (Fig. 2.14), coincident with *Titf-1* expression, and its expression in the thyroid continues until adult life. In the kidney, Pax-8 is expressed together with Pax-2 in the nephrogenic cords and the mesonephric tubules on E-10.5. Subsequently, both are expressed in mesenchymal condensations and the epithelial structures of the nephric ducts. In the nervous system, both Pax-8 and Pax-2 are expressed at the midbrain/hindbrain boundary and in the spinal cord on E-11.5.

The role of Pax-8 in thyroid development has been elucidated from the phenotype of *Pax-8*-null mice. These mice are growth retarded, likely due to thyroid deficiency (95), and they die at an early age unless given thyroid hormone. At birth, they have low serum T_4 concentrations, and their thyroid glands are very small and lack follicles; most of the cells are C-cells. The cells express TTF-1 but do not contain thyroglobulin or TPO, as determined by immunohistochemistry. These findings indicate that Pax-8 plays a role in the development of the follicular cells but not C-cells. In these null mice, at E-10.5 to E-11.0, the thyroid anlagen that derives from the endodermal cells of the primitive pharynx is present, but at E-11.5 they do not expand laterally, as occurs in wild type mice, and the lobar structure is completely missing. The absence of Pax-8 is compatible with the initial events of thyroid development but not later stages, such as formation of thyroid follicles and functional differentiation in thyroid cells (96).

The presence of Pax-8, Pax-5, and Pax-2 in fish suggests that these genes originated from a common ancestral gene. Pax-2.1 is required for the development of thyroid follicles in zebrafish (97), animals in which it should be easy to study the molecular mechanisms involved in thyroid organogenesis.

From the prior information, the temporal expression of the thyroid-specific transcription factors during thyroid development take place before specific thyroid genes are expressed. A schematic representation of the initial mechanisms that govern thyroid gland formation (i.e., budding, specification of cells, cell migration, and follicle formation) is shown in Figure 2.14.

Other Transcription Factors Involved in Thyroid Development

The identification of other transcription factors controlling thyroid development has been elucidated from the detailed study of mice in which different genes were knocked out. Some of these factors bind to the promoter region of the *Titf-1* gene, and therefore regulate transcription of that gene.

Hox *Gene*

The *Hox* genes encode a class of transcription factors that contain a highly conserved DNA-binding motif, the *An-tennapedia* homeodomain. Humans and mice have multiple *Hox* genes distributed in four groups, named Hox-A, Hox-B, Hox-C, and Hox-D, located on four separate chromosomes. These genes are thought to specify positional identity according to the Hox code (98). The genes of the third group are expressed in the anterior neuroectoderm, branchial arches, and their derivatives, including the thyroid bud. Hox-3 is expressed in a region in which thyroid is included, and it binds and activates TTF-1; thus, it is possible that this gene carries positional information contributing to turning on the expression of the *Titf-1* gene (99). Mice in which the *Hox-3* gene is knocked out have a poorly developed thyroid gland and abnormal development of the thymus and parathyroid glands (100,101). Hox-5 has a role in thyroid organogenesis; *Hox-5*-null mice have manifestations of hypothyroidism, including transient growth retardation and delayed eye opening and ear elevation. Thyroid gland morphogenesis begins normally, but formation of thyroid follicles and processing of thyroglobulin are impaired (102).

Hex *Gene*

The homeobox *Hex* gene is expressed in the anterior visceral endoderm and rostral endoderm in early mouse embryos. Later, Hex transcripts can be detected in the liver, thyroid, and endothelial precursor cells (103). *Hex*$^{-/-}$ embryos, which die during mid-gestation, have variable truncations of the forebrain, liver, and thyroid dysplasia. Unlike *Hox* genes, which are barely expressed in the thyroid gland of adult animals, the Hex gene is expressed in thyroid follicular cells of adult mice, in which it acts as a repressor of thyroglobulin gene expression (92). Hex expression falls in thyroid cell lines transformed with oncogenes as well as in human thyroid cancer cells (104). TTF-1 increases Hex promoter activity. Moreover, Hex and TTF-1 interact to increase *Hex* gene expression, demonstrating the existence of direct cross-regulation between thyroid transcription factors.

Hepatocyte Nuclear Factor-3 (FOXE-2) Gene

The fork head transcription factor hepatocyte nuclear factor (HNF)-3 (also known as FOXE-2) is expressed early in the primitive endoderm and is decisive for organogenesis of the liver (58,105). It binds *in vitro* to the TPO promoter at the same binding site at which TTF-2 binds (106). However, whether this factor is important in thyroid development is not known. This factor is also expressed in the lungs, in which it binds to the promoter region of the *Titf-1* gene (84).

Eya *Gene*

The *Eya* (*Eyes absent*) gene regulates organogenesis in both vertebrates and invertebrates, and has an important role in the morphogenesis of organs derived from the pharyngeal region, including the thymus, parathyroid glands, and thyroid gland. Eya-1 is expressed in the third and fourth pharyngeal regions and ultimobranchial bodies. *Eya-1*-null mice have thyroid hypoplasia, with severe reduction in the number of C-cells and the size of the thyroid lobes, and the C-cells and thyroid cells lobes do not fuse together. These results suggest that Eya-1 controls critical early inductive events involved in the morphogenesis of the thyroid gland and other organs derived from the pharyngeal region.

Mutations in the *TTF-1, TTF-2,* and *Pax-8* genes have been described in humans with congenital hypothyroidism (see section on congenital hypothyroidism in Chapter 75) (44,107). Thyroid malformations or dysfunction have not been described in humans with *Hox, Hex,* or *Eya* gene mutations.

Other Signals Involved in Early Steps of Thyroid Development

TSH is the main regulator of thyroid function in adults, in whom it stimulates almost every aspect of thyroid hormone biosynthesis, including increases in thyroglobulin synthesis and TPO and NIS activity (see Chapter 4, and section on biological actions of TSH in Chapter 10). TSH also stimulates thyroid proliferation, aggregation of thyroid cells into follicles, and maintenance of follicular architecture. In rats, there is a temporal correlation between expression of TSHRs and the formation of thyroid follicles.

In mouse embryos, TSHR messenger RNA is expressed by E-15 (80), and its expression increases on E-17 or E-18. At this stage, thyroid-specific genes (thyroglobulin, TPO, and NIS) are up-regulated and colloid formation begins (108). Studies of mice in which the genes for TSH or TSHR were knocked out have revealed that TSH signaling is not a global regulator of thyroid function during development (72). TSH and TSHR are required for expression of some of the genes involved in thyroid hormone biosynthesis, such as TPO and NIS, but not for the onset of thyroglobulin expression. Knock-in mice, in which there is early expression of a constitutively activated form of TSHR, do not express TPO or NIS at an earlier stage, suggesting that additional mechanisms are involved in TSH-controlled gene expression. Thyroid gland size is not altered in *TSH*-null or *TSHR*-null mice, indicating that different signals control thyroid gland size and growth during embryogenesis and adult life. In fact, other growth factors such as insulin-like growth factor-1 and epidermal growth factor can promote thyroid-cell proliferation in culture (70,71). Moreover, these two growth factors are expressed during embryonic life (109,110) and could be the primary regulators of thyroid growth at that time.

In *TSHR*-null mice the thyroid glands are small, and consist of small follicles filled with colloid, suggesting that TSH signaling maintains rather than initiates folliculogen-

esis (72), although other studies suggests a role for TSH in the initiation of folliculogenesis (111). If activation of the TSH/TSHR pathway occurs in mice at E-15, and the expression of thyroid transcription factors TTF-1, TTF-2, and Pax-8, starts at E-8.5, then signals different from TSH must be involved in early thyroid development as well as in thyroid migration and final organogenesis. Despite the considerable information that is available about the morphogenic signals involved in pituitary development, there is little information about the inductive signals responsible for formation and growth of the thyroid anlagen and the signals that control migration and final organogenesis. These signals may involve a stimulus from the adjacent mesenchyme, because transplants of the presumptive thyroid region form typical thyroid tissue only when mesenchyme is present (112). The fact that fibroblast growth factor and its receptor regulate patterning of the pharyngeal region suggests that this pathway could be one of the initial steps directing the formation of the thyroid anlagen (113). Shh may also be involved, because *Shh*-null mice have thyroid ectopia or hemiagenesis (114).

INFLUENCE OF THE MATERNAL ENVIRONMENT ON FETAL THYROID FUNCTION

The maturation of the human fetal hypothalamic–pituitary–thyroid unit is complex, and the role of the maternal environment is still somewhat uncertain. Neither TSH nor TRH crosses the placenta in sufficient amounts to increase thyroid function, although high doses of exogenous TRH administered to pregnant women can increase fetal serum TSH concentrations (115). For years it was thought that very little maternal T_4 and T_3 reached the fetus during most of development, because the placenta contains a high level of type 3 deiodinase, which catalyzes the conversion of T_4 to reverse T_3 and T_3 to 3,3′-diiodothyronine (T_2), both of which are biologically inactive (see Chapters 7 and 74) (116). Nonetheless, T_4 and T_3 can be detected in embryonic and fetal fluids very early in the first trimester (6 weeks gestation), and the concentrations steadily increase thereafter (117). Therefore, fetal tissues are exposed to concentrations of T_4 and T_3 that are biologically relevant in adults long before the onset of active T_4 and T_3 secretion by the fetal thyroid gland at about mid-gestation. Furthermore, some maternal T_4 and T_3 reaches the fetus until delivery, because at birth athyreotic infants have serum T_4 and T_3 concentrations that are 20% to 50% of the concentrations in normal infants (118). In rats, T_4 and T_3 are found on E-9, well before the onset of thyroid function at E-18, and maternal thyroidectomy delays fetal development, including slowing the increase in T_4 and T_3 content in the fetal thyroid (119). Thus, in rats, maternal T_4 and T_3 affect the fetus at early stages, and it is likely that this is true for humans as well. Indeed, serum-free T_4 concentrations are lower in premature neonates than in normal fetuses *in utero* (120), and postnatal maturation of thyroid function is delayed in comparison with term infants who were not prematurely cut off from maternal T_4.

Another important aspect of fetal thyroid development that depends on the placenta is the provision of sufficient iodine for T_4 and T_3 production. Iodine is actively transported across the placenta, and fetal serum iodide concentrations at mid-gestation are considerably higher than those in maternal serum. Maternal iodine deficiency leads to neurological cretinism (see Chapter 49).

REFERENCES

1. Treier M, Rosenfeld MG. The hypothalamic-pituitary axis: co-development of two organs. *Curr Opin Cell Biol* 1996;8:833.
2. Rosenfeld MG, Briata P, Dasen J, et al. Multistep signaling and transcriptional requirements for pituitary organogenesis in vivo. *Recent Prog Horm Res* 2000;55:1.
3. Scully KM, Rosenfeld MG. Pituitary development: regulatory codes in mammalian organogenesis. *Science* 2002;295:2231.
4. Dasen JS, Rosenfeld MG. Signaling and transcriptional mechanisms in pituitary development. *Annu Rev Neurosci* 2001;24:327.
5. Sheng HZ, Moriyama K, Yamashita T, et al. Multistep control of pituitary organogenesis. *Science* 1997;278:1809.
6. Gleiberman AS, Fedtsova NG, Rosenfeld MG. Tissue interactions in the induction of anterior pituitary: role of the ventral diencephalon, mesenchyme, and notochord. *Dev Biol* 1999; 213:340.
7. Kawamura K, Kikuyama S. Induction from posterior hypothalamus is essential for the development of the pituitary proopiomelacortin (POMC) cells of the toad (Bufo japonicus). *Cell Tissue Res* 1995;279:233.
8. Kimura S, Hara Y, Pineau T, et al. The T/ebp null mouse: thyroid-specific enhancer-binding protein is essential for the organogenesis of the thyroid, lung, ventral forebrain, and pituitary. *Genes Dev* 1996;10:60.
9. Hogan BL. Bone morphogenetic proteins in development. *Curr Opin Genet Dev* 1996;6:432.
10. Ericson J, Norlin S, Jessell TM, et al. Integrated FGF and BMP signaling controls the progression of progenitor cell differentiation and the emergence of pattern in the embryonic anterior pituitary. *Development* 1998;125:1005.
11. Winnier G, Blessing M, Labosky PA, et al. Bone morphogenetic protein-4 is required for mesoderm formation and patterning in the mouse. *Genes Dev* 1995;9:2105.
12. Olson LE, Rosenfeld MG. Perspective: genetic and genomic approaches in elucidating mechanisms of pituitary development. *Endocrinology* 2002;143:2007.
13. Treier M, Gleiberman AS, O'Connell SM, et al. Multistep signaling requirements for pituitary organogenesis in vivo. *Genes Dev* 1998;12:1691.
14. Takuma N, Sheng HZ, Furuta Y, et al. Formation of Rathke's pouch requires dual induction from the diencephalon. *Development* 1998;125:4835.
15. Ruiz I, Altaba A, Palma V, Dahmane N. Hedgehog-Gli signalling and the growth of the brain. *Nat Rev Neurosci* 2002;3:24.
16. Treier M, O'Connell S, Gleiberman A, et al. Hedgehog signaling is required for pituitary gland development. *Development* 2001; 128:377.
17. Martinez Arias A. Wnts as morphogens? The view from the wing of *Drosophila*. *Nat Rev Mol Cell Biol* 2003;4:321.
18. Eastman Q, Grosschedl R. Regulation of LEF-1/TCF transcription factors by Wnt and other signals. *Curr Opin Cell Biol* 1999; 11:233.
19. Clevers H. Inflating cell numbers by Wnt. *Mol Cell* 2002;10:1260.
20. Kioussi C, Briata P, Baek SH, et al. Identification of a Wnt/Dvl/ beta-catenin–Pitx2 pathway mediating cell-type-specific proliferation during development. *Cell* 2002;111:673.
21. Watkins-Chow DE, Camper SA. How many homeobox genes does it take to make a pituitary gland? *Trends Genet* 1998;14:284.
22. Dasen JS, Rosenfeld MG. Combinatorial codes in signaling and synergy: lessons from pituitary development. *Curr Opin Genet Dev* 1999;9:566.
23. Dosen JS, Rosenfeld MG. Signaling mechanisms in pituitary morphogenesis and cell fate determination. *Curr Opin Cell Biol* 1999;11:669.
24. Sheng HZ, Zhadanov AB, Mosinger B Jr, et al. Specification of pituitary cell lineages by the LIM homeobox gene Lhx3. *Science* 1996;272:1004.
25. Szeto DP, Rodriguez-Esteban C, Ryan AK, et al. Role of the bicoid-related homeodomain factor Pitx1 in specifying hindlimb morphogenesis and pituitary development. *Genes Dev* 1999;13:484.
26. Semina EV, Reiter R, Leysens NJ, et al. Cloning and characterization of a novel bicoid-related homeobox transcription factor gene, RIEG, involved in Rieger syndrome. *Nat Genet* 1996;14:392.
27. Bach I, Rhodes SJ, Pearse RV 2nd, et al. P-Lim, a LIM homeodomain factor, is expressed during pituitary organ and cell commitment and synergizes with Pit-1. *Proc Natl Acad Sci USA* 1995;92:2720.
28. Wu W, Cogan JD, Pfaffle RW, et al. Mutations in PROP1 cause familial combined pituitary hormone deficiency. *Nat Genet* 1998;18:147.
29. Deladoey J, Fluck C, Buyukgebiz A, et al. "Hot spot" in the PROP1 gene responsible for combined pituitary hormone deficiency. *J Clin Endocrinol Metab* 1999;84:1645.
30. Rosenbloom AL, Almonte AS, Brown MR, et al. Clinical and biochemical phenotype of familial anterior hypopituitarism from mutation of the PROP1 gene. *J Clin Endocrinol Metab* 1999;84:50.
31. Pernasetti F, Toledo SP, Vasilyev VV, et al. Impaired adrenocorticotropin-adrenal axis in combined pituitary hormone deficiency caused by a two-base pair deletion (301–302delAG) in the prophet of Pit-1 gene. *J Clin Endocrinol Metab* 2000;85:390.
32. Dasen JS, Barbera JP, Herman TS, et al. Temporal regulation of a paired-like homeodomain repressor/TLE corepressor complex and a related activator is required for pituitary organogenesis. *Genes Dev* 2001;15:3193.
33. Bentley CA, Zidehsarai MP, Grindley JC, et al. Pax6 is implicated in murine pituitary endocrine function. *Endocrine* 1999; 10:171.
34. Kioussi C, O'Connell S, St-Onge L, et al. Pax6 is essential for establishing ventral-dorsal cell boundaries in pituitary gland development. *Proc Natl Acad Sci U S A* 1999;96:14378.
35. Andersen B, Rosenfeld MG. POU domain factors in the neuroendocrine system: lessons from developmental biology provide insights into human disease. *Endocr Rev* 2001;22:2.
36. Bodner M, Castrillo JL, Theill LE, et al. The pituitary-specific transcription factor GHF-1 is a homeobox-containing protein. *Cell* 1988;55:505.
37. Ingraham HA, Chen RP, Mangalam HJ, et al. A tissue-specific transcription factor containing a homeodomain specifies a pituitary phenotype. *Cell* 1988;55:519.
38. Li S, Crenshaw EB III, Rawson EJ, et al. Dwarf locus mutants lacking three pituitary cell types result from mutations in the POU-domain gene pit-1. *Nature* 1990;347:528.

39. Palomino T, Sanchez-Pacheco A, Pena P, et al. A direct protein-protein interaction is involved in the cooperation between thyroid hormone and retinoic acid receptors and the transcription factor GHF-1. *FASEB J* 1998;12:1201.

40. Dasen JS, O'Connell SM, Flynn SE, et al. Reciprocal interactions of Pit1 and GATA2 mediate signaling gradient-induced determination of pituitary cell types. *Cell* 1999;97:587.

41. Stone JA, Figueroa RE. Embryology and anatomy of the neck. *Neuroimaging Clin N Am* 2000;10:55.

42. Hoyes AD, Kershaw DR. Anatomy and development of the thyroid gland. *Ear Nose Throat J* 1985;64:318.

43. Pintar JE. Normal development of hypothalamic-pituitary-thyroid axis. In: Braverman LE, Utiger RD, eds. *Werner's and Ingbar's The thyroid: a fundamental and clinical text,* 8th ed. Philadelphia: Lippincott Williams & Wilkins, 2000:7.

44. Macchia PE. Recent advances in understanding the molecular basis of primary congenital hypothyroidism. *Mol Med Today* 2000;6:36.

45. Van Vliet G. Development of the thyroid gland: lessons from congenitally hypothyroid mice and men. *Clin Genet* 2003;63:445.

46. Capen CC. Thyroid anatomy. In: Braverman LE, Utiger RD, eds. *Werner's and Ingbar's The thyroid: a fundamental and clinical text,* 8th ed. Philaldelphia: Lippincott Williams & Wilkins, 2000:20.

47. Yap AS, Manley SW. Microtubule integrity is essential for apical polarization and epithelial morphogenesis in the thyroid. *Cell Motil Cytoskeleton* 2001;48:201.

48. Toda S, Matsumura S, Yonemitsu N, et al. Effects of various types of extracellular matrices on adhesion, proliferation, differentiation, and c-fos protein expression of porcine thyroid follicle cells. *Cell Struct Funct* 1995;20:345.

49. Tepass U. Adherens junctions: new insight into assembly, modulation and function. *Bioessays* 2002;24:690.

50. Fagman H, Grande M, Edsbagge J, et al. Expression of classical cadherins in thyroid development: maintenance of an epithelial phenotype throughout organogenesis. *Endocrinology* 2003;144:3618.

51. Ericson LE, Nilsson M. Structural and functional aspects of the thyroid follicular epithelium. *Toxicol Lett* 1992;64/65:365.

52. Takasu S, Ohno S, Komiya I, et al. Requirements of follicle structure for thyroid hormone synthesis: cytoskeletons and iodine metabolism in polarized monolayer cells on collagen gel and in double layered, follicle-forming cells. *Endocrinology* 1992; 131:1143.

53. Ramsdem JD. Angiogenesis in the thyroid gland. *J Endocrinol* 2000;166: 475.

54. Zaret KS. Liver specification and early morphogenesis. *Mech Dev* 2000;92:83.

55. Edlund H. Pancreatic organogenesis: developmental mechanisms and implication for therapy. *Nat Rev Genet* 2002;3:524.

56. Collins WT, Capen CC. Ultrastructural and functional alterations of the rat thyroid gland produced by polychlorinated biphenyls compared with iodide excess and deficiency, and thyrotropin and thyroxine administration. *Virchows Arch* 1980;33:213.

57. Nilsson M, Ericson LE. Graded response in the individual thyroid follicle cell to increasing doses of TSH. *Mol Cell Endocrinol* 1986;44:165.

58. Ericson LE, Engström G. Quantitative electron microscopic studies on exocytosis and endocytosis in the thyroid follicle cell. *Endocrinology* 1978;103:883.

59. Many M-C, Denef J-F, Haumont S, et al. Morphological and functional changes during thyroid hyperplasia and involution in C3H mice: effects of iodine and 3,5,38-triiodothyronine during involution. *Endocrinology* 1985;116:798.

60. Vassart G, Bacolla A, Brocas H, et al. Structure, expression and regulation of the thyroglobulin gene. *Mol Cell Endocrinol* 1985;40:89.

61. De La Vieja A, Dohan O, Levy O, Carrasco N. Molecular analysis of the sodium/iodide symporter: impact on thyroid and extrathyroid pathophysiology. *Physiol Rev* 2000;80:1083.

62. Dohan O, De la Vieja A, Paroder V, et al. The sodium/iodide symporter (NIS): characterization, regulation, and medical significance. *Endocr Rev* 2003;24:48.

63. Yoshida A, Taniguchi S, Hisatome I, et al. Pendrin is an iodide-specific apical porter responsible for iodide efflux from thyroid cells. *J Clin Endocrinol Metab* 2002;87:3356.

64. Everett LA, Green ED. A family of mammalian anion transporters and their involvement in human genetic diseases. *Hum Mol Genet* 1999;8:1883.

65. Kimura S, Kotani T, McBride OW, et al. Human thyroid peroxidase: complete cDNA and protein sequence, chromosome mapping, and identification of two alternately spliced mRNAs. *Proc Natl Acad Sci USA* 1987;84:5555.

66. De Deken X, Wang D, Dumont JE, et al. Characterization of ThOX proteins as components of the thyroid H(2)O(2)–generating system. *Exp Cell Res* 2002;273:187.

67. Moreno JC, Keijser R, Aarraas, et al. Cloning and characterization of a novel thyroidal gene encoding proteins with a conserved nitroreductase domain. *J Endocrinol Invest* 2002;25 [Suppl]:23.

68. Vassart G, Dumont JE. The thyrotropin receptor and the regulation of thyrocyte function and growth. *Endocr Rev* 1992; 13: 596.

69. Szkudlinski MW, Fremont V, Ronin C, et al. Thyroid-stimulating hormone and thyroid-stimulating hormone receptor structure-function relationships. *Physiol Rev* 2002;82:473.

70. Medina DL, Santisteban P. Thyrotropin-dependent proliferation of in vitro rat thyroid cell systems. *Eur J Endocrinol* 2000; 143: 161.

71. Kimura T, Van Keymeulen A, Golstein J, et al. Regulation of thyroid cell proliferation by TSH and other factors: a critical evaluation of in vitro models. *Endocr Rev* 2001;22:631.

72. Postiglione MP, Parlato R, Rodriguez-Mallon A, et al. Role of the thyroid-stimulating hormone receptor signaling in development and differentiation of the thyroid gland. *Proc Natl Acad Sci USA* 2002;99:15462.

73. Guazzi S, Price M, De Felice M, et al. Thyroid nuclear factor 1 (TTF-1) contains a homeodomain and displays a novel DNA binding specificity. *EMBO J* 1990;9:3631.

74. Zannini M, Francis-Lang H, Plachov D, et al. Pax-8, a paired domain-containing protein, binds to a sequence overlapping the recognition site of a homeodomain and activates transcription from two thyroid-specific promoters. *Mol Cell Biol* 1992; 12: 4230.

75. Zannini M, Avantaggiato V, Biffali E, et al. TTF-2, a new forkhead protein, shows a temporal expression in the developing thyroid which is consistent with a role in controlling the onset of differentiation. *EMBO J* 1997;16:3185.

76. Damante G, Di Lauro R. Thyroid-specific gene expression. *Biochim Biophys Acta* 1994;1218:255.

77. Damante G, Tell G, Di Lauro R. A unique combination of transcription factors controls differentiation of thyroid cells. *Prog Nucleic Acid Res Mol Biol* 2001;66:307.

78. Laughon A. DNA binding specificity of homeodomains. *Biochemistry* 1991;30:11357.

79. De Felice M, Damante G, Zannini M, et al. Redundant domains contribute to the transcriptional activity of the thyroid transcription factor 1. *J Biol Chem* 1995;270:26649.

80. Lazzaro D, Price M, de Felice M, et al. The transcription factor TTF-1 is expressed at the onset of thyroid and lung morpho-

genesis and in restricted regions of the foetal brain. *Development* 1991;113:1093.

81. Minoo P, Hamdan H, Bu D, et al. TTF-1 regulates lung epithelial morphogenesis. *Dev Biol* 1995;172:694.

82. Suzuki K, Kobayashi Y, Katoh R, et al. Identification of thyroid transcription factor-1 in C cells and parathyroid cells. *Endocrinology* 1998;139:3014.

83. Sussel L, Marin O, Kimura S, et al. Loss of Nkx2. 1 homeobox gene function results in a ventral to dorsal molecular respecification within the basal telencephalon: evidence for a transformation of the pallidum into the striatum. *Development* 1999; 126:3359.

84. Costa RH, Kalinichenko VV, Lim L. Transcription factors in mouse lung development and function. *Am J Physiol Lung Cell Mol Physiol* 2001;280:L823.

85. Kaestner KH, Knochel W, Martinez DE. Unified nomenclature for the winged helix/forkhead transcription factors. *Genes Dev* 2000;14:142.

86. Clark KL, Halay ED, Lai E, et al. Co-crystal structure of the HNF-3/fork head DNA-recognition motif resembles histone H5. *Nature* 1993;364:412.

87. Cirillo LA, Lin FR, Cuesta I, et al. Opening of compacted chromatin by early developmental transcription factors HNF3 (FoxA) and GATA-4. *Mol Cell* 2002;9:279.

88. Dathan N, Parlato R, Rosica A, et al. Distribution of the titf2/foxe1 gene product is consistent with an important role in the development of foregut endoderm, palate, and hair. *Dev Dyn* 2002;224:450.

89. De Felice M, Ovitt C, Biffali E, et al. A mouse model for hereditary thyroid dysgenesis and cleft palate. *Nat Genet* 1998; 19: 395.

90. Walther C, Guenet JL, Simon D, et al. Pax: a murine multigene family of paired box-containing genes. *Genomics* 1991;11:424.

91. Xu W, Rould MA, Jun S, et al. Crystal structure of a paired domain-DNA complex at 2. 5 A resolution reveals structural basis for Pax developmental mutations. *Cell* 1995;80:639.

92. Pellizzari L, D'Elia A, Rustighi A, et al. Expression and function of the homeodomain-containing protein Hex in thyroid cells. *Nucleic Acids Res* 2000;28:2503.

93. Di Palma T, Nitsch R, Mascia A, et al. The paired domain-containing factor Pax8 and the homeodomain-containing factor TTF-1 directly interact and synergistically activate transcription. *J Biol Chem* 2003;278:3395.

94. Dahl E, Koseki H, Balling R. Pax genes and organogenesis. *Bioessays* 1997;19:755.

95. Mansouri A, Chowdhury K, Gruss P. Follicular cells of the thyroid gland require Pax8 gene function. *Nat Genet* 1998;19:87.

96. Pasca di Magliano M, Di Lauro R, Zannini M. Pax8 has a key role in thyroid cell differentiation. *Proc Natl Acad Sci USA* 2000;97:13144.

97. Wendl T, Lun K, Mione M, et al. Pax2.1 is required for the development of thyroid follicles in zebrafish. *Development* 2002; 129:3751.

98. Kessel M, Drescher U, Gruss P. The murine homeo domain protein Hox 1.1. *Ann N Y Acad Sci* 1987;511:88.

99. Guazzi S, Lonigro R, Pintonello L, et al. The thyroid transcription factor-1 gene is a candidate target for regulation by Hox proteins. *EMBO J* 1994;13:3339.

100. Manley NR, Capecchi MR. The role of Hoxa-3 in mouse thymus and thyroid development. *Development* 1995;121:1989.

101. Manley NR, Capecchi MR. Hox group 3 paralogs regulate the development and migration of the thymus, thyroid, and parathyroid glands. *Dev Biol* 1998;195:1.

102. Meunier D, Aubin J, Jeannotte L. Perturbed thyroid morphology and transient hypothyroidism symptoms in Hoxa5 mutant mice. *Dev Dyn* 2003;227:367–378.

103. Martinez Barbera JP, Clements M, Thomas P, et al. The homeobox gene Hex is required in definitive endodermal tissues for normal forebrain, liver and thyroid formation. *Development* 2000;127:2433.

104. D'Elia AV, Tell G, Russo D, et al. Expression and localization of the homeodomain-containing protein HEX in human thyroid tumors. *J Clin Endocrinol Metab* 2002;87:1376.

105. Zaret KS. Regulatory phases of early liver development: paradigms of organogenesis. *Nat Rev Genet* 2002;3:499.

106. Sato K, Di Lauro R. Hepatocyte nuclear factor 3 beta participates in the transcriptional regulation of the thyroperoxidase promoter. *Biochem Biophys Res Commun* 1996;220:86.

107. Pohlenz J, Dumitrescu A, Zundel D, et al. Partial deficiency of thyroid transcription factor 1 produces predominantly neurological defects in humans and mice. *J Clin Invest* 2002;109: 469.

108. Brown RS, Shalhoub V, Coulter S, et al. Developmental regulation of thyrotropin receptor gene expression in the fetal and neonatal rat thyroid: relation to thyroid morphology and to thyroid-specific gene expression. *Endocrinology* 2000;141: 340.

109. Partanen AM. Epidermal growth factor and transforming growth factor-alpha in the development of epithelial-mesenchymal organs of the mouse. *Curr Top Dev Biol* 1990;24:31.

110. Bondy CA, Werner H, Roberts CT Jr, et al. Cellular pattern of insulin-like growth factor-I (IGF-I) and type I IGF receptor gene expression in early organogenesis: comparison with IGF-II gene expression. *Mol Endocrinol* 1990;4:1386.

111. Beamer WG, Cresswell LA. Defective thyroid ontogenesis in fetal hypothyroid (hyt/hyt) mice. *Anat Rec* 1982;202:387.

112. Dossal WE. Effects of depletion and substitution of perivascular mesenchyme upon the development of the thyroid primordium. *J Elisha Mitchell Sci Soc* 1957;73:244.

113. Trokovic N, Trokovic R, Mai P, et al. Fgfr1 regulates patterning of the pharyngeal region. *Genes Dev* 2003;17:141.

114. Fagman H, Grände M, Gritli-Linde A, et al. Genetic deletion of sonic hedgehog causes hemiagenesis and ectopic development of the thyroid in mouse. *Am J Pathol* 2004;164:1865.

115. Martino E, Grasso S, Bambini G, et al. Ontogenetic development of pancreatic thyrotropin-releasing hormone in human foetuses and in infants. *Acta Endocrinol (Copenh)* 1986;112: 372.

116. Roti E. Regulation of thyroid-stimulating hormone (TSH) secretion in the fetus and neonate. *J Endocrinol Invest* 1988; 11:145.

117. Calvo RM, Jauniaux E, Gulbis B, et al. Fetal tissues are exposed to biologically relevant free thyroxine concentrations during early phases of development. *J Clin Endocrinol Metab* 2002; 87:1768.

118. Vulsma T, Gons MH, de Vijlder JJ. Maternal-fetal transfer of thyroxine in congenital hypothyroidism due to a total organification defect or thyroid agenesis. *N Engl J Med* 1989;321:13.

119. Morreale de Escobar G, Obregon MJ, Escobar del Rey F. Is neuropsychological development related to maternal hypothyroidism or to maternal hypothyroxinemia? *J Clin Endocrinol Metab* 2000;85:3975.

120. Morreale de Escobar G, Ares S. The hypothyroxinemia of prematurity. *J Clin Endocrinol Metab* 1998;83:713.

ANATOMY AND PATHOLOGY
OF THE THYROTROPHS

MUBARAK AL-GAHTANY
MUBARAK AL-SHRAIM
KALMAN KOVACS
EVA HORVATH

It had long been known that the pituitary gland regulates the functional activity of the thyroid gland and produces a hormone called thyroid-stimulating hormone, or thyrotropin (TSH), but it was only about 50 years ago that the adenohypophysial cell type that produces TSH was morphologically identified. In studies of the pituitaries of rats that had altered function of the thyroid and other glands, using periodic acid-Schiff (PAS) and various trichrome, aldehyde fuchsin (AF), and aldehyde thionin (AT) staining techniques, several investigators delineated the thyrotrophs in the rat pituitary anterior lobe (1,2). Subsequently, the fine structural features of rat thyrotrophs were revealed by transmission electron microscopy, and the ultrastructural alterations resulting from functional changes were disclosed (3). Several attempts were also made, through the application of these and other staining procedures, to identify the thyrotrophs in the human pituitary, but it became possible to do this after the introduction of immunocytochemistry and electron microscopy.

DEVELOPMENT AND ANATOMY

The thyrotrophs can be detected by immunocytochemistry during the 12th week of gestation in the anteromedial zone of the fetal pituitary (4). They become recognizable at about the same time as the gonadotrophs, after the appearance of the somatotrophs and corticotrophs and before that of the lactotrophs. Biologically active TSH is detected in the pituitary at 14 weeks of gestation. The thyrotrophs also develop in anencephalic fetuses, and tissue culture studies indicate that their differentiation and maturation are independent of the presence of hypothalamic hormones (5,6). During development, two populations of thyrotrophs cells are generated. A lineage not dependent on the presence of the transcription factor Pit-1 appears first in the rostral part of the gland and disappears by birth. The definitive Pit-1-dependent thyrotrophs appear later in the

dorsal region of the gland and persist in the adult (7). In rats, mitoses of thyrotrophs contribute to the proliferation of the pituitary gland during the early postnatal period (8). Mitosis also has been demonstrated in the thyrotrophs of thyroidectomized adult rats and may be regulated by thyroxine (T_4) and thyrotropin-releasing hormone (TRH) (9,10).

Several pituitary transcription factors and other factors have been identified that play important roles in the processes that direct organogenesis, cell commitment, proliferation, and differentiated function. Any or all of these substances are candidates for mutations causing pituitary dysfunction. Transcription factors like Pit-1, GATA-2, and PROP1 play a major role in the differentiation and maturation of thyrotrophs (11–15). These factors also play a role in cell-specific gene expression and regulation of the gene products, namely TSH (16,17). Other factors that may play a role in thyrotroph maturation and function include cleaved-prolactin variant and neurotensin (NT) (18,19). The autocrine/paracrine regulation of TSH secretion is evidenced by the pituitary bombesin-like peptide termed neuromedin B, which acts as a local regulator of TSH secretion. Neuromedin B is up-regulated by thyroid hormones and down-regulated by TRH (20,21).

In the human pituitary, the thyrotrophs represent 1% to 5% of all adenohypophysial cells. They are not randomly located throughout the gland, but are concentrated in the anteromedial portion of the mucoid wedge of the anterior lobe; thus, they are not in proximity to the posterior lobe. In this well-demarcated area, the thyrotrophs are the predominant cell type (Fig. 3.1) (22). They contain PAS-, AF- and AT-positive cytoplasmic granules, but they are less basophilic and less PAS-positive than the corticotrophs. They do not stain with acidophilic dyes, lead hematoxylin, erythrosin, or carmoisin. Immunocytochemistry is the most reliable method to reveal the presence of thyrotrophs by light microscopy (Fig. 3.2). In situ hybridization reveals the presence of estrogen receptor

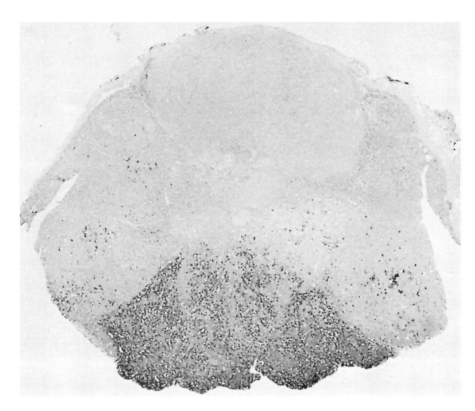

FIGURE 3.1. Photomicrograph of a human pituitary gland, showing thyrotrophs concentrated in the anteromedial portion of the gland. The section was immunostained for thyrotropin (TSH) using the avidin-biotin-peroxidase method (magnification ×6).

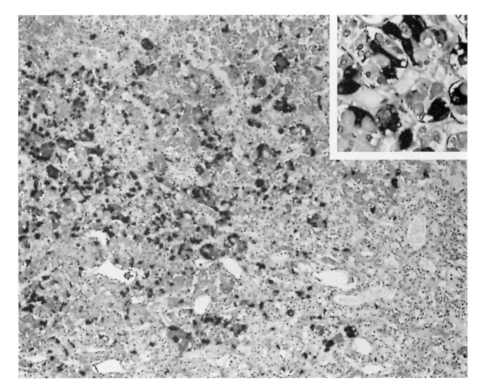

FIGURE 3.2. Low-magnification (×250) and high-magnification (×400, inset) photomicrographs of an area of the anterior lobe of a human pituitary gland rich in thyrotropin (TSH)-immunoreactive cells with long cytoplasmic processes (avidin-biotin-peroxidase method).

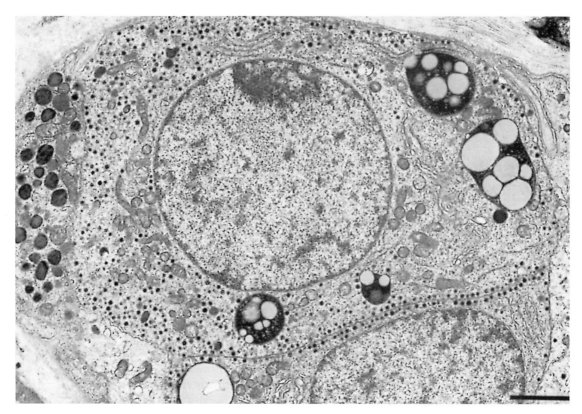

FIGURE 3.3. Electron photomicrograph of normal human thyrotrophs with euchromatic nuclei, well-developed cytoplasm, small secretory granules (100–200 nm), many of which are adjacent to the plasma membrane, and large phagolysosomes (magnification ×11,000; bar = 2 μm).

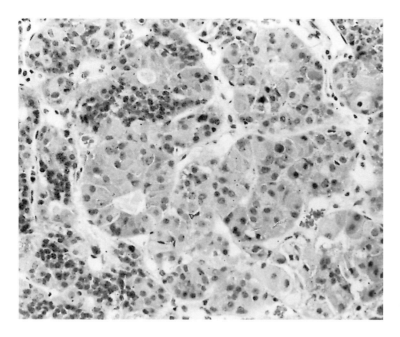

FIGURE 3.4. Photomicrograph of thyrotroph hyperplasia in the pituitary of a patient with hypothyroidism, showing large acinar structures formed by columnar cells possessing abundant, slightly vacuolated cytoplasm (hematoxylin and eosin, magnification ×220).

mRNA in nontumorous and adenomatous thyrotrophs (23).

CYTOLOGY

By electron microscopy, the thyrotrophs are medium-sized or large, elongated cells with conspicuous cytoplasmic processes and centrally located spherical or ovoid nuclei (Fig. 3.3). The cytoplasm is abundant, and its rough-surfaced endoplasmic reticulum consists of randomly distributed, slightly dilated cisternae. The Golgi complex is located in the perinuclear area; its prominence varies depending on the hormonal activity of the cell. The mitochondria are rod shaped with regular transverse cristae and a moderately electron-dense matrix. Phagolysosomes are common. The secretory granules are small, most often measuring 100 to 200 nm. They are spherical, vary slightly in electron density, and are membrane bound with an electron-lucent halo between the electron-dense core and the limiting membrane. Secretory granule extrusions are not seen.

Immunocytochemistry shows strong immunoreactivity for the β-subunit of TSH and for the α-subunit, but not for other hormones (22). Immunoelectron microscopy confirms that the thyrotrophs contain TSH localized in the secretory granules. In the rat pituitary, a few cells that contain both immunoreactive growth hormone and TSH can be identified (24), suggesting a close link between somatotrophs and thyrotrophs, and raising the possibility that somatotrophs can transform to thyrotrophs. Consistent with this suggestion, in the pituitaries of rats made hypothyroid by administration of propylthiouracil, some somatotrophs degranulate and transform into thyroidectomy cells, exhibiting the ultrastructural signs of active secretion (25). Transdifferentiation of somatotrophs to thyrotrophs has also been found in the pituitary of humans with protracted primary hypothyroidism (26). These findings support the assumption that different adenohypophysial cell types cannot be conclusively separated and that under special conditions, one cell type may transform to another cell type and become able to produce the hormone characteristic of the latter cell type. Thus, the "one cell, one hormone" theory that dominated our thinking for several decades, which recognized five distinct cell types producing the six adenohypophysial hormones, is no longer accepted (22, 27,28).

Thyrotrophs are present throughout life, and there are no major sex differences in their number, distribution, immunocytochemical profile, and histologic and ultrastructural features. They do not regress in old age, but continue to produce and release TSH (29). Indeed, the thyrotrophs are more prominent in older people in whom the incidence of subclinical and overt hypothyroidism is higher than in young or middle-aged people.

EFFECT OF THYROID DISORDERS ON PITUITARY MORPHOLOGY

Hypothyroidism

Changes in the secretion of TSH markedly affect the morphology of the thyrotrophs. In patients with long-standing primary hypothyroidism, the thyrotrophs increase in number and size (30) (Figs. 3.4 and 3.5). Reticulin stains show enlarged acinar structures without compression of surrounding tissue (Fig. 3.6). The large thyrotrophs have an abundant vacuolated cytoplasm and long, prominent cytoplasmic processes, and they contain many large, strongly PAS-positive cytoplasmic globules, which are in fact large lysosomes. These latter structures, however, may occur in other conditions and in other cell types as well (24,31,32).

Thyrotroph hyperplasia may be diffuse or nodular; the thyrotroph area within the anterior lobe enlarges, and the thyrotrophs extend to other parts of the anterior lobe. The extent of thyrotroph hypertrophy and hyperplasia may be sufficient to cause radiologically detectable enlargement of the pituitary and occasionally even optic nerve compression. Massive thyrotroph hyperplasia due to primary hypothyroidism thus may be difficult to distinguish clinically from a pituitary tumor causing central (secondary) hypothyroidism. Also, several patients with marked thyrotroph hyperplasia have been misdiagnosed as having prolactin-secreting pituitary adenomas because patients with long-standing primary hypothyroidism may have amenorrhea, galactorrhea, and hyperprolactinemia as well as pituitary enlargement (33,34).

By electron microscopy, the hypertrophic and hyperplastic thyrotrophs of patients with hypothyroidism show different degrees of dilatation and vesiculation of the endoplasmic reticulum, a prominent Golgi complex, and normal mitochondria. Also, compared with normal thyrotrophs, the secretory granules are less numerous and are similar in size or are slightly enlarged (Fig. 3.7). No exocytosis is seen (24).

In hypothyroid rats, the thyrotrophs also are large and have pale, vacuolated cytoplasm. Neurofilaments (NF-H) are seen in the thyrotrophs of hypothyroid rats, and discontinuation of antithyroid treatment leads to disappearance of the filaments (35). Electron microscopy reveals prominent endoplasmic reticulum membranes and Golgi complexes. The endoplasmic reticulum is dilated and vesiculated. The secretory granules in these thyrotrophs are small and sparse, measuring 50 to 150 nm (24). These stimulated cells are called thyroidectomy or thyroid deficiency cells and are assumed to represent hyperactive cells

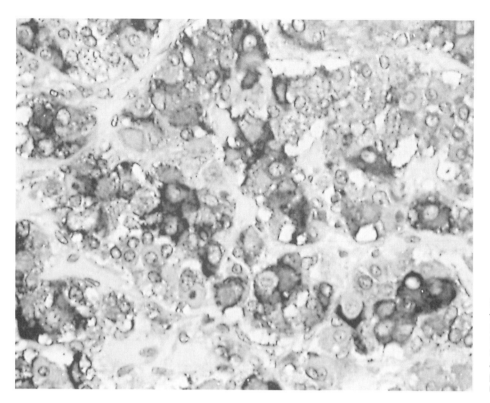

FIGURE 3.5. Photomicrograph of thyrotroph hyperplasia in the pituitary of a patient with hypothyroidism. The enlarged acini contain numerous cells intensely or moderately immuno-stained for thyrotropin (TSH) (avidin-biotin-peroxidase method, magnification ×250).

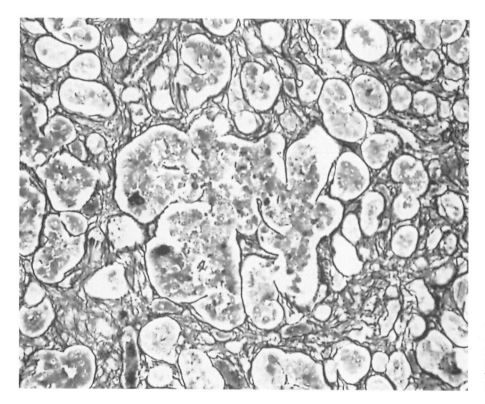

FIGURE 3.6. Reticulin-stained section of thyrotroph hyperplasia in the pituitary of a patient with hypothyroidism, showing enlarged acinar structures and loosened reticulin network (magnification ×100).

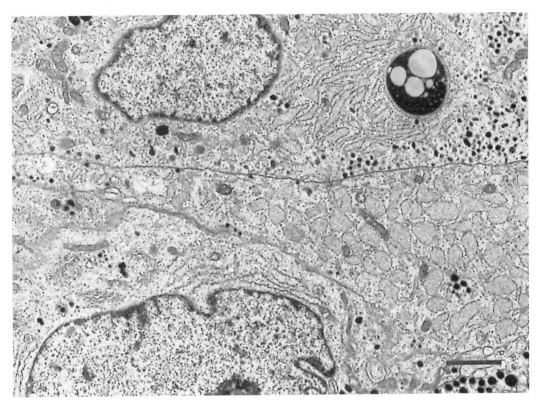

FIGURE 3.7. Electron photomicrograph of stimulated thyrotrophs in the pituitary of a patient with hypothyroidism. The rough endoplasmic reticulum is well developed and dilated or vesiculated. A lactotroph is shown at the bottom of the micrograph (magnification ×9,000; bar = 2 µm).

due to protracted stimulation secondary to the lack of negative feedback action of thyroid hormone (24). Occasionally, thyrotroph hyperplasia may progress to adenoma formation, suggesting that protracted stimulation may not only increase TSH synthesis and release, as well as cell proliferation, but also cause neoplastic transformation (34).

In humans and animals with primary hypothyroidism, thyroid hormone therapy results in regression of the morphologic changes in the pituitary, indicating that the hypertrophy and hyperplasia of thyrotrophs are reversible. This reversal is partly due to reversal of transdifferentiation and partly due to apoptosis (36).

The morphology of thyrotrophs in TRH deficiency has not yet been described in humans. In this situation, TSH secretion is decreased, and one would expect this decrease to be accompanied by morphologic changes that reflect decreased functional activity. A recent study of mice with congenital TRH deficiency revealed that TRH is not essential for fetal thyroid development, but is essential for normal postnatal thyrotroph function, including normal feedback regulation of the TSH gene by thyroid hormone (37,38).

In patients with a rare familial form of dwarfism characterized by hypothyroidism and prolactin deficiency, the pituitary contains no somatotrophs, lactotrophs, and thyrotrophs (see section on congenital hypothyroidism in Chapter 75) (39). This syndrome is caused by mutation of the *pit-1* gene (40,41). The simultaneous absence of these cells confirms the close lineal relationship among these three types of adenohypophysial cells.

Thyrotoxicosis

Pituitary morphology has not been studied much in patients with thyrotoxicosis. In 1966, Murray and Ezrin (42) described the light microscopic features of thyrotrophs in patients with thyrotoxicosis caused by Graves' disease. Using conventional histology as well as AT staining, they demonstrated regression of thyrotrophs in these patients. Well-granulated thyrotrophs could not be identified, and the cells resembling thyrotrophs were small and had small nuclei, a thin rim of cytoplasm, and a few AT-positive vesicles. Immunocytochemical studies confirmed the reversible involution of thyrotrophs in patients with Graves' disease (43).

Other Conditions

In other endocrine or nonendocrine diseases, the thyrotrophs are not altered. For example, in patients with primary adrenal insufficiency or primary hypogonadism, the number, size, distribution, and morphologic appearance of

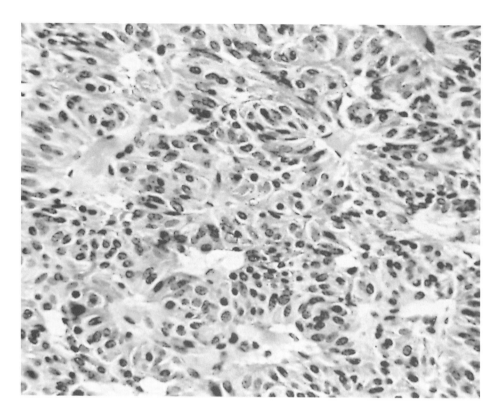

FIGURE 3.8. Photomicrograph of a thyrotroph adenoma. The chromophobic cells are disposed in pseudorosettes around vessels (hematoxylin and eosin, magnification ×250).

the thyrotrophs are normal. Similarly, the thyrotrophs are normal in patients with pituitary tumors not associated with TSH hypersecretion.

Thyrotroph Adenomas

Thyrotroph adenomas are the rarest type of anterior pituitary tumor (31,44,45), and one case of a thyrotroph carcinoma has been described (46). It is not clear why adenomas arise less frequently in thyrotrophs than in other cell types. Thyrotroph adenomas may develop in association with thyrotoxicosis or hypothyroidism (47–50), and the adenomas in both types of patients have similar morphologic features.

At the time of discovery, thyrotroph adenomas in patients with thyrotoxicosis range in size from microadenomas to large macroadenomas that occupy the entire sella turcica and may extend above it or invade neighboring structures. The adenomas are usually well demarcated from the surrounding pituitary tissue, because they are surrounded by a pseudocapsule that consists of condensed reticulin fibers and a few rows of compressed nontumorous adenohypophysial cells. The adenoma cells are chromophobic (Fig. 3.8) and contain a few small PAS-positive cytoplasmic granules or, occasionally, large PAS-positive lysosomal globules. Immunocytochemistry demonstrates the presence of TSH in the cytoplasm of the adenoma cells (Fig. 3.9) in most tumors, but in some tumors the ade-

noma cells cannot be immunostained, suggesting either loss of TSH during fixation and embedding or production of an abnormal TSH that is not immunoreactive (22). Nontumorous and adenomatous thyrotrophs express pit-1, the transcription factor responsible for the development and maturation of thyrotrophs. Although it plays no major role in the pathogenesis of thyrotroph adenomas, the invariable expression of the pit-1 protein in TSH-positive adenomas suggest that it plays a role in differentiation of the adenoma cells (51–53).

By electron microscopy, thyrotroph adenomas are composed of middle-sized or large, usually well-differentiated, moderately polar, elongated cells that have spherical nuclei showing focal pleomorphism and prominent nucleoli as well as abundant cytoplasm with long cytoplasmic processes (Fig. 3.10). The cytoplasm contains well-developed rough endoplasmic reticulum membranes. The Golgi complexes, poorly represented in some tumors but well developed in others, are located in the perinuclear area and are composed of sacs, vesicles, and a few immature secretory granules. The mitochondria are ovoid or spherical, with transverse cristae and a moderately electron-dense matrix. The secretory granules are mostly spherical and usually small, measuring 100 to 200 nm in diameter (Fig. 3.10); occasionally, adenomas have larger secretory granules (up to 400 nm). The secretory granules accumulate in the cytoplasmic processes and are often located in a single row underneath the plasmalemma, but granule exocytosis is not seen.

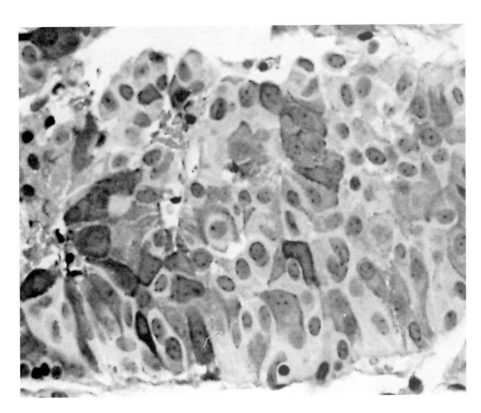

FIGURE 3.9. Photomicrograph of a thyrotroph adenoma. Most cells contain immunoreactive thyrotropin (TSH) (avidin-biotin-peroxidase method, magnification ×250).

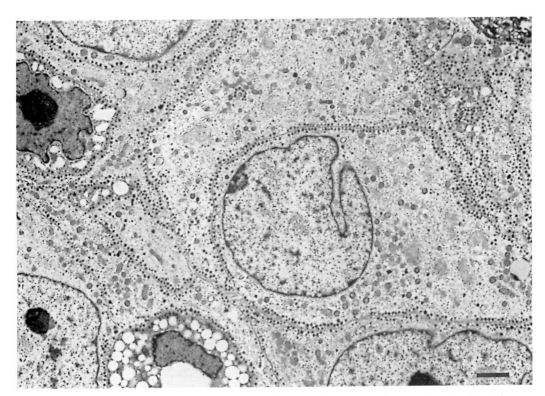

FIGURE 3.10. Electron photomicrograph of a thyrotroph adenoma, showing thyrotrophs with indented nuclei containing large nucleoli and long cytoplasmic processes. Small secretory granules are present at the periphery of the cytoplasm (magnification ×5,000; bar = 2 μm).

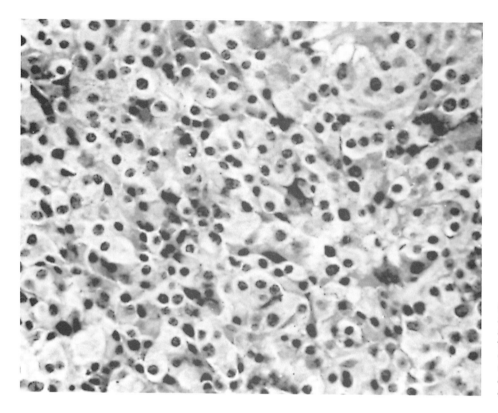

FIGURE 3.11. Photomicrograph of a glyco-protein-producing pituitary adenoma containing scattered thytropin (TSH)-immunoreactive cells (avidin-biotin-peroxidase method, magnification ×250). This tumor also contained growth hormone and α-subunit (not shown).

Thyrotroph adenomas rarely contain thyroidectomy cells. In a few tumors, however, usually in hypothyroid or euthyroid patients, the adenoma cells have the appearance of typical thyroidectomy cells. The importance of thyroidectomy cells in thyrotroph adenomas is not known, but the finding could reflect the absence of thyroid hormone receptors in the tumors. The absence of thyroidectomy cells in most tumors may reflect immaturity or the absence of TRH receptors (54).

With the wider use of immunocytochemistry and electron microscopy, it has become evident that TSH-producing cells occur often in other hormone-secreting pituitary

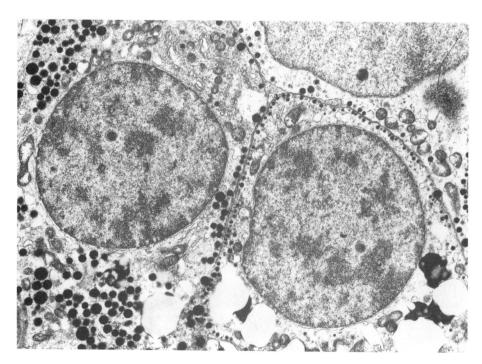

FIGURE 3.12. Electron micrograph of a plurihormonal adenoma containing cells with features of thyrotrophs (*TSH*) and somatotrophs (*GH*). The thyrotrophs contain small secretory granules lined up along the cell membranes (*right*). The cell with randomly arranged large secretory granules (*left*) is a somatotroph (magnification ×11,000).

adenomas (27,31,55,56), especially adenomas that contain growth hormone, TSH, and α-subunit. Most of these tumors are composed of densely granulated somatotrophs and are associated with acromegaly (57). There are also adenomas that contain growth hormone or prolactin, or both, along with TSH and α-subunit, with the structural features of glycoprotein-producing adenomas (31) (Fig. 3.11). Ultrastructurally, they are monomorphic adenomas that consist of cells with the characteristics of thyrotrophs (31,58). Such tumors may be associated with acromegaly and thyrotoxicosis (31,57,58). Plurihormonal adenomas composed of different cell types indicating multidirectional differentiation have also been described (Fig. 3.12) (59); usually, the expressed hormones are not secreted in clinically important amounts. Null cell adenomas and oncocytomas often have a few scattered cells or groups of cells that contain immunoreactive TSH (31). These clinically nonfunctioning tumors are thought to be derived from an uncommitted precursor cell, which may undergo multidirectional differentiation and produce various hormones, including TSH.

REFERENCES

1. Halmi NS. Two types of basophils in anterior pituitary of rat and their respective cytophysiological significance. *Endocrinology* 1950;47:289.
2. Purves HD. Cytology of the adenohypophysis. In: Harris GW and Donovan BT, eds. *The pituitary gland.* Vol 1. London: Butterworths, 1966:147.
3. Farquhar MG, Rinehart JF. Cytologic alterations in the pituitary gland following thyroidectomy: an electron microscopic study. *Endocrinology* 1954;55:857.
4. Asa SL, Kovacs K, Singer W. Human fetal adenohypophysis: morphologic and functional analysis in vitro. *Neuroendocrinology* 1991;53:562.
5. Dubois PM, Begeot M, Dubois MP, et al. Immunocytological localization of LH, FSH, TSH and their subunits in the pituitary of normal and anencephalic human fetuses. *Cell Tissue Res* 1978;191:249.
6. Dubois PM, Hemming FJ. Fetal development and regulation of pituitary cell types. *J Electron Microsc Tech* 1991;19:2.
7. Pulichino AM, Vallette-Kasic S, Tsai JP, et al. Tpit determines alternate fates during pituitary cell differentiation. *Genes Dev* 2003;17:738.
8. Taniguchi Y, Yasutaka S, Kominami R, et al. Mitoses of thyrotrophs contribute to the proliferation of the rat pituitary gland during the early postnatal period. *Anat Embryol (Berl)* 2002; 206:67.
9. Quintanar-Stephano A, Valverde R, Kovacs K. Mitotic counts in rat adenohypophysial thyrotrophs and somatotrophs: effects of short-term thyroidectomy, thyroxine, and thyrotropin-releasing hormone. *Endocr Pathol* 1999;10:335.
10. Quintanar-Stephano A, Valverde C. Mitogenic effects of thyroxine and TRH on thyrotrophs and somatotrophs of the anterior pituitary gland in thyroidectomized rats. *J Endocrinol* 1997; 154:149.
11. Li S, Crenshaw EB III, Ranson EJ, et al. Dwarf locus mutants lacking three pituitary cell types result from mutations in the POU-domain gene pit-1. *Nature* 1990;347:528.
12. Pfaffle RW, DiMattia GE, Parks JS, et al. Mutation of the POU-specific domain of pit-1 and hypopituitarism without pituitary hypoplasia. *Science* 1992;257:1118.
13. Asa SL, Ezzat S. Molecular basis of pituitary development and cytogenesis. In: Kontogeorges G and Kovacs K, eds. *Molecular pathology of the pituitary: frontiers in hormone research.* Basel: Karper 2004;32:1.
14. Rosenbloom AL, Almonte AS, Brown MR, et al. Clinical and biochemical phenotype of familial anterior hypopituitarism from mutation of the PROP1 gene. *J Clin Endocrinol Metab* 1999;84:50.
15. Parks JS, Adess ME, Brown MR. Genes regulating hypothalamic and pituitary development. *Acta Paediatr Suppl* 1997;423:28.
16. Hashimoto Y, Cisternino M, Cohen LE. A novel nonsense mutation in the Pit-1 gene: evidence for a gene dosage effect. *J Clin Endocrinol Metab* 2003;88:1241.
17. Asa SL, Ezzat S. Molecular determinants of pituitary cytodifferentiation. *Pituitary* 1999;1:159.
18. Andries M, Jacobs GF, Tilemans D, et al. In vitro immunoneutralization of a cleaved prolactin variant: evidence for a local paracrine action of cleaved prolactin in the development of gonadotrophs and thyrotrophs in rat pituitary. *J Neuroendocrinol* 1996;8:123.
19. Bello AR, Hernandez G, Gonzalez M, et al. Immunoreactive neurotensin in gonadotrophs and thyrotrophs is regulated by sex steroid hormones in the female rat. *J Neuroendocrinol* 1999;11: 785.
20. Pazos-Moura CC, Ortiga-Carvalho TM, Gaspar DM. The autocrine/paracrine regulation of thyrotropin secretion. *Thyroid* 2003;13:167.
21. Persani L. Hypothalamic thyrotropin-releasing hormone and thyrotropin biological activity. *Thyroid* 1998;8:941.
22. Kovacs K and Horvath E. Tumors of the pituitary gland. In: Hartman WH, ed. *Atlas of tumor pathology,* 2nd ed. Washington, DC: Armed Forces Institute of Pathology, 1986.
23. Stefaneanu L, Kovacs K, Horvath E, et al. In situ hybridization study of estrogen receptor messenger ribonucleic acid in human adenohypophysial cells and pituitary adenomas. *J Clin Endocrinol Metab* 1994;78:83.
24. Horvath E, Kovacs K. Fine structural cytology of the adenohypophysis in rat and man. *J Electron Microsc Tech* 1988;8:401.
25. Horvath E, Lloyd RV, Kovacs K. Propylthiouracyl-induced hypothyroidism results in reversible transdifffferentiation of somatotrophs into thyroidectomy cells: a morphologic study of the rat pituitary including immunoelectron microscopy. *Lab Invest* 1990;63:511.
26. Vidal S, Horvath E, Kovacs K, et al. Transdifferentiation of somatotrophs to thyrotrophs in the pituitary of patients with protracted primary hypothyroidism. *Virchows Arch* 2000;436: 43.
27. Kovacs K, Horvath E, Asa SL, et al. Pituitary cells producing more than one hormone: human pituitary adenomas. *Trends Endocrinol Metab* 1989;1:95.
28. Thapar K, Stefaneanu L, Kovacs K, et al. Plurihormonal pituitary tumors: beyond the one cell-one hormone theory. *Endocr Pathol* 1993;4:1.
29. Sano T, Kovacs K, Scheithauer BW, et al. Aging and the human pituitary gland. *Mayo Clin Proc* 1993;68:971.
30. Scheithauer BW, Kovacs K, Randall RV, et al. Pituitary gland in hypothyroidism: histologic and immunocytologic study. *Arch Pathol Lab Med* 1985;109:499.
31. Horvath E and Kovacs K. The adenohypophysis. In: Kovacs K, Asa SL, eds. *Functional endocrine pathology.* Boston: Blackwell, 1991:247.
32. Alkhani AM, Cusimano M, Kovacs K, et al. Cytology of pituitary thyrotroph hyperplasia in protracted primary hypothyroidism. *Pituitary* 1999;1:291.

33. Khalil A, Kovacs K, Sima AAF, et al. Pituitary thyrotroph hyperplasia mimicking prolactin-secreting adenoma. *J Endocrinol Invest* 1984;7:399.

34. Al-Gahtany M, Horvath E, Kovacs K. Pituitary hyperplasia. *Hormones* 2003;2:149.

35. Salinas E, Quintanar JL. Neurofilaments in thyrotrophs of hypothyroid rats: an immunohistochemical study. *Endocr Pathol* 2000;11:195.

36. Kulig E, Camper SA, Kuecker S, et al. Remodeling of hyperplastic pituitaries in hypothyroid us-subunit knockout mice after thyroxine and 17β-estradiol treatment: role of apoptosis. *Endocr Pathol* 1998;9:261.

37. Shibusawa N, Yamada M, Hirato J, et al. Requirement of thyrotropin-releasing hormone for the postnatal functions of pituitary thyrotrophs: ontogeny study of congenital tertiary hypothyroidism in mice. *Mol Endocrinol* 2000;14:137.

38. Yamada M, Saga Y, Shibusawa N, et al. Tertiary hypothyroidism and hyperglycemia in mice with targeted disruption of the thyrotropin-releasing hormone gene. *Proc Natl Acad Sci USA* 1997;4:10862.

39. Asa SL, Kovacs K, Halasz A, et al. Absence of somatotrophs, lactotrophs, and thyrotrophs in the pituitary of two dwarfs with hypothyroidism: deficiency of pituitary transcription factor-1? *Endocr Pathol* 1992;3:93.

40. Ingraham HA, Albert VR, Chen R, et al. A family of POU-domain and pit-1 tissue-specific transcription factors in pituitary and neuroendocrine development. *Annu Rev Physiol* 1990;52:773.

41. Simmons DM, Voss JW, Ingraham HA, et al. Pituitary cell phenotypes involve cell-specific pit-1 mRNA translation and synergistic interactions with other classes of transcription factors. *Genes Dev* 1990;4:695.

42. Murray S, Ezrin C. Effects of Graves' disease on the "thyrotroph" of the adenohypophysis. *J Clin Endocrinol Metab* 1966;26:287.

43. Scheithauer BW, Kovacs KT, Young WF Jr, et al. The pituitary gland in hyperthyroidism. *Mayo Clin Proc* 1992;67:22.

44. Klibanski A, Zervas NT. Diagnosis and management of hormone-secreting pituitary adenomas. *N Engl J Med* 1991;324:822.

45. Thapar K, Kovacs K, Laws ER Jr, et al. Pituitary adenomas: current concepts in classification, histopathology, and molecular biology. *Endocrinologist* 1993;3:39.

46. Mixson AJ, Friendman TC, Katz DA, et al. Thyrotropin-secreting pituitary carcinoma. *J Clin Endocrinol Metab* 1993;76: 529.

47. Beckers A, Abs R, Mahler C, et al. Thyrotropin-secreting pituitary adenomas: report of seven cases. *J Clin Endocrinol Metab* 2003;72:477.

48. Gesundheit N, Petrick PA, Nissim M, et al. Thyrotropin-secreting pituitary adenomas: clinical and biochemical heterogeneity. case reports and follow-up of nine patients. *Ann Intern Med* 1989;111:827.

49. Mindermann T, Wilson CB. Thyrotropin-producing pituitary adenomas. *J Neurosurg* 1993;79:521.

50. Wynne AG, Charib H, Scheithauer BW, et al. Hyperthyroidism due to inappropriate secretion of thyrotropin. *Am J Med* 1992; 92:15.

51. Lloyd RV, Chandler WF, Horvath E, et al. Pituitary specific transcription factor messenger ribonucleic expression in adenomatous and nontumorous human pituitary tissues. *Lab Invest* 1993;69:570.

52. Pellegrini I, Barlier A, Gunz G, et al. Pit-1 gene expression in the human pituitary and pituitary adenomas. *J Clin Endocrinol Metab* 1994;79:189.

53. Sanno N, Teramoto A, Matsuno A, et al. Expression of human Pit-1 product in the human pituitary and pituitary adenomas. Immunohistochemical studies using an antibody against synthetic human Pit-1 product. *Arch Pathol Lab Med* 1996;120:73.

54. Chanson P, Li JY, Le Dafniet M, et al. Absence of receptors for thyrotropin (TSH)-releasing hormone in human TSH-secreting pituitary adenoma associated with hyperthyroidism. *J Clin Endocrinol Metab* 1988;66:447.

55. Felix I, Asa SL, Kovacs K, et al. Recurrent plurihormonal bimorphous pituitary adenomas producing growth hormone, thyrotropin, and prolactin. *Arch Pathol Lab Med* 1994;118:66.

56. Terzolo M, Orlandi F, Basetti M, et al. Hyperthyroidism due to a pituitary adenoma composed of two different cell types, one secreting alpha-subunit alone and another cosecreting alpha-subunit and thyrotropin. *J Clin Endocrinol Metab* 1991;72:415.

57. Scheithauer BW, Horvath E, Kovacs K, et al. Plurihormonal pituitary adenomas. *Semin Diagn Pathol* 1986;3:69.

58. Kovacs K, Horvath E, Ezrin C, et al. Adenoma of the human pituitary producing growth hormone and thyrotropin: a histologic, immunocytologic and fine-structural study. *Virchows Arch* 1982;395:59.

59. Horvath E, Kovacs K, Scheithauer BW, et al. Pituitary adenomas producing growth hormone, prolactin and one or more glycoprotein hormones: a histologic, immunohistochemical and ultrastructural study of four surgically-removed tumors. *Ultrastruct Pathol* 1983;5:171.

THYROID SYNTHESIS AND SECRETION

4

THYROID HORMONE SYNTHESIS

4A   THYROID IODINE TRANSPORT

NANCY CARRASCO

Iodine [or iodide (I^-) in its ionized form] is an essential nutrient, primarily because of the role it plays as an indispensable component of the two thyroid hormones triiodothyronine (T_3) and thyroxine (T_4). The thyroid hormones are iodothyronines, i.e., the result of two coupled iodotyrosines, and are the only iodine-containing hormones in vertebrates. Without iodine there is no biosynthesis of thyroid hormones. Therefore, thyroid function ultimately depends on an adequate supply of iodine. A remarkably efficient and specialized system has evolved in the thyroid that ensures that most of the ingested dietary I^- (the only source of I^-) is accumulated in the gland and thus made available for T_3 and T_4 biosynthesis. The importance of this becomes more apparent when one considers that I^- is rather scarce in the environment. Endemic goiter and cretinism caused primarily by insufficient dietary supply of I^- remain a major health problem in many parts of the world, affecting millions of people (1). This situation dramatizes the health value of I^- as a nutrient and the consequences to society of its environmental scarcity.

Iodine was discovered in 1811 by Courtois, who isolated it by treating seaweed ash with sulphuric acid (2). The ability of the thyroid to concentrate I^- was first reported as early as the 19th century (3,4). The thyroid gland was found to be capable of concentrating I^- by a factor of 20 to 40 with respect to its concentration in the plasma under physiological conditions. Hence the existence of a thyroid I^- transporter was inferred, and some of its properties were elucidated over the years [see (5–7) for reviews]. Briefly, I^- accumulation in the thyroid has long been shown to be an active transport process that occurs against the I^- electrochemical gradient, stimulated by thyrotropin (TSH), and blocked by the well-known "classic" competitive inhibitors, the anions thiocyanate and perchlorate. Eventually, it was determined that the thyroid I^- transporter is a sodium-iodide (Na^+/I^-) symporter (NIS) (8–12), i.e., an intrinsic plasma membrane transport protein that couples the inward "downhill" translocation of Na^+ with the inward "uphill" translocation of I^- (Fig. 4A.1). The driving force for the process is the inwardly directed Na^+ gradient generated by the Na^+/K^+ adenosine triphos-

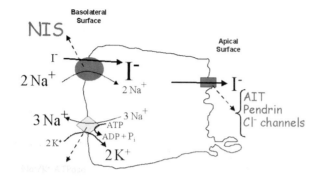

FIGURE 4A.1. Iodide (I⁻) transport in thyroid follicular cells. The basolateral surface of the cell is shown on the left side of the figure and the apical surface on the right. *Circle:* active accumulation of I⁻, mediated by the sodium-iodide symporter; *diamond:* Na^+/K^+ adenosine triphosphatase; *rectangle:* I⁻ efflux into the colloid, mediated by apical iodide transporter, pendrin, or Cl⁻ channels.

phate (ATP)-ase (Fig. 4A.1). The ability of the thyroid to accumulate I⁻ via NIS provided the basis for diagnostic scintigraphic imaging of the thyroid with radioiodide and has served as an effective means for pharmacologic doses of radioiodide to target and destroy hyperfunctioning thyroid tissue, such as in Graves' disease, or I⁻-transporting thyroid cancer cells. Therefore, the study of NIS is of great relevance to thyroid pathophysiology. Nevertheless, no molecular information on NIS was available until 1996, when after a decades-long search by numerous investigators, the DNA encoding rat NIS was finally isolated by expression cloning in *Xenopus laevis* oocytes (13). This development marked the beginning of the molecular characterization of NIS.

NIS mediates the first and key step in the process of supplying I⁻ to the gland for thyroid hormone biosynthesis, that is, the active transport of I⁻ against its electrochemical gradient across the basolateral plasma membrane into the cytoplasm of the follicular cells (I⁻ uptake) (Fig. 4A.1). I⁻ is then translocated across the apical membrane into the colloid, located in the follicular lumen (I⁻ efflux). I⁻ efflux into the follicular lumen has been suggested to be mediated by a different plasma membrane transporter putatively located on the apical side of the follicular cells, facing the colloid. The identity of this transporter has yet to be unequivocally established. Two different proteins, pendrin (14) and the apical iodide transporter (AIT) (15), have been proposed to play the role of mediator of I⁻ efflux. However, it is also possible that I⁻ efflux is mediated by Cl⁻ channels or transporters (Fig. 4A.1).

This chapter focuses on the most recent NIS research at the molecular level, which has become an exciting new field in thyroidology, and on the impact this research is having on our understanding of thyroidal and extrathyroidal physiology and disease.

POSSIBLE ROLE OF SODIUM-IODIDE SYMPORTER IN HUMAN EVOLUTION

In a fascinating and provocative report, Dobson (16) suggested that the geographical distribution of the environmental supply of iodine and hominid adaptations to it may have played a major role in human evolution. Dobson suggested that the anatomical characteristics of Neanderthals were remarkably similar to those of modern humans who suffer from cretinism as a result of iodine deficiency. He argues persuasively that these observations support the notion that a single genetic alteration, which resulted in a better ability to trap I⁻ in the thyroid, may explain the differences between Neanderthals and modern humans, and may account for the eventual replacement of Neanderthal populations by modern humans. In light of Dobson's article, it seems conceivable that the development of numerous characteristic and essential traits of modern humans, most notably brain development and intelligence, may have resulted in part from improved thyroidal I⁻ transport. Although it remains to be demonstrated, if such a single genetic alteration indeed occurred, and had the described effect, it could have involved, precisely, the gene that encodes NIS.

MOLECULAR CHARACTERIZATION OF SODIUM-IODIDE SYMPORTER

Identification of the Sodium-Iodide Symporter DNA

A promising development in the search for the NIS molecule was the expression of perchlorate-sensitive Na^+/I^- symport activity in *X. laevis* oocytes by microinjection of poly A⁺ RNA isolated from FRTL-5 cells, a highly functional line of rat thyroid-derived cells (11). A sevenfold increase of I⁻ accumulation over background was observed 6 to 7 days after injection. Poly A⁺ RNA was subsequently fractionated by sucrose gradient centrifugation, and fractions were assayed for their ability to induce I⁻ accumulation in oocytes. The poly A⁺ RNA encoding NIS was found in fractions containing messenger RNA that were 2.8 to 4.0 kb in length (11). Thus, the oocyte system was shown to be of potential value for the possible expression cloning of the cDNA that encodes NIS in the absence of oligonucleotides, based on protein sequence data or anti-NIS antibodies. After a few years, this cloning strategy was successful.

Dai et al (13) generated several cDNA libraries from poly A⁺ RNA of FRTL-5 cells and subjected them to expression screening in *X. laevis* oocytes. The library was size-fractionated, and the fraction containing inserts from 2.5 to 4.5 kb was screened. The poly A⁺ RNA encoding NIS was found in a fraction containing messages of 2.8 to 4.0 kb in length (11). The expression cloning of NIS was carried out by measuring perchlorate-sensitive Na$^+$/I$^-$ symport activity in oocytes microinjected with cRNAs made *in vitro* from pools containing decreasing numbers of cDNA clones. The cloning of NIS marked the beginning of its molecular characterization, as discussed later in the chapter.

Primary Sequence and Secondary Structure Model of Sodium-Iodide Symporter

The complete nucleotide sequence of the cloned NIS cDNA and the deduced amino-acid sequence are presented in the Dai et al study (13). Beginning with Met at position 1, a long, open-reading frame codes for a protein of 618 amino acids (relative molecular mass, 65,196). The hydropathic profile and initial secondary structure predictions of the protein led Dai et al (13,17) to suggest an intrinsic membrane protein with 12 putative transmembrane segments. However, this model has subsequently been revised, as detailed later in the chapter. The NH$_2$ terminus was originally placed on the cytoplasmic side, given the absence of a signal sequence. The COOH terminus, which was also predicted to be on the cytoplasmic side, was found to contain a large hydrophilic region of ~70 amino acids. Levy et al demonstrated experimentally the intracellular orientation of the COOH terminus by showing that an anti-COOH terminus antibody to its epitope only after cell permeabilization (18). Three potential Asn-glycosylation sites were identified in the deduced amino acid sequence at positions 225, 485, and 497. The first was located in a predicted intracellular hydrophilic loop, while the last two were located in the last hydrophilic loop, a segment predicted to be on the extracellular face of the membrane.

Levy et al (19) obtained conclusive evidence that, contrary to previous suggestions (20), neither partial nor total lack of *N*-linked glycosylation impairs the activity, stability, or targeting of NIS. Using site-directed mutagenesis, Levy et al (19) substituted both separately and simultaneously the Asn residues (amino acids 225, 485, and 497) with Gln in all three putative *N*-linked glycosylation consensus sequences of NIS and assessed the effects of the mutations. All mutants were active and displayed 50% to 100% of wild-type NIS activity, including the completely nonglycosylated triple mutant. The half-life of nonglycosylated NIS was similar to wild-type NIS, and the K$_m$ value for I$^-$ (~20 to 30 mM) in nonglycosylated NIS was virtually identical to that of wild-type NIS. These findings demonstrate that, to a considerable extent, function, targeting, and stability of NIS are present even in the total absence of *N*-linked glycosylation (19). Therefore, a bacterial expression system in which no *N*-linked glycosylation occurs might be used to overproduce NIS for structural studies.

Levy et al (19) also demonstrated that the putative *N*-linked glycosylation site at N225, which had originally been predicted to face intracellularly, is indeed glycosylated. Therefore, it is now clear that the hydrophilic loop that contains this sequence faces the extracellular milieu rather than the cytosol. They have proposed a 13-transmembrane-segment model to be the most likely secondary structure for NIS (Fig. 4A.2). In contrast to the original model, in which the NH$_2$ terminus was predicted to face the cytosol on account of the lack of a signal sequence in NIS, in the current model both the NH$_2$ terminus and the hydrophilic loop containing N225 are predicted to be on the extracellular side, and the COOH terminus faces the cytosol.

Levy et al (19) subsequently demonstrated unequivocally that the NH$_2$ terminus faces the external milieu, as proposed in the current model. This conclusion was reached using two independent experimental approaches. First, these authors introduced a FLAG epitope at the NH$_2$ terminus. COS cells transfected with FLAG-containing NIS displayed I$^-$ uptake undistinguishable from that of COS cells transfected with wild-type NIS. Immunofluorescence experiments demonstrated positive immunoreactivity with anti-FLAG antibodies (Ab) in nonpermeabilized COS cells transfected with FLAG-containing NIS. Positive immunoreactivity in nonpermeabilized cells indicates that the NH$_2$ terminus faces externally. In contrast, immunoreactivity using anti-COOH Ab requires permeabilization because the COOH terminus faces the cytosol (18,20). The second technique took advantage of a previous observation that nonglycosylated NIS is active. The *N*-linked glycosylation amino acid sequence NNSS was introduced into the NH$_2$ terminus of unglycosylated NIS (21). They observed glycosylation of NIS at the NH$_2$ terminus upon transfection of NNSS-containing NIS into COS cells, thus proving that the NH$_2$ terminus faces the

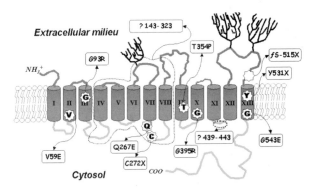

FIGURE 4A.2. Model of the secondary structure of the human sodium-iodide symporter. Iodide transport defect–causing mutations are shown in the *rounded rectangles*, which contain the WT amino acid letter, its position, and the letter of the amino acid causing the mutation. X, stop codon; fS, frame shift; δ, deletion.

lumen of the endoplasmic reticulum during biosynthesis and therefore faces the external milieu upon reaching the plasma membrane.

Sodium-Iodide Symporter Mechanism and Stoichiometry

Eskandari et al (22) have examined the mechanism, stoichiometry, and specificity of NIS by means of electrophysiological, tracer-uptake, and electron microscopic methods in *X. laevis* oocytes expressing NIS. These authors obtained electrophysiological recordings using the two microelectrode voltage clamp technique. They showed that an inward steady-state current (i.e., a net influx of positive charge) is generated in NIS-expressing oocytes upon addition of I^- to the bathing medium, leading to depolarization of the membrane. Since the recorded current is attributable to NIS activity, this observation confirms that NIS activity is electrogenic. Simultaneous measurements of tracer fluxes and currents revealed that two Na^+ ions are transported with one anion, demonstrating unequivocally a 2:1 Na^+/I^- stoichiometry. Therefore, the observed inward steady-state current is due to a net influx of Na^+ ions.

Eskandari et al (22) determined that the turnover rate of NIS is ~36 s^{-1}, and reported that expression of NIS in oocytes led to a ~2.5-fold increase in the density of plasma membrane protoplasmic face intramembrane particles, as ascertained by freeze-fracture electron microscopy. This is the first direct electron microscopy visualization of ostensible NIS molecules present in the oocyte plasma membrane. Moreover, on the basis of their kinetic results, these authors proposed an ordered simultaneous transport mechanism in which Na^+ binds to NIS before I^-, where transport of both ions is simultaneous, binding is ordered and sequential.

Specificity of Sodium-Iodide Symporter

Similar steady-state inward currents were generated by a wide variety of anions in addition to I^- (including ClO_3^-, SCN^-, $SeCN^-$, NO_3^-, Br^-, IO_4^-, and BrO_3^-), indicating that these anions are also transported by NIS. However, perchlorate (ClO_4^-), the most widely characterized inhibitor of thyroidal I^- uptake, was found surprisingly to not generate a current, strongly suggesting that it is not transported (22). Yoshida et al (23) have reported, similarly, that perchlorate did not induce an inward current in Chinese hamster ovary (CHO) cells stably expressing NIS, as measured using the whole-cell patch-clamp technique. The most likely interpretation of these observations is that perchlorate is not transported by NIS, although the unlikely possibility that perchlorate is translocated by NIS on a 1:1 Na^+/ClO_4^- stoichiometry cannot be ruled out. To

unequivocally elucidate whether perchlorate is translocated or not by NIS, flux experiments would need to be performed with perchlorate labeled with ^{36}Cl. However, the low specific activity and exorbitant cost of ^{36}Cl make such experiments practically impossible. Yoshida et al (24) thereafter showed that perchlorate elicits no change in the membrane current in the highly functional rat thyroid cell line FRTL-5, as revealed by the whole-cell patch-clamp technique, thus strongly suggesting that perchlorate is not transported into FRLT-5 cells and supporting both their previous observations in CHO cells (23) and Eskandari et al's (22) results in oocytes. Therefore, currently available data indicate that perchlorate is a potent inhibitor of NIS that acts as a blocker, not a substrate.

REGULATION OF THE SODIUM-IODIDE SYMPORTER

Regulation of Sodium-Iodide Symporter Transcription

Three different transcription factors have been implicated in thyroid-specific gene transcription (25,26): (a) thyroid transcription factor-1 (TTF-1), a homeodomain (HD)-containing protein present in the developing thyroid, lung, forebrain, and pituitary, as well as in the adult thyroid and lung; (b) TTF-2, a fork head protein detected in developing thyroid, anterior pituitary, and adult thyroid; and (c) Pax-8, a nuclear protein member of the murine family of paired-domain (PD)–containing genes, present in the developing thyroid, kidney, and midbrain boundary, as well as in the adult thyroid and kidney. Specific combinations of these factors have been proposed to regulate transcription of the thyroid-specific proteins thyroglobulin (Tg), thyroid peroxidase (TPO), and thyrotropin receptor (TSHR).

Genomic Organization of the Human Sodium-Iodide Symporter

The cDNA-encoding human NIS (hNIS) was identified on the expectation that hNIS would be highly homologous to rat NIS (rNIS). Using primers to the rNIS cDNA sequence (specifically rNIS nucleotide sequences 362 to 480 and 671 to 900), Smanik et al (27) amplified a cDNA fragment of hNIS from human papillary thyroid carcinoma tissue by PCR, utilized this cDNA fragment to screen a human thyroid cDNA library, and isolated a single cDNA clone encoding hNIS. The nucleotide sequence of hNIS revealed an open reading frame of 1929 nucleotides, which encodes a protein of 643 amino acids. Human NIS exhibits 84% identity and 93% similarity to rNIS, and it differs from rNIS only in that it has a 5 amino acid insertion between the last two hydrophobic domains (amino acids 485 to 488 and 499) and a 20 amino acid insertion in the COOH terminus (amino acids 618 to 637). Subsequently, Smanik et al (28) examined the expression, exon-intron organization, and chromosome mapping of hNIS. Fifteen exons encoding hNIS were found to be interrupted by 14 introns (Fig. 4A.3), and the hNIS gene was mapped to chromosome 19p. The human NIS promoter has been sequenced by three different groups (29–31).

Analysis of the Rat and Human Sodium-Iodide Symporter Promoters

It has long been established that TSH stimulates NIS activity via the cyclic adenosine monophosphate (cAMP) pathway (20,32,33) and, more recently, that it up-regulates NIS messenger RNA (mRNA) levels (34). However, to fully understand these mechanisms, it is necessary to study the transcriptional regulation of NIS. As for rNIS, Endo et al (35) localized a TTF-1 binding site between -245 and -230 bp, in the proximal rNIS promoter (2 kb), that confers thyroid-specific transcription, but only exerts a modest effect. The same group (36) subsequently identified, in the 5'-flaking region between -1968 and +1 bp, a novel TSH-responsive element (TRE) between -420 and -385 bp upstream of the TTF-1 site in the rNIS promoter that up-regulated two- to threefold NIS expression. The TSH effect is cyclic AMP-mediated and thyroid-specific. The protein that binds this site is different from TTF-1, TTF-2, Pax-8, or other known transcription factors. The authors named the putative binding protein in the TRE site NTF-1 (NIS TSH-responsive factor-1). However, as the TSH up-regula-

tion of NIS via this TRE site is lower than the regulation that the same group reported previously (~sixfold) (34), they have suggested that other transcription-binding sequences may be present upstream from the region they studied.

A thorough characterization of the upstream enhancer of the rNIS gene was reported by Ohno et al (37). These authors showed that the rNIS regulatory region contains a non-thyroid-specific promoter between -564 and -2 bp, and an enhancer located between -2264 and -2495 bp that recapitulates the most relevant aspects of NIS regulation (Fig. 4A.4). This rNIS enhancer mediates thyroid-specific gene expression by the interaction of Pax-8 with a novel cyclic AMP-dependent pathway. The NIS upstream enhancer (NUE) stimulates transcription in a thyroid-specific and cyclic AMP-dependent manner. NUE contain: two Pax-8–binding sites (PA and PB); two TTF-1 binding sites (TA and TB), which have no effect on rNIS transcription; and a degenerate cyclic AMP-responsive element (CRE) sequence (5'-TGACGCA-3'), which is important for NUE transcriptional activity (Fig. 4A.4). Interestingly, the same degenerate CRE sequence has been implicated in tissue-specific cyclic AMP response of other promoters, such as the β-hydroxylase (38), prohormone convertase 1 (39), and proenkephalin genes (40). In NUE, both Pax-8 and the unidentified CRE-like binding factor act synergistically to obtain full

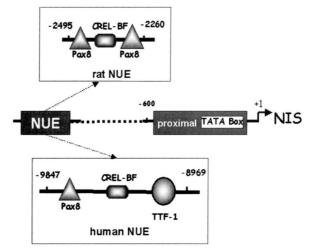

FIGURE 4A.4. Diagram of the sodium-iodide symporter (NIS) promoter indicating the major transcription start site (+1), the TATA box, the proximal promoter, and the NIS upstream enhancer (NUE). The rat proximal promoter contains a thyroid transcription factor-1 (TTF-1) binding site and a thyrotropin (TSH)-responsive element where a putative transcription factor NIS TSH-responsive factor-1 interacts. The rat NIS upstream enhancer (NUE) **(top)** contains two Pax-8 binding sites and a degenerative cyclic AMP-response-element sequence (CRE); and the human NUE **(bottom)** contains one Pax-8 binding site, one TTF-1 binding site, and one CRE-like binding site, which are important for full TSH/cyclic AMP-dependent transcription.

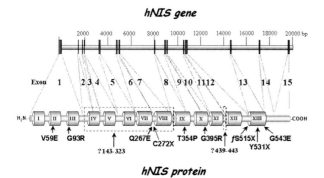

FIGURE 4A.3. Correlation of the structural organization of the human sodium-iodide symporter (hNIS) gene with the NIS protein. Exons in the hNIS gene are represented by *gray rectangles*. The putative 13 transmembrane segments in the protein are represented by *roman numerals*. Exons are connected to the corresponding amino acid region of the protein by dotted lines. Localization of the iodide transport defect mutations is indicated under the schematic representation of the hNIS protein.

TSH/cyclic AMP-dependent transcription. However, this enhancer is also able to mediate cyclic AMP-dependent transcription by a novel protein kinase A (PKA)-independent mechanism (37).

Transcriptional regulation of the Tg, TPO, and TSHR genes by TSH/forskolin is mediated by cyclic AMP. However, no CRE sequences have been identified for any of these, except the TSHR gene. Thus, the novel PKA-independent mechanism reported by Ohno et al (37) is highly significant, as it establishes a direct relationship between thyroid-specific transcription factors and the TSH/cyclic AMP regulation in rNIS. This picture clearly separates rNIS gene regulation from that of true thyroid-restricted genes (Tg and TPO) and also from TSHR, a notion consistent with the fact that NIS is not exclusively expressed in the thyroid gland.

Recently, a thyroid-specific, TSH-responsive, far-upstream (-9847 to -8968) enhancer in the human NIS gene—highly homologous to the rat NUE—has been reported by two groups (41,42). It contains putative Pax-8 and TTF-1 binding sites and a CRE-like sequence. The TTF-1 binding site is not required for full activity (41,42) (Fig. 4A.4).

Regulation of Sodium-Iodide Symporter in the Thyroid by Thyrotropin

TSH is the primary hormonal regulator of thyroid function overall and has long been known to stimulate thyroidal I⁻ accumulation. Most actions of TSH take place through activation of adenylyl cyclase via the guanosine triphosphate (GTP) binding protein Gα. This cascade of events is initiated by the interaction of TSH with its receptor (i.e., TSHR) on the basolateral membrane of the follicular cells. Early observations made prior to the isolation of the NIS cDNA suggested that TSH stimulation of I⁻ accumulation results, at least in part, from the cyclic AMP-mediated increased biosynthesis of NIS (32,33). Once the rat NIS cDNA was isolated (13) and anti-NIS Ab were generated, Levy et al demonstrated in rats that NIS protein expression is up-regulated by TSH *in vivo* (18). Consistent with these findings is a later observation by Uyttersprot et al (43) that the expression of NIS mRNA in dog thyroid (~3.9 kb) is dramatically up-regulated by goitrogenic treatment [i.e., propylthiouracil (PTU) treatment, which leads to high TSH serum levels *in vivo*].

Up-regulation of thyroid NIS expression and I⁻ uptake activity by TSH has been demonstrated not only in rats *in vivo* (18), but in rat thyroid-derived FRTL-5 cells (33) and human thyroid primary cultures (44,45). Marcocci et al (46), Kogai et al (34), and Ohno et al (37) have all shown that TSH up-regulates I⁻ uptake activity by a cyclic AMP-mediated increase in NIS transcription. After TSH withdrawal, a reduction of both intracellular cyclic AMP levels

and I⁻ uptake activity is observed in FRTL-5 cells (33). This is a reversible process, as I⁻ uptake activity can be restored either by TSH or agents that increase cyclic AMP (33,37). To investigate NIS biogenesis, Levy et al (18) carried out metabolic labeling and immunoprecipitation experiments in the presence of TSH and observed that NIS is synthesized as a precursor (~56 kDa) (19). After a 60-minute chase period, a broad, fully processed polypeptide band (~90 kDa) also became apparent.

Kaminsky et al (32) made the surprising observation that I⁻ uptake activity is present in membrane vesicles (MV) prepared from FRTL-5 cells that, when intact, had completely lost I⁻ uptake activity due to prolonged TSH deprivation (Fig. 4A.5). This suggests that mechanisms other than transcription may also operate to regulate NIS activity in response to TSH.

Kogai et al (44) have shown that TSH markedly stimulates NIS mRNA and protein levels in both monolayer and follicle-forming human primary thyrocyte cultures, whereas significant stimulation of I⁻ uptake is observed only in follicles. These interesting observations indicate that, in addition to TSH stimulation, cell polarization and spatial organization are crucial for proper NIS activity, and suggest that NIS may be regulated by such posttranscriptional events as subcellular distribution. Riedel et al (47) have demonstrated conclusively by immunoblot analysis that NIS is present in FRTL-5 cells as late as 10 days after TSH withdrawal and that *de novo* NIS biosynthesis requires TSH (47). Therefore, it is clear that any NIS molecules detected in TSH-deprived FRTL-5 cells had to be synthesized prior to TSH withdrawal. This is consistent with NIS being a protein with an exceptionally long half-life, as suggested by Kogai et al (34) and Paire et al (20). Riedel et al (47) determined by pulse-chase analysis that the NIS half-life is ~5 days in the presence and ~3 days in the absence of TSH. Even though the NIS half-life in the absence of TSH is 40% shorter than in its presence, persistence of significant I⁻ uptake activity in MV from cells deprived of TSH (47).

Riedel et al (47) later observed that 3 days after TSH deprivation, intracellular NIS decreases at a slower rate than plasma membrane NIS, supporting the notion that active NIS molecules, initially located in the plasma membrane while TSH is present, are redistributed to intracellular compartments in response to TSH withdrawal. This model explains the presence of NIS activity in MV from cells deprived of TSH that, when intact, have no NIS activity (Fig. 4A.5). Clearly, TSH regulates I⁻ uptake by modulating the subcellular distribution of NIS without apparently influencing the intrinsic functional status of the NIS molecules. Riedel et al (47) have also shown that NIS is phosphorylated *in vivo* and that serines are the main amino acid residues in which phosphorylation takes place in NIS, independently of TSH presence. However, the phosphopeptide map of NIS obtained when TSH was present was

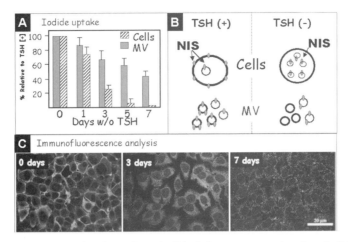

FIGURE 4A.5. Thyrotropin (TSH) regulates iodide (I⁻) transport and sodium-iodide symporter (NIS) expression in thyroid cells. **A:** I⁻ transport activity. FRTL-5 cells were kept in the presence or absence of TSH for the indicated number of days. I⁻ transport was measured in intact cells (*dashed bars*) and in membrane vesicles (MV) prepared from those cells (*filled bars*). I⁻ transport measured in cells maintained in the presence of TSH and in their MV was defined as 100%. I⁻ transport corresponding to Days 1, 3, 5, and 7 after TSH removal was expressed as the percentage of I⁻ transport relative to Day 0. **B:** Schematic model to illustrate the presence of NIS activity in MV from cells deprived of TSH that, when intact, exhibit no NIS activity. This model supports the notion that active NIS molecules, initially located at the plasma membrane while TSH is present, are redistributed to intracellular compartments in response to TSH withdrawal. NIS molecules are represented as *cylinders*. The plasma membrane is shown in thicker lines than the intracellular compartments. **C:** NIS is redistributed to intracellular compartments during TSH deprivation. NIS staining was performed in FRTL-5 cells with anti-rat NIS antibodies. Cells were maintained in the presence or absence of TSH for the indicated number of days. NIS immunofluorescence in these cells was analyzed by confocal microscopy.

markedly different from that of when TSH was absent (47). In conclusion, TSH not only stimulates NIS transcription and biosynthesis, it is also required for targeting NIS to and/or retaining it at the plasma membrane.

Regulation of Sodium-Iodide Symporter by Iodide

The main factor regulating the accumulation of I⁻ in the thyroid (i.e., NIS activity) other than TSH has long been considered to be I⁻ itself. As early as 1944, Morton et al (48) reported that the biosynthesis of thyroid hormones by sheep thyroid slices was inhibited by high doses of I⁻. Wolff and Chaikoff reported in 1948 (49) that organic binding of I⁻ in rat thyroid was blocked when plasma I⁻ concentrations reached a critical high threshold, a phenomenon known as the acute Wolff-Chaikoff effect. These authors observed further that approximately 2 days later, in the presence of continued high plasma I⁻ concentrations, an "escape," or adaptation, from the acute effect occurred, so that the level of I⁻ organification was restored and normal hormone biosynthesis resumed (50). The mechanism responsible for the acute Wolff-Chaikoff effect has yet to be fully elucidated, but it has been proposed to be the result of organic iodocompounds acting as mediators (51–53). The mechanism for the "escape" from the

acute Wolff-Chaikoff effect was proposed by Braverman and Ingbar (54) to be due to a decrease in I⁻ transport, which would presumably lead to sufficiently low intracellular I⁻ concentrations to remove inhibition of I⁻ organification.

The Wolff-Chaikoff effect and the ensuing "escape" constitute a highly specialized intrinsic autoregulatory system that protects the thyroid from the deleterious effects of I⁻ overload, while at the same time ensuring adequate I⁻ uptake for hormone biosynthesis. The level of I⁻ capable of inhibiting I⁻ organification and concomitantly stopping thyroid hormone synthesis is determined by the ratio of organified to nonorganified intracellular I⁻ content, which in turn depends on the previous I⁻ supply.

Isolation of the NIS cDNA has spurred a renewed impetus to investigate the regulatory role played by I⁻ on NIS function. As described earlier, *in vivo* studies carried out by Uyttersprot et al (43) showed that I⁻ inhibited the expression of both TPO and NIS mRNAs in dog thyroid. These observations support the proposed mechanism to explain the "escape" from the Wolff-Chaikoff effect (i.e., that it is due to a decrease in I⁻ uptake possibly caused by downregulation of NIS expression). Eng et al (55) reported that both NIS mRNA and NIS protein levels decreased significantly after either 1 or 6 days of I⁻ administration in rats. NIS mRNA levels were already significantly reduced at 6 hours after injection of a single dose of I⁻. In contrast, a significant decrease of NIS protein levels was detected at only 24 hours. These findings were not correlated with NIS activity by thyroid scintigraphy. The conclusion of this study was that the decrease in active I^- transport, that is, the basis for the "escape," occurs between 6 and 24 hours by a mechanism that at least in part involves a decrease in NIS transcription.

Eng et al (56) later investigated the effect of I^- on NIS mRNA and protein expression in FRTL-5 cells. Incubation of FRTL-5 cells with I^- (10^{-3} M) did not affect NIS mRNA levels, but NIS protein levels decreased significantly in a dose-dependent manner. This conflicts with the authors' previous *in vivo* observations (55) and with the findings of Spitzweg et al (57), who reported a 50% decrease in NIS mRNA levels in FRTL-5 cells incubated with I^- (10^{-4} M). When I^- was administered during TSH stimulation (72 hours after TSH deprivation), the increase in NIS protein levels was less pronounced in the I^--treated cells than in the controls. Performing pulse-chase experiments, the authors found that the half-life of the NIS protein was shorter in the I^--treated cells, suggesting increased NIS protein turnover in these cells. However, the half-life of NIS indicated in this study in normal untreated FRTL-5 cells was <24 hours, which is much shorter than the 4 to 5 days reported by several other groups (18,20,34,47). In summary, the authors (50,56) concluded that high doses of I^- administered *in vivo* lead to decreases in both NIS mRNA and protein levels by a mechanism that is likely to be at least in part transcriptional, whereas their studies *in vitro* suggested that the I^--induced decrease in NIS protein levels appears to be due at least in part to an increase in NIS protein turnover.

Clearly, NIS regulation is complex. Whereas NIS is located both at the plasma membrane and in intracellular organelles, I^- uptake is mediated only by NIS molecules at the plasma membrane (32,47). The subcellular distribution of NIS is regulated mainly by TSH (32,47). Hence, studies parallel of NIS mRNA and protein expression, and the cellular distribution and function of NIS, both *in vitro* and *in vivo,* are needed to better understand the regulatory effects exerted by I^- on NIS.

Sodium-Iodide Symporter Regulation by Thyroglobulin

As discussed earlier, NIS activity is up-regulated by TSH. Kohn's group (58) reported the intriguing observation that Tg acts as a potent suppressor of NIS mRNA levels and thyroid-restricted genes (i.e., Tg, TPO, and TSHR) in FRTL-5 cells, and suggested that Tg could counterbalance the effect of TSH on these genes. The notion of Tg acting as a NIS suppressor is surprising because of the characteristics of the Tg molecule. Tg is synthesized as a 12S molecule that forms a 19S dimer and a 27S tetramer (59,60).

Using 19S follicular Tg (at concentrations known to exist in the follicular lumen) these researchers (61) indicated that follicular Tg suppressed TSH-increased NIS activity *in vitro* and *in vivo*, and regulated the Tg, TPO, and TSHr genes at the transcriptional level (61). Purified 12S, 19S, and 27S follicular Tg suppression of thyroid-restricted gene expression was dependent on the ability of the Tg to bind to thyrocytes (62). This binding was blocked by an antibody against the thyroid apical membrane asialoglycoprotein receptor, a phosphoprotein that is critical for ATP-mediated inactivation of receptor-mediated endocytosis (62).

CURRENT AND FUTURE CLINICAL RELEVANCE OF THE SODIUM-IODIDE SYMPORTER

Sodium-Iodide Symporter in Thyroid Cancer

Thyroid cancer remnants and metastases have long been successfully treated with radioiodide, after thyroidectomy. Although I^- uptake in most thyroid cancers is decreased relative to the surrounding normal tissue, uptake is still sufficient to enable administered radioiodide to destroy remnant tumor cells and metastases. A clear understanding of the cause of diminished I^- uptake in thyroid cancer will certainly have major implications for the treatment of this disease. The fundamental issue is whether I^- uptake is reduced in thyroid cancer cells as a result of a decrease in NIS expression, or by some other mechanism, such as a defect in NIS targeting to the plasma membrane. NIS expression in thyroid cancer has been investigated at both the RNA and protein levels by several groups (63–68). First, no mutations were found in NIS by direct sequencing by PCR of NIS cDNA obtained from papillary carcinomas, ruling out that a mutation might be impairing NIS function in these tumors (66). Second, variable levels of NIS mRNA expression in thyroid carcinomas have been found by molecular biologic methods, which (63–68) provide information only on the level but not the stability of the NIS mRNA. Given that there is great interest in increasing NIS function in thyroid cancer, some investigators have attempted to induce NIS expression in thyroid carcinoma cell lines by means of demethylation treatment and with transretinoic acid. However, the results have been inconclusive (69,70).

Since NIS is a membrane protein with a long half-life (19) and with a complex transcriptional, posttranscriptional, and posttranslational regulation, the presence or absence of the NIS transcript and the levels observed are not sufficiently revealing on the levels of expression of the NIS protein, and even less on whether NIS is properly targeted to the plasma membrane, the only location where it is functional. It is relevant to point out that the coexistence of marked differences in mRNA and protein levels has been reported with such other proteins as the transferrin receptor (71,72). The expression of the NIS protein can be ascertained by immunoblot analysis and immunohistochemistry. Whereas immunoblot analysis does provide information on the expression of the NIS protein, it is a technique that requires a relatively large amount of tissue, which is rarely available, and has the disadvantage that it does not reveal the subcellular localization of the protein. Immunohistochemistry, does give an indication of the subcellular localization of NIS. Saito et al (73) investigated papillary and follicular cancers by immunoblot analysis and immunohistochemistry, and reported overexpression of the NIS protein in the majority of tumors. Dohán et al (74) have also investigated NIS protein expression by immunohistochemistry in a large sample of differentiated thyroid carcinomas and found that as many as 70% overexpressed NIS protein compared to the surrounding normal tissue (Fig. 4A.6). Significantly, NIS was localized mainly intracellularly in most of the tumors, strongly suggesting that the decrease in I⁻ uptake in most thyroid carcinomas is not due to low NIS expression but to alterations in NIS trafficking (Fig. 4A.6) (74). This was somewhat surprising, because a lower NIS expression could have been expected in the face of the established lower NIS activity in these cells.

The finding that the NIS protein is actually overexpressed in thyroid cancer cells suggests that the mechanism for the decrease in activity is not a simple impairment of NIS protein expression. These results have been confirmed and extended by Wapnir et al (75), who analyzed a very large number of tissue microarrays and conventional sections and found NIS protein expression in 75% of benign

thyroid nodules and 73% of thyroid cancers. Furthermore, Tonacchera et al (76) have reported that 54% of benign nonfunctional thyroid nodules overexpressed hNIS protein, as compared to normal surrounding tissue; significantly, NIS was located intracellularly in these nodules as well.

In short, currently available data indicating that the decrease of I⁻ transport activity coexists with NIS overexpression, but with a predominantly intracellular localization, underscore the importance of elucidating the molecular mechanisms underlying the proper targeting to and retention of NIS at the plasma membrane.

Iodide Efflux

To be therapeutically effective, radioiodide has to remain within the thyroid cancer cells for a sufficiently long time. The major determinants of I⁻ retention in thyroid cells are NIS-mediated I⁻ uptake, I⁻ organification, and I⁻ efflux. Based on the thus far sparse investigations on I⁻ organification in thyroid cancer, it seems that organification is impaired in these tumors. Several groups have tried to identify the mediator of apical I⁻ efflux in thyroid epithelial cells. Two recently cloned molecules are the main candidates, pendrin and apical iodide transporter (AIT), although neither has been conclusively proven to be the mediator of apical I⁻ efflux.

In 1997, a gene defective in Pendred's syndrome (PDS) was identified by positional cloning (77). PDS is characterized by sensorineural (most often prelingual) deafness and goiter with defective I⁻ organification. In PDS, goiter can develop at any age or may be absent, whereas deafness is generally present (78). Pendrin has been localized on the apical membrane of the thyroid epithelial cells by immunohistochemistry (79). In heterologous expression systems, pendrin has been shown to transport iodide, chloride, formate, and nitrate (14).

The organification defect characteristic of PDS was attributed to defective pendrin-mediated apical iodide transport into the colloid, where organification occurs (Fig. 4A.1). Surprisingly, although *Pds*-knockout mice are completely deaf, they do not have a pathologic thyroidal phenotype (78); therefore, pendrin's function as the AIT remains to be further investigated.

Using a cloning strategy based on NIS sequence homologies, a 610 amino acid protein-coding gene was recently cloned from a human kidney cDNA library. The newly identified protein shares both a strikingly high identity (46%) and similarity (70%) to hNIS (15). This protein, called the human AIT (hAIT), has been localized to the apical membrane of thyroid epithelial cells; however, a thorough molecular and kinetic characterization is required to unequivocally establish whether hAIT mediates "downhill" movements of I⁻ from the cytosol to the colloid.

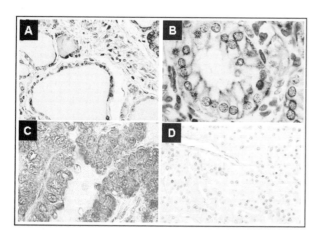

FIGURE 4A.6. Immunohistochemical analysis of sodium-iodide symporter (NIS) protein expression in thyroid carcinomas. **A:** Normal thyroid (400× magnification). **B:** Thyroid tissue from a patient with Graves' hyperthyroidism showing a distinct basolateral staining pattern (1,000× magnification). **C:** Papillary carcinoma tissue showing strong intracellular staining (1,000× magnification). **D:** Papillary carcinoma with negative NIS expression (400× magnification).

Stunning

Radioiodide is the cornerstone of the treatment of metastatic thyroid cancer. The optimal therapeutic radioiodide dose is calculated on the basis of the scintigraphic image obtained upon administration of a radioiodide test dose. This test dose must be properly adjusted so as to prevent uptake inhibition of the subsequently administered therapeutic dose of $^{131}I^-$. The interference of radioiodide test doses with uptake of subsequent therapeutic doses is called "stunning," the molecular mechanism of which is unknown (80) (see Chapter 12).

To investigate stunning, Nilsson et al (81) exposed pig thyrocyte primary cultures [grown in a bicameral chamber, where vectorial (basal to apical) I^- transport can be assessed] to increasing doses of $^{131}I^-$ or stable, nonradioactive $^{127}I^-$ (1 to 100 Gy, iodide $<10^{-9}$ *M*) for 48 hours in the presence of TSH and methimazole (MMI). Basal to apical I^- transport was then measured using $^{125}I^-$. Immediately after exposure to radioiodide, active I^- transport was similar to the control. However, 3 days after $^{131}I^-$ exposure, basal to apical I^- transport decreased in a radioiodide dose-dependent manner. Based on these observations, the authors concluded that stunning of I^- accumulation after radioiodide exposure is due to selective inhibition of the I^- transporting mechanism.

Iodide Transport Defect

The molecular analysis of some of the NIS mutations detected in patients with congenital I^- transport defect has provided important structural information about the symporter. Iodide transport defects—caused by NIS mutations—are conditions characterized (if untreated) by hypothyroidism, goiter, low thyroid I^- uptake, and low saliva/plasma I^- ratio. Eleven NIS mutations have been identified so far: V59E, G93R, Q267E, C272X, G395R, T354P, frame-shift 515X, Y531X, G543E, δ143 to 323, and δ439 to 443 (82–91). They are either nonsense, alternative splicing, frame-shift, deletion, or missense mutations of the NIS gene (Fig. 4A.2).

The T354P, G395R, and Q267E NIS mutant molecules have been investigated at the molecular level. Both mutant T354P and G395R NIS proteins are synthesized and properly targeted to the plasma membrane. The detailed molecular analysis of mutation T354P, carried out by Levy et al (92), revealed that a hydroxyl group at the β-carbon at position 354 is essential for NIS function. Dohán et al (93), thorough structure/function analysis of the G395R mutation, showed that the presence of an uncharged amino acid residue with a small side chain at position 395 is required for NIS function, and that the presence of charge or of a long side-chain at position 395 results in decreased turnover rate of the transporter, without affecting its ion-binding affinity. Based on flow cytometry data, it

was at first suggested that the Q267E mutation results in impaired plasma membrane trafficking of the mutated NIS protein (94). However, De la Vieja et al (95), using several experimental approaches, have recently shown that the Q267E mutant NIS is modestly active and properly targeted to the plasma membrane. The mutant protein has a lower V_{max} for iodide as compared to the wild-type protein, which could result in the lower transport rate. In contrast to T354P, G395R, and Q267E, G543E NIS matures only partially, and it is the only mutant identified thus far that is not targeted properly to the cell surface, apparently because of faulty folding (95). Therefore, the G543 residue plays significant roles in NIS maturation and trafficking. Remarkably, NIS activity was rescued by small neutral amino acid substitutions at this position, suggesting that G543 is in a tightly packed region of NIS. Clearly, the detailed molecular analysis of NIS mutations will continue to reveal substantial structure/function information on NIS.

NIS in Extrathyroidal Tissues

The field of I^- transport systems outside the thyroid has changed considerably since the extensive review published on the topic in 1961 by Brown-Grant (96). The main vertebrate nonthyroid tissues reported to actively accumulate I^- are salivary glands, gastric mucosa, and lactating mammary gland (Fig. 4A.7). Many of these transport systems exhibit functional similarities with their thyroid counterpart, notably a susceptibility to inhibition by thiocyanate and perchlorate. However, they also display important differences: (a) nonthyroid I^- transporting tissues do not have the ability to organify accumulated I^- (with the possible exception of the lactating mammary gland); therefore, they behave like MMI-treated thyroid tissue; (b) TSH exerts no regulatory influence on nonthyroid I^- accumulation; (c) at least salivary glands and gastric mucosa concentrate thiocyanate, unlike the thyroid, where thiocyanate is metabolized after uptake and therefore not concentrated.

NIS is clearly regulated and processed differently in each tissue. The cloning of human NIS cDNAs has been reported from gastric mucosa, parotid glands, and mammary glands, all of which exhibited full identity to thyroid hNIS cDNA. Whereas hNIS gene expression has been detected in many other tissues by (27,97–102), the molecular biologic techniques used yield a large number of false positives due to their high sensitivity (103). Therefore, the detection of the NIS amplified product in a given tissue cannot be regarded as sufficient evidence that NIS is functionally expressed in that tissue. A thorough characterization of NIS protein expression is necessary to properly evaluate the significance of results ob-

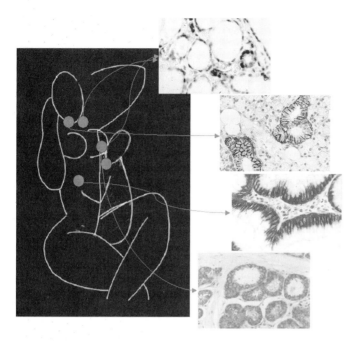

FIGURE 4A.7. Immunohistochemical analysis of sodium-iodide symporter protein expression in tissues that exhibit active I⁻ transport. Shown from **top** to **bottom** are thyroid, salivary gland, stomach, and lactating mammary gland.

tained by these techniques. Still, even with the use of a wide variety of techniques (Northern analysis, DWA amplification, Western analysis, and immunohistochemistry), different groups have often obtained inconsistent and sometimes conflicting results on whether or not NIS is expressed in a particular tissue. Hence, once NIS protein expression has been demonstrated, a correlation with Na⁺-dependent, perchlorate-sensitive, active I⁻ accumulation in that tissue must be established. By these criteria, and taking into consideration the results mentioned earlier, NIS is expressed and active in extrathyroidal tissues previously known to exhibit NIS activity, such as salivary glands, gastric mucosa, and lactating mammary gland. NIS expression in different tissues is shown in Figure 4A.8. Electrophoretically, NIS migrates as a broad band, which is characteristic of extremely hydrophobic, polytopic membrane proteins. The significance of the detection of the amplified NIS product in other human and rat tissues remains to be ascertained.

Sodium-Iodide Symporter in Breast Cancer

As indicated earlier, NIS is differently regulated and subjected to distinct posttranslational modifications in each tissue where it is expressed (104–106). Physiologically, I⁻ transport in the mammary gland occurs during late pregnancy and lactation, resulting in the transfer of I⁻ to the milk. An adequate supply of I⁻ for sufficient thyroid hormone production is essential for proper development of the newborn's nervous system, skeletal muscle, and lungs. In contrast, no I⁻ transport is observed in normal breast tissue in the absence of pregnancy and lactation.

Using *in vivo* scintigraphic imaging and immunoblot analysis, Tazebay et al (106) demonstrated functional expression of NIS in experimental mammary adenocarcinomas in nongestational and nonlactating female transgenic mice carrying either an activated *ras* oncogene (*c-Ha-ras*) or overexpressing the *Neu* oncogene (*c-erbB-2*) (107). When Tazebay et al (106) studied through immunohistochemical analysis human breast tissue specimens for NIS expression, they found that 87% of the invasive breast cancers and 83% of the ductal carcinomas *in situ* expressed

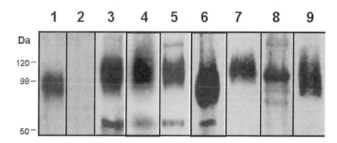

FIGURE 4A.8. Immunoblot analysis of sodium-iodide symporter (NIS)-expressing cell lines *(lanes 1 through 5)* and human tissues *(lanes 6 through 9)*. *Lane 1:* FRTL-5 cells. *Lane 2:* FRT cells. *Lane 3:* COS-7 cells transiently transfected with rat NIS (rNIS) cyclic DNA (cDNA). *Lane 4:* COS-7 cells transiently transfected with human NIS cDNA. *Lane 5:* MCF-7 cells. *Lane 6:* Thyroid. *Lane 7:* Salivary gland (parotid). *Lane 8:* Breast tissue from a pregnant woman in the third trimester. *Lane 9:* Gastric mucosa. Membrane fractions from the cell lines or from homogenized tissues were separated by 9% SDS-PAGE, then electroblotted to nitrocellulose, and probed by 0.5 μg/mL affinity-purified polyclonal anti-rNIS antibodies (Ab) *(lanes 1 through 3)* or by hNIS Ab *(lanes 4 through 9)*, followed by horseradish-peroxidase (HRP)-labeled goat anti-rabbit Ab. Immunoreactive bands were visualized by enhanced chemiluminescence.

NIS, as compared with only 23% of the extratumoral samples adjacent to or in the vicinity of the tumors and to none of the normal samples from reductive mammoplasties (76). More recently, Wapnir et al (75) examined the immunohistochemical profile of NIS in thyroid, breast, and other carcinomas using high density tissue microarrays and conventional sections. The results confirmed the findings stated above: NIS expression was demonstrated in whole tissue sections in 76% of invasive breast carcinoma and 88% of ductal carcinoma *in situ* samples. The majority of normal breast cores were negative (87%), as were 70% of normal/nonproliferative samples analyzed. Plasma membrane immunoreactivity was observed in gestational breast tissues, and in some *in situ* ductal carcinomas and invasive ductal carcinomas.

Because all the above studies in human samples were carried out by immunohistochemistry, the findings demonstrate only NIS expression, but not necessarily NIS functional expression in human breast cancer. Hence, in a significant first step addressing this issue, Moon et al (108) have reported pertechnetate accumulation in primary breast tumors in humans *in vivo*. Pertechnetate ($^{99m}TcO_4$) is a radioisotope widely used for diagnostic imaging, also transported by NIS, with the advantage of having a shorter half-life ($t_{1/2}$ 6 hours) than ^{131}I ($t_{1/2}$ 8 days). These authors studied 25 cancer patients by scintigraphy and found active uptake by the tumors in 4 patients. This is a highly meaningful result, not only because it demonstrates the existence of I^- transport activity in a significant percentage of human breast cancer patients *in vivo*, but also because the observation was made in patients whose thyroid glands were not down-regulated (i.e., in these patients thyroid NIS was still expressed, and therefore there was avid thyroidal I^- uptake; this decreased the amount of radioisotope available for uptake by breast tumors). It is possible that a larger proportion of I^--accumulating breast cancer tumors might have been detected by scintigraphy if the availability of the radioisotope to tumoral tissue had been optimized by thyroid suppression.

In conclusion, although more extensive studies in humans are necessary, functional expression of NIS in breast cancer has been documented both in mice and humans. This suggests strongly that NIS is up-regulated with high frequency during malignant transformation in breast cancer. Therefore, endogenous NIS has tremendous potential to serve as the conduit for radioiodide in the diagnosis and treatment of this devastating disease.

Sodium-Iodide Symporter Gene Transfer

Given the high efficacy and low rate of side effects of NIS-mediated radioiodide therapy in thyroid cancer, it is extremely desirable to develop strategies to apply this therapy in other cancers. For this purpose, cancers may be divided into two groups, namely those that express endogenous NIS (with full, partial, or no activity) and those that do not. To date, the only cancer other than thyroid cancer shown to express functional endogenous NIS molecules is breast cancer. For both thyroid and breast cancer, it appears to be advantageous to identify ways to increase activation of endogenous NIS, such as by prodding more NIS molecules to be targeted to the plasma membrane instead of being retained in intracellular compartments (47). For cancers that do not express endogenous NIS, ectopic NIS may be introduced by a variety of gene transfer techniques, as explained later in the chapter (109–111).

Whether a tumor expresses functional NIS endogenously or ectopically (by gene transfer), NIS function makes it possible to image, monitor, and treat the tumor with radioiodide, just as in differentiated thyroid cancer. Compared with other genes that have been transferred, NIS offers the unique advantage that it can be used both as a reporter and a therapeutic gene, as has been shown by *in vivo* imaging of NIS-bearing tumors in various animal models (109–112). Functional expression of NIS can be detected by using available techniques to monitor the radioactive tracers transported by NIS, such as ^{125}I, ^{123}I, ^{124}I, or $^{99m}TcO_4^-$. Each of these tracers offers its own advantages and disadvantages in terms of its half-life, availability, price, and so on.

Human and rat NIS have been introduced into several different tumor cell lines under the control of tissue-specific or general promoters using different transfer methodologies, such as liposomal transfection, electroporation, or adenoviral or retroviral transduction (104,105). As expected, functional NIS expression was detected *in vitro* in these cells. All authors concluded that *in vivo* gene therapy experiments have to be the next step. However, the most difficult problem to overcome is the targeted delivery of the NIS gene to the tumors *in vivo*. Thus far, three *in vivo* studies in mice have yielded promising results (109–111).

Using NIS-containing recombinant adenovirus, Cho et al (109) have recently shown that hNIS can be functionally expressed in xenografted human glioma in rats. These authors observed significant radioiodide retention in the tumors over 24 hours. They administered 3×4 mCi (in 2-day intervals) of ^{131}I for 2 weeks following tumor implantation, and observed longer survival in animals bearing NIS-expressing tumors. Spitzweg et al (114) introduced NIS in a recombinant adenovirus into a human prostate carcinoma cell line under the regulation of the prostate specific antigen promoter. They reported a mean retention time of 5.6 hours in NIS-expressing prostate carcinoma xenografts in nude mice and a remarkable decrease (>80%) of the size of these xenografts after a single intraperitoneal injection of 3 mCi ^{131}I. Dingli and colleagues (110) expressed NIS in a myeloma cell line using transcriptionally targeted lentiviral vector, where the therapeutic or reporter gene is under the control of minimal immunoglobulin promoter and enhancer elements (immuno-globulin κ-light chain enhancer elements). These authors also investigated the so-called bystander effect. β-particles emitted during the decay of ^{131}I can travel a distance of 0.2 to 2.4 mm. Therefore, the isotope is capable of destroying the "bystanding" non-NIS-expressing cells. Dingli et al (110) also treated myeloma xenografts containing variable numbers of radioiodide-transporting, NIS-transduced and nontransduced tumor cells. The result was striking: all tumors in which 50% to 100% of the cells expressed NIS completely regressed 2 weeks after a single dose of 1 mCi ^{131}I.

The above results provide strong evidence against the widely held notion that radioiodide therapy is likely to be ineffective in nonthyroidal cells that, while functionally expressing NIS (whether endogenously or by targeted transfection), lack the ability to organify I^-. The reasoning was that the absence of organification resulted in the isotope not being retained in the cells for a sufficiently long time. Yet, in several studies (109–113), radioiodide treatment was effective even in the absence of I^- organification.

The therapeutic potential of other radioisotopes transported by NIS is currently under investigation. Astatide (^{211}At), an α-emitter with high linear energy transfer (97 keV/μM) and a short tissue range (79 μm), has been shown to be transported by NIS in a perchlorate-sensitive manner in the UVW human glioma cell line stably transfected with hNIS cDNA (114).

^{188}ReO$_4$, a β-emitter (E$_{average}$ = 0.764 MeV) (^{131}I E = 0.134 MeV, optimal tissue range: 2.6 to 5 mm), has been suggested as an alternative to ^{131}I for breast cancer treatment. ReO$_4$ was not transported in NIS-expressing *X. laevis* oocytes (22); however, Van Sande et al (115) have reported its accumulation in FRTL-5 cells and in COS-7 cells stably transfected with hNIS. In MDCK cells permanently transfected with hNIS, it has been shown that the K$_m$ for ReO$_4$ is similar to that of iodide, but the V$_{max}$ and consequently the accumulated isotope in the cells is about half (116). These new NIS-transported radioisotopes can be potentially useful in various clinical settings, but for now we lack the experience in using them the same way we do after having accumulated over 60 years of employing radioiodide in thyroid cancer.

CONCLUDING REMARKS AND FUTURE PERSPECTIVES

The thyroid's ability to actively take up I^-, first detected as early as the 19th century, has long been regarded as one of the most distinctive and significant attributes of the gland, even before NIS was identified as the thyroid I^- transporter. For over six decades, this ability has been key to the evaluation of thyroid function and the diagnosis and treatment of thyroid disease. Once it was identified, NIS was

quite naturally expected to prove to be a thyroid-specific protein with major physiological and medical significance, probably not expressed in any other tissues. As NIS was demonstrated to be the single mediator of active I^- uptake in several other I^--transporting tissues, most notably the lactating mammary gland, it becomes apparent that NIS may have medical applications beyond the thyroid. Remarkably, NIS is now seen as the key to extend the use of radioiodide and possibly related isotopes to a wide variety of cancers beyond the thyroid, as effective anticancer therapy. The discovery that endogenous NIS is functionally expressed in breast cancer, especially, places NIS squarely at the center of some of the current efforts to combat the deadliest malignancy in women. In addition, available findings on the transfer of the NIS gene to a variety of cancers, from prostate to glioma, suggest that radioiodide may also be eventually used against cancers that do not express NIS endogenously. There is no question that the continued elucidation of NIS structure/ function relations, regulation, and mechanistic information will provide additional insights of ample physiological and pathophysiological importance.

REFERENCES

1. World Health Organization. *Iodine deficiency disorders* (Facts Sheet No. 121.) Geneva: 1996.
2. Courtois M. Decouverte d'une substance nouvelle dans le varech. *Ann Chem* 1813;88:310.
3. Baumann E. Uber das Thyrojodin. *Munch Med Wschr* 1896;43:309–312.
4. Baumann E. Uber den Jodgehalt der Schilddrüsen von Menchen und tieren. *Z Physiol Chem* 1896;22:1–17.
5. Carrasco N. Iodide transport in the thyroid gland. *Biochim Biophys Acta* 1993;1154:65–82.
6. Halmi N. Thyroidal iodide transport. *Vitam Horm* 1961;19:133–163.
7. Wolff J. Transport of iodide and other anions in the thyroid gland. *Physiol Rev* 1964;44:45–90.
8. Iff HW, Wilbrandt W. The dependency of iodine accumulation in thyroid slices on the ionic composition of the incubation medium and its influence by cardiac glycosides. *Biochim Biophys Acta* 1963;78:711–725.
9. Kaminsky SM, Levy O, Garry MT, et al. Inhibition of the Na+/I- symporter by harmaline and 3-amino-1-methyl-5H-pyrido(4,3-b)indole acetate in thyroid cells and membrane vesicles. *Eur J Biochem* 1991;200:203–207.
10. O'Neill B, Magnolato D, Semenza G. The electrogenic, Na+-dependent I- transport system in plasma membrane vesicles from thyroid glands. *Biochim Biophys Acta* 1987;896:263–274.
11. Vilijn F, Carrasco N. Expression of the thyroid sodium/iodide symporter in *Xenopus laevis* oocytes. *J Biol Chem* 1989;264:11901–11903.
12. Weiss SJ, Philp NJ, Grollman EF. Iodide transport in a continuous line of cultured cells from rat thyroid. *Endocrinology* 1984;114:1090–1098.
13. Dai G, Levy O, Carrasco N. Cloning and characterization of the thyroid iodide transporter. *Nature* 1996;379:458–460.
14. Scott DA, Wang R, Kreman TM, et al. The Pendred syndrome gene encodes a chloride-iodide transport protein. *Nat Genet* 1999;21:440–443.

15. Rodriguez AM, Perron B, Lacroix L, et al. Identification and characterization of a putative human iodide transporter located at the apical membrane of thyrocytes. *J Clin Endocrinol Metab* 2002;87:3500–3503.

16. Dobson J. The iodine factor in health and evolution. *Geographical Review* 1998;88:1–28.

17. Dai G, Levy O, Amzel LM, et al. The mediator of thyroidal iodide accumulation: the sodium/iodide symporter. In: Konings WN, Kaback HR, Lolkema JS, eds. *Handbook of biological physics*. Vol. II. *Transport processes in eukaryotic and prokaryotic organisms*. Amsterdam: Elsevier Science, 1996:343–367.

18. Levy O, Dai G, Riedel C, et al. Characterization of the thyroid Na+/I- symporter with an anti-COOH terminus antibody. *Proc Natl Acad Sci U S A* 1997;94:5568–5573.

19. Levy O, De la Vieja A, Ginter CS, et al. N-linked glycosylation of the thyroid Na+/I- symporter (NIS). Implications for its secondary structure model. *J Biol Chem* 1998;273:22657–22663.

20. Paire A, Bernier-Valentin F, Selmi-Ruby S, et al. Characterization of the rat thyroid iodide transporter using anti-peptide antibodies: relationship between its expression and activity. *J Biol Chem* 1997;272:18245–18249.

21. De la Vieja A, Ginter C, Carrasco N. Topology of the sodium/iodide symporter: 12th International Thyroid Congress; Kyoto, Japan. *Endocrine J* 2000:162.

22. Eskandari S, Loo DD, Dai G, et al. Thyroid Na+/I- symporter. Mechanism, stoichiometry, and specificity. *J Biol Chem* 1997; 272:27230–27238.

23. Yoshida A, Sasaki N, Mori A, et al. Different electrophysiological character of I-, ClO4-, and SCN- in the transport by Na+/I- symporter. *Biochem Biophys Res Commun* 1997;231:731–734.

24. Yoshida A, Sasaki N, Mori A, et al. Differences in the electrophysiological response to I- and the inhibitory anions SCN- and ClO4-, studied in FRTL-5 cells. *Biochim Biophys Acta* 1998;1414:231–237.

25. Damante G, Di Lauro R. Thyroid-specific gene expression. *Biochim Biophys Acta* 1994;1218:255–266.

26. Missero C, Cobellis G, De Felice M, et al. Molecular events involved in differentiation of thyroid follicular cells. *Mol Cell Endocrinol* 1998;140:37–43.

27. Smanik PA, Liu Q, Furminger TL, et al. Cloning of the human sodium Iodide symporter. *Biochem Biophys Res Commun* 1996; 226:339–345.

28. Smanik PA, Ryu KY, Theil KS, et al. Expression, exon-intron organization, and chromosome mapping of the human sodium iodide symporter. *Endocrinology* 1997;138:3555–3558.

29. Behr M, Schmitt TL, Espinoza CR, et al. Cloning of a functional promoter of the human sodium/iodide-symporter gene. *Biochem J* 1998;331[Pt 2]:359–363.

30. Ryu KY, Tong Q, Jhiang SM. Promoter characterization of the human Na+/I- symporter. *J Clin Endocrinol Metab* 1998;83: 3247–3251.

31. Venkataraman GM, Yatin M, Ain KB. Cloning of the human sodium-iodide symporter promoter and characterization in a differentiated human thyroid cell line, KAT-50. *Thyroid* 1998; 8:63–69.

32. Kaminsky SM, Levy O, Salvador C, et al. Na(+)-I- symport activity is present in membrane vesicles from thyrotropin-deprived non-I(-)-transporting cultured thyroid cells. *Proc Natl Acad Sci U S A* 1994;91:3789–3793.

33. Weiss SJ, Philp NJ, Ambesi-Impiombato FS, et al. Thyrotropin-stimulated iodide transport mediated by adenosine 3′,5′-monophosphate and dependent on protein synthesis. *Endocrinology* 1984;114:1099–1107.

34. Kogai T, Endo T, Saito T, et al. Regulation by thyroid-stimulating hormone of sodium/iodide symporter gene expression and protein levels in FRTL-5 cells. *Endocrinology* 1997;138:2227–2232.

35. Endo T, Kaneshige M, Nakazato M, et al. Thyroid transcription factor-1 activates the promoter activity of rat thyroid Na+/I- symporter gene. *Mol Endocrinol* 1997;11:1747–1755.

36. Ohmori M, Endo T, Harii N, et al. A novel thyroid transcription factor is essential for thyrotropin-induced up-regulation of Na+/I- symporter gene expression. *Mol Endocrinol* 1998; 12:727–736.

37. Ohno M, Zannini M, Levy O, et al. The paired-domain transcription factor Pax8 binds to the upstream enhancer of the rat sodium/iodide symporter gene and participates in both thyroid-specific and cyclic-AMP-dependent transcription. *Mol Cell Biol* 1999;19:2051–2060.

38. Swanson DJ, Zellmer E, Lewis EJ. The homeodomain protein Arix interacts synergistically with cyclic AMP to regulate expression of neurotransmitter biosynthetic genes. *J Biol Chem* 1997;272:27382–27392.

39. Jansen E, Ayoubi TA, Meulemans SM, et al. Cell type-specific protein-DNA interactions at the cAMP response elements of the prohormone convertase 1 promoter. Evidence for additional transactivators distinct from CREB/ATF family members. *J Biol Chem* 1997;272:2500–2508.

40. Comb M, Mermod N, Hyman SE, et al. Proteins bound at adjacent DNA elements act synergistically to regulate human proenkephalin cAMP inducible transcription. *Embo J* 1988; 7:3793–3805.

41. Schmitt TL, Espinoza CR, Loos U. Characterization of a thyroid-specific and cyclic adenosine monophosphate-responsive enhancer far upstream from the human sodium iodide symporter gene. *Thyroid* 2002;12:273–279.

42. Taki K, Kogai T, Kanamoto Y, et al. A thyroid-specific far-upstream enhancer in the human sodium/iodide symporter gene requires Pax-8 binding and cyclic adenosine 3′,5′-monophosphate response element-like sequence binding proteins for full activity and is differentially regulated in normal and thyroid cancer cells. *Mol Endocrinol* 2002;16:2266–2282.

43. Uyttersprot N, Pelgrims N, Carrasco N, et al. Moderate doses of iodide in vivo inhibit cell proliferation and the expression of thyroperoxidase and Na+/I- symporter mRNAs in dog thyroid. *Mol Cell Endocrinol* 1997;131:195–203.

44. Kogai T, Curcio F, Hyman S, et al. Induction of follicle formation in long-term cultured normal human thyroid cells treated with thyrotropin stimulates iodide uptake but not sodium/iodide symporter messenger RNA and protein expression. *J Endocrinol* 2000;167:125–135.

45. Saito T, Endo T, Kawaguchi A, et al. Increased expression of the Na+/I- symporter in cultured human thyroid cells exposed to thyrotropin and in Graves' thyroid tissue. *J Clin Endocrinol Metab* 1997;82:3331–3336.

46. Marcocci C, Cohen JL, Grollman EF. Effect of actinomycin D on iodide transport in FRTL-5 thyroid cells. *Endocrinology* 1984;115:2123–2132.

47. Riedel C, Levy O, Carrasco N. Post-transcriptional regulation of the sodium/iodide symporter by thyrotropin. *J Biol Chem* 2001;276:21458–21463.

48. Morton ME, Chaikoff IL, Rosenfeld S. Inhibiting effect of inorganic iodide on the formation in vitro thyroxine and diiodotyrosine by surviving thyroid tissue. *Journal of Biological Chemistry* 1944;154:381–387.

49. Wolff J, Chaikoff IL. Plasma inorganic iodide as a homeostatic regulator of thyroid function. *Journal of Biological Chemistry* 1948;174:555–564.

50. Wolff J, Chaikoff IL, Goldberg RC, et al. The temporary nature of the inhibitory action of excess iodide on organic iodide synthesis in the normal thyroid. *Endocrinology* 1949;45:504.

51. Dugrillon A. Iodolactones and iodoaldehydes—mediators of iodine in thyroid autoregulation. *Exp Clin Endocrinol Diabetes* 1996;104[Suppl 4]:41–45.

52. Panneels V, Van den Bergen H, Jacoby C, et al. Inhibition of H_2O_2 production by iodoaldehydes in cultured dog thyroid cells. *Mol Cell Endocrinol* 1994;102:167–176.

53. Panneels V, Van Sande J, Van den Bergen H, et al. Inhibition of human thyroid adenylyl cyclase by 2-iodoaldehydes. *Mol Cell Endocrinol* 1994;106:41–50.

54. Braverman LE, Ingbar, SH. Changes in thyroidal function during adaptation to large doses of iodide. *J Clin Invest* 1963;42:1216–1231.

55. Eng PH, Cardona GR, Fang SL, et al. Escape from the acute Wolff-Chaikoff effect is associated with a decrease in thyroid sodium/iodide symporter messenger ribonucleic acid and protein. *Endocrinology* 1999;140:3404–3410.

56. Eng PH, Cardona GR, Previti MC, et al. Regulation of the sodium iodide symporter by iodide in FRTL-5 cells. *Eur J Endocrinol* 2001;144:139–144.

57. Spitzweg C, Joba W, Morris JC, et al. Regulation of sodium iodide symporter gene expression in FRTL-5 rat thyroid cells. *Thyroid* 1999;9:821–830.

58. Suzuki K, Lavaroni S, Mori A, et al. Autoregulation of thyroid-specific gene transcription by thyroglobulin. *Proc Natl Acad Sci U S A* 1998;95:8251–8256.

59. Palumbo G, Tecce MF. Molecular organization of 19 S calf thyroglobulin. *Arch Biochem Biophys* 1984;233:169–173.

60. Suzuki K, Mori A, Saito J, et al. Follicular thyroglobulin suppresses iodide uptake by suppressing expression of the sodium/iodide symporter gene. *Endocrinology* 1999;140:5422–5430.

61. Kohn LD, Suzuki K, Nakazato M, et al. Effects of thyroglobulin and pendrin on iodide flux through the thyrocyte. *Trends Endocrinol Metab* 2001;12:10–16.

62. Ulianich L, Suzuki K, Mori A, et al. Follicular thyroglobulin (TG) suppression of thyroid-restricted genes involves the apical membrane asialoglycoprotein receptor and TG phosphorylation. *J Biol Chem* 1999;274:25099–25107.

63. Arturi F, Russo D, Giuffrida D, et al. Sodium-iodide symporter (NIS) gene expression in lymph-node metastases of papillary thyroid carcinomas. *Eur J Endocrinol* 2000;143:623–627.

64. Arturi F, Russo D, Schlumberger M, et al. Iodide symporter gene expression in human thyroid tumors. *J Clin Endocrinol Metab* 1998;83:2493–2496.

65. Lazar V, Bidart JM, Caillou B, et al. Expression of the Na+/I-symporter gene in human thyroid tumors: a comparison study with other thyroid-specific genes. *J Clin Endocrinol Metab* 1999;84:3228–3234.

66. Russo D, Manole D, Arturi F, et al. Absence of sodium/iodide symporter gene mutations in differentiated human thyroid carcinomas. *Thyroid* 2001;11:37–39.

67. Ryu KY, Senokozlieff ME, Smanik PA, et al. Development of reverse transcription-competitive polymerase chain reaction method to quantitate the expression levels of human sodium iodide symporter. *Thyroid* 1999;9:405–409.

68. Tanaka K, Otsuki T, Sonoo H, et al. Semi-quantitative comparison of the differentiation markers and sodium iodide symporter messenger ribonucleic acids in papillary thyroid carcinomas using RT-PCR. *Eur J Endocrinol* 2000;142:340–346.

69. Schmutzler C, Winzer R, Meissner-Weigl J, et al. Retinoic acid increases sodium/iodide symporter mRNA levels in human thyroid cancer cell lines and suppresses expression of functional symporter in nontransformed FRTL-5 rat thyroid cells. *Biochem Biophys Res Commun* 1997;240:832–838.

70. Venkataraman GM, Yatin M, Marcinek R, et al. Restoration of iodide uptake in dedifferentiated thyroid carcinoma: relationship to human Na+/I-symporter gene methylation status. *J Clin Endocrinol Metab* 1999;84:2449–2457.

71. Cazzola M, Skoda RC. Translational pathophysiology: a novel molecular mechanism of human disease. *Blood* 2000;95:3280–3288.

72. Hentze MW, Kuhn LC. Molecular control of vertebrate iron metabolism: mRNA-based regulatory circuits operated by iron, nitric oxide, and oxidative stress. *Proc Natl Acad Sci U S A* 1996;93:8175–8182.

73. Saito T, Endo T, Kawaguchi A, et al. Increased expression of the sodium/iodide symporter in papillary thyroid carcinomas. *J Clin Invest* 1998;101:1296–1300.

74. Dohán O, Baloch Z, Banrevi Z, et al. Rapid communication: predominant intracellular overexpression of the Na(+)/I(-) symporter (NIS) in a large sampling of thyroid cancer cases. *J Clin Endocrinol Metab* 2001;86:2697–2700.

75. Wapnir IL, van de Rijn M, Nowels K, et al. Immunohistochemical profile of the sodium/iodide symporter in thyroid, breast, and other carcinomas using high density tissue microarrays and conventional sections. *J Clin Endocrinol Metab* 2003;88:1880–1888.

76. Tonacchera M, Viacava P, Agretti P, et al. Benign nonfunctioning thyroid adenomas are characterized by a defective targeting to cell membrane or a reduced expression of the sodium iodide symporter protein. *J Clin Endocrinol Metab* 2002;87:352–357.

77. Everett LA, Glaser B, Beck JC, et al. Pendred syndrome is caused by mutations in a putative sulphate transporter gene (PDS). *Nat Genet* 1997;17:411–422.

78. Everett LA, Belyantseva IA, Noben-Trauth K, et al. Targeted disruption of mouse Pds provides insight about the inner-ear defects encountered in Pendred syndrome. *Hum Mol Genet* 2001;10:153–161.

79. Mian C, Lacroix L, Bidart JM, et al. Sodium/iodide symporter in thyroid cancer. *Exp Clin Endocrinol Diabetes* 2001;109:47–51.

80. Yeung HW, Humm JL, Larson SM. Radioiodine uptake in thyroid remnants during therapy after tracer dosimetry. *J Nucl Med* 2000;41:1082–1085.

81. Nilsson M, Lindencrona U, Himmelman J, et al. Radiation-induced stunning of iodide accumulation is caused by specific inhibition of iodide transport: 12th International Thyroid Congress; Kyoto, Japan. *Endocrine J* 2000;47:185.

82. Fujiwara H. Congenital hypothyroidism caused by a mutation in the Na+/I-symporter. *Nat Genet* 1997;17:122.

83. Fujiwara H, Tatsumi K, Miki K, et al. Recurrent T354P mutation of the Na+/I- symporter in patients with iodide transport defect. *J Clin Endocrinol Metab* 1998;83:2940–2943.

84. Kosugi S, Bhayana S, Dean HJ. A novel mutation in the sodium/iodide symporter gene in the largest family with iodide transport defect. *J Clin Endocrinol Metab* 1999;84:3248–3253.

85. Kosugi S, Inoue S, Matsuda A, et al. Novel, missense and loss-of-function mutations in the sodium/iodide symporter gene causing iodide transport defect in three Japanese patients. *J Clin Endocrinol Metab* 1998;83:3373–3376.

86. Kosugi S, Okamoto H, Tamada A, et al. A novel peculiar mutation in the sodium/iodide symporter gene in Spanish siblings with iodide transport defect. *J Clin Endocrinol Metab* 2002;87:3830–3836.

87. Kosugi S, Sato Y, Matsuda A, et al. High prevalence of T354P sodium/iodide symporter gene mutation in Japanese patients with iodide transport defect who have heterogeneous clinical pictures. *J Clin Endocrinol Metab* 1998;83:4123–4129.

88. Matsuda A, Kosugi S. A homozygous missense mutation of the sodium/iodide symporter gene causing iodide transport defect. *J Clin Endocrinol Metab* 1997;82:3966–3971.

89. Pohlenz J, Medeiros-Neto G, Gross JL, et al. Hypothyroidism in a Brazilian kindred due to iodide trapping defect caused by a homozygous mutation in the sodium/iodide symporter gene. *Biochem Biophys Res Commun* 1997;240:488–491.

90. Pohlenz J, Rosenthal IM, Weiss RE, et al. Congenital hypothyroidism due to mutations in the sodium/iodide symporter. Identification of a nonsense mutation producing a downstream cryptic 3' splice site. *J Clin Invest* 1998;101:1028–1035.

91. Tonacchera M, Agretti P, de Marco G, et al. Congenital hypothyroidism due to a new deletion in the sodium/iodide symporter protein. *Clin Endocrinol (Oxf)* 2003;59:500–506.

92. Levy O, Ginter CS, De la Vieja A, et al. Identification of a structural requirement for thyroid Na+/I- symporter (NIS) function from analysis of a mutation that causes human congenital hypothyroidism. *FEBS Lett* 1998;429:36–40.

93. Dohán O, Gavrielides MV, Ginter C, et al. Na(+)/I(-) symporter activity requires a small and uncharged amino acid residue at position 395. *Mol Endocrinol* 2002;16:1893–1902.

94. Pohlenz J, Duprez L, Weiss RE, et al. Failure of membrane targeting causes the functional defect of two mutant sodium iodide symporters. *J Clin Endocrinol Metab* 2000;85:2366–2369.

95. De la Vieja A, Ginter C, Carrasco N. The Q267E mutation in the sodium/iodide symporter (NIS) causes congenital iodide transport defect (ITD) by decreasing the NIS turnover number. *J Cell Sci* 2004;117:677.

96. Brown-Grant K. Extra thyroidal iodide concentrating mechanisms. *Physiol Rev* 1961;41:189–213.

97. Ajjan RA, Kamaruddin NA, Crisp M, et al. Regulation and tissue distribution of the human sodium iodide symporter gene. *Clin Endocrinol (Oxf)* 1998;49:517–523.

98. Cho JY, Leveille R, Kao R, et al. Hormonal regulation of radioiodide uptake activity and Na+/I- symporter expression in mammary glands. *J Clin Endocrinol Metab* 2000;85:2936–2943.

99. Lacroix L, Mian C, Caillou B, et al. Na(+)/I(-) symporter and Pendred syndrome gene and protein expressions in human extra-thyroidal tissues. *Eur J Endocrinol* 2001;144:297–302.

100. Perron B, Rodriguez AM, Leblanc G, et al. Cloning of the mouse sodium iodide symporter and its expression in the mammary gland and other tissues. *J Endocrinol* 2001;170:185–196.

101. Spitzweg C, Dutton CM, Castro MR, et al. Expression of the sodium iodide symporter in human kidney. *Kidney Int* 2001;59:1013–1023.

102. Spitzweg C, Joba W, Eisenmenger W, et al. Analysis of human sodium iodide symporter gene expression in extrathyroidal tissues and cloning of its complementary deoxyribonucleic acids from salivary gland, mammary gland, and gastric mucosa. *J Clin Endocrinol Metab* 1998;83:1746–1751.

103. Foley KP, Leonard MW, Engel JD. Quantitation of RNA using the polymerase chain reaction. *Trends Genet* 1993;9:380–385.

104. De La Vieja A, Dohan O, Levy O, et al. Molecular analysis of the sodium/iodide symporter: impact on thyroid and extrathyroid pathophysiology. *Physiol Rev* 2000;80:1083–1105.

105. Dohan O, De la Vieja A, Paroder V, et al. The sodium/iodide symporter (NIS): characterization, regulation, and medical significance. *Endocr Rev* 2003;24:48–77.

106. Tazebay UH, Wapnir IL, Levy O, et al. The mammary gland iodide transporter is expressed during lactation and in breast cancer. *Nat Med* 2000;6:871–878.

107. Guy CT, Cardiff RD, Muller WJ. Induction of mammary tumors by expression of polyomavirus middle T oncogene: a transgenic mouse model for metastatic disease. *Mol Cell Biol* 1992;12:954–961.

108. Moon DH, Lee SJ, Park KY, et al. Correlation between 99mTc-pertechnetate uptakes and expressions of human sodium iodide symporter gene in breast tumor tissues. *Nucl Med Biol* 2001;28:829–834.

109. Cho JY, Xing S, Liu X, et al. Expression and activity of human Na+/I- symporter in human glioma cells by adenovirus-mediated gene delivery. *Gene Ther* 2000;7:740–749.

110. Dingli D, Diaz RM, Bergert ER, et al. Genetically targeted radiotherapy for multiple myeloma. *Blood* 2003;102:489–496.

111. Spitzweg C, Zhang S, Bergert ER, et al. Prostate-specific antigen (PSA) promoter-driven androgen-inducible expression of sodium iodide symporter in prostate cancer cell lines. *Cancer Res* 1999;59:2136–2141.

112. Groot-Wassink T, Aboagye EO, Glaser M, et al. Adenovirus biodistribution and noninvasive imaging of gene expression in vivo by positron emission tomography using human sodium/iodide symporter as reporter gene. *Hum Gene Ther* 2002;13:1723–1735.

113. Spitzweg C, Dietz AB, O'Connor MK, et al. In vivo sodium iodide symporter gene therapy of prostate cancer. *Gene Ther* 2001;8:1524–1531.

114. Carlin S, Mairs RJ, Welsh P, et al. Sodium-iodide symporter (NIS)-mediated accumulation of [(211)At]astatide in NIS-transfected human cancer cells. *Nucl Med Biol* 2002;29:729–739.

115. Van Sande J, Massart C, Beauwens R, et al. Anion selectivity by the sodium iodide symporter. *Endocrinology* 2003;144:247–252.

116. Zuckier L, Dohan O, Li Y, et al. Kinetics of perrhenate uptake and comparative biodistribution of perrhenate, pertechnetate and iodide by NIS-expressing tissues in vivo. *J Nucl Med* 2004;45:500.

4B   THYROID HORMONE SYNTHESIS

PETER KOPP

Thyroid hormone biosynthesis, storage, and secretion require a series of highly regulated steps. Iodide, the rate-limiting substrate for thyroid hormone synthesis, is actively transported into thyroid follicular cells (thyrocytes) by the sodium-iodide symporter (NIS) at the basolateral membrane (Fig. 4B.1). At the apical membrane of the cells, iodide efflux into the follicular lumen is mediated, at least in part, by pendrin (PDS/SLC26A4). On the luminal side of the apical membrane, iodide is oxidized by thyroid peroxidase (TPO), a reaction that requires the presence of hydrogen peroxide (H_2O_2). H_2O_2 is generated by a calcium-dependent flavoprotein enzyme system that includes the

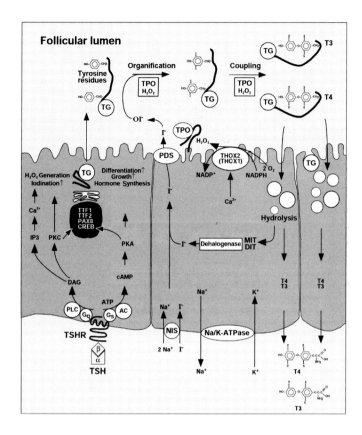

FIGURE 4B.1. Thyroid hormone synthesis, secretion, and major signaling pathways in thyrocytes. *AC*, adenylyl cyclase; *cAMP*, cyclic adenosine monophosphate; *DAG*, diacylglycerol; *DIT*, diiodotyrosine; *MIT*, monoiodotyrosine; *NIS*, sodium-iodide symporter; *PDS*, pendrin; *PKA*, protein kinase A; *PKC*, protein kinase C; *PLC*, phospholipase C; *TG*, thyroglobulin; *TPO*, thyroid peroxidase; *TSH*, thyrotropin; *TSHR*, thyrotropin receptor.

nicotinamide adenine dinucleotide phosphate (NADPH) oxidase THOX2. In the follicular lumen, thyroglobulin serves as matrix for the synthesis of thyroxine (T_4) and triiodothyronine (T_3). In a first step, TPO catalyzes the iodination of selected tyrosyl residues in thyroglobulin, a process referred to as iodination or organification. This results in the formation of mono- and diiodotyrosines (MIT, DIT). In the subsequent coupling reaction, which is also catalyzed by TPO, two iodotyrosines are coupled to form T_4 or T_3. Iodinated thyroglobulin is stored as colloid in the follicular lumen. In response to demand for thyroid hormone secretion, thyroglobulin is internalized into the follicular cell by micro- and macropinocytosis and digested in lysosomes. Subsequently, the thyronines T_4 (~80%) and T_3 (~20%) are released into the blood stream. MIT and DIT are deiodinated by an intracellular iodotyrosine dehalogenase, and the released iodide is recycled for hormone synthesis.

Thyroid hormone synthesis is dependent on the nutritional availability of iodine, and it is predominantly regulated by thyrotropin (thyroid-stimulating hormone, TSH). TSH binds to its cognate receptor, a member of the family of G (guanine nucleotide-binding) protein-coupled seven-transmembrane receptors, which is expressed at the basolateral membrane (Fig. 4B.1) (see section on the thyrotropin receptor in Chapter 10). Binding of TSH to its receptor leads primarily to coupling to $G\alpha_s$ and subsequent activation of adenylyl cyclase. The resulting increase in cyclic adenosine monophosphate (cyclic AMP) formation leads to phosphorylation of protein kinase A and activation of tar-

gets in the cytosol and the nucleus. The TSH-dependent cyclic AMP cascade is the major regulator of growth, differentiation, and hormone secretion of thyrocytes. At higher concentrations of TSH, stimulation of $G\alpha_{9/11}$ and the phospholipase C-dependent inositol phosphate Ca^{2+}/diacylglycerol pathway activates H_2O_2 generation and iodination.

In addition to TSH, iodide uptake is inversely regulated by the intracellular iodide concentration, and the organification process is transiently blocked by high intracellular iodide concentrations. These autoregulatory mechanisms protect the thyroid from iodide excess while ensuring adequate iodide uptake for hormone synthesis.

Previous versions of this chapter by Taurog provided comprehensive reviews of the mechanisms underlying thyroid hormone synthesis, with particular emphasis on the biochemical characteristics of thyroid peroxidase and the mechanisms of action of antithyroid drugs (1,2). Other recent detailed reviews include chapters by Gentile et al (3) and Dunn (4) in other books.

IODIDE UPTAKE INTO THE THYROID

Under physiological conditions, the thyroid iodide concentration is 20 to 40 times higher than the serum iodide concentration, and iodide uptake occurs against a cell-to-plasma electrochemical gradient of about –40 mV (5). The dependence of iodide uptake on a sodium gradient created by Na+,K+-adenosine triphospatase led to the prediction that iodide uptake is mediated by NIS (5–9), a prediction confirmed by the cloning of the symporter, which mediates iodide uptake at the basolateral membrane (8–10). The properties of NIS are discussed in more detail in the preceding section of this chapter.

The Gene and Protein Structure of the Sodium-Iodide Symporter

The ability of thyroid cells to concentrate iodide was recognized as early as 1896 (11), a century before the cloning of NIS (10,12). Human NIS is encoded by a single-copy gene with 15 exons that is located on chromosome 19p13 (13). NIS, officially designated as Solute Carrier 5A (SLC5A), belongs to a family of transporters that requires an electrochemical sodium gradient as the driving force for solute transport. Human NIS is a 643-amino-acid protein, which is thought to have 13 transmembrane domains with an extracellular amino terminus and an intracellular carboxy terminus (14, 15). Mature human NIS is a glycoprotein of ~108 kDa (15). Partial or total deglycosylation does not impair the activity, stability, or membrane targeting of NIS (15).

Functional Characterization of the Sodium-Iodide Symporter

Consistent with findings in FRTL-5 cells (7), the Michaelis-Menten constant (K_m) of NIS expressed in *Xenopus* oocytes is ~36 µ*M* (10). Electrophysiological studies in oocytes demonstrate that NIS is electrogenic, resulting in an inwardly directed influx of positive charge upon addition of iodide to the extracellular perfusing solution (16). The inward steady-state current is due to the influx of sodium, and the stoichiometry of sodium to iodide is 2:1 (16). Based on kinetic results, it is thought that sodium binds to NIS before iodide, and that this is followed by a simultaneous transport of both ions (16).

Both perchlorate and thiocyanate cause rapid release of intracellular iodide across the basolateal membrane if organification is blocked by propylthiouracil (PTU) (17,18).

This phenomenon is the basis for the perchlorate discharge test, which is used to evaluate intrathyroidal iodide organification (18). These anions inhibit iodide uptake through competitive inhibition (16). It is, however, controversial whether perchlorate itself serves as a substrate for NIS. In contrast to thiocyanate, perchlorate does not elicit an inward current, suggesting that perchlorate is not transported by NIS despite its potent inhibitory action on iodide uptake (16,19,20). This conclusion contrasts with studies using tetrahedral oxyanions in transfected cells, which suggest that NIS may mediate uptake of perchlorate (21).

Regulation of Iodide Uptake and Sodium-Iodide Symporter Function and Expression

TSH, acting through the cyclic AMP pathway, stimulates iodide accumulation in the thyroid (22,23). The increase in iodide uptake is the consequence of increased transcription of NIS and posttranscriptional stimulation of NIS activity. TSH up-regulates NIS mRNA and protein expression *in vivo* and *in vitro* (14,24–26). Consistent with an expression pattern that is not restricted to the thyroid, the structure of the promoter region of the NIS gene differs from those of the *Tg* (thyroglobulin) and *TPO* genes (Fig. 4B.2) (27–29).

TSH also modulates NIS protein turnover; in the presence of TSH, the half-life of NIS in FRTL-5 thyroid cells is ~5 days, in its absence it decreases to ~3 days (30). Aside from increasing NIS synthesis, TSH also regulates posttranslational events such as the subcellular distribution of NIS, specifically the targeting to and retention of NIS in the basolateral membrane. In the absence of TSH, NIS remains in the cell, and little reaches the plasma membrane.

In addition to TSH, iodide accumulation and organification are directly regulated by iodide itself (31–33). Negative regulation of the expression of NIS mRNA occurs in thyroid tissue of dogs fed moderate doses of iodide for 2 days (34). High doses of iodide block thyroid hormone synthesis through inhibition of the organification process, the Wolff-Chaikoff effect (31). This transient blockade of

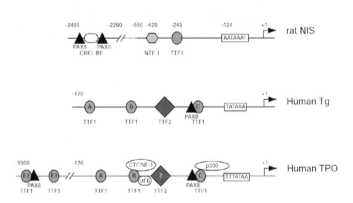

FIGURE 4B.2. Schematic structure of the promoter regions of the *NIS* (sodium-iodide symporter), *Tg* (thyroglobulin), and *TPO* (thyroid peroxidase) genes showing the sites where different transcription factors bind to the DNA. (From Dohán O, De la Vieja A, Paroder V, et al. The sodium/iodide symporter (NIS): characterization, regulation, and medical significance. *Endocr Rev* 2003;24:48, and Damante G, Di Lauro R. Thyroid-specific gene expression. *Biochim Biophys Acta* 1994;1218 255, modified with permission.)

organification is dependent on the intracellular iodide concentration (31,32). The escape from the acute Wolff-Chaikoff effect involves a decrease in iodide transport, which leads to intracellular iodide concentrations that are too low to maintain the inhibitory effect (35). At the molecular level, an iodide-induced down-regulation of NIS expression, possibly an increase in NIS protein turnover, and a decrease in NIS activity contribute to this complex autoregulatory phenomenon induced by an increase in intracellular iodide concentrations (34,36–38). The down-regulation of NIS expression and activity is thyroid-specific, independent of TSH, and may be associated with formation of inactive NIS dimers (39). Thyroglobulin down-regulates NIS transcription (40,41), as do several cytokines, including transforming growth factor-β, tumor necrosis factor-α, interleukin-1, and interferon-γ (9,42).

Mutations in the Sodium-Iodide Symporter Gene

Congenital hypothyroidism can be caused by developmental defects of the thyroid, collectively referred to as thyroid dysgenesis, or by inborn errors of one of the steps required for thyroid hormone synthesis, referred to as thyroid dyshormonogenesis (see Chapter 48 and see section on congenital hypothyroidism in Chapter 75) (43–45). Among patients with thyroid dyshormonogenesis, a few have an iodide-trapping defect (46). The thyroid gland (and other tissues that contain NIS) does not concentrate iodine; therefore, thyroid and salivary uptake of radioiodine is very low, and the saliva/serum radioiodide ratio is very low (46). The thyroid may be normal in size at birth, but it enlarges soon thereafter unless the infant is given high doses of iodine or T$_4$. After the *NIS* gene was cloned, several patients with hypothyroidism caused by this defect were found to be homozygous or compound heterozygous for inactivating NIS mutations (8,9,47). Some of the mutations decrease NIS function by substituting key functional amino acid residues (48), and others lead to misfolding and retention of NIS in intracellular compartments (see the preceding section of this chapter) (49).

IODIDE EFFLUX FROM THE THYROID

Compared with the mechanisms mediating iodide uptake at the basolateral membrane, iodide efflux at the apical membrane is less well characterized (Fig. 4B.1). Iodide efflux is stimulated by TSH in both poorly polarized FRTL-5 cells (50) and polarized porcine thyrocytes (51,52). In primary porcine thyrocytes grown in a transwell system, bidirectional measurements indicate that TSH stimulates iodide efflux at the apical membrane, while efflux in the basal direction does not change (52). This rapid effect of TSH facilitates the transport of iodide into the follicular lumen.

Electrophysiological studies performed with inverted plasma membrane vesicles suggest the existence of two apical channels for iodide efflux (53). One of these channels has a high permeability and specificity for iodide (K_m ~70 μ*M*), and the second channel has a lower affinity for iodide (K_m ~33 mM) (53). However, the identity of these channels has not been established at the molecular level. The demonstration of iodide transport by the anion channel pendrin, together with the phenotype in patients with Pendred's syndrome, suggest that pendrin is one of the channels promoting apical iodide efflux (54–58). Whether the recently identified channel referred to as human apical iodide transporter (hAIT/SLC5A8) is involved in apical iodide efflux (59) or transport of other anions in thyrocytes is not known.

Cloning of the Pendrin (PDS/SLC26A4) Gene

Pendred's syndrome is an autosomal recessive disorder defined by sensorineural deafness, goiter, and impaired iodide organification (60–62). After Pendred's syndrome was linked to chromosome 7q22–31.1 (63,64), the *PDS* gene, now designated as *SLC26A4*, was cloned (54). The *PDS/SLC26A4* gene encompasses 21 exons and contains an open reading frame of 2,343 base pairs (Fig. 4B.3). The SLC26A family contains several transporters of sulfate or other anions and the motor protein prestin (SLC26A5), which is expressed in outer hair cells (Table 4B.1) (65–67). The genes encoding pendrin, prestin (SCLC26A5), and DRA/CLD (down-regulated in adenoma/congenital chloride diarrhea, SLC26A3) are located in close vicinity on chromosome 7q21–31 and have a very similar genomic structure, suggesting a common ancestral gene.

Protein Structure of Pendrin

Pendrin is a highly hydrophobic membrane protein consisting of 780 amino acids (Fig. 4B.3) (54). It contains a conserved, albeit slightly variant sulfate transport motif. Initially, pendrin was thought to have 11 transmembrane domains with an intracellular amino terminus and an extracellular carboxy terminus (54), but more recent studies suggest there are 12 transmembrane domains and an intracellular carboxy terminus (68). The intracellular location of both the amino terminus and the carboxy terminus has been confirmed by the analysis of pendrin fusion proteins (58). Pendrin is a glycoprotein with three putative extracellular *N*-glycosylation sites (68,69). In extracts of human thyroid membranes studied under denaturing conditions, pendrin is a single molecular species of ~110 to 115 kDa; deglycosylation leads to a reduction in molecular mass to ~85 kDa (69).

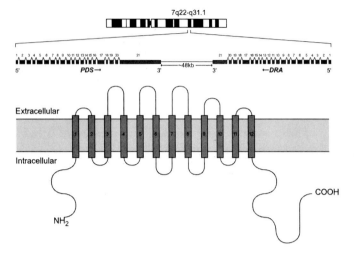

FIGURE 4B.3. Chromosomal location and structure of the *PDS/SLC26A4* gene and current model of the secondary structure of the pendrin *(PDS)* protein. (From Everett LA, Glaser B, Beck JC, et al. Pendred syndrome is caused by mutations in a putative sulphate transporter gene (PDS). *Nature Genet* 1997; 17:411; Everett LA, Green ED. A family of mammalian anion transporters and their involvement in human genetic diseases. *Hum Mol Genet* 1999;8:1883; and Royaux IE, Suzuki K, Mori A, et al. Pendrin, the protein encoded by the Pendred syndrome gene (PDS), is an apical porter of iodide in the thyroid and is regulated by thyroglobulin in FRTL-5 cells. *Endocrinology* 2000;141:839, modified with permission.)

Expression and Regulation of Pendrin

Pendrin mRNA, assessed by Northern analysis, is primarily detected in the thyroid (54), but small amounts of both pendrin mRNA and protein are in the endolymphatic system of the inner ear (70,71), β-intercalated cells of the renal cortical collecting duct (72–74), syncytiotrophoblast cells of the placenta (75), endometrium (76), and mammary glands of pregnant and lactating mice (77). Very low levels of pendrin mRNA have also been found in lung, prostate, and testis (78).

Immunolocalization studies reveal that pendrin is located at the apical membrane of thyrocytes (68,79). The immunostaining is heterogeneous within and among normal thyroid follicles (79). In thyroid tissue from patients with Graves' disease, immunostaining revealed higher pendrin protein expression than in normal thyroid tissue, suggesting a correlation between pendrin abundance and increased iodide organification (68,80). In hyperfunctioning thyroid adenomas, the levels of pendrin mRNA were normal, but immunostaining and Western blot analysis revealed more pendrin, as compared with normal thyroid tissue (79,81). In follicular adenomas, the levels of pendrin mRNA and protein were similar to those in normal thyroid tissue (69,82). In hypofunctioning adenomas, the levels of pendrin mRNA were normal, but the pendrin content of the adenomas, as detected by immunostaining, was highly variable (79,81). In FRTL-5 cells, low concentrations of thyroglobulin, but

TABLE 4B.1. SELECTED MEMBERS OF THE SOLUTE CARRIER FAMILY 26A

Gene Symbol	Alternative Gene Symbols	Protein	Major Expression	Anion Transport/ Function	Chromosome Location	Human Disease
SCL26A2	DTDST	Diastrophic dysplasia	Ubiquitous	Sulfate Chloride Oxalate	5q32-q33.1	Diastrophic dysplasia Achondrogenesis IB Atelosteogenesis II
SCL26A3	DRA or CLD	Down-regulated in adenoma	Ileum Colon Seminal vesicle	Sulfate Chloride Bicarbonate Hydroxide Oxalate	7q21–31	Congenital chloride diarrhea
SCL26A4	PDS	Pendrin	Inner ear Thyroid Kidney	Iodide Chloride Bicarbonate Hydroxide Formate	7q21–31	Pendred's syndrome Enlarged vestibular aqueduct Recessive deafness
SCL26A5	PRES	Prestin	Outer hair-cells	Motor protein	7q21–31	Sensorineural deafness

CLD, chloride diarrhea; DFNB4, autosomal recessive deafness 4; DTDST, diastrophic dysplasia sulfate transporter; SCL, Solute Carrier.

not TSH, insulin, interferon-α, or iodide, increased pendrin mRNA levels (68). This contrasts with the negative effect of thyroglobulin on the levels of expression of the *NIS, TPO, Tg,* and *TSH receptor* genes (40,41).

In differentiated thyroid carcinomas, pendrin mRNA and protein expression were low (69,79,80,83) and did not correlate with NIS expression (83,84). Pendrin mRNA was also scarce in thyroid cancer cell lines (68). Consistent with this low or absent expression, aberrant hypermethylation of the promoter region of the *PDS* gene was found in the majority of thyroid cancers (85).

Functional Characterization of Pendrin

Pendrin, expressed in *Xenopus* oocytes and S f9 insect cells, and present in cultured thyrocytes from patients with Pendred's syndrome, is unable to transport sulfate despite its homology with sulfate transporters (Fig. 4B.4) (55,86). In *Xenopus* oocytes, pendrin mediated uptake of chloride and iodide in a sodium-independent manner (55). The apical localization of pendrin in thyrocytes (68,79), together with its ability to transport iodide in oocytes and the impaired iodide organification found in patients with Pendred's syndrome (55), suggested a possible role in iodide transport into the follicular lumen (65,68). Functional studies in transfected cells subsequently demonstrated that the protein can indeed mediate iodide efflux (56,57). Further evidence that pendrin mediated apical iodide efflux was obtained in a model system with polarized Madin-Darby canine kidney (MDCK) cells expressing NIS and pendrin (Fig. 4B.5) (58). Consistent with the partial organification defect present in patients with Pendred's syndrome, naturally occurring mutations of pendrin lead to impaired apical transport of iodide into the follicular lumen of thyroid follicles (56,58,87).

The function of pendrin is not limited to iodide transport. In *Xenopus* oocytes, pendrin acts as a chloride/formate exchanger (88). In transfected HEK-293 cells, pendrin facilitates exchange of chloride with bicarbonate, hydroxide, and formate (72). Perfused renal tubules isolated from alkali-loaded normal mice secrete bicarbonate, whereas tubules from alkali-loaded *Pds-/-* mice do not, confirming that pendrin is a chloride/base exchanger (73). A physiological role for pendrin in bicarbonate secretion is also suggested by its differential regulation by acid-base and electrolyte status (89,90). In mice, acid-loading results in reduction of the pendrin content in cortical-collecting duct cells, and it is relocalized from the apical membrane to the cytosol (89,90). Conversely, bicarbonate loading results in an increase in pendrin in the membranes of these cells (90). Based on the enlargement of the endolymphatic system in patients with Pendred's syndrome and *Pds* null mice (91, 92), pendrin is thought to be involved in anion and fluid transport and maintenance of the endocochlear potential in the inner ear (71,91,92).

Pendred's Syndrome and Its Allelic Variants

Pendred's syndrome was first recognized by Vaughan Pendred in 1896 (see Chapter 48) (93). The incidence of Pendred's syndrome is thought to be as high as 7.5 to 10 in 100,000 people, and it is probably the most common form of syndromic deafness, accounting for about 10% of all patients with hereditary deafness (94,95).

The first insights into the pathophysiology of Pendred's syndrome followed recognition that these patients have a partial defect in the organification of iodide (96). Despite this defect, many patients with Pendred's syndrome are clinically and biochemically euthyroid unless dietary iodine intake is low (61,62). Furthermore, the prevalence of goiter may be lower in patients with this syndrome who

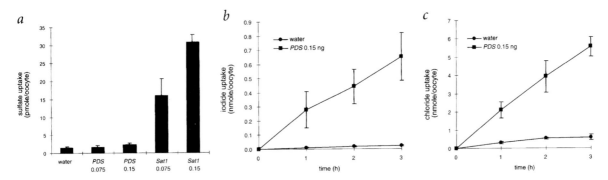

FIGURE 4B.4. Time course of anion transport by pendrin in *Xenopus* oocytes injected with PDS/SLC26A4 complementary RNA. Pendrin, in contrast to the rat sulfate transporter Sat1, is unable to promote uptake of (^{35}S)-Na$_2$SO$_4$ **(a)**, but does promote uptake of (^{125}I)-tetramethylammonium iodide **(b)** and (^{36}C)-tetramethylammonium chloride **(c)**. (From Scott DA, Wang R, Kreman TM, et al. The Pendred syndrome gene encodes a chloride-iodide transport protein. *Nature Genet* 1999; 21:440, with permission.)

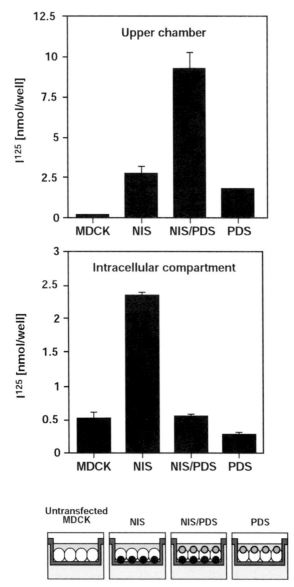

FIGURE 4B.5. Transport of iodide by cells expressing NIS, pendrin (PDS), or both. Polarized MDCK cells expressing sodium-iodide symporter (NIS), pendrin, or NIS and pendrin growing in a bicameral cells were exposed to a solution containing (^{125}I)-iodide in the lower chamber. There was a large increase in intracellular iodide in the cells expressing NIS. In cells expressing NIS and pendrin, the intracellular iodide content was low, and there was a large increase in iodide transport into the upper chamber. Cells expressing only pendrin accumulated little iodide in the intracellular compartment, but iodide did reach the upper chamber in increased amounts, as compared with wild-type MDCK cells. (From Gillam MP, Sidhaye A, Lee EJ, et al. Functional characterization of pendrin in a polarized cell system: evidence for pendrin-mediated apical iodide efflux. *J Biol Chem* 2004;279: 13004, with permission.)

live in iodine-replete regions (97,98). *Pds* knockout mice do not have thyroid enlargement or abnormal serum thyroid hormone production (92). These findings suggest that iodide may enter the lumen of thyroid follicles independent of pendrin, either by means of another iodide-trans-

porting channel or nonspecific anion channels assisted by the electrochemical gradient between the cytoplasm of thyrocytes and the lumen (53).

Patients with Pendred's syndrome from consanguineous families are homozygous for *PDS* gene mutations, whereas sporadic cases typically have compound heterozygous mutations (62). Mutations in the *PDS* gene display impressive allelic heterogeneity, and more than 75 mutations have already been identified (54,99–104). In many instances, the mutated pendrin protein is retained in an intracellular compartment, usually the endoplasmic reticulum (56,58, 105), indicating that the mutations result in aberrant folding of the protein, thus preventing full maturation and insertion into the cell membrane. Other mutated pendrin molecules are normally inserted into the membrane but cannot normally mediate iodide efflux, suggesting that the mutations involve amino acid residues that are important for iodide transport (56).

Mutations in the *PDS* gene are found not only in patients with classic Pendred's syndrome, but also in patients with familial enlargement of the vestibular aqueduct (106,107), suggesting that the incidence of sensorineural hearing impairment associated with alterations in this gene may even be higher than previously thought. Limited functional studies in oocytes suggest that the mutations found in Pendred's syndrome result in complete loss of chloride and iodide transport, whereas the mutations found in nonsyndromic hearing loss have some transport activity (87). However, the same mutation may be associated with variable phenotypic expression, suggesting that other genetic and environmental factors modify the effects of the mutation (56).

THYROGLOBULIN

Thyroglobulin, a large glycoprotein dimer secreted into the follicular lumen, serves as the matrix for the synthesis of T_4 and T_3, and as the storage form of the hormones and iodide (see Chapter 5). When T_4 and T_3 are needed, thyroglobulin is taken up by the thyrocytes and digested in lysosomes, and T_4 and T_3 are released into the blood stream (Fig. 4B.1).

Structure of the Thyroglobulin Gene and Protein

Thyroglobulin is encoded by a single-copy gene of 270 kb located on human chromosome 8q24.2–8q24.3 (108–111). It contains 48 exons separated by introns of up to 65 kb (108,112,113). The promoter region of the gene has remarkable structural similarity with the promoter region of the *TPO* gene and is regulated by the transcription factors TTF-1, TTF-2, and Pax-8 (Fig. 4B.2) (28,29). The full-length human mRNA contains a 41-nucleotide 5′-untranslated segment preceding an open reading frame of

8,307 bases, and a 3′-untranslated region ranging from 101 to 120 base pairs (114,115).

The thyroglobulin monomer consists of a 19-amino-acid signal peptide followed by 2,749 residues containing 66 tyrosine residues (115). After translation of the mRNA, thyroglobulin monomers are transported to the endoplasmic reticulum (ER), where they are folded and undergo dimerization. The dimers are then glycosylated. Mature thyroglobulin migrates to the apical membrane in small secretory vesicles and is secreted into the follicular lumen (116,117). In the follicular lumen, thyroglobulin is present as a 19S dimeric glycoprotein of 660 kDa (118).

Analysis of the primary structure of thyroglobulin for internal homology led to its division into four major regions. The type 1 repetitive region has 11 segments that contain a cysteine-rich consensus sequence CWCV(D), a sequence found in many proteins (119–121). These segments may bind and inhibit cysteine proteases, a feature that could play a role in the processing and degradation of thyroglobulin (see later in the chapter) (119,120). In the mature protein lacking the signal peptide, these segments are located between amino acids 12 and 1191 and amino acids 1492 and 1546. The type 2 repetitive region, composed of three elements, is located between amino acids 1437 and 1484. The type 3 repetitive region is characterized by five elements between residues 1584 and 2168. The carboxy-terminal region of the thyroglobulin monomer, encompassing residues 2192 to 2716, shares remarkable homology with acetylcholinesterase (121,122). Overall, this structure has been interpreted to indicate the possibility of a convergent origin of the *Tg* gene from different ancestral DNA sequences (123).

The maturation of thyroglobulin is controlled by several molecular chaperones such as BiP, GRP94, Erp72, and calnexin (see Chapter 5) (124). Thyroglobulin monomers contain 20 potential glycosylation sites; among them, 16 are known to be glycosylated (4,125), and about 10% of the molecular weight is accounted for by carbohydrates. Other secondary modifications of the protein include sulfation and phosphorylation (126,127). Consensus sequences required for tyrosine sulfation are present at most of the hormonogenic sites within thyroglobulin, and sulfation may play a role in hormone formation (128).

Mutations in the Thyroglobulin Gene

Recessive mutations in the *Tg* gene have been identified in several animal species and humans with goiter and overt or subclinical hypothyroidism (see Chapter 48) (129–131). The patients typically have very low serum thyroglobulin concentrations (132). Most have had homozygous inactivating mutations in the *TG* gene (130,131); rare patients have had different mutations in each allele (compound heterozygous genotype) (133). Some of these mutations result

in synthesis of thyroglobulin molecules that are retained in the endoplasmic reticulum and thus fall into the class of ER storage diseases (124,134,135).

THYROID PEROXIDASE

In order to serve as an iodinating agent, iodide must be oxidized to a higher oxidation state, a step that is dependent on the presence of H_2O_2 and is catalyzed by TPO. TPO, a glycoprotein with a prosthetic heme group, is located in the apical membrane. In addition to catalyzing the oxidation of iodide, TPO is also essential for the incorporation of iodide into tyrosine residues in thyroglobulin (organification) and coupling of the iodotyrosines to form T_4 and T_3 (Fig. 4B.1).

The purification and the biochemical properties of TPO were discussed in detail in the previous versions of this chapter by Taurog (1,2). The cloning of TPO and its role as an autoantigen in autoimmune thyroid disease, which is discussed in Chapter 14, have been reviewed by McLachlan and Rapoport (136).

The Gene and Protein Structure of Thyroid Peroxidase

The human *TPO* gene is located on chromosome 2pter-p12 (137,138), spans about 150 kb, and consists of 17 exons separated by 16 introns (139). The first cDNAs encoding TPO were isolated from human and porcine cDNA libraries (137,140,141). The full-length human TPO cDNA encodes a protein of 933 amino acids (137). In addition to the full-length mRNA encoding full-length TPO (TPO1), several shorter transcripts of unknown biological importance have been identified (137,142,143). The most abundant alternative transcript lacks 171 nucleotides, secondary to deletion of exon 10, which encompasses codons 533 to 590 (TPO2) (137,144). The encoded protein lacks enzymatic activity (144). In immunoblot analyses, TPO appears as a doublet of 110 and 105 kDa, a phenomenon that is not explained by translation of TPO2 (145).

The amino terminus of TPO is located in the lumen of thyroid follicles, and the extracellular domain forms a loop created by two (human) or one (porcine) intramolecular disulfide bonds, which is followed by a single membrane-spanning domain in close proximity to its carboxy terminus (146,147). Introduction of a stop codon immediately upstream of the putative transmembrane domain (amino acids 846 to 870) results in a soluble protein that is secreted into the medium and retains enzymatic activity (148). Human TPO has five potential glycosylation sites, and about 10% of its weight is carbohydrate (2). The location and nature of the *N*-linked oligosaccharide units have been determined only for porcine TPO (149).

The prosthetic heme group, a *bis*-hydroxylated heme that is distinct from the heme b (protoporphyrin IX) found in many other hemoproteins, is covalently bound to glutamine 399 and aspartate 238 of the apoprotein (150). Amino-acid side chains directly linked to the iron atom or positioned in its immediate proximity are critical for modulating enzyme reactivity and specificity. These side chains are provided by two histidine residues located on opposite sides of the heme moiety, a proximal histidine coordinately linked to the iron center, and a distal histidine located in proximity of the peroxide-binding pocket (150–152). Based on sequence alignment with myeloperoxidase (MPO), the distal histidine in TPO is located at position 239, and the proximal histidine at position 494 (150,152). The distal histidine and a nearby arginine residue at position 396 are thought to be involved in the formation of compound I, a two-electron oxidized form of TPO (see later in chapter) (150,152). TPO2 is enzymatically inactive (144), presumably because it lacks asparagine 579, which forms a stabilizing hydrogen bond with the proximal histidine 494 (150,152).

All mammalian peroxidases belong to the same gene family (152). TPO has a high degree of sequence similarity with MPO (140,153–155) and other mammalian peroxidases (156–158). The first 735 amino acids of TPO have 42% sequence identity with MPO (141), and the homology between TPO and MPO in the vicinity of the heme group is as high as 74% (140). Based on sequence analyses, which have revealed domains homologous to epidermal growth factor, complement C4b, and mitochondrial cytochrome C oxidase I, the *TPO* gene may be a mosaic gene (141). The structure of MPO has been solved at 3 Å resolution (159), and more recently at 1.8 Å resolution (160,161). Theoretical three-dimensional structures have been proposed for other mammalian peroxidases using the MPO model as a scaffold (151), but the three-dimensional structure of TPO has not been modeled (2). TPO, analogous to MPO (159), may form a disulfide-linked dimer in its native form, based on immunoblot experiments under nonreducing conditions (162,163), a model that has been questioned (145).

Proper folding and membrane insertion are essential for enzyme activity. Immunohistochemical studies localize TPO at the apical membrane (164), and abundant immunopositivity is also found in the cytoplasm (165). Stimulation with TSH acutely increases TPO immunoreactivity at the apical membrane and increases enzymatic activity (166,167). Thus, TPO is probably brought to the apical through the secretory pathway. The sorting and trafficking of TPO are cell type-dependent (168). In stably transfected heterologous cell systems, TPO is often largely retained in intracellular compartments (168–171). In contrast, it reaches the plasma membrane efficiently in stably transfected rat PCCl3 thyroid cells (168). These findings suggest that continuous membrane insertion of TPO requires the presence of thyroid-specific factors.

Functional Characterization of Thyroid Peroxidase

Before the cloning of the TPO cDNA, catalytically active TPO was purified by solubilizing membrane fractions of thyroid tissue with detergent and limited proteolytic digestion (146,147), eventually combined with immunoaffinity chromatography (172,173). The catalytic activity of these preparations was determined using several assay procedures, including guaiacol oxidation, iodide oxidation, iodination of albumin, and coupling of DIT to form T_4 within thyroglobulin (146). After the molecular cloning of TPO cDNAs, recombinant TPO has been expressed in mammalian cells, insect cells, and yeast [for review, see reference 136]. Recombinant TPO preparations have been particularly useful for immunologic studies, although many have diminished catalytic activity (2,174). Eukaryotic cells may be more suitable as an expression system for obtaining a functional and soluble recombinant TPO, presumably because of their ability to glycosylate the protein fully (174).

Expression and Regulation of Thyroid Peroxidase

The activity of TPO is increased by TSH *in vivo* (175, 176), and this stimulatory effect is the consequence of increased synthesis of TPO (177). The mechanisms leading to stimulation of TPO synthesis vary in different model systems. TSH and other stimulators of the cyclic AMP signaling pathway increase TPO mRNA abundance in cultured thyroid cells (178–182). In FRTL-5 cells, the increase in TPO mRNA levels is due to an increase in mRNA stability (180,181), whereas transcriptional stimulation accounts for the increase in canine thyroid cells (179,183).

TSH-induced stimulation of *TPO* gene transcription does not require the presence of insulin or insulin-like growth factor 1 (179,180), whereas both stimulators are required for transcription of the *Tg* gene (180). Phorbol esters, interferon-γ, and interleukin-1α and -1β inhibit TSH-induced TPO mRNA expression in cultured human thyroid cells (184–186). In contrast to TSH, follicular thyroglobulin decreases the expression of TTF-1, TTF-2, and Pax-8, actions that decrease the expression of the genes for TPO as well as for NIS, thyroglobulin, and the TSH receptor (40,41).

TSH and forskolin rapidly increase TPO promoter activity without the requirement for protein synthesis (187). This stimulation correlates with an increase in TTF-2 binding to the TPO promoter (188) but does not involve TTF-1 or a cyclic AMP response element (28,189). The structure of the promoter region of the human *TPO* gene resembles that of the *Tg* gene promoter, and it contains a TATA box, three binding sites for TTF-1, and a binding site for Pax-8 and TTF-2 in the region between −170 to +1 base pairs relative to the transcriptional start site (Fig. 4B.2)

(28). As in the *Tg* gene promoter, the Pax-8 and the TTF-1 binding sites overlap, and *in vitro* the binding of the two transcription factors to DNA is mutually exclusive (190). However, Pax-8 and TTF-1 combine with each other, and the combination synergistically activates the *Tg* gene promoter (Fig. 4B.2) (191). This particular mechanism may not apply to the TPO promoter (191), although the two transcription factors have synergistic actions on TPO transcription (192). CTF/NF-1, a member of the CCAAT-binding transcription-factor family, which is inducible by cyclic AMP and insulin, cooperates with TTF-2 in increasing the activity of the promoter region of the *TPO* gene (193). Moreover, the carboxy terminus of Pax-8 associates with the nuclear coactivator p300 to increase *TPO* gene transcription (194). This suggests that the stimulatory effect of TSH on TPO mRNA expression may be mediated through p300 or CBP (CREB-binding protein), because the TPO promoter does not contain a cyclic AMP response element (28,189,194). A thyroid-specific enhancer region has been identified 5.5 kb upstream of the transcriptional start site in the human *TPO* gene (28,195). This region has overlapping binding sites for TTF-1 and Pax-8 that may be mutually exclusive (196,197), suggesting that the ratio of TTF-1 to Pax-8 may be important in the regulation of *TPO* gene expression (197).

Mutations in Thyroid Peroxidase

Recessive TPO defects are among the most frequent causes of inborn abnormalities of thyroid hormone synthesis (see Chapter 48) (198–200). The decrease or absence of TPO activity results in a partial or total iodide organification defect, so that affected patients have a substantial discharge of radioiodine after the administration of perchlorate. A survey from the Netherlands confirmed that *TPO* gene defects are the most common cause of severe defects in iodine organification (201). Of the patients available for molecular studies, 37% were homozygous and 46% were compound heterozygous for mutations affecting the exons or intron/exon boundaries of the *TPO* gene. In a small percentage, only one abnormal allele could be identified, and only one of the families did not have a TPO mutation. One patient had a partial maternal isodisomy of chromosome 2p resulting in homozygosity for an inactivating *TPO* gene mutation (201).

THE HYDROGEN PEROXIDE–GENERATING SYSTEM

H_2O_2 is an essential and limiting factor in the oxidation of iodide, its organification, and the coupling reaction (Fig. 4B.1) (202). The H_2O_2-generating system is localized at the apical membrane (203,204), and its generation in-

volves the oxidation of NADPH by an NADPH oxidase (205–208). This enzyme system contains a membrane-bound flavoprotein using FAD as a cofactor (209,210), and it requires micromolar concentrations of calcium (204,206, 211–213). A functional NADPH oxidase that generates H_2O_2 in a Ca^{2+}-dependent manner has been solubilized from plasma membranes of porcine thyroid tissue (210); sequence information derived from this protein led to cloning of a partial cDNA (214).

Cloning of the Thyroid Oxidase Genes

Two cDNAs encoding thyroidal NADPH oxidases have been cloned (214,215). The two oxidases are commonly referred to as THOX1 and THOX2, for "thyroid" oxidase; their official designations are DUOX1 and DUOX2, an eponym derived from "dual" oxidase. Human and porcine cDNA sequences encoding the carboxy-terminal region of an NADPH oxidase (initially called p138Tox) were isolated by reverse transcription-polymerase chain reaction (RT-PCR) using degenerate primers derived from peptide microsequences obtained from purification of a flavoprotein-containing oxidase (210,214). Two full-length cDNAs encoding thyroid NADPH oxidases were cloned using a strategy assuming a homology between the NADPH oxidase systems in thyrocytes and granulocytes (215). The probes used to screen thyroid cDNA libraries were based on gp91Phox (NOX2), a heme-binding oxidase that is part of the enzyme system responsible for the production of superoxide (O_2^-) in granulocytes (216,217). THOX2 was also detected as an abundant transcript in thyroid cells using serial analysis of gene expression (218).

The two *THOX* genes are closely linked and located on chromosome 15q15 (214,215). They both consist of 33 exons; the *THOX1* gene spans about 36 kb, and the *THOX2* gene spans about 22 kb (214,215). Human THOX1 has an open reading frame of 1,551 amino acids, THOX2 of 1,548 residues (215). The protein p138Tox corresponds to THOX2 but lacks the first 338 amino acids (214).

The Protein Structure of Thyroid Oxidases

THOX genes encode two closely related proteins that have 83% homology. They are related not only to gp91Phox (NOX2) found in granulocytes (216), but also to MOX1, a superoxide-generating oxidase present in nonphagocytic cells (219), and a *Caenorhabditis elegans* protein (215). Analysis of the secondary structure, and comparison with the model proposed for gp91Phox (NOX2) (216), predicts seven putative transmembrane domains, two everted finger motifs in the first intracellular loop, four NADPH-binding sites, and one FAD-binding site (Fig. 4B.6) (214,215). The intracellular location of the everted finger domains, which are calcium-binding sites, is consistent with the activation

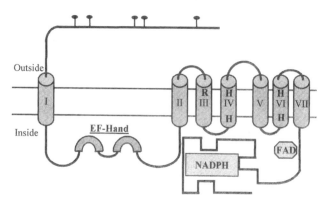

FIGURE 4B.6. Proposed structure of THOX proteins with seven transmembrane domains, two putative Ca^{2+}-binding EF-finger motifs in the first intracellular loop, and cytosolic FAD- and NADPH-binding sites. (From De Deken X, Wang D, Many MC, et al. Cloning of two human thyroid cDNAs encoding new members of the NADPH oxidase family. *J Biol Chem* 2000;275:23227, with permission.)

of the H_2O_2 generation system by cytosolic Ca^{2+} in thyroid membranes (208,211), intact follicles (204), and thyroid slices (202,220).

As predicted from analysis of the primary structure, which suggests the presence of five possible glycosylation sites (215), the THOX proteins are glycosylated (221,222). Western blots reveal two proteins with a molecular weight of ~180 kDa to 190 kDa. Only the 190-kDa form is resistant to endoglycosidase H digestion, suggesting that it is the completely processed form. After complete deglycosylation, the size of the protein is reduced to ~160 kDa (221).

The amino termini of both THOX proteins have a homology of ~43% with TPO. Remarkably, this domain of THOX1 and its *C. elegans* homologue have peroxidase activity (223). The finding of a peroxidase activity domain and an NADPH oxidase domain in the same protein led to their official designation as dual oxidases (223). The carboxy-terminal part of THOX1 and THOX2 are highly homologous to the mammalian oxidases gp91Phox (NOX2) and p65Mox (NOX1), and contain the putative intracellular FAD- and NADPH-binding sites. The four histidine residues and arginine residue thought to be involved in heme binding in gp91Phox (NOX2) are conserved (216).

Expression and Regulation of Thyroid Oxidases

The mRNAs for THOX1 and THOX are almost exclusively detected in thyroid tissue (214,215,224). A very small amount of THOX2 mRNA has been found in the stomach (215) and possibly the trachea (225), and an expressed sequence tag for THOX2 has been found in a pancreas library (218). THOX2 transcripts were also detected in the intestinal tract (duodenum, small intestine, colon) of adult rats by RT-PCR analysis (224).

The levels of THOX1 and THOX2 mRNA increase in response to stimulation of the cyclic AMP pathway in human, porcine, canine and rat thyroid cells *in vitro* (214,215,224). The stimulation is greater in dog than in human thyroid tissue (215). In rats treated with methimazole (MMI), the levels of THOX2 mRNA are reduced (224), a finding that contrasts with the change in cultured cells (214,215,224). Treatment of thyroid cells and follicles with iodide inhibits H_2O_2 generation and NADPH activity *in vitro* (213,226). While treatment of porcine thyroid follicles with iodide downregulates the levels of NIS and TPO mRNA, it does not affect the level of THOX2 mRNA (222). However, it does antagonize the cyclic AMP-induced glycosylation of THOX2 to its mature form, possibly explaining the decrease in H_2O_2 generation (222). This phenomenon may contribute to the mechanisms underlying the antithyroid effect of high iodine concentrations (Wolff-Chaikoff effect) (222).

Immunohistochemical analyses demonstrate THOX protein at the apical membrane of thyrocytes and colocalization with TPO (215,225). The fraction of THOX proteins reaching the apical membrane is, however, modest (221), similar to TPO (227). The low content of THOX proteins at the apical membrane may serve to limit the generation of oxidative agents (221). The THOX proteins and TPO are barely inserted into the membrane of nonthyroidal cells (168,170,171); in nonthyroidal cells transfected with THOX1 and THOX2 cDNAs, the expressed proteins remain restricted to intracellular compartments (221). In addition, a finding that contrasts with the observations in thyrocytes, they are present only as a 180-kDa form (221).

The levels of THOX mRNA are variable in benign and malignant human thyroid tissues (225,228). In thyroid tissue from patients with Graves' disease, only a few cells are stained with anti-THOX antibodies (225). In multinodular goiters, the average number of positive cells is similar to that of normal thyroid tissue, but in hypofunctioning tissue THOX is more abundant (225). In general, as determined by immunostaining, the thyroid tissue content of NIS and THOX is inversely related (225).

Cotransfection of THOX proteins with TPO and p22Phox, one of the proteins required for NADPH oxidase activity of gp91Phox (NOX2), into CHO cells does not result in insertion of THOX or TPO into the cell membrane, and does not result in H_2O_2 generation (221). Similarly, transfection of THOX cDNAs into PLB-XCGD cells, a human myeloid cell line devoid of NADPH oxidase activity, does not result in H_2O_2 generation (221). These findings indicate that additional components are required to achieve membrane targeting and full enzymatic activity of THOX (221).

Mechanism of Hydrogen Peroxide Generation

The biochemical mechanisms resulting in H_2O_2 generation are controversial (2). The H_2O_2-generating system in-

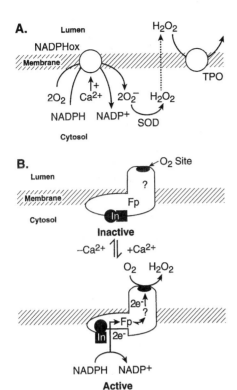

FIGURE 4B.7. Proposed mechanisms of hydrogen peroxide (H_2O_2) formation in thyrocytes. Two substantially different mechanisms are shown. **A:** NADPH oxidase in the apical membrane interacts with NADPH, Ca^{2+}, and O_2 to generate superoxide anions (O_2^-) on the cytosolic side of the membrane. Through the action of superoxide dismutase (*SOD*), the O_2^- is converted to H_2O_2, which traverses the apical membrane to react with TPO. (From Nakamura Y, Makino R, Tanaka T, Ishimura Y, Ohtaki S. 1991 Mechanism of H_2O_2 production in porcine thyroid cells: evidence for intermediary formation of superoxide anion by NADPH-dependent H_2O_2-generating machinery. *Biochemistry* 1991;30:4880, with permission.) **B:** NADPH oxidase in the apical membrane is a complex flavoprotein, which is activated by Ca^{2+}. Activation occurs when Ca^{2+} binds to an inhibitory protein or to an autoinhibitory domain. The activated flavoprotein transfers electrons from NADPH to O_2 in some as yet undisclosed manner to form H_2O_2 directly on the luminal side of the apical membrane. (From Dème D, Doussiere J, De Sandro V, et al. The Ca^{2+}/NADPH-dependent H_2O_2 generator in thyroid plasma membrane: inhibition by diphenyleneiodonium. *Biochem J* 1994;301:75, with permission.)

volves a Ca^{2+}-dependent NADPH oxidase—most likely THOX2—but it is unclear whether H_2O_2 is formed directly or through a process that includes the formation of O_2^- as an intermediate step. In one proposed model, O_2 is first oxidized to O_2^- and then converted to H_2O_2 by a superoxide dismutase (Fig. 4B.7) (206,229,230). In this model, both steps are thought to occur on the cytosolic side of the membrane, and the H_2O_2 then traverses to the luminal side of the membrane, where it reacts with TPO. In a second model, O_2 is directly converted to H_2O_2 by a complex Ca^{2+}-dependent NADPH oxidase system containing a flavoprotein (Fig. 4B.7) (209,231–234). The secondary structure of the THOX proteins is consistent

with the functional domains predicted by this model (214, 215). Further functional characterization of the THOX proteins, together with the isolation of additional components of this enzyme system, will provide a more thorough understanding of the mechanisms underlying H_2O_2 generation.

Regulation of Hydrogen Peroxide Activity

The generation of H_2O_2 is Ca^{2+}-dependent, and it is rapidly activated by agents stimulating the phosphatidyl-inositol pathway (204,212,226,235,236). In addition, TSH stimulates the production of H_2O_2 through the cyclic AMP pathway. Chronic TSH stimulation was initially reported to decrease H_2O_2 generation in porcine and FRTL-5 cells (236), but in more recent studies performed in canine and porcine cells, TSH and other stimulators of the cyclic AMP pathway clearly increased H_2O_2 generation (Fig. 4B.8) (213,233). This effect requires protein synthesis, since co-incubation with cycloheximide partially inhibits the TSH-mediated stimulation (233). In particulate fractions obtained from human and porcine thyroid tissue, the Ca^{2+}- and NADPH-dependent H_2O_2-generating activity is inducible by TSH and down-regulated by transforming growth factor-β (208). These tissues also have a small amount of Ca^{2+}-independent, NADH-dependent H_2O_2-generating activity that is not stimulated by TSH or forskolin, but whether this weak constitutive activity is exerted by THOX1 or another unidentified enzyme is not known (208).

H_2O_2 generation is inhibited by high concentrations of iodide (220,226), and iodohexadecanal, an intermediary that may be involved in autoregulatory processes in the thyroid (237,238). In contrast, low concentrations of iodide mildly stimulate H_2O_2 generation in thyroid tissue from several species (239). This effect is more pronounced in thyroid tissue previously deprived of iodide. The concentration-dependent control of H_2O_2 generation by iodide permits efficient hormone synthesis when iodide is scarce, while avoiding excessive hormone synthesis when iodide is abundant (239).

Defects in Hydrogen Peroxide Generation

Confirmation for the physiological role of THOX2 in H_2O_2 generation comes from patients with congenital hypothyroidism who have *THOX2* gene mutations (see Chapter 48) (240). One patient with severe permanent hypothyroidism and a total iodide organification defect had a homozygous nonsense mutation in the *THOX2* gene. Three other patients had transient congenital hypothyroidism and a partial iodide organification defect; they had monoallelic nonsense mutations in the *THOX2*

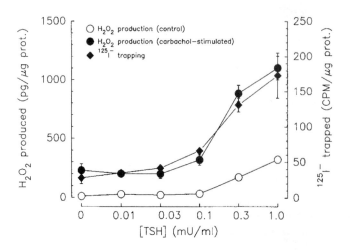

FIGURE 4B.8. Hydrogen peroxide generation and basal (^{125}I)-iodide uptake in canine thyrocytes cultured for 5 days in medium containing varying concentrations of thyrotropin (TSH). The Ca^{2+}-phosphatidylinositol cascade was stimulated with carbachol. (From Raspé E, Dumont JE. Tonic modulation of dog thyrocyte H_2O_2 generation and I⁻ uptake by thyrotropin through the cyclic adenosine 3',5'-monophosphate cascade. *Endocrinology* 1995;136:965.)

gene. All four mutations resulted in severe truncations of THOX2, eliminating the putative H_2O_2-generating domain. No mutations were found in the *THOX1* gene. The finding of biallelic mutations in the patient with a total iodide organification defect provides strong evidence that THOX2 is essential for normal H_2O_2 and thyroid hormone synthesis. The fact that THOX1 is unable to compensate for the deficiency in THOX2 suggests that the enzymes have different functional roles. The milder, transient hypothyroidism in the patients with monoallelic THOX2 mutations indicates that two functioning alleles are needed to meet the large requirements for thyroid hormone synthesis early in life (240). Whether these patients are at risk for subclinical or overt hypothyroidism during other periods when thyroid secretion increases, for example during pregnancy, is unknown.

Deficient H_2O_2 generation has been proposed as the explanation for euthyroid goiter and decreased iodide organification in a few sporadic patients, because *in vitro* addition of an H_2O_2-generating system to thyroid homogenates or slices from these patients restored normal organification (241,242). In two siblings with hypothyroidism, goiter, and decreased iodide organification, very low NADPH oxidase activity was detected in thyroid tissue, suggesting impaired H_2O_2 generation, but the molecular defect is not known (243).

IODINATION AND THYROID HORMONE SYNTHESIS

The synthesis of thyroid hormone occurs at the apical membrane. Iodide is oxidized by TPO in the presence of H_2O_2 (Fig. 4B.1). The iodination of selected tyrosyl residues of thyroglobulin, a reaction referred to as organification, then leads to the formation of the monoiodotyrosine (MIT) and diiodotyrosine (DIT). Lastly, two iodotyrosyls

couple to form the thyronines T_4 and T_3. Iodination and coupling are both catalyzed by TPO, and, although presented as sequential steps, they occur simultaneously.

Oxidation of Thyroid Peroxidase to Compound I and Compound II

The heme in native peroxidases is in the ferric form (FeIII) (Fig. 4B.9). The reaction product of TPO or other peroxidases with H_2O_2, a two-electron reaction resulting in the reduction of H_2O_2 to H_2O and oxidation of the enzyme, is referred to as compound I (TPO-O) (244). One electron is removed from the iron, giving rise to an oxyferryl (FeIV=O) intermediate, and the second electron is removed from the porphyrin ring, a state referred to as π-cation radical. A second, unstable form of compound I, which probably does not occur in the thyroid, is a protein radical in which the second electron is withdrawn from an aromatic amino acid of the apoprotein (245). The one-electron reduction of compound I generates compound II, and a further one-electron reduction brings the enzyme back to its native state (Fig. 4B.9).

Oxidation of Iodide

In order to become an iodinating agent, iodide must be oxidized. The nature of the iodinating species has not been determined with certainty; several models have been proposed (2). An early model was based on a one-electron oxidation that generated radicals of iodine and tyrosine bound to TPO, which then formed MIT, and in a subsequent reaction DIT (246,247). It is more likely that iodide is oxidized in a two-electron reaction to form either hypoiodite (OI⁻) (248–250), hypoiodous acid (HOI) (251,252), or iodinium (I⁺) (253–256).

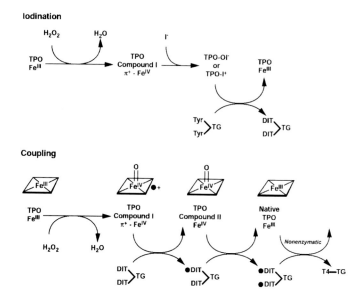

FIGURE 4B.9. Oxidation of iodide, organification, and coupling. The heme in native peroxidases is in the ferric form (Fe^{III}). The reaction product of thyroid peroxidase (TPO) with hydrogen peroxide (H_2O_2), a two-electron reaction that results in the reduction of H_2O_2 to H_2O and oxidation of the enzyme, is referred to as compound I (TPO-O). One electron is removed from the iron, giving rise to an oxyferryl ($FeIV=O$) intermediate; the second electron is removed from the porphyrin ring, a state referred to as π-cation radical. Although the nature of the iodinating species (OI^-, HOI, or I^+) has not been determined with certainty, iodide is then oxidized in a two-electron reaction, and selected tyrosyls are iodinated. In the coupling reaction, successive one-electron oxidations of hormonogenic tyrosyl residues in thyroglobulin (TG), mediated by compound I and compound II of TPO, are proposed to result in the formation of diiodotyrosine radicals, before two iodotyrosyls are coupled in a nonenzymatic reaction to form thyroxine (or triiodothyronine). DIT, diiodotyrosine; Tyr, tyrosine.

Iodination and Coupling of Tyrosyl Residues

In the iodination reaction, only a subset of the 132 tyrosyl residues of the thyroglobulin dimer are iodinated, giving rise to MIT and DIT (118,257–259). During the coupling reaction, a tyrosyl residue donates its iodinated phenyl group to become the outer ring of the iodothyronine amino acid at an acceptor site, leaving dehydroalanine at the donor site (245,260). The location of the hormonogenic iodotyrosyl residues within thyroglobulin creates an optimal spatial alignment, facilitating the coupling reaction, and is highly conserved among various species (see Chapter 5) (4,118,258,259,261). The main hormonogenic acceptor sites in human thyroglobulin are at positions 5, 1291, 2554, 2568, and 2747 (4,118,258,259). Donor sites include tyrosine residues 130, 847, and 1448. The most important T_4-forming site is located at tyrosine 5, and tyrosine 130 is the dominant donor site (262).

Iodination and the intramolecular coupling reaction have been studied *in vitro* using reconstituted systems containing TPO, thyroglobulin, radiolabeled iodide, and an H_2O_2-generating glucose/glucose-oxidase system (Fig. 4B.10) (2,245,247,256). Peroxidase-catalyzed iodination of selected tyrosine residues within thyroglobulin probably occurs on the enzyme (2,248–250,252,263). As in thyroglobulin from normal thyroid glands, MIT and DIT are the most abundant iodinated residues in these *in vitro* systems (264). Evidence for the catalytic role of TPO in the coupling reaction was obtained by incubating thyroglobulin labeled with iodine-131 with or without TPO (265). In the presence of TPO, the formation of T_4 and T_3 is significantly increased at the expense of a decrease in DIT and to a lesser extent in MIT (265). Analogous to rats fed an iodide-deficient diet (266), T_3 forma-

tion is more pronounced at lower iodide concentrations (265). The coupling reaction is stimulated by low concentrations of free DIT (265,267), a phenomenon thought to be caused by oxidation of free DIT, which then facilitates electron transfer from peptide-linked DIT to the prosthetic heme group (268,269). Formation of T_4 decreases with increasing iodide concentrations, which may play a role in the autoregulatory effect of iodide on thyroid function (245).

While iodination may be catalyzed by the π-cation radical of compound I and coupling by the protein radical (270), it is more likely that both reactions are catalyzed by the π-cation radical form of compound I, at least under conditions of normal iodide intake (245). As summarized in Figure 4B.9, successive one-electron oxidations of hormonogenic tyrosyl residues in thyroglobulin, mediated by compound I and compound II of TPO, are proposed to result in the formation of DIT radicals (245,269,271). Lastly, in a nonenzymatic reaction, two iodotyrosyls, positioned in optimal spatial location, form an unstable quinol ether bond, which is rapidly rearranged to form an iodothyronine, leaving dehydroalanine at the position of the donor iodotyrosyl contributing the outer ring (Fig. 4B.11). In the formation of T_4, the outer ring comes from a DIT residue, whereas in the formation of T_3 it comes from MIT.

Inhibition of Thyroid Peroxidase by Thionamide Drugs

The mechanisms underlying the inhibitory effects of thionamides on TPO-catalyzed iodination has been comprehensively reviewed by Taurog (2), and their role in the treatment of patients with thyrotoxicosis, which is discussed in Chapter 45, have been reviewed by Cooper (272).

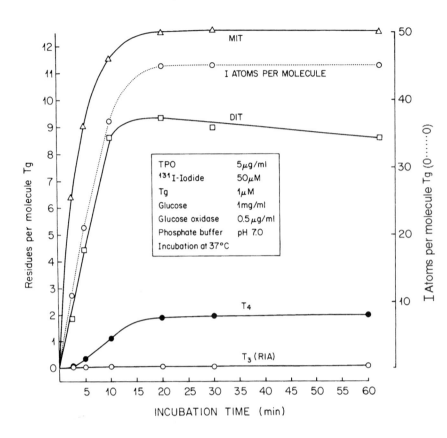

FIGURE 4B.10. Time course of iodination and of formation of diiodotyrosine, mono-iodotyrosine, thyroxine (T_4), and triiodothyronine (T_3) in thyroglobulin iodinated under the conditions indicated. The thyroglobulin contained 0.038% iodine (two atoms iodine per molecule). The value for A_{410}/A_{280} for thyroid peroxidase was 0.38. The reaction was started by addition of glucose oxidase (100 U/mg). (From Taurog A. Hormone synthesis: thyroid iodine metabolism. In: Braverman L, Utiger R, eds. *Werner and Ingbar's The thyroid: a fundamental and clinical text*, 8th ed. Philadelphia: Lippincott, Williams & Wilkins, 2000:61, with permission.)

The thionamides PTU, MMI, and carbimazole (CBZ), which is converted to MMI *in vivo* (273), are concentrated severalfold in the thyroid gland (274–277). The uptake of these drugs is stimulated by TSH and inhibited by iodide (2,278). Thionamides inhibit iodination and coupling (275,279,280). *In vitro*, low doses of MMI and PTU inhibit TPO-catalyzed iodination of thyroglobulin transiently and reversibly, whereas the effect of higher doses is irreversible (Fig. 4B.12) (279,280). The inhibitory effect of thionamides is also dependent on the ratio between drug and iodide concentration. While it is irreversible at lower iodide concentrations, it is only transient at high iodide concentrations (280). Under conditions of reversible inhibition, thionamides are rapidly metabolized to higher oxidation products (281–283). Iodination resumes once metabolism of the drug is complete. Under these conditions, thionamides are competitive inhibitors by competing with tyrosyls for oxidized iodide; oxidation of the drug is the favored reaction. Conversely, thionamides are only partially oxidized at high drug/iodide ratios (284). In this situation, TPO is inactivated, presumably by covalent binding of an oxidized form of the drug to the prosthetic heme group of the enzyme, and as a result iodination is irreversibly blocked (284). Data obtained from rats fed an iodide-deficient diet are consistent with this *in vitro* model, in that intrathyroidal me-tabolism of radiolabeled PTU and MMI is decreased (275).

Thionamides have a more pronounced effect on iodothyronine formation than on iodotyrosine formation (285). This does not necessarily imply a specific inhibitory effect on coupling, since the formation of T_4 requires preceding DIT formation. However, under selected *in vitro* conditions, such as low concentrations of iodide, TPO or H_2O_2, PTU and MMI may have an inhibitory effect on coupling without inhibiting iodination (285).

CELLULAR UPTAKE AND PROTEOLYSIS OF THYROGLOBULIN

Iodinated thyroglobulin is stored as colloid in the follicular lumen. In response to demand for thyroid hormone secretion, further processing of thyroglobulin requires its reentry into thyroid cells through vesicular internalization, i.e., micropinocytosis (Fig. 4B.1) (Chapter 5). Micropinocytosis may be initiated by both nonselective fluid-phase uptake and by receptor-mediated endocytosis (286–289). Fusion of the thyroglobulin-containing vesicles with lysosomes results in proteolytic breakdown of the thyroglobulin and release of T_4, T_3, and the iodotyrosines (4).

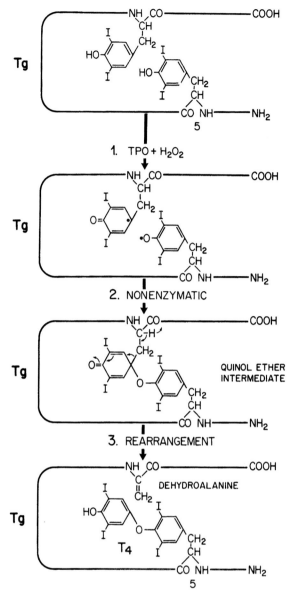

FIGURE 4B.11. Proposed scheme for coupling of diiodotyrosyl residues to form thyroxine within a thyroglobulin (Tg) molecule. The major hormonogenic site at tyrosyl residue 5 is indicated. (From Taurog A. Hormone synthesis: thyroid iodine metabolism. In: Braverman L, Utiger R, eds. *Werner and Ingbar's The thyroid: a fundamental and clinical text,* 8th ed. Philadelphia: Lippincott, Williams & Wilkins, 2000:61, with permission.)

Digestion of thyroglobulin with lysosomal extracts results in the preferential release of hormone-rich fractions (290). Several endopeptidases have been identified in the thyroid. They include cathepsins D, B, L, and H (291). Inhibition of these enzymes blocks degradation of thyroglobulin, suggesting that they are important in thyroglobulin breakdown (292). After cleavage of thyroglobulin by endopeptidases, it undergoes further degradation by exopeptidases such as dipeptidyl-peptidases I and II, lysosomal

dipeptidase I, and *N*-acetyl-L-phenolalanyl-L-tyrosine hydrolase (292). Digestion of thyroglobulin *in vitro* with the endopeptidase cathepsin B and the exopeptidase lysosomal dipeptidase I results first in the release of the dipeptide T_4-glutamine, corresponding to the amino-terminal hormonogenic site 5 and glutamine at position 6, and subsequent release of T_4 (293). The cysteine-rich type I motif of thyroglobulin, which has been identified as a potent inhibitor of cysteine proteases (120), may play an autoregulatory role in the digestion of thyroglobulin (119).

Aside from degradation of thyroglobulin in lysosomes, it can also be recycled back into the follicular lumen (294). The recycling of immature forms of thyroglobulin back to the apical membrane after endocytosis is thought to involve an asialoglycoprotein receptor (295). Thyroglobulin can also be transported from the apical to the basolateral membrane, where it is released into the bloodstream (296, 297). This transepithelial transport or transcytosis is mediated by megalin, a receptor located on the apical membrane of the thyrocytes (288,289).

Ultimately, after degradation of thyroglobulin in the lysosomal pathway, T_4 and T_3 are secreted into the bloodstream at the basolateral membrane. Specific thyroidal channels mediating the transport of thyroid hormone across the basolateral membrane have not been identified.

DEIODINATION OF MONOIODOTYROSINE AND DIIODOTYROSINE

Minimal amounts of iodotyrosines, MIT and DIT, are released into the circulation, even though they are more abundant than T_4 and T_3 in thyroglobulin. The majority of these iodotyrosines are deiodinated by an intrathyroidal dehalogenase, and the iodide is recycled for hormone synthesis. This dehalogenase is thought to be an NADPH-dependent flavoprotein (298). An mRNA sequence encoding a putative iodotyrosine dehalogenase protein (DEHAL1), isolated from a thyroid mRNA library, has been identified (Genbank AY259176, AY259177) (299); the protein has not yet been characterized.

Dehalogenase Deficiency

Patients with congenital hypothyroidism and goiter caused by a defective iodotyrosine dehalogenase system have been identified (see Chapter 48). In these patients, MIT and DIT are not deiodinated, but rather leak into the circulation and are excreted in the urine. This leads to substantial loss of iodide, and, if the iodine supply is scarce, to goiter and hypothyroidism (300). The diagnosis of a defective dehalogenase can be formally established by administration of radiolabeled DIT. It is normally deiodinated, but in patients with a defective dehalogenase, most is excreted unal-

REVERSIBLE INHIBITION   IRREVERSIBLE INHIBITION

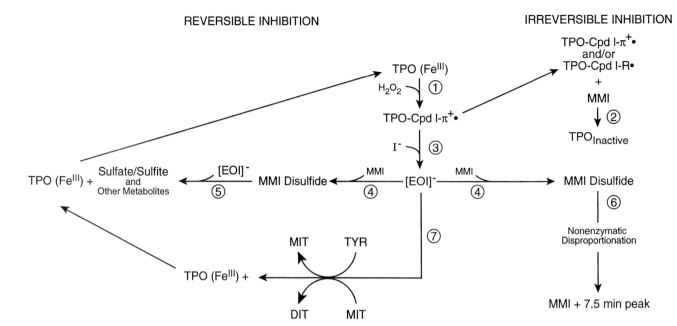

FIGURE 4B.12. Scheme for mechanism of inhibition of thyroid peroxidase (TPO)–catalyzed iodination by methimazole (MMI). The reactions associated with reversible inhibition of iodination are shown **on the left,** irreversible inhibition **on the right.** The relative rates of reactions 2 and 3 determine whether inhibition of iodination is reversible or irreversible. If reaction 2 is predominant, TPO will be inactivated and inhibition of iodination will be irreversible. The inactivation probably involves covalent binding of an oxidized form of MMI to the heme group of compound I *(CpdI).* If reaction 3 is predominant, this will lead to extensive drug oxidation, permitting iodination to begin after the drug has been metabolized. Reactions 4 and 7 indicate that oxidized iodide (EOI)⁻ acts both to oxidize MMI and to iodinate tyrosyl residues in thyroglobulin. Reversible inhibition depends on competition between MMI and tyrosyl for (EOI)⁻. Drug oxidation is the preferred reaction, and as long as sufficient drug is present, (EOI)⁻ is diverted from iodination to drug oxidation. (From Taurog A. Hormone synthesis: thyroid iodine metabolism. In: Braverman L, Utiger R, eds. *Werner and Ingbar's The thyroid: a fundamental and clinical text,* 8th ed. Philadelphia: Lippincott, Williams & Wilkins, 2000:61, with permission.)

tered in the urine. These patients can be treated with large doses of iodide, as well as with T_4. The disorder is inherited as an autosomal recessive trait.

ACKNOWLEDGMENT

Supported by 1R01DK63024–01 from NIH/NIDDK.

REFERENCES

1. Taurog A. Hormone synthesis: thyroid iodine metabolism. In: Braverman L, Utiger R, eds. *Werner and Ingbar's the thyroid: a fundamental and clinical text*, 7th ed. Philadelphia: Lippincott-Raven, 1996:47.
2. Taurog A. Hormone synthesis: thyroid iodine metabolism. In: Braverman L, Utiger R, eds. *Werner and Ingbar's the thyroid: a fundamental and clinical text*, 8th ed. Philadelphia: Lippincott, Williams & Wilkins, 2000:61.
3. Gentile F, Di Lauro R, Salvatore G. Biosynthesis and secretion of thyroid hormones. In: De Groot L, ed. *Endocrinology*. Philadelphia: WB Saunders, 1995:517.
4. Dunn J. Biosynthesis and secretion of thyroid hormones. In: DeGroot L, Jameson J, eds. *Endocrinology*. Philadelphia: WB Saunders, 2001:1290.
5. Wolff J. Transport of iodide and other anions in the thyroid gland. *Physiol Rev* 1964;44:45.
6. Saito K, Yamamoto K, Takai T, et al. The sodium-dependent iodide transport by phospholipid vesicles reconstituted with the thyroid plasma membrane. *J Biochem (Tokyo)* 1982;92:2001.
7. Weiss SJ, Philp NJ, Grollman EF. Iodide transport in a continuous line of cultured cells from rat thyroid. *Endocrinology* 1984;114:1090.
8. De La Vieja A, Dohan O, Levy O, et al. Molecular analysis of the sodium/iodide symporter: impact on thyroid and extrathyroid pathophysiology. *Physiol Rev* 2000;80:1083.
9. Dohán O, De la Vieja A, Paroder V, et al. The sodium/iodide symporter (NIS): characterization, regulation, and medical significance. *Endocr Rev* 2003;24:48.
10. Dai G, Levy O, Carrasco N. Cloning and characterization of the thyroid iodide transporter. *Nature* 1996;379:458.
11. Baumann E. Aüber den Jodgehalt der SchilddrÜsen von Menschen und Tieren. *Hoppe Seylers Z Physiol Chem* 1896;22:1.

12. Smanik PA, Liu Q, Furminger TL, et al. Cloning of the human sodium iodide symporter. *Biochem Biophys Res Commun* 1996; 226:339.

13. Smanik PA, Ryu KY, Theil KS, et al. Expression, exon-intron organization, and chromosome mapping of the human sodium iodide symporter. *Endocrinology* 1997;138:3555.

14. Levy O, Dai G, Riedel C, et al. Characterization of the thyroid Na$^+$/I$^-$ symporter with an anti-COOH terminus antibody. *Proc Natl Acad Sci U S A* 1997;94:5568.

15. Levy O, De la Vieja A, Ginter CS, et al. N-linked glycosylation of the thyroid Na$^+$/I$^-$ symporter (NIS): implications for its secondary structure model. *J Biol Chem* 1998;273:22657.

16. Eskandari S, Loo DD, Dai G, et al. Thyroid Na$^+$/I$^-$ symporter: mechanism, stoichiometry, and specificity. *J Biol Chem* 1997; 272:27230.

17. Barker HM. The blood cyanates in the treatment of hypertension. *JAMA* 1936;106:762.

18. Hilditch TE, Horton PW, McCruden DC, et al. Defects in intrathyroid binding of iodine and the perchlorate discharge test. *Acta Endocrinol (Copenh)* 1982;100:237.

19. Yoshida A, Sasaki N, Mori A, et al. Different electrophysiological character of I$^-$, ClO$_4^-$, and SCN$^-$ in the transport by Na$^+$/I$^-$ symporter. *Biochem Biophys Res Commun* 1997;231:731.

20. Yoshida A, Sasaki N, Mori A, et al. Differences in the electrophysiological response to I- and the inhibitory anions SCN- and ClO-4, studied in FRTL-5 cells. *Biochim Biophys Acta* 1998;1414:231.

21. Van Sande J, Massart C, Beauwens R, et al. Anion selectivity by the sodium iodide symporter. *Endocrinology* 2003;144:247.

22. Weiss SJ, Philp NJ, Ambesi-Impiombato FS, et al. Thyrotropin-stimulated iodide transport mediated by adenosine 3′,5′-monophosphate and dependent on protein synthesis. *Endocrinology* 1984;114:1099.

23. Vassart G, Dumont JE. The thyrotropin receptor and the regulation of thyrocyte function and growth. *Endocr Rev* 1992;13:596.

24. Kogai T, Endo T, Saito T, et al. Regulation by thyroid-stimulating hormone of sodium/iodide symporter gene expression and protein levels in FRTL-5 cells. *Endocrinology* 1997;138:2227.

25. Saito T, Endo T, Kawaguchi A, et al. Increased expression of the Na$^+$/I$^-$ symporter in cultured human thyroid cells exposed to thyrotropin and in Graves' thyroid tissue. *J Clin Endocrinol Metab* 1997;82:3331.

26. Kogai T, Curcio F, Hyman S, et al. Induction of follicle formation in long-term cultured normal human thyroid cells treated with thyrotropin stimulates iodide uptake but not sodium/iodide symporter messenger RNA and protein expression. *J Endocrinol* 2000;167:125.

27. Jhiang SM, Cho JY, Ryu KY, et al. An immunohistochemical study of Na+/I- symporter in human thyroid tissues and salivary gland tissues. *Endocrinology* 1998;139:4416.

28. Damante G, Di Lauro R. Thyroid-specific gene expression. *Biochim Biophys Acta* 1994;1218:255.

29. Kambe F, Seo H. Thyroid-specific transcription factors. *Endocr J* 1997;44:775.

30. Riedel C, Levy O, Carrasco N. Post-transcriptional regulation of the sodium/iodide symporter by thyrotropin. *J Biol Chem* 2001;276:21458.

31. Wolff J, Chaikoff I. Plasma inorganic iodide as homeostatic regulator of thyroid function. *J Biol Chem* 1948;174:555.

32. Wolff J, Chaikoff I, Goldberg R, et al. The temporary nature of the inhibitory action of excess iodide on organic iodide synthesis in the normal thyroid. *Endocrinology* 1949;45:504.

33. Grollman EF, Smolar A, Ommaya A, et al. Iodine suppression of iodide uptake in FRTL-5 thyroid cells. *Endocrinology* 1986; 118:2477.

34. Uyttersprot N, Pelgrims N, Carrasco N, et al. Moderate doses of iodide in vivo inhibit cell proliferation and the expression of thyroperoxidase and Na$^+$/I$^-$ symporter mRNAs in dog thyroid. *Mol Cell Endocrinol* 1997;131:195.

35. Braverman LE, Ingbar SH. Changes in thyroidal function during adaptation to large doses of iodide. *J Clin Invest* 1963;42:1216.

36. Spitzweg C, Joba W, Morris JC, et al. Regulation of sodium iodide symporter gene expression in FRTL-5 rat thyroid cells. *Thyroid* 1999;9:821.

37. Eng PH, Cardona GR, Fang SL, et al. Escape from the acute Wolff-Chaikoff effect is associated with a decrease in thyroid sodium/iodide symporter messenger ribonucleic acid and protein. *Endocrinology* 1999;140:3404.

38. Eng PH, Cardona GR, Previti MC, et al. Regulation of the sodium iodide symporter by iodide in FRTL-5 cells. *Eur J Endocrinol* 2001;144:139.

39. Carrasco N Surprising new mechanistic insights into the escape from the Wolff-Chaikoff effect: the downregulaton of NIS-mediated I- transport by I- is thyroid-specific but TSH-independent, correlates with NIS dimerization, and is absent in thyroid and mammary cancer cells. Sixth International Workshop on Resistance to Thyroid Hormone, Miami Beach, FL, 2003.

40. Suzuki K, Lavaroni S, Mori A, et al. Autoregulation of thyroid-specific gene transcription by thyroglobulin. *Proc Natl Acad Sci U S A* 1998;95:8251.

41. Suzuki K, Mori A, Saito J, et al. Follicular thyroglobulin suppresses iodide uptake by suppressing expression of the sodium/iodide symporter gene. *Endocrinology* 1999;140:5422.

42. Jhiang SM. Regulation of sodium/iodide symporter. *Rev Endocr Metab Disord* 2000;1:205.

43. Gillam MP, Kopp P. Genetic regulation of thyroid development. *Curr Opin Pediatr* 2001;13:358.

44. Kopp P. Perspective: genetic defects in the etiology of congenital hypothyroidism. *Endocrinology* 2002;143:2019.

45. Van Vliet G. Development of the thyroid gland: lessons from congenitally hypothyroid mice and men. *Clin Genet* 2003;63:445.

46. Wolff J. Congenital goiter with defective iodide transport. *Endocr Rev* 1983;4:240.

47. Fujiwara H, Tatsumi K, Miki K, et al. Congenital hypothyroidism caused by a mutation in the Na$^+$/I$^-$ symporter. *Nat Genet* 1997;16:124.

48. Levy O, Ginter CS, De la Vieja A, et al. Identification of a structural requirement for thyroid Na$^+$/I$^-$ symporter (NIS) function from analysis of a mutation that causes human congenital hypothyroidism. *FEBS Lett* 1998;429:36.

49. Pohlenz J, Duprez L, Weiss RE, et al. Failure of membrane targeting causes the functional defect of two mutant sodium iodide symporters. *J Clin Endocrinol Metab* 2000;85:2366.

50. Weiss SJ, Philp NJ, Grollman EF. Effect of thyrotropin on iodide efflux in FRTL-5 cells mediated by Ca^{2+}. *Endocrinology* 1984;114:1108.

51. Nilsson M, Bjorkman U, Ekholm R, et al. Iodide transport in primary cultured thyroid follicle cells: evidence of a TSH-regulated channel mediating iodide efflux selectively across the apical domain of the plasma membrane. *Eur J Cell Biol* 1990;52:270.

52. Nilsson M, Bjorkman U, Ekholm R, et al. Polarized efflux of iodide in porcine thyrocytes occurs via a cAMP-regulated iodide channel in the apical plasma membrane. *Acta Endocrinol (Copenh)* 1992;126:67.

53. Golstein P, Abramow M, Dumont JE, et al. The iodide channel of the thyroid: a plasma membrane vesicle study. *Am J Physiol* 1992;263:C590.

54. Everett LA, Glaser B, Beck JC, et al. Pendred syndrome is caused by mutations in a putative sulphate transporter gene (PDS). *Nature Genet* 1997;17:411.

55. Scott DA, Wang R, Kreman TM, et al. The Pendred syndrome gene encodes a chloride-iodide transport protein. *Nature Genet* 1999;21:440.

56. Taylor JP, Metcalfe RA, Watson PF, et al. Mutations of the *PDS* gene, encoding pendrin, are associated with protein mislocalization and loss of iodide efflux: implications for thyroid dysfunction in Pendred syndrome. *J Clin Endocrinol Metabol* 2002;87:1778.

57. Yoshida A, Taniguchi S, Hisatome I, et al. Pendrin is an iodide-specific apical porter responsible for iodide efflux from thyroid cells. *J Clin Endocrinol Metabol* 2002;87:3356.

58. Gillam MP, Sidhaye A, Lee EJ, et al. Functional characterization of pendrin in a polarized cell system: evidence for pendrin-mediated apical iodide efflux. *J Biol Chem* 2004;279:13004.

59. Rodriguez AM, Perron B, Lacroix L, et al. Identification and characterization of a putative human iodide transporter located at the apical membrane of thyrocytes. *J Clin Endocrinol Metab* 2002;87:3500.

60. Fraser GR, Morgans ME, Trotter WR. The syndrome of sporadic goitre and congenital deafness. *Q JM* 1960;29:279.

61. Medeiros-Neto G, Stanbury JB. Pendred's syndrome: association of congenital deafness with sporadic goiter. In: Medeiros-Neto G, Stanbury JB, eds. *Inherited disorders of the thyroid system.* Boca Raton, FL: CRC Press, 1994:81.

62. Kopp P. Pendred's syndrome and genetic defects in thyroid hormone synthesis. *Rev Endocr Metabol Dis* 2000;1/2:109.

63. Sheffield VC, Kraiem Z, Beck JC, et al. Pendred syndrome maps to chromosome 7q21–34 and is caused by an intrinsic defect in thyroid iodine organification. *Nature Genet* 1996;12:424.

64. Coyle B, Coffrey R, Armour JAL, et al. Pendred syndrome (goitre and sensorineural hearing loss) maps to chromosome 7 in the region containing the nonsyndromic deafness gene DFNB4. *Nature Genet* 1996;12:421.

65. Everett LA, Green ED. A family of mammalian anion transporters and their involvement in human genetic diseases. *Hum Mol Genet* 1999;8:1883.

66. Zheng J, Shen W, He DZ, et al. Prestin is the motor protein of cochlear outer hair cells. *Nature* 2000;405:149.

67. Liu XZ, Ouyang XM, Xia XJ, et al. Prestin, a cochlear motor protein, is defective in non-syndromic hearing loss. *Hum Mol Genet* 2003;12:1155.

68. Royaux IE, Suzuki K, Mori A, et al. Pendrin, the protein encoded by the Pendred syndrome gene (PDS), is an apical porter of iodide in the thyroid and is regulated by thyroglobulin in FRTL-5 cells. *Endocrinology* 2000;141:839.

69. Porra V, Bernier-Valentin F, Trouttet-Masson S, et al. Characterization and semiquantitative analyses of pendrin expressed in normal and tumoral human thyroid tissues. *J Clin Endocrinol Metab* 2002;87:1700.

70. Everett LA, Morsli H, Wu DK, et al. Expression pattern of the mouse ortholog of the Pendred's syndrome gene (Pds) suggests a key role for pendrin in the inner ear. *Proc Natl Acad Sci U S A* 1999;96:9727.

71. Royaux IE, Belyantseva IA, Wu T, et al. Localization and functional studies of pendrin in the mouse inner ear provide insight about the etiology of deafness in Pendred syndrome. *J Assoc Res Otolaryngol* 2003;4:394.

72. Soleimani M, Greeley T, Petrovic S, et al. Pendrin: an apical Cl⁻/OH⁻/HCO₃⁻ exchanger in the kidney cortex. *Am J Physiol Renal Physiol* 2001;280:F356.

73. Royaux IE, Wall SM, Karniski LP, et al. Pendrin, encoded by the Pendred syndrome gene, resides in the apical region of renal intercalated cells and mediates bicarbonate secretion. *Proc Natl Acad Sci U S A* 2001;98:4221.

74. Wall SM, Hassell KA, Royaux IE, et al. Localization of pendrin in mouse kidney. *Am J Physiol Renal Physiol* 2003;284:F229.

75. Bidart JM, Lacroix L, Evain-Brion D, et al. Expression of Na⁺/I⁻ symporter and Pendred syndrome genes in trophoblast cells. *J Clin Endocrinol Metab* 2000;85:4367.

76. Suzuki K, Royaux IE, Everett LA, et al. Expression of PDS/Pds, the Pendred syndrome gene, in endometrium. *J Clin Endocrinol Metab* 2002 87:938.

77. Rillema JA, Hill MA. Prolactin regulation of the pendrin-iodide transporter in the mammary gland. *Am J Physiol Endocrinol Metab* 2003;284:E25.

78. Lacroix L, Mian C, Caillou B, et al. Na⁺/I⁻ symporter and Pendred syndrome gene and protein expressions in human extra-thyroidal tissues. *Eur J Endocrinol* 2001;144:297.

79. Bidart JM, Mian C, Lazar V, et al. Expression of pendrin and the Pendred syndrome (PDS) gene in human thyroid tissues. *J Clin Endocrinol Metab* 2000;85:2028.

80. Mian C, Lacroix L, Alzieu L, et al. Sodium iodide symporter and pendrin expression in human thyroid tissues. *Thyroid* 2001;11:825.

81. Russo D, Bulotta S, Bruno R, et al. Sodium/iodide symporter (NIS) and pendrin are expressed differently in hot and cold nodules of thyroid toxic multinodular goiter. *Eur J Endocrinol* 2001;145:591.

82. Kondo T, Nakamura N, Suzuki K, et al. Expression of human pendrin in diseased thyroids. *J Histochem Cytochem* 2003;51:167.

83. Arturi F, Russo D, Bidart JM, et al. Expression pattern of the pendrin and sodium/iodide symporter genes in human thyroid carcinoma cell lines and human thyroid tumors. *Eur J Endocrinol* 2001;145:129.

84. Gerard AC, Daumerie C, Mestdagh C, et al. Correlation between the loss of thyroglobulin iodination and the expression of thyroid-specific proteins involved in iodine metabolism in thyroid carcinomas. *J Clin Endocrinol Metab* 2003;88:4977.

85. Xing M, Tokumaru Y, Wu G, et al. Hypermethylation of the Pendred syndrome gene SLC26A4 is an early event in thyroid tumorigenesis. *Cancer Res* 2003;63:2312.

86. Kraiem Z, Heinrich R, Sadeh O, et al. Sulfate transport is not impaired in Pendred syndrome thyrocytes. *J Clin Endocrinol Metabol* 1999;84:2574.

87. Scott DA, Wang R, Kreman TM, et al. Functional differences of the PDS gene product are associated with phenotypic variation in patients with Pendred syndrome and non-syndromic hearing loss (DFNB4). *Hum Mol Genet* 2000;9:1709.

88. Scott DA, Karniski LP. Human pendrin expressed in *Xenopus laevis* oocytes mediates chloride/formate exchange. *Am J Cell Physiol* 2000;278:C207.

89. Petrovic S, Wang Z, Ma L, et al. Regulation of the apical Cl⁻/HCO₃⁻ exchanger pendrin in rat cortical collecting duct in metabolic acidosis. *Am J Physiol Renal Physiol* 2003;284:F103.

90. Wagner CA, Finberg KE, Stehberger PA, et al. Regulation of the expression of the Cl⁻/anion exchanger pendrin in mouse kidney by acid-base status. *Kidney Int* 2002;62:2109.

91. Reardon W, OMahoney CF, Trembath R, et al. Enlarged vestibular aqueduct: a radiological marker of pendred syndrome, and mutation of the PDS gene. *Q JM* 2000;93:99.

92. Everett LA, Belyantseva IA, Noben-Trauth K, et al. Targeted disruption of mouse Pds provides insight about the inner-ear defects encountered in Pendred syndrome. *Hum Mol Genet* 2001;10:153.

93. Pendred V. Deaf-mutism and goitre. *Lancet* 1896;ii:532.

94. Fraser GR. Association of congenital deafness with goitre (Pendred's syndrome). *Ann Hum Genet* 1965;28:201.

95. Nilsson LR, Borgfors N, Gamstorp I, et al. Non-endemic goitre and deafness. *Acta Paed* 1964;53:117.

96. Morgans ME, Trotter WR. Association of congenital deafness with goitre: the nature of the thyroid defect. *Lancet* 1958;1: 607.

97. Gausden E, Coyle B, Armour JA, et al. Pendred syndrome: evidence for genetic homogeneity and further refinement of linkage. *J Med Genet* 1997;34:126.

98. Sato E, Nakashima T, Miura Y, et al. Phenotypes associated with replacement of His by Arg in the Pendred syndrome gene. *Eur J Endocrinol* 2001;145:697.

99. Coyle B, Reardon W, Herbrick JA, et al. Molecular analysis of the PDS gene in Pendred syndrome (sensorineural hearing loss and goitre). *Hum Mol Genet* 1998;7:1105.

100. Van Hauwe P, Everett LA, Coucke P, et al. Two frequent missense mutations in Pendred syndrome. *Hum Mol Genet* 1998; 7:1099.

101. Fugazzola L, Mannavola D, Cerutti N, et al. Molecular analysis of the Pendred's syndrome gene and magnetic resonance imaging studies of the inner ear are essential for the diagnosis of true Pendred's syndrome. *J Clin Endocrinol Metab* 2000;85:2469.

102. Gonzalez Trevino O, Karamanoglu Arseven O, Ceballos C, et al. Clinical and molecular analysis of three Mexican families with Pendred's syndrome. *Europ J Endocrinol* 2001;144:1.

103. Park H-J, Shaukat S, Liu X-Z, et al. Origins and frequencies of *SLC26A4 (PDS)* mutations in east and south Asians: global implications for the epidemiology of deafness. *J Med Genet* 2003; 40:242.

104. Tsukamoto K, Suzuki H, Harada D, et al. Distribution and frequencies of PDS (SLC26A4) mutations in Pendred syndrome and nonsyndromic hearing loss associated with enlarged vestibular aqueduct: a unique spectrum of mutations in Japanese. *Eur J Hum Genet* 2003;24:24.

105. Rotman-Pikielny P, Hirschberg K, Maruvada P, et al. Retention of pendrin in the endoplasmic reticulum is a major mechanism for Pendred syndrome. *Hum Mol Genet* 2002;11: 2625.

106. Li XC, Everett LA, Lalwani AK, et al. A mutation in PDS causes non-syndromic deafness. *Nature Genet* 1998;18:215.

107. Usami S, Abe S, Weston MD, et al. Non-syndromic hearing loss associated with enlarged vestibular aqueduct is caused by *PDS* mutations. *Hum Genet* 1999;104:188.

108. Mendive FM, Rivolta CM, Moya CM, et al. Genomic organization of the human thyroglobulin gene: the complete intron-exon structure. *Eur J Endocrinol* 2001;145:485.

109. Baas F, Bikker H, Geurts van Kessel A, et al. The human thyroglobulin gene: a polymorphic marker localized distal to C-MYC on chromosome 8 band q24. *Hum Genet* 1985;69:138.

110. Rabin M, Barker PE, Ruddle FH, et al. Proximity of thyroglobulin and c-myc genes on human chromosome 8. *Somat Cell Mol Genet* 1985;11:397.

111. Berge-Lefranc JL, Cartouzou G, Mattei MG, et al. Localization of the thyroglobulin gene by in situ hybridization to human chromosomes. *Hum Genet* 1985;69:28.

112. Mendive FM, Rivolta CM, Vassart G, et al. Genomic organization of the 3′ region of the human thyroglobulin gene. *Thyroid* 1999;9:903.

113. Moya CM, Mendive FM, Rivolta CM, et al. Genomic organization of the 5′ region of the human thyroglobulin gene. *Eur J Endocrinol* 2000;143:789.

114. Malthiery Y, Lissitzky S. Primary structure of human thyroglobulin deduced from the sequence of its 8448-base complementary DNA. *Eur J Biochem* 1987;165:491.

115. van de Graaf SA, Pauws E, de Vijlder JJ, et al. The revised 8307 base pair coding sequence of human thyroglobulin transiently expressed in eukaryotic cells. *Eur J Endocrinol* 1997;136: 508.

116. Kim PS, Arvan P. Hormonal regulation of thyroglobulin export from the endoplasmic reticulum of cultured thyrocytes. *J Biol Chem* 1993;268:4873.

117. Arvan P, Kim PS, Kuliawat R, et al. Intracellular protein transport to the thyrocyte plasma membrane: potential implications for thyroid physiology. *Thyroid* 1997;7:89.

118. Dunn JT, Dunn AD. Thyroglobulin: chemistry, biosynthesis, and proteolysis. In: Braverman LE, Utiger RD, eds. *Werner & Ingbar's The thyroid: a fundamental and clinical text,* 8th ed. Philadelphia: Lippincott Williams & Wilkins, 2000:91.

119. Molina F, Bouanani M, Pau B, et al. Characterization of the type-1 repeat from thyroglobulin, a cysteine-rich module found in proteins from different families. *Eur J Biochem* 1996;240: 125.

120. Yamashita M, Konagaya S. A novel cysteine protease inhibitor of the egg of chum salmon, containing a cysteine-rich thyroglobulin-like motif. *J Biol Chem* 1996;271:1282.

121. Mercken L, Simons MJ, De Martynoff G, et al. Presence of hormonogenic and repetitive domains in the first 930 amino acids of bovine thyroglobulin as deduced from the cDNA sequence. *Eur J Biochem* 1985;147:59.

122. Swillens S, Ludgate M, Mercken L, et al. Analysis of sequence and structure homologies between thyroglobulin and acetylcholinesterase: possible functional and clinical significance. *Biochem Biophys Res Commun* 1986;137:142.

123. Parma J, Christophe D, Pohl V, et al. Structural organization of the 5′ region of the thyroglobulin gene. Evidence for intron loss and "exonization" during evolution. *J Mol Biol* 1987;196:769.

124. Kim PS, Arvan P. Endocrinopathies in the family of endoplasmic reticulum (ER) storage diseases: disorders of protein trafficking and the role of ER molecular chaperones. *Endocr Rev* 1998;19:173.

125. Yang SX, Pollock HG, Rawitch AB. Glycosylation in human thyroglobulin: location of the N-linked oligosaccharide units and comparison with bovine thyroglobulin. *Arch Biochem Biophys* 1996;327:61.

126. Sakurai S, Fogelfeld L, Schneider AB. Anionic carbohydrate groups of human thyroglobulin containing both phosphate and sulfate. *Endocrinology* 1991;129:915.

127. Blode H, Heinrich T, Diringer H. A quantitative assay for tyrosine sulfation and tyrosine phosphorylation in peptides. *Biol Chem Hoppe Seyler* 1990;371:145.

128. Venot N, Nlend MC, Cauvi D, et al. The hormonogenic tyrosine 5 of porcine thyroglobulin is sulfated. *Biochem Biophys Res Commun* 2002;298:193.

129. Ricketts MH, Simons MJ, Parma J, et al. A nonsense mutation causes hereditary goitre in the Afrikander cattle and unmasks alternative splicing of thyroglobulin transcripts. *Proc Natl Acad Sci U S A* 1987;84:3181.

130. Ieiri T, Cochaux P, Targovnik HM, et al. A 3′ splice site mutation in the thyroglobulin gene responsible for congenital goiter with hypothyroidism. *J Clin Invest* 1991;88:1901.

131. van de Graaf SA, Ris-Stalpers C, Pauws E, et al. Up to date with human thyroglobulin. *J Endocrinol* 2001;170:307.

132. Medeiros-Neto G, Targovnik HM, Vassart G. Defective thyroglobulin synthesis and secretion causing goiter and hypothyroidism. *Endocr Rev* 1993;14:165.

133. Caron P, Moya CM, Malet D, et al. Compound heterozygous mutations in the thyroglobulin gene (1143delC and 6725G>A [R2223H]) resulting in fetal goitrous hypothyroidism. *J Clin Endocrinol Metab* 2003;88:3546.

134. Targovnik HM, Vono J, Billerbeck AE, et al. A 138-nucleotide deletion in the thyroglobulin ribonucleic acid messenger in a congenital goiter with defective thyroglobulin synthesis. *J Clin Endocrinol Metab* 1995;80:3356.

135. Medeiros-Neto G, Kim PS, Yoo SE, et al. Congenital hypothyroid goiter with deficient thyroglobulin. Identification of an endoplasmic reticulum storage disease with induction of molecular chaperones. *J Clin Invest* 1996;98:2838.

136. McLachlan SM, Rapoport B. The molecular biology of thyroid peroxidase: cloning, expression and role as autoantigen in autoimmune thyroid disease. *Endocr Rev* 1992;13:192.

137. Kimura S, Kotani T, McBride OW, et al. Human thyroid peroxidase: complete cDNA and protein sequence, chromosome mapping, and identification of two alternately spliced mRNAs. *Proc Natl Acad Sci U S A* 1987;84:5555.

138. de Vijlder JJ, Dinsart C, Libert F, et al. Regional localization of the gene for thyroid peroxidase to human chromosome 2pter-p12. *Cytogenet Cell Genet* 1988;47:170.

139. Kimura S, Hong YS, Kotani T, et al. Structure of the human thyroid peroxidase gene: comparison and relationship to the human myeloperoxidase gene. *Biochemistry* 1989;28:4481.

140. Magnusson RP, Gestautas J, Taurog A, et al. Molecular cloning of the structural gene for porcine thyroid peroxidase. *J Biol Chem* 1987;262:13885.

141. Libert F, Ruel J, Ludgate M, et al. Thyroperoxidase, an autoantigen with a mosaic structure made of nuclear and mitochondrial gene modules. *Embo J* 1987;6:4193.

142. Nagayama Y, Seto P, Rapoport B. Characterization, by molecular cloning, of smaller forms of thyroid peroxidase messenger ribonucleic acid in human thyroid cells as alternatively spliced transcripts. *J Clin Endocrinol Metab* 1990;71:384.

143. Ferrand M, Le Fourn V, Franc JL. Increasing diversity of human thyroperoxidase generated by alternative splicing. Characterized by molecular cloning of new transcripts with single- and multispliced mRNAs. *J Biol Chem* 2003;278:3793.

144. Niccoli P, Fayadat L, Panneels V, et al. Human thyroperoxidase in its alternatively spliced form (TPO2) is enzymatically inactive and exhibits changes in intracellular processing and trafficking. *J Biol Chem* 1997;272:29487.

145. Cetani F, Costagliola S, Tonacchera M, et al. The thyroperoxidase doublet is not produced by alternative splicing. *Mol Cell Endocrinol* 1995;115:125.

146. Taurog A, Dorris ML, Yokoyama N, et al. Purification and characterization of a large, tryptic fragment of human thyroid peroxidase with high catalytic activity. *Arch Biochem Biophys* 1990;278:333.

147. Yokoyama N, Taurog A. Porcine thyroid peroxidase:relationship between the native enzyme and an active, highly purified tryptic fragment. *Mol Endocrinol* 1988;2:838.

148. Foti D, Kaufman KD, Chazenbalk GD, et al. Generation of a biologically active, secreted form of human thyroid peroxidase by site-directed mutagenesis. *Mol Endocrinol* 1990;4:786.

149. Rawitch AB, Pollock HG, Yang SX. Thyroglobulin glycosylation: location and nature of the N-linked oligosaccharide units in bovine thyroglobulin. *Arch Biochem Biophys* 1993;300:271.

150. Taurog A, Wall M. Proximal and distal histidines in thyroid peroxidase: relation to the alternatively spliced form, TPO-2. *Thyroid* 1998;8:185.

151. De Gioia L, Ghibaudi E, Laurenti E, et al. A theoretical three-dimensional model for lactoperoxidase and eosinophil peroxidase, built on the scaffold of the myeloperoxidase X-ray structure. *J Biol Inorg Chem* 1996;1:476.

152. Taurog A. Molecular evolution of thyroid peroxidase. *Biochimie* 1999;81:557.

153. Johnson KR, Nauseef WM, Care A, et al. Characterization of cDNA clones for human myeloperoxidase: predicted amino acid sequence and evidence for multiple mRNA species. *Nucleic Acids Res* 1987;15:2013.

154. Morishita K, Kubota N, Asano S, et al. Molecular cloning and characterization of cDNA for human myeloperoxidase. *J Biol Chem* 1987;262:3844.

155. Kimura S, Ikeda-Saito M. Human myeloperoxidase and thyroid peroxidase, two enzymes with separate and distinct physiological functions, are evolutionarily related members of the same gene family. *Proteins* 1988;3:113.

156. Dull TJ, Uyeda C, Strosberg AD, et al. Molecular cloning of cDNAs encoding bovine and human lactoperoxidase. *DNA Cell Biol* 1990;9:499.

157. Kiser C, Caterina CK, Engler JA, et al. Cloning and sequence analysis of the human salivary peroxidase-encoding cDNA. *Gene* 1996;173:261.

158. Sakamaki K, Tomonaga M, Tsukui K, et al. Molecular cloning and characterization of a chromosomal gene for human eosinophil peroxidase. *J Biol Chem* 1989;264:16828.

159. Zeng J, Fenna RE. X-ray crystal structure of canine myeloperoxidase at 3 A° resolution. *J Mol Biol* 1992;226:185.

160. Fiedler TJ, Davey CA, Fenna RE. X-ray crystal structure and characterization of halide-binding sites of human myeloperoxidase at 1. 8 A° resolution. *J Biol Chem* 2000;275:11964.

161. Blair-Johnson M, Fiedler T, Fenna R. Human myeloperoxidase: structure of a cyanide complex and its interaction with bromide and thiocyanate substrates at 1.9 A resolution. *Biochemistry* 2001;40:13990.

162. Baker JR, Arscott P, Johnson J. An analysis of the structure and antigenicity of different forms of human thyroid peroxidase. *Thyroid* 1994;4:173.

163. Nishikawa T, Rapoport B, McLachlan SM. Exclusion of two major areas on thyroid peroxidase from the immunodominant region containing the conformational epitopes recognized by human autoantibodies. *J Clin Endocrinol Metab* 1994;79:1648.

164. Nilsson M, Molne J, Karlsson FA, et al. Immunoelectron microscopic studies on the cell surface location of the thyroid microsomal antigen. *Mol Cell Endocrinol* 1987;53:177.

165. Pinchera A, Mariotti S, Chiovato L, et al. Cellular localization of the microsomal antigen and the thyroid peroxidase antigen. *Acta Endocrinol* 1987;281:57.

166. Bjorkman U, Ekholm R, Ericson LE. Effects of thyrotropin on thyroglobulin exocytosis and iodination in the rat thyroid gland. *Endocrinology* 1978;102:460.

167. Chiovato L, Vitti P, Lombardi A, et al. Expression of the microsomal antigen on the surface of continuously cultured rat thyroid cells is modulated by thyrotropin. *J Clin Endocrinol Metab* 1985;61:12.

168. Zhang X, Arvan P. Cell type-dependent differences in thyroid peroxidase cell surface expression. *J Biol Chem* 2000;275:31946.

169. Penel C, Gruffat D, Alquier C, et al. Thyrotropin chronically regulates the pool of thyroperoxidase and its intracellular distribution: a quantitative confocal microscopic study. *J Cell Physiol* 1998;174:160.

170. Fayadat L, Niccoli-Sire P, Lanet J, et al. Human thyroperoxidase is largely retained and rapidly degraded in the endoplasmic reticulum. Its N-glycans are required for folding and intracellular trafficking. *Endocrinology* 1998;139:4277.

171. Fayadat L, Siffroi-Fernandez S, Lanet J, et al. Degradation of human thyroperoxidase in the endoplasmic reticulum involves two different pathways depending on the folding state of the protein. *J Biol Chem* 2000;275:15948.

172. Nakagawa H, Kotani T, Ohtaki S, et al. Purification of thyroid peroxidase by monoclonal antibody-assisted immunoaffinity chromatography. *Biochem Biophys Res Commun* 1985;127:8.

173. Ohtaki S, Kotani T, Nakamura Y. Characterization of human thyroid peroxidase purified by monoclonal antibody-assisted chromatography. *J Clin Endocrinol Metab* 1986;63:570.

174. Guo J, McLachlan SM, Hutchison S, et al. The greater glycan content of recombinant human thyroid peroxidase of mammalian than of insect cell origin facilitates purification to homogeneity of enzymatically protein remaining soluble at high concentration. *Endocrinology* 1998;139:999.

175. Nagataki S, Uchimura H, Masuyama Y, et al. Thyrotropin and thyroidal peroxidase activity. *Endocrinology* 1973;92:363.

176. Yamamoto K, DeGroot LJ. Peroxidase and NADPH-cytochrome C reductase activity during thyroid hyperplasia and involution. *Endocrinology* 1974;95:606.

177. Nagasaka A, Hidaka H. Quantitative modulation of thyroid iodide peroxidase by thyroid stimulating hormone. *Biochem Biophys Res Commun* 1980;96:1143.

178. Chazenbalk G, Magnusson RP, Rapoport B. Thyrotropin stimulation of cultured thyroid cells increases steady state levels of the messenger ribonucleic acid for thyroid peroxidase. *Mol Endocrinol* 1987;1:913.

179. Gerard CM, Lefort A, Libert F, et al. Transcriptional regulation of the thyroperoxydase gene by thyrotropin and forskolin. *Mol Cell Endocrinol* 1988;60:239.

180. Isozaki O, Kohn LD, Kozak CA, et al. Thyroid peroxidase: rat cDNA sequence, chromosomal localization in mouse, and regulation of gene expression by comparison to thyroglobulin in rat FRTL-5 cells. *Mol Endocrinol* 1989;3:1681.

181. Damante G, Chazenbalk G, Russo D, et al. Thyrotropin regulation of thyroid peroxidase messenger ribonucleic acid levels in cultured rat thyroid cells: evidence for the involvement of a nontranscriptional mechanism. *Endocrinology* 1989;124:2889.

182. Nagayama Y, Yamashita S, Hirayu H, et al. Regulation of thyroid peroxidase and thyroglobulin gene expression by thyrotropin in cultured human thyroid cells. *J Clin Endocrinol Metab* 1989;68:1155.

183. Gerard CM, Lefort A, Christophe D, et al. Control of thyroperoxidase and thyroglobulin transcription by cAMP: evidence for distinct regulatory mechanisms. *Mol Endocrinol* 1989;3:2110.

184. Collison KS, Banga JP, Barnett PS, et al. Activation of the thyroid peroxidase gene in human thyroid cells: effect of thyrotrophin, forskolin and phorbol ester. *J Mol Endocrinol* 1989;3:1.

185. Ashizawa K, Yamashita S, Nagayama Y, et al. Interferon-gamma inhibits thyrotropin-induced thyroidal peroxidase gene expression in cultured human thyrocytes. *J Clin Endocrinol Metab* 1989;69:475.

186. Ashizawa K, Yamashita S, Tobinaga T, et al. Inhibition of human thyroid peroxidase gene expression by interleukin 1. *Acta Endocrinol (Copenh)* 1989;121:465.

187. Abramowicz MJ, Vassart G, Christophe D. Thyroid peroxidase gene promoter confers TSH responsiveness to heterologous reporter genes in transfection experiments. *Biochem Biophys Res Commun* 1990;166:1257.

188. Aza-Blanc P, Di Lauro R, Santisteban P. Identification of a cis-regulatory element and a thyroid-specific nuclear factor mediating the hormonal regulation of rat thyroid peroxidase promoter activity. *Mol Endocrinol* 1993;7:1297.

189. Abramowicz MJ, Vassart G, Christophe D. Functional study of the human thyroid peroxidase gene promoter. *Eur J Biochem* 1992;203:467.

190. Zannini M, Francis-Lang H, Plachov D, et al. Pax-8, a paired domain-containing protein, binds to a sequence overlapping the recognition site of a homeodomain and activates transcription from two thyroid-specific promoters. *Mol Cell Biol* 1992;12:4230.

191. Di Palma T, Nitsch R, Mascia A, et al. The paired domain-containing factor Pax8 and the homeodomain-containing factor TTF-1 directly interact and synergistically activate transcription. *J Biol Chem* 2003;278:3395.

192. Miccadei S, De Leo R, Zammarchi E, et al. The synergistic activity of thyroid transcription factor 1 and Pax 8 relies on the promoter/enhancer interplay. *Mol Endocrinol* 2002;16:837.

193. Ortiz L, Aza-Blanc P, Zannini M, et al. The interaction between the forkhead thyroid transcription factor TTF-2 and the constitutive factor CTF/NF-1 is required for efficient hormonal regulation of the thyroperoxidase gene transcription. *J Biol Chem* 1999;274:15213.

194. De Leo R, Miccadei S, Zammarchi E, et al. Role for p300 in Pax 8 induction of thyroperoxidase gene expression. *J Biol Chem* 2000;275:34100.

195. Kikkawa F, Gonzalez FJ, Kimura S. Characterization of a thyroid-specific enhancer located 5. 5 kilobase pairs upstream of the human thyroid peroxidase gene. *Mol Cell Biol* 1990;10:6216.

196. Mizuno K, Gonzalez FJ, Kimura S. Thyroid-specific enhancer-binding protein (T/EBP): cDNA cloning, functional characterization, and structural identity with thyroid transcription factor TTF-1. *Mol Cell Biol* 1991;11:4927.

197. Esposito C, Miccadei S, Saiardi A, et al. PAX 8 activates the enhancer of the human thyroperoxidase gene. *Biochem J* 1998; 331:37.

198. Abramowicz MJ, Targovnik HM, Varela V, et al. Identification of a mutation in the coding sequence of the human thyroid peroxidase gene causing congenital goiter. *J Clin Invest* 1992;90:1200.

199. Bikker H, Vulsma T, Baas F, et al. Identification of five novel inactivating mutations in the thyroid peroxidase gene by denaturing gradient gel electrophoresis. *Hum Mutat* 1995;6:9.

200. Pannain S, Weiss RE, Jackson CE, et al. Two different mutations in the thyroid peroxidase gene of a large inbred Amish kindred: power and limits of homozygosity mapping. *J Clin Endocrinol Metab* 1999;84:1061.

201. Bakker B, Bikker H, Vulsma T, et al. Two decades of screening for congenital hypothyroidism in the Netherlands: TPO gene mutations in total iodide organification defects (an update). *J Clin Endocrinol Metab* 2000;85:3708.

202. Corvilain B, van Sande J, Laurent E, et al. The H_2O_2-generating system modulates protein iodination and the activity of the pentose phosphate pathway in dog thyroid. *Endocrinology* 1991;128:779.

203. Ekholm R. Iodination of thyroglobulin. An intracellular or extracellular process? *Mol Cell Endocrinol* 1981;24:141.

204. Bjorkman U, Ekholm R. Generation of H_2O_2 in isolated porcine thyroid follicles. *Endocrinology* 1984;115:392.

205. Virion A, Michot JL, Deme D, et al. NADPH-dependent H_2O_2 generation and peroxidase activity in thyroid particular fraction. *Mol Cell Endocrinol* 1984;36:95.

206. Nakamura Y, Ogihara S, Ohtaki S. Activation by ATP of calcium-dependent NADPH-oxidase generating hydrogen peroxide in thyroid plasma membranes. *J Biochem* 1987;102:1121.

207. Dupuy C, Kaniewski J, Deme D, et al. NADPH-dependent H_2O_2 generation catalyzed by thyroid plasma membranes. Studies with electron scavengers. *Eur J Biochem* 1989;185:597.

208. Leseney AM, Deme D, Legue O, et al. Biochemical characterization of a Ca^{2+}/NAD(P)H-dependent H_2O_2 generator in human thyroid tissue. *Biochimie* 1999;81:373.

209. Dème D, Doussiere J, De Sandro V, et al. The Ca^{2+}/NADPH-dependent H_2O_2 generator in thyroid plasma membrane: inhibition by diphenyleneiodonium. *Biochem J* 1994;301:75.

210. Gorin Y, Ohayon R, Carvalho DP, et al. Solubilization and characterization of a thyroid Ca^{2+}-dependent and NADPH-dependent $K_3Fe(CN)_6$ reductase. Relationship with the NADPH-dependent H_2O_2-generating system. *Eur J Biochem* 1996;240:807.

211. Dème D, Virion A, Hammou NA, et al. NADPH-dependent generation of H₂O₂ in a thyroid particulate fraction requires Ca²⁺. *FEBS Lett* 1985;186:107.

212. Raspé E, Laurent E, Corvilain B, et al. Control of the intracellular Ca²⁺-concentration and the inositol phosphate accumulation in dog thyrocyte primary culture: evidence for different kinetics of Ca²⁺-phosphatidylinositol cascade activation and for involvement in the regulation of H₂O₂ production. *J Cell Physiol* 1991;146:242.

213. Raspé E, Dumont JE. Tonic modulation of dog thyrocyte H₂O₂ generation and I⁻ uptake by thyrotropin through the cyclic adenosine 3′,5′-monophosphate cascade. *Endocrinology* 1995;136:965.

214. Dupuy C, Ohayon R, Valent A, et al. Purification of a novel flavoprotein involved in the thyroid NADPH oxidase: cloning of the porcine and human cDNAs. *J Biol Chem* 1999;274:37265.

215. De Deken X, Wang D, Many MC, et al. Cloning of two human thyroid cDNAs encoding new members of the NADPH oxidase family. *J Biol Chem* 2000;275:23227.

216. Yu L, Quinn MT, Cross AR, et al. Gp91(phox) is the heme binding subunit of the superoxide-generating NADPH oxidase. *Proc Natl Acad Sci U S A* 1998;95:7993.

217. Babior BM. NADPH oxidase: an update. *Blood* 1999;93:1464.

218. Moreno JC, Pauws E, van Kampen AH, et al. Cloning of tissue-specific genes using serial analysis of gene expression and a novel computational substraction approach. *Genomics* 2001;75:70.

219. Suh YA, Arnold RS, Lassegue B, et al. Cell transformation by the superoxide-generating oxidase Mox1. *Nature* 1999;401:79.

220. Corvilain B, Laurent E, Lecomte M, et al. Role of the cyclic adenosine 3′,5′-monophosphate and the phosphatidylinositol-Ca²⁺ cascades in mediating the effects of thyrotropin and iodide on hormone synthesis and secretion in human thyroid slices. *J Clin Endocrinol Metab* 1994;79:152.

221. De Deken X, Wang D, Dumont JE, et al. Characterization of ThOX proteins as components of the thyroid H₂O₂-generating system. *Exp Cell Res* 2002;273:187.

222. Morand S, Chaaraoui M, Kaniewski J, et al. Effect of iodide on nicotinamide adenine dinucleotide phosphate oxidase activity and Duox2 protein expression in isolated porcine thyroid follicles. *Endocrinology* 2003;144:1241.

223. Edens WA, Sharling L, Cheng G, et al. Tyrosine cross-linking of extracellular matrix is catalyzed by Duox, a multidomain oxidase/peroxidase with homology to the phagocyte oxidase subunit gp91phox. *J Cell Biol* 2001;154:879.

224. Dupuy C, Pomerance M, Ohayon R, et al. Thyroid oxidase (THOX2) gene expression in the rat thyroid cell line FRTL-5. *Biochem Biophys Res Commun* 2000;277:287.

225. Caillou B, Dupuy C, Lacroix L, et al. Expression of reduced nicotinamide adenine dinucleotide phosphate oxidase (ThoX, LNOX, Duox) genes and proteins in human thyroid tissues. *J Clin Endocrinol Metab* 2001;86:3351.

226. Corvilain B, Van Sande J, Dumont JE. Inhibition by iodide of iodide binding to proteins: the "Wolff-Chaikoff" effect is caused by inhibition of H₂O₂ generation. *Biochem Biophys Res Commun* 1988;154:1287.

227. Kuliawat R, Lisanti MP, Arvan P. Polarized distribution and delivery of plasma membrane proteins in thyroid follicular epithelial cells. *J Biol Chem* 1995;270:2478.

228. Lacroix L, Nocera M, Mian C, et al. Expression of nicotinamide adenine dinucleotide phosphate oxidase flavoprotein DUOX genes and proteins in human papillary and follicular thyroid carcinomas. *Thyroid* 2001;11:1017.

229. Nakamura Y, Ohtaki S, Makino R, et al. Superoxide anion is the initial product in the hydrogen peroxide formation catalyzed by NADPH oxidase in porcine thyroid plasma membrane. *J Biol Chem* 1989;264:4759.

230. Nakamura Y, Makino R, Tanaka T, et al. Mechanism of H₂O₂ production in porcine thyroid cells: evidence for intermediary formation of superoxide anion by NADPH-dependent H₂O₂-generating machinery. *Biochemistry* 1991;30:4880.

231. Dupuy C, Deme D, Kaniewski J, et al. Ca²⁺ regulation of thyroid NADPH-dependent H₂O₂ generation. *FEBS Lett* 1988;233:74.

232. Dupuy C, Virion A, Ohayon R, et al. Mechanism of hydrogen peroxide formation catalyzed by NADPH oxidase in thyroid plasma membrane. *J Biol Chem* 1991;266:3739.

233. Carvalho DP, Dupuy C, Gorin Y, et al. The Ca²⁺- and reduced nicotinamide adenine dinucleotide phosphate-dependent hydrogen peroxide generating system is induced by thyrotropin in porcine thyroid cells. *Endocrinology* 1996;137:1007.

234. Gorin Y, Leseney AM, Ohayon R, et al. Regulation of the thyroid NADPH-dependent H₂O₂ generator by Ca²⁺: studies with phenylarsine oxide in thyroid plasma membrane. *Biochem J* 1997;321:383.

235. Bjorkman U, Ekholm R. Accelerated exocytosis and H₂O₂ generation in isolated thyroid follicles enhance protein iodination. *Endocrinology* 1988;122:488.

236. Bjorkman U, Ekholm R. Hydrogen peroxide generation and its regulation in FRTL-5 and porcine thyroid cells. *Endocrinology* 1992;130:393.

237. Ohayon R, Boeynaems JM, Braekman JC, et al. Inhibition of thyroid NADPH-oxidase by 2-iodohexadecanal in a cell-free system. *Mol Cell Endocrinol* 1994;99:133.

238. Panneels V, Van den Bergen H, Jacoby C, et al. Inhibition of H₂O₂ production by iodoaldehydes in cultured dog thyroid cells. *Mol Cell Endocrinol* 1994;102:167.

239. Corvilain B, Collyn L, van Sande J, et al. Stimulation by iodide of H₂O₂ generation in thyroid slices from several species. *Am J Physiol Endocrinol Metab* 2000;278:E692.

240. Moreno JC, Bikker H, Kempers MJ, et al. Inactivating mutations in the gene for thyroid oxidase 2 (THOX2) and congenital hypothyroidism. *N Engl J Med* 2002;347:95.

241. Kusakabe T. Deficient cytochrome b₅ reductase activity in nontoxic goiter with iodide organification defect. *Metabolism* 1975;24:1103.

242. Niepomniszcze H, Targovnik HM, Gluzman BE, et al. Abnormal H₂O₂ supply in the thyroid of a patient with goiter and iodine organification defect. *J Clin Endocrinol Metab* 1987;65:344.

243. Figueiredo MD, Cardoso LC, Ferreira AC, et al. Goiter and hypothyroidism in two siblings due to impaired Ca⁺²/NAD(P)H-dependent H₂O₂-generating activity. *J Clin Endocrinol Metab* 2001;86:4843.

244. Dawson JH. Probing structure-function relations in heme-containing oxygenases and peroxidases. *Science* 1988;240:433.

245. Taurog A, Dorris ML, Doerge DR. Mechanism of simultaneous iodination and coupling catalyzed by thyroid peroxidase. *Arch Biochem Biophys* 1996;330:24.

246. Pommier J, Deme D, Nunez J. Effect of iodide concentration on thyroxine synthesis catalysed by thyroid peroxidase. *Eur J Biochem* 1973;37:406.

247. Nunez J, Pommier J. Formation of thyroid hormones. *Vitam Horm* 1982;39:175.

248. Morrison M, Schonbaum GR. Peroxidase-catalyzed halogenation. *Annu Rev Biochem* 1976;45:861.

249. Magnusson RP, Taurog A, Dorris ML. Mechanisms of thyroid peroxidase- and lactoperoxidase-catalyzed reactions involving iodide. *J Biol Chem* 1984;259:13783.

250. Magnusson RP, Taurog A, Dorris ML. Mechanism of iodide-dependent catalic activity of thyroid peroxidase and lactoperoxidase. *J Biol Chem* 1984;259:197.

251. Dunford HB, Ralston IM. On the mechanism of iodination of tyrosine. *Biochem Biophys Res Commun* 1983;116:639.

252. Sun W, Dunford HB. Kinetics and mechanism of the peroxidase-catalyzed iodination of tyrosine. *Biochemistry* 1993;32:1324.

253. Morris DR, Hager LP. Mechanism of the inhibition of enzymatic halogenation by antithyroid agents. *J Biol Chem* 1966;241:3582.

254. Ohtaki S, Nakagawa H, Kimura S, et al. Analyses of catalytic intermediates of hog thyroid peroxidase during its iodinating reaction. *J Biol Chem* 1981;256:805.

255. Nakamura M, Yamazaki I, Nakagawa H, et al. Steady state kinetics and regulation of thyroid peroxidase-catalyzed iodination. *J Biol Chem* 1983;258:3837.

256. Ohtaki S, Nakagawa H, Nakamura M, et al. Thyroid peroxidase: experimental and clinical integration. *Endocr J* 1996;43:1.

257. Malthiery Y, Marriq C, Berge-Lefranc JL, et al. Thyroglobulin structure and function: recent advances. *Biochimie* 1989;71:195.

258. Lamas L, Anderson PC, Fox JW, et al. Consensus sequences for early iodination and hormonogenesis in human thyroglobulin. *J Biol Chem* 1989;264:13541.

259. Xiao S, Dorris ML, Rawitch AB, et al. Selectivity in tyrosyl iodination sites in human thyroglobulin. *Arch Biochem Biophys* 1996;334:284.

260. Gavaret JM, Nunez J, Cahnmann HJ. Formation of dehydroalanine residues during thyroid hormone synthesis in thyroglobulin. *J Biol Chem* 1980;255:5281.

261. Kim PS, Dunn JT, Kaiser DL. Similar hormone-rich peptides from thyroglobulins of five vertebrate classes. *Endocrinology* 1984;114:369.

262. Dunn AD, Corsi CM, Myers HE, et al. Tyrosine 130 is an important outer ring donor for thyroxine formation in thyroglobulin. *J Biol Chem* 1998;273:25223.

263. Dème D, Pommier J, Nunez J. Specificity of thyroid hormone synthesis. The role of thyroid peroxidase. *Biochim Biophys Acta* 1978;540:73.

264. Taurog A, Riesco G, Larsen PR. Formation of 3,3′-diiodothyronine and 3′,5′,3-triiodothyronine (reverse T3) in thyroid glands of rats and in enzymatically iodinated thyroglobulin. *Endocrinology* 1976;99:281.

265. Taurog A, Nakashima T. Dissociation between degree of iodination and iodoamino acid distribution in thyroglobulin. *Endocrinology* 1978;103:633.

266. Abrams GM, Larsen PR. Triiodothyronine and thyroxine in the serum and thyroid glands of iodine-deficient rats. *J Clin Invest* 1973;52:2522.

267. Dème D, Fimiani E, Pommier J, et al. Free diiodotyrosine effects on protein iodination and thyroid hormone synthesis catalyzed by thyroid peroxidase. *Eur J Biochem* 1975;51:329.

268. Virion A, Deme D, Pommier J, et al. The role of iodide and of free diiodotyrosine in enzymatic and non-enzymatic thyroid hormone synthesis. *Eur J Biochem* 1981;118:239.

269. Taurog A, Dorris M, Doerge DR. Evidence for a radical mechanism in peroxidase-catalyzed coupling. I. Steady-state experiments with various peroxidases. *Arch Biochem Biophys* 1994;315:82.

270. Virion A, Courtin F, Deme D, et al. Spectral characteristics and catalytic properties of thyroid peroxidase-H2O2 compounds in the iodination and coupling reactions. *Arch Biochem Biophys* 1985;242:41.

271. Doerge DR, Taurog A, Dorris ML. Evidence for a radical mechanism in peroxidase-catalyzed coupling. II. Single turnover experiments with horseradish peroxidase. *Arch Biochem Biophys* 1994;315:90.

272. Cooper DS. Antithyroid drugs in the management of patients with Graves' disease: an evidence-based approach to therapeutic controversies. *J Clin Endocrinol Metab* 2003;88:3474.

273. Nakashima T, Taurog A. Rapid conversion of carbimazole to methimazole in serum; evidence for an enzymatic mechanism. *Clin Endocrinol (Oxf)* 1979;10:637.

274. Marchant B, Lees JF, Alexander WD. Antithyroid drugs. *Pharmacol Ther* 1978;3:305.

275. Nakashima T, Taurog A, Riesco G. Mechanism of action of thioureylene antithyroid drugs: factors affecting intrathyroidal metabolism of propylthiouracil and methimazole in rats. *Endocrinology* 1978;103:2187.

276. Shiroozu A, Taurog A, Engler H, et al. Mechanism of action of thioureylene antithyroid drugs in the rat: possible inactivation of thyroid peroxidase by propylthiouracil. *Endocrinology* 1983;113:362.

277. Kampmann JP, Hansen JM. Clinical pharmacokinetics of antithyroid drugs. *Clin Pharmacokinet* 1981;6:401.

278. Lang JC, Lees JF, Alexander WD, et al. Effect of variations in acute and chronic iodine intake on the accumulation and metabolism of [^{35}S]methimazole by the rat thyroid gland. Differences from [35S]propylthiouracil. *Biochem Pharmacol* 1983;32:241.

279. Taurog A. The mechanism of action of the thioureylene antithyroid drugs. *Endocrinology* 1976;98:1031.

280. Engler H, Taurog A, Luthy C, et al. Reversible and irreversible inhibition of thyroid peroxidase-catalyzed iodination by thioureylene drugs. *Endocrinology* 1983;112:86.

281. Taurog A, Dorris ML, Guziec FS, Jr. Metabolism of ^{35}S- and ^{14}C-labeled 1-methyl-2-mercaptoimidazole in vitro and in vivo. *Endocrinology* 1989;124:30.

282. Taurog A, Dorris ML. A reexamination of the proposed inactivation of thyroid peroxidase in the rat thyroid by propylthiouracil. *Endocrinology* 1989;124:3038.

283. Taurog A, Dorris ML, Guziec FS, Jr., et al. Metabolism of ^{35}S- and ^{14}C-labeled propylthiouracil in a model in vitro system containing thyroid peroxidase. *Endocrinology* 1989;124:3030.

284. Doerge DR. Mechanism-based inhibition of lactoperoxidase by thiocarbamide goitrogens: identification of turnover and inactivation pathways. *Biochemistry* 1988;27:3697.

285. Engler H, Taurog A, Dorris ML. Preferential inhibition of thyroxine and 3,5,3′-triiodothyronine formation by propylthiouracil and methylmercaptoimidazole in thyroid peroxidase-catalyzed iodination of thyroglobulin. *Endocrinology* 1982;110:190.

286. Bernier-Valentin F, Kostrouch Z, Rabilloud R, et al. Coated vesicles from thyroid cells carry iodinated thyroglobulin molecules: first indication for an internalization of the thyroid prohormone via a mechanism of receptor-mediated endocytosis. *J Biol Chem* 1990;265:17373.

287. Kostrouch Z, Bernier-Valentin F, Munari-Silem Y, et al. Thyroglobulin molecules internalized by thyrocytes are sorted in early endosomes and partially recycled back to the follicular lumen. *Endocrinology* 1993;132:2645.

288. Marino M, McCluskey RT. Role of thyroglobulin endocytic pathways in the control of thyroid hormone release. *Am J Physiol Cell Physiol* 2000;279:C1295.

289. Marino M, Pinchera A, McCluskey RT, et al. Megalin in thyroid physiology and pathology. *Thyroid* 2001;11:47.

290. Tokuyama T, Yoshinari M, Rawitch AB, et al. Digestion of thyroglobulin with purified thyroid lysosomes:preferential release of iodoamino acids. *Endocrinology* 1987;121:714.

291. Dunn AD, Crutchfield HE, Dunn JT. Proteolytic processing of thyroglobulin by extracts of thyroid lysosomes. *Endocrinology* 1991;128:3073.

292. Dunn AD, Crutchfield HE, Dunn JT. Thyroglobulin processing by thyroidal proteases. Major sites of cleavage by cathepsins B, D, and L. *J Biol Chem* 1991;266:20198.

293. Dunn AD, Myers HE, Dunn JT. The combined action of two thyroidal proteases releases T4 from the dominant hormone-forming site of thyroglobulin. *Endocrinology* 1996;137:3279.

294. Miquelis R, Courageot J, Jacq A, et al. Intracellular routing of GLcNAc-bearing molecules in thyrocytes: selective recycling through the Golgi apparatus. *J Cell Biol* 1993;123:1695.

295. Ulianich L, Suzuki K, Mori A, et al. Follicular thyroglobulin (TG) suppression of thyroid-restricted genes involves the apical membrane asialoglycoprotein receptor and TG phosphorylation. *J Biol Chem* 1999;274:25099.

296. Herzog V. Transcytosis in thyroid follicle cells. *J Cell Biol* 1983;97:607.

297. Druetta L, Bornet H, Sassolas G, et al. Identification of thyroid hormone residues on serum thyroglobulin: clue to the source of circulating thyroglobulin in thyroid diseases. *Eur J Endocrinol* 1999;140:457.

298. Rosenberg IN, Goswami A. Purification and characterization of a flavoprotein from bovine thyroid with iodotyrosine deiodinase activity. *J Biol Chem* 1979;254:12318.

299. Moreno JC. Identification of novel genes involved in congenital hypothyroidism using serial analysis of gene expression. *Horm Res* 2003;60:96.

300. Medeiros-Neto G, Stanbury JB. The iodotyrosine deiodinase defect. In: Medeiros-Neto G, Stanbury JB, eds. *Inherited disorders of the thyroid system.* Boca Raton, FL: CRC Press, 1994:139.

5

THYROGLOBULIN STRUCTURE, FUNCTION, AND BIOSYNTHESIS

PETER ARVAN
BRUNO DI JESO

Thyroglobulin (Tg) is the most highly expressed protein in the thyroid gland. Its vastly higher abundance than other proteins in thyroid extracts tends to yield an exaggerated estimate of its expression relative to that of other thyroid proteins, because most Tg in the thyroid gland is in fact extracellular, having been secreted into the lumen of thyroid follicles, where it is stored as colloid. Nevertheless, even when extracellular storage is not considered, Tg is still the predominant thyroid protein, and is the most important one, because its encoded structure provides for the coupling reaction that underlies the biosynthesis of the active thyroid hormones thyroxine (T_4) and triiodothyronine (T_3) (see section on thyroid hormone synthesis in Chapter 4).

Tg has a number of remarkable features. First, it falls within the top 1% of all proteins in terms of the molecular mass of its monomeric structure (~330 kDa). Approximately 10% of this mass (i.e., ~30 kDa) consists of covalently bound carbohydrates, the result of posttranslational modifications as Tg passes along the intracellular secretory pathway of thyroid follicular cells (thyrocytes). Indeed, Tg has long served as a model protein for analysis of the carbohydrate side-chain structures that are formed during N-linked glycoprotein processing (1). In addition, the polypeptide backbone of Tg, amounting to ~90% of its total molecular mass (i.e., ~300 kDa), consists of a signal peptide sequence plus ~2750 residues (± 5 residues, depending upon the species) (2). The secreted polypeptide contains at least 66 tyrosine residues (in human Tg, with additional tyrosines in other species). The percentage of tyrosine residues in Tg that become iodinated normally varies with the dietary iodine supply, but it is not unusual for 20% of them to contain iodine, with three quarters of these as residues of monoiodotyrosine (MIT) and diiodotyrosine (DIT) that are not used for the formation of T_4 and T_3 (3). Thus, Tg protein serves as the primary internal reservoir of recycling iodine in the body, upon which future biosynthesis of thyroid hormones is based.

PHYLOGENY AND ONTOGENY OF THYROGLOBULIN

The appearance of Tg in evolution is associated with thyroid hormone biosynthesis. A colloid-filled follicular lumen surrounded by thyrocytes (presumably a response to decreasing availability of iodide as animals migrated away from the sea to a terrestial environment) and the Tg protein are present in all vertebrates (4). During mammalian embryonic thyroid folliculogenesis (5), as well as folliculogenesis in reconstituted mammalian thyrocyte cultures and in vivo models, intracellular lumens (membrane-bound internal cavities) form within thyrocytes. The cells then associate with one another, after which the intracellular lumens are externalized to form a central, apical extracellular space, which is a hallmark of Tg storage (6). The intracellular lumens have a close physical relationship with the Golgi complex through which newly synthesized Tg traverses (7), and iodination of Tg can occur within them (8), resulting in thyroid hormone formation [nevertheless, their quantitative contribution to overall iodination or hormonogenesis is probably insignificant, because the intracellular availability of hydrogen peroxide in vertebrates is limited (9)]. Although not well studied, some sea-dwelling prevertebrates have specialized pharyngeal epithelial cells that do not aggregate to form obvious follicles (perhaps such cells bear weak evolutionary relationships to salivary epithelial cells that exhibit basolateral iodide uptake and do not enclose an apical lumen), but do form Tg-like iodoproteins (10). Any such means to produce and secrete iodoproteins would not efficiently conserve iodide. Nevertheless, even in prevertebrates, formation of T_4 and T_3 is likely to be linked to a Tg evolutionary precursor (11), and within hagfish or lamprey eels, Tg-like protein is already present (12) along with demonstrable follicles. These findings suggest evolutionarily conserved roles for Tg protein in iodine storage (particularly in land-dwelling and freshwater organisms) and iodothyronine formation. Cloning and sequencing of Tg-like complementary DNA (cDNA) derived from prevertebrates could provide valuable new insights into the evolutionary origins of T_4-forming sites and the domain structure of Tg molecules.

THE THYROGLOBULIN GENE AND ITS MESSENGER RNA

The functionality of the Tg messenger RNA (mRNA) was initially established when a 33S thyroidal mRNA fraction injected into *Xenopus* oocytes resulted in production of immunoreactive Tg protein in the eggs (13), while a similar 33S thyroidal mRNA fraction obtained from a strain of Dutch goats with congenital goiter did not result in production of detectable Tg protein (14). The complete Tg mRNA sequence was eventually deduced by sequencing of fragments of bovine Tg cDNA (2) and those of other species (Fig. 5.1), which allowed for many structural insights (15) and confirmed that there is only one Tg gene in mammals. The human Tg gene spans approximately 300 kB on the long arm of chromosome 8, of which only ~3% represents the exons [48 of them (16)], separated in many instances by large intronic sequences. Mutations within introns as well as imprecision in the mRNA splicing mechanism have led to the possibility of production of Tg splice variants with no change in Tg exon sequence (2,17–19). Alternative splicing is also promoted by increasing thyrotropin (TSH) stimulation (20). This might serve as an evolutionary adaptation to the high frequency of variations in the Tg coding sequence in the population (21), some of which might be less competent for hormonogenesis (22). Nevertheless, TSH action on its receptor is not an absolute requirement for Tg production (23), although there are requirements for the transcription factors TTF-1, TTF-2 (24), and Pax-8 (25), in conjunction with other factors (26). There are also reports of patients with congenital goiter whose thyrocytes may not maintain a sufficient steady-state level of Tg mRNA (27,28). While this could represent a class of transcriptional defects (29), active translation (polyribosome formation) is one of the critical features promoting mRNA stability. Therefore, poorly translated Tg mRNAs (from splice forms, or from exon sequence changes bearing frame-shifts and/or premature termination codons) are likely to correlate with low mRNA abundance of those forms.

The development of Tg cDNA expression vectors for mammalian cells (30) has allowed the study of full-length recombinant versions leading to Tg secretion from heterologous cells (31). Such an approach overlooks the complexity of Tg mRNA splicing, although it increases focus on the exon sequences. It is important to note that the Tg protein has never been studied by x-ray crystallography, because crystals of the pure protein have not been obtained, perhaps due to the numerous posttranslational modifications of Tg (see later in the chapter). Thus, insights into the internal structure of the Tg protein have been limited largely to primary sequence analysis—although negative-staining electron microscopy has demonstrated that a major form of Tg isolated from thyroid gland is dimeric (32).

REGIONAL STRUCTURE OF THYROGLOBULIN DOMAINS DEDUCED FROM THE PRIMARY SEQUENCE

The (12S) Tg monomer in all vertebrates is comprised mainly of four regions (Fig. 5.2), the first three containing distinct cysteine-rich repeats (2). Region I, found within the first ~1200 residues, contains 10 of the 11 so-called "Tg type 1 repeats" of roughly 60 amino acids each. Each repeat surrounds a central WCV (Trp-Cys-Val) sequence plus at least three additional cysteines (one expanding the motif to CWCV, in which each of the two Cys residues are partnered into different disulfide bonds), thereby shaping and stabilizing the domain. Type 1A repeats have a total of six cysteine residues in the domain (three disulfide bonds), which are also found in several other proteins, including equistatin and the thyropin family of cysteine protease inhibitors (33,34), entactin/nidogen (35), insulin-like growth factor-binding protein-6 (IGFBP-6) (36), and the carcinoma-associated antigen GA733–2 (37). Type 1B repeats have only four cysteine residues (38). The disulfide bond pattern Cys_1-Cys_2, Cys_3-Cys_4, Cys_5-Cys_6 prevails in all Tg type 1A repeats (37) and the sequence homology between different proteins bearing the repeat (Fig. 5.3) suggests that this domain has evolved with a common fold designed to be protease resistant and to function as a protease inhibitor/regulator (39). Region II (Fig. 5.2) contains the 11th Tg type 1 repeat, while region III contains the so-called type 3 repeat units that have little or no homology with other proteins in existing databases (2). Because cysteine side chains are internally located within the various Tg repeats, they form a series of domains internally "stapled together" (via disulfide bridges) while being tethered end-to-end with intervening peptide sequences. Consistent with such a view, limited digestion using a variety of proteases tends to cleave between the repeats, liberating them intact from the parent Tg molecule (40).

The fourth and most carboxyl-terminal region, the acetylcholinesterase (AChE) region, (Fig. 5.2) Tg has 31% identity and 47% similarity to the entire length of acetylcholinesterase (41,42). All six cysteine residues involved in cholinesterase intrachain disulfide bonding are conserved in Tg (43), and it is likely that these two proteins share a common folding pattern in their respective tertiary structures.

Altogether, human (and bovine) Tg has 122 cysteines (mouse Tg has 121 Cys residues). When studied by nonreducing SDS-PAGE, the mobility of monomeric Tg in-

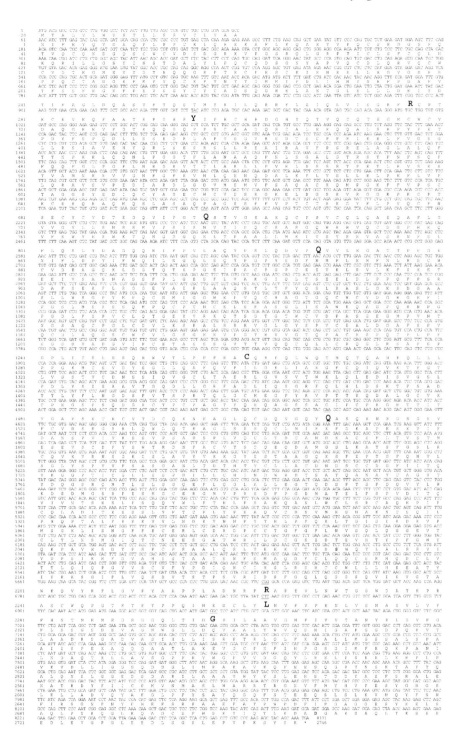

FIGURE 5.1. The nucleotide and encoded 2746 amino-acid sequence of murine thyroglobulin (Tg) (described in single-letter code), derived from Genbank accession number AF076186. In addition, the location of selected point mutations in the coding sequence of Tg associated with thyroid pathology in several different species has been identified on this map by the normal amino acid presented in enlarged, bold type. In order, from amino to carboxyl terminus, this includes: a premature stop codon at position 277 in human Tg (260), a premature stop codon at position 296 in goat Tg (261), a premature stop codon at position 697 in bovine Tg (106), a Glu to His change in exon 10 in human (126,127), a Cys to Arg substitution at position 1263 in human Tg (124), a stop codon at position 1510 in human Tg (28), an Arg to His substitution at position 2223 in human Tg (123), a Leu to Pro substitution at position 2263 in murine Tg (112), and a Gly to Arg substitution at position 2320 in rat Tg (120,121).

creases dramatically, indicating that its molecular radius decreases progressively as a function of time after Tg biosynthesis (44), in comparison with the mobility of the same Tg molecules that have been fully "opened" (i.e., linearized) by reducing all disulfide bonds with dithiothreitol (Fig. 5.4). These results indicate that the vast majority of cysteine thiols are involved in intradomain disulfide pairing within the four major regions of Tg (45). That few unpaired Cys residues remain (46) may explain why Tg homodimers are not covalently associated during transit through the intracellular secretory pathway of thyrocytes (47,48). Nevertheless, extracellular Tg may begin to form intermolecular disulfide bridges when it reaches the oxidizing/iodinating environment of the follicular lumen, resulting in cross-linked dimers (19S), tetramers (27S), and higher order assemblies (49).

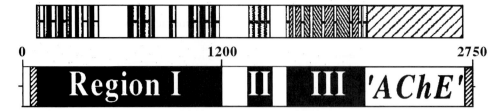

FIGURE 5.2. Sketch of the regional structure **(below)**, including repeat domains **(above)**, in the primary sequence of Tg. Note that the region and domain alignments are not drawn precisely to scale. As shown in the sketch **(below)**, the amino-acid sequence of Tg begins with a cleavable signal peptide *(open box)*, the conserved thyroxine hormonogenic site A (see text) *(hatched box)*, the ten type 1 (A+B) repeat domain units contained in region I, the Cys-rich region II which comprises the 11th type 1 repeat, the region III with repeat units that do not closely match known sequences in the database, and the acetylcholinesterase-homology region followed by the hormonogenic site C (see text) *(hatched box)*.

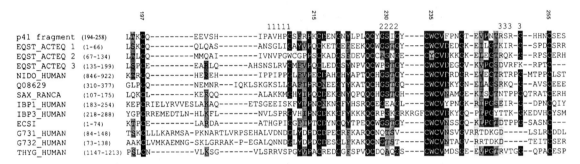

FIGURE 5.3. An alignment of polypeptide sequences containing thyroglobulin (Tg) type 1 repeats, showing the relative positioning of the conserved Cys residues. The last sequence shown is derived from human Tg.

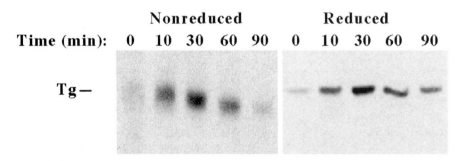

FIGURE 5.4. Kinetic resolution of the maturation of intrachain disulfide bonds of thyroglobulin (Tg). As disulfide bonds are formed within newly synthesized Tg and the structure of the various repeat domains is reorganized, the molecular radius of Tg decreases. When subjected to acrylamide gel electrophoresis under nonreducing conditions, this Tg penetrates further into the gel *(lower band)*. When the Tg protein is intentionally denatured and all disulfide bonds are disrupted, and the protein subjected to electrophoresis under reducing conditions, the penetration of the newly synthesized Tg is unchanged at all times shown. (From Di Jeso B, Ulianich L, Pacifico F, et al. The folding of thyroglobulin in the calnexin/calreticulin pathway and its alteration by a loss of Ca2+ from the endoplasmic reticulum. *Biochem J* 2003;370:449, with permission.)

THYROGLOBULIN TRANSLATION AND INITIAL POLYPEPTIDE FOLDING

The initial stages of Tg biosynthesis are similar to those of other secretory glycoproteins. During translation, nascent Tg polypeptide chains, while still emerging from the ribosome-studded polyribosomes, are directed to the cytosolic side of the endoplasmic reticulum by virtue of the Tg signal peptide sequence that promotes association with the signal recognition particle and its receptor in the membranes of the endoplasmic reticulum (50). From there, the nascent Tg polypeptide is translocated into the lumen of the endoplasmic reticulum via the intramembrane Sec61 protein complex, with assistance from molecular chaperones on the lumenal side (51). After translocation of ~100 amino acids, the Tg signal peptide is excised by a specific protease (52), while ongoing translation is coupled to the translocation of the large remaining nascent polypeptide.

Immediately upon entry into the endoplasmic reticulum, the linear Tg polypeptide begins to be converted into a native three-dimensional structure. This process is more extensive than coupled translation-translocation, in the sense that while a small peptide hormone precursor such as proinsulin achieves its native state after no more than a few minutes within the endoplasmic reticulum (53), for Tg this takes about an hour. During this process (54), many of the repeat domains are likely to be buried interiorly within the tertiary structure of Tg, based on the fact that it requires progressively increasing concentrations of reducing agents *in vitro* to gain access to these domains in the native structure (55). Few of the details of the Tg folding process are known, but the basic steps are likely to be similar to those of other secretory glycoproteins. For example, at an estimated translation rate of 6.5 amino acids per second, one can deduce that it should take ~7 minutes for the entire nascent Tg polypeptide to be delivered into the endoplasmic reticulum. In this case, many of the repeating units of region I of Tg will have been engaged in folding for several minutes before some of the downstream domains of Tg arrive within the lumen of the endoplasmic reticulum. Thus, initial folding of the type 1 repeats is likely to be independent of later downstream domains encoded in the Tg sequence. Along the same lines, when the domain of Tg homologous to AChE reaches the endoplasmic reticulum, its initial folding is likely to be independent from that of the N-terminal domains of Tg that are already beyond their earliest stages of folding. Quite possibly, regional folding may even be sequential (56).

The slowness with which nascent Tg buries its many cysteine side-chains while forming a compact structure (Fig. 5.4) suggests that there is ample opportunity for mispairing of Tg disulfides, and indeed there is evidence that some nascent Tg complexes have mispaired intermolecular disulfide bonds (54,57,58). These disulfide-linked complexes are apparently "on-pathway" in normal Tg folding, because their disappearance correlates with the appearance of Tg monomers (and later, dimers). Resolution of disulfide mispairings is likely to require the involvement of protein disulfide isomerase (PDI) or other members of the superfamily of endoplasmic reticulum oxidoreductases (59–62).

Additional molecular chaperones of the endoplasmic reticulum also play distinct roles in facilitating the early folding of nascent Tg. One member of the heat-shock protein-70 family, known as BiP (63), has been identified repeatedly in protein interactions with Tg both *in vitro* and within the endoplasmic reticulum (57,64–69). BiP is a glucose-regulated protein (GRP), i.e., it is transcriptionally and translationally up-regulated when the extracellular glucose concentration is low (70), when glycosylation is compromised by energy depletion (71) [such as in states of compromised blood flow (68)], or when misfolded Tg or other secretory proteins begin to accumulate in the endoplasmic reticulum for any other reason (such as alterations in redox environment or lumenal calcium concentrations) (72,73). GRP94, a member of the heat-shock protein-90 family that is located in the endoplasmic reticulum and regulated like BiP, also associates with nascent Tg (67). Neither BiP nor GRP94 actively participate in the process of folding Tg (31,74); rather they reversibly associate with newly synthesized Tg molecules, with preferential binding to short hydrophobic sequences, to prevent other inappropriate hydrophobic interactions. Merely by limiting the opportunity for "off-pathway" folding events, the association of the endoplasmic reticulum chaperones promotes "on-pathway" folding of Tg, thus improving the overall yield of native Tg. As this is crucial to the success of secretory protein production in all cells, several (but not all) endoplasmic-reticulum chaperone proteins are essential for life among eukaryotes (75), and the control of their expression is tightly regulated (76,77). Additional chaperones that interact with Tg during its maturation in the endoplasmic reticulum are still being discovered, such as GRP170 (69) and ERp29 (78).

ASPARAGINE-LINKED GLYCOSYLATION AND ITS ROLE IN THYROGLOBULIN FOLDING

Potential asparagine (N)-linked carbohydrate acceptor sites are encoded by the sequence Asn-Xxx-Ser/Thr (Xxx is any amino acid), each of which may accept transfer of a pre-assembled "core oligosaccharide" containing 14 monosaccharide units attached to the asparagine side chain. There are 20 such potential acceptor sites in the sequence of human Tg (and mouse Tg); on average, 16 of these sites are actually utilized by oligosaccharyl transferase (79). This varies between species and amongst the population of Tg molecules within a single species (80), e.g., bovine Tg has a lesser degree of N-glycosylation (81).

Initial Processing of N-linked Glycans of Tg

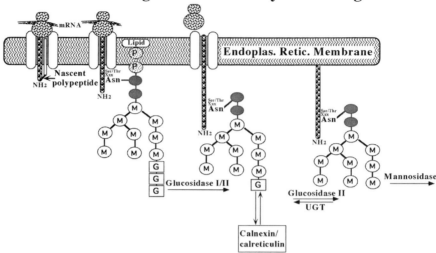

FIGURE 5.5. Early N-linked carbohydrate-processing events on newly synthesized thyroglobulin (Tg). As the nascent Tg polypeptide enters the lumen of the endoplasmic reticulum, a high fraction of its encoded potential Asn-linked glycosylation acceptor sites bind covalently to a 14-unit oligosaccharide from a lipid-linked donor. Three terminal glucose residues *(G)* on one branch of the oligosaccharide structure are the site of attack of endoplasmic-reticulum glucosidases I and II. A monoglucosylated oligosaccharide is the site of binding of the endoplasmic reticulum lectin chaperones calreticulin or calnexin. These lectin chaperones are also associated with the thiol reductase ERp57, which assists in the formation/isomerization of Tg disulfide bonds, further facilitating Tg folding (see text). If a glycosylated Tg domain remains unfolded after the sole remaining glucose residue has been removed, this domain serves as a potential substrate for UDP-glycoprotein glucosyl transferase (UGT). UGT re-adds a single glucose residue to the carbohydrate structure, restoring its capacity to bind calreticulin/calnexin and associated ERp57. Ultimately, for Tg that is properly folded, mannose *(M)* trimming by mannosidases begins in the endoplasmic reticulum and continues in the Golgi complex. For Tg that is misfolded, mannose trimming by endoplasmic-reticulum mannosidase I precedes a process of endoplasmic reticulum-associated degradation that occurs via the ubiquitin-proteasome system (see text).

One critical link between N-glycosylation and Tg stability stems from the discovery that a family of endoplasmic-reticulum chaperones known as calreticulin and calnexin function as lectins, that is, they recognize sugars (82). Calreticulin is abundantly expressed in the lumen of the endoplasmic reticulum, while calnexin is an abundant integral membrane protein whose lumenal domain is highly homologous to calreticulin (83). The initially added N-linked core glycan has a $(GlcNAc)_2(Man)_9(Glc)_3$ structure in which the nine mannose (Man) residues form a three-pronged branching structure, and all three glucose (Glc) residues are stacked at the terminus of one branch (Fig. 5.5). This is followed by stepwise removal of all three terminal glucose residues via the sequential actions of the endoplasmic-reticulum glucosidases I and II. During the short period when the core oligosaccharide structure has a single terminal glucose, it is a substrate for binding to calreticulin or calnexin. Both chaperone lectins have the same oligosaccharide-binding specificity, although only one lectin may be bound to the carbohydrate at any one time. Ultimately, removal of the final glucose residue destroys the calreticulin/calnexin binding site. However, if the domain in Tg (or other substrate glycoprotein) has not folded, it can be recognized by UDP-Glc glycoprotein glucosyl transferase (UGT) (Fig. 5.5), a critically important enzyme that adds a single glucose residue back to the same site on the core oligosaccharide (84,85). This in turn re-forms the calreticulin/calnexin binding site, so that chaperone association may proceed again, in a cyclical manner, until the domain has folded to the point that it is no longer a substrate for re-glucosylation by UGT (because UGT is active only on unfolded Tg and not on properly folded Tg) (86,87). Meanwhile, mannosidase activities of the endoplasmic reticulum initiate trimming of Man residues from the other oligosaccharide branches (1), an event that usually occurs in preparation for further modifications that will take place when Tg reaches the Golgi complex (see later in the chapter). The binding of Tg to calnexin under normal conditions is relatively modest (65), because some calnexin dissociation occurs cotranslationally (65,88) and also because calreticulin may be a more important lectin-chaperone for Tg (44).

An additional special feature of calreticulin or calnexin binding is that it brings the folding of nascent Tg into proximity with ERp57, a thiol reductase member of the

PDI superfamily that catalyzes formation/isomerization of disulfide bonds (89). Thus, ERp57 disulfide-isomerase function is also dependent upon the same early steps in N-linked carbohydrate processing. Because formation/ isomerization of mispaired disulfide bonds is of great importance in the folding of newly synthesized Tg, the activity of ERp57 and the proper processing of the N-glycans of Tg (90) must be viewed as key steps ensuring an adequate rate and efficiency of this process. At the conclusion of the extended period of intrachain disulfide bond formation, which may be rate limiting in achieving proper regional domain structures, the tertiary structure of nascent Tg monomers is now suitable for homodimerization, and this proceeds before exit from the endoplasmic reticulum (54, 57,64,91).

These considerations provide a molecular explanation for the established relationship between N-linked glycosylation and the stability of Tg, which in turn affects the efficiency of Tg iodination (92,93). In relation to this, perturbations of divalent cation concentrations in the secretory pathway, particularly those of Ca^{2+} (and perhaps Mn^{2+}) may destabilize Tg structure (94). Some of this effect may be indirect, because calcium depletion from the endoplasmic reticulum alters carbohydrate processing (95--97), reduces Tg binding to calreticulin and calnexin (44), and greatly inhibits export of Tg from this compartment (91). This may be caused by a diminished rate of isomerization/formation of the Tg disulfide bonds needed for folding; under improper glycosylation conditions, increased residence time of newly synthesized Tg in the endoplasmic reticulum correlates with its prolonged association with BiP and GRP94 (44,57,69).

CONGENITAL GOITROUS HYPOTHYROIDISM DUE TO THYROGLOBULIN MISFOLDING

Even without global effects on the environment of the endoplasmic reticulum, mutations altering the amino acid sequence of Tg could yield phenotypes similar to those described earlier. Patients and animals with congenital goiter and hypothyroidism who have abnormal Tg molecules have been described (98,99). In some instances, the endoplasmic reticulum in the thyrocytes was dilated or swollen (100,101), with little or no stainable Tg in the colloid (102), but knowledge of the specific molecular defects at the genetic level was lacking (103). The finding of nonfunctional Tg mRNA was a first step in this direction (14). These disorders are inherited as autosomal recessive traits in virtually all humans and animals. The mating, without inbreeding, of phenotypically unaffected heterozygotes yielding affected compound heterozygous progeny is such a rare event that it may initially be confused with autosomal dominant inheritance (104) (see Chapters 20 and 48).

Patients with these disorders may have normal or low levels of Tg, depending on how well their Tg mRNA can be translated (105,106).

Unlike the Tg splicing and frame-shift mutants that have been described (21), there are relatively few descriptions of single missense mutations (amino acid substitutions). Thus, what have been called "Tg synthesis defects" are not typically explained by mutations in the coding region of the Tg gene (22). Only a few particular examples of these defects are described here.

The homozygous *cog* mutation in mice results in the murine version of cretinism with microcephaly and hypomyelination (107). In addition, the animals are runts, with little or no detectable 19S Tg in their thyroid gland (108). Instead, a peak at 12S extends to above the 27S position, indicating defective dimerization and formation of abnormal Tg complexes, and very little Tg is iodinated (108–110). Serum TSH concentrations are very high, and there is massive thyrocyte hyperplasia and hypertrophy, with a swollen endoplasmic reticulum and increased expression of multiple molecular chaperones (111). The folding and dimerization defect, which is to some extent ameliorated at lower temperature (111), is the result of a single L2263P (leucine→proline) substitution in the AChE-homology domain of Tg (112). The misfolded mutant protein is primarily retained within the endoplasmic reticulum until the carbohydrate is trimmed by the endoplasmic-reticulum mannosidase I (112A), after which it is translocated back to the cytosol (113) for degradation by the ubiquitin-proteasome system.

A similar situation seems to prevail in dwarf (*rdw/rdw*) rats. These rats were initially thought to have growth hormone deficiency (114,115), but in fact their growth failure is secondary to congenital hypothyroidism (116,117). Although their serum TSH concentrations are not as high as those of *cog/cog* mice, the thyroid glands of *rdw/rdw* rats also have massive expansion of the endoplasmic reticulum (118) (Fig. 5.6), which contains high levels of multiple molecular chaperones (119). There is likely to be a similar defect in Tg folding and dimerization as in *cog/cog* mice, as the mutation in rat Tg proved to be due to a single G2320R (glycine→arginine) substitution (120), less than 60 residues away from the site of the *cog* mutation within the AChE-homology domain that blocks Tg secretion (121). The *rdw/rdw* rats have little thyroid gland enlargement, suggesting that accumulation of the mutant Tg protein may limit thyroid growth (122).

In humans, single Tg amino-acid substitutions involved in congenital hypothyroid goiter have been reported only rarely. One mutation was in the AChE-homology domain (123); others have involved replacement of a conserved cysteine residue. The homozygous C1263R mutant resulted in only mild hypothyroidism, indicating that the mutant Tg protein can be iodinated and serve as a substrate

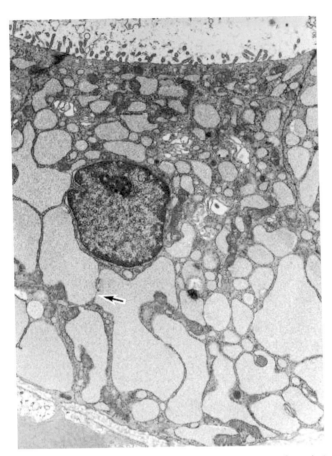

FIGURE 5.6. Electron photomicrograph a thyrocyte of a *rdw/rdw* rat, showing enlarged endoplasmic reticulum–derived vacuoles that overcrowd the remaining cytoplasm *(arrow)*. Thyrocytes from some humans with congenital goiter due to defective Tg synthesis have a similar appearance (5,600× magnification). (From Sakai Y, Yamashina S, Furudate SI. Missing secretory granules, dilated endoplasmic reticulum, and nuclear dislocation in the thyroid gland of rdw rats with hereditary dwarfism. *Anat Rec* 2000;259:60, with permission.)

for hormonogenesis (124). Given the importance of intrachain disulfide bonding within Tg (Fig. 5.4), folding defects associated with replacement of single Cys residues are easy to rationalize.

Simple goiter without hypothyroidism has also been associated with production of defective Tg (125), such as the missense mutation resulting in a glutamine to histidine substitution within exon 10 of the Tg gene (126,127). A variant type of adenomatous goiter, without hypothyroidism, has been attributed to the C1995S (cysteine→ serine) mutation (128). By analogy to the *cog/cog* mice, which as adults have normal serum T$_4$ concentrations (108), humans in whom the Tg is only slightly defective may, by increasing the total number of thyrocytes contributing to hormonogenesis, compensate for the reduced efficiency of hormonogenesis within individual thyrocytes, so that euthyroidism is achieved at the expense of goiter.

POSTTRANSLATIONAL MODIFICATIONS OF THYROGLOBULIN IN LATER STEPS OF THE SECRETORY PATHWAY

As Tg migrates to the Golgi complex, roughly two-thirds of the N-linked core glycans become modified to a "complex glycan" structure (129). This includes additional trimming of mannose residues from the core glycan branches by alpha-mannosidase-II and endomannosidase (130), followed by addition to these branches of other carbohydrates (131), including N-acetylglucosamine, galactose, fucose, sialic acid (132,133), or sulfate (134,135) or phosphate (136,137). [Independently of this, sulfation and phosphorylation may also occur directly on the Tg polypeptide backbone (136,138,139)].

In addition, human Tg has been reported to undergo "O-linked" glycosylation; in this case, the carbohydrate is attached to the side chain of serine or threonine (1). Such O-linked carbohydrate has various structures, including typical glycosaminoglycan chains that may also be sulfated (140,141).

Knowledge of these additional post-translational modifications of Tg has helped to identify normal and abnormal Tg maturation at defined points along the secretory pathway. As an example, both protein and carbohydrate sulfation are thought to occur primarily within the trans-Golgi network (142). Therefore, perturbed secretion of Tg that had been radiolabeled with ^{35}S-methionine might represent delayed export from the endoplasmic reticulum, whereas perturbed secretion of Tg that had been radiolabeled with ^{35}S-sulfate might represent a delay in a late Golgi or post-Golgi step of the Tg secretory pathway. A similar investigative tool involves *in vitro* digestion of Tg with endoglycosidase H (endo H), which will cleave N-linked oligosaccharides representative of the initial core carbohydrate structure within the endoplasmic reticulum. As Tg contains carbohydrates amounting to ~30kDa of its molecular mass, endo H digestion of Tg that has been confined to the endoplasmic reticulum compartment results in a substantial decrease in molecular mass, observed as an increased mobility of the Tg band by SDS-PAGE. By contrast, when the mannose-trimmed core oligosaccharide becomes modified in the Golgi complex by addition of N-acetylglucosamine (the first of the "complex sugars" to be added), that oligosaccharide can no longer be digested by endo H. Consequently, on endo H digestion, Tg that has migrated to the Golgi compartment loses much less molecular mass, corresponding to only the ~one-third of N-linked core glycans that did not become modified to a "complex glycan" structure. The ratio of this endo H-resistant Tg to endo H-sensitive Tg in the steady state, as well as the rate of acquisition of endo H-resistance in kinetic studies, are both useful indicators of the efficiency of Tg export from the endoplasmic reticulum. Typically, in congenital goitrous hypothyroidism due to a mutation in Tg

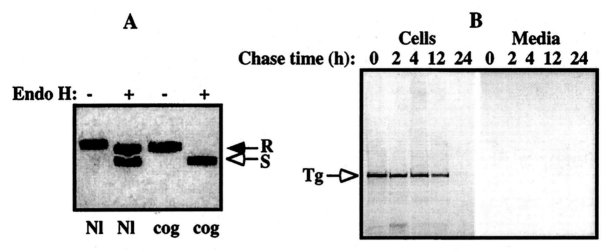

FIGURE 5.7. Thyroglobulin (Tg) glycans normally acquire resistance to digestion with endoglycosidase H upon exit from the endoplasmic reticulum, but defective Tg that does not migrate to the Golgi complex remains persistently endo H-sensitive. **A:** Newly synthesized Tg in normal *(Nl)* murine thyroid tissue comprises both post-Golgi, endo H-resistant Tg *(R)* and pre-Golgi, endo H-sensitive Tg *(S)*. In thyrocytes from *cog/cog* mice the newly synthesized Tg does not acquire endo H-resistance, being comprised entirely of endo H-sensitive molecules. **B:** Consistent with its inability to exit the endoplasmic reticulum, newly-synthesized Tg from *cog/cog* thyrocytes in primary culture disappears from the cells over a one-day period (by a process of endoplasmic reticulum–associated degradation) without being detectably secreted into the extracellular space. (From Kim PS, Hossain SA, Park YN, et al. A single amino acid change in the acetylcholinesterase-like domain of thyroglobulin causes congenital goiter with hypothyroidism in the *cog/cog* mouse: a model of human ER storage diseases. *Proc Natl Acad Sci U S A* 1998;95:9909, with permission).

that affects its folding, the Tg protein never acquires endo H-resistance (Fig. 5.7).

The biological functions of the aforementioned post-translational modifications of Tg glycans (or polypeptide) in the Golgi complex are not clear. One hypothesis is that carbohydrate modifications may control the intracellular targeting of Tg in later stages of the intracellular secretory or endocytotic pathways. For example, Tg that is secreted to the apical side of thyrocytes (i.e., the lumenal side) may have in some of its carbohydrate side chains the lysosomal recognition marker mannose-6-phosphate (143). If so, endocytotic degradation of Tg, which is essential for hormonogenesis, might be directed initially by the well-known mannose 6-phosphate receptors (144); however, this hypothesis has not been confirmed. A second hypothesis is that biosynthetic sulfation (or phosphorylation) of tyrosyl residues could alter the capacity of Tg for subsequent iodination and hormonogenesis (145,146). Such a view is not easily reconciled with the very low degree of tyrosine sulfation or phosphorylation in Tg (134), although, theoretically, these ions could be displaced from Tg at the time of iodination or coupling (147). There are other hypotheses (some described below), but the general view of these Golgi-type post-translational modifications is that they have further structural effects on Tg, such as facilitating multimerization (148), and surface charge effects that increase the solubility of Tg (48).

TSH clearly regulates the carbohydrate processing of Tg, affecting both the number of N-linked glycosylation sites that are initially utilized and the subsequent modifications of those glycans to a complex structure (135,149, 150). This may include an increase in the number of oligosaccharides bearing galactose and sialic acid, as well as alterations of sulfation. Perhaps the most interesting of these changes is in respect to the domain structure of Tg. Specifically, in region I (the first ~1200 amino acids) of bovine Tg there are 6 sequential N-linked glycans, and these bear complex or hybrid-type oligosaccharides (at positions 91, 464, 476, 835, 928, and 1121) (81). The situation appears essentially identical in human Tg (79). Thus, a TSH-stimulated increase in the number of complex oligosaccharide units is likely to have a more profound structural effect on the C-terminal half of the Tg molecule. Future studies should focus on the last two or three N-glycosylation sites of Tg [i.e., positions 2104 and 2277 of bovine Tg and positions 2275 and 2562 of human Tg, which are ordinarily high mannose units (79, 81)], because changes in glycosylation near the C-terminus of Tg might create structural alterations that would increase the exposure of the C-terminal iodination site and thereby help to account for the increase in production of T_3 that results from increased TSH secretion or the action of TSH receptor-stimulating antibodies in patients with Graves' thyrotoxicosis.

THYROGLOBULIN TRAFFICKING IN THE EXOCYTOTIC PATHWAY

Thyrocytes are highly polarized epithelial cells with distinct apical and basolateral regions (151). The secretion of newly synthesized proteins by these cells is directed to both regions (152,153), but Tg is transported almost completely through the apical region into the follicular lumen (154). The apical targeting and storage of Tg is known to go awry in Graves' disease, thyroiditis, and many thyroid cancers. Still, very little is known about the molecular mechanisms of sorting that allow for normal Tg targeting to the apical surface of the cells for iodination, even while other proteins are selectively targeted basolaterally (155–160). The apical secretory pathway of polarized epithelial cells may be created in the trans-Golgi network by the creation and merging (in the plane of the membrane) of lipid-protein microdomains known as rafts, which serve as a platform upon which apical secretory proteins can be ferried (161). These rafts are especially enriched in glycosphingolipids. Two key features of the rafts are that they are not solubilized at 4°C in the presence of 1% Triton X-100 (unlike other membranes as well as a large fraction of cellular proteins that are soluble in the presence of this non-ionic detergent), and because they are lipid-rich they rise to the top of a sucrose-flotation gradient. Several newly synthesized apical-plasma-membrane proteins are recovered in the raft fraction (162). The raft fraction has been used as a source of antigen to identify novel proteins that may be involved mechanistically in membrane transport to the apical cell surface. One such protein, VIP17 (163), also known as MAL (164), is a membrane protein whose expression in some epithelial cells is correlated with the efficiency of apical-plasma-membrane protein delivery (165). MAL is expressed in human thyrocytes both at the mRNA and protein level (where it is restricted to the apical zone of thyroid follicles), as well as in some thyroid-cell culture lines such as FRT, in which it is recovered in the raft fraction (166). These features raise the possibility of Tg transport via a raft pathway from the Golgi complex to the thyroid follicular lumen (163).

In PC Cl3 thyrocytes, the steady-state pool size of Tg in the Golgi complex or in post-Golgi compartments is small, as compared with that in the endoplasmic reticulum. Nevertheless, from the endo H-resistant Tg pool (i.e., Tg having passed through the Golgi complex), most is recovered in Triton X-100 insoluble rafts, in spite of the fact that secreted Tg is completely soluble in Triton X-100 (167). The endo H-resistant portion of recombinant Tg expressed in heterologous epithelial cells is also recovered in a raft fraction, and depletion of MAL from these cells inhibits apical secretion of Tg (168). These findings suggest that Tg may be actively selected for apical delivery by association with one or more other raft components. Although the mechanism of this selection is unknown, it

may be mediated by one or more novel lectins (169). One such lectin isolated from the raft fraction, known as VIP36, specifically binds N-acetylgalactosamine (170, 171), raising again the idea that carbohydrate modifications of Tg occurring in the Golgi could serve as recognition signals for post-Golgi protein trafficking. One potentially serious problem with this model is that treatment of thyrocytes with various inhibitors of carbohydrate processing (e.g., castanospermine) does not prevent the apical secretion of Tg (90,172). Additionally, several basolaterally secreted thyroid proteins also have N-linked glycans (55,160), and it remains to be proven that carbohydrate processing of these proteins in the Golgi is appreciably different from that of apically secreted glycoproteins.

The sheer abundance of Tg is likely to stoichiometrically overwhelm the expression level of any putative Tg sorting receptor for apical secretion. However, if Tg were to undergo higher-order self-assembly while still within the Golgi complex (which presently is merely speculation) (148), such a mechanistic problem might be circumvented. In fact, such a mechanism appears to exist in other peptide hormone-producing endocrine cells that must package high concentrations of a subset of newly synthesized protein products into secretory granules (173). Tg has certain features that suggest it might be incorporated into classical secretory granules, including the presence in thyrocytes of Tg secretory compartments that have been described as apical vesicles or secretory granules (174,175). In addition, Tg exocytosis is to some extent acutely stimulated by TSH both *in vivo* (176) and in primary thyrocyte cultures (156–158, 160,177). Moreover, in filter-polarized thyrocyte monolayers, certain heterologous (recombinant) peptide hormones are also secreted apically (153). The recent observations that an increasing number of classical secretory granule proteins also may utilize the raft mechanism for their Golgi-based sorting makes such a possibility plausible for Tg as well (172–182).

IODINATION AND IODOTYROSYL COUPLING WITHIN THYROGLOBULIN

After exocytosis, especially after stimulation with TSH (175,183), Tg that has fully matured within the secretory pathway undergoes iodination in the lumen of the thyroid follicles. It is nearly impossible to study iodination and hormonogenesis in human Tg *in vivo*. While this can be done *in vivo* in animals (especially rodents), there are likely to be differences in Tg structure (e.g., glycosylation) and iodination among different species. Normally (as described above), only a subset of the tyrosine residues of Tg becomes iodinated (184), and the fraction that is iodinated is further diminished in iodide-poor environments (see section on iodine deficiency in Chapter 11). It is important to understand how the iodination sites are selected, because it has long been recognized that iodination of Tg provides a much higher yield of the hormonally active iodothyronines, T_4 and T_3, than iodination of any other protein, and that most of the specificity of the iodination sites (and subsequent coupling to form iodothyronines) is somehow encoded in the structure of Tg itself (13).

While denatured Tg can be readily iodinated *in vitro*, it is no longer competent for hormonogenesis (185,186), indicating that there are stringent steric requirements within Tg that allow thyroid peroxidase to catalyze efficiently not only iodination but also formation of T_4 and T_3 from the iodotyrosyl residues (13). By contrast, T_4 and T_3 synthesis *in vitro* can be catalyzed not only by thyroid peroxidase but also by myeloperoxidase (187) and lactoperoxidase (188), although the efficiency of hormonogenesis and maintenance of the integrity of Tg structure varies with the conditions used. Provided certain critical domains of Tg are in the native state, iodination of isolated (iodine-poor) Tg *in vitro* probably provides a relatively faithful estimation of the iodotyrosyl selectivity that occurs *in vivo* (189). Using this methodology, efforts have been directed to explore the hypothesis that hormonogenic sites occur at limited and fixed positions in the Tg protein, involving discrete donor and acceptor sites that have relatively precise physical and spatial relationships. For identification of most sites of iodination and hormonogenesis, there has been good agreement between studies of Tg iodinated *in vivo* and *in vitro*. Site identification has rested largely on the sequencing of peptides after limited proteolytic digestion of Tg to find iodotyrosines and iodothyronines and their neighboring amino acids, in order to identify the iodopeptide location within the context of the complete Tg sequence. Because the coupling reaction involves iodophenyl transfer from a donor MIT or DIT residue to an acceptor DIT residue, this method is relatively straightforward for locating the acceptor residues, but it will not identify donor iodotyrosine residues. For donor residue identification, it is necessary to identify the dehydroalanine residues that remain within the polypeptide chain after transfer of the iodophenyl moiety to a DIT residue (190–194).

The conclusion of these studies is that, from the many tyrosines in the Tg molecule, three specific tyrosine residues located near the amino and carboxyl ends of the protein are the primary acceptor sites for hormonogenesis, including positions 5 ("site A"), 2554 ("site B") and 2747 ("site C") of human Tg, respectively (195). Site A (Tyr5) is the predominant hormonogenic site. It is the most conserved between species, the first to become iodinated in some species, and normally is reserved for formation of T_4 (196–201). Site B (Tyr2554) is the second most highly utilized site for T_4 formation, comprising one-fourth to one-fifth of the T_4 content of Tg (3). Site C (position 2747) tends to be favored for T_3 formation [with even greater pre-

dominance in certain rodent species (197)], although it may account for as much as one-seventh of T_4 formation in human Tg (3). In addition to these three sites there are four ancillary hormonogenic sites, termed sites "D" (position 1291), "G" (position 2568), "N" (position 685), and "R" (equivalent to position 632 although not present in human Tg) that may be favored in certain species under certain conditions, but which tend to be more variable than the three primary iodination sites (3).

The variability of specific tyrosine sites for iodination and hormonogenesis is likely to reflect at least three features: tyrosine exposure on the outer surface of Tg; the amino acids flanking the iodination sites, which may provide a biochemical basis favoring iodination and coupling; and the physical proximity of paired "donor" and "acceptor" iodotyrosines, thereby promoting the coupling reaction. It seems plausible that positioning tyrosines near the ends of the protein is likely to increase their surface exposure, although a definitive statement awaits three-dimensional structural analyses of Tg. As regards flanking information, *in vitro* iodination of human Tg reveals three patterns of neighboring amino acids that favor both early tyrosine iodination as well as T_4 formation: Asp/Glu-Tyr; Ser/Thr-Tyr-Ser; and Glu-X-Tyr (195). With respect to proximity of iodotyrosyl pairs, increasing evidence suggests that the donor sites may be closely positioned within the same regions of Tg as their paired acceptor sites (202). Evidence from *in vitro* iodination of full-length bovine Tg suggests that Tyr130 is an important outer ring donor for T_4 formation at Tyr5 (194). Although not completely physiological (203), coupling between Tyr5 and Tyr130 can also be achieved by *in vitro* iodination of a fragment containing only the first 171 residues of human Tg (192), which is facilitated by N-glycosylation in this domain (204). Mutagenic replacement of 4 of the 5 other tyrosines in the vicinity with phenylalanine (at positions 29, 89, 97, and 192) does not dminish the content of T_4 generated *in vitro* in such a fragment (205). T_4 formation has also been demonstrated in a fragment of rat Tg just large enough to encode iodination sites B and C (206). These findings increase the likelihood that the primary donor and acceptor tyrosine sites are near each other within the same monomer of the Tg homodimer.

THYROGLOBULIN ACTIVITY IN COLLOID BEFORE INTERNALIZATION INTO THYROCYTES

The state of the Tg in the colloid may vary, depending upon the levels of TSH and iodination (207–209). At the time of exocytosis, Tg is actively iodinated and hormone formation is occurring (210). The proximity of these newly completed Tg molecules to the surface of the apical plasma membrane makes them most readily available for endocytotic internalization. Especially with TSH stimulation (or in Graves' disease), the newly-secreted and iodinated molecules contribute maximally to the pool of iodinated Tg that provides most of the soon-to-be-secreted T_4 and T_3; this has come to be known as the "last come, first served" hypothesis (211,212).

Tg also undergoes further structural changes upon iodination and storage in colloid (213). As reviewed above, Tg initially forms noncovalently bound homodimers. To the extent that higher order noncovalent Tg complexes are formed (148), they tend to be quantitatively dissociated under the conditions of sample preparation used for the analysis of oligomerization of cellular Tg by sucrose gradient or native gel electrophoresis. Indeed, noncovalently bound Tg homodimers are relatively easily dissociated by heating, changes of ionic strength, or in the presence of increasing concentrations of various detergents. On the other hand, upon TSH stimulation of Tg secretion into colloid (214), and especially in conjunction with iodination, Tg dimers (215) and higher order oligomers (216) are stabilized. The stability of tetrameric Tg (27S by sucrose velocity gradient) is directly correlated with increasing iodine content (3). This could be due to direct structural modification of Tg by iodide, but more likely is due to secondary structural events within the oxidative environment of the colloid; specifically, interchain covalent cross linking primarily via disulfide bonds (49) and secondarily via N-epsilon-amino lysine cross linking (217) and formation of dityrosine bridges (218,219). Such iodide-rich, multimeric Tg is curiously devoid of T_4 and T_3 (220), possibly because hormone-rich iodopeptides have already been released from the remaining Tg protein by proteolysis (221). In any event, SDS-PAGE analysis of colloidal Tg under reducing conditions reveals the presence of many iodinated Tg fragments, including a variety of overlapping N-terminal fragments that include the primary "site A" for T_4 formation (189). The generation of these and other Tg fragments within the colloidal space has been attributed both to direct peptide bond cleavage during the oxidative process of iodination (221–223), as well as possible cleavage by secreted proteases (224–226) with discrete and distinct cleavage sites. Most of these cleavage fragments are likely to remain associated within the parent molecule under nonreduced conditions because of the extensive disulfide bonded structure of Tg.

THYROGLOBULIN BINDING AND INTERNALIZATION

Tg has the potential to interact with a number of additional proteins, not only within the endoplasmic reticulum but also in later compartments of the secretory pathway. Tg interacts with receptor proteins in the apical plasma membrane, followed by endocytotic internalization. In addition, there may be a sufficiently high concentration of soluble, newly iodinated Tg molecules that an ample number should be available for fluid-phase endocytosis, requiring no receptors, after which they are directed to lysosomes for complete proteolytic digestion, including liberation of T_4 and T_3 (227). In this case, the high-affinity apical receptors for Tg could be used for apical recycling of Tg, presumably for the purpose of increasing the ultimate efficiency of its iodination (228); for transcytosis to the basolateral (bloodstream) side of the cell (229) [a process which is less easily linked to normal thyroid hormonogenesis (230)]; or for selective uptake of a subset of colloidal Tg molecules en route to lysosomes (231). Given the very large size of Tg, it is not surprising that several peptides derived from the Tg molecule have the capability for binding to surface molecules of thyrocytes and other cells (232). The more difficult question is the physiological importance of such binding (233).

N-acetylglucosamine receptors (228,234,235) may be important in endocytotic routing of poorly-iodinated Tg molecules (236), although recently this notion was modified to suggest modulation or recognition of protein determinants on extracellular Tg (237) by the cell-surface protein disulfide isomerase (PDI) (238). Alternatively, cell-surface PDI-like activity might function in conjunction with the oxidizing environment of the follicular lumen to promote disulfide-linked multimerization of Tg (239); or extracellular PDI might (in conjunction with other extracellularly located chaperones) work oppositely, to solubilize multimeric colloidal Tg (240).

Megalin is another endocytotic receptor for Tg. Initially, it was was thought that megalin-mediated Tg endocytosis might be involved in thyroid hormone synthesis (241). Later studies suggested that Tg does not dissociate from megalin at the low pH of endosomes (242), but rather that megalin binding to Tg facilitates apical-to-basal transcytosis of Tg (243). Addition of receptor-associated protein (RAP) inhibits Tg binding to megalin (241), presumably by a direct interaction between RAP and Tg (244). Tg also contains short heparin-binding sequences, and heparin treatment inhibits Tg binding by megalin (245,246), which may signify a role for one or more heparan-sulfate proteoglycans in the internalization process (247). These experiments have been mostly conducted in cultures of rat thyroid FRTL5 cells, but megalin is expressed in normal thyroid tissue. In rats with aminotriazole-induced goiters, the thyroid content of megalin is increased, suggesting TSH-dependent regulation (243).

Tg binding to the surface of FRTL5 cells has been reported to alter the expression of several thyroid differentiation markers (248–250). This effect may be mediated by apical binding of Tg (251), specifically, via an apical version of the asialoglycoprotein receptor (252). Nevertheless, as Tg displays to the cell surface many potential binding sites, it is not clear whether this effect of Tg binding is actually restricted to this receptor, restricted to thyrocytes (253), or requires that Tg be present under native conditions (254). Overall, these studies are intriguing, but need to be pursued further to determine whether Tg is a physiological regulator of the expression of markers of thyroid differentiation *in vivo*.

PROTEOLYTIC DIGESTION OF THYROGLOBULIN IN THE ENDOSOME-LYSOSOME SYSTEM

Ultimately, Tg is exposed to cathepsins within lysosomes to liberate T_4 and T_3 from the Tg backbone. Early studies of the endocytotic degradation of Tg were done in collagenase-digested porcine thyroid follicles using [^{125}I]Tg (255). Although confounded by the possibility of Tg binding to the basolateral surface (256), Western blotting with anti-Tg of lysosomes isolated from the thyrocytes revealed slightly smaller-than-normal dimeric Tg which dissociated into fragments upon SDS-PAGE under reducing conditions (257), consistent with early limited proteolysis. Indeed, extracts of thyroid lysosomes can themselves generate such fragments from pure Tg (258). It is difficult to establish the fraction of such fragments that are generated before endocytosis (224,225) versus the fraction generated within the endosome-lysosome system, especially because lysosomes themselves may, under stimulation, undergo exocytosis (226).

In vitro analyses have established that cysteine proteinases mediate proteolytic processing of Tg (3). Individual Tg type 1 repeats are themselves substrates for lysosomal cysteine proteases (33), even as they may function as inhibitors of these enzymes (34). Studies in mice with genetic deficiency of various cathepsins (B, K, or L) have revealed impaired proteolysis of Tg in mice deficient for cathepsin B or cathepsin L, but not cathepsin K-deficient mice (259). Of particular interest, cathepsin K(-/-)/L(-/-) double-mutant mice had low serum free T_4 concentrations, suggesting that either or both of these enzymes may participate in liberation of T_4 from the Tg backbone.

ACKNOWLEDGEMENTS

The authors acknowledge funding from NIH DK40344 and from Ministero dellâ Université Ricerca Scientifica Grant No. 2002063745. The authors also thank Drs. E. Consiglio, S. Formisano, Y. N. Park, and P. Kim for helpful discussions and support.

REFERENCES

1. Spiro M. Synthesis and processing of thyroglobulin carbohydrate units. In: MC Eggo, GN Burrow, eds. *Thyroglobulin: the prothyroid hormone.* New York: Raven Press, 1985;103.
2. Mercken L, Simons MJ, Swillens S, et al. Primary structure of bovine thyroglobulin deduced from the sequence of its 8,431-base complementary DNA. *Nature* 1985;316:647.
3. Dunn JT, Dunn AD. Thyroglobulin: chemistry, biosynthesis, and proteolysis. In: LE Braverman, RD Utiger, eds. *Werner & Ingbar's the thyroid: a fundamental and clinical text.* Philadelphia: Lippincott Williams & Wilkins, 2000:91.
4. Brisson A, Marchelidon J, Lachiver F. Comparative studies on the amino acid composition of thyroglobulins from various lower and higher vertebrates: phylogenetic aspect. *Comp Biochem Physiol B Biochem Mol Biol* 1974;49:51.
5. Shepard TH. Development of the human fetal thyroid. *Gen Comp Endocrinol* 1968;10:174.
6. Yap AS, Stevenson BR, Keast JR, et al. Cadherin-mediated adhesion and apical membrane assembly define distinct steps during thyroid epithelial polarization and lumen formation. *Endocrinology* 1995;136:4672.
7. Alluchon-Gerard MJ. Morphogenese ultrastructurale et differenciation fonctionnelle du follicule thyroidien de la Rousette. *Arch Anat Microsc Morphol Exp* 1979;68:43.
8. Ericson L. Intracellular lumens in thyroid follicle cells of thyroxine-treated rats. *J Ultrastruct Res* 1979;69:297.
9. Nilsson M. Iodide handling by the thyroid epithelial cell. *Exp Clin Endocrinol Diabetes* 2001;109:13.
10. Suzuki S, Kondo Y. Demonstration of thyroglobulin-like iodinated proteins in the branchial sac of tunicates. *Gen Comp Endocrinol* 1971;17:402.
11. Thorndyke MC. Evidence for a 'mammalian' thyroglobulin in endostyle of the ascidian Styela clava. *Nature* 1978;271:61.
12. Suzuki S, Gorbman B, Rolland M, and et al. Thyroglobulins of cyclostomes and an elasmobranch. *Gen Comp Endocrinol* 1975;26:59.
13. Lissitzky S. Biosynthesis and secretion of thyroglobulin. *Ann Endocrinol (Paris)* 1981;42:363.
14. de Vijlder JJ, van Ommen GJ, van Voorthuizen WF, et al. Nonfunctional thyroglobulin messenger RNA in goats with hereditary congenital goiter. *J Mol Appl Genet* 1981;1:51.
15. Malthiery Y, Marriq C, Berge-Lefranc JL, et al. Thyroglobulin structure and function: recent advances. *Biochimie* 1989;71:195.
16. Mendive FM, Rivolta CM, Vassart G, et al. Genomic organization of the 3' region of the human thyroglobulin gene. *Thyroid* 1999;9:903.
17. Ieiri T, Cochaux P, Targovnik HM, et al. A 3' splice site mutation in the thyroglobulin gene responsible for congenital goiter with hypothyroidism. *J Clin Invest* 1991;88:1901.
18. Bertaux F, Noel M, Lasmoles F, et al. Identification of the exon structure and four alternative transcripts of the thyroglobulin-encoding gene. *Gene* 1995;156:297.
19. Targovnik HM, Rivolta CM, Mendive FM, et al. Congenital goiter with hypothyroidism caused by a 5' splice site mutation in the thyroglobulin gene. *Thyroid* 2001;11:685.
20. Graves PN, Davies TF. A second thyroglobulin messenger RNA species (rTg-2) in rat thyrocytes. *Mol Endocrinol* 1990;4:155.
21. van de Graaf SA, Ris-Stalpers C, Pauws E, et al. Up to date with human thyroglobulin. *J Endocrinol* 2001;170:307.
22. van de Graaf SA, Cammenga M, Ponne NJ, et al. The screening for mutations in the thyroglobulin cDNA from six patients with congenital hypothyroidism. *Biochimie* 1999;81:425.
23. Marians RC, Ng L, Blair HC, et al. Defining thyrotropin-dependent and -independent steps of thyroid hormone synthesis by using thyrotropin receptor-null mice. *Proc Natl Acad Sci U S A* 2002;99:15776.
24. Damante G, Tell G, Di Lauro R. A unique combination o f transcription factors controls differentiation of thyroid cells. *Prog Nucleic Acid Res Mol Biol* 2001;66:307.
25. Pasca di Magliano M, Di Lauro R, Zannini M. Pax8 has a key role in thyroid cell differentiation. *Proc Natl Acad Sci U S A* 2000;97:13144.
26. Mascia A, Nitsch L, Di Lauro R, et al. Hormonal control of the transcription factor Pax8 and its role in the regulation of thy-

roglobulin gene expression in thyroid cells. *J Endocrinol* 2002; 172:163.

27. Targovnik H, Propato F, Varela V, et al. Low levels of thyroglobulin messenger ribonucleic acid in congenital goitrous hypothyroidism with defective thyroglobulin synthesis. *J Clin Endocrinol Metab* 1989;69:1137.

28. Targovnik, HM, Medeiros-Neto G, Varela V, et al. A nonsense mutation causes human hereditary congenital goiter with preferential production of a 171-nucleotide-deleted thyroglobulin ribonucleic acid messenger. *J Clin Endocrinol Metab* 1993;77:210.

29. Gonzalez-Sarmiento R, Corral J, Mories MT, et al. Monoallelic deletion in the 5′ region of the thyroglobulin gene as a cause of sporadic nonendemic simple goiter. *Thyroid* 2001;11:789.

30. van de Graaf SA, Pauws E, de Vijlder JJ, et al. The revised 8307 base pair coding sequence of human thyroglobulin transiently expressed in eukaryotic cells. *Eur J Endocrinol* 1997;136:508.

31. Muresan Z, Arvan P. Thyroglobulin transport along the secretory pathway. Investigation of the role of molecular chaperone, GRP94, in protein export from the endoplasmic reticulum. *J Biol Chem* 1997;272:26095.

32. Berg G, Ekholm R. Electron microscopy of low iodinated thyroglobulin molecules. *Biochim Biophys Acta* 1975;386:422.

33. Pungercic G, Dolenc I, Dolinar M, et al. Individual recombinant thyroglobulin type-1 domains are substrates for lysosomal cysteine proteinases. *Biol Chem* 2002;383:1809.

34. Galesa K, Pain R, Jongsma MA, et al. Structural characterization of thyroglobulin type-1 domains of equistatin. *FEBS Lett* 2003;539:120.

35. Durkin ME, Chakravarti S, Bartos BB, et al. Amino acid sequence and domain structure of entactin. Homology with epidermal growth factor precursor and low density lipoprotein receptor. *J Cell Biol* 1988;107:2749.

36. Neumann GM, Bach LA. The N-terminal disulfide linkages of human insulin-like growth factor-binding protein-6 (hIGFBP-6) and hIGFBP-1 are different as determined by mass spectrometry. *J Biol Chem* 1999;274:14587.

37. Chong JM, Speicher DW. Determination of disulfide bond assignments and N-glycosylation sites of the human gastrointestinal carcinoma antigen GA733–2 (CO17–1A, EGP, KS1–4, KSA, and Ep-CAM). *J Biol Chem* 2001;276:5804.

38. Mercken L, Simons MJ, De Martynoff G, et al. Presence of hormonogenic and repetitive domains in the first 930 amino acids of bovine thyroglobulin as deduced from the cDNA sequence. *Eur J Biochem* 1985;147:59.

39. Guncar G, Pungercic G, Klemencic I, et al. Crystal structure of MHC class II-associated p41 Ii fragment bound to cathepsin L reveals the structural basis for differentiation between cathepsins L and S. *EMBO J* 1999;18:793.

40. Gentile F, Salvatore G. Preferential sites of proteolytic cleavage of bovine, human, and rat thyroglobulin. The use of limited proteolysis to detect solvent exposed regions of the primary structure. *Eur J Biochem* 1993;218:603.

41. Swillens S, Ludgate M, Mercken L, et al. Analysis of sequence and structure homologies between thyroglobulin and acetylcholinesterase: possible functional and clinical significance. *Biochem Biophys Res Commun* 1986;137:142.

42. Mori N, Itoh N, Salvaterra PM. Evolutionary origin of cholinergic macromolecules and thyroglobulin. *Proc Natl Acad Sci U S A* 1987;84:2813.

43. MacPhee-Quigley K, Vedvick TS, Taylor P, et al. Profile of the disulfide bonds in acetylcholinesterase. *J Biol Chem* 1986;261: 13565.

44. Di Jeso B, Ulianich L, Pacifico F, et al. The folding of thyroglobulin in the calnexin/calreticulin pathway and its alteration by a loss of Ca2+ from the endoplasmic reticulum. *Biochem J* 2003;370:449.

45. Veneziani BM, Giallauria F, Gentile F. The disulfide bond pattern between fragments obtained by the limited proteolysis of bovine thyroglobulin. *Biochimie* 1999;81:517.

46. Andreoli M, Sena L, Edelhoch H, et al. The noncovalent subunit structure of human thyroglobulin. *Arch Biochem Biophys* 1969;134:242.

47. Schneider AB, Bornet H, Edelhoch H. The effects of low temperature on the conformation of thyroglobulin. *J Biol Chem* 1971;246:2672.

48. Tarutani O, Kondo T, Shulman S. Properties of carbohydrate-stripped thyroglobulin. III. Solubility characteristics of thyroglobulin. *Biochim Biophys Acta* 1977;492:284.

49. Berndorfer U, Wilms H, Herzog V. Multimerization of thyroglobulin (TG) during extracellular storage: isolation of highly cross-linked TG from human thyroids. *J Clin Endorinol Metab* 1996;81:1918.

50. Stroud RM, Walter P. Signal sequence recognition and protein targeting. *Curr Opin Struct Biol* 1999;9:754.

51. Sanders SL, Whitfield KM, Vogel JP, et al. Sec61p and BiP directly facilitate polypeptide translocation into the ER. *Cell* 1992;69:353.

52. Rutkowski T, Lingappa VR. Membrane targeting of proteins. In: *Cell Biology* www.ergito.com. 2002, Chapter 2.

53. Huang XF, Arvan P. Intracellular transport of proinsulin in pancreatic b-cells: structural maturation probed by disulfide accessibility. *J Biol Chem* 1995;270:20417.

54. Kim PS, Arvan P. Folding and assembly of newly synthesized thyroglobulin occurs in a pre-Golgi compartment. *J Biol Chem* 1991;266:12412.

55. Prabakaran D, Kim PS, Dixit VM, et al. Oligomeric assembly of thrombospondin in the endoplasmic reticulum of thyroid epithelial cells. *Eur J Cell Biol* 1996;70:134.

56. Netzer WJ, Hartl FU. Recombination of protein domains facilitated by co-translational folding in eukaryotes. *Nature* 1997; 388:343.

57. Kim P, Bole D, Arvan P. Transient aggregation of nascent thyroglobulin in the endoplasmic reticulum: relationship to the molecular chaperone, BiP. *J Cell Biol* 1992;118:541.

58. Kim PS, Kim KR, Arvan P. Disulfide-linked aggregation of thyroglobulin normally occurs during nascent protein folding. *Am J Physiol* 1993;265:C704.

59. Mazzarella RA, Srinivasan M, Haugejorden SM, et al. ERp72, an abundant luminal endoplasmic reticulum protein, contains three copies of the active site sequences of protein disulfide isomerase. *J Biol Chem* 1990;265:1094.

60. Rupp K, Birnbach U, Lundstrom J, et al. Effects of CaBP2, the rat analog of ERp72, and of CaBP1 on the refolding of denatured reduced proteins. Comparison with protein disulfide isomerase. *J Biol Chem* 1994;269:2501.

61. Molinari M, Helenius A. Glycoproteins form mixed disulphides with oxidoreductases during folding in living cells. *Nature* 1999;402:90.

62. Anelli T, Alessio M, Mezghrani A, et al. ERp44, a novel endoplasmic reticulum folding assistant of the thioredoxin family. *EMBO J* 2002;21:835.

63. Munro S, Pelham HR. An hsp70-like protein in the ER: identity with the 78kd glucose-regulated protein and immunoglobulin heavy chain binding protein. *Cell* 1986;46:291.

64. Kim PS, Arvan P. Hormonal regulation of thyroglobulin export from the endoplasmic reticulum of cultured thyrocytes. *J Biol Chem* 1993;268:4873.

65. Kim PS, Arvan P. Calnexin and BiP act as sequential molecular chaperones during thyroglobulin folding in the endoplasmic reticulum. *J Cell Biol* 1995;128:29.

66. Nigam SK, Goldberg AL, Ho S, et al. A set of endoplasmic reticulum proteins possessing properties of molecular chaper-

ones includes Ca2+ binding proteins and members of the thio-redoxin superfamily. *J Biol Chem* 1994;269:1744.

67. Kuznetsov G, Chen LB, Nigam SK. Several endoplasmic reticulum stress proteins, including ERp72, interact with thyroglobulin during its maturation. *J Biol Chem* 1994;269:22990.

68. Kuznetsov G, Bush KT, Zhang PL, et al. Perturbations in maturation of secretory proteins and their association with endoplasmic reticulum chaperones in a cell culture model for epithelial ischemia. *Proc Natl Acad Sci U S A* 1996;93:8584.

69. Kuznetsov G, Chen LB, Nigam SK. Multiple molecular chaperones complex with misfolded large oligomeric glycoproteins in the endoplasmic reticulum. *J Biol Chem* 1997;272:3057.

70. Kaufman RJ, Scheuner D, Schroder M, et al. The unfolded protein response in nutrient sensing and differentiation. *Nat Rev Mol Cell Biol* 2002;3:411.

71. Spiro RG, Spiro MJ, Bhoyroo VD. Studies on the regulation of the biosynthesis of glucose-containing oligosaccharide-lipids. *J Biol Chem* 1983;258:9469.

72. Lee AS. Mammalian stress response: induction of the glucose-regulated protein family. *Curr Opin Cell Biol* 1992;4:267.

73. Leonardi A, Vito P, Mauro C, et al. Endoplasmic reticulum stress causes thyroglobulin retention in this organelle and triggers activation of nuclear factor-kappa B via tumor necrosis factor receptor-associated factor 2. *Endocrinology* 2002;143:2169.

74. Muresan Z, Arvan P. Enhanced binding of the molecular chaperone, BiP, slows thyroglobulin export from the endoplasmic reticulum. *Mol Endocrinol* 1998;12:458.

75. Rose MD, Misra LM, Vogel JP. KAR2, a karyogamy gene, is the yeast homolog of the mammalian BiP/GRP78 gene. *Cell* 1989;57:1211.

76. Kaufman RJ. Orchestrating the unfolded protein response in health and disease. *J Clin Invest* 2002;110:1389.

77. Harding HP, Calfon M, Urano F, et al. Transcriptional and translational control in the mammalian unfolded protein response. *Annu Rev Cell Dev Biol* 2002;18:575.

78. Sargsyan E, Baryshev M, Szekely L, et al. Identification of ERp29, an endoplasmic reticulum lumenal protein, as a new member of the thyroglobulin folding complex. *J Biol Chem* 2002;277:17009.

79. Yang SX, Pollock HJ, Rawitch AB. Glycosylation in human thyroglobulin: location of the N-linked oligosaccharide units and comparison with bovine thyroglobulin. *Arch Biochem Biophys* 1996;327:61.

80. Franc JL, Mallet B, Lanet J, et al. The number of oligosaccharides borne by porcine thyroglobulin is variable. *Endocrinology* 1994;134:885.

81. Rawitch AB, Pollock HG, Yang SX. Thyroglobulin glycosylation: location and nature of the N-linked oligosaccharide units in bovine thyroglobulin. *Arch Biochem Biophys* 1993;300:271.

82. Helenius A, Trombetta ES, Hebert DN, et al. Calnexin, calreticulin and the folding of glycoproteins. *Trends Cell Biol* 1997;7:193.

83. Wada I, Imai S, Kai M, et al. Chaperone function of calreticulin when expressed in the endoplasmic reticulum as the membrane-anchored and soluble forms. *J Biol Chem* 1995;270:20298.

84. Parodi AJ, Mendelzon DH, Lederkremer GZ. Transient glucosylation of protein-bound Man9GlcNAc2, Man8GlcNAc2, and Man7GlcNAc2 in calf thyroid cells. A possible recognition signal in the processing of glycoproteins. *J Biol Chem* 1983;258:8260.

85. Trombetta SE, Ganan SA, Parodi AJ. The UDP-Glc-glycoprotein glucosyltransferase is a soluble protein of the endoplasmic reticulum. *Glycobiology* 1991;1:155.

86. Sousa MC, Ferrero-Garcia MA, Parodi AJ. Recognition of the oligosaccharide and protein moieties of glycoproteins by the UDP-Glc:glycoprotein glucosyltransferase. *Biochemistry* 1992;31:97.

87. Sousa M, Parodi AJ. The molecular basis for the recognition of misfolded glycoproteins by the UDP-Glc:glycoprotein glucosyltransferase. *EMBO J* 1995;14:4196.

88. Chen W, Helenius J, Braakman I, et al. Cotranslational folding and calnexin binding during glycoprotein synthesis. *Proc Natl Acad Sci U S A* 1995;92:6229.

89. Oliver JD, van der Wal FJ, Bulleid NJ, et al. Interaction of the thiol-dependent reductase ERp57 with nascent glycoproteins. *Science* 1997;275:86.

90. Franc JL, Giraud A, Lanet J. Effects of deoxymannojirimycin and castanospermine on the polarized secretion of thyroglobulin. *Endocrinology* 1990;126:1464.

91. Di Jeso B, Pereira R, Consiglio E, et al. Demonstration of a Ca2+ requirement for thyroglobulin dimerization and export to the Golgi complex. *Eur J Biochem* 1998;252:583.

92. Eggo MC, Burrow GN. Glycosylation of thyroglobulin—its role in secretion, iodination, and stability. *Endocrinology* 1983;113:1655.

93. Mallet B, Lejeune PJ, Baudry N, et al. N-glycans modulate in vivo and in vitro thyroid hormone synthesis. Study at the N-terminal domain of thyroglobulin. *J Biol Chem* 1995;270:29881.

94. Formisano S, Di Jeso B, Acquaviva R, et al. Calcium-induced changes in thyroglobulin conformation. *Arch Biochem Biophys* 1983;227:351.

95. Choudhury P, Liu Y, Bick RJ, et al. Intracellular association between UDP-glucose:glycoprotein glucosyltransferase and an incompletely folded variant of alpha1-antitrypsin. *J Biol Chem* 1997;272:13446.

96. Di Jeso B, Formisano S, Ulianich L. Perturbation of cellular calcium delays the secretion and alters the glycosylation of thyroglobulin in FRTL-5 cells. *Biochem Biophys Res Commun* 1997;234:133.

97. Di Jeso B, Formisano S, Consiglio E. Depletion of divalent cations within the secretory pathway inhibits the terminal glycosylation of complex carbohydrates of thyroglobulin. *Biochimie* 1999;81:497.

98. Riesco G, Bernal J, Sanchez-Franco F. Thyroglobulin defect in a human congenital goiter. *J Clin Endocrinol Metab* 1974;38:33.

99. Monaco F, Grimaldi S, Dominici R, et al. Defective thyroglobulin synthesis in an experimental rat thyroid tumor: iodination and thyroid hormone synthesis in isolated tumor thyroglobulin. *Endocrinology* 1975;97:347

100. Michel-Bechet M, Cotte G, Codaccioni JL, et al. Ultrastructure thyroidienne et perturbations biochimiques de l'hormonogenese. *Acta Anat (Basel)* 1969;73:389.

101. Medeiros-Neto G, Targovnik H, Knobel M, et al. Qualitative and quantitative defects of thyroglobulin resulting in congenital goiter. Absence of gross gene deletion of coding sequences in the TG gene structure. *J Endocrinol Invest* 1989;12:805.

102. Medeiros-Neto G, Kim PDS, Yoo SE, et al. Congenital hypothyroid goiter with deficient thyroglobulin. Identification of an endoplasmic reticulum storage disease (ERSD) with induction of molecular chaperones. *J Clin Invest* 1996;98:2838.

103. Lissitzky S, Torresani J, Burrow GN, et al. Defective thyroglobulin export as a cause of congenital goiter. *Clin Endocrinol (Oxf)* 1975;4:363.

104. Baas F, Bikker H, van Ommen GJ, et al. Unusual scarcity of restriction site polymorphism in the human thyroglobulin gene. A linkage study suggesting autosomal dominance of a defective thyroglobulin allele. *Hum Genet* 1984;67:301.

105. Cabrer B, Brocas H, Perez-Castillo A, et al. Normal level of thyroglobulin messenger ribonucleic acid in a human congenital goiter with thyroglobulin deficiency. *J Clin Endocrinol Metab* 1986;63:931.

106. Ricketts MH, Simons MJ, Parma J, et al. A nonsense mutation causes hereditary goitre in the Afrikander cattle and unmasks alternative splicing of thyroglobulin transcripts. *Proc Natl Acad Sci U S A* 1987;84:3181.

107. Sugisaki T, Beamer WG, Noguchi T. Microcephalic cerebrum with hypomyelination in the congenital goiter mouse (cog). *Neurochem Res* 1992;17:1037.

108. Adkison LR, Taylor S, Beamer WG. Mutant gene-induced disorders of structure, function and thyroglobulin synthesis in congenital goitre (cog/cog) in mice. *J Endocrinol* 1990;126: 51.

109. Basche M, Beamer WG, Schneider AB. Abnormal properties of thyroglobulin in mice with inherited congenital goiter (cog/cog). *Endocrinology* 1989;124:1822.

110. Fogelfeld L, Harel G, Beamer WG, et al. Low-molecular-weight iodoproteins in the congenital goiters of cog/cog mice. *Thyroid* 1992;2:329.

111. Kim PS, Kwon OY, Arvan P. An endoplasmic reticulum storage disease causing congenital goiter with hypothyroidism. *J Cell Biol* 1996;133:517.

112. Kim PS, Hossain SA, Park YN, et al. A single amino acid change in the acetylcholinesterase-like domain of thyroglobulin causes congenital goiter with hypothyroidism in the cog/cog mouse: a model of human ER storage diseases. *Proc Natl Acad Sci U S A* 1998;95:9909.

112A. Tokunaga F, Brostrom C, Kiode T, et al. Endoplasmic reticulum (ER)-associated degradation of misfolded N-linked glycoproteins is suppressed upon inhibition of ER mannosidase I. *J Biol Chem* 2000;275:40757.

113. Hosokawa N, Wada I, Hasegawa K, et al. A novel ER alpha-mannosidase-like protein accelerates ER-associated degradation. *EMBO Rep* 2001;2:415.

114. Koto M, Sato T, Okamoto M, et al. rdw rats; a new hereditary dwarf model in the rat. *Jikken Dobutsu* 1988;37:21.

115. Umezu M, Fujimura T, Sugawara S, et al. Pituitary and serum levels of prolactin (PRL), thyroid stimulating hormone (TSH) and serum thyroxine (T4) in hereditary dwarf rats (rdw/rdw). *Jikken Dobutsu* 1993;42:211.

116. Ono M, Harigai T, Furudate S. Pituitary-specific transcription factor Pit-1 in the rdw rat with growth hormone- and prolactin-deficient dwarfism. *J Endocrinol* 1994;143:479.

117. Umezu M, Kagabu S, Jiang J, et al. Evaluation and characterization of congenital hypothyroidism in rdw dwarf rats. *Lab Anim Sci* 1998;48:496.

118. Sakai Y, Yamashina S, Furudate SI. Missing secretory granules, dilated endoplasmic reticulum, and nuclear dislocation in the thyroid gland of rdw rats with hereditary dwarfism. *Anat Rec* 2000;259:60.

119. Oh-Ishi M, Omori A, Kwon JY, et al. Detection and identification of proteins related to the hereditary dwarfism of the rdw rat. *Endocrinology* 1998;139:1288.

120. Hishinuma A, Furudate S, Oh-Ishi M, et al. A novel missense mutation (G2320R) in thyroglobulin causes hypothyroidism in rdw rats. *Endocrinology* 2000;141:4050.

121. Kim PS, Ding M, Menon S, et al. A missense mutation G2320R in the thyroglobulin gene causes non-goitrous congenital primary hypothyroidism in the WIC-rdw rat. *Mol Endocrinol* 2000;14:1944.

122. Kim PS, Arvan P. Endocrinopathies in the family of endoplasmic reticulum (ER) storage diseases: disorders of protein trafficking and the role of ER molecular chaperones. *Endocr Rev* 1998;19:173.

123. Caron P, Moya CM, Malet D, et al. Compound heterozygous mutations in the thyroglobulin gene (1143delC and 6725G—>A [R2223H]) resulting in fetal goitrous hypothyroidism. *J Clin Endocrinol Metab* 2003;88:3546.

124. Hishinuma A, Kasai K, Masawa N, et al. Missense mutation (C1263R) in the thyroglobulin gene causes congenital goiter with mild hypothyroidism by impaired intracellular transport. *Endocr J* 1998;45:315.

125. Ohyama Y, Hosoya T, Kameya T, et al. Congenital euthyroid goitre with impaired thyroglobulin transport. *Clin Endocrinol (Oxf)* 1994;41:129.

126. Corral J, Martin C, Perez R, et al. Thyroglobulin gene point mutation associated with non-endemic simple goitre. *Lancet* 1993;341:462.

127. Perez-Centeno C, Gonzalez-Sarmiento R, Mories MT, et al. Thyroglobulin exon 10 gene point mutation in a patient with endemic goiter. *Thyroid* 1996;6:423.

128. Hishinuma A, Takamatsum J, Ohyama Y, et al. Two novel cysteine substitutions (C1263R and C1995S) of thyroglobulin cause a defect in intracellular transport of thyroglobulin in patients with congenital goiter and the variant type of adenomatous goiter. *J Clin Endocrinol Metab* 1999;84:1438.

129. Ronin C, Fenouillet E, Hovsepian S, et al. Biosynthesis of thyroglobulin carbohydrate chains. In: Eggo MC, Burrow GN, eds. *Thyroglobulin: the prothyroid hormone.* New York: Raven Press, 1985:95.

130. Zuber C, Spiro MJ, Guhl B, et al. Golgi apparatus immunolocalization of endomannosidase suggests post-endoplasmic reticulum glucose trimming: implications for quality control. *Mol Biol Cell* 2000;11:4227.

131. Arima T, Spiro MJ, Spiro RG. Studies on the carbohydrate units of thyroglobulin. *J Biol Chem* 1972;247:1825.

132. Yamamoto K, Tsuji T, Irimura T, et al. The structure of carbohydrate unit B of porcine thyroglobulin. *Biochem J* 1981;195: 701.

133. Grollman EF, Saji M, Shimura Y, et al. Thyrotropin regulation of sialic acid expression in rat thyroid cells. *J Biol Chem* 1993;268:3604.

134. Spiro MJ, Spiro RG. Biosynthesis of sulfated asparagine-linked complex carbohydrate units of calf thyroglobulin. *Endocrinology* 1988;123:56.

135. Desruisseau S, Franc JL, Gruffat D, et al. Glycosylation of thyroglobulin secreted by porcine cells cultured in chamber system: thyrotropin controls the number of oligosaccharides and their anionic residues. *Endocrinology* 1994;134:1676.

136. Consiglio E, Acquaviva AM, Formisano S, et al. Characterization of phosphate residues on thyroglobulin. *J Biol Chem* 1987;262:10304.

137. Sakurai S, Fogelfeld L, Ries A, et al. Anionic complex-carbohydrate units of human thyroglobulin. *Endocrinology* 1990;127: 2056.

138. Herzog V. Secretion of sulfated thyroglobulin. *Eur J Cell Biol* 1986;39:399.

139. Spiro M J, Gorski KM. Studies on the posttranslational migration and processing of thyroglobulin: use of inhibitors and evaluation of the role of phosphorylation. *Endocrinology* 1986; 119:1146.

140. Schneider AB, McCurdy A, Chang T, et al. Metabolic labeling of human thyroglobulin with [^{35}S]sulfate: incorporation into chrondroitin 6-sulfate and endoglycosidase-F-susceptible carbohydrate units. *Endocrinology* 1988;122:2428.

141. Fogelfeld L, Schneider AB. Inhibition of chondroitin sulfate incorporation into human thyroglobulin by p-nitrophenyl-b-D-xylopyranoside. *Endocrinology* 1990;126:1064.

142. Baeuerle PA, Huttner WB. Tyrosine sulfation is a trans-Golgi-specific protein modification. *J Cell Biol* 1987;105:2655.

143. Herzog V, Neumuller W, Holzmann B. Thyroglobulin, the major and obligatory exportable protein of thyroid follicle cells, carries the lysosomal recognition marker mannose-6-phosphate. *EMBO J* 1987;6:555.

144. Kasper D, Dittmer F, von Figura K, et al. Neither type of mannose 6-phosphate receptor is sufficient for targeting of lysosomal enzymes along intracellular routes. *J Cell Biol* 1996;134: 6150623.

145. Nlend MC, Cauvi D, Venot N, et al. Sulfated tyrosines of thyroglobulin are involved in thyroid hormone synthesis. *Biochem Biophys Res Commun* 1999;262:193.

146. Nlend MC, Cauvi D, Venot N, et al. Thyrotropin regulates tyrosine sulfation of thyroglobulin. *Eur J Endocrinol* 1999;141: 61.

147. Venot N, Nlend MC, Cauvi D, et al. The hormonogenic tyrosine 5 of porcine thyroglobulin is sulfated. *Biochem Biophys Res Commun* 2002;298:193.

148. Shifrin S, Consiglio E, Kohn LD. Effect of the complex carbohydrate moiety on the structure of thyroglobulin. *J Biol Chem* 1983;258:3780.

149. Ronin C, Fenouillet E, Hovsepian S, et al. Regulation of thyroglobulin glycosylation. *J Biol Chem* 1986;261:7287.

150. Di Jeso B, Liguoro D, Ferranti P, et al. Modulation of the carbohydrate moiety of thyroglobulin by thyrotropin and calcium in Fisher rat thyroid line-5 cells. *J Biol Chem* 1992;267:1938.

151. Chambard M, Verrier B, Gabrion J, et al. Polarization of thyroid cells in culture: evidence for the basolateral localization of the iodide "pump" and of the thyroid-stimulating hormone receptor-adenyl cyclase complex. *J Cell Biol* 1983;96:1172.

152. Mauchamp J, Chambard M, Verrier B, et al. Epithelial cell polarization in culture: orientation of cell polarity and expression of specific functions, studied with cultured thyroid cells. *J Cell Sci Suppl* 1987;8:345.

153. Prabakaran D, Ahima RS, Harney JW, et al. Polarized targeting of epithelial cell proteins in thyrocytes and MDCK cells. *J Cell Sci* 1999;112:1247.

154. Bjorkman U, Ekholm R, Elmqvist LG, et al. Induced unidirectional transport of protein into the thyroid follicular lumen. *Endocrinology* 1974;95:1506.

155. Ericson LE. Exocytosis and endocytosis in the thyroid follicle cells. *Mol Cell Endocrinol* 1981;22:1.

156. Chambard M, Mauchamp J, Chabaud O. Synthesis and apical and basolateral secretion of thyroglobulin by thyroid cell monolayers on permeable substrate: modulation by thyrotropin. *J Cell Physiol* 1987;133:37.

157. Chambard M, Depetris D, Gruffat D, et al. Thyrotrophin regulation of apical and basal exocytosis of thyroglobulin by porcine thyroid monolayers. *J Mol Endocrinol* 1990;4:193.

158. Arvan P, Lee J. Regulated and constitutive protein targeting can be distinguished by secretory polarity in thyroid epithelial cells. *J Cell Biol* 1991;112:365.

159. Desruisseau-Gonzalvez S, Delori P, Gruffat D, et al. Polarized secretion of tissue-plasminogen activator in cultured thyroid cells. *Vitro Cell Dev Biol-Animal* 1993;29:161.

160. Prabakaran D, Kim PS, Kim KR, et al. Polarized secretion of thrombospondin is opposite to thyroglobulin in thyroid epithelial cells. *J Biol Chem* 1993;268:9041.

161. Scheiffele P, Roth MG, Simons K. Interaction of influenza virus haemagglutinin with sphingolipid-cholesterol membrane domains via its transmembrane domain. *EMBO J* 1997;16: 5501.

162. Danielsen EM. Involvement of detergent-insoluble complexes in the intracellular transport of intestinal brush border enzymes. *Biochemistry* 1995;34:1596.

163. Cheong KH, Zacchetti D, Schneeberger EE, et al VIP17/ MAL, a lipid raft-associated protein, is involved in apical transport in MDCK cells. *Proc Natl Acad Sci U S A* 1999;96: 6241.

164. Puertollano R, Alonso MA. MAL, an integral element of the apical sorting machinery, is an itinerant protein that cycles between the trans-Golgi network and the plasma membrane. *Mol Biol Cell* 1999;10:3435.

165. Puertollano R, Martin-Belmonte F, Millan J, et al. The MAL proteolipid is necessary for normal apical transport and accurate sorting of the influenza virus hemagglutinin in Madin-Darby canine kidney cells. *J Cell Biol* 1999;145:141.

166. Martin-Belmonte F, Kremer L, Albar JP, et al. Expression of the MAL gene in the thyroid: the MAL proteolipid, a component of glycolipid-enriched membranes, is apically distributed in thyroid follicles. *Endocrinology* 1998;139:2077.

167. Martin-Belmonte F, Alonso MA, Zhang X, et al. Thyroglobulin is selected as luminal protein cargo for apical transport via detergent-resistant membranes in epithelial cells. *J Biol Chem* 2000;275:41074.

168. Martin-Belmonte F, Arvan P, Alonso MA. MAL mediates apical transport of secretory proteins in polarized epithelial Madin-Darby canine kidney cells. *J Biol Chem* 2001;276: 49337.

169. Scheiffele P, Peranen J, Simons K. N-glycans as apical sorting signals in epithelial cells. *Nature* 1995;378:96.

170. Fiedler K, Parton RG, Kellner R, et al. VIP36, a novel component of glycolipid rafts and exocytic carrier vesicles in epithelial cells. *EMBO J* 1994;13:1729.

171. Fiedler K, Simons K. Characterization of VIP36, an animal lectin homologous to leguminous lectins. *J Cell Sci* 1996;109:271.

172. Franc JL, Hovsepian S, Fayet G, et al. Inhibition of N-linked oligosaccharide processing does not prevent the secretion of thyrogloblulin. A study with swainsonine and deoxynojirimicin. *Eur J Biochem* 1986;157:225.

173. Arvan P, Zhang BY, Feng L, et al. Lumenal protein multimerization in the distal secretory pathway/secretory granule. *Curr Opin Cell Biol* 2002;14:448.

174. Novikoff AB, Novikoff PM, Ma M, et al. Cytochemical studies of secretory and other granules associated with the endoplasmic reticulum in rat thyroid epithelial cells. In: Ceccarelli B, Clementi F, Meldolesi J, eds. *Advances in cytopharmacology.* New York: Raven Press, 1974:349.

175. Bjorkman U, Ekholm R, Ericson LE. Effects of thyrotropin on thyroglobulin exocytosis and iodination in the rat thyroid gland. *Endocrinology* 1978;102:460.

176. Yi X, Yamamoto K, Shu L, et al. Effects of propyithiouracil (ptu) administration on the synthesis and secretion of thyroglobulin in the rat thyroid gland: a quantitative immunoelectron microscopic study using immunogold technique. *Endocr Path* 1997;8:315.

177. Desruisseau S, Alquier C, Depetris D, et al. Hormonal regulation of some steps of thyroglobulin synthesis and secretion in bicameral cell culture. *J Cell Physiol* 1994;160:336.

178. Dhanvantari S, Loh YP. Lipid raft association of carboxypeptidase E is necessary for its function as a regulated secretory pathway sorting receptor. *J Biol Chem* 2000;275:29887.

179. Blazquez M, Thiele C, Huttner WB, et al. Involvement of the membrane lipid bilayer in sorting prohormone convertase 2 into the regulated secretory pathway. *Biochem J* 2000;349:843.

180. Blazquez M, Docherty, Shennan KI. Association of prohormone convertase 3 with membrane lipid rafts. *J Mol Endocrinol* 2001;27:107.

181. Schmidt K, Schrader M, Kern HF, et al. Regulated apical secretion of zymogens in rat pancreas. Involvement of the glycosylphosphatidylinositol-anchored glycoprotein GP-2, the lectin ZG16p, and cholesterol-glycosphingolipid-enriched microdomains. *J Biol Chem* 2001;276:14315.

182. Zhang CF, Dhanvantari S, Lou H, et al. Sorting of carboxypeptidase E to the regulated secretory pathway requires interaction of its transmembrane domain with lipid rafts. *Biochem J* 2003; 369:453.

183. Bjorkman U, Ekholm R. Accelerated exocytosis and H_2O_2 generation in isolated thyroid follicles enhance protein iodination. *Endocrinology* 1988;122:488.

184. Dunn JT. The amino acid neighbors of thyroxine in thyroglobulin. *J Biol Chem* 1970;245:5954.

185. Turakulov I, Saatov T, Babaev TA, et al. Synthesis of iodoamino acids during in vitro thyroglobulin iodination in different states of its molecule. *Biokhimiia* 1976;41:1004.

186. Maurizis JC, Marriq C, Rolland M, et al. Thyroid hormone synthesis and reactivity of hormone-forming tyrosine residues of thyroglobulin. *FEBS Lett* 1981;132:29.

187. Taurog A, Dorris ML. Myeloperoxidase-catalyzed iodination and coupling. *Arch Biochem Biophys* 1992;296:239.

188. Magnusson RP, Taurog A, Dorris ML. Mechanism of thyroid peroxidase- and lactoperoxidase-catalyzed reactions involving iodide. *J Biol Chem* 1984;259:13783.

189. Dunn JT, Kim PS, Dunn AD. Favored sites for thyroid hormone formation on the peptide chains of human thyroglobulins. *J Biol Chem* 1982;257:88.

190. Palumbo G. Thyroid hormonogenesis. Identification of a sequence containing iodophenyl donor site(s) in calf thyroglobulin. *J Biol Chem* 1987;262:17182.

191. Ohmiya Y, Hayashi H, Kondo T, et al. Location of dehydroalanine residues in the amino acid sequence of bovine thyroglobulin. *J Biol Chem* 1990;265:9066.

192. Marriq C, Lejeune PJ, Venot N, et al. Hormone formation in the isolated fragment 1–171 of human thyroglobulin involves the couple tyrosine 5 and tyrosine 130. *Mol Cell Endocrinol* 1991;81:155.

193. Gentile F, Ferranti P, Mamone G, et al. Identification of hormonogenic tyrosines in fragment 1218–1591 of bovine thyroglobulin by mass spectrometry. *J Biol Chem* 1997;272:639.

194. Dunn AD, Corsi CM, Myers HE, et al. Tyrosine 130 is an important outer ring donor for thyroxine formation in thyroglobulin. *J Biol Chem* 1998;273:25223.

195. Dunn JT, Dunn AD. The importance of thyroglobulin structure for thyroid hormone biosynthesis. *Biochimie* 1999;81:505.

196. Dunn JT, Anderson PC, Fox JW, et al. The sites of thyroid hormone formation in rabbit thyroglobulin. *J Biol Chem* 1987; 262:16948.

197. Fassler CA, Dunn JT, Anderson PC, et al. Thyrotropin alters the utilization of thyroglobulin's hormonogenic sites. *J Biol Chem* 1988;263:17366.

198. Gavaret JM, Deme D, Nunez J, et al. Sequential reactivity of tyrosyl residues of thyroglobulin upon iodination catalyzed by thyroid peroxidase. *J Biol Chem* 1977;252:3281.

199. Palumbo G, Gentile F, Condorelli GL, et al. The earliest site of iodination in thyroglobulin is residue number 5. *J Biol Chem* 1990;265:8887.

200. Rawitch AB, Chernoff SB, Litwer MR, et al. Thyroglobulin structure-function. The amino acid sequence surrounding thyroxine. *J Biol Chem* 1983;258:2079.

201. Rawitch AB, Litwer MR, Gregg J, et al. The isolation of identical thyroxine containing amino acid sequences from bovine, ovine and porcine thyroglobulins. *Biochem Biophys Res Comm* 1984;118:423.

202. Erregragui K, Prato S, Miquelis R, et al. Antigenic mapping of human thyroglobulin–topographic relationship between antigenic regions and functional domains. *Eur J Biochem* 1997;244:801.

203. Xiao S, Pollock HG, Taurog A, et al. Characterization of hormonogenic sites in an N-terminal, cyanogen bromide fragment of human thyroglobulin. *Arch Biochem Biophys* 1995;320:96.

204. Baudry N, Lejeune PJ, Niccoli P, et al. Dityrosine bridge formation and thyroid hormone synthesis are tightly linked and are both dependent on N-glycans. *FEBS Lett* 1996;396:223.

205. den Hartog MT, Sijmons CC, Bakker O, et al. Importance of the content and localization of tyrosine residues for thyroxine formation within the N-terminal part of human thyroglobulin. *Eur J Endocrinol* 1995;132:611.

206. Asuncion M, Ingrassia R, Escribano J, et al. Efficient thyroid hormone formation by in vitro iodination of a segment of rat thyroglobulin fused to Staphylococcal protein A. *FEBS Lett* 1992;297:266.

207. Anderberg B, Enestrom S, Gillquist J, et al. Protein composition in single follicles, homogenates and fine-needle aspiration biopsies from normal and diseased human thyroid. *Acta Endocrinol (Copenh)* 1981;96:328.

208. Smeds S. On the distribution of thyroglobin and larger iodoproteins in single rat thyroid follicles. *Pflugers Arch* 1977; 372:145.

209. Smeds S, Anderberg B. Change of the protein composition of the thyroid colloid during treatment with propylthiouracil and thyroxine: a microgel electrophoretic study of single rat thyroid follicles. *Biochim Biophys Acta* 1978;542:47.

210. Ekholm R. Biosynthesis of thyroid hormones. *Int Rev Cytol* 1990;120:243.

211. Schneider PB. Thyroidal iodine heterogeneity: "last come, first served" system of iodine turnover. *Endocrinology* 1964; 74:973.

212. Matsukawa S, Hosoya T. Process of iodination of thyroglobulin and its maturation. II. Properties and distribution of thyroglobulin labeled in vitro or in vivo with radioiodine, 3H-tyrosine, or 3H-galactose in rat thyroid glands. *J Biochem (Tokyo)* 1979;86:199.

213. Saboori AM, Rose NR, Bresler HS, et al. Iodination of human thyroglobulin (Tg) alters its immunoreactivity. I. Iodination alters multiple epitopes of human Tg. *Clin Exp Immunol* 1998; 113:297.

214. Dunn JT, Ray SC. Changes in thyroglobulin structure after TSH administration. *J Biol Chem* 1975;250:5801.

215. Matsukawa S, Hosoya T. Process of iodination of thyroglobulin and its maturation. I. Properties and distribution of thyroglobulin labeled with radioiodine in pig thyroid slices. *J Biochem* 1979;85:1009.

216. Frati L, Bilstad J, Edelhoch H, et al. Biosynthesis of the 27S thyroid iodoprotein. *Arch Biochem Biophys* 1974;162:126.

217. Saber-Lichtenberg Y, Brix K, Schmitz A, et al. Covalent cross-linking of secreted bovine thyroglobulin by transglutaminase. *FASEB J* 2000;14:1005.

218. Herzog,V, Berndorfer U, Saber Y. Isolation of insoluble secretory product from bovine thyroid: extracellular storage of thyroglobulin in covalently cross-linked form. *J Cell Biol* 1992; 118:1071.

219. Leonardi A, Acquaviva R, Marinaccio M, et al. Presence of dityrosine bridges in thyroglobulin and their relationship with iodination. *Biochem Biophys Res Communun* 1994;202:38.

220. Baudry N, Lejeune PJ, Delom F, et al. Role of multimerized porcine thyroglobulin in iodine storage. *Biochem Biophys Res Commun* 1998;242:292.

221. Dunn JT, Kim PS, Dunn AD, et al. The role of iodination in the formation of hormone-rich peptide from thyroglobulins. *J Biol Chem* 1983;258:9093.

222. Kim PS, Dunn JT, Kaiser DL. Similar hormone-rich peptides from thyroglobulins of five vertebrate classes. *Endocrinology* 1984;114:369.

223. Duthoit C, Estienne V, Delom F, et al. Production of immunoreactive thyroglobulin C-terminal fragments during thyroid hormone synthesis. *Endocrinology* 2000;141:2518.

224. Brix K, Lemansky P, Herzog V. Evidence for extracellularly acting cathepsins mediating thyroid hormone liberation in thyroid epithelial cells. *Endocrinology* 1996;137:1963.

225. Metaye T, Kraimps JL, Goujon JM, et al. Expression, localization, and thyrotropin regulation of cathepsin D in human thyroid tissues. *J Clin Endocrinol Metab* 1997;82:3383.

226. Linke M, Jordans S, Mach L, et al. Thyroid stimulating hormone upregulates secretion of cathepsin B from thyroid epithelial cells. *Biol Chem* 2002;383:773.

227. Marino M, McCluskey RT. Role of thyroglobulin endocytic pathways in the control of thyroid hormone release. *Am J Physiol* 2000;279:C1295.

228. Bastiani P, Papandreou MJ, Blanck O, et al. On the relationship between completion of N-acetyllactosamine oligosaccharide units and iodine content of thyroglobulin: a reinvestigation. *Endocrinology* 1995;136:4204.

229. Herzog V. Transcytosis in thyroid follicle cells. *J Cell Biol* 1983;97:607.

230. Romagnoli P, Herzog V. Transcytosis in thyroid follicle cells: regulation and implications for thyroglobulin transport. *Exp Cell Res* 1991;194:202.

231. Montuori N, Pacifico F, Mellone S, et al. The rat asialoglycoprotein receptor binds the amino-terminal domain of thyroglobulin. *Biochem Biophys Res Comm* 2000;268:42.

232. Siffroi-Fernandez S, Delom F, Nlend MC, et al. Identification of thyroglobulin domain(s) involved in cell-surface binding and endocytosis. *J Endocrinol* 2001;170:217.

233. Hatipoglu BA, Schneider AB. Selective endocytosis of thyroglobulin: a review of potential mechanisms for protecting newly synthesized molecules from premature degradation. *Biochimie* 1999;81:549.

234. Miquelis R, Courageot J, Jacq A, et al. Intracellular routing of GlcNAc-bearing molecules in thyrocytes: selective recycling through the Golgi apparatus. *J Cell Biol* 1993;123:1695.

235. Blanck O, Perrin C, Mziaut H, et al. Molecular cloning, cDNA analysis, and localization of a monomer of the N-acetylglucosamine-specific receptor of the thyroid, NAGR1, to chromosome 19p13.3–13.2. *Genomics* 1994;21:18.

236. Thibault V, Blanck O, Courageot J, et al. The N-acetylglucosamine-specific receptor of the thyroid: purification, further characterization, and expression patterns on normal and pathological glands. *Endocrinology* 1993;132:468.

237. Mziaut H, Bastiani P, Balivet T, et al. Carbohydrate and protein determinants are involved in thyroglobulin recognition by FRTL 5 cells. *Endocrinology* 1996;137:1370.

238. Mezghrani A, Courageot J, Mani JC, et al. Protein-disulfide isomerase (PDI) in FRTL5 cells. pH-dependent thyroglobulin/PDI interactions determine a novel PDI function in the post-endoplasmic reticulum of thyrocytes. *J Biol Chem* 2000;275:1920.

239. Klein M, Gestmann I, Berndorfer U, et al. The thioredoxin boxes of thyroglobulin: possible implications for intermolecular disulfide bond formation in the follicle lumen. *Biol Chem* 2000;381:593.

240. Delom F, Mallet B, Carayon P, et al. Role of extracellular molecular chaperones in the folding of oxidized proteins. Refolding of colloidal thyroglobulin by protein disulfide isomerase and immunoglobulin heavy chain-binding protein. *J Biol Chem* 2001;276:21337.

241. Zheng G, Marino M, Zhao J, et al. Megalin (gp330): a putative endocytic receptor for thyroglobulin (Tg). *Endocrinology* 1998;139:1462.

242. Marino M, Lisi S, Pinchera A, et al. Targeting of thyroglobulin to transcytosis following megalin-mediated endocytosis: evidence for a preferential pH-independent pathway. *J Endocrinol Invest* 2003;26:222.

243. Marino M, Zheng G, Chiovato L, et al. Role of megalin (gp330) in transcytosis of thyroglobulin by thyroid cells. A novel function in the control of thyroid hormone release. *J Biol Chem* 2000;275:7125.

244. Marino M, Chiovato L, Lisi S, et al. Binding of the low density lipoprotein receptor-associated protein (RAP) to thyroglobulin (Tg): putative role of RAP in the Tg secretory pathway. *Mol Endocrinol* 2001;15:1829.

245. Lisi S, Pinchera A, McCluskey RT, et al. Binding of heparin to human thyroglobulin (Tg) involves multiple binding sites including a region corresponding to a binding site of rat Tg. *Eur J Endocrinol* 2002;146:591.

246. Marino M, Zheng G, McCluskey RT. Megalin (gp330) is an endocytic receptor for thyroglobulin on cultured fisher rat thyroid cells. *J Biol Chem* 1999;274:12898.

247. Marino M, Pinchera A, McCluskey RT, et al. Megalin in thyroid physiology and pathology. *Thyroid* 2001;11:47.

248. Suzuki K, Lavaroni S, Mori A, et al. Autoregulation of thyroid-specific gene transcription by thyroglobulin. *Proc Natl Acad Sci U S A* 1998;95:8251.

249. Suzuki K, Mori A, Lavaroni S, et al. In vivo expression of thyroid transcription factor-1 RNA and its relation to thyroid function and follicular heterogeneity: identification of follicular thyroglobulin as a feedback suppressor of thyroid transcription factor-1 RNA levels and thyroglobulin synthesis. *Thyroid* 1999;9:319.

250. Royaux IE, Suzuki K, Mori A, et al. Pendrin, the protein encoded by the Pendred syndrome gene (PDS), is an apical porter of iodide in the thyroid and is regulated by thyroglobulin in FRTL-5 cells. *Endocrinology* 2000;141:839.

251. Suzuki K, Mori A, Saito J, et al. Follicular thyroglobulin suppresses iodide uptake by suppressing expression of the sodium/iodide symporter gene. *Endocrinology* 1999;140:5422.

252. Ulianich L, Suzuki K, Mori A, et al. Follicular thyroglobulin (TG) suppression of thyroid-restricted genes involves the apical membrane asialoglycoprotein receptor and TG phosphorylation. *J Biol Chem* 1999;274:25099.

253. Sellitti DF, Suzuki K, Doi SQ, et al. Thyroglobulin increases cell proliferation and suppresses Pax-8 in mesangial cells. *Biochem Biophys Res Comm* 2001;285:795.

254. Huang SS, Cerullo MA, Huang FW, et al. Activated thyroglobulin possesses a transforming growth factor-beta activity. *J Biol Chem* 1998;273:26036.

255. Rousset B, Selmi S, Alquier C, et al. In vitro studies of the thyroglobulin degradation pathway: endocytosis and delivery of thyroglobulin to lysosomes, release of thyroglobulin cleavage products—iodotyrosines and iodothyronines. *Biochimie* 1989;71:247.

256. Gire V, Kostrouch Z, Bernier-Valentin F, et al. Endocytosis of albumin and thyroglobulin at the basolateral membrane of thyrocytes organized in follicles. *Endocrinology* 1996;137:522.

257. Rousset B, Selmi S, Bornet H, et al. Thyroid hormone residues are released from thyroglobulin with only limited alteration of the thyroglobulin structure. *J Biol Chem* 1989;264:12620.

258. Dunn AD, Crutchfield HE, Dunn JT. Proteolytic processing of thyroglobulin by extracts of thyroid lysosomes. *Endocrinology* 1991;129:3073.

259. Friedrichs B, Tepel C, Reinheckel T, et al. Thyroid functions of mouse cathepsins B, K, and L. *J Clin Invest* 2003;111:1733.

260. van de Graaf SA, Ris-Stalpers C, Veenboer GJ, et al. A premature stop codon in thyroglobulin messenger RNA results in familial goiter and moderate hypothyroidism. *J Clin Endocrinol Metab* 1999;84:2537.

261. Veenboer GJ, de Vijlder JJ. Molecular basis of the thyroglobulin synthesis defect in Dutch goats. *Endocrinology* 1993;132:377.

PERIPHERAL HORMONE METABOLISM

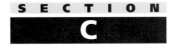

6

THYROID HORMONE TRANSPORT PROTEINS AND THE PHYSIOLOGY OF HORMONE BINDING

SALVATORE BENVENGA

This chapter includes part of the data published in the eighth edition of the text by Robbins (1). Because the sterol hormone–binding proteins (SHBP) also bind thyroid hormone (TH), they do contribute to TH binding in serum. Since TH and sterol-derived hormones are hydrophobic, they must be associated with proteins for transport in blood and delivery to distant sites of action. Multiple plasma proteins are involved in the transport of these hormones. For example, cortisol has cortisol-binding globulin (CBG) as a major carrier, and albumin and sex hormone–binding globulin (SHBG) as minor carriers (2). The opposite is true for dihydrotestosterone, whereas estradiol (E_2) has both albumin and SHBG as a major and CBG as a minor carrier (2). Of the total circulating $1,25(OH)_2D_3$ and less potent $25(OH)D$, 85% and 90% are bound to the α_2-globulin vitamin D–binding protein (VDBP) and the remainder to albumin, a VDBP homologue (3). However, about half of the intestinal absorbed vitamin D is carried by lipoproteins (4).

There are three conventional major carriers for TH (Fig. 6.1) [thyroxine-binding globulin (TBG), transthyretin (TTR), and albumin (Table 6.1)], plus a number of minor carriers (5) (Table 6.2), some of which are also SHBP. TBG and CBG belong to the family of the serine protease inhibitors (SERPINs). In human plasma, the free fraction of TH [~0.03% of total thyroxine (T_4) and ~0.3% of the biologically more potent triiodothyronine (T_3)] is lower than free steroid hormones (> 1%), similar to the free fraction of $25(OH)D$ (0.03%) and the more potent $1,25(OH)_2D_3$ (0.4%). To add to the parallelism between TH and vitamin D, VDBP in the Emydidae family of turtles is a high-affinity binder of both vitamin D and T_4 (6). Finally, considering that one TBG homologue, lipoproteins, and TTR are carriers of retinoids (or the retinoid precursor retinol), then it is of interest that such diverse hormones, which share the ancestors of the corresponding nuclear receptors, also share a number of plasma carriers. Indeed, nine hydrophobic repeats in domain 3 of α-fetoprotein (AFP)—a homologue of albumin and VDBP that binds TH, steroid hormones, and retinoids (7,8)—has structural homology with the heptad dimerization repeats of the nuclear receptor superfamily (9).

THYROXINE-BINDING GLOBULIN

TBG is the major plasma carrier of TH in most of the large mammals. Of 100,000 molecules of circulating TBG, approximately 20,000 are occupied by T_4 as compared to approximately 300 of TTR and 3 of albumin. Unlike TTR

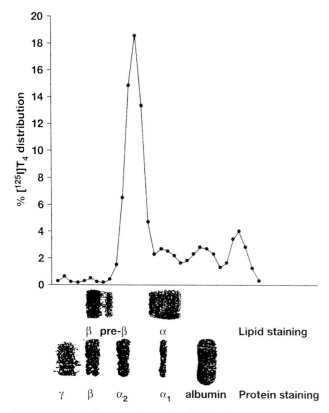

FIGURE 6.1. Iodine 125 thyroxine (T_4) binding to serum proteins as assessed by zone electrophoresis on agarose gel in a euthyroid adult. Three aliquots from the same incubation mixture (serum plus radiolabeled T_4) were run: one aliquot for counting radioactivity, one for protein staining (Coomassie blue), and one for lipid staining (Oil-red-o). Note the inter-α position of the highest peak of radioactivity (i.e., the TBG peak) and that the α1 tail of the thyroxine-binding globulin peak overlaps the left part of the α-lipoprotein area (i.e., high-density lipoprotein). The most anodal and cathodal radioactive peaks are transthyretin and immunoglobulin, respectively. (From Benvenga S, Lapa D, Trimarchi F. Thyroxine binding to members and nonmembers of the serine protease inhibitor family. *J Endocrinol Invest* 2002;25:32–38, with permission.)

and albumin, TBG is a glycoprotein. The four carbohydrate chains contain the following oligosaccharide residues per TBG molecule: 10 of sialic acid, 9 to 13 each of galactose and mannose, and about 20 of glucosamine. The carbohydrate moiety contributes, with TH, to its molecular stability and is responsible for TBG microheterogeneity in the pI (isoelectri point) 4.2 to 5.0 range (the greater the sialic acid content, the greater the anodal mobility). TBG crystallographic structure has not yet been determined, unlike that of other homologues [e.g., α_1-antitrypsin (α_1-AT)]. Based on α_1-AT structure, the T_4 binding site of TBG is in a β-barrel formed by three strands of sheet C (amino acids 212–223, 279–286, and 357–368) and four strands of sheet B (amino acids 220–225, 233–242, 245–252, and 370–379), particularly important being Phe249. Segments 215–291 and 365–395 are the part of human TBG most conserved in mammal TBG (> 95%

similarity) (10), and indeed, the acid dissociation constant (K_a) for T_4 of mammal and hTBG match (10). For compounds affecting TH binding to TBG and other carriers, see Chapters 11 and 13.

The large discrepancy between zone electrophoresis (ZE) and radioimmunoprecipitation (RIP) (Table 6.1) is seen because TBG migration overlaps with other α-globulins, whereas TTR and albumin do not comigrate with other proteins. At an average concentration of 2 mg/dL in a serum containing 7.0 g/dL total protein and 0.98 g/dL total α-globulins, TBG accounts for only 0.2% of the total plasma α-globulins. Thus, a number of other α-globulins could bind TH and be confused with TBG in ZE. This is the case of high-density lipoproteins (HDLs), the α-migrating lipoproteins (Fig. 6.1), which bind approximately 3% of circulating T_4. Other binders are the TBG homologues α_1-AT, α_1-chymotrypsin (α_1-ACT), antithrombin III (AT-III), and CBG, and the nonhomologous α_1-acid glycoprotein (AGP) and SHBG, a β-globulin (5) (Table 6.2). Additional T_4 carriers could include AFP (7–9) and lipocalins (see later section Additional Proteins). SERPINs have one TH site with relative affinity $T_4 > T_3$, but K_a for T_4 is much lower than in TBG (5). Conservation of most residues in the β-strand 3B, including TBG Phe249, occurs in these SERPINs and TBG.

Recently the binding of E_2, progesterone, testosterone, cortisol, aldosterone, and all-*trans*-retinoic acid to the inhibitory SERPINs AT-III, heparin cofactor II, plasminogen activator inhibitor I, and protein C inhibitor (PCI) was studied. Only all-*trans*-retinoic acid bound to PCI (fivefold more than buffer vs. twofold for the other hormones), specifically with a dissociation constant (K_d) of 2.4 μM and one site per mole (11). All *trans*-retinoic acid is also bound by plasma lipoproteins (12).

TRANSTHYRETIN

TTR circulates as a homotetramer of known crystallographic structure. The four subunits are arranged symmetrically around a cylindrical channel. The central β-barrel where TH binds is formed by eight strands (strands A–H) (Fig. 6.2), corresponding to amino acids 11–19, 29–32, 42–49, 53–55, 67–74, 91–97, 105–112, and 115–121. Strands G and H contribute 6/10 residues of the TH binding surface. The TH sites of the homotetramer are two, but only one is occupied due to the much lower K_a of the second site, as a result of negativity cooperativity. Crystallography studies have shed light on the structural basis for negative cooperativity (13). The primary site has a larger diameter than the second site, and T_4 (or other ligand) binding is followed by a slight collapse of the outer and inner parts of this site, and concomitant opening of the second site. Binding of the second ligand is then followed by collapse of the second site. However, this second col-

TABLE 6.1. MAIN CHARACTERISTICS OF THE MAJOR PROTEIN TRANSPORTERS OF THYROID HORMONES IN HUMANS

	TBG	TTR	Albumin
Gene			
Family	SERPINS	Transthyretin	Alb/αFP/VDBP
Chromosome	Xq22.2	18q12.1	4q11-q13
Coding exons	5	4	15
Protein			
Site of synthesis	L	L, P islets, CP, R, K	L
Molecular mass (kd)	54	54 (tetramer)	65
Residues (n)[a]	395	127	595
Electrophoretic mobility[b]	α-globulin	Prealbumin	Albumin
Serum concentration	~12–30 mg/L	~150–400 mg/L	~3.5–5.0 g/dL
	~0.22–0.56 μM	~2.8–7.4 μM	~540–770 μM
Half-life (days)	5	2	15
Binding sites			
K_a for T_4 (M^{-1})			
Primary	No. 1, ~1.0×10^{10}	No. 1, ~7.0×10^7	No. 1, ~7.0×10^5
Secondary		No. 1, ~7.0×10^5	No. 1–5, ~5.0×10^4
K_a for T_3 (M^{-1})			
Primary	No. 1, ~5.0×10^8	No. 1, ~1.0×10^7	No. 1, ~1.0×10^5
Secondary		No. 1, ~5.0×10^5	No. 1–5, ~7.0×10^3
% Serum T_4 carried[c]			
Electrophoresis	64[d] (68)	13 (11)	9 (20)
Immunoprecipitation	49[d]	12	7
% Serum T_3 carried (electrophoresis)	80	9	11
Other ligands		Retinol-binding protein	Steroids, vitamin D, ions, lipids, drugs, etc.

αFP, α-fetoprotein; CP, choroid plexus; K, kidney; K_a, affinity constant; L, liver; P, pancreas; R, retina; T_3, triiodothyronine; T_4, thyroxine; TBG, thyroxine-binding globulin; TTR, transthyretin; VDBP, vitamin D–binding protein.
[a]Mature protein. The corresponding precursors are 415, 147, and 609 residues long.
[b]TBG peaks between α_1 and α_2 (inter-α globulin zone). The coexistence of the normal and variant (alloalbumin) protein causes the appearance of a bifid albumin peak (bisalbuminemia) in heterozygotes but no perturbation of thyroid homeostasis.
[c]Percentages for T_3 and those in parentheses for T_4 are from the 8th edition of this chapter (1). The other percentages for T_4 at electrophoresis and immunoprecipitation are from reference 5. For comparative purposes with some steroids, albumin binds 6.3%, 21%, and 60.8% of circulating cortisol, dihydrotestosterone, and estradiol, respectively (2).
[d]The large discrepancy between zone electrophoresis (ZE) and radioimmunoprecipitation (RIP) is seen because other α-migrating proteins bind T_4 (see reference 5 and Table 6.2). Assuming that the two α-globulins not tested by RIP in reference 5 bind ~0.7% of T_4 each, the average proportion of circulating T_4 carried by α_1-AT, α_1-ACT, AT-III, cortisol-binding globulin, and high-density lipoprotein would add up to 6.3%. Hence, the 64% carried by TBG at ZE (5) is overestimated by at least 6%. If the 49% proportion of serum T_4 bound by TBG at RIP is correct, then there still is 9% of T_4 (58% − 49% = 9%), which is carried by other alpha-globulins to be indentified.

lapse is more limited, so that the second molecule of ligand is bound less tightly (13). TTR is predominantly a retinol-binding protein (RBP), because RBP is carried by one in three molecules of TTR, and there are four RBP binding sites, but only one is likely to be occupied. The RBP and TH sites are independent. RBP, in turn, binds retinol (vitamin A) in a 1:1 molar ratio. Retinol, retinoids, carotenoids, and 1% to 2% of TTR itself are carried by lipoproteins (12,14,15). Interaction with TH is affected by several compounds, the strongest and most selective inhibitor being the flavonoid EMD 21388. A number of environmental pollutants also interfere with TH binding to TTR and/or TBG and albumin (16–18).

TTR is the sole member of its family, a gene of much more ancient lineage than TBG. Indeed, TTR is present in marsupials, rodents, insectivora, birds, reptiles, amphibians, and fish, and open-reading frames for TTR gene–like

nucleotide sequences were found in bacteria, yeast and the nematode *Cunninghamella elegans* (19). Of interest, TTR of birds, reptiles, amphibians, and fish binds T_3 preferentially (19). The switch to the preferential binding of T_4 in mammals was due to selective pressure on the N-terminus of TTR, which became shorter and more hydrophilic during evolution (19). Similar to TBG and apolipoproteins (apos), the T_4 binding domain is the part best conserved in the phylum. In nonhuman animals, plasma TTR binds more TH than does TBG, but regardless of species, TTR is the major TH transport protein in the cerebrospinal fluid (CSF) (19). The vast majority of TTR in CSF derives from central nervous system synthesis (19). This synthesis (which is restricted to the choroid plexus, except for very little in the meninges) is absent in amphibians and fish, namely in species without a neocortex, but it does exist in species as ancient as reptiles, which are the first species

TABLE 6.2. MINOR THYROID HORMONE PLASMA CARRIERS

	Lipoprotein[a]					
	VLDL	**LDL**	**HDL**	**Ig**	**SERPIN**[b]	**Others**[c]
% T_4, GFC	0.04	0.3	2.9	ND	ND	ND
ZE	0.15	1.2	8.6	2	ND	ND
RIP	1.7 (VLDL + LDL)		3.5	4 (2 IgG, 2 IgM)	2.8	~0.6
% T_3, GFC	0.02	0.05	6.0	ND	ND	ND
ZE	ND	ND	ND	2	ND	ND
RIP	ND	ND	ND	4 (2 IgG, 2 IgM)	ND	ND
K_a for T_4 (M^{-1})[d]	10^6	4×10^6	10^6	10^6–10^{10}	~2×10^6	ND
K_a for T_3 (M^{-1})	$\leq 10^5$	$\leq 10^5$	$\leq 10^5$	10^5–10^9	< K_a for T_4	ND
Synthesis[e]	L	From VLDL	L, I, P	B-lymphocytes	L	L

GFC, gel filtration chromatography; HDL, high-density lipoprotein; I, intestine; Ig, immunoglobulin; K_a, affinity constant; L, liver; LDL, low-density lipoprotein; ND, not determined; P, plasma; RIP, radioimmunoprecipitation; T_3, triiodothyronine; T_4, thyroxine; VLDL, very low-density lipoprotein; ZE, zone electrophoresis.

[a]Chylomicrons, which are synthesized in the intestine, are not listed because normally they are present only in postprandial plasma. Their structural apo is apoB-48, which consists of the first 2152 residues of the full-length apoB-100 (4536 residues). Thus, apoB-48 contains the first two of the three thyroid hormone–binding sites of apoB-100 [amino acids 380–392, 1310–1338 and 4223–4510 (data from reference 32)]. Chylomicrons also contain apoA-I, A-IV, and, by transfer from the HDL, apoE and the apoCs.

[b] The following SERPINs were tested and demonstrated to be T_4 binders in reference 5: α_1-antitrypsin (α_1-AT), α_1-antichymotrypsin (α_1-ACT), antithrombin III (AT-III) and corticosteroid-binding globulin (CBG). The first two were also tested by RIP, with ^{125}I-T_4 binding averaging 1.0% and 0.4% of total activity added to human serum, and Scatchard analysis (K_a = 1.9 and 1.0 × 10^6 M^{-1} and number of binding sites 0.9 and 1.0, respectively). The listed value of 2.8% by RIP assumes that AT-III and CBG bind 0.7% each. Binding to α_1-AT, α_1-ACT, and the non-SERPIN α_1-acid glycoprotein, which are all positive acute-phase reactants, should be much greater than listed here during stressful conditions and nonthyroid illnesses, because serum levels of the three proteins increase considerably. Under the same conditions, serum levels of TTR and albumin, and sometimes TBG, decrease. For comparison with corticosteroids, CBG binds 89.7% of circulating cortisol (2), 4% of testosterone, 2% of progesterone, and < 0.1% of estradiol (5).

[c]These other non-SERPIN proteins were tested and demonstrated to be T_4 binders in reference 5: α_1-acid glycoprotein (orosomucoid) and the β-globulin sex hormone–binding globulin (SHBG). The former only was tested by RIP, and an average of 0.30% of ^{125}I-T_4 was bound. The listed value of 0.6% assumes a similar value for SHBG. However, as explained in the text and Table 6.1, other α-globulins that are minor thyroid hormone plasma carriers should exist. For comparison with some steroids, SHBG binds 0.2%, 37.3%, and 78.4% of circulating cortisol, estradiol, and dihydrotestosterone, respectively (2).

[d]Concerning lipid-free apos, only K_a for T_4 of human apoA-1 and apoE has been experimentally determined by Scatchard analysis (34). Depending on the apo preparations used, K_a for T_4 was 4.4 to 7.5 × 10^7 M^{-1} (apoA-1), and 2.4 to 4.0 ×10^7 M^{-1}(apoE). K_a of bovine apoA-1 or rabbit apoE matched the corresponding human apo (34).

[e]Tissue synthesis of apos is always in the liver, except apoA-IV and B-48 (intestine). ApoA-I is also synthesized in the intestine and brain, and apoE is in a variety of tissues (brain, in particular).

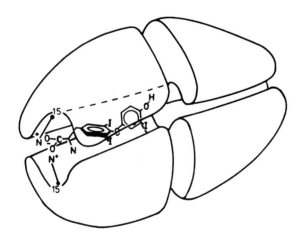

FIGURE 6.2. Schematic drawing of the transthyretin tetramer with triiodothyronine occupying one of the two identical sites in the binding channel. The 3' iodine is in the distal configuration. The side chain carboxylate is shown at the channel entrance interacting with the ϵ-amino group of lysine 15. (From Jorgensen EC. Thyroid hormones and analogs. II. Structure activity relationships. In: Li CH, ed. *Hormonal proteins and peptides.* Vol. 6. New York: Academic, 1978:107, with permission. Drawn from the crystallographic data of Blake and colleagues.)

showing traces of a cortex (19). Also expressed in the ependymal cells of the choroid plexus, but primarily in neurons of the adult brain, is the TBG homologue neuroserpin. Variants of this axonal-secreted protein cause an autosomal-dominant form of dementia (20). Neuroserpin is likely to be a low-affinity TH carrier, and impairment of TH binding could favor the intraneuronal polymerization of neuroserpin (21).

Local amino acid sequence homology exists between the tail of TTR (amino acids 90–127) and the glucagon-secretin family of gastrointestinal hormones (22), while two TTR segments (amino acids 18–53 and 72–117) share homology with the amyloid-related proteins (ARP), including the amyloidogenetic A4 segment of the amyloid β-protein precursor (AβPP) associated with Alzheimer's disease (23). The homology with ARP is relevant, because native TTR and several TTR variants are involved in senile amyloidosis and familial amyloid polyneuropathy, respectively. Finally, amino acids 38–57 of the β-subunit of human luteinizing hormone (LH) are homologous with residues 10–30 of TTR (24).

ALBUMIN

This multiligand protein is also of ancient lineage. It is composed of three repeated domains (amino acids 25–205, 212–397, and 404–595 in humans), each containing two subdomains (A and B). Using crystallographic analysis, four T_4 sites were identified in subdomains 2A, 3A, and 3B (25). A fifth site is in the cleft between domains 1 and 2, created by the conformational changes on albumin induced by binding of the fatty acids (26). Fatty acids inhibit TH binding to plasma proteins; on albumin they bind in hydrophobic pockets that are distributed asymmetrically (26). Important for the high affinity of the site in subdomain 2A is Arg218. As mentioned above, albumin binds sterol-derived hormones, and its homologue VDBP binds both T_4 and vitamin D in turtles of the Emydidae family (7), whereas the homologue AFP binds TH, steroid hormones, and vitamins (7–9).

LIPOPROTEINS

Gel filtration chromatography (GFC) of human plasma demonstrated binding of T_4 (~3%), T_3 (~6%), and reverse T_3 (rT_3) (~0.2%) to all classes of lipoproteins: chylomicrons, very low-density lipoproteins (VLDLs), low-density lipoproteins (LDLs), and high-density lipoproteins (HDLs) (27,28) (Table 6.2). However, there might be dissociation of TH from lipoproteins during GFC, because ZE and RIP give higher binding values (28). HDL, the major lipoproteins binder, encompasses a broad spectrum of particles between the approximately 60,000 to 450,000 molecular weight range. Distribution of TH between the numerous HDL subfractions is affected by thyroid status (29,30). For example, in euthyroid plasmas, T_4 and T_3 are associated with HDL subfractions of 111,000 ± 34,000 and 148,000 ± 31,000 (mean ± SD), respectively. However, in hypothyroid plasmas, the corresponding HDL subfractions have molecular weights of 176,000 ± 24,000 and 94,000 ± 30,000 (29). Interestingly, one HDL particle has the same molecular weight as albumin, has very little lipid, and its only protein moiety is apoA-1 (31). The association of TH with lipoprotein lipids has not been quantified. TH, though, binds specifically to apoA-I, apoA-II, apoA-IV, apoB-100, apoC-I, apoC-II, apoC-III, and apoE (27,28,32–34). The K_a for TH of the lipoproteins (i.e., the lipid-associated apos) is one to two orders of magnitude lower, because lipids inhibit TH binding to apos. Unlike with TBG (35), several types of lipids inhibit this binding.

The non-apoB-100 apos contain a single TH site of 10^7 M^{-1} binding affinity (27,34), with relative affinity $T_4 = rT_3 > T_3$. The TH site is N-terminal, in the exon 3-coded

region (exon 2 for apoA-IV), which contains β-sheet structure. There is remarkable local homology in the TH binding domains of apos and TBG, TTR, and albumin (34). The homologous sequences are amino acids 292–348 and 497–534 of albumin, 72–122 of TTR (a segment that contains 6 of the 10 residues that form the TH binding surface, and strands F, G, and H of the binding channel), and 231–273 and 349–395 of TBG, corresponding to β-strands B2, B3, B4, and C2. Apos, including apoB100, share the hydrophobic motif Y,L/I/M/,X,X,V/L/I, the first two residues being conserved in TBG, TTR, and albumin. Particularly, Y matches F_{249} of TBG. This motif (located, for instance, at position 18–22 in apoA-I and 36–40 in apoE) is well conserved in the phyla, and it is believed to represent the core of the TH binding site (33,35). ApoB-100 contains three TH sites, one in each of three nonoverlapping fragments generated from the natural cleavage by circulating enzymes (32). Experimental data indicated TH sites at amino acids 380–392, 1310–1338, and 4223–4510 (32), in keeping with the sequences 360–406, 1303–1344, and 4281–4341 found by homology search (33).

In the trout, lipoproteins (HDL > LDL > VLDL) are the major T_4 and T_3 carriers (36), but unlike human lipoproteins, the K_a values for T_4 and T_3 are similar (36).This recalls the evolutionary changes in TH affinity of TTR (19). Lipoproteins also bind the lipid-soluble vitamins (4, 14,37) and steroids (38) (see also S. Benvenga, unpublished observation).

IMMUNOGLOBULINS

Immunoglobulins (Igs) are minor TH carriers (Table 6.2 and Fig. 6.1). Unlike ZE, RIP permits discrimination between Ig classes (39,40). Above each one's laboratory cutoff point (i.e., the greatest proportion of TH bound to any Ig class in healthy persons), the serum is said to contain TH autoantibodies (THAbs). These can be T_3Ab (approximately half of the cases), T_4Ab (approximately one fourth of the cases), or T_3 plus T_4Ab (approximately one fourth of the cases). Traditionally, THAbs are considered to be IgG, though other Ig classes were not always investigated. Cases of IgA, IgM (41), and IgE THAbs were reported (42). In one patient, THAbs also bound steroids (41,43).

ADDITIONAL PROTEINS

Other minor proteins binding TH include AGP (5), which belongs to the lipocalin family and also includes proteins such as α_1-microglobulin, tear prealbumin (a cysteine proteinase inhibitor), and apoD. Lipocalins adopt a β-barrel tertiary structure and are carriers of small hydrophobic ligands. The retinol binder, choroid plexus–secreted lipocalin

1 has functional homology with TTR (44). ApoD, which circulates predominantly associated with the HDL, is homologous with RBP and binds progestational hormones (45).

PATHOPHYSIOLOGY

Changes in Serum Levels of Thyroxine-Binding Globulin, Transthyretin, and Albumin

Mean serum levels are given in Table 6.1. TBG and TTR are age and gender dependent, but in opposite ways (46–51). TBG is highest in neonates (~28 mg/L) and progressively declines to approximately 19 mg/L at 10 to 15 years (46), with a significant decrease between Tanner stages 1 and 5 (47). TBG remains substantially stable thereafter, with values in premenopausal women greater than in men, because of the increased half-life that derives from the estrogen-induced sialylation of TBG (47). Interestingly, in one man with endogenous hyperestrogenemia and hypertestosteronemia, the androgen antagonized the E_2 effect on TBG but failed in the E_2 effect on PRL and TSH (49). Pregnancy, contraceptive pills, estrogen receptor modulators, 5-fluorouracil, liver diseases, acute intermittent porphyria, hypothyroidism, and inherited TBG excess (TBG-E) increase serum TBG; androgens, corticosteroids, hyperthyroidism, terminal illnesses, and inherited TBG deficiency (TBG-D) decrease or tend to decrease serum TBG.

Serum TTR in newborns averages 110 mg/L and progressively increases to approximately 300 mg/L at 10 to 14 years (50). After 50 years, TTR levels decrease and average 200 mg/L in octogenarians (51); in adulthood men have higher levels than women. In addition to androgen administration, TTR excess has been reported in pancreatic endocrine tumors (52), chronic renal failure (53), and as a compensatory mechanism in analbuminemia (inherited deficiency of albumin). In maintenance dialysis patients, serum TTR of less than 300 mg/L predicts increased risk for morbidity and mortality (53). Serum TTR decreases in severe nonthyroid illnesses, protein-calorie malnutrition, and inherited α_1-AT deficiency (54). Persistently or progressively low serum TTR is predictive of death (54,55). Causes of proteinuria decrease serum TBG, TTR, and albumin but increase lipoproteins. Changes in serum levels of albumin and minor carriers are irrelevant for thyroidologists.

Concentrations of TBG, TTR, and albumin in human CSF are 0.0028, 0.42, and 2.3 μmol/L, with a total protein concentration in human CSF that is approximately 0.5% that in human plasma (19). FT_4 in human CSF is approximately 70 pmol/L or approximately 1.7% of total T_4 in human CSF (19).

Inherited Abnormalities of Protein Concentration or Thyroid Hormone–Binding Affinity

Changes in either plasma concentration or TH affinity of TBG affect plasma levels of T_4, and sometimes T_3, in the same direction: hypothyroxinemia when the concentration or K_a of TBG decreases, hyperthyroxinemia when concentration increases. Increased affinity of TBG for TH has not been reported yet. Due to the much lower amount of TH transported by either TTR or albumin, compared with TBG, only an increased protein concentration (never described for albumin) or an increased affinity (which can occur for either TTR or albumin) can enhance plasma levels of T_4. Reduced protein concentration and even absence of either protein does not cause hypothyroxinemia. Congenital or acquired absence of TTR has not been reported, unlike congenital absence of albumin (analbuminemia). Importantly, all the inherited or acquired variations in transport proteins leave unchanged both FT_4 and FT_3, in accordance with the clinical euthyroid status (euthyroid hypothyroxinemia or hyperthyroxinemia).

TBG-D can be partial (e.g., TBG-PD San Diego or TBG-PD Montreal) or complete (e.g., TBG-CD Buffalo). A catalog of the TBG mutations is available online (56). Some mutations, though, are associated with normal or mildly decreased serum TBG levels. These variants are TBG-poly (Leu283Phe), TBG-slow (Asp171Asn), TBG-Chicago (Tyr309Phe), and the not yet characterized TBG-C1 and TBG-F (56). These five TBG variants represent TBG polymorphism because of their enhanced presence in certain populations. For instance, allele frequency ranges from 16% to 31% for TBG-poly in French Canadians, Japanese, and Han Chinese of Taiwan, and from 2% to 16% for TBG-slow in Pacific Islanders and Black populations of African origin (56,57). TBG-D and TBG-E are inherited as X-linked traits, with a single exception (56). Most often, TBG-D are frame shifts or stop codons, resulting in synthesis of a truncated protein, and they occur at several positions. Based on neonatal screening programs for congenital hypothyroidism, TBG-CD is more frequent in Japanese than in whites (1:1200–1:1900 vs. 1:5000 to 1:13,000) (58). A particular form of TBG-D is due to reduced glycosylation of TBG and other glycoproteins as well (58). TBG-E is rarer (1:6000 to 1:40,000), and its molecular basis is TBG gene amplification (duplication, triplication) (56). An unexpected frequency of association between TBG-E and hyperthyroidism, greater than between TBG-D and hyperthyroidism, has been noted (59).

In addition to TBG-E, another cause of familial euthyroid hyperthyroxinemia (FEH) is the increased T_4 affinity of either TTR or albumin (familial dysalbuminemic hyperthyroxinemia, FDH) (60), FDH being the most frequent cause of FEH. FDH prevalence is 0.01% to 1.8%, depending on the ethnic group, with the highest prevalence in

Hispanics (61). FDH is caused by a change of Arg218 of albumin to either His or Pro, the latter also producing increased serum T_3. Increased affinity for either TH arises because Arg218, which contacts the TH bound in subdomain 2A, causes a localized conformational change, relaxing steric restrictions on TH binding at this site (25). Another mutation, Leu66Pro, causes euthyroid hypertriiodothyroninemia because of a 40-fold increase in the K_a for T_3 with a negligible increase of the K_a for T_4 (56). Similar to FDH, mutations of TTR with increased TH affinity are autosomal dominant. Such mutations concern Ala109 or Thr119 (56), whereas wild-type TTR can be associated with senile amyloidosis. Mutations at numerous codons other than 109 and 119, the most common being Val30Met, are associated with familial amyloid polyneuropathy (FAP) (62), and mutations at codons (Val30, Leu58, Ser77, Ile84, Val122) decrease TH affinity (56). Prevalence of FAP is 1:100,000 to 1:1,000,000 (62), but FAP due to TTR mutations is the most common association with autosomal-dominant systemic amyloidosis. Interestingly, mutations of apos (apoA-1 and apoSAA) can result in other inherited amyloidoses (63). ApoA-1 Gly$_{26}$Arg causes a TTR-like FAP. ApoA-1, apoSAA, and murine apoA-2 (which is involved in amyloidosis-associated accelerated senescence of the mouse) share local homology with the other amyloid proteins (23). Genetic polymorphism of TTR exists in monkeys but not humans (56). In contrast, there are numerous polymorphic forms of albumin, from very slow to very fast.

Significance of Thyroid Hormone Binding to Plasma Proteins

Studies on patients with a defective gene product or equivalent knock-out mice have illuminated the functions of a particular protein. This is not the case for any of the TH plasma carrier proteins, in contrast with other hormone carriers. For instance, in the rare inherited CBG deficiency, there is an unusually high frequency of hypotension, chronic fatigue, and obesity (64,65). In contrast, patients with TBG complete deficiency or analbuminemia are entirely normal. However, analbuminemic patients and rats have a compensatory increase of other proteins, including TTR, Ig, α_1-AT, α_2-macroglobulin, transferrin, and ceruloplasmin, but most of all lipoproteins (66). This increase in lipoproteins is associated with increased lipogenesis and gene expression of several apos. TTR null mice have normal thyroid and retinoid status (67), including normal TH entry into and distribution in the brain (67), and normal retinal anatomy and function (68). These findings are surprising considering that the choroid plexus has the highest concentration of TTR messenger RNA in the body (4.4 µg/g wet weight tissue, compared with 0.4 µg/g in liver) (69) and that TTR is the most abundant transcript in human retinal pigment epithelium (70). Considering the

conservation of the TH-binding domain of a given protein across species, functions presumably exist. In apos, the highly conserved TH-binding motif Y,L/I/M,X,X,V/I/L is spared by natural mutations (34), which contrasts with the occurrence of mutations in the TH-binding domain of the major TH carriers. Based on a number of data (71–110), certain functions can be hypothesized, for some of which details are given (Table 6.3).

Two functions are apparent: to limit the urinary loss of TH and to act as a buffer counterbalancing sudden fluctuations in thyroid gland secretion. A third function is to constitute an extracellular reservoir that circulates continuously (in the blood and other fluids such as CSF), steadily releasing free TH and making TH available to tissues for replacing the TH used (74). A fourth function is temporary and local, occurring at sites of inflammation (75–78). Unrelated to inflammation, apoB-100 and apoE are attacked by plasma enzymes so that both intact and fragmented forms of the two apos circulate in plasma (27,32).

Because sterol hormone delivery to target cells has been described for CBG, SHBG, and VDBP through specific sites on the plasma membrane (79), a fifth function might be facilitation of TH transport (entry or exit) across cells (76,80,81) (Fig. 6.3). Albumin, TTR, or TBG inhibits TH entry (80–82), although cell uptake of TTR and TBG was described by others (76,83). The superiority of a minor carrier protein (lipoprotein) over the major carrier proteins was also observed with vitamin D, because its uptake by liver cells was greatest when vitamin D_3 was presented to the cells on LDL and least when presented on VDBP (84). Delivery to certain tissues of another lipid-soluble vitamin, vitamin E, is also dependent on LDL interaction with the LDL-R (85), whereas HDL is important for vitamin E efflux from cells (86). The permissive effect of albumin on T_3 efflux has been known since the mid 1980s (87). Unlike TH entry, TH exit is facilitated by all proteins, and in a nonsaturable fashion (88) (Fig. 6.3). Importantly, if from the extracellular mixture containing all proteins only a single protein at a time is removed, the efflux of either T_4 or T_3 remains unaffected (88). These data indicate that redundancy of TH plasma carriers compensate for the absence of single proteins.

Particular functions may be attributed to the presence of lipoprotein receptors or apos in certain tissues or fluids, as reviewed previously (27). These functions include enterohepatic circulation of TH (27), distribution of TH in the nervous system mainly for reparative and seasonal biorhythm regulation purposes (27,90–96), and TH transport across the placenta or oocytes (27,97–103). In the placenta, SHBG or apos stimulate secretion of human chorionic gonadotropin or human placental lactogen (104,105).

Considering that TH exerts numerous nongenomic effects (106), most of which are best served by T_4, and that part of the LDL-facilitated T_4 cell entry does not have access to cell nuclei (81), a number of nongenomic effects

TABLE 6.3. SELECTED POSSIBLE FUNCTIONS OF THYROID HORMONE (TH)–BINDING PROTEINS

Function	Comments (with example references)
Prevention of the urinary loss of TH	Albumin, VDBP, and TTR are internalized by megalin (83), a multiligand endocytotic receptor of the LDL-R family that is expressed on the apical surface of several resorptive epithelia, including KPTs. KPTs contain TTR, apos, and a novel apoA-1 binding protein that might be responsible for apoA-1 resorption (83).
Uniform distribution of TH to all cells of a tissue	In rat liver, distribution of T_4 is taken up uniformly by all cells of the hepatic lobule when the organ is perfused with a solution of TBG, TTR, and albumin (74). Perfusion with albumin alone suffices for this purpose.
Accumulation of free TH at sites of inflammation	SERPINs have an exposed reactive site loop for cleavage by serine proteases such as neutrophil-derived elastase. As a result of cleavage, the hormone affinity decreases, and free hormone is liberated (75,76). T_4 released is locally degraded to DIT and other metabolites with bactericidal properties (75). LDL and HDL, which have antiviral and antimicrobial activities (77,78), are attacked by the same elastase (27). Either lipoprotein favors elastase release from neutrophils (27).
Facilitation of TH entry into cells	Facilitation of TH entry reported for TBG in blood mononuclear cells (27,76). TTR uptake reported for several human or animal cells (76,83), and this uptake is increased in the presence of high T_4 or T_3 concentrations (76). LDL–TH complexes are internalized via the LDL-R, and human skin fibroblasts internalize up to 50% more T_4 than they would if cells were exposed to the same concentration of T_4 but without LDL (80). Only two thirds of T_4 internalized via LDL/LDL-R have access to the cell nuclei (81). In contrast, HDL facilitates uptake of a lesser extra-quota of T_4 (up to +25%), and independently from HDL-R (81). All of this extra-quota of T_4 has access to the cell nuclei. There could be an interplay between TTR and lipoprotein, as part of circulating TTR is transported by lipoprotein. Lipoproteins inhibit TTR uptake, and TTR uptake is partly mediated by megalin (a member of the LDL-R family) (83).
Facilitation of TH exit from cells	All TH plasma carriers favor both T_4 and T_3 exit from cells (88). On a molar basis, the order of potency is TBG > TTR > albumin > LDL > HDL, but at ambient concentration, the effect of lipoprotein (HDL > LDL) is comparable with that of the nonlipoproteins (TBG = TTR = albumin). Lipoproteins are so effective because their lipids permit a better interaction with the lipids of plasma membrane. All proteins act as sink for the extruded TH, thus maintaining the physical gradient from outside to inside the cells that drives the passive efflux of TH.
Enterohepatic circulation of TH	LDL-R and HDL-R are present in the liver and intestine (27). Apos are synthesized in the intestine, liver, and epithelial cells of the bile ducts, and are present in the bile (27). TH stimulates apo expression of both liver and intestine apos (27). HDL transports bilirubin.
TH distribution in the central and peripheral nervous system, mainly for reparative purposes	SERPINs (including TBG, α_1-AT, α_1-ACT), TTR, albumin (and the albumin homologues AFP and VDBP), apos, and other TH-binding proteins (e.g., α_1-AGP, Ig) are present in CSF (19,27,90–93). TTR, albumin, AFP, apos, α_1-AT, 1-ACT, and α_1-AGP are synthesized in the brain (19,27,90–94,96); LDL-R are also expressed in brain (27). Apos and LDL-R genes are overexpressed, so that the corresponding protein products accumulate after either cranial or peripheral nerve injury and subsequent nerve repair and regeneration (27,94).
Regulation of hibernation and seasonal rhythms	(a) Regulation of hibernation. In the golden-mantled ground squirrel, four mRNAs vary seasonally, augmenting in the winter (hibernation) compared with summer. These mRNAs are TBG (15-fold), cathepsin H (5-fold), α_2-macroglobulin (4.5-fold), and apoA-1 (2.6-fold) (95). mRNA of albumin did not change, while TTR was not tested. (b) Regulation of the annual transition in reproductive function of seasonally breeding animals through regulation of T_4 access to specific hypothalamic areas. In Siberian hamsters, expression of TBG, TTR, and albumin genes is associated with reproductive refractoriness to short day lengths (96). Down-regulation of these genes is associated with reduced hypothalamic T_4 uptake, which is reversed by long-day photoperiod treatments that restored responsiveness to short days. Circulating T_4 did not vary with states of photoresponsiveness.
Transport across placenta and/or oocytes of TH	Maternal serum levels of TBG, CBG, SHBG, and lipoprotein increase in pregnancy (27,97). Synthesis in or uptake by placenta, oocytes, or yolk sac of hormone transport proteins has been shown (98–103). Expression of the apos precedes that of the major TH transport proteins in the yolk sac (103).
Nongenomic effects	A clear background exists for apos. In addition to the enterohepatic circulation of TH (see above), TH binding to apos may protect plasma lipoprotein from oxidation (107), contribute to vasodilatation, and stimulate enzyme activity (LCAT, LpL) for which apos have activating properties (108). TH exert several nongenomic effects (106), including interference with oxidation (109), promotion of vasodilatation (110) and stimulation of certain apo-associated enzyme activities (LCAT, LpL) (27,108).

α_1-ACT, α_1-antichymotrypsin; α_1-AGP, α_1-acid glycoprotein; α_1-AT, α_1-antitrypsin; AFP, alpha-fetoprotein; apos, apoliproteins; CBG, corticosteroid-binding globulin; CSF, cerebrospinal fluid; DIT, diiodothyrosine; HDL, high-density lipoprotein; HDL-R, HDL receptor; Ig, immunoglobulin; KPT, kidney proximal tubule; LCAT, lecithin-cholesterol-acyltransferase; LDL-R, low-density lipoprotein receptor; LpL, lipoprotein lipase; SERPINs, serine protease inhibitors; SHBG, sex hormone–binding globulin; T_3, triiodothyronine; T_4, thyroxine; TBG, thyroxine-binding globulin; TH, thyroid hormone; TTR, transthyretin; VDBP, vitamin D–binding protein.

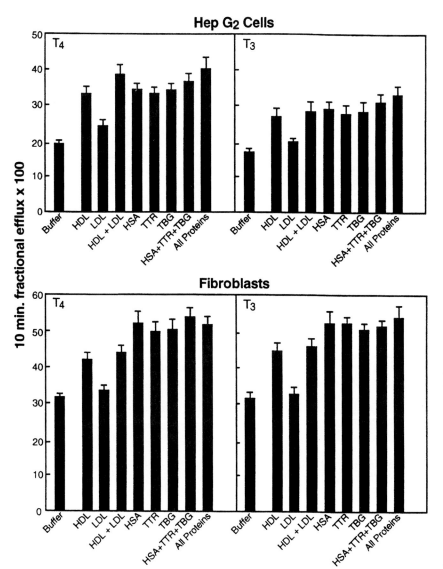

FIGURE 6.3. Ten-minute fractional efflux (mean ± SD) of radiolabeled thyroxine or tri-iodothyronine from human hepatocytes (HepG$_2$ cells) or human skin fibroblasts in the absence (buffer) or presence of individual proteins or mixture of proteins. The protein concentrations approximate the ambient concentrations for hepatocytes (plasma) and fibroblasts (interstitial fluid). (From Benvenga S, Robbins J. Thyroid hormone efflux from monolayer cultures of human fibroblasts and hepatocytes. Effect of lipoproteins and other thyroxine transport proteins. *Endocrinology* 1998;139:4311–4318, with permission.) Note that the effect of high-density lipoprotein (HDL) and HDL plus low-density lipoprotein (LDL) is disproportionately similar to that produced by the three major thyroid hormone–binding proteins when tested either individually or combined. Independently of cell and hormone, the effect given by all proteins (i.e., HDL + LDL + human serum albumin + transthyretin + thyroxine-binding globulin) did not change when each of these five proteins was removed one at a time (not shown).

can be hypothesized (Table 6.3). Overall, the nongenomic actions summarized in Table 6.3 would have an antiatherogenic effect (107), and the apo-TH binding could potentiate individual antiatherogenic properties of the HDL apos and TH (108–110).

THAbs are considered the rarest thyroid autoantibodies (39,40), their rate of detection being low even when investigated in isolated IgG (111). Contributing to the rarity is the fact that THAbs can be transient (40,112,113). However, prevalence of THAb at our center has increased steadily, particularly in patients with autoimmune thyroid diseases (114). Surprisingly, prevalence in autoimmune thyroid diseases is lower than in primary Sjögren's syndrome and rheumatoid arthritis (114). THAbs have iodinated thyroglobulin as the autoantigen (40) and can be induced by viruses (113), drugs (115), or other insults (40).

In summary, the major TH transport proteins, while they individually may be absent without endangering health, together contribute importantly to thyroid homeostasis. On the other hand, TBG, TTR, and minor transport proteins such as lipoproteins also have additional physiologic and pathophysiologic functions, both real and potential, that further investigation will elucidate.

ACKNOWLEDGMENTS

I am appreciative of the helpful discussions with professor Francesco Trimarchi (Head, Sezione di Endocrinologia and Director, Dipartimento di Medicina e Farmacologia Clinica, University of Messina School of Medicine) and Dr. Jacob Robbins (Scientist Emeritus, NIH).

REFERENCES

1. Robbins J. Thyroid hormone transport proteins and the physiology of hormone binding. In: Braverman LE, Utiger RD, ed. *Werner & Ingbar's The thyroid. A fundamental and clinical text*, 8th ed. Philadelphia: Lippincott Williams & Wilkins, 2000: 105–120.
2. Dunn JF, Nisula BC, Rodbard D. Transport of steroid hormones: binding of 21 endogenous steroids to both testosterone-binding and corticosteroid-binding globulin in human plasma. *J Clin Endocrinol Metab* 1981;53:58–68.
3. Bringhurst FR, Demay MB, Kronenberg HM. Hormones and disorders of mineral metabolism. In: Larsen PR, Kronenberg HM, Melmed S, Polonsky KS, eds. *Williams textbook of endocrinology*, 10th ed. Philadelphia: WB Saunders, 2003:1303–1371.
4. Haddad JG . Human plasma transport of vitamin D after its endogenous synthesis. *J Clin Invest* 1993;91:2552–2555.
5. Benvenga S, Lapa D, Trimarchi F. Thyroxine binding to members and nonmembers of the serine protease inhibitor family. *J Endocrinol Invest* 2002;25:32–38.
6. Whitworth DJ, Hunt L, Licht P. Widespread expression of the mRNA encoding a novel vitamin D/thyroxine dual binding protein in the turtle Trachemys scripta. *Gen Comp Endocrinol* 2000;118:354–358.
7. Herve F, Grigorova AM, Rajkowski K, et al. Differences in the binding of thyroid hormones and indoles by rat alpha-1-fetoprotein and serum albumin. *Eur J Biochem* 1982;122:609–612.
8. Aussel C. Presence of three different binding sites for retinoids, bilirubin and estrogen or arachidonic acid on rat alpha-fetoprotein. *Tumor Biol* 1985;6:179–193.
9. Mizejewski GJ. An apparent dimerization motif in the third domain of alpha-fetoprotein: molecular mimicry of the steroid/thyroid nuclear receptor superfamily. *Bioassay* 1993;15:427–432.
10. Janssen OE, Lahner H, Grasberger H, et al. Characterization and primary structures of bovine and porcine thyroxin-binding globulin. *Mol Cell Endocrinol* 2002;186:27–35.
11. Jerabek I, Zechmeister-Machhart M, Binder BR, et al. Binding of retinoic acid by the inhibitory serpin protein C inhibitor. *Eur J Biochem* 2001;268:5989–5996.
12. Wasan K, Ramaswamy M, Ng SP, et al. Differences in the lipoprotein distribution of free and liposome-associated all-trans-retinoic acid in human, dog, and rat plasma are due to variations in lipoprotein lipid and protein content. *Antimicrob Agents Chemother* 1998;42:1646–1653.
13. Neuman P, Cody V, Wojtczak. Structural basis of negative co-operativity in transthyretin. *Acta Biochim Pol* 2001;48:867–875.
14. Parker RS. Absorption, metabolism, and transport of carotenoids. *FASEB J* 1996;10:542–551.
15. Sousa MM, Berglund MM, Saraiva MJ. Transthyretin in high density lipoproteins: association with apolipoprotein A-I. *J Lipid Res* 2000;41:58–65.
16. Brucker-Davis F. Effects of environmental synthetic chemical on thyroid function. *Thyroid* 1998;8:827–856.
17. Zheng W, Deane R, Redzic Z, et al. Transport of L-[125]thyroxine by in situ perfused ovine choroid plexus: inhibition by lead exposure. *J Toxicol Environ Health A* 2003;66:435–451.
18. Yamauchi K, Ishihara A, Fukazawa H, et al. Competitive interactions of chlorinated phenol compounds with 3,3′,5-triiodothyronine binding to transthyretin: detection of possible thyroid-disrupting chemicals in environmental waste water. *Toxicol Appl Pharmacol* 2003;187:110–117.
19. Schreiber G. The evolutionary and integrative roles of transthyretin in thyroid hormone homeostasis. *J Endocrinol* 2002; 175:61–73.
20. Davis RL, Shrimpton AE, Carrel RW, et al. Association between conformational mutations in neuroserpin and onset and severity of dementia. *Lancet* 2002;359:2242–2247.
21. Benvenga S. Conformational mutations in neuroserpin and familial dementias [Letter]. *Lancet* 2002;360:1696.
22. Jornvall H, Carlstrom A, Pettersson T, et al. Structural homologies between prealbumin, gastrointestinal prohormones and other proteins. *Nature* 1981;291:261–263.
23. Benvenga S, Campennì A, Facchiano A. Internal repeats of prion protein and AβPP, and reciprocal similarity with the amyloid-related proteins. *Amyloid* 1999;6:250–255.
24. Milius RP, Keutman HT, Ryan RJ. Molecular modeling of residues 38–57 of the beta-subunit of human lutotropin. *Mol Endocrinol* 1990;4:859–868.
25. Petitpas I, Petersen CE, Ha CE, et al. Structural basis of albumin-thyroxine interactions and familial dysalbuminemic hyperthyroxinemia. *Proc Natl Acad Sci USA* 2003;100:6440–6445.
26. Curry S, Mandelkow H, Brick P, et al. Crystal structure of human serum albumin complexed with fatty acid reveals an asymmetrical distribution of binding sites. *Nat Struct Biol* 1998;5:827–835.
27. Benvenga S, Robbins J. Lipoprotein-thyroid hormone interaction. *Trends Endocrinol Metab* 1993;4:194–198.
28. Benvenga S, Lapa D, Trimarchi F. Re-evaluation of the thyroxine-binding to human plasma lipoproteins using three techniques. *J Endocrinol Invest* 2001;24:RC16–RC18.
29. Benvenga S, Robbins J. Altered thyroid hormone binding to plasma lipoprotein in hypothyroidism. *Thyroid* 1996;6:595–600.
30. Benvenga S, Robbins J. Altered thyroid hormone binding to plasma lipoproteins in the syndrome of resistance to thyroid hormones. *Biochimie* 1999;81:545–548.
31. Benvenga S. The 27-kilodalton thyroxine (T$_4$)-binding protein is human apolipoprotein A-I: identification of a 68-kilodalton high density lipoprotein that binds T$_4$. *Endocrinology* 1989; 124:1265–1269.
32. Benvenga S, Cahnmann HJ, Robbins J. Localization of the thyroxine binding sites in apolipoprotein B100 of human low density lipoproteins. *Endocrinology* 1990;127:2241–2246.
33. Benvenga S, Cahnmann HJ, Rader D, et al. Thyroid hormone binding to isolated apolipoproteins A-II, C-I, C-II and C-III. Homology in thyroxine binding sites. *Thyroid* 1994;4:261–267.
34. Benvenga S. A thyroid hormone binding motif is evolutionarily conserved in apolipoproteins. *Thyroid* 1997;7:605–611.
35. Benvenga S, Li Calzi L, Robbins J. Effect of free fatty acids and nonlipid inhibitors of thyroid hormone binding in the immunoradiometric assay of thyroxin-binding globulin. *Clin Chem* 1987;33:1752–1755.
36. Babin PJ. Binding of thyroxine and 3,5,3′-triiodothyronine to trout plasma lipoproteins. *Am J Physiol* 1992;262:E712–E720.
37. Stoker A, Azzi A. Tocopherol binding proteins: their function and significance. *Antioxid Redox Signal* 2000;2:397–404.
38. Vilhlma V, Tiitien A, Yliorkala O, et al. Quantitative determination of estradiol fatty acid esters in lipoprotein fractions of human blood. *J Clin Endocrinol Metab* 2003;88:2552–2555.
39. Benvenga S, Trimarchi F, Robbins J. Circulating thyroid hormone autoantibodies. *J Endocrinol Invest* 1987;605:619.
40. Benvenga S, Bartolone L, Squadrito S, et al. Thyroid hormone autoantibodies elicited by diagnostic fine needle biopsy. *J Clin Endocrinol Metab* 1997;82:4217–4223.
41. Trimarchi F, Benvenga S, Fenzi G, et al. Immunoglobulin binding of thyroid hormones in a case of Waldenström's

macroglobulinemia. *J Clin Endocrinol Metab* 1982;54:1045–1050.

42. Benvenga S, Trimarchi F, Barbera C, et al. Circulating immunoglobulin E (IgE) antibodies in a euthyroid patient with multinodular goiter and allergic rhinitis. *J Endocrinol Invest* 1984;7:47–50.

43. Benvenga S, Trimarchi F, Barbera C, et al. Abnormal cortisol binding in a case of Waldenström's macroglobulinemia [Letter]. *N Engl J Med* 1980;303:1179–1180.

44. Lepperdinger G. Amphibian choroid plexus lipocalin, Cpl1. *Biochem Biophys Acta* 2000;1482:1119–1126.

45. Rassart E, Bediran A, Do Carmo S, et al. Apolipoprotein D. *Biochem Biophys Acta* 2000;1482:185–198.

46. Camargo Neto U, Rubin R. Thyroxine-binding globulin in neonates and children [Letter]. *West J Med* 2001;175:306.

47. Elmlinger MW, Kuhnel W, Lambrecht HG, et al. Reference intervals from birth to adulthood of serum thyroxine (T$_4$), triiodothyronine (T$_3$), free T$_3$, free T$_4$, thyroxine-binding globulin (TBG) and thyrotropin (TSH). *Clin Chem Lab Med* 2001; 39:973–979.

48. Ain KB, Mori Y, Refetoff S. Reduced clearance rate of thyroxine-binding globulin (TBG) with increased sialylation: A mechanism for estrogen induced elevation of serum TBG concentration. *J Clin Endocrinol Metab* 1987;65:689–696.

49. Benvenga S, Smedile G, Lo Giudice F, et al. Euthyroid hyperthyrotropinemia secondary to hyperestrogenemia in a male with congenital adrenal hyperplasia. *Horm Metab Res* 2000;32:321–325.

50. Benvenga S, De Luca F, Pandullo E, et al. Changes in radioimmunoassayable thyroxine-binding prealbumin serum levels from birth to adulthood. *Horm Metab Res* 1986;18:73.

51. Benvenga S, Morgante L, Bartalena L, et al. Radioimmunoassay of the thyroxine-binding prealbumin. *Ann Clin Lab Sci* 1986;16:231–240.

52. Maye P, Bisetti A, Burger A, et al. Hyperprealbuminemia, euthyroid hyperthyroxinemia, Zollinger-Ellison-like syndrome and hypercorticism in a pancreatic endocrine tumour. *Acta Endocrinol (Copenh)* 1989;120:87–91.

53. Cano NJ. Metabolism and clinical interest of serum transthyretin (prealbumin) in dialysis patients. *Clin Chem Lab Med* 2002;1313–1319.

54. Schlossmacher P, Hasselmann M, Meyer N, et al. The prognostic value of nutritional and inflammatory indices in critically ill patients with acute respiratory failure. *Clin Chem Lab Med* 2002;40:1339–1343.

55. Benvenga S, Morgante L, Bartalena L, et al. Serum thyroid hormone binding proteins in patients with completed stroke. *Ann Clin Res* 1986;18:203–207.

56. Refetoff S. Defects of thyroid hormone transport in serum. In: deGroot LJ, Hennemann G, eds. *www.thyroidmanager.com.*

57. Su CC, Wu YC, Chiu CY, et al. Two novel mutations in the gene encoding thyroxine-binding globulin (TBG) as a cause of complete TBG deficiency in Taiwan. *Clin Endocrinol* 2003;58:409–414.

58. Domigues R, Bugalho MJ, Garrao A, et al. Two novel variants in the thyroxine-binding globulin (TBG) gene behind the diagnosis of TBG deficiency. *Eur J Endocrinol* 2002;146:485–490.

59. Benvenga S, LiCalzi L. Graves' disease and thyroxine-binding globulin excess [Letter]. *Arch Intern Med* 1989;149:705.

60. Ruiz M, Rajatavin R, Young R, et al. Familial dysalbuminemic hyperthyroxinemia: a new syndrome potentially confused with thyrotoxicosis. *N Engl J Med* 1982;306:635–639.

61. De Cosimo DR, Fang SL, Braverman LE. Prevalence of familial dysalbuminemic hyperthyroxinemia in Hispanics. *Ann Intern Med* 1987;107:780–781.

62. Benvenga S, Bartolone L, Musolino R, et al. Homozygous transthyretin Leu64: a very rare transthyretin mutation associated with amyloidosis but not euthyroid hyperthyroxinemia. *J Endocr Genet* 1999;1:101–104.

63. Genschel J, Haas R, Propsting MJ, et al. Apolipoprotein A-I induced amyloidosis. *FEBS Lett* 1998;430:145–149.

64. Torpy DJ, Bachmann AW, Grice JE, et al. Familial corticosteroid-binding globulin deficiency due to a novel null mutation: association with fatigue and relative hypotension. *J Clin Endocrinol Metab* 2001;86:3692–3700.

65. Joyner JM, Hutley LJ, Bachmann AW, et al. Greater replication and differentiation of preadipocytes in inherited corticosteroid-binding globulin deficiency. *Am J Physiol Endocrinol Metab* 2003;284:E1049–E1054.

66. Kang J, Holland M, Jones H. Coordinate augmentation in expression of genes encoding transcription factors and liver secretory proteins in hypo-oncotic states. *Kidney Int* 1999;56: 452–460.

67. Palha JA, Nissanov J, Fernandes R, et al. Thyroid hormone distribution in the mouse brain: the role of transthyretin. *Neuroscience* 2002;113:837–847.

68. Bui BV, Armitage JA, Fletcher EL, et al. Retinal anatomy and function of the transthyretin null mice. *Exp Eye Res* 2001;73:651–659.

69. Schreiber G. The evolution of transthyretin synthesis in the choroid plexus. *Clin Chem Lab Med* 2002;40:1200–1210.

70. Buraczynska M, Mears AJ, Zareparsi S, et al. Gene expression profile of native human retinal pigment epithelium. *Invest Ophthalmol Vis Sci* 2002;43:603–607.

71. Sousa MM, Norden AG, Jacobsen C, et al. Evidence for the role of megalin in renal uptake of transthyretin. *J Biol Chem* 2000;275:38176–38181.

72. Ritter M, Buechler C, Boettcher A, et al. Cloning and characterization of a novel apolipoprotein A-I binding protein, AI-BP, secreted by cells of the kidney proximal tubules in response to HDL or ApoA-I. *Genomics* 2002;79:693–670.

73. Willnow TE, Nykjaer A. Pathways for kidney-specific uptake of the steroid hormone 25-hydroxy vitamin D$_3$. *Curr Opin Lipidol* 2002;13:255–260.

74. Mendel CM, Weisinger RA, Jones AL et al. Thyroid-hormone binding proteins in plasma facilitate uniform distribution of thyroxine within tissues: a perfused rat liver study. *Endocrinology* 1987;120:1742–1749.

75. Janssen OE, Golcher HM, Grasberger H, et al. Characterization of T$_4$-binding globulin cleaved by human leukocyte elastase. *J Clin Endocrinol Metab* 2002;87:1217–1222.

76. Schussler GC. The thyroxine-binding proteins. *Thyroid* 2000; 10:141–149.

77. Concha MI, Molina S, Oyarzun C, et al. Local expression of apolipoprotein A-1 gene and possible role for HDL in primary defence in the carp skin. *Fish Shellfish Immunol* 2003;14:259–273.

78. Motizuki M, Satoh T, Takei T, et al. Structure-activity analysis of an antimicrobial peptide derived from bovine apolipoprotein A-II. *J Biochem (Tokyo)* 2002;132:115–119.

79. Rossner W. The functions of corticosteroid-binding globulin and sex-hormone binding globulin: recent advances. *Endocr Rev* 1990;11:80–91.

80. Benvenga S, Robbins J. Enhancement of thyroxine entry into low density lipoprotein (LDL) receptor-competent fibroblasts by LDL: an additional mode of entry of thyroxine into cells. *Endocrinology* 1990;126:933–940.

81. Benvenga S, Alesci S, Trimarchi F. High-density lipoprotein-facilitated entry of thyroid hormones into cells: a mechanism different from the low-density lipoprotein-facilitated entry. *Thyroid* 2002;12:547–556.

82. Sarne DH, Refetoff S. Normal cellular uptake of thyroxine from serum of patients with familial dysalbuminemic hyperthyroxinemia or elevated thyroxine-binding globulin. *J Clin Endocrinol Metab* 1988;67:1166–1170.

83. Sousa MM, Saraiva MJ. Internalization of transthyretin. Evidence of a novel yet unidentified receptor-associated protein (RAP)-sensitive receptor. *J Biol Chem* 2001;276:14420–14425.

84. Haddad G, Jennings AS, Aw TC. Vitamin D uptake and metabolism by perfused rat liver: influences of carrier proteins. *Endocrinology* 1988;123:498–504.

85. Aten RF, Kolodecik TR, Behrman HR. Ovarian vitamin E accumulation: evidence for a role of lipoproteins. *Endocrinology* 1994;135:533–539.

86. Oram JF, Vaughan AM, Stocker R. ATP-binding cassette transporter A1 mediates cellular secretion of alpha-tocopherol. *J Biol Chem* 2001;276:39898–39902.

87. Hennemann G, Krennin EP, Bernard P, et al. Regulation of influx and efflux of thyroid hormones in rat hepatocytes: possible physiological significance of the plasma membrane in the regulation of thyroid hormone activity. *Horm Metab Res Suppl* 1984;141:1–6.

88. Benvenga S, Robbins J. Thyroid hormone efflux from monolayer cultures of human fibroblasts and hepatocytes. Effect of lipoproteins and other thyroxine transport proteins. *Endocrinology* 1998;139:4311–4318.

89. Harper KD, McLeod JF, Kowalski MA et al. Vitamin D binding protein sequesters monomeric actin in the circulation of the rat. *J Clin Invest* 1987;79:1365–1370 (erratum in 1987;80:277).

90. Davidsson P, Folkesson S, Christiansson M, et al. Identification of proteins in human cerebrospinal fluid using liquid-phase isoelectric focusing as a prefractionation step followed by two-dimensional gel electrophoresis and matrix-assisted laser desorption/ionisation mass spectrometry. *Rapid Commun Mass Spectrom* 2002;16:2083–2088.

91. Puppione DL, MacDonald MH. Characterization of lipoproteins in cerebrospinal fluid of mares during pregnancy and lactation. *Am J Vet Res* 2002;63:886–889.

92. Pitas RE, Boyles JK, Lee SH, et al. Lipoproteins and their receptors in the central nervous system. Characterization of the lipoproteins in the cerebrospinal fluid and identification of apolipoprotein B,E (LDL) receptors in the brain. *J Biol Chem* 1987;262:14352–14360.

93. Aldred AR, Brack CM, Schreiber G. The cerebrospinal expression of plasma protein genes in different species. *Comp Biochem Physiol B* 1995;111:1–15.

94. Ignatius MJ, Gebicke-Hartner PJ, Pate Skene JH, et al. Expression of apolipoprotein E during nerve degeneration and regeneration. *Proc Natl Acad Sci U S A* 1986;83:1125–1129.

95. Epperson LE, Martin SL. Quantitative assessment of ground squirrel mRNA levels in multiple stages of hibernation. *Physiol Genom* 2002;10:93–102.

96. Prendergast BJ, Mosinger B Jr, Kolattukudy PE, et al. Hypothalamic gene expression in reproductively photoresponsive and photorefractory Siberian hamsters. *Proc Natl Acad Sci U S A* 2002;99:16291–16296.

97. Ekins R. Hypothesis. Role of serum thyroxine-binding proteins and maternal thyroid hormones in foetal development. *Lancet* 1985;1:1129–1132.

98. Anahory T, Dechaud H, Bennes R, et al. Identification of new proteins in follicular fluid of mature human follicles. *Electrophoresis* 2002;23:1197–1202.

99. Vieira AV, Sanders EJ, Schneider WJ. Transport of serum transthyretin into chicken oocytes. A receptor-mediated mechanism. *J Biol Chem* 1995;270:2952–2956.

100. McLeod JF, Cooke NE. The vitamin D–binding protein, alpha-fetoprotein, albumin multigene family: detection of transcripts in multiple tissues. *J Biol Chem* 1989;264:21760–21769.

101. Douglas GC, Moreira-Cali P, King BF, et al. Uptake of ^{125}I-labeled alpha2-macroglobulin and albumin by human placental syncytiotrophoblast *in vitro*. *J Cell Biochem* 1988;68:427–435.

102. Malassine A, Besse C, Roche A, et al. Ultrastructural visualization of the internalization of low density lipoproteins by human placental cells. *Histochemistry* 1987;87:457–464.

103. Shi WK, Hopkins B, Thomson S, et al. Synthesis of apolipoproteins, alphafoetoprotein, albumin and transferrin by the human foetal yolk sac and other foetal organs. *J Embryol Exp Morphol* 1985;85:191–206.

104. Quepio G, Deas M, Arranz C, et al. Sex hormone binding globulin stimulates chorionic gonadotropin secretion from human cytotrophoblasts in culture. *Hum Reprod* 1998;13:1368–1373.

105. Handwerger S, Quarford S, Barret J, et al. Apolipoprotein A-I, A-II and C-I stimulate placental lactogen release from human placental tissue. A novel action of high density lipoprotein apolipoproteins. *J Clin Invest* 1987;79:625–628.

106. Davis PJ, Tillmann HC, Davis FB, et al. Comparison of the mechanisms of nongenomic actions of thyroid hormone and steroid hormones. *J Endocrinol Invest* 2002;25:377–388.

107. Diekman T, Demacker PNM, Kastelein JJP, et al. Increased oxidizability of low density lipoproteins in hypothyroidism. *J Clin Endocrinol Metab* 1998;83:1752–1755.

108. Mahley RW, Weisgraber KH, Farese RV. Disorders of lipid metabolism. In: Larsen PR, Kronenberg HM, Melmed S, et al., eds. *Williams textbook of endocrinology*, 10th ed. Philadelphia: WB Saunders, 2003:1642–1705.

109. Hanna AN, Feller DR, Witiak DT, et al. Inhibition of low density lipoprotein oxidation by thyronine and probucol. *Biochem Pharmacol* 1993;45:753–762.

110. Schmidt BMW, Martin M, Georgens AC, et al. Nongenomic cardiovascular effects of triiodothyronine in euthyroid male volunteers. *J Clin Endocrinol Metab* 2002;87:1681–1686.

111. Li Calzi L, Benvenga S, Battiato S, et al. Autoantibodies to thyroxine and triiodothyronine in the immunoglobulin G fraction of serum. *Clin Chem* 1988;34:2561–2562.

112. Benvenga S, Trimarchi F. Thyroid hormone autoantibodies in Hashimoto's thyroiditis: often transient, but also increasingly frequent. *Thyroid* 2003;13:995–996.

113. Shimon I, Pariente C, Shlomo-David J, et al Transient elevation of triiodothyronine caused by triiodothyronine autoantibody associated with acute Epstein-Barr virus infection. *Thyroid* 2003;13:211–215.

114. Ruggeri RM, Galletti M, Mandolfino MG, et al Thyroid hormone autoantibodies in primary Sjögren syndrome and rheumatoid arthritis are more prevalent than in autoimmune thyroid disease, becoming progressively more frequent in these diseases. *J Endocrinol Invest* 2002;25:447–454.

115. Chan BW, Chow CC, Cockram CS. Discrepant thyroid function tests in a patient treated with interferon-alpha [Letter]. *J R Soc Med* 2002;95:606.

INTRACELLULAR PATHWAYS OF IODOTHYRONINE METABOLISM

ANTONIO C. BIANCO
P. REED LARSEN

Thyroxine (T_4), the main product of the thyroid gland, is a prohormone that must be activated by deiodination to triiodothyronine (T_3) in order to initiate thyroid action. This deiodination reaction occurs in the phenolic or outer ring of the T_4 molecule and is catalyzed by two deiodinases, type 1 (D1) and type 2 (D2) (Fig. 7.1). In humans, approximately 80% of the T_3 that is produced each day is produced by extrathyroidal deiodination of T_4, demonstrating the critical importance of this pathway for thyroid hormone homeostasis. In normal humans, this occurs primarily via D2, because their serum T_3 concentrations do not decline much when they are given propylthiouracil (PTU), a specific inhibitor of D1. In contrast, in rodents, both D1 and D2 contribute about equally to extrathyroidal T_3 production. As a counterpoint to the activation pathway, both T_4 and T_3 can be irreversibly inactivated by deiodination of their tyrosyl ring (inner ring deiodination), a reaction catalyzed by either D1 or type 3 deiodinase (D3), the third member of the deiodinase group. About 40% of the T_4 and nearly all of the T_3 that is produced each day is deiodinated by inner ring deiodination, mostly via D3 (Fig. 7.1). Therefore, the deiodinases have the capacity to promote or terminate thyroid hormone action, constituting a critical mechanism to vary thyroid status in different organs (1).

Iodine availability is likely to have been a major factor in the evolutionary pressure leading to the selection of the deiodinases as important regulators of thyroid hormone homeostasis and biologic activity. T_3 is the short-lived biologically active molecule (half-life ~1 day in humans) that is responsible for most if not all thyroid action in tissues. If T_3 were the main product of thyroid secretion, its production would fluctuate according to the availability of iodine. Rather, the human thyroid secretes large amounts of T_4, a long-lived molecule (half-life ~7 days) that binds to circulating proteins and accumulates in a large extrathyroidal pool, approximately 770 μg (1 μmol) in adult humans. Appropriate changes in deiodinase activity accommodate variations in iodine availability by adapting to modifications in serum T_4 concentrations in order to maintain constant serum T_3 concentrations (1).

STRUCTURE OF THE DEIODINASES

The three deiodinase proteins (D1, D2, and D3) are structurally similar (~50% sequence identity). All are integral membrane proteins of 29 to 33 kd, and they are especially similar in the region surrounding the active catalytic center (2–4). Because of inherent difficulties in the crystallization of membrane-anchored proteins, further insight into the structures of these proteins has been obtained through the use of hydrophobic cluster analysis (5), which is based on protein folding and two-dimensional transposition of sequences, allowing resolution of a sequence into its secondary structures centered on the so-defined hydrophobic clusters.

Based on this type of analysis, the three deiodinases have a single transmembrane segment, which is present near the N-terminus, and several well-conserved clusters, typical of α-helixes or β-strands, suggesting that they correspond to core secondary structures of the deiodinases. A striking common feature is the similarity of the deiodinases with various members of the thioredoxin (TRX) family, proteins that contain in their three-dimensional structure a fold defined by βαβ and ββα motifs (Fig. 7.2). The deiodinases contain extra elements, not found in the canonical thioredoxin fold, that interrupt the relationship between the βαβ and ββα motifs. These intervening sequences correspond to distinct secondary structural elements added to the canonical thioredoxin fold, a feature also present in other proteins of the thioredoxin family (6). A unique aspect of the deiodinases, however, is that one of these intervening sequences has striking similarity to α-L-iduronidase (IDUA; 47% identity with D1 and D3 and 60% with D2), a lysosomal enzyme that cleaves α-iduronic acid residues from the glycosaminoglycans heparan sulfate and dermatan sulfate (7) (Fig. 7.2). This structural similarity between the deiodinases and iduronidase may reflect the similarity of their substrates, T_4 (or T_3) and sulfated α-L-iduronic acid, respectively.

The three-dimensional model predicts that the active center of the three deiodinases is a pocket defined by the β_1-α_1-β_2 motifs of the thioredoxin fold and the IDUA-like insertion (Fig. 7.3). The most striking feature of this pocket

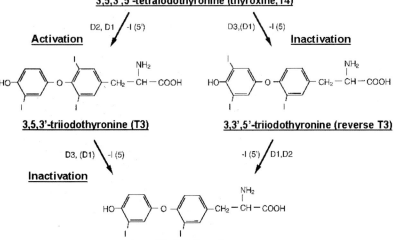

3,5,3',5'-tetraiodothyronine (thyroxine,T4)

D2, D1 ‑I (5')　**Activation**　　　D3, (D1) ‑I (5)　**Inactivation**

3,5,3'-triiodothyronine (T3)　　　**3,3',5'-triiodothyronine (reverse T3)**

D3, (D1) ‑I (5)　**Inactivation**　　　‑I (5') D1,D2

3,3'-diiodothyronine

FIGURE 7.1. Structures and interrelationships between the principal iodothyronines activated or inactivated by the selenodeiodinases.

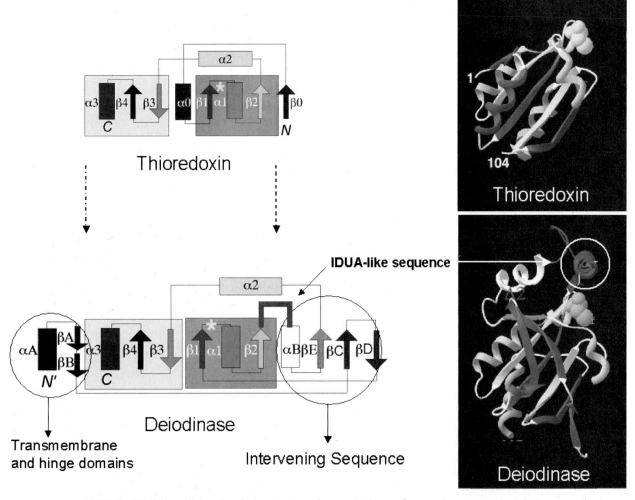

FIGURE 7.2. Three-dimensional structures and organization of secondary structure of the archetype thioredoxin enzyme and the rough model of the deiodinases deduced from the alignment revealed by hydrophobic cluster analysis. The transmembrane, hinge, and intervening sequences are circled. (Modified from Callebaut I, Curcio-Morelli C, et al. The iodothyronine selenodeiodinases are thioredoxin-fold family proteins containing a glycoside hydrolase-clan GH-A-like structure. *J Biol Chem* 2003;278:36887, with permission.)

Proposed D2 active center

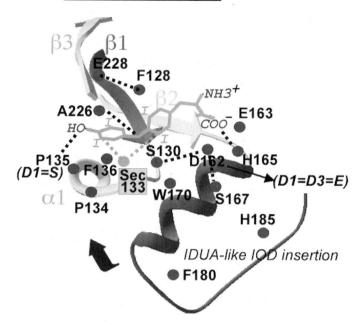

Conserved positions in the deiodinase active center

D1	D2	D3
F121	F128	F139
S123	S130	S141
Sec126	Sec133	Sec144
S128	P135	P146
F129	F136	F147
E155	D162	E173
E156	E163	E174
H158	H165	H176
S160	S167	S178
W163	W170	W181
H174	H185	H193
S212	A226	Y231
E214	E228	E233

FIGURE 7.3. Schematic representation of the putative active site of deiodinases deduced from sequence alignment and from the associated modeling (see Fig. 7.2). The positions shown are those of type 2 deiodinase (D2), and the table contains the corresponding positions and residues in D1 and D3. The iduronidase (*IDUA*)-like insertion likely constitutes a cap that may cover the active site after ligand binding. (Modified from Callebaut I, Curcio-Morelli C, Mornon JP, et al. The iodothyronine selenodeiodinases are thioredoxin-fold family proteins containing a glycoside hydrolase-clan GH-A-like structure. *J Biol Chem* 2003;278:36887, with permission.)

is the presence of the rare amino acid selenocysteine, which is critical for the catalytic activity of the three deiodinases. The presence of selenocysteine was first identified when rodent D1 complementary DNA (cDNA) was found to contain UGA that encoded selenocysteine; in the vast majority of messenger RNAs (mRNAs), UGA is a stop codon (8).

The cis-acting sequences that allow for the incorporation of selenocysteine rather than a stop codon consist of the seleocysteine codon (UGA) itself and a specific RNA stem-loop located in the 3'-untranslated region of the mRNA. Only in the presence of the stem-loop structure and in several trans-acting factors are UGA codons "recoded" to

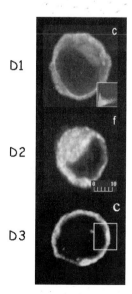

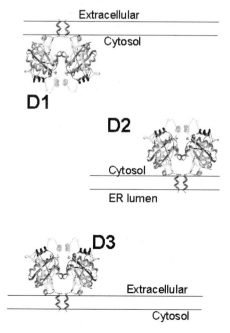

FIGURE 7.4. Subcellular localization and topology of D1, D2, and D3. Left panel: Immunofluorescence confocal microscopy of HEK-293 cells transiently expressing one of the deiodinases as indicated. D1 is visible in the periphery of the cell, and does not colocalize with BiP, an endoplasmic reticulum marker visible around the nucleus. D2 is visible colocalized with BiP, whereas D3 is visible in the cell border. Right panel: Schematic representation of type 1 deiodinase (D1), D2, and D3 dimers with their respective orientations and subcellular localization. (From Toyoda N, Berry MJ, Harney JW, et al. Topological analysis of the integral membrane protein, type 1 iodothyronine deiodinase (D1). *J Biol Chem* 1995;270:12310; Baqui MM, Gereben B, Harney JW, et al. Distinct subcellular localization of transiently expressed types 1 and 2 iodothyronine deiodinases as determined by immunofluorescence confocal microscopy. *Endocrinology* 2000; 141:4309; and Baqui MM, Botero D, Gereben B, et al. Human type 3 iodothyronine selenodeiodinase is located in the plasma membrane and undergoes rapid internalization to endosomes. *J Biol Chem* 2003;278:1206, with permission.)

specify selenocysteine. The stem-loop sequence is termed the Selenocysteine (sec) insertion sequence, or SECIS, element; it is present in all three deiodinases and all other eukaryotic selenoproteins (9).

All three deiodinases can form homodimers when transiently expressed (10,11) (Fig. 7.4). This is supported by the finding of catalytic activity in the higher-molecular-weight forms (~65 kd) (12,13). However, these higher-molecular-weight forms of the deiodinases may reflect associations with other cellular proteins not primarily involved in their catalytic function, but which could, for example, regulate their half-life, intracellular transport, or subcellular localization. It is not clear that dimerization occurs or that it is necessary for function when the enzymes are expressed at endogenous levels.

TOPOLOGY AND SUBCELLULAR LOCALIZATION

The D1 and D2 monomers are integral membrane proteins oriented with a small amino-terminal extension in the extracellular space (D1) or lumen of the endoplasmic reticulum (D2), and a single transmembrane domain exiting the membrane at about position 40 (14,15). This puts the active center of both D1 and D2 in the cytosol. D3 is also an integral membrane protein, but its orientation is opposite, so that its active center is the extracellular space (Fig. 7.4).

The location of mature D1 in the plasma membrane has been demonstrated in several types of cells that normally contain D1, including thyroid and kidney cells, and in cells transiently expressing the enzyme (10,16–18). Using confocal laser microscopy of human and mouse cells, transiently expressed FLAG-tagged D1 was also localized to the plasma membrane. D1 does not colocalize with the endoplasmic reticulum protein BiP, as does D2 (15). This plasma membrane localization has been confirmed by labeling of D1 with cell-impermeable reagents (19). D2, on the other hand, is an endoplasmic reticulum protein. Immunofluorescent confocal microscopy of human and mouse cells transiently expressing FLAG-tagged D2 revealed colocalization of D2 with BiP. Endogenously expressed D2 also colocalizes with BiP in MSTO-211H cells (20).

Using similar techniques, endogenously and transiently expressed FLAG-tagged D3 was identified in the plasma membrane. It colocalizes with the α-subunit of Na$^+$,K$^+$-ATPase, the early endosomal marker EEA-1, and clathrin, but not with endoplasmic-reticulum proteins. Most of the D3 is extracellular (Fig. 7.4), and its extracellular portion can be covalently labeled with a cell-impermeant probe, confirming its plasma membrane location. There is constant internalization of D3 that is blocked by sucrose-containing medium, and exposing cells to a weak base such as primaquine increases the pool of internalized D3, suggest-

ing that D3 is recycled between plasma membrane and early endosomes. Such recycling could account for the longer half-life of D3 (12 hours), as compared with D1 (8 hours) or D2 (1 hour) (19).

A plasma membrane location for D1 could be viewed teleologically as allowing ready access of circulating T$_4$ to the enzyme as well as facilitating the entry of the T$_3$ produced from T$_4$ into the extracellular fluid. The plasma membrane localization of D1 contrasts with the localization of D2 in the endoplasmic reticulum in the same cell types (15). This differential subcellular localization of D1 and D2 may explain the small contribution of T$_3$ generated by D1 and the large contribution of T$_3$ generated by D2 to intranuclear T$_3$ (21–24). The extracellular location of D3 makes it readily accessible to extracellular, and therefore circulating T$_4$ and T$_3$, explaining its capacity for rapid inactivation of circulating T$_4$ and T$_3$ in patients with hemangiomas and its blockade of the access of maternal thyroid hormones to the fetus.

STRUCTURE-FUNCTION RELATIONSHIPS OF DEIODINASES AND MECHANISM OF DEIODINATION

The deiodination of iodothyronines by D1, D2, and D3 is a reductive dehalogenation that *in vitro* requires a reducing agent, such as dithiothreitol, as cofactor. An endogenous cofactor capable of sustaining multiple rounds of iodothyronine deiodination has not yet been identified. Based on major differences in substrate preference, reaction kinetics, and sensitivity to various inhibitors, it was assumed that the substrate-binding pockets of these enzymes were fundamentally different. However, the structural model described above predicts a conserved structure for all three deiodinases, particularly for the active center, the accuracy of which is supported by the substantial perturbations in enzyme function that result from changes of single amino acids in the binding pocket (5) (Fig. 7.3).

D1 has a relatively low affinity for T$_4$ [Michaelis-Menten constant (K_m), 1–2 μM], and its catalytic activity is bisubstrate in nature, with a thiol-containing cofactor serving as the second substrate with "ping-pong" kinetics (25) (Fig. 7.5). D2 and D3, on the other hand, have relatively high affinity for T$_4$ and T$_3$, respectively (K_m, 1–4 nM), and both have sequential reaction kinetics, suggesting that the iodothyronine and the thiol-containing cofactor interact with the enzyme simultaneously before the reaction takes place (25). Regardless of the reaction kinetics, the selenocysteine residue in the active center of the three deiodinases probably acts as a nucleophile catalyzing the removal of iodine. The critical role of selenocysteine in this function was ascertained through characterization of the kinetic properties of the wild-type selenoenzymes (D1, D2, and D3) and

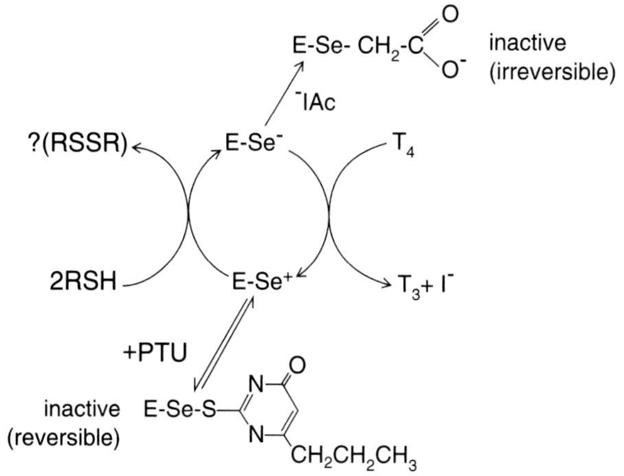

FIGURE 7.5. Mechanism of type 1 deiodinase (D1)-catalyzed thyroxine (T_4) conversion to triiodothyronine (T_3). The steps in the enzymatic reaction cycle at which iodoacetic acid (IAc) and propylthiouracil (PTU) are thought to inhibit catalysis are indicated. (From Leonard JL, Rosenberg IN. Thyroxine 5′-deiodinase activity of rat kidney: observations on activation by thiols and inhibition by propylthiouracil. *Endocrinology* 1978;103:2137, with permission.)

the corresponding cysteine (Cys) mutants, which have lower affinity for the substrates and decreased turnover rates (2,11,26).

D1, D2, and D3 differ in their sensitivity to PTU. D1 is quite sensitive [inhibition constant (K_i), 5 μM; in vitro at 10 μM dithiothreitol], but D2 and D3 are not (K_i, >1 mM). PTU probably inhibits D1 by competing with the endogenous thiol-containing cofactor for a putative selenenyl iodide (E-Se-I) intermediate (25) (Fig. 7.5). Supporting this interpretation is the fact that PTU inhibition is uncompetitive with the first D1 substrate (iodothyronine), but competitive with the second (e.g., dithiothreitol) (25). Because of the PTU insensitivity, D2- or D3-catalyzed deiodination proceeds by removal of an iodonium (I^+) ion by the endogenous cofactor, resulting in an enzyme-thyronine intermediate [D2-T_3 (or reverse T_3)] complex and a cofactor-Se-I complex (27). In this regard, it is notable that the sequence Thr-Sec-Pro-Pro/Ser-Phe is identical in D1, D2, and D3, but that in all D1 sequences, excepting the PTU-insensitive D1 of the blue tilapia (*Oreochromis aureus*), the uncharged polar side chain of the Ser residue substitutes for the nonpolar side chain of Pro at position 128 (28). The existence of this natural variation prompted the creation of the Ser128Pro D1, Pro135Ser D2, and Pro146Ser D3 proteins (Fig. 7.3). Remarkably, replacement of Pro135 with Ser in D2 results in a two orders of magnitude increase in K_m (T_4) to approximately 250 nM, approximately 10-fold lower than that of D1 for T_4, and the enzyme operates with ping-pong kinetics. Furthermore, the Pro135Ser D2-catalyzed deiodination is two orders of magnitude more sensitive to PTU (K_i, 4.0 μM), although PTU inhibition is noncompet-

itive with dithiothreitol. Thus, the substitution of Ser for Pro135 in D2 results in changes in the enzyme that make its kinetics more similar to those of D1, indicating a critical influence of the amino acid occupying this position on enzyme function. Similar observations were made with the Pro146Ser D3 protein, which has a fivefold higher K_m (T_3) and is highly sensitive to inhibition by PTU (K_i, 1.0 μM). As mentioned above, Ser128Pro D1 catalyzed deiodination is resistant to PTU (K_i, >1 mM), suggesting that there is no longer an accessible E-Se-I intermediate, again illustrating the pivotal role of this position in the active center of the deiodinase molecule.

The presence of Pro in the 128/135/146 positions of D1, D2, and D3 may result in tighter binding of the substrate in the D2 (and D3) binding pockets, perhaps explaining the approximately 1000-fold higher affinity of D2 and D3 for T_4, as compared with D1. This could reflect an interaction between the phenolic hydroxyl group of T_4 and the Pro residue at these positions, and explain why sulfate conjugation of the phenolic hydroxyl group dramatically increases the maximum velocity (V_{max})/K_m and changes the T_4 deiodination site from an outer to an inner ring iodine (29).

Three conserved amino acids with charged polar side chains mark the transition between the β_2-strand and the α-helix in the IDUA-like insertion, Glu/Asp155, Glu156, and His158 (D1 residues). When the invariant Glu156 (D1), Glu163 (D2), and Glu174 (D3) were replaced with Ala, the resulting enzymes had no deiodinase activity. Replacement of Glu156 with Asp in D1 supported deiodination, but with an approximately 4.5-fold higher K_m (rT_3), whereas a similar substitution at position 163 in D2 did not alter the K_m (T_4). Thus, the acidic amino acids in this region of the deiodinase pocket are important for substrate binding or enzyme function, although the length of the side chain can vary. This is further supported by mutational studies of His at position 158 in D1 (30). Its mutation to Asn, Gln, or Phe resulted in complete loss of deiodinase activity. Replacement of the corresponding His165 in D2 with Asn also resulted in loss of deiodinase activity. According to the model, residues in this acidic pocket could interact with either the amino or the carboxyl group in the alanine side chain of the iodothyronines, a hypothesis supported by previous studies indicating that the positively charged T_4 analogue (3,5,3′,5′-tetraiodothyroethylamine), which lacks a carboxyl group, is not a substrate for D1 (31). In addition, the compounds with the highest affinity for D1 (lowest apparent K_m values) are those that lack positively charged functional groups (NH_3^+), such as tetraiodothyroacetic acid. Furthermore, the K_m (T_4) values for D- and L-T_4 are similar (31). These results argue that the carboxyl group in the iodothyronines interacts with the NH_3 group of His in the 158 position of D1 and that the other acidic residues in this pocket act to reduce the ionization of the His residue. The critical role played by the IDUA-like insertion is further strengthened by the complete loss of deiodinase activity when the conserved Trp163 in D1 and the corresponding Trp170 in D2 are replaced with Ala.

SPECIFIC PROPERTIES OF THE DEIODINASES

Type 1 Deiodinase

PTU-inhibitable, D1-catalyzed conversion of T_4 to T_3 supplies approximately 20% to 30% of the T_3 in the serum in normal humans, but 50% or more in patients with thyrotoxicosis. D1 is the only selenodeiodinase that can function as either an outer (5′)- or inner (5)-ring iodothyronine deiodinase, D2 and D3 being exclusively outer and inner ring deiodinases, respectively (32). The molecular basis for these differences is not known.

The gene (*Dio1*) for human D1 is on chromosome 1 p32-p33, in a region syntenic with mouse chromosome 4, the location of mouse *Dio1* (33). The complete cDNA sequences have been determined for rat, human, mouse, dog, chicken, and tilapia D1 (8,28,34–37). The size of the mRNAs for these D1s is about 2 to 2.1 kb, and all contain a UGA codon in the region encoding the active center, which is highly conserved among species. By Northern analysis, D1 is expressed in many tissues of most vertebrates, but not in amphibia (38–40). In rats, these include the liver, kidneys, central nervous system, anterior pituitary gland, thyroid gland, intestine, and placenta. In humans, D1 activity is notably absent from the central nervous system, but is present in the liver, kidneys, thyroid and pituitary (41,42).

Regulation of D1 Synthesis

Changes in D1 activity have been investigated in developing rats; in general, D1 activity is low in all tissues of fetal rats. It appears soon after birth in the intestine, liver, kidneys, cerebrum, cerebellum, and gonads (43). The age-related changes in D1 mRNA content are similar, indicating that the changes in activity arise at a pretranslational level. The mechanism for the age-related changes in D1 expression is unknown. The physiologic benefit of the low D1 activity in the fetus is presumably low serum T_3 concentrations, thus permitting changes in intracellular T_3 to be determined by the developmentally programmed changes in D2 and D3 activity (44).

Thyroid Hormone

Thyroid hormone–induced increases in D1 activity and mRNA content are well documented in rats, mice, and humans (8,45). The increases are due to increased transcription, which in the human *Dio1* gene can be attributed to the presence of two thyroid hormone-response elements (TREs) in the 5′-flanking region of the gene (46–48). Studies in thyroid receptor (TR) knockout mice indicate that the T_3-induced D1 stimulation is largely mediated by the β subtype of the receptor (49). Given this finding, the responsiveness of the human *Dio1* gene to T_3 would be expected to be greatest in patients with thyrotoxicosis. In fact, the D1 mRNA content of peripheral blood mononuclear cells is increased in proportion to the degree of thyrotoxicosis (42). This increase can explain the acute decrease in serum T_3 concentrations that occurs in response to PTU in patients with thyrotoxicosis (50).

Cytokines

Interleukin-1 (IL-1), IL-6, tumor necrosis factor-α (TNF-α), and other cytokines are potential mediators of the alterations in thyroid function that occur in patients with severe nonthyroidal illness (see section on nonthyroidal illness in Chapter 11) (51–53). TNF-α, IL-1β, and interferon-γ decrease D1 activity and mRNA in rodent thyroid (FRTL5) cells (54). The effects of TNF-α have been examined in hepatocytes and HepG2 cells with contradictory results. TNF-α decreased the stimulatory effect of T_3 on D1 mRNA production in HEPG2 cells, an action that is blocked by nuclear factor kappa B (55). In dispersed rat hepatocytes, IL-1β and IL-6 blocked T_3 stimulation of D1 mRNA and activity; however, TNF-α had no effect (56). The effect of IL-1β was blocked by coexpression of the nuclear steroid receptor coactivator-1 (SRC-1), but not by CREB binding protein (CBP) or CBP-associated factor (pCAF). Because IL-1 did not alter the amount of SRC-1 in hepatocytes, the effect was attributed to competition between IL-1 and T_3-stimulated transcriptional events for limiting quantities of SRC-1. More recent studies describing decreases in D1 activity in liver and D2 activity in skeletal muscle and increases in D3 activity in liver and skeletal muscle in patients dying of multiple organ failure and related conditions are discussed in the section on nonthyroidal illness in Chapter 11.

Nutritional Influences on D1 Expression

A decrease in serum T_3 concentrations relative to those of T_4 and an increase in serum reverse T_3 concentrations during fasting in humans was one of the earliest indications that the peripheral metabolism of thyroid hormones in humans was modulated by physiologic or pathophysiologic events (57). Similar changes occur in virtually all acutely ill and many chronically ill patients (58,59). Because thyroidal secretion accounts for only about 20% of daily T_3 production in humans, the illness-associated decrease in serum T_3 concentrations must be caused, largely if not completely, by decreased T_4 to T_3 conversion by D1 or D2 or by increased T_3 clearance by D3 (60,61).

Early studies of liver D1 activity in rats suggested that the decrease in T_4 conversion to T_3 that occurred during fasting might be caused by a decrease in the thiol cofactor that serves as the cosubstrate for D1-catalyzed T_4 to T_3 conversion (62,63). However, this cofactor has not been identified. Although rats have been studied extensively as a model for the effects of fasting (and illness) on T_4 to T_3 conversion in humans, they are a poor model for the effects of fasting in humans because of their low body fat content and the fact that, unlike humans, their serum TSH and T_4 concentrations decrease rapidly when they are starved (64). Also, despite reduced hepatic D1 activity, total body conversion of T_4 to T_3 is not reduced during starvation in rats (65,66). The marked fasting-induced reduction in serum TSH, T_4, and T_3 concentrations (i.e., central hypothyroidism) in rats is probably due, at least in part, to leptin deficiency (67). Prefeeding rats with a high-fat diet to induce obesity results in less urinary nitrogen loss and a lesser decline in serum T_4 and T_3 concentrations during starvation, and serum T_3 concentrations actually increase if the period of starvation is prolonged (64). In contrast, in humans, serum T_3 concentrations decrease rapidly to about 50% of baseline during fasting, and they remain low for up to 3 weeks of fasting, but serum T_4 and TSH concentrations change little (68).

Selenium Availability

A decrease in hepatic D1 activity of Se-deficient rats and the demonstration that D1 could be labeled with ^{75}Se were the first clues that this trace element was critical to the function of D1 (69–72). However, the effects of Se deficiency on the synthesis of intracellular selenoproteins, such as the selenodeiodinases, depend on the tissue being examined. For example, in Se-deficient rats, thyroidal D1 activity is preserved, while that in the liver declines precipitously (73), serum T_4 concentrations increase, and serum T_3 concentrations do not change (74). Se deficiency also decreases D1 activity in the kidneys; this is accompanied by a decrease in D1 mRNA, which does not occur in the liver (75). Se deficiency can occur in patients receiving diets that are restricted in protein content, such as those given for phenylketonuria, and has also been found in elderly patients (76–79). In Se-deficient humans, serum T_4 concentrations and the serum ratio of T_4 to T_3 are slightly increased, but serum TSH concentrations are normal. In one endemic goiter region in Africa, there is an accompanying Se deficiency (80,81). When Se was supplied to these iodine-deficient people, their thyroid function deteriorated, as evidenced by an increase in serum TSH concentrations and a decrease in serum T_3 concentrations, suggesting that the reduction in D1 activity during Se deficiency can pro-

tect against iodine deficiency, presumably by reducing inner ring deiodination of T_4 or T_3 (82,83).

Type 2 Deiodinase

Type 2 deiodinase is an obligate outer ring selenodeiodinase that catalyzes the conversion of T_4 to T_3. The K_m of D2 for T_4 is in the nanomolar range under *in vitro* conditions in the presence of 20 mM dithiothreitol. The presence of considerable D2 activity in human skeletal muscle, unexpected because it is absent in rats and mice, provides a plausible source for a substantial fraction of the extrathyroidally generated T_3 in human serum (26). T_4 causes a posttranslational decrease in D2 activity, due to stimulation of proteolysis of D2 via the ubiquitin-proteasome pathway (84–86).

Gene Structure and Chromosomal Localization

The *Dio2* gene is present as a single copy located on the long arm of chromosome 14 (14q24.3) in humans (87,88). It is about 15 kb in size, and the coding region is divided into two exons by an intron of approximately 7.4 kb. The exon/intron junction is located in codon 75, and is at the same position in the human and mouse *Dio2* genes (87, 89,90). For the human gene, there are three transcriptional start sites, 707, 31, and 24 nucleotides 5′ to the initiator codon ATG. The longest 5′-untranslated region of human D2 mRNA contains an intron of approximately 300 bp that can be alternatively spliced (90). Other splicing variants involving the coding region have also been identified (91). The human, mouse, and rat *Dio2* 5′-flanking regions have been isolated and functionally characterized. All contain a functional cyclic adenosine monophosphate (cyclic AMP) response element, but only human *Dio2* has binding sites for thyroid transcription factor-1 (TTF-1) (90,92,93).

D2 mRNA and Protein

Human, mouse, and chicken D2 cDNAs containing intact 3′-untranslated regions (5- to 7.5-kb) have been identified using GenBank searches and library screening. These D2 cDNAs encode functional D2 proteins, as determined by expression in *Xenopus laevis* oocytes (89,94, 95). Rat and human D2 mRNAs are approximately 7.5 kb, and chicken cDNA is approximately 6 kb (26,94–96). A detailed analysis involving nuclease mapping, primer extension, and Northern blots indicated that human D2 mRNA exists as four different transcripts in thyroid, brain, and possibly other tissues (90). The longest transcript is approximately 7.5 kb, starts 708 nucleotides upstream from the initiator ATG codon, and is the only transcript found in placenta. A shorter (approximately 7.2-kb)-minor D2 species uses the same transcriptional start site, but the approximately 300-bp intron is spliced out. Two shorter transcripts of approximately 6.8 kb, differing by only seven nucleotides, use 3′ transcriptional start sites close to the translation initiation site. It is not known whether the rat and mouse genes use the same two major transcriptional start sites, but this is likely to be so for D2 in rat brain (26,90,96). The deduced amino acid sequences of the chicken, mouse, rat, and human D2 enzymes contain two selenocysteine residues. The first is in the active center of the enzyme, whereas the second is located close to the carboxy-terminus. In fish and frog D2, there is only one selenocysteine codon, which is located in the active center of the enzyme (26,89,95–98). Truncating the C-terminal amino acids, including the C-terminal selenocysteine, in human D2 has no effect on D2 enzyme kinetics or activity (99).

Tissue Distribution

In rats, D2 activity is predominantly expressed in the pituitary, brain, and brown adipose tissue (24,100–104). D2 activity is also present in the gonads, pineal, thymus, and uterus of rats, mammary gland of mice, and vascular smooth muscle cells in humans (43,105–109). High levels of D2 mRNA and activity are found in the mouse cochlea at the eighth postnatal day, suggesting a role for D2 in generating T_3 for cochlear development (110). In the cerebral cortex of neonatal rats, D2 mRNA is present in astrocytes (111) and tanycytes; the latter are specialized ependymal cells lining the third ventricle that have multiple cellular processes that express D2 mRNA and that extend to the median eminence (111–114). A monosynaptic pathway has also been identified between the arcuate nucleus, which contains D2, and the paraventricular nucleus, which contains thyrotropin-releasing hormone (TRH) (115).

In humans, D2 mRNA or activity is expressed not only in vascular smooth muscle cells, but also in the thyroid, heart, brain, spinal cord, skeletal muscle, and placenta, and small amounts of D2 mRNA have been detected in the kidneys and pancreas (26,90,96,116–118). Thyroid tissue contains relatively more D2 mRNA than D2 activity, with the exception of thyroid tissue in patients with thyrotoxicosis caused by Graves' disease and follicular adenomas, in which both D2 mRNA and activity are present in large amounts (116). The discrepancy between D2 mRNA and activity is probably due to substrate-induced D2 ubiquitination. D2 mRNA sequences are also present in libraries from prostate, breast, and uterus, but none of these tissues have D2 activity (94). D2 mRNA or activity is present in human pituitary glands and brain tumors (116,119,120), and D2 activity has been found in human keratinocytes (121) and mesothelioma cells (20).

Regulation of D2 Synthesis

The *Dio2* gene is regulated in part by a cyclic AMP-mediated pathway. Cold exposure increases D2 mRNA and activity in brown adipose tissue in rodents, and α_1- or β-adrenergic antagonist agents block this effect (104,122). In isolated brown adipocytes, the increase of D2 activity during catecholamine treatment is actinomycin D sensitive (123–125). In addition, D2 activity in brown adipose tissue is induced by norepinephrine, isoproterenol, insulin, and glucagon, and it is inhibited by growth hormone (126,127). Cyclic AMP increases D2 activity in mesothelioma cells (20) and in rat astroglial cells (101,128), as does both nicotine and cyclic guanosine monophosphate (cyclic GMP) (129,130). As noted above, D2 mRNA and activity are increased in thyroid tissue from patients with Graves' thyrotoxicosis, and forskolin increases D2 mRNA in dispersed human thyroid cells (90,116). It is therefore not surprising that human, rat, and mouse *Dio2* contains a cyclic AMP response element approximately 90 nucleotides upstream of the transcriptional start site (90,92,93,131). The promoter activity of human *Dio2* increases 10-fold when cells are cotransfected with *Dio2* and the α-catalytic subunit of protein kinase A. Mutation of the latter element abolishes the effect and decreases basal expression of *Dio2* by approximately 90% (90).

Although there is a high level of D2 mRNA in human thyroid tissue, no D2 mRNA or activity is present in FRTL-5 rat thyroid cells, and in adult rat thyroid tissue D2 mRNA levels are very low and D2 activity is undetectable (93,116,132). Expression of the *Dio2* gene in human thyroid tissue is under the control of TTF-1 but is not affected by Pax-8 (93). The human *Dio2* gene has two TTF-1 binding sites, which are not present in the rat *Dio2* gene, despite an overall 73% cross-species homology. The lack of these sites may explain the very low expression of D2 mRNA and activity in rat thyroid tissue.

Regulation of Degradation of D2

D2 is the critical T_3-generating deiodinase due to its substantial responsiveness to physiologic signals. For example, D2 responsiveness to cyclic AMP constitutes the basis for the adrenergic stimulation of D2 activity in brown adipose tissue, and human skeletal muscle and thyroid tissue. This links D2 expression with the sympathetic nervous system and widens the spectrum of environmental and endogenous stimuli that can potentially influence adaptive T_3 production (see reference 1 for review).

Several transcriptional and posttranslational mechanisms have evolved to ensure tight control of tissue levels of D2, which is inherent to its homeostatic function. The D2 mRNA in higher vertebrates is more than 6 kb in length, containing long 5′ and 3′ untranslated regions. The D2 5′ untranslated regions are greater than 600 nucleotides in length, and they contain three to five short open reading frames, which reduce D2 expression by as much as fivefold (133). Alternative splicing is another mechanism that regulates the level of D2 synthesis, because mRNA transcripts similar in size to the major 6- to 7-kb D2 mRNAs, but not encoding an active enzyme, are present in both human and chicken tissues (133).

The ratios of D2 activity to D2 mRNA level in tissues vary, indicating substantial posttranslational regulation of D2 expression (134). In fact, the decisive property of D2 that characterizes its homeostatic behavior is a half-life of approximately 40 minutes that can be further reduced to approximately 25 minutes by exposure to physiologic concentrations of its substrate, T_4, or extended to approximately 300 minutes when cells are grown in medium lacking T_4 (135–142). This constitutes a rapid, potent regulatory feedback loop that efficiently controls T_3 production and intracellular T_3 concentrations based on how much T_4 is available. The potency of the T_4 in inducing loss of D2 activity mirrors the enzyme's affinity for the substrate, indicating that enzyme–substrate interaction must occur in order to induce loss of D2 activity.

At the molecular level, D2 activity is regulated by conjugation to ubiquitin, a protein of approximately 8 kd. The ubiquitinated D2 is subsequently recognized and degraded by proteasomes (143,144) (Fig. 7.6). The first evidence for this process was obtained in GH4C1 cells, in which the half-life of endogenous D2 was noted to be stabilized by MG132, a proteasome inhibitor (84). Substrate-induced loss of D2 activity was also inhibited by MG132 in these cells, indicating that both pathways affecting loss of D2 activity were mediated by the proteasomes. This implies that the loss of D2 activity is at least partially due to proteolysis of D2, a premise that was confirmed when the levels of immunoprecipitable D2 were found to parallel D2 activity, both under basal conditions and after exposure to T_4 (85). In subsequent studies it became clear that D2 is ubiquitinated (86), and the various enzymes involved in this process were identified. In studies in which human D2 was expressed in yeast, Ubc6p and Ubc7p were identified as the ubiquitin conjugases involved in ubiquitination of D2 (145), and it is now clear that these conjugases play a role in ubiquitination of human D2 (146,147).

Fusion of the 8–amino acid FLAG sequence to the carboxyl-, but not the amino-, terminus of D2 prolongs its activity and increases the size of the ubiquitin-D2 pool by 20- to 30-fold (86), suggesting that D2 ubiquitination is reversible, because not all Ub-D2 undergoes proteolysis. Enzymatic deubiquitination of ubiquitin-D2 occurs *in vitro* (148) and could explain recycling *in vivo*. D2 was recently identified as a substrate for the deubiquitinating enzymes VDU1 and VDU2 (149). Confocal studies indicate that both VDUs colocalize with D2, itself an integral endoplasmic-reticulum membrane protein. The physical colocalization of VDU with D2 provides the opportunity for deubiquitination of D2.

VDU1-catalyzed D2 deubiquitination is an important part of the adaptive mechanism that regulates thyroid hormone action. In stimulated brown fat tissue, D2 increases intracellular T_3 production, resulting in isolated tissue thyrotoxicosis (150–152). This is an important mechanism for cold acclimatization in rodents; mice with targeted inactivation of the D2 gene develop hypothermia and marked weight loss during cold exposure due to impaired thermogenesis in brown adipose tissue (151,153). Increased VDU1-catalyzed deubiquitination of ubiquitin-D2, and therefore rescue of D2 from proteasomal degradation, is an integral part of this mechanism. In brown adipose tissue, VDU1 mRNA levels are markedly up-regulated by cold exposure or norepinephrine, which amplifies the transcriptional increase in D2 activity, and hence T_3 production increases by approximately 2.5-fold. Although ubiquitination is known to play a physiologic role in several cellular processes (154–158), enzyme reactivation due to deubiquitination is unusual.

The availability of a reversible ubiquitination-dependent mechanism to control the activity of D2 constitutes a biochemical and physiologic advantage that allows for rapid control of thyroid hormone activation. The finding that VDU1 and VDU2 are coexpressed with D2 in many human tissues, including brain, heart, and skeletal muscle (1,159), suggests that the importance of this mechanism may extend well beyond thermal homeostasis to include brain development, cardiac performance, glucose utilization, and energy expenditure.

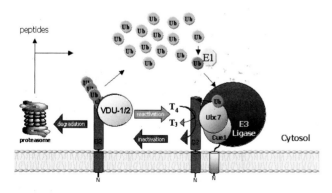

FIGURE 7.6. Representation of ubiquitination and proteasomal degradation of type 2 deiodinase (D2). *Ub,* ubiquitin; *E1,* enzyme that activates Ub; *E2,* Ub conjugase; *Ubc6 and Ubc7,* E2s involved in D2 ubiquitination; *Cue1,* endoplasmic reticulum–docking protein for Ubc7; *asterisk in the D2 molecule,* selenocysteine-containing active center; isopeptidase catalyzes D2 deubiquitination.

Type 3 Deiodinase

D3, acting by inner ring deiodination, is the major T_3- and T_4-inactivating enzyme, although D1 also has some activity as an inner ring deiodinase (160). D3, which has almost exclusively inner ring deiodination activity, catalyzes the conversion of T_4 to reverse T_3 and the conversion of T_3 to 3,3'-diiodothyronine (T_2), both of which are biologically inactive (Fig. 7.1). That reverse T_3 and T_2 do not support thyroid hormone–dependent gene expression is illustrated by the severe consumptive hypothyroidism that occurs in patients with hemangiomas, in whom tumor overexpression of D3 results in very high serum reverse T_3 concentrations, and the blockade of metamorphosis that occurs in tadpoles overexpressing D3 (161,162).

D3 contributes to thyroid hormone homeostasis by protecting tissues from an excess of thyroid hormone. It was identified in monkey hepatocarcinoma cells (NCLP6E), and the first physiologic studies were performed in the central nervous systems of rats (163–166). In humans, D3 is present in not only the central nervous system, but also skin and placenta; it is also present in fetal liver and in the uterus of pregnant rats (167). The highest activity found to date is in hemangioma-type tumors in humans (162). In amphibians, D3 plays a critical role in development (168); it is present in tadpoles from premetamorphosis to the onset of the metamorphic climax, after which it declines to barely detectable levels. In mammals, D3 is critical for thyroid hormone homeostasis, because it protects the fetus from premature exposure to excessive amounts of thyroid hormone, which can result in malformations, altered growth, mental retardation, and even death. In fetal and neonatal animals, D3 expression is highly regulated in tissue-specific patterns that are likely to be critical to the coordinated regulation of thyroid hormone effects on development.

Gene Structure and Chromosomal Localization

The *Dio3* gene is located on human chromosome 14q32 and mouse chromosome 12F1 (169). A unique feature of the human and mouse *Dio3* gene is that it has no introns (3), which is a rarity among eukaryotes (169,170). The gene is preferentially expressed (imprinted) from the paternal allele in mice (171). The *Dio3* gene likely belongs to the same cluster of imprinted genes in mouse chromosome 12 and human chromosome 14, and as such it might play a role in the phenotypic abnormalities associated with uniparental disomy of those chromosomes, a condition in which gene expression is altered due to abnormal genomic imprinting (172).

Human D3 mRNA contains 2066 nucleotides. There are 220 bp in the 5'-untranslated region, an 834-bp open reading frame, and a 3'-untranslated region of 1012 bp (173). All D3 cDNAs identified to date include a selenocysteine-encoding TGA codon, as well as SECIS element in the 3'-untranslated region. There is a high degree of identity between the *Dio3* gene in human and other species, particularly in the putative active center where the

selenocysteine is located. The conservation of this enzyme from tadpoles to humans implies that its role in regulating thyroid hormone inactivation during embryologic development is essential. The most common form of D3 mRNA in most tissues is 2.3 kb, but there are at least four differently sized mRNAs in the central nervous system of rats, and thyroid hormone causes increases in the relative intensity of these mRNAs (174).

Tissue Distribution

D3 has been identified in various tissues in several animal species, among which rats have been studied most extensively. In adult rats, D3 is found predominantly in the central nervous system and skin. In neonatal rats, it is found not only in these tissues, but also in skeletal muscle, liver, and intestine (43,164,175–178). In particular, using *in situ* hybridization analysis, D3 mRNA has been identified throughout the brain in adult rats, especially in hippocampal pyramidal neurons, granule cells of the dentate nucleus, and layers II to VI of the cerebral cortex (174). It is noteworthy that these regions also contain the highest concentrations of thyroid receptors in the brain, and they have critical roles in learning, memory, and higher cognitive functions (179–181). Furthermore, the distribution of D3 mRNA in the central nervous system changes during the early stages of development. At postnatal day 0, D3 is selectively expressed in the bed nucleus of the stria terminalis, the preoptic area, and other areas related anatomically and functionally to the bed nucleus, such as the central amygdala; all of these areas are involved in the sexual differentiation of the brain (182). D3 expression in these areas was transient and was no longer detected at postnatal day 10. The overall pattern of distribution of D3 in the brain of rats strongly suggests that it is primarily expressed in neurons, but it is also present in astrocytes (183–185).

Very high levels of D3 activity and mRNA have been identified in hemangiomas in infants. In infants with very large tumors, the result is hypothyroidism, caused by very rapid deiodination of T_4 and T_3 (162). This syndrome, termed consumptive hypothyroidism, has also been described in an adult with a large hepatic hemangiopericytoma (186).

D3 activity has also been detected in the retina in rat fetuses and, in lesser amounts, in adults (187). In *Xenopus laevis*, the localized expression of D3 in the cells of the marginal zone of the retina accounts for the asymmetric growth of the retina (188). As noted above, D3 is highly expressed in the skin of adult rats (43,189), and in them skin contains more reverse T_3 than any other tissue, suggesting that the high levels of D3 activity in homogenates of skin accurately reflect the activity of this enzyme *in vivo* (189). In this regard, T_4 applied to normal human skin is largely converted to reverse T_3 (190).

Large amounts of D3 are present in the placenta of rats, guinea pigs, and humans, and it is by far the predominant deiodinase present in this tissue (176,191–194). High levels of D3 are also present in the uterus of pregnant rats, initially in decidual cells and later in the single-cell layer of the epithelium (195). The levels of D3 are highest at the implantation site, nearly double the highest values obtained for placental tissue (196). In humans, the highest levels of D3 are in the endometrium (Fig. 7.7), and it is also found in fetal skin, tracheal and bronchiolar epithelium, mesothelium, and intestinal epithelium (197).

Regulation of D3 Synthesis

Thyroid Hormone

Parallels between D3 activity and thyroid status have been demonstrated in several species, although the underlying molecular mechanisms remain obscure. In *Xenopus laevis* tadpoles, administration of T_3 before the climax of metamorphosis results in a rapid and marked increase in D3 activity (39). In rats, D3 activity in the central nervous system is increased by thyroid hormone administration and decreased by hypothyroidism (164). In *in situ* hybridization histochemical studies, D3 gene expression within the central nervous system increased 4- to 50-fold in rats made thyrotoxic, with the greatest increase in the cerebellum. Conversely, D3 mRNA is not detectable in Northern blots of brain tissue of hypothyroid rats (174). Whether the dramatic increase in D3 mRNA in rats given T_3 is due to increases in gene transcription, mRNA stabilization, or a combination of these factors is not known. In *X. laevis*, this T_3 effect is not blocked by inhibition of protein synthesis. The promoter regions of the *Dio3* gene are stimulated by

T_3, but the magnitude of this stimulation is modest as compared with the effect of T_3 on D3 activity. Regulation of D3 activity by thyroid hormone has also been demonstrated in cultured astroglial cells. In these cells, the addition of 10 nM T_3 (or T_4) to the culture medium caused a slow increase in D3 activity, which reached a plateau in 48 hours (198).

Sex Steroids

D3 is expressed in the uterus, and the content increases during pregnancy. In rats, uterine D3 activity increases immediately after implantation, or artificial decidualization of the uterus in pseudopregnant rats, whereas the increases in activity are minimal in the nondecidualized uterine horn in the latter rats. In spontaneously cycling female rats, D3 activity was three to eight times higher during estrus, as compared with diestrus. Furthermore, the uterine levels of D3 activity were synergistically increased in ovariectomized rats given estradiol and progesterone in various combinations. Thus, estradiol and progesterone regulate thyroid hormone metabolism in the uterus, and the implantation process is a potent stimulus for the induction of D3 activity in this organ.

Nonthyroidal Illness

Most critically ill patients have low serum T_3 and high serum reverse T_3 concentrations (see section on nonthyroidal illness in Chapter 11). In patients with multiple organ system failure and other serious illnesses who died, hepatic D1 activity was low, and hepatic and skeletal muscle D3 activity was high (61). These findings suggest that T_4 and T_3 metabolism is altered in tissue-specific ways in illness, particularly with respect to reducing T_3 formation or increasing T_3 degradation. Similarly, D3 activity was increased in cardiac muscle of rats with cardiac hypertrophy and failure (199); among these rats, right ventricular D3 activity was significantly higher in those animals in which hypertrophy progressed to heart failure, as compared with the animals in which it did not. The induction of D3 in cardiac muscle would be expected to result in reduced intracellular concentrations of T_3, which might reduce cardiac work and therefore help maintain cardiac compensation.

Extracellular Receptor Kinase–Activated Pathways

In cultured rat astroglial cells, factors that alter cellular processes through signaling cascades originating at the plasma membrane increase D3 activity. For example, D3 activity increases markedly and rapidly after exposure of the cells to 12-*O*-tetradecanoyl phorbol-13-acetate (TPA), fibroblast growth factor, epidermal growth factor, platelet-derived growth factor, and cyclic AMP analogues (200). The stimulatory effects of TPA and fibroblast growth factor on D3 mRNA and activity appear to be mediated at least partially by activation of the MEK/ERK signaling cascade (201).

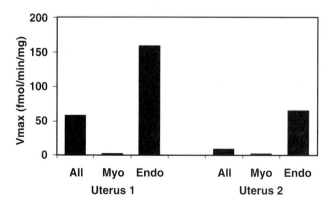

FIGURE 7.7. Type 3 deiodinase (D3) activity in the uterus and its myometrial and endometrial components. The endometrial (*Endo*) and myometrial (*Myo*) layers of the uterus from two nonpregnant women were dissected and assayed for D3 activity in the presence of 1 mM propylthiouracil. The values shown are maximum velocity, as determined by Lineweaver-Burke analysis.

NONDEIODINATIVE METABOLISM OF IODOTHYRONINES

Iodothyronines are mostly metabolized by deiodination. There are other pathways of metabolism, such as ether bond cleavage [mainly of T_4 in leukocytes (202)], deamination and decarboxylation of the alanine side chain (203,204), sulfoconjugation mediated by cytosolic phenol sulfotransferases in several tissues (205), and glucuronidation and O-methylation, which renders the products more hydrophilic and thereby facilitates their excretion by bile, feces, and urine (206).

Sulfoconjugation is the most important alternative iodothyronine metabolic pathway. The sulfotransferases of liver are normally involved in inactivation and detoxification reactions, with a preference for lipophilic substrates (207,208). Sulfation of iodothyronines facilitates rapid inner ring deiodination by D1 but not by D3. All iodothyronines except reverse T_3, the preferred substrate of D1, are sulfated to some extent (205).

Iodothyronines with two iodine atoms at the phenolic ring are preferentially conjugated with glucuronic acid, whereas iodothyronines that contain only one iodine atom in the phenolic ring are sulfated with the following preference: $3'\text{-}T_1 = 3,3'\text{-}T_2 > T_3 > rT_3 > T_4$ (166,205,207,209–211). T_3 can be sulfated by human cytosolic liver phenol sulfotransferase (EC 2.8.2.1), with K_m values in the 100 mM range, considerably greater than that for D1 (212). Biliary and urinary excretion of iodothyronine sulfates is a minor route for thyroid hormone elimination in humans. Considerable amounts of iodothyronine sulfates are detectable in plasma and bile after inhibition of D1 by PTU in rats (205,213,214). Moreover, at a high substrate concentration (> 1 mM) *in vitro,* metabolism proceeds mainly by sulfation, whereas at lower concentrations (< 0.1 mM), sulfation is the rate-limiting step; no sulfates accumulate because of the rapid deiodination of the sulfated iodothyronines. Thus far, the cellular capacity for conjugation seems to be unsaturable, in contrast to enzymic monodeiodination (29,166,209). In human hepatocarcinoma cells (HepG2 cells), inner ring deiodination of T_3 is reduced, due to deficient T_3 sulfation, which appears to be an obligatory step before deiodination of T_3 (215).

Rats with selenium deficiency have high serum T_3 sulfate concentrations and increased enterohepatic cycling of T_3 sulfate, and the serum half-life of T_3 is prolonged, as compared with normal rats (216). Under these conditions, sulfoconjugation might lead to greater availability of the active hormone. Sulfoconjugates of T_4, T_3, rT_3, and $3,3'\text{-}T_2$ have been identified in human serum and amniotic fluid by specific radioimmunoassays (217–221). These conjugates are normal components of maternal and fetal serum and amniotic fluid. Their production and metabolism are regulated by the hormonal state, nonthyroidal illness, and drugs that inhibit deiodinase activity; sulfoconjugates of maternal origin may contribute to fetal thyroid economy.

PHYSIOLOGIC ROLES OF THE SELENODEIODINASES

D2 and Regulation of Thyrotropin Secretion

The main secretory product of the thyroid gland is T_4, and serum T_4 is a more important regulator of TSH secretion than serum T_3. Because T_3 is the biologically active thyroid hormone, T_4 sensing must be preceded by its conversion to T_3. The first evidence that there was a PTU-insensitive pathway for T_4 to T_3 conversion was that T_4 very rapidly (within 30 minutes) inhibited TSH secretion in rats with hypothyroidism, and the inhibitory effect was not blocked by PTU (24,222–224). Subsequent studies in which combinations of $^{125}\text{I-}T_4$ and $^{131}\text{I-}T_3$ were injected revealed $^{125}\text{I-}T_3$ bound to thyroid hormone receptors in the nuclei of pituitary cells within 15 minutes after injection of $^{125}\text{I-}T_4$. This could not be explained by accumulation of $^{125}\text{I-}T_3$ from serum, and was not inhibited by pretreatment with PTU (21,24). Pretreatment with iopanoic acid blocked both the generation of pituitary nuclear $^{125}\text{I-}T_3$ and the biologic effect of T_4 on TSH release (225).

The presence of D2 can account for the requirement for physiologic concentrations of both T_4 and T_3 for normal secretion of TSH. This requirement can account for the increase in TSH secretion that occurs in the early stages of iodine deficiency, when only T_4, but not T_3, production is decreased (226). Furthermore, normal serum concentrations of both T_3 and T_4 are required to suppress TRH mRNA production in the paraventricular nucleus of the hypothalamus and to normalize serum TSH concentrations in thyroidectomized rats (227–229). However, no D2 activity is present in this region of the hypothalamus; it is instead concentrated in the arcuate nucleus and median eminence (112,230). Subsequent *in situ* hybridization studies revealed that D2 is localized in the tanycytes (111,113,114). These specialized ependymal cells have their cell bodies in the inferior portion of the third ventricle, and they are probably where T_4 is converted to T_3, providing T_3 that is released into the hypothalamic-pituitary portal system and carried to the thyrotrophs of the pituitary to regulate TSH secretion.

Triiodothyronine Homeostasis

The thyroid secretes T_4 and T_3 in a proportion determined by the T_4/T_3 ratio in thyroglobulin (15/1 in humans), as modified by the minimal thyroidal conversion of T_4 to T_3 (231). Thus, the prohormone T_4 is the major secreted iodothyronine in iodine-sufficient subjects; the molar ratio of secreted T_4 to T_3 is about 11 to 1 due to intrathyroidal T_4 to T_3 conversion via D1 and D2 (116,232,233). As noted above, most T_3 production occurs in various extrathyroidal tissues via 5'-deiodination of T_4 catalyzed by D1 and D2. The serum concentrations of free T_4 and T_3 are constant, but the concentrations of T_4 and T_3 in cells vary according the amounts of each hormone that are transported or diffuse into the cells, and the type and activity of the deiodinases in the cells. These deiodinases can increase (D2) or decrease (D3) the intracellular concentrations of T_3 and consequently the nuclear content of thyroid receptor-T_3 complexes independently of the serum T_4 and T_3 concentrations. As a result, the impact of T_4 and T_3 in serum on thyroid hormone action varies in different tissues. In liver and kidney, for example, the saturation of the thyroid receptors is approximately 50%, whereas in the central nervous system it is close to 95%. Lastly, tissue T_3 concentrations change throughout development, partially as a result of changes in the activity of D2 and D3. The deiodinases also modulate the thyroid status of individual tissues in response to iodine deficiency, hypothyroidism, and thyrotoxicosis. Cells lacking the capacity to alter the rate of deiodination of T_4 and T_3 are the most affected, because their thyroid status will be determined primarily by the serum free T_3 concentration. On the other hand, in cells expressing D2 or D3, changes in the activity of these enzymes mitigate fluctuations in serum free T_4 and T_3 concentrations, constituting a potent mechanism for maintaining thyroid homeostasis.

The relative contributions of the two sources of T_3, thyroid secretion and extrathyroidal deiodination of T_4, can be quantified by determining the T_4 to T_3 conversion rate, which is, on average, about 35% to 40% in normal humans (60). Hence, with a normal T_4 production rate of approximately 110 nmol/day (85 µg/day), approximately 40 nmol (25 µg) of T_3 are produced by peripheral deiodination of T_3 and the remaining 10 nmol (6 µg) are released by the thyroid (Fig. 7.8).

Both D1 and D2 contribute to extrathyroidal production of T_3, but assessing the contribution of the two deiodinases *in vivo* is difficult. In patients with primary hypothyroidism receiving constant doses of T_4, administration of PTU in a dose of 1000 mg daily for 7 to 8 days caused a 20% to 30% decrease in serum T_3 concentrations (234, 235). In another study, conversion of radiolabeled T_4 to T_3 in serum was not reduced in patients given 1200 mg/day of PTU (236). The results of these studies suggest that D1-catalyzed T_3 production is not a major component of extrathyroidal T_3 production in normal humans. However, in patients with thyrotoxicosis, the contribution from D1 is higher, about 50% (50), due to an increase in D1 activity. Fractional conversion of T_4 to T_3 is increased when serum T_4 concentrations are low, indicative of increased D2 activity, because D1-catalyzed T_3 production is decreased (50, 237–239). It is difficult to define which compartments or tissues contribute the most to extrathyroidal T_3 production in humans (240); depending on the assumptions used, one can obtain estimates suggesting that as much as 81% or as little as 15% of T_3 derives from rapidly equilibrating (D1-containing) tissues, with the remainder coming from slowly equilibrating (D2-containing) tissues.

The relative contributions of the D1 and D2 pathways to whole-body T_3 production can be assessed more accurately in rats. In normal rats treated chronically with high doses of PTU to inhibit D1 activity, the T_4 to T_3 conversion rate is reduced by 50% (241). Accordingly, in T_4-treated thyroidectomized rats, treatment with PTU results in a 50% decrease in serum T_3 concentrations (223). The results of compartmental analyses of T_4 to T_3 conversion rates in rats are similar, assuming that T_4 to T_3 conversion in the rapidly equilibrating pool occurs via D1 and more delayed conversion via D2 (242). Taken together, these data indicate that D1 catalyzes about half of the daily extrathyroidal T_3 production from T_4 in rats. This estimate of 50% in rats is clearly higher than the estimate of approximately 25% in humans from the above-mentioned PTU studies (Fig. 7.8).

There are several implications of the above calculations. Based on the data available, D2-catalyzed 5′-deiodination of T_4 appears to be a more important source of T_3 than does D1-catalyzed 5′-deiodination of T_4 in humans. Until recently, D2 activity was believed to be restricted mainly to the central nervous system and pituitary. The identification of D2 mRNA and activity in skeletal muscle and heart suggests a more important role for D2 in T_3 production (26,243). The fact that only approximately 20% of serum T_3 comes from thyroidal secretion, as opposed to about 40% in rats, also indicates a need for more widespread T_4 to T_3 conversion in humans.

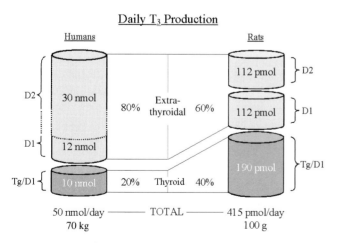

FIGURE 7.8. Daily triiodothyronine (T_3) production in humans and rats. The dotted lines in the cylinder representing human extrathyroidal production reflect the uncertainty about the contributions of type 1 deiodinase (D1) and type 2 deiodinase (D2) to this pool. Values given are based on studies cited in the text. Estimates for rats are normalized to 100 g body weight. To convert nmol to µg, multiply by 0.65, and to convert pmol to µg, multiply by 0.00065.

Intracellular Triiodothyronine Homeostasis

Serum T_3 equilibrates rapidly with most tissues. Both T_4 and T_3 are carried across the plasma membrane by stereospecific energy-dependent transporters (244,245), and they may also diffuse into cells. At equilibrium, one can estimate the nuclear T_3 derived from serum T_3 from the ratio of nuclear to serum T_3 and the serum T_3 concentration. Measurements of the maximum binding capacity of the thyroid receptors for T_3 allow calculation of the degree of saturation of the receptors, which is normally 40% to 50% in most tissues (246). Thus, changes in serum T_3 concentrations during thyrotoxicosis or hypothyroidism are mirrored by changes in the occupancy of the thyroid receptors in those tissues, and it is the latter that determines the intensity of the biologic actions of thyroid hormone. However, in selected tissues, especially pituitary gland, brain, and brown adipose tissue, additional T_3 is provided by intracellular T_4 to T_3 conversion (24,247). This has been termed $T_3(T_4)$ to differentiate it from $T_3(T_3)$, the nuclear T_3 derived directly from serum T_3. These tissues contain D2, and in them the T_3 generated by D2-catalyzed T_4 deiodination supplements that from serum as though it were derived from a kinetically different pool. As a result, thyroid receptor occupancy by T_3 is much higher (70%–90%), and 50% to 80% of this receptor-bound T_3 is T_3 (T_4) (21,23,248).

These differences have been confirmed using constant infusions of radiolabeled T_3 and T_4 (249–252) and direct quantitation of nuclear T_3 (253). Other tissues (e.g., liver, kidney) in which serum T_3 is the only source of nuclear T_3 contain mostly D1. As discussed above, confocal microscopic studies of transiently expressed D2 suggest that it is located in the endoplasmic reticulum in the perinuclear region, and T_3 formed in this region might have preferential access to the nucleus. D1, however, is distributed in the periphery of the cell, typical of a plasma membrane protein. The rapid exit of T_3 from D1-containing tissues and its retention in D2-containing tissues explain the three- to four-fold higher ratio of nuclear to cytoplasmic free T_3 in brain than in liver, kidney, or heart (254). The consequence of the presence of D2 is that the impact of changes in T_4 production on cellular T_3 content can be dampened at a prereceptor level by compensatory alterations in D2 activity.

Iodine Deficiency and Hypothyroidism

Iodine availability can be rate limiting for thyroidal T_4 and T_3 production, and multiple thyroidal and extrathyroidal mechanisms have evolved to mitigate the consequences of iodine deficiency (see the section on thyroid iodine transport in Chapter 4 and the section on iodine deficiency in Chapter 11) (255). Accordingly, in iodine-deficient rats, growth, O_2 consumption, and thermal homeostasis are similar to those of normal rats, despite approximately 10-fold higher serum TSH concentrations and very low serum T_4 concentrations (256,257). However, if iodine deficiency is severe and prolonged, signs of hypothyroidism do eventually develop, with reduced O_2 consumption and reduced

activity of T_3-dependent enzymes (258–260). It is difficult to distinguish between compensated iodine deficiency and hypothyroidism, except by measurements of T_3 actions, because serum TSH concentrations are high at all stages.

Iodine deficiency results in a series of physiologic adaptations in the hypothalamic–pituitary–thyroid axis, similar to those that occur in hypothyroidism, which maintain serum and tissue T_3 concentrations in the normal range, delaying the onset of hypothyroidism. The earliest thyroidal adaptation is a decrease in diiodotyrosine formation, with a consequent decrease in thyroidal T_4 synthesis, whereas thyroidal T_3 synthesis is maintained (226,261). TSH secretion increases as serum T_4 concentrations decrease, increasing thyroidal iodide transport and the subsequent steps of thyroid hormone production (226,261). This stimulation helps to maintain thyroid hormone production, but with continuing iodine deficiency the ratio of diiodotyrosine to monoiodotyrosine in thyroglobulin decreases by approximately 3-fold and the ratio of T_4 to T_3 decreases by approximately 25-fold; the latter is due to a decrease in thyroidal T_4 content, not to an increase in T_3 content. The ratio of T_4 to T_3 in the serum of iodine-deficient subjects is also low, due to hypothyroxinemia, not an increase in serum T_3 concentrations. Thus, the hallmarks of iodine deficiency, and the early phase of primary hypothyroidism, are low serum T_4, normal serum T_3, and high serum TSH concentrations (261–263).

The extrathyroidal adaptations to iodine deficiency or primary hypothyroidism are more complex and involve a high degree of tissue specificity. As noted above, the overall fractional conversion of T_4 to T_3 is increased in patients with hypothyroidism (237). This increase is due to an increase in D2 activity, and its effect is to maintain extrathyroidal T_3 production (26,96,243). In rats, the fractional T_4 to T_3 conversion rate is not substantially changed by hypothyroidism, but extrathyroidal T_3 production shifts from being relatively PTU sensitive (~50%) to being PTU insensitive (264), indicating that the relative contribution of D2-catalyzed T_4 conversion to T_3 increases substantially.

In tissues that express D2, the activity of this enzyme is increased during iodine deficiency or hypothyroidism, thus increasing the local fractional conversion of T_4 to T_3, and mitigating the decrease in serum T_4 concentrations (22,73, 265–267). This has been particularly well documented for the brain; because of the negative regulation of *Dio2* gene transcription by thyroid hormone (268), D2 mRNA increases in iodine-deficient animals in all regions of the brain that contain D2, and D2 activity increases even more (267), similar to what occurs in hypothyroid rats (134). This increase in D2 activity is explained by the hypothyroxinemia of iodine deficiency per se acting at a posttranslational level, as noted above in the sections on regulation of D2 synthesis and degradation.

In hypothyroidism, there is not only an increase in fractional conversion of T_4 to T_3, but the clearance of T_3 from the brain also is reduced. This is because D3 is a T_3-dependent gene, and its activity correlates with thyroid status. In both fetal and adult rats with iodine deficiency, overall brain D3 activity decreases by 50% (73,164,174,269,270). However, in specific brain regions, such as the cerebral cortex, hippocampus, and cerebellum, D3 activity decreases by 80% to 90% (73). The consequences of the decrease in D3 activity are twofold. First, the residence time of T_3 within the tissue is prolonged (271). Second, because T_4 is also a substrate for D3, relatively more of it will be available within the tissue for conversion to T_3 by D2. Particularly in tissues like the brain, in which the exchange of T_3 with serum is slow and most of the T_3 is generated *in situ*, it is likely that fluctuations in the rate of T_3 degradation have a greater influence on tissue levels of T_3 than in tissues in which cellular T_3 is in more rapid equilibrium with serum, such as the liver and kidney (272).

The increased fractional production of T_3 from T_4 by D2 combined with the prolonged residence time of T_3 mitigates the effects of severe iodine deficiency and hypothyroidism. This has been demonstrated in mild to moderate hypothyroidism using tracer studies (273). These predictions were confirmed directly by measuring thyroid hormone concentrations in various regions of the CNS in iodine-deficient rats (265). As expected, tissue T_4 concentrations were markedly decreased, whereas tissue T_3 concentrations were reduced by only 50%. This illustrates the effectiveness of these compensatory mechanisms.

Embryonic Development

Thyroid hormone is critically important for the coordination of developmental processes in all vertebrate species. During embryogenesis, thyroid hormone acts primarily to promote differentiation and thus attenuate proliferation. As a result, either insufficient levels of T_3 or premature exposure of the embryo to high T_3 concentrations result in abnormal development (274). As an example, exposure of neonatal rats to excess thyroid hormone causes accelerated morphogenesis of pyramidal neurons and their dendritic spines in the cerebrum and a persistent reduction in total number of neurons (275). The best characterized action by which thyroid hormone influences developmental processes is via changes in gene expression initiated by the binding of T_3 to its receptors (276,277). During development in experimental animals, two deiodinases (D3 and D2) exert the major control of T_3 concentrations (43). As mentioned earlier, fetal serum T_3 concentrations are very low, and during early development D3 is the predominant deiodinase expressed in most rat tissues, and its activity in these tissues is much higher than in adult rats. In human fetuses, D3 is also present in the liver, and its content decreases near the end of gestation (167). This pattern suggests that D3 plays a major role in preventing premature exposure of fetal tissues to T_3.

Conversely, D2 is expressed in most mammalian tissues for a limited period of time during development. This sug-gests that there is a tissue-specific program of T_3-dependent differentiation. This has been found during tadpole metamorphosis, and it likely occurs during neuronal and glial maturation and cochlear maturation in rats (39,110, 278–281). Finally, D1 activity is generally lower during fetal development than at later stages of life (282). This also would result in lower serum T_3 concentrations at that time of life.

Deiodinases in Mammalian Development

Precisely timed D2 expression is fundamental during critical periods of mammalian development. In rat brain, D2 increases rapidly after birth, reaching its highest level around day 28. It then declines, reaching adult levels by day 50 (165). The cochlea is among the organs most sensitive to thyroid deficiency, as is evident from the deafness that is associated with endemic cretinism. In rats, complete cochlear maturation and the onset of auditory function require the presence of T_3 between the late embryonic stage and the second postnatal week. So far, little is known about the mechanisms that control this temporal regulation. Analysis of cochlear homogenates from 2- to 8-day old rat pups revealed a striking peak of D2 activity peak at about 7 days, followed by an abrupt decline by day 10, a few days before the onset of hearing (110). Relative to serum, cochlear tissue has a high ratio of T_3 to T_4, supporting a role for D2 in increasing local T_3 concentrations. D2 mRNA is localized in connective tissue near the region where dendritic and axonal projections of the cochlear nerve connect with the hair cells. D2 expression is complementary to, rather than coincident with, that of the β subtype of the thyroid receptor, suggesting a paracrine rather than endocrine mode of signaling in cochlear tissue. D2-deficient mice have defective auditory function, retarded differentiation of the cochlear inner sulcus and sensory epithelium, and deformity of the tectorial membrane. The similarity of this phenotype to that caused by thyroid receptor mutations suggests that D2 controls the T_3 signal that activates thyroid receptors in the cochlea (283).

Maternal-Fetal Physiology

In humans, the capacity to synthesize thyroid hormones does not appear until 10 to 12 weeks of gestation (see Chapter 74). However, human fetuses have thyroid receptors containing T_3 at an earlier time (284); this T_3 must come from the maternal circulation, via the placenta and the coelomic and amniotic fluids (285). At 6 to 12 weeks' gestation, the average total T_4 concentrations are 11.3, 0.07, and 0.002 μg/dL (146, 0.96, and 0.02 n*M*), respectively, in maternal serum, coelomic fluid, and amniotic fluid, suggesting a marked gradient of T_4 from mother to fetus. The gradient for reverse T_3 is in the opposite direction, its concentrations being 3.8 and 15 times higher in the coelomic fluid and amniotic fluid, respectively, as compared with maternal serum (285). Also during the second and third trimesters, there are marked maternal-to-fetal gradients of free T_4 and T_3 (286,287).

D2 and D3 activity appear in fetal tissues at midgestation, whereas D1 is not evident until later (44). Accordingly, fetal serum T_3 concentrations are very low before 30 weeks; thereafter they increase slightly, due to an increase in D1 activity in fetal tissues. The serum concentrations of sulfated iodothyronine concentrations are high in fetuses; although T_3 sulfate does not bind to thyroid receptors, local desulfation, if it occurred, would provide a local source of T_3 in fetal tissues (217,220,288,289). The pattern of circulating iodothyronines in the fetus, which is characterized by low serum T_3 and high reverse T_3 concentrations, is due to the combination of high D3 activity and low D1 activity in fetal tissues throughout most of gestation.

Triiodothyronine Modulation of Placental Thyroid Hormone Transfer

The placenta is the pathway for maternal-fetal thyroid hormone transfer, and therefore can be an important determinant of the thyroid status of the fetus. Placental D3 activity increases with gestational age in rats and humans (176, 192,290,291). In the first trimester, when the placenta and the surface area available for transfer are small, the activity of D3 per unit of placental tissue is high. At term, the activity per unit is lower, but because the placenta is much larger total placental D3 activity is higher. In rats, unlike humans, placental D3 activity increases about twofold from embryonic day 14 until day 16 or 17, after which it decreases (176,292, 293). As mentioned above, placenta also contains D2; however, at all gestational ages, placental D3 activity is approximately 200-fold higher than is that of D2. In placental tissue, there is no direct correlation between D2 activity and mRNA levels, and although D3 activity is always higher than D2 activity, their mRNA levels are comparable (291).

The cellular localization of D2 and D3 in placental tissue also differs. D2 activity is higher in the chorionic and decidual membranes of the placenta than in the amniotic membranes, whereas D3 is found mostly in trophoblasts (194). However, given the low levels of D2 at all gestational ages, fluctuations in D2 activity are not likely to have a major effect on fetal serum T_3 concentrations.

The physiologic consequence of the high placental D3 activity is clear. Placental tissue actively deiodinates T_4 to reverse T_3 and T_3 to 3,3′-diiodothyronine, some of which is further deiodinated to 3′-monoiodothyronine (191). In isolated perfused human placental lobules, little of the T_4 added to the maternal side appears on the fetal side. In contrast, reverse T_3 concentrations rise progressively on both sides. Addition of the deiodinase inhibitor iopanoic

acid to the maternal perfusate results in an increase in T_4 and a decrease in reverse T_3 on the fetal side, providing direct evidence that human placental D3 is a major factor controlling transfer of maternal T_4 to the fetus (294).

The uterus of pregnant rats also contains high levels of D3 activity, initially in decidual cells and later in the single-cell layer of the epithelium (195). D3 activity is highest at the implantation site, and the activity there is almost double the highest value found in the placenta. These changes precede the appearance of thyroid receptor mRNA (295). Throughout gestation, D3 activity remains higher in the uterus than in the placenta, and is 10 times higher than in the entire fetus. D3 activity has also been detected in amniotic fluid (195). High uterine and placental D3 activity also protects against high T_3 concentrations, which can induce structural abnormalities in the cephalic and branchial arches (296).

The presence of D3 in the endometrium and placenta villae as well as every epithelial surface of the human fetus constitutes a barrier to inappropriate transfer of maternal T_4 and T_3 to the fetus (197). This barrier is so potent that instillation of 700 µg of T_4 into amniotic fluid at term results in little increase in umbilical cord serum T_3 concentrations of infants born 24 hours later (297). The high level of D3 activity in the uterus and placenta contributes to the need for more T_4 in women with hypothyroidism when they are pregnant (298).

Paradoxically, despite inactivation of T_4 and T_3 by the uterus and placenta, neonates with congenital hypothyroidism often have little evidence of hypothyroidism at birth. Among infants with a complete defect in thyroid iodide organification, cord serum T_4 concentrations are 20% to 50% of those in normal infants, indicating there is substantial transplacental passage of T_4. The concentrations decrease rapidly after birth in these infants (299). These results indicate that a steep maternal-fetal gradient of T_4 overcomes the placental barrier, permitting maternal T_4 to enter the fetal circulation.

THE DEIODINASES IN HUMAN PATHOPHYSIOLOGY
Nonthyroidal Illness

Extrathyroidal conversion of T_4 to T_3 is decreased in patients with virtually all nonthyroidal illness, as discussed above and in the section on nonthyroidal illness in Chapter 11.

Consumptive Hypothyroidism

As noted above, high levels of D3 are expressed in hemangiomas. If these tumors are sufficiently large, the rate of T_4 and T_3 deiodination can exceed thyroidal production of the hormones, even in the presence of intense TSH stimulation. The first patient documented to have this condition was a 3-month-old infant who had severe hypothyroidism, with high serum TSH, undetectable T_4 and T_3, and high reverse T_3 concentrations. To reverse the hypothyroidism rapidly, the infant was given T_3 and T_4 intravenously in doses sufficient to reduce TSH secretion to normal. The respective daily doses were 96 µg of T_3 and 50 µg of T_4 (162), doses that would cause overt thyrotoxirosis in not only normal infants but also normal adults (300). Remarkably, even during the infusions, serum T_3 concentrations barely reached the normal range, serum T_4 was never detectable, and serum reverse T_3 concentrations were very high, providing direct evidence of excessive inner ring deiodination. D3 activity was subsequently identified in the infant's hemangioma at levels eight times that in the placenta, and in situ hybridization localized the D3 mRNA to hemangioma cells. Other patients with this unique syndrome have now been reported (301).

The relationship between infantile hemangiomas and D3 expression is important because it identifies a cause of hypothyroidism at a critical age for neurologic development. Although large hepatic hemangiomas can be fatal, a substantial fraction of these infants survive with therapy and the natural propensity of these tumors to regress. If hypothyroid, these patients may require high doses of T_4 in addition to therapy directed at their hemangiomas.

D3 Expression and the Requirement for Thyroxine in Normal Pregnancy

Most pregnant women with hypothyroidism need an increase in T_4 dose of approximately 40% to maintain normal serum TSH concentrations (299,302). The need for an increase begins early in pregnancy and persists until delivery (303), and its existence indicates that T_4 and T_3 production must increase in normal pregnant women. The causes of this need for more T_4 and T_3 include an increase in uterine D3 activity and the presence of placental D3 activity, transfer of T_4 and T_3 to the fetus, and the estrogen-induced increase in serum thyroxine-binding globulin concentrations.

Overexpression of Deiodinases and Excess Triiodothyronine Production

In patients with thyrotoxicosis, there is a disproportionate increase in the production rate of T_3 and serum T_3 concentrations, as compared with those of T_4, by a factor of two (50). The human *Dio1* gene promoter is T_3-responsive, and D1 mRNA levels are increased in thyroid tissue and mononuclear leukocytes in patients with thyrotoxicosis (42,304,305). In these patients, PTU—which blocks D1, but not D2, activity—results in a more rapid acute decrease in serum T_3 concentrations than does methimazole, which has no effect of either D1 or D2 activity (50). These

results indicate that D1-catalyzed T_4 to T_3 conversion is increased in patients with thyrotoxicosis (234–236). This has led to the recommendation that patients with severe thyrotoxicosis be treated with large doses of PTU or other drugs that block T_4 conversion to T_3 (see Chapter 45) (306–309).

In patients with Graves' thyrotoxicosis, thyroidal D2 mRNA is increased despite high serum T_4 and T_3 concentrations (116). This is presumably due to the effect of TSH receptor–stimulating antibodies to activate the cyclic AMP-dependent *Dio2* gene, which overwhelms the negative transcriptional effect of T_3 on this gene. Therefore, some of the relative excess of T_3 production in patients with thyrotoxicosis is caused by an increase in thyroidal D2 activity (116).

Another consequence of thyroid overexpression of D2 is illustrated by three athyreotic patients with widespread follicular carcinoma of the thyroid in whom the ratio of T_3 to T_4 in serum was persistently high, in the absence of autonomous production of T_3 by the tumor. In one patient, the tumor contained a high level of D2 activity, and resection of the tumor resulted in a normal T_4 to T_3 ratio in serum. In two other patients, treatment with T_4 in doses sufficient to suppress TSH secretion was associated with high normal serum T_3 and subnormal free T_4 values (310). These findings indicate that increases in T_4 conversion to T_3, presumably caused by increased D2 activity, can alter serum T_4 and T_3 concentrations.

CONCLUSION

Many tissues contain deiodinase activity, and it is now clear that these enzymes are important determinants of thyroid hormone homeostasis in both health and disease. Two deiodinases catalyze the intracellular conversion of T_4 to T_3, and a third catalyzes intracellular conversion of T_4 and T_3 to biologically inactive products. Variations in the activity of these enzymes, as a result of thyroid and other disorders, can affect thyroid hormone availability and therefore thyroid hormone action, in many tissues.

ACKNOWLEDGMENT

This work was supported by National Institutes of Health Grants DK36256, DK44128, and DK58538.

REFERENCES

1. Bianco AC, Salvatore D, Gereben B, et al. Biochemistry, cellular and molecular biology and physiological roles of the iodothyronine selenodeiodinases. *Endocr Rev* 2002;23:38.
2. Berry MJ, Kieffer JD, Harney JW, et al. Selenocysteine confers the biochemical properties of the type I iodothyronine deiodinase. *J Biol Chem* 1991;266:14155.

3. Croteau W, Whittemore SL, Schneider MJ, et al. Cloning and expression of a cDNA for a mammalian type III iodothyronine deiodinase. *J Biol Chem* 1995;270:16569.

4. Buettner C, Harney JW, Larsen PR. The role of selenocysteine 133 in catalysis by the human type 2 iodothyronine deiodinase. *Endocrinology* 2000;141:4606.

5. Callebaut I, Curcio-Morelli C, Mornon JP, et al. The iodothyronine selenodeiodinases are thioredoxin-fold family proteins containing a glycoside hydrolase-clan GH-A-like structure. *J Biol Chem* 2003;278:36887.

6. Martin JL. Thioredoxin—a fold for all reasons. *Structure* 1995; 3:245.

7. Coutinho PM, Henrissat B. Carbohydrate-active enzymes. http://afmb.cnrs-mrs.fr/CAZY, accessed 9 August 2004.

8. Berry MJ, Banu L, Larsen PR. Type I iodothyronine deiodinase is a selenocysteine-containing enzyme. *Nature* 1991;349:438.

9. Berry MJ, Banu L, Chen YY, et al. Recognition of UGA as a selenocysteine codon in type I deiodinase requires sequences in the 3′ untranslated region. *Nature* 1991;353:273.

10. Leonard JL, Visser TJ, Leonard DM. Characterization of the subunit structure of the catalytically active type I iodothyronine deiodinase. *J Biol Chem* 2000;276:2600.

11. Curcio-Morelli C, Gereben B, Zavacki AM, et al. *In vivo* dimerization of types 1, 2, and 3 iodothyronine selenodeiodinases. *Endocrinology* 2003;144:3438.

12. Leonard JL, Rosenberg IN. Solubilization of a phospholipid-requiring enzyme, iodothyronine 5′-deiodinase, from rat kidney membranes. *Biochim Biophys Acta* 1981;659:205.

13. Safran M, Leonard JL. Comparison of the physicochemical properties of type I and type II iodothyronine 5′-deiodinase. *J Biol Chem* 1991;266:3233.

14. Toyoda N, Berry MJ, Harney JW, et al. Topological analysis of the integral membrane protein, type 1 iodothyronine deiodinase (D1). *J Biol Chem* 1995;270:12310.

15. Baqui MM, Gereben B, Harney JW, et al. Distinct subcellular localization of transiently expressed types 1 and 2 iodothyronine deiodinases as determined by immunofluorescence confocal microscopy. *Endocrinology* 2000;141:4309.

16. Leonard JL, Rosenberg IN. Subcellular distribution of thyroxine 5′-deiodinase in the rat kidney: a plasma membrane location. *Endocrinology* 1978;103:274.

17. Kohrle J, Rasmussen UB, Rokos H, et al. Selective affinity labeling of a 27-kd integral membrane protein in rat liver and kidney with *N*-bromoacetyl derivatives of L-thyroxine and 3,5,3′-triiodo-L-thyronine. *J Biol Chem* 1990;265:6146.

18. Prabakaran D, Ahima RS, Harney JW, et al. Polarized targeting of epithelial cell proteins in thyrocytes and MDCK cells. *J Cell Sci* 1999;112:1247.

19. Baqui MM, Botero D, Gereben B, et al. Human type 3 iodothyronine selenodeiodinase is located in the plasma membrane and undergoes rapid internalization to endosomes. *J Biol Chem* 2003;278:1206.

20. Curcio C, Baqui MMA, Salvatore D, et al. The human type 2 iodothyronine deiodinase is a selenoprotein highly expressed in a mesothelioma cell line. *J Biol Chem* 2001;276:30183.

21. Silva JE, Larsen PR. Contributions of plasma triiodothyronine and local thyroxine monodeiodination to triiodothyronine to nuclear triiodothyronine receptor saturation in pituitary, liver, and kidney of hypothyroid rats: further evidence relating saturation of pituitary nuclear triiodothyronine receptors and the acute inhibition of thyroid-stimulating hormone release. *J Clin Invest* 1978;61:1247.

22. Larsen PR, Silva JE, Kaplan MM. Relationships between circulating and intracellular thyroid hormones: physiological and clinical implications. *Endocr Rev* 1981;2:87.

23. Silva JE, Dick TE, Larsen PR. The contribution of local tissue thyroxine monodeiodination to the nuclear 3,5,3′-triiodothyronine in pituitary, liver, and kidney of euthyroid rats. *Endocrinology* 1978;103:1196.

24. Silva JE, Larsen PR. Pituitary nuclear 3,5,3′-triiodothyronine and thyrotropin secretion: an explanation for the effect of thyroxine. *Science* 1977;198:617.

25. Leonard JL, Visser TJ. Biochemistry of deiodination. In: Hennemann G, ed. *Thyroid hormone metabolism.* New York: Marcel Dekker, 1986:189.

26. Salvatore D, Bartha T, Harney JW, et al. Molecular biological and biochemical characterization of the human type 2 selenodeiodinase. *Endocrinology* 1996;137:3308.

27. Kuiper GG, Klootwijk W, Visser TJ. Substitution of cysteine for a conserved alanine residue in the catalytic center of type II iodothyronine deiodinase alters interaction with reducing cofactor. *Endocrinology* 2002;143:1190.

28. Sanders JP, Van der Geyten S, Kaptein E, et al. Characterization of a propylthiouracil-insensitive type I iodothyronine deiodinase. *Endocrinology* 1997;138:5153.

29. Otten MH, Mol JA, Visser TJ. Sulfation preceding deiodination of iodothyronines in rat hepatocytes. *Science* 1983;221:81.

30. Berry MJ. Identification of essential histidine residues in rat type I iodothyronine deiodinase. *J Biol Chem* 1992;267:18055.

31. Kohrle J, Hesch RD. Biochemical characteristics of iodothyronine monodeiodination by rat liver microsomes: the interaction between iodothyronine substrate analogs and the ligand binding site of the iodothyronine deiodinase resembles that of the TBPA-iodothyronine ligand binding. *Horm Metab Res* 1984;14:42(suppl).

32. Fekkes D, Hennemann G, Visser TJ. Evidence for a single enzyme in rat liver catalyzing the deiodination of the tyrosyl and the phenolic ring of iodothyronines. *Biochem J* 1982;201:673.

33. Jakobs TC, Koehler MR, Schmutzler C, et al. Structure of the human type I iodothyronine 5′-deiodinase gene and localization to chromosome 1p32-p33. *Genomics* 1997;42:361.

34. Mandel SJ, Berry MJ, Kieffer JD, et al. 1992 Cloning and *in vitro* expression of the human selenoprotein, type I iodothyronine deiodinase. *J Clin Endocrinol Metab* 1992;75:1133.

35. Maia AL, Berry MJ, Sabbag R, et al. Structural and functional differences in the dio1 gene in mice with inherited type 1 deiodinase deficiency. *Mol Endocrinol* 1995;9:969.

36. Toyoda N, Harney JW, Berry MJ, et al. Identification of critical amino acids for 3,5,3′-triiodothyronine deiodination by human type 1 deiodinase based on comparative functional-structural analyses of the human, dog, and rat enzymes. *J Biol Chem* 1994; 269:20329.

37. Van der Geyten S, Sanders JP, Kaptein E, et al. Expression of chicken hepatic type I and type III iodothyronine deiodinases during embryonic development. *Endocrinology* 1997;138:5144.

38. Galton VA. Iodothyronine 5′-deiodinase activity in the amphibian *Rana catesbeiana* at different stages of the life cycle. *Endocrinology* 1988;122:1746.

39. Becker KB, Stephens KC, Davey JC, et al. The type 2 and type 3 iodothyronine deiodinases play important roles in coordinating development in *Rana catesbeiana* tadpoles. *Endocrinology* 1997;138:2989.

40. St. Germain DL, Galton VA. The deiodinase family of selenoproteins. *Thyroid* 1997;7:655.

41. Campos-Barros A, Hoell T, Musa A, et al. Phenolic and tyrosyl ring iodothyronine deiodination and thyroid hormone concentrations in the human central nervous system. *J Clin Endocrinol Metab* 1996;81:2179.

42. Nishikawa M, Toyoda N, Yonemoto T, et al. Quantitative measurements for type 1 deiodinase messenger ribonucleic acid in

human peripheral blood mononuclear cells: mechanism of the preferential increase of T_3 in hyperthyroid Graves' disease. *Biochem Biophys Res Commun* 1998;250:642.

43. Bates JM, St. Germain DL, Galton VA. Expression profiles of the three iodothyronine deiodinases, D1, D2, and D3, in the developing rat. *Endocrinology* 1999;140:844.

44. Burrow GN, Fisher DA, Larsen PR. Maternal and fetal thyroid function. *N Engl J Med* 1994;331:1072.

45. Berry MJ, Kates AL, Larsen PR. Thyroid hormone regulates type I deiodinase messenger RNA in rat liver. *Mol Endocrinol* 1990;4:743.

46. Toyoda N, Zavacki AM, Maia AL, et al. A novel retinoid X receptor-independent thyroid hormone response element is present in the human type 1 deiodinase gene. *Mol Cell Biol* 1995; 15:5100.

47. Jakobs TC, Schmutzler C, Meissner J, et al. The promoter of the human type I 5'-deiodinase gene-mapping of the transcription start site and identification of a DR+4 thyroid-hormone–responsive element. *Eur J Biochem* 1997;247:288.

48. Zhang C, Kim S, Harney JW, et al. Further characterization of thyroid hormone response elements in the human type 1 iodothyronine deiodinase gene. *Endocrinology* 1998;139: 1156.

49. Amma LL, Campos-Barros A, Wang Z, et al. Distinct tissue-specific roles for thyroid hormone receptors beta and alpha1 in regulation of type 1 deiodinase expression. *Mol Endocrinol* 2001;15:467.

50. Abuid J, Larsen PR. Triiodothyronine and thyroxine in hyperthyroidism: comparison of the acute changes during therapy with antithyroid agents. *J Clin Invest* 1974;54:201.

51. Chopra IJ, Sakane S, Chua Teco GN. A study of the serum concentration of tumor necrosis factor-α in thyroidal and nonthyroidal illnesses. *J Clin Endocrinol Metab* 1991;72: 1113.

52. Boelen A, Platvoet-Ter Schiphorst MC, Wiersinga WM. Association between serum interleukin-6 and serum 3,5,3'- triiodothyronine in nonthyroidal illness. *J Clin Endocrinol Metab* 1993;77:1695.

53. van der Poll T, Romijn JA, Wiersinga WM, et al. Tumor necrosis factor: a putative mediator of the sick euthyroid syndrome in man. *J Clin Endocrinol Metab* 1990;71:1567.

54. Pekary AE, Berg L, Santini F, et al. Cytokines modulate type I iodothyronine deiodinase mRNA levels and enzyme activity in FRTL-5 rat thyroid cells. *Mol Cell Endocrinol* 1994;101:R31.

55. Nagaya T, Fujieda M, Otsuka G, et al. A potential role of activated NF-kappa B in the pathogenesis of euthyroid sick syndrome. *J Clin Invest* 2000;106:393.

56. Yu J, Koenig RJ. Regulation of hepatocyte thyroxine 5'-deiodinase by T_3 and nuclear receptor coactivators as a model of the sick euthyroid syndrome. *J Biol Chem* 2000;275:38296.

57. Portnay GI, O'Brien JT, Bush J, et al. The effect of starvation on the concentration and binding of thyroxine and triiodothyronine in serum and on the response to TRH. *J Clin Endocrinol Metab* 1974;39:191.

58. Burrows AW, Shakespear RA, Hesch RD, et al. Thyroid hormones in the elderly sick: "T_4 euthyroidism." *BMJ* 1975;4:437.

59. Kaplan MM, Larsen PR, Crantz FR, et al. Prevalence of abnormal thyroid function test results in patients with acute medical illnesses. *Am J Med* 1992;72:9.

60. Larsen PR, Davies TF, Hay ID. The thyroid gland. In: Wilson JD, Foster DW, Kronenberg HM, et al., eds. *Williams textbook of endocrinology,* 9th ed. Philadelphia: WB Saunders, 1998:389.

61. Peeters RP, Wouters PJ, Kaptein E, et al. Reduced activation and increased inactivation of thyroid hormone in tissues of critically ill patients. *J Clin Endocrinol Metab* 2003;88:3202.

62. Harris ARC, Fang SL, Vagenakis AG, et al. Effect of starvation, nutrient replacement, and hypothyroidism on *in vitro* hepatic T_4 to T_3 conversion in the rat. *Metabolism* 1978;27: 1680.

63. Harris ARC, Fang SL, Hinerfeld L, et al. The role of sulfhydryl groups on the impaired hepatic 3',3,5-triiodothyronine generation from thyroxine in the hypothyroid, starved, fetal and neonatal rodent. *J Clin Invest* 1979;63:516.

64. Goodman MN, Larsen PR, Kaplan MM, et al. Starvation in the rat. II. Effect of age and obesity on protein sparing and fuel metabolism. *Am J Physiol* 1980;239:E277.

65. Kinlaw WB, Schwartz HL, Oppenheimer JH. Decreased serum triiodothyronine in starving rats is due primarily to diminished thyroidal secretion of thyroxine. *J Clin Invest* 1984;75:1238.

66. Safran M, Kohrle J, Braverman LE, et al. Effect of biological alterations of type I 5'deiodinase activity on affinity labeled membrane proteins in rat liver and kidney. *Endocrinology* 1990; 126:826.

67. Legradi G, Emerson CH, Ahima RS, et al. Leptin prevents fasting-induced suppression of prothyrotropin-releasing hormone messenger ribonucleic acid in neurons of the hypothalamic paraventricular nucleus. *Endocrinology* 1997;138:2569.

68. Vignati L, Finley RJ, Hagg S, et al. Protein conservation during prolonged fast: a function of triiodothyronine levels. *Trans Assoc Am Physicians* 1978;91:169.

69. Beckett GJ, Beddows SE, Morrice PC, et al. Inhibition of hepatic deiodination of thyroxine is caused by selenium deficiency in rats. *Biochem J* 1987;248:443.

70. Beckett GJ, MacDougal DA, Nicol F, et al. Inhibition of type I and II iodothyronine deiodinase activity in rat liver, kidney and brain produced by selenium deficiency. *Biochem J* 1989;259: 887.

71. Arthur JR, Nicol F, Beckett GJ. Hepatic iodothyronine 5'-deiodinase. The role of selenium. *Biochem J* 1990;272:537.

72. Behne D, Kyriakopoulos A, Meinhold H, et al. Identification of type I iodothyronine 5'-deiodinase as a selenoenzyme. *Biochem Biophys Res Commun* 1990;173:1143.

73. Meinhold H, Campos-Barros A, Behne D. Effects of selenium and iodine deficiency on iodothyronine deiodinases in brain, thyroid and peripheral tissue. *Acta Med Aust* 1992;19:8.

74. Meinhold H, Campos-Barros A, Walzog B, et al. Effects of selenium and iodine deficiency on type I, type II and type III iodothyronine deiodinases and circulating thyroid hormones in the rat. *Exp Clin Endocrinol* 1993;101:87.

75. DePalo D, Kinlaw WB, Zhao C, et al. Effect of selenium deficiency on type I 5'-deiodinase. *J Biol Chem* 1994;269:16223.

76. Calomme M, Vanderpas J, Francois B, et al. Effects of selenium supplementation on thyroid hormone metabolism in phenylketonuria subjects on a phenylalanine restricted diet. *Biol Trace Elem Res* 1995;47:349.

77. Jochum F, Terwolbeck K, Meinhold H, et al. Effects of a low selenium state in patients with phenylketonuria. *Acta Paediatr* 1997;86:775.

78. Lombeck I, Jochum F, Terwolbeck K. Selenium status in infants and children with phenylketonuria and in maternal phenylketonuria. *Eur J Pediatr* 1996;155 (suppl):140.

79. Kauf E, Dawczynski H, Jahreis G, et al. Sodium selenite therapy and thyroid-hormone status in cystic fibrosis and congenital hypothyroidism. *Biol Trace Elem Res* 1994;40:247.

80. Vanderpas JB, Contempre B, Duale NL, et al. Iodine and selenium deficiency associated with cretinism in northern Zaire. *Am J Clin Nutr* 1990;52:1087.

81. Goyens P, Golstein J, Nsombola B, et al. Selenium deficiency as a possible factor in the pathogenesis of myxoedematous endemic cretinism. *Acta Endocrinol (Copenh)* 1987;114:497.

82. Contempre B, Dumont JE, Ngo B, et al. Effect of selenium supplementation in hypothyroid subjects of an iodine and selenium deficient area: the possible danger of indiscriminate supplementation of iodine-deficient subjects with selenium. *J Clin Endocrinol Metab* 1991;73:213.

83. Contempre B, Duale NL, Dumont JE, et al. Effect of selenium supplementation on thyroid hormone metabolism in an iodine and selenium deficient population. *Clin Endocrinol (Oxf)* 1992; 36:579.

84. Steinsapir J, Harney J, Larsen PR. Type 2 iodothyronine deiodinase in rat pituitary tumor cells is inactivated in proteasomes. *J Clin Invest* 1998;102:1895.

85. Steinsapir J, Bianco AC, Buettner C, et al. Substrate-induced down-regulation of human type 2 deiodinase (hD_2) is mediated through proteasomal degradation and requires interaction with the enzyme's active center. *Endocrinology* 2000;141:1127.

86. Gereben B, Goncalves C, Harney JW, et al. Selective proteolysis of human type 2 deiodinase: a novel ubiquitin-proteasomal mediated mechanism for regulation of hormone activation. *Mol Endocrinol* 200;14:1697.

87. Celi FS, Canettieri G, Mentuccia D, et al. Structural organization and chromosomal localization of the human type II deiodinase gene. *Eur J Endocrinol* 200;143:267.

88. Araki O, Murakami M, Morimura T, et al. Assignment of type II iodothyronine deiodinase gene (DIO2) to human chromosome band 14q24.2 & q24.3 by in situ hybridization. *Cytogenet Cell Genet* 1999;84:73.

89. Davey JC, Schneider MJ, Becker KB, et al. Cloning of a 5.8 kb cDNA for a mouse type 2 deiodinase. *Endocrinology* 1999; 140:1022.

90. Bartha T, Kim SW, Salvatore D, et al. Characterization of the 5′-flanking and 5′-untranslated regions of the cyclic adenosine 3′,5′-monophosphate-responsive human type 2 iodothyronine deiodinase gene. *Endocrinology* 2000;141:229.

91. Ohba K, Yoshioka T, Muraki T. Identification of two novel splicing variants of human type II iodothyronine deiodinase mRNA. *Mol Cell Endocrinol* 2001;172:169.

92. Song S, Adachi K, Katsuyama M, et al. Isolation and characterization of the 5′-upstream and untranslated regions of the mouse type II iodothyronine deiodinase gene. *Mol Cell Endocrinol* 2000;165:189.

93. Gereben B, Salvatore D, Harney JW, et al. The human, but not rat, dio2 gene is stimulated by thyroid transcription factor-1 (TTF-1). *Mol Endocrinol* 2001;15:112.

94. Buettner C, Harney JW, Larsen PR. The 3′-untranslated region of human type 2 iodothyronine deiodinase mRNA contains a functional selenocysteine insertion sequence element. *J Biol Chem* 1998;273:33374.

95. Gereben B, Bartha T, Tu HM, et al. Cloning and expression of the chicken type 2 iodothyronine 5′-deiodinase. *J Biol Chem* 1999;274:13768.

96. Croteau W, Davey JC, Galton VA, et al. Cloning of the mammalian type II iodothyronine deiodinase: a selenoprotein differentially expressed and regulated in human and rat brain and other tissues. *J Clin Invest* 1996;98:405.

97. Davey JC, Becker KB, Schneider MJ, et al. Cloning of a cDNA for the type II iodothyronine deiodinase. *J Biol Chem* 1995; 270:26786.

98. Valverde C, Croteau W, Lafleur GJ, Jr, et al. Cloning and expression of a 5′-iodothyronine deiodinase from the liver of *Fundulus heteroclitus*. *Endocrinology* 1997;138:642.

99. Salvatore D, Harney JW, Larsen PR. Mutation of the Secys residue 266 in human type 2 selenodeiodinase alters ^{75}Se incorporation without affecting its biochemical properties. *Biochimie* 1999;81:1.

100. Cheron RG, Kaplan MM, Larsen PR. Physiological and pharmacological influences on thyroxine to 3,5,3′-triiodothyronine conversion and nuclear 3,5,3′-triiodothyronine binding in rat anterior pituitary. *J Clin Invest* 1979;64:1402.

101. Leonard JL. Dibutyryl cAMP induction of type 5′deiodinase activity in rat brain astrocytes in culture. *Biochem Biophys Res Commun* 1988;151:1164.

102. Visser TJ, Leonard JL, Kaplan MM, et al. Kinetic evidence suggesting two mechanisms for iodothyronine 5′-deiodination in rat cerebral cortex. *Proc Natl Acad Sci USA* 1982; 79:5080.

103. Crantz FR, Larsen PR. Rapid thyroxine to 3,5,3′-triiodothyronine conversion and nuclear 3,5,3′-triiodothyronine binding in rat cerebral cortex and cerebellum. *J Clin Invest* 19980;65:935.

104. Silva JE, Larsen PR. Adrenergic activation of triiodothyronine production in brown adipose tissue. *Nature* 1983;305:712.

105. Molinero P, Osuna C, Guerrero JM. Type II thyroxine 5′-deiodinase in the rat thymus. *J Endocrinol* 195;146:105.

106. Song S, Sorimachi K, Adachi K, et al. Biochemical and molecular biological evidence for the presence of type II iodothyronine deiodinase in mouse mammary gland. *Mol Cell Endocrinol* 2000;160:173.

107. Kamiya Y, Murakami M, Araki O, et al. Pretranslational regulation of rhythmic type II iodothyronine deiodinase expression by beta-adrenergic mechanism in the rat pineal gland. *Endocrinology* 199;140:1272.

108. Galton VA, Martinez E, Hernandez A, et al. The type 2 iodothyronine deiodinase is expressed in the rat uterus and induced during pregnancy. *Endocrinology* 2001;142:2123.

109. Mizuma H, Murakami M, Mori M. Thyroid hormone activation in human vascular smooth muscle cells: expression of type II iodothyronine deiodinase. *Circ Res* 2001;88:313.

110. Campos-Barros A, Amma LL, Faris JS, et al. Type 2 iodothyronine deiodinase expression in the cochlea before the onset of hearing. *Proc Natl Acad Sci USA* 2000;97:1287.

111. Guadano-Ferraz A, Obregon MJ, St. Germain DL, et al. The type 2 iodothyronine deiodinase is expressed primarily in glial cells in the neonatal rat brain. *Proc Natl Acad Sci USA* 1997; 94:10391.

112. Riskind PN, Kolodny JM, Larsen PR. The regional hypothalamic distribution of type II 5′-monodeiodinase in euthyroid and hypothyroid rats. *Brain Res* 1987;420:194.

113. Tu HM, Kim SW, Salvatore D, et al. Regional distribution of type 2 thyroxine deiodinase messenger ribonucleic acid in rat hypothalamus and pituitary and its regulation by thyroid hormone. *Endocrinology* 1997;138:3359–3368.

114. Fekete C, Mihaly E, Herscovici S, et al. DARPP-32 and CREB are present in type 2 iodothyronine deiodinase-producing tanycytes: implications for the regulation of type 2 deiodinase activity. *Brain Res* 2000;862:154.

115. Diano S, Naftolin F, Goglia F, et al. Monosynaptic pathway between the arcuate nucleus expressing glial type II iodothyronine 5′-deiodinase mRNA and the median eminence-projective TRH cells of the rat paraventricular nucleus. *J Neuroendocrinol* 1998;10:731.

116. Salvatore D, Tu H, Harney JW, et al. 1996 Type 2 iodothyronine deiodinase is highly expressed in human thyroid. *J Clin Invest* 1996;98:962.

117. Murakami M, Araki O, Hosoi Y, et al. Expression and regulation of type II iodothyronine deiodinase in human thyroid gland. *Endocrinology* 2001;142:2961.

118. Imai Y, Toyoda N, Maeda A, et al. Type 2 iodothyronine deiodinase expression is upregulated by protein kinase A–dependent pathway and is downregulated by the protein kinase C–depen-

dent pathway in cultured human thyroid cells. *Thyroid* 2001; 11:899.

119. Itagaki Y, Yoshida K, Ikede H, et al. Thyroxine 5'-deiodinase in human anterior pituitary tumors. *J Clin Endocrinol Metab* 1990;71:340.

120. Murakami M, Araki O, Morimura T, et al. Expression of type II iodothyronine deiodinase in brain tumors. *J Clin Endocrinol Metab* 2000;85:4403.

121. Kaplan MM, Pan C, Gordon PR, et al. Human epidermal keratinocytes in culture convert thyroxine to 3,5,3'-triiodothyronine by type II iodothyronine deiodination: a novel endocrine function of the skin. *J Clin Endocrinol Metab* 1988;66:815.

122. Salvatore D, Bartha T, Larsen PR. The guanosine monophosphate reductase gene is conserved in rats and its expression increases rapidly in brown adipose tissue during cold exposure. *J Biol Chem* 1998;273:31092.

123. Mills I, Raasmaja A, Moolten N, et al. Effect of thyroid status on catecholamine stimulation of thyroxine 5'-deiodinase in brown adipocytes. *Am J Physiol* 1989;256:E74.

124. Raasmaja A, Larsen PR. Alpha 1- and beta-adrenergic agents cause synergistic stimulation of the iodothyronine deiodinase in rat brown adipocytes. *Endocrinology* 1989;125:2502.

125. Noronha M, Raasmaja A, Moolten N, et al. Triiodothyronine causes rapid reversal of alpha 1/cyclic adenosine monophosphate synergism on brown adipocyte respiration and type II deiodinase activity. *Metabolism* 1991;40:1327.

126. Silva JE, Larsen PR. Hormonal regulation of iodothyronine 5'-deiodinase in rat brown adipose tissue. *Am J Physiol* 1986;251: E639.

127. Silva JE, Larsen PR. Interrelationships among thyroxine, growth hormone, and the sympathetic nervous system in the regulation of 5'-iodothyronine deiodinase in rat brown adipose tissue. *J Clin Invest* 1986;77:1214.

128. Pallud S, Lennon AM, Ramauge M, et al. Expression of the type II iodothyronine deiodinase in cultured rat astrocytes is selenium-dependent. *J Biol Chem* 1997;272:18104.

129. Gondou A, Toyoda N, Nishikawa M, et al. Induction of type 2 deiodinase activity by cyclic guanosine 3',5'-monophosphate in cultured rat glial cells. *Thyroid* 1998;8:615.

130. Gondou A, Toyoda N, Nishikawa M, et al. Effect of nicotine on type 2 deiodinase activity in cultured rat glial cells. *Endocr J* 1999;46:107.

131. Canettieri G, Celi FS, Baccheschi G, et al. Isolation of human type 2 deiodinase gene promoter and characterization of a functional cyclic adenosine monophosphate response element. *Endocrinology* 2000;141:1804.

132. Borges M, Ingbar SH, Silva JE. Iodothyronine deiodinase activities in FRTL5 cells: predominance of type I 5'-deiodinase. *Endocrinology* 1990;126:3059.

133. Gereben B, Kollar A, Harney JW, et al. The mRNA structure has potent regulatory effects on type 2 iodothyronine deiodinase expression. *Mol Endocrinol* 2002;16:1667.

134. Burmeister LA, Pachucki J, St. Germain DL. Thyroid hormones inhibit type 2 iodothyronine deiodinase in the rat cerebral cortex by both pre- and posttranslational mechanisms. *Endocrinology* 1997;138:5231.

135. Leonard JL, Kaplan MM, Visser TJ, et al. Cerebral cortex responds rapidly to thyroid hormones. *Science* 1981;214:571.

136. Koenig RJ, Leonard JL, Senator D, et al. Regulation of thyroxine 5'-deiodinase activity by 3,5,3'-triiodothyronine in cultured rat anterior pituitary cells. *Endocrinology* 1984;115:324.

137. Silva JE, Leonard JL. Regulation of rat cerebrocortical and adenohypophyseal type II 5'-deiodinase by thyroxine, triiodothyronine, and reverse triiodothyronine. *Endocrinology* 1985;116: 1627.

138. Halperin Y, Shapiro LE, Surks MI. Down-regulation of type II L-thyroxine, 5'-monodeiodinase in cultured GC cells: different pathways of regulation by L-triiodothyronine and 3,3',5'-triiodo-L-thyronine. *Endocrinology* 1994;135:1464.

139. Leonard JL, Silva JE, Kaplan MM, et al. Acute posttranscriptional regulation of cerebrocortical and pituitary iodothyronine 5'-deiodinases by thyroid hormone. *Endocrinology* 1984;114: 998.

140. Obregon MJ, Larsen PR, Silva JE. The role of 3,3',5'-triiodothyronine in the regulation of type II iodothyronine 5'-deiodinase in the rat cerebral cortex. *Endocrinology* 1986;119: 2186.

141. St. Germain DL. The effects and interactions of substrates, inhibitors, and the cellular thiol-disulfide balance on the regulation of type II iodothyronine 5'-deiodinase. *Endocrinology* 1988;122:1860–1868.

142. Leonard JL, Siegrist-Kaiser CA, et al. Regulation of type II iodothyronine 5'-deiodinase by thyroid hormone: inhibition of actin polymerization blocks enzyme inactivation in cAMP-stimulated glial cells. *J Biol Chem* 1990;265:940.

143. Coux O, Tanaka K, Goldberg AL. Structure and functions of the 20S and 26S proteasomes. *Annu Rev Biochem* 1996;65:801.

144. Hershko A, Ciechanover A. The ubiquitin system. *Annu Rev Biochem* 1998;67:425.

145. Botero D, Gereben B, Goncalves C, et al. Ubc6p and Ubc7p are required for normal and substrate-induced endoplasmic reticulum-associated degradation of the human selenoprotein type 2 iodothyronine monodeiodinase. *Mol Endocrinol* 2002; 16:1999.

146. Tiwari S, Weissman AM. Endoplasmic reticulum (ER)-associated degradation of T cell receptor subunits: involvement of ER-associated ubiquitin-conjugating enzymes (E2s). *J Biol Chem* 2001;276:16193.

147. Kim BW, Zavacki AM, Curcio-Morelli C, et al. ER-associated degradation of the human type 2 iodothyronine deiodinase (D$_2$) is mediated via an association between mammalian UBC7 and the carboxyl region of D$_2$. *Mol Endocrinol* 2003;17:2603.

148. Bianco AC, Harney J, Larsen PR, Identification of ubiquitinated forms of human type 2 deiodinase (hD$_2$). 72nd Annual Meeting, American Thyroid Association, Palm Beach, FL, 1999, p 5.

149. Curcio-Morelli C, Zavacki AM, Christofollete M, et al. Deubiquitination of type 2 iodothyronine deiodinase by pVHL-interacting deubiquitinating enzymes regulates thyroid hormone activation. *J Clin Invest* 2003;112:189.

150. Bianco AC, Silva JE. Cold exposure rapidly induces virtual saturation of brown adipose tissue nuclear T$_3$ receptors. *Am J Physiol* 1988;255:E496.

151. de Jesus LA, Carvalho SD, Ribeiro MO, et al. The type 2 iodothyronine deiodinase is essential for adaptive thermogenesis in brown adipose tissue. *J Clin Invest* 2001;108:1379.

152. Bianco AC, Silva JE. Intracellular conversion of thyroxine to triiodothyronine is required for the optimal thermogenic function of brown adipose tissue. *J Clin Invest* 1987;79:295.

153. Christoffolete MA, Linardi CCG, de Jesus LA, et al. Mice with targeted disruption of the Dio2 gene have cold-induced overexpression of uncoupling protein 1 gene but fail to increase brown adiose tissue lipogenesis and adaptive thermogenesis. *Diabetes* 2004;53:577.

154. Huang Y, Baker RT, Fischer-Vize JA. Control of cell fate by a deubiquitinating enzyme encoded by the fat facets gene. *Science* 1995;270:1828.

155. Moazed D, Johnson D. A deubiquitinating enzyme interacts with SIR4 and regulates silencing in *S. cerevisiae*. *Cell* 1996;86: 667.

156. Zhu Y, Carroll M, Papa FR, et al. DUB-1, a deubiquitating enzyme with growth-suppressing activity. *Proc Natl Acad Sci U S A* 1996;93:3275.

157. Naviglio S, Mattecucci C, Matoskova B, et al. UBPY: a growth-regulated human ubiquitin isopeptidase. *EMBO J* 1998;17:3241.

158. Park KC, Kim JH, Choi EJ, et al. Antagonistic regulation of myogenesis by two deubiquitinating enzymes, UBP45 and UBP69. *Proc Natl Acad Sci U S A* 2002;99:9733.

159. Li Z, Na X, Wang D, et al. Ubiquitination of a novel deubiquitinating enzyme requires direct binding to von Hippel-Lindau tumor suppressor protein. *J Biol Chem* 2002;277:4656.

160. Moreno M, Berry MJ, Horst C, et al. Activation and inactivation of thyroid hormone by type I iodothyronine deiodinase. *FEBS Lett* 1994;344:143.

161. Huang H, Marsh-Armstrong N, Brown DD. Metamorphosis is inhibited in transgenic *Xenopus laevis* tadpoles that overexpress type III deiodinase. *Proc Natl Acad Sci U S A* 1999;96:962.

162. Huang SA, Tu HM, Harney JW, et al. Severe hypothyroidism caused by type 3 iodothyronine deiodinase in infantile hemangiomas. *N Engl J Med* 2000;343:185.

163. Sato K, Robbins J. Thyroid hormone metabolism in cultured monkey hepatocarcinoma cells. *J Biol Chem* 1980;255:7347.

164. Kaplan MM, Yaskoski KA. Phenolic and tyrosyl ring deiodination of iodothyronines in rat brain homogenates. *J Clin Invest* 1980;66:551.

165. Kaplan MM, Yaskoski KA. Maturational patterns of iodothyronine phenolic tyrosyl ring deiodinase activities in rat cerebrum, cerebellem and hypothalamus. *J Clin Invest* 1981;67:1208.

166. Sorimachi K, Robbins J. Metabolism of thyroid hormones by cultured monkey hepatocarcinoma cells: nonphenolic ring deiodination and sulfation. *J Biol Chem* 1977;252:4458.

167. Richard K, Hume R, Kaptein E, et al. Ontogeny of iodothyronine deiodinases in human liver. *J Clin Endocrinol Metab* 1998;83:2868.

168. Berry DL, Rose CS, Remo BF, et al. The expression pattern of thyroid hormone response genes in remodeling tadpole tissues defines distinct growth and resorption gene expression programs. *Dev Biol* 1998;203:24.

169. Hernandez A, Park JP, Lyon GJ, et al. Localization of the type 3 iodothyronine deiodinase (DIO3) gene to human chromosome 14q32 and mouse chromosome 12F1. *Genomics* 1998;53:119.

170. Hernandez A, Lyon GJ, Schneider MJ, et al. Isolation and characterization of the mouse gene for the type 3 iodothyronine deiodinase. *Endocrinology* 1999;140:124.

171. Hernandez A, Martinez ME, Croteau W, et al. Complex organization and structure of sense and antisense transcripts expressed from the DIO3 gene imprinted locus. *Genomics* 2004;83:413.

172. Hernandez A, Fiering S, Martinez E, et al. The gene locus encoding iodothyronine deiodinase type 3 (Dio3) is imprinted in the fetus and expresses antisense transcripts. *Endocrinology* 2002;143:4483.

173. Salvatore D, Low SC, Berry M, et al. Type 3 iodothyronine deiodinase: cloning, *in vitro* expression, and functional analysis of the placental selenoenzyme. *J Clin Invest* 1995;96:2421.

174. Tu HM, Legradi G, Bartha T, et al. Regional expression of the type 3 iodothyronine deiodinase messenger ribonucleic acid in the rat central nervous system and its regulation by thyroid hormone. *Endocrinology* 1999;140:784.

175. Bates JM, Spate VL, Morris JS, et al. Effects of selenium deficiency on tissue selenium content, deiodinase activity, and thyroid hormone economy in the rat during development. *Endocrinology* 2000;141:2490.

176. Roti E, Braverman LE, Fang S-L, et al. Ontogenesis of placental inner ring thyroxine deiodinase and amniotic fluid 3,3'5'-triidothyronine concentration in the rat. *Endocrinology* 1982;111:959.

177. Kaplan MM, McCann UD, Yaskoski KA, et al. Anatomical distribution of phenolic and tyrosyl ring iodothyronine deiodinases in the nervous system of normal and hypothyroid rats. *Endocrinology* 1981;109:397.

178. Galton VA, McCarthy PT, St Germain DL. The ontogeny of iodothyronine deiodinase systems in liver and intestine of the rat. *Endocrinology* 1991;128:1717.

179. Squire LR. Mechanisms of memory. *Science* 1986;342:1612.

180. Puymirat J, Miehe M, Marchand R, et al. Immunocytochemical localization of thyroid hormone receptors in the adult rat brain. *Thyroid* 1991;1:173.

181. Puymirat J. Thyroid receptors in the rat brain. *Prog Neurobiol* 1992;39:281.

182. Escamez MJ, Guadano-Ferraz A, Cuadrado A, et al. Type 3 iodothyronine deiodinase is selectively expressed in areas related to sexual differentiation in the newborn rat brain. *Endocrinology* 1999;140:5443.

183. Leonard JL, Larsen PR. Thyroid hormone metabolism in primary cultures of fetal rat brain cells. *Brain Res* 1985;327:1.

184. Cavalieri RR, Gavin LA, Cole R, et al. Thyroid hormone deiodinases in purified primary glial cell cultures. *Brain Res* 1986;364:382.

185. Mori K, Yoshida K, Kayama T, et al. Thyroxine 5-deiodinase in human brain tumors. *J Clin Endocrinol Metab* 1993;77:1198.

186. Huang SA, Fish SA, Dorfman DM, et al. A 21-year-old woman with consumptive hypothyroidism due to a vascular tumor expressing type 3 iodothyronine deiodinase. *J Clin Endocrinol Metab* 2002;87:4457.

187. McCann UD, Shaw EA, Kaplan MM. Iodothyronine deiodination reaction types in several rat tissues: effects of age, thyroid status, and glucocorticoid treatment. *Endocrinology* 1984;114:1513.

188. Marsh-Armstrong N, Huang H, Remo BF, et al. Asymmetric growth and development of the *Xenopus laevis* retina during metamorphosis is controlled by type III deiodinase. *Neuron* 1999;24:871.

189. Huang TS, Chopra IJ, Beredo A, et al. Skin is an active site for the inner ring monodeiodination of thyroxine to 3,3',5'-triiodothyronine. *Endocrinology* 1985;117:2106.

190. Santini F, Vitti P, Chiovato L, et al. Role for inner ring deiodination preventing transcutaneous passage of thyroxine. *J Clin Endocrinol Metab* 2003;88:2825.

191. Castro MI, Braverman LE, Alex S, et al. Inner-ring deiodination of 3,5,3'-triiodothyronine in the *in situ* perfused guinea pig placenta. *J Clin Invest* 1985;76:1921.

192. Roti E, Fang SL, Green K, et al. Human placenta is an active site of thyroxine and 3,3',5-triiodothyronine tyrosyl ring deiodination. *J Clin Endocrinol Metab* 1981;53:498.

193. Fay M, Roti E, Fang SL, et al. The effects of propylthiouracil, iodothyronines, and other agents on thyroid hormone metabolism in human placenta. *J Clin Endocrinol Metab* 1984;58:280.

194. Hidal JT, Kaplan MM. Characteristics of thyroxine 5'-deiodination in cultured human placental cells: regulation by iodothyronines. *J Clin Invest* 1985;76:947.

195. Galton VA, Martinez E, Hernandez A, et al. Pregnant rat uterus expresses high levels of the type 3 iodothyronine deiodinase. *J Clin Audiometry* 1999;103:979.

196. Wasco EC, Martinez E, Grant KS, et al. Determinants of iodothyronine deiodinase activities in rodent uterus. *Endocrinology* 2000;144:4253.

197. Huang SA, Dorfman DM, Genest DR, et al. Type 3 iodothyronine deiodinase is highly expressed in the human uteroplacental unit and in fetal epithelium. *J Clin Endocrinol Metab* 2003;88:1384.

198. Esfandiari A, Courtin F, Lennon AM, et al. Induction of type III deiodinase activity in astroglial cells by thyroid hormones. *Endocrinology* 1992;131:1682.

199. Wassen FW, Schiel AE, Kuiper GG, et al. Induction of thyroid hormone-degrading deiodinase in cardiac hypertrophy and failure. *Endocrinology* 2002;143:2812.

200. Courtin F, Liva P, Gavaret JM, et al. Induction of 5-deiodinase activity in astroglial cells by 12-O-tetradecanoylphorbol 13-acetate and fibroblast growth factors. *J Neurochem* 1991;56:1107.

201. Pallud S, Ramauge M, Gavaret JM, et al. Regulation of type 3 iodothyronine deiodinase expression in cultured rat astrocytes: role of the Erk cascade. *Endocrinology* 1999;40:2917.

202. Klebanoff SJ, Green WL. Degradation of thyroid hormones by phagocytosing human leukocytes. *J Clin Invest* 1973;52:60.

203. Visvanathan A, Shanmugasundaram KR. Alterations in L-triiodothyronine aminotransferase activity in hypothyroid rats—effects of administration of iodobenzene and L-thyroxine. *Ind J Exp Biol* 1984;22:442.

204. Pittman CS, Shimizu T, Burger A, et al. The nondeiodinative pathways of thyroxine metabolism: 3,5,3′,5-tetraiodothyroacetic acid turnover in normal and fasting human subjects. *J Clin Endocrinol Metab* 1980;50:712.

205. Visser TJ. Role of sulfation in thyroid hormone metabolism. *Chem Biol Interact* 1994;92:293.

206. Visser TJ. Importance of deiodination and conjugation in the hepatic metabolism of thyroid hormone. In: Greer MA, ed. *The thyroid gland.* New York: Raven, 1990:255.

207. Sekura RD, Sato K, Cahnmann HJ, et al. Sulfate transfer to thyroid hormones and their analogs by hepatic aryl sulfotransferases. *Endocrinology* 1981;108:454.

208. Anderson RJ, Babbitt LL, Liebentritt DK. Human liver triiodothyronine sulfotransferase: copurification with phenol sulfotransferases. *Thyroid* 1995;5:61.

209. Sato K, Robbins J. Thyroid hormone metabolism in primary cultured rat hepatocytes. Effects of glucose, glucagon, and insulin. *J Clin Invest* 1981;68:475.

210. de Herder WW, Bonthuis F, Rutgers M, et al. Effects of inhibition of type I iodothyronine deiodinase and phenol sulfotransferase on the biliary clearance of triiodothyronine in rats. *Endocrinology* 1998;122:153.

211. Sorimachi K, Robbins J. Effects of propylthiouracil and methylmercaptoimidazol on metabolism of thyroid hormones by cultured monkey hepatocarcinoma cells. *Horm Metab Res* 1979;11:39.

212. Young WF Jr. Human liver tyrosylsulfotransferase. *Gastroenterology* 1990;99:1072.

213. Rooda SJE, Kaptein E, Visser TJ. Serum triiodothyronine sulfate in man measured by radioimmunoassay. *J Clin Endocrinol Metab* 1989;69:552.

214. Rooda SJE, Kaptein E, Rutgers M, et al. Increased plasma 3,5,3′-triiodothyronine sulfate in rats with inhibited type I iodothyronine dediodinase activity, as measured by radioimmunoassay. *Endocrinology* 1989;124:740.

215. van Stralen PG, van der Hoek HJ, Docter R, et al. Reduced T_3 deiodination by the human hepatoblastoma cell line HepG2 caused by deficient T_3 sulfation. *Biochim Biophys Acta* 1993;1157:114.

216. Chanoine JP, Safran M, Farwell AP, et al. Effects of selenium deficiency on thyroid hormone economy in rats. *Endocrinology* 1992;131:1787.

217. Wu SY, Huang WS, Polk D, et al. Identification of thyroxine sulfate (T_4S) in human serum and amniotic fluid by a novel T_4S radioimmunoassay. *Thyroid* 1992;2:101.

218. Chopra IJ, Santini F, Hurd RE, et al. A radioimmunoassay for measurement of thyroxine sulfate. *J Clin Endocrinol Metab* 1993;76:145.

219. Santini F, Cortelazzi D, Baggiani AM, et al. A study of the serum 3,5,3′-triiodothyronine sulfate concentration in normal and hypothyroid fetuses at various gestational stages. *J Clin Endocrinol Metab* 1993;76:1583.

220. Wu S-Y, Huang W-S, Polk D, et al. The development of a radioimmunoassay for reverse triiodothyronine sulfate in human serum and amniotic fluid. *J Clin Endocrinol Metab* 1993;76:1625.

221. LoPresti JS, Nicoloff JT. 3,5,3′-Triiodothyronine (T_3) sulfate: a major metabolite in T_3 metabolism in man. *J Clin Endocrinol Metab* 1994;78:688.

222. Frumess RD, Larsen PR. Correlation of serum triiodothyronine (T_3) and thyroxine (T_4) with biologic effects of thyroid hormone replacement in propylthiouracil-treated rats. *Metabolism* 1975;24:547.

223. Larsen PR, Frumess RD. Comparison of the biological effects of thyroxine and triiodothyronine in the rat. *Endocrinology* 1977;100:980.

224. Silva JE, Larsen PR. Peripheral metabolism of homologous thyrotropin in euthyroid and hypothyroid rats: acute effects of thyrotropin-releasing hormone, triiodothyronine, and thyroxine. *Endocrinology* 1978;102:1783.

225. Larsen PR, Dick TE, Markovitz BP, et al. Inhibition of intrapituitary thyroxine to 3,5,3′-triiodothyronine conversion prevents the acute suppression of thyrotropin release by thyroxine in hypothyroid rats. *J Clin Invest* 1979;64:117.

226. Riesco G, Taurog A, Larsen R, et al. Acute and chronic responses to iodine deficiency in rats. *Endocrinology* 1977;100:303.

227. Segerson TP, Kauer J, Wolfe H, et al. Thyroid hormone regulates TRH biosynthesis in the paraventricular nucleus of the rat hypothalamus. *Science* 1987;238:78.

228. Connors JM, Hedge GA. Feedback effectiveness of periodic versus constant triiodothyronine replacement. *Endocrinology* 1980;106:911.

229. Connors JM, Hedge GA. Feedback regulation of thyrotropin by thyroxine under physiological conditions. *Am J Physiol* 1981;240:E308.

230. Kakucska I, Rand W, Lechan RM. Thyrotropin-releasing hormone (TRH) gene expression in the hypothalamic paraventricular nucleus is dependent upon feedback regulation by both triiodothyronine and thyroxine. *Endocrinology* 1992;130:2845.

231. Izumi M, Larsen PR. Triiodothyronine, thyroxine, and iodine in purified thyroglobulin from patients with Graves' disease. *J Clin Invest* 1977;59:1105.

232. Larsen PR. Thyroidal triiodothyronine and thyroxine in Graves' disease: correlation with presurgical treatment, thyroid status, and iodine content. *J Clin Endocrinol Metab* 1975;41:1098.

233. Laurberg P. Mechanisms governing the relative proportions of thyroxine and 3,5,3′-triiodothyronine in thyroid secretion. *Metabolism* 1984;33:379.

234. Geffner DL, Azukizawa M, Hershman JM. Propylthiouracil blocks extrathyroidal conversion of thyroxine to triiodothyronine and augments thyrotropin secretion in man. *J Clin Invest* 1975;55:224.

235. Saberi M, Sterling FH, Utiger RD. Reduction in extrathyroidal triiodothyronine production by propylthiouracil in man. *J Clin Invest* 1975;55:218.

236. LoPresti JS, Eigen A, Kaptein E, et al. Alterations in 3,3′5′-triiodothyronine metabolism in response to propylthiouracil, dexamethasone, and thyroxine administration in man. *J Clin Invest* 1989;84:1650.

237. Inada M, Kasagi K, Kurata S, et al. Estimation of thyroxine and triiodothyronine distribution and of the conversion rate of thyroxine to triiodothyronine in man. *J Clin Invest* 1975;55:1337.

238. Lum SM, Nicoloff JT, Spencer CA, et al. Peripheral tissue mechanism for maintenance of serum triiodothyronine values in a thyroxine-deficient state in man. *J Clin Invest* 1984;73:570.

239. Nicoloff JT, Lum SM, Spencer CA, et al. Peripheral autoregulation of thyroxine to triiodothyronine conversion in man. *Horm Metab Res* 1984;14:74(suppl.).

240. Pilo A, Iervasi G, Vitek F, et al. Thyroidal and peripheral production of 3,5,3'-triiodothyronine in humans by multicompartmental analysis. *Am J Physiol* 1990;258:E715.

241. Oppenheimer JH, Schwartz HL, Surks MI. Propylthiouracil inhibits the conversion of L-thyroxine to L-triiodothyronine: an explanation of the antithyroxine effect of propylthiouracil and evidence supporting the concept that triiodothyronine is the active thyroid hormone. *J Clin Invest* 1972;51:2493.

242. Nguyen TT, Chapa F, DiStefano JJ 3rd. Direct measurement of the contributions of type I and type II 5'-deiodinases to whole body steady state 3,5,3'-triiodothyronine production from thyroxine in the rat. *Endocrinology* 1998;139:4626.

243. Hosoi Y, Murakami M, Mizuma H, et al. Expression and regulation of type II iodothyronine deiodinase in cultured human skeletal muscle cells. *J Clin Endocrinol Metab* 1999;84:3293.

244. Friesema EC, Docter R, Moerings EP, et al. Identification of thyroid hormone transporters. *Biochem Biophys Res Commun* 1999;254:497.

245. Hennemann G, Docter R, Friesema ECH, et al. Plasma membrane transport of thyroid hormones and its role in thyroid hormone metabolism and bioavailability. *Endocr Rev* 2001;22:451.

246. Oppenheimer JH. Thyroid hormone action at the cellular level. *Science* 1979;203:971.

247. Silva JE, Leonard JL, Crantz FR, et al. Evidence for two tissue specific pathways for in vivo thyroxine 5' deiodination in the rat. *J Clin Invest* 1982;69:1176.

248. Bianco AC, Silva JE. Nuclear 3,5,3'-triiodothyronine (T_3) in brown adipose tissue: receptor occupancy and sources of T_3 as determined by *in vivo* techniques. *Endocrinology* 1897;120:55.

249. van Doorn JD, Roelfsema F, van der Heide D. Contribution from local conversion of thyroxine to 3,5,3'-triiodothyronine to cellular 3,5,3'-triiodothyronine in several organs in hypothyroid rats at isotope equilibrium. *Acta Endocrinol (Copenh)* 1982;101:386.

250. van Doorn JD, van der Heide D, Roelfsema F. Sources and quantity of 3,5,3'-triiodothyronine in several tissues of the rat. *J Clin Invest* 1983;72:1778.

251. van Doorn JD, Roelfsema F, van der Heide D. Concentrations of thyroxine and 3,5,3'-triiodothyronine at 34 different sites in euthyroid rats as determined by an isotopic equilibrium technique. *Endocrinology* 1985;117:1201.

252. Eales JG, McLeese JM, Holmes JA, et al. Changes in intestinal and hepatic thyroid hormone deiodination during spontaneous metamorphosis of the sea lamprey, *Petromyzon marinus. J Exp Zool* 2000;286:305.

253. Larsen PR, Bavli SZ, Castonguay M, et al. Direct radioimmunoassay of nuclear 3,5,3' triiodothyronine in rat anterior pituitary. *J Clin Invest* 1980;65:675.

254. Oppenheimer JH, Schwartz HL. Stereospecific transport to triiodothyronine from plasma to cytosol and from cytosol to nucleus in rat liver, kidney, brain and heart. *J Clin Invest* 1985;75:147.

255. Dunn JT. Global IDD status. *IDD Newsletter* 1999;15:17.

256. Silva JE. Disposal rates of thyroxine and triiodothyronine in iodine-deficient rats. *Endocrinology* 1972;91:1430.

257. Pazos-Moura CC, Moura EG, Dorris ML, et al. Effect of iodine deficiency and cold exposure on thyroxine 5'-deiodinase activity in various rat tissues. *Am J Physiol* 1991;260:E175.

258. Okamura K, Taurog A, Krulich L. Hypothyroidism in severely iodine-deficient rats. *Endocrinology* 1981;109:464.

259. Santisteban P, Obregon MJ, Rodriguez-Pena A, et al. Are iodine-deficient rats euthyroid? *Endocrinology* 1982;110:1780.

260. Obregon MJ, Santisteban P, Rodriguez-Pena A, et al. Cerebral hypothyroidism in rats with adult-onset iodine deficiency. *Endocrinology* 1984;115:614.

261. Riesco G, Taurog A, Larsen PR. Variations in the response of the thyroid gland of the rat to different low-iodine diets: correlation with iodine content of diet. *Endocrinology* 1976;99:270.

262. Greer MA, Grimm Y, Studer H. Qualitative changes in the secretion of thyroid hormones induced by iodine deficiency. *Endocrinology* 1968;83:1193.

263. Abrams GM, Larsen PR. Triiodothyronine and thyroxine in the serum and thyroid glands of iodine-deficient rats. *J Clin Invest* 1873;52:2522.

264. Silva JE, Gordon MB, Crantz FR, et al. Qualitative and quantitative differences in the pathways of extrathyroidal triiodothyronine generation between euthyroid and hypothyroid rats. *J Clin Invest* 1984;73:898.

265. Campos-Barros A, Meinhold H, Walzog B, et al. Effects of selenium and iodine deficiency on thyroid hormone concentrations in the central nervous system of the rat. *Eur J Endocrinol* 1997;136:316.

266. Guadano-Ferraz A, Escamez MJ, Rausell E, et al. Expression of type 2 iodothyronine deiodinase in hypothyroid rat brain indicates an important role of thyroid hormone in the development of specific primary sensory systems. *J Neurosci* 1999;19:3430.

267. Peeters R, Fekete C, Goncalves C, et al. Regional physiological adaptation of the central nervous system deiodinases to iodine deficiency. *Am J Physiol Endocrinol Metab* 2001;281:E54.

268. Kim SW, Harney JW, Larsen PR. Studies of the hormonal regulation of type 2 5'-iodothyronine deiodinase messenger ribonucleic acid in pituitary tumor cells using semiquantitative reverse transcription-polymerase chain reaction. *Endocrinology* 1998;139:4895.

269. St. Germain DL, Schwartzman RA, Croteau W, et al. A thyroid hormone-regulated gene in *Xenopus laevis* encodes a type III iodothyronine 5-deiodinase. *Proc Natl Acad U S A* 1994;91:7767.

270. Schroder-van der Elst JP, van der Heide D, Morreale de Escobar G, et al. Iodothyronine deiodinase activities in fetal rat tissues at several levels of iodine deficiency: a role for the skin in 3,5,3'-triiodothyronine economy? *Endocrinology* 1998;139:2229.

271. Silva JE, Matthews PS. Production rates and turnover of triiodothyronine in rat developing cerebral cortex and cerebellum. *J Clin Invest* 1984;74:1035.

272. Crantz FR, Silva JE, Larsen PR. An analysis of the sources and quantity of 3,5,3'-triiodothyronine specifically bound to nuclear receptors in rat cerebral cortex and cerebellum. *Endocrinology* 1982;110:367.

273. Silva JE, Larsen PR. Comparison of iodothyronine 5'-deiodinase and other thyroid-hormone-dependent enzyme activities in the cerebral cortex of hypothyroid neonatal rat: evidence for adaptation to hypothyroidism. *J Clin Invest* 1982;70:1110.

274. Porterfield SP, Hendrich CE. The role of thyroid hormones in prenatal and neonatal neurological development—current perspectives. *Endocr Rev* 1993;14:94.

275. Pasquini JM, Adamo AM. Thyroid hormones and the central nervous system. *Dev Neurosci* 1994;16:1.

276. Brent GA. The molecular basis of thyroid hormone action. *N Engl J Med* 1994;331:847.

277. Zhang J, Lazar MA. The mechanism of action of thyroid hormones. *Annu Rev Physiol* 2000;62:439.

278. Kaplan MM, Shaw EA. Type II iodothyronine 5′-deiodination by human and rat placenta *in vitro. J Clin Endocrinol Metab* 1984;59:253.

279. Kaplan MM. Regulatory influences on iodothyronine deiodination in animal tissues. In: Hennemann G, ed. *Thyroid hormone metabolism.* New York: Marcel Dekker, 1986:231.

280. Marsh-Armstrong N, Cai L, Brown DD. Thyroid hormone controls the development of connections between the spinal cord and limbs during Xenopus laevis metamorphosis. *Proc Natl Acad Sci U S A* 2004;101:165.

281. Cai L, Brown DD. Expression of type II iodothyronine deiodinase marks the time that a tissue responds to thyroid hormone-induced metamorphosis in *Xenopus laevis. Dev Biol* 2004;266:87.

282. Huang T, Chopra IJ, Boado R, et al. Thyroxine inner ring monodeiodinating activity in fetal tissues of the rat. *Pediatr Res* 1988;23:196.

283. Ng L, Goodyear RJ, Woods CA, et al. Hearing loss and retarded cochlear development in mice lacking type 2 iodothyronine deiodinase. *Proc Natl Acad Sci U S A* 2004;101:3474.

284. Thorpe-Beeston JG, Nicolaides KH, McGregor AM. Fetal thyroid function. *Thyroid* 1992;2:207.

285. Contempre B, Jauniaux E, Calvo R, et al. Detection of thyroid hormones in human embryonic cavities during the first trimester of pregnancy. *J Clin Endocrinol Metab* 1993;77:1719.

286. Fisher DA, Lehman H, Lackey C. Placental transport of thyroxine. *J Clin Endocrinol* 1964;24:393.

287. Abuid J, Klein AH, Foley TP Jr, et al. 1974 Total and free triiodothyronine and thyroxine in early infancy. *J Clin Endocrinol Metab* 1974;39:263.

288. Chopra IJ, Wu SY, Chua Teco GN, et al. A radioimmunoassay for measurement of 3,5,3′-triiodothyronine sulfate: studies in thyroidal and non-thyroidal disease, pregnancy and neonatal life. *J Clin Endocrinol Metab* 1992;75:189.

289. Santini F, Chopra IJ, Wu SY, et al. Metabolism of 3,5,3′-triiodothyronine sulfate by tissues of the fetal rat: a consideration of the role of desulfation of 3,5,3′-triiodothyronine sulfate as a source of T3. *Pediatr Res* 1992;31:541.

290. Koopdonk-Kool JM, deVijlder JJM, Veenboer GJM, et al. Type II and Type III deiodinase activity in human placenta as a function of gestational age. *J Clin Endocrinol Metab* 1996;81:2154.

291. Stulp MR, de Vijlder JJ, Ris-Stalpers C. Placental iodothyronine deiodinase III and II ratios, mRNA expression compared to enzyme activity. *Mol Cell Endocrinol* 1998;142:67.

292. Yoshida K, Suzuki M, Sakurada T. Changes in thyroxine monodeiodination in rat liver, kidney and placenta during pregnancy. *Acta Endocrinol (Copenh)* 1984;107:495.

293. Remesar X, Arola L, Palou A, et al. Activities of enzymes involved in amino-acid metabolism in developing rat placenta. *Eur J Biochem* 1980;110:289.

294. Mortimer RH, Galligan JP, Cannell GR, et al. Maternal to fetal thyroxine transmission in the human term placenta is limited by inner ring deiodination. *J Clin Endocrinol Metab* 1996;81:2247.

295. Bradley DJ, Towle HC, Young WSI. Spatial and termporal expression of a- and b-thyroid hormone receptor mRNAs, including the b2-subtype, in the developing mammalian nervous system. *J Neurosci* 1992;12:2288.

296. Kraft JC, Willhite CC, Juchau MR. Embryogenesis in cultured whole rat embryos after combined exposures to 3,3′,5-triiodo-L-thyronine (T3) plus all-trans-retinoic acid and to T3 plus 9-cis-retinoic acid. *J Craniofac Genet Dev Biol* 1994;14:75.

297. Klein AH, Hobel CJ, Sack J, et al. Effect of intraamniotic fluid thyroxine injection on fetal serum and amniotic fluid iodothyronine concentrations. *J Clin Endocrinol Metab* 1978;47:1034.

298. Mandel SJ, Larsen PR, Seely EW, et al. Increased need for thyroxine during pregnancy in women with primary hypothyroidism. *N Engl J Med* 1990;323:91.

299. Vulsma T, Gons MH, DeVijlder JMM. Maternal fetal transfer of thyroxine in congenital hypothyroidism due to a total organification defect of thyroid dysgenesis. *N Engl J Med* 1989;321:13.

300. LaFranchi S. Congenital hypothyroidism: etiologies, diagnosis, and management. *Thyroid* 1999;9:735.

301. Ayling RM, Davenport M, Hadzic N, et al. Hepatic hemangioendothelioma associated with production of humoral thyrotropin-like factor. *J Pediatr* 2001;138:932.

302. Kaplan MM. Monitoring thyroxine treatment during pregnancy. *Thyroid* 1992;2:147.

303. Alexander EK, Marqusee E, Lawrence J, et al. Timing and magnitude of increases in levothyroxine requirements during pregnancy in women with hypothyroidism. N Engl J Med 2004;241.

304. Ishii H, Inada M, Tanaka K, et al. Triiodothyronine generation from thyroxine in human thyroid: enhanced conversion in Graves' thyroid tissue. *J Clin Endocrinol Metab* 1981;52:1211.

305. Sugawara M, Lau R, Wasser HL, et al. Thyroid T4 5′-deiodinase activity in normal and abnormal human thyroid glands. *Metabolism* 1984;33:332.

306. Wu SY, Shyh TP, Chopra IJ, et al. Comparison sodium ipodate (oragrafin) and propylthiouracil in early treatment of hyperthyroidism. *J Clin Endocrinol Metab* 1982;54:630.

307. Burgi H, Wimpfheimer C, Burger A, et al. Changes of circulating thyroxine, triiodothyronine and reverse triiodothyronine after radiographic contrast agents. *J Clin Endocrinol Metab* 1976;43:1203.

308. Croxson MS, Hall TD, Nicoloff JT. Combination drug therapy for treatment of hyperthyroid Graves' disease. *J Clin Endocrinol Metab* 1977;45:623.

309. Laurberg P, Torring J, Weeke J. A comparison of the effects of propylthiouracil and methimazol on circulating thyroid hormones and various measures of peripheral thyroid hormone effects in thyrotoxic patients. *Acta Endorinol (Copenh)* 1985;108:51.

310. Kim BW, Daniels GH, Harrison BJ, et al. Overexpression of type 2 iodothyronine deiodinase in follicular carcinoma as a cause of low circulating free thyroxine levels. *J Clin Endocrinol Metab* 2003;88:594.

THYROID HORMONE ACTION

8

GENOMIC AND NONGENOMIC ACTIONS OF THYROID HORMONES

PAUL M. YEN

Thyroid hormone (TH) (e.g., L-triiodothyronine, T_3; L-tetraiodothyronine, T_4) regulates a wide range of cellular and physiologic activities such as growth, development, metabolism (1–3). TH has prominent effects during gestation and early childhood. In humans, TH's critical role in development is demonstrated by the distinctive neurological and physical deficits that occur in cretins from iodine-deficient areas. TH also has important effects on growth and development in the latter stages of childhood. However, unlike its early developmental-specific effects, growth and eumetabolism are restored after the institution of TH treatment. TH's primary effects in adults are mostly metabolic. These effects include changes in oxygen consumption, protein, carbohydrate, lipid, and vitamin metabolism. Dramatic clinical improvement and correction of metabolic derangements in hypothyroidism occur with TH therapy. Taken together, the clinical and metabolic manifestations of hypo- and hyperthyroidism highlight TH's myriad effects on many different pathways and target organs.

Since the initial description of TH effects on metabolic rate more than 100 years ago, (4) many theories have been proposed to explain its mechanism of action. They have included uncoupling of oxidative phosphorylation, stimulation of energy expenditure by the activation of Na+-K+ adenosinetriphosphatase (ATPase) activity, and direct modulation of TH transporters and enzymes in the plasma membrane and mitochondria (5). While TH may have some activities at nongenomic sites such as the plasma membrane, cytoplasm, and mitochondrion, it appears that TH exerts its major effects at the genomic level. In 1966, Tata et al. proposed that TH increased gene expression with concomitant increases in protein synthesis and enzyme activity (6). In the early 1970s, the Samuels and Oppenheimer groups identified high-affinity nuclear-binding sites for TH (Kd [dissociation constant] approximately 10^{-10} M for T_3) (7,8). The receptor-binding affinity of various THs and analogues correlated with their biologic potencies, suggesting that most biologic effects were mediated by a nuclear receptor (1).

During the past 15 years, much progress has been made in our understanding of the molecular mechanisms involved in TH regulation of gene transcription due to the cloning of the thyroid hormone receptor (TR) isoforms (9,10), identification of regulatory DNA elements in TH-responsive genes (3,11), and generation of TR isoform knockout mice (12,13). A general schema has emerged for TH effects on gene transcription (Fig. 8.1). Circulating free TH enters the cell, most likely via plasma membrane transporters. Additionally, the more biologically active T_3 may be converted intracellularly from circulating serum T_4 in some tissues by iodothyronine 5'-deiodinases (see later in this chapter). TH then enters the nucleus, where it binds to the nuclear TRs with high affinity and specificity. TR is a ligand-regulated transcription factor that is intimately associated with chromatin and heterodimerizes with another member of the nuclear receptor superfamily, retinoid X re-

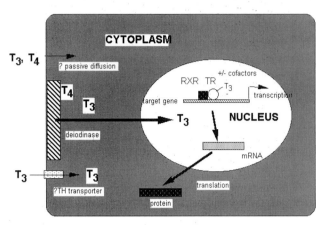

FIGURE 8.1. General model for thyroid hormone action in the nucleus.

ceptors (RXRs). TR/RXR, in turn, is bound to target DNA sequences known as TH-response elements (TREs), generally located in the promoter regions of target genes. The formation of a liganded TR/DNA complex, and subsequent recruitment of transcriptional coactivators, leads to activation of the target gene, with attendant increases in messenger RNA (mRNA) and protein expression. Additionally, TH can negatively regulate some target genes. This chapter will focus on the major aspects of transcriptional regulation by TH, as well as describe some of its nongenomic effects.

THYROID HORMONE METABOLISM AND NUCLEAR BINDING OF THYROID HORMONES

Both T_4 and T_3 are synthesized by the thyroid gland, with T_4 as the major product. In many respects, T_4 can be considered a prohormone for the more potent hormone, T_3. Indeed, most of the intracellular TH bound to nuclear receptors is in the form of T_3. The major pathway for the production of circulating T_3 is via 5′ deiodination of the outer ring of T_4 by deiodinases (14,15). Type I deiodinase is found in peripheral tissues such as liver and kidney, and is responsible for the conversion of the majority of T_4 to T_3 in circulation. Type II deiodinase has high affinity for T_4 (Kd in the nanomolar range) and is found primarily in the pituitary gland, brain, and brown fat, where conversion of T_4 to T_3 modulates the intracellular concentration of T_3. Thus, tissues that contain type II deiodinase can respond differently to a given circulating concentration of T_4 (by intracellular conversion to T_3) than organs that can only respond to T_3. Type III deiodinase, which is found primarily in placenta, brain, and skin, in combination with Type I deiodinase, converts T_4 to reverse triiodothyronine (rT_3), leading to the inactivation of TH. These deiodinases have recently been cloned and shown to be selenoproteins (16).

Additionally, rT_3 and T_3 can be further deiodinated in the liver and are sulfo- and glucuronide conjugated before excreted in the bile (17). Enterohepatic circulation of TH occurs as intestinal flora deconjugate some of these TH metabolites and promote their reuptake.

T_3 binds to its receptors with approximately 10- to 15-fold higher affinity than T_4 (1). The dissociation constants for liver nuclear receptors measured *in vitro* are 2×10^{-9} M for T_4 and 2×10^{-10} M for T_3. Nuclear receptors are approximately 75% saturated with TH in the brain and pituitary, and 50% saturated with TH in the liver and kidney. Of note, TR occupancy varies among different tissues, and thus provides a mechanism for fine adjustment of circulating TH levels to nuclear receptor concentration. In contrast to the related steroid hormone receptors, TRs are mostly nuclear, both in the absence and presence of TH (3,11). In fact, TRs are tightly associated with chromatin (18–20), consistent with their proposed role as DNA-binding proteins that regulate gene expression.

Thyroid Hormone Receptors

In 1986, the Vennstrom and Evans laboratories identified and cloned the TR isoforms, TRα and TRβ (9,10). These ground-breaking studies ushered in the molecular era for our understanding of TRs and TH action. It was quickly noted that the TRs are the cellular homologues (c-erbA) of v-erbA, a viral oncogene product involved in chick erythroblastosis. Furthermore, TRs are members of the nuclear hormone receptor (NR) superfamily that include the steroid, vitamin D, retinoic acid, peroxisomal proliferator, and "orphan" (unknown ligand and/or DNA target) receptors (3,21). TRs act as ligand-regulatable transcription factors that bind both ligand and DNA-enhancer elements or TREs located in the promoters of target genes. TRs have a central DNA-binding domain (DBD) that contains two "zinc-finger" motifs that intercalate with the major and minor grooves of TRE nucleotides sequences, and a carboxy-terminal ligand-binding domain (LBD) (Fig. 8.2). The hinge region between these two domains is a stretch of multiple lysines that are important for nuclear localization of the receptor. (3,22,23). Recent X-ray crystallographic studies of the liganded rat TRα-1 and human TRβ LBDs demonstrate that TH is buried in a hydrophobic "pocket" lined by discontinuous stretches of amino acids with addi-

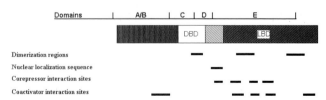

FIGURE 8.2. General organization of major thyroid hormone receptor domains and functional subregions.

tional hydrophobic interfaces likely contributing to RXR heterodimerization (24,25). The LBD is composed of 12 amphipathic helices, with specific helices providing the contact surfaces for protein-protein interactions with coactivators and corepressors (helices 3, 5, 6, 12 and 3, 4, 5, 6, respectively) (26–29). Ligand-binding induces major conformational changes in the TR LBD, particularly in helix 12, which affect TR interaction with coactivators and corepressors, respectively.

There are two gene-encoding TR isoforms (*Thra* and *Thrb*) located on human chromosomes 17 and 3, respectively (3,22,23). These genes generate several major TR isoforms, TRβ-1,α-1,α-2, which bind TH with similar affinity and mediate TH-regulated transcription (Fig. 8.3). The TR α isoforms, which range from 400 to slightly over 500 amino acids in length among mammalian species, contain highly conserved DBDs and LBDs.

The *Thra* gene encodes two different proteins, TRα-1 and c-erbAa-2, which are generated by alternative-splicing of Tra mRNA. In the rat and human, these proteins are identical to amino acid residues 1 through 370; however, their respective sequences diverge markedly thereafter (Fig. 8.3). Consequently, c-erbAα-2 cannot bind T$_3$, as it contains a 122-amino-acid carboxy-terminus that replaces a region in TRα-1 LBD required for TH binding. Additionally, c-erbAa-2 binds TREs weakly but cannot transactivate TH-responsive genes. On certain target genes, c-erbAα-2 may act as a dominant negative inhibitor of TH action, possibly by competing for binding to TREs (30,31). Furthermore, the anatagonist activity of c-erbAα-2 may be modulated by its phosphorylation state (32). The TRα-1 and c-erbAα-2 system, then, represents one of the first examples in mammalian species in which multiple mRNAs generated by alternative splicing encode proteins that may be antagonistic to each other. A second TRα variant, c-erbAα2V, in which the first 39 amino acids of the divergent sequence are missing, has been identified (33); however, its function is currently unknown. Yet another surprising aspect of the TRα gene is the use of the opposite strand to generate another gene product, rev-erbA. The mRNA of rev-erbA contains a 269-nucleotide stretch, which is complementary to the c-erbAα-2 mRNA due to its transcription from the DNA strand opposite of that

used to generate TRα-1 and c-erbAα-2 (34,35). This protein also is a member of the NR superfamily. It is primarily expressed in fat and muscle, can bind to TREs and retinoic acid response elements and can repress transcription of target genes containing these elements (36–38). Nonetheless, rev-erbA should be considered an orphan receptor since its cognate ligand and function are not known. One potential role for rev-erbA may be the regulation of TRα mRNA splicing increased levels of rev-erbA mRNA correspond with increased TRα-1 mRNA (relative to c-erbAα-2) (39–41). It also may help promote adipogenesis (40).

The *Thrb* gene encodes two major TRβ isoforms (42,43). This gene contains two promoter regions, and by their alternate use, one or both of the coding mRNAs are transcribed (44). The resultant TRβ isoforms are designated as TRβ-1 and TRβ-2. The amino acid sequences of the DNA-binding, hinge-region, and ligand-binding domains of these two TR isoforms are identical; however, the amino-terminal regions are divergent (Fig. 8.3). Both TRβ isoforms have high homologue with TRα-1 DBD and LBD. They bind TREs and TH with high affinity and specificity, and mediate TH-dependent transcription. TRβ-2 is expressed selectively in tissues, and its expression may be regulated by factors such as the pituitary-specific transcription factors, Pit-1 (44).

Both TRα-1 and TRβ-1 mRNAs and proteins are expressed in almost all TRα-1 muscle and brown fat, whereas TRβ-1 mRNA has highest expression in brain, liver, and kidney (45,46). The c-erbAα-2 mRNA is most prevalent in testis and brain. In contrast, TRβ-2 mRNA and protein are expressed tissue-selectively in the anterior pituitary gland and hypothalamus, as well as in the developing brain and inner ear (45–50). In the chick and mouse, TRβ-2 mRNA also is expressed in the developing retina (51). Additionally, several short forms of TRα and TRβ generated by alternative-splicing of mRNA or by use of internal transcriptional start sites have been found in embryonic stem cells and fetal bone cells. These short forms may have biological significance in certain tissues, as some of them block wild-type TR transcriptional activity (dominant negative activity) (52,53).

Regulation of the TR isoform mRNAs varies and is cell-type dependent. In the intact rat pituitary, T$_3$ decreases

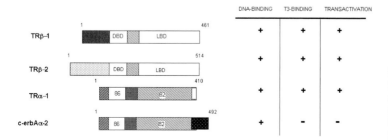

FIGURE 8.3. Comparison of amino acid homologies and their functional properties among thyroid hormone receptor (TR) isoforms' length of receptors is indicated just above receptor diagrams, and percentage of amino acid homology with TRβ-2 is included in the receptor diagrams.

TRβ-2 mRNA, modestly decreases TRα-1 mRNA, and slightly increases rat TRβ-1 mRNA (45). These net changes reduce total T₃ binding by 30% in the T₃-treated rat pituitary. With the exception of TRβ-1 in the brain, where c-erbAα-2 levels are unaffected, T₃ slightly decreases TRα-1 and c-erbAα-2 mRNA in almost all tissues. T₃ has minimal effect on TRβ-1 mRNA expression in nonpituitary tissues. Additionally, TRH from the hypothalmus decreases TRβ-2 mRNA, slightly decreases TRα-1 mRNA, and minimally affects TRβ-1 mRNA in GH3 cells (54). Retinoic acid reduces the negative regulation by T₃ in these cells (55,56). Additionally, in patients with nonthyroidal illness who had decreased circulating free T₃ and T₄ levels, TRα and TRβ mRNAs were increased in peripheral mononuclear cells and liver biopsy specimens (57). It is possible that compensatory TR induction may help maintain a eumetabolic intracellular state in these patients.

The amino acid sequences of TR isoforms are highly conserved among mammalian species (43), which suggests that TR isoforms may have specialized functions (58). The evidence for isoform-specific function at individual target genes has been limited despite distinct phenotypes observed when TR isoforms are knocked out in mice (12,13). Recent studies have suggested that TRβ-1 may exhibit isoform-specific regulation of the TRH and myelin basic protein genes, and TRβ-2 may play an important role in the regulation of the growth hormone and TSHB gene expression in the pituitary (59–63). However, complementary DNA (cDNA) microarray studies, in TR isoform knockout mice, suggest that TRα and TRβ provide compensatory transcriptional regulation of target genes (64). Taken together, these data suggest that total TR, rather than specific TR isoform expression, may be the key determinant for transcription levels of target genes, at least in the liver. Future studies with TR knockout mice, RNA silencing, isoform-specific ligands, and antagonists may help resolve the issue of TR isoform-specificity and potentially identify isoform-specific pathways (12,65–68). It is possible that they provide novel therapies for diseases such as hypercholesterolemia and obesity, while minimizing cardiac side effects, as the heart contains mostly TRα-1 (69).

THYROID HORMONE RESPONSE ELEMENTS

TRs bind to TREs, which are typically located in the upstream promoter regions of target genes. In positively regulated target genes, TREs generally contain two or more hexamer half-site sequence of AGGT(C/A)A arranged in tandem (70). TRs bind to TREs, which have considerable degeneracy in primary nucleotide sequences of half-sites, as well as the number, spacing, and orientation of their half-sites (70,71) (Fig. 8.4). In particular, they can bind to TREs in which half-sites are arranged as direct repeats, inverted palindromes, and palindromes that contain optimal spac-

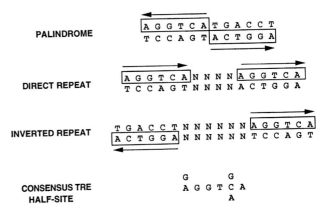

FIGURE 8.4. Conformation of thyroid response elements (TREs). The TREs shown are **(top to bottom)** a palindrome, a direct repeat + 4 nucleotide spacer (N), and an inverted repeat +6N spacer. N is any nucleotide (A, G, C, or T). The conformations shown are idealized with respect to the constancy of the ACCTCA core sequence and the spacing of the half-sites. As discussed in the text, TREs have a great deal of diversity of sequence and conformation. (From Chin WW. Current concepts of thyroid hormone action: progress notes for the clinician. *Thyroid Today* 1992;15:1, with permission.)

ing of four, six, or zero nucleotides between half-sites, respectively. Of the approximately 20 to 30 natural positive TREs that have been characterized thus far, direct repeats occur most frequently, followed by inverted palindrome and infrequently palindromes (3,70) (Table 8.1). TR heterodimerization with RXR facilitates binding to a wide repertoire of nucleotide sequences and motifs (71), as RXR proteins enhance TR binding to DNA and reduce the rate of receptor dissociation from DNA (72). The specificity and affinity for the TR/RXR heterodimer is determined by sequences within the half-site, the length of the spacer region, and the sequence context within the spacer region.

TRs can interact with a wide variety of other nuclear receptors and transcriptional adaptor proteins (see next section); however, the RXR proteins (a, b, g) are its most important heterodimeric partners (71). RXR also heterodimerizes with the retinoic acid and vitamin D receptors, and promotes binding to their respective hormone response elements. TR/RXR binds to direct repeat TREs with half-site spacing of four nucleotides, whereas vitamin D and retinoic acid receptors bind to response elements with half-site spacing of three or five nucleotides, respectively. The proposed 3-4-5 rule for nuclear receptor specificity on hormone response elements underscores the role of spacing between half-sites as a critical determinant of nuclear receptor binding (73,74). RXR binds to the 5′ sequence, and TR binds to the 3′ sequence in direct repeat TREs (75–77). The DBDs interact with the major grooves of the half-sites on the same face of DNA (78). The carboxy-terminal end of the TR DBD forms an α-helical structure that interacts with the spacer region in the DNA minor groove between the TRE half-sites. Although protein-protein contacts between the RXR and TR DBDs

TABLE 8.1. NATURALLY OCCURRING THYROID HORMONE RESPONSE ELEMENTS

Gene	Sequence	Position
Positive TREs		
Rat growth hormone	AAGGTAAGATCAGGGACGTGACCGC	−190 to −166
Rat myelin basic protein	AGACCTCGGCTGAGGACACGGCGG	−186 to −163
Rat α-myosin heavy chain	CTGGAGGTGACAGGAGGACAACAGCCCTGA	−130 to −159
Rat malic enzyme	AGGACGTTGGGGTTAGGGGAGGACAGTG	−287 to −260
Rat *S14*	TRE1: TACTTGGGGCCTGGCAGC	−2700 to −2683
	TRE2: GTCTAGGGGCCTGAGATG	−2797 to −2814
	TRE3: GGTCAAGGGCCTGGCCAG	−2616 to −2633
Pcp-2	AGGCCTTCTCAGGTCAGAGACCAGGAGA	−295 to −268
SERCA2	TRE1: GCGGAGGCAAGCCAAGGACACCAG	−481 to −458
	TRE2: GCCGCGACCGCGTAAGGTCGGGCT	−310 to −287
	TRE3: CGCGCGGCCTCGATCCGGGTTACTGG	−219 to −194
Synthetic TRE palindrome, based on rat growth hormone	TCAGGTCATGACCTGA	
Negative TREs		
Rat TSH β-subunit	AGTGCAAAGTAAGGTAGGTCTCTACCCGGC	+15 to +44
	TGAACAGAGTCTGGGTCATCACAGCATTAAC	−22 to +4
	CGCCAGTGCAAAGTAAG	+11 to +27
Rat α-subunit	TGGGCTTAGGTGCAGGTGGGAGCATGCAATTTGTATT	−74 to −38
Human TSH β-subunit	TTTGGGTCACCACAGCATCTGCTCACCAATGCAAAGTAAGGTAGGT	−3 to +43
	Domain 1 (+1 to +17) GGGTCACCACAGCATCT	
	Domain 2 (+28 to +37) GCAAACTAAG	
Human α-subunit	GCAGGTGAGGACTTCA	−22 to −7
Mouse TSH β-subunit	TGAACGGAGAGTGGGTCATCACAGCA	−22 to +3
Human growth hormone	Multiple putative half sites in this region, whole region confers repression in transfections, regions bind in gel shifts, no accurate localization yet	+2021 to +2175

Concentrations of TR protein were calculated as the product of the fractional distribution of the TR protein determined by immunoprecipitation with specific antiserum and the total nuclear binding capacity.
TRE, thyroid hormone response element; TSH, thyrotropin.
From Schwartz HL, Lazar MA, Oppenheimer JH. Widespread distribution of immunoreactive thyroid hormone β₂ receptor in the nuclei of extrapituitary rat tissues. *J Biol Chem* 1994;269:24777.

contribute to dimerization, their LBDs probably contain the most critical interaction sites (79,80). The dimerization surface of TR appears to involve residues located in helices 10 and 11 (24).

T_3 enhances the formation of TR/RXR heterodimers in solution (81). In *in vitro* studies, unliganded TRs can bind as homodimers and heterodimers to TREs, whereas liganded TRs bind primarily as heterodimers (3). Thus, it is likely that TR/RXR heterodimers play the major role in T_3-mediated transcription. The RXRs bind a stereoisomer of all *trans*retinoic acid, 9-*cis* retinoic acid (82,83). In combination with T_3, 9-cis RA can enhance transcriptional activity of some target genes (3,84).

TRANSCRIPTIONAL REGULATION BY THYROID HORMONE RECEPTORS

A number of TH-responsive target genes have been characterized over the years and are shown in Table 8.1. Recently, cDNA microarrays were used to study TH regulation of hepatic genes in mice and have led to the identification of a large number of novel target genes (both positively and

negatively regulated) (85,86). These studies showed that TH affected gene expression in a wide range of cellular pathways and functions, including gluconeogenesis, lipogenesis, insulin signaling, adenylate cyclase signaling, cell proliferation, and apoptosis. Although many of the TH-responsive genes were regulated directly by TRs, others were probably regulated indirectly through intermediary genes. Indirect gene regulation by TH can occur whenever the time course for transcriptional induction is slow (hours) and whenever protein synthesis inhibitors block TH induction. Although TH acts mainly at the level of transcription, it also can affect mRNA stability and translational efficiency (87,88). Thus, TH regulation of protein expression needs to be considered at multiple levels.

THYROID HORMONE RECEPTOR–INTERACTING COREPRESSORS/BASAL REPRESSION

Unliganded TRs not only bind to TREs but repress (or silence) basal transcription of positively regulated target genes in cotransfection studies. This feature of TRs stands in contradistinction to steroid hormone receptors, which are transcriptionally inactive in the absence of ligand (22, 89). These initial observations on repression of basal transcription by TRs were puzzling at first, as it was not known whether they represented a genuine feature of TRs or were due to overexpression of TRs and titration of critical cofactors (squelching) in the cotransfection studies. However, our understanding of the mechanism for basal repression by unliganded TRs was greatly aided by the cloning and characterization of two major corepressors called nuclear receptor corepressor (NCoR) and silencing mediator for retinoic acid receptor (RAR) and TR (SMRT) (90–92). These 270 kD proteins preferentially interact with unliganded TR and RAR and repress basal transcription of target genes in the absence of their cognate ligands (Figs. 8.5, 8.6). Upon ligand addition, they dissociate from NRs.

These corepressors have three transferable repression domains and two carboxy-terminal α-helical interaction domains. These latter interaction domains contain consensus LXXI/HIXXXI/L sequences, which resemble the LXXLL sequences that enable coactivators to interact with NRs (93). Of note, these sequences allow both corepressors and coactivators to interact with similar amino acid residues on helices 3,5, and 6 of the TR ligand-binding domain. Differences in the length and specific sequences of the corepressor and coactivator interaction sites, combined with ligand-induced conformational changes in the conserved AF-2 region of helix 12, help determine whether corepressor or coactivator binds to TR (93). Additionally, corepressors can bind to RXR as helix 12 of RXR masks a corepressor binding site in RXR, which becomes available after heterodimerization with TR (94).

Recently, it has been shown that corepressors can form a larger complex with other repressors, such as Sin 3 and histone deacetylases (HDACs), that are mammalian homologues of well-characterized yeast transcriptional repressors RPD1 and RPD3 (3,22,93). Thus, histone deacetylation

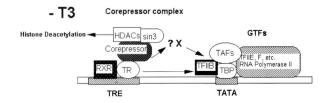

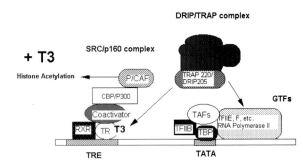

FIGURE 8.6. Molecular model for basal repression in the absence of L-triiodothyronine (T₃) and transcriptional activation in the presence of T₃. *X* refers to possible additional cofactors that remain to be identified. See text for details. CBP, cyclic adenosine monophosphate response element–binding protein; DRIP, vitamin D receptor–interacting protein; GTFs, general transcription factors; HDAC, histone deacetylase; P/CAF, p300/CBP-associated factor; RXR, retinoid X receptor; SRC, steroid receptor coactivator; TAF, TATA-binding protein-associated factor; TBP, TATA-binding protein; TF, transcription factor; TR, thyroid hormone receptor; TRAP, TR-associated protein; TRE, thyroid hormone response element.

of chromatin near the TREs of target genes may help maintain chromatin structure in a state that shuts down basal transcription. Studies examining TRβA promoter in a Xenopus oocyte system show that simultaneous chromatin assembly and TR/RXR binding are required for basal repression of transcription (95). Addition of T₃ relieves this repression and also causes chromatin remodeling. Thus, it is likely that histone deacetylation and acetylation upon ligand addition modulates the chromatin stucture and nucleosome positioning that is critical for target gene transcription. Additionally, DNA methylation may play a role in basal repression as methyl-CpG-binding proteins can associate with a corepressor complex containing Sin 3 and histone deacetylase (96). Finally, unliganded TR can interact directly with the basal transcription factor, TFIIB (97,98), which may promote silencing in some circumstances.

The fact that the TR alters the level of gene transcription in the absence and presence of T₃ has important implications for TH physiology. At low hormone concentrations, such as in hypothyroidism, the unliganded receptor is predicted to repress expression rather than function as an inactive receptor. In some respects, this model is borne out by targeted deletion of the TRα and TRβ genes. The phenotypes of these

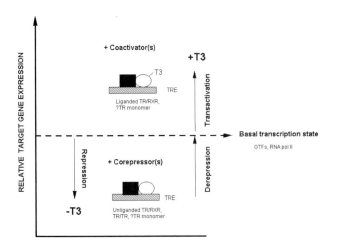

FIGURE 8.5. Model for repression, derepression, and transcriptional activation by thyroid hormone receptor.

knockout mice are, for the most part, milder than the clinical features observed in congenital hypothyroidism (12,13). Deletion of the receptor may eliminate its ability to function as a repressor in the absence of hormone and allow a milder phenotype due to basal levels of transcription.

THYROID HORMONE RECEPTOR–INTERACTING COACTIVATORS/TRANSCRIPTIONAL ACTIVATION

A growing number of cofactors have been shown to interact with liganded NRs and enhance transcriptional activation (3,21). At present, the precise roles of all these putative coactivators and their respective contribution to ligand-regulated transcription are not known. However, it appears there are at least two major coactivator complexes involved in ligand-dependent transcriptional activation of NRs in mammals: the steroid receptor coactivator (SRC) complex and the vitamin D receptor–interacting protein/ TR-associated protein (DRIP/TRAP) complex (Fig. 8.6). O'Malley and coworkers used the yeast two-hybrid system to identify the first member of SRC family, SRC-1 (99). This 160 kD protein interacts directly with NRs, including TRs, and enhances their ligand-dependent transcription. Subsequent work has shown there are at least two other related members of the SRC family, SRC-2 and SRC-3, that also can enhance transcription by liganded NRs (21). The SRCs contain multiple NR interaction sites that contain a signature LXXLL sequence motif, in which X represents any amino acid. This sequence has been shown to be important for coactivator binding to coactivator interaction sequences in the TR LBD (helices 3, 5, 6, and 12) (100, 101). SRCs also interact with the CREB-binding protein (CBP) (the coactivator for cyclic adenosinemonophosphate-stimulated transcription) as well as the related protein, p300 (which interacts with the viral coactivator E1A) (21). CBP/p300 can serve as coactivators for CREB, p53, AP-1, and NF-κ B, and thus may function as integrator molecules for multiple cell-signaling pathways (102).

CBP/p300 can also interact with PCAF (p300/CBP-associated factor), the mammalian homologue of a yeast transcriptional activator, general control nonrepressed protein 5, GCN5 (21,102). Like GCN5, PCAF has histone acetyltransferase activity (HAT), which, in the case of PCAF, is directed primarily toward H3 and H4 histones. PCAF itself is part of a preformed complex that contains TBP associated factors (TAFs), which can interact with SRC-1 and SRC-3. CBP also is part of a stable complex with RNA polymerase II (RNA pol II) (103). Thus, PCAF and CBP possess dual roles as adaptors of nuclear receptors to the basal transcriptional machinery and as enzymes that can alter chromatin structure (HAT activity).

The DRIP/TRAP complex contains approximately 15 subunits, ranging from 70 to 230 kD, which directly or indirectly interact with liganded VDRs and TRs (104,105). A critical subunit in this coactivator complex is DRIP205/TRAP220, which contains a LXXLL motif similar to those found in SRCs, and appears to anchor the rest of the subunit proteins to the NR. It is noteworthy that none of the DRIP/TRAP subunits are members of the SRC family or their associated proteins. Additionally, the DRIP/TRAP complex does not appear to have intrinisic HAT activity. Several DRIP/TRAP components, however, are mammalian homologues of the yeast Mediator complex, which associates with RNA Pol II (104, 105). This suggests that TR recruitment of the DRIP/ TRAP complex may help recruit or stabilize RNA Pol II holoenzyme. Recently, another coactivator, TR-binding protein (TRBP), interacts with TR via a LXXLL motif (106). It also can interact with both CBP/p300 and DRIP130, as well as with a DNA-dependent protein kinase (107). The precise interplay between TRBP and the other major coactivator complexes is currently not known.

Recent chromatin immunoprecipitation assays of proteins bound to hormone response elements (HREs) suggest that there may be a sequential, perhaps cyclical, recruitment of different coactivator complexes to HREs (108–110). Recently, it has been shown that glucocorticoid and progesterone receptors (GRs and PRs) preferentially recruit different SRC coactivators on the MMTV promoter (111). Thus, it is likely that both temporal recruitment pattern and the particular coactivator recruitment may play key roles in determining the specificity and strength of hormonal response on a given target gene.

In the current model of TR action (Fig. 8.6), p160/SRC complex may initiate transcriptional activity by recruiting cofactors with HAT activity to ligand-bound NRs followed by DRIP/TRAP complex, which can then recruit RNA pol II holoenzyme to promote transcription of target genes. CBP can acetylate ACTR (SRC-3) and promote its dissociation from NRs; thus, acetylation of components of the p160/SRC complex may facilitate the exchange of complexes (112). Recently, it also has been shown that mammalian homologues of Sw-1/Snf, BRG-1 and BRM-1, can associate with NRs *in vitro* and activate transcription (113). It is possible that these chromatin remodeling proteins with ATPase activity also may be involved in transcriptional activation, particularly in the early stages.

NEGATIVE REGULATION BY THYROID HORMONE RECEPTORS

In contrast to positively regulated target genes, negatively regulated genes can be stimulated in the absence of TH and repressed in response to the ligand. Regulation of TRH and the TSHβ and glycoprotein hormone α-subunit genes have been studied most extensively as models of negatively regulated genes. From a physiological perspective, negative regulation of these genes represents a critical aspect of feedback control of hypothalamic/pituitary/thyroid axis. The T_3-responsive regions of these negatively regulated genes have been localized to the proximal promoter regions (70,114–116). However, TR binding to putative TREs in these promoters is relatively weak in comparison to the binding sites in positively regulated genes.

The mechanism(s) for negative transcriptional regulation by TH is not well understood, and several different mechanisms may be operative. First, negative regulation may involve receptor interference with the actions of other transcription factors or components of the basal transcriptional machinery (117). For instance, TR can inhibit the activity of AP-1, a heterodimeric transcription factor composed of Jun and Fos (118). T_3-mediated repression of the prolactin promoter has been proposed to occur by preventing AP-1 binding (119). The TR also interacts with other classes of transcription factors, including NF-1, Oct-1, Sp-1, p53, Pit-1, and CTCF (120–124). Thus, it is possible that TR binding to such enhancers leads to a reduction in target gene transcription. Second, negative regulation may occur by TR directly binding to DNA sequences of the target gene. A negative TRE (nTRE) of the TSHβ gene resides in an exon downstream of the start site of transcription (114), raising the possibility that it occludes the formation of a transcription complex. Lastly, liganded TRs may potentially recruit positive cofactors off DNA (squelching), which, in turn, could lead to decreased transcription of target genes.

Corepressors and coactivators also may be involved in the control of negatively regulated target genes. In contrast to the basal repression of unliganded TR in the case of positively regulated genes, corepressors cause basal activation of the TSH and TRH genes (62,114,115). Coactivators also play an apparently paradoxical role in T_3-dependent repression of negatively regulated genes (125). On the other hand, it appears that HDACs are recruited by TRs during ligand-dependent negative regulation in some instances (126). Cofactor-associated changes in histone acetylation and alterations in chromatin structure may therefore be involved in negative regulation by TR. It is interesting to note that not all negatively regulated target genes are activated in the absence of ligand, suggesting that cofactor may be differentially recruited on promoters of target genes (64). Last, there may be TR isoform specificity in the negative regulation of some target genes, particularly TRβ-2 action on TSH subunits and TRβ-1 on TRH (61,127,128).

RESISTANCE TO THYROID HORMONE

In the syndrome of resistance to thyroid hormone (RTH), affected individuals are usually clinically euthyroid and have thyroid function tests that show elevated circulating free TH levels with concomitant, inappropriately "normal" or elevated TSH levels. RTH is an autosomal dominant disorder in almost all inherited cases (129,130). Patients with RTH typically have mutations in one of three different regions of the TRβ LBD (referred to as "hot spots"). These mutations often reduce the TH-binding affinity of the mutant TR (67,129). Additionally, the mutant TR exerts dominant negative activity on wild-type TRs by blocking TH-regulated transcription of target genes. Dimerization and DNA-binding of the mutant TR are required for dominant negative activity, as formation of inactive heterodimers or homodimers on TREs are necessary to actively compete for DNA-binding with wild-type TRs (131). Recently, several studies have shown that TRβs containing mutations in the AF-2 region of the LBD have dominant negative activity (132–134). These mutants typically have normal T_3-binding affinity but are unable to interact with coactivators. Thus, mutant TRs that cannot interact with coactivators can also cause RTH. Additionally, mutant TRs that have defective release from corepressors in the presence of TH have strong dominant negative activity (135–137). In most cases, decreased T_3-binding affinity correlates with decreased corepressor release. Taken together, these findings suggest that transcriptionally inactive TRs, which have either reduced corepressor release or coactivator interaction, are able to mediate dominant negative activity.

Several patients with clinical features of RTH and who do not have TRβ or TRβ mutations have recently been described (138). It is possible that mutations in cofactors or their inappropriate expression may have caused the RTH phenotype observed in these patients. In this connection, Weiss et al have shown that loss of a coactivator, SRC-1, can lead to mild RTH in mice (139).

There also have been several somatic TR mutations described in human tumors. Somatic mutations in TRα and TRβ have been found in hepatic, renal cell, and thyroid carcinomas (140,141). It is not known whether these mutant TRs directly contribute to oncogenesis or are a secondary phenomenon. Recently, a somatic TRβ mutation and an aberrantly spliced TRβ-2 mRNA have been identified in TSH-secreting adenomas (142,143). These resultant aberrant TRs have dominant negative activity and likely cause dysregulation of TSHb and glycoprotein hormone, a subunit expression in these tumors.

THYROID HORMONE RECEPTOR ISOFORM KNOCKOUT AND KNOCKIN MICE

Several mouse models of RTH have been developed in which transgenic mice express dominant-negative mutant TRs ubiquitously or in selective tissues. Recently, targeted gene inactivation [knockout (KO)] of TR isoforms and targeted gene expression of mutant TRs in the appropriate TRα or TRβ gene loci [knockins (KIs)] have provided insight on TH effects on development, metabolism, and physiology, as well as on RTH (12,144–147).

Transgenic mice with ubiquitous expression of v-erbA and a natural frameshift TRβ-1 mutation have been generated (148,149). The mice that expressed v-erbA had multiple abnormalities including hypothyroidism (due to follicular disorganization in the thyroid), inappropriate TSH response, enlarged seminal vesicles, hepatomas, decreased fertility, and reduced adipose tissue. Since v-erbA has dominant negative activity on retinoic acid–mediated transcription, it is possible that some of these effects may be due to blockade of RAR-, in addition to T_3-, mediated transcription. The transgenic mice that expressed the mutant TRβ-1 had elevated T_3, inappropriately normal TSH, behavioral abnormalities, decreased fertility, and decreased weight. These findings resembled some of the clinical features of RTH patients with this mutation. Mutant TRβs have also been selectively targeted to tissues such as pituitary, heart, and liver, and have exhibited RTH in these tissues while maintaining TH sensitivity in other tissues (12).

Several different TRα KO mice with different phenotypes have been generated (150,151). The TRα gene structure is complex, as it encodes TRα-1, c-erbAα-2 (which cannot bind T_3), and rev-erbA (generated from the opposite strand encoding TRα); thus, the site of homologous recombination determines which isoforms will be knocked out (34). Transgenic mice that lack both TRα-1 and c-erbAα-2 (TRα$^{-/-}$) have a more severe phenotype with hypothyroidism, intestinal malformation, growth retardation, and early death shortly after weaning (150). Transgenic mice that lack only TRα-1 (TRα-1$^{-/-}$) have a milder phenotype with decreased body temperature and heart rate, and prolonged QT interval on EKG (151). These findings suggest a major role for TRα-1 in regulating cardiac function. Although the differences between the two phenotypes could be due to specific functions of c-erbAa-2 , this is unlikely, as the specific KO of c-erbAa-2 did not affect survival of the pups (12). Short TRα isoforms generated from internal transcriptional start sites, which can block TR transcriptional activity, have been described (52); thus, it is likely that these short TR isoforms may be responsible for the more severe phenotype of the TRα$^{-/-}$ KO mice. Indeed, a TRα KO that lacks all TRα isoforms, including the short TR isoforms (TRα%), has a milder phenotype than TRα$^{-/-}$ (152). Interestingly, TH stimulation of some target genes was increased in these mice, perhaps due to the absence of c-erbA α-2, which inhibits normal TH-mediated transcription.

TRβ KO mice that lack both TRβ-1 and TRβ-2 (TRβ$^{-/-}$) have been generated. These mice have elevated serum TSH and T_4 levels, thyroid hyperplasia, and hearing defects (153,154), and thus resemble the index cases of RTH who also had deletions of TRβ (155). TSH elevation occurs in hypothyroid TRβ$^{-/-}$ mice, but suppression of TSH by TH is impaired (156). Additionally, these findings implicate TRβ in the development of the auditory system (154). Recently, TRβ-2 has been selectively knocked out (127). These mice had elevated levels of TH and TSH, implicating TRβ-2 as an important regulator of TSH. Interestingly, these mice did not have any hearing defects, suggesting that TRβ-2 may not be absolutely required for auditory development, or that its function may be compensated by other TR isoforms, particularly TRβ-1.

The relatively mild phenotypes of both the TRα and TRβ KO mice suggests the two isoforms may have redundant transcriptional activity and compensate for each other in most target genes. Indeed, microarray studies of hepatic gene expression in the TR isoform KO mice show a similar pattern (64). Additionally, overexpression of TRα was able to rescue the hearing deficits in TRβ KO mice (157). Taken together, these findings suggest that TR expression levels, rather than isoform-specific function or tissue-specific expression may be the key determinant of TH action in a given tissue. Double TRα-1 $^{-/-}$/TRβ$^{-/-}$ and TRα%/TRβ$^{-/-}$ KOs have been generated and surprisingly, are viable (158,159). They have markedly elevated T_4, T_3, and TSH levels and large goiters. They also have growth retardation and decreased fertility, as well as impaired bone development and reduced bone mineral content. Of note, the double KO mice have a milder phenotype than congenitally hypothyroid mice. Thus, the absence of TRs does not give the same phenotype as absence of hormone, as basal repression of target genes may be occurring in the latter condition (64). In this connection, recent microarray studies comparing the gene expression profiles of these mice show that different sets of target genes are regulated by these mice.

Two groups recently have generated KI mouse models in which mutant TRs are introduced into the endogenous TRβ gene locus (144,145). When a frameshift mutant TRβ PV was introduced, the heterozygous mice had elevated serum T_4 and TSH, mild goiter, hypercholesterolemia, impaired weight gain, abnormal bone development, and resembled patients with RTH (144). Homozygous mice had markedly elevated serum T_4 and TSH and a much more severe phenotype. Interestingly, homozygous mice had an increased incidence of thyroid cancer, suggesting that dominant negative activity by mutant TR may contribute to oncogenesis in this tissue (160). When a dominant negative TRβ mutant was introduced into the TRβ gene locus, abnormalities in cerebellar development and function in mutant TRβ-1 KO mice were observed that were not present in TRβ KO mice. These findings implicate corepressors in mediating the deleterious effects by unliganded TR in the hypothyroid brain (145). Recently, three groups have generated KO mice expressing different mutant TRαs (corresponding to natural TRβ mutations) in the endogenous TRβ gene locus (146,147,161). These mice had decreased growth and decreased TH levels. The difference between the observed phenotypes of TRα and TRβ mutant KOs raises the possibility of isoform-specific effects on basal repression and dominant negative activity. Interestingly, one knockin TRα-1 mouse had increased visceral adiposity, insulin resistance, and decreased catecholamine-induced lipolysis (161). The reasons for these differences among the TRα KO mice remain to be elucidated. Recently, a KO mouse expressing a mutant TRβ that cannot bind DNA was generated. This model should be useful in distinguishing signaling and developmental patterns due to protein-protein interactions of TRs (e.g., AP-1) from those that require TR binding to TREs of target genes (162,163).

NONGENOMIC EFFECTS OF THYROID HORMONE

The major effects of T_3 are mediated by nuclear TR regulation of target gene transcription. However, nongenomic effects by T_3 and T_4 also have been documented, although the precise mechanisms for these effects are not well understood (5). Evidence suggesting these nongenomic effects include the lack of dependence on nuclear TRs; structure–function relationships of TH analogues that are different than their affinities for TRs; rapid onset of action (typically seconds to minutes); occurrence in the face of transcriptional blockade; and utilization of membrane-signaling pathways, typically involving kinases or calmodulin, that have not been implicated directly in nuclear TR function.

Transport of T_3 across plasma and nuclear membranes has been studied extensively. T_3 is lipophilic and generally thought to diffuse passively across the plasma and nuclear membranes. However, there is evidence for facilitated transport across plasma membranes and high-affinity TH-binding sites in the plasma membranes of different cells (164–168). In one study of human erythrocytes, T_3 is concentrated 55-fold inside cells. Furthermore, a 58-fold higher concentration of L-T_3 and a fourfold higher concentration of D-T_3 in the nucleus than in the cytoplasm, using isotope dilution methods, suggest there may be a stereospecific transporter of T_3 into the nucleus, although it is possible that differences in TR concentration also contribute to this difference (165,169). Several proteins have been suggested as putative TH transporters. One potential transporter may be the multidrug resistance P glycoprotein, which can modulate TH concentration when overexpressed in cells (168). Other transporters, such as the organic anion, monocarboxylate, and System L transporters, have been shown to import TH into hepatocytes (170–174). Of note, patients with mutations in the monocarboxylate transporter 8 have severely impaired neurological development as well as RTH (175,176).

Other potential targets of T_3 in the plasma membrane are calcium ATPase, adenylate cyclase, and glucose transporters (164–167,177–180). In the last case, T_3 enhances uptake of sugars in a variety of tissues via a mechanism that does not require new protein synthesis, suggesting a direct effect on the plasma membrane transport system (177,178, 181). Additionally, T_3 binds to an endoplasmic reticulum

associated protein, prolyl hydroxylase, and to a subunit of pyruvate kinase when the enzyme is monomeric but not tetrameric (182–184). It is not known whether T_3 modulates the activities of these enzymes or whether these enzymes may be involved in other functions related to T_3 action such as transport or storage. In this connection, T_4 inhibits deiodinase type II activity by an allosteric mechanism and may promote targeting of a substrate-binding subunit to endosomes (185). Additionally, deiodinase type II can be proteosomally degraded in the presence of T_4 and rT_3 (186).

Nongenomic effects by TH on cell structure proteins have also been observed. Actin depolymerization blocks type II deiodinase inactivation by T_4 in cAMP-stimulated glial cells, suggesting that an intact actin-cytoskeleton is required for down-regulation of deiodinase activity (185, 187). Surprisingly, T_4, but not T_3, promotes actin polymerization in astrocytes (188) and may influence the down-regulation of type II deiodinase activity by a secondary mechanism such as targeting to lysosomes (185,187). Additionally, regulation of actin polymerization may contribute to TH effects of TH on neuronal arborization, axonal transport, and cell-cell contacts during central nervous system development. In this connection, it has been shown that T_4 is required for integrin clustering and attachment to laminin by integrin in astrocytes (189).

TH may have direct effects on mitochondria and may account for some of the known T_3 effects on mitochondrial activity and cellular energy state. Sterling and colleagues have suggested the site of TH action in mitochondria is the adenine nucleotide translocase of the inner mitochondrial membrane (190,191). However, this work has been difficult to confirm, as there are conflicting reports on the site of TH action in mitochondria (5,192,193). Of note, a 43 kD protein related to TRα-1 LBD has been described in mitochondria that also could bind to TREs and mitochondrial DNA sequences (194,195). Transfection of TRα-1 in CV-1 cells resulted in mitochondrial localization and stimulation of mitochondrial activity. These results raise the intriguing possibility that there may be specific mitochondrial receptors for T_3 that may also serve as transcription factors in mitochondria.

TH can modulate kinase activities in the cell; thus, there can be cross-talk among plasma membrane receptors, intracellular signaling pathways, and even TRs. Lin and co-workers have observed that the antiviral effects of interferon α can be potentiated by T_4 and T_3 (196). These effects were rapid and did not require protein synthesis, as they were not blocked by cycloheximide treatment, and required PKC and PKA activation. The authors also recently showed that T_4 can activate mitogen-activated protein kinase, phosphorylate p53, and TRβ-1 (197,198). In the latter case, it is possible that phosphorylation of TRβ-1 may help promote corepressor release from the unliganded receptor TRβ-1.

The foregoing data suggest that THs may have rapid nongenomic activities. However, the precise molecular mechanisms, including putative membrane and intracellular receptors, remain to be elucidated. Moreover, it is not known whether any of these effects may be mediated by the classical TRs since there is evidence for nuclear-cytoplasmic shuttling of TRs and other NRs (169,199,200). Recently, a novel metabolite of TH has been described, which does not bind to nuclear TRs but is an agonist for an orphan G protein–coupled receptor (201). Rodents injected with this metabolite had decreased temperature and cardiac output, suggesting this metabolite may oppose actions of TH. Discovery of natural and synthetic TH analogues that can distinguish between nongenomic and nuclear TR-mediated pathways will prove useful in determining nongenomic functions of THs.

SUMMARY

Much has been learned about the molecular mechanisms of nuclear TH action in recent years. With the availability of new techniques, such as microarray and proteomic studies, structural biology approaches, chromatin immunoprecipitation assays, *in vitro* transcriptional systems, and genetically altered animal models, much new information is anticipated for the future. It is hoped that such information will not only provide a better understanding of the molecular pathophysiology of diseases caused by abnormal levels of circulating TH, but could lead to the development of specific agonists, antagonists, and transcriptional modifiers that could potentially serve as valuable therapeutic agents.

REFERENCES

1. Oppenheimer JH, Schwartz HL, Mariash CN, et al. Advances in our understanding of thyroid hormone action at the cellular level. *Endocr Rev* 1987;8:288–308.
2. Brent GA. The molecular basis of thyroid hormone action. *N Engl J Med* 1994;331:847–853.
3. Yen PM. Physiological and molecular basis of thyroid hormone action. *Physiol Rev* 2001;81:1097–1142.
4. Magnus-Levey A. Ueber den respiratorischen gasweschsel unter dem einfluss der thyroidea sowie unter vershiedenen pathologische zustand. *Ber Klin Wschr* 1895;32:650.
5. Davis PJ, Davis FB. Nongenomic actions of thyroid hormone. *Thyroid* 1996;6:497–504.
6. Tata JR, Widnell CC. Ribonucleic acid synthesis during the early action of thyroid hormones. *Biochemical Journal* 1966;98:604–629.
7. Oppenheimer JH, Koerner D, Schwartz HL, et al. Specific nuclear triiodothyronine binding sites in rat liver and kidney. *J Clin Endocrinol Metab* 1972;35:330–333.
8. Samuels HH, Tsai JS. Thyroid hormone action in cell culture: demonstration of nuclear receptors in intact cells and isolated nuclei. *Proc Natl Acad Sci USA* 1973;70:3488–3492.
9. Sap J, Munoz A, Damm K. The c-erbA protein is a high affinity receptor for thyroid hormone. *Nature* 1986;324:635–640.
10. Weinberger C, Thompson CC, Ong ES, et al. The c-erbA gene encodes a thyroid hormone receptor. *Nature* 1986;324:641–646.
11. Harvey CB, Williams GR. Mechanism of thyroid hormone action. *Thyroid* 2002;12:441–446.
12. Forrest, D, Vennstrom B. Functions of thyroid hormone receptors in mice. *Thyroid* 2000;10:41–52.
13. Flamant, F, Samarut J. Thyroid hormone receptor: lessons from knockout and knock-in mice. *Trends in Endocrinology and Metabolism* 2003;14:85–90.
14. Braverman LE, Ingbar SH, Sterling K. Conversion of thyroxine (T_4) to triiodothyronine (T_3) in athyreotic human subjects. *J Clin Invest* 1970;49:855–864.
15. Kohrle, J. The selenoenzyme family of deiodinase isozymes controls local thyroid hormone availability. *Reviews in Endocrine and Metabolic Disorders* 2000;1:49–58.
16. Larsen, PR, Berry MJ. Nutritional and hormonal regulation of thyroid hormone deiodinases. *Annu Rev Nutr* 1995;15:323–352.
17. Engler D, Burger AG. The deiodination of the iodothyronines and of their derivatives in man. *Endocr Rev* 1984;5:151–184.
18. Perlman AJ, Stanley F, Samuels HH. Thyroid hormone nuclear receptor. Evidence for multimeric organization in chromatin. *J Biol Chem* 1982;257:930–938.
19. Jump DB, Seelig S, Schwartz HL, et al. Association of the thyroid hormone receptor with rat liver chromatin. *Biochemistry* 1981;20:6781–6789.
20. MacLeod KM, Baxter JD. Chromatin receptors for thyroid hormones. Interactions of the solubilized proteins with DNA. *J Biol Chem* 1976;251:7380–7387.
21. McKenna NJ, Lanz RB, O'Malley BW. Nuclear receptor coregulators: cellular and molecular biology. *Endocr Rev* 1999;20:321–344.
22. Zhang J, Lazar MA. The mechanism of action of thyroid hormones. *Annu Rev Physiol* 2000;62:439–466.
23. Cheng SY. Multiple mechanisms for regulation of the transcriptional activity of tyroid hormone receptors. *Reviews in Endocrine and Metabolic Disorders* 2000;1/2:9–18.
24. Wagner RL, Apriletti JW, McGrath ME, et al. A structural role for hormone in the thyroid hormone receptor. *Nature* 1995;378: 690–697.
25. Ribeiro RC, Feng W, Wagner RL, et al. Definition of the surface in the thyroid hormone receptor ligand binding domain for association as homodimers and heterodimers with retinoid × receptor. *J Biol Chem* 2001;276:14987–14995.
26. Perissi V, Staszewski LM, McInerney EM, et al. Molecular determinants of nuclear receptor-corepressor interaction. *Genes Dev* 1999;13:3198–3208.
27. Nagy L, Kao HY, Love JD, et al. Mechanism of corepressor binding and release from nuclear hormone receptors. *Genes Dev* 1999;13:3209–3216.
28. Feng W, Ribeiro RC, Wagner RL, et al. Hormone-dependent coactivator binding to a hydrophobic cleft on nuclear receptors. *Science* 1998;280:1747–1749.
29. Hu X, Lazar MA. The CoRNR motif controls the recruitment of corepressors by nuclear hormone receptors. *Nature* 1999; 402: 93–96.
30. Koenig RJ, Lazar MA, Hodin RA, et al. Inhibition of thyroid hormone action by a non-hormone binding c-erbA protein generated by alternative mRNA splicing. *Nature* 1989;337:659–661.
31. Lazar MA, Hodin RA, Chin WW. Human carboxyl-terminal variant of a-type c-erbA inhibits trans-activation by thyroid hormone receptors without binding thyroid hormone. *Proc Natl Acad Sci USA* 1989;86:7771–7774.

32. Katz D, Reginato MJ, Lazar MA. Functional regulation of thyroid hormone receptor variant TR alpha 2 by phosphorylation. *Mol Cell Biol* 1995;15:2341–2348.

33. Mitsuhashi TG, Tennyson GE, Nikodem VM. Alternative splicing generates messages encoding rat c-erbA proteins that do not bind thyroid hormone. *Proc Natl Acad Sci USA* 1988;85: 5804–5808.

34. Lazar MA, Hodin RA, Darling DS, et al. A novel member of the thyroid/steroid hormone receptor family is encoded by the opposite strand of the rat c-erbAa transcriptional unit. *Mol Cell Biol* 1989;9:1128–1136.

35. Miyajima N, Horiuchi R, Shibuya Y, et al. Two erbA homologs encoding proteins with different T_3 binding capacities are transcribed from opposite DNA strands of the same genetic locus. *Cell* 1989;57:31–39.

36. Spanjaard RA, Nguyen VP, Chin WW. Rat Rev-erbA alpha, an orphan receptor related to thyroid hormone receptor, binds to specific thyroid hormone response elements. *Mol Endocrinol* 1994;8:286–295.

37. Harding HP, Lazar MA. The monomer-binding orphan receptor Rev-Erb represses transcription as a dimer on a novel direct repeat. *Mol Cell Biol* 1995;15:4791–4802.

38. Zamir I, Harding HP, Adkins GB, et al. A nuclear hormone receptor corepressor mediates transcriptional silencing by receptors with distinct repression domains. *Mol Cell Biol* 1996;16: 5458–5465.

39. Lazar MA, Hodin RA, Cardona GR, et al. Gene expression from the c-erbAa/Rev-erbAa genomic locus: potential regulation of alternative splicing by complementary transcripts from opposite DNA strands. *J Biol Chem* 1990;265:12859–12863.

40. Chawla A, Lazar MA. Induction of Rev-ErbA alpha, an orphan receptor encoded on the opposite strand of the alpha-thyroid hormone receptor gene, during adipocyte differentiation. *J Biol Chem* 1993;268:16265–16269.

41. Jeannin E, Robyr D, Desvergne B. Transcriptional regulatory patterns of the myelin basic protein and malic enzyme genes by the thyroid hormone receptors alpha1 and beta1. *J Biol Chem* 1998;273:24239–24248.

42. Hodin RA, Lazar MA, Wintman BI, et al. Identification of a novel thyroid hormone receptor that is pituitary-specific. *Science* 1989;244:76–79.

43. Lazar MA. Thyroid hormone receptors: multiple forms, multiple possibilities. *Endocr Rev* 1993;14:348–399.

44. Wood WM, Dowding JM, Bright TM, et al. Thyroid hormone receptor beta2 promoter activity in pituitary cells is regulated by Pit-1. *J Biol Chem* 1996;271:24213–24220.

45. Hodin RA, Lazar MA, Chin WW. Differential and tissue-specific regulation of the multiple rat c-erbA mRNA species by thyroid hormone. *J Clin Invest* 1990;85:101–105.

46. Strait KA, Schwartz HL, Perez-Castillo A, Oppenheimer J.H. Relationship of c-erbA mRNA content to tissue triiodothyronine nuclear binding capacity and function in developing and adult rats. *J Biol Chem* 1990;265:10514–10521.

47. Yen PM, Sunday ME, Darling DS, et al. Isoform-specific thyroid hormone receptor antibodies detect multiple thyroid hormone receptors in rat and human pituitaries. *Endocrinology* 1992;130:1539–1546.

48. Bradley DJ, Towle HC, Young WS. Alpha and beta thyroid hormone receptor (TR) gene expression during auditory neurogenesis: evidence for TR isoform-specific transcriptional regulation *in vivo*. *Proc Natl Acad Sci USA* 1994;91:439–443.

49. Bradley DJ, Towle HC, Young WS. Spatial and temporal expression of a- and b-thyroid hormone receptor mRNAs, including the b2–subtype, in the developing mammalian system. *J Neurosci* 1992;12:2288–2302.

50. Cook CB, Kakucska I, Lechan RM, et al. Expression of thyroid hormone receptor b2 in rat hypothalamus. *Endocrinology* 1992;130:1077–1079.

51. Sjoberg M, Vennstrom B, Forrrest D. Thyroid hormone receptors in chick retinal development: differential expression of mRNAs for alpha and N-terminal variant beta receptors. *Development* 1992;114:39–47.

52. Chassande O, Fraichard A, Gauthier K, et al. Identification of transcripts initiated from an internal promoter in the c-erbA alpha locus that encode inhibitors of retinoic acid receptor-alpha and triiodothyronine receptor activities. *Mol Endocrinol* 1997; 11:1278–1290.

53. Williams GR. Cloning and characterization of two novel thyroid hormone receptor (beta) variants. Mol Cell Biol 2000; 20:8329–8342.

54. Jones KE, Chin WW. Differential regulation of thyroid hormone receptor messenger ribonucleic acid levels by thyrotropin-releasing hormone. *Endocrinology* 1991;128:1763–1768.

55. Jones KE, Yaffe BM, Chin WW. Regulation of thyroid hormone receptor b-2 mRNA levels by retinoic acid. *Mol Cell Endocrinol* 1993;91:113–118.

56. Davis KD, Lazar MA. Selective antagonism of thyroid hormone action by retinoic acid. *J Biol Chem* 1992;267:3185–3189.

57. Williams GR, Franklyn JA, Neuberger JM, et al. Thyroid hormone receptor expression in the "sick euthyroid" syndrome. *Lancet* 1989;2:1477–1481.

58. Darling DS, Carter RL, Yen PM, et al. Different dimerization activities of a and b thyroid hormone receptor isoforms. *J Biol Chem* 1993;268:10221–10227.

59. Lazar MA. Sodium butyrate selectively alters thyroid hormone receptor gene expression in GH3 cells. *J Biol Chem* 1990;265: 17474–17477.

60. Farsetti A, Desvergne B, Hallenbeck P, et al. Characterization of myelin basic protein thyroid hormone response element and its function in the context of native and heterologous promoter. *J Biol Chem* 1992;267:15784–15788.

61. Lezoualc'h F, Hassan AH, Giraud P, et al. Assignment of the beta-thyroid hormone receptor to 3,5,3′-triiodothyronine-dependent inhibition of transcription from thyrotropin-releasing hormone promoter in chick hypothalamic neurons. *Mol Endocrinol* 1992;6:1797–1804.

62. Hollenberg AN, Monden T, Wondisford FE. Ligand-independent and -dependent functions of thyroid hormone receptor isoforms depend upon on their distinct amino terminal. *J Biol Chem* 1995;270:14272–14280.

63. Abel ED, Kaulbach HC, Campos-Barros A, et al. Novel insight from transgenic mice into thyroid hormone resistance and the regulation of thyrotropin. *J Clin Invest* 1999;103: 271–279.

64. Yen PM, Feng X, Flamant F, et al. Effects of ligand and thyroid hormone receptor isoforms on hepatic gene expression profiles of thyroid hormone receptor knockout mice. *EMBO Rep* 2003; 4:581–587.

65. Ball SG, Ikeda M, Chin WW. Deletion of the thyroid hormone beta1 receptor increases basal and triiodothyronine-induced growth hormone messenger ribonucleic acid in GH3 cells. *Endocrinology* 1997;138:3125–3132.

66. Chiellini G, Apriletti JW, al Yoshihara H, et al. A high-affinity subtype-selective agonist ligand for the thyroid hormone receptor. *Chem Biol* 1998;5:299–306.

67. Yen PM. Molecular basis of resistance to thyroid hormone. *Trends in Endocrinology Metabolism* 2003;14:327–333.

68. Baxter JD, Goede P, Apriletti JW, et al. Structure-based design and synthesis of a thyroid hormone receptor (TR) antagonist. *Endocrinology* 2002;143:517–524.

69. Dillmann WH. Cellular action of thyroid hormone on the heart. *Thyroid* 2002;12:447–452.

70. Williams GR, Brent GA. Thyroid hormone response elements. In: Weintraub B, ed. *Molecular endocrinology: basic concepts and clinical correlations.* New York: Raven Press, 1995:217–239.

71. Glass CK. Differential recognition of target genes by nuclear receptor monomers, dimers and heterodimers. *Endocr Rev* 1994;15:391–407.

72. Yen PM, Brubaker JH, Apriletti JW, et al. Roles of T_3 and DNA-binding on thyroid hormone receptor complex formation. *Endocrinology* 1994;134:1075–1081.

73. Umesono K, Murakami K, Thompson CC, et al. Direct repeats as selective response elements for the thyroid hormone, retinoic acid, vitamin D3 receptors. *Cell* 1991;65:1255–1266.

74. Naar AM, Boutin JM, Lipkin SM, et al. The orientation and spacing of core DNA-binding motifs dictate selective transcriptional responses to three nuclear receptors. *Cell* 1991;65:1255–1266.

75. Kurokawa R, Soderstrom M, Horlein A, et al. Polarity-specific activities of retinoic acid receptors determined by a co-repressor. *Nature* 1995;377:451–454.

76. Perlmann T, Rangarajan PN, Umesono K, et al. Determinants for selective RAR and TR recognition of direct repeat HREs. *Genes Dev* 1993;7:1411–1422.

77. Yen PM, Ikeda M, Wilcox EC, et al. Half-site arrangement of hybrid glucocorticoid and thyroid hormone response elements specifies thyroid hormone receptor complex binding to DNA and transcriptional activity. *J Biol Chem* 1994;269:12704–12709.

78. Rastinejad F, Perlmann T, Evans RM, et al. Structural determinants of nuclear receptor assembly on DNA direct repeats. *Nature* 1995;375:203–211.

79. Nagaya T, Jameson JL. Distinct dimerization domains provide antagonist pathways for thyroid hormone receptor action. *J Biol Chem* 1993;268:24278–24282.

80. Au-Fliegner M, Helmer E, Casanova J, et al. The conserved ninth C-terminal heptad in thyroid hormone and retinoic acid receptors mediates diverse responses by affecting heterodimer but not homodimer formation. *Mol Cell Biol* 1993;13:5725–5737.

81. Collingwood TN, Butler A, Tone Y, et al. Thyroid hormone-mediated enhancement of heterodimer formation between thyroid hormone receptor beta and retinoid × receptor. *J Biol Chem* 1997;272:13060–13065.

82. Levin AA, Sturzenbecker LJ, Kaxmer S, et al. 9-cis retinoic acid stereoisomer binds and activates the nuclear receptor RXRa. *Nature* 1992;355:359–361.

83. Heyman RA, Mangelsdorf DJK, Dyk JA, et al. 9-cis retinoic acid is a high affinity ligand for the retinoid × receptor. *Cell* 1992;68:397–440.

84. Rosen ED, O'Donnell AL, Koenig RJ. Ligand-dependent synergy of thyroid hormone and retinoid × receptors. *J Biol Chem* 1992;267:22010–22013.

85. Feng X, Jiang Y, Meltzer P, et al. Thyroid hormone regulation of hepatic genes *in vivo* detected by complementary DNA microarray. *Mol Endocrinol* 2000;14:947–955.

86. Flores-Morales A, Gullberg H, Fernandez L, et al. Patterns of liver gene expression governed by TRbeta. *Mol Endocrinol* 2002;16:1257–1268.

87. Krane IM, Spindel ER., Chin WW. Thyroid hormone decreases the stability and the poly(A) tract length of rat thyrotropin beta-subunit messenger RNA. *Mol Endocrinol* 1991; 5:469–475.

88. Leedman PJ, Stein AR, Chin WW. Regulated specific protein binding to a conserved region of the 3′-untranslated region of thyrotropin beta-subunit mRNA. *Mol Endocrinol* 1995;9:375–387.

89. Brent GA, Dunn MK, Harney JW, et al. Thyroid hormone aporeceptor represses T_3-inducible promoters and blocks activity of the retinoic acid receptor. *New Biologist* 1989;1:329–336.

90. Horlein AJ, Naar AM, Heinzel T, et al. Ligand-independent repression by the thyroid hormone receptor mediated by a nuclear co-repressor. *Nature* 1995;377:397–404.

91. Chen JD, Evans RM. A transcriptional co-repressor that interacts with nuclear hormone receptors. *Nature* 1995;377:454–457.

92. Seol W, Choi HS, Moore DD. Isolation of proteins that interact specifically with the retinoid × receptor: two novel orphan receptors. *Mol Endocrinol* 1995;9:72–85.

93. Hu I, Lazar MA. Transcriptional repression by nuclear hormone receptors. *Trends in Endocrinology Metabolism* 2000;11:6–10.

94. Zhang J, Hu X, Lazar MA. A novel role for helix 12 of retinoid × receptor in regulating repression. *Mol Cell Biol* 1999;19: 6448–6457.

95. Wong J, Shi YB, Wolffe AP. A role for nucleosome assembly in both silencing and actiation of the xenopus TR beta A gene by the thyroid hormone receptor. *Genes Dev* 1996;9:2696–1711.

96. Nan X, Ng HH, Johnson CA, et al. Transcriptional repression by the methyl-CpG-binding protein MeCP2 involves a histone deacetylase complex. *Nature* 1998;393:386–389.

97. Baniahmad A, Ha I, Reinberg D, et al. Interaction of human thyroid hormone receptor b with transcription factor TFIIB may mediate target gene derepression and activation by thyroid hormone. *Proc Natl Acad Sci USA* 1993;90:8832–8836.

98. Hadzic E, Desai-Yajnik V, Helmer E, et al. A 10 amino acid sequence in the N-terminal A/B domain of thyroid hormone receptor alpha is essential for transcriptional activation and interaction with the general transcription factor TFIIB. *Mol Cell Biol* 1995;15:4507–4517.

99. Onate SA, Tsai SY, Tsai MJ, et al. Sequence and characterization of a coactivator for the steroid hormone receptor superfamily. *Science* 1995;270:1354–1357.

100. McInerney EM, Rose DW, Flynn SE, et al. Determinants of coactivator LXXLL motif specificity in nuclear receptor transcriptional activation. *Genes Dev* 1998;12:3357–3368.

101. Heery DM, Kalkhoven E, Hoare S, et al. A signature motif in transcriptional co-activators mediates binding to nuclear receptors. *Nature* 1997;387:733–736.

102. Torchia J, Glass C, Rosenfeld MG. Co-activators and co-repressors in the integration of transcriptional responses. *Curr Opin Cell Biol* 1998;10:373–383.

103. Nakajima T, Uchida C, Anderson SF, et al. RNA helicase A mediates association of CBP with RNA polymerase II. *Cell* 1997;90:1107–1112.

104. Ito M, Roeder RG. The TRAP/SMCC/Mediator complex and thyroid hormone receptor function. *Trends in Endocrinology Metabolism* 2001;12:127–134.

105. Rachez C, Freedman LP. Mediator complexes and transcription. *Curr Opin Cell Biol* 2001;13:274–280.

106. Ko L, Cardona GR, Chin WW. Thyroid hormone receptor-binding protein, an LXXLL motif-containing protein, functions as a general coactivator. *Proc Natl Acad Sci USA* 2000;97: 6212–6217.

107. Ko L, Chin WW. Nuclear receptor coactivator thyroid hormone receptor-binding protein (TRBP) interacts with and stimulates its associated DNA-dependent protein kinase. *J Biol Chem* 2003;278:11471–11479.

108. Sharma D, Fondell JD. Ordered recruitment of histone acetyltransferases and the TRAP/mediator complex to thyroid hor-

mone-responsive promoters *in vivo*. *Proc Natl Acad Sci USA* 2002;99:7934–7939.

109. Shang Y, Hu X, DiRenzo J, et al. Cofactor dynamics and sufficiency in estrogen receptor-regulated transcription. *Cell* 2000; 103:843–852.

110. Reid G, Hubner MR, Metivier R, et al. Cyclic, proteasome-mediated turnover of unliganded and liganded ERalpha on responsive promoters is an integral feature of estrogen signaling. *Mol Cell* 2003;11:695–707.

111. Li X, Wong J, Tsai SY, et al. Progesterone and glucocorticoid receptors recruit distinct coactivator complexes and promote distinct patterns of local chromatin modification. *Mol Cell Biol* 2003;23:3763–3773.

112. Chen H, Lin RJ, Schiltz RL, et al. Nuclear receptor coactivator ACTR is a novel histone acetyltransferase and forms a multimeric activation complex with P/CAF and CBP/p300. *Cell* 1997;90:569–580.

113. DiRenzo J, Shang Y, Phelan M, et al. BRG-1 is recruited to estrogen-responsive promoters and cooperates with factors involved in histone acetylation. *Mol Cell Biol* 2000;20:7541–7549.

114. Bodenner DL, Mroczynski MA, Weintraub BD, et al. A detailed functional and structural analysis of a major thyroid hormone inhibitory element in the human thyrotropin beta-subunit gene. *J Biol Chem* 1991;266:21666–21673.

115. Chatterjee VK, Lee JK, Rentoumis A, et al. Negative regulation of the thyroid-stimulating hormone alpha gene by thyroid hormone: receptor interaction adjacent to the TATA box. *Proc Natl Acad Sci USA* 1989;86:9114–9118.

116. Hollenberg AN, Monden T, Flynn TR, et al. The human thyrotropin-releasing hormone gene is regulated by thyroid hormone through two distinct classes of negative thyroid hormone response elements. *Mol Endocrinol* 1995;9:540–550.

117. Madison LD, Ahlquist JA, Rogers SD, et al. Negative regulation of the glycoprotein hormone a subunit gene promoter by thyroid hormone: mutagenesis of a proximal receptor binding site preserves transcriptional repression. *Mol Cell Endocrinol* 1993;94:129–136.

118. Zhang XK, Wills KN, Husmann M, et al. Novel pathway for thyroid hormone receptor action through interaction with Jun and Fos oncogene activities. *Mol Cell Biol* 1991;11:6016–6025.

119. Pernasetti, F, Caccavelli L, Van de Weerdt C, et al. Thyroid hormone inhibits the human prolactin gene promoter by interfering with activating protein-1 and estrogen stimulations. *Mol Endocrinol* 1997;11:986–996.

120. Tansey WP, Catanzaro DF. Sp1 and thyroid hormone receptor differentially activate expression of human growth hormone and chorionic somatomammotropin genes. *J Biol Chem* 1991; 266:9805–9813.

121. Schaufele F, West BL, Reudelhuber TL. Overlapping Pit-1 and Sp1 binding sites are both essential to full rat growth hormone gene promoter activity despite mutually exclusive Pit-1 and Sp1 binding. *J Biol Chem* 1990;265:17189–17196.

122. Barrera-Hernandez G, Zhan Q, Wong R, et al. Thyroid hormone receptor is a negative regulator in p53–mediated signaling pathways. *DNA Cell Biol* 1998;17:743–750.

123. Qi JS, Yuan Y, Desai-Yajnik V, et al. Regulation of the mdm2 oncogene by thyroid hormone receptor. *Mol Cell Biol* 1999; 19:864–872.

124. Lutz M, Burke LJ, LeFevre P, et al. Thyroid hormone-regulated enhancer blocking: cooperation of CTCF and thyroid hormone receptor. *EMBO J* 2003;22:1579–1587.

125. Tagami T, Madison LD, Nagaya T, et al. Nuclear receptor corepressors activate rather than suppress basal transcription of genes that are negatively regulated by thyroid hormone. *Mol Cell Biol* 1997;17:2642–2648.

126. Sasaki S, Lesoon-Wood LA, Dey A, et al. Ligand-induced recruitment of a histone deacetylase in the negative-feedback regulation of the thyrotropin beta gene. *EMBO J* 1999;18:5389–5398.

127. Abel ED, Boers ME, Pazos-Moura C, et al. Divergent roles for thyroid hormone receptor beta isoforms in the endocrine axis and auditory system. *J Clin Invest* 1999;104:291–300.

128. Langlois M.F, Zanger K, Monden T, et al. A unique role of the beta-2 thyroid hormone receptor isoform in negative regulation by thyroid hormone: mapping of a novel amino-terminal domain important for ligand-independent activation. *J Biol Chem* 1997;272:24927–24933.

129. Refetoff S, Weiss RA, Usala SJ. The syndromes of resistance to thyroid hormone. *Endocr Rev* 1993;14:348–399.

130. Beck-Peccoz P, Chatterjee VK. The variable clinical phenotype in thyroid hormone resistance syndrome. *Thyroid* 1994;4:225–232.

131. Yen PM, Sugawara A, Refetoff S, et al. New insights on the mechanism(s) of the dominant negative effect of mutant thyroid hormone receptor in generalized resistance to thyroid hormone. *J Clin Invest* 1992;90:1825–1831.

132. Collingwood TN, Rajanayagam O, Adams M, et al. A natural transactivation mutation in the thyroid hormone b receptor: impaired interaction with putative transcriptional mediators. *Proc Natl Acad Sci USA* 1997;94:248–253.

133. Liu Y, Takeshita A, Misiti S, et al. Lack of coactivator interaction can be a mechanism for dominant negative activity by mutant thyroid hormone receptors. *Endocrinology* 1998;139: 4197–4204.

134. Tagami T, Gu WX, Peairs PT, et al. A novel natural mutation in the thyroid hormone receptor defines a dual functional domain that exchanges nuclear receptor corepressors and coactivators. *Mol Endocrinol* 1998;12:1888–1902.

135. Yoh SM, Chatterjee VK, Privalsky ML. Thyroid hormone resistance manifests as an aberrant interaction between mutant T_3 receptors and transcriptional corepressors. *Mol Endocrinol* 1997;11:470–480.

136. Tagami T, Jameson JL. Nuclear corepressors enhance the dominant negative activity of mutant receptors that cause resistance to thyroid hormone. *Endocrinology* 1998;139:640–650.

137. Safer JD, Cohen RN, Hollenberg AN, et al. Defective release of corepressor by hinge mutants of the thyroid hormone receptor found in patients with resistance to thyroid hormone. *J Biol Chem* 1998;273:30175–30182.

138. Pohlenz J, Weiss RE, Macchia PE, et al. Five new families with resistance to thyroid hormone not caused by mutations in the thyroid hormone receptor beta gene. *J Clin Endocrinol Metab* 1999;84:3919–3928.

139. Weiss RE, Xu J, Ning G, et al. Mice deficient in the steroid receptor co-activator 1 (SRC-1) are resistant to thyroid hormone. *EMBO J* 1999;18:1900–1904.

140. Lin K-H, Zhu X-G, Shieh H-Y, et al. Identification of naturally occurring dominant negative mutants of thyroid hormone a1 and b1 receptors in a human hepatocellular carcinoma cell lines. *Endocrinology* 1996;137:4073–4081.

141. Yen P, Cheng S. Somatic thyroid hormone receptor mutations in man. *J Endocrinol Invest* 2003;26:780–787.

142. Ando S, Sarlis NJ, Krishnan J, et al. Aberrant alternative splicing of thyroid hormone receptor in a TSH-secreting pituitary tumor is a mechanism for hormone resistance. *Mol Endocrinol* 2001;15:1529–1538.

143. Ando S, Sarlis NJ, Oldfield EH, et al. Somatic mutation of TR-beta can cause a defect in negative regulation of TSH in a TSH-secreting pituitary tumor. *J Clin Endocrinol Metab* 2001;86: 5572–5576.

144. Kaneshige M, Kaneshige K, Zhu X, et al. Mice with a targeted mutation in the thyroid hormone beta receptor gene exhibit

impaired growth and resistance to thyroid hormone. *Proc Natl Acad Sci USA* 2000;97:13209–13214.

145. Hashimoto K, Curty FH, Borges PP, et al. An unliganded thyroid hormone receptor causes severe neurological dysfunction. *Proc Natl Acad Sci USA* 2001;98:3998–4003.

146. Kaneshige M, Suzuki H, Kaneshige K, et al. A targeted dominant negative mutation of the thyroid hormone alpha 1 receptor causes increased mortality, infertility, dwarfism in mice. *Proc Natl Acad Sci USA* 2001;98:15095–15100.

147. Tinnikov A, Nordstrom K, Thoren P, et al. Retardation of postnatal development caused by a negatively acting thyroid hormone receptor alpha1. *EMBO J* 2002;21:5079–5087.

148. Barlow C, Meister B, Lardelli M, et al. Thyroid abnormalities and hepatocellular carcinoma in mice transgenic for v-erbA. *EMBO J* 1994;13:4241–4250.

149. Wong R, Vasilyev VV, Ting YT, et al. Transgenic mice bearing a human mutant thyroid hormone beta 1 receptor manifest thyroid function anomalies, weight reduction, hyperactivity. *Mol Med* 1997;3:303–314.

150. Fraichard A, Chassande O, Plateroti M, et al. The T$_3$R alpha gene encoding a thyroid hormone receptor is essential for postnatal development and thyroid hormone production. *EMBO J* 1997;16:4412–4420.

151. Wikstrom L, Johansson C, Salto C, et al. Abnormal heart rate and body temperature in mice lacking thyroid hormone receptor alpha 1. *Embo J* 1998;17:455–461.

152. Macchia PE, Takeuchi Y, Kawai T, et al. Increased sensitivity to thyroid hormone in mice with complete deficiency of thyroid hormone receptor alpha. *Proc Natl Acad Sci USA* 2001;98:349–354.

153. Forrest D, Hanebuth E, Smeyne RJ, et al. Recessive resistance to thyroid hormone in mice lacking thyroid hormone receptor beta: evidence for tissue-specific modulation of receptor function. *EMBO J* 1996;15:3006–3015.

154. Forrest D, Erway LC, Ng L, et al. Thyroid hormone receptor beta is essential for development of auditory function. *Nat Genet* 1996;13:354–357.

155. Refetoff S, DeWind LT, DeGroot LJ. Familial syndrome combining deaf-mutism, stippled epiphyses, goiter and abnormally high PBI: possible target organ refractoriness to thyroid hormone. *J Clin Endocrinol Metab* 1967;27:279–294.

156. Weiss RE, Forrest D, Pohlenz J, et al. Thyrotropin regulation by thyroid hormone in thyroid hormone receptor beta-deficient mice. *Endocrinology* 1997;138:3624–3629.

157. Ng L, Rusch A, Amma LL, et al. Suppression of the deafness and thyroid dysfunction in Thrb-null mice by an independent mutation in the Thra thyroid hormone receptor alpha gene. *Hum Mol Genet* 2001;10:2701–2708.

158. Gothe S, Wang Z, Ng L, et al. Mice devoid of all known thyroid hormone receptors are viable but exhibit disorders of the pituitary-thyroid axis, growth, bone maturation. *Genes Dev* 1999;13:1329–1341.

159. Gauthier K, Chassande O, Plateroti M, et al. Different functions for the thyroid hormone receptors TRalpha and TRbeta in the control of thyroid hormone production and post-natal development. *EMBO J* 1999;18:623–631.

160. Suzuki H, Willingham MC, Cheng SY. Mice with a mutation in the thyroid hormone receptor beta gene spontaneously develop thyroid carcinoma: a mouse model of thyroid carcinogenesis. *Thyroid* 2002;12:963–969.

161. Liu YY, Schultz JJ, Brent GA. A thyroid hormone receptor alpha gene mutation (P398H) is associated with visceral adiposity and impaired catecholamine-stimulated lipolysis in mice. *J Biol Chem* 2003;278:38913–38920.

162. Shibusawa N, Hashimoto K, Nikrodhanond AA, et al. Thyroid hormone action in the absence of thyroid hormone receptor DNA-binding *in vivo*. *J Clin Invest* 2003;112:588–597.

163. Saatcioglu F, Deng T, Karin M. A novel cis element mediating ligand-independent activation by c-erbA: implications for hormonal regulation. *Cell* 1993;75:1095–1105.

164. Lakshmanan M, Goncalves E, Lessly G et al. The transport of thyroxine into mouse neuroblastoma cells, NB41A3: the effect of L-system amino acids. *Endocrinology* 1990;126:3245–3250.

165. Osty J, Valensi P, Samson M, et al. Transport of thyroid hormones by human erythrocytes: kinetic characterization in adults and newborns. *J Clin Endocrinol Metab* 1990;71:1589–1595.

166. Samson M, Osty J, Blondeau JP. Identification by photoaffinity labeling of a membrane thyroid hormone-binding protein associated with the triiodothyronine transport system in rat erythrocytes. *Endocrinology* 1993;132:2470–2476.

167. Mooradian AD, Schwartz HL, Mariash CN, et al. Transcellular and transnuclear transport of 3,5,3′-triiodothyronine in isolated hepatocytes. *Endocrinology* 1985;117:2449–2456.

168. Ribeiro RCJ, Cavalieri RR, Lomri N, et al. Thyroid hormone export regulates cellular hormone content and response. *J Biol Chem* 1996;271:17147–17151.

169. Baumann CT, Maruvada P, Hager GL, et al. Nuclear cytoplasmic shuttling by thyroid hormone receptors. multiple protein interactions are required for nuclear retention. *J Biol Chem* 2001;276:11237–11245.

170. Abe T, Kakyo M, Tokui T, et al. Identification of a novel gene family encoding human liver-specific organic anion transporter LST-1. *J Biol Chem* 1999;274:17159–17163.

171. Friesema EC, Docter R, Moerings EP, et al. Identification of thyroid hormone transporters. *Biochem Biophys Res Commun* 1999;254:497–501.

172. Friesema EC, Ganguly S, Abdalla A, et al. Identification of monocarboxylate transporter 8 as a specific thyroid hormone transporter. *J Biol Chem* 2003;278:40128–40135.

173. Ritchie JW, Shi YB, Hayashi Y, et al. A role for thyroid hormone transporters in transcriptional regulation by thyroid hormone receptors. *Mol Endocrinol* 2003;17:653–661.

174. Pizzagalli F, Hagenbuch B, Stieger B, et al. Identification of a novel human organic anion transporting polypeptide as a high affinity thyroxine transporter. *Mol Endocrinol* 2002;16:2283–2296.

175. Friesema E, Gruters A, Halestrap A, et al. Mutations in a thyroid hormone transporter in young boys with sever psychomotor retardation and high serum T$_3$ levels: a novel mechanism of thyroid hormone resistance. In: 6th International Workshop on Resistance to Thyroid Hormone; 13–15 September 2003; Miami, FL. Abstract 2.

176. Dumitrescu AM, Liao XH, Best TB, et al. A novel syndrome combining thyroid and neurological abnormalities is associated with mutations in a monocarboxylate transporter gene. *Am J Hum Genet* 2004;74:168–175.

177. Segal J, Ingbar SH. 3,5,3′-triiodothyronine increases 3′,5′-monophosphate concentration and sugar uptake in rat thymocytes by stimulating adenylate cyclase activity: studies with the adenylate cyclase inhibitor MDL 12330A. *Endocrinology* 1989;124:2166–2171.

178. Segal J, Ingbar SH. Studies on the mechanism by which 3,5,3′triiodothyronine stimulates 2–deoxyglucose uptake in rat thymocytes *in vitro*. Role of calcium and adenosine 3′,5′-monophosphate. *J Clin Invest* 1981;68:103–110.

179. Davis PJ, Blas SD. *In vitro* stimulation of human red blood cell Ca2+-ATPase by thyroid hormone. *Biochem Biophys Res Commun.* 1981;99:1073–1080.

180. Davis FB, Davis PJ, Blas SD. Role of calmodulin in thyroid hormone stimulation of *in vitro* human erythrocyte Ca2+-ATPase activity. *J Clin Invest* 1983;71:579–586.

181. Segal J, Gordon A. The effects of actinomycin D, puromycin, cycloheximide, hydroxyurea on 3'5'3–triiodo-L-thyronine stimulated 2–deoxy-D-glucose uptake in chick embryo heart cells *in vitro*. *Endocrinology* 1977;101:150–156.

182. Cheng SY, Gong QH, Parkison C, et al. The nucleotide sequence of a human cellular thyroid hormone binding protein present in endoplasmic reticulum. *J Biol Chem* 1987;262:11221–11227.

183. Kato H, Fukuda T, Parkison C, et al. Cytoplasmic thyroid hormone-binding protein is a monomer of pyruvate kinase. *Proc Natl Acad Sci U S A* 1990;86:7681–7685.

184. Ashizawa K, McPhie P, Lin KH, et al. An *in vitro* novel mechanism of regulating the activity of pyruvate kinase M2 by thyroid hormone and fructose 1,6 bisphosphate. *Biochemistry* 1991;30:7105–7111.

185. Farwell AP, Safran M, Dubord S, et al. Degradation and recycling of the substrate-binding subunit of type II iodothyronine 5'deiodonase in astrocytes. *J Biol Chem* 1996;271:16369–16374.

186. Steinsapir J, Bianco AC, Buettner C, et al. Substrate-induced down-regulation of human type 2 deiodinase (hD2) is mediated through proteasomal degradation and requires interaction with the enzyme's active center. *Endocrinology* 2000;141:1127–1135.

187. Farwell AP, DiBenedetto DJ., Leonard JL. Thyroxine targets different pathways of internalization of type II iodothyronine 5'-deiodinase in astrocytes. *J Biol Chem* 1993;268:5055.

188. Siegrist-Kaiser CA, Juge-Aubry C, Tranter MP, et al. Thyroxine-dependent modulation of actin polymerization in cultured astrocytes: a novel extranuclear action of thyroid hormone. *J Biol Chem* 1990;265:5296–5302.

189. Farwell AP, Tranter MP, Leonard JL. Thyroxine-dependent regulation of integrin-laminin interactions in astrocytes. *Endocrinology* 1995;136:3909–3915.

190. Sterling K, Brenner MA. Thyroid hormone action: effect of triiodothyronine on mitochondrial adenine nucleotide translocase *in vivo* and *in vitro*. *Metabolism* 1995;44:193–199.

191. Romani A, Marfella C, Lakshmanan M. Mobilization of Mg2+ from rat heart and liver mitochondria following the interaction of thyroid hormone with adenine nucleotide translocase. *Thyroid* 1996;6:513–519.

192. Lanni A, Moreno M, Lombardi A, et al. Rapid stimulation *in vitro* of rat liver cytochrome oxidase activity by 3,5-diiodo-L-thyronine and by 3,3'-diiodo-L-thyronine. *Mol Cell Endocrinol* 1994;99:89–94.

193. Hafner RP, Brown GC, Brand MD. Thyroid hormone control of state-3 respiration in isolated rat liver mitochondria. *Biochemical J* 1990;265:731–734.

194. Wrutniak C, Cassar-Malek I, Marchal S, et al. A 43 kD protein related to c-erb A alpha 1 is located in the mitochondrial matrix of rat liver. *J Biol Chem* 1995;270:16347–16354.

195. Casas F, Rochard P, Rodier A, et al. A variant form of the nuclear triiodothyronine receptor c-erbA alpha1 plays a direct role in regulation of mitochondrial RNA synthesis. *Mol Cell Biol* 1999;19:7913–7924.

196. Lin H-Y, Thacore HR, Davis PJ, et al. Thyroid hormone potentiates the antiviral action of interferon-gamma in culutured human cells. *J Clinl Endocrinol Metab* 1994;79:62–65.

197. Shih A, Lin HY, Davis FB, et al. Thyroid hormone promotes serine phosphorylation of p53 by mitogen-activated protein kinase. *Biochemistry* 2001;40:2870–2878.

198. Davis PJ, Shih A, Lin HY, et al. Thyroxine promotes association of mitogen-activated protein kinase and nuclear thyroid hormone receptor (TR) and causes serine phosphorylation of TR. *J Biol Chem* 2000;275:38032–38039.

199. Bunn CF, Neidig JA, Freidinger KE, et al. Nucleocytoplasmic shuttling of the thyroid hormone receptor alpha. *Mol Endocrinol* 2001;15:512–533.

200. Maruvada P, Baumann CT, Hager GL, et al. Dynamic shuttling and intranuclear mobility of nuclear hormone receptors. *J Biol Chem* 2003;278:12425–12432.

201. Scanlan T. TR agonists and antagonists. In: 6th International Workshop on Resistance to Thyroid Hormone; 2003; Miami, Fl. 4.

THYROID HORMONE STRUCTURE–FUNCTION RELATIONSHIPS

VIVIAN CODY

Studies of the thyroid hormones continue to provide new insights into the molecular events that control their biosynthesis, transport, and mechanism of action. Thyroid hormones are protein bound during transport in the general circulation, at the cell membrane, and at the cell nucleus. Therefore, their molecular interactions with proteins are of paramount interest. Most recently, emphasis has been focused on thyroid hormone protein interactions of transthyretin (TTR), its retinol-binding protein complex, thyroxine-binding globulin (TBG), and the hormone-binding domain of the thyroid nuclear receptor.

The major product of the thyroid gland, thyroxine (T_4) (3′,5′,3,5-tetraiodo-L-thyronine), was first isolated by Kendall in 1914 (Fig. 9.1) (1). Its correct composition, however, was not established until 1927, by Harington and Barger (2). Although thyroid hormones elicit a multitude of biologic responses, the specific nature of their actions remains unclear. The impetus to synthesize and test many analogues stemmed from attempts to define those features essential for T_4-like activity (3,4). A number of hypotheses have been proposed to relate the various structural features of thyroid hormones to the expression of their biologic effects (Table 9.1). Among the proposals suggested, the following are considered of key importance: (a) the unique role of iodine, for both its steric and its electronic properties; (b) the diphenyl ether linkage in controlling conformation; and (c) the 4′-hydroxyl and side-chain composition for receptor binding. Investigation of these hypotheses has been carried out using techniques such as nuclear magnetic resonance (NMR), spectroscopy, and X-ray crystallography to elucidate their structure–activity relationships.

For example, it is well known that hypothyroidism is accompanied by high serum levels of low-density lipoprotein cholesterol and, potentially, an increased risk of atherosclerosis, whereas thyrotoxicosis is associated with decreased cholesterol levels. Thyroid hormones could not be used therapeutically to lower serum cholesterol because of their potential to induce cardiac side effects. Thus, modification of the thyroid hormone molecule was carried out to produce analogues that could differentiate between liver-selective actions and cardiotoxic effects (4). These studies revealed that the introduction of specific arylmethyl groups at the 3′-position of triiodothyronine (T_3) resulted in analogues that are liver-selective, cardiac-sparing thyromimetic compounds.

More recent efforts have extended this concept to the design of thyromimetics with tissue-selective actions. For example, thyromimetics have been synthesized to be selective for the β-form of the thyroid hormone receptor (THRβ) (5), while other analogues elicit a T_3 response from mutant forms of the thyroid receptor (TRβ R320C) (6). These analogues suggest that such "pharmacological rescue" agents have potential for the treatment of thyroid disease. Another example of the design of thyromimetics that could overcome mutational diseases is that involving treatment of amyloid formation of TTR. Rational design efforts have identified several structurally diverse molecules that can bind and stabilize TTR under fibrillogenic conditions (7,8).

STRUCTURE AND STEREOCHEMICAL CHARACTERISTICS

The thyronine nucleus constitutes the basic structural unit of thyroid hormones. By varying the degree of iodination, all known thyroid hormone structures can be derived (Fig. 9.2). Depending on the reference point, the molecule can be described as a substituted alanine amino acid or, in terms of the diphenyl ether moiety, with substituents in the 4′- and 1- positions (Fig. 9.1).

The thyroid literature does not conform to the standard International Union of Pure and Applied Chemistry nomenclature, but uses instead the substituted diphenyl ether system. Because the thyronine nucleus has five single bonds (Fig. 9.1), rotation about these bonds results in a number of conformations, many of which have been observed in the solid state (9–11). This flexibility, quantitatively described by the magnitudes of these rotations, is

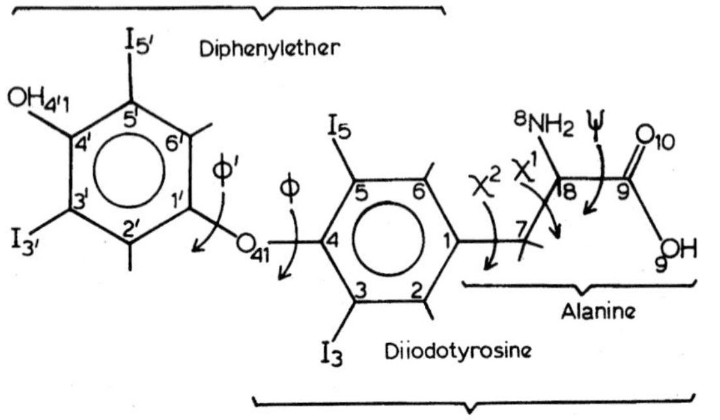

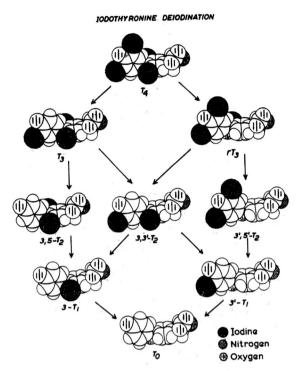

FIGURE 9.1. Thyroxine with torsion angles and molecular components. (From Cody V. Thyroid hormone interactions: molecular conformation, protein binding, and hormone action. *Endocr Rev* 1980;1:140, with permission.)

FIGURE 9.2. Spatial representation of thyroxine deiodination cascade. (From Auf'mkolk M, Koehrle J, Hesch RD, et al. Inhibition of rat liver iodothyronine deiodinase: interactions of aurone with the iodothyronine deiodinase binding site. *J Biol Chem* 1986;261:11623, with permission.)

controlled by (a) ring-substitution effects, (b) ether bridge substitutions, (c) side-chain composition, and (d) hydrogen-bonding effects.

A major structural feature of the thyroid hormones is that the two phenyl rings are joined by a bridging ether oxygen with an angle of 120 degrees. Early in the study of the thyroid hormones, it became evident that these substances possessed special stereochemical characteristics and that their three-dimensional features must be considered. Examination of space-filling models of the thyroid hormones revealed that the bulky orthoiodine atoms near the ether bridge caused the two aromatic ring systems to be nearly perpendicular, and that these bulky groups hindered rotation about the phenyl ether bonds. Structural data for the thyroid hormones showed that the minimal steric interaction between the orthotyrosyl iodine atoms and the phenolic orthohydrogen atoms was maintained when one ring is coplanar with, and the other perpendicular to, the plane of the two ether bonds (9). This gave rise to a skewed conformation of the hormone and the concept of pre-

ferred, if not somewhat rigid, orientations of the molecule (Fig. 9.3). These stereochemical properties also revealed that the 3'-iodine of the hormone 3,5,3'-triiodo-thyronine (T_3) possessed two positional isomers—distal and proximal—depending on whether the phenolic ring iodine atom was oriented away from or near the tyrosyl ring, respectively. Activity measurements of rigid analogues re-

TABLE 9.1. RELATIVE BINDING AFFINITIES AND BIOLOGIC POTENCIES OF SELECTED THYROID HORMONE ANALOGS

Compound	Thyroxine-binding Globulin (%)	Transthyretin (%)	Membrane (%)	Nuclear (%)	Potency[a] (%)
T_3	100.0	39.3	96.6	12.5	18.1
D-T_4	4.0	0.95	63.0	—	3.0
T_4-propionic acid	3.6	76.4	23.0	—	3.0
T_4-acetic acid	1.7	100.0	30.3	—	0.25
S-bridge T_4	63.0	—	—	—	—
CH_2-bridge T_4	35.0	—	—	2.6	—
T_3	9.0	1.4	100.0	100.0	100.0
rT_3	38.0	3.1	67.5	0.1	< 0.1

[a]Potency is percentage of T_3 (triiodothyronine; 3',3,5-triiodothyronine).
T_4, thyroxine; D-T_4, detiorotomes; S-bridge T_4, s replaces ether O between rings in T_4; CH_2-bridge T_4, CH_2 replaces ether O between rings in T_4; rT_3, reverse triiodothyronine.
From Cody V. Thyroid–hormone interactions: molecular conformation, protein binding, and hormone action. *Endocr Rev* 1980;1:140, with permission.

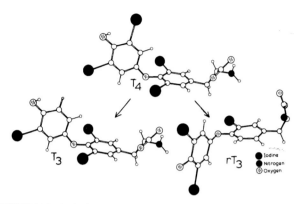

FIGURE 9.3. Deiodination products of thyroxine to skewed tri-iodothyronine (T_3) and antiskewed reverse (3',5',3-)triiodothyronine (rT_3). (From Cody V, Koehrle J, Auf'mkolk M, Hesch RD. Structure-activity relationships of flavonoid deiodinase inhibitors and enzyme active site models. In: Cody V, Middleton E Jr, Harborne JB, eds. *Plant flavonoids in biology and medicine: biochemical, pharmaceutical and structure-activity relationships.* New York: Alan R. Liss, 1986:373, with permission.)

vealed that a distal T_3 conformation was the more active analogue.

Crystallographic analysis of thyroid hormones shows that a skewed diphenyl ether conformation is observed in the structures of all 3,5-disubstituted hormone analogues (9–11). As mentioned earlier, the bulk of the tyrosyl ring substituents forces the diphenyl ether to adopt a skewed conformation (i.e., φ = 0 degrees, φ' = 90 degrees), whereas removal of one of these substituents releases this constraint, permitting an antiskewed conformation (i.e., the tyrosyl ring is perpendicular to, and bisecting, the phenolic ring φ = 90 degrees and φ' = 0 degrees), as observed in the crystal structure of 3',5',3-triiodothyronine (rT_3) (12) (Fig. 9.3). T_4 cannot adopt an antiskewed conformation because the bulk of the tyrosyl ring iodine atom would be placed into the electron density of the phenolic ring. Therefore, the active hormones T_4 and T_3, as well as 3,5-T_2, can adopt only a skewed conformation, whereas those with at least one tyrosyl ring iodine can have either a skewed or antiskewed conformation (13).

All the thyroid hormone–binding proteins have a requirement for a diphenyl ether moiety, because those derivatives of T_4 that contain only one ring or have a biphenyl connection do not possess activity or binding affinity. The need for the bridging atom to be oxygen is not absolute. Studies of various oxygen bridge–substituted analogues (C-X-C, where X = CH_2, S) showed that the sulfur- and methylene-bridged analogues had substantial binding affinity and activity. Thus, one role of the oxygen bridge is to maintain the appropriate relative orientation of the iodophenyl substituents (14).

The conformational space available to the thyroid hormone side chain is defined by three torsion angles: χ^1, χ^2, and ψ (Fig. 9.1). From the set of all accessible conforma-

tions, only specific subsets are predicted to be favored energetically, and most of these have been observed (9,11,15). These features play a role in differentiating the binding affinity of hormone analogues for their various hormone-binding proteins. For example, T_4 has the strongest binding affinity for TBG, whereas the metabolite tetraiodothyroacetic acid has the strongest binding affinity for TTR (see Table 9.1).

Under normal physiologic conditions, the thyroid hormone amino acid is a zwitterion; the amine has a net positive charge, and the carboxylic oxygen atoms have a net negative charge. As a result of the differences in pKa of the 4'-OH in T_3 and T_4 (8.47 and 6.73, respectively), the 4'-OH of T_4 is about 80% ionized at physiologic pH, whereas in T_3 it is about 10% ionized. Because many protein-substrate interactions are by way of receptor interactions, it is important to understand the nature of the hydrogen bonding in these structures. A study of the hydrogen bonding observed in the crystal structures of thyroid hormones shows that there is a high degree of directional specificity in the location of the hydrogen bond donors and acceptors (10). One unique property of iodine is its polarizability, which is reflected in its predisposition to form short intermolecular contact distances of the type I . . . I and I . . . O in the crystal lattice (16). The propensity for iodine to form such short intermolecular contacts may explain hormone-binding selectivity to the various T_4-binding proteins.

PROTEIN-BINDING INTERACTIONS

Sequence analysis showed that TTRs from various species are more than 86% identical to those from humans (17). In the case of rat TTR, there are 22 residues that differ from the human sequence, most of which are distal from the ligand-binding domain. Structure–activity data show that thyroid hormone analogues have different binding affinities for TTR, depending on their substituent patterns (Table 9.1). In addition, many pharmacologic agents and natural products, such as plant flavonoids, nonsteroidal analgesic drugs, inotropic bipyridines, and organohalogen environmental agents, are strong competitors for T_4 binding to TTR, with binding affinities much greater than T_4. For example, structure–activity correlations indicated that certain plant flavonoids that exhibit strong TTR binding can also exhibit various antihormonal properties, including inhibition of the enzyme iodothyronine deiodinase (13, 18). These data further revealed that aurones are the most potent inhibitors of enzyme activity and strong competitors for T_4 binding to TTR (18). Computer graphic modeling of the binding interactions with TTR suggested that the best structural homology between thyroid hormones and flavonoids involved the phenolic ring of both classes of compound (19,20). Studies of T_4 displacement from TTR further revealed that a synthetic plant flavonoid, EMD 21388 (3-methyl-4',6-dihydroxy-3',5'-dibromo-flavone), is the strongest competitor for T_4 binding to human TTR (21,22), and showed that this T_4 antagonist alters the circulating total and percentage of free thyroid hormones and serum thyrotropin concentrations (23).

To verify this structure–activity data, the crystal structures of a number of ligand complexes with human or rat TTR have been studied (7,8,24–37). Most crystals of human TTR ligand complexes are isomorphous with the orthorhombic $P2_12_12$ cell reported previously for native TTR (38,39) and have two independent monomers in the asymmetric unit of the crystal lattice. The presence of a crystallographic twofold axis through the center of the binding domains requires that the ligand either possess molecular twofold symmetry or have a 50% statistical disorder. Because T_4 does not possess twofold symmetry, it must occupy this site with a statistical disorder. On the other hand, crystals of rat TTR crystallize in a tetragonal space group $P4_32_12$, with a complete tetramer in the asymmetric unit of the lattice (40). Data for the rat TTR-T_4 complex (30) revealed electron density in the binding domain and provide the first opportunity to examine the hormone-binding interactions in a unique environment.

LIGAND-BINDING MODES

Structural data for the hTTR-T_4 complex (39) revealed that T_4 binds in a "forward" mode, with its 4'-OH buried deep within the channel running through the tetrameric protein, and has its amino acid side-chain near the channel entrance interacting with Lys-15 and Glu-54. Recently, the TTR-T_4 complex was determined to be a cocrystallized hormone complex (28). These data showed that T_4 binds deeper in the channel and displaces the bound water observed in the crystals soaked with T_4 (39). Although the orientation is similar, the hormone is rotated such that it shares common binding sites for the 3- and 3'-iodine atoms. These data verify that T_4 binding does not affect the main chain conformation significantly but results in local rearrangements of residue side-chains in the binding channel.

The orientation of the weak binding metabolite 3,3'-T_2 (26) differs significantly from that of T_4. As shown in Figure 9.4, it binds deeper in the channel than T_4, and in this orientation, 3,3'-T_2 occupies the binding domain in a completely different manner from T_4. The binding affinity of 3,3'-T_2, which is 100-fold lower than that of T_4, reflects the lack of the second pair of iodine atoms interacting in the channel.

The thyroid hormone metabolite T_4 acetic acid (Table 9.1), a tight binder of TTR, shows multiple binding modes in structures with human and rat TTR (24,30). These data revealed the hormone metabolite binds with a mixed population of both "forward" and "reverse" orientations in one binding domain, and two, alternate "forward" binding po-

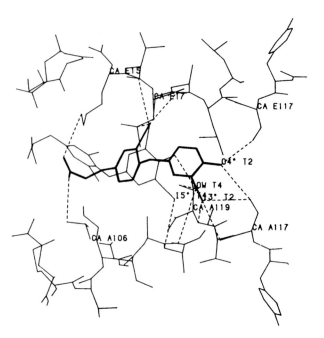

FIGURE 9.4. Position of thyroxine *(light line)* and 3,3'-T_2 *(thick line)* bound in their respective transthyretin complexes. The one-letter code symbols label the residues forming the binding site. (From Wojtczak A, Luft JR, Cody V. Mechanism of molecular recognition: crystal structure of 3,3'diiodo-L-thyronine human transthyretin complex and mutant interactions. *J Biol Chem* 1992;267:353, with permission.)

sitions in the second domain. These added intermolecular interactions may reflect the tight binding affinity of this metabolite for TTR.

Structural results show that flavones bind to TTR in a manner different from T_4. Data for the structure of the hTTR–EMD21388 complex revealed that bromoflavone binds deeper in the channel than T_4; the bromine atoms occupy symmetric sites in both a "forward" mode (Fig. 9.5) and "reverse" mode, with the bromophenolic ring near the channel entrance in TTR (24,32). A bromoaurone analogue binds in a similar manner (25). The observation of two alternative binding orientations for EMD 21388 may explain its greater binding affinity for TTR (22). Similar results have been observed for the organohalogens, tri- and pentabromophenol, that were observed to bind exclusively in the "reverse" mode (35). Solution NMR data on TTR also indicated that thyroid hormones may bind in more than one mode (41).

Biochemical data for the competitive inhibition of T_4 binding by bipyridine inotropic agents revealed that the potent cardioactive positive inotrope milrinone, a 2-methyl-5-cyano-bipyridine, has a binding affinity of 59% that of T_4, whereas its less potent parent inotrope, amrinone, the 5-amino-bipyridine analogue, was a weak competitor (42,43). Structural results for the TTR-milrinone complex showed that the 5-cyano group binds in the same site as the 5'-iodo group of the hormone (27). Modeling

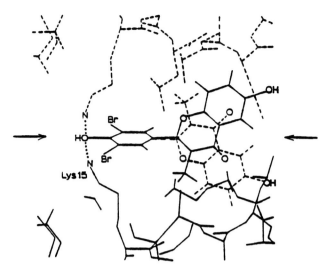

FIGURE 9.5. Representation of EMD 21388 in the "reverse" binding mode of human transthyretin. The close contact between the flavone 4′-OH and NZ of Lys-15 (lysine) near the channel entrance is shown. (From Cody V, Wojtczak A, Ciszak E, et al. Differences in inhibitor and substrate binding in transthyretin crystal complexes. In: Gordon A, Gross J, Hennemann G, eds. *Progress in thyroid research.* Rotterdam: Balema, 1991:793, with permission.)

amrinone binding in the milrinone site revealed that the 5-amino group cannot participate in the same interactions as the 5-cyano group, thereby weakening its binding affinity.

TRANSTHYRETIN VARIANTS AND AMYLOIDIC DISEASE

Increased efforts have been made to understand the mechanisms underlying TTR tetramer stability and their relationship to the formation of amyloid fibrils that characterize amyloid diseases, including familial amyloid polyneuropathy (FAP), senile systemic amyloidosis, and Alzheimer's disease (44–55). Recent data showed that wild-type and variant TTR form amyloid fibrils that are the causative agents in FAP and senile systemic amyloidosis diseases. To date, more than 70 single amino acid variants of the 127 residue monomer of TTR have been implicated in FAP disease (44); however, structural studies of TTR variants have failed to identify major differences that could explain their amyloidogenicity (46–49). Several hypotheses have been proposed based on monomeric or dimeric amyloidogenic intermediates to explain fibril formation from TTR monomers. One model proposes head-to-tail polymerization of monomeric intermediates (44,53). Another model is based on the formation of linear aggregates of TTR molecules, each linked by a pair of disulfide bonds involving Cys-10 (46,48,55). In this case, the intermediate is a dimer. A third model is based on data from two engineered amyloidogenic mutants and requires dimers that are associ-

ated by antiparallel organization of the F and H strands of the native protein. This model requires the destabilization of the tetramer prior to fibril formation (44,45). Yet another model invokes proteolytic cleavage as the initiation step in fibril formation (45,52).

Although the mechanism of tetramer stabilization is still unclear, it has been shown that ligand binding stabilizes tetramer formation in all variant species (44,50). Therefore, one means of intervention for disease treatment could involve binding of nonthyromimetic analogues that can stabilize the TTR tetramer and possibly delay the onset of fibril formation. To this end, numerous compounds have been screened (5–8,50). Structural data for the TTR complex with flufenemic acid showed that it mediates intersubunit hydrophobic interactions and intersubunit hydrogen bonds that stabilize the normal tetrameric fold (50). Data for the TTR complex with another analgesic analogue, VCP-6, which has 628% the affinity of T_4, showed that the molecule forms strong hydrogen bond interactions of its 2-carboxylate with Lys-15 and with the 3,5-dichloro atoms in symmetric hydrophobic pockets near the tetramer interface (Fig. 9.6) (36,37). These results suggest that the strategy of stabilization by strong competitors may prove fruitful. Comparison of the environment near the 22 residues in the rat sequence that differ from those in humans also

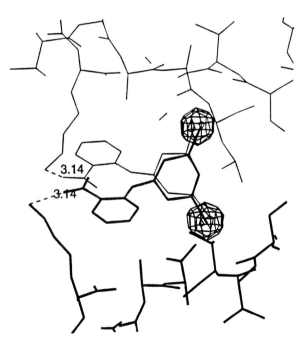

FIGURE 9.6. Representation of VCP-6 bound to human transthyretin (TTR). The close contact between the 2-carboxylate and NZ of Lys-15 near the channel entrance is shown. Different electron density (Fo-Fc, 3σ) shows position of 3′,5′-chlorine atoms near the center of the tetramer. Light lines are a twofold symmetry-related monomer that makes up binding domain A. Hydrogen bonding to Lys-15 and close contacts of chlorine atoms in hydrophobic pockets result in tight binding affinity of VCP-6 to TTR.

permit evaluation of their influence on hormone-binding interactions and tetramer assembly.

REFERENCES

1. Kendall EC. *Thyroxine*. American Chemical Society Monograph Series, No. 47. New York: Chemical Catalogue Company, 1929.
2. Harington CR, Barger G. Chemistry of thyroxine. III. Constitution and synthesis of thyroxine. *Biochem J* 1927;21:169–183.
3. Jorgensen EC, Stereochemistry of thyroxine and analogues. *Mayo Clin Proc* 1964;39:560–568.
4. Leeson PD, Emmett JC, Shah VP, et al. Selective thyromimetics. Cardiac-sparing thyroid hormone analogues containing 3'-arylmethyl substituents. *J Med Chem* 1989;32:320–336.
5. Yoshihara HAI, Apriletti JW, Baxter JD, et al. Structural determinants of selective thyromimetics. *J Med Chem* 2003;46:3152–3161.
6. Ye HF, O'Reilly KE, Koh JT. A Subtype-selective thyromimetic designed to bind a mutant thyroid hormone receptor implicated in resistance to thyroid hormone. *J Am Chem Soc* 2001;123:1521–1522.
7. Oza VB, Smith C, Raman P, et al. Synthesis, structure and activity of diclofenac analogues as transthyretin amyloid fibril formation inhibitors. *J Med Chem* 2002;45:321–332.
8. Razavi H, Palaninathan SK, Powers ET, et al. Benzoxazoles as transthyretin amyloid fibril inhibitors: synthesis, evaluation, and mechanism of action. *Angew Chem In. Ed* 2003;42:2758–2761.
9. Cody V. Thyroid hormone interactions: molecular conformation, protein binding, and hormone action. *Endocr Rev* 1980;1:140–169.
10. Cody V. Structure of thyroxine: role of thyroxine hydroxyl in protein binding. *Acta Crystallogr* 1981;SectB37:1685–1693.
11. Cody V. Triiodothyronine: molecular structure and biologic function. In: Chopra IJ, ed. *Triiodothyronines in health and disease*. New York: Springer-Verlag, 1981:15–57.
12. Okabe N, Fujiwara T, Yamagata Y, et al. The crystal structure of a major metabolite of thyroid hormone: 3',5',3-triiodo-L-thyronine. *Biochim Biophys Acta* 1982;717:179–181.
13. Cody V, Koehrle J, Auf'mkolk M, et al. Structure–activity relationships of flavonoid deiodinase inhibitors and enzyme active site models. In: Cody V, Middleton E Jr, Harborne JB, eds. *Plant flavonoids in biology and medicine: biochemical, pharmaceutical and structure-activity relationships*. New York: Alan R. Liss, 1986:373–382.
14. Cody V. Conformational effects of ether bridge substitution in thyroid hormone analogues. *Endocr Res Commun* 1982;9:55.
15. Cody V. Thyroid hormone structure-activity relationships: molecular structure of 3,5,3'-triiodothyropropionic acid. *Endocr Res* 1988;14:165–176.
16. Cody V, Murray-Rust P. Iodine . . . X(O,N,S) intermolecular contacts: models of thyroid hormone-protein binding interactions using information from the Cambridge Crystallogr Data Files. *J Mol Struc* 1984;112:189–199.
17. Sundelin J, Melhus H, Das S, et al. The primary structure of rabbit and rat prealbumin and a comparison with the ternary structure of human prealbumin. *J Biol Chem* 1985;260:6481–6485.
18. Auf'mkolk M, Koehrle J, Hesch RD, et al. Inhibition of rat liver iodothyronine deiodinase: interactions of aurone with the iodothyronine deiodinase binding site. *J Biol Chem* 1986;261:11623–11630.
19. Cody V, Luft JR, McCourt M, et al. Conformational analysis of flavonoids: crystal and molecular structure of 3',5'-dibromo-3-methyl-6,4'-dihydroxyflavone (1:2) triphenylphosphine oxide complex. *Struc Chem* 1991;2:601–606.
20. Ciszak E, Cody V, Luft JR, et al. Flavonoid conformational analysis: comparison of the molecular structure of (z)-4,4',6-triacetoxyaurone and (z)-3',5'-dibromo-2,4,4',6-tetrahydroxyaurone monohydrate by crystallographic and molecular orbital methods. *J Mol Struc (Theochem)* 1991;251:345–357.
21. Koehrle J, Fang SL, Yang Y, et al. Rapid effects of the flavonoid EMD 21388 on serum thyroid hormone binding and thyrotropin regulation in the rat. *Endocrinology* 1989;125:532–537.
22. Rosen HN, Murrell JR, Liepnieks JJ, et al. Threonine-for-alanine substitution at position 109 of transthyretin differentially alters TTR's affinity for iodothyronines. *Endocrinology* 1994;134:27–34.
23. Safran M, Koehrle J, Braverman LE, et al. Effect of biological alternations of type I 5'-deiodinase activity on affinity labeled membrane proteins in rat liver and kidney. *Endocrinology* 1990;126:826–831.
24. Cody V, Wojtczak A, Ciszak E, et al. Differences in inhibitor and substrate binding in transthyretin crystal complexes. In: Gordon A, Gross J, Hennemann G, eds. *Progress in thyroid research*. Rotterdam: Balema, 1991:793–799.
25. Ciszak E, Luft JR, Cody V. Crystal structure determination at 2.3 Å resolution of human transthyretin-3',5'-dibromo-2',4,4',6-tetrahydroxyaurone complex. *Proc Natl Acad Sci USA* 1992;89:6644–6648.
26. Wojtczak A, Luft JR, Cody V. Mechanism of molecular recognition: crystal structure of 3,3'-diiodo-L-thyronine human transthyretin complex and mutant interactions. *J Biol Chem* 1992;267:353–357.
27. Wojtczak A, Luft JR, Cody V. Structural aspects of inotropic bipyridine binding: crystal structure determination to 1.9 Å of the human serum transthyretin-milrinone complex. *J Biol Chem* 1993;268:6202–6206.
28. Wojtczak A, Cody V, Luft JR, Pangborn W. Structures of human transthyretin complexed with thyroxine at 2.0 Å resolution and 3',3'-Dinitro-N-acetyl-L-thyronine at 2.2 Å resolution. *Acta Crystallogr* 1996;SectionD52:758–765.
29. Wojtczak A, Neumann P, Cody V. Crystal structure of a new polymorphic form of human transthyretin at 3.0Å resolution reveals a mixed complex between unliganded and T4-Bound tetramers of TTR. *Acta Crystallogr* 2001;SectionD57:957–967.
30. Wojtczak A, Cody V, Luft JR, et al. Crystal structure of rat transthyretin (rTTR) complex with thyroxine at 2.5 Å resolution. First non-biased insight into thyroxine binding reveals different hormone orientation in two binding sites. *Acta Cryst* 2001;SectionD57:1061–1070.
31. Muziol T, Cody V, Luft JR, et al. Complex of rat transthyretin with tetraiodothyroacetic acid refined to 2.1 and 1.8Å resolution. *Acta Biochim Pol* 2001;48:877–884.
32. Muziol T, Cody V, Wojtczak A. Comparison of binding interactions of dibromoflavonoids in transthyretin. *Acta Biochim Pol* 2001;48:885–892.
33. Neumann P, Cody V, Wojtczak A. Structural basis of negative cooperativity in transthyretin. *Acta Biochim Pol* 2001;48:867–875.
34. De LaPaz P, Burridge JM, Oatley SJ, et al. Multiple modes of binding thyroid hormones and other iodothyronines to human plasma transthyretin. In: Beddell CR, ed. *The design of drugs to macromolecular targets*. New York: John Wiley and Sons, 1992:119–171.
35. Ghosh M, Meerts IATM, Cook A, et al. Structure of human transthyretin complexed with bromophenols: a new mode of binding. *Acta Cryst* 2000;SectionD56:1085–1095.
36. Cody V, Luft JR, Pangborn W, et al. Molecular recognition: modes of ligand binding to human transthyretin. *Chem Design Automation News* 1995;39–40.
37. Cody V. Mechanisms of molecular recognition: crystal structure analysis of human and rat transthyretin inhibitor complexes. *Clin Chem Lab Med* 2002;40:1237–1243.

38. Blake CCF, Geisow MJ, Oatley SJ, et al. Structure of prealbumin: secondary, tertiary and quaternary interactions determined by fourier refinement at 1.8A. *J Mol Biol* 1978;121:339–356.
39. Blake CCF, Oatley SJ. Protein-DNA and protein-hormone interactions in prealbumin: a model of the thyroid hormone nuclear receptor? *Nature* 1977;268:115–120.
40. Wojtczak A. Crystal structure of rat transthyretin at 2.5 Å resolution: first report on a unique tetrameric structure: *Acta Biochim Polonica* 1997;44:505–517.
41. Reid DG, MacLachlan LK, Voyle M, et al. A proton and fluorine nuclear magnetic resonance and fluorescence study of the binding of some natural and synthetic thyromimetics to prealbumin (transthyretin). *J Biol Chem* 1989;264:2013–2023.
42. Mylotte KM, Cody V, Davis PJ, et al. Milrinone and thyroid hormone stimulate myocardial membrane Ca^{2+}-ATPase activity and share structural homologies. *Proc Natl Acad Sci USA* 1985;82:7974–7978.
43. Davis PJ, Cody V, Davis FB, et al. Milrinone, a non-iodinated bipyridine, competes with thyroid hormone for binding sites on human serum prealbumin (TBPA). *Biochem Pharmacol* 1987;36:3635–3640.
44. Kelly JW. Alternative conformations of amyloidogenic proteins govern their behavior. *Curr Opin Struct Biol* 1996;6:11–17.
45. Nettleton EJ, Sunde M, Lai Z, et al. Protein subunit interactions and structural integrity of amyloidogenic transthyretins: evidence from electrospray mass spectrometry. *J Mol Biol* 1998;281:553–564.
46. Quintas A, Saraiva MJM, Brito RMM. The amyloidogenic potential of transthyretin variants correlates with their tendency to aggregate in solution. *FEBS Lett* 1997;418:297–300.
47. Schormann N, Murrell JR, Benson MD. Tertiary structures of amyloidgenic and non-amyloidogenic transthyretin variants: new model for amyloid fibril formation. Amyloid. *Int J Exp Clin Invest* 1998;5:175–187.
48. Blake CCF, Serpell L. Synchrotron X-ray studies suggest that the core of the transthyretin amyloid fibril is a continuous β-sheet helix. *Structure* 1996;4:989–998.
49. Peterson SA, Klabunde T, Lashuel HA, et al. Inhibiting transthyretin conformational changes that lead to amyloid fibril formation. *Proc Natl Acad Sci USA* 1998;95:12956–12969.
50. Baures PW, Peterson SA, Kelly JW. Discovering transthyretin amyloid fibril inhibitors by limited screening. *Bioorg Med Chem* 1998;6:1389–1401.
51. Eneqvist T, Andersson K, Olofsson A, et al. The β-slip: a novel concept in transthytetin amyloidosis. *Mol Cell* 2000;6:1207–1218.
52. Eneqvist T, Olofsson A, Ando Y, et al. Disulfide-bond formation in the transthyretin mutant Y114C prevents amyloid fibril formation in vivo and in vitro. *Biochemistry* 2002;41:13143–13151.
53. Hammarstrom P, Sekijima Y, White JT, et al. D18G transthyretin is monomeric, aggregation prone, and not detectable in plasma and cebrebrospinal fluid: a prescription for central nervous system amyloidosis. *Biochemistry* 2003;42:6656–6663.
54. Hammarstrom P, Wiseman RL, Powers ET, et al. Prevention of transthyretin amyloid disease by changing protein misfolding energetics. *Science* 2003;299;713–716.
55. Zhang Q, Kelly JW. Cys 10 mixed disulfides make transthyretin more amyloidogenic under mildly acidic conditions. *Biochemistry* 2003;42:8756–8761.

FACTORS THAT CONTROL THYROID FUNCTION

10

THYROTROPIN

10A   CHEMISTRY AND BIOSYNTHESIS OF THYROTROPIN

RONALD N. COHEN
FREDRIC E. WONDISFORD

Thyrotropin (thyroid-stimulating hormone, TSH) is the main regulator of thyroid hormone biosynthesis and secretion. Therefore, its availability and actions are critical determinants of thyroid function.

CHEMISTRY

TSH is one of four related glycoprotein hormones synthesized either by the anterior lobe of the pituitary gland or by the placenta. TSH, pituitary luteinizing hormone (LH), pituitary follicle-stimulating hormone (FSH), and chorionic gonadotropin (CG) consist of two noncovalently linked α- and β-subunits (1). The amino acid sequence of the α-subunit is common to all four of these hormones within any mammalian species. The β-subunit of each hormone has a different amino acid sequence, and this subunit carries the specific information relating to receptor binding and expression of hormonal activity; however, free β-subunits are devoid of bioactivity and require noncovalent combination with the common α-subunit to express this information.

Thyroid-stimulating activity has been extracted from virtually all mammalian pituitary glands, as well as in those of lower vertebrates. The best chemical information has been derived from a study of bovine, porcine, and human TSH (1). TSH preparations purified from pituitary glands by various chromatographic procedures contain heterogeneous but closely related components, which have variable biologic activity. These components can be separated by gel electrophoresis, isoelectric focusing, or chromatofocusing. The molecular weights of these various components of mammalian TSH are in the range of 28,000 to 30,000 daltons. Differences in molecular weight are attributed to heterogeneity of the oligosaccharide chains, heterogeneity at the amino terminus, and the extent of amidation of glutamic and aspartic acid residues.

The human α-subunit contains a protein core of 92 amino acid residues, while the bovine α-subunit contains 96 amino acids. The heterogeneity of the amino terminus of the α-subunits of the different glycoprotein hormones is probably artifactual, since *in vitro* studies (see later in the chapter) suggest that processing of the precursor protein yields a single product. The α-subunits contain 10 half-cystine residues, all of which are in disulfide linkage, as are those in the β-subunits. Knowledge of the specific location of the disulfide bonds in both subunits has been advanced by X-ray crystallographic analysis of the closely related gly-coprotein, human CG (2,3). The three-dimensional structure of TSH likely contains the cysteine knot motif and basic folding patterns found in human CG.

The β-subunits dissociated from intact human TSH prepared from pituitaries have a protein core of 112 amino acids; however, the complementary DNA for human TSH-β predicts a protein of 118 amino acids, 6 more than present in the isolated protein. When the linear sequences of β-subunits from different species are aligned to juxtapose half-cystine residues (12 in number), many regions of similar or identical sequences are apparent. From such relationships, and the fact that each can recombine with the common α-subunit, it seems probable that the three-dimensional structures of different β-subunits are similar. Indeed, evidence from chemical modification studies indicate that the regions around amino acid residues 51 to 57 and 75 to 80 of the β-subunit are among those involved in interaction with the common α-subunit. Based on the similarities in sequences between the β-subunits, all probably evolved from a single gene precursor.

Both the α- and β-subunits of TSH, as well as of LH, FSH, and CG, contain covalently linked carbohydrate chains. For TSH, LH, and FSH, these chains are linked to asparagine residues (N-linked), and for the β-subunit of human CG there are additional linkages to serine residues (O-linked). Moreover, the free α-subunit that is secreted also contains an additional site of O-glycosylation (4). In human TSH the sugar residues include mannose, fucose, N-acetylglucosamine, galactose, N-acetylgalactosamine, and sialic acid. Moreover, TSH and LH contain an unusual sulfate group that terminates certain chains; such sulfation is found only to a small extent in FSH, and not at all in CG (5,6). The sugar residues are three oligosaccharide units, all of which are heterogeneous and whose specific structures

may vary with the developmental and endocrine state (7). Recombinant human TSH has been produced in large amounts (see later in the chapter), and the biologic properties of particular isoforms of TSH and clinical use of TSH are being investigated (8–11).

GENES ENCODING THE SUBUNITS OF THYROTROPIN

Chromosome Localization

The gene encoding the common α-subunit of human CG, FSH, LH, and TSH, and the genes encoding their respective β-subunits are all located on different chromosomes. The location of the common α-subunit and specific β-subunit on different chromosomes raises interesting questions about how their expression is coordinately regulated during the synthesis of each hormone. Moreover, the gene for the β-subunit of CG is the only β-subunit gene of this family that exists in more than one copy; at least two of the seven copies on chromosome 19 are actively transcribed.

Structure of the Common α-Subunit Gene

The α-subunit gene has been isolated from a variety of species, including cows (12), mice (13), rats (14), and humans (15). The organization of each gene is similar in that it contains four exons and three introns, and all are of approximately the same size. The human gene is 9.4 kilobases (kb) in length and contains three introns of 6.4 kb, 1.7 kb, and 0.4 kb. Intron 1 is located between the 5'-untranslated region contained in exons 1 and 2; intron 2 interrupts the α-subunit peptide-coding region in codon 6; and intron 3 is between codons 67 and 68 of the peptide (Fig. 10A.1). In rats and cows, intron 2 interrupts the peptide-coding region within amino acid 10, resulting in a mature α-subunit peptide that is four amino acids longer than the human α-subunit peptide (96 amino acids vs. 92 amino acids).

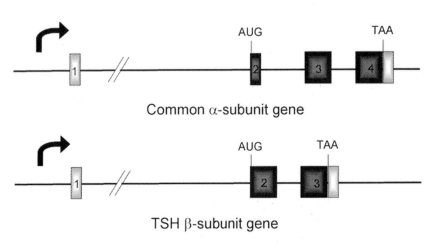

Common α-subunit gene

TSH β-subunit gene

FIGURE 10A.1. Schematic representation of the genes for the subunits of human thyrotropin (TSH). The genes for the α- and β-subunits have four and three exons *(numerals)*, respectively, represented by *boxes* separated by introns *(thin lines)*. The coding exons are denoted by *black boxes*, and the untranslated regions are represented by *white boxes*. The translation start *(AUG)* and stop *(TAA)* codons are shown in their relative position below each gene; the start of transcription is denoted by a *bent arrow*.

A single transcription start site has been found in each of these genes by mapping studies of pituitary RNA. Upstream of these start sites are consensus TATA boxes, thought to be important for correct and efficient transcription by RNA polymerase II (16). In the human α-subunit gene, the TATA box is -26 base pairs (bp) from the transcription start site (15). In addition, there is considerable homology among these species in other 5′-flanking regions, including a palindromic sequence of TGACGTCA in the human α-subunit gene that confers responsiveness to cyclic adenosine monophosphate (cyclic AMP) (17,18). However, the palindrome is altered in the other species to TGATGTCA; at least in cows, this change reduces its cyclic AMP responsiveness dramatically (19).

Structure of the Thyrotropin β-Subunit Gene

The TSH-β-subunit gene has been isolated from rats (20), humans (21–23), and mice (24,25). The rat and human genes contain three exons. The mouse gene contains five exons: the two additional exons are 5′-untranslated regions; these are unique due to changes in the sequence of the gene in mice (21). With this exception, the organization of these genes is quite similar in that there are 5′-untranslated exons(s) separated from the TSH-β coding region by a large first intron (Fig. 10A.1). The first exon of the human TSH-β gene is 37 bp and is untranslated, while the second exon encodes the leader peptide and first 34 amino acids of the mature TSH-β peptide; the third exon contains the remaining coding region (amino acids 35 to 118) and 3′-untranslated sequences.

The start of transcription has been determined in the rat, mouse, and human TSH-β genes. Both the rat and mouse genes contain two transcriptional start sites approximately 40 base pairs (bp) apart, as assessed by primer extension or S1 nuclease analysis of pituitary RNA (20,24, 25). Most transcription initiates from the downstream site (90% to 99%), and both sites are preceded by consensus TATA box sequences. Transcription from the downstream site is dramatically increased in hypothyroid rats and mice, while transcription from the upstream site is either unaffected or reduced by thyroid hormone (20,24,25).

The TSH-β gene in humans contains only one transcriptional start site in a location similar to that of the downstream site in the TSH-β gene in rats and mice (21–23). This difference may be due to an alteration in the upstream TATA box, which is changed from TATATAA in the rat and mouse gene to TGTATAA in the human gene. There may be an additional start site in the human gene (26). However, based on RNA mapping studies done in one TSH-secreting adenoma, this site does not correspond to the upstream TATA box in the human TSH-β gene.

Central Hypothyroidism Due to Thyrotropin-β-Subunit Gene Abnormalities or Alterations in Thyrotroph Development

Several kindreds with central hypothyroidism and undetectable or at least inappropriately low serum TSH concentrations due to mutations in the TSH β-subunit gene have been described (27,28). Two affected members of a Japanese family had a point mutation in exon 2 that changed a glycine residue to an arginine residue (G29R) (27). This mutation is in a region that is highly conserved among glycoprotein subunit genes (CAGY) and is thought to be important in subunit combination (Fig. 10A.2). This mutation resulted in synthesis of a TSH-β-subunit that could not associate with the α-subunit, and therefore no TSH heterodimer was produced.

Two related Greek families have been described in which affected family members had a mutation in the β-subunit of TSH that caused premature termination of synthesis of the subunit (E12X) (28). A Turkish family was found to have a different mutation that also resulted in premature termination of synthesis of the subunit (Q49X) (29). In another family a mutation was found in the second intron of the β-subunit gene (G29R) that predicts skipping of exon 2 and generation of a 25 amino-acid nonsense peptide from an aberrant start site in exon 3 (30). A Brazilian kindred with central hypothyroidism was described in which there was a frame-shift deletion in codon 105 (C105Vfs114X) of the β-subunit gene (31). This mutation substantially reduced TSH secretion, although some TSH was detected in the serum of the affected patients. Based on the crystallographic structure of the related hormone, CG, the mutation interferes with a disulfide bond that stabilizes

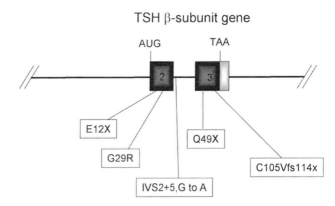

FIGURE 10A.2. Point mutations of the human thyrotropin (TSH) β-subunit gene in patients with familial TSH deficiency. Three point mutations in this gene have been described (see text). Two of these mutations (E12X and G29R) occur in exon 2, and predict either a truncated TSH-β subunit or one with an amino-acid change in the CAGY region. The *single letters* define the wild-type amino acid (preceding the number of the amino acid) and the substituted amino acid (after the number of the amino acid); *fs*, frame shift.

the αβ heterodimer of TSH (2). This mutation may be the most frequent β-subunit mutation (32). All of these disorders are autosomal recessive in inheritance, and affected family members do not produce TSH with biologic activity (Fig. 10A.2) (see Chapter 51).

Central hypothyroidism can also be caused by defects in pituitary development, which results in impaired formation or survival of thyrotrophs and expression of TSH (see Chapter 2). In general, pituitary organogenesis is characterized by the orderly expression of cell-specific transcription factors (Fig. 10A.3), including Pit-1, Prophet of Pit-1 (Prop-1), P-Lim (Lhx-3), Ptx, Hesx-1 (Rpx), and thyrotroph embryonic factor (TEF) (for review see reference 33).

TEF is expressed in the region of developing thyrotrophs, at the time of onset of expression of the β-subunit of TSH (34). TEF binds to sites in the promoter region of the β-subunit gene to regulate expression of the gene. In contrast, Pit-1 is expressed after the initiation of expression of the TSH-β-subunit gene (35). However, Pit-1 is required for thyrotroph survival and expression of the TSH-β-subunit gene. While there are Pit-1–dependent and Pit-1–independent thyrotrophs in the developing anterior pituitary, the latter population disappears before birth (35,36). Pit-1 also regulates the expression of growth hormone and prolactin, and is required for normal somatotroph and lactotroph function. In mice, Pit-1 mutations result in TSH, growth hormone, and prolactin deficiency and pituitary hypoplasia (37). Pit-1 mutations in humans cause analogous defects, a syndrome termed combined pituitary hormone deficiency (Fig. 10A.4) (38,39). A well-characterized Pit-1 mutation implicated in hypopituitarism in humans is the R271W mutation (40), which leads to production of a mutant Pit-1 that binds DNA but does not transactivate appropriately. These patients have hypothyroidism, but may have inappropriately normal serum TSH concentrations. They have a blunted serum TSH response to thyrotropin-releasing hormone (TRH),

suggesting the importance of Pit-1 in the TRH signaling pathway (see later in the chapter).

Not all Pit-1 mutations leading to combined pituitary hormone deficiency impair transactivation of the TSH subunit, growth hormone, and prolactin genes. The K216E mutation binds to DNA and transactivates normally (41) but binds poorly to retinoic acid receptors (RAR), leading to defective retinoic acid induction of the Pit-1 gene enhancer. This defect, in turn, causes impaired pituitary development (41).

Prop-1 gene expression precedes the expression of Pit-1, and appears to be required for the development of Pit-1–dependent cell lines. Ames mice, which have hormonal defects similar to those in Snell and Jackson dwarf mice, have a mutation in the alpha helix of the homeodomain of the Prop-1 gene (42). Similar to Snell and Jackson dwarf mice, analogous defects have been found in some patients with congenital combined pituitary hormone deficiency (43–45). These patients have central hypothyroidism as well as growth hormone and prolactin deficiency, similar to patients with Pit-1 mutations. However, patients with mutations in Prop-1 also tend to have LH and FSH deficiency. One common Prop-1 mutation is a 2-bp deletion (A301G302) (45), which results in impaired DNA binding (43).

PRETRANSLATIONAL REGULATION OF THYROTROPIN BIOSYNTHESIS

Thyroid Hormone

Thyroid hormone receptors (TR) are cellular homologues of the viral erythroblastic leukemia oncogene (v-erbA) (Fig. 10A.5). TRs are derived from two separate gene loci in mammals: α and β (see Chapter 8) (46). The α locus in humans is located on chromosome 17 (17q11.2) and the β locus on chromosome 3 (3p24.3). The TR-α gene undergoes alternative splicing, generating two isoforms: TR-α1

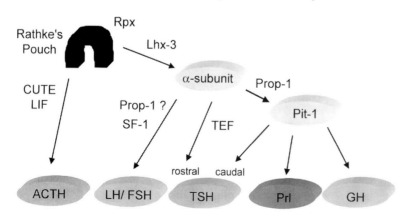

Anterior Pituitary Development

FIGURE 10A.3. Schematic representation of development of the anterior pituitary gland. The sequential expression of transcription factors leads to cell-specific expression of pituitary hormones. *ACTH*, corticotropin; *CUTE*, corticotroph upstream transcription binding protein; *GH*, growth hormone; *Prl*, prolactin; *Prop-1*, Prophet of Pit-1; *SF-1*, steroidogenic factor-1; and *TEF*, thyrotroph embryonic factor.

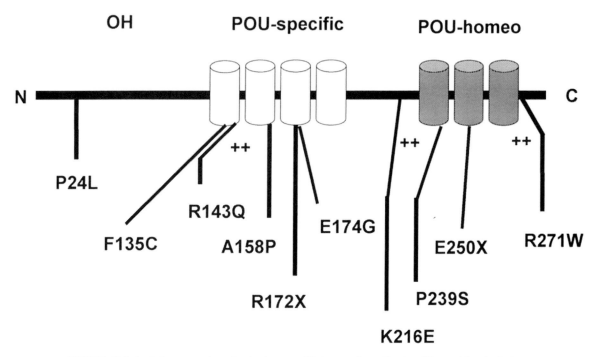

FIGURE 10A.4. Point mutations in the human Pit-1 gene in patients with combined pituitary hormone deficiency, as defined using the single-letter code for amino acids. POU-specific and POU-homeodomains, and the corresponding α-helices, are outlined in relation to indicated mutations in the Pit-1 gene. ++, lysine- and arginine-rich domains; *N*, the amino terminus of the Pit-1 protein; and *C*, the carboxyl terminus of the Pit-1 protein.

and TR-α2. TR-α1 is a bona fide TR, whereas alternative splicing of the C-terminus of TR-α2 generates a non–triiodothyronine (T_3)-binding isoform. The TR-β gene generates two major isoforms due to alternative promoter utilization: TR-β1 and TR-β2. This results in two β receptors, each with a different amino terminus.

TRs are variably expressed in mammals. In general, TR-α1 and TR-β1 are ubiquitously expressed. TR-α1 is most

highly expressed in the brain and heart, whereas TR-β1 is most highly expressed in the liver. In contrast, TR-β2 expression is limited principally to the hypothalamus, pituitary, cochlea, and retina (47). Differences in the expression patterns as well as structure of TRs suggest that one or both of these characteristics may determine thyroid hormone action in particular tissues.

TRs are members of the nuclear hormone receptor superfamily. TRs share in common with other members of this superfamily a conserved DNA-binding region, which contains two coordinated zinc molecules. Carboxy-terminal to the DNA-binding domain is the ligand-binding domain, which determines ligand-binding specificity. This domain is not highly conserved among different members of this superfamily. Similarly, the amino terminus domain, N-terminal to the DNA-binding domain, is not conserved in the superfamily. In addition to known ligands for members of this superfamily, other receptors known as orphan receptors have been described for which no ligands have been identified.

TRs bind to DNA as a homodimer or a heterodimer with the retinoid X receptor, also known as RXR (48). TR homodimers dissociate after binding T_3, whereas TR-RXR heterodimers do not. This has led to the suggestion that TR-RXR heterodimers are the most important determinants of T_3 action. In the absence of T_3, TRs bind constitutively to a class of proteins termed nuclear corepressors. These proteins share the characteristic of recruiting histone

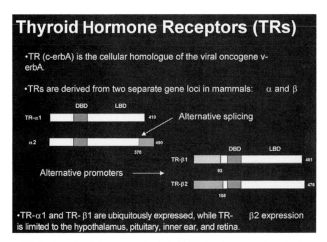

FIGURE 10A.5. Schematic drawing of the human thyroid hormone receptors. *DBD*, DNA-binding domain; *LBD*, ligand-binding domain.

deacetylase enzymes to the transcription complex, which results in histone deacetylation and increased chromatin packing (49). When T_3 binds to its receptors, the nuclear corepressors are released and nuclear coactivators are recruited. These include principally the p160 class of coactivators, named because of their molecular weight, as well as the cointegrator class of cofactors (CBP and p300). These proteins have intrinsic histone acetylase activity, which results in histone acetylation and unwrapping of the chromatin. Presumably, this looser configuration of chromatin allows easier access to RNA polymerase II, and transcription is increased. TRs are among the few members of the nuclear receptor superfamily that bind nuclear corepressors in the absence of ligand. This unique property suggests that it may control gene expression in a way that is unique from receptors that do not bind corepressors in this manner.

Thyroid hormone inhibits the synthesis and secretion of TSH at the level of the pituitary and indirectly at the level of the hypothalamus by reducing the secretion of TRH (50–53). In animals, thyroid hormone administration results in a dramatic decrease in the levels of messenger RNA (mRNA) for the common α- and TSH-β-subunits due to a reduction in transcription of the respective genes (50,51). However, the magnitude and rapidity of suppression varies among the subunits. In mouse TSH-secreting tumor cells exposed to T_3, the level of TSH-β mRNA fell more rapidly (50% inhibition at 4 hours) and to a greater extent (>95% suppression at 4 hours) than that of the common α-subunit. In addition, after prolonged T_3 exposure TSH-β-subunit mRNA was undetectable, whereas the level of α-subunit mRNA remains at approximately 25% of control levels (see section on regulation of thyrotropin secretion in this chapter) (50).

In addition to the expected suppression of TSH secretion by thyroid hormone, paradoxical increases in TSH secretion have been noted soon after initiation of thyroid hormone replacement, followed by later suppression of TSH secretion. In one study, administration of a low dose of T_3 to patients with hypothyroidism resulted in an increase in the serum TSH response to TRH (54). This effect may be due to a generalized defect in protein synthesis, corrected by low doses of T_3, or stimulation of expression of TSH subunit genes, perhaps by T_3 activation of a stimulatory cis-acting element.

The mechanisms underlying negative regulation of the TRH- and TSH-subunit genes by thyroid hormone are not clear. The thyroid hormone-inhibitory elements in these genes have unique properties, as compared with thyroid hormone-stimulatory elements (for review see reference 55). First, most of the inhibitory elements in these genes do not bind RXRs, and, unlike stimulating TR elements, RXRs antagonize TR binding to these elements (56). The exception is an important negative thyroid hormone re-

sponse element in the TRH gene promoter that binds TR monomers, TR homodimers, and TR-RXR heterodimers (57). Although some models suggest that negative regulation by thyroid hormone can occur in the absence of TR binding to DNA, newer *in vitro* and *in vivo* studies have clearly demonstrated that this binding is essential for thyroid hormone inhibition (58,59)

Studies in mice in which one or several of the TR isoforms were deleted have revealed that not all TR isoforms are involved in the production of TSH (60–64). The most important isoform controlling TSH production is TR-β2 (62). In the hypothalamus, it is perhaps the only isoform responsible for negative regulation of the TRH gene (65). It is also the most important isoform for negative regulation in the pituitary, although the TR-α1 and TR-β1 isoforms play some role at the extremes of serum thyroid hormone concentrations. Based on these studies, it seems clear that the main locus for the set point at which serum thyroid hormone concentrations control TSH secretion is the hypothalamus, due to the ability of TRH to modify the biological activity of TSH. In contrast, the main locus for coarse control of TSH synthesis is the pituitary (Fig. 10A.6).

In contrast to many mouse TR knockout models of resistance to thyroid hormone, human forms of this syndrome are caused by point mutations in the TR-β gene, except for one case (reviewed in 66) (see Chapter 81). This syndrome is characterized by mild-to-marked elevations in serum thyroxine (T_4) and T_3 concentrations and inappropriately normal or slightly high serum TSH concentrations resulting from resistance to thyroid hormone action in the hypothalamus and pituitary. Point mutations in the hinge region and ligand-binding domain of the gene for TR-β have been found in several hundred families; in contrast, no patients with mutations in the TR-α gene have been identified. Studies of mice in which the TR-β gene was knocked out provide an explanation for this curious finding in patients with thyroid hormone resistance. Mice with homozygous deletions of the TR-β gene have central resistance to thyroid hormone, indicating that the TR-α receptors cannot substitute for TR-β receptors in the regulation of TSH secretion (67,68). Thus, given the TR isoform–specific regulation of the pituitary, it is not surprising that TR mutations in patients with thyroid hormone resistance are found only in the gene for the β isoform of the TR. Moreover, a somatic mutation of the TR-β gene conferring thyroid hormone resistance was detected in a TSH-secreting pituitary tumor (69).

Steroid Hormones

TSH subunit gene expression is altered by steroid hormones, including glucocorticoids, estrogen, and testosterone. In humans, high doses of dexamethasone decrease serum TSH concentrations (70); dexamethasone also decreases TSH secretion in patients with TSH-secreting pituitary

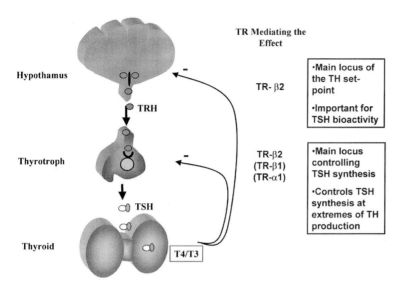

TR Mediating the
Effect

TR-β2

·Main locus of
the TH set-
point

·Important for
TSH bioactivity

TR-β2
(TR-β1)
(TR-α1)

·Main locus
controlling
TSH synthesis

·Controls TSH
synthesis at
extremes of TH
production

Hypothamus

TRH

Thyrotroph

TSH

Thyroid

T4/T3

FIGURE 10A.6. Schematic diagram of the hypothalamic–pituitary–thyroid axis. Thyroid hormone–inhibition of thyrotropin (TSH) secretion occurs both in the hypothalamus, where the hormones inhibit TSH secretion, and in the thyrotroph cells of the pituitary gland, where the hormones directly inhibit TSH secretion (central feedback). The role of individual thyroid hormone receptor *(TR)* isoforms in each compartment is summarized on the **right side** of the figure.

adenomas. In mice with thyrotropic tumors, dexamethasone decreased TSH secretion, but the levels of TSH-subunit mRNA in the tumor did not change (71). Therefore, dexamethasone may exert its effect on TSH-subunit biosynthesis at a translational or posttranslational level.

In animals and humans, estrogen administration does not alter basal or TRH-stimulated serum TSH concentrations (72). In hypothyroid rats, however, high doses of estradiol augment thyroid hormone-stimulated suppression of synthesis of α- and β-subunit mRNA (72). In animals, testosterone has similar effects, perhaps caused by its peripheral conversion to estrogen. Steroid hormones are not major regulators of TSH secretion under normal conditions, but they may play a role during some pathologic conditions such as hypothyroidism.

Thyrotropin-Releasing Hormone

In humans, TRH is the major positive regulator of TSH secretion. In animals, TRH stimulates the transcriptional activity of the TSH-subunit genes three- to fivefold (73). The stimulatory effect of TRH is augmented in hypothyroidism, which may be explained, at least in part, by an increase in the number of TRH receptors on the thyrotrophs (74). Alternatively, TRH may augment the effect of hypothyroidism to increase expression of the genes for the common α- and TSH β-subunits. There are cis-acting elements in the gene for the β-subunit of TSH in humans located between -128 and +8 bp in relation to the transcription start site (75). One element is located between -128 and -91 bp, and the second element is located from -28 to +8 bp and includes the TATA box and transcription start site. The upstream element in the human gene and the equivalent region in the rat gene bind the pituitary-specific transcription factor Pit-1 and mediate both TRH and cyclic AMP responsiveness of this gene through changes in the state of the Pit-1 protein (76). As noted above, mutations in Pit-1 result in loss of somatotroph, lactotroph, and thyrotroph function (combined pituitary hormone deficiency). In some families, only TRH-stimulation of TSH or prolactin secretion is impaired, and basal secretion of these hormones is normal, further implicating Pit-1 in the TRH signaling pathway. In fact, cyclic AMP-response element (CREB)-binding protein (CBP) and Pit-1 synergistically activate prolactin gene expression in response to TRH, suggesting a specific role for Pit-1 and CBP in TRH action (77,78).

In mice, deletion of the TRH gene results in central hypothyroidism (79). These animals have slightly high serum TSH concentrations, suggesting that TRH is not absolutely necessary for TSH production. However, their TSH has decreased biologic activity. Patients with TRH-receptor mutations have been described who also have hypothyroidism (see Chapter 48) (80,81).

In addition, in mice in which a mutant TR was expressed in the pituitary, thyroid hormone feedback at the pituitary, but not at the hypothalamus, was impaired (62). These mice had high serum TSH concentrations and high levels of TSH-β mRNA in the pituitary, but only a small increase in serum T_4 concentrations, indicating that the biological activity of the TSH was reduced. Because the mutant receptor was not expressed in the hypothalamus, T_3 feedback at this level was intact. In fact, in situ hybridization suggested that TRH gene expression was decreased compared with control animals. When TRH was replaced, serum T_4 concentrations increased significantly, suggesting that in thyroid hormone resistance syndromes resistance occurs at the levels of both the pituitary and hypothalamus (central resistance).

Cyclic AMP

Elevation of intracellular cyclic AMP levels increases the levels of mRNA of the common α- and TSH- β-subunits. The hypothalamic hormone arginine vasopressin stimulates TSH release from the thyrotrophs (82). It also stimulates TSH-subunit gene expression via an increase in cyclic AMP levels; however, it is unclear at present whether the vasopressin receptor in pituitary thyrotrophs is coupled to adenylyl cyclase. The TSH- β-subunit gene in humans has DNA sequences that mediate cyclic AMP induction located predominantly between -128 and -28 bp of the gene (75). This region does not contain DNA sequences homologous to the cyclic AMP-responsive element that binds the transacting factor, CREB, which mediates activation of the gene for the common α-subunit. Pit-1 interacts with CBP (77,82), and CBP and Pit-1 synergistically activate protein kinase A-dependent prolactin gene expression, suggesting a role for Pit-1 in cyclic AMP-mediated gene expression in the pituitary. The regions of CBP responsible for this protein kinase A effect are distinct from those involved in TRH stimulation of the prolactin gene (77).

Dopamine

Dopamine rapidly decreases basal and TRH-stimulated TSH secretion in man by approximately 50% (83). In rat pituitary cells, dopamine decreases TSH-subunit gene transcription by about 50% in 15 minutes, and inhibition is maximal (75% inhibition) in 30 minutes (73). Dopamine may act to decrease intracellular cyclic AMP levels and thus interfere with cyclic AMP-mediated stimulation of TSH-subunit gene expression. Endogenous dopamine may exert some tonic control of TSH secretion, because

dopamine antagonist drugs increase serum TSH concentrations transiently in normal subjects and patients with hypothyroidism (84,85).

Summary of Pretranslation Regulation of the Human Common α- and TSH-β-subunit Gene Expression

Figure 10A.7 is a schematic representation of a thyrotroph cell and the regulatory pathways that appear to be important in modifying TSH-subunit gene expression. Thyroid hormone is the major negative regulator of TSH-subunit gene expression; dopamine and somatostatin are less-important negative regulatory hormones. Thyroid hormone inhibits gene expression by binding to DNA cis-acting elements via a nuclear TR, and presumably interacts with the transcription initiation complex through protein–protein interactions. Somatostatin and presumably dopamine reduce intracellular cyclic AMP levels, via an *inhibitory* guanyl nucleotide-binding protein, and thus reduce TSH-subunit gene expression.

TRH is the major positive regulator of TSH-subunit gene expression and acts through a guanyl nucleotide-binding protein to activate phospholipase C. Phospholipase C hydrolyzes phosphatidylinositol 4,5-bisphosphate (PIP2) to diacylglycerol (DAG) and inositol 1,4,5 triphosphate (IP3). DAG activates protein kinase C, which, in turn, phosphorylates and presumably activates transacting nuclear factors responsible for TSH-subunit gene expression. IP3 releases Ca^{++} from intracellular pools and raises intracellular Ca^{++} levels. Another positive regulator of TSH-subunit gene expression is vasopressin, which may act via a *stimulatory* guanyl nucleotide-binding protein to increase intracellular cyclic AMP levels. Cyclic AMP then

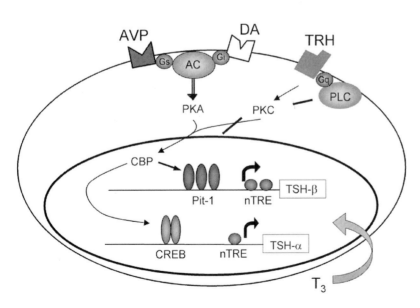

FIGURE 10A.7. Overview of the regulation of expression of the gene for the β-subunit of thyrotropin (TSH) within the thyrotroph cells of the pituitary gland (see text for details). *AC,* adenylyl cyclase; *CBP,* CREB-binding protein; *CREB,* cyclic adenosine monophosphate-response element; *DA,* dopamine; *Gi,* inhibitory guanine-nucleotide-binding protein; *Gs,* stimulatory guanine nucleotide-binding protein; *nTRE,* negative thyroid hormone-response element; *PKA,* protein kinase A; *PKC,* protein kinase C; *PLC,* phospholipase C; and *TR,* thyroid hormone receptor.

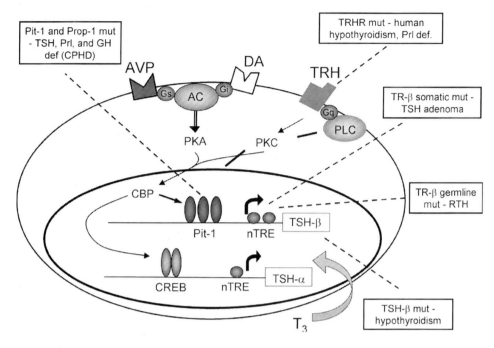

FIGURE 10A.8. Overview of molecular defects in the expression of genes for the subunits of TSH within the thyrotroph cells of the anterior pituitary gland. *AC*, adenylyl cyclase; *AVP*, arginine vasopressin; *CPHD*, combined pituitary hormone deficiencies; *CBP*, CREB-binding protein; *CREB*, cyclic adenosine monophosphate-response element; *Gi*, inhibitory guanine nucleotide-binding protein; *Gs*, stimulatory guanine nucleotide-binding protein; *mut*, mutation; *nTRE*, negative thyroid hormone-response element; *PKA*, protein kinase A; *PKC*, protein kinase C; and *TRHR*, thyrotropin-releasing hormone receptor.

activates protein kinase A (PKA) and cellular proteins are phosphorylated. One such protein is CREB, the cyclic AMP-response DNA-binding protein that has been shown to activate common α-subunit gene transcription. Protein kinase A activates TSH-β-subunit gene expression through a CREB-independent mechanism that is mediated, in part, by Pit-1. Human disorders that directly alter thyrotroph function are summarized in Fig. 10A.8.

POSTTRANSLATIONAL PROCESSING OF THYROTROPIN

In Vitro Translation of Thyrotropin-β-Subunit and α-Subunit Messenger RNA

The posttranslational processing of TSH was initially studied in cell-free translation systems, which were important to define the initial translation products, termed presubunits (86,87). Such pre–α- and pre–β-subunits contain the subunit proteins as well as amino-terminal leader or signal peptides necessary for translocation across the membrane of the endoplasmic reticulum.

α-Subunit mRNA was extracted from mouse thyrotropic tumors and translated in wheat germ or reticulocyte lysate cell-free systems devoid of the enzymes necessary for the proteolytic cleavage of polypeptide precursors or glycosylation (86,87). The major translation product, pre–α-subunit, had an apparent molecular weight of 14,000 to 17,000 daltons. Even though it did not contain carbohydrate, its molecular weight was about 3,000 dal-

tons greater than the protein portion of the standard α-subunit, suggesting the presence of a signal peptide

Detection of the TSH β-subunit precursor, pre-β, in cell-free translation mixtures of mouse tumor mRNA was also achieved, though this proved to be more difficult than detection of pre–α-subunits (88). Gel electrophoresis of the β precursor disclosed an apparent molecular weight of 15,000 (or 2,500 daltons greater than the protein portion of standard TSH-β-subunits), again consistent with the presence of a signal peptide.

Biosynthesis of Thyrotropin in Intact Cells

Cell-free mRNA translation studies were important to define the initial precursor forms of TSH subunits, because these forms are rapidly processed *in vivo*. Studies of TSH biosynthesis in intact cells, however, were necessary to elucidate the steps of posttranslational processing of TSH, including the glycosylation and combination of TSH subunits, and the subsequent processing of the oligosaccharides (89).

After incubation of mouse thyrotropic tumor tissue with ^{35}S-methionine for 10 minutes, most α-subunits had a molecular weight of 18,000 daltons, while a few had a molecular weight of 21,000 daltons (90). When the pulse incubation was followed by chase incubations, the 18,000-dalton form of the α-subunit was progressively converted to the 21,000-dalton form. Treatment with endoglycosidase H converted both the 18,000- and 21,000-dalton molecular weight forms to an 11,000-dalton form, consistent with the weight of the protein portion of standard α-subunits, suggesting that the 11,000-, 18,000-, and 21,000-dalton forms of the α-subunit have 0, 1, and 2 asparagine-linked oligosaccharide chains, respectively.

[35]S-methionine-labeled β-subunits accumulated as an 18,000-dalton form, which was then converted to an 11,000-dalton form after endoglycosidase H treatment. Thus, it appeared that the 11,000- and 18,000-dalton forms had 0 and 1 asparagine-linked oligosaccharide units, respectively (90). Approximately 20% of the β-subunits combined with excess α-subunits after a 20-minute pulse incubation. Analyses of subcellular fractionations disclosed that combination of α- and β-subunits began in the rough endoplasmic reticulum, and that the combining subunits had high-mannose, endoglycosidase H–sensitive oligosaccharides (91). TSH-subunit precursors were processed slowly to forms with mature complex oligosaccharides that were resistant to endoglycosidase H. TSH and excess free α-subunits, but no free β-subunits, were released into the medium after a 60- to 240-minute chase, and most had endoglycosidase H–resistant oligosaccharide chains.

The free α-subunits that were secreted had a slightly higher molecular weight than the form of α-subunit that combined with β-subunits. Free α-subunits from bovine pituitaries were found to be glycosylated at an additional site: the threonine at position 43 (92). This residue is located in a domain of the α-subunit thought to contact the β-subunit during heterodimer formation (1). Apparently, free α-subunits bearing this O-linked oligosaccharide are no longer able to bind to β-subunits. The physiologic importance of such noncombining forms of α-subunits is unclear.

Processing of High-Mannose Precursor Oligosaccharides

The subunits of TSH are cotranslationally glycosylated with oligosaccharides containing three glucose and nine mannose residues, termed high-mannose precursors. The oligosaccharides are preassembled in the rough endoplasmic reticulum, in which they are linked by phosphates at the reducing terminus to a long organic molecule containing approximately 20 units of polyprene, the dolichol phosphate carrier. Asparagine residues in nascent peptides destined to become glycosylated in an N-linked fashion are present in the sequence: asparagine-(X)-serine or asparagine-(X)-threonine, where X is any amino acid. There is a cotranslational en bloc transfer of the oligosaccharide from the dolichol carrier to the asparagine in the nascent α- or β-subunit. Two glucose residues are then quickly trimmed by a glucosidase, followed by a slower cleavage of the third glucose by another glucosidase. Mannose residues are then progressively cleaved by two mannosidases until a three-unit "core" remains, followed by addition of N-

acetylglucosamine (GlcNAc) and other sugars by specific glycosyltransferases, to form complex oligosaccharides. For the pituitary glycoprotein hormones, TSH and LH, such complex oligosaccharides may terminate in either sulfate or sialic acid residues and yield heterogeneous forms with one sulfate (S1), two sulfates (S2), one sialic acid (N1), two sialic acids (N2), three sialic acids (N3), or one sulfate and one sialic acid (S-N). Processing of the high-mannose oligosaccharides of the TSH subunits is relatively slow compared with other glycoproteins (90,93). The rate of trimming of mannose residues appears to be much faster for free α-subunits than for TSH β-subunits.

Terminal Sulfation and Sialylation of Complex Oligosaccharides

The presence of an unusual terminal constituent on TSH oligosaccharides was suggested by studies showing that TSH, unlike CG, was partially resistant to neuraminidase digestion. Subsequently, sulfate was detected as a component of certain complex oligosaccharides of α-subunits of bovine TSH and LH and human LH, but not human CG (94). The negatively charged sulfate was thought to play some functional role comparable to that of the negatively charged sialic acid. Later studies revealed metabolic incorporation of ^{35}S-sulfate into the oligosaccharides of the α- and β-subunits of bovine and ovine LH (95,96). Similarly, subunits of mouse TSH could be metabolically labeled with sulfate and sialic acid, there was differential sulfation of α- and β-subunits of TSH, and the sulfate moieties proved to be entirely linked to carbohydrate chains (97, 98).

The sulfate moiety in TSH and LH oligosaccharides is covalently linked to N-acetylgalactosamine residues, in contrast to the usual terminal structure of complex oligosaccharides, in which sialic acid is bound to galactose residues (99). Bovine pituitary tissue contains a N-acetylgalactosamine transferase that specifically recognizes the β-subunits of TSH and LH, as well as the common α-subunit (100). A pituitary sulfotransferase is responsible for transfer of the sulfate moiety to the oligosaccharide and does not require subunit peptide determinants for recognition. This enzyme, like the N-acetylgalactosamine transferase, is absent from the placenta, which explains why only pituitary glycoprotein hormones contain the unusual N-acetylgalactosamine sulfate terminal residues.

The structures and distributions of heterogeneous forms of sulfated and sialylated oligosaccharides on TSH as well as various other glycoprotein hormones have been determined (98,101). For bovine TSH, 48% of the oligosaccharides contained S2, 32% contained S1, 18% were neutral, and 2% contained S-N; no complex oligosaccharides contained sialic acid residues exclusively. In contrast, the complex oligosaccharide structure of human TSH was somewhat different: 25% contained S1, 21% contained S-N, 18% were neutral, 12% contained N2, and 5% contained N1.

In addition to terminal sulfation and sialylation, TSH oligosaccharides contain variable amounts of fucose linked to the innermost N-acetylglucosamine residue (101). In general, β-subunits of TSH contain about twice as much fucose as α-subunits. Although fucosylation is normally thought to occur primarily in the Golgi apparatus, in pituitaries from hypothyroid mice a major proportion of the fucosylation occurs in the rough endoplasmic reticulum (102). In normal subjects, intravenous infusion of TRH causes the acute release of TSH isoforms that are more highly fucosylated than the TSH present before TRH administration (103).

DEVELOPMENTAL AND ENDOCRINE REGULATION OF THYROTROPIN GLYCOSYLATION

The high-mannose oligosaccharides of TSH are differentially processed in mouse pituitary glands, depending on the thyroid state of the animals or level of TRH stimulation (93,104). *In vitro*, TRH stimulates the production of TSH enriched in biantennary complex oligosaccharides, as opposed to more complicated triantennary forms. This effect is closely coupled with TSH secretion, and intracellular forms of TSH do not vary in carbohydrate structure. *In vivo*, rats with hypothalamic or thyroidal hypothyroidism also have changes in the oligosaccharide structure of TSH (105–108). Animals with lesions of the paraventricular nucleus of the hypothalamus, which results in TRH deficiency, secreted TSH with fewer biantennary structures, as compared with normal animals. In contrast, thyroidectomized animals secreted TSH with more complex triantennary structures. Administration of TRH to the animals with hypothalamic lesions resulted in secretion of TSH with an increase in multiantennary structures so that their TSH was similar to that of normal animals. The differences between *in vitro* and *in vivo* TRH administration on the carbohydrate structure of TSH indicates that static exposure of cultured cells to TRH results in a pattern of glycosylation that differs from the resulting pulsatile pattern of TRH secretion *in vivo*. In TRH-knockout mice, the TSH that is secreted has decreased biological activity, presumably as a result of alterations in glycosylation (79).

The pattern of sulfation and sialylation of the oligosaccharides of TSH that is secreted varies during maturation of the pituitary–thyroid axis in rats (109–111). During the neonatal period, the amounts of sialylated oligosaccharides increased, as compared with sulfated oligosaccharides, as did all forms of complex oligosaccharides containing three or more negatively charged terminal moieties. In the neonatal period, hypothyroidism of even a few days or weeks duration resulted in major increases in the sialylated as compared with sulfated oligosaccharides. This change, present in both α- and β-subunits, was particularly striking in the latter. Moreover, there was a major increase in β-subunits containing three or more charged oligosaccharide units. Similar increases in the proportion of sialylated compared with sulfated oligosaccharides in TSH were found in adult hypothyroid rats, but, as compared with neonatal rats, the appearance of these changes was slow.

In humans, the sialylation of TSH varies among those who are normal and those with various thyroid disorders, in particular primary and central hypothyroidism (112, 113). Patients with severe nonthyroidal illness secrete forms of TSH with altered binding to concanavalin-A, suggesting increased amounts of multiantennary complex chains (114). In patients with TSH-secreting pituitary adenomas, the TSH and free α-subunits that are secreted vary considerably in oligosaccharide content (115,116), which changes if tumoral secretion of TSH falls in response to octreotide therapy (117,118) (see Chapter 24).

Thus, the complex carbohydrate structure of TSH can be altered by a variety of developmental, endocrine, and cellular factors. Although the functional effect of changes in the carbohydrate structure of TSH have not been completely elucidated, it is very clear that certain structure changes are associated with changes in the biologic activity of TSH or its metabolic clearance.

BIOACTIVITY AND METABOLIC CLEARANCE OF THYROTROPIN

Heterogeneous forms of TSH may have different degrees of biological activity in a variety of *in vivo* and *in vitro* bioassays (reviewed in 7). These differences in activity are primarily due to differences in carbohydrate composition, as noted previously. The role of the complex oligosaccharide moieties in TSH action has been determined by studies in which chemical or enzymatic deglycosylation was used to remove complex side-chains. In initial studies, bovine or human TSH preparations were deglycosylated with anhydrous hydrogen fluoride or trifluoromethane sulfonic acid (119–121). Although deglycosylated TSH had receptor-binding properties similar to those of the native hormone, its biological activity both *in vitro* and *in vivo* was markedly decreased. Moreover, the deglycosylated TSH competitively inhibited the action of native TSH (120). Most studies have confirmed the link between TSH oligosaccharide structure and bioactivity, and have established that the oligosaccharides of the α-subunit are particularly important for bioactivity (122–124).

TSH isohormones separated by isoelectric focusing have different bioactivity, but the chemical basis of the difference has remained unclear. Incubation of rat pituitary glands with TRH *in vitro* led to secretion of TSH with increased bioactivity (125). Because other studies (described earlier in the chapter) demonstrated that TRH alters the carbohydrate structure of TSH, it seems reasonable to conclude that such altered bioactivity is related to changes in carbohydrate. In fact, serum TSH from some patients with central hypothyroidism had a low ratio of biologic to immunologic activity, as compared with TSH from normal subjects (126). In some of the patients, chronic TRH administration resulted in secretion of TSH with more biological activity, as detected not only *in vitro*, but also by a rise in the patients' serum T_4 concentrations (126). Increases in the ratio of biologic to immunologic activity have also been found in the serum TSH of patients with TSH-secreting pituitary adenomas (127) and patients with resistance to thyroid hormone (128). However, a change in the ratio of biologic to immunologic activity of TSH in serum does not necessarily prove that its bioactivity has changed, because the ratio would also change if the hormone's immunologic activity changed.

The oligosaccharide content of TSH not only affects its bioactivity, but also its metabolic clearance. In humans, the half-time of disappearance of TSH varies with thyroid state—being slower in patients with hypothyroidism and faster in patients with thyrotoxicosis (129). In rats, the kidney is the major organ of clearance, with the thyroid being of secondary importance, and there is little hepatic clearance; chemically deglycosylated TSH is cleared more rapidly than is native TSH (130). Moreover, serum or pituitary TSH from hypothyroid rats is cleared more slowly than that from normal rats when injected into normal rats. These results suggest that the clearance of TSH varies according to both the thyroid status of the TSH 'donor' and the thyroid status of the animal in which the clearance studies are done. Presumably, the slower metabolic clearance rate of the TSH of hypothyroid rats is related to its increased sialylation (110,111). With respect to recombinant human TSH, sialylation is an important determinant of the hormone's metabolic clearance rate and *in vivo* bioactivity (10).

THREE-DIMENSIONAL CONFORMATION OF THYROTROPIN

While the exact structure of TSH is not known, the structure of human CG, as determined by crystallography, is known (3,4). Modeling of the structure of TSH based on the structure of CG has been extremely valuable in under-

standing its structure–function relationships (for review see reference 131); for example, it has allowed the location of the disulfide bonds within the subunits to be determined—crucial information for a meaningful model to be constructed. Based on a double alkylation method, TSH contains disulfide bonds analogous to human CG (132). Each TSH subunit has three loops (L1-L3) and a central cystine-knot structure (Fig. 10A.9). Two loops from the same subunit are on one side of the knot and a long loop is on the other side. The α-subunit loop 2 (αL2) loop is unique in that it contains a two-turn α helix. In the β-subunit of TSH, three disulfide bridges are involved in forming the cystine-knot, one bridge links two β-hairpin loops, and two bridges form the seat belt where the β-subunit wraps around the α-subunit. Moreover, one of the α-subunit oligosaccharides known to be more important for signal transduction, the oligosaccharide at Asn52, lies near TSH-subunit residues believed to be vital for receptor binding. However, differences in not only amino acid content but also glycosylation between human CG and TSH could affect their structures. Finally, TSH may undergo a conformational change when bound to its receptor.

The use of computer modeling, site-directed mutagenesis, and antibodies or synthetic peptides has enabled inves-

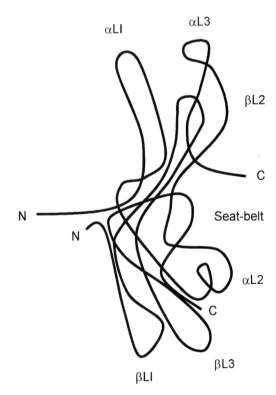

FIGURE 10A.9. Diagram of the structure of human thyrotropin (TSH) based on human chorionic gonadotropin crystallography and TSH structure–function studies. The seat-belt region is where the β-subunit wraps around loop 2 of the α-subunit (αL2) and stabilizes the TSH heterodimer. α*L*, α-subunit loop; β*L*, β-subunit loop.

tigators to make inferences about the three-dimensional conformation of TSH, the subunit contact domains, and the receptor-binding domains of the two subunits (133–142). For example, based on a mutagenesis approach, the seat-belt region appears to regulate the specificity of glycoprotein hormone receptor recognition (143). In particular, when the seat-belt region of TSH-β is replaced by the corresponding region of CG, the chimeric protein binds to the CG/LH receptor, but not the TSH receptor. Conversely, when the seat-belt region of CG is replaced by the corresponding region of TSH, CG/LH receptor recognition is abolished, and the chimeric protein binds to the TSH receptor. In contrast, when the seat-belt region of TSH is exchanged with that of FSH, the chimeric protein does not bind to the FSH receptor (143), suggesting that other regions also mediate the specificity of receptor interactions.

Mutagenesis experiments have also implicated domains in the α-subunit responsible for TSH action. For example, bovine TSH has greater biologic activity than human TSH, and they differ in amino acids 11 to 20 of the α-subunit. Replacement of amino acids 11, 13, 16, or 20 of the human α-subunit with lysine (all are present as lysine in the bovine α-subunit), and joining the mutant α-subunit with the β-subunit of human TSH, generates TSH molecules with greater receptor-binding affinity and biological activity than human TSH (144).

Mutagenesis of individual residues within amino acids 33 to 44 of the α-subunit has demonstrated the importance of this region for glycoprotein hormone assembly and action (145). In particular, Pro38 is important for heterodimerization with TSH-β and FSH-β. In contrast, Phe33 and Arg35 mediate heterodimerization with FSH-β, but not TSH-β, and Ala36 mediates heterodimeriztion with CG-β. Mutations of Arg35 impair the ability of TSH to stimulate cyclic AMP production in thyroid tissue, and residues Arg42-Ser43-Lys44 are important for TSH-receptor binding. Therefore, changes in the amino-terminal portion of the α-subunit generate mutants with altered capacity for heterodimerization and receptor binding, and altered *in vitro* bioactivity (144,145).

Mutations in the carboxyl-terminal portion of the α-subunit, residues 89 to 92, also cause decreased TSH receptor binding and bioactivity (146). In contrast, mutations in the cystine knot region of the α-subunit impaired secretion and heterodimer formation, but did not decrease *in vitro* bioactivity (147). Fusion of the α- and β-subunits created a single protein with longer half-life than native TSH, but normal receptor binding (148,149). Fusion of LH-β with the α-subunit also generated a mutant protein with increased stability (150). These data suggest that heterodimer dissociation is important in determining the *in vivo* half-life of glycoprotein hormones (148). These mutant hormones may be useful in generating other glycoprotein hormone analogs with novel properties.

RECOMBINANT HUMAN THYROTROPIN

Recombinant human TSH has been produced by transfection of the gene for the common α-subunit and the gene for the β-subunit of human TSH into human embryonic kidney cells or Chinese hamster ovary cells (151–153). The recombinant TSH was more highly sialylated than TSH extracted from human pituitary glands, and it also contained no N-acetylgalactosamine, implying the absence of terminal sulfate moieties [both are present in pituitary TSH (9)]. The absence of N-acetylgalactosamine and sulfate was expected, since only the pituitary contains the specific enzymes for transfer of these moieties to carbohydrate chains. The maximum stimulatory activity of recombinant human TSH was similar to that of pituitary TSH in two different *in vitro* bioassays (153); however, the recombinant preparation was slightly less potent as judged by the concentration required for half-maximal response. This decreased potency was clearly related to the increased sialic acid content, because the activity of the TSH increased after treatment with neuraminidase. In rats, the rate of metabolic clearance of recombinant human TSH was slower, by half, than that of pituitary TSH, which resulted in greater than 10-fold higher serum concentrations 3 hours after intravenous TSH administration (153). The slower metabolic clearance rate was again related to the increased sialic acid content, since neuraminidase-treated TSH was cleared considerably faster. All these differences can be related to the higher degree of sialylation of recombinant human TSH, as compared with standard pituitary TSH.

It is possible to produce recombinant human TSH in large quantities (10). Unlike natural human TSH extracted and purified derived from pools of human pituitaries obtained at autopsy, recombinant TSH is more homogeneous and free of other contaminating pituitary hormones and growth factors as well as artifactual proteolytic cleavage products. The heterogeneity of the recombinant hormone is primarily related to six to nine different isoforms, differing in the number of terminal sialic acid residues present in the carbohydrate chains (10).

Recombinant TSH is also valuable clinically and has provided a new diagnostic agent for the evaluation of patients with thyroid carcinoma (see Chapter 14 and section on radioiodine and other treatments and outcomes in Chapter 70).

REFERENCES

1. Pierce JG, Parsons TF. Glycoprotein hormones: structure and function. *Annu Rev Biochem* 1981;50:465.
2. Lapthorn AJ, Harris DC, Littlejohn A, et al. Crystal structure of human chorionic gonadotropin. *Nature* 1994;369:455.
3. Wu H, Lustbader JW, Liu Y, et al. Structure of human chorionic gonadotropin at 2.6A resolution from MAD analysis of the selenomethionyl protein. *Structure* 1994;2:545.

4. Magner JA. Thyroid-stimulating hormone: biosynthesis, cell biology, and bioactivity. *Endocr Rev* 1990;11:354.

5. Green ED, Baenziger JU. Asparagine-linked oligosaccharides on lutropin, follitropin, and thyrotropin. I. structural elucidation of the sulfated and sialylated oligosaccharides on bovine, ovine, and human pituitary glycoprotein hormones. *J Biol Chem* 1988;263:25.

6. Green ED, Baenziger JU. Asparagine-linked oligosaccharides on lutropin, follitropin, and thyrotropin. II. Distributions of sulfated and sialylated oligosaccharides on bovine, ovine, and human pituitary glycoprotein hormones. *J Biol Chem* 1988;263:36.

7. Persani L. Hypothalamic thyrotropin-releasing hormone and thyrotropin biological activity. *Thyroid* 1998;8:941.

8. Cole ES, Lee K, Lauziere K, et al. Recombinant human thyroid stimulating hormone: development of a biotechnology product for detection of metastatic lesions of thyroid carcinoma. *Biotechnology* 1993;11:1014.

9. Szkudlinski MW, Thotakura NR, Bucci I, et al. Purification and characterization of recombinant human thyrotropin (TSH) isoforms produced by Chinese hamster ovary cells: the role of sialylation and sulfation in TSH bioactivity. *Endocrinology* 1993; 133:1490.

10. Braverman LE, Pratt BM, Ebner S, et al. Recombinant human thyrotropin stimulates thyroid function and radioactive iodine uptake in the rhesus monkey. *J Clin Endocrinol Metab* 1992; 74:1135.

11. Ladenson PW, Braverman LE, Mazzaferri EL, et al. Comparison of administration of recombinant human thyrotropin with withdrawal of thyroid hormone for radioactive iodine scanning in patients with thyroid carcinoma. *N Engl J Med* 1997;337: 888.

12. Goodwin RG, Moncman CL, Rottman FM, et al. Characterization and nucleotide sequence of the gene for the common α-subunit of the bovine pituitary glycoprotein hormones. *Nucleic Acids Res* 1983;11:6873

13. Gordon DF, Wood WM, Ridgway EC. Organization and nucleotide sequence of the mouse α-subunit gene of the pituitary glycoprotein hormones. *DNA* 1988;7:679

14. Burnside J, Buckland PR, Chin WW. Isolation and characterization of the gene encoding the α-subunit of the rat pituitary glycoprotein hormones. *Gene* 1988;70:67.

15. Fiddes JC, Goodman HM. The gene encoding the common alpha subunit of the four human glycoprotein hormones. *J Mol Appl Genet* 1981;1:3.

16. Breathnach R, Chambon P. Organization and expression of eucaryotic split genes coding for proteins. *Annu Rev Biochem* 1981;50:349.

17. Deutsch PJ, Jameson JL, Habener JF. Cyclic AMP responsiveness of human gonadotropin α gene transcription is directed by a repeated 10-bp enhancer. *J Biol Chem* 1987;262:12169.

18. Silver BJ, Bokar JA, Virgin JB, et al. Cyclin AMP regulation of the human glycoprotein hormone α-subunit is mediated by an 18-bp element. *Proc Natl Acad Sci U S A* 1987;84: 2198.

19. Bokar JA, Keri RA, Farmerie TA, et al. Expression of the glycoprotein hormone α-subunit gene in the placenta requires a functional cyclic AMP response element, whereas a different cis-acting element mediates pituitary-specific expression. *Mol Cell Biol* 1989;9:5113.

20. Carr FE, Need LR, Chin WW. Isolation and characterization of the rat thyrotropin β-subunit gene: differential regulation of two transcriptional start sites by thyroid hormone. *J Biol Chem* 1987;262:981.

21. Wondisford FE, Radovick S, Moates JM, et al. Isolation and characterization of the human thyrotropin β-subunit gene. *J Biol Chem* 1988;262:12538

22. Guidon PT, Whitfield GK, Porti D, et al. The human thyrotropin β-subunit gene differs in 5' structure from murine TSHβ genes. DNA 1988;7:691.

23. Tatsumi K, Hayashizaki Y, Hiraoka Y, et al. The structure of the human thyrotropin β-subunit gene. *Gene* 1988;73:489

24. Wolf D, Kourides IA, Gurr JA. Expression the gene for the β-subunit of mouse thyrotropin results in multiple mRNAs differing in their 5' untranslated region. *J Biol Chem* 1987;262: 16596.

25. Gordon DF, Wood WM, Ridgway EC. Organization and nucleotide sequence of the gene encoding the beta subunit of murine thyrotropin. DNA 1988;7:17.

26. Samuels MH, Wood WM, Gordon DF, et al. Clinical and molecular studies of a thyrotropin-secreting pituitary adenoma. *J Clin Endocrinol Metab* 1989;68:1211.

27. Hayashizaki Y, Hiraoka Y, Endo Y, et al. Thyroid-stimulating hormone (TSH) deficiency caused by a single base substitution in the CAGYC region of the β-subunit. *EMBO J* 1989; 8:2291.

28. Dacou-Voutetakis C, Feltquate DM, Drakopoulou M, et al. Familial hypothyroidism caused by a nonsense mutation in the thyroid-stimulating hormone β-subunit gene. *Am J Hum Genet* 1990;16:988.

29. Vuissoz JM, Deladoey J, Buyukgebiz A, et al. New autosomal recessive mutation of the TSH-beta subunit gene causing central isolated hypothyroidism. *J Clin Endocrinol Metab* 2001; 86:4468.

30. Pohlenz J, Dumitrescu A, Aumann U, et al. Congenital secondary hypothyroidism caused by exon skipping due to a homozygous donor splice site mutation in the TSH beta subunit gene. *J Clin Endocrinol Metab* 2002; 87:336.

31. Medeiros-Neto G, Herodotou DT, Rajan S, et al. A circulating, biologically inactive thyrotropin caused by a mutation in the beta subunit gene. *J Clin Invest* 1996;97:1250.

32. Deladoey J, Vuissoz JM, Domene HM, et al. Congenital secondary hypothyroidism due to a mutation C105Vfs114X thyrotropin-beta mutation: genetic study of five unrelated families from Switzerland and Argentina. *Thyroid* 2003;13:553.

33. Cohen LE, Radovick S. Molecular basis of combined pituitary hormone deficiencies. *Endocr Rev* 2002;23:431.

34. Drolet DW, Scully KM, Simmons DM, et al. TEF, a transcription factor expressed specifically in the anterior pituitary during embryogenesis, defines a new class of leucine zipper proteins. *Genes Dev* 1991;5:1739.

35. Lin SC, Li S, Drolet DW, et al. Pituitary ontogeny of the Snell dwarf mouse reveals Pit-1-independent and Pit-1-dependent origins of the thyrotrope. *Development* 1994;120:515.

36. Cohen LE, Wondisford FE, Radovick S. Role of Pit-1 in the gene expression of growth hormone, prolactin, and thyrotropin. *Endocrinol Metab Clin North Am* 1996; 25:523.

37. Li S, Crenshaw EB, Rawson EJ, et al. Dwarf locus mutants lacking three pituitary cell types result from mutations in the POU-domain pit-1. *Nature* 1990;347:528.

38. Radovick S, Nations M, Du Y, et al. A mutation in the POU-homeodomain of Pit-1 responsible for combined pituitary hormone deficiency. *Science* 1992;257:1115.

39. Pfaffle RW, DiMattia GE, Parks JS, et al. Mutation of the POU-specific domain of Pit-1 and hypopituitarism without pituitary hypoplasia. *Science* 1992;257:1118.

40. Cohen LE, Wondisford FE, Salvatoni A, et al. A "hot spot" in the Pit-1 gene responsible for combined pituitary hormone deficiency: clinical and molecular correlates. *J Clin Endocrinol Metab* 1995; 80:679.

41. Cohen LE, Zanger K, Brue T, et al. Defective retinoic acid regulation of the Pit-1 gene enhancer: a novel mechanism of combined pituitary hormone deficiency. *Mol Endocrinol* 1999;13: 476.

42. Sornson MW, Wu W, Dasen JS, et al. Pituitary lineage determination by the prophet of Pit-1 homeodomain factor defective in Ames dwarfism. *Nature* 1996;384:327.

43. Wu W, Cogan JD, Pfaffle RW, et al. Mutations in PROP1 cause familial combined pituitary hormone deficiency. *Nat Genet* 1998;18:147.

44. Fluck C, Deladoey, Rutishauser K, et al. Phenotypic variability in familial combined pituitary hormone deficiency caused by a PROP1 gene mutation resulting in the substitution of Arg–Cys at Codon 120 (R120C). *J Clin Endocrinol Metab* 1998;83:3727.

45. Cogan JD, Wu W, Phillips JA, et al. The PROP1 2-base pair deletion is a common cause of combined pituitary hormone deficiency. *J Clin Endocrinol Metab* 1998;83:3346.

46. Lazar M.A. Thyroid hormone receptors: multiple forms, multiple possibilities. *Endocr Rev* 1993 14:184.

47. Bradley DJ, Towle HC, Young WS 3rd. Alpha and beta thyroid hormone receptor (TR) gene expression during auditory neurogenesis: evidence for TR isoform-specific transcriptional regulation in vivo. *Proc Natl Acad Sci U S A* 1994;91:439.

48. Yen PM. Physiological and molecular basis of thyroid hormone action. *Physiol Rev* 2001;81:1097.

49. Jepsen K, Rosenfeld MG. Biological roles and mechanistic actions of co-repressor complexes. *J Cell Sci* 2002;115:689.

50. Shupnik MA, Chin WW, Habener JF, et al. Transcriptional regulation of the thyrotropin subunit genes by thyroid hormone. *J Biol Chem* 1985;260:2900.

51. Gurr JA, Kourides IA. Thyroid hormone regulation of thyrotropin α and β-subunit gene transcription. *DNA* 1985;4:301.

52. Segerson TP, Kauer J, Wolfe HC, et al. Thyroid hormone regulates TRH biosynthesis in the paraventricular nucleus of the rat hypothalamus. *Science* 1987;238:78.

53. Taylor T, Wondisford FE, Blaine T, et al. The paraventricular nucleus of the hypothalamus has a major role in thyroid hormone feedback regulation of thyrotropin synthesis and secretion. *Endocrinology* 1990;126:317.

54. Ridgway EC, Kourides IA, Chin WW, et al. Augmentation of pituitary thyrotropin response to TRH during subphysiological triiodothyronine therapy in hypothyroidism. *Clin Endocrinol (Oxf)* 1979;10:343.

55. Wondisford FE. Thyroid hormone action: insight from transgenic mouse models. *J Investig Med* 2003;51:215.

56. Cohen O, Flynn TR, Wondisford FE. Ligand-dependent antagonism by retinoid X receptors of inhibitory thyroid hormone response elements. *J Biol Chem* 1995;270:13899.

57. Hollenberg AN, Monden T, Flynn TR, et al. The human thyrotropin-releasing hormone gene is regulated by thyroid hormone through two distinct classes of negative thyroid hormone response elements. *Mol Endocrinol* 1995;9:540.

58. Shibusawa N, Hollenberg AN, Wondisford FE. Thyroid hormone receptor DNA binding is required for both positive and negative gene regulation. *J Biol Chem* 2003 278:732.

59. Shibusawa N, Hashimoto K, Nikrodhanond AA, et al. Thyroid hormone action in the absence of thyroid hormone receptor DNA-binding in vivo. *J Clin Invest* 2003;112:588.

60. Forrest D, Erway LC, Ng L, et al. Thyroid hormone receptor beta is essential for development of auditory function. *Nat Genet* 1996;13:354.

61. Weiss RE, Forrest D, Pohlenz J, et al. Thyrotropin regulation by thyroid hormone in thyroid hormone receptor beta-deficient mice. *Endocrinology* 1997;138:3624.

62. Abel ED, Boers ME, Pazos-Moura C, et al. Divergent roles for thyroid hormone receptor beta isoforms in the endocrine axis and auditory system. *J Clin Invest* 1999;104:291.

63. Gauthier K, Chassande O, Plateroti M, et al. Different functions for the thyroid hormone receptors TR alpha and TR beta in the control of thyroid hormone production and post-natal development. *EMBO J* 1999;18:623.

64. Gothe S, Wang Z, Ng L, et al. Mice devoid of all known thyroid hormone receptors are viable but exhibit disorders of the pituitary-thyroid axis, growth, and bone maturation. *Genes Dev* 1999;13:1329.

65. Abel ED, Ahima R, Boer ME, et al. Critical role for thyroid hormone receptor β-2 in the regulation of TRH neurons in the paraventricular hypothalamus. *J Clin Invest* 2001;107:1017.

66. Weiss RE, Refetoff S. Resistance to thyroid hormone. *Rev Endocrinol Metab Disord* 2000;1:97.

67. Hashimoto K, Curty FH, Borges PP, et al. An unliganded thyroid hormone receptor causes severe neurological dysfunction. *Proc Natl Acad Sci U S A* 2001;98:3998.

68. Kaneshige M, Kaneshige K, Zhu X, et al. Mice with a targeted mutation in the thyroid hormone beta receptor gene exhibit impaired growth and resistance to thyroid hormone. *Proc Natl Acad Sci U S A* 2000;97:13209.

69. Ando S, Sarlis NJ, Krishnan J, et al. Aberrant alternative splicing of thyroid hormone receptor in a TSH-secreting pituitary tumor is a mechanism for hormone resistance. *Mol Endocrinol* 2001;15:1529.

70. Re RN, Kourides IA, Ridgway EC. The effect of glucocorticoid administration on human pituitary secretion of thyrotropin and prolactin. *J Clin Endocrinol Metab* 1976;43:338.

71. Ross DS, Ellis MF, Milbury P, et al. A comparison of changes in plasma thyrotropin β and α-subunits, and mouse thyrotropic tumor thyrotropin β and α-subunit mRNA concentrations after in vivo dexamethasone or T3 administration. *Metabolism* 1987;36:799.

72. Ahlquist JAO, Franklyn JA, Wood DF, et al. Hormonal regulation of thyrotropin synthesis and secretion. *Horm Metab Res Suppl* 1987;17:86.

73. Shupnik MA, Greenspan SL, Ridgway EC. Transcriptional regulation of thyrotropin subunit genes by thyrotropin-releasing hormone and dopamine in pituitary cell culture. *J Biol Chem* 1986; 261:12675.

74. Perrone MH, Hinkle PM. Regulation of pituitary receptors for thyrotropin-releasing hormone by thyroid hormones. *J Biol Chem* 1978;253:5168.

75. Weintraub BD, Wondisford FE, Farr EA, et al. Pre-translational and post-translational regulation of TSH synthesis in normal and neoplastic thyrotrophs. *Horm Res* 1989;32:22.

76. Steinfelder HJ, Radovick S, Wondisford FE. Hormonal regulation of the thyrotropin β subunit gene by phosphorylation of the pituitary-specific transcription factor Pit-1. *Proc Natl Acad Sci U S A* 1992;89:5942.

77. Zanger K, Cohen LE, Hashimoto K, et al. A novel mechanism for cyclic adenosine 3′,5′-monophosphate regulation of gene expression by CREB-binding protein. *Mol Endocrinol* 1999; 13: 268.

78. Hashimoto K, Zanger K, Hollenberg AN, et al. cAMP response element-binding protein-binding protein mediates thyrotropin-releasing hormone signaling on thyrotropin subunit genes. *J Biol Chem* 2000;275:33365.

79. Yamada M, Saga Y, Shibusawa N, et al. Tertiary hypothyroidism and hyperglycemia in mice with targeted disruption of the thyrotropin-releasing hormone gene. *Proc Natl Acad Sci U S A* 1997;94:10862.

80. Collu R, Tang J, Castagne J, et al. A novel mechanism for isolated central hypothyroidism: inactivating mutations in the thyrotropin-releasing hormone receptor gene. *J Clin Endocrinol Metab* 1997;82:1561.

81. Collu R. Genetic aspects of central hypothyroidism. *J Endocrinol Invest* 2000 ;23:125.

82. Xu L, Lavinsky RM, Dasen JS, et al. Signal-specific co-activator domain requirements for Pit-1 activation. *Nature* 1998; 395:301.

83. Cooper DS, Klibanski A, Ridgway EC. Dopaminergic modulation of TSH and its subunits; in vivo and in vitro studies. *Clin Endocrinol (Oxf)* 1983;18:265.

84. Scanlon WF, Weightman DR, Shale DJ, et al. Dopamine is a physiological regulator of thyrotropin secretion in man. *Clin Endocrinol (Oxf)* 1979;10:7.

85. Lee E, Chen P, Rao H, et al. Effect of acute high dose dobutamine administration on serum thyrotrophin (TSH). *Clin Endocrinol (Oxf)* 1999;50:487.

86. Chin WW, Habener JF, Kieffer JD, et al. Cell-free translation of the messenger RNA coding for the α-subunit of thyroid-stimulating hormone. *J Biol Chem* 1978;253:7985.

87. Kourides IA, Weintraub BD. mRNA directed biosynthesis of α subunit of thyrotropin: translation in cell-free and whole-cell systems. *Proc Natl Acad Sci U S A* 1979;76:298.

88. Giudice LC, Weintraub BD. Evidence for conformational differences between precursor and processed forms of TSH-β-subunit. *J Biol Chem* 1979;254:12679.

89. Chin WW, Maloof F, Habener JF. Thyroid-stimulating hormone biosynthesis. *J Biol Chem* 1981;256:3059.

90. Weintraub BD, Stannard BSD, Magner JA, et al. Glycosylation and post-translational processing of thyroid-stimulating hormone: clinical implications. *Recent Prog Horm Res* 1985;41: 577.

91. Magner JA, Weintraub BD. Thyroid-stimulating hormone subunit processing and combination in microsomal subfractions of mouse pituitary tumor. *J Biol Chem* 1982;257:6709.

92. Parsons TF, Bloomfield GA, Pierce JG. Purification of an alternative form of the α subunit of the glycoprotein hormones from bovine pituitaries and identification of its O-linked oligosaccharides. *J Biol Chem* 1983;258:240.

93. Ronin C, Stannard BS, Weintraub BD. Differential processing and regulation of thyroid-stimulating hormone subunit carbohydrate chains in thyrotropic tumors and in normal and hypothyroid pituitaries. *Biochemistry* 1985;24:562.

94. Parsons TF, Pierce JG. Oligosaccharide moieties of glycoprotein hormones: bovine lutropin resists enzymatic deglycosylation because of terminal O-sulfated N-acetylhexosamines. *Proc Natl Acad Sci U S A* 1980;77:7089.

95. Hortin G, Natowicz M, Pierce J, et al. Metabolic labeling of lutropin with [35S]sulfate. *Proc Natl Acad Sci U S A* 1981;78: 7468.

96. Anumula KR, Bahl OP. Biosynthesis of lutropin in ovine pituitary slices: incorporation of [35S]sulfate in carbohydrate units. *Arch Biochem Biophys* 1993;220:645.

97. Gesundheit N, Magner JA, Chen T, et al. Differential sulfation and sialylation of secreted mouse thyrotropin (TSH) subunits: regulation by TSH-releasing hormone. *Endocrinology* 1986; 119:455.

98. Gesundheit N, Gyves PW, DeCherney GS, et al. Characterization and charge distribution of the asparagine-linked oligosaccharides on secreted mouse thyrotropin and free α subunits. *Endocrinology* 1989;124:2967.

99. Baenziger JU, Green ED. Pituitary glycoprotein hormone oligosaccharides: structure, synthesis and function of the asparagine-linked oligosaccharides on lutropin, follitropin and thyrotropin. *Biochim Biophys Acta* 1988;947:287.

100. Smith PL, Baenziger JU. A pituitary N-acetylgalactosamine transferase that specifically recognizes glycoprotein hormones. *Science* 1988;242:930.

101. Hiyama J, Weisshaar G, Renwick AG. The asparagine-linked oligosaccharides at individual glycosylation sites in human thyrotropin. *Glycobiology* 1992;2:401.

102. Magner JA, Novak W, Papagiannes E. Subcellular localization of fucose incorporation into mouse thyrotropin and free α subunits: studies employing subcellular fractionation and inhib-

itors of the intracellular translocation of proteins. *Endocrinology* 1986;119:1315.

103. Magner JA, Kane J, Chou ET. Intravenous thyrotropin (TSH)-releasing hormone releases human TSH that is structurally different than basal TSH. *J Clin Endocrinol Metab* 1992;74:1306.

104. Gesundheit N, Fink DL, Silverman LA, et al. Effect of thyrotropin-releasing hormone on the carbohydrate structure of secreted mouse thyrotropin: analysis by lectin affinity chromatography. *J Biol Chem* 1987;262:5197.

105. Taylor T, Gesundheit N, Gyves PW, et al. Hypothalamic hypothyroidism caused by lesions in rat paraventricular nuclei alters the carbohydrate structure of secreted thyrotropin. *Endocrinology* 1988;122:283.

106. Taylor T, Gesundheit N, Weintraub BD. Effects of in vivo bolus versus continuous TRH administration on TSH secretion, biosynthesis, and glycosylation in normal and hypothyroid rats. *Mol Cell Endocrinol* 1986;46:253.

107. Taylor T, Weintraub BD. Altered thyrotropin (TSH) carbohydrate structures in hypothalamic hypothyroidism created by paraventricular nuclear lesions are corrected by in vivo TSH-releasing hormone. *Endocrinology* 1989;125:2198.

108. Taylor T, Wondisford FE, Blaine T, et al. The paraventricular nucleus of the hypothalamus has a major role in thyroid feedback regulation of thyrotropin synthesis and secretion. *Endocrinology* 1990;126:317.

109. Gyves PW, Gesundheit N, Stannard BS, et al. Alterations in the glycosylation of secreted thyrotropin during ontogenesis: analysis of sialylated and sulfated oligosaccharides. *J Biol Chem* 1989;264:6104.

110. Gyves PW, Gesundheit N, Thotakura NR, et al. Changes in the sialylation and sulfation of secreted thyrotropin in congenital hypothyroidism. *Proc Natl Acad Sci U S A* 1990;87: 3792.

111. DeCherney GS, Gesundheit N, Gyves PW, et al. Alterations in the sialylation and sulfation of secreted mouse thyrotropin in primary hypothyroidism. *Biochem Biophys Res Commun* 1989; 159:755.

112. Papandreou M-J, Persani L, Asteria C, et al. Variable carbohydrate structures of circulating thyrotropin as studied by lectin affinity chromatography in different clinical conditions. *J Clin Endocrinol Metab* 1993;77:393.

113. Papandreou M-J, Asteria C, Pettersson K, et al. Concanavalin A affinity chromatography of human serum gonadotropins: evidence for changes of carbohydrate structure in different clinical conditions. *J Clin Endocrinol Metab* 1993;76:1008.

114. Lee HL, Suhl J, Pekary AE, et al. Secretion of thyrotropin with reduced concanavalin-A-binding activity in patients with severe nonthyroidal illness. *J Clin Endocrinol Metab* 1987;65:942.

115. Magner JA, Klibanski A, Fein H, et al. Ricin and lentil lectin-affinity chromatography reveals oligosaccharide heterogeneity of thyrotropin secreted by 12 human pituitary tumors. *Metabolism* 1992;41:1009.

116. Sergi I, Medri G, Papandreou M-J, et al. Polymorphism of thyrotropin and alpha subunit in human pituitary adenomas. *J Endocrinol Invest* 1993;16:45.

117. Chanson P, Weintraub BD, Harris AG. Octreotide therapy for thyroid-stimulating hormone-secreting pituitary adenomas: a follow-up of 52 patients. *Ann Intern Med* 1993;119: 236.

118. Francis TB, Smallridge RC, Kane J, et al. Octreotide changes serum thyrotropin (TSH) glycoisomer distribution as assessed by lectin chromatography in a TSH macroadenoma patient. *J Clin Endocrinol Metab* 1993;77:183.

119. Amir SM, Kubota K, Tramontano D, et al. The carbohydrate moiety of bovine thyrotropin is essential for full bioactivity but not for receptor recognition. *Endocrinology* 1987;120: 345.

120. Amr S, Menezes-Ferreira MM, Shimohigashi Y, et al. Activities of deglycosylated thyrotropin at the thyroid membrane receptor adenylate cyclase system. *J Endocrinol Invest* 1986;8:537.

121. Thotakura NR, LiCalzi L, Weintraub BD. The role of carbohydrate in thyrotropin action assessed by a novel method of enzymatic deglycosylation. *J Biol Chem* 1990;265:11527.

122. Endo Y, Tetsumoto T, Nagasaki H, et al. The distinct roles of α and β subunits of human thyrotropin in the receptor-binding and postreceptor events. *Endocrinology* 1990;127:149.

123. Thotakura NR, Szkudlinski MW, Weintraub BD. Structure-function studies of oligosaccharides of recombinant human thyrotrophin by sequential deglycosylation and resialylation. *Glycobiology* 1994;4:525.

124. Beck-Peccoz P, Persani L. Variable biological activity of thyroid-stimulating hormone. *Acta Endocrinol (Copenh)* 1994;131:331.

125. Menezes-Ferreira MM, Petrick PA, Weintraub BD. Regulation of thyrotropin (TSH) bioactivity by TSH-releasing hormone and thyroid hormone. *Endocrinology* 1986;118:2125.

126. Beck-Peccoz, Amr S, Menezes-Ferreira MM, et al. Decreased receptor binding of biologically inactive thyrotropin in central hypothyroidism: effect of treatment with thyrotropin-releasing hormone. *N Engl J Med* 1985;312:1085.

127. Nissim M, Lee KO, Petrick PA, et al. A sensitive thyrotropin (TSH) bioassay based on iodide uptake in rat FRTL-5 thyroid cells: comparison with the adenosine 3′,5′-monophosphate response to human serum TSH and enzymatically deglycosylated bovine and human TSH. *Endocrinology* 1987;121:1278.

128. Persani L, Asteria C, Tonacchera M, et al. Evidence for the secretion of thyrotropin with enhanced bioactivity in syndromes of thyroid hormone resistance. *J Clin Endocrinol Metab* 1994;78:1034.

129. Ridgway EC, Weintraub BD, Maloof F. Metabolic clearance and production rates of human thyrotropin. *J Clin Invest* 1974;53:895.

130. Constant RB, Weintraub BD. Differences in the metabolic clearance of pituitary and serum thyrotropin (TSH) derived from euthyroid and hypothyroid rats: effects of chemical deglycosylation of pituitary TSH. *Endocrinology* 1986;119:2720.

131. Szkudlinski MW, Fremont V, Ronin C, et al. Thyroid-stimulating hormone and thyroid-stimulating hormone receptor structure-function relationships. *Physiol Rev* 2002;82:473.

132. Fairlie WD, Stanton PG, Hearn MT. The disulphide bond structure of thyroid-stimulating hormone beta subunit. *Biochem J* 1996;314:449.

133. Reichert Jr LE, Dattatreyamurty B, Grasso P, et al. Structure-function relationships of the glycoprotein hormones and their receptors. *Trends Pharmacol Sci* 1991;12:199.

134. Combarnous Y. Molecular basis of the specificity of binding of glycoprotein hormones to their receptors. *Endocr Rev* 1992;13:670.

135. Keutmann HT. Receptor-binding regions in human glycoprotein hormones. *Mol Cell Endocrinol* 1992;186:C1.

136. Reed DK, Ryan RJ, McCormick DJ. Residues in the subunit of human choriotropin that are important for interaction with the lutropin receptor. *J Biol Chem* 1991;266:14251.

137. Leinung MC, Reed DK, McCormick DJ, et al. Further characterization of the receptor-binding region of the thyroid-stimulating hormone α subunit: A comprehensive synthetic peptide study of the α subunit 26–46 sequence. *Biochemistry* 1991;88:9707.

138. Liu C, Roth KE, Shepard BAL, et al. Site-directed alanine mutagenesis of Phe33, Arg35, and Arg42-Ser43-Lys44 in the human gonadotropin α subunit. *J Biol Chem* 1993;268:21613.

139. Xia H, Chen F, Puett D. A region in the human glycoprotein hormone α subunit important in holoprotein formation and receptor binding. *Endocrinology* 1994;134:1768.

140. Yoo J, Zeng H, Ji I, et al. COOH-terminal amino acids of the α subunit play common and different roles in human choriogonadotropin and follitropin. *J Biol Chem* 1993;28:13034.

141. Leinung MC, Bergert ER, McCormick DJ, et al. Synthetic analogs of the carboxyl-terminus of β-thyrotropin: The importance of basic amino acids in receptor binding activity. *Biochemistry* 1992;31:10094.

142. Freeman SL, McCormick DJ, Ryan RJ, et al. Inhibition of TSH bioactivity by synthetic TSH beta peptides. *Endocr Res* 1992;18:1.

143. Grossman M, Szkudlinski MW, Wong R, et al. Substitution of the seat-belt region of the thyroid-stimulating hormone (TSH) β subunit with the corresponding regions of choriogonadotropin or follitropin confers luteotropic but not follitropic activity to chimeric TSH. *J Biol Chem* 1997;272:15532.

144. Szkudlinski MW, Teh NG, Grossman M, et al. Engineering human glycoprotein hormone superactive analogues. *Nat Biotechnol* 1996;14:1257.

145. Grossman M, Szkudlinski MW, Dias JA, et al. Site-directed mutagenesis of amino acids 33–44 of the common α subunit reveals different structural requirements for heterodimer expression among the glycoprotein hormones and suggests that cyclic adenosine 3′,5′-monophosphate production and growth promotion are potentially dissociable functions of human thyrotropin. *Mol Endocrinol* 1996;10:769.

146. Grossman M, Szkudlinski MW, Zeng H, et al. Role of the carboxy-terminal residues of the α subunit in the expression and bioactivity of human thyroid-stimulating hormone. *Mol Endocrinol* 1995;9:948.

147. Sato A, Perlas E, Ben-Menahem D, et al. Cystine knot of the gonadotropin α-subunit is critical for intracellular behavior but not for in vitro biological activity. *J Biol Chem* 1997;272:18098.

148. Grossman M, Wong R, Szkudlinski MW, et al. Human thyroid-stimulating hormone (hTSH) subunit gene fusion produces hTSH with increased stability and serum half-life and compensates for mutagenesis-induced defects in subunit association. *J Biol Chem* 1997;272:21312.

149. Fares FA, Yamabe S, Ben-Menahem D, et al. Conversion of thyrotropin heterodimer to a biologically active single-chain. *Endocrinology* 1998;139:2459.

150. Garcia-Campayo V, Sato A, Hirsch B, et al. Design of stable biologically active recombinant lutropin analogs. *Nat Biotech* 1997;15:663.

151. Wondisford FE, Usala SJ, DeCherney SG, et al. Cloning of the human thyrotropin beta subunit gene and transient expression of biologically active human thyrotropin after gene transfection. *Mol Endocrinol* 1988;2:32.

152. Watanabe S, Hayashizaki Y, Endo Y, et al. Production of human thyroid-stimulating hormone in Chinese hamster ovary cells. *Biochem Biophys Res Commun* 1989;149:1149.

153. Thotakura NR, Desai RK, Bates LG, et al. Biological activity and metabolic clearance of a recombinant human thyrotropin produced in Chinese hamster ovary cells. *Endocrinology* 1991;128:341.

10B   THE THYROTROPIN RECEPTOR

GILBERT VASSART
SABINE COSTAGLIOLA

Thyrotropin (TSH) is a glycoprotein hormone composed of two subunits, an α-subunit that is common to TSH, luteinizing hormone (LH), follicle-stimulating hormone (FSH), and chorionic gonadotropin (CG), and a unique β-subunit. The β-subunits of these hormones, although differing in biologic activity (when combined with an α-subunit), are encoded by genes that have a common ancestor but have evolved by gene duplication (paralogous genes) and, as such, have structural similarity (Fig. 10B.1). The corresponding receptors for TSH, FSH, and LH/CG also have structural similarity and are encoded by paralogous genes.

STRUCTURE OF THE THYROTROPIN RECEPTOR

The receptors for TSH, FSH, and LH/CG are members of the rhodopsin-like G protein–coupled receptor family. As such, the TSH receptor has a "serpentine" domain containing seven transmembrane regions with many (but not all) of the features typical of this receptor family. In addition, and this is a hallmark of the subfamily of glycoprotein hormone receptors (1–3), it has a large (about 400 amino-acid residues) amino-terminal extracellular domain that contains sites that selectively bind TSH with high affinity (4).

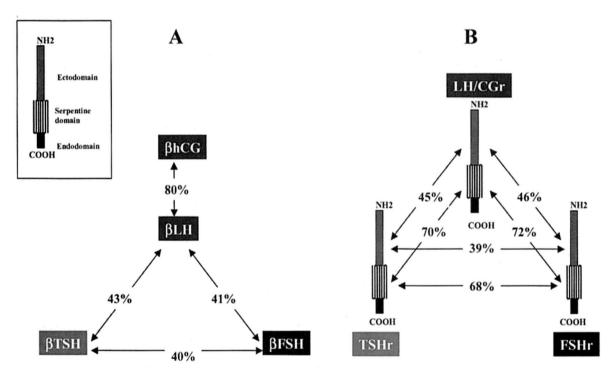

FIGURE 10B.1. Both the β-subunits of the glycoprotein hormones and the glycoprotein hormone receptors are encoded by paralogous genes. **A:** Similarity of the amino acid sequences of the β-subunits of human chorionic gonadotropin (*hCG*), luteinizing hormone (*LH*), thyrotropin (*TSH*), and follicle-stimulating hormone (FSH). **Inset:** Diagram of the general structure of the receptor for these hormones, showing the ectodomain (extracellular domain), serpentine domain (transmembrane domain), and endodomain (intracellular domain). **B:** Similarity of the amino-acid sequences of the receptors (*r*) for LH/CG, TSH, and FSH. Sequence identities are indicated separately for the extracellular and serpentine domains of the three receptors. The pattern of shared similarities suggests coevolution of the hormones and the extracellular domain of their receptors, resulting in specificity barriers. The high similarity of the serpentine domains of the receptors is compatible with a conserved mechanism of intramolecular signal transduction. (Reproduced from Vassart G, Pardo L, Costagliola S. Molecular dissection of the glycoprotein hormone receptors. *Trends Biochem Sci* 2004;29:119, with permission.)

The higher sequence identity of the serpentine domains of the glycoprotein hormone receptors (~70%) as compared with the extracellular domains (~40%) (Fig. 10B.1) suggest that the former are interchangeable modules capable of activating guanine nucleotide-binding (G) proteins (mainly $G\alpha_s$) after specific binding of the individual hormones to their receptors (5). Unlike other rhodopsin-like G-protein-coupled receptors, the glycoprotein hormones bind to their respective extracellular domains with high affinity in the absence of the serpentine domain (6–8). The intramolecular transduction of the signal between these two portions of the receptors involves mechanisms specific to the glycoprotein hormone receptor family. The relatively high sequence identity between the hormone-binding domains of the TSH and LH/CG receptors opens the possibility of CG stimulation of thyroid secretion during normal and especially molar or twin pregnancies, when serum CG concentrations are several orders of magnitude higher than are serum TSH concentrations. This provides an explanation for cases of gestational thyrotoxicosis (see Chapters 26 and 80).

The TSH receptor contains six sites for N-glycosylation, of which four are effectively glycosylated (8). The functional role of the individual carbohydrate chains is still debated. It is likely that they contribute to the routing and stabilization of the receptor as it passes through the membrane system of the cell and is inserted into the cell membrane. Alone among the glycoprotein hormone receptors, the extracellular domain of the TSH receptor is cleaved, severing it from the serpentine domain (see reference 4 for review). This phenomenon has been related to the presence in the extracellular domain of the receptor of a 50-amino-acid insertion for which there is no counterpart in the FSH receptor or LH/CG receptor. The initial cleavage step, due to the action of a metalloprotease, takes place at about position 314 (within the 50-amino-acid insertion) from the amino terminus of the receptor, and is followed by removal of approximately 50 amino acids from the amino-terminal end of the serpentine-containing portion of the receptor (9,10). The amino-terminal end of the receptor is bound to the extracellular end of the serpentine domain by disulfide bonds. The functional importance of this TSH receptor-specific postranslational modification remains unclear. Whereas all wild-type TSH receptors on the surface of thyroid follicular cells seem to be in cleaved form, noncleavable mutant constructs are functionally undistinguishable from cleaved receptors, when expressed in transfected cells (4). When transiently or permanently transfected in nonthyroid cells, wild-type human TSH receptors are present at the cell surface as a mixture of monomers and cleaved dimers.

The TSH receptor is specifically inserted into the basolateral membrane of thyroid follicular cells. This phenomenon involves signals encoded in the primary structure of the protein, because it is conserved when the receptor is expressed in MDCK cells, a polarized cell of nonthyroid origin (11).

The possibility that TSH receptors are present on the cell surface as dimers of cleaved dimers was raised after demonstration that most rhodopsin-like G protein–coupled receptors do dimerize (12). Functional complementation of receptors with mutations in the extracellular and the serpentine domains has been observed after cotransfection of FSH receptor constructs into cells (13), demonstrating the possibility of dimerization for glycoprotein hormone receptors. Preliminary data have been provided for dimerization of the TSH receptor (14), but definitive demonstration of the functional importance of dimerization of this receptor is lacking.

THYROTROPIN RECEPTOR GENE

The gene coding for the human TSH receptor has been localized on the long arm of chromosome 14 (14q31) (15, 16). It is more than 60 kilobases (kb) long and is organized into 10 exons. The extracellular domain is encoded by a series of 9 exons, each of which corresponds to one or an integer number of leucine-rich repeat segments. The carboxyl-terminal part of the extracellular domain, the serpentine domain, and the intracellular carboxyl-terminal end of the receptor are encoded by a single large exon (17), in keeping with the fact that the genes for many G protein–coupled receptors have no introns. A likely evolutionary scenario derives from this gene organization: the glycoprotein hormone receptor genes would have evolved from the condensation of an intronless classic G protein–coupled receptor with a mosaic gene encoding a protein with leucine-rich repeat segments (17). Triplication of this ancestral gene and subsequent divergence led to the receptors for TSH, FSH, and LH/CG. The existence of 10 exons in both the TSH and FSH receptor genes (as opposed to the 11-exon LH/CG-receptor gene) suggests the following evolutionary steps: first, duplication of an ancestral glycoprotein hormone receptor gene, yielding the LH/CG-receptor gene and the ancestors of the TSH- and FSH-receptor genes. After losing one intron, the latter duplicated subsequently into the TSH and FSH receptor genes.

The promoter region of the human and rat TSH receptor gene has been cloned and sequenced (17,18). It has the characteristics of "housekeeping" genes in that it is GC-rich and devoid of TATA boxes; in rats it stimulates transcription from multiple start sites (18) and contains a functional recognition site for thyroid transcription factor (TTF)-1 (19). Expression of the TSH receptor gene is largely thyroid specific. Constructs made of a chloramphenicol acetyltransferase reporter gene under control of the 5'-flanking region of the rat TSH receptor gene are expressed when transfected into FRTL5 cells and FRT cells, but not into nonthyroid cells such as HeLa or rat liver (BRL) cells (18). However, TSH receptor messenger RNA (mRNA) has been clearly demonstrated in adipose tissue of guinea pigs (20) and after differentiation of preadipocytes into adipocytes (21,22). TSH receptors may also be present in lymphocytes, extraocular tissue, cartilage, and bone, but their functional importance in these tissues is uncertain (23). Expression of the TSH receptor in thyroid cells is extremely robust. It is moderately up-regulated by TSH *in vitro* and down-regulated by iodide *in vivo* (24).

RECOGNITION OF THE RECEPTOR BY THYROTROPIN

Three-dimensional structures are available for CG and FSH (25–27), but only structural models are available for TSH (see preceding section of this chapter) and for the ex-

tracellular domains of the TSH and other glycoprotein hormone receptors. The extracellular domains of all three glycoprotein hormone receptors are composed of a central portion containing leucine-rich repeats flanked by cysteine-rich domains (Fig. 10B.2). The leucine-rich repeat segments are composed of 20 to 25 amino acids formed into a β strand and an α helix, connected by a turn. When assembled sequentially in a protein, the leucine-rich repeat segments determine a horseshoe-like structure with the β strands forming a concave inner surface (Fig. 10B.2). This surface constitutes the binding interface in the first protein containing leucine-rich repeat segments that was crystallized: the ribonuclease inhibitor (28). The leucine-rich repeat-containing portion of the TSH receptor con-

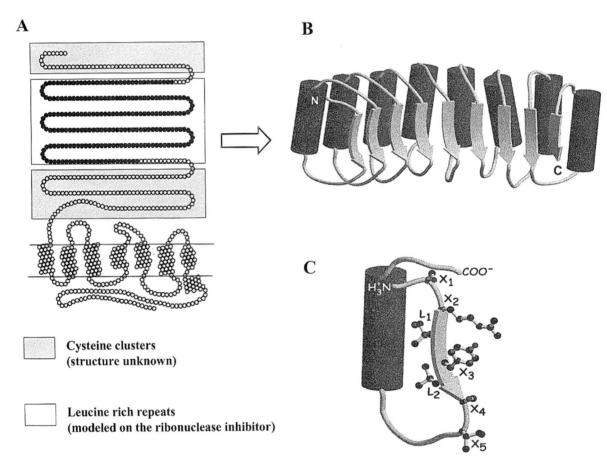

Cysteine clusters (structure unknown)

Leucine rich repeats (modeled on the ribonuclease inhibitor)

FIGURE 10B.2. Schematic representations of the structure of the thyrotropin (TSH) receptor. **A:** Two-dimensional representation with indication of the various domains. The two shaded boxes correspond to the amino-terminal and the cysteine-rich carboxyl-terminal portions of the extracellular domain, flanking nine leucine-rich repeats. **B:** Repeats are composed of 20 to 24 amino acids forming a β strand followed by an α helix. In proteins that contain leucine-rich repeat segments, the repeat segments are arranged with their β strands and α helices parallel to a common axis and organized spatially to form a horseshoe-shaped molecule, with the β strands and α helices making the concave and convex surfaces of the horseshoe, respectively. *N*, amino terminus; *C*, carboxyl terminus. **C:** Representation of a single leucine-rich repeat segment. The inner surface of the horseshoe is composed of seven residues: $X_1X_2L_1X_3L_2X_4X_5$. The side chains of the leucine residues are pointing inside the hydrophobic core of the protein and are important for its stability. The side chains of the X residues are predicted to be exposed, making the surface available for interaction with the ligands. (Reproduced from Smits G, Campillo M, Govaerts C, et al. Glycoprotein hormone receptors: determinants in leucine-rich repeats responsible for ligand specificity. *EMBO J* 2003;22:2692, with permission.)

tains nine such segments, and it has been modeled on the known three-dimensional structure of the ribonuclease inhibitor (29). The model predicts that nonleucine residues $(X_{1,2,3,4,5})$ (Fig. 10B.2) point outward and are available for interaction with TSH, immediately suggesting that they might be implicated in recognition specificity.

Replacement by site-directed mutagenesis of the X_i residues in the leucine-rich repeat portion of the TSH receptor with their counterparts in the LH/CG receptor provide strong support for the above model (30). Exchanging eight amino acids of the TSH receptor for the corresponding amino acids in the LH/CG receptor resulted in a mutant receptor that bound human CG as well as the wild-type LH/CG receptor. While gaining sensitivity to human CG, the mutant receptor retained normal sensitivity to TSH, making it a dual-specificity receptor. It is necessary to exchange 12 additional amino-acid residues to transform fully this mutant receptor into a bona fide LH/CG receptor (30). From an evolutionary point of view, these observations indicate that the specificity of hormone receptors is based on both attractive and repulsive residues, and that residues at different homologous positions have been selected to achieve this result in the different receptors.

Inspection of electrostatic surface maps of models of the wild-type TSH and LH/CG receptors and some of the mutants is revealing in this respect (30). The LH/CG receptor has an acidic groove in the middle of its horseshoe, extending to the lower part of it (corresponding to the carboxyl-terminal ends of the β strands). Generation of a similar distribution of charges in the dual-specificity and reverse-specificity TSH receptor mutants suggests that this is important for recognition of human CG. Attempts to correlate charge distributions in the wild-type and mutant TSH receptors with those of residues in TSH and human CG suggest that the "seat-belt" portion of the β subunits of the hormones, known to play a key role in recognition specificity (see preceding section and references 31–33), might face the bottom border of the horseshoe. The importance of electrostatic bonds in TSH–TSH receptor interactions has long been known, from the observation that efficient binding *in vitro* required low salt concentrations.

In addition to the hormone-specific interactions genetically encoded in the primary structure of glycoprotein hormone receptors and their ligands, there are important non-hormone-specific ionic interactions involving sulfated tyrosine residues present in the extracellular domains of all three receptors (34). In the TSH receptor, both tyrosine residues of a conserved Tyr-Asp-Tyr motif located close to the border between the extracellular domain and the first transmembrane helix are sulfated (Fig. 10B.3). Sulfation of the first tyrosine of the motif contributes importantly to the affinity of the receptor for TSH, without interfering with specificity (34).

ACTIVATION OF THE SERPENTINE PORTION OF THE THYROTROPIN RECEPTOR

Being a member of the G protein–coupled receptor family, the serpentine domain of the TSH receptor is likely to share with rhodopsin common mechanisms of activation (35,36). However, sequence variations in this domain of the glycoprotein hormone receptors suggest the existence of idiosyncrasies associated with hormone-specific mechanisms of activation (Fig. 10B.3). In addition, many gain-of-function somatic mutations have been found in this domain of the TSH receptor (37–39) (see Chapter 25); according to the available data, mutations of more than 30 residues result in constitutive activation of the TSH receptor. Many somatic mutations affecting a given residue have been found repeatedly; therefore, it is likely that we are getting close to having a saturation map for spontaneous gain-of-function mutations. Attempts have been made to translate this map into mechanisms of transition between inactive and active conformations of the receptor, in the light of structural data for rhodopsin. Three sequence patterns affected by gain-of-function mutations deserve special mention and may help in understanding how the TSH receptor is activated.

The first pattern is centered on an aspartate in position 6.44 (Asp633), at the cytoplasmic side of transmembrane helix VI. [The standardized numbering system of Ballesteros and Weinstein is used to identify residues in the transmembrane segments of different receptors. Each residue is identified by two numbers: the first, 1 through 7,

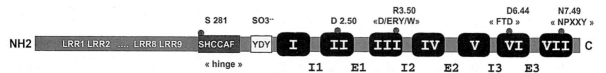

FIGURE 10B.3. Linear representation of the thyrotropin (TSH) receptor. Sequences common to all rhodopsin-like G protein–coupled receptors and sequences specific to the glycoprotein hormone receptor gene family are both implicated in activation of the TSH receptor. Key residues are indicated (*dots*), as are conserved motifs: SO3⁻ denotes postranslational sulfation of the indicated tyrosine residues (34). The boxes containing Roman numerals denote transmembrane helices; I1-I3 and E1-E3, intracellular and extracellular loops, respectively; and LRR, leucine-rich repeats.

corresponds to the helix in which it is located; the second indicates its position relative to the most conserved residue in that helix, arbitrarily assigned to 50 (40)]. When mutated to a variety of amino acids the result is constitutive activation (38,41). This suggests that the gain of function results from the breakage of one or more bonds, rather than the creation of novel interactions, by the mutated residue, and the main partner of Asp6.44 was identified as Asn7.49 in transmembrane helix VII. The results of site-directed mutagenesis studies suggested that, in the inactive conformation of the TSH receptor, the side chain of Asp7.49 is normally "sequestered" by both Thr6.43 and Asp6.44, and that the active conformations require establishment of novel interactions of N7.49, probably involving Asp in position 2.50 (41,42).

In the second pattern, glutamate 3.49 and arginine 3.50 of the highly conserved "D/ERY/W" motif at the bottom of transmembrane helix III form an ionic lock with aspartate 6.30 at the cytoplasmic end of transmembrane helix VI. Disruption of this ionic lock (e.g., by mutations affecting Asp6.30) leads to constitutively active mutant receptors (42). Thus, the movements of transmembrane helix III and transmembrane helix VI at the cytoplasmic side of the membrane is necessary for receptor activation (43).

The third pattern involves serine 281, which belongs to a YPSHCCAF sequence located at the carboxyl-terminal end of the leucine-rich repeat segment in the extracellular domain of the receptor (Fig. 10B.3). Mutation of this serine residue activates the TSH receptor constitutively (44), and this segment, sometimes referred to as the "hinge" motif, plays an important role in activation of all three glycoprotein hormone receptors (45). The functional effect of substitutions of S281 in the TSH receptor likely results in a local loss of structure, because the more destructuring the substitutions, the stronger the activation (45,46). This observation, together with the finding that mutation of specific residues in the extracellular loops of the TSH receptor cause constitutive activation (47), led to the hypothesis that activation of the receptor could involve the rupture of an inhibitory interaction between the extracellular domain and the serpentine domain (44).

INTERACTION BETWEEN THE EXTRACELLULAR AND SERPENTINE DOMAINS OF THE THYROTROPIN RECEPTOR

Mutant TSH receptor constructs devoid of the extracellular domain are partially activated, confirming the inhibitory effect of the extracellular domain on the serpentine domain (48,49). However, cyclic AMP production in cells transfected with truncated constructs was increased much less than after full stimulation of the wild-type recep-

tor by TSH or after mutation of Ser281 (48). These results led to the following model for activation of the TSH receptor (48) (Fig. 10B.4). In the resting state, the extracellular domain inhibits the activity of an inherently active rhodopsin-like serpentine domain. Upon activation, by binding of TSH, or secondary to mutation of S281 in the hinge region, the extracellular domain switches from inverse agonist to full agonist of the serpentine domain. The ability of the strongest S281 mutants to activate the receptor fully in the absence of TSH suggests that the ultimate agonist of the serpentine domain would be the "activated" extracellular domain, with no need for a direct interaction between TSH and the serpentine domain.

ACTIVATION BY CHORIONIC GONADOTROPIN

The sequence similarity between TSH and human CG, and between their receptors, allows for some degree of promiscuous activation of the TSH receptor by CG during the first trimester of pregnancy, when serum CG concentrations are highest. The inverse relationship between serum TSH and CG concentrations in most pregnant women is a clear indication that their thyroid gland is stimulated by CG (50) (see Chapter 80). Although most pregnant women are euthyroid, thyrotoxicosis may occur if CG production is excessive (as occurs in twin pregnancies or chorionic tumors (see Chapter 26), or in rare women who have a mutant TSH receptor with increased sensitivity to CG (51).

ACTIVATION BY THYROTROPIN-RECEPTOR ANTIBODIES

The serum antibodies found in most patients with Graves' thyrotoxicosis and some patients with hypothyroidism caused by chronic autoimmune thyroiditis can stimulate or block the TSH receptor, respectively (see Chapters 15, 23, and 47). The epitopes recognized by TSH receptor–stimulating antibodies and the mechanisms leading to activation of the receptor are still ill defined. This situation should change shortly, now that monoclonal antibodies with thyroid-stimulating activity have been produced in mice and hamsters and isolated from the serum of patients with Graves' thyrotoxicosis (52–55). Although most TSH receptor–stimulating antibodies do compete with TSH for binding to the receptor (56), the precise targets of TSH and the antibodies are likely to be different. The sulfated tyrosine residues, which are important for TSH binding, are not implicated in recognition of TSH receptor by TSH receptor–stimulating antibodies (34). Also, most TSH recep-

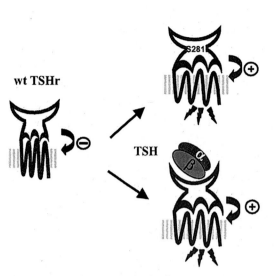

S281L mutation converts the ectodomain into a full agonist of the serpentine

wt TSHr

TSH

High affinity interaction with TSH is postulated to have the same effect

FIGURE 10B.4. Model for activation of the thyrotropin (TSH) receptor. Interactions between the extracellular domain and the serpentine domain are implicated in the activation mechanism. The TSH receptor is represented with its extracellular domain containing a concave, hormone-binding structure facing upward and a transmembrane serpentine domain. The basal state of the receptor is characterized by an inhibitory interaction between the extracellular domain and the serpentine domain [indicated by the (-) sign]. In the absence of the agonist, the extracellular domain would function as a tethered inverse agonist of the serpentine domain. Mutation of Ser281 in the extracellular domain into leucine switches the extracellular domain from an inverse agonist into a full agonist of the serpentine domain [indicated by the (+) sign]. Binding of TSH (indicated by the $\alpha\beta$ dimeric structure) to the extracellular domain is proposed to have a similar effect, converting it into a full agonist of the serpentine domain. The serpentine domain in the basal state is shown as a compact structure. The fully activated serpentine domain is shown as a relaxed structure with arrows indicating activation of Gα within the cell. *Wt TSHr*, wild-type TSH receptor.

tor–stimulating antibodies stimulate cyclic AMP accumulation in cells transfected with TSH receptors more slowly than does TSH (57). The recent availability of highly purified TSH receptor–stimulating antibody preparations from individual patients should allow these differences between the antibodies and TSH to be explored directly (56).

DOWN-REGULATION OF THE THYROTROPIN RECEPTOR

Desensitization of some G protein–coupled receptors involves phosphorylation of specific residues by G protein receptor kinases (homologous desensitization) or protein kinase A (heterologous desensitization) (58). Acute desensitization of the receptor in the presence of TSH, presumably by phosphorylation, is weak and delayed (59). When compared with other G protein–coupled receptors, the TSH receptor contains few serine or threonine residues in its intracellular loops and intracellular carboxyl-terminal domain that can be phosphorylated, which probably accounts for the limited desensitization after stimulation by TSH. Weak down-regulation, confounded by the long life of both TSH receptor mRNA and protein, does occur

but has little functional role (60). The persistence of thyrotoxicosis in patients with TSH-secreting pituitary adenomas and in patients with Graves' disease is *in vivo* evidence of the weakness of down-regulation of the TSH receptor.

REFERENCES

1. Dias JA, Van Roey P. Structural biology of human follitropin and its receptor. *Arch Med Res* 2001;32:510.
2. Szkudlinski MW, Fremont V, Ronin C, et al. Thyroid-stimulating hormone and thyroid-stimulating hormone receptor structure-function relationships. *Physiol Rev* 2002;82:473.
3. Ascoli M, Fanelli F, Segaloff DL. The lutropin/choriogonadotropin receptor, a 2002 perspective. *Endocr Rev* 2002;23:141.
4. Rapoport B, Chazenbalk GD, Jaume JC, et al. The thyrotropin (TSH) receptor: interaction with TSH and autoantibodies. *Endocr Rev* 1998;19:673.
5. Vassart G, Dumont JE. The thyrotropin receptor and the regulation of thyrocyte function and growth. *Endocr Rev* 1992;13:596.
6. Schmidt A, MacColl R, Lindau-Shepard B, et al. Hormone-induced conformational change of the purified soluble hormone binding domain of follitropin receptor complexed with single chain follitropin. *J Biol Chem* 2001;276:23373.

7. Remy JJ, Nespoulous C, Grosclaude J, et al. Purification and structural analysis of a soluble human chorionogonadotropin hormone-receptor complex. *J Biol Chem* 2001;276:1681.

8. Cornelis S, Uttenweiler-Joseph S, Panneels V, et al. Purification and characterization of a soluble bioactive amino-terminal extracellular domain of the human thyrotropin receptor. *Biochemistry* 2001;40:9860.

9. Couet J, Sar S, Jolivet A, et al. Shedding of human thyrotropin receptor ectodomain. Involvement of a matrix metalloprotease. *J Biol Chem* 1996;271:4545.

10. de Bernard S, Misrahi M, Huet JC, et al. Sequential cleavage and excision of a segment of the thyrotropin receptor ectodomain. *J Biol Chem* 1999;274:101.

11. Beau I, Misrahi M, Gross B, et al. Basolateral localization and transcytosis of gonadotropin and thyrotropin receptors expressed in Madin-Darby canine kidney cells. *J Biol Chem* 1997; 272:5241.

12. Angers S, Salahpour A, Bouvier M. Dimerization: an emerging concept for G protein-coupled receptor ontogeny and function. *Annu Rev Pharmacol Toxicol* 2002;42:409.

13. Lee C, Ji I, Ryu K, et al. Two defective heterozygous luteinizing hormone receptors can rescue hormone action. *J Biol Chem* 2002;277:15795.

14. Latif R, Graves P, Davies TF. Ligand-dependent inhibition of oligomerization at the human thyrotropin receptor. *J Biol Chem* 2002;277:45059.

15. Libert F, Passage E, Lefort A, et al. Localization of human thyrotropin receptor gene to chromosome region 14q3 by *in situ* hybridization. *Cytogenet Cell Genet* 1990;54:82.

16. Rousseau-Merck MF, Misrahi M, Loosfelt H, et al. Assignment of the human thyroid stimulating hormone receptor (TSHR) gene to chromosome 14q31. *Genomics* 1990;8:233.

17. Gross B, Misrahi M, Sar S, et al. Composite structure of the human thyrotropin receptor gene. *Biochem Biophys Res Commun* 1991;177:679.

18. Ikuyama S, Niller HH, Shimura H, et al. Characterization of the 5′-flanking region of the rat thyrotropin receptor gene. *Mol Endocrinol* 1992;6:793.

19. Civitareale D, Castelli MP, Falasca P, et al. Thyroid transcription factor 1 activates the promoter of the thyrotropin receptor gene. *Mol Endocrinol* 1993;7:1589.

20. Roselli-Rehfuss L, Robbins LS, Cone RD. Thyrotropin receptor messenger ribonucleic acid is expressed in most brown and white adipose tissues in the guinea pig. *Endocrinology* 1992;130:1857.

21. Bell A, Gagnon A, Grunder L, et al. Functional TSH receptor in human abdominal preadipocytes and orbital fibroblasts. *Am J Physiol Cell Physiol* 2000;279:C335.

22. Crisp MS, Lane C, Halliwell M, et al. Thyrotropin receptor transcripts in human adipose tissue. *J Clin Endocrinol Metab* 1997;82:2003.

23. Abe E, Marians RC, Yu W, et al. TSH is a negative regulator of skeletal remodeling. *Cell* 2003;115:151.

24. Uyttersprot N, Pelgrims N, Carrasco N, et al. Moderate doses of iodide *in vivo* inhibit cell proliferation and the expression of thyroperoxidase and Na$^+$/I$^-$ symporter mRNAs in dog thyroid. *Mol Cell Endocrinol* 1997;131:195.

25. Lapthorn AJ, Harris DC, Littlejohn A, et al. Crystal structure of human chorionic gonadotropin. *Nature* 1994;369:455.

26. Wu H, Lustbader JW, Liu Y, et al. Structure of human chorionic gonadotropin at 2.6 A resolution from MAD analysis of the selenomethionyl protein. *Structure* 1994;2:545.

27. Fox KM, Dias JA, Van Roey P. Three-dimensional structure of human follicle-stimulating hormone. *Mol Endocrinol* 2001;15:378.

28. Kobe B, Deisenhofer J. Crystal structure of porcine ribonuclease inhibitor, a protein with leucine-rich repeats. *Nature* 1993;366:751.

29. Kajava AV, Vassart G, Wodak SJ. Modeling of the three-dimensional structure of proteins with the typical leucine-rich repeats. *Structure* 1995;3:867.

30. Smits G, Campillo M, Govaerts C, et al. Glycoprotein hormone receptors: determinants in leucine-rich repeats responsible for ligand specificity. *EMBO J* 2003;22:2692.

31. Grossmann M, Weintraub BD, Szkudlinski MW. Novel insights into the molecular mechanisms of human thyrotropin action: structural, physiological, and therapeutic implications for the glycoprotein hormone family. *Endocr Rev* 1997;18:476.

32. Moyle WR, Campbell RK, Myers RV, et al. Co-evolution of ligand-receptor pairs. *Nature* 1994;368:251.

33. Dias JA, Zhang Y, Liu X. Receptor binding and functional properties of chimeric human follitropin prepared by an exchange between a small hydrophilic intercysteine loop of human follitropin and human lutropin. *J Biol Chem* 1994; 269:25289.

34. Costagliola S, Panneels V, Bonomi M, et al. Tyrosine sulfation is required for agonist recognition by glycoprotein hormone receptors. *EMBO J* 2002;21:504.

35. Palczewski K, Kumasaka T, Hori T, et al. Crystal structure of rhodopsin: a G protein-coupled receptor. *Science* 2000;289:739.

36. Ridge KD, Abdulaev NG, Sousa M, et al. Phototransduction: crystal clear. *Trends Biochem Sci* 2003;28:479.

37. Parma J, Duprez L, Van Sande J, et al. Somatic mutations in the thyrotropin receptor gene cause hyperfunctioning thyroid adenomas. *Nature* 1993;365:649.

38. Parma J, Duprez L, Van Sande J, et al. Diversity and prevalence of somatic mutations in the TSH receptor and Gs alpha genes as a cause of toxic thyroid adenomas. *J Clin Endocrinol Metab* 1997;82:2695.

39. Refetoff S, Dumont JE, Vassart G. Thyroid disorders. In: Scriver CR, ed. *The metabolic and molecular bases of inherited diseases,* 8th ed. New York: McGraw-Hill, 2000:4029.

40. Ballesteros JA, Weinstein H. Integrated methods for modeling G-protein coupled receptors. *Methods Neurosci* 1995;25:366.

41. Govaerts C, Lefort A, Costagliola S, et al. A conserved ASN in transmembrane helix 7 is an on/off switch in the activation of the TSH receptor. *J Biol Chem* 2001;276:22991.

42. Claeysen S, Govaerts C, Lefort A, et al. A conserved Asn in TM7 of the TSH receptor is a common requirement for activation by both mutations and its natural agonist. *FEBS Lett* 2002;517:195.

43. Ballesteros JA, Jensen AD, Liapakis G, et al. Activation of the beta 2-adrenergic receptor involves disruption of an ionic lock between the cytoplasmic ends of transmembrane segments 3 and 6. *J Biol Chem* 2001;276:29171.

44. Duprez L, Parma J, Costagliola S, et al. Constitutive activation of the TSH receptor by spontaneous mutations affecting the N-terminal extracellular domain. *FEBS Lett* 1997;409:469.

45. Nakabayashi K, Kudo M, Kobilka B, et al. Activation of the luteinizing hormone receptor following substitution of Ser-277 with selective hydrophobic residues in the ectodomain hinge region. *J Biol Chem* 2000;275:30264.

46. Ho SC, Van Sande J, Lefort A, et al. Effects of mutations involving the highly conserved S281HCC motif in the extracellular domain of the thyrotropin (TSH) receptor on TSH binding and constitutive activity. *Endocrinology* 2001;142:2760.

47. Parma J, Van Sande J, Swillens S, et al. Somatic mutations causing constitutive activity of the TSH receptor are the major cause of hyperfunctional thyroid adenomas: identification of additional mutations activating both the cAMP and inisitolphosphate-Ca^{++} cascades. *Mol Endocrinol* 1995;9:725.

48. Vlaeminck V, Ho SC, Rodien P, et al. Activation of the cAMP pathway by the TSH receptor involves switching of the ectodomain from a tethered inverse agonist to an agonist. *Mol Endocrinol* 2002;16:736.

49. Zhang M, Tong KP, Fremont V, et al. The extracellular domain suppresses constitutive activity of the transmembrane domain of

the human TSH receptor: implications for hormone-receptor interaction and antagonist design. *Endocrinology* 2000;141:3514.

50. Glinoer D. The regulation of thyroid function in pregnancy: pathways of endocrine adaptation from physiology to pathology. *Endocr Rev* 1997;18:404.

51. Rodien P, Bremont C, Sanson ML, et al. Familial gestational hyperthyroidism caused by a mutant thyrotropin receptor hypersensitive to human chorionic gonadotropin. *N Engl J Med* 1998; 339:1823.

52. Sanders J, Jeffreys J, Depraetere H, et al. Thyroid-stimulating monoclonal antibodies. *Thyroid* 2002;12:1043.

53. Sanders J, Evans M, Premawardhana LD, et al. Human monoclonal thyroid stimulating autoantibody. *Lancet* 2003;362:126.

54. Ando T, Latif R, Pritsker A, et al. A monoclonal thyroid-stimulating antibody. *J Clin Invest* 2002;110:1667.

55. Costagliola S, Franssen JD, Bonomi M ,et al. Generation of a mouse monoclonal TSH receptor antibody with stimulating activity. *Biochem Biophys Res Commun* 2002;299:891.

56. Morgenthaler NG, Minich WB, Willnich M, et al. Affinity purification and diagnostic use of TSH receptor autoantibodies from human serum. *Mol Cell Endocrinol* 2003;212:73.

57. Van Sande J, Costa MJ, Massart C, et al. Kinetics of thyrotropin-stimulating hormone (TSH) and thyroid-stimulating antibody binding and action on the TSH receptor in intact TSH receptor-expressing CHO cells. *J Clin Endocrinol Metab* 2003; 88:5366.

58. Lefkowitz RJ, Cotecchia S, Kjelsberg MA, et al. Adrenergic receptors: recent insights into their mechanism of activation and desensitization. *Adv Second Messenger Phosphoprotein Res* 1993; 28:1.

59. Delbeke D, Van Sande J, Swillens S, et al. Cooling enhances adenosine $3':5'$ monophosphate accumulation in thyrotropin stimulated dog thyroid slices. *Metabolism* 1982;31:797.

60. Maenhaut C, Brabant G, Vassart G, et al. *In vitro* and *in vivo* regulation of thyrotropin receptor mRNA levels in dog and human thyroid cells. *J Biol Chem* 1992;15:3000.

10C BIOLOGICAL ACTIONS OF THYROTROPIN

STEPHEN W. SPAULDING

Thyrotropin (TSH) is the major regulator of thyroid hormone synthesis and secretion. TSH is best known for actions that are mediated by cyclic $3',5'$-adenosine monophosphate (cyclic AMP), but TSH regulates many other signaling pathways. When stimulated, TSH receptors usually couple with large G-protein $\alpha\beta\gamma$ -heterotrimers that activate adenylyl cyclase, but TSH receptors can also associate with $\alpha\beta\gamma$- heterotrimers that stimulate small guanosine triphosphatases, phospholipid metabolism, phosphatidylinositide 3 (PI3)-kinase, and other signaling pathways. After activation, various pathways can be down-regulated, permitting tight control of hormone production as well as of growth and death of thyroid follicular cells (thyrocytes). Many of the signaling pathways in thyrocytes are also regulated by other hormones, growth factors, and cytokines, in addition to receiving signals from the colloid, from adjacent cells, and from the extracellular matrix. Studies of normal rodents have provided much understanding of the actions of TSH, and studies of gene-knockout mice are providing new insights, but certain aspects of signaling, cell regeneration, and death differ between rodents and humans (1,2). Some responses to TSH vary between species and even between strains of animal (3). *In vitro* models can provide information not otherwise obtainable, but paracrine factors and direct connections with neighboring cells and structures are missing or distorted, and there is substantial variation in TSH responses between *in vitro* models. It is important to emphasize, however, that pathways found to be regulated by TSH in such experimental models have proven to be important clinically as causes of thyroid autonomy, and of benign and malignant tumors.

EFFECTS OF THYROTROPIN ON THYROID TRANSCRIPTION FACTORS AND THYROID DEVELOPMENT

Although TSH is a tonic regulator of growth and function of the adult thyroid, it is not required for early thyroid development (see Chapter 2). Before any TSH or TSH receptors are expressed in the embryo, thyroid precursor cells express a combination of three transcription factors found uniquely in thyrocytes: TTF-1 (thyroid transcription factor-1 or Titf1), TTF-2 (or Foxe1), and Pax-8 (paired box gene 8). TTF-1 and Pax-8 are phosphoproteins required for the development of thyrocyte precursor cells, while TTF-2 is needed for correct migration of the cells. During normal thyroid development, TSH and its receptor first appear at about the 16th embryonic day in rats and mice, after which small follicular structures appear and thyroid hormone production begins. In mutant mice in which the TSH receptor has been "knocked out," full maturation of the thyroid is impaired, although some follicle formation occurs in late embryonic life. These mice survive only if they are treated with thyroid hormone (4). The thyroid vestigium in these animals contains very little sodium-iodide symporter protein or thyroid peroxidase, but noniodinated thyroglobulin is present. If forskolin is added to normal thyroid precursor tissue from 15-day rodent embryos in order to directly activate adenylyl cyclase and increase cyclic AMP production, follicular structures form and iodine-concentrating activity is induced prematurely (5). Similarly, if the thyroid vestigium from TSH-receptor knockout mice is incubated with forskolin, some organified iodine can be detected, indicating that signaling mechanisms required for iodide uptake and organification have been preserved, even in the absence of a TSH receptor, and confirming the importance of cyclic AMP for the normal function of the thyroid (6).

In addition to playing essential roles in thyroid development, TTF-1 and Pax-8 are involved in regulating the expression of several thyroid-specific genes. In FRTL-5 (Fisher rat thyrocyte cell line-5) cells, TSH decreases TTF-1 expression and down-regulates expression of the TSH receptor gene—whose promoter contains TTF-1 binding sites but no Pax-8 binding site—but only if serum and insulin are present in the culture medium (7). In contrast, TSH increases Pax-8 expression and up-regulates the expression of the thyroglobulin gene—whose promoter contains an overlapping binding site for both Pax-8 and TTF-1—regardless of whether serum and insulin are present (7). TTF-1 and Pax-8 can exist as a complex and act synergistically to promote transcription from the rat thyroglobulin gene promoter in rat PCCl3 thyrocytes (8).

Patients with a mutation in one TTF-1 allele have high serum TSH concentrations, and some are overtly hypothyroid. Similarly, mice with one defective TTF-1 allele also have high serum TSH concentrations (9). Despite the high levels of TSH, their serum thyroxine (T_4) levels remain somewhat low, but administering exogenous TSH can normalize the T_4 (9). Their thyroid glands contain diminished levels of TSH receptor and thyroglobulin messenger RNA (mRNA), whereas expression of other thyroid-specific genes is not significantly decreased. Thus biallelic expression of TTF-1 is necessary for the thyroid to be fully responsive to TSH (9). Although both TTF-1 and Pax-8 are phosphoproteins, and cyclic AMP and protein kinase A (PKA) are involved in their regulation (10), it appears that the effect of PKA may not be mediated by directly phosphorylating them (11).

Pax-8 and TTF-1 activities are influenced by their redox state (12,13). In FRTL-5 cells, TSH increases the DNA-binding activity of endogenous Pax-8 and TTF-1 by reducing their oxidized forms, accompanied by increased expression of thioredoxin (13). Thioredoxin is a major intrathyroidal antioxidant that restores binding activity to these and other redox-regulated transcription factors (13). Ref-1 (redox factor-1) repairs DNA damaged by oxidative stress, and also regulates the redox state and DNA-binding activity of transcription factors like AP-1, NF-κB, and p53, in addition to protein kinase A TTF-1 and Pax-8. Ref-1 associates with thioredoxin in the nucleus, reducing

oxidized Pax-8 and increasing its binding to the promoter regions of the sodium-iodide symporter and thyroglobulin genes (12,14). TSH increases Ref-1 levels in FRTL-5 cells by a cyclic AMP-mediated mechanism (15,16), and also causes translocation of Ref-1 from the cytoplasm to the nucleus of FRTL-5 cells (16) Clinically, histochemical studies indicate that Ref-1 levels are high in hyperfunctioning thyroid adenomas, particularly in the nuclear fraction (16). Some of the effects of TSH on AP-1 target genes may be mediated by actions of Ref-1 on the redox state of the different components that can comprise AP-1 dimers (15,17). Ref-1 may also guard cells from apoptosis by protecting them from oxidative stressors like hydrogen peroxide (H_2O_2), which may be another response regulated by this mediator of TSH action (see later in the chapter).

HOW THYROTROPIN ACTIVATES ITS G-PROTEIN HETEROTRIMERS

When TSH binds to its transmembrane receptor, it induces a change in the receptor that activates αβγ heterotrimers on the inner surface of the basolateral plasma membrane of thyrocytes (Fig. 10C.1). Activation causes a guanosine triphosphate (GTP) molecule to replace the guanosine diphosphate (GDP) molecule that is bound to the Gα-subunit associated with a Gβγ-dimer in the basal state. The activated GTP-containing Gα-subunit then dissociates from the Gβγ-dimer, permitting the free Gα-subunit and membrane-bound Gβγ-dimer to interact with various downstream effectors. The specific pathway that is activated by a given TSH molecule is determined by the particular α-, β-, and γ-subunits that comprise the heterotrimer to which the TSH receptor has coupled. The duration of the signals produced by a given Gα-subunit could simply depend on when its intrinsic GTPase hydrolyzes the GTP back to GDP, which inactivates the Gα-subunit and permits it to re-associate with whatever Gβγ-dimer is available. However, other proteins can regulate both the rate at which GTP initially displaces the GDP from an inactive Gα-subunit, as well as the rate at which the GTP is hydrolyzed. The dose and duration of the TSH stimulus, the extent of glycosylation of the TSH, and the structure of the receptor also affect the responses. If the duration of TSH stimulation is protracted, the thyroid may react by decreasing the expression of TSH receptors and heterotrimer components. When G-coupled receptors are occupied by ligand, they can be phosphorylated by G-protein receptor kinases, which can down-regulate the response to subsequent stimuli by permitting the binding of arrestins that promote internalization and degradation of the receptors. Uncoupled G-protein heterotrimers are also able to interact with other receptors in thyroid plasma membranes, such as those for catecholamines, lysophosphatidic

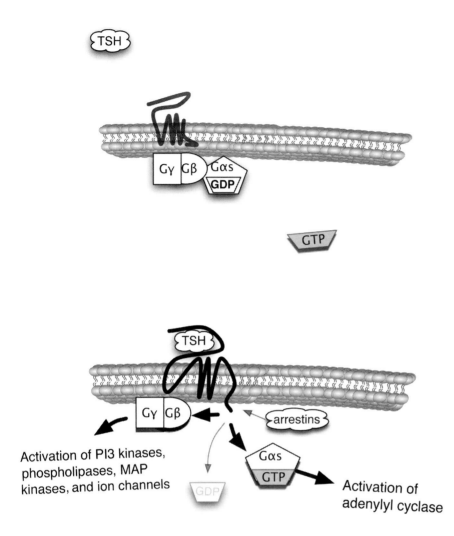

FIGURE 10C.1. Regulation of the thyrotropin (TSH) receptor and G-protein heterotrimers. **Top diagram:** In the basal state, the TSH receptor does not contain a ligand, while the inactive Gα-subunit in the heterotrimer contains a guanosine diphosphate (GDP) molecule. **Bottom diagram:** TSH binds to and activates the receptor, and causes guanosine triphosphate (GTP) to replace the GDP on the Gα-subunit. The activated Gα-subunit dissociates from the Gβγ-subunit dimer, which then interacts with various downstream effectors. The heterotrimer shown in the diagram contains a $G\alpha_s$-subunit, which activates adenylyl cyclases. However, other heterotrimers may contain $G\alpha_{i/o}$-subunits that can inhibit adenylyl cyclases, $G\alpha_{q/11}$-subunits that can activate phospholipases, or $G\alpha_{s12/13}$-subunits that can activate phospholipases or guanosine exchange factors that activate small GTPases. An activated receptor is susceptible to phosphorylation by receptor kinases, which then permits arrestin proteins to bind that promote receptor internalization and degradation.

acid, prostaglandins, and cholinergic and purinergic agents (18).

EFFECTS OF THYROTROPIN ON ADENYLYL CYCLASES, CYCLIC ADENOSINE MONOPHOSPHATE–DEPENDENT PROTEIN KINASES, AND PHOSPHODIESTERASES

Under basal conditions, a stimulatory Gα protein ($G\alpha_s$) is the predominant Gα isoform in the thyroid. $G\alpha_s$ stimulates adenylyl cyclases and increases production of cyclic AMP, which not only activates cyclic AMP-dependent PKAs, but also independently activates guanine nucleotide exchange proteins activated by cyclic AMP (EPAC) proteins that regulate certain small GTPases. Cyclic nucleotides are degraded by phosphodiesterases. One action of TSH is to increase the activity of cyclic AMP-specific phosphodiesterases, which creates a negative feedback loop that limits the cyclic AMP response to TSH as well as to other factors that stimulate cyclic AMP production in the thyroid. Clinically, patients who have autonomous thyroid adenomas that contain an activating mutation—either in the TSH receptor gene or in the $G\alpha_s$ gene—commonly express a higher level of cyclic AMP phosphodiesterase activity in the tumor than is present in the surrounding normal thyroid tissue (19), which suggests that some cells in the adenomas retain the homeostatic tendency to limit cyclic AMP-dependent responses. In FRTL-5 cells, TSH rapidly increases phosphodiesterase activity via cyclic AMP-dependent phosphorylation of the enzyme (20), while longer exposure to TSH increases the transcription of phosphodiesterases as well (21). Transfecting these cells with a constitutively active mutant $G\alpha_s$ causes phosphodiesterase-4 activities to increase, as determined by the selective inhibitor rolipram (22). Rolipram has no effect on the proliferation of wild-type cells, but in cells expressing the constitutively active mutant $G\alpha_S$, rolipram causes TSH-independent proliferation, indicating that cyclic AMP plays a key role in the proliferation of FRTL-5 cells (22). It is important to note, however, that "immortalized" thyrocyte cell lines may respond to TSH differently than thyrocytes grown in primary culture, to say nothing of thyroid tissue *in vivo*. Thus, for example, FRTL-5 cells are known to dedifferentiate with increasing number of cell passages (23), may be tetraploid (24), and can harbor mutations in important genes (23,25).

Cyclic AMP activates cyclic AMP-dependent PKAs by binding to the regulatory subunit dimer in the holoenzyme (Fig. 10C.2). The dimerization region on R-subunits also

permits them to bind to AKAPs (A-kinase anchoring proteins), which are scaffolding proteins that tether different PKA isoforms in specific locations within the cell. When the four cyclic AMP, binding sites on the R-subunit dimer are occupied, catalytic C-subunits are released, which then incorporate phosphate groups on certain serine or threonine residues in neighboring substrates, modulating their interactions with other proteins. The CREB, CREM, and ATF-1 family of transcription factors are important nuclear substrates of PKA, although they are phosphorylated by other kinases as well. Phosphorylation by PKA permits CREB dimers to bind to cyclic AMP-response elements (CREs) in various genes, and to recruit components of the transcription complex, thereby activating cyclic AMP-responsive genes. Inducible cyclic AMP early repressor

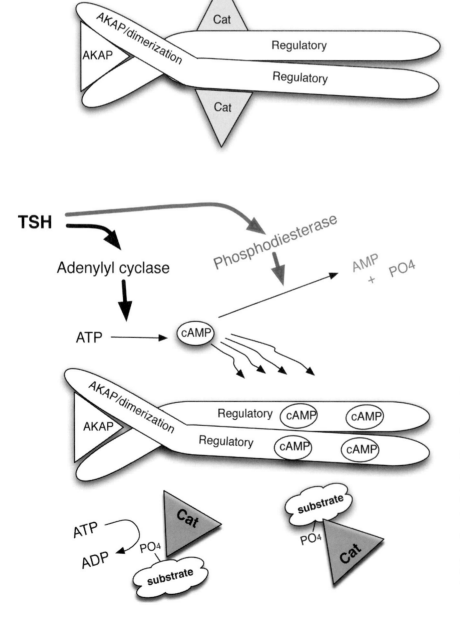

FIGURE 10C.2. Regulation of cyclic and cyclic AMP-dependent protein kinases (PKA). **Top diagram:** In the basal state, PKA heterotrimers consist of a regulatory subunit dimer and two catalytic *(Cat)* subunits, and may be tethered in specific subcellular locations by binding to A-kinase anchoring proteins (AKAP). **Bottom diagram:** Thyrotropin (TSH) activates adenylyl cyclase and converts adenosine triphosphate to cyclic AMP. When all the cyclic AMP binding sites on PKA are occupied, catalytic subunits are released so they can phosphorylate nearby substrates. Subsequently, TSH activates cyclic AMP-specific phosphodiesterases that degrade the cyclic AMP, allowing catalytic subunits to reassociate with regulatory subunit dimers.

(ICER) is a cyclic AMP-inducible antagonistic transcription factor that is produced from an alternative promoter in the CREM gene, and which down-regulates its own expression. In hypophysectomized rats, injection of TSH initially raises the level of TSH receptor mRNA, but it falls as ICER mRNA levels peak (26). TSH also transiently increases ICER levels in primary dog thyrocytes, which correlates with down-regulation of TSH receptors (27).

Clinically, some thyroid adenomas bear somatic mutations in the TSH-receptor gene that act in a dominant fashion to activate the receptor in the absence of ligand (see Chapter 25). However, mutations that inactivate the receptor act in a recessive fashion, so both alleles of the gene must be affected before clinical TSH resistance or hypothyroidism occur (see Chapter 48). Mutations in the TSH-receptor gene may alter the basal level of activity of the receptor or the ability of the receptor to couple with certain $G\alpha$- subunits, selectively affecting, for example, the ability of TSH to generate inositol phosphate signals (28,29).

When a dominant negatively acting isoform of CREB is experimentally targeted to the mouse thyroid, the mice are born hypothyroid (10). The thyroid glands of these mice are poorly developed despite the high serum TSH levels, and they express only low levels of the mRNAs encoding the TSH receptor, thyroglobulin, thyroid peroxidase, and the transcription factors Pax-8, TTF-1, and TTF-2, indicating the importance of CREB in both the growth and the function of the thyroid (10). The state of CREB phosphorylation also mediates thyrocyte responsiveness to TSH stimulation. When TSH-starved FRTL-5 cells are given TSH, there is an initial burst in cyclic AMP-dependent transcription that then decreases gradually over a period of hours, reflecting a progressive dephosphorylation of CREB by protein phosphatase 1 (30). More prolonged exposure to TSH causes decreased translation of PKA catalytic subunits, further desensitizing the response to cyclic AMP (30). Finally, chronically high levels of TSH decrease the density of TSH receptors in the thyrocytes of rats *in vivo*, as well as in FRTL-5 cells *in vitro* (31).

Still another way that a change in the cyclic AMP responsiveness of thyrocytes will occur is if TSH activates a receptor that couples with a G-protein heterotrimer containing a $G\alpha_{i/o}$-subunit, which inhibits adenylyl cyclases (32).

EFFECTS OF THYROTROPIN ON G-PROTEIN HETEROTRIMERS ACTING VIA OTHER PATHWAYS

In addition to regulating cyclic AMP pathways, TSH receptors can couple with G-protein heterotrimers containing $G\alpha_{q/11}$- subunits, which activate phospholipases that generate inositol phosphates and diacylglycerol, which in turn activate Ca++/phospholipid-dependent kinases (PKC). Higher concentrations of TSH are needed to activate these $G\alpha$-isoforms than are needed to activate $G\alpha_s$. If a receptor couples with a heterotrimer containing a $G\alpha_{12}$-subunit, it can affect small GTPases by interacting with proteins that activate guanosine exchange factors, as well as other pathways (33). It is important to note that when TSH stimulates the release of any of the $G\alpha$-isoforms, it simultaneously releases $G\beta\gamma$-dimers that then interact with other proteins. The $G\beta\gamma$-dimers, which are prenylated and remain membrane-bound, can activate certain phospholipases, phosphatidylinositol-3-kinases (PI3-kinases) and small GTPases.

EFFECTS OF THYROTROPIN ON SMALL GUANINE TRIPHOSPHATASES

Small guanosine triphosphatases (GTPase) are molecular switches that regulate membrane trafficking of receptors, transporters, and ion channels, as well as regulating the activity of many kinases (Fig. 10C.3). Clinical and experimental data show that several small GTPases play important roles in thyroid differentiation, proliferation, apoptosis and tumorogenesis. Inactive small GTPases contain GDP, but if the GDP is replaced by GTP, the proteins become active. The switch to the active state is regulated by guanosine exchange factors that promote the displacement of GDP by GTP (34), while inactivation is enhanced by GTPase-activating proteins. Several hundred of these regulatory molecules have effects on different small GTPases. Their activities in turn can be regulated by cyclic AMP, Ca++, diacylglycerol, and redox conditions, as well as by other small GTPase regulators. Small GTPases often undergo prenylation, which promotes their association with membranes.

Ras small GTPases are protooncogenes located predominantly in membranes, and are of clinical importance, since mutations in Ki-Ras, N-Ras, and Ha-Ras are found in multinodular goiters, microfollicular adenomas, and papillary and follicular carcinomas (35,36). When activated, Ras proteins regulate Raf kinase as well as PI3-kinase–signaling cascades. Posttranslational modifications of Ras proteins affect their association with other proteins, with intracellular membranes, and the signaling pathways they regulate. Experimentally, when an oncogenic Ha-Ras mutant is expressed in normal human thyrocytes, it causes proliferation but does not affect differentiated function (37). In rat thyroid cell lines, however, experimental expression of a constitutively active Ras causes apoptosis (38) and dedifferentiation (37,39). In FRTL-5 cells, TSH induces proliferation via PKA-mediated phosphorylation of Ras, which stimulates its interaction with PI3-kinase (40). Cyclic AMP also stimulates proliferation of Wistar rat thyrocytes. Active GTP-Ras must be present before TSH can stimulate proliferation of these cells, and this response is independent of PKA and tyrosine kinase activities (41,42). TSH and cyclic AMP also stimulate proliferation of cultured dog thyrocytes; however, both agents actually reduce

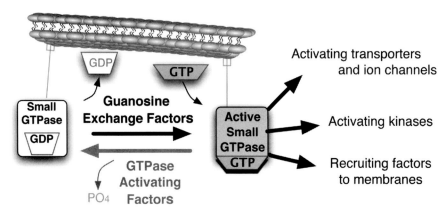

FIGURE 10C.3. Regulation of small guanosine triphosphatase (GTPase) proteins. Small GTPases are commonly membrane-associated due to their covalent modification by various kinds of prenylation (indicated with a *trident*). In the basal state, a small GTPase contains a guanosine diphosphate (GDP) molecule. Activation occurs when GTP displaces the GDP, which can be promoted by various guanosine exchange factors. Activated small GTPases can recruit factors to membranes, and can activate kinases and transporters. Subsequently, the protein's intrinsic GTPase activity hydrolyzes the GTP back to GDP, which can be accelerated by various GTPase activating factors.

the level of GTP-Ras-GTP (43). These varied effects of TSH on Ras may reflect species and strain differences reported in Ras and in the proteins that interact with Ras.

The Rap proteins (Rap-1a, -1b, and Rap-2) are small GTPases (Fig. 10C.4) that affect tyrosine kinases and integrin-mediated cell adhesion. The Rap phosphoproteins are homologous to Ras, and they bind to many of the proteins to which Ras binds, but counteract some of the transforming effects of Ras. TSH activates Rap activity in a number of thyroid cell lines. Expressing a constitutively active Rap-1a mutant in Wistar rat thyrocytes causes differentiation, while cells expressing a dominant negative mutant Rap-1 no

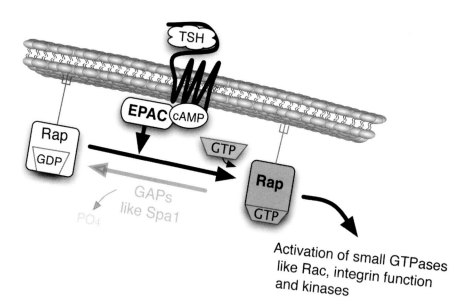

FIGURE 10C.4. Regulation of the small guanosine triphosphatase (GTPase) Rap-1. Activation of the small GTPase Rap-1 causes membrane recruitment and activation of various kinases and other small GTPases, and alters membrane signaling. GTP-Rap-1 levels can be increased via guanosine exchange factors, and can be decreased by GTPase activating proteins such as Rap-1 glyceraldehyde-3-phosphate (GAP). TSH and cyclic adenosine monophosphate (cyclic AMP) activate Rap-1 in Wistar rat thyrocytes, presumably via guanine nucleotide exchange proteins activated by cyclic AMP and not via protein kinases (PKA), although PKA can phosphorylate Rap-1. TSH stabilizes Rap-1 GAP, and this effect is mediated by PKA, possibly via its action on phosphoprotein phosphatase. If TSH is removed from the medium, Rap-1 GAP levels decrease due to phosphorylation by glycogen synthase kinase 3β, which causes proteasomal degradation of Rap-1 GAP.

longer proliferate in response to TSH (41). The activation of Rap-1 is mimicked by cyclic AMP but does not require PKA, although PKA does shorten the duration of Rap-1 activation, whereas blocking PKA prolongs the activation of Rap-1 by TSH (41). PKA stabilizes Rap-1GAP, a GTPase activator of Rap that is a tumor suppressor, and if TSH is removed from Wistar rat cells, the level of Rap-1GAP falls (41,42). In PCCl3 rat thyrocytes that overexpress Rap-1GAP, PKA no longer can inhibit Akt (42a). In FRTL-5 cells, TSH also increases Rap-GTP levels by a cyclic AMP-mediated effect that does not involve PKA (43). TSH and forskolin activate Rap in primary cultures of dog thyrocytes, however carbachol, phorbol esters, insulin, and epidermal growth factor also have the same effect, and these agents do not activate PKA (43). Furthermore, microinjecting Rap-1b alone or in combination with a catalytic subunit of PKA into dog thyrocytes does not affect their proliferation or differentiation (43). A synthetic transgene that can be switched from a constitutively active form of Rap1b to a dominant negative form has been targeted to the mouse thyroid (43a). The constitutively active transgene perchlovate for 6 months causes nodules to form in the hyperplastic goiters that normally occur. These nodules express the constitutively active protein. If the goitrogens are removed, those findings reversed within 2 months, but if the goitrogens are continued for a year, frank invasion of the capsule, blood vessels and surrounding tissue occurs. Switching the transgene to the dominant negative form reduces the size of goiters produced by the goitrogens and the amount of cell proliferation, indicating Rap1b can have an oncogenic effect when linked to the mitogenic action of chronically elevated cyclic AMP levels (43a). While TSH and cyclic AMP do influence Rap activity, it is af-

fected by other pathways as well. The non-PKA mediated effects of cyclic AMP on Rap may be mediated by EPAC proteins, which bind cyclic AMP directly, and which promote the displacement of GDP by GTP and thus activate Rap. EPAC-1 mRNA is known to be expressed at high levels in the thyroid (34), while EPAC-2 can be expressed in several isoforms due to alternative mRNA splicing, so the relative importance of different EPAC-mediated effects could underlie some of the differences in the actions of cyclic AMP that are not mediated by PKA.

EFFECTS OF THYROTROPIN ON RAF KINASES

The Raf protein kinases (e.g., B-Raf and Raf-1) are phosphoproteins that become recruited to membranes by binding to activated small GTPases like GTP-Ras (Fig. 10C.5). The phosphorylation and dephosphorylation of Raf regulates its affinity for GTP-Ras, although phosphoprotein-binding proteins can regulate the access of GTP-Ras to these phosphorylated sites. Once Raf has been recruited to the membrane, its activity is regulated by membrane receptors that signal through kinases such as PI3-kinase and Akt. Activated Raf is a mitogen-activated protein (MAP) kinase kinase kinase (MAPKKK) that phosphorylates and activates MEK (MAPK/ERK kinase or MAPKK), which in turn activates MAP kinases. Many papillary thyroid carcinomas contain a specific mutation in B-Raf, indicating obvious clinical importance. In FRTL-5 cells, forskolin activates and recruits B-Raf to membranes, where it co-localizes with Rap-1 and subsequently activates ERK (44). In-

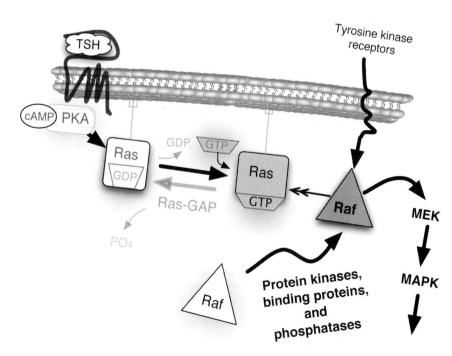

FIGURE 10C.5. Regulation of Raf kinases. The Raf protein kinase family can be recruited to the plasma membrane by activated small guanosinetriphosphatases, like Rap and Ras. The ability of Raf to be recruited depends on the state of certain phosphorylated sites on Raf, and access to them can be blocked if the sites are occupied by phosphoprotein-binding proteins. Once Rafs have been recruited to membranes, they are activated by various kinases, and in turn activate nitrogen-activated protein (MAP) kinase cascades.

terestingly, these effects of forskolin are not mediated by PKA (44).

EFFECTS OF THYROTROPIN ON PHOSPHATIDYLINOSITIDE-3-KINASES AND SOME PHOSPHOINOSITIDE-DEPENDENT KINASES

PI3-kinases are heterodimers that can contain one of several possible noncatalytic subunits that suppress the activity of a catalytic subunit (Fig. 10C.6). One type of noncatalytic subunit contains SH-2 or SH-3 domains that bind to phosphotyrosine residues produced when membrane tyrosine kinase receptors are activated, while another type of noncatalytic subunit of PI3-kinase binds to the Gβγ-dimers that become available on the plasma membrane when G-coupled receptors are activated. Since PI3-kinases can be activated both by G-protein–coupled receptors (like TSH receptors) and receptor tyrosine kinases (like insulin and IGF-1 receptors), these two kinds of signals intersect, and differences in signaling responses can arise (45). Once PI3-kinase holoenzymes are bound at the membrane, their conformation changes and the activated catalytic subunit then phosphorylates proteins and lipids in the plasma membrane. The lipid kinase activity increases the membrane levels of several phosphatidylinositol 3′phosphates, which have differing affinity and selectivity for proteins with pleckstrin homology domains. Proteins that contain these domains include Akt, phosphoinositide-dependent kinase-1, and phospholipase-C isoforms, which can also be activated once they become membrane associated. The major lipid phosphatase responsible for down-regulating the signaling of phosphatidylinositol phosphates is PTEN, which is a tumor suppressor as well as a regulator of cell migration and cell size. Clinically, PTEN is silenced in several types of thyroid tumor.

PI3-kinases mediate various actions of TSH in FRTL-5 and Wistar rat thyrocyte cell lines (40,45–50). Since PI3-kinases can phosphorylate proteins like insulin regulatory substrate-1, TSH can activate pathways that are also regulated by insulin and insulin-like growth factor 1 (IGF-1) (45,46). TSH also induces IGF-1 production in FRTL-5 cells, as well as potentiating IGF-1–mediated proliferation via PI3-kinase, tyrosine kinase, and MAPK pathways (45,46). Anti-TSH receptor–immunocomplexes prepared from FRTL-5 cells contain PI3-kinase activity, and treating the cells with TSH increases the amount of PI3-kinase precipitated, as well as the amount of phosphotyrosine present. Additional evidence for the important role played by PI3-kinase in mediating the action of cAMP in these cells was provided by the use of the PI3-kinase inhibitor wortmannin, which blocked cyclic AMP-mediated phosphotyrosine production (46,47). PKA stimulates formation of a complex between PI3-kinase and Ras (40), and increases the phosphorylation and amount of PI3-kinase regulatory subunit that precipitates with anti-TSH receptor antibody in FRTL-5 cells (47). IGF-1 and TSH are synergistic in causing FRTL-5 cell proliferation, but in contrast, IGF-1 blocks the induction of sodium-iodine symporter mRNA by TSH and cyclic AMP (48). The inhibitory effect of IGF-1 on the symporter can be eliminated by blocking PI3-kinase, but is not affected by inhibiting PKA, PKC, or MEK (48). In Wistar rat thyrocytes, PI3-kinase is required for cyclic AMP to stimulate mitogenesis, and this involves both PKA-dependent and -independent pathways (49,50). Although TSH amplifies insulin and IGF-1 signaling in primary cultures of dog thyrocytes, it does not change PI3-kinase activity (51).

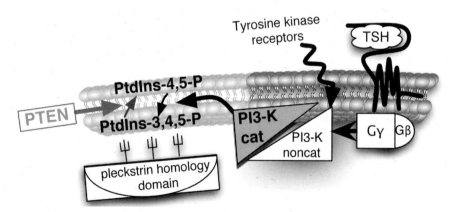

FIGURE 10C.6. Regulation of phosphatidylinositide-3-kinases (PI3-kinases). In the basal state, PI3-kinases are heterodimers containing a catalytic subunit *(Cat)* that is suppressed by a noncatalytic subunit. When TSH stimulates a receptor, it releases Gβγ dimers that can recruit one type of noncatalytic subunit to the plasma membrane and activate its associated catalytic subunit. Membrane receptor tyrosine kinases can recruit another type of noncatalytic subunit to the plasma membrane and also activate its associated catalytic subunit. The activated PI3-kinase catalytic subunits then phosphorylate proteins as well as lipids in the plasma membrane. By increasing the levels of phosphatidylinositol-3-phosphate molecules in membranes, PI3-kinases attract proteins with pleckstrin homology domains (shown as *three tridents*), permitting those proteins to be activated as well. Subsequently, the lipid phosphatase PTEN turns off this signal.

One of the kinases with a pleckstrin domain that is attracted by increased phosphatidylinositol phosphate levels in membranes is 3-phosphoinositide-dependent protein kinase-1. Once it is located in the membrane, it can be activated by various kinases: when phosphorylated by PI3-kinase, it can undergo subcellular translocation. TSH alters the subcellular distribution of this kinase in FRTL-5 cells via both PI3-kinase and PKA mediated pathways (47). 3-phosphoinositide-dependent protein kinase-1 then acts by phosphorylating the activation loop of members of the PKA, PKC, and cyclic GMP-dependent kinase families.

S6K is another pleckstrin domain–containing kinase that is phosphorylated by many kinase pathways: SK6 in turn phosphorylates the 40S ribosomal protein S6 and the initiation factor 4E-binding protein-1 required for cells to traverse from G1 to S phase. If FRTL-5 cells are maintained in medium without any TSH, insulin, or serum, the addition of TSH stimulates p70-S6K activity, but this response can be blocked either by inhibitors of PKA or of PI3-kinase (47). In Wistar rat thyrocytes, TSH and cyclic AMP stimulate S6K both by Rap-1A– and cyclic AMP-dependent pathways (49,50). In primary dog thyrocytes, TSH rapidly activates p70-S6K but does not affect p90-S6K (51).

The mammalian target of rapamycin (mTOR) is yet another pleckstrin domain–containing kinase whose phosphorylation is regulated by small GTPases. The mammalian target of rapamycin senses nutrient levels, receives mitogenic signals, and transmits signals to S6K to regulate cell proliferation. Rapamycin, a specific inhibitor of mTOR, blocks TSH/cAMP-mediated phosphorylation of S6K in FRTL-5 cells, and causes cell cycle arrest, implicating mTOR in this action of TSH (48).

Protein kinase B (also called PKB) kinases are phosphoproteins located in cytosol in a relatively inactive form under basal conditions. Increasing the membrane level of phosphatidylinositol phosphates causes Akts to bind to the membrane, which alters the structure of the Akts and permits their activation (52,53). In FRTL-5 cells and human thyroid cancer cells, TSH does not affect Akt phosphorylation, although insulin does (55,56). Akt is involved in FRTL-5 cell proliferation: expressing a constitutively active Akt-1 mutant in these cells increases basal DNA synthesis, and serum or insulin/IGF-1 are no longer needed for TSH to induce DNA synthesis (55). In Wistar rat thyrocytes (grown with insulin but without serum), TSH causes phosphorylation of Akt. Expressing a constitutively active Rap increases TSH-mediated phosphorylation of Akt in these cells (53). In contrast, in rat PCCl3 cells (grown with insulin but without serum), TSH inhibits Akt activity via PKA, presumably via PKA-mediated phosphorylation and activation of Rap-1b (54). When a constitutively active form of Rap is expressed in PCCl3 cells it decreases Akt phosphorylation, and potentiates the inhibitory effect of forskolin on Akt phosphorylation (54). These three different effects of TSH on Akt in three rat thyrocyte models could reflect the different ways that these immortalized cells were obtained: Wistar cells were cloned from fibroblasts of thyroids from immature rats, PCCl3 cells were cloned from 18-month-old rats, and FRTL-5 cells were obtained by culturing young rat thyroid cells in low levels of calf serum. If vascular cells are treated with H_2O_2, Akt becomes oxidized, and its phosphorylation is affected (this action of H_2O_2 on Akt appears to be mediated by PI3-kinase, since it is blocked by wortmannin) (52).

EFFECTS OF THYROTROPIN ON THE REGULATION OF THYROID PEROXIDASE, H_2O_2 PRODUCTION, AND REDOX BALANCE

TSH regulates thyroid peroxidase expression via cyclic AMP pathways, whereas H_2O_2 production involves Ca^{++}/phosphoinositol pathways in all species. In dog thyrocytes, TSH and cyclic AMP agonists stimulate the production of H_2O_2 (57), and high doses of TSH can increase H_2O_2 production in FRTL-5 cells as well (13). It is noteworthy that exogenous H_2O_2 can induce apoptosis in FRTL-5 cells (58), and a variety of factors are involved in controlling the toxic effects of H_2O_2, lipid hydroperoxides, and free radicals. TSH increases the expression of Ref-1 (15), the transcription factor that repairs DNA damaged by oxidative stress, and Ref-1 also protects cells from oxidative apoptotic stimuli. Changes in the redox state of a cell alter the activity of CHOP, a transcription factor that monitors endoplasmic reticulum stress and which also can regulate apoptosis. CHOP is expressed in rat thyroids, as well as in FRTL-5 and PCCl3 cells. If TSH is removed from the culture medium of FRTL-5 cells, CHOP levels fall unless forskolin is present (59). This protective effect of forskolin on CHOP levels involves PKA, mTOR, and the level of reactive oxygen species (59). In FRTL-5 cells, TSH increases the expression of antioxidants like peroxiredoxin-1 and thioredoxin (13,58). Thioredoxin reductase is induced by Ca^{++}/phosphoinositol pathways, but not by cyclic AMP in human thyrocytes (60). Duox-2 is a flavoprotein involved in H_2O_2 production, and which is regulated by TSH and cyclic AMP in pig (61), human, and dog thyrocytes (62). Insulin also increases Duox-2 mRNA expression in FRTL-5 cells grown in TSH-free low-serum medium, but the addition of insulin switches the stimulatory action of forskolin on Duox-2 to an inhibitory one (63). This illustrates how a hormone that does not directly act via cyclic AMP can dramatically alter a thyrocyte's response to cyclic AMP.

EFFECTS OF THYROTROPIN ON MITOGEN-ACTIVATED PROTEIN KINASES AND JANUS KINASE/SIGNAL TRANSDUCER AND ACTIVATOR OF TRANSCRIPTION PATHWAYS

Many kinds of stress can activate MAPKKK/MAPKK/MAP kinase cascades, and thus regulate cell growth, transformation, and apoptosis. The downstream cascades can be divided into three subfamilies: p38 MAPKs and the JNKs (c-jun N-terminal kinases) (both associated with regulation in response to cellular stresses), and the ERKs (extracellular signal–regulated kinases), which are associated with regulation of cell proliferation and differentiation, although the actions of the subfamilies can overlap.

When pig thyrocytes are cultured with TSH, they form follicle-like structures. If the TSH is removed, this stress causes the cells to migrate and become confluent monolayers. The loss of higher organization and the migration can be prevented if TSH or cyclic AMP agonists are added to the culture medium (64). The loss of organization involves activation-specific phosphorylation of ERK, which accumulates in the thyrocyte nuclei. ERK inhibitors block the migratory responses, and PI3-kinase inhibitors block the initiation of cell movement, but not the activation of ERK, suggesting that two pathways are involved in the cell migration that is tonically inhibited by the presence of TSH or cyclic AMP (64).

TSH and cyclic AMP agonists also cause a rapid but transient phosphorylation of ERK in FRTL-5 cells (45). The importance of this response was confirmed by inhibiting MEK (MAPKK), which blocks MEK-dependent phosphorylation of ERK as well as cyclic AMP-mediated DNA synthesis (45). The cyclic AMP-mediated DNA synthesis and ERK reponses were not blocked by the PKA inhibitor H89, whereas H89 does inhibit p38 MAP kinase phosphorylation in response to TSH (65). This cyclic AMP-dependent activation of p38 MAP kinase appears to involve reactive oxygen species (65). In dog and human thyrocytes, insulin must be present in order for TSH or cyclic AMP to be mitogenic, and its action is also inhibited when MEK is inhibited (66).

When cytokine receptors in the plasma membrane are activated, they attract the cytoplasmic tyrosine kinase JAK (Janus kinase), creating docking sites for SH-2–containing proteins like the STATs (signal transducer and activator of transcription). Several cytokines are known to alter thyrocyte growth and function, and TSH and cyclic AMP influence these actions of cytokines. As has been observed for other heterotrimeric G-protein–coupled receptors, activation of the TSH receptor can alter the tyrosine phosphorylation and activation of STATs. In FRTL-5 cells, TSH causes tyrosine phosphorylation of STAT-3, induces the formation of a STAT-3/DNA complex (67), and induces the expression of the feedback inhibitor SOCS-1 (suppressor of cytokine signaling-1), a target gene of STAT-3 (68). Expression of a dominant negative STAT-3 inhibited the action of TSH on SOCS-1 expression, confirming that TSH is acting via JAK/STAT signaling (67). The action of TSH and forskolin on STAT-3 phosphorylation can be blocked by inhibitors of PKC, but not by inhibitors of PKA (69).

EFFECTS OF THYROTROPIN ON PHOSPHOLIPASES, CALCIUM, AND PROTEIN KINASE C (PKC)

TSH activates $G\alpha_q$-containing heterotrimers to stimulate isoforms of phospholipase A, C, and D, and provides diacylglycerol (DAG) and inositol 1,4,5-trisphosphate, which can mobilize intracellular pools of Ca2+ to activate PKC. Cross regulation and indirect effects have made it difficult to establish which are the primary actions of TSH. For example, the activity and subcellular location of phospholipase D is regulated by multiple pathways, including phospholipids, small GTPases, PKC, as well as via indirect effects through tyrosine kinases. The phosphatidic acid that phospholipase D produces acts as a cofactor in a number of signaling cascades, in addition to being converted to DAG by phosphatidic acid phosphatases. Phospholipases also release arachidonic and linoleic acids that can be metabolized by lipoxygenase to form free radicals and lipid peroxides, which provide another inflammatory stress that can induce apoptosis. Arachidonate also may be converted to prostanoids. The stimulation of phospholipase D activity by TSH appears to involve both cyclic AMP and PKC, since inhibitors of PKC and PKA have separate inhibitory actions on TSH-mediated phospholipase D activity (70).

EFFECTS OF THYROTROPIN ON VASCULAR ELEMENTS AND BLOOD FLOW IN THE THYROID

TSH stimulates blood flow in the thyroid by increasing nitric oxide synthase and nitric oxide production (71). Chronic TSH stimulation increases the vascularity of the thyroid gland, TSH increases the expression of FGF-1 (fibroblast growth factor 1) and in primary cultures of human thyrocytes (72). If a dominant negative FGF-1 mutation is expressed in FRTL-5 cells, it inhibits the actions of TSH on cell growth and iodide uptake, and if it is expressed in mice, it reduces the goiter and the vascular growth produced by a low iodine diet plus perchlorate, indicating that FGF receptor–signaling affects several thyroid responses (73). Adding FGF-2 to human thyrocytes increases their growth but inhibits their iodide uptake (72). Vascular endothelial growth factor (VEGF) isoforms have different effects in different models, but in primary cultures of human thyrocytes, VEGF stimulates nitric oxide release (74). Histochemical studies show that thyroid follicles with a cuboidal epithelium are metabolically active, and express TSH receptor, sodium-iodine symporter, pendrin, thyroid peroxidase, and thyroglobulin that contains T_4, whereas follicles with a flat epithelium are metabolically inactive and express little of these substances. The capillary networks that surround active follicles contain nitric oxide synthase III and endothelin, but the capillaries around flat follicles do not, suggesting there is a paracrine connection that communicates the activity of epithelial cells to the neighboring vascular cells (75). Thyrocytes are known to produce angiogenic factors, including IGF-I and angiopoietins, but the primary regulators of thyroid vascularity remain to be established. Interestingly, if rats are given a low iodine diet plus goitrogens to raise the circulating level of TSH, the vascular endothelium begins to proliferate before the thyrocytes (76). Chronic TSH stimulation of rats causes thrombospondin, an inhibitor of angiogenesis, to disappear progressively from thyroid endothelial cells and stroma (77).

EXAMPLES OF OTHER HORMONES INVOLVED IN THYROIDAL RESPONSES TO THYROTROPIN

Thyroid hormones can act on the thyroid gland directly, and on the other hand, TSH and cyclic AMP increase nuclear level of triiodothyronine (T_3) receptors as well as increasing the activity of deiodinases in human thyrocytes, responses that can be inhibited by activating PKB (78). The nuclear T_3 receptor is involved in the growth of the thyroid, and if one gives T_3 to hypophysectomized rats, the density of TSH receptors expressed on the thyroid increases, representing another way that thyroid hormone can affect the function of the thyroid directly (31). Studies *in vivo* (79) and in FRTL-5 cells (80) indicate that epidermal growth factor acts as an autocrine factor produced within the thyroid in response to changes in thyroid hormone levels.

Somatostatin is commonly added to culture media to promote thyrocyte differentiation *in vitro*, but the somatostatin gene is expressed in FRTL-5 cells and is regulated by TSH, indicating it is an autocrine inhibitory factor (81). Adding exogenous somatostatin to FRTL-5 cells inhibits the proliferative responses both to TSH and to insulin, while it increases the expression of p27^{kip1}, the cyclin-dependent kinase cell cycle inhibitor (81). Somatostatin also lessens TSH-mediated activation of adenylyl cyclase, and inhibits PI3-kinase in a PKA-independent fashion in these cells (82). In PCCl3 cells, somatostatin inhibits the proliferation by activating a membrane phosphotyrosine phosphatase, which prevents the activation of MAP kinase and stabilizes p27^{kip1} (83,84).

EFFECTS OF THYROTROPIN ON APOPTOSIS

When a goiter undergoes involution, organized cell death is involved (85). Apoptosis occurs in both stromal as well as vascular cells if a normal level of iodine is added to the diet of rats that have been fed a low iodine diet plus methimazole (86). In rats with methimazole-induced goiter, withdrawal of the methimazole initially inhibits cell proliferation, while apoptosis becomes evident about a week later (87).

TSH and cyclic AMP agonists protect FRTL-5 cells from apoptosis that normally would be induced by actinomycin D or H_2O_2 (88). The extracellular matrix is an important regulator of cell development and survival. If serum is removed from the incubation medium of FRTL-5 cells, TSH must be present in order to prevent apoptosis. This action involves increased cell adhesion and is mediated in part by PKA (89). If serum is removed from the incubation medium, human thyrocytes degrade extracellular matrix, lose integrin-fibronectin interactions, and apoptosis ensues. Adding an inhibitor of PI3-kinase promotes apoptosis in this model (90). TSH protects Wistar rat thyrocytes from nitroprusside-induced apoptosis, and this effect involves PKA and S6K (91). Rap-1 also plays a role, since in cells expressing a constitutively active Rap-1, the apoptotic effect of nitroprusside is accentuated, whereas cells expressing a dominant negative Rap-1 resist the apoptotic effect of nitroprusside (91).

EFFECTS OF THYROTROPIN ON REGULATORS OF THE CELL CYCLE

TSH affects various members of the complex network of cell cycle activators and inhibitors, but no single common pathway applies for all models. It is commonly held that cyclin-dependent kinases (CDKs) need to be activated before cells can enter the S phase of the cell cycle, and that the level of the cyclin inhibitor protein p27^{kip1} must decrease to allow CDK activation. In FRTL-5 cells, TSH does cause the expected decrease in p27^{kip1} and increases cyclin D1 levels, whereas phosphodiesterase inhibitors curtail the cyclin D1 response to TSH and IGF-1 (21). Cyclic AMP is involved in the proliferation of synchronized FRTL-5 cells: the levels of RI and RII isoforms of PKA both change with the cell cycle, and experimentally altering these regulatory subunit responses affects cell cycle progression (92). The predominant cyclin D isoform in many thyrocytes is cyclin D3, and this isoform appears to be important clinically because it is overexpressed in most follicular adenomas (93). In rats given propylthiouracil, cyclin D3 levels increase within 5 days, while in PCCl3 cells grown in serum alone, adding TSH increases cyclin D3 synthesis within 6 hours (93). Cyclin D3 also plays a role in TSH-mediated proliferation of primary cultures of dog thyrocytes, since proliferation is suppressed when cyclin D3 is neutralized by microinjecting antibody to cyclin D3 (94). If TSH, serum or insulin are added to starved WRT or PCCl3 cells, there is no increase in cell proliferation (94a). However if serum is combined with either TSH or forskolin, the cells proliferate rapidly. Adding the full complement of growth factors causes CDK2 levels to increase at 3 hours, followed by an increase in cyclin D1 and then in cyclin D3. Although total p27^{kip1} levels decreased only slightly at 15 hours, nuclear staining of p27^{kip1} in WRT cells decreased within 6 hours. TSH or forskolin did not deplete nuclear p27^{kip1}, but they accelerated and potentiated this effect of serum. The disappearance of nuclear p27^{kip1} staining correlated with progression of cells from G1 to S (94a).

EFFECTS OF THYROTROPIN ON THYROTROPIN RECEPTORS IN NONTHYROID TISSUES AND CELL LINES

Functional TSH receptors are expressed in several nonthyroid tissues in which the actions of TSH are not mediated by cyclic AMP. For example, the action of TSH on neurotransmitter-induced ion currents in submucosal glands from human trachea is blocked by tyrosine kinase inhibitors, and is not mimicked by cyclic AMP (95). In abdominal preadipocytes and orbital fibroblasts, TSH increases S6K activity, and this response can be blocked by wortmannin, the inhibitor of PI3-kinase (96). Studies in TSH receptor knockout mice suggest that TSH may have a direct effect on osteoclast formation that is mediated by JNK phosphorylation, and may affect osteoblast differentiation and type 1 collagen formation via Wnt and VEGF signaling pathways (97). If 3T3-L1 preadipocytes are grown without serum, TSH acts as a survival factor (98). TSH has no effect on cyclic AMP levels in these cells, but it increases phosphotyrosine and phosphatidylinositol phosphate levels—presumably via PI3-kinase, since TSH increases the level of activated S6K and Akt, and since these responses can be blocked by PI3-kinase inhibitors (98).

EFFECTS OF THYROTROPIN ON THYROTROPIN RECEPTORS EXPRESSED EXPERIMENTALLY IN CELLS

Many nonthyroid cells have been transfected to express TSH receptors, and in some cells TSH activates pathways that are not prominent in thyroid models, probably because in the spectrum of proteins expressed is different from the spectrum expressed in thyrocytes. Furthermore, only a low level of TSH receptor is normally expressed in thyrocytes, whereas experimental expression of a high level of TSH receptor may drive interactions that would not occur normally. This is also true when PKA subunits are overexpressed in cells (99). Nonetheless, the results obtained by such studies can be interesting. For example, cyclic AMP normally suppresses the growth of wild-type mouse NIH-3T3 fibroblasts. These fibroblasts express a relatively low level of the RIIβ isoform of A-kinase, and if RIIβ is overexpressed, the cells undergo apoptosis, which can be reversed by adding 8-Br cyclic AMP. If wild-type NIH-3T3 fibroblasts are transfected with a human TSH receptor gene under control of a tetracycline repressor gene and then tetracycline is removed, TSH causes cyclic AMP levels to rise and cell growth is inhibited, as would be expected. However, if both TSH receptors and RIIβ are expressed in these cells, TSH

actually stimulates growth, which appears to involve CREB phosphorylation, Rap-1, Akt, and ERK activity (100).

SUMMARY

As different mechanisms of action of TSH are uncovered in different models, we are obtaining a deeper understanding of the way different signaling pathways come together to control thyroid function, growth, and apoptosis. The clinical insights we have obtained from such studies have provided a deeper understanding of several thyroid diseases and of diseases in other organs as well.

REFERENCES

1. Hamad NM, Elconin JH, Karnoub AE, et al. Distinct requirements for Ras oncogenesis in human versus mouse cells. *Genes Dev* 2002;16:2045–57.
2. Smogorzewska A, de Lange T. Different telomere damage signaling pathways in human and mouse cells. *EMBO J* 2002;21:4338–48.
3. Pohlenz J, Maqueem A, Cua K, et al. Improved radioimmunoassay for measurement of mouse thyrotropin in serum: strain differences in thyrotropin concentration and thyrotroph sensitivity to thyroid hormone. *Thyroid* 1999;9:1265–71.
4. Postiglione MP, Parlato R, Rodriguez-Mallon A, et al. Role of the thyroid-stimulating hormone receptor signaling in development and differentiation of the thyroid gland. *Proc Natl Acad Sci U S A* 2002;99:15462–7.
5. Pic P, Michel-Bechet M, el Atiq F, et al. Forskolin stimulates cAMP production and the onset of the functional differentiation in the fetal rat thyroid *in vitro*. *Biol Cell* 1986;57:231–7.
6. Marians RC, Ng L, Blair HC, et al. Defining thyrotropin-dependent and -independent steps of thyroid hormone synthesis by using thyrotropin receptor-null mice. *Proc Natl Acad Sci USA* 2002;99:15776–81.
7. Medina DL, Suzuki K, Pietrarelli M, et al. Role of insulin and serum on thyrotropin regulation of thyroid transcription factor-1 and PAX8 genes expression in FRTL-5 thyroid cells. *Thyroid* 2000;10:295–303.
8. Di Palma T, Nitsch R, Mascia A, et al. The paired domain-containing factor Pax8 and the homeodomain-containing factor TTF1 directly interact and synergistically activate transcription. *J Biol Chem* 2003;278:3395–3402.
9. Moeller LC, Kimura S, Kusakabe T, et al. Hypothyroidism in TTF1 haploinsufficiency is caused by reduced expression of the TSH receptor. *Mol Endocrinol* 2003;17:2295–2302.
10. Nguyen LQ, Kopp P, Martinson F, et al. A dominant negative CREB (cAMP response element-binding protein) isoform inhibits thyrocyte growth, thyroid-specific gene expression, differentiation, and function. *Mol Endocrinol* 2000;14:1448–1461.
11. Feliciello A, Allevato G, Musti AM, et al. Thyroid transcription factor 1 phosphorylation is not required for PKA-dependent transcription of the thyroglobulin promoter. *Cell Growth Differ* 2000;11:649.
12. Puppin C, Arturi F, Ferretti E, et al. Transcriptional regulation of human NIS gene: a role for Redox factor-1. *Endocrinology* 2004;145:1290.
13. Kambe F, Nomura Y, Okamoto T, et al. Redox regulation of thyroid-transcription factors, PAX8 and TTF1, is involved in

their increased DNA-binding activities by thyrotropin in rat thyroid FRTL-5 cells. *Mol Endocrinol* 1996;10:801–812.

14. Cao X, Kambe F, Ohmori S, et al. Oxidoreductive modification of two cysteine residues in paired domain by Ref-1 regulates DNA-binding activity of PAX8. *Biochem Biophys Res Commun* 2002;297:288–293.

15. Asai T, Kambe F, Kikumori T, et al. Increase in Ref-1 mRNA and protein by thyrotropin in rat thyroid FRTL-5 cells. *Biochem Biophys Res Commun* 1997;236:71–74.

16. Russo D, Celano M, Bulotta S, et al. APE/Ref-1 is increased in nuclear fractions of human thyroid hyperfunctioning nodules. *Mol Cell Endocrinol* 2002;194:71–76.

17. Kambe F, Miyazaki T, Seo H. Differential induction of fos and jun family genes by thyrotropin in rat thyroid FRTL-5 cells. *Thyroid* 1996;6:123–128.

18. Iacovelli L, Franchetti R, Grisolia D, et al. Selective regulation of G protein-coupled receptor-mediated signaling by G protein-coupled receptor kinase 2 in FRTL-5 cells: analysis of thyrotropin, alpha(1β)-adrenergic, and A (1) adenosine receptor-mediated responses. *Mol Pharmacol* 1999;56:316–324.

19. Persani L, Lania A, Alberti L, et al. Induction of specific phosphodiesterase isoforms by constitutive activation of the cAMP pathway in autonomous thyroid adenomas. *J Clin Endocrinol Metab* 2000;85:2872–2878.

20. Oki N, Takahashi SI, Hidaka H, et al. Short term feedback regulation of cAMP in FRTL-5 thyroid cells. Role of PDE4D3 phosphodiesterase activation. *J Biol Chem* 2000;275:10831–10837.

21. Takahashi SI, Nedachi T, Fukushima T, et al. Long-term hormonal regulation of the cAMP-specific phosphodiesterases in cultured FRTL-5 thyroid cells. *Biochim Biophys Acta* 2001;1540:68–81.

22. Nemoz G, Sette C, Hess M, et al. Activation of cyclic nucleotide phosphodiesterases in FRTL-5 thyroid cells expressing a constitutively active Gsα. *Mol Endocrinol* 1995;9:1279–1287.

23. Green LM, Murray DK, Tran DT, et al. A spontaneously arising mutation in connexin32 with repeated passage of FRTL-5 cells coincides with increased growth rate and reduced thyroxine release. *J Mol Endocrinol* 2001;27:145–163.

24. Tasevski V, Benn D, Peters G, et al. The Fischer rat thyroid cell line FRTL-5 exhibits a nondiploid karyotype. *Thyroid* 1998;8:623–626.

25. Derwahl M, Seto P, Rapoport B. An abnormal splice donor site in one allele of the thyroid peroxidase gene in FRTL5 rat thyroid cells introduces a premature stop codon: association with the absence of functional enzymatic activity. *Mol Endocrinol* 1990;4:793–799.

26. Lalli E, Sassone-Corsi P. Thyroid-stimulating hormone (TSH)-directed induction of the CREM gene in the thyroid gland participates in the long-term desensitization of the TSH receptor. *Proc Natl Acad Sci USA* 1995;92:9633–9637.

27. Uyttersprot N, Costagliola S, Dumont JE, et al. Requirement for cAMP-response element (CRE) binding protein/CRE modulator transcription factors in thyrotropin-induced proliferation of dog thyroid cells in primary culture. *Eur J Biochem* 1999;259:370–378.

28. Arseven OK, Wilkes WP, Jameson JL, et al. Substitutions of tyrosine 601 in the human thyrotropin receptor result in increase or loss of basal activation of the cyclic adenosine monophosphate pathway and disrupt coupling to Gq/11. *Thyroid* 2000;10:3–10.

29. Wonerow P, Chey S, Fuhrer D, et al. Functional characterization of five constitutively activating thyrotrophin receptor mutations. *Clin Endocrinol (Oxf)* 2000;53:461–468.

30. Armstrong R, Wen W, Meinkoth J, et al. A refractory phase in cyclic AMP-responsive transcription requires down regulation of PKA. *Mol Cell Biol* 1995;15:1826–1832.

31. Denereaz N, Lemarchand-Beraud T. Severe but not mild alterations of thyroid function modulate the density of thyroid-stimulating hormone receptors in the rat thyroid gland. *Endocrinology* 1995;136:1694–1700.

32. Holzapfel HP, Bergner B, Wonerow P, et al. Expression of G(alpha)(s) proteins and TSH receptor signalling in hyperfunctioning thyroid nodules with TSH receptor mutations. *Eur J Endocrinol* 2002;147:109–116.

33. Shi CS, Lee SB, Sinnarajah S, et al. Regulator of G-protein signaling 3 (RGS3) inhibits Gβγ 2-induced inositol phosphate production, mitogen-activated PKA activation, and Akt activation. *J Biol Chem* 2001;276:24293–24300.

34. Kawasaki H, Springett GM, Mochizuki N, et al. A family of cAMP-binding proteins that directly activate Rap1. *Science* 1998;282:2275–2279.

35. Namba H, Rubin SA, Fagin JA. Point mutations of Ras oncogenes are an early event in thyroid tumorigenesis. *Mol Endocrinol* 1990;4:1474–1479.

36. Vasko V, Ferrand M, Di Cristofaro J, et al. Specific pattern of Ras oncogene mutations in follicular thyroid tumors. *J Clin Endocrinol Metab* 2003;88:2745–2752.

37. Gire V, Wynford-Thomas D. Ras oncogene activation induces proliferation in normal human thyroid epithelial cells without loss of differentiation. *Oncogene* 2000;19:737–744.

38. Cheng G, Lewis AE, Meinkoth JL. Ras stimulates aberrant cell cycle progression and apoptosis in rat thyroid cells. *Mol Endocrinol* 2003;17:450–459.

39. Francis-Lang H, Zannini M, De Felice M, et al. Multiple mechanisms of interference between transformation and differentiation in thyroid cells. *Mol Cell Biol* 1992;12:5793–5800.

40. Ciullo I, Diez-Roux G, Di Domenico M, et al. cAMP signaling selectively influences Ras effectors pathways. *Oncogene* 2001;20:1186–1192.

41. Tsygankova OM, Kupperman E, Wen W, et al. Cyclic AMP activates Ras. *Oncogene* 2000;19:3609–3615.

42. Tsygankova OM, Feshchenko E, Klein P, et al. TSH/cAMP and GSK3 beta elicit opposing effects on Rap1GAP stability. *J Biol Chem* 2004;279:5501–7.

42a. Lou L, Urbani J, Ribeiro-Neto F, et al. cAMP inhibition of Akt is mediated by activated and phosphorylated Rap1b. *J Biol Chem* 2002;277:32799–32806.

43. Dremier S, Vandeput F, Zwartkruis FJ, et al. Activation of the small G protein Rap1 in dog thyroid cells by both cAMP-dependent and -independent pathways. *Biochem Biophys Res Commun* 2000;267:7–11.

43a. Ribiero-Neto F, Leon L, Urbani-Brocard, et al. cAMP-dependent oncogenic action of Rap1b in the thyroid gland. *J Biol Chem* 2004 e-pub Aug 26.

44. Iacovelli L, Capobianco L, Salvatore L, et al. Thyrotropin activates mitogen-activated protein kinase pathway in FRTL-5 by a PKA-independent mechanism. *Mol Pharmacol* 2001;60:924–933.

45. Ariga M, Nedachi T, Akahori M, et al. Signalling pathways of insulin-like growth factor-I that are augmented by cAMP in FRTL-5 cells. *Biochem J* 2000;348[Pt 2]:409–416.

46. Nedachi T, Akahori M, Ariga M, et al. Tyrosine kinase and phosphatidylinositol 3-kinase activation are required for cyclic adenosine 3′,5′-monophosphate-dependent potentiation of deoxyribonucleic acid synthesis induced by insulin-like growth factor-I in FRTL-5 cells. *Endocrinology* 2000;141:2429–2438.

47. Suh JM, Song JH, Kim DW, et al. Regulation of the phosphatidylinositol 3-kinase, Akt/protein kinase B, FRAP/mammalian target of rapamycin, and ribosomal S6 kinase 1 signaling pathways by thyroid-stimulating hormone (TSH) and stimulating type TSH receptor antibodies in the thyroid gland. *J Biol Chem* 2003;278:21960–21971.

48. Garcia B, Santisteban P. PI3K is involved in the IGF-I inhibition of TSH-induced sodium-iodide symporter gene expression. *Mol Endocrinol* 2002;16:342–352.

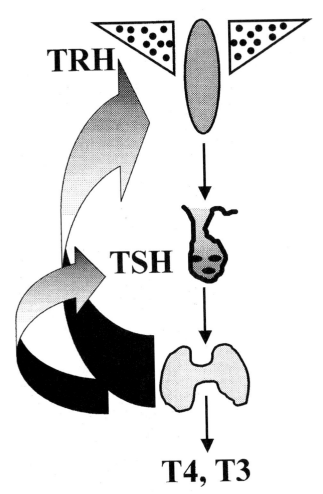

TRH

TSH

T4, T3

FIGURE 10D.1. Schematic diagram of the hypothalamic–pituitary–thyroid axis. Thyrotropin-releasing hormone (TRH) is synthesized in neurons within the paraventricular nucleus of the hypothalamus that project to the median eminence. At the median eminence, TRH is released into the hypothalamic–pituitary portal circulation and carried to the pituitary, where it activates TRH-1 receptors on the thyrotroph cells of the pituitary to synthesize and release thyrotropin (TSH). TSH acts on the thyroid via TSH receptors to stimulate the synthesis and secretion of thyroxine (T$_4$) and triiodothyronine (T$_3$). T$_4$ and T$_3$ inhibit TRH and TSH secretion, closing the feedback loop.

eminence. The most important hypothalamic regulator of TSH secretion is TRH. However, other hypothalamic neuropeptides and transmitters such as somatostatin and dopamine may also regulate TSH secretion. TRH neurons project from the paraventricular nucleus (located on either side of the third ventricle) to the median eminence, where TRH is released and carried through the portal system to the pituitary (1).

The thyrotroph cells of the pituitary originate from a common pituitary stem cell and differentiate early in embryonic development (see Chapter 2). TRH is not required for the normal development of the thyrotrophs (2). The thyrotrophs share lineage with other pituitary cell types, including lactotrophs and somatotrophs, as demonstrated

by mutations in the transcription factor Pit-1, which lead to defects in all three cell types (3–5). In addition, the thyrotrophs share lineage with the gonadotroph cells, based on upon their shared expression of the common α-subunit of TSH, luteinizing hormone (LH), and follicle-stimulating hormone (FSH), and the key role of the transcription factor Prophet of *Pit-1* (PROP-1) in both gonadotroph and thyrotroph development in humans (6). It is clear that development of the thyrotrophs requires the action of several transcription factors (7).

REGULATION OF THYROTROPIN SECRETION

Like other pituitary hormones, TSH secretion is pulsatile, with 6 to 18 pulses per 24 hours in adult humans (8,9). The frequency and amplitude of the pulses are reasonably constant during the day, but there is an increase in both frequency and amplitude in the late evening and early morning (10 PM to 2 to 4 AM) (10–13). As a result, serum TSH concentrations are about twofold higher during this period than during the rest of the day. This nocturnal surge of TSH secretion appears soon after birth and wanes with age. The mechanisms underlying TSH pulsatility and its nocturnal accentuation are not known, but likely include pulsatile TRH secretion and some input from the suprachiasmatic nucleus of the hypothalamus, which plays a role in many circadian rhythms in mammals (14). The pulsatility, especially at night, of TSH secretion decreases during fasting and nonthyroidal illness (15,16).

Thyrotropin-Releasing Hormone

Production of TRH in the paraventricular nucleus of the hypothalamus is essential for normal TSH secretion. TRH-knockout mice have central hypothyroidism, with slightly high serum TSH concentrations, but the biological activity of the TSH is decreased (17). In addition, mice with TRH deficiency and resistance to thyroid hormone have lower serum TSH concentrations than do mice with only resistance to thyroid hormone (18). Similarly, in humans TRH deficiency results in a decrease in both the amount of TSH that is secreted and its biological activity (19). While isolated TRH deficiency has not been found in humans, a patient with central hypothyroidism was found to be a compound heterozygote for mutations of the TRH receptor, with both mutant receptors being nonfunctional, confirming the essential role of TRH in humans (20).

Structure and Synthesis of Thyrotropin-Releasing Hormone

TRH is a tripeptide (pyroGlu-His-ProNH$_2$) that is produced by the processing of a larger prohormone in the hypothalamus and elsewhere in the central nervous system

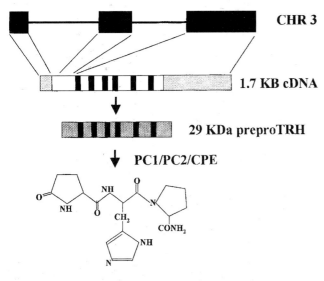

CHR 3

1.7 KB cDNA

29 KDa preproTRH

PC1/PC2/CPE

TRH (pyroGlu-His-Pro-NH₂)

FIGURE 10D.2. Structures of the thyrotropin-releasing hormone (TRH) gene, preproTRH, and TRH. The gene encoding human preproTRH is present on chromosome (*CHR*) 3 and is encoded by three exons. The first exon codes for the 5′-untranslated region, and exons 2 and 3 code for the full 29 kDa preproTRH. The 3′-untranslated region is also coded for in exon 3. Human preproTRH contains six copies of the TRH progenitor sequence (*black boxes*), which are cleaved and further modified (see text) to yield mature TRH. *PC*, prohormone convertase; *CPE*, carboxypeptidase E.

(Fig. 10D.2) (1,21). It was the first hypothalamic hormone to be identified (22,23). The complementary DNA (cDNA) sequence of murine and rat TRH encodes for a preprohormone (preproTRH) of approximately 29 kilodaltons (kDa), which includes five copies of the sequence of the TRH prohormone, whereas in humans the cDNA contains six copies (24–26). The hormone cDNA sequence is flanked by codons that encode pairs of basic amino acids that allow for processing of the progenitor TRH sequence (Gln-His-Pro-Gly) by two convertases, PC-1 and PC-2, and carboxypeptidase E (27,28). The progenitor TRH sequence is subsequently modified via cyclization at the N-terminus and amidation at the C-terminus to yield mature TRH (29,30).

TRH mRNA also encodes several other peptides between the progenitor TRH sequences that can be isolated from the mammalian hypothalamus. TRH peptide 160–169, which lies between the third and fourth TRH progenitor sequences, has been isolated from rat hypothalamic tissue. This peptide can potentiate TRH-mediated TSH release from the anterior pituitary through a receptor separate from the TRH receptor that is probably located on nonendocrine cells of the pituitary (31–33). Rat TRH peptides 83–106 and 178–199 are both increased during suckling; they may contribute to prolactin release by blocking hypothalamic dopamine release (34). Several

other pro–TRH-derived peptides have been isolated, including TRH-Gly, the direct precursor to TRH, but their role *in vivo* is not known (35). Related TRH peptides have also been identified in the human hypothalamus and placenta, but because the intervening sequences are different from those in rats, the sequences of these peptides are different (36,37), and their biological activity, if any, is not known.

Based on the role of processing in producing mature TRH, it is clear that TRH production can be controlled through the regulation of enzymes such as PC-1 and PC-2 and carboxypeptidase E. Indeed, both PC-1 and PC-2 are down-regulated by thyroid hormone, consistent with their key regulatory role in the production of TRH (38,39). Mice that are deficient in carboxypeptidase E have less mature TRH and more of its precursor forms than normal mice (28). A single human patient with defective PC-1 has been described; this patient had defective processing of several hormones, including insulin, and mild primary, not central, hypothyroidism (40,41).

TRH is rapidly deamidated after its release to TRH-free acid and histidyl-proline-diketopiperazine (His-Pro-DKP), a stable cyclized metabolite (30,42). The principal enzymes that degrade TRH are three forms of pyroglutamyl aminopeptidase (PAP I, PAP II, and thyroliberase), which yield His-Pro-DKP, and prolyl endopeptidase, which yields the TRH-free acid. PAP I is a cytosolic enzyme that has broad substrate specificity and has a role in the metabolism of other neuropeptides (42,43). In contrast, PAP II (also known as TRH-degrading enzyme) is present in synaptosomal fractions of neural tissue and in pituitary cell membranes (44–47). Furthermore, PAP II has a substrate specificity restricted to TRH and TRH-like peptides, which, together with its tissue distribution, suggests that it is the major peptidase that removes the amino-terminal pyroglutamate residue from TRH (42,48). His-Pro-DKP, which has a variety of endocrine and neural actions, was only reduced by 50% in the hypothalamus and cerebral cortex of TRH-knockout mice, suggesting that it has other sources (49). The third PAP enzyme, thyroliberase, is present in serum and appears to catabolize TRH there. It is similar to PAP II, but because it is not membrane bound it may regulate TRH concentrations during transport through the portal system. This enzyme may be a proteolytic product of the PAPII gene, which also is expressed in the liver (50). Thyroid hormone increases PAP II activity in the pituitary (44). Furthermore, TRH itself appears to down-regulate PAP II activity in the pituitary (51). Thus, the bioavailability of TRH can be modified at the protein level through changes in both its processing and its degradation.

The Thyrotropin-Releasing Hormone Gene

The structure of the murine, rat, and human TRH genes are identical. Each consists of three exons and two introns

(Fig. 10D.2). The sequences of the exons are well conserved among the species, whereas the sequences of the introns are less conserved. The first exon encodes the 5'-untranslated region, while the coding sequence for the preprohormone and the 3'-untranslated region are on exons 2 and 3. The promoter is immediately adjacent to exon 1, as demonstrated by the presence of a TATA box within 25 base pairs (bp) of the transcription start site. In the hypothalamus, the content of TRH mRNA is highest in the paraventriclar nucleus and the lateral hypothalamic area. It is also found in the preoptic region, the olfactory lobes, the periaqueductal gray region, and the medullary raphe neurons in the brainstem, which contain much of the TRH found in the spinal cord. In addition, TRH mRNA is present in peripheral tissues, including the heart and the pancreas, where TRH may play a role in glucose homeostasis (17). In areas of the brain outside the paraventricular nucleus, TRH mRNA and its derived peptides have several functions, including regulation of gastric motility and gastric acid secretion through activation of vagal outflow (52).

The cell bodies of the TRH neurons (hypophysiotropic neurons) that control TSH secretion are located in the paraventricular nucleus. This nucleus has two major groups of neurons: a magnocellular group that is located laterally and expresses oxytocin and vasopressin, and a parvocellular group that is located medially. TRH neurons are found throughout the parvocellular group, but only those TRH neurons in certain anatomic subdivisions project to the median eminence to regulate thyrotroph function (1). The hypophysiotropic group of TRH neurons is also defined by coexpression of the mRNA encoding the cocaine- and amphetamine-related neuropeptide (CART) (53,54) and by their ability to regulate preproTRH mRNA levels, as discussed later in the chapter. The role of TRH neurons in the paraventricular nucleus that do not express CART and do not project to the median eminence is not clear. A separate group of medial parvocellular neurons of the paraventricular nucleus contain corticotropin-releasing hormone, the key hypothalamic regulator of corticotropin (ACTH) secretion. Corticotropin-releasing hormone is also present in other areas of the paraventricular nucleus during stress (55).

The underlying mechanism allowing for cell-specific TRH gene expression is not known. However, the transcription factor simple-minded (Sim)-1 is required for the formation of all paraventricular-nucleus neurons *in vivo*, and mice that lack Sim-1 have little development of the paraventricular nucleus and also the supraoptic nucleus of the hypothalamus (56,57). It is likely that Sim-1 and its partner, the transcription factor arylhydrocarbon receptor nuclear translocator (Arnt)-2 act upstream of another transcription factor, Brn-2, to allow appropriate development of these two hypothalamic nuclei (58,59). In addition, the transcription factor orthopedia (Otp) is also critical for the

development of the paraventricular nucleus; it acts before Sim-1 in the developing hypothalamus (60,61). The factors that cause the development of separate TRH neurons from other neuropeptide-expressing neurons in the paraventricular nucleus are not known, but it is likely that still-unidentified cell-specific factors are needed for the development of these neurons, perhaps by interacting directly with regulatory elements in the TRH promoter which are required for its hypothalamic expression (62).

Regulation of the Expression of the Thyrotropin-Releasing Hormone Gene

TRH gene expression is dynamically regulated in the medial and periventricular regions of the paraventricular nucleus in order to regulate TSH secretion and subsequently thyroid secretion in response to many conditions, including illness, starvation, cold, and thyroid disease. An understanding of the mechanisms involved can be discerned through an examination of both the milieu in which the hypophysiotropic TRH neurons lie and the regulatory elements present within the promoter region of the TRH gene.

The TRH neurons in the paraventricular nucleus receive input from other regions of the brain as well as from the circulation. The major afferent connections to these neurons include catecholamine neurons from the brain stem (63) and neurons from the arcuate nucleus (1,64). Catecholamine signaling likely plays an important role in the up-regulation of TRH gene expression during cold exposure (65), while input from the arcuate nucleus plays a critical role in the down-regulation of TRH gene expression during starvation and illness. Indeed, insight into the regulation of TRH neurons by inputs from the arcuate nucleus has shed considerable light on the importance of pathways via which energy expenditure regulates the axis.

Regulation by Pathways Important in Energy Expenditure

In rodents, fasting results in a rapid fall in serum TSH and thyroid hormone concentrations (66,67), caused, in part, by down-regulation of TRH gene expression in the paraventricular nucleus (68,69). Administration of the adipocyte hormone leptin, the production of which also falls during fasting, prevents the fasting-induced fall in thyroid secretion by preventing the fall in TRH mRNA levels (70,71). Thus, leptin is a key regulator of TRH gene expression (Fig. 10D.3). The actions of leptin in the hypothalamus are mediated by the long-form of the leptin receptor (ObRb), a member of the cytokine receptor family that is coupled to the janus kinase 2/signal transducer of activated transcription 3 (JAK-2/STAT-3) signaling cascade (72). The ObRb is expressed strongly in the arcuate nucleus and, in a more limited way, in the paraventricular nucleus (73–75), and is thus poised to regulate TRH ex-

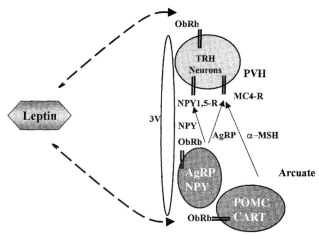

FIGURE 10D.3. Schematic diagram of the actions of leptin on thyrotropin-releasing hormone (TRH) gene expression. Leptin, produced in adipocytes, crosses the blood–brain barrier and regulates TRH gene expression via the melanocortin system in the arcuate nucleus, whose neurons project to TRH neurons in the paraventricular nucleus. In addition, leptin regulates TRH gene expression directly in TRH neurons. *AgRP*, agouti-related protein; *CART*, cocaine- and amphetamine-related neuropeptide; *α-MSH*, α-melanocyte-stimulating hormone; *MC4-R*, melanocortin-4 receptors; *NPY*, neuropeptide Y; *NPY1,5-R*, neuropeptide-1 and -5 receptors; *ObRb*, leptin receptor; *POMC*, proopiomelanocortin; *PVH*, paraventricular nucleus; *3V*, third ventricle. (Adapted from Bjorbaek C, Hollenberg AN. Leptin and melanocortin signaling in the hypothalamus. *Vitam Horm* 2002;65:281, with permission.)

pression both indirectly and directly (76,77). Lesions of the arcuate nucleus prevent the effects of leptin on TRH gene expression (78).

Two neuronal groups within the arcuate nucleus express leptin receptors and project to the TRH neurons in the paraventricular nucleus. The neurons in the first group contain both pro-opiomelanocortin (POMC) and CART (79–81). In the arcuate nucleus, unlike the pituitary, POMC is processed primarily to α-melanocyte-stimulating hormone (MSH), a potent anorexigenic peptide, which signals through both the melanocortin (MC)-3 and -4 receptors. TRH neurons in the paraventricular nucleus have MC-4 receptors and are directly innervated by α-MSH nerve terminals (82,83). In addition, central administration of α-MSH prevents the fasting-induced suppression of TSH and thyroid secretion (76,77). The second group of arcuate-nucleus neurons that have leptin receptors synthesize the neuropeptides agouti-related peptide (AgRP) and neuropeptide Y (NPY). These neurons also directly contact TRH neurons in the paraventricular nucleus. In contrast to POMC, both AgRP and NPY are orexigenic peptides and are down-regulated by leptin and up-regulated during fasting (84–86). Both AgRP, an MC-4–receptor antagonist (and possibly an inverse agonist), and NPY (through NPY receptor–isoforms expressed on TRH neurons), when administered centrally, can cause central hypothyroidism by down-regulating TRH mRNA expression in the paraventricular nucleus (87–90). In summary, the arcuate nucleus serves to integrate leptin signaling and as-

sist in the regulation of TRH gene expression, as well as regulate food intake and energy expenditure (91).

The direct and indirect actions of leptin on TRH neurons to regulate TSH and thyroid secretion in situations of nutritional stress are probably mediated by changes in TRH gene transcription. The proximal regions of the promoter regions of the rodent and human TRH genes are structurally similar (Fig. 10D.4). Both of the genes have a TATAA box within 25 bp of the transcriptional start site and a region termed Site 4 between 60 and 52 bp upstream of the start site. First identified as a thyroid hormone receptor (TR)–binding site (see later in the chapter) (25,92), Site 4 is critical for basal activity of the TRH promoter in mammalian cell lines. In addition, Site 4 can bind the cyclic adenosine monophosphate (cyclic AMP) response element–binding protein (CREB), which is downstream in the signaling cascade induced by α-MSH via MC-4 receptors. Thus, modulation of CREB activity via α-MSH, AgRP, and NPY signaling should allow for varying degrees of TRH gene expression. In addition to Site 4, the TRH gene has a conserved STAT-binding site between 150 and 140 bp upstream of the start site. This site interacts with STAT3 and mediates transcriptional responses to leptin signaling via the ObRb (64,93). Thus, the promoter region of the TRH gene has sites whereby multiple inputs can be integrated to control TRH gene expression.

While most of the studies of nutritional regulation of TRH production, or at least gene expression, have been performed in rodents, there is increasing evidence that similar mechanisms affect TRH production and therefore TSH and thyroid secretion in humans during food deprivation and illness. Humans with mutations of the leptin receptor have central hypothyroidism, although humans who have a defective leptin gene do not (94). Furthermore, controlled caloric restriction in humans leading to weight loss results in a decline in serum thyroid hormone concentrations that can be reversed by leptin (95). Also, acute fasting in humans leads to a decrease in pulsatile TSH secretion, which also can be reversed by administration of leptin (15,96). However, humans with MC-4-receptor mutations, the most common genetic form of obesity, have normal serum TSH and thyroid hormone concentrations (97, 98).

Regulation of Expression of the Thyrotropin-Releasing Hormone Gene by Nonthyroidal Illness

Many changes in pituitary-thyroid function occur in nonthyroidal illness, including a decrease in TSH secretion (see section on nonthyroidal illness in Chapter 11). One cause of the decrease in TSH secretion is a decrease in TRH secretion, as manifested by a decrease in TRH gene expression in the paraventricular nucleus (16,99). The frequent presence of anorexia in these patients suggests that the leptin and melanocortin signaling pathways may play a role in

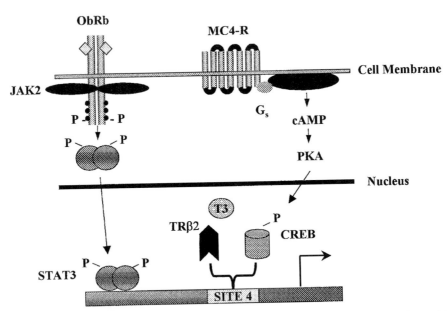

FIGURE 10D.4. Activation of the thyrotropin-releasing hormone (TRH) promoter by multiple signaling pathways. The TRH promoter responds to leptin, melanocortin, and T$_3$ via a number of cis-acting elements. Binding of leptin to its receptor (*ObRb*) activates JAK2, leading to its phosphorylation and subsequent recruitment and phosphorylation (*P*) of STAT3. Phosphorylated STAT3 homodimers enter the nucleus and bind directly to the promotor region of the TRH gene to stimulate its expression. The proopiomelanocortin (*POMC*)-derived peptide, melanocyte-stimulating hormone (α-*MSH*), activates TRH transcription via protein kinase A (*PKA*) by binding to the melanocortin-4 receptor (*MC4-R*) on TRH neurons. PKA phophorylates cyclic AMP response element–binding protein (*CREB*) bound to Site 4 in the TRH promoter, which leads to TRH transcription. In contrast, triiodothyronine binds to the β2 isoform of TR (thyroid receptor), which also acts through Site 4 to down-regulate TRH gene expression. *JAK2*, janus-kinase 2; *STAT3*, signal transducer of activated transcription 3. Together they form the JAK2/STAT3 signaling cascade.

the decrease. However, it is also likely that cytokines such as interleukin-1, and -1β, tumor necrosis factor, and interferon contribute to the decrease. MC-4–receptor knockout mice do not develop cachexia in response to cytokine administration or an increased tumor burden, suggesting that the melanocortin signaling pathway plays an important role in the response. However, increased expression of arcuate-nucleus neuropeptides during cachexia does not by itself explain low TRH gene expression or, for that matter, decreased food intake. It is likely that interactions between the cytokine-signaling pathways and the melanocortin system contribute to the central suppression of TRH gene expression in the paraventricular nucleus during nonthyroidal illness, or that other cytokine-activated pathways are involved (100–102).

Regulation of Thyrotropin-Releasing Hormone Gene Expression by Thyroid Hormone

An important component of the control of TSH secretion is inhibition of TRH gene expression in the paraventricular nucleus by thyroid hormone, principally T$_3$. Conversely, TRH gene expression increases in response to low serum T$_4$ and T$_3$ concentrations (103,104). TRH mRNA levels in other regions of the hypothalamus are not regulated by T$_3$.

In terms of serum hormone, T$_4$ may be more important than T$_3$ (105), with the T$_3$ being produced locally from T$_4$ by the action of type 2 iodothyronine deiodinase (D2), the principal deiodinase present in the central nervous system (see Chapter 7). This is supported by the finding that D2-knockout mice maintain TSH secretion in the presence of high serum T$_4$ concentrations (106). D2 is not expressed in the TRH neurons in the paraventricular nucleus, but it is present in specialized cells termed tanycytes that line the third ventricle and whose processes extend to the TRH neurons. It is likely that T$_4$ is converted to T$_3$ in the tanycytes, and the T$_3$ is then released to act on the neurons (107,108).

T$_3$ regulates TRH gene expression at the level of transcription via the nuclear thyroid hormone receptor (TR) (Fig. 10D.4). There are three TR-isoforms, α1, β1, and β2, which bind T$_3$ and mediate transcriptional regulation (see Chapter 8). The TRβ-isoforms are alternatively spliced products of a single gene and differ structurally only in the amino terminus, while TRα1 is the product of a separate gene but functions in the same way as the TRβ-isoforms (109,110). The greatest difference in each of the isoforms may be in their cell-specific expression patterns (111). Mice devoid of both TRβ-isoforms have normal or slightly high serum TSH and high T$_4$ and T$_3$ concentrations, findings that resemble those found in patients with resistance to thyroid hormone (see Chapter 81), consistent with the predominant expression of TRβ-isoforms in the pituitary and hypothalamus (112,113). The values are similar in mice with selective ablation of the β2-isoform, demonstrating the requirement for this isoform for negative regulation by T_3 of TRH gene expression (114); this isoform is also required for the normal development of color vision due to its unique expression in the retina (115). In contrast to the TRH gene, T_3 regulation of the genes for the α- and β-subunits of TSH is mediated not only via the β2 isoform of the TR, but also to some extent via the β1- and α1-isoforms (116,117).

On genes that are positively regulated by the TRs, the TR isoforms bind to thyroid hormone response elements present in the regulatory regions of target genes as either homo- or heterodimers with retinoid-X-receptors (RXR). In the absence of T_3, or in the hypothyroid state, the TR isoforms repress gene transcription by recruiting nuclear corepressor molecules, which in turn recruit a multiprotein complex that modifies chromatin through histone deacetylation, leading to transcriptional repression (118–122). The presence of T_3 leads to a conformational change in the TR, which results in release of the corepressor complex and the sequential recruitment of coactivators, which result in histone acetylation and transcriptional activation (123–125).

The molecular mechanism by which the TR isoforms inhibit gene transcription is less clear. *In vitro*, genes repressed by T_3 are activated in the absence of T_3 and subsequently repressed by the addition of T_3, the mirror image of the process in positively regulated genes. Proposed mechanisms for this effect include interference with other transcription factors (independent of DNA binding) by T_3–TR complexes, and interaction of the T_3–TR complexes with specific negative thyroid hormone response elements to cause down regulation. Recent studies have demonstrated that negative regulation of TRH and TSH α- and β-subunit gene expression requires binding of the β isoform of TR to DNA (126). Indeed, the promoter regions of both the TRH and TSHβ-subunit genes have TR-binding sites, which are required for negative regulation (25,92,127,128). The TR-binding site in the promoter region of the TRH gene includes Site 4, which is required for basal and cyclic AMP-stimulated activity of the promoter. Taken together, it is likely that negative regulation of the TRH gene by T_3 requires binding of TR-β2 to Site 4 and the recruitment of coregulators such as members of the steroid receptor coactivator family (129).

REGULATION OF THYROTROPIN SECRETION FROM THE PITUITARY

TSH secretion is regulated not only by TRH, but also by thyroid hormone and other factors acting directly on the thyrotrophs (Fig. 10D.1). These inputs arise from either the peripheral circulation or other regions of the hypothalamus. Regulators from the periphery include thyroid hormones, glucocorticoids, and retinoids. Other hypothalamic peptides and neurotransmitters that regulate TSH secretion include somatostatin and dopamine. These signals are integrated in the thyrotrophs to determine TSH secretion.

Action of Thyrotropin-Releasing Hormone on the Pituitary

Once TRH reaches the pituitary it acts to increase the synthesis and secretion of TSH from the thyrotrophs (Fig. 10D.5). [TRH also stimulates prolactin secretion, and it stimulates growth hormone secretion in some patients with somatotroph adenomas (acromegaly) and FSH or LH secretion in some patients with gonadotroph adenomas (130–132).] In normal subjects, intravenous administration of TRH in doses of 50 to 500 μg results in a dose-dependent 4- to 20-fold rise in serum TSH concentrations within 15 to 30 minutes, followed by a small rises in serum T_3 concentrations in 1.5 to 3 hours and small rises in serum T_4 concentrations in 4 to 8 hours (133,134). Before the development of sensitive TSH assays and hypothalamic-pituitary imaging techniques, the TRH stimulation test

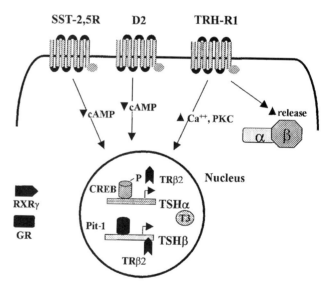

FIGURE 10D.5. Regulation of thyrotropin (TSH) secretion in the thyrotrophs of the pituitary gland. TSH secretion is regulated via multiple cell-surface and nuclear receptors on the thyrotrophs. The receptors include thyrotropin-releasing hormone 1 (TRH-1) and sst-2 and sst-5 (somatostatin) receptors in the cell membrane, which act via cyclic AMP (cAMP) or protein kinase C (*PKC*) or calcium ions to alter the expression of the genes for the subunits of TSH. In addition, activation of TRH receptors stimulates release of stored TSH. Within the nucleus, the β2 isoform of thyroid receptor (*TR*), retinoid-X-receptor g (*RXRγ*), and glucocorticoid receptor (*GR*) regulate transcription of the genes for the α- and β-subunits of TSH (TSHα and TSHβ). All of these pathways probably interact with the transcription factors cAMP response element binding-protein (*CREB*) and pituitary transcription factor 1 (Pit-1).

was a useful test for the diagnosis of thyrotoxicosis (no rise in serum TSH) and differentiation of hypothalamic from pituitary hypothyroidism (delayed rise vs. no rise in serum TSH) (135). TRH stimulation of prolactin secretion is also dose-dependent, and the response is supranormal in patients with hypothyroidism (136,137).

The actions of TRH on the thyrotrophs are mediated by binding of TRH to cell-surface receptors, in particular type 1 TRH receptors (TRH-R1) (138). A second TRH receptor (TRH-R2) has been identified in rodents but is not known to have a role in humans (139,140). A third receptor was identified in *Xenopus laevis,* but its affinity for TRH is so low that it is probably not a TRH receptor (141). The two TRH receptors are, for the most part, expressed in separate regions of the central nervous system, with TRH-R1 being principally expressed in the anterior pituitary as well as in the hypothalamus, autonomic nervous system, and portions of the brainstem. In contrast, TRH-R2 is more extensively expressed in the thalamus, subthalamic area, and cortex (142,143).

Both TRH receptors are members of the G-protein–coupled receptor family, and both are coupled to guanine nucleotide-binding (G) proteins ($G_{q/11}$) to mediate signal transduction. TRH and its analogs bind to both receptors with similar affinity (143). TRH binding to the receptor activates phospholipase C in the cells, leading to the production of inositol 1,4,5-trisphosphate and an increase in intracellular calcium, which in turn leads to activation of protein kinase C. The TRH receptors may also couple to other G proteins and activate other intracellular signaling pathways (143,144). The activation of these signaling cascades leads to the transcriptional regulation of target genes; these include the genes for the α- and β-subunits of TSH in the thyrotrophs and the gene for prolactin in the lactotrophs (145). TRH-receptor signaling is further regulated by receptor internalization after TRH binding, which leads to either degradation or recycling of the receptor to the cell membrane (146–148).

Activation of TRH-R1 receptors in the pituitary appears to control transcription by regulating the interaction of several transcription factors and coactivators with the promoter regions of the target genes. The promoter of the gene for the α-subunit of TSH is regulated by both CREB and Lim-1 (149,150), the activity of which is increased by TRH through the recruitment of the cofactor CREB-binding protein (CBP) (151,152). In contrast, the gene for the β-subunit of TSH is regulated primarily through direct binding of the transcription factors Pit-1 and GATA-2. Pit-1 in turn recruits CBP in a TRH-dependent fashion (151,153). Pit-1 is also a key regulator of prolactin gene expression, and TRH signaling increases transcription of the prolactin gene through this pathway.

The paradoxical stimulatory effect of TRH on growth hormone secretion in patients with somatotroph adenomas is probably due to the expression of receptors of the TRH-R1 type in these adenomas (154–156); TRH-R1 mRNA can be detected in the adenomas of patients whose serum growth hormone concentrations increase in response to TRH (157). Some somatotroph adenomas also have an aberrantly spliced variant of TRH-R1 lacking the sixth and seventh transmembrane domains that would be predicted not to bind TRH, but this probably inactive isoform is not found in adenomas that respond to TRH (157).

TRH stimulates not only the expression of the genes for the subunits of TSH, but also the posttranslational glycosylation of TSH, which contributes significantly to its biological activity (18,158,159). Some patients with central hypothyroidism have slightly high serum TSH concentrations that increase in both amount and bioactivity after the administration of TRH (see Chapter 51). Similarly, TRH-knockout mice also have slightly high serum TSH concentrations that increase in response to TRH, but their TSH has decreased thyroid-stimulating activity (17).

The Effect of Thyroid Hormones in the Thyrotrophs

Since the advent of serum TSH assays in the late 1960s and the development of the TRH stimulation test it has been clear that TSH secretion is very tightly controlled by T_4 and T_3, and that very small changes in serum T_4 and T_3 concentrations have large effects on TSH secretion (Fig. 10D.6) (160–162). Indeed, there is a log/linear relationship between serum TSH and free T_4 concentrations at all levels of thyroid secretion (163) (see Chapter 13). The sensitivity of the thyrotrophs to small changes in serum thyroid hormone concentrations underscores the importance of the latter as the most important regulator of TSH secretion in humans.

As discussed previously, T_3 plays a critical role in TRH gene expression. In addition, T_3 acting on the thyrotrophs regulates the expression of the genes for both TSH subunits and the TRH receptor (TRH-R1). The actions of T_3 to regulate both hypothalamic and pituitary gene expression allow for the very close control of TSH secretion, which is expressed clinically in the log/linear relationship described above. While the molecular mechanism underlying T_3 regulation of TRH signaling in the pituitary is unclear, experimental data suggests that T_3 may both inhibit TRH-R1 mRNA expression and decrease the level of TRH-R1 protein in the thyrotrophs (164–166).

T_3, in conjunction with TR isoforms, inhibits the transcription of the genes for the α- and β-subunits of TSH in the thyrotrophs *in vivo* (167). At least in mice, all TR isoforms are present in the thyrotrophs and contribute to the regulation of TSH, though among them β-isoforms are probably the most important (Fig. 10D.7) (113,114,116, 117,168). Indeed, mutations in the ligand-binding domain of the β-isoform have been found in TSH-secreting pituitary adenomas (169,170).

While the β-isoforms are required for T_3 responsiveness, the molecular mechanism by which T_3 inhibits the genes

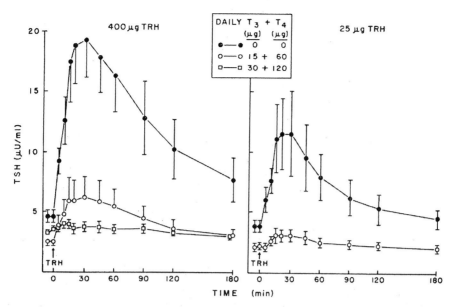

FIGURE 10D.6. Mean (±SE) serum thyrotropin (TSH) concentrations before and after intravenous administration of thyrotropin-releasing hormone (TRH) in eight normal subjects before and during administration of two combinations of triiodothyronine (T_3) plus thyroxine (T_4) **(inset)**, each given for 3 to 4 weeks. The low T_3 plus T_4 combination reduced basal serum TSH concentrations and especially the serum TSH responses to 400 μg of TRH (all eight subjects) and 25 μg of TRH (six subjects). The higher T_3 plus T_4 combination abolished the serum TSH response to 400 μg of TRH (the response to 25 μg of TRH was not tested after this T_3 plus T_4 dose). At the time of the three studies, the subjects' mean serum T_3 and T_4 concentrations were: base line, serum T_3 119 ng/dL (1.8 nmol/L) and T_4 6.9 μg/dL (89 nmol/L); low T_3 plus T_4 combination, serum T_3 110 ng/dL (1.7 nmol/L) and T_4 7.0 μg/dL (90 nmol/L); and high T_3 plus T_4 combination, serum T_3 141 ng/dL (2.2 nmol/L) and T_4 7.8 μg/dL (101 nmol/L). (From Snyder PJ, Utiger RD. Inhibition of thyrotropin response to thyrotropin-releasing hormone by small quantities of thyroid hormones. *J Clin Invest* 1972;51:2077, with permission.)

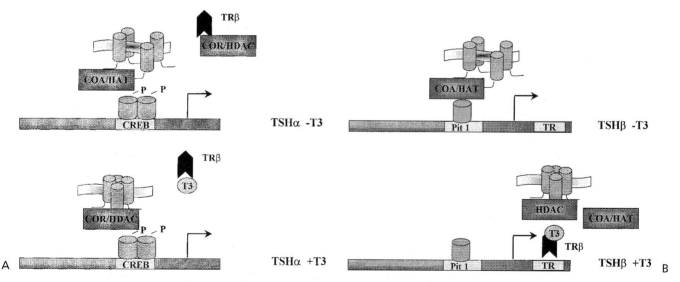

FIGURE 10D.7. Mechanisms of negative regulation of the genes for the α- and β-subunits of TSH by T_3. **A:** The gene for the α-subunit appears to be regulated by the thyroid receptor (TR) via a mechanism that does not involve TR binding to DNA. In this model, the TR alone [absence of triiodothyronine (T_3)] increases α-subunit gene expression by removing corepressors (*COR*) and histone deacetylase (*HDAC*) from the promoter, leading to activation of transcription by coactivators (*COA*) and increased histone acetylase (*HAT*) activity. In the presence of T_3, the corepressors remain bound to the promoter, leading to histone deacetylation and repression. **B:** In contrast, inhibition of the gene for the β-subunit requires binding of complexes of T_3 and TR to a site in exon 1. This binding recruits histone deacetylase activity either directly or via corepressors. Alternatively, the T_3–TR complexes may recruit captivators that may paradoxically function to repress transcription. *CREB*, cyclic AMP response element-binding protein.

for the subunits of TSH appears to be different. The promoter region of the gene for the α-subunit has a TR-binding site just downstream from its TATA box (171), but this site is probably not used; instead T_3 inhibition is achieved through protein–protein interactions between the TR and coregulators, which mediate the response of the promotor to cyclic AMP (172). In the absence of T_3, TR binds to a repression complex containing corepressor molecules and histone deacetylases, leading to activation. The presence of T_3 prevents the repression complexes from interacting with the TR, allowing the complex to remain on the promoter, which leads to repression (173).

In contrast, the promoter region of the gene for the β-subunit of TSH contains a negative thyroid hormone response element that binds TR isoforms. This element is located in exon 1, just downstream from the transcription start site; it appears to bind the TR as a monomer to mediate T_3-dependent repression (128). RXR antagonizes negative regulation by T_3 by competing with the TR for binding to the response element. The negative thyroid hormone response element and a region surrounding it have been termed the Z-region, and this region appears to bind β-isoforms of TR and histone deacetylases only in the presence of T_3. The Z-region is present in several other genes, including the gene for the α-subunit of TSH, but its role in these other genes is not known (174).

The molecular mechanisms governing negative regulation of the TSH subunit genes by T_3 are becoming clearer; they are multiple, and they are not as straightforward as positive regulation. *In vivo*, T_3-mediated negative regulation of TRH and TSH-subunit gene expression is prolonged, because TSH gene expression and indeed TSH secretion that has been inhibited by T_3 can remain low for prolonged periods. The mechanism underlying this long-term effect is unknown.

Retinoids and Thyrotropin Secretion

The role of vitamin A analogues in the regulation of TSH secretion was noted in 1999 when patients with cutaneous T-cell lymphoma who were being treated with a novel RXR ligand, bexarotene, developed reversible central hypothyroidism (175). Heterodimeric complexes of RXR and one of the isoforms of TR mediate many actions of T_3, although the complexed RXR usually binds little if any of its own ligand. In the case of bexarotene, the inhibition of TSH secretion is probably due solely to inhibition of TSH-β gene expression by RXRγ, the principal RXR isoform in the thyrotrophs (175,176). RXRγ knockout mice are resistant to thyroid hormone; they have high serum TSH and thyroid hormone concentrations (177). The interaction of RXRγ with the TSH-β promoter is probably through a separate response element that binds RXR homodimers; RXR ligands inhibit TSH secretion in mice in which the TRβ gene is knocked out (178). In rodents, RXR ligands inhibit TSH secretion within two hours after their administration, before there are any changes in TSH-subunit gene expression or protein levels (179). Thus, the effects of retinoids on the thyrotrophs are multifactorial. Whether endogenous RXR ligands regulate TSH secretion is not known.

Glucocorticoids and Thyrotropin Secretion

TSH secretion is inhibited by high doses of glucocorticoids and endogenous hypercortisolemia, and some patients have mild central hypothyroidism. In contrast, patients with Addison's disease tend to have slightly high serum TSH concentrations. Glucocorticoids act in the paraventricular nucleus to inhibit TRH gene expression *in vivo* (180), although the mechanism is unclear, and glucocorticoids stimulate TRH gene expression in primary cultures of hypothalamic tissue (181,182). In addition, glucocorticoids inhibit TSH secretion in cultured pituitary cells; this effect may be due to an increase in secretion of annexin-1 by the folliculostellate cells of the pituitary, which then inhibits TSH release (183).

Glucocorticoids may contribute to regulation of TSH secretion in normal subjects. In patients with Addison's disease, continuous administration of hydrocortisone in doses that mimicked the normal diurnal variation of serum cortisol concentrations resulted in normal serum TSH concentrations, including normal nocturnal pulses of TSH secretion (184). In normal subjects, administration of metyrapone, which blocks cortisol secretion, resulted in an increase in serum TSH concentrations and reduced nocturnal TSH secretion (185). Thus, small changes in endogenous cortisol secretion can alter TSH secretion, probably by perturbing TRH synthesis and release.

The doses of glucocorticoid needed to inhibit TSH secretion in humans have not been well defined, but it is clear that even prolonged administration of high doses does not cause hypothyroidism. The reason is that the potent effect of low serum T_4 and T_3 concentrations to raise TSH secretion overcomes the glucocorticoid-induced inhibition of TSH secretion. The same phenomenon probably explains why none of the other substances that inhibit TSH secretion (see following sections) cause hypothyroidism.

Somatostatin and Thyrotropin Secretion

Somatostatin is an inhibitor of growth hormone secretion that was identified initially as a 14-amino-acid– and subsequently also as a 28-amino-acid–secreted peptide (186–188). It is synthesized in neurons in the periventricular and arcuate nucleus as well as in nonneural tissue, most notably the pancreas (189). The actions of somatostatin are mediated through five receptors (sst-1 through -5), which are G-protein coupled and signal in part through inhibition of adenylyl cyclase and a reduction in intracellular levels of cyclic AMP (Fig 10D.5) (189). The five receptors bind the secreted forms of somatostatin equally well, but they are expressed differently and likely differ in their signaling capabilities in different tissues.

Early studies of the pituitary actions of somatostatin revealed that it inhibited not only growth hormone but also TSH release, and incubation of pituitary tissue *in vitro* with antisomatostatin antibodies and administration of the antibodies *in vivo* increased release of TSH (190–192). In humans, intravenous administration of high doses of somatostatin reduces serum TSH concentrations and blocks TRH-mediated stimulation of TSH release. This effect is of little if any importance in the overall regulation of TSH secretion. Growth hormone itself can reduce TSH secretion, probably by increasing endogenous somatostatin release.

Long-term administration of somatostatin analogues, for example in patients with acromegaly, does not cause hypothyroidism. However, these analogues (as well as somatostatin itself) do inhibit TSH secretion in patients with TSH-secreting pituitary adenomas, and long-term analogue therapy may result in a decrease in adenoma size. The efficacy of octreotide and other long-acting analogues of somatostatin in patients with TSH-secreting pituitary adenomas is based upon the compounds' high affinity for sst-2 and sst-5 receptors, which appear to be preferentially expressed in these tumors (193–197). These analogues are now the principal medical therapy for patients with TSH-secreting adenomas (see Chapter 24) (198,199).

Catecholamines and Thyrotropin Secretion

Networks of catecholamine-containing fibers make contact with TRH neurons in the paraventricular nucleus, and they may also make contact with the nerve terminals of TRH-secreting neurons in the median eminence. The majority of these neurons originate in discrete regions of the brain stem (55,200). Stimulation of the α-adrenergic signaling system increases TSH release via α2-adrenergic receptors, and inhibition of the same system blocks TSH release (134,201–203). The effect of cold exposure is the best example of the role of the catecholamine system in the regulation of TSH secretion. Both TRH release and TRH mRNA synthesis in the paraventricular nucleus increase within 1 hour after exposure to cold (65,204–206); this response can be blocked by α-adrenergic antagonist drugs (65). Activation of this pathway probably explains the rapid increase in TSH secretion that occurs soon after birth in humans (see Chapter 74) (207,208). Cold has little effect on TSH secretion in adults.

Dopamine-containing neurons of the arcuate nucleus that project to the median eminence are important regulators of prolactin secretion, and they may also play a role in TSH secretion (209). Dopamine blocks TSH release from pituitary cells, probably acting via the A_2 isoform of the dopamine receptor to inhibit intracellular cyclic AMP accumulation. In addition, in cultured rat pituitary cells, do-

pamine inhibits the expression of the genes for the α- and β-subunits of TSH (210,211). In humans, intravenous administration of dopamine inhibits TSH secretion, and this is one cause of the low serum TSH concentrations often present in patients with severe nonthyroidal illness (see section on nonthyroidal illness in Chapter 11). The acute administration of metoclopramide or domperidone, both dopamine receptor antagonists, can lead to a rise in serum TSH concentrations, while the acute administration of bromocriptine, a dopamine receptor agonist, lowers serum TSH concentrations (209,212–214). The effects of these drugs are not clinically important, in that long-term therapy has no effect on TSH secretion.

CLINICAL ASSESSMENT OF THYROTROPIN SECRETION

The first assays for serum TSH were not sufficiently sensitive to detect TSH in the serum of all normal subjects. That is no longer the case, and assays are now available that detect far less TSH than is present in all normal subjects. As a result, measurement of serum TSH has become the standard test to screen for thyroid dysfunction. However, there are some clinical situations in which a patient's serum TSH concentration is not a reliable indicator of clinical status (see Chapter 13).

Thyrotoxicosis

Measurement of serum TSH is an excellent screening test for thyrotoxicosis. However, because of the log/linear relationship between serum TSH and free T_4 concentrations, serum TSH concentrations may be low in patients with normal serum free T_4 concentration (see Chapter 79). Furthermore, the serum free T_4 and TSH values are often dissociated during treatment, with the former falling to normal or even below normal, but the latter remaining low (see Chapter 45) (215, 216).

Inappropriate Thyrotropin Secretion

Serum TSH concentrations may be inappropriately high or normal in patients with normal or high serum free T_4 concentrations. This can occur when the patient has serum heterophile antibodies; these antibodies interfere in TSH assays to raise the value (217). It also occurs in patients with a TSH-secreting pituitary adenoma (see Chapter 24), in patients with resistance to thyroid hormone (see Chapter 81), and in patients who take a large dose of T_4 just before testing (218). All these situations are rare; among 7908 consecutive serum samples submitted to the laboratory of a large tertiary care hospital, the free T_4 concentration was high and the TSH concentration was >1 mU/L in 18 samples (from 17 patients) (219).

Nonthyroidal Illness

A substantial proportion of patients with nonthyroidal illness have abnormal serum TSH concentrations. Some of them have low serum TSH and low free T_4 concentrations (220), or what might be called illness-related central hypothyroidism. During recovery, their serum TSH concentrations may be high transiently (221). The mechanisms underlying the suppression of TSH secretion in these patients are probably multiple, and include cytokines, glucocorticoids, and possibly the leptin-signaling pathway. A major question is whether this central hypothyroidism is a beneficial or harmful adaptation to illness. This problem is discussed in detail in the section on nonthyroidal illness in Chapter 11.

REFERENCES

1. Lechan RM, Hollenberg AN. Thyrotropin-releasing hormone (TRH). In: Henry HL, Norman AW, eds. *Encyclopedia of hormones.* New York: Elsevier Science, 2003:510.
2. Shibusawa N, Yamada M, Hirato J, et al. Requirement of thyrotropin-releasing hormone for the postnatal functions of pituitary thyrotrophs: ontogeny study of congenital tertiary hypothyroidism in mice. *Mol Endocrinol* 2000;14:13.
3. Vallette-Kasic S, Pellegrini-Bouiller I, Sampieri F, et al. Combined pituitary hormone deficiency due to the F135C human Pit-1 (pituitary-specific factor 1) gene mutation: functional and structural correlates. *Mol Endocrinol* 2001;15:411.
4. Radovick S, Nations M, Du Y, et al. A mutation in the POU-homeodomain of Pit-1 responsible for combined pituitary hormone deficiency. *Science* 1992;257:1115,
5. Cohen LE, Wondisford FE, Radovick S. Role of Pit-1 in the gene expression of growth hormone, prolactin, and thyrotropin. *Endocrinol Metab Clin North Am* 1996;25:523.
6. Wu W, Cogan JD, Pfaffle RW, et al. Mutations in PROP1 cause familial combined pituitary hormone deficiency. *Nat Genet* 1998;18:147.
7. Burrows HL, Douglas KR, Seasholtz AF, et al. Genealogy of the anterior pituitary gland: tracing a family tree. *Trends Endocrinol Metab* 1999;10:343.
8. Patel YC, Alford FP, Burger HG. The 24-hour plasma thyrotrophin profile. *Clin Sci* 1972;43:71.
9. Vanhaelst L, Van Cauter E, Degaute JP, et al. Circadian variations of serum thyrotropin levels in man. *J Clin Endocrinol Metab* 1972;35:479.
10. Brabant G, Ranft U, Ocran K, et al. Thyrotropin—an episodically secreted hormone. *Acta Endocrinol (Copenh)* 1986;112: 315.
11. Greenspan SL, Klibanski A, Schoenfeld D, et al. Pulsatile secretion of thyrotropin in man. *J Clin Endocrinol Metab* 1986; 63:661.
12. Samuels MH, Veldhuis JD, Henry P, et al. Pathophysiology of pulsatile and copulsatile release of thyroid-stimulating hormone, luteinizing hormone, follicle-stimulating hormone, and alpha-subunit. *J Clin Endocrinol Metab* 1990;71:425.
13. Brabant G, Prank K, Ranft U, et al. Physiological regulation of circadian and pulsatile thyrotropin secretion in normal man and woman. *J Clin Endocrinol Metab* 1990;70:403.
14. Kalsbeek A, Fliers E, Franke AN, et al. Functional connections between the suprachiasmatic nucleus and the thyroid gland as revealed by lesioning and viral tracing techniques in the rat. *Endocrinology* 2000;141:3832.
15. Romijn JA, Adriaanse R, Brabant G, et al. Pulsatile secretion of thyrotropin during fasting: a decrease of thyrotropin pulse amplitude. *J Clin Endocrinol Metab* 1990;70:1631–1636.
16. Romijn JA, Wiersinga WM. Decreased nocturnal surge of thyrotropin in nonthyroidal illness. *J Clin Endocrinol Metab* 1990; 70:35.
17. Yamada M, Saga Y, Shibusawa N, et al. Tertiary hypothyroidism and hyperglycemia in mice with targeted disruption of the thyrotropin-releasing hormone gene. *Proc Natl Acad Sci USA* 1997;94:10862.
18. Abel ED, Kaulbach HC, Campos-Barros A, et al. Novel insight from transgenic mice into thyroid hormone resistance and the regulation of thyrotropin. *J Clin Invest* 1999;103:271.
19. Beck-Peccoz P, Amr S, Menezes-Ferreira MM, et al. Decreased receptor binding of biologically inactive thyrotropin in central hypothyroidism. Effect of treatment with thyrotropin-releasing hormone. *N Engl J Med* 1985;312:1085.
20. Collu R, Tang J, Castagne J, et al. A novel mechanism for isolated central hypothyroidism: inactivating mutations in the thyrotropin-releasing hormone receptor gene. *J Clin Endocrinol Metab* 1997;82:1561.
21. Lechan RM, Wu P, Jackson IM, et al. Thyrotropin-releasing hormone precursor: characterization in rat brain. *Science* 1986; 231:159.
22. Boler J, Enzmann F, Folkers K, et al. The identity of chemical and hormonal properties of the thyrotropin releasing hormone and pyroglutamyl-histidyl-proline amide. *Biochem Biophys Res Commun* 1969;37:705.
23. Burgus R, Dunn TF, Desiderio D, et al. Synthetic polypeptide derivatives with TRF hypophysiotropic activity. New data. *CR Acad Sci Hebd Seances Acad Sci D* 1969;269:226.
24. Lee SL, Stewart K, Goodman RH. Structure of the gene encoding rat thyrotropin releasing hormone. *J Biol Chem* 1988; 263:16604.
25. Satoh T, Yamada M, Iwasaki T, et al. Negative regulation of the gene for the preprothyrotropin-releasing hormone from the mouse by thyroid hormone requires additional factors in conjunction with thyroid hormone receptors. *J Biol Chem* 1996; 271:27919.
26. Yamada M, Radovick S, Wondisford F, et al. Cloning and structure of human genomic DNA and hypothalamic cDNA encoding human prepro thyrotropin-releasing hormone. *Mol Endocrinol* 1990;4:551.
27. Schaner P, Todd RB, Seidah NG, et al. Processing of prothyrotropin-releasing hormone by the family of prohormone convertases. *J Biol Chem* 1997;272:19958.
28. Nillni EA, Xie W, Mulcahy L, et al. Deficiencies in pro-thyrotropin-releasing hormone processing and abnormalities in thermoregulation in Cpefat/fat mice. *J Biol Chem* 2002;277: 48587.
29. Nillni EA, Luo LG, Jackson IM, et al. Identification of the thyrotropin-releasing hormone precursor, its processing products, and its coexpression with convertase 1 in primary cultures of hypothalamic neurons: anatomic distribution of PC1 and PC2. *Endocrinology* 1996;137:5651.
30. Nillni EA, Sevarino KA. The biology of pro-thyrotropin-releasing hormone-derived peptides. *Endocr Rev* 1999;20:599.
31. Valentijn K, Bunel DT, Liao N, Pelletier G, et al. Release of pro-thyrotropin-releasing hormone connecting peptides PS4 and PS5 from perifused rat hypothalamic slices. *Neuroscience* 1991;44:223.
32. Roussel JP, Hollande F, Bulant M, et al. A prepro-TRH connecting peptide (prepro-TRH 160–169) potentiates TRH-induced TSH release from rat perifused pituitaries by stimulating

dihydropyridine- and omega-conotoxin-sensitive Ca2+ channels. *Neuroendocrinology* 1991;54:559.

33. Pekary AE. Is Ps4 (prepro-TRH [160–169]) more than an enhancer for thyrotropin-releasing hormone? *Thyroid* 1998;8:963.

34. Nillni EA, Aird F, Seidah NG, et al. PreproTRH(178–199) and two novel peptides (pFQ7 and pSE14) derived from its processing, which are produced in the paraventricular nucleus of the rat hypothalamus, are regulated during suckling. *Endocrinology* 2001;142:896.

35. Yamada M, Iwasaki T, Satoh T, et al. Activation of the thyrotropin-releasing hormone (TRH) receptor by a direct precursor of TRH, TRH-Gly. *Neurosci Lett* 1995;196:109.

36. Mori M, Yamada M, Satoh T, et al. Different posttranslational processing of human preprothyrotropin-releasing hormone in the human placenta and hypothalamus. *J Clin Endocrinol Metab* 1992;75:1535.

37. Yamada M, Konaka S, Satoh T, et al. Human thyrotropin-releasing hormone-associated peptide 3 (hTAP-3) in serum. *Endocr J* 1999;46:675.

38. Li QL, Jansen E, Brent GA, et al. Regulation of prohormone convertase 1 (PC1) by thyroid hormone. *Am J Physiol Endocrinol Metab* 2001;280:E160.

39. Li QL, Jansen E, Brent GA, et al. Interactions between the prohormone convertase 2 promoter and the thyroid hormone receptor. *Endocrinology* 2000;141:3256.

40. O'Rahilly S, Gray H, Humphreys PJ, et al. Impaired processing of prohormones associated with abnormalities of glucose homeostasis and adrenal function. *N Engl J Med* 1995;333:1386.

41. Jackson RS, Creemers JW, Ohagi S, et al. Obesity and impaired prohormone processing associated with mutations in the human prohormone convertase 1 gene. *Nat Genet* 1997;16:303.

42. Cummins PM, O'Connor B. Pyroglutamyl peptidase: an overview of the three known enzymatic forms. *Biochim Biophys Acta* 1998;1429:1.

43. Cummins PM, O'Connor B. Bovine brain pyroglutamyl aminopeptidase (type-1): purification and characterisation of a neuropeptide-inactivating peptidase. *Int J Biochem Cell Biol* 1996;28:883.

44. Bauer K. Adenohypophyseal degradation of thyrotropin releasing hormone regulated by thyroid hormones. *Nature* 1987;330:375.

45. Horsthemke B, Leblanc P, Kordon C, et al. Subcellular distribution of particle-bound neutral peptidases capable of hydrolyzing gonadoliberin, thyroliberin, enkephalin and substance P. *Eur J Biochem* 1984;139:315.

46. O'Connor B, O'Cuinn G. Localization of a narrow-specificity thyroliberin hydrolyzing pyroglutamate aminopeptidase in synaptosomal membranes of guinea-pig brain. *Eur J Biochem* 1984;144:271.

47. Garat B, Miranda J, Charli JL, et al. Presence of a membrane bound pyroglutamyl amino peptidase degrading thyrotropin releasing hormone in rat brain. *Neuropeptides* 1985;6:27.

48. Vargas MA, Cisneros M, Herrera J, et al. Regional distribution of pyroglutamyl peptidase II in rabbit brain, spinal cord, and organs. *Peptides* 1992;13:255.

49. Yamada M, Shibusawa N, Hashida T, et al. Abundance of cyclo (His-Pro)-like immunoreactivity in the brain of TRH-deficient mice. *Endocrinology* 1999;140:538.

50. Schmitmeier S, Thole H, Bader A, et al. Purification and characterization of the thyrotropin-releasing hormone (TRH)-degrading serum enzyme and its identification as a product of liver origin. *Eur J Biochem* 2002;269:1278.

51. Vargas MA, Cisneros M, Joseph-Bravo P, et al. Thyrotropin-releasing hormone-induced down-regulation of pyroglutamyl aminopeptidase II activity involves L-type calcium channels and cam kinase activities in cultures of adenohypophyseal cells. *J Neuroendocrinol* 2002;14:184.

52. Martinez V, Barrachina MD, Ohning G, et al. Cephalic phase of acid secretion involves activation of medullary TRH receptor subtype 1 in rats. *Am J Physiol Gastrointest Liver Physiol* 2002;283:G1310.

53. Elias CF, Lee CE, Kelly JF, et al. Characterization of CART neurons in the rat and human hypothalamus. *J Comp Neurol* 2001;432:1.

54. Elias CF, Lee C, Kelly J, et al. Leptin activates hypothalamic CART neurons projecting to the spinal cord. *Neuron* 1998;21:1375.

55. Sawchenko PE, Brown ER, Chan RK, et al. The paraventricular nucleus of the hypothalamus and the functional neuroanatomy of visceromotor responses to stress. *Prog Brain Res* 1996;107:201.

56. Michaud JL, Rosenquist T, May NR, et al. Development of neuroendocrine lineages requires the bHLH-PAS transcription factor SIM1. *Genes Dev* 1998;12:3264.

57. Michaud JL, Boucher F, Melnyk A, et al. Sim1 haploinsufficiency causes hyperphagia, obesity and reduction of the paraventricular nucleus of the hypothalamus. *Hum Mol Genet* 2001;10:1465.

58. Keith B, Adelman DM, Simon MC. Targeted mutation of the murine arylhydrocarbon receptor nuclear translocator 2 (Arnt2) gene reveals partial redundancy with Arnt. *Proc Natl Acad Sci U S A* 2001;98:6692.

59. Michaud JL, DeRossi C, May NR, et al. ARNT2 acts as the dimerization partner of SIM1 for the development of the hypothalamus. *Mech Dev* 2000;90:253.

60. Acampora D, Postiglione MP, Avantaggiato V, et al. Progressive impairment of developing neuroendocrine cell lineages in the hypothalamus of mice lacking the Orthopedia gene. *Genes Dev* 1999;13:2787.

61. Wang W, Lufkin T. The murine Otp homeobox gene plays an essential role in the specification of neuronal cell lineages in the developing hypothalamus. *Dev Biol* 2000;227:432.

62. Balkan W, Tavianini MA, Gkonos PJ, et al. Expression of rat thyrotropin-releasing hormone (TRH) gene in TRH-producing tissues of transgenic mice requires sequences located in exon 1. *Endocrinology* 1998;139:252.

63. Sawchenko PE, Swanson LW. The organization of noradrenergic pathways from the brainstem to the paraventricular and supraoptic nuclei in the rat. *Brain Res* 1982;257:275.

64. Harris M, Aschkenasi C, Elias CF, et al. Transcriptional regulation of the thyrotropin-releasing hormone gene by leptin and melanocortin signaling. *J Clin Invest* 2001;107:1.

65. Arancibia S, Rage F, Astier H, et al. Neuroendocrine and autonomous mechanisms underlying thermoregulation in cold environment. *Neuroendocrinology* 1996;64:257.

66. Spencer CA, Lum SM, Wilber JF, et al. Dynamics of serum thyrotropin and thyroid hormone changes in fasting. *J Clin Endocrinol Metab* 1983;56:883.

67. Hugues JN, Burger AG, Pekary AE, et al. Rapid adaptations of serum thyrotrophin, triiodothyronine and reverse triiodothyronine levels to short-term starvation and refeeding. *Acta Endocrinol (Copenh)* 1984;105:194.

68. Blake NG, Eckland DJ, Foster OJ, et al. Inhibition of hypothalamic thyrotropin-releasing hormone messenger ribonucleic acid during food deprivation. *Endocrinology* 1991;129:2714.

69. Blake NG, Johnson MR, Eckland DJ, et al. Effect of food deprivation and altered thyroid status on the hypothalamic-pituitary-thyroid axis in the rat. *J Endocrinol* 1992;133:183.

70. Ahima RS, Prabakaran D, Mantzoros C, et al. Role of leptin in the neuroendocrine response to fasting. *Nature* 1996;382:250.

71. Legradi G, Emerson CH, Ahima RS, et al. Leptin prevents fasting-induced suppression of prothyrotropin-releasing hormone

messenger ribonucleic acid in neurons of the hypothalamic paraventricular nucleus. *Endocrinology* 1997;138:2569.

72. Tartaglia LA, Dembski M, Weng X, et al. Identification and expression cloning of a leptin receptor, OB-R. *Cell* 1995;83:1263.

73. Mercer JG, Hoggard N, Williams LM, et al. Coexpression of leptin receptor and prepronoeuropeptide Y mRNA in arcuate nucleus of mouse hypothalamus. *J Neuroendocrinol* 1996;8:733.

74. Mercer JG, Hoggard N, Williams LM, et al. Localization of leptin receptor mRNA and the long form splice variant (Ob-Rb) in mouse hypothalamus and adjacent brain regions by in situ hybridization. *FEBS Lett* 1996;387:113.

75. Elmquist JK, Bjorbaek C, Ahima RS, et al. Distributions of leptin receptor mRNA isoforms in the rat brain. *J Comp Neurol* 1998;395:535.

76. Fekete C, Legradi G, Mihaly E, et al. alpha-Melanocyte-stimulating-hormone is contained in nerve terminals innervating thyrotropin-releasing hormone synthesizing neurons in the hypothalamic paraventricular nucleus and prevents fasting induced suppression of prothyrotropin-releasing hormone gene expression. *J Neurosci* 2000;20:1550.

77. Kim MS, Small CJ, Stanley SA, et al. The central melanocortin system affects the hypothalamo-pituitary thyroid axis and may mediate the effect of leptin. *J Clin Invest* 2000;105:1005.

78. Legradi G, Emerson CH, Ahima RS, et al. Arcuate nucleus ablation prevents fasting-induced suppression of ProTRH mRNA in the hypothalamic paraventricular nucleus. *Neuroendocrinology* 1998;68:89.

79. Schwartz MW, Seeley RJ, Campfield LA, et al. Identification of targets of leptin action in rat hypothalamus. *J Clin Invest* 1996;98:1101.

80. Schwartz MW, Seeley RJ, Woods SC, et al. Leptin increases hypothalamic pro-opiomelanocortin mRNA expression in the rostral arcuate nucleus. *Diabetes* 1997;46:2119.

81. Cheung CC, Clifton DK, Steiner RA. Proopiomelanocortin neurons are direct targets for leptin in the hypothalamus. *Endocrinology* 1997;138:4489.

82. Kielar D, Clark JS, Ciechanowicz A, et al. Leptin receptor isoforms expressed in human adipose tissue. *Metabolism* 1998;47:844.

83. Kishi T, Aschkenasi CJ, Lee CE, et al. Expression of melanocortin 4 receptor mRNA in the central nervous system of the rat. *J Comp Neurol* 1994;457:213–35.

84. Stephens TW, Basinski M, Bristow PK, et al. The role of neuropeptide Y in the antiobesity action of the obese gene product. *Nature* 1995;377:530.

85. Schwartz MW, Baskin DG, Bukowski TR, et al. Specificity of leptin action on elevated blood glucose levels and hypothalamic neuropeptide Y gene expression in ob/ob mice. *Diabetes* 1996;45:531.

86. Mizuno TM, Mobbs CV. Hypothalamic agouti-related protein messenger ribonucleic acid is inhibited by leptin and stimulated by fasting. *Endocrinology* 1999;140:814.

87. Mihaly E, Fekete C, Tatro JB, et al. Hypophysiotropic thyrotropin-releasing hormone-synthesizing neurons in the human hypothalamus are innervated by neuropeptide Y, agouti-related protein, and alpha-melanocyte-stimulating hormone. *J Clin Endocrinol Metab* 2000;85:2596.

88. Fekete C, Kelly J, Mihaly E, et al. Neuropeptide Y has a central inhibitory action on the hypothalamic-pituitary-thyroid axis. *Endocrinology* 2001;142:2606.

89. Fekete C, Sarkar S, Rand WM, et al. Agouti-related protein (AGRP) has a central inhibitory action on the hypothalamic-pituitary-thyroid (HPT) axis: comparisons between the effect of AGRP and neuropeptide Y on energy homeostasis and the HPT axis. *Endocrinology* 2002;143:3846.

90. Fekete C, Sarkar S, Rand WM, et al. Neuropeptide Y1 and Y5 receptors mediate the effects of neuropeptide Y on the hypothalamic-pituitary-thyroid axis. *Endocrinology* 2002;143:4513.

91. Bjorbaek C, Hollenberg AN. Leptin and melanocortin signaling in the hypothalamus. *Vitam Horm* 2002;65:281.

92. Hollenberg AN, Monden T, Flynn TR, et al. The human thyrotropin-releasing hormone gene is regulated by thyroid hormone through two distinct classes of negative thyroid hormone response elements. *Mol Endocrinol* 1995;9:540.

93. Nillni EA, Vaslet C, Harris M, et al. Leptin regulates prothyrotropin-releasing hormone biosynthesis. Evidence for direct and indirect pathways. *J Biol Chem* 2000;36124.

94. Clement K, Vaisse C, Lahlou N, et al. A mutation in the human leptin receptor gene causes obesity and pituitary dysfunction. *Nature* 1998;392:398.

95. Rosenbaum M, Murphy EM, Heymsfield SB, et al. Low dose leptin administration reverses effects of sustained weight-reduction on energy expenditure and circulating concentrations of thyroid hormones. *J Clin Endocrinol Metab* 2002;87:2391.

96. Chan JL, Heist K, DePaoli AM, et al. The role of falling leptin levels in the neuroendocrine and metabolic adaptation to short-term starvation in healthy men. *J Clin Invest* 2003;111:1409.

97. Farooqi IS, Yeo GS, Keogh JM, et al. Dominant and recessive inheritance of morbid obesity associated with melanocortin 4 receptor deficiency. *J Clin Invest* 2000;106:271.

98. Farooqi IS, Keogh JM, Yeo GS, et al. Clinical spectrum of obesity and mutations in the melanocortin 4 receptor gene. *N Engl J Med* 2003;348:1085.

99. Fliers E, Guldenaar SE, Wiersinga WM, et al. Decreased hypothalamic thyrotropin-releasing hormone gene expression in patients with nonthyroidal illness. *J Clin Endocrinol Metab* 1997;82:4032.

100. Marks DL, Butler AA, Turner R, et al. Differential role of melanocortin receptor subtypes in cachexia. *Endocrinology* 2003;144:1513.

101. Wisse BE, Frayo RS, Schwartz MW, et al. Reversal of cancer anorexia by blockade of central melanocortin receptors in rats. *Endocrinology* 2001;142:3292.

102. Wisse BE, Schwartz MW, Cummings DE. Melanocortin signaling and anorexia in chronic disease states. *Ann N Y Acad Sci* 2003;994:275.

103. Segerson TP, Kauer J, Wolfe HC, et al. Thyroid hormone regulates TRH biosynthesis in the paraventricular nucleus of the rat hypothalamus. *Science* 1987;238:78.

104. Dyess EM, Segerson TP, Liposits Z, et al. Triiodothyronine exerts direct cell-specific regulation of thyrotropin-releasing hormone gene expression in the hypothalamic paraventricular nucleus. *Endocrinology* 1988;123:2291.

105. Kakucska I, Rand W, Lechan RM. Thyrotropin-releasing hormone gene expression in the hypothalamic paraventricular nucleus is dependent upon feedback regulation by both triiodothyronine and thyroxine. *Endocrinology* 1992;130:2845.

106. Schneider MJ, Fiering SN, Pallud SE, et al. Targeted disruption of the type 2 selenodeiodinase gene (DIO2) results in a phenotype of pituitary resistance to T4. *Mol Endocrinol* 2001;15:2137.

107. Tu HM, Kim SW, Salvatore D, et al. Regional distribution of type 2 thyroxine deiodinase messenger ribonucleic acid in rat hypothalamus and pituitary and its regulation by thyroid hormone. *Endocrinology* 1997;138:3359.

108. Diano S, Naftolin F, Goglia F, et al. Fasting-induced increase in type II iodothyronine deiodinase activity and messenger ribonucleic acid levels is not reversed by thyroxine in the rat hypothalamus. *Endocrinology* 1998;139:2879.

109. Lazar MA. Thyroid hormone receptors: multiple forms, multiple possibilities. *Endocr Rev* 1993;14:184.

110. Hollenberg AN. Thyroid hormone receptor isoforms, nuclear corepressors and coactivators and their role in thyroid hormone action. *Curr Opin Endocrinol Diabetes* 1998;5:314.

111. Forrest D, Vennstrom B. Functions of thyroid hormone receptors in mice. *Thyroid* 2000;10:41.

112. Cook CB, Kakucska I, Lechan RM, et al. Expression of thyroid hormone receptor beta 2 in rat hypothalamus. *Endocrinology* 1992;130:1077.

113. Forrest D, Erway LC, Ng L, et al. Thyroid hormone receptor beta is essential for development of auditory function. *Nat Genet* 1996;13:354.

114. Abel ED, Ahima RS, Boers ME, et al. Critical role for thyroid hormone receptor beta2 in the regulation of paraventricular thyrotropin-releasing hormone neurons. *J Clin Invest* 2001; 107:1017.

115. Ng L, Hurley JB, Dierks B, et al. A thyroid hormone receptor that is required for the development of green cone photoreceptors. *Nat Genet* 2001;27:94.

116. Gauthier K, Chassande O, Plateroti M, et al. Different functions for the thyroid hormone receptors TRalpha and TRbeta in the control of thyroid hormone production and post-natal development. *EMBO J* 1999;18:623.

117. Gothe S, Wang Z, Ng L, et al. Mice devoid of all known thyroid hormone receptors are viable but exhibit disorders of the pituitary-thyroid axis, growth, and bone maturation. *Genes Dev* 1999;13:1329.

118. Alland L, Muhle R, Hou H Jr, et al. Role for N-CoR and histone deacetylase in Sin3-mediated transcriptional repression. *Nature* 1997;387:49.

119. Heinzel T, Lavinsky RM, Mullen TM, et al. A complex containing N-CoR, mSin3 and histone deacetylase mediates transcriptional repression. *Nature* 1997;387:43.

120. Nagy L, Kao HY, Chakravarti D, et al. Nuclear receptor repression mediated by a complex containing SMRT, mSin3A, and histone deacetylase. *Cell* 1997;89:373.

121. Guenther MG, Lane WS, Fischle W, et al. A core SMRT corepressor complex containing HDAC3 and TBL1, a WD40-repeat protein linked to deafness. *Genes Dev* 2000;14:1048.

122. Guenther MG, Yu J, Kao GD, et al. Assembly of the SMRT-histone deacetylase 3 repression complex requires the TCP-1 ring complex. *Genes Dev* 2002;16:3130.

123. Onate SA, Tsai SY, Tsai MJ, et al. Sequence and characterization of a coactivator for the steroid hormone receptor superfamily. *Science* 1995;270:1354.

124. Fondell JD, Ge H, Roeder RG. Ligand induction of a transcriptionally active thyroid hormone receptor coactivator complex. *Proc Natl Acad Sci U S A* 1996;93:8329.

125. Glass CK, Rosenfeld MG. The coregulator exchange in transcriptional functions of nuclear receptors. *Genes Dev* 200;14:121.

126. Shibusawa N, Hashimoto K, Nikrodhanond AA, et al. Thyroid hormone action in the absence of thyroid hormone receptor DNA-binding in vivo. *J Clin Invest* 2003;112:588.

127. Wondisford FE, Radovick S, Moates JM, et al. Isolation and characterization of the human thyrotropin beta-subunit gene. Differences in gene structure and promoter function from murine species. *J Biol Chem* 1988;263:12538.

128. Bodenner DL, Mroczynski MA, Weintraub BD, et al. A detailed functional and structural analysis of a major thyroid hormone inhibitory element in the human thyrotropin beta-subunit gene. *J Biol Chem* 1991;266:21666.

129. Weiss RE, Xu J, Ning G, et al. Mice deficient in the steroid receptor co-activator 1 (SRC-1) are resistant to thyroid hormone. *EMBO J* 1999;18:1900.

130. Faglia G, Beck-Peccoz P, Ferrari C, et al. Plasma growth hormone response to thyrotropin-releasing hormone in patients with active acromegaly. *J Clin Endocrinol Metab* 1973;36:1259.

131. Irie M, Tsushima T. Increase of serum growth hormone concentration following thyrotropin-releasing hormone injection in patients with acromegaly or gigantism. *J Clin Endocrinol Metab* 1972;35:97.

132. Snyder PJ. Gonadotroph cell adenomas of the pituitary. *Endocr Rev* 1985;6:552.

133. Anderson MS, Bowers CY, Kastin AJ, et al. Synthetic thyrotropin-releasing hormone. A potent stimulator of thyrotropin secretion in man. *N Engl J Med* 1971;285:1279.

134. Jackson IMD. Thyrotropin-releasing hormone. *N Engl J Med* 1982;306:145.

135. Spencer CA, Schwarzbein D, Guttler RB, et al. Thyrotropin (TSH)-releasing hormone stimulation test responses employing third and fourth generation TSH assays. *J Clin Endocrinol Metab* 1993;76:494.

136. Bowers CY, Friesen HG, Hwang P, et al. Prolactin and thyrotropin release in man by synthetic pyroglutamyl-histidyl-prolinamide. *Biochem Biophys Res Commun* 1971;45:1033.

137. Hershman JM, Pittman JA Jr. Control of thyrotropin secretion in man. *N Engl J Med* 1971;285:997.

138. Straub RE, Frech GC, Joho RH, et al. Expression cloning of a cDNA encoding the mouse pituitary thyrotropin-releasing hormone receptor. *Proc Natl Acad Sci U S A* 1990;87:9514.

139. Itadani H, Nakamura T, Itoh J, et al. Cloning and characterization of a new subtype of thyrotropin-releasing hormone receptors. *Biochem Biophys Res Commun* 1998;250:68.

140. Cao J, O'Donnell D, Vu H, et al. Cloning and characterization of a cDNA encoding a novel subtype of rat thyrotropin-releasing hormone receptor. *J Biol Chem* 1998;273:32281.

141. Lu X, Bidaud I, Ladram A, et al. Pharmacological studies of thyrotropin-releasing hormone (TRH) receptors from *Xenopus laevis*: is xTRHR3 a TRH receptor? *Endocrinology* 2003;144:1842.

142. Heuer H, Schafer MK, O'Donnell D, et al. Expression of thyrotropin-releasing hormone receptor 2 (TRH-R2) in the central nervous system of rats. *J Comp Neurol* 2000;428:319.

143. Sun Y, Lu X, Gershengorn MC. Thyrotropin-releasing hormone receptors—similarities and differences. *J Mol Endocrinol* 2003;30:87

144. Gershengorn MC, Osman R. Molecular and cellular biology of thyrotropin-releasing hormone receptors. *Physiol Rev* 1996;76:175.

145. Carr FE, Shupnik MA, Burnside J, et al. Thyrotropin-releasing hormone stimulates the activity of the rat thyrotropin beta-subunit gene promoter transfected into pituitary cells. *Mol Endocrinol* 1989;3:717.

146. Ashworth R, Yu R, Nelson EJ, et al. Visualization of the thyrotropin-releasing hormone receptor and its ligand during endocytosis and recycling. *Proc Natl Acad Sci USA* 1995;92:512.

147. Cook LB, Zhu CC, Hinkle PM. Thyrotropin-releasing hormone receptor processing: role of ubiquitination and proteasomal degradation. *Mol Endocrinol* 2003;17:1777.

148. Zhu CC, Cook LB, Hinkle PM. Dimerization and phosphorylation of thyrotropin-releasing hormone receptors are modulated by agonist stimulation. *J Biol Chem* 2002;277:28228.

149. Roberson MS, Schoderbek WE, Tremml G, et al. Activation of the glycoprotein hormone alpha-subunit promoter by a LIM-homeodomain transcription factor. *Mol Cell Biol* 1994;14:2985.

150. Bach I, Rhodes SJ, Pearse RV 2nd, et al. P-Lim, a LIM homeodomain factor, is expressed during pituitary organ and cell commitment and synergizes with Pit-1. *Proc Natl Acad Sci USA* 1995;92:2720.

151. Hashimoto K, Zanger K, Hollenberg AN, et al. cAMP response element-binding protein-binding protein mediates thyrotropin-releasing hormone signaling on thyrotropin subunit genes. *J Biol Chem* 2000;275:33365.

152. Zanger K, Radovick S, Wondisford FE. CREB binding protein recruitment to the transcription complex requires growth factor-dependent phosphorylation of its GF box. *Mol Cell* 2001;7:551.

153. Dasen JS, O'Connell SM, Flynn SE, et al. Reciprocal interactions of Pit1 and GATA2 mediate signaling gradient-induced determination of pituitary cell types. *Cell* 1999;97:587.

154. Yamada M, Monden T, Satoh T, et al. Pituitary adenomas of patients with acromegaly express thyrotropin-releasing hormone messenger RNA: cloning and functional expression of the human thyrotropin-releasing hormone receptor gene. *Biochem Biophys Res Commun* 1993;195:737.

155. Yamada M, Hashimoto K, Satoh T, et al. A novel transcript for the thyrotropin-releasing hormone receptor in human pituitary and pituitary tumors. *J Clin Endocrinol Metab* 1997;82:4224.

156. Ehrchen J, Peters A, Ludecke DK, et al. Analysis of thyrotropin-releasing hormone-signaling components in pituitary adenomas of patients with acromegaly. *J Clin Endocrinol Metab* 2000;85:2709.

157. Igarashi-Migitaka J, Yamada S, Hara M, et al. Gene expression study of thyrotropin releasing hormone (TRH) receptor using RT-PCR: relationship to clinical and immunohistochemical phenotypes in a series of human pituitary adenomas. *Endocr J* 2003;50:459.

158. Taylor T, Gesundheit N, Gyves PW, et al. Hypothalamic hypothyroidism caused by lesions in rat paraventricular nuclei alters the carbohydrate structure of secreted thyrotropin. *Endocrinology* 1988;122:283.

159. Mori M, Kobayashi I, Kobayashi S. Thyrotrophin-releasing hormone does not accumulate glycosylated thyrotrophin, but changes heterogeneous forms of thyrotrophin within the rat anterior pituitary gland. *J Endocrinol* 1986;109:227.

160. Reichlin S, Utiger RD. Regulation of the pituitary-thyroid axis in man: relationship of TSH concentration to concentration of free and total thyroxine in plasma. *J Clin Endocrinol Metab* 1967;27:251.

161. Snyder PJ, Utiger RD. Inhibition of thyrotropin response to thyrotropin-releasing hormone by small quantities of thyroid hormones. *J Clin Invest* 1972;51:2077.

162. Vagenakis AG, Rapoport B, Azizi F, et al. Hyperresponse to thyrotropin-releasing hormone accompanying small decreases in serum thyroid hormone concentrations. *J Clin Invest* 1974;54:913.

163. Spencer CA, LoPresti JS, Patel A, et al. Applications of a new chemiluminometric thyrotropin assay to subnormal measurement. *J Clin Endocrinol Metab* 1990;70:453.

164. Hinkle PM, Perrone MH, Schonbrunn A. Mechanism of thyroid hormone inhibition of thyrotropin-releasing hormone action. *Endocrinology* 1981;108:199.

165. Hinkle PM, Goh KB. Regulation of thyrotropin-releasing hormone receptors and responses by L-triiodothyronine in dispersed rat pituitary cell cultures. *Endocrinology* 1982;110:1725.

166. Yamada M, Monden T, Satoh T, et al. Differential regulation of thyrotropin-releasing hormone receptor mRNA levels by thyroid hormone in vivo and in vitro (GH3 cells). *Biochem Biophys Res Commun* 1992;184:367.

167. Shupnik MA, Chin WW, Habener JF, et al. Transcriptional regulation of the thyrotropin subunit genes by thyroid hormone. *J Biol Chem* 1985;260:2900.

168. Abel ED, Boers ME, Pazos-Moura C, et al. Divergent roles for thyroid hormone receptor beta isoforms in the endocrine axis and auditory system. *J Clin Invest* 1999;104:291.

169. Ando S, Sarlis NJ, Oldfield EH, et al. Somatic mutation of TR-beta can cause a defect in negative regulation of TSH in a TSH-secreting pituitary tumor. *J Clin Endocrinol Metab* 2001;86:5572.

170. Ando S, Sarlis NJ, Krishnan J, et al. Aberrant alternative splicing of thyroid hormone receptor in a TSH-secreting pituitary tumor is a mechanism for hormone resistance. *Mol Endocrinol* 2001;15:1529.

171. Chatterjee VK, Lee JK, Rentoumis A, et al. Negative regulation of the thyroid-stimulating hormone alpha gene by thyroid hormone: receptor interaction adjacent to the TATA box. *Proc Natl Acad Sci U S A* 1989;86:9114.

172. Tagami T, Park Y, Jameson JL. Mechanisms that mediate negative regulation of the thyroid-stimulating hormone alpha gene by the thyroid hormone receptor. *J Biol Chem* 1999;274:22345.

173. Hollenberg AN. Negative regulation by thyroid hormone. *Hot Thyroidology* 2002;2.

174. Sasaki S, Lesoon-Wood LA, Dey A, et al. Ligand-induced recruitment of a histone deacetylase in the negative-feedback regulation of the thyrotropin beta gene. *EMBO J* 1999;18:5389.

175. Sherman SI, Gopal J, Haugen BR, et al. Central hypothyroidism associated with retinoid X receptor-selective ligands. *N Engl J Med* 1999;340:1075.

176. Haugen BR, Brown NS, Wood WM, et al. The thyrotrope-restricted isoform of the retinoid-X receptor-gamma1 mediates 9-cis-retinoic acid suppression of thyrotropin-beta promoter activity. *Mol Endocrinol* 1997;11:481.

177. Brown NS, Smart A, Sharma V, et al. Thyroid hormone resistance and increased metabolic rate in the RXR-gamma-deficient mouse. *J Clin Invest* 2000;106:73.

178. Macchia PE, Jiang P, Yuan YD, et al. RXR receptor agonist suppression of thyroid function: central effects in the absence of thyroid hormone receptor. *Am J Physiol Endocrinol Metab* 2002;283:E326.

179. Liu S, Ogilvie KM, Klausing K, et al. Mechanism of selective retinoid X receptor agonist-induced hypothyroidism in the rat. *Endocrinology* 2002;143:2880.

180. Kakucska I, Qi Y, Lechan RM. Changes in adrenal status affect hypothalamic thyrotropin-releasing hormone gene expression in parallel with corticotropin-releasing hormone. *Endocrinology* 1995;136:2795.

181. Luo LG, Bruhn T, Jackson IM. Glucocorticoids stimulate thyrotropin-releasing hormone gene expression in cultured hypothalamic neurons. *Endocrinology* 1995;136:4945.

182. Luo LG, Jackson IM. Glucocorticoids stimulate TRH and c-fos/c-jun gene co-expression in cultured hypothalamic neurons. *Brain Res* 1998;791:56.

183. John CD, Christian HC, Morris JF, et al. Kinase-dependent regulation of the secretion of thyrotrophin and luteinizing hormone by glucocorticoids and annexin 1 peptides. *J Neuroendocrinol* 2003;15:946.

184. Samuels MH. Effects of variations in physiological cortisol levels on thyrotropin secretion in subjects with adrenal insufficiency: a clinical research center study. *J Clin Endocrinol Metab* 2000;85:1388.

185. Samuels MH. Effects of metyrapone administration on thyrotropin secretion in healthy subjects—a clinical research center study. *J Clin Endocrinol Metab* 2000;85:3049.

186. Krulich L, Dhariwal AP, McCann SM. Stimulatory and inhibitory effects of purified hypothalamic extracts on growth hormone release from rat pituitary in vitro. *Endocrinology* 1968;83:783.

187. Ling N, Burgus R, Rivier J, et al. The use of mass spectrometry in deducing the sequence of somatostatin—a hypothalamic polypeptide that inhibits the secretion of growth hormone. *Biochem Biophys Res Commun* 1973;50:127.

188. Brazeau P, Vale W, Burgus R, et al. Hypothalamic polypeptide that inhibits the secretion of immunoreactive pituitary growth hormone. *Science* 1973;179:77.

189. Patel YC. Somatostatin and its receptor family. *Front Neuroendocrinol* 1999;20:157.

190. Vale W, Brazeau P, Rivier C, et al. Somatostatin. *Recent Prog Horm Res* 1975;31:365.
191. Arimura A, Schally AV. Increase in basal and thyrotropin-releasing hormone (TRH)-stimulated secretion of thyrotropin (TSH) by passive immunization with antiserum to somatostatin in rats. *Endocrinology* 1976;98:1069.
192. Ferland L, Labrie F, Jobin M, et al. Physiological role of somatostatin in the control of growth hormone and thyrotropin secretion. *Biochem Biophys Res Commun* 1976;68:149.
193. Lamberts SW, Krenning EP, Reubi JC. The role of somatostatin and its analogs in the diagnosis and treatment of tumors. *Endocr Rev* 1991;12:450.
194. Chanson P, Weintraub BD, Harris AG. Octreotide therapy for thyroid-stimulating hormone-secreting pituitary adenomas. A follow-up of 52 patients. *Ann Intern Med* 1993;119:236.
195. Lamberts SW, van der Lely AJ, de Herder WW, et al. Octreotide. *N Engl J Med* 1996;334:246.
196. Bertherat J, Brue T, Enjalbert A, et al. Somatostatin receptors on thyrotropin-secreting pituitary adenomas: comparison with the inhibitory effects of octreotide upon in vivo and in vitro hormonal secretions. *J Clin Endocrinol Metab* 1992;75:540.
197. Greenman Y, Melmed S. Expression of three somatostatin receptor subtypes in pituitary adenomas: evidence for preferential SSTR5 expression in the mammosomatotroph lineage. *J Clin Endocrinol Metab* 1994;79:724.
198. Beck-Peccoz P, Brucker-Davis F, Persani L, et al. Thyrotropin-secreting pituitary tumors. *Endocr Rev* 1996;17:610.
199. Beck-Peccoz P, Persani L. Medical management of thyrotropin-secreting pituitary adenomas. *Pituitary* 2002;5:83.
200. Sawchenko PE. Toward a new neurobiology of energy balance, appetite, and obesity: the anatomists weigh in. *J Comp Neurol* 1998;402:435.
201. Krulich L, Giachetti A, Marchlewska-Koj A, et al. On the role of the central noradrenergic and dopaminergic systems in the regulation of TSH secretion in the rat. *Endocrinology* 1977;100:496.
202. Krulich L, Mayfield MA, Steele MK, et al. Differential effects of pharmacological manipulations of central alpha 1- and alpha 2-adrenergic receptors on the secretion of thyrotropin and growth hormone in male rats. *Endocrinology* 1982;110:796.
203. Tapia-Arancibia L, Arancibia S, Astier H. Evidence for alpha 1-adrenergic stimulatory control of in vitro release of immunoreactive thyrotropin-releasing hormone from rat median eminence: in vivo corroboration. *Endocrinology* 1985;116:2314.
204. Arancibia S, Tapia-Arancibia L, Astier H, et al. Physiological evidence for alpha 1-adrenergic facilitatory control of the cold-induced TRH release in the rat, obtained by push-pull cannulation of the median eminence. *Neurosci Lett* 1989;100:169.
205. Arancibia S, Tapia-Arancibia L, Assenmacher I, et al. Direct evidence of short-term cold-induced TRH release in the median eminence of unanesthetized rats. *Neuroendocrinology* 1983;37:225.
206. Hefco E, Krulich L, Illner P, et al. Effect of acute exposure to cold on the activity of the hypothalamic-pituitary-thyroid system. *Endocrinology* 1975;97:1185.
207. Fisher DA, Odell WD. Acute release of thyrotropin in the newborn. *J Clin Invest* 1969;48:1670.
208. Fisher DA, Schoen EJ, La Franchi S, et al. The hypothalamic-pituitary-thyroid negative feedback control axis in children with treated congenital hypothyroidism. *J Clin Endocrinol Metab* 2000;85:2722.
209. Cooper DS, Klibanski A, Ridgway EC. Dopaminergic modulation of TSH and its subunits: in vivo and in vitro studies. *Clin Endocrinol (Oxf)* 1983;18:265.
210. Shupnik MA, Greenspan SL, Ridgway EC. Transcriptional regulation of thyrotropin subunit genes by thyrotropin-releasing hormone and dopamine in pituitary cell culture. *J Biol Chem* 1986;261:12675.
211. Greenspan SL, Shupnik MA, Klibanski A, et al. Divergent dopaminergic regulation of TSH, free alpha-subunit, and TSH-beta in pituitary cell culture. *Metabolism* 1986;35:843.
212. Scanlon MF, Weightman DR, Shale DJ. Dopamine is a physiological regulator of thyrotrophin (TSH) secretion in normal man. *Clin Endocrinol (Oxf)* 1979;10:7.
213. Samuels MH, Kramer P. Effects of metoclopramide on fasting-induced TSH suppression. *Thyroid* 1996;6:85.
214. Pinto LP, Hanna FW, Evans LM, et al. The TSH response to domperidone reflects the biological activity of prolactin in macroprolactinaemia and hyperprolactinaemia. *Clin Endocrinol (Oxf)* 2003;59:580.
215. Toft AD, Seth J, Hunter WM, et al. Plasma-thyrotrophin and serum-thyroxine in patients becoming hypothyroid in the early months after iodine-131. *Lancet* 1974;1:704.
216. Toft AD, Irvine WJ, Sinclair I, et al. Thyroid function after surgical treatment of thyrotoxicosis. A report of 100 cases treated with propranolol before operation. *N Engl J Med* 1978;298:643.
217. Kahn BB, Weintraub BD, Csako G, et al. Factitious elevation of thyrotropin in a new ultrasensitive assay: implications for the use of monoclonal antibodies in "sandwich" immunoassay. *J Clin Endocrinol Metab* 1988;66:526.
218. Beckett GJ, Toft AD. First-line thyroid function tests—TSH alone is not enough. *Clin Endocrinol (Oxf)* 2003;58:20.
219. Mitchell DR, Parvin CA, Gronowski AM. Rules-based detection of discrepancies between TSH and free T4 results. *Clin Chim Acta* 2003;332:89.
220. Nicoloff JT, Spencer CA. The use and misuse of the sensitive thyrotropin assays. *J Clin Endocrinol Metab* 1990;71:553.
221. Hamblin PS, Dyer SA, Mohr VS, et al. Relationship between thyrotropin and thyroxine changes during recovery from severe hypothyroxinemia of critical illness. *J Clin Endocrinol Metab* 1986;62:717.

INTRINSIC AND EXTRINSIC VARIABLES

11A AGE-RELATED CHANGES IN THYROID SECRETION

CLARK T. SAWIN*

It is natural to wonder, as we get older, whether or not there is some change with age that might be reversed and thereby prolong our lives or, at least, make the later years more pleasant. Some of the ancients thought that the changes seen in older persons were due to a gradual drying out or cooling of the body; possible remedies were thus the addition of moisture or warmth to one's daily regimen, although neither seemed to actually slow the aging process (1).

This type of reasoning by analogy persisted into the late 19th and early 20th centuries. A prime example is the similarity and equation of the clinical findings in severe hypothyroidism and the changes that occur as we age. In the 1870s and 1880s, many saw the new and striking description of myxoedema (2,3), then the term for what we now call hypothyroidism, as a kind of premature aging. When, in 1888, the Clinical Society of London published its famous report (4), which concluded that the cause of this peculiar disorder was a "destructive change of the thyroid gland," Victor Horsley, who had done the experimental thyroidectomies for the report, had already concluded that "the symptoms of mere senility may be accounted for by the loss of the functions of the thyroid body" (5). With this background, it is no great surprise that, after the discovery of the successful therapy of hypothyroidism with thyroid extract in 1891 (6), others used the same therapy to try to prevent aging or at least to prevent one of its concomitants, atherosclerotic disease, until well into the 20th century (7–10). When there were no specific tests of thyroid function, such attempts were reasonable.

The underlying assumption of this type of thinking is that hypothyroidism is a natural consequence of becoming older. If this were so, then one ought to be able to show a clear decrease in thyroid function in all, or almost all, older persons. If, on the other hand, the presence of hypothyroidism in older persons is an incidental disease and so a confounder in the study of the aging process rather than its consequence, then there may or may not be a decrease in thyroid function as we age. As with most studies of aging, the reality may be that the problem of whether or not thyroid secretion falls with age is not, strictly speaking, soluble. For example, if there are two variables, age and disease, neither of which can be held constant and each of which might affect the thyroid gland, any change in glandular function might be due to either or both variables, and one may not be able to distinguish the effects of the two. The problem is common in epidemiology (e.g., the definition of endemic goiter largely depends on an arbitrary selection of a prevalence rate above which goiter is considered endemic, i.e., all are subject to it, and below which it is not, i.e., goiter is sporadic and peculiar to an individual).

Why should any thyroid changes be a problem if the thyroid gland slows down only in old persons? The answer is clear: life span is increasing in many countries, and any systematic or episodic change in thyroid function that affects longevity or the quality of life is important. Note, for example, that a person 80 years old will, on average, live 7 or 9 more years (men or women, respectively) (11).

The remainder of this chapter discusses issues related to changes in thyroid function with increasing age in humans. The conclusions need to be somewhat tentative because of the confounders just noted; further, almost all the data are cross-sectional, the definition of "normal" or "healthy" is rarely explicit, and cohort or survival effects are usually not addressed. Better answers would come from careful longitudinal studies of the same persons followed for many years, but as yet there are no such studies.

SERUM THYROXINE CONCENTRATIONS

The serum concentration of thyroxine (T_4), the principal circulating thyroid hormone, seems to change little with

---

*Deceased.

increasing age. This was first shown indirectly with measurement of the serum concentration of protein-bound iodine (PBI), which measures mainly T_4 (12,13), and then with assays of serum total T_4 and estimates of serum free T_4 concentrations (13–15). The data are sometimes confounded by the inadvertent inclusion of those with subclinical hypothyroidism, with a resulting decrease in the mean serum T_4 or free T_4 concentration (16–18). Other data that show a slight increase in serum T_4 in women (19) or in free T_4 estimates in men and women (14,20,21) are less easy to explain, but are likely of little clinical relevance in view of the generally unchanged or perhaps slightly lower serum thyrotropin (thyroid-stimulating hormone, TSH) concentrations in older persons (see later in the chapter). In a few instances of a lower serum free T_4 index in older persons, the hypothesis has been raised of a resetting downward of the feedback threshold by which thyroid hormones shut off the secretion of TSH (22); however, the evidence for this idea is thin.

It is also possible that a lessened secretion of T_4 in older persons might be due to a fall in the ability of the thyroid gland to respond to stimulation by TSH. Thyroid cell membranes from old rats, for example, seem to have a decreased response of adenylyl cyclase to TSH that matches the lower response of thyroid hormone secretion to TSH in this species (23). However, in humans, the response of serum thyroid hormones to TSH is the same in older and younger adults (24), and there is no decrease in the binding of TSH to human thyroid tissue from older persons (25). Further, if there were a fall in thyroid sensitivity to TSH in older persons, one would expect a rise in serum TSH, which seems not to occur in the absence of hypothyroidism (see later in the chapter).

Overall, there is no clinically important change in the serum concentration of T_4 in older persons.

THYROID RADIOIODINE UPTAKE AND THYROXINE TURNOVER

Despite the stability of serum T_4 concentration throughout the human age span, thyroid uptake of radioiodine is lower in older compared with younger men (26). This finding suggests that thyroid hormone secretion decreases with advancing age, a conclusion supported with the demonstration of a decrease in T_4 degradation in older men in the presence of a constant serum concentration of T_4 (12). The only way the serum level could remain constant in the face of a decreased metabolic clearance of T_4 have a concomitant decrease in T_4 secretion from the thyroid gland. An early systematic review confirmed these conclusions for both men and women (27). The clinical corollary that one would expect with a decreased secretion of thyroid hor-

mone with older age is that the replacement dose of T_4 in patients with primary hypothyroidism should be lower, on average, in older than in younger persons. In fact, this is so (28–30), although the phenomenon may be somewhat dependent on the cause of the hypothyroidism (31).

In sum, T_4 secretion decreases with older age but the serum concentration does not.

SERUM TRIIODOTHYRONINE CONCENTRATIONS

If there is less T_4 secreted in older persons, the serum concentration of triiodothyronine (T_3) might also be lower because most of the circulating T_3 derives from circulating T_4. Much would depend on the conversion rate of T_4 to T_3 and on the clearance of T3 itself.

At first, the data showed that older persons did have a lower serum concentration of T_3 and, when estimated, of free T_3 (16,17,32–35), although perhaps the findings might have applied only to men (36). Then came the recognition that illness sufficient to cause admission to a nursing home or to hospital is a common cause of a low serum concentration of T_3 whereas, when selected for good overall health, older persons have no decrease in the serum level of T_3 (37,38). More recent data indicate that, while there is a slightly lower serum concentration of total T_3 in older men (though perhaps not in older women), age has no effect on the concentration of free T_3 (20) and few healthy older persons have a value of serum free T_3 outside the reference range for younger adults (39).

Data on healthy centenarians indicate that these truly old persons do indeed have a lower level of serum T_3 but that the decrease does not occur until about the age of 80 years (40,41) and stays within the reference range, although even at this age some have not found such a decrease (42). Even here, however, the interpretation of the data is not clear, because there is almost certainly selection bias in comparing centenarians to middle-aged adults. Those who reach 100 years of age are a small group of survivors and are not typical of the population of persons over age 60 years. For example, there is a clear increase in the prevalence of thyroid antibodies above the age of 60 to 70 years, although this is not found in centenarians (43); the best interpretation is that few with thyroid antibodies reach 100 years of age.

On balance, there is probably a slight fall in the serum concentration of T_3 with increasing age, but it is unlikely to be of clinical importance. If an individual has a clearly low serum T_3 concentration, it is more likely due to nonthyroid illness and the associated blunting of the conversion of serum T_4 to T_3.

SERUM THYROTROPIN CONCENTRATIONS

Because part of the definition of "normal" often includes a serum concentration of TSH that is within the reference range for younger adults, it is not easy to say whether or not older persons have a high or low serum TSH level; persons with such levels are often excluded in a population study. Further, the prevalence of subclinical hypothyroidism rises with increasing age, especially in women; unless hypothyroidism is specifically sought and excluded prior to a study, the results will likely show a higher serum concentration of TSH in older compared with younger persons. Ideal studies might examine the serum TSH concentrations in older persons matched with younger persons on the basis of comparable serum concentrations of T_4 and T_3 and would follow, as noted earlier, the same population for some years; such studies are not available.

The available information is conflicting. Basal serum concentrations of TSH can be unchanged in older persons (24,35,38,44), slightly higher in older women (45) or in older men (18), or slightly lower in both older men and women (21,41).

Perhaps more relevant to the issue of a change in TSH secretion with age is the finding that, with multiple measurements made over 24 hours, the mean serum concentration of TSH is slightly but clearly lower in older men compared to younger ones, although the values in the older men generally remained within the reference range for younger adults (44). Further, there is a blunting of the nocturnal rise in TSH secretion in older men (46).

What of the serum TSH response to thyrotropin-releasing hormone (TRH) in older persons? This would be important to study because the rise in serum TSH after giving TRH is proportional to the basal level of TSH. Because changes in the basal level may be difficult to detect because of excessive noise in the assay, the magnified concentrations of TSH after TRH may better reflect the true basal value. Here, most data indicate that at least some older persons have a lesser response of serum TSH to TRH than do younger persons (21,35), although the decreased response may be found only in older women (38) or only in older men (32,45). Occasionally, investigators have not found any difference in the TSH response to TRH in older men (18). Some have attributed a diminished response of serum TSH to TRH in older persons to the presence of unsuspected nodular goiter and a mild degree of thyroid autonomy rather than to older age per se (47).

That there is some decrease in TSH secretion in older age is supported by the observation that serum concentrations of TSH in primary hypothyroidism are not as high in older persons as in younger ones (48). That this in turn might be related to a decrease in TRH secretion by the hypothalamus has some experimental support, in that TRH secretion *in vitro* is lower than expected in hypothalamic tissue excised from older rats (49).

Physiologically, a lower TRH and TSH secretion in older age makes sense in view of the lesser need for T_4 secretion as a result of the decreased T_4 turnover noted earlier. A clinical corollary of this idea is seen in the small but significant percentage of older persons who have a clearly low serum TSH concentration compared to younger adults but who do not have thyrotoxicosis (50).

Thus, there is probably a small decrease in TSH secretion in older persons that may be related to the decreased clearance of T_4. This slight fall in TSH secretion is generally within the reference range for younger adults and is probably of little clinical importance.

THYROID HORMONE ACTION

Whether or not there is some change in the action of thyroid hormone in older persons, at least on selected tissues, is an old speculation that has only modest support. The issue is raised because how else can one explain the notable differences in the clinical presentation of thyrotoxicosis in older persons compared to younger ones (51,52), wherein it is often difficult to detect the disorder in older persons despite comparable elevations in serum thyroid hormone concentrations?

There is some evidence in older rats that there is a decrease in the sensitivity of some tissues, especially the heart, to thyroid hormone, and that this decrease is related to a parallel age-related diminution in β-adrenergic responsiveness (53). It is possible, though by no means proven, that a similar mechanism operates in humans. The opposite speculation, i.e., that there is an increase in tissue sensitivity to thyroid hormones in older persons, has also been raised, as in the mention earlier of a possible resetting of the pituitary's response to thyroid hormones. While there is little evidence for a change in tissue sensitivity to thyroid hormones, why the clinical presentation of thyrotoxicosis differs in older persons remains unexplained.

SCREENING AND CASE-FINDING

Physicians rarely do true "screening," which is the testing of an entire community or population; they usually do "case-finding," which is testing for a disease in patients who come to them with a complaint of one kind or another. In the case of thyroid failure, the presence of a risk factor for thyroid dysfunction (Tables 11A.1–11A.2) is sufficient reason to test for such dysfunction at any age and, of course, age itself is a risk factor for hypothyroidism. Because the clinical findings of hypothyroidism in older persons are vague and nonspecific, because the only reliable way to make the specific diagnosis is to measure serum TSH, because the number of older persons with hypothyroidism is

TABLE 11A.1. RISK FACTORS FOR HYPOTHYROIDISM

History:

Age >60 y
Other autoimmune disease
    Addison's disease
    Pernicious anemia
    Diabetes mellitus (type 1)
Subacute thyroiditis (overt or silent)
Head/neck cancer (treated)
Family member with thyroid disease

Medication use:

Lithium carbonate
Amiodarone
Iodine (any form)

Routine tests (if previously done):

Hypercholesterolemia

Thyroid tests (if previously done):

Slightly raised serum TSH concentration
High serum antithyroid peroxidase antibody concentration

TSH, thyrotropin.

TABLE 11A.2. RISK FACTORS FOR THYROTOXICOSIS

History:

Family member with thyroid disease
Known goiter
Cigarette smoking (Graves' disease)

Current findings:

Atrial fibrillation
Goiter
Osteopenia
Congestive heart failure

Medication:

Amiodarone
Iodine (any form)
Lithium

Routine tests:

Radiographic contrast agent

Thyroid tests:

Low serum TSH concentration

TSH, thyrotropin.

reasonably high, and because there is an effective treatment, one could argue that on these grounds alone all older persons should be tested for hypothyroidism, i.e., that they should be screened. Nevertheless, a recent complete assessment of the available evidence does not support such screening of all older persons as a routine practice (54).

SUMMARY

In general, there is little systematic change in thyroid function with increasing age in hymans. In older persons, there is a modest decrease in T_4 secretion without a change in the circulating level of the hormone, a slight fall in circulating T_3 concentration after the age of 80 years or so, and perhaps a slight fall in the secretion of TSH. There is no change in the thyroid gland's response to TSH in older persons and no proven decrease in tissue response to thyroid hormones. All of these changes, except possibly the fall in serum T_3 concentrations, are generally within the reference ranges for younger adults, which can therefore be used to diagnose thyroid dysfunction in older persons. Thus, age-related changes in thyroid function in older persons do not have major effects on the tests used to detect thyroid disease. When there are abnormalities in these tests that would indicate disease in younger adults, thyroid dysfunction should be presumed present in older persons unless proven otherwise. There is as yet no solid explanation for

the different clinical appearances of thyroid dysfunction in older persons as compared to younger ones. There are no firm data to support routine testing ("screening") of all older persons for thyroid dysfunction, principally because data to support benefit are lacking; however, vigorous case-finding is sensible.

When a younger adult is treated with T_4 for hypothyroidism for many years, there should be consideration of a decrease in the dose when that person reaches the age of 60 years or so.

REFERENCES

1. Birren JE. History of gerontology. In: *Encyclopedia of gerontology*, Vol. 1. New York: Academic Press, 1996:655.
2. Gull WW. On a cretinoid state supervening in adult life in women. *Trans Clin Soc London* 1874;7:180.
3. Ord WM. On myxoedema, a term proposed to be applied to an essential condition in the "cretinoid" affection occasionally observed in middle-aged women. *Med-Chir Trans* 1878; 61:57.
4. Ord WM, Cavafy J, Durham AE, et al. Report of a committee of the Clinical Society of London nominated December 14, 1883, to investigate the subject of myxoedema. *Trans Clin Soc Lond* 1888;21[Suppl]:1–215.
5. Horsley V. Relation of the thyroid gland to general nutrition. *Lancet* 1886;1:3.
6. Murray GR. Note on the treatment of myxoedema by hypodermic injections of an extract of the thyroid gland of a sheep. *BMJ* 1891;2:796.

7. Barnes BO. Prophylaxis of ischaemic heart-disease by thyroid therapy. *Lancet* 1959;2:149.

8. Wren JC. Symptomatic atherosclerosis: prevention or modification by treatment with desiccated thyroid. *J Am Geriatr Soc* 1971;19:7.

9. Starr P. Atherosclerosis, hypothyroidism, and thyroid hormone therapy. *Adv Lipid Res* 1978;16:345.

10. Lev-Ran A. Thyroid hormones and prevention of atherosclerotic heart disease: an old-new hypothesis. *Perspect Biol Med* 1994;37:487.

11. Manton KG, Vaupel JW. Survival after the age of 80 in the United States, Sweden, France, England and Japan. *N Engl J Med* 1995;333:1232.

12. Gregerman RI, Gaffney GW, Shock NW, et al. Thyroxine turnover in euthyroid man with special references to changes with age. *J Clin Invest* 1962;41:2065.

13. Braverman LE, Dawber NA, Ingbar SH. Observations concerning the binding of thyroid hormones in sera of normal subjects of varying ages. *J Clin Invest* 1966;45:1273.

14. Blum CJ, Lafont C, Ducasse M, et al. Thyroid function tests in ageing and their relation to associated nonthyroidal disease. *J Endocrinol Invest* 1989;12:307.

15. Runnels BL, Garry PJ, Hunt WC, et al. Thyroid function in a healthy elderly population: implications for clinical evaluation. *J Gerontol A Biol Sci Med Sci* 1991;46:B39.

16. Herrmann J, Rusche HJ, Kroll HJ, et al. Free triiodothyronine (T3) and thyroxine (T4) serum levels in old age. *Horm Metab Res* 1974;6:239.

17. Lipson A, Nickoloff EL, Hsu TH, et al. A study of age-dependent changes in thyroid function tests in adults. *J Nucl Med* 1979;20:1124.

18. Harman SM, Wehmann RE, Blackman MC. Pituitary-thyroid hormone economy in healthy aging men: basal indices of thyroid function and thyrotropin responses to constant infusions of thyrotropin releasing hormone. *J Clin Endocrinol Metab* 1984;58:320.

19. Britton KE, Ellis SM, Miralles JM, et al. Is "T4 toxicosis" a normal biochemical finding in elderly women? *Lancet* 1975;2:141.

20. Hershman JM, Pekary AE, Berg L, et al. Serum thyrotropin and thyroid hormone levels in elderly and middle-aged euthyroid persons. *J Am Geriatr Soc* 1993;41:823.

21. Monzani F, Del Guerra P, Caraccio N, et al. Age-related modifications in the regulation of the hypothalamic-pituitary-thyroid axis. *Horm Res* 1996;46:107.

22. Lewis GF, Alessi CA, Imperial JG, et al. Low serum free thyroxine index in ambulating elderly is due to a resetting of the threshold of thyrotropin feedback suppression. *J Clin Endocrinol Metab* 1991;73:843.

23. Reymond F, Dénéréaz N, Lemarchand-Béraud T. Thyrotropin action is impaired in the thyroid gland of old rats. *Acta Endocrinol* 1992;126:55.

24. Szabolcs I, Szilágyi G, Góth M, et al. Plasma triiodothyronine response to thyrotropin releasing hormone, thyrotropin and propranolol in old age. *Exp Gerontol* 1981;16:309.

25. Durica S, Zakula Z, Isenovic E, et al. Age-related changes of TSH receptors in thyroid tissues obtained from euthyroid patients. *Arch Gerontol Geriatr* 1993;17:203.

26. Gaffney OW, Gregerman RI, Shock NW. Relationship of age to the thyroidal accumulation, renal excretion and distribution of radioiodide in euthyroid man. *J Clin Endocrinol Metab* 1962;22:784.

27. Oddie TH, Meade JH, Fisher DA. An analysis of published data on thyroxine turnover in human subjects. *J Clin Endocrinol* 1966;26:425.

28. Rosenbaum RL, Barzel US. Levothyroxine replacement dose for primary hypothyroidism decreases with age. *Ann Intern Med* 1982;96:53.

29. Sawin CT, Herman T, Molitch ME, et al. Aging and the thyroid. Decreased requirement for thyroid hormone in older hypothyroid patients. *Am J Med* 1983;75:206.

30. Davis FB, LaMantia RS, Spaulding SW, et al. Estimation of a physiologic replacement dose of levothyroxine in elderly patients with hypothyroidism. *Arch Intern Med* 1984;144:1752.

31. Kabadi UM. Influence of age on optimal daily levothyroxine dosage in patients with primary hypothyroidism grouped according to etiology. *South Med J* 1997;90:920.

32. Snyder PJ, Utiger RD. Response to thyrotropin releasing hormone (TRH) in normal man. *J Clin Endocrinol Metab* 1972;34:380.

33. Rubenstein HA, Butler VP, Werner SC. Progressive decrease in serum triiodothyronine concentrations with human aging: radioimmunoassay following extraction of serum. *J Clin Endocrinol Metab* 1973;37:247.

34. Caplan RH, Wickus G, Glasser JE, et al. Serum concentrations of the iodothyronines in elderly subjects: decreased triiodothyronine (T3) and free T3 index. *J Am Geriatr Soc* 1981;29:19.

35. Jacques C, Schlienger JL, Kissel C, et al. TRH-induced TSH and prolactin responses in the elderly. *Age Ageing* 1987;16:181.

36. Snyder PJ, Utiger RD. Thyrotropin response to thyrotropin releasing hormone in normal females over forty. *J Clin Endocrinol Metab* 1972;34:1006.

37. Olsen T, Laurberg P, Weeke J. Low serum triiodothyronine and high serum reverse triiodothyronine in old age: an effect of disease not age. *J Clin Endocrinol Metab* 1978;47:1111.

38. Kaiser FE. Variability of response to thyrotropin-releasing hormone in normal elderly. *Age Ageing* 1987;16:345.

39. Goichot B, Schlienger JL, Grunenberger F, et al. Thyroid hormone status and nutrient intake in the free-living elderly. Interest of reverse triiodothyronine assessment. *Eur J Endocrinol* 1994;130:244.

40. Pénzes L, Gergely I. Thyroid hormones in the light of general health status of Hungarian centenarians. *Age* 1989;12:137.

41. Mariotti S, Barbesino G, Caturegli P, et al. Complex alteration of thyroid function in healthy centenarians. *J Clin Endocrinol Metab* 1993;77:1130.

42. Maugeri D, Russo MS, Di Stefano F, et al. Thyroid function in healthy centenarians. *Arch Gerontol Geriatr* 1997;25:211.

43. Marioth S, Sansoni P, Barbesino G, et al. Thyroid and other organ-specific autoantibodies in healthy centenarians. *Lancet* 1992;339:1506.

44. Van Coevorden A, Laurent E, Decoster C, et al. Decreased basal and stimulated thyrotropin secretion in healthy elderly men. *J Clin Endocrinol Metab* 1989;69:177.

45. Erfuth EM, Norden NE, Hedner P, et al. Normal reference interval for thyrotropin response to thyroliberin: dependence on age, sex, free thyroxin index, and basal concentrations of thyrotropin. *Clin Chem* 1984;30:196.

46. Greenspan SL, Klibanski A, Rowe JW, et al. Age-related alterations in pulsatile secretion of TSH: role of dopaminergic regulation. *Am J Physiol* 1991;260:E486.

47. Croxson MS, Wilson TM, Ballantyne GH. TRH testing, T4-thyrotoxicosis and the aging thyroid gland. *N Z Med J* 1981;93:417.

48. Wiener R, Utiger RD, Lew R, et al. Age, sex, and serum thyrotropin concentrations in primary hypothyroidism. *Acta Endocrinol (Copenh)* 1991;124:364.

49. Pekary AE, Mirell CJ, Turner LF, et al. Hypothalamic secretion of thyrotropin releasing hormone declines in aging rats. *J Gerontol* 1987;42:447.

50. Sawin CT, Geller A, Kaplan MM, et al. Low serum thyrotropin (thyroid-stimulating hormone) in older persons without thyrotoxicosis. *Arch Intern Med* 1991;151:165.
51. Trivalle C, Doucet J, Chassagne P, et al. Differences in the signs and symptoms of thyrotoxicosis in older and younger patients. *J Am Geriatr Soc* 1996;44:50.
52. Martin FIR, Deam DR. Thyrotoxicosis in elderly hospitalized patients. Clinical features and treatment outcomes. *Med J Aust* 1996;164:200.
53. Mooradian AD, Wong NCW. Age-related changes in thyroid hormone action. *Eur J Endocrinol* 1994;131:451.
54. Surks, MI, Ortiz E, Daniels GH, et al. Subclinical thyroid disease. Scientific review and guidelines for diagnosis and management. *JAMA* 2004;291:228–238.

11B ENVIRONMENTAL INFLUENCES UPON THYROID HORMONE REGULATION

H. LESTER REED

The environment in which humans live and work can be defined as a complex of climatic, terrestrial, and biotic factors that act upon an organism to determine its form and survival. Accumulating evidence over the past three decades now supports the concept that human physiology acclimates to changing environmental factors, such as temperature (1,2), photoperiod (3), altitude (4), gravity (5,6), season (7–10), and time zone (11). Understanding the influences of these changes upon thyroid hormone economy may help with our insight into a seasonal presentation of thyroid cancer (12,13), interpreting repeated measures of thyroid function, planning clinical studies, and predicting the hormone changes for pregnancy and nonthyroidal illness (see Chapter 80). These extrinsic influences on iodothyronine homeostasis may be characterized as direct, which include cold (14–16) and warm (17) temperature, photoperiod (3), altitude (18), and microgravity (6); or more interactive, which include exercise (19), sleep (20,21), nutrition (22), age (see preceding section), pregnancy (see Chapter 80), illness, depression, and toxic or geographic radiation exposure (see Chapter 70). Under usual circumstances, humans cannot completely isolate themselves from many direct factors, such as temperature (22,23), photoperiod (3,9–11), and altitude (18,24–26).

Although detailed studies are possible using small rodents, these models often lack similarity to humans with respect to such basic homeostatic mechanisms as thermal regulation (27,28). Therefore, this review will include human studies and will only reference alternate animal studies when no other data are available. The present review will not address whether the human thyroidal responses to the described environmental changes are adaptive or maladaptive.

EFFECTS OF ENVIRONMENTAL TEMPERATURE

Cold

Physiologic Cold Adaptation

When tested during a cold air tolerance test (1,15,29), humans show physiologic cold adaptation after repeated exposure to either cold water (15) or air (29,30). These characteristics include a decrease in skin and rectal temperature (15), as well as in the threshold for shivering and the blood pressure response with cold air (29). Human adaptation to cold may be observed when only the face, hands, or feet are repeatedly exposed to cold temperatures (15, 31).

Thyroid Hormone Responses to Brief Cold Climate Chamber Exposures

Serum iodothyronines and thyrotropin (thyroid-stimulating hormone, TSH) do not change dramatically in adults (32) exposed up to 120 minutes of cold air to when they have not been previously exposed to cold (cold naive) (7,16,30). If the subjects walk at 3 miles per hour in 5°C air for 6 hours, serum total triiodothyronine (T_3) and total thyroxine (T_4) increase only during the cold air exercise period without a change in TSH (33). These increases are not common with the same amount of or even more severe exercise at 20° to 24°C (see Table 11B.1). After correcting for changes in plasma volume, free T_3 and free T_4 decline following 115 minutes of resting while exposed to cold air without changes in T_3, T_4, or TSH (15,30). Neonates, however, unlike adults, have substantial thermogenic brown adipose tissue (see Chapter 74) and, in contrast to adults, have an increase in serum TSH during cold air exposure (16,32).

Thyroid Hormone Responses to Repeated Cold Chamber Exposures

Subjects undergoing multiple (14,15,30,34) (-20° to 10°C) or extended (10° to 12°C) air exposure for 4 hours to 14 days have changes in both thyroid hormone kinetic and static values. Ingbar and Bass originally reported that in seminude men exposed to cold (11° to 16°C) for 12 to 14 days, organic iodide production more than doubled and radiolabeled T_4 degradation increased (16,32). Men exposed briefly to cold air (4°C) twice a day (14) increase their T_3 plasma clearance rate (PCR) and T_3 plasma appearance rate (PAR) by approximately 18% after the first

14 days. All of these men had similar increases in T_3 PCR and PAR, and all developed cold adaptation, even though half received oral T_3 to suppress TSH and free T_4 by approximately 50% (14), suggesting that cold-induced T_3 PCR and PAR have little dependence on serum TSH and free T_4 (14). Following 40 exposures of the legs to cold (4°C) water for 5 to 60 minutes, each over for 30 days, a 115-minute cold air test showed both cold adaptation physiology and decreases in serum T_3 (15). This decrease is in general agreement with longer cold air tests (30,34,35) but not shorter ones (29) (Table 11B.1). Factory workers with occupational exposure for approximately 3.5 hours to severe cold (-40° to -20°C) or continuous moderate exposure (-10° to 8°C) for 8 hr/day show a decline in serum T_3 by 10% with cold exposure, whereas only with the most severe temperature did T_4 decrease (34). Serum T_4 was decreased before their daily duties only in the severely cold-

TABLE 11B.1. EFFECTS OF COLD ON THYROID FUNCTION

Cold Exposure Testing	During Initial[a] Exposure (0°–5°C)	Following Multiple[b] Exposures (20°–24°C)	During Field[c] Exposures (20°–24°C)	Field Time Course[d] (Approx. No. Days)	Seasonal Peak Change (Month)
Conditions:	Chamber[e]	Ambient[f]	Ambient		
T_3	≈(↑[g])	≈	≈/↓(4%[h])	5–30	↑(5%)[III[i]] (Jan.)
free T_3	↓	≈/↓	≈/↑(7%)[k]	35–60[k]	↑(6%)[IV] (Mar.)
					↑5–60%
UT_3	N/A	N/A	N/A	N/A	↑(23%) (Feb.)
T_4	≈(↑[g])	≈	↓(4%)	60–140	↑(Nov.-Jan.)
free T_4	≈/↓	≈	≈/↓	60–140	↑(Mar.)
			↑	5–60	
TBG	≈	≈	≈/↑	60–120	N/A
TSH	≈	≈	↑(15%–30%)	70–140	↑(14%)[II] (Dec.)
Tg	N/A	N/A	↑(17%–30%)	70–140	N/A
T_3 PAR	N/A	↑	↑↑	14–30	N/A
T_3 PCR	N/A	↑	↑↑(15%–180%)	14–30	↑(15%)[I] (Sep.)
$T_3 V_d$	N/A	≈	↑↑(100%–300%)	70–140	NA
T_4 PAR	N/A	↑	≈	12–14	NA
Adapted[j]	No	Yes	Yes	10–14	Sep.
Reference no.	14,29,33,34,82	14–16,29, 30,32,34	16,34, 37–40,46	15,16,23,31, 38–42,99,101	23,48,98

↑, increased; ↓, decreased; ≈, no change; FT$_3$, free triiodothyronine; FT$_4$, free thyroxine; N/A, not available; PAR, plasma appearance rate; PCR, plasma clearance rate; TBG, thyroxine-binding globulin; Tg, thyroglobulin; TSH, thyrotropin; TT$_3$, total T$_3$; TT$_4$, total T$_4$; UT$_3$, urinary T$_3$; V$_d$, distribution volume.
[a]Subjects never exposed to experimental cold-air testing.
[b]Subjects with repeated exposures to cold air in an environmental chamber.
[c]Subjects tested after cold exposure from their occupation or geographic relocation.
[d]Per changes in the "During field" category.
[e]Studies during a cold-air challenge test.
[f]Studies conducted after cold-air challenge.
[g]Change summarized as increased (↑), decreased (↓), or no change (≈).
[h]Percentages indicate change from the annual mean.
[i]Roman numerals indicate the northern hemisphere seasonal time sequence.
[j]The presence or absence of hypothermic cold adaptation.
[k]Studies in references 34 and 38.
The comparisons of changes are between conditions of either before and after the chamber studies, before and after the geographic relocation, between cold-exposed and non-cold-exposed occupations, and percentage change from the annual mean.

exposed group while the free T_4 and free T_3 values were generally elevated and did not change much with cold exposure in this severely cold exposed group (34). Specific occupational controls and study protocol, subject sex, lack of plasma volume status correction, and free hormone analogue assay differences may account for the discrepancy in free T_4 and free T_3 values when compared with other studies (15,29,35). The study also reported reverse T_3 (rT_3) to follow the same pattern as the T_3 and T_4 decline, thus arguing against the notion that the decline in T_3 (15,16, 29,34) is from a decrease in PAR or inhibition of iodothyronine 5'-deiodinase type 1 (5'-D1) activity as seen with fasting (22,36) or illness.

Thyroid Hormone Responses to Cold Climate Environmental Field Studies

Results from early field studies are in contrast to more recent publications describing polar residents (35,37–40) or occupational exposure (34) (Table 11B.2). These prior studies may have been confounded by sleep deprivation (20), dietary changes (22), and plasma volume shifts (15). Extended residence in Antarctica and other high latitude environments is associated with exposures to extremes of photoperiod, low relative humidity, social isolation, and low temperatures, along with seasonal variability (7,31, 41–43). Humans living in these conditions for approximately 5 months develop cold adaptation (16,35), even though only the hands and face may be directly exposed to outdoor temperatures (15). Furthermore, energy requirements increase by approximately 40%, and appear to be divided between a decrease in exercise efficiency by 22% to 25% and an increase in resting metabolic rate by 11% to 19% (44). Body temperature declines within the first month when compared with measurements taken before deployment to Antarctica (16,31,35,37,40,44). Indigenous populations at high latitudes have basal metabolic rates (BMR) that are approximately 12% higher (42) and energy requirements approximately 35% higher (43) than mid latitude standards. The BMR variances are correlated to serum thyroid hormones in some of these populations (42).

T_3 is a likely candidate to mediate some of these effects (14,16). Much of the 24-hour energy expenditure is dependent on skeletal muscle (36), the thermogenic effects of thyroid hormones are becoming more clear (27,28,42,45). T_3 is concentrated in muscle, along with theoretical mechanisms of uncoupling energy use (27,28,45). Serum TSH and thyroglobulin (46) increase by about 30% above baseline after 2 to 4 months in Antarctica (16,31,39,40,47), although they retain sensitivity to T_3 (40) and T_4 (44,46). These hormonal changes are associated with a more than doubling in the T_3 distribution volume (Vd), PAR, and PCR (37). Small changes in T_4 kinetics suggest an approximate 17% decline in the T_4 Vd without an increase in the T_4 PAR (37). A small decline in free T_4 (~6%) and can be detected using serial measurements after arrival in Antarctica (39,44,47). These observations suggest a change in T_3 kinetics and distribution, initiating a chain of effects that are time dependent (Table 11A.1) (16) and eventually replacing in an equimolar fashion approximately 17% of the T_4 pool with T_3, thus more than doubling the T_3 pool (7,

TABLE 11B.2. EFFECTS OF ALTITUDE ON THYROID FUNCTION[a]

Altitude	2,315–3,048 m	3,500 m	3,750–3,810 m	4,300 m	5,080–5,400 m	6,300 m
T_3	≈	↑(17%-80%)	↑	N/A	↑(16%)	↑(12%)
free T_3	↑	N/A	↑	N/A	≈	↑[b]
T_4	≈/↓	↑(70%–128%)	↑	↑(PAR)	↑(27%)	↑(44%)
free T_4	↑	N/A	↑	N/A	↑(28%)	↑(28%)
T_4:T_3	≈	↑	N/A	N/A	↑	↑
TSH	≈	≈	N/A	N/A	↑(69%) ([c]↓)	↑(50%)
TSH_{TRH}	≈	N/A	N/A	N/A	↑(~60%)	
TBG	N/A	≈	N/A	N/A	↑(23%)	↑(19%)
$RAIU_{24h}$	N/A	N/A	↑(80%–100%)	↑(50%)	N/A	N/A
TER	N/A	N/A	N/A	↑(6%)	N/A	N/A
Reference no.	24,25,59	18	26,60	61,62,69	26,63	26,63

↑, increased; ↓, decreased; ≈, no change; free T_3, free triiodothyronine, free T_4, free thyroxine; N/A, not available; $RAIU_{24h}$, 24-hour thyroidal radioactive iodine uptake; TBG, thyroxine-binding globulin; Tg, thyroglobulin; TER, total energy requirements; TRH, thyrotropin-releasing hormone; TSH, thyrotropin; TSH_{TRH}, TSH response to a TRH stimulus; T_3, total T_3; T_4, total T_4.
[a]Thyroid hormone responses to altitude derived from hypobaric chamber studies and field conditions.
[b]Altitude adapted at 6,300 m.
[c]Acute change within 17 days.

16,37); hence, the term "polar T_3 syndrome" (15,35,37). Both the increased T_3 PCR and cold adaptation seem independent (14,29) of low serum free T_4 and TSH, and the TSH response (34) that subsequently occurs (39). The TSH change may be insufficient in some settings to return free T_4 to basal concentrations (16,39,41,44,48). Within the first 4 months of Antarctic residence, memory declines by approximately 13%, a decrement that returns to baseline with the administration of T_4 (44). A placebo group continues to display this same decrease in cognition over the next 7 months of Antarctic residence, and the cognitive decline was correlated with a decrease in serum free T_4 (44). Elevations in serum TSH, in both U.S. (49) and Chinese Antarctic expeditioners (47), are associated with increases in anxiety and derepression.

Military troops operating in circumpolar locations who are involved in physical exercise with marginal nutritional intake and partial sleep deprivation have declines in serum T_3 and T_4 regardless of their housing conditions (38,50). free T_3 and free T_4 are increased after 5 to 10 days (38) and decreased after 60 days (50). T_3 PCR and Vd are increased, and TSH is insufficient after 60 days to return free T_4 to predeployment concentrations (50). In contrast, soldiers stationed at high latitudes who are relatively sedentary and living in heated quarters show a seasonal change in both total and free T_3 and T_4 that extends the seasonal change in T_3 observed at temperate climates (23,41) (Table 11B.1, Fig. 11B.1). Multifactorial influences such as undernutrition (51), sleep deprivation, and exercise (33) possibly interact to influence the effects of photoperiod and temperature inherent to these high-latitude residents. An element of mild tissue-specific or thyroid receptor isoform-specific (45) hypothyroxinemia (16) may develop in the brain (44) along with a decrease in nuclear T_3 binding (52) during cold exposure. In addition, possibly similar hepatic changes may occur (39) and neither inhibit the T_3 kinetic changes of cold exposure (14) or the development of cold adaptation (15,29).

Possible Cellular Mechanisms

Human leukocyte nuclear T_3 receptor binding increases three- to fivefold when serum free T_4 concentrations are decreased during multiple cold exposures (53). Human cytosolic T_3-binding proteins retain binding with cold (54). These observations support an interrelationship between cold exposure and the possible expansion of T_3 Vd (15,37,39). Muscle isoforms of calcium adenosine triphos-

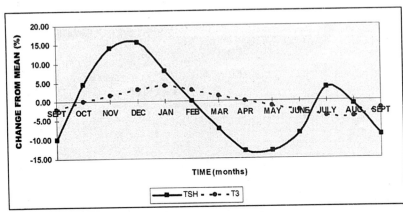

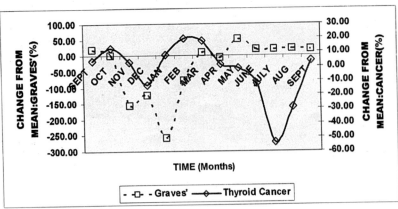

FIGURE 11B.1. Upper panel: The seasonal periodicity for the northern hemisphere of human serum thyrotropin (TSH) *(filled square)* and triiodothyronine (T_3) *(filled circle)* as cosinor functions repeated at 366 (*p*<0.00004) days for T_3 and 169 (*p*<0.007) days for TSH are shown. The TSH annual maximum (acrophase) precedes the T_3 acrophase by 30 days (*p*<0.0002). **Lower panel:** The season incidence of the presentation for thyroid cancer in Sweden and Norway for over 6,060 patients *(open diamond)* (*p*<0.001); and the seasonal presentation for Graves' disease in Arizona, USA *(open square)*, where 47% of the variability is due to seasonal temperature. (From Maes M, Mommen K, Hendrickx D, et al. Components of biological variation, including seasonality, in blood concentrations of TSH, TT$_3$, FT$_4$, PRL, cortisol and testosterone in healthy volunteers. *Clin Endocrinol (Oxf)* 1997; 46:587; Lambe M, Blomqvist P, Bellocco R. Seasonal variation in the diagnosis of cancer: a study based on national cancer registration in Sweden. *Br J Cancer* 2003;88: 1358–1360; Akslen LA, Sothern RB. Seasonal variation in the presentation and growth of thyroid cancer. *Br J Cancer* 1998;77:1174–1179; and Westphal SA. Seasonal variation in the diagnosis of Graves' disease. *Clin Endocrinol (Oxf)* 1994; 41:27, with permission.)

phatase (ATPase) (SERCA2a) changes with T_3 (55), the uncoupling of ATP synthesis in human muscle by T_3 (27), and the role of adaptive thermogenesis by thyroid hormone receptor isoforms (28,45) all support a molecular mechanism in humans for augmenting thermogenesis from muscle with exposure to cold. Uncoupling protein isoforms may be responsive to T_3, adding possible controls (28). Hormone delivery and tissue uptake in response to cold were studied by Margarity et al, who reported that local T_3 production and receptor binding decrease in the brain of cold exposed rats (52), while from other reports, peripheral tissues have increased T_3 availability and binding (28).

Heat

Physiologic and Thyroid Hormone Responses to Heat Exposure

Human physiologic adaptation to heat involves an expansion of the plasma compartment, increased rate of sweat loss, and an increase in aldosterone, which have been well described (2). In contrast to cold exposure, the human thyroid axis during exposure to heat has been studied much less. Thyroidal uptake of iodine-131 (^{131}I) is decreased in warm environments (56), although some of this decrement may be accounted for by an expanded extracellular volume. Heat-naive subjects exposed to 60 minutes of 35°C air have an elevation in rectal temperature, a decrease in serum T_3, and an increase in rT_3 without changes in T_4, suggesting a decrease in 5′-deiodinase type 1 activity (17). Saini et al reported that although the nocturnal surge of TSH was attenuated at 35°C, it was not statistically different, whereas 24-hour elevations in plasma renin activity (PRA) occurred during 6 days of heat exposure (2). Chronic residence at equatorial latitudes may affect the sleep-associated inhibition of nocturnal TSH secretion. In a warm climate study, 17% of the annual cases of thyrotoxicosis were identified in the northern hemisphere in the month of May (57), highlighting a possible interaction with circannual patterns of changing thyroid status and heat intolerance (Fig. 11B.1). A 72-kDa protein called heat shock protein (HSP) has been implicated in enhanced cytoprotective mechanisms following acclimation. The full expression of HSP seems to occur when a fall in T_3 and T_4 exceed 30% to 40% (58).

EFFECTS OF ALTITUDE AND HYPOXIA

Humans residing at or being transported to high altitudes of 2,315 (24), 3,000 (59), 3,500 (18), 3,810 (60), 4,300 (61,62), 5,400 (63), and 6,300 (63) meters are exposed to graded changes in low partial pressures of oxygen, hypobaric conditions, cold temperatures, low relative humidity, increased ultraviolet radiation, high winds, and often extreme physical exertion during altitude acclimation (4). Some studies have tried to isolate these factors by using hypobaric chamber experiments (18,59,60), whereas others have evaluated field conditions (62–64) or studied subjects who reside for extended periods at high altitudes (25,26).

Simulated Altitude in Environmental Chambers

Intermittent (4 to 8 hr/day) exposure to simulated altitude in thermoneutral hypobaric environmental chambers (18, 59,60,65) mostly supports the notion that elevations of up to 3,500 m increase serum T_4 and T_3 concentrations (18) and thyroidal ^{131}I uptake (60) without changes in thyroxine-binding globulin (TBG) (18). Additionally, in these chamber studies, T_4 administration and subsequent TSH suppression does not appear to negate increases in T_4 and T_3 observed below 4,500 m (Table 11B.2) (18).

Altitude Field Studies

In a 5-day study in which humans were transported rapidly to 2,315 m, the subjects had a mild hypoxic response of increased serum erythropoietin concentration, whereas serum free T_4, free T_3, and TSH remained unchanged. In contrast, individuals residing at 2,600 m (25) and 3,750 m (26) have increased free T_3 and free T_4 compared with sea-level residents, but without changes in TSH (25). Athletes training at 1,100 to 2,700 m have only increased free T_3 (66), suggesting the interaction of exercise and altitude exposure and perhaps temperature (19,33,67). Field studies conducted at higher elevations of 4,300 m (61,62) and 5,400 to 6,300 m (63) showed increases in serum T_4, free T_4, and T_3 without changes in free T_3 unless the subjects were chronically exposed to the high altitudes (26), findings that are in general agreement with chamber studies (18,60). A decreased peripheral T_4 conversion from undernutrition associated with exercise (51,68) and an increased BMR of 6% at 4,300 m (69) may modify the augmented free T_3 response (51,63,69, 70). This blunted response recovers with free T_3 increased over low-altitude controls if climbers remain at 6,300 m for an extended period without further exertion (51). Changes in TBG are found in some (63) but not all (18) reports. Thyroidal ^{131}I uptake (61) and T_4 degradation (62) are increased at 4,300 m. At 5,000 and 6,300 m, serum TSH and the results of a thyrotropin-releasing hormone (TRH) challenge test, respectively, were elevated over preascent responses (63), in contrast to observations at lower elevations (18,25). Changes

TABLE 11B.3. EFFECTS OF EXERCISE AND NUTRITION ON THYROID FUNCTION

	↑Energy Intake[a]	↓Energy Intake[b]	Exercise and Low Energy Intake	Exercise and Balanced Energy Intake[c]
T_3	↑(≈)	↓↓	↓	≈(↓),([d],↑)
free T_3	↑	↓↓	↓	≈(↓)
rT_3	↓(↓)	↑(↑)	↑	≈(↓)
T_4	≈ (≈)	≈ (≈/↓)	↑	≈(↓),([d],↑)
free T_4	N/A (≈)	↑(↑)	↑	≈(↓)
TSH	≈ (≈)	≈ (↓)	≈	≈(↓),([d],↑)
T_3 PAR	↑	↓↓	N/A	↑
T_3 PCR	↑	↓	N/A	↑
$T_3 V_d$	↑	N/A	N/A	↓
T_4 PAR	≈	≈/↓	N/A	≈
T_4 PCR	≈	≈/↓	N/A	N/A
rT_3 PCR	↑↑	↓↓	N/A	N/A
RAIU	N/A	N/A	N/A	↑
TV	N/A	N/A	↓	N/A
Weight	↑	↓	↓	≈
Reference no:	22	22,36,71, 83	68,85	19,33,67,80, 84,87

↑, increased; ↓, decreased; ≈, no change; free T_3 free triiodothyronine, free T_4, free thyroxine; N/A, not available; PAR, plasma appearance rate; PCR, plasma clearance rate; RAIU, thyroidal radioactive iodine uptake; TSH, thyrotropin; T_3, total T_3; T_4, total T_4.
[a]Extended overnutrition for 3 to 7 months.
[b]Extended fasting for 2.3 to 14 days or energy restriction for up to 2 years.
[c]Amenorrheic athletic women.
[d]Special combined conditions of walking 3 mph for 6 hr in 5°C air while wet (33).

in plasma volume and binding proteins cannot account for all the reported hormone elevation (18), and some researchers speculate that a decrease in extravascular binding may occur (64). The discordant responses of serum free T_4 and TSH at high altitudes support the concept that the hypothalamic–pituitary feedback of T_4 may be altered near 5,400 m (63,65) (Table 11B.3). Possibilities to explain these findings would include an inhibition of pituitary 5′-deiodinase type 2 activity, a decrease in nuclear binding and local production of central nervous system T_3, as happens with cold exposure in some species, or suppression of TSH by cortisol at lower altitudes (25,52,70,71).

EFFECTS OF MICROGRAVITY AND EXAGGERATED GRAVITY

Acceleration results from impaired cerebral blood flow when the inertial vector is in a head-to-foot direction [positive z-axis orientation of the gravitational vector (+Gz)] (72). A human centrifuge can isolate this stimulus from other aviation-related conditions such as hypoxia and microgravity (5,72). Serum TSH does not change with about 1 minute of 1- to 6-Gz stress (72). This degree of Gz stim-

ulus decreases plasma volume (72) and is accompanied by an increase in PRA and serum T_4 without changes in T_3 (5). Working at 4 to 11 atmospheres pressure during simulated saturation diving decreases T_4 by 10% and T_3 by 20%, while increasing plasma volume by only 5% (73).

Microgravity is encountered routinely on space shuttle flights (6), and a G stress of 1 to 3 has been documented on Apollo flights during reentry into the earth's atmosphere (74). Early flights lasting 8 to 13 days are associated with elevated serum T_4 values. These elevated values, obtained 2 hours after an ocean landing, do not appear to result from a decreased plasma volume, and they returned to preflight concentrations over 14 days (74). Later reports suggest serum TSH is elevated and T_4 and T_3 decreased during spaceflight (75,76). However, in a recent survey of all US spaceflights, McMonigal et al report that iodinated water sources on early missions were associated with elevations in TSH (77). During flights since 1998, where total iodine exposure has been reduced to 8 mg over 17 days, serum TSH values were no longer elevated (77). T_3 administration appears to allow the "bed rest" model to more closely approximate weightlessness (78), supporting a possible role of thyroid hormones during spaceflight, but more work is needed in this area.

EFFECTS OF EXERCISE

A negative energy balance, which may have genetic and geographic contributions (42,43), results if nutrient intake is not increased during physical training (69,79). Four-day fixed energy expenditures with small deficits in energy availability will lower serum free T_3 by approximately 9% and, with further negative energy balance, will increase free T_4 by 11% and rT_3 by 22% (68). Female competitive rowers who intensively train over a 20-week period while consuming adequate nutrition can show a decrease in TSH and free T_3 temporarily during the first 5 weeks of resistance training (80). During further endurance training, these values return to normal gradually; the fall in TSH strongly correlates with a fall in leptin (80). Strenuous training protocols in men are associated with declines in T_4, T_3, and TSH, as well as a declining trend in free T_4 (81,82). These situations are very similar to periods of energy restriction without exercise during which small decreases in energy intake will reduce serum T_3 (22) and more severe restriction will lower serum TSH (71). An exercise-mediated negative energy balance does not appear to change declines in free T_4 and free T_3 with acute cold exposure (82). With continued energy restriction for up to 2 years, T_3 remains reduced by 19% and body weight by 17% (82). However, by replacing calories either during short 3.5-hour bicycle exercise (79), extensive aerobic exercise (51), or following 2 years of restriction (83), serum T_3 can return to baseline quickly. Castellani et al report that a eucaloric 7-day exercise protocol with cold and wet exposure increases T_3 and T_4 during the cold exposure exercise period only (33). These values return to baseline after the exercise period (33), suggesting that the combination of temperature and exercise can interact to affect thyroid economy differently than either one individually.

During 4 to 6 weeks of aerobic training, T_3 PAR increases by approximately 10%, PCR increases by approximately 9% (19), thyroidal iodide uptake increases (84), and body weight does not change (19). With extensive exercise over 6 months, a fall in body weight is highly correlated with a decrease in thyroid volume measured by ultrasound (85). In contrast, the T_4 degradation rate decreases by approximately 9% during this type of aerobic training, and serum free T_4 tends to decline by 7% but does not reach a level of significance (19). Male athletes have an approximate 30% increase in T_3 PAR, PCR, and Vd, with no difference in serum T_3, T_4, or TSH when compared with sedentary controls (67) (Table 13.3).

Athletic men do not have dramatic changes in serum T_4, T_3, or TSH (67,85), whereas women, depending on their menstrual and gonadal status, have decreases in serum T_4, free T_4, T_3, and free T_3 when compared with sex-matched sedentary controls. TSH stimulation by TRH is not different in trained men (86), but may be blunted in athletic women with hypothalamic–pituitary ovarian dysfunction (87).

When the increased energy requirements with exercise are corrected, T_3 PAR, PCR, and radioiodine uptake (RAIU) increase and are similar, but not identical, to results of overfeeding studies (22). Furthermore, hypothalamic–pituitary–thyroid axis changes with extreme exercise may occur in amenorrheic women (87) and in men who have low testosterone production (51).

EFFECTS OF PHOTOPERIOD, SLEEP, AND CIRCADIAN RHYTHMS

The circadian pattern of TSH appears as a combination of the ultradian rhythm and factors such as photoperiod (3), serum T_4 and T_3 (71), sleep (20,21), and energy restriction (71, see Chapter 13). This circadian TSH oscillation is linked closely with body temperature (3) and is regulated in part by TRH (see Chapter 13). The TSH and body temperature rhythm can be reset by a pulse of light (5,000 lux) or sleep deprivation (3), and natural sleep can suppress the circadian TSH peak (20). By the second day of a shift-work change, the circadian pattern of TSH can be reset (88). The typical nocturnal surge in TSH rises 70% (3) (see Chapter 13) over the 24-hour mean, whereas the ratio of T_3:T_4 has a nocturnal increase of only 8% (89). Furthermore, the changing T_3:T_4 ratio is eliminated by fasting and unaltered by T_4 suppression of TSH, suggesting a peripheral mechanism for this rhythm (89). Thyroid receptor TRβ1 undergoes a diurnal variation with a 25% increase in binding capacity when studied in rat hepatic tissue, possibly related to a nocturnal feeding pattern (90). Pharmacologic sleep facilitation has limited effectiveness after 24 hours in normalizing nocturnal elevations in serum TSH following an intentional phase shift (90). Acutely, both total and partial sleep deprivation will raise serum TSH, T_4, free T_4, and T_3, although the patterns are slightly different with the degree of deprivation (20,21). Chronically, a partial sleep debt of 4 hours per night for 6 nights decreases the 24-hour profile of TSH by 33% and increases salivary cortisol by 20% compared with sleep restoration (91).

EFFECTS OF CIRCANNUAL RHYTHMS

Mid-latitude residents who are exposed to changing patterns of light and temperature demonstrate physiologic and endocrine seasonal rhythms for thyroid cancer presentation (12,13), cerebral and myocardial infarction (7,8), blood pressure (7), serum cholesterol (7), calcium metabolism (9), glucocorticoid activity (92), female (7) and male (93) gonadal hormones, sperm number (94), and mood disorders (10).

Seasonal Rhythm of Thyrotropin in Hypothyroid and Euthyroid Subjects

The serum TSH response to TRH increases during the winter in hypothyroid patients taking a fixed dose of T_4 (7,95). In early studies, euthyroid subjects were not reported to have increased serum TSH or TRH-stimulated TSH, or altered 24-hour circadian TSH profiles (7), during the winter season (16). Also, when the intersubject variation was large, no seasonal difference in TSH was found (96). However, when 24-hour circadian patterns were studied in the same elderly euthyroid women, serum TSH had a clear circannual pattern, but this was not seen in men near the same age (97). With the improved TSH assay and better control of study populations to eliminate subclinical thyroid disease, this issue has been clarified with a study of 8,310 euthyroid subjects in Italy, stratified by age and sex (98). Men and women over 41 years of age had a serum TSH peak in December, which represents an increase of approximately 30% over the trough summer value (98). Using monthly samplings and a cosinor analysis, a serum TSH change of 29% was also described between a spring minimum and winter maximum in Belgium subjects with a mean age of 39 years (23). In this study, there was a circannual rhythm (peak or acrophase, December 11; $p<0.004$), as well as two underlying harmonic rhythms of 104 and 169 days for TSH (Fig. 11B.1). The December peak was confirmed by Hassi et al, who reported on approximately 28% elevation in serum TSH over the seasonal mesor for men 26 to 40 years old who live in Finland (48). The changes in TSH are linked to luminosity 7 days before the blood sample ($p<0.001$). The circadian and ultradian TSH rhythms may obscure a smaller amplitude seasonal rhythm unless attention is directed to intrasubject variability (23) and sampling time.

Seasonal Rhythm of Thyroxine and Triiodothyronine in Euthyroid and Hypothyroid Subjects

It is unknown whether these circannual patterns of TSH secretion are a primary response of the hypothalamic–pituitary axis to changing light and ambient temperature (7) or whether they reflect small declines in either the Vd or serum T_4 (7,95). Investigations of T_3 and T_4 report serum T_3 elevation (23,35), urinary T_3 elevation (7,48), or no change in serum T_3 during the autumn and winter months. Little change in T_4 and no clear or consistent circannual pattern of free T_4 was found with most mid-latitude winter studies (23,98). The reported 8.2% winter elevation for Belgian residents in total T_3 (acrophase, January 10) was preceded by an elevation of TSH by 30 days ($p<0.0001$) and inversely related to temperature but not luminosity (Fig. 11B.1) (23). Hassi et al have extended this observa-

tion in Finland by showing a small decline in serum free T_3 and increase in urinary T_3 in winter (February) by 32% over the annual mean (48). They correlated these seasonal increases to preceding declines in temperature but not luminosity (48). The PCR of T_3 increases within 14 days after repeated cold air exposure (14). Kinetic studies in euthyroid subjects at mid-latitudes (Bethesda, MD; USA) suggest that T_3 PCR increases by approximately 30% between spring–summer trough values and autumn–winter peaks (99) (Table 11B.2). This increase in T_3 PCR precedes and possibly initiates a small and nearly undetectable decline in free T_4 (14). Indigenous populations (42) and other residents (44) living at high latitudes have increased energy requirements. The BMR of these indigenous peoples are about 12% higher than expected, and these variations in BMR are positively correlated with serum free T_4 (1). Small changes in serum TSH have been linked to corresponding changes in BMR during clinical studies (28), which could support the broader environmental observation by Leonard et al (42).

Circannual Changes of Thyroid Size, Iodine Content, Thyroid Cancer Presentation, and Growth

The intrathyroidal iodine content studied in Belgian subjects using X-ray fluorescence had a peak in April and a trough in September (100). The approximate 40% increase in these subjects' thyroidal iodine during April was not thought to be from differences in dietary iodine between winter and summer (100). The seasonal TSH profile reported in Belgium and Finland shows a peak in December (23,48) (Fig. 11B.1). Thyroidal size measured by serial ultrasonography increases by approximately 23% from summer to winter without a change in serum T_4, T_3, or TSH in Denmark (101), however with a reduced serum thyroglobulin in winter, when gland size is greater (96). Thyroid cancer presents more frequently, with a larger size and higher indicators of proliferation in late autumn and winter compared with summer in Norway and Sweden (12,13) (Figure 11B.1). This difference of more than a 60% increase of winter suggests an environmental trigger such as TSH (13).

REFERENCES

1. Bittel J. The different types of general cold adaptation in man. *Int J Sports Med* 1992;13[suppl]:172.
2. Saini J, Brandenberger G, Libert JP, et al. Nocturnal pituitary hormone and renin profiles during chronic heat exposure. *J Appl Physiol* 1993;75:294.
3. Allan JS, Czeisler CA. Persistence of the circadian thyrotropin rhythm under constant conditions and after light-induced shifts of circadian phase. *J Clin Endocrinol Metab* 1994;79:508.
4. West JB. Human physiology at extreme altitudes on Mount Everest. *Science* 1984;223:784.

5. Vangelova KK, Zlatev RZ. Changes in some biochemical and physiological indexes after hypergravity. *Rev Environ Health* 1994;10:33.

6. Tipton CM, Greenleaf JE, Jackson CG. Neuroendocrine and immune system responses with space flight. *Med Sci Sports Exerc* 1996;28:988.

7. Reed HL. Circannual changes in thyroid hormone physiology: the role of cold environmental temperatures. *Arch Med Res* 1995;54[Suppl 2]:9.

8. Ornato JP, Peberdy MA, Chandra NC, et al. Seasonal pattern of acute myocardial infarction in the National Registry of Myocardial Infarction. *J Am Coll Cardiol* 1996;28:1684.

9. Storm D, Eslin R, Porter ES, et al. Calcium supplementation prevents seasonal bone loss and changes in biochemical markers of bone turnover in elderly New England women: a randomized placebo-controlled trial. *J Clin Endocrinol Metab* 1998;83:3817.

10. Wehr TA, Rosenthal NE. Seasonality and affective illness. *Am J Psychiatry* 1989;146:829.

11. Hirschfeld U, Moreno-Reyes R, Akseki E, et al. Progressive elevation of plasma thyrotropin during adaptation to simulated jet lag: effects of treatment with bright light or zolpidem. *J Clin Endocrinol Metab* 1996;81:3270.

12. Lambe M, Blomqvist P, Bellocco R. Seasonal variation in the diagnosis of cancer: a study based on national cancer registration in Sweden. *Br J Cancer* 2003;88:1358–1360.

13. Akslen LA, Sothern RB. Seasonal variation in the presentation and growth of thyroid cancer. *Br J Cancer* 1998;77:1174–1179.

14. Reed HL, D'Alesandro MM, Kowalski KR, et al. Multiple cold air exposures change oral triiodothyronine kinetics in normal men. *Am J Physiol* 1992;263:E85.

15. Savourey G, Caravel J, Barnavol B, et al. Thyroid hormone changes in a cold air environment after local cold acclimation. *J Appl Physiol* 1994;76:1963.

16. Do NV, LeMar H, Reed HL. Thyroid hormone responses to environmental cold exposure and seasonal change: a proposed model. *Trends Endocrinol Metab* 1996;3:7.

17. Epstein Y, Udassin R, Sack J. Serum 3,5,38-triiodothyronine and 3,38,58-triiodothyronine concentrations during acute heat load. *J Clin Endocrinol Metab* 1979;49:677

18. Sawhney RC, Malhotra AS. Thyroid function in sojourners and acclimatised low landers at high altitude in man. *Horm Metab Res* 1991;23:81.

19. Balsam A, Leppo LE. Effect of physical training on the metabolism of thyroid hormones in man. *J Appl Physiol* 1975;38:212.

20. Baumgartner A, Dietzel M, Saletu B, et al. Influence of partial sleep deprivation on the secretion of thyrotropin, thyroid hormones, growth hormone, prolactin, luteinizing hormone, follicular stimulating hormone, and estradiol in healthy women. *Psychiatry Res* 1993;48:153.

21. Parker DC, Rossman LG, Pekary AE, et al. Effect of 64-hour sleep deprivation on the circadian waveform of thyrotropin (TSH): further evidence of sleep-related inhibition of TSH release. *J Clin Endocrinol Metab* 1987;64:157.

22. Danforth E, AG Burger. The impact of nutrition on thyroid hormone physiology and action. *Annu Rev Nutr* 1989;9:201.

23. Maes M, Mommen K, Hendrickx D, et al. Components of biological variation, including seasonality, in blood concentrations of TSH, TT_3, FT_4, PRL, cortisol and testosterone in healthy volunteers. *Clin Endocrinol (Oxf)* 1997;46:587.

24. Gunga HC, Kirsch K, Rücker L, et al. Time course of erythropoietin, triiodothyronine, thyroxine, and thyroid stimulating hormone at 2,315 m. *J Appl Physiol* 1994;76:1068.

25. Ramirez G, Herrera R, Pineda D, et al. The effects of high altitude on hypothalamic-pituitary secretory dynamics in men. *Clin Endocrinol (Oxf)* 1995;43:11.

26. Basu M, Pal K, Malhotra AS, et al. Free and total thyroid hormones in humans at extreme altitude. *Int J Biometeorol* 1995;39:17.

27. Silva JE. The multiple contributions of thyroid hormone to heat production. *J Clin Invest* 2001;108;35–37.

28. Silva JE. The thermogenic effect of thyroid hormone and its clinical implications. *Ann Intern Med* 2003;139:205–213.

29. Hesslink RL, D'Alesandro MM, Armstrong DW, et al. Human cold air habituation is independent of thyroxine and thyrotropin. *J Appl Physiol* 1992;72:2134.

30. Leppäluoto J, Korhonen I, Hassi J. Habituation of thermal sensations, skin temperatures, and norepinephrine in men exposed to cold air. *J Appl Physiol* 2001;90:1211–1218.

31. Sawhney RC, Malhotra AS, Nair CS, et al. Thyroid function during a prolonged stay in Antarctica. *Eur J Appl Physiol* 1995;72:127.

32. Fregly MJ. Activity of the hypothalamic–pituitary–thyroid axis during exposure to cold. *Pharmacol Ther* 1989;41:85.

33. Castellani JW, Young AJ, Stulz DA, et al. Pituitary-adrenal and pituitary-thyroid hormone responses during exercise-cold exposure after 7 days exhaustive exercise. *Aviat Space Environ Med* 2002;73:544–550.

34. Solter M, Brkic K, Petek M, et al. Thyroid hormone economy in response to extreme cold exposure in healthy factory workers. *J Clin Endocrinol Metab* 1989;68:168.

35. Reed HL, Brice D, Shakir KM, et al. Decreased free fraction of thyroid hormones after prolonged Antarctic residence. *J Appl Physiol* 1990;69:1467.

36. LoPresti JS, Gray D, Nicoloff JT. Influence of fasting and refeeding on 3,3',5-triiodothyronine metabolism in man. *J Clin Endocrinol Metab* 1991;72:130.

37. Reed HL, Silverman ED, Shakir KM, et al. Changes in serum triiodothyronine (T_3) kinetics after prolonged antarctic residence: the polar T_3 syndrome. *J Clin Endocrinol Metab* 1990;70:965.

38. Hackney AC, Hodgdon JA. Thyroid hormone changes during military field operations: effects of cold exposure in the arctic. *Aviat Space Environ Med* 1992;63:606.

39. Harford RR, Reed HL, Morris MT, et al. Relationship between changes in serum thyrotropin and total and lipoprotein cholesterol with prolonged antarctic residence. *Metabolism* 1993;42:1159.

40. Reed HL, Ferreiro JA, Shakir KM, et al. Pituitary and peripheral hormone responses to T_3 administration during antarctic residence. *Am J Physiol* 1988;254:E733.

41. Levine M, Duffy L, Moore DC, et al. Acclimation of a nonindigenous sub-Arctic population: seasonal variation in thyroid function in interior Alaska. *Comp Biochem Physiol A Mol Integr Physiol* 1995;111:209.

42. Leonard W, Sorensen MV, Galloway VA, et al. Climatic influences on basal metabolic rates among circumpolar populations. *Am J Human Biol* 2002;1:609–620.

43. Leonard WR, Galloway VA, Ivakine E, et al. Nutrition, thyroid function and basal metabolism of the Evenki of central siberia. *Int J Circumpolar Health* 1999;58:281–295.

44. Reed HL, Reedy KR, Palinkas LA, et al. Impairment in cognitive and exercise performance during prolonged Antarctic residence: effect of thyroxine supplementation in the polar triiodothyronine syndrome. *J Clin Endocrinol Metab* 2001;86:110–116.

45. Ribeiro MO, Carvalho SD, Schultz JJ, et al. Thyroid hormone—sympathetic interaction and adaptive thermogenesis are thyroid hormone receptor isoform—specific. *J Clin Invest* 2001;108:97–105.

46. Xu C, Zhu G, Xuc Q, et al. The elevation in serum thyroglobulin during prolonged Antarctic residence: effect of thyroxine supplementation in the Polar T3 Syndrome. In: Program and abstracts book of the Endocrine Society 83rd Meeting; 2001; Denver, CO. *J Clin Endocrinol Metab* 2004;89:1529–1533.

47. Chengli X, Guangjin Z, Quanfu X, et al. Effect of the Antarctic environment on hormone levels and mood of the 16th Chinese expeditioners. *Int J Circumpolar Health* 2003;62:255–267.

48. Hassi J, Sikkliä K, Ruokonen A, et al. The pituitary-thyroid axis in healthy men living under subarctic climatological conditions. *J Endocrinology* 2001;169:195–203.

49. Palinkas LA, Reed HL, Reedy KR, et al. Circannual pattern of hypothalamic-pituitary-thyroid (HPT) function and mood during extended antarctic residence. *Psychoneuroendocrinology* 2001;26:421–431.

50. Kowalski K, Reed L, Lopez A, et al. Changes in energy intake and triiodothyronine (T$_3$) kinetics with extended arctic winter operations. *FASEB J* 1991;4:A393(abst).

51. Friedl KE, Moore RJ, Hoyt RW, et al. Endocrine markers of semistarvation in healthy lean men in a multistressor environment. *J Appl Physiol* 2000;88:1820–1830.

52. Margarity M, Valcana T. Effect of cold exposure on thyroid hormone metabolism and nuclear binding in rat brain. *Neurochem Res* 1999;24:423–426.

53. D'Alesandro MM, Malik M, Reed HL, et al. Changes in triiodothyronine (T$_3$) mononuclear leukocyte receptor kinetics after T$_3$ administration and multiple cold air exposures. *Receptor* 1994;4:259.

54. Fanjul AN, Farias RN. Novel cold-sensitive cytosolic 3,5,38-triiodo-L-thyronine-binding proteins in human red blood cell. *J Biol Chem* 1991;266:16145.

55. Simonides WS, Thelen MH, van der Linden CG, et al. Mechanism of thyroid-hormone regulated expression of SERCA genes in skeletal muscle: implications for thermogenesis. *Biosci Rep* 2001;21:139–154.

56. Lewitus Z, Hasenfrantz J, Toor M, et al. ^{131}I uptake studies under hot climatic conditions. *J Clin Endocrinol Metab* 1964; 24:1084.

57. Westphal SA. Seasonal variation in the diagnosis of Graves' disease. *Clin Endocrinol (Oxf)* 1994;41:27.

58. Horowitz M. From molecular and cellular to integrative heat defense during exposure to chronic heat. *Comp Biochem Physiol A Mol Integr Physiol* 2002;131:475–483.

59. Vaernes RJ, Owe JO, Myking O. Central nervous reactions to a 6.5-hour altitude exposure at 3048 meters. *Aviat Space Environ Med* 1984;55:921.

60. Rawal SB, Singh MV, Tyagi AK, et al. Thyroidal handling of radioiodine in sea level residents exposed to hypobaric hypoxia. *Eur J Nucl Med* 1993;20:16.

61. Moncola F, Guerra-García R, Subauste C, et al. Endocrine studies at high altitude. I. Thyroid function in sea level natives exposed for two weeks to altitude of 4300 meters. *J Clin Endocrinol Metab* 1966;26:1237.

62. Surks MI, Beckwitt HJ, Chidsey CA. Changes in plasma thyroxine concentration and metabolism, catecholamine excretion and basal oxygen consumption in man during acute exposure to high altitude. *J Clin Endocrinol Metab* 1967;27:789.

63. Mordes JP, Blume FD, Boyer S, et al. High-altitude pituitary–thyroid dysfunction on Mount Everest. *N Engl J Med* 1983; 308:1135.

64. Rastogi GK, Malhotra MS, Srivastava MC, et al. Study of the pituitary-thyroid functions at high altitude in man. *J Clin Endocrinol Metab* 1977;44:447.

65. Savourey G, Garcia N, Caravel JP, et al. Pre-adaptation, adaptation and de-adaptation to high altitude in humans: hormonal and biochemical changes at sea level. *Eur J Appl Physiol* 1998; 77:37.

66. Koistinen P, Martikkala V, Karpakka J, et al. The effects of moderate altitude on circulating thyroid hormones and thyrotropin in training athletes. *J Sports Med Phys Fitness* 1996;36:108.

67. Rone JK, Dons RF, Reed HL. The effect of endurance training on serum triiodothyronine kinetics in man: physical conditioning marked by enhanced thyroid hormone metabolism. *Clin Endocrinol (Oxf)* 1992;37:325.

68. Loucks AB, Heath EM. Induction of low-T$_3$ syndrome in exercising women occurs at a threshold of energy availability. *Am J Physiol* 1994;266:R817.

69. Mawson JT, Braun B, Rock PB, et al. Women at altitude: energy requirement at 4,300 m. *J Appl Physiol* 2000;88:272–281.

70. Hackney AC, Feith S, Pozos R, et al. Effects of high altitude and cold exposure on resting thyroid hormone concentrations. *Aviat Space Environ Med* 1995;66:325.

71. Samuels MH, McDaniel PA. Thyrotropin levels during hydrocortisone infusions that mimic fasting-induced cortisol elevations: a clinical research center study. *J Clin Endocrinol Metab* 1997;82:3700.

72. Mills FJ, Marks V. Human endocrine responses to acceleration stress. *Aviat Space Environ Med* 1982;53:537.

73. Mateev G, Djarova T, Ilkov A, et al. Hormonal and cardiorespiratory changes following simulated saturation dives to 4 and 11 ATA. *Undersea Biomedical Research* 1990;17:1–11.

74. Sheinfeld M, Leach CS, Johnson PC. Plasma thyroxine changes of the Apollo crewmen. *Aviat Space Environ Med* 1975; 46:47.

75. Strollo F. Adaptation of the human endocrine system to microgravity in the context of integrative physiology and ageing. *Pflügers Arch* 2000;441[suppl]:R85–R90.

76. Leach CS, Johnson PC, Driscoll TB. Prolonged weightlessness effect on postflight plasma thyroid hormones. *Aviat Space Environ Med* 1977;48:595–597.

77. McMonigal KA, Braverman LE, Dunn JT, et al. Thyroid function changes related to use of iodinated water in the U.S. space program. *Aviat Space Environ Med* 2000;71:1120–1125.

78. Lovejoy JC, Smith SR, Zachwieja JJ, et al. Low-dose T3 improves the bed rest model of simulated weightlessness in men and women. *Am J Physiol* 1999;277:E370.

79. O'Connell M, Robbins DC, Horton ES, et al. Changes in serum concentrations of 3,3',5-triiodothyronine and 3,5,3'-triiodothyronine during prolonged moderate exercise. *J Clin Endocrinol Metab* 1979;49:242.

80. Sinsch C, Lormes W, Petersen KG, et al. Training intensity influences leptin and thyroid hormones in highly trained rowers. *Int J Sports Med* 2002;23:422–447.

81. Pakarinen A, Häkkinen K, Alen M. Serum thyroid hormones, thyrotropin and thyroxine binding globulin in elite athletes during very intense strength training of one week. *J Sports Med Phys Fitness* 1991;31:142.

82. Tikuisis P, Ducharme B, Moroz D, et al. Physiological responses of exercised-fatigued individuals exposed to wet-cold conditions. *J Appl Physiol* 1999; 86:1319–1328.

83. Walford RL, Mock D, Verdery R, et al. Calorie restriction in Biosphere 2: alterations in physiologic, hematologic, hormonal, and biochemical parameters in humans restricted for a 2-year period. *J Gerontol A Biol Sci Med* 2002;57:B211–B224.

84. Rawal SB, Singh MV, Tyagi AK. Effect of yogi exercises in thyroid function in subjects resident at sea level upon exposure to high altitude. *Int J Biometeorol* 1994;38:44.

85. Wesche MFT, Wiersinga WM. Relation between lean body mass and thyroid volume in competition rowers before and

during intensive physical training. *Horm Metab Res* 2001;33: 423–427.

86. Smallridge RC, Whorton NE, Burman KD, et al. Effects of exercise and physical fitness on the pituitary–thyroid axis and on prolactin secretion in male runners. *Metabolism* 1985;34:949.

87. Loucks AB, Laughlin GA, Mortola JF, et al. Hypothalamic–pituitary–thyroidal function in eumenorrheic and amenorrheic athletes. *J Clin Endocrinol Metab* 1992;75:514.

88. Goichot B, Weibel L, Chapotot F, et al. Effect of the shift of sleep-wake cycle on three robust endocrine markers of the circadian clock. *Am J Physiol* 1998;E243–E248.

89. Nimalasuriya A, Spencer CA, Lin SC, et al. Studies on the diurnal pattern of serum 3,5,38-triiodothyronine. *J Clin Endocrinol Metab* 1986;62:153.

90. Zandieh BZ, Schiphorst MP, van Beeren HC, et al. TRβ1 protein is preferentially expressed in the pericentral zone of rat liver and exhibits marked diurnal variation. *Endocrinology* 2002;143:979–984.

91. Spiegel K, Leproult R, van Cauter E. Impact of sleep debt on metabolic and endocrine function. *Lancet* 1999;354:1435–1439.

92. Walker BR, Best R, Noon JP, et al. Seasonal variation in glucocorticoid activity in healthy men. *J Clin Endocrinol Metab* 1997;82:4015.

93. Svartberg J, Jorde R, Sundsfjord J, et al. Seasonal variation of testosterone and waist to hip ratio in men: the Trømso Study. *J Clin Endocrinol Metab* 2003;88:3099–3104.

94. Kraus A, Krause W. Seasonal variation inhuman seminal parameters. *Eur J Obstet* 2002;101:175–178.

95. Hamada N, Ohno M, Morii H, et al. Is it necessary to adjust the replacement dose of thyroid hormone to the season in patients with hypothyroidism? *Metabolism* 1984;33:215.

96. Feldt-Rasmussen U, Hegedüs L, Perrild H, et al. Relationship between serum thyroglobulin, thyroid volume and serum TSH in healthy non-goitrous subjects and the relationship to seasonal variations in iodine intake. *Thyroidology* 1989;3:115.

97. Nicolau GY, Lakatua D, Sackett-Lundeen L, et al. Circadian and circannual rhythms of hormonal variables in elderly men and women. *Chronobiol Int* 1984;1:301.

98. Simoni M, Velardo A, Montanini V, et al. Circannual rhythm of plasma thyrotropin in middle-aged and old euthyroid subjects. *Horm Res* 1990;33:184.

99. Reed HL, D'Alesandro MM, Kowalski KR, et al. Circannual cycling of triiodothyronine kinetics in normal subjects. In: *Program of the Endocrine Society 73rd Annual Meeting*. Washington, DC: Endocrine Society, 1991;1244.

100. Jonckheer M, Coomans D, Broeckaert I, et al. Seasonal variation of stable intrathyroidal iodine in nontoxic goiter disclosed by x-ray fluorescence. *J Endocrinol Invest* 1982;5:27.

101. Hegedüs L, Rasmussen N, Knudsen N. Seasonal variation in thyroid size in healthy males. *Horm Metab Res* 1987;19:391.

11C EFFECTS OF DRUGS AND OTHER SUBSTANCES ON THYROID HORMONE SYNTHESIS AND METABOLISM

CHRISTOPH A. MEIER
ALBERT C. BURGER

Various drugs and other substances are known to interfere with thyroid hormone homeostasis. Although the action of some compounds on thyroid hormone secretion and metabolism are considered to be adverse effects, the inhibitory effect of certain molecules (e.g., thionamides, perchlorate, and iodinated compounds) is exploited clinically for the treatment of thyrotoxicosis. Pharmacologic agents may influence thyroid hormone homeostasis at four different levels (Fig. 11C.1 and Table 11C.1). First, they may alter the synthesis and/or secretion of thyroid hormones. Second, they may change the serum concentrations of thyroid hormones by altering either the level of binding proteins or by competing for their hormone binding sites. Third, they may modify the cellular uptake and metabolism of thyroid hormones. Lastly, they may interfere with hormone action at the target tissue level. Although most drug-induced changes in thyroid hor-

mone homeostasis are transient, they may hinder the interpretation of thyroid function tests. However, with improvements in the quality of routine measurements of serum-free thyroid hormone and thyroid-stimulating hormone (thyrotropin; TSH) concentrations, the latter difficulties have decreased in importance.

SUBSTANCES INTERFERING WITH THYROID HORMONE SYNTHESIS

In the early part of the twentieth century, the prevalence of severe to moderate iodine deficiency in developed countries was still widespread. Goiter formation was therefore ubiquitous, yet its degree varied despite similar levels of iodine deficiency. This also has been observed more recently in

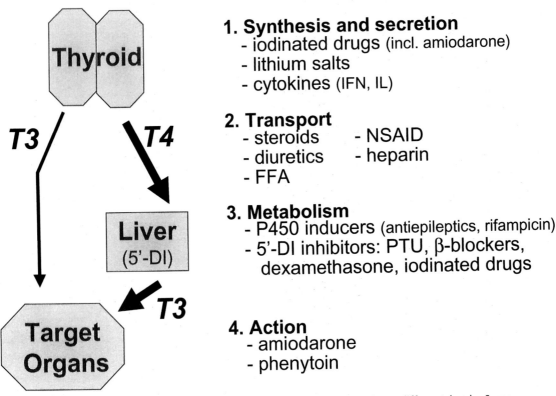

1. Synthesis and secretion
- iodinated drugs (incl. amiodarone)
- lithium salts
- cytokines (IFN, IL)

2. Transport
- steroids   - NSAID
- diuretics   - heparin
- FFA

3. Metabolism
- P450 inducers (antiepileptics, rifampicin)
- 5'-DI inhibitors: PTU, β-blockers, dexamethasone, iodinated drugs

4. Action
- amiodarone
- phenytoin

FIGURE 11C.1. Drugs may perturb thyroid hormone homeostasis at different levels. Some drugs, such as amiodarone and phenytoin, have several mechanisms of interaction. *FFA,* free fatty acids; *IFN,* interferon; *IL,* interleukin; *NSAID,* nonsteroidal anti-inflammatory drugs; *5'-DI,* 5'-monodeiodinase type 1.

developing countries. Low iodine intake is a good experimental condition for discovering additional factors leading to goiter formation, and it is probable that in the presence of high iodine intake many substances interfering with thyroid hormone synthesis would not have been discovered so easily. The development of large goiters in rabbits fed cabbage led to the discovery of the precursor of the presently used thionamides. Of the ionic antithyroid compounds, precursors of thiocyanate are present in cassava, which led to severe endemic goiter in Congo; however, they can also be found in maize, bamboo shoots, and sweet potatoes. Mechanistically, the thionamides interfere with the process of hormone synthesis, whereas the ionic compounds mainly but not exclusively inhibit the active transport of iodide.

THIONAMIDES (ANTITHYROID DRUGS)

Three compounds of this class are the most widely used antithyroid drugs. In the United States, propylthiouracil (PTU) and methimazole (MMI) are the most frequently used antithyroid drugs, whereas in Europe carbimazole is the main antithyroid drug (Table 11C.1). Carbimazole dif-

fers from MMI by a carboxy side chain, which is cleaved off during the first liver passage, converting carbimazole to MMI (See Chapter 45).

All three compounds are completely absorbed, and their metabolism is little affected by liver or kidney disease (Table 11C.1) (1). The thyroid avidly concentrates these compounds. This uptake is more pronounced in very active glands, as in iodine deficiency or hyperthyroidism. The thyroid also plays an important role in the degradation of these drugs (2,3). In rat ^{35}S-labeled metabolites of PTU can be detected up to 40 hours after injection. *In vitro* studies indicate that the intrathyroidal degradation of PTU and MMI is strongly influenced by the intrathyroidal iodide content (Fig. 11C.2). The serum half-life is <6 hours for MMI and <2 hours for PTU (Table 11C.2. Clinical studies have shown effects of MMI lasting as long as 24 to 36 hours, and a single dose of PTU was effective for more than 12 hours. This correlates well with the intrathyroidal presence of ^{35}S-labeled metabolites of these drugs. The intrathyroidal mechanism of action of the three drugs is similar. They inhibit hormone synthesis by thyroid peroxidase (TPO). This synthesis can be separated into two steps, whereby initially a tyrosine residue of thyroglobulin (Tg) is

TABLE 11C.1. COMPOUNDS INTERFERING WITH THYROID FUNCTION

	Organ	Site of Action	Mode of Action	Dose/Day	Remarks
PTU	Thyroid	Thyroid peroxidase	Competitive inhibition of iodination	50–600 mg	
	Liver, thyroid	Deiodinase type 1	Inhibition	600 mg	
Methimazole, carbimazole	Thyroid	Thyroid peroxidase	Inhibition	5–60 mg	
Thiocyanate	Thyroid	Na/I symporter	Steric inhibition		
Perchlorate	Thyroid	Na/I symporter	Steric inhibition	1 g	
Iodine	Thyroid	Na/I symporter, thyroid peroxidase and secretion	Steric inhibition of iodination and independent block of secretion		Transient effect (except after ^{131}I treatment) as discussed in this chapter
Radiographic contrast agents	Thyroid	Na/I symporter, thyroid peroxidase and secretion	Steric inhibition of iodination and independent block of secretion		
Amiodarone	Thyroid	Na/I symporter, thyroid peroxidase and secretion	Steric inhibition of iodination and independent block of secretion		Transient effect (except after ^{131}I treatment) as discussed in this chapter
	Liver, brain, thyroid	Deiodinase types 1 and 2	Inhibition		
Iopanoic acid	Thyroid	Na/I symporter, thyroid peroxidase and secretion	Steric inhibition of iodination and independent block of secretion	2 g first day, then 0.5 g/day	
	Liver, brain, thyroid	Deiodinase types 1 and 2	Inhibition		
Iopodate	Thyroid	Na/I symporter, thyroid peroxidase and secretion	Steric inhibition of iodination and independent block of secretion	2 g first day, then 0.5 g	
	Liver, brain, thyroid	Deiodinase types 1 and 2	Inhibition		
Goitrin	Thyroid	Thyroid peroxidase		Not used	
Flavenoids	Transthyretin and monodeiodination	Binding site for T_4	Displacement	Not used	
Cytokines (IFN-γ, IL-2, GM-CSF)	Immune system	Follicular cell	Stimulation or inhibition		
Lithium	Thyroid	Thyroid secretion	Inhibition	Serum levels used in psychiatric disease	
Salicylates	Transthyretin	Binding site of T_4	Displacement	> 2 g	
Furosemide	Transthyretin			0.5–1 g	
Heparin	TBG and transthyretin	Binding site of T_4	Displacement		
Free fatty acids	TBG and transthyretin	Binding site of T_4	Displacement	> 3.5 mM	
Cholestyramine	Small intestine	Absorption	Chelation		
Phenytoin	Small intestine and liver	Liver metabolism	Conjugation	200–300 mg/day	
Propranolol	Liver, peripheral β-blockade	Monodeiodinase type 1	Inhibition	> 240 mg/day	
Aluminum hydroxyde	Small intestine	Absorption	Chelation		
Ferrous sulfate	Small intestine	Absorption	Chelation		
Charcoal	Small intestine	Absorption	Chelation		
Sucralfate	Small intestine	Absorption	Chelation		
Phenobarbital	Liver	Hepatocyte	Conjugation	100 mg/day	
Carbamazepine	Liver	Hepatocyte	Conjugation	200–800 mg/day	
Rifampine	Liver	Hepatocyte	Conjugation	400–1200 mg/day	
Dexamthasone	? (liver)	Hepatocyte	Deiodination	2–12 mg/day	

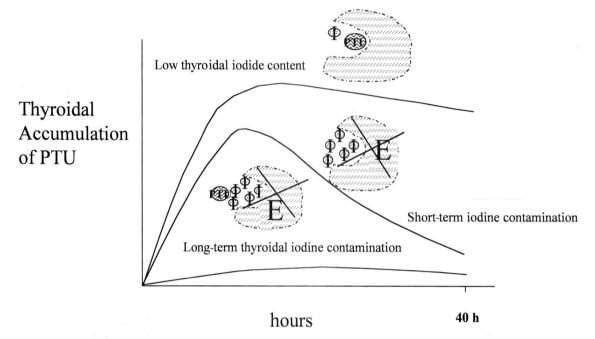

Thyroidal Accumulation of PTU and Interference in T4 Synthesis

FIGURE 11C.2. Schematic presentation of the intrathyroidal metabolism of propylthiouracil (PTU). In the presence of low intrathyroidal iodine concentrations, the PTU and/or its metabolites remain in the thyroid for a much longer time than in serum. With an iodide load, PTU is more rapidly metabolized, and during chronic iodine contamination, its uptake is also decreased.

iodinated followed by a coupling reaction, also under the control of TPO, resulting in the formation of an ether bond between two diiodotyrosines of Tg and the formation of thyroxine (T$_4$) and, to a minor extent, of triiodothyronine (T$_3$) (See section Thyroid Hormone Synthesis in Chapter 4). Both reactions are inhibited by thionamides. There is a marked competition between iodide and the thionamides for the active site of TPO. The mechanism of this competition is complex. There is competitive inhibition for the active site, and the residence time of PTU or MMI is inversely related to the intrathyroidal iodide concentration. *In vitro* the degradation of ^{35}S-labeled PTU was extremely slow in iodine deficiency and accelerated with increasing iodide concentrations (2,3). In situations of severe iodine

TABLE 11C.2. PHARMACOKINETICS OF ANTITHYROID DRUGS

	Methimazole (carbimazole)	PTU	Perchlorate
Absorption	Rapid and complete	Rapid and complete	Rapid and complete
Serum half-life	4–6 h	< 2 h	4–6 h
Excretion		Renal	
Intrathyroidal concentrations	High and prolonged	High and prolonged Decreased with iodine excess	High and short-lived
Duration of action	24 h (15 mg)	> 12 h (300 mg)	4–8 h
Transplacental passage	Minimal	Minimal	?
Passage into breast milk	Minimal	Minimal	?

excess, these are the two major mechanisms leading to the loss of efficiency of these drugs. It is also likely that iodine excess reduces the capacity of the thyroid to concentrate the thionamides.

Side Effects

All three thionamide drugs have similar side effects. At least 5% of patients initially complain of pruritus, and more rarely of an urticarial rash and drug fever. These symptoms often appear during early treatment and with high doses. Reducing the dose is in general helpful, but an occasional patient may have to stop treatment or to switch from one drug to the other. In an occasional patient the drugs, particularly PTU, can be cause a bitter taste, which does not disappear with time. Carbimazole and MMI may cause cholestatic jaundice. PTU occasionally increases serum aminotransferases and can cause fulminant hepatic failure has been reported (4).

The major serious complication of these drugs is agranulocytosis (< 500 neutrophils/mm^3). It is rare complication and probably occurs with all three drugs in < 0.25% of cases. Its onset is usually abrupt. Due to the rapid appearance of agranulocytosis, monitoring of the white blood cell count is not helpful. Patients must, however, seek medical care in case of a sore throat and fever and stop treatment until the white blood cell count is determined. Stopping antithyroid drug treatment is sufficient to permit complete recovery in almost all patients.

PTU-induced antineutrophil cytoplasmic antibody (ANCA)–related vasculitis and nephritis have also been reported, and it has been suggested that in patients treated with PTU the presence of ANCA should be monitored (5–7).

Special Indications and Differences between Propylthiouracil and Methimazole

PTU differs in two clinically relevant aspects from MMI and carbimazole. Probably due to its very short plasma half-life, its transplacental effects are minor, and it is also excreted less in maternal milk. Therefore, PTU is the drug of choice in pregnancy (8–10), although this remains somewhat controversial (see Chapter 80). In the postpartum period, MMI is also very safe, and its tolerance is even better documented than PTU (11). Only PTU has an inhibitory effect on deiodinase type 1 activity (12). In cases of severe iodine contamination, PTU probably has an advantage over MMI because of its extra thyroidal action. However, in humans this effect can only be achieved by large doses of PTU, and it results in only a 30% reduction of serum T$_3$ levels; in practice, therefore, the therapeutic advantage is small.

In vitro, MMI and PTU have an immunosuppressive effect. The relevance of this effect on remission rates is debated, but a difference has not been detected in the cure and relapse rates of patients with Graves' hyperthyroidism (13,14).

IONIC INHIBITORS

The molecular mechanism of iodide trapping by the thyroid has been elucidated through the cloning of the thyroid sodium iodide (Na$^+$/I$^-$) symporter (NIS) (15,16). Two anionic compounds, perchlorate and thiocyanate, are of some clinical relevance. These are bulky anions, which sterically resemble iodide. Their mode of action is to compete with iodide for the symporter, and perchlorate is a more potent inhibitor than thiocyanate. Perchlorate is also able to discharge intrathyroidal iodide rapidly and may have additional actions, such as actions inhibiting the transport of iodide from the cell into the lumen of the follicles. Perchlorate can accumulate in the follicular cell; as for iodide, its accumulation is dependent on TSH stimulation. The trapping of iodide is closely linked to countertransport of Na$^+$, and here, too, perchlorate could have an inhibitory action (17). The peak blood levels occur approximately 3 hours after oral intake, and its intrathyroidal concentration peaks at 4 to 6 hours. Its duration of action has not been studied in detail, but it is believed to be short, and is therefore preferably given two to four times daily.

The first reports of the clinical use of perchlorate date to the 1950s. Its use for treatment of thyrotoxicosis when irreversible aplastic bone marrow suppression was reported. Other side effects are rashes, drug fever, lymphadenopathy, and agranulocytosis, but these complications are likely to be less frequent than with thionamides. Rare cases of nephrotic syndrome also have been reported. The appearance of aplastic anemia limited the use of this drug to few specific clinical conditions. In case of congenital goiters due to genetic defects of thyroid hormone synthesis, the perchlorate discharge test is the diagnostic standard for revealing an abnormally large pool of intracellular iodide that has not been incorporated into thyroglobulin. This metabolic block can be mimicked by thionamides, which induce a functional block at the level of TPO (see Chapter 4). There are two variations of the perchlorate discharge test. The classical test uses only 1 g perchlorate, which is given 2 hours after administration of iodine-123 (^{123}I). Uptake of ^{123}I is measured just before administering perchlorate and 1 and 2 hours later. In normal thyroids the discharge should not exceed 15% of the accumulated thyroidal dose. A modification of this test has been introduced in order to reveal partial organification defects. In this case, 500 µg iodide administered at the same time as the ^{123}I. This leads to a transient increase in intracellular free iodide, and perchlorate can reveal small defects that are not seen with the classical test. This modification has been applied to demonstrate mild organification defects in autoimmune thyroiditis. Perchlorate also has been used for short-term inhibition of thyroidal radioactive iodide accumulation after administration of contrast media for angiographic studies and computed axial tomography. Perchlorate is also indicated for the treatment of severe cases of amiodarone- or iodine-induced thyrotoxicosis, which can be a life-threatening situation. The addition of 0.5 g perchlorate twice daily to high-dose PTU or MMI treatment has shortened the period of thyrotoxicosis (see Chapter 51). In contrast to perchlorate, thiocyanate is not used in clinical medicine.

ENVIRONMENTAL CONTAMINANTS WITH GOITROGENIC ACTION

Isothiocyanates and thiocyanates or their precursors are substances that can be found in various geographic regions in plants of the Cruciferae family. In Africa cassava contains large amounts of thiocyanate and is responsible for aggravating goiter formation in iodine-deficient areas (18–21). Thiocyanate is also found in high concentrations in tobacco and waste water effluents of coal conversion processes. The most potent goitrogenic substance, L-5-vinyl-2-thiooxazolidone, known as goitrin, is found in yellow turnips and Brassica seeds. This substance inhibits thyroid hormone synthesis, and its mechanism of action resembles that of the thionamides. The concentrations of these goitrogens as contaminants of food and drinking waters are nevertheless too low to induce goiter if iodine intake is sufficient.

In recent years there has been great interest in flavonoids. These compounds are present in most fruits and vegetables, and they are particularly abundant in subtropical and arid areas. They may aggravate goiter formation in areas with coexistent iodine deficiency. These substances have complex actions, and synthetic analogues have been tested (22–24). One of these substances, EMD 21388, decreased deiodinase type 1 activity, and it very efficiently displaced T_4 from transthyretin, resulting in an increase in free T_4 concentrations.

Other substances of potential goitrogenic action are phenols, ubiquitous contaminants of drinking and waste water (25). Their toxic effects are well documented experimentally at high concentrations. Such concentrations are unlikely to be obtained under present environmental conditions, but if present could impart fetal and neonatal development (26). One of them, resorcinol, was used as a dermatologic ointment and resulted in goiter formation. Polyvinylfluoride products contain phthalate esters that, in very high concentrations, are able to produce goiters in rats (27). It is unlikely that the environmental concentrations, cause goiters in rats (27). It is unlikely that the environmental concentrations of these substances are sufficient to increase goiter size in iodine-deficient areas in humans.

IODINE AND IODINATED DRUGS

Thyroid hormone secretion can be either increased or decreased in response to iodinated drugs, such as radiographic contrast media and amiodarone (Table 11C.1). Although the inhibitory effect of iodine on thyroidal hormone synthesis and secretion is usually spontaneously reversible after several days, TSH and free T_4 levels may transiently change for 1 to 2 weeks following an acute iodine load. Long-standing iodine-induced thyrotoxicosis and hypothyroidism occur less frequently and are described elsewhere in this chapter.

Amiodarone in particular induces thyrotoxicosis and hypothyroidism. Although amiodarone-induced thyrotoxicisosis is particularly prevalent (10%) in iodine-deficient regions and in patients with underlying thyroid disease, such as nodular autonomy or Graves' disease, can also occur in patients with no preexisting thyroid disease (28–31). There are two forms of amiodarone-induced thyrotoxicosis: (a) type I, which is similar to classical iodine-induced excess of hormone synthesis in patients with preexisting thyroid abnormalities (32), and (b) type II, which resembles subacute destructive thyroiditis with excess hormone release in patients with no history of prior thyroid disease, possibly due to a direct cytotoxic effect of amiodarone (33–37). The latter form is characterized by a low 24-hour thyroidal radioactive iodine uptake and high serum interleukin-6 (IL-6) levels, the latter reflecting a thyroid-destructive process (35). However, high IL-6 concentrations have not been found by others, and C-reactive protein levels have not been found to be helpful in the differential diagnosis between type I and type II (37a). Color flow Doppler sonography may be able to distinguish between these two entities (38). The therapeutic response of both forms is similar (39). Amiodarone-induced thyroid gland dysfunction, including thyrotoxicosis and hypothyroidism, is discussed in detail elsewhere in this chapter. The inhibitory effects of amiodarone on thyroid hormone deiodination and the peripheral actions of thyroid hormone also are discussed in detail later in the chapter.

CYTOKINES

Several cytokines alter thyroid hormone secretion and metabolism (40,41). Administration of interferons, interleukins, and granulocyte-macrophage colony-stimulating factor has been associated with a high frequency of transient thyrotoxicosis and hypothyroidism (40,42–48) (Table 11C.1). Although these cytokines may elicit either the appearance of thyroid antibodies or an increase in thyroid antibody titers, these changes are not always associated with thyroid dysfunction, which also may occur in the absence of antibodies, possibly through direct effects on the thyroid gland. In addition, the pattern of antibodies after cytokine therapy appears to be different from that in patients with endogenous autoimmune thyroid disease (49).

About 5% of patients receiving treatment with interferon-α for hepatitis C develop thyroid dysfunction, mostly autoimmune thyroiditis, and more rarely Graves' disease (50–52). Similarly, patients with multiple sclerosis and treated with interferon-β are at risk of developing thyroid dysfunction (53). However, the appearance of thyroid antibodies without thyroid dysfunction during interferon-α therapy is much more common, and it is not influenced by the concomitant administration of ribavirin (54). The occurrence of transient thyrotoxicosis followed by a hypothyroid phase, typical for silent thyroiditis, has also been reported (55–57). It is notable that patients with hepatitis C have an increased risk for thyroid autoimmunity even before undergoing antiviral treatment (51,58). Moreover, positive thyroid antibodies at baseline are a clear risk factor for developing hypothyroidism during treatment (51). While it is tempting to screen for thyroid antibodies in patients with hepatitis C, its impact on patient management is unclear. Given the low incidence of hypothyroidism in these patients and the fact that most patients develop subclinical hypothyroidism, this author prefers to measure serum TSH before and after completion (usually 1 year) of treatment for hepatitis C, and to perform an additional TSH measurement 6 months late only in patients with symptoms of thyroid dysfunction. Others suggest more frequent measurements of thyroid function (58a). Thyroid dysfunction usually appears after 3 months of treatment and may persist even after its discontinuation (59). It is important to recognize that patients with a history of thyroid dysfunction during interferon-α therapy remain susceptible to developing iodine-induced thyroid disease later (60).

Interferons, interleukin-1 (IL-1) ,and tumor necrosis factor-α are also known to inhibit iodine organification and hormone release, as well as to modulate thyroglobulin production and thyrocyte growth (61–64). In contrast to interferon-α and interleukin-2 (IL-2), interferon-γ increases the expression of the major histocompatibility complex class II molecules on the cell surface, which is thought to be an important event in the initiation of autoimmune diseases (65,66). IL-2 is used experimentally in the immunotherapy of cancer, which results in transient thyroid dysfunction in 15% to 40% of patients (44). Thyroid function sometimes normalizes during therapy, but always after stopping the cytokine treatment.

SUBSTANCES INHIBITING THYROID HORMONE SECRETION

Lithium, used in the treatment of bipolar depression, is associated with subclinical and overt hypothyroidism in up to 34% and 15% of patients, respectively, and can appear abruptly even after many years of treatment (67). Therefore, patients should be regularly examined for symptoms and signs of thyroid dysfunction, and thyroid function tests should be performed once or twice a year (68,69). The inhibitory effect of lithium occurs mainly at the level of hormone secretion, although effects on iodine trapping, release, and coupling have been described. In contrast to lithium-induced hypothyroidism, lithium-associated thyrotoxicosis is not common and occurs mainly after the long-term use of this drug (70). Although the mechanisms are unclear, the induction of antibodies and of ophthalmopathy has been reported, and histologic features of either autoimmune or destructive thyroiditis have been reported in some cases (71–73). Finally, transient euthyroid hyperthyroxinemia has been reported after the discontinuation of lithium treatment (74).

The inhibitory effect of lithium on the secretion of thyroid hormone and iodine may be of some therapeutic use in the treatment of severe thyrotoxicosis (e.g., after amiodarone), as well as for enhancement of the efficacy of radioactive iodine in Graves' hyperthyroidism (75,76) or differentiated thyroid cancer (76A).

SUBSTANCES ALTERING THYROID HORMONE TRANSPORT

Alterations in Concentrations of Thyroxine Hormone–Binding Globulin

The three major serum T_4- and T_3-binding proteins are thyroxine-binding globulin (TBG); transthyretin, formerly called thyroxine-binding prealbumin; and albumin. In addition, the high-density lipoproteins transport 3% to 6% of the circulating T_4 and T_3, and high-affinity binding sites have been demonstrated on one of the apoproteins, apoprotein A-I (77–79).

In humans, approximately 0.02% of the circulating T_4 and about 0.1% of circulating T_3 are free; hence, the serum total T_4 and T_3 concentrations are equivalent to the concentrations of bound T_4 and T_3 (80). The bound hormones represent a circulating reservoir and are usually not directly accessible to the tissues. Little evidence suggests that substantial amounts of protein-bound T_4 or T_3 can be taken up by cells (80,81). There may be some exceptions to this rule. For example, the choroid plexus synthesizes and secretes transthyretin into the cerebrospinal fluid. This represents a transport mechanism for T_4. In addition, glial cells have specific receptors for transthyretin, so there may be uptake of T_4 bound to protein into these cells (82–84). For most tissues, however, the circulating free T_4 and T_3 concentrations determine delivery of T_4 and T_3 and are considered responsible for the cellular effects of thyroid hormones.

Further details on the physiology and abnormalities of the thyroid hormone–binding proteins and the clinical understanding of these perturbations in thyroid hormone transport are discussed in detail in Chapters 6 and 13 and elsewhere in this chapter.

DRUGS THAT COMPETE WITH THYROXINE- AND TRIIODOTHYRONINE-BINDING SITES ON SERUM THYROID HORMONE–BINDING PROTEINS

Many drugs inhibit the binding of T_4 and T_3 to their binding sites on serum transport proteins *in vitro* (85,86) (Table 11C.1). These effects require high concentrations of such drugs, and the effects do not occur *in vivo*. The following paragraphs describe the effects of drugs that result in *in vivo* alteration of serum thyroid hormone levels. When such alterations occur, serum total T_4 and T_3 concentrations decline, but the free hormone concentrations do not.

Nonsteroidal Anti-inflammatory Drugs

Salicylates are important drugs in this category because of their widespread use in clinical medicine. Salicylates inhibit T_4 and T_3 binding to both TBG and transthyretin, resulting in a fall in serum T_4 and T_3 concentrations (87,88). Other nonsteroidal antiinflammatory drugs also displace T_4 from its binding sites, particularly fenclofenac, but this drug is no longer available in most countries (89).

Diuretics

Furosemide has been reported to inhibit T_4 binding (90). The effect does not occur with oral doses of < 100 mg, but is found consistently with very large intravenous doses of furosemide.

Flavons

These naturally occurring substances are structurally similar to thyroid hormones. A synthetic flavonoid (EMD 21388) has been designed to optimize its competitive effect for thyroid hormone binding, and in rats it has proven to be a potent inhibitor of T_4 binding to transthyretin. Its effects on T_3 are less marked. It does not compete for T_4 binding to TBG. The flavonoid-induced alterations of free hormone levels in rats affect TSH feedback regulation and tissue transfer and elimination of thyroid hormones. EMD is also an inhibitor of deiodination. Naturally occurring flavonoids may have similar but less dramatic effects on thyroid function (24,84).

HEPARIN AND FATTY ACIDS

Although the addition of heparin to serum does not increase serum free T_4 levels, it causes transient increases in free T_4 levels *in vivo*, particularly when equilibrium dialysis

was used for its measurement (91,92). These findings have been confirmed with enoxaparin (93). The authors proposed a 10-hour delay in measuring free T_4 after an intravenous injection of 2,000 U enoxaparin. These recommendations may depend on the type of heparin and free T_4 method, but caution in interpretation of free T_4 values in these circumstances remains necessary. It is thought that large doses of heparin alter the distribution of T_4 between plasma and its rapidly exchangeable tissue pools so as to increase the former and decrease the latter (94,95). These changes are of diagnostic, but not clinical, consequence because heparin-treated patients do not become thyrotoxic. The underlying pathogenesis of the heparin effect is thought to be lipoprotein lipase activation both *in vivo* and *in vitro*, with hydrolysis of triglycerides to free fatty acids (FFAs). *In vitro* activation of the lipoprotein lipase can be minimized by rapid and careful pre-analytical handling and by avoiding repeated freezing and thawing. To be effective, serum FFA levels have to exceed 2.5 to 3 mEq/L. *In vivo*, such concentrations occur rarely. They may be encountered during hemodialysis and intravenous hyperalimentation, particularly if serum albumin levels are low and if the patient is treated with heparin (92). It is claimed that some newer analogue methods for measuring serum free T_4 or T_3 are unaffected by heparin–lipase–FFA effects.

ALTERATIONS OF THYROID HORMONE METABOLISM AND ACTION

Drugs can alter thyroid hormone availability not only by means of changes in the free serum hormone concentration, but also by modulating the cellular uptake, metabolism, and nuclear actions of the hormone.

THYROID HORMONE UPTAKE

The inhibition of thyroid hormone uptake by drugs may occur at the intestinal level, thereby leading to decreased serum hormone levels, or in target tissues, potentially resulting in cellular hypothyroidism, despite normal serum levels. However, the physiologic relevance of cellular thyroid hormone transport systems is still controversial (96–98).

Absorption

Several drugs are known to reduce the absorption of T_4 from the gut, such as cholestyramine, calcium carbonate, aluminum hydroxide, ferrous sulfate, activated charcoal, and sucralfate (99–102). Although normally 80% of a dose of T_4 is absorbed within 6 hours, this value decreases when these substances are taken simultaneously, resulting in lower serum T_4 and higher TSH levels. This problem can be circumvented by separating the intake of both drugs by several hours. The malabsorption of T_4 in the presence of these substances may be due to either the formation of an insoluble complex or an inhibition of hormone transport by intestinal cells.

Cellular Uptake

Amiodarone is the best known drug that inhibits cellular thyroid hormone uptake. A selective decrease in hepatic T_4 transport was demonstrated in hepatocytes and perfused rat liver, and impaired T_3 uptake was observed in an anterior pituitary cell line (103,104). In addition, amiodarone inhibits T_4 and T_3 deiodination and binding of T_3 to nuclear receptors, as described later in the chapter. Benzodiazepines also inhibit cellular T_3 uptake, possibly due to their conformational similarity with this hormone (105). Hepatic and muscle T_3 uptake seem to a calcium-dependent process, as inferred from the inhibition of T_3 uptake by various calcium channel blockers, such as nifedipine, verapamil, and diltiazem (106). Finally, furosemide and some nonsteroidal anti-inflammatory drugs compete for cytosolic T_3-binding sites in cultured cells (107). However, whether the *in vitro* observations for these various drugs are quantitatively relevant *in vivo* remains to be demonstrated.

DRUGS THAT ALTER THE INTRACELLULAR METABOLISM OF IODOTHYRONINES

Drugs That Induce the Hepatic p450 Complex (Mixed-Function Oxygenases)

Many lipophilic drugs are made water soluble by oxidation and conjugation in the liver before their elimination from the body by enzymes that are part of the type II metabolic processes (108). The type I metabolic processes include enzymes responsible for the oxidative and reducing reactions and belong to the cytochrome p450 complex, which consists of more than 100 isoenzymes. Some of these enzymes (CYP3A) can be induced by the antiepileptic drug phenytoin, phenobarbital, and carbamazepine, as well as the antituberculous drug rifampicin (Table 11C.1).

Antiepileptic Drugs

It has been known for 30 years that the administration of phenytoin causes alterations in serum thyroid hormone levels (109–112). Serum thyroid hormone levels can decrease markedly during phenytoin (and rifampicin therapy); the effects on serum TSH are, however, minor. Similar but less important effects have been reported for carbamazepine. It may potentiate the effects of the other antiepileptic drugs when used in combination with them (113).

Phenytoin is of particular interest because its effects are not limited to the induction of hepatic drug metabolism. Early *in vitro* studies indicated that high levels of phenytoin displaced T_4 and T_3 from TBG. However, the *in vivo*

serum concentrations do not reach such levels, and the free fractions of T_4 and T_3 that would result from a displacing drug do not occur in such patients. Nevertheless, the serum total and free T_4 levels are clearly decreased in euthyroid phenytoin-treated patients, whereas in most reports the serum total and free T_3 concentrations are unchanged or even slightly increased. The decreased serum T_4 levels are not typical of the other drugs inducing the mixed function oxygenases, which do not change serum levels of total and free T_4 and suggest more complex functions of phenytoin. For instance, it has been reported that phenytoin decreases serum TSH levels and inhibits the TSH response to thyrotropin releasing hormone (TRH) (114,115). These findings and others have led to the hypothesis that phenytoin may interfere with cellular uptake of T_3 and may have agonistic nuclear effects (116,117). Since serum TSH levels in euthyroid subjects are in the normal range, hypothyroidism is almost certainly not present. However, serum TSH levels increase in T_4 treated hypothyroid patients. Because the metabolic clearance rate and the hepatic metabolism of T_4 increases in patients treated with phenytoin, it is likely that in normal subjects thyroidal secretion increases in order to compensate for the hepatic losses, whereas hypothyroid patients need increased doses of T_4 (118).

Rifampicin

Although the effects of phenytoin and the other antiepileptic drugs have received the most attention, the antituberculosis drug rifampicin is one of the most potent inducers of hepatic mixed-function oxygenases. Significant decreases in serum total and free T_4 and reverse T_3 (rT_3) concentrations have been described in some but not other studies. Rifampicin acts like phenytoin on intracellular thyroid hormone metabolism, but it does not inhibit T_4 and T_3 binding to serum-binding proteins (119–121). T_4 kinetic data show that rifampicin increases the clearance rate of T_4; in normal subjects, T_4 secretion increases to compensate for the increase in T_4 clearance, T_4 to T_3 conversion does not change, and T_3 production is normal. That T_4 secretion increases is also suggested by the increase in thyroid volume that occurs during rifampicin treatment (122). Therefore, in hypothyroid T_4-treated patients, serum TSH levels must be monitored. One T_4-treated hypothyroid patient developed marked hypothyroidism during rifampicin treatment (123).

Neither phenytoin nor rifampicin has much effect on T_3 metabolism. This was shown more clearly in studies in rats given the most potent inducer of mixed function oxygenases, nafenopin (124). In rats, this drug greatly increases the metabolic clearance rate of T_4 and its hepatic disposal without changing the T_3 kinetics. This difference is best explained by the fact that glucuronidation of T_4 is increased, whereas T_3 is preferentially a substrate for sulfation, which is not increased by the induction of mixed-function oxygenases.

In summary, drugs that increase the activity of the hepatic p450 enzymatic system result in a decrease in serum total T_4 concentrations. This is due primarily to an acceleration of the hepatic metabolism of T_4 and results in a decrease in its plasma half-life or, more specifically, in an increase in its metabolic clearance rate. In euthyroid subjects there is also a slight increase in T_4 production, with the consequence that serum T_4 levels do not change. Basal serum TSH concentrations increase slightly but not significantly. These findings suggest that the function of the pituitary–thyroid axis can compensate in euthyroid patients, and this is in accordance with the clinical impression of euthyroidism in these subjects. However, in T_4-treated patients, with hypothyroidism, the T_4 dose often needs to be raised.

Drugs That Inhibit the Deiodination of Thyroxine

Deiodination involves the sequential removal of iodine atoms from T_4 and is the most important metabolic pathway of this iodothyronine (125, 126). This topic is discussed in detail in Chapter 7. Deiodination of the outer phenolic ring (5'-deiodination) of iodothyronines is different than that of the inner ring (5-deiodination). Outer-ring deiodination is responsible not only for the conversion of T_4 to T_3, but also for the degradation of rT_3. At least two enzymes are known to catalyze this reaction: one present primarily in liver, kidney, heart, muscle, and thyroid, called 5'-deiodinase type 1; the other predominating in brain cortex, cerebellum, anterior pituitary, and placenta, called 5'-deiodinase type 2. 5'-deiodinase type 1 is reduced in hypothyroidism and catabolic states. It can be inhibited by several drugs (see later in the chapter), including PTU.

5'-deiodinase type 2 has a different tissue distribution, and its regulation is opposite to 5'-deiodinase type 1. For example, its activity is reduced in thyrotoxicosis and increased in hypothyroidism. It is not affected by catabolic states, and so far the only known specific inhibitors are T_4 and rT. It can be inhibited by iodinated contrast agents, but these agents are not specific inhibitors because they do not directly block the catalytic site. PTU does not inhibit type 2 deiodinase, and this property is used for determining its specific activity (127).

Only one deiodinating enzyme has been demonstrated for the inner ring, 5-deiodinase type 3. It is found in the brain, skin, subcutaneous tissue, and placenta. All three enzymes are selenoproteins (128) (See Chapter 7).

Drugs inhibiting deiodination can be divided into two groups: those that are iodinated and those that are not. The iodinated drugs are more potent *in vivo* and inhibit 5'-deiodinase type 1 and 2 as well as 5'-deiodinase type 3 activities; the noniodinated drugs inhibit mainly 5'-deiodinase type 1 activity. Both types of compounds exert their effects predominantly on the process of 5'-deiodination, and this results in a decrease in serum T_3 concentrations. Reverse T_3 concentrations are increased to a variable extent by the action of these agents. The increase in its serum concentration can mainly be explained by inhibition of its metabolism, which depends on 5'-deiodinase type 1. Dexamethasone is an exception; it also increases production of rT_3 (129).

Noniodinated Drugs

The most important drugs in the noniodinated class are PTU, the synthetic glucocorticoid dexamethasone, and the β-receptor antagonist propranolol.

Propylthiouracil
PTU was the first drug shown to inhibit the conversion of T_4 to T_3 in peripheral tissues, but it is not the most potent (130). When it is administered in doses of 450 to 600 mg/day to T_4-treated hypothyroid patients, serum T_3 concentrations decrease by 25% to 30% within 48 hours and remain at this level as long as PTU is given (131). Basal serum TSH concentrations increase slightly, and the serum TSH response to TRH is augmented. In untreated euthyroid subjects, serum rT_3 concentrations increase initially but tend to decline slowly if the drug is continued (132,133). All values return to pretreatment levels when the drug is discontinued. Therapeutically, this effect is exploited in the treatment of iodine-induced thyrotoxicosis, where antithyroid drugs are less potent inhibitors of thyroid hormone synthesis and this additional action is most welcome. A PTU analogue, anilino-thiouracil, has been demonstrated to inhibit 5'-deiodinase type 1 but does not affect thyroid hormonogenesis in rats (134).

Dexamethasone
Dexamethasone has multiple effects on thyroid physiology in humans. Large doses given acutely or moderate doses administered for a prolonged period suppress the secretion of TSH by the anterior pituitary in normal and hypothyroid individuals and therefore decrease thyroid hormone secretion (135,136). In addition, large doses of dexamethasone decrease serum T_3 concentrations in normal subjects and in hypothyroid patients receiving T_4 therapy (117,137). This latter effect is predominantly due to an inhibitory action on 5'-deiodination (138,139). Kinetic data on the *in vivo* effects of dexamethasone, however, are not identical to those of PTU; dexamethasone increases serum rT_3 levels by increasing rT_3 production, whereas PTU increases rT_3 by decreasing its plasma clearance (129). In patients with thyrotoxicosis caused by Graves' disease, large doses of dexamethasone decrease serum concentrations of T_4 (140). This is due to a decrease in T_4

secretion (whether this is by a direct thyroidal effect or by decreasing thyroid-stimulating immunoglobulin production is not known). Other glucocorticoids in comparable doses have similar effects, but none have been studied as extensively as dexamethasone. Clinically, the effect of dexamethasone on thyroid hormone metabolism is helpful in rapidly decreasing serum T_3 concentrations in preparation of thyrotoxic patients for surgery, and its antiinflammatory effect is useful in a subset of patients with amiodarone-induced thyrotoxicosis (see earlier in this chapter).

These above findings are supported by the observations that treatment of rats for 5 days with dexamethasone reduces the rate of T_4 to T_3 conversion and the rate of rT_3 degradation *in vitro* in liver homogenates. In contrast to other potent inhibitors of the deiodination reaction, however, the addition of dexamethasone to rat liver homogenates *in vitro* has no effect on the rate of T_4 to T_3 conversion (86).

Propranolol

Beta-receptor antagonists are useful drugs in the symptomatic treatment of thyrotoxicosis (see Chapter 45). These drugs reduce pulse rate, tremor, anxiety, and hyperreflexia, and they are particularly useful in the treatment of thyrotoxic crisis (141–147) (see Chapter 43). The mechanisms by which decreased sympathetic nervous system activity alleviates these symptoms and signs are far from clear. Studies in thyrotoxic patients have shown that propranolol has no demonstrable effect on thyroid iodine release or T_4 turnover (148). When given in moderate to high doses to euthyroid and/or thyrotoxic subjects, it induces a modest reduction in serum free T_3 concentrations and a small increase in rT_3 concentrations. This action of propranolol on T_4 metabolism *in vivo* is not shared by the β-receptor antagonists metoprolol or atenolol, or the mixed β- and α-receptor antagonist labetalol (145,149). These drugs are nevertheless effective in the relief of the symptomatology of thyrotoxicosis.

The effects of propranolol on the extrathyroidal metabolism of T_4, T_3, and rT_3 have been evaluated by noncompartmental kinetic methods. The results indicate that the reduction in serum T_3 is mainly due to a reduction in its generation from T_4. The increase in serum rT_3 is largely due to reduction in its metabolic clearance rate, and its generation rate from T_4 is unchanged. The disposal rate of T_4 is reduced, suggesting that its bioavailability to tissues is reduced by the drug.

In vitro studies have shown that the racemic form of propranolol and other β-adrenergic antagonists (149) inhibit T_4 conversion to T_3 and rT_3 degradation in rat liver homogenates, isolated intact liver cells, and renal tubules. The latter results suggested that the major site of action of propranolol might be at the cell membrane (150,151). Generation of T_3 from T_4 in isolated rat renal tubules is in-

hibited not only by DL-propranolol but also by the D- and L-isomers of propranolol. Because D-propranolol is devoid of β-receptor antagonist properties, DL-propranolol is thought to affect T_4 5′-deiodination by its ability to stabilize cell membranes. This latter action is akin to that exerted by quinidine; indeed, quinidine also inhibits T_4 3′-deiodination in this system. Alternatively, propranolol could block T_4 transport into cells (96,97), although the effect of propranolol did not appear to be due to an alteration in the cellular uptake of T_4 by the renal tubules.

In summary, propranolol, as well as other β-receptor antagonists, alleviates the peripheral manifestations of thyrotoxicosis. This clinical benefit far exceeds the modest reduction in serum T_3 concentrations caused by the drug, and other related drugs have the same clinical benefits without altering serum T_3 concentrations. These results indicate that the clinical benefits of β-receptor antagonists are not related to their ability to inhibit T_4 to T_3 conversion.

Iodinated Drugs

Drugs considered in this section include the iodinated radiographic contrast agents and the antiarrhythmic drug amiodarone.

All iodinated agents affect thyroid function by their large iodine content. Some of these compounds, all of which are lipid soluble, are used for cholecystography, namely iopanoic acid, sodium ipodate, and tyropanoate, also inhibit T_4 deiodination (152,153). When given to normal subjects, they significantly increase serum free T_4 and rT_3 and decrease serum free T_3 concentrations (152). However, the extent of the changes varies from one compound to another. In contrast to these lipid-soluble substances, water-soluble contrast agents such as those used for arteriography and venography do not affect deiodination. The lipid-soluble agents can be useful for the treatment of severe thyrotoxicosis (154).

In people with normal thyroid function, most changes of serum thyroid hormone levels are due to alterations in their metabolism. This can be illustrated in normal subjects receiving 0.2 mg T_4 daily in whom serum TSH levels were suppressed. Iopanoic acid caused significant increases in serum total and free T_4 levels and decreases in serum T_3 and rT_3 concentrations similar to those in normal subjects not receiving T_4 (Fig. 11C.3). The increase in serum T_4 concentrations is mainly a reflection of a decreased disposal rate. In addition, kinetic studies have shown that these drugs can acutely discharge T_4 from hepatic (and possibly renal) storage sites (155). For example, in normal subjects who received an intravenous injection of ^{125}I-T_4, tyropanoate and, to a lesser extent, ipodate led to a 50% to 60% reduction in hepatic radioactivity within 4 hours. This reduction was accompanied by a 57% to 70% increase in serum radioactiv-

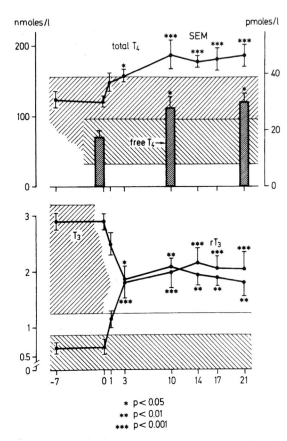

FIGURE 11C.3. Effect of iopanoic acid on serum thyroid hormone levels in four normal subjects maintained on 0.2 mg thyroxine (T_4) per day. Iopanoic acid was given on Days 0, 7, and 14. Serum total and free T_4 and reverse triiodothyronine (T_3) concentrations rapidly increased above the normal range **(upper and lower panels)**, and serum T_3 concentrations decreased by ~40%. The normal range for each hormone is indicated by the *hatched bars*. (From Burgi H, Wimpfheimer C, Burger A, et al. Changes of circulating thyroxine, triiodothyronine, and reverse triiodothyronine after radiographic contrast agents. *J Clin Endocrinol Metab* 1976;43:1203, with permission.)

ity, as well as an increase in serum T_4 concentrations. The plasma clearance rate of T_4 decreased. In euthyroid subjects, changes in thyroid secretion also occur during the readaptation of thyroid homeostasis. There is an initial increase in serum TSH concentration, likely due to a dual effect of these inhibitors, which inhibit 5'-deiodinase type 2 as well as 5'-deiodinase type 1. Serum TSH levels subsequently return to normal.

In addition to the radiographic contrast agents, the antiarrhythmic drug amiodarone is known to interfere with thyroid function. Besides causing thyroid dysfunction, as discussed earlier in this chapter, it induces in every euthyroid subject alterations in thyroid hormone metabolism, due to the ability of the drug to inhibit T_4 deiodination (156–158). The changes in serum T_4, T_3, rT_3, and TSH concentrations are similar to those caused by the iodinated

radiographic contrast agents, and the magnitude of these alterations is dose dependent. In normal subjects given 400 mg amiodarone (150 mg organic iodine) for 3 weeks, serum total and free T_4 concentrations increased, again due to a decrease in the T_4 metabolic clearance rate. The results of kinetic studies suggest decreased transfer of T_4 from the plasma pool to the rapidly exchangeable tissue pools, such as the liver (159). The T_3 plasma clearance rate was only slightly decreased (160). Therefore, the decreased serum T_3 levels mainly reflect the decreased conversion of T_4 to T_3. This observation is substantiated by the observed changes in thyroid function tests after the acute intravenous administration of amiodarone. Serum TSH levels increased from the first day of therapy, followed by a decrease in T_3 level after the second day, whereas free and total T_4 levels did not increase until the fourth day of treatment (161).

After the first 2 weeks, the thyroid escapes from this inhibition, and under the drive of increased TSH secretion, T_4 production tends to increase. This has been demonstrated to occur for iopanoic acid, which induces effects on thyroid hormone metabolism similar to those of amiodarone. However, T_4 secretion does not increase sufficiently to restore serum T_3 to pretreatment levels. This suggests that inhibition of intrapituitary conversion is less than in the periphery. These effects have attracted much attention, and it has been postulated that some of the antiarrhythmic effects of this drug might be due to a hypothyroid state of the heart. Experiments in rats support this hypothesis, even though in these studies only tissue T_3 content and not the actual saturation of the T_3 receptor with T_3 was measured (162). In addition, amiodarone and/or its main metabolite desethylamiodarone is a weak antagonist of thyroid hormone action (163,164). Despite these experimental studies, most clinical studies do not support the hypothesis that the antiarrhythmic effect of amiodarone is due its action on thyroid hormone metabolism or action (165,166).

In clinical practice, amiodarone is used for long-term treatment. After several weeks of treatment with a moderate dose (200 or 100 mg/day), serum thyroid hormone levels tend to remain within the normal limits, even though serum free T_4 levels are higher and serum T_3, free T_3, and TSH levels are lower than before treatment. In some patients, however, particularly those treated with higher doses of amiodarone, serum free T_4 levels can be as high as in moderate thyrotoxicosis (158). When T_4 kinetic parameters are compared in chronically treated subjects with normal TSH levels with those of thyrotoxic Graves' disease patients, striking differences are found. Thus, the T_4 production rate of the amiodarone-treated group is significantly lower than that of the thyrotoxic group, and the disappearance of injected ^{125}I-T_4 is significantly delayed (Fig. 11C.4). These findings demonstrate that, despite increased serum total and free T_4 concentrations, T_4 kinetics in amiodarone-treated patients more closely approximate

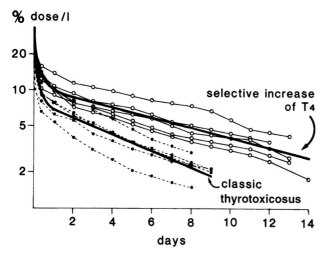

FIGURE 11C.4. The disappearance of serum ¹²⁵I-thyroxine (T₄) in four patients with classic thyrotoxicosis *(open circle)* and five patients with selective increases in serum total and free T₄ concentrations *(dots)* due to a reduced clearance rate of T₄ during amiodarone treatment without evidence of hyperthyrodism. (From Lambert MJ, Burger AG, Galeazzi RL, et al. Are selective increases in serum thyroxine (T4) due to iodinated inhibitors of T₄ monodeiodination indicative of hyperthyroidism? *J Clin Endocrinol Metab* 1982;55:1058, with permission.)

those of a euthyroid subject. In addition, these patients have normal serum T₃ and/or free T₃ levels. These patients often have no obvious clinical stigmata of thyrotoxicosis, and the peripheral tissues may not be frankly thyrotoxic. Nevertheless, the suppressed serum TSH suggests the escape of thyroidal secretion from the normal feedback control mechanism.

Clinical Use of Iodinated Inhibitors of Deiodination

These agents have been used successfully in the treatment of severe forms of thyrotoxicosis caused by Graves' disease or toxic multinodular goiter (167–169). Most studies have used the more rapidly cleared ipodate, which decreases serum T₃ levels to within the normal range in a short period of time (2–6 days) (170,171). Serum T₄ levels decrease more slowly than with potassium iodide treatment, probably reflecting the decrease in T₄ plasma clearance rate induced by ipodate. The therapeutic use of these agents is mainly restricted to preoperative treatment; during long-term treatment, escape from the iodide inhibition of thyroidal secretion often occurs (172). Another rare indication may be thyrotoxicosis factitia (173); their long half-life makes this unwise (174,175).

In summary, the lipid-soluble radiographic contrast agents and amiodarone induce alterations in thyroid hormone levels by actions on the peripheral tissues, on thyroidal secretion, and probably on the pituitary gland. These actions result in elevations in serum T₄ and rT₃ concentrations, transient increases in TSH concentrations, and decreases in T₃ concentrations. These findings may be explained by inhibition of T₄ and rT₃ 3'-deiodination in many tissues (liver, kidney, brain), and by the liberation of T₄ (and rT₃) from hepatic and renal storage pools. In contrast to their effects in normal subjects, in thyrotoxic patients these agents cause a decrease in serum T₄ concentrations as well as a decrease in serum T₃ levels. In addition, these agents, particularly amiodarone, are prone to induce thyroid dysfunction, which is particularly difficult to treat.

Effects on Thyroid Hormone Action in the Nucleus

Amiodarone decreases thyroid hormone synthesis, secretion, and deiodination. In addition, desethylamiodarone, the major metabolite of amioderone, is a noncompetitive inhibitor of T₃ binding to *Escherichia coli*–expressed T₃-receptor protein, with an IC50 of 2×10^{-5} M and preferential binding to unoccupied receptors (176,177). However, at higher concentrations (>2 m*M*) amiodarone appears to a competitive antagonist (178). This observation might explain the decreased nuclear receptor T₃-binding capacity in the myocardium of amiodarone-treated rats, as well as the antagonistic effect of amiodarone treatment on pituitary growth hormone expression and cardiac b-adrenoreceptor density (103,179–182). No data exist to support the notion of selective target tissue resistance to T₃ in amiodarone-treated patients. Although an elevation of serum TSH levels during amiodarone treatment has been described in patients on a constant replacement dose of T₄, this finding is most compatible with an amiodarone-induced decrease in pituitary and peripheral deiodination. However, a contribution from decreased cellular uptake and nuclear action cannot be excluded (183,184). In contrast, phenytoin, in addition to its effects on thyroid hormone metabolism, as described earlier, has been considered as a partial thyroid hormone agonist (114,115).

REFERENCES

1. El Sheikh M, McGregor AM. Antithyroid drugs: their mechanism of action and clinical use. In: Weetman AP, Grossman A, eds. *Pharmacotherapeutics of the thyroid gland.* New York: Springer-Verlag New York, 1998:189–201.
2. Taurog A, Dorris ML, Guziec FS, et al. Metabolism of 35S- and 14C-labeled propylthiouracil in a model in vitro system containing thyroid peroxidase. *Endocrinology* 1989;124:3030–3037.
3. Engler H, Taurog A, Luthy C, et al. Reversible and irreversible inhibition of thyroid peroxidase-catalyzed iodination by thioureylene drugs. *Endocrinology* 1983;112:86–95.
4. Ruiz JK, Rossi GV, Vallejos HA, et al. Fulminant hepatic failure associated with propylthiouracil. *Ann Pharmacother* 2003;37:224–228.

5. Casis FC, Perez JB. Leukocytoclastic vasculitis: a rare manifestation of propylthiouracil allergy. *Endocr Pract* 2000;6:329–332.

6. Gunton JE, Stiel J, Clifton-Bligh P, et al. Prevalence of positive anti-neutrophil cytoplasmic antibody (ANCA) in patients receiving anti-thyroid medication. *Eur J Endocrinol* 2000;142:587.

7. Sato H, Hattori M, Fujieda M, et al. High prevalence of anti-neutrophil cytoplasmic antibody positivity in childhood onset Graves' disease treated with propylthiouracil. *J Clin Endocrinol Metab* 2000;85:4270–4273.

8. Burrow GN, Fisher DA, Larsen PR. Maternal and fetal thyroid function. *N Engl J Med* 1994;331:1072–1078.

9. Becks GP, Burrow GN. Thyroid disease and pregnancy. *Med Clin North Am* 1991;75:121–150.

10. Wing DA, Millar LK, Koonings PP, et al. A comparison of propylthiouracil versus methimazole in the treatment of hyperthyroidism in pregnancy. *Am J Obstet Gynecol* 1994;170:90–95.

11. Azizi F, Khoshniat M, Bahrainian M, et al. Thyroid function and intellectual development of infants nursed by mothers taking methimazole. *J Clin Endocrinol Metab* 2000;85:3233–3238.

12. Leonard JL, Rosenberg IN. Thyroxine 5′-deiodinase activity of rat kidney: observations on activation by thiols and inhibition by propylthiouracil. *Endocrinology* 1978;103:2137–2144.

13. Reinwein D, Benker G, Lazarus JH, et al. A prospective randomized trial of antithyroid drug dose in Graves' disease therapy: European Multicenter Study Group on Antithyroid Drug Treatment. *J Clin Endocrinol Metab* 1993;76:1516–1521.

14. Lucas A, Salinas I, Rius F, et al. Medical therapy of Graves' disease: does thyroxine prevent recurrence of hyperthyroidism? *J Clin Endocrinol Metab* 1997;82:2410–2413.

15. Vieja A, Dohan O, Levy O, et al . Molecular analysis of the sodium/iodide symporter: Impact on thyroid and extrathyroid pathophysiology. *Physiol Rev* 2000;80:1083–1105.

16. Dohan O, De la Vieja A, Paroder V, et al. The sodium/iodide Symporter (NIS): characterization, regulation, and medical significance. *Endocr Rev* 2003;24:48–77.

17. Wolf J. Perchlorate and the thyroid gland. *Pharmacol Rev* 1998;50:89–105.

18. Delange F. The role of goitrogenic factors distinct from iodine deficiency in the etiology of goiter [in French]. *Ann Endocrinol (Paris)* 1988;49:302–305.

19. Moreno-Reyes R, Boelaert M, el Badawi S, et al. Endemic juvenile hypothyroidism in a severe endemic goitre area of Sudan. *Clin Endocrinol (Oxf)* 1993;38:19–24.

20. Vanderpas J, Bourdoux P, Lagasse R, et al. Endemic infantile hypothyroidism in a severe endemic goitre area of central Africa. *Clin Endocrinol (Oxf)* 1984;20:327–340.

21. Bourdoux P, Delange F, Gerard M, et al. Evidence that cassava ingestion increases thiocyanate formation: a possible etiologic factor in endemic goiter. *J Clin Endocrinol Metab* 1978;46:613–621.

22. Kohrle J, Brabant G, Hesch RD. Metabolism of the thyroid hormones. *Horm Res* 1987;26:58–78.

23. Schroder-van der Elst JP, van der Heide D, Kohrle J. In vivo effects of flavonoid EMD 21388 on thyroid hormone secretion and metabolism in rats. *Am J Physiol* 1991;261:227–232.

24. Abend SL, Fang SL, Alex S, et al. Rapid alteration in circulating free thyroxine modulates pituitary type II 5′ deiodinase and basal thyrotropin secretion in the rat. *J Clin Invest* 1991;88:898–903.

25. Winneke G, Walkowiak J, Lilienthal H. PCB-induced neurodevelopmental toxicity in human infants and its potential mediation by endocrine dysfunction. *Toxicology* 2002;181/182:161–165.

26. Moriyama K, Tagami T, Akamizu T, et al. Thyroid hormone action is disrupted by bisphenol A as an antagonist. *J Clin Endocrinol Metab* 2002;87:5185–5190.

27. Muakkassah-Kelly SF, Krinke AL, Malinowski W, et al. The effect of short term feeding of the antioxidant triethyleneglycol-bis-3(3-tert-butyl-4-hydroxy-5-methyl)propionate on serum thyrotropin and thyroid hormones in the male rat. *Toxicol Appl Pharmacol* 1991;107:129–140.

28. Martino E, Safran M, Aghini-Lombardi F, et al. Environmental iodine intake and thyroid dysfunction during chronic amiodarone therapy. *Ann Intern Med* 1984; 101:28–34.

29. Trip, MD, Wiersinga, W, and Plomp, TA. Incidence, predictability, and pathogenesis of amiodarone-induced thyrotoxicosis and hypothyroidism. *Am J Med* 1991; 91:507–511.

30. Vorperian VR, Havighurst TC, Miller S, et al. Adverse effects of low dose amiodarone: a meta-analysis [see comments]. J Am Coll Cardiol 1997;30:791–798.

31. Harjai KJ, Licata AA. Effects of amiodarone on thyroid function [see comments]. *Ann Intern Med* 1997; 126:63–73.

32. Martino E, Bartalena L, Mariotti S, et al. Radioactive iodine thyroid uptake in patients with amiodarone-iodine-induced thyroid dysfunction. *Acta Endocrinol (Copenh)*. 1988;119:167–173.

33. Roti E, Minelli R, Gardini E, et al. Thyrotoxicosis followed by hypothyroidism in patients treated with amiodarone: a possible consequence of a destructive process in the thyroid. *Arch Intern Med* 1993;153:886–892.

34. Smyrk TC, Goellner JR, Brennan MD, et al. Pathology of the thyroid in amiodarone-induced thyrotoxicosis. *Am J Surg Pathol*. 1987;11:197–204.

35. Bartalena L, Grasso L, Brogioni S, et al. Serum interleukin-6 in amiodarone-induced thyrotoxicosis. *J Clin Endocrinol Metab* 1994; 78:423–427.

36. Chiovato L, Martino E, Tonacchera M, et al. Studies on the in vitro cytotoxic effect of amiodarone. *Endocrinology* 1994;134:2277–2282.

37. Bartalena, L, Brogioni, S, Grasso, L et al. Treatment of amiodarone-induced thyrotoxicosis, a difficult challenge: results of a prospective study. *J Clin Endocrinol Metab* 1996;81:2930–2933.

37a. Pearce EN, Bogazzi F, Martino E, et al. The prevalence of elevated serum C-reactive protein levels in inflammatory and non-inflammatory thyroid disease. *Thyroid* 2003;13:643–648.

38. Bogazzi F, Bartalena L, Brogioni S, et al. Color flow Doppler sonography rapidly differentiates type I and type II amiodarone-induced thyrotoxicosis. *Thyroid* 1997;7:541–545.

39. Osman F, Franklyn JA, Sheppard MC, et al. Successful treatment of amiodarone-induced thyrotoxicosis. *Circulation* 2002; 105:1275–11277.

40. Vial T, Descotes J. Immune-mediated side-effects of cytokines in humans. *Toxicology* 1995;105:31–57.

41. Ajjan RA, Watson PF, Weetman AP. Cytokines and thyroid function. *Adv Neuroimmunol* 1996;6:359–386.

42. Burman P, Totterman TH, Orberg K, et al. Thyroid autoimmunity in patients on long term therapy with leukocyte-derived interferon. *J Clin Endocrinol Metab* 1986; 63:1086–1090.

43. Reichlin S. Neuroendocrine-immune interactions. *N Engl J Med* 1993;329:1246–1253.

44. Atkins MB, Mier JW, Parkinson DR, et al. Hypothyroidism after treatment with interleukin-2 and lymphokine-activated killer cells. *N Engl J Med* 1988;318:1557–1563.

45. Hoekman K, von Blomberg-van der Flier B, Wagstaff J, et al. Reversible thyroid dysfunction during treatment with GM-CSF. *Lancet* 1991;338:541–542.

46. van Hoff ME, Howell A. Risk of thyroid dysfunction during treatment with G-CSF. *Lancet* 1992;340:1169.

47. Miossec P. Cytokine-induced autoimmune disorders. *Drug Saf* 1997;17:93–104.

48. Sachithanandan S, Clarke G, Crowe J, et al. Interferon-associated thyroid dysfunction in anti-D-related chronic hepatitis C. *J Interferon Cytokine Res* 1997;17:409–411.

49. Schuppert F, Rambusch E, Kirchner H, et al. Patients treated with interferon-alpha, interferon-beta, and interleukin-2 have a different thyroid autoantibody pattern than patients suffering from endogenous autoimmune thyroid disease. *Thyroid* 1997; 7:837–842.

50. Russo MW, Fried MW. Side effects of therapy for chronic hepatitis C. *Gastroenterology* 2003; 124:1711–1719.

51. Deutsch M, Dourakis S, Manesis EK, et al. Thyroid abnormalities in chronic viral hepatitis and their relationship to interferon alfa therapy. *Hepatology* 1997;26:206–210.

52. Villanueva RB, Brau N. Graves' ophthalmopathy associated with interferon-alpha treatment for hepatitis C. *Thyroid* 2002; 12:737–738.

53. Rotondi M, Mazziotti G, Biondi B, et al. Long-term treatment with interferon-beta therapy for multiple sclerosis and occurrence of Graves' disease. *J Endocrinol Invest* 2000;23: 321–324.

54. Carella C, Mazziotti G, Morisco F et al. The addition of ribavirin to interferon-alpha therapy in patients with hepatitis C virus-related chronic hepatitis does not modify the thyroid autoantibody pattern but increases the risk of developing hypothyroidism. *Eur J Endocrinol* 2002;146:743–749.

55. Schwartzentruber DJ, White DE, Zweig MH, et al. Thyroid dysfunction associated with immunotherapy for patients with cancer. *Cancer* 1991;68:2384–2390.

56. Vialettes B, Guillerand MA, Viens P, et al. Incidence rate and risk factors for thyroid dysfunction during recombinant interleukin-2 therapy in advanced malignancies. *Acta Endocrinol (Copenh)* 1993;129:31–38.

57. Vassilopoulou-Sellin R, Sella A, Dexeus FH, et al. Acute thyroid dysfunction (thyroiditis) after therapy with interleukin-2. *Horm Metab Res* 1992;24:434–438.

58. Huang MJ, Tsai SL, Huang BY, et al. Prevalence and significance of thyroid autoantibodies in patients with chronic hepatitis C virus infection: a prospective controlled study. *Clin Endocrinol (Oxf)* 1999;50:503–509.

58a.Pearce, En, Farwell, AP, Braverman, LE. Thyroiditis. *N Engl J Med* 2003;348:2646–55.

59. Carella C, Mazziotti G, Morisco F, et al. Long-term outcome of interferon-alpha-induced thyroid autoimmunity and prognostic influence of thyroid autoantibody pattern at the end of treatment. *J Clin Endocrinol Metab* 2001;86:1925–1929.

60. Minelli R, Braverman LE, Giuberti T, et al. Effects of excess iodine administration on thyroid function in euthyroid patients with a previous episode of thyroid dysfunction induced by interferon-alpha treatment. *Clin Endocrinol (Oxf)* 1997;47:357–361.

61. Sato K, Satoh T, Shizume K, et al. Inhibition of 125I organification and thyroid hormone release by interleukin-1, tumor necrosis factor-alpha, and interferon-gamma in human thyrocytes in suspension culture. *J Clin Endocrinol Metab* 1990;70: 1735–1743.

62. Mooradian AD, Reed RL, Osterweil D, et al. Decreased serum triiodothyronine is associated with increased concentrations of tumor necrosis factor. *J Clin Endocrinol Metab* 1990;71:1239–1242.

63. Chopra IJ, Sakane S, Teco GN. A study of the serum concentration of tumor necrosis factor-alpha in thyroidal and nonthyroidal illnesses. *J Clin Endocrinol Metab* 1991;72:1113–1116.

64. Yamazaki K, Kanaji Y, Shizume K, et al. Reversible inhibition by interferons alpha and beta of 125I incorporation and thyroid hormone release by human thyroid follicles in vitro. *J Clin Endocrinol Metab* 1993;77:1439–1441.

65. Kraiem Z, Sobel E, Sadeh O, et al. Effects of gamma-interferon on DR antigen expression, growth, 3,5,3'- triiodothyronine secretion, iodide uptake, and cyclic adenosine 3',5'-monophosphate accumulation in cultured human thyroid cells. *J Clin Endocrinol Metab* 1990;71:817–824.

66. Kasuga Y, Matsubayashi S, Akasu F, et al. Effects of recombinant human interleukin-2 and tumor necrosis factor-alpha with or without interferon-gamma on human thyroid tissues from patients with Graves' disease and from normal subjects xenografted into nude mice. *J Clin Endocrinol Metab* 1991; 72:1296–1301.

67. Lazarus JH. The effects of lithium therapy on thyroid and thyrotropin-releasing hormone. *Thyroid* 1998;8:909–913.

68. Davies PH, Franklyn JA. The effects of drugs on tests of thyroid function. *Eur J Clin Pharmacol* 1991;40:439–451.

69. Kirov G. Thyroid disorders in lithium-treated patients. *J Affect Disord* 1998;50:33–40.

70. Barclay ML, Brownlie BE, Turner JG, et al. Lithium associated thyrotoxicosis: a report of 14 cases, with statistical analysis of incidence. *Clin Endocrinol (Oxf)* 1994;40:759–764.

71. Bocchetta A, Bernardi F, Pedditzi M, et al. Thyroid abnormalities during lithium treatment. *Acta Psychiatr Scand* 1991;83: 193–198.

72. Mizukami Y, Michigishi T, Nonomura A, et al. Histological features of the thyroid gland in a patient with lithium induced thyrotoxicosis. *J Clin Pathol* 1995; 48:582–584.

73. Miller KK, Daniels GH. Association between lithium use and thyrotoxicosis caused by silent thyroiditis. *Clin Endocrinol (Oxf)* 2001;55:501–508.

74. Stratakis CA, Chrousos GP. Transient elevation of serum thyroid hormone levels following lithium discontinuation. *Eur J Pediatr* 1996;155:939–941.

75. Bogazzi F, Bartalena L, Brogioni S, et al. Comparison of radioiodine with radioiodine plus lithium in the treatment of Graves' hyperthyroidism. *J Clin Endocrinol Metab* 1999;84: 499–503.

76. Dickstein G, Shechner C, Adawi F, et al. Lithium treatment in amiodarone-induced thyrotoxicosis. *Am J Med* 1997;102:454–458.

76a.Koong SS, Reynolds JC, Movius EG, et al. Lithium as a potential adjuvant to 131I therapy of metastatic well differentiated thyroid cancer. *J Clin Endocrinol Metab* 1999;84:912–916.

77. Benvenga S, Cahnmann HJ, Gregg RE, et al. Characterization of the binding of thyroxine to high density lipoproteins and apolipoproteins A-I. *J Clin Endocrinol Metab* 1989;68:1067–1072.

78. Benvenga S, Cahnmann HJ, Robbins J. Localization of the thyroxine binding sites in apolipoprotein B-100 of human low density lipoproteins. *Endocrinology* 1990;127:2241–2246.

79. Benvenga S, Cahnmann HJ, Robbins J. Characterization of thyroid hormone binding to apolipoprotein-E: localization of the binding site in the exon 3-coded domain. *Endocrinology* 1993;133:1300–1305.

80. Mendel CM. The free hormone hypothesis: a physiologically based mathematical model. *Endocr Rev* 1989;10:232–274.

81. Mendel CM, Cavalieri RR, Weisiger RA. Uptake of thyroxine by the perfused rat liver: implications for the free hormone hypothesis. *Am J Physiol* 1988;255:E110–E119.

82. Divino CM, Schussler GC. Receptor-mediated uptake and internalization of transthyretin. *J Biol Chem* 1990;265:1425–1429.

83. Harms PJ, Tu GF, Richardson SJ, et al. Transthyretin (prealbumin) gene expression in choroid plexus is strongly conserved during evolution of vertebrates. *Comp Biochem Physiol B Biochem Mol Biol* 1991;99:239–249.

84. Chanoine JP, Alex S, Fang SL, et al. Role of transthyretin in the transport of thyroxine from the blood to the choroid plexus, the cerebrospinal fluid, and the brain. *Endocrinology* 1992;130: 933–938.

85. Wenzel KW. Disturbances of thyroid function tests by drugs. *Acta Med Austriaca* 1996;23:57–60.

86. Cavalieri RR. Effects of drugs on human thyroid hormone metabolism. In: Hennemann G, ed. *Thyroid hormone metabolism.* New York: Marcel Dekker Inc, 1986.

87. Ratcliffe WA, Hazelton RA, Thompson JA. Effect of fenclofenac on thyroid-function tests. *Lancet* 1980;1:432–430.

88. Baranetsky NG, Chertow BS, Webb MD, et al. Combined phenytoin and salicylate effects on thyroid function tests. *Arch Int Pharmacodyn Ther* 1986;284:166–176.

89. Humphrey MJ, Capper SJ, Kurtz AB. Fenclofenac and thyroid hormone concentrations. *Lancet* 1980;1:487–480.

90. Lim CF, Bai Y, Topliss DJ, et al. Drug and fatty acid effects on serum thyroid hormone binding. *J Clin Endocrinol Metab* 1988;67:682–688.

91. Wang YS, Hershman JM, Smith V, et al. Effect of heparin on free thyroxin as measured by equilibrium dialysis and ultrafiltration. *Clin Chem* 1986;32:700.

92. Mendel CM, Frost PH, Kunitake ST, et al. Mechanism of the heparin-induced increase in the concentration of free thyroxine in plasma. *J Clin Endocrinol Metab* 1987;65:1259–1264.

93. Jain R, Uy HL. Increase in serum free thyroxine levels related to intravenous heparin treatment. *Ann Intern Med* 1996;124: 74–75.

94. Saeed-Uz-Zafar M, Miller JM, Breneman GM, et al. Observations on the effect of heparin on free and total thyroxine. *J Clin Endocrinol Metab* 1971; 32:633–630.

95. Schwartz HL, Schadlow AR, Faierman D, et al. Heparin administration appears to decrease cellular binding of thyroxine. *J Clin Endocrinol Metab* 1973;36:598–590.

96. Krenning EP, Docter R. Plasma membrane transport of thyroid hormone. In: *Thyroid hormone metabolism.* Hennemann G, ed. New York: Marcel Dekker Inc. 1986:131–186.

97. Pontecorvi A, Robbins J. The plasma membrane and thyroid hormone entry into cells. *Trends Endocrinol Metab* 1989;1: 90–94.

98. Dejong M, Visser TJ, Bernard BF, et al. Transport and metabolism of iodothyronines in cultured human hepatocytes. *J Clin Endocrinol Metab* 1993;77:139–143.

99. Northcutt RC, Stiel JN, Hollifield JW, et al. The influence of cholestyramine on thyroxine absorption. *JAMA* 1969;208: 1857–1861.

100. Liel Y. Levothyroxine therapy. *Ann Intern Med* 1994;120:619–620.

101. Shakir KM, Chute JP, Aprill BS, et al. Ferrous sulfate-induced increase in requirement for thyroxine in a patient with primary hypothyroidism. *South Med J* 1997;90:637–639.

102. Sherman SI, Tielens ET, Ladenson PW. Sucralfate causes malabsorption of L-thyroxine. *Am J Med* 1994;96:531–535.

103. Norman MF, Lavin TN. Antagonism of thyroid hormone action by amiodarone in rat pituitary tumor cells. *J Clin Invest* 1989;83:306–313.

104. de Jong M, Docter R, Van der Hoek H, et al. Different effects of amiodarone on transport of T4 and T3 into the perfused rat liver. *Am J Physiol* 1994;266:E44–E49.

105. Kragie L, Forrester ML, Cody V, et al. Computer-assisted molecular modeling of benzodiazepine and thyromimetic inhibitors of the HepG2 iodothyronine membrane transporter. *Mol Endocrinol* 1994;8:382–391.

106. Topliss DJ, Scholz GH, Kolliniatis E, et al. Influence of calmodulin antagonists and calcium channel blockers on triiodothyronine uptake by rat hepatoma and myoblast cell lines. *Metabolism* 1993;42:376–380.

107. Barlow JW, Curtis AJ, Raggatt LE, et al. Drug competition for intracellular triiodothyronine-binding sites. *Eur J Endocrinol* 1994;130:417–421.

108. Nebert DW, Russell DW. Clinical importance of the cytochromes P450. *Lancet* 2002;360:1155–11562.

109. Yeo PP, Bates D, Howe JG, et al. Anticonvulsants and thyroid function. *BMJ* 1978;1:1581–1583.

110. Cavalieri RR, Gavin LA, Wallace A, et al. Serum thyroxine, free T4, triiodothyronine, and reverse-T3 in diphenylhydantoin-treated patients. *Metabolism* 1979;28:1161–1165.

111. Kozlowski BW, Taylor ML, Baer MT, et al. Anticonvulsant medication use and circulating levels of total thyroxine, retinol binding protein, and vitamin A in children with delayed cognitive development. *Am J Clin Nutr* 1987;46:360–368.

112. Larkin JG, Macphee GJ, Beastall GH, et al. Thyroid hormone concentrations in epileptic patients. *Eur J Clin Pharmacol* 1989;36:213–216.

113. Rootwelt K, Ganes T, Johannessen SI. Effect of carbamazepine, phenytoin and phenobarbitone on serum levels of thyroid hormones and thyrotropin in humans. *Scand J Clin Lab Invest* 1978;38:731–736.

114. Surks MI, Ordene KW, Mann DN, et al. Diphenylhydantoin inhibits the thyrotropin response to thyrotropin-releasing hormone in man and rat. *J Clin Endocrinol Metab* 1983;56: 940–945.

115. Smith PJ, Surks MI. Multiple effects of 5,5′-diphenylhydantoin on the thyroid hormone system. *Endocr Rev* 1984;5: 514–524.

116. Zemel LR, Biezunski DR, Shapiro LE, et al. 5,5′-Diphenylhydantoin decreases the entry of 3,5,3′-triiodo-L- thyronine but not L-thyroxine in cultured GH-producing cells. *Acta Endocrinol* 1988;117:392–398.

117. Gingrich SA, Smith PJ, Shapiro LE, et al. 5,5′-Diphenylhydantoin (phenytoin) attenuates the action of 3,5,3′- triiodo-L-thyronine in cultured GC cells. *Endocrinology* 1985;116:2306–2313.

118. Surks MI. Hypothyroidism and phenytoin. *Ann Intern Med* 1985;102:871.

119. Ohnhaus EE, Studer H. The effect of different doses of rifampicin on thyroid hormone metabolism. *Br J Clin Pharmacol* 1980;9:285–286.

120. Ohnhaus EE, Burgi H, Burger A, et al. The effect of antipyrine, phenobarbitol and rifampicin on thyroid hormone metabolism in man. *Eur J Clin Invest* 1981;11:381–387.

121. Ohnhaus EE, Studer H. A link between liver microsomal enzyme activity and thyroid hormone metabolism in man. *Br J Clin Pharmacol* 1983;15:71–76.

122. Christensen HR, Simonsen K, Hegedus L, et al. Influence of rifampicin on thyroid gland volume, thyroid hormones, and antipyrine metabolism. *Acta Endocrinol (Copenh)* 1989;121:406–410.

123. Isley WL. Effect of rifampin therapy on thyroid function tests in a hypothyroid patient on replacement L-thyroxine. *Ann Intern Med* 1987;107:517–518.

124. Kaiser CA, Seydoux J, Giacobino JP, et al. Increased plasma clearance rate of thyroxine despite decreased 5'-monodeiodination: study with a peroxisome proliferator in the rat. *Endocrinology* 1988;122:1087–1093.
125. Engler D, Burger AG. The deiodination of the iodothyronines and of their derivatives in man. *Endocr Rev* 1984;5:151–184.
126. Danforth E, Burger AG. The impact of nutrition on thyroid hormone physiology and action. *Annu Rev Nutr* 1989;9:201–227.
127. Visser TJ, Leonard JL, Kaplan MM, et al. Different pathways of iodothyronine 5'-deiodination in rat cerebral cortex. *Biochem Biophys Res Commun* 1981;101:1297–1304.
128. Bianco AC, Salvatore D, Gereben B, et al. Biochemistry, cellular and molecular biology, and physiological roles of the iodothyronine selenodeiodinases. *Endocr Rev* 2002;23:38–89.
129. LoPresti JS, Eigen A, Kaptein E, et al. Alterations in 3,3'5'-triiodothyronine metabolism in response to propylthiouracil, dexamethasone, and thyroxine administration in man. *J Clin Invest* 1989;84:1650–1656.
130. Geffner DL, Azukizawa M, Hershman JM. Propylthiouracil blocks extrathyroidal conversion of thyroxine to triiodothyronine and augments thyrotropin secretion in man. *J Clin Invest* 1975;55:224–220.
131. Saberi M, Sterling FH, Utiger RD. Reduction in extrathyroidal triiodothyronine production by propylthiouracil in man. *J Clin Invest* 1975;55:218–223.
132. Kaplan MM, Schimmel M, Utiger RD. Changes in serum 3,3',5'-triiodothyronine (reverse T3) concentrations with altered thyroid hormone secretion and metabolism. *J Clin Endocrinol Metab* 1977;45:447–456.
133. Westgren U, Melander A, Wahlin E, et al. Divergent effects of 6-propylthiouracil on 3,3',5'-triiodothyronine (RT3) serum levels and in man. *Acta Endocrinol (Copenh)* 1977;85:345–350.
134. Nogimori T, Braverman LE, Taurog A, et al. A new class of propylthiouracil analogs: comparison of 5'-deiodinase inhibition and antithyroid activity. *Endocrinology* 1986;118:1598–1605.
135. Wilber JF, Utiger RD. The effect of glucocorticoids on thyrotropin secretion. *J Clin Invest* 1969;48:2096–2090.
136. Nicoloff JT, Fisher DA, Appleman MDJ. The role of glucocorticoids in the regulation of thyroid function in man. *J Clin Invest* 1970;49:1922–1920.
137. Duick DA, Warren DW, Nicoloff JT, et al. Effect of single-dose dexamethasone on the concentration of serum triiodothyronine in man. *J Clin Endocrinol Metab* 1974;39:1151–1150.
138. Chopra IJ, Williams DE, Orgiazzi J, et al. Opposite effects of dexamethasone on serum concentrations of 3,3',5'-triiodothyronine (reverse T3) and 3,3'5-triiodothyronine (T3). *J Clin Endocrinol Metab* 1975;41:911–920.
139. Burr WA, Ramsden DB, Griffiths RS, et al. Effect of a single dose of dexamethasone on serum concentrations of thyroid hormones. *Lancet* 1976;2:58–61.
140. Williams DE, Chopra IJ, Orgiazzi J, et al. Acute effects of corticosteroids on thyroid activity in Graves' disease. *J Clin Endocrinol Metab* 1975;41:354–361.
141. Verhoeven RP, Visser TJ, Docter R, et al. Plasma thyroxine, 3,3',5-triiodothyronine and 3,3',5'-triiodothyronine during beta-adrenergic blockade in hyperthyroidism. *J Clin Endocrinol Metab* 1977;44:1002–1005.
142. Lotti G, Delitala G, Devilla L, et al. Reduction of plasma triiodothyronine (T3) induced by propranolol. *Clin Endocrinol (Oxf)* 1977;6:405–410.
143. Saunders J, Hall SE, Crowther A, et al. The effect of propranolol on thyroid hormones and oxygen consumption in thyrotoxicosis. *Clin Endocrinol (Oxf)* 1978;9:67–72.
144. Kallner G, Ljunggren JG, Tryselius M. The effect of propranolol on serum levels of T4, T3 and reverse-T3 in hyperthyroidism. *Acta Med Scand* 1978;204:35–37.
145. Murchison LE, How J, Bewsher PD. Comparison of propranolol and metoprolol in the management of hyperthyroidism. *Br J Clin Pharmacol* 1979;8:581–587.
146. Feely J, Isles TE, Ratcliffe WA, et al. Propranolol, triiodothyronine, reverse triiodothyronine and thyroid disease. *Clin Endocrinol (Oxf)* 1979;10:531–538.
147. Faber J, Friis T, Kirkegaard C, et al. Serum T4, T3 and reverse T3 during treatment with propranolol in hyperthyroidism, L-T4 treated myxedema and in normal man. *Horm Metab Res* 1979;11:34–36.
148. Wartofsky L, Dimond RC, Noel GL, et al. Failure of propranolol to alter thyroid iodine release, thyroxine turnover, or the TSH and PRL responses to thyrotropin-releasing hormone in patients with thyrotoxicosis. *J Clin Endocrinol Metab* 1975;41:485–490.
149. Shulkin BL, Peele ME, Utiger RD. Beta-adrenergic antagonist inhibition of hepatic 3,5,3'-triiodothyronine production. *Endocrinology* 1984;115:858–861.
150. Heyma P, Larkins RG, Higginbotham L, et al. D-propanolol and DL-propanolol both decrease conversion of L-thyroxine to L-triiodothyronine. *BMJ* 1980;281:24–20.
151. Heyma P, Larkins RG, Campbell DG. Inhibition by propanolol of 3,5,3'-triiodothyronine formation from thyroxine in isolated rat renal tubules: an effect independent of beta-adrenergic blockade. *Endocrinology* 1980; 106:1437–1430.
152. Burgi H, Wimpfheimer C, Burger A, et al. Changes of circulating thyroxine, triiodothyronine and reverse triiodothyronine after radiographic contrast agents. *J Clin Endocrinol Metab* 1976;43:1203–1210.
153. Suzuki H, Kadena N, Takeuchi K, et al. Effects of three-day oral cholecystography on serum iodothyronines and TSH concentrations: comparison of the effects among some cholecystographic agents and the effects of iopanoic acid on the pituitary-thyroid axis. *Acta Endocrinol (Copenh)* 1979;92:477–488.
154. Brown RS, Cohen JH, Braverman LE. Successful treatment of massive acute thyroid hormone poisoning with iopanoic acid. *J Pediatr* 1998;132:903–905.
155. Felicetta JV, Green WL, Nelp WB. Inhibition of hepatic binding of thyroxine by cholecystographic agents. *J Clin Invest* 1980;65:1032–1040.
156. Burger A, Dinichert D, Nicod P, et al. Effect of amiodarone on serum triiodothyronine, reverse triiodothyronine, thyroxin, and thyrotropin. A drug influencing peripheral metabolism of thyroid hormones. *J Clin Invest* 1976;58:255–259.
157. Melmed S, Nademanee K, Reed AW, et al. Hyperthyroxinemia with bradycardia and normal thyrotropin secretion after chronic amiodarone administration. *J Clin Endocrinol Metab* 1981;53:997–990.
158. Lambert MJ, Burger AG, Galeazzi RL et al. Are selective increases in serum thyroxine (T4) due to iodinated inhibitors of T$_4$ monocodination indicative of hyperthyroidism? *J Clin Endocrinol Metab* 1982;55:1058–1065.
159. Kaptein EM, Egodage PM, Hoopes MT, et al. Amiodarone alters thyroxine transfer and distribution in humans. *Metabolism* 1988;37:1107–1113.
160. Zaninovich AA, Bosco SC, Fernandez-Pol AJ. Amiodarone does not affect the distribution and fractional turnover of triiodothyronine from the plasma pool, but only its generation from thyroxine in extrathyroidal tissues. *J Clin Endocrinol Metab* 1990;70:1721–1724.
161. Iervasi G, Clerico A, Manfredi C et al. Acute effects of intravenous amiodarone on sulphate metabolites of thyroid hormones in arrhythmic patients. *Clin Endocrinol (Oxf)* 1997;47:699–705.

162. Schroder van der Elst JP, van der Heide D. Thyroxine, 3,5,3′-triiodothyronine, and 3,3′,5′-triiodothyronine concentrations in several tissues of the rat: effects of amiodarone and desethylamiodarone on thyroid hormone metabolism (corrected) (published erratum appears in Endocrinology 1991 Jan; 128 (1):393). *Endocrinology* 1990;127:1656–1664.

163. van Beeren HC, Bakker O, Wiersinga WM. Desethylamiodarone interferes with the binding of co-activator GRIP-1 to the beta 1-thyroid hormone receptor. *FEBS Lett* 2000;481:213–216.

164. van Beeren HC, Bakker O, Wiersinga WM. Desethylamiodarone is a competitive inhibitor of the binding of thyroid hormone to the thyroid hormone alpha 1-receptor protein. *Mol Cell Endocrinol* 1995;112:15–19.

165. Polikar R, Goy JJ, Schlapfer J, et al. Effect of oral triiodothyronine during amiodarone treatment for ventricular premature complexes. *Am J Cardiol* 1986;58:987–991.

166. Lambert M, Burger AG, De Nayer P, et al. Decreased TSH response to TRH induced by amiodarone. *Acta Endocrinol (Copenh)* 1988;118:449–452.

167. Wu SY, Chopra IJ, Solomon DH, et al. Changes in circulating iodothyronines in euthyroid and hyperthyroid subjects given ipodate (Oragrafin), an agent for oral cholecystography. *J Clin Endocrinol Metab* 1978;46:691–697.

168. Wu SY, Chopra IJ, Solomon DH, et al. The effect of repeated administration of ipodate (Oragrafin) in hyperthyroidism. *J Clin Endocrinol Metab* 1978;47:1358–1362.

169. Karpman BA, Rapoport B, Filetti S, et al. Treatment of neonatal hyperthyroidism due to Graves' disease with sodium ipodate. *J Clin Endocrinol Metab* 1987;64:119–123.

170. Roti E, Robuschi G, Gardini E, et al. Comparison of methimazole, methimazole and sodium ipodate, and methimazole and saturated solution of potassium iodide in the early treatment of hyperthyroid Graves' disease. *Clin Endocrinol (Oxf)* 1988;28:305–314.

171. Berghout A, Wiersinga WM, Brummelkamp WH. Sodium ipodate in the preparation of Graves' hyperthyroid patients for thyroidectomy. *Horm Res* 1989;31:256–250.

172. Martino E, Balzano S, Bartalena L, et al. Therapy of Graves' disease with sodium ipodate is associated with a high recurrence rate of hyperthyroidism. *J Endocrinol Invest* 1991;14:847–851.

173. Cohen JH, Ingbar SH, Braverman LE. Thyrotoxicosis due to ingestion of excess thyroid hormone: update 1994. *Endocr Rev* 1994;10:364–375.

174. Van Reeth O, Unger J. Effects of amiodarone on serum T3 and T4 concentrations in hyperthyroid patients treated with propylthiouracil. *Thyroid* 1991;1:301–306.

175. Van Reeth O, Decoster C, Unger J. Effect of amiodarone on serum T4 and T3 levels in hyperthyroid patients treated with methimazole. *Eur J Clin Pharmacol* 1987;32:223–227.

176. Bakker O, van Beeren HC, Wiersinga WM. Desethylamiodarone is a noncompetitive inhibitor of the binding of thyroid hormone to the thyroid hormone beta 1-receptor protein. *Endocrinology* 1994;134:1665–1670.

177. van Beeren HC, Bakker O, Wiersinga WM. Structure-function relationship of the inhibition of the 3,5,3′-triiodothyronine binding to the alpha1- and beta1-thyroid hormone receptor by amiodarone analogues. *Endocrinology* 1996;137:2807–2814.

178. Drvota V, Carlsson B, Haggblad J et al. Amiodarone is a dose-dependent noncompetitive and competitive inhibitor of T3 binding to thyroid hormone receptor subtype beta 1, whereas disopyramide, lignocaine, propafenone, metoprolol, dl-sotalol, and verapamil have no inhibitory effect. *J Cardiovasc Pharmacol* 1995;26:222–226.

179. Gotzsche LBH, Orskov H. Cardiac triiodothyronine nuclear receptor binding capacities in amiodarone-treated, hypo- and hyperthyroid rats. *Eur J Endocrinol* 1994;130:281–290.

180. Paradis P, Lambert C, Rouleau J. Amiodarone antagonizes the effects of T3 at the receptor level: an additional mechanism for its in vivo hypothyroid-like effects. *Can J Physiol Pharmacol* 1991;69:865–870.

181. Perret G, Yin YL, Nicolas P, et al. Amiodarone decreases cardiac beta-adrenoceptors through an antagonistic effect on 3,5,3′ triiodothyronine. *J Cardiovasc Pharmacol* 1992;19:473–478.

182. Gotzsche LBH. Beta-adrenergic receptors, voltage-operated Ca2+ -channels, nuclear triiodothyronine receptors and triiodothyronine concentration in pig myocardium after long-term low-dose amiodarone treatment. *Acta Endocrinol (Copenh)* 1993;129:337–347.

183. Figge HL, Figge J. The effects of amiodarone on thyroid hormone function: a review of the physiology and clinical manifestations. *J Clin Pharmacol* 1990;30:588–595.

184. Figge J, Dluhy RG. Amiodarone-induced elevation of thyroid stimulating hormone in patients receiving levothyroxine for primary hypothyroidism. *Ann Intern Med* 1990;113:553–555.

11D   NONTHYROIDAL ILLNESS

WILLIAM M. WIERSINGA

Changes in the function of the hypothalamic–pituitary–thyroid axis and in thyroid hormone transport and metabolism are common in patients with nonthyroidal illness. Illness in this context comprises virtually all nonthyroidal disorders, surgical and nonsurgical trauma, and inadequate caloric intake. Many patients with nonthyroidal illness also receive drugs that affect thyroid hormone regulation and metabolism, but for the sake of clarity pharmacologic in-

terference is not considered an intrinsic part of the spectrum of changes in hypothalamic–pituitary–thyroid function that occurs in these patients.

The effects of illness are not confined to the thyroid axis; in fact, illness induces temporary changes in many neuroendocrine systems (1). The changes in thyroid function are therefore only one component of the neuroendocrine response to illness and can be viewed as part of the general adaptation to stress. It is thus reasonable to assume that these changes contribute to the maintenance of homeostasis in patients with any illness.

The changes in hypothalamic–pituitary–thyroid function are sometimes referred to as the sick euthyroid syndrome. This name is not appropriate, for several reasons. First, there is no single syndrome, but rather a constellation of changes of widely varying magnitude. Second, it is not clear that the patients are in fact euthyroid in those tissues that are targets for the action of thyroid hormone (2,3). The changes to be described here in humans and animals have been reviewed extensively (3–7); those that occur in animals are discussed here only to clarify aspects of the changes for which data from humans are lacking. Although these changes are heterogeneous, as is most evident from the particular changes in patients with specific disease entities, the majority of illnesses induce a rather uniform pattern of changes.

DESCRIPTION OF NONTHYROIDAL ILLNESS

Changes in Serum Thyroid Hormone and Thyrotropin Concentrations

Serum Triiodothyronine and Reverse Triiodothyronine Concentrations

A fall in serum triiodothyronine (T_3) concentrations and a rise in serum reverse triiodothyronine (rT_3) concentrations are the most common changes in patients with nonthyroidal illness, which is often referred to as the low T_3 syndrome. Fasting induces these changes in serum T_3 and rT_3 concentrations within 24 to 36 hours, and the values return rapidly to baseline upon refeeding. The composition of the food is relevant: refeeding with glucose is more effective in restoring normal values than refeeding with equicaloric amounts of protein or fat (4). Similarly, serum T_3 concentrations fall and serum rT_3 concentrations rise within a few hours after initiation of general anesthesia and surgery, and return to normal in several days if the postoperative course is uncomplicated.

The low serum T_3/high rT_3 pattern is found in patients with most acute and chronic illnesses, including infectious diseases, infiltrative and metabolic disorders, cardiovascular diseases, pulmonary diseases, gastrointestinal diseases, cancer, burns, and trauma. Serum rT_3 concentrations increase to supranormal values in patients with mild illnesses and do not increase much more in patients with more severe illnesses. In contrast, serum T_3 concentrations decrease further as the severity of illness increases (Fig. 11D.1). Serum T_3 concentrations are low or even undetectable in patients with critical illnesses, and they are persistently low in patients with chronic illnesses. The severity of the illness is in general reflected by the magnitude of the changes in serum T_3 and rT_3 concentrations. For example,

there is an inverse relationship between serum T_3 concentrations and glycosylated hemoglobin values in patients with diabetes mellitus and between serum T_3 concentrations and serum creatinine concentrations in patients with renal insufficiency. Similarly, in patients who have a myocardial infarction, the size of the infarction is inversely related to the fall in serum T_3 concentrations and directly related to the rise in serum rT_3 concentrations.

In general, serum free T_3 concentrations fall to a lesser extent than do serum total T_3 concentrations, but the results of measurements of serum free T_3 in patients with nonthyroidal illness depend greatly on the assay used. Indirect methods in which the fraction of serum T_3 that is unbound is measured give low values (8,9) more often than when serum free T_3 is measured directly (direct measurement of free T_3 after physical separation from bound T_3) (10,11).

Serum Thyroxine and Free Thyroxine Concentrations

Serum thyroxine (T_4) concentrations do not change during fasting in healthy subjects, but they decrease in patients with

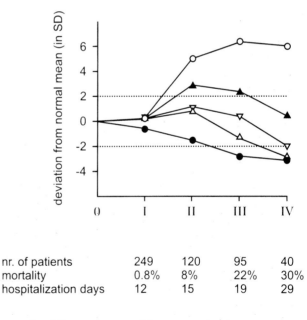

nr. of patients	249	120	95	40
mortality	0.8%	8%	22%	30%
hospitalization days	12	15	19	29

severity of illness   mild ⟶ moderate ⟶ severe

FIGURE 11D.1. Serum thyroid hormone concentrations (*filled circle*, triiodothyronine (T_3); *open circle*, reverse T_3 (rT_3); *open triangle*, thyroxine (T_4); *upside down open triangle*, free T_4 index; *closed triangle*, free T_4, measured by equilibrium dialysis) in 504 newly hospitalized patients, divided as follows: group I, all values within the normal reference range; group II, serum rT_3 values high but serum T_3 and T_4 values normal; group III, serum T_3 values low but serum T_4 values normal; group IV, serum T_3 and T_4 values low. The hospitalization days are given as median days for the survivors. (From Docter R, Krenning EP, de Jong M, et al. The sick euthyroid syndrome: changes in thyroid hormone serum parameters and hormone metabolism. *Clin Endocrinol (Oxf)* 1993;39:499, with permission.)

protein-calorie malnutrition. Patients with mild to moderate nonthyroidal illnesses usually have normal serum T_4 concentrations. Some severely ill patients have low serum T_4 concentrations (Fig. 11D.1), and among them, serum T_4 concentrations are inversely correlated with the mortality rate.

There is uncertainty about serum free T_4 concentrations in patients with nonthyroidal illness; the results vary depending on the method of measurement (see Chapter 13). When measured directly, using methods that involve initial physical separation of free T_4 from protein-bound T_4 by equilibrium dialysis or ultrafiltration with minimal dilution of serum so as not to alter the equilibrium between free and bound T_4, and quantification by radioimmunoassay, serum free T_4 concentrations are usually normal or even high in patients with nonthyroidal illness, even in those who are critically ill and have low serum total T_4 concentrations (11). In contrast, the serum free T_4 values are normal or low when measured indirectly, by two-step immunoassays in which free T_4 is immunoextracted from serum, analogue immunoassays that use labeled analogues of T_4 that bind to T_4 antibodies but not to serum thyroid hormone–binding proteins, or index methods in which free T_4 values are calculated as the product of the serum total T_4 concentration and a test of the number of unoccupied serum protein-binding sites (thyroid hormone–binding ratio or T_3-resin uptake) (Fig. 11D.1) (12–14). None of these methods for measuring serum free T_4 is completely free of methodologic artifacts.

The issue is further complicated by the decrease in serum protein concentrations (especially the concentrations of transthyretin and albumin) that occur in some patients with severe nonthyroidal illnesses. The analogue methods may give falsely low values for serum free T_4 due to differences in serum proteins between patients with nonthyroidal illness and the standard serum used in the assays. The two-step serum free T_4 assays are better validated, but vulnerable to an *in vitro* effect of heparin (which falsely raises measured serum free T_4 values) or the influence of sample dilution (which attenuates the effect of inhibitors of binding). Furthermore, the serum of some patients with nonthyroidal illness contains substances that inhibit the binding of T_4 to serum binding proteins, which may explain in part results suggesting that T_4 binding is decreased in some of the patients (15,16). Based on the most reliable

assays, it appears that most patients with nonthyroidal illness, even critically ill patients, have serum free T_4 concentrations that are within the normal reference range.

Serum Thyrotropin Concentrations

Serum thyrotropin (TSH) concentrations are normal in most patients with nonthyroidal illness, but may increase to slightly above the normal range (10 to 20 mU/L) for a few days soon after recovery begins (17,18). However, some critically ill patients who have low serum T_4 concentrations also have low serum TSH concentrations (19), although the serum TSH concentrations are rarely as low as in patients with thyrotoxicosis. The serum TSH response to thyrotropin-releasing hormone (TRH) is usually proportional to the baseline serum TSH concentration. Thus, critically ill patients with low basal serum TSH concentrations have low serum TSH responses to TRH, and both findings are indicative of a poor prognosis (20). Additionally, critically ill patients are often treated with infusions of dopamine or high doses of glucocorticoids, both of which lower serum TSH concentrations, even in normal subjects (see section on regulation of thyrotropin secretion in Chapter 10).

Changes in Thyroid Hormone Kinetics

Kinetic studies of thyroid hormone production and metabolism have been conducted in normal subjects during fasting and in patients with chronic renal failure, cirrhosis, diabetes mellitus, mild illness, and critical illness. The results can be summarized as follows (21). In patients with low serum T_3 concentrations, the production rate of T_3 is decreased, but its metabolic clearance rate is unchanged. The decrease in T_3 production is due to decreased extrathyroidal deiodination of T_4 to T_3, which normally provides ~80% of the daily T_3 production (Fig. 11D.2). The fractional rate of transport of T_3 into tissues is unaltered. For rT_3, the production rate is unchanged, but the metabolic clearance rate is decreased, due to decreased extrathyroidal deiodination of rT_3 to 3,3'-diiodothyronine. For T_4 the metabolic clearance rate is usually normal, but it may be increased in patients with severe illnesses who have low serum T_4 concentrations, due at least in part to decreased production of one

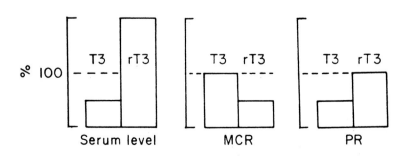

FIGURE 11D.2. Effect of nonthyroidal illness on serum concentrations, metabolic clearance rate (*MCR*), and production rate (*PR*) of triiodothyronine (T_3) and reverse T_3 (rT_3; expressed as a percentage of the values in normal subjects). (From Doctor R, Krenning EP, de Jong M, et al. The sick euthyroid syndrome: changes in thyroid hormone serum parameters and hormone metabolism. *Clin Endocrinol (Oxf)* 1993;39:499, with permission.)

Changes in Peripheral Thyroid Hormone Metabolism

In biopsies taken from intensive-care-unit patients immediately after death, liver iodothyronine deiodinase type 1 (D1) activity was decreased, whereas iodothyronine 5′-deiodinase type 3 (D3) activity was increased in liver and skeletal muscle (see Chapter 7) (35). Their premortem serum T_3/rT_3 ratio correlated positively with the D1 activity and negatively with the D3 activity in the liver; the levels of D1 and D3 mRNA levels corresponded with the activity of the respective enzyme. The fall in D1 activity, in accord with findings in tissues from starved and sick animals (36), will decrease the extrathyroidal conversion of T_4 to T_3 and of rT_3 to 3,3′-diiodothyronine, thereby contributing to low serum T_3 concentrations and high serum rT_3 concentrations. The remarkable induction of the activity of D3, which degrades T_3 to 3,3′-diiodothyronine, thereby further decreases the availability of T_3. D3 is not detectable in normal liver or muscle, but is found in cardiac muscle in animals with heart failure (37).

The changes in iodothyronine deiodination also affect the serum concentrations of diiodothyronines (38,39). Nondeiodinative pathways of iodothyronine degradation are frequently increased in patients with nonthyroidal illness; serum concentrations of T_3 sulfate are increased (40,41), although those of T_4 sulfate are normal (42). There may be increases in the products of ether-link cleavage, such as diiodotyrosine, and in the products of oxidative deamination of the alanine side chain of T_4 and T_3, which are, respectively, tetraiodothyroacetic acid and triiodothyroacetic acid, in patients with nonthyroidal illness (43).

There are few data on T_3-nuclear receptors in patients with nonthyroidal illness (see Chapter 8). Liver T_3-nuclear receptor-α_1 and -β_1 mRNA and protein levels in patients with hepatic diseases were unchanged, as compared with normal liver (44). In contrast, the number of receptors, but not their affinity, was decreased in the livers of animals that were fasted or had diabetes or cancer (7), and lipopolysaccharide injection in mice caused a major fall in T_3-nuclear receptor-α_1, -α_2 and -β_1 mRNA and protein expression in liver, and binding of the T_3-nuclear receptor/retinoid X receptor heterodimers to DNA was reduced (45). The factors that cause these changes are unknown.

The thyroid hormone content of tissues is decreased in patients with nonthyroidal illness. The mean T_3 concentrations in the cerebral cortex, liver, kidney, and lung were lower by 46% to 76% in patients who died of nonthyroidal illness, as compared with those who died suddenly, but the values in heart and skeletal muscle were similar (31). The mean T_4 concentration in the liver was 66% lower in the patients with nonthyroidal illness, but the values in the cerebral cortex were similar in the two groups.

Thyroid Hormone Action in Tissue

Most if not all of the changes described earlier would seem to indicate that nonthyroidal illness leads to reduction in thyroid hormone production, especially in the production of T_3, and therefore that the availability of T_3 in tissues should be reduced. This raises the important but still incompletely answered question of what the level of thyroid hormone action is in the tissues of patients with nonthyroidal illness. During fasting, oxygen consumption and protein breakdown decrease so that energy is saved and organ function may be preserved. The lower T_3 production rate during fasting might contribute to this useful metabolic adaptation; similar changes occur in hypothyroidism. Prolongation of the Achilles tendon reflex relaxation time in patients with anorexia nervosa and of the pulse-wave arrival time during hypocaloric feeding are compatible with a hypothyroid-like state in undernutrition (Table 11D.1) (46,47).

TABLE 11D.1. SIMILARITIES AND DISSIMILARITIES BETWEEN CHANGES IN INTERMEDIARY METABOLISM AND PERIPHERAL TISSUE FUNCTION TESTS DURING FASTING, HYPOTHYROIDISM, AND ILLNESS

	Fasting	Hypothyroidism	Illness
Resting energy expenditure	↓	↓	↑
Glucose utilization	↓	↓	↑
Proteolysis	↓	↓	↑
Lipolysis	↑	↓	↑
Fat oxidation	↑	↓	↑
Pulse-wave arrival time (QKd) (ref. 46)	↑	↑	=
Achilles tendon reflex half-relaxation time (ref. 47)	↑	↑	=
Serum angiotensin-converting enzyme (ref. 48)		↓	↓
Serum sex hormone-binding globulin (ref. 49)		↓	=
Serum osteocalcin (ref. 49)		↓	=
Erythrocyte Na+,K+-ATPase (ref. 50)		↑	↑

↑, Increase; ↓, decrease; =, no change; Na+,K+-ATPase, sodium, potassium-adenosine triphosphatase; QKd, time interval between Q-wave on electrocardiogram and arrival of pulse wave in brachial artery.

In contrast, the illness-induced changes in glucose, protein, and fat metabolism are opposite to those that occur in hypothyroidism (48–50). In theory, then, the occurrence of the low T_3 syndrome could be a beneficial adaptation to illness, serving to minimize its catabolic effects.

PATHOGENESIS OF CHANGES IN THYROID FUNCTION IN NONTHYROIDAL ILLNESS

Inhibition of Iodothyronine 5'-Deiodinase

The decreased rate of extrathyroidal production of T_3 and decreased metabolic clearance rate of rT_3 during fasting and illness can be explained by a decrease in activity of D1, which catalyses both the 5'-monodeiodination of T_4 to T_3 and of rT_3 to 3,3'-diiodothyronine. The decrease in D1 activity may be due to inhibition by drugs such as high doses of glucocorticoids and propranolol or amiodarone. The increase of cortisol secretion during illness does not appear to contribute to the decrease in D1 activity, because there is no consistent relationship between serum cortisol and T_3 concentrations in patients with nonthyroidal illness, and the decrease in serum T_3 concentrations after abdominal hysterectomy persists despite abolition of the postoperative increase in serum cortisol by afferent nerve blockade (51).

The decrease in liver D1 activity of patients with critical illness (35) might be causally related to cytokines, in view of the capacity of interleukin (IL)-1β, IL-6, tumor necrosis factor (TNF)-α, and interferon-γ to decrease D1 mRNA *in vitro* (52). Indeed, IL-1 and IL-6 inhibit the T_3-induced induction of D1 mRNA and enzyme acitivity in cultured rat hepatocytes; this transcriptional effect can be partially overcome by exogenous steroid receptor coactivator-1 (SRC-1) (53). The proposed mechanism is competition for limiting amounts of nuclear receptor coactivators between the D1 promotor and the promoters of cytokine-induced genes. TNF-α impairs T_3-dependent induction of D1 gene expression by activation of nuclear factor-kappa B, (NF-kB), possibly via sequestration of common cofactors shared between NF-kB and thyroid hormone receptors (54).

Inhibition of Plasma Membrane Transport of Iodothyronines

T_4 and T_3 enter cells by active, energy-dependent transport across the plasma membrane of the cells. Several biologic compounds inhibit cell uptake of T_4 and T_3, as determined by incubation of cultured rat hepatocytes with radioiodine-labeled T_4 or T_3 and subsequent measurements of iodide and T_4 or T_3 conjugates in the medium. This system allows discrimination between inhibition of transport (lowered iodide production without accumulation of conjugates) and inhibition of deiodination (lowered iodide production with accumulation of sulfates and glucuronides). In these cultures, the furan fatty acid 3-carboxy-4-methyl-5-propyl-

2-furan propanoic acid (CMPF), indoxyl sulfate, and hippuric acid all inhibit iodide production, and conjugates do not accumulate. The serum of patients with chronic renal insufficiency has similar effects; the serum concentrations of CMPF and indoxyl sulfate (but not of hippuric acid) in these patients are above the minimum concentration required for *in vitro* inhibition of iodide production by these compounds (55). It follows that CMPF and indoxyl sulfate may be responsible for the low T_3 syndrome in patients with chronic renal insufficiency by inhibiting cellular uptake and subsequent deiodination of T_4. These compounds do not affect the uptake of T_4 or T_3 by cultured rat anterior pituitary cells, nor do they interfere with TSH release (56). Thus, the uptake of thyroid hormones into the pituitary is regulated differently than uptake into the liver.

Bilirubin and nonesterified fatty acids like oleic acid also inhibit T_4 transport into hepatocytes. Inhibition of T_4 transport by the serum of critically ill patients with high serum bilirubin concentrations correlated with the molar ratio of bilirubin to albumin and that of nonesterified fatty acids to albumin (57). There may be other inhibitors of T_4 transport into cells as well. In a study of serum samples from patients with mild, moderate, or severe nonthyroidal illness, the degree of inhibition of T_4 transport into rat hepatocytes was inversely correlated with the patients' serum T_3 concentrations (58).

The liver is a major site for production of T_3 and clearance of rT_3, and inhibition of transport of T_4 and rT_3 (which share the same transport mechanism) into the liver might thus contribute to the characteristic decreases in production of T_3 and clearance of rT_3 that occur in patients with nonthyroidal illness. This fits with data indicating that cellular uptake of thyroid hormones is rate limiting for subsequent intracellular metabolism and nuclear binding, and with the observed reduction of the fractional transfer rate of T_4 from plasma to tissues in patients with nonthyroidal illness (59). Further support for this hypothesis comes from studies in human subjects in whom the low T_3 syndrome caused by caloric deprivation was associated with decreased T_3 and especially T_4 uptake into the liver (60,61). The decrease in uptake, which is an energy-dependent process, could well be due to a low adenosine triphosphate (ATP) content in the liver, as has been demonstrated in starvation and nonthyroidal illness by magnetic resonance spectroscopy (62). Fructose, which lowers hepatic ATP content, indeed decreases hepatic T_4 uptake (63).

Inhibition of Thyroxine Binding to Serum Proteins

Serum concentrations of thyroxine-binding globulin (TBG), the main carrier protein for T_4, are usually normal in patients with nonthyroidal illness, but some patients have slightly low concentrations. The serum concentrations of the two other carrier proteins, transthyretin and albumin, can be low as well. These decreases result in lower serum total T_4 (and T_3) concentrations but should not affect serum free T_4 concentrations under equilibrium conditions. The rapid decrease of TBG (a member of the serpin superfamily) during sepsis and cardiopulmonary bypass might be due to cleavage by inflammatory serine proteases; the smaller TBG cleavage product has a reduced affinity for T_4 (64,65).

Another cause of decreased serum binding of T_4 is the presence of inhibitors of binding. Both protein and non-protein inhibitors of T_4 binding to TBG or the other thyroid hormone–binding proteins have been found in the serum of patients with nonthyroidal illness in different studies (15,16,66–68). The non-protein-binding inhibitors include furosemide, fenclofenac, and salicylate. High doses of these drugs are competitive inhibitors of T_4 binding to TBG. They therefore acutely raise serum free T_4 concentrations, which inhibits TSH secretion, so that serum free T_4 concentrations return to normal; serum T_4 concentrations decrease because the protein-binding sites are occupied by the drug (see Chapter 13).

Nonesterified fatty acids also have been proposed as a nonprotein inhibitor of T_4 binding. Addition of nonesterified fatty acids to normal human serum increases the free T_4 fraction by inhibiting T_4 binding to albumin, but only if the molar ratio of nonesterified fatty acids to albumin is higher than 5:1, a value rarely reached even in critically ill patients (69). Heparin is a weak inhibitor of T_4 binding to TBG. Its action is indirect, via activating serum lipoprotein lipase that then breaks down triglycerides to nonesterified fatty acids (and glycerol) *in vitro*, and can be prevented by adding protamine to the serum *in vitro* (70). Thus, these substances are unlikely to affect T_4 binding appreciably *in vivo*.

Inhibitory Effects of Cytokines

Cytokines are important mediators of the acute phase response to tissue injury. It is thus plausible to suppose that cytokines cause some of the changes in hypothalamic–pituitary–thyroid function that occur in patients with nonthyroidal illness. Indeed, some cytokines, such as IL-1, IL-6, TNF-α, and interferon-γ inhibit the synthesis or secretion of TSH, thyroglobulin, T_3, and thyroid hormone–binding proteins and decrease D1 mRNA and the binding capacity of T_3-nuclear receptors *in vitro* in cultured human and animal cells (52,71). IL-1 and TNF-α act mainly in a paracrine and autocrine fashion; their serum concentrations are mostly undetectable or low, even during illness, and no quantitative relationships have been found between serum T_3 or T_4 concentrations and the serum concentrations of either of these cytokines in patients with nonthyroidal illness (72–74). Similarly, serum T_3 concentrations are not correlated with serum interferon-γ, IL-8, and IL-10 concentra-

tions in these patients (75). In contrast, IL-6 is a systemic cytokine that has endocrine actions, and there is an inverse correlation between serum T_3 and IL-6 concentrations in patients with nonthyroidal illness (Fig. 11D.5) (74,76–78).

Soluble forms of membrane-bound cytokine receptors or receptor antagonists have the ability to modulate cytokine activity and are generated in response to the same inflammatory stimuli that induce cytokine production, and the serum concentrations of these proteins reflect the degree of activation of the cytokine network. Serum T_3 concentrations are negatively correlated with the serum concentrations of solu-

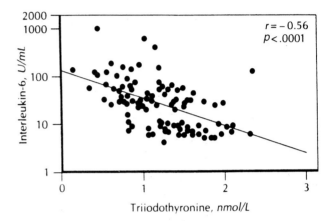

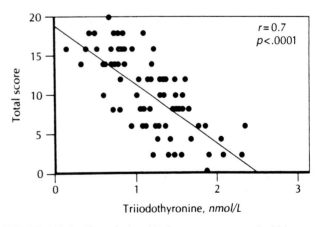

FIGURE 11D.5. The relationship between serum triiodothyronine (T_3) and serum interleukin (IL)-6 concentrations **(top)** and a cytokine score, derived from the summation of serum IL-6, soluble tumour necrosis factors (TNF) receptors (sTNFaRp55 and sTNFaRp75), soluble IL-2 receptor, and IL-1 receptor antagonist concentrations in individual serum samples **(bottom)** in consecutive hospitalized patients with nonthyroidal disease. To convert serum T_3 values to ng/dL, multiply by 65.1. (From Boelen A, Platvoet-ter Schiphorst M, Wiersinga WM. Association between serum interleukin-6 and serum 3,5,3'-triiodothyronine in nonthyroidal illness. *J Clin Endocrinol Metab* 1993;77:1695; and Boelen A, Platvoet-ter Schiphorst MC, Wiersinga WM. Soluble cytokine receptors and the low 3,5,3'-triiodothyronine syndrome in patients with nonthyroidal disease. *J Clin Endocrinol Metab* 1995;80:971, with permission.)

ble TNF receptors (sTNFaRp55 and sTNFaRp75), soluble IL-2 receptors, and IL-1 receptor antagonist in patients with nonthyroidal illness (79). A cytokine score composed of the serum concentrations of soluble cytokine receptors and IL-6 is strongly inversely correlated with serum T_3 concentrations in these patients (Fig. 11D.5). The serum concentrations of C-reactive protein, an acute-phase protein induced by IL-6, also are inversely correlated with serum T_3 concentrations in such patients (74,78).

Administration of single doses of TNF-α, interferon-α, or IL-6 to normal subjects results within hours in a 12% to 25% decrease in serum T_3 concentrations, a 36% to 72% increase in serum rT_3 concentrations, and a 13% to 32% decrease in serum TSH concentrations, whereas serum total and free T_4 concentrations change little (80–82). A single dose of interferon-γ had no effect (83). Despite the resemblance of these changes to those that occur in patients with nonthyroidal illness, the findings do not prove that cytokines cause the changes in patients with nonthyroidal illness. Furthermore, administration of cytokines causes an influenza-like illness, with headache, nausea, and fever, which may cause the hormonal changes via other mechanisms. Chronic administration of cytokines to humans or experimental animals also results in transient changes in thyroid hormone metabolism and regulation, possibly explained by the capacity of cytokines—which operate both as a cascade and as a network—to modulate the production of other cytokines and cytokine receptors.

Administration of bacterial endotoxin to normal subjects is followed by a fall in serum T_3, free T_4, and TSH concentrations, and a rise in serum rT_3 concentrations. Blocking the action of IL-1 by coadministration of IL-1 receptor antagonist or the action of TNF-α by administration of recombinant dimeric TNF receptors has no effect on the endotoxin-induced changes (84,85). The results of studies of immunoneutralization of cytokines in animals have also been inconclusive (86). The best evidence to date for a causal role of cytokines in the pathogenesis of the changes in nonthyroidal illness comes from experiments with IL-6 knock-out mice (87), in which the decrease in serum T_3 concentrations during induced illness is less than that of normal mice; hepatic D1 activity does not change in the knock-out mice but decreases in normal mice.

Inhibition of Thyrotropin-Releasing Hormone and Thyrotropin Secretion

The changes in the relationship between serum TSH and serum thyroid hormone concentrations in patients with nonthyroidal illness indicate a decrease in the sensitivity of TSH secretion to decreases in serum T_4 and T_3 concentrations. A decrease in sensitivity is further suggested by the smaller than normal increase in serum TSH concentrations

in response to the small decreases in serum T_4 and T_3 concentrations induced by administration of inorganic iodide that occurs in patients with nonthyroidal illness (88). The cause of the change in sensitivity of the thyrotroph cells is not known, but the decrease in TRH gene expression in the paraventricular nucleus of the hypothalamus in patients with nonthyroidal illness is correlated with the decrease in serum TSH concentrations (30). Changes in brain thyroid-hormone metabolism or in serum cortisol and leptin concentrations, as well as induction of cytokines, could be involved in the down-regulation of TRH (see section on regulation of thyrotropin secretion in Chapter 10).

In humans, T_3-nuclear receptors are found in the hypothalamic paraventricular nucleus and infundibular nucleus (the human homologue of the rat arcuate nucleus). Iodothyronine-5'-deiodinase type 2 (D2) is—at least in rats—not expressed in the paraventricular nucleus, but is present in the arcuate nucleus in tanycytes, specialized ependymal cells lining the wall of the third ventricle near the median eminence of the hypothalamus. In fasted rats, D2 activity in the arcuate nucleus is upregulated: the increase of locally produced T_3 is likely responsible for lower TRH synthesis in the paraventricular nucleus, but which neurons of the arcuate nucleus projecting to the paraventricular nucleus mediate this effect is unknown (89). In systemic illness induced by bacterial lipopolysaccharide in rats, D2 activity increased markedly in the anterior pituitary and in tanycytes; the locally generated T_3 may suppress the synthesis of pituitary TSH as well as that of TRH (90).

Adrenalectomy in rats results in an increase in TRH mRNA in the paraventricular nucleus, and administration of glucocorticoid reverses the increase (91). However, the hypercortisolism of critically ill patients probably does not contribute to the fall in TRH production, because TRH production remains low when adrenalectonized animals treated with corticosterone are given lipopolysaccharide (92).

The adipocyte-derived hormone leptin has been recognized as an important mediator of neuroendocrine changes during illness. Leptin binds to leptin receptors in the infundibular nucleus where neuropeptide-Y (NPY)-containing cells are key targets. NPY, agouti-related protein (AGRP), and α-melanocyte stimulating hormone (α-MSH) neurons project directly from the infundibular nucleus to hypophysiotropic TRH neurons in the paraventricular nucleus (93). NPY and AGRP (both suppressed by leptin) inhibit and α-MSH (induced by leptin) stimulates TRH gene expression (83,94,95). In starved animals, the fall in serum leptin concentrations is associated with a decrease of TRH mRNA in the paraventricular nucleus, and administration of leptin reverses the decrease in TRH mRNA (96). This effect is mediated via the arcuate nucleus, because ablation of the arcuate nucleus prevents the decrease in hypothalamic TRH and serum T_4 concentrations during fasting and prevents the reversal of these changes by leptin (97). In humans, however, administration of leptin only partially prevents the starvation-induced decrease in serum TSH concentrations, and does not prevent the fall in serum T_3 concentrations or the rise in rT_3 concentrations (98).

In patients with systemic illness serum leptin concentrations are often increased, like they do acutely in response to administration of TNF-α or IL-1, but the increase is not related to serum T_3 and T_4 concentrations (99,100). In rats, endotoxin increases serum leptin concentrations and propiomelanocortin but not NPY gene expression in the arcuate nucleus, which together would increase rather than decrease hypothalamic TRH production. Furthermore, serum leptin is negatively correlated with NPY mRNA expression in the infundibular nucleus of critically ill patients, and the NPY expression is—in contrast to the situation in food-deprived rodents—positively correlated with TRH mRNA expression in the paraventricular nucleus (101). There is thus no evidence that leptin is involved in the changes in peripheral thyroid hormone metabolism; leptin may be

partially responsible for the decrease in TSH secretion during fasting, but probably has no role in systemic illness.

The role of cytokines (especially IL-1β) in the activation of the hypothalamic–pituitary–adrenal axis is well known. Cytokines also affect TRH production, at least in rats. The hypothalamic content of TRH mRNA decreases after administration of IL-1, inappropriate for the decrease in serum T_3 and T_4 concentrations that occurs at the same time (102). Interleukin-1β decreases the release of TSH (but not of other anterior pituitary hormones) in cultured rat anterior pituitary cells, an effect not mediated by thyroid hormone uptake or T_3 nuclear receptor occupancy (103). The effect of TNF-α on TSH release is disputed. Interleukin-6 decreases TSH secretion, possibly by a direct effect on the thyrotrophs.

There are few studies on the handling of thyroid hormones in the pituitary during nonthyroidal illness, but the available data do not indicate that thyroid hormone uptake is altered (56). Up-regulation of D2 activity in the medio-

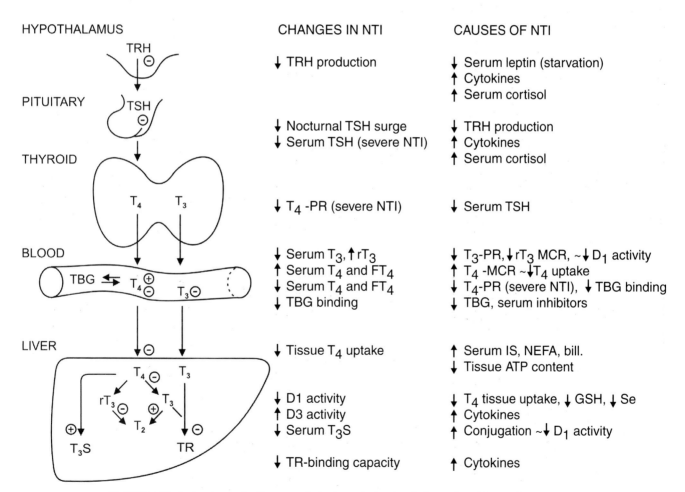

FIGURE 11D.6. A schematic diagram of the hypothalamic–pituitary–thyroid axis showing the changes that occur in patients with nonthyroidal illness (*NTI*) and the causes of those changes (for explanation, see text). *bil*, bilirubin; *D1*, iodothyronine 5′-deiodinase type 1; *D3*, iodothyronine 5-deiodinase type 3; *GSH*, glutathione; *IS*, indoxyl sulfate; *MCR*, metabolic clearance rate; *NEFA*, nonesterified fatty acids; *PR*, production rate; *Se*, selenium; *TR*, thyroid receptor; *T_3S*, triiodothyronine (T_3) sulfate.

basal hypothalamus and anterior pituitary, as found during critical illness, may contribute to suppression of production of TRH and TSH, respectively, and it is tempting to speculate that cytokines are involved. Experimental data support the notion that cytokines induce D2 activity in tanycytes via NF-kB binding sites in the promoter region of the D2 gene (54).

The down-regulation at the hypothalamus–pituitary level provides an explanation for the decreased sensitivity of TSH secretion to low serum T_3 and T_4 concentrations in patients with nonthyroidal illness. Specifically, decreased TRH secretion is the likely cause of the decreased nocturnal TSH surge and the release of TSH of reduced biologic activity, phenomena akin to the changes in some patients with central hypothyroidism.

The changes in hypothalamic–pituitary–thyroid function that occur in patients with nonthyroidal illness thus occur as a result of changes in both the central and peripheral compartments of the thyroid endocrine system (Fig. 11D.6). Although a persistent decrease in TRH and TSH secretion might lead to a decrease in T_4 production, the peripheral changes develop independent of changes in the hypothalamus and pituitary. It follows that the factors mediating the various changes are operative simultaneously both centrally and peripherally.

CLINICAL IMPORTANCE OF THE CHANGES IN THYROID FUNCTION IN NONTHYROIDAL ILLNESS

Prognostic Importance

The magnitude of the changes that occur in patients with nonthyroidal illness in general reflects the severity of the illness, and several of the individual changes have been linked to outcome in different studies. In general, the prognosis is poorer in patients with lower serum T_3, T_4, or TSH concentrations or higher serum rT_3 concentrations. In a study of critically ill patients admitted to an intensive care unit, the sensitivity and specificity in predicting mortality were 75% and 80%, respectively, for a serum T_4 concentration of <3.1 µg/dL (40 nmol/L), 56% and 100% for an 8 AM serum cortisol concentration of >30 µg/dL (830 nmol/L), and 100% and 82% for the combination (104).

Diagnosis of Thyroid Disease in Nonthyroidal Illness

The prevalence of nonthyroidal illness depends on what groups of patients are evaluated. Among patients admitted to hospital medical services, the prevalence of a low serum T_3 concentration is ~50%, that of a low serum T_4 concen-

tration is ~15% to 20%, and that of an abnormal (low or high) serum TSH concentration ~10%. The changes are less frequent among outpatients and more frequent among patients admitted to intensive care units.

The high prevalence of changes among hospitalized patients hampers the diagnosis of thyrotoxicosis or hypothyroidism among them, and therefore argues against screening them for thyroid dysfunction. In patients clinically suspected to have thyroid disease, the single most useful test is measurement of serum TSH. A normal result virtually excludes thyrotoxicosis or hypothyroidism (as it does among outpatients) (105,106).

A high serum TSH concentration is compatible with primary hypothyroidism, but also with nonthyroidal illness, if the elevation is slight (Fig. 11D.7). The combination of high serum TSH and low T_4 concentrations increases the likelihood of hypothyroidism, but also can be found in patients recovering from a nonthyroidal illness. The finding of a high ratio of T_3 to T_4 in serum, a low thyroid hormone–binding ratio, and a low serum rT_3 concentration favor the presence of hypothyroidism, because the opposite changes occur in nonthyroidal illness, but the diagnostic accuracy of any of these measurements is limited (107). Furthermore, in patients with hypothyroidism the high serum TSH concentrations may decrease, even into the normal range, during an acute illness, especially in those patients given dopamine or high doses of glucocorticoids (108).

A low serum TSH value in any patient raises the possibility of thyrotoxicosis, especially if the serum free T_4 concentration is high. This combination of test results is unfortunately also found in patients with nonthyroidal illness. However, the greater the extent of TSH suppression, the greater the likelihood of thyrotoxicosis (Fig. 11D.7). The combination of thyrotoxicosis and nonthyroidal illness may cause T_4-thyrotoxicosis because the illness causes a decrease in serum T_3 concentrations in patients with thyrotoxicosis just as it does in any other patient (Fig. 11D.8).

In some of these situations, history, physical examination, and the presence of high serum thyroid antibody concentrations can provide further clues to the presence or absence of thyroid disease. In many patients, however, no definite diagnosis can be established, and the most prudent policy is to repeat the thyroid function tests after the nonthyroidal illness has improved.

Thyroid Hormone Treatment of Patients with Nonthyroidal Illness

In obese subjects starting a hypocaloric diet, maintenance of baseline serum T_3 concentrations by administration of T_3 prevents the occurrence of hypothyroid-like effects such as a

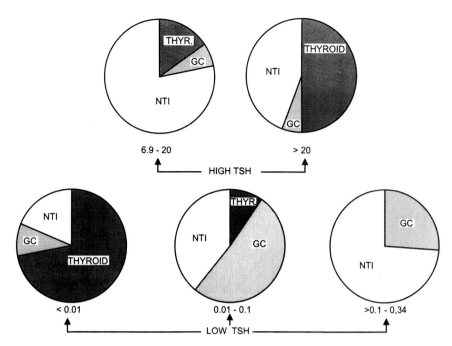

FIGURE 11D.7. The proportion of patients with thyroid disease (*Thyr. or Thyroid*), nonthyroidal illness (*NTI*), and receiving glucocorticoid therapy (*GC*) among a large group of hospitalized patients, subdivided according to five ranges of serum thyrotropin TSH concentrations. (From Stockigt JR. Guidelines for diagnosis and monitoring of thyroid disease: nonthyroidal illness. *Clin Chem* 1996;42:188, modified with permission; and Spencer CA. Clinical utility and cost-effectiveness of sensitive thyrotropin assays in ambulatory and hospitalized patients. *Mayo Clin Proc* 1988;63: 1214, with permission.)

decrease in pulse rate and oxygen consumption and prolongation of the pulse-wave arrival time (46,109). In fasting normal subjects, prevention of the decrease in serum T_3 concentrations by exogenous T_3 administration increases protein breakdown and inhibits TSH secretion (110). These results suggest that the occurrence of the low T_3 syndrome during periods of inadequate caloric intake has pro-

tective value in conserving energy and limiting proteolysis. However, administration of T_3 during more prolonged fasting does not increase proteolysis, but does increase hepatic glucose appearance (109,111,112). The role of insulin might be important in this respect, because decreasing insulin secretion during fasting is a critical determinant of the shift from carbohydrate- to fat-based metabolism.

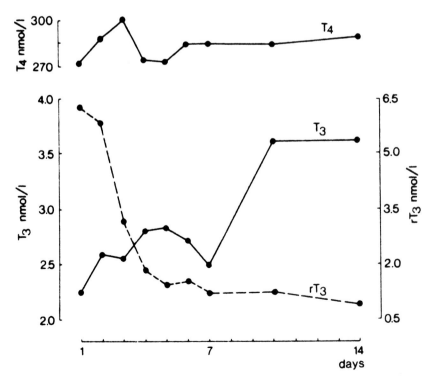

FIGURE 11D.8. Serum thyroxine (T_4), triiodothyronine (T_3), and reverse T_3 (rT_3) concentrations in a patient with thyrotoxicosis hospitalized for treatment of pneumonia. The initial values represented the biochemical pattern of T_4-thyrotoxicosis, but with recovery from the pneumonia they evolved to those of classical thyrotoxicosis with high serum T_4 and T_3 concentrations. Serum thyrotropin values were undetectable at all times. To convert serum T_4 values to µg/dL, multiply by 0.078; and to convert serum T_3 and rT_3 values to ng/dL, multiply by 65.1.

In severely ill patients with serum T_4 concentrations <5.0 µg/dL (65 nmol/L), intravenous administration of replacement doses of T_4 (1.5 µg/kg/day) for 2 weeks did not reduce mortality as compared with untreated patients; during treatment the patients given T_4 had serum T_3 concentrations similar to those in the other group, but their serum T_4 concentrations were higher and their serum TSH concentrations were lower (113). Likewise, administration of T_3 to patients with severe burns did not reduce mortality despite restoration of normal serum free T_3 index values (114), and T_4 given intravenously to patients with acute renal failure actually increased mortality (115). In patients with chronic renal insufficiency, T_3 administration increased proteolysis (116). Finally, administration of T_4 or T_3 to animals with nonthyroidal illness has no clinically beneficial effect and may in fact increase mortality (117–119). Taken together, the results of these studies argue against thyroid-hormone treatment of patients with nonthyroidal illness, including those with low serum TSH and T_4 concentrations, and instead suggest that the changes are beneficial adaptations to illness.

In general, the acute-phase response to illness is not uniformly beneficial: when extreme, it can be fatal, as for example in patients with septic shock. The possibility remains that the changes may represent maladaptation. In adult patients undergoing coronary artery bypass surgery, serum T_3 concentrations decrease by ~40% within minutes or hours after the operation. In studies in which supraphysiologic doses of T_3 were given starting immediately after completion of bypass surgery, resulting in supranormal serum T_3 concentrations, the cardiac index was slightly higher and systemic vascular resistance was slightly lower in the patients given T_3, as compared with placebo. The need for inotropic drugs or mechanical assistance, the incidence of atrial fibrillation, and postoperative morbidity and mortality were lower in some but not all studies (120–123). In children with congenital heart disease T_3 treatment, as compared with placebo, after cardiac surgery

also increased cardiac output and decreased systemic vascular resistance (124,125). The overall utility of T_3 administration after cardiac surgery is still not fully established.

Lastly, co-infusion of growth hormone–releasing peptide (GHRP-2) plus TRH (but not TRH alone) in protracted critical illness induced restoration of pulsatile growth hormone and TSH release, near-normal serum T_4 and T_3 values, and a shift toward anabolic metabolism (126). This interesting finding corroborates the neuroendocrine component of nonthyroidal illness.

SPECIFIC TYPES OF NONTHYROIDAL ILLNESS

Chronic Renal Insufficiency

Serum T_3 concentrations are low, but serum rT_3 concentrations may not be high in patients with chronic renal insufficiency (Table 11D.2). This poses a conceptual problem because hepatic uptake of rT_3 as well as that of T_4 is thought to be inhibited in these patients. Serum free T_3 and free T_4 concentrations are lower in the patients than in normal subjects, independent of the assay method used, and increase slightly after hemodialysis (126,127). After transplantation, serum T_3 concentrations reflect graft function (128). A high frequency of goiter, up to 43% in one study, has been described in patients with chronic renal insufficiency, and has been attributed to high serum inorganic iodide concentrations (129).

Liver Disease

Patients with cirrhosis have changes in serum thyroid hormone and TSH concentrations similar to those of patients with nonthyroidal illness in general. In those with infectious hepatitis, serum T_4 and T_3 concentrations are often

TABLE 11D.2. CHANGES IN SERUM THYROID HORMONE AND THYROTROPIN CONCENTRATIONS IN PATIENTS WITH NONTHYROIDAL ILLNESS

	Serum T_3	Serum rT_3	Serum T_4	Serum free T_4	Serum TSH
Fasting	↓	↑	=	=	↓
Mild illness	↓	↑	=	=,↑	=
Critical illness	↓	↑	↓	=,↓	↓
Surgical trauma, burns	↓	↑	↓	↓	=,↓
Chronic renal failure	↓	=	=,↓	=,↓	=,↓
Hepatitis	=,↑	=,↑	=,↑	=,↓	=
HIV infection	=	↓	=	=,↓	=,↑
Depression	=,↓	=,↑	=,↑	=,↑	=,↓

=, no change; ↑ or ↓; direction of change compared with values in normal subjects; HIV, human immunodeficiency virus; rT_3, reverse triiodothyronine; T_4, thyroxine; TSH, thyrotropin.

high, due to an increase in serum TBG concentrations; their serum free T_4 and T_3 concentrations are usually normal. The findings are similar in patients with chronic active hepatitis and primary biliary cirrhosis, except in those with substantial hepatic insufficiency, in whom the concentrations decrease.

Human Immunodeficiency Virus Infection

Patients with asymptomatic human immunodeficiency virus (HIV) infection or those with the acquired immunodeficiency syndrome (AIDS) who have no opportunistic infections or hepatic dysfunction have normal serum T_4 and T_3 concentrations. Their serum free T_4 index values and free T_4 concentrations are normal or slightly low (130,131). Some of the patients have slightly high serum TBG concentrations, which tend to be inversely related to the percentage of CD4 cells, and serum TBG values have been used as a surrogate marker for disease progression (132). Serum TSH concentrations can be slightly high as well, but the small changes in TBG and TSH are different from those in nonthyroidal illness, and their pathogenesis and relevance are unknown. The prevalence of subclinical hypothyroidism may be increased in patients with HIV infection, especially in patients receiving highly active antiretroviral therapy (HAART) (133–135). The HAART-associated lipodystrophy characterized by peripheral fat wasting and central adiposity is apparently not related to thyroid function (136).

Patients with AIDS complicated by *Pneumocystis carinii* infections or other serious infections have the typical findings of patients with other severe nonthyroidal illness (137).

Psychiatric Disease

Patients with posttraumatic stress disorder may have slightly high serum T_4, T_3, and TBG concentrations, but their serum free T_4 and free T_3 concentrations are normal (138). Among patients with acute psychosis who are hospitalized, ~10% have some abnormality in thyroid function, including high or low serum TSH concentrations and high serum T_4 concentrations (139,140). The changes are somewhat dependent on the particular psychiatric disorder; patients with substance abuse are more likely to have high serum TSH concentrations, whereas those with mood disorders tend to have high serum T_4 concentrations (with low, normal, or high serum TSH concentrations). The tests usually become normal in 7 to 10 days.

Patients with rapid cycling bipolar disorder may have slightly low serum T_4 concentrations and high serum TSH concentrations. Those with major depression tend to have higher than average serum T_4 and free T_4 concentrations (although the values are usually within the respective normal ranges) and low basal and TRH-stimulated serum TSH concentrations (141), in line with a decreased TRH mRNA in the paraventricular nucleus (142). The hypercortisolism and hyperthyroxinemia in patients with depression may inhibit D2 activity in the brain, resulting in low intracerebral T_3 content. This may exaggerate the decrease in brain serotonin concentrations that occurs in depressed patients. Such a mechanism may explain why administration of T_3 might be effective in patients with depression refractory to tricyclic antidepressant drugs, as has been reported in some but not all studies (143,144). A recent study, however, found that the efficacy and the rapidity of the response to selective serotonin reuptake inhibitors was not increased by adding T_3 (145).

CONCLUSION

Patients with nonthyroidal illness have many changes in hypothalamic–pituitary–thyroid function, the magnitude of which roughly correlates with the severity of the illness. The changes include central down-regulation by inhibition of the hypothalamus–pituitary–thyroid axis and peripheral down-regulation by inhibition of the extrathyroidal production of T_3. The central and peripheral changes can occur independently of each other. The pathogenesis of these changes is almost certainly multifactorial, with various mechanisms simultaneously operative at different levels. Overall, the changes are apparently geared to limit the impact of T_3 on its target organs, which from a teleologic point of view might be a beneficial adaptation during starvation and illness to conserve energy and substrates and minimize excessive tissue catabolism. Although severe nonthyroidal illness may represent maladaptation, the limited data available suggest that administration of thyroid hormone to patients with nonthyroidal illness does not improve the outcome of their illness, but high doses of T_3 given directly after cardiac surgery may have some clinical utility. The ill-chosen term "nonthyroidal illness syndrome" might better be replaced by thyroid hormone adaptation syndrome.

REFERENCES

1. Van den Berghe G, de Zegher F, Bouillon R. Acute and prolonged critical illness as different neuroendocrine paradigms. *J Clin Endocrinol Metab* 1998;83:1827.
2. Chopra IJ. Euthyroid sick syndrome: is it a misnomer? *J Clin Endocrinol Metab* 1997;82:329.
3. DeGroot LJ. Dangerous dogmas in medicine: the nonthyroidal illness syndrome. *J Clin Endocrinol Metab* 1999;84:151.
4. Wartofsky L, Burman KD. Alterations in thyroid function in patients with systemic illness: the "euthyroid sick syndrome." *Endocr Rev* 1982;3:164.
5. Wartofsky L. The low T_3 or "sick euthyroid syndrome": update 1994. *Endocr Rev* 1994;3:248.

6. Docter R, Krenning EP, de Jong M, et al. The sick euthyroid syndrome: changes in thyroid hormone serum parameters and hormone metabolism. *Clin Endocrinol (Oxf)* 1993;39:499.

7. Tibaldi JM, Surks MI. Animal models of nonthyroidal disease. *Endocr Rev* 1985;6:87.

8. Mak YT, Chan ELP, Chan A, et al. Free triiodothyronine in sera of acutely ill general medical patients: a prognostic indicator? *Clin Chem* 1992;38:414.

9. Sapin R, Schlienger JL, Kaltenbach G, et al. Determination of free triiodothyronine by six different methods in patients with non-thyroidal illness and in patients treated with amiodarone. *Ann Clin Biochem* 1995;32:314.

10. Faber J, Siersbaek-Nielsen K. Serum free 3,5,3'-triiodothyronine (T$_3$) in non-thyroidal somatic illness, as measured by ultrafiltration and immunoextraction. *Clin Chim Acta* 1996; 256:115.

11. Chopra IJ. Simultaneous measurement of free thyroxine and free 3,5,3'-triiodothyronine in undiluted serum by direct equilibrium dialysis/radioimmunoassay: evidence that free triiodothyronine and free thyroxine are normal in many patients with the low triiodothyronine syndrome. *Thyroid* 1998; 8:249.

12. Surks MI, Hupart KH, Pan C, et al. Normal free thyroxine in critical nonthyroidal illnesses measured by ultrafiltration of undiluted serum and equilibrium dialysis. *J Clin Endocrinol Metab* 1988;67:1031.

13. Wong TK, Pekary AE, Hoo GS, et al. Comparison of methods for measuring free thyroxine in nonthyroidal illness. *Clin Chem* 1992;38:720.

14. Docter R, Toor H van, Krenning EP, et al. Free thyroxine assessed with three assays in sera of patients with nonthyroidal illness and of subjects with abnormal concentrations of thyroxine-binding proteins. *Clin Chem* 1993;39:1668.

15. Chopra IJ, Teco GNC, Nguyen AH, et al. In search of an inhibitor in non-thyroidal illnesses. *J Clin Endocrinol Metab* 1979;49:63.

16. Oppenheimer JH, Schwartz HL, Mariash CN, et al. Evidence for a factor in the sera of patients with non-thyroidal disease which inhibits iodothyronine binding to solid matrices, serum proteins, and rat hepatocytes. *J Clin Endocrinol Metab* 1982; 54:757.

17. Hamblin PS, Dyer SA, Mohr VS, et al. Relationship between thyrotropin and thyroxine changes during recovery from severe hypothyroxinemia of critical illness. *J Clin Endocrinol Metab* 1986;62:717.

18. Feelders RA, Swaak AJG, Romijn JA, et al. Characteristics of recovery from the euthyroid sick syndrome induced by tumor necrosis factor alpha in cancer patients. *Metabolism* 1999;48: 324.

19. Wehman RE, Gregerman RI, Burns WH, et al. Suppression of thyrotropin in the low-thyroxine state of severe nonthyroidal illness. *N Engl J Med* 1985;312:546.

20. Sumita S, Ujike Y, Namiki A, et al. Suppression of the thyrotropin response to thyrotropin-releasing hormone and its association with severity of critical illness. *Crit Care Med* 1994; 22:1603.

21. Kaptein EM. Thyroid hormone metabolism in illness. In: Hennemann G, ed. *Thyroid hormone metabolism.* New York: Marcel Dekker Inc, 1986:297.

22. Romijn JA, Adriaanse R, Brabant G, et al. Pulsatile secretion of thyrotropin during fasting: a decrease of thyrotropin pulse amplitude. *J Clin Endocrinol Metab* 1990;71:1631.

23. Bartalena L, Martino E, Brandi LS, et al. Lack of nocturnal serum thyrotropin surge after surgery. *J Clin Endocrinol Metab* 1990;70:293.

24. Wheatly T, Clark PMS, Clark JDA, et al. Abnormalities of thyrotropin (TSH) evening rise and pulsatile release in haemodialysis patients: evidence for hypothalamic-pituitary changes in chronic renal failure. *Clin Endocrinol (Oxf)* 1989;31:39.

25. Arem R, Deppe S. Fatal nonthyroidal illness may impair nocturnal thyrotropin levels. *Am J Med* 1990;88:258.

26. Romijn JA, Wiersinga WM. Decreased nocturnal surge of thyrotropin in nonthyroidal illness. *J Clin Endocrinol Metab* 1990; 70:35.

27. Bartalena L, Cossu E, Grasso L, et al. Relationship between nocturnal serum thyrotropin peak and metabolic control in diabetic patients. *J Clin Endocrinol Metab* 1993;76:983.

28. Adriaanse R, Romijn JA, Brabant G, et al. Pulsatile thyrotropin secretion in nonthyroidal illness. *J Clin Endocrinol Metab* 1993; 77:1313.

29. Adriaanse R, Brabant G, Endert E, et al. Pulsatile thyrotropin release in patients with untreated pituitary disease. *J Clin Endocrinol Metab* 1993;77:205.

30. Fliers E, Guldenaar SEF, Wiersinga WM, et al. Decreased hypothalamic thyrotropin-releasing hormone gene expression in patients with nonthyroidal illness. *J Clin Endocrinol Metab* 1997;82:4032.

31. Arem R, Wiener GG, Kaplan SG, et al. Reduced tissue thyroid hormone levels in fatal illness. *Metabolism* 1993;42: 1102.

32. Lee H-Y, Suhl J, Pekary AE, et al. Secretion of thyrotropin with reduced concanavalin-A binding activity in patients with severe nonthyroidal illness. *J Clin Endocrinol Metab* 1987;65: 942.

33. Magner J, Roy P, Fainter L, et al. Transiently decreased sialylation of thyrotropin (TSH) in a patient with the euthyroid sick syndrome. *Thyroid* 1997;7:55.

34. DeJongh FE, Jöbsis AC, Elte JWF. Thyroid morphology in lethal non-thyroidal illness: a post-mortem study. *Eur J Endocrinol* 2000;144:221.

35. Peeters RP, Wouters PJ, Kaptein E, et al. Reduced activation and increased inactivation of thyroid hormone in tissues of critically ill patients. *J Clin Endocrinol Metab* 2003;88: 3202.

36. Bianco AC, Salvatore D, Gereben B, et al. Biochemistry, cellular and molecular biology, and physiological roles of the iodothyronine selenodeiodinases. *Endocr Rev* 2002;23:38.

37. Wassen FW, Schiel AE, Kuiper GG, et al. Induction of thyroid hormone-degrading deiodinase in cardiac hypertrophy and failure. *Endocrinology* 2002;143:2812.

38. Pinna G, Hiedra L, Meinhold H, et al. 3,3'-diiodothyronine concentrations in the sera of patients with nonthyroidal illnesses and brain tumors and of healthy subjects during acute stress. *J Clin Endocrinol Metab* 1998;83:3071.

39. Pinna G, Meinhold H, Hiedra L, et al. Elevated 3,5-diiodothyronine concentrations in the sera of patients with nonthyroidal illness and brain tumors. *J Clin Endocrinol Metab* 1997;82: 1535.

40. Chopra IJ, Wu SY, Chua Teco GN, et al. A radioimmunoassay of 3,5,3'-triiodothyronine sulfate: studies in thyroidal and nonthyroidal diseases, pregnancy, and neonatal life. *J Clin Endocrinol Metab* 1992;75:189.

41. Santini F, Chiovato L, Bartalena L, et al. Study of serum 3,5,3'-triiodothyronine sulfate concentration in patients with systemic nonthyroidal illness. *Eur J Endocrinol* 1996;134:45.

42. Chopra IJ, Santini F, Hurd RE, et al. A radioimmunoassay for measurement of thyroxine sulfate. *J Clin Endocrinol Metab* 1993;76:145.

43. Meinhold H, Gramm HJ, Meissner W, et al. Elevated serum diiodotyrosine (DIT) in severe infections and sepsis: DIT, a

possible new marker of leukocyte activity. *J Clin Endocrinol Metab* 1991;72:945.

44. Chamba A, Neuberger J, Strain A, et al. Expression and function of thyroid hormone receptor variants in normal and chronically diseased human liver. *J Clin Endocrinol Metab* 1996;81:360.

45. Beigneux AP, Moser AH, Shigenaga JK, et al. Sick euthyroid syndrome is associated with decreased TR expression and DNA binding in mouse liver. *Am J Physiol Endocrinol Metab* 2003; 284:E228.

46. Osburn RC, Mayers EA, Rodbard D, et al. Adaptation to hypocaloric feeding: physiological significance of the fall in serum T_3 as measured by pulse wave arrival time (QKd). *Metabolism* 1983;32:9.

47. Croxson MS, Ibbertson HK. Low serum triiodothyronine (T_3) and hypothyroidism in anorexia nervosa. *J Clin Endocrinol Metab* 1977;44:167.

48. Brent GA, Hershman JM, Reed AW, et al. Serum angiotensin-converting enzyme in severe nonthyroidal illness associated with low serum thyroxine concentration. *Ann Intern Med* 1984;100:680.

49. Seppel T, Becker A, Lippert F, et al. Serum sex hormone-binding globulin and osteocalcin in systemic nonthyroidal illness associated with low thyroid hormone concentrations. *J Clin Endocrinol Metab* 1996;81:1663.

50. Dasmahapatra A, Cohen MP, Grossman SD, et al. Erythrocyte sodium/potassium adenosine triphosphatase in thyroid disease and nonthyroidal illness. *J Clin Endocrinol Metab* 1985;61: 110.

51. Brandt MR, Kehlet H, Skovsted L, et al. Rapid decrease in plasma triiodothyronine during surgery and epidural analgesia independent of afferent neurogenic stimuli and cortisol. *Lancet* 1976;2:1333.

52. Jakobs TC, Mentrup B, Schnutzler C, et al. Proinflammatory cytokines inhibit the expression and function of human type I 5′-deiodinase in HepG2 hepatocarcinoma cells. *Eur J Endocrinol* 2002;146:559.

53. Yu J, Koenig RJ. Regulation of hepatocyte thyroxine 5′-deiodinase by T3 and nuclear receptor coactivators as a model of the sick euthyroid syndrome. *J Biol Chem* 2000;275:38296.

54. Nagaya T, Fujieda M, Otsuka G, et al. A potential role of activated NF-kB in the pathogenesis of the sick euthyroid syndrome. *J Clin Invest* 2000;106:393.

55. Lim C-F, Bernard BF, de Jong M, et al. A furan fatty acid and indoxyl sulfate are the putative inhibitors of thyroxine hepatocyte transport in uremia. *J Clin Endocrinol Metab* 1993;76: 318.

56. Everts ME, Lim CF, Moerings EPCM, et al. Effects of a furan fatty acid and indoxyl sulfate on thyroid hormone uptake in cultured anterior pituitary cells. *Am J Physiol* 1995; 268:E974.

57. Lim C-F, Docter R, Visser TJ, et al. Inhibition of thyroxine transport into cultured rat hepatocytes by serum of nonuremic critically ill patients: effects of bilirubin and nonesterified fatty acids. *J Clin Endocrinol Metab* 1993;76:1165.

58. Vos RA, Jong M de, Bernard BF, et al. Impaired thyroxine and 3,5,3′-triiodothyronine handling by rat hepatocytes in the presence of serum of patients with nonthyroidal illness. *J Clin Endocrinol Metab* 1995;80:2364.

59. Hennemann G, Everts ME, de Jong M, et al. The significance of plasma membrane transport in the bioavailability of thyroid hormone. *Clin Endocrinol (Oxf)* 1998;48:1.

60. Lim C-F, Docter R, Krenning EP, et al. Transport of thyroxine into cultured hepatocytes: effects of mild non-thyroidal illness and caloric restriction in obese subjects. *Clin Endocrinol (Oxf)* 1994;40:79.

61. Van der Heijden JTM, Docter R, Van Toor H, et al. Effect of caloric deprivation on the thyroid hormone tissue uptake and the generation of the low-T_3 syndrome. *Am J Physiol* 1986; 251:E156.

62. Hennemann G, Docter R, Friesema ECH, et al. Plasma membrane transport of thyroid hormones and its role in thyroid hormone metabolism and bioavailability. *Endocr Rev* 2001; 22:451.

63. De Jong M, Docter R, Bernard HF, et al. T_4 uptake into the perfused rat liver and liver T_4 uptake in humans are inhibited by fructose. *Am J Physiol* 1994;266:E768.

64. Jirasakuldech B, Schussler GC, Yap MG, et al. A characteristic serpin cleavage product of thyroxine-binding globulin appears in sepsis sera. *J Clin Endocrinol Metab* 2000;85:3996.

65. Afandi B, Schussler GC, Arafeh AH, et al. Selective consumption of thyroxine-binding globulin during cardiac bypass surgery. *Metabolism* 2000;49:270.

66. Mendel CM, Laughton CW, McMahon FA, et al. Inability to detect an inhibitor of thyroxine-serum protein binding in sera from patients with nonthyroidal illness. *Metabolism* 1991;40:491.

67. Chopra IJ, Huang T-S, Beredo A, et al. Serum thyroid hormone binding inhibitor in nonthyroidal illnesses. *Metabolism* 1986;35:152.

68. Willcox RB, Nelson JC, Tomei RT. Heterogeneity in affinities of serum proteins for thyroxine among patients with nonthyroidal illness as indicated by the serum free thyroxine response to serum dilution. *Eur J Endocrinol* 1994;131:9.

69. Mendel CM, Frost PH, Cavalieri RR. Effect of free fatty acids on the concentration of free thyroxine in human serum: the role of albumin. *J Clin Endocrinol Metab* 1986;63:1394.

70. Mendel CM, Frost PH, Kunitaka ST, et al. Mechanism of the heparin-induced increase in the concentration of free thyroxine in plasma. *J Clin Endocrinol Metab* 1987;65:1259.

71. Wolf M, Hansen N, Greten H. Interleukin-1β, tumor necrosis factor-α, and interleukin 6 decrease nuclear thyroid hormone receptor capacity in a liver cell line. *Eur J Endocrinol* 1994; 131:307.

72. Moordian AD, Reed RL, Osterweil D, et al. Decreased serum triiodothyronine is associated with increased concentrations of tumor necrosis factor. *J Clin Endocrinol Metab* 1990;71:1239.

73. Chopra IJ, Sakane S, Chua Teco GN. A study of the serum concentration of tumor necrosis factor-α in thyroidal and nonthyroidal illness. *J Clin Endocrinol Metab* 1991;72:1113.

74. Hashimoto H, Igarashi N, Yachie A, et al. The relationship between serum levels of interleukin-6 and thyroid hormone in children with acute respiratory infection. *J Clin Endocrinol Metab* 1994;78:288.

75. Boelen A, Platvoet-ter Schiphorst MC, Wiersinga WM. Relationship between serum 3,5,3′-triiodothyronine and serum interleukin-8, interleukin-10 or interferon-γ in patients with nonthyroidal illness. *J Endocrinol Invest* 1996;19:480.

76. Boelen A, Platvoet-ter Schiphorst M, Wiersinga WM. Association between serum interleukin-6 and serum 3,5,3′-triiodothyronine in nonthyroidal illness. *J Clin Endocrinol Metab* 1993; 77:1695.

77. Bartalena L, Brogioni S, Grasso L, et al. Relationship of the increased serum interleukin-6 concentration to changes of thyroid function in nonthyroidal illness. *J Endocrinol Invest* 1994; 17:269.

78. Davies PH, Black EG, Sheppard MC, et al. Relation between serum interleukin-6 and thyroid hormone concentrations in 270 hospital in-patients with non-thyroidal illness. *Clin Endocrinol (Oxf)* 1996;44:199.

79. Boelen A, Platvoet-ter Schiphorst MC, Wiersinga WM. Soluble cytokine receptors and the low 3,5,3′-triiodothyronine syn-

drome in patients with nonthyroidal disease. *J Clin Endocrinol Metab* 1995;80:971.

80. Poll T van der, Romijn JA, Wiersinga WM, et al. Tumor necrosis factor: a putative mediator of the sick euthyroid syndrome in man. *J Clin Endocrinol Metab* 1990;71:1567.

81. Corssmit EPM, Heijligenberg R, Endert E, et al. Acute effects of interferon-α administration on thyroid hormone metabolism in healthy men. *J Clin Endocrinol Metab* 1995;80:3140.

82. Stouthard JML, van der Poll T, Endert E, et al. Effects of acute and chronic interleukin-6 administration on thyroid hormone metabolism in humans. *J Clin Endocrinol Metab* 1994;79:1342.

83. Metz J de, Romijn JA, Endert E, et al. Administration of interferon-γ in healthy subjects does not modulate thyroid hormone metabolism. *Thyroid* 2000;10:87.

84. Van der Poll T, van Zee KJ, Endert E, et al. Interleukin-1 receptor blockade does not affect endotoxin-induced changes in plasma thyroid hormone and thyrtropin concentrations in man. *J Clin Endocrinol Metab* 1995;80:1341.

85. Van der Poll T, Endert E, Coyle SM, et al. Neutralization of TNF does not influence endotoxin-induced changes in thyroid hormone metabolism in humans. *Am J Physiol* 1999;276:R357.

86. Boelen A, Platvoet-ter Schiphorst MC, Wiersinga WM. Immunoneutralization of interleukin-1, tumor necrosis factor, interleukin-6 or interferon does not prevent the LPS-induced sick euthyroid syndrome in mice. *J Endocrinol* 1997;153:115.

87. Boelen A, Maas MAW, Lowik CWGM, et al. Induced illness in interleukin-6 (IL-6) knock-out mice: a causal role of IL-6 in the development of the low 3,5,3'-triiodothyronine syndrome. *Endocrinology* 1996;137:5250.

88. Maturlo SJ, Rosenbaum RL, Pan C, et al. Variable thyrotropin response to thyrotropin-releasing hormone after small decreases in plasma free thyroid hormone concentrations in patients with nonthyroidal diseases. *J Clin Invest* 1980;66:451.

89. Diano S, Naftolin F, Goglin F, et al. Fasting-induced increase in type II iodothyronine deiodinase activity and messenger ribonucleic acid level is not reversed by thyroxine in the rat hypothalamus. *Endocrinology* 1998;139:2879.

90. Fekete C, Gereben B, Doleschall M, et al. Lipopolysaccharide induces type 2 iodothyronine deiodinase in the mediobasal hypothalamus: implications for the nonthyroidal illness syndrome. *Endocrinology* 2004;145:1649.

91. Kakucska I, Qi Y, Lechan RM. Changes in adrenal status affect hypothalamic thyrotropin-releasing hormone gene expression in parallel with corticotropin-releasing hormone. *Endocrinology* 1995;136:2795.

92. Kondo K, Harbuz MS, Levy A, et al. Inhibition of the hypothalamic-pituitary-thyroid axis in response to lipopolysaccharide is independent of changes in circulating corticosteroids. Suppression of thyrotropin-releasing hormone gene expression by interleukin-1 beta in the rat: implications for nonthyroidal illness. *Neuroimmunomodulation* 1997;4:188.

93. Mihaly E, Fekete C, Tatro JB, et al. Hypophysiotropic thyrotropin releasing hormone-synthesizing neurons in the human hypothalamus are innervated by neuropeptide Y, agouti-related protein, and alpha-melanocyte-stimulating hormone. *J Clin Endocrinol Metab* 2000;85:2596.

94. Fekete C, Sarkar S, Rand WM, et al. Agouti-related protein (AGRP) has a central inhibitory action on the hypothalamic-pituitary thyroid (HPT) axis; comparisons between the effect of AGRP and neuropeptide Y on energy homeostasis and the HPT axis. *Endocrinology* 2002;143:3846.

95. Fekete C, Legradi G, Mihaly E, et al. Alpha-melanocyte-stimulating hormone is contained in nerve terminals innervating thyrotropin-releasing hormone-synthesizing neurons in hypothalamic paraventricular nucleus and prevents fasting-induced suppresion of prothyrotropin-releasing hormone gene expression. *J Neurosci* 2000;20:1550.

96. Legradi G, Emerson CH, Ahima RS, et al. Leptin prevents fasting-induced suppression of prothyrotropin-releasing hormone messenger ribonucleic acid in neurons of the hypothalamic paraventricular nucleus. *Endocrinology* 1997;138:2569.

97. Legradi G, Emerson CH, Ahima RS, et al. Arcuate nucleus ablation prevents fasting-induced suppression of proTRH mRNA in the hypothalamic paraventricular nucleus. *Neuroendocrinology* 1998;68:89.

98. Chan JL, Heist K, DePaoli AM, et al. The role of falling leptin levels in the neuroendocrine and metabolic adaptation to short-term starvation in healthy men. *J Clin Invest* 2003;111:1409.

99. Bornstein SR, Torpy DJ, Chrousos GP, et al. Leptin levels are elevated despite low thyroid hormone levels in the "euthyroid sick" syndrome. *J Clin Endocrinol Metab* 1997;82:4278.

100. Van den Berghe G, Wouters P, Carlsson L, et al. Leptin levels in protracted critical illness: effects of growth hormone-secretagogues and thyrotropin-releasing hormone. *J Clin Endocrinol Metab* 1998;83:3062.

101. Fliers E, Unmehopa U, Manniesing S, et al. Decreased neuropeptide Y (NPY) expression in the infundibular nucleus of patients with nonthyroidal illness. *Peptides* 2001;22:459.

102. Kakucska I, Romero LI, Clark BD, et al. Suppression of thyrotropin-releasing hormone gene expression by interleukin-1b in the rat: implications for nonthyroidal illness. *Neuroendocrinology* 1994;59:127.

103. Wassen FNJS, Moerings EPCM, van Toor H, et al. Effects of interleukin-1b on thyrotropin secretion and thyroid hormone uptake in clutured rat anterior pituitary cells. *Endocrinology* 1996;137;1591.

104. Arem R, Thornby JI, Deppe SA. Comparison of thyroid hormone and cortisol measurements with APACHE II and TISS scoring systems as predictors of mortality in the medical intensive care unit. *J Intens Care Med* 1997;12:12.

105. Spencer CA. Clinical utility and cost-effectiveness of sensitive thyrotropin assays in ambulatory and hospitalized patients. *Mayo Clin Proc* 1988;63:1214.

106. Franklyn JA, Black EG, Betteridge J, et al. Comparison of second and third generation methods for measurement of serum thyrotropin in patients with overt hyperthyroidism, patients receiving thyroxine therapy, and those with nonthyroidal illness. *J Clin Endocrinol Metab* 1994;78:1368.

107. Burmeister LA. Reverse T₃ does not reliably differentiate hypothyroid sick syndrome from euthyroid sick syndrome. *Thyroid* 1995;5:435.

108. Hooper MJ. Diminished TSH secretion during acute nonthyroidal illness in untreated primary hypothyroidism. *Lancet* 1976;1:48.

109. Nair KS, Halliday D, Ford GC, et al. Effect of triiodothyronine on leucine kinetics, metabolic rate, glucose concentration and insulin secretion rate during two weeks of fasting in obese women. *Int J Obesity* 1989;13:487.

110. Gardner DF, Kaplan MM, Stanley CA, et al. Effect of triiodothyronine replacement on the metabolic and pituitary responses to starvation. *N Engl J Med* 1979;300:579.

111. Burman KD, Wartofsky L, Dinterman RE, et al. The effect of T₃ and reverse T₃ administration on muscle protein catabolism during fasting as measured by 3-methylhistidine excretion. *Metabolism* 1979;28:805.

112. Byerley LO, Heber D. Metabolic effects of triiodothyronine replacement during fasting in obese subjects. *J Clin Endocrinol Metab* 1996;81:968.

113. Brent GA, Hershman JM. Thyroxine therapy in patients with severe nonthyroidal illnesses and low serum thyroxine concentration. *J Clin Endocrinol Metab* 1986;63:1.

114. Becker RA, Vaughan GM, Ziegler MG, et al. Hypermetabolic low triiodothyronine syndrome of burn injury. *Crit Care Med* 1982;10:870.

115. Acker CG, Singh AR, Flick RP, et al. A trial of thyroxine in acute renal failure. *Kidney Int* 2000;57:293.

116. Lim VS, Tsalikian E, Flanigan MJ. Augmentation of protein degradation by L-triiodothyronine in uremia. *Metabolism* 1989;38:1210.

117. Little JS. Effect of thyroid hormone supplementation on survival after bacterial infection. *Endocrinology* 1985;117:1431.

118. Chopra IJ, Huang TS, Boado R, et al. Evidence against benefit from replacement doses of thyroid hormone in nonthyroidal illness (NTI): studies using turpentine oil-injected rats. *J Endocrinol Invest* 1987;10:559.

119. Dulchavaky SA, Kennedy PR, Geller ER, et al. T$_3$ preserves respiratory function in sepsis. *J Trauma* 1991;31:753.

120. Klemperer JD, Klein I, Gomez M, et al. Thyroid hormone treatment after coronary-artery bypass surgery. *N Engl J Med* 1995;333:1522.

121. Klemperer JD, Klein IL, Ojaman K, et al. Triiodothyronine therapy lowers the incidence of atrial fibrillation after cardiac operations. *Ann Thorac Surg* 1996;61:1323.

122. Bennett-Guerrero E, Jimenez JL, White WD, et al. Cardiovascular effects of intravenous triiodothyronine in patients undergoing coronary artery bypass graft surgery: a randomized, double-blind, placebo-controlled trial. *JAMA* 1996;275:687.

123. Mullis-Jansson SL, Argeneiano M, Corwin S, et al. A randomized double-blind study of the effect of triiodothyronine on cardiac function and morbidity after coronary-bypass surgery. *J Thorac Cardiovasc Surg* 1999;117:1128.

124. Chowdhury D, Parnell V, Ojamaa K, et al. Usefulness of triiodothyronine (T$_3$) treatment after surgery for complex congenital heart disease in infants and children. *Am J Cardiol* 1999;84:1107.

125. Bettendorf M, Schmidt KG, Grulich-Henn J, et al. Triiodothyronine treatment in children after cardiac surgery: a double-blind, randomised, placebo-controlled study. *Lancet* 2000;356:529.

126. Van den Berghe G, Wouters P, Weekers F, et al. Reactivation of pituitary hormone release and metabolic improvement by infusion of growth hormone-releasing peptide and thyrotropin-releasing hormone in patients with protracted critical illness. *J Clin Endocrinol Metab* 1999;84:1311.

127. Iitaka M, Kawasaki S, Sakurai S-I, et al. Serum substances that interfere with thyroid hormone assays in chronic renal failure. *Clin Endocrinol (Oxf)* 1998;48:739.

128. Reinhardt W, Misch C, Jockenhövel F, et al. Triiodothyronine (T$_3$) reflects renal graft function after renal transplantation. *Clin Endocrinol (Oxf)* 1997;46:563.

129. Kaptein EM. Thyroid hormone metabolism and thyroid diseases in chronic renal failure. *Endocr Rev* 1996;17:45.

130. LoPresti JS, Fried JC, Spencer CA, et al. Unique alterations of thyroid hormone indices in the acquired immunodeficiency syndrome (AIDS). *Ann Intern Med* 1989;110:970.

131. Hommes MJT, Romijn JA, Endert E, et al. Hypothyroid-like regulation of the pituitary–thyroid axis in stable human immunodeficiency virus infection. *Metabolism* 1993;42:556.

132. Hirschfeld S, Lane L, Cutler GB, et al. Thyroid abnormalities in children infected with human immunodeficiency virus. *J Pediatr* 1996;128:70.

133. Grappin M, Piroth L, Verges B, et al. Increased prevalence of subclinical hypothyroidism in HIV patients treated with highly active antiretroviral therapy. *AIDS* 2000;14:1070.

134. Calza L, Manfredi R, Chiodo F. Subclinical hypothyroidism in HIV-infected patients receiving highly active antiretroviral therapy. *J Acquired Immune Deficiency Syndromes* 2002;31:361.

135. Beltran S, Lescure FX, Desailloud R, et al. Increased prevalence of hypothyroidism among human immunodeficiency virus-infected patients: a need for screening. *Clin Inf Dis* 2003;37:579.

136. Renard E, Fabre J, Paris F, et al. Syndrome of body fat redistribution in HIV-1-infected patients: relationships to cortisol and catecholamines. *Clin Endocrinol (Oxf)* 1999;51:223.

137. Koutkia P, Mylonakis E, Levin RM. Human immunodeficiency virus infection and the thyroid. *Thyroid* 2002;12:577.

138. Mason J, Southwick S, Yehuda R, et al. Elevation of serum free triiodothyronine, total triiodothyronine, thyroxine-binding globulin, and total thyroxine levels in combat-related posttraumatic stress disorder. *Arch Gen Psychiatry* 1994;51:629.

139. Nader S, Warner MD, Doyle S, et al. Euthyroid sick syndrome in psychiatric inpatients. *Biol Psychiatry* 1996;40:1288.

140. Arem R, Cusi K. Thyroid function testing in psychiatric illness. Usefulness and limitations. *Trends Endocrinol Metab* 1997;8:282.

141. Kirkegaard C, Faber J. The role of thyroid hormones in depression. *Eur J Endocrinol* 1998;138:1.

142. Alkemade A, Unmehopa UA, Brouwer JP, et al. Decreased thyrotropin-releasing hormone gene expression in the hypothalamic paraventricular nucleus of patients with major depression. *Mol Psychiatry* 2003;8:838.

143. Aronson R, Offman H, Joffe RT, et al. Triiodothyronine augmentation in the treatment of refractory depression. A meta-analysis. *Arch Gen Psychiatry* 1996;53:842.

144. Altshuler LL, Bauer M, Frye MA, et al. Does thyroid supplementation accelerate tricyclic antidepressant response? A review and meta-analysis of the literature. *Am J Psych* 2001;158:1617.

145. Fliers E, Appelhof BC, Brouwer JP, et al. Effect of triiodothyronine (T3) addition to paroxetine in major depressive disorder: a randomized clinical trial. In: Program and abstracts of the Endocrine Society's 85th Annual Meeting; 2003; Philadelphia, PA. Abstract S-19.2.

11E   IODINE DEFICIENCY

FRANÇOIS M. DELANGE
JOHN T. DUNN*

Iodine is a trace element present in the human body in minute amounts (15 to 25 mg), almost exclusively in the thyroid gland (1). It is an essential component of the thyroid hormones, thyroxine (T_4) and triiodothyronine (T_3), comprising 65% and 59% of their respective weights. Thyroid hormones, in turn, regulate metabolic processes in most cells, and play a determining role in the process of early growth and development of most organs, especially the brain (2). In humans, most of the growth and development of the brain occur during fetal life and the first 2 to 3 postnatal years (3). Consequently, iodine deficiency, if severe enough to affect thyroid hormone synthesis during this critical period, will result in hypothyroidism and brain damage. The clinical consequence will be irreversible mental retardation (4).

The daily dietary intake of iodine recommended by the World Health Organization/International Council for Control of Iodine Deficiency Disorders/United Nations Emergency Children's Fund (WHO/ICCIDD/UNICEF) is 90 µg for age 0 to 59 months, 120 µg for age 6 to 12 years, 150 µg for adolescents and adults, and 200 µg during pregnancy and lactation (5). Fairly similar recommendations have been made by the Food and Nutrition Board of the U.S. National Academy of Sciences, but higher for pregnancy (220 µg) and lactation (290 µg). A recent summary of these and other national and international guidelines has been published (6)

When these physiologic requirements of iodine are not met in a given population, a series of functional and developmental consequences occur (Table 11E.1), including thyroid function abnormalities and, when iodine deficiency is severe, endemic goiter and cretinism (7,8), decreased fertility rate, and increased perinatal death and infant mortality (9). These complications, which hinder the development of the affected populations, are grouped under the general heading of iodine deficiency disorders (IDD) (10).

Broad geographic areas exist where the population's daily intake of iodine is below the recommended dietary allowance, and the population is affected by IDD (7,8,11). These areas frequently are mountainous because the soils lowest in iodine are those that were covered longest by qua-

ternary glaciers. When these glaciers melted, most of the iodine leached out of the ground beneath (12). The most important goitrous areas in the world today include the Himalayas and the Andes, but iodine deficiency also occurs in lowlands far from the oceans, such as in the central parts of Africa, central Asia, and central and eastern Europe.

In 1999, IDD represented a significant public health problem for 2.225 billion people (38% of the world population) in 130 countries (Table 11E.2), and 740 million had a goiter (11). In 1994, 43 million were believed to be mentally handicapped as a result of iodine deficiency (13), which, therefore, is the most prevalent preventable cause of impaired intellectual development in the world. WHO and ICCIDD keep databases on the current global status of iodine nutrition, by country (13a,13b). In a recent tabu-

TABLE 11E.1. SPECTRUM OF IODINE DEFICIENCY DISORDERS

Fetus
  Spontaneous abortions
  Stillbirths
  Congenital anomalies
  Increased perinatal and infant mortality
  Endemic cretinism
Neonate
  Goiter
  Overt or subclinical hypothyroidism
  Cretinism
Infant/Child/Adolescent
  Goiter
  Subclinical or overt hypothyroidism
  Mental retardation
  Retarded physical development
  Increased susceptibility of the thyroid gland to nuclear
    radiation
Adult
  Goiter and its complications
  Hypothyroidism
  Endemic mental retardation
  Decreased fertility
  Spontaneous hyperthyroidism in the elderly
  Increased susceptibility of the thyroid to nuclear radiation

From Hetzel BS. Iodine deficiency disorders (IDD) and their eradication. *Lancet* 1983:ii:1126; Stanbury JB, Ermans AE, Bourdoux P, et al. Iodine-induced hyperthyroidism: occurrence and epidemiology. *Thyroid* 1998;8:83; and Laurberg P, Nohr SB, Pedersen KM, et al. Thyroid disorders in mild iodine deficiency. *Thyroid* 2000;10:951, with permission.

*Deceased.

TABLE 11E.2. POPULATIONS AFFECTED BY IODINE DEFICIENCY AND BY GOITER AS OF 1999

WHO Region	Population, Million	Population Affected by Iodine Deficiency, Million (%)	Population Affected by Goiter, Million (%)
Africa	612	295 (48.2)	124 (20.3)
Americas	788	196 (24.9)	39 (4.9)
Eastern Mediterranean	473	348 (73.6)	152 (32.7)
Europe	869	275 (31.6)	130 (15.0)
Southeast Asia	1,477	599 (40.6)	172 (11.6)
Western Pacific	1,639	513 (31.3)	124 (7.6)
Total	5,858	2,225 (38.4)	741 (12.6)

From WHO/UNICEF/ICCIDD. *Progress towards the elimination of iodine deficiency disorders (IDD).* Geneva: World Health Organization; 1999. Publication WHO/NHD/99.4, modified with permission.

lation 50% of the world's population were thought to live in countries with iodine deficiency (14). The true extent is not fully known, however, because many countries have inadequate monitoring systems.

Although the disorders that result from iodine deficiency are preventable by appropriate iodine delivery, they continue to occur because of various socioeconomic, cultural, and political limitations to adequate iodine supplementation (11).

The objective of this chapter is to review present knowledge about the thyroid disorders induced by iodine deficiency. Endemic cretinism and mental retardation are discussed in Chapter 49. As indicated in Table 11E.3, three different degrees of severity of IDD have been considered: mild, moderate, and severe. Although the basic mechanisms of adaptation to iodine deficiency are similar among them, this discussion separates severe IDD complicated by cretinism, as seen typically in remote areas of developing countries, and mild to moderate IDD, as seen typically in Europe. Special emphasis is placed on the pediatric aspects of adaptation to iodine deficiency: neonates and young infants are the most important targets of iodine deficiency because it causes irreversible brain damage and mental retardation from thyroid failure during fetal and early postnatal life (see Chapter 49). Extensive reviews are available on endemic goiter, the disorders induced by iodine deficiency and its treatment (7,8,15–22), including its pediatric aspects (23,24).

SEVERE IODINE DEFICIENCY DISORDERS

Epidemiology

The following definitions were proposed by WHO/UNICEF/ICCIDD for public health studies conducted in the field (5).

TABLE 11E.3. CLASSIFICATION OF GOITER ENDEMIAS BY SEVERITY

Variables	Target Population	Mild Iodine Deficiency	Moderate Iodine Deficiency	Severe Iodine Deficiency
Median urinary iodine, µg/L	SAC	50–99.0	20–49.0	<20.0
Prevalence of goiter, % (Grade >0)	SAC	5.0–19.9	20.0–29.9	≥30.0
Frequency of thyroid volume >97th percentile by ultrasound, %	SAC	5.0–19.9	20.0–29.9	≥30.0
Frequency of serum TSH >5m U/L whole blood, %	Newborns	3.0–19.9	20.0–39.9	≥40.0

SAC, school-aged children; Tsk, thyrotropin.
Adapted from WHO/UNICEF/ICCIDD. *Assessment of the iodine deficiency disorders and monitoring their elimination.* Geneva: World Health Organization; 2001. Publication WHO/NHD/01.1; and WHO/UNICEF/ICCIDD. *Indicators for assessing iodine deficiency disorders and their control through salt iodization.* Geneva: World Health Organization; 1994. Publication WHO/NUT/94.6, with permission.

Goiter

A thyroid gland each of whose lobes has a volume greater than the terminal phalanx of the thumb of the person examined will be considered goitrous. Under this condition the thyroid is enlarged by a factor of at least 4 to 5.

The following simplified classification of goiter by palpation has been proposed:

Grade 0: No palpable or visible goiter.
Grade 1: A goiter that is palpable but not visible when the neck is in the normal position (i.e., the thyroid is not visibly enlarged). Nodules in a thyroid that is otherwise not enlarged fall into this category.
Grade 2: A swelling in the neck that is clearly visible when the neck is in a normal position and is consistent with an enlarged thyroid when the neck is palpated.

This clinical classification is still appropriate for field surveys in remote areas where no other methods are available. However, the use of transportable ultrasonographic equipment in field studies has shown that the clinical assessment of thyroid size is imprecise for small goiters, especially in young children. In these circumstances, misclassification between grades 0 and 1 can be as high as 40% (13,25–27), and, consequently, the goiter rate can be incorrect. Therefore, measurement of thyroid volume by ultrasonography is highly recommended (5), especially in endemic areas where the visible goiter rate is low. Results of ultrasonography from a study population should be compared with normative data. Values proposed by WHO/ICCIDD (28) on the basis of data collected in Europe (29) were overestimated by some 30% (30), but reliable new values have recently been obtained by an international team applying standardized methodology in six study areas on five continents with long-standing iodine sufficiency (31).

Endemic Goiter

An area is arbitrarily defined as an endemic goiter area if more than 5% of the children aged 6 to 12 years have a goiter. The figure 5% was chosen because a higher prevalence usually implies an environmental factor, while a prevalence of less than 5% is common even when all known environmental risk factors are absent.

Goiter endemics should be described not only by the frequency of goiter but also by the severity of iodine deficiency. Table 11E.3 shows recommendations for classification of goiter endemias based on public health surveys.

The present definitions are deliberately less severe and elaborate than those used in clinical endocrinology, to avoid overestimation of severity and to facilitate comparison of results obtained in different parts of the world by health workers who are not necessarily endocrinologists.

In epidemiologic surveys, the most rigorous method for evaluating the prevalence of goiter is to examine the entire population in a likely area. This is often difficult to organize, especially in urban areas. Many surveys are limited, therefore, to particular age groups, most typically children in school (11).

Goiter prevalence is critically influenced by age and sex (Fig. 11E.1). In severe endemias, goiter appears very early. Its prevalence increases sharply and peaks during puberty and child-bearing years. From the age of 10 years onward, the prevalence is higher in girls than in boys. In both sexes, it decreases during adulthood, but more sharply in men than in women.

Etiology

Iodine Deficiency

Low dietary iodine intake is the main factor responsible for the development of endemic goiter (5,7,8,18–22,32,33). When iodine supplementation is introduced in an endemic area, the goiter incidence always declines markedly. The

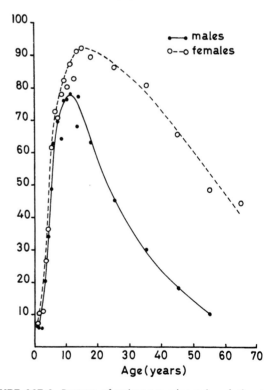

FIGURE 11E.1. Pattern of goiter prevalence in relation to age and sex in the inhabitants of Idjwi Island endemic goiter area, Democratic Republic of Congo. (From Delange F. Endemic goitre and thyroid function in Central Africa. *Monographs in pediatrics.* Basel: S. Karger AG, 1974:1, modified with permission.)

long-term persistence of a significant goiter prevalence in spite of correction of iodine deficiency suggests the additional role of a naturally occurring goitrogen (34).

Goiter develops in iodine-deficient environments among populations that consume locally grown foods. The iodine content of most foodstuffs is low; the highest being found in sea fish and shellfish and, to a lesser extent, in milk, eggs, and meat, depending on the diet of the livestock and poultry (35). Fruits and vegetables usually have a very low iodine content. The iodine content of foodstuffs varies greatly, depending on country, season, and method of cooking. The iodine content of drinking water is too low to serve as a consistent contributor.

A rigorous assessment of food iodine content is extremely difficult, for methodological reasons. Iodine balance studies have shown that adults are in equilibrium with their iodine environment and that the fecal excretion of iodine is usually negligible (5 μg/day) (35). Therefore, most estimates of dietary iodine intake are based on measurements of iodine excretion in urine. In nonendemic areas, the daily urinary excretion of iodine is at least 100 μg (5). In endemic areas it is usually much lower and varies from 75 to 3 μg/day (see reviews in references 6,7,18–22,33). Complete 24-hour collection of urine is often difficult in field investigations. An alternative procedure is measuring the ratio between the concentrations of iodine and creatinine in casual urine samples (36,37) or even the concentration of iodine alone, provided that the observation covers at least 50 to 100 randomly selected samples (5,38).

The etiologic role of iodine deficiency in endemic goiter also has been confirmed by an enormous amount of experimental work in animals (39,40). In several regions, it has been possible to demonstrate geographic superimpostion of human endemic goiter and enzootic goiter (33,39, 41).

The correction of iodine deficiency usually is followed by the disappearance of endemic goiter (see treatment and prophylaxis).

Other Goitrogenic Factors

Iodine deficiency is not the sole cause of endemic goiter. Indeed, the disease has been found in regions where there is no iodine deficiency (42,43) or even where iodine excess is present (44–46). Conversely, some other regions with extremely severe iodine deficiency are free of endemic goiter (34,47–49). These data strongly suggest that goitrogenic factors in the diet or environment, other than iodine deficiency, can play a critical role in the etiology of the disease (34,50–55). Table 11E.4 summarizes data from goiter endemias where such environmental goitrogenic factors have been demonstrated.

Natural goitrogens were first found in vegetables of the genus *Brassica* (53) (of the Cruciferae family) that cause goiter in animals. Their antithyroid action is related to the presence of thioglucosides, which, after digestion, release thiocyanate and isothiocyanate (52,56,57). A particular thioglucoside, goitrin (L-5-vinyl-2 thiooxazolidone), is present in certain Cruciferae growing as weeds in pastures in Finland and Tasmania (42,57). Goitrin has potent thionamide-like properties (52). It can probably reach humans by ingestion of milk (53,58).

Another important group of naturally occurring goitrogens is the cyanoglucosides, which have been found in several staples (cassava, maize, bamboo shoots, sweet potatoes, lima beans) (47,51,54,57). After ingestion, they release cyanide, which is detoxified by conversion to thiocyanate, a powerful goitrogenic agent that acts acutely by inhibiting thyroid iodide transport and, at higher doses, competes with iodide in the organification process (59, 60,61).

Cassava (manioc), one of the basic foodstuffs in tropical areas, has definite goitrogenic properties in rats (59,62). Its role in the etiology of endemic goiter, in association with iodine deficiency, has been clearly demonstrated in Africa (50,51,63,64), and confirmed in Malaysia (65) and Brazil (66). The chronic consumption of poorly detoxified cassava in these areas induces a marked increase in the serum concentration of thiocyanate which, in association with iodine deficiency, impairs thyroid function, characterized by low serum T_4 and high thyrotropin (TSH) concentrations, and produces goiter (64). Improved detoxification of cassava results in normalization of serum thiocyanate and of thyroid function (67).

The determining factor in the goitrogenic action of cassava is the balance between the dietary supplies of iodine and of thiocyanate. Goiter develops when the urinary iodine/thiocyanate ratio, used as an index of this balance, decreases below a critical threshold of about 3 μg iodine per mg thiocyanate (51). This can occur when thiocyanate is excessive in overt iodine deficiency, or even with an almost normal iodine supply when the thiocyanate overload is very high (68). Experimentally, acute thiocyanate overload inhibits thyroidal uptake of iodine-131 (^{131}I), but chronic administration of cassava or of small doses of thiocyanate in iodine-deficient rats does not decrease thyroidal uptake of ^{131}I in spite of high concentrations of thiocyanate. A marked inhibition of thyroidal iodide uptake may be detected, however, in the same animals if iodine organification is blocked by propylthiouracil (59). These findings agree with previous observations that a moderate increase in the thiocyanate concentration markedly accelerates the exit rate of iodide from the gland but does not affect unidirectional iodide clearance (69). These observations account both for the clinical observation of a very high thyroidal uptake of radioiodine in iodine-deficient subjects with abnormally high serum thiocyanate levels and for the fact that iodine supplementation completely reverses the goitrogenic effect of cassava.

TABLE 11E.4. GOITER ENDEMIAS ATTRIBUTED TO GOITROGENS IN FOOD AND TO CHEMICAL AND BACTERIAL POLLUTION OF THE WATER-EXPOSURE PATHWAY

Locality	Source	Vehicle	Active Ingredient
Europe			
Finland	Grass, weeds	Milk	L-5-Vinyl-2-thiooxazolidone (goitrin)
England (Sheffield area)	Grass	Milk	(?)
Spain (Navarro)	Grass	Milk	Thiocyanate
Spain (Avila)	Walnuts		(?)
Ex-Czecoslovakia (Bohemia-Moravia)	Grass (*Brassicae*)	Milk	Goitrin
Ex-Yugoslavia (Krk Island)	Grass (*Brassicae*)	Milk	Goitrin
Greece	*Escherichia coli*	Water	Thyroid antibodies (?)
North America			
West Virginia	*Escherichia coli*	Water	(?)
Eastern Kentucky	Coals and gram-negative bacteria	Water	Phenolic and phtalate ester derivatives (?)
South America			
Colombia	Shales and coals, humic substances, and gram-negative bacteria	Water	Resorcinol, phtalate ester derivatives, and disulfides
Venezuela	Various rocks and soils	Water	Lithium
Chile	Piñon nuts		(?)
Brazil	Palm tree fruit (*Babassu*)		Phenolic derivatives (?)
Africa			
Nigeria	Cassava		Thionamide-like goitrogen
Zaire	Cassava		Cyanogenic glucoside (linamarin → thiocyanate)
Sudan	Millet		Flavonoids and thiocyanate
Asia			
Lebanon	Onions, garlic		(?)
Japan	Seaweeds		Iodide and polyhydroxyphenols (?)
Malaysia	Cassava		Linamarin → thiocyanate
China	Seaweeds		Iodide
Oceania			
Tasmania	Grass, weeds		Isothiocyanate (cheilorine)

?, active ingredient not known.
Data from Gaitan E. *Environmental goitrogenesis.* Boca Raton: CRC Press, 1989:1–250; and Delange F, Ermans AM. Endemic goiter and cretinism. Naturally occurring goitrogens. *Pharmacol Ther* 1976;1:57–93.

Pathophysiology: Adaptation of Thyroid Function to Iodine Deficiency

Endemic goiter is a disease of adaptation that develops in response to dietary iodine deficiency. This classic concept was established in 1954 by Stanbury and colleagues (70) and has been confirmed since by an enormous number of clinical and experimental observations (6,7,17–23,33,71).

When iodine intake is abnormally low, adequate secretion of thyroid hormones may still be achieved by marked modifications of thyroid activity. This adaptation includes stimulation of the trapping mechanism as well as of the subsequent steps in the intrathyroidal metabolism of iodine, leading to preferential synthesis and secretion of T_3. These responses are triggered and maintained by increased secretion of TSH. The morphologic consequence of prolonged TSH stimulation is the development of goiter, making it appear to be the mechanism of adaptation to iodine deficiency (70). However, large goiters may no longer be considered adaptive in view of their decreased ability to synthesize thyroid hormones (72).

Increased Stimulation by Thyrotropin

High serum TSH levels have been reported often, but not systematically, in humans with chronic iodine deficiency (73–77). Moreover, within a given area, striking and large variations in serum TSH levels occur in adults independently of the presence or absence of goiter (73,74,76). The lack of systematic correlation between goiter and TSH levels suggests that differences in the duration of high TSH levels and in thyroid responsiveness to TSH, as well as other factors (e.g., growth hormone, epidermal growth and fibroblast factors, insulin, cortisone, cyclic GMP, or other intrathyroidal mechanisms) may determine whether goiter develops (78).

Increase in Iodide Trapping

The fundamental mechanism by which the thyroid gland adapts to an insufficient iodine supply is to increase the trapping of iodide. This results in the accumulation within

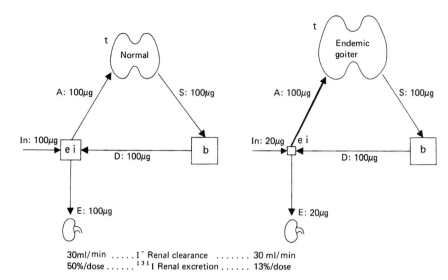

30ml/min .....I⁻ Thyroidal clearance 155ml/min
50%/dose......¹³¹I Thyroid uptake 87%/dose

30ml/min .....I⁻ Renal clearance ....30 ml/min
50%/dose......¹³¹I Renal excretion 13%/dose

FIGURE 11E.2. Kinetics of iodide in a normal subject (**left**) and in a goitrous subject living in an iodine-deficient area (**right**). Respective iodine intakes *(In)* are 100 µg/day and 20 µg/day. The three iodine compartments are intrathyroid iodine *(t)*; hormonal ("bound") extrathyroid iodine *(b)*; and extrathyroid iodide *(ei)*. Transfer rates of iodine are expressed in µg/day; ei, renewal of extrathyroid iodide originating from intake and from hormonal degradation *(D)*; *A*, accumulation rate within the thyroid; *S*, secretion rate; *E*, urinary excretion rate. ¹³¹iodine thyroid uptake *(U)* is the fraction of ¹³¹I tracer accumulated in the thyroid and *1-U*, the fraction of ¹³¹I excreted in urine. Thyroid and renal clearances of iodide are expressed in mL/min. The schema is based on the three-compartment model of iodine metabolism proposed by Riggs. (From Riggs DS. Quantitative aspects of iodine metabolism in man. *Pharmacol Rev* 1952;4:284, with permission.)

the gland of a larger percentage of the ingested exogenous iodide and a more efficient reuse of iodide released by the thyroid or generated by the degradation of thyroid hormones (70,79). The increased iodide trapping is the result of both TSH stimulation and TSH-independent stimulation of iodide trapping by the thyroid sodium-iodide symporter (80).

For any adequate adjustment of iodide supply to the thyroid, iodide trapping must fulfill two conditions. First, it must reduce the amount of iodine excreted in the urine to that of iodine intake, this condition being required to preserve preexisting iodine stores. Second, it must ensure the accumulation in the thyroid of definite amounts of iodide per day (about 100 µg). This latter parameter is extremely important because it quantitatively controls all further steps of intrathyroidal iodine metabolism, including the secretion rate of the thyroid hormones. Two examples of adjustment of iodide trapping are shown in Figure 11E.2, the first for a presumably normal subject (iodine supply: 100 µg/day) and the second for a goitrous subject living in an endemic area (iodine supply: 20 µg/day) (81). In the normal subject, renewal of the extrathyroidal iodide compartment is 200 µg/day, half of which originates from iodine intake *(In)* and the other half from peripheral degradation of the thyroid hormones. Thyroid iodide clearance *(Clt)* is adjusted to 30 mL/min and thus equals renal iodide clearance *(Clr)*. The fraction of the iodide compartment taken up by the thyroid gland *(IU)* is given by the following equation: $IU = IClt / (IClt + IClr)$. The amount of iodide taken up by the gland *(A)* and excreted in urine *(E)* per day are thus, respectively, *IU* and $I(1 - U)$. In a normal

subject: $U = 30/(30 + 30) = 0.5$, and *A* and *E* are both 100 µg/day (200 µg × 0.5). In a patient with goiter, renewal of the extrathyroidal iodide compartment is only 120 µg/day, reflecting the reduction of iodide intake (20 µg/day). Thyroid clearance is adjusted to 155 mL/min, and the resulting value of *U* is $155/(155 + 30) = 0.83$, *A* being equal to 120 µg × 0.83 = 100 µg and *E* = 120 µg × 0.17 = 20 µg.

Thus, despite a drastic reduction in the iodide supply, renal iodide excretion does not exceed iodine intake, and adequate amounts of iodine accumulate in the gland. It is obvious that this oversimplified scheme accounts neither for the qualitative changes of thyroid secretion nor for the iodide spillage observed in endemic goiter (82). The fraction of extrathyroidal iodide taken up by the gland thus appears as the main determining factor for the distribution of both exogenous and endogenous iodide. The *U* fraction does not, however, give a reliable estimate of the true modification of the trapping mechanism. As shown in Figure 11E.2, the adaptation from a normal iodine supply to a poor one enhances the value of *U* from 50% to 87%, that is by a factor of 1.7. This situation is achieved only by a tremendous augmentation of thyroid clearance, which increases from 30 to 155 mL/min, an increase by a factor of 5.7.

For practical purposes, *U* is given with a good approximation by the ¹³¹I thyroidal uptake. Absolute iodine uptake *(A)* is generally estimated from the daily renal excretion of iodide *(E)* according to the formula: $A = EU/(1-U)$. This equation is based on the assumption that the distribution of extrathyroidal stable iodide during 24 hours is the same as the distribution of a single tracer dose of ¹³¹I (70). The ratio between thyroidal accumulation and renal excre-

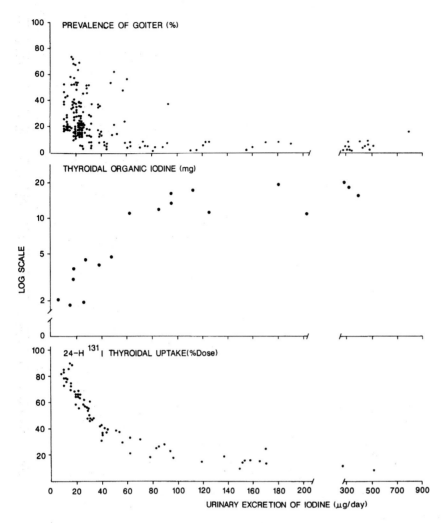

FIGURE 11E.3. Relationship between the daily urinary excretion of iodine and the prevalence of goiter, the hormonal iodine content of the thyroid (exchangeable organic iodine pool determined by kinetic studies), and thyroidal uptake of radioiodine. (From Schaefer AE. Status of salt iodization in PAHO member countries. In: Dunn JT, Medeiros-Neto GA, eds. *Endemic goiter and cretinism: continuing threats to world health.* Washington, DC; Pan American Health Organization (PAHO); 1974. Scientific No. 292:242; Delange F, Bourdoux P, Chanoine JP, et al. Physiopathology of iodine nutrition during pregnancy, lactation and early postnatal life. In: Berger H, ed. *Vitamins and minerals in pregnancy and lactation.* New York: Raven Press, 1988:205; and Tovar E, Maisterrena JA, Chavez A. Iodine nutrition levels of schoolchildren in rural Mexico. In: Stanbury JB, ed. *Endemic goiter.* Washington, D.C.: Pan American Health Organization (PAHO); 1969. Scientific No. 193: 411, with permission.)

tion is the same for ^{127}I and ^{131}I; therefore, the equation from which the formula mentioned earlier is derived: A/E = U (1-U).

Increased thyroidal uptake of ^{131}I and reduction of urinary iodine excretion are the main markers of a goiter endemia caused by iodine deficiency. A clear-cut inverse relationship between both parameters was demonstrated in 1954 (70), has been confirmed in a large number of goiter endemias (33), and is further illustrated in Figure 11E.3. It indicates that as soon as the iodine supply decreases below the physiological requirement of 100 µg per day in adults, the thyroid uptake of radioiodine increases, indicating an accelerated clearance rate of iodide by the thyroid.

Under these conditions, in spite of a decrease in the serum concentration of iodide, the absolute uptake of iodide by the thyroid remains normal (79) and its organic iodine content remains within the limits of normal (i.e., 15 to 25 mg), as long as the iodine intake remains above a threshold of about 50 µg/day. Below this critical level, in spite of a further increase of thyroid clearance, the absolute

uptake of iodide diminishes and the iodine content of the thyroid decreases. Goiter, the visible consequence of iodine deficiency, starts to develop only when the iodine intake is still lower, although for low iodine intake, the prevalence of goiter markedly varies from one area to another (83–85).

Because of the relationship between thyroidal uptake and urinary iodine excretion, it has been suggested that the estimation of urinary ^{127}I excretion, and therefore of the iodine intake, could be directly deduced, with considerable accuracy, from the value of the ^{131}I thyroidal uptake (86).

Modifications of Intrathyroidal Iodine Metabolism

Under experimental conditions, increased TSH stimulation induced by iodine deficiency provokes a marked acceleration of all steps of intrathyroidal iodine metabolism, with a consequently faster turnover of this compartment and an increase in its heterogeneity (87). A similar pattern

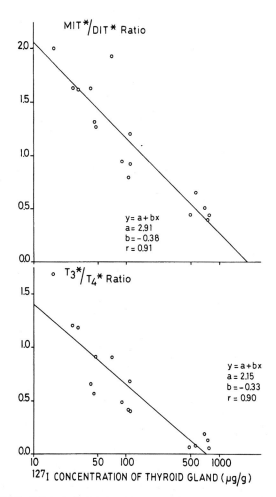

FIGURE 11E.4. Relationship between monoiodotyrosine (MIT)*/ diiodotyrosine (DIT)* and triiodothyronine (T₃)*/thyroxine (T₄)* ratios in the hydrolysates of rat thyroids and corresponding concentrations of ^{127}I in the thyroid tissue. Each point corresponds to the mean value of five animals. Rats were fed a low iodine diet for 15 to 20 days with, in some groups, an iodine supplement of 5 µg/day. *, radioactive compound. (From Delange F, Ermans AM. Iodine deficiency. In: Braverman LE, Utiger RD, eds. *The thyroid: A fundamental and clinical text*. Philadelphia: JB Lippincott Co, 1991:368, with permission.)

TABLE 11E.5. WEIGHT, IODINE CONTENT, AND IODOAMINO ACID DISTRIBUTION IN THE THYROID AND IN THE SERUM OF NORMAL AND IODINE-DEFICIENT ADULT RATS

	Mean±SD	
Variables	**Normal Rats (n=12)**	**Iodine-Deficient Rats (n=10)**
Thyroid		
Weight (mg/100 g)	4.1±0.7	12.0±3.0
Iodine content (ng/mg thyroid wt)	880.0±180.0	21.0±30.0
MIT*/DIT* ratio	0.42±0.07	2.00±0.30
T₃*/T₄* ratio	0.12±0.01	1.80±0.90
T₃/T₄ ratio (M)	0.12±0.03	1.01±0.90
Serum		
T₄ (µg/dL)	4.2±0.6	<0.5
T₃ (ng/dL)	44.0±9.0	43.0±6.0

DIT, diiodotyrosine; MIT, monoiodotyrosine; T_3, triiodothyronine; T_4, thyroxine; ^{125}I-labeled.
Results are calculated from the percentages of ^{125}I found in each iodocompound in thyroid hydrolysates 24 hours after injection of ^{125}I. From Abrams GM, Larsen PR. Triiodothyronine and thyroxine in the serum and thyroid glands of iodine-deficient rats. *J Clin Invest* 1973;52:2522, with permission.

is observed in endemic goiter, but only in a restricted number of subjects, generally children and adolescents (88). In most goitrous subjects, ^{131}I distribution reveals a slow-release pattern: plasma protein-bound ^{131}I is as low as in subjects with normal thyroid uptake living in nongoitrous areas, and the biologic half-life of thyroidal ^{131}I is long. These observations would suggest that in these highly stimulated glands, intrathyroidal iodine would turn over at a subnormal rate. A possible explanation for this finding (87) is that the glands with apparently slow secretion could have access to a large endogenous source of stable iodine not in equilibrium with the compartment labeled by the exogenous tracer. This unlabeled iodine could dilute the tracer and render the fast turnover undetectable by isotope studies.

Studies in rats show that thyroid hyperplasia induced by iodine deficiency is associated with an altered pattern of tracer iodine distribution in the gland, characterized by an increase in poorly iodinated compounds, monoiodotyrosine (MIT) and T_3, and a decrease in diiodotyrosine (DIT) and T_4 (87,89). Figure 11E.4 indicates that the increases in the MIT/DIT and T_3/T_4 ratios are closely related to the degree of iodine depletion of the gland. Table 11E.5 confirms these findings by showing that the iodine depleted glands of iodine-deficient rats have a dramatic reduction of T_4 and a markedly increased T_3/T_4 ratio.

Corresponding information about human endemic goiter is more limited. In them, the amount of iodine is markedly reduced and the MIT/DIT ratio is increased. There is also, as in sporadic goiter, an increased DIT/T_4 ratio, suggesting reduced efficiency of the coupling reaction (87).

The main features of intrathyroidal metabolism in endemic goiter appear to be as follows (71,72,87): because of a large thyroidal iodine pool that is not in equilibrium with the compartment labeled by the exogenous tracer, iodination of the large amounts of thyroglobulin (Tg) accumulated within the colloid remains low. The subsequent abnormal configuration of Tg is responsible for reduced efficiency of iodothyronine synthesis. Only a small fraction of the large iodine stores is, therefore, actually moving along the normal pathway of hormone synthesis and secretion, while a considerable percentage seems to be wasted, accounting for the tremendous morphological, functional

TABLE 11E.6. COMPARISON OF EPIDEMIOLOGIC AND BIOCHEMICAL DATA[a] EXPLORING THYROID FUNCTION AND ENDEMIC GOITER IN BRUSSELS, BELGIUM, AND THE IDJWI ISLAND AND UBANGI AREAS OF THE DEMOCRATIC REPUBLIC OF CONGO

Variables	Mean±SE (n)	
	Belgium	Congo
Daily urinary excretion of iodine (μg/d)	51.2 ± 5.8 (38)	15.5 ± 1.3 (243)
Prevalence of goiter (%)	3	77
Serum concentration of:		
T_4 (μg/dL)	8.1 ± 0.1 (125)	4.9 ± 0.2 (358)
T_3 (ng/dL)	144 ± 3 (124)	166 ± 3 (299)
TSH (μU/mL)	1.7 ± 1.1 (255)	18.6 ± 2.1 (365)
PB ^{131}I 24 h (% dose/L)	0.06 ± 0.01 (27)	0.17 ± 0.02 (105)
Thyroidal uptake of ^{131}I 24 h (% dose)	46.4 ± 1.1 (255)	65.2 ± 0.9 (167)
Thyroidal organic iodine exchangeable pool (mg)	15.8 ± 3.5 (12)	1.6 ± 0.2 (30)

PB, protein-bound; T_3, triiodothyronine; T_4, thyroxine; TSH, thyrotropin.
The differences between the two groups are highly significant ($p<0.0001$) for all variables.
Adapted from from Delange F. Adaptation to iodine deficiency during growth: etiopathogenesis of endemic goiter and cretinism. In: Delange F, Fisher D, Malvaux P, eds. *Pediatric thyroidology.* Basel: S. Karger AG, 1985:295; Delange F, Iteke FB, Ermans AM. *Nutritional factors involved in the goitrogenic action of cassava.* Ottawa: International Development Research Centre, 1982:1; Ermans AM, Kinthaert J, Delcroix C, et al. Metabolism of intrathyroidal iodine in nomal men. *J Clin Endocrinol Metab* 1968;28:169; Dumont JE, Ermans AM, Bastenie PA. Thyroidal function in a goiter endemic. IV. Hypothyroidism and endemic cretinism. *J Clin Endocrinol Metab* 1963;23:325; and Camus M, Ermans AM, Bastenie PA. Alterations of iodine metabolism in asymptomatic thyroiditis. *Metabolism* 1968;17:1064.

and biochemical heterogeneity of endemic goiter. These different metabolic anomalies are particularly evident in large colloid goiters, which, therefore, represent maladaptation to iodine deficiency (72).

Thyrotropin Stimulation and Alterations in Circulating Thyroid Hormones

Clinically, euthyroid adults in areas of severe iodine deficiency have a low serum T_4, high TSH, and normal or high T_3 (73,74,76,77,90–92) (Table 11E.6). The mechanisms responsible for this pattern are unclear but may include thyroidal secretion of T_4 and T_3 in the same ratio they have within the gland (87,89,93–95), preferential secretion of T_3 (96) or increased peripheral conversion of T_4 to T_3. The shift to increased T_3 secretion and serum T_3/T_4 ratios may play an important role in the adaptation to iodine deficiency, since T_3 has about 4 times the metabolic potency of T_4 but requires only 75% as much iodine for synthesis (96). It is only under conditions of extreme thyroid failure, as are found in myxedematous endemic cretinism (see Chapter 49), that both serum T_4 and T_3 are low and serum TSH is dramatically elevated. In less severe goiter endemias, serum T_4 and T_3 levels are only slightly abnormal or remain normal. Under these conditions, basal TSH and TSH response to the intravenous injection of thyrotropin-releasing hor-

mone (TRH) are often exaggerated, indicating an increase in pituitary TSH reserve (97), a condition often reported as subclinical hypothyroidism (98). This condition represents mild thyroid failure and should be treated (99).

In severe endemic goiter, an inverse relation exists between serum T_4 and TSH, but not for serum T_3, which is the most active thyroid hormone (87). This paradoxical finding is explained, in part, by the fact that the direct effect of T_4 on TSH suppression results from intrapituitary T_4 to T_3 conversion and the subsequent binding of T_3 to the nucleus of the thyrotrophs, while, in other tissues, the largest part of intracellular T_3 originates from serum T_3 (100). These findings account for the observation in endemic goiter that normal serum T_3 levels enable a patient to maintain an overall euthyroid status, but pituitary stimulation persists as long as the serum T_4 level is low.

In endemic goiter, the serum concentration of thyroxine-binding globulin (TBG) is normal unless its synthesis is decreased by the concomitant presence of protein malnutrition (101). The serum concentration of Tg is markedly elevated (102–106). Serum Tg correlates with serum TSH and is not higher in goitrous than in nongoitrous subjects. Finally, the incidence of positive anti-Tg and antimicrosomal antibodies (anti-TP0) is very low (102,107–109), but may increase after iodine prophylaxis (107) (see also section below on side effects of iodine supplementation).

Morphologic Changes

Morphologic changes in patients with endemic goiter are mainly nodular enlargement of the thyroid gland with striking macroscopic and microscopic heterogeneity (110,111). Diffuse enlargement is rarely found in severe endemic goiter and then only in young subjects. At this stage, the characteristic hyperplastic picture induced experimentally by iodine deficiency may be observed: parenchyma is abundant, follicular epithelium is high with papillary infolding, and colloid is decreased. A later stage is the formation of small nodules of different size and consistency throughout the entire thyroid gland. At this time, histologically, the major part of the gland has extremely distended vesicles with a flattened epithelium filled with colloid, but a few thyroid follicles show a typical pattern of stimulation.

CLINICAL ASPECTS AND DIAGNOSIS

The symptoms of endemic goiter do not differ from those found in nontoxic sporadic goiter; the differential diagnosis is established mainly by epidemiologic criteria. In individual patients, all types of thyroid enlargement may be observed, from the small, solitary thyroid nodule without any appreciable hyperplasia of the rest of the gland, to a huge multinodular goiter. Complications are those described for sporadic goiter (see Chapter 69). The most common are deviation and compression of the trachea, venous distension, the development of a collateral venous circulation on the chest, and thyroid hormone insufficiency. Hypothyroidism is often difficult to demonstrate on clinical grounds or from biologic data, because, as mentioned earlier, the serum T_4 concentration is often low, the TSH concentration high, and the ^{131}I thyroid uptake high (>50% at 24 hours) in clinically euthyroid subjects living in goitrous areas. Scintigraphy of the thyroid reveals the marked heterogeneity of the goiters and often cold or hot nodules.

The presence of hard thyroid nodules may suggest the diagnosis of thyroid cancer. An increase in the absolute number of thyroid cancers in endemic goiter remains controversial (112–114); however, the mortality rate from thyroid cancer may be higher because enlarged thyroids are already frequent in the population and may delay concern about individual nodules.

PEDIATRIC ASPECTS OF ADAPTATION TO IODINE DEFICIENCY

Sequential Development of the Mechanisms of Adaptation to Iodine Deficiency during Growth

Pathogenesis of Endemic Goiter

The view that endemic goiter constitutes the most efficient mechanism of adaptation to iodine deficiency is based, with a few exceptions (47,115–118), on information obtained from adults. Therefore, in an attempt to define the metabolic history of endemic goiter, a study was conducted

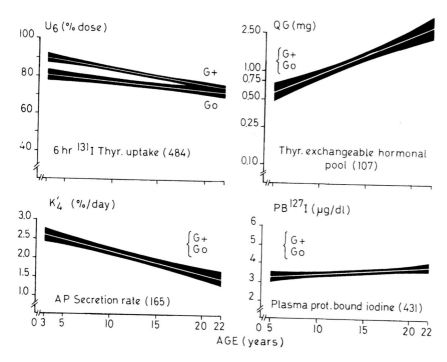

FIGURE 11E.5. Changes with age of the 6-hour thyroidal uptake of radioiodine *(U6)*, the thyroidal iodine exchangeable hormonal pool *(Qg)*, the apparent secretion rate of radioiodine by the thyroid *(K′4)* and the serum concentration of protein-bound iodine *(PBI)* in goitrous *(G+)* and non-goitrous *(Go)* inhabitants of the Idjwi Island endemic goiter area, Democratic Republic of Congo. Values recorded as mean±SE. The number of patients is shown in parentheses. (From Delange F. Adaptation to iodine deficiency during growth: etiopathogenesis of endemic goiter and cretinism. In: Delange F, Fisher D, Malvaux P, eds. *Pediatric thyroidology.* Basel: S. Karger AG, 1985:295; and Delange F. Endemic goitre and thyroid function in Central Africa. *Monographs in pediatrics.* Basel: S. Karger AG, 1974:1, with permission.)

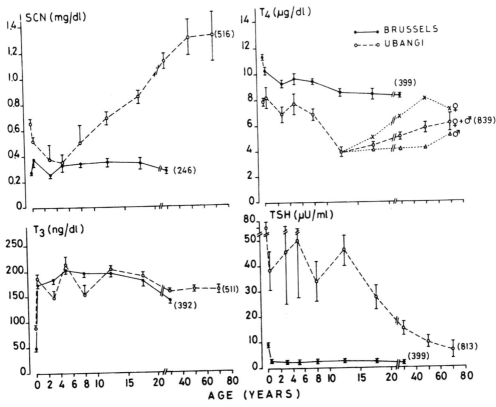

FIGURE 11E.6. Changes with age of the serum concentrations of thyroxine, triiodothyronine, thyrotropin, and thiocyanate *(SCN)* in the Ubangi endemic goiter area, Democratic Republic of Congo (○), and in Brussels (●). Values recorded as mean±SE. The number of patients is shown in parentheses. (From Delange F. Adaptation to iodine deficiency during growth: etiopathogenesis of endemic goiter and cretinism. In: Delange F, Fisher D, Malvaux P, eds. *Pediatric thyroidology.* Basel: S. Karger AG, 1985:295, with permission.)

(23,32) on how thyroid function changed with age, from 3 to 22 years, in goitrous and nongoitrous inhabitants of the Idjwi Island endemic goiter area in the Democratic Republic of Congo (Fig. 11E.5). Thyroidal uptake of radioiodine reached its maximum value in the earliest years of life and then declined progressively until adulthood. Uptake was higher in goitrous than in nongoitrous subjects. The thyroid exchangeable hormonal iodine pool increased progressively with age. The value was about 0.5 mg iodine in young infants; it increased progressively with age but reached only 2.5 mg in adults, which is 4 to 10 times lower than in adults in nonendemic areas. Conversely, the renewal rate of intrathyroidal radioactive iodine (apparent secretion rate, $K'4$) was extremely high in infancy and decreased with age.

This study demonstrates that the acceleration in the main steps of iodine kinetics is more marked in childhood and adolescence than in adulthood, and that it progressively decreases during growth. Subjects from another part of Idjwi Island, with a similar degree of iodine deficiency but no goiter (32), showed that (a) the radioiodine thyroidal uptake also was increased but to a lesser extent, (b) the iodine stores

in the thyroid were much lower, and (c) the plasma protein-bound iodine was higher. These data suggest that goiter is by no means the optimal mechanism of adaptation to iodine deficiency, confirming the view that goiter represents, rather, maladaptation to iodine deficiency (72).

AGE-RELATED MODIFICATIONS OF THYROTROPIN REGULATION

In clinically euthyroid subjects residing in a severe endemic goiter area in the Ubangi region of the Democratic Republic of Congo, the youngest infants unexpectedly had the highest values of serum TSH, although they also had the highest T_4 values (Fig. 11E.6) (119). For a given value of T_4, the TSH level was about twice as high in the 4- to 15-year-old group as in the 16- to 20-year-old group (Fig. 11E.7). These variations in the serum TSH/T_4 ratio as a function of age are poorly understood and could reflect the increase in thyroidal iodine with age. They also could be explained by changes with age in the T_4 turnover rate (120)

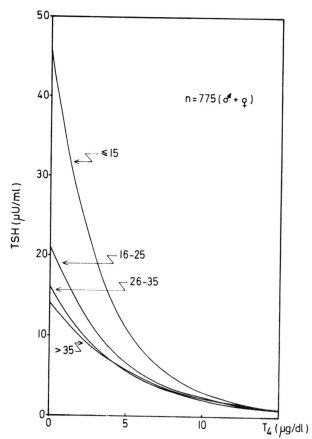

FIGURE 11E.7. Computed correlation curves between thyrotropin (TSH) and thyroxine (T_4) serum concentrations in 840 inhabitants of the Ubangi endemic goiter area (Democratic Republic of Congo). The curves are derived from the linear inverse correlations ($p<0.001$) between log TSH and T_4 in four age groups (younger than 15 years, 16 to 25 years, 26 to 35 years, and older than 35 years). (From Bourdoux P, Ermans AM. Factors influencing the levels of circulating T4, T3 and TSH in human beings submitted to severe iodine deficiency. *Ann Endocrinol (Paris)* 1981;42:40A, with permission.)

or by changes in thyroid gland sensitivity to TSH, including progressive development of thyroid autonomy (121).

Thyroid Function in Early Life

Results from systematic screening for congenital hypothyroidism in the neonates in iodine-deficient areas have provided much useful information (24). In such areas, the alterations of thyroid function in neonates are much more frequent and severe than in adults. A large number of neonates and young infants have the biochemical features of thyroid failure that are found in western countries only in permanent sporadic congenital hypothyroidism.

The most extreme situation has been reported from the Democratic Republic of Congo (122–124), where thyroid failure in neonates results from the combined action of io-

dine deficiency and thiocyanate overload during late fetal life (see Chapter 49). In this area (Fig. 11E.8), cord serum TSH and T_4 levels in unselected newborns were frequently outside the normal range. Eleven percent of the neonates had both a cord serum TSH above 100 µU/mL and a cord serum T_4 below 3.1 µg/dL (40 nmol/L), indicating severe congenital hypothyroidism according to the criteria used in western countries, where the incidence of the condition is only 0.025%. A similar frequency of biochemical hypothyroidism has been found in the same area in young infants (125), indicating that the findings in neonates were not due to nonspecific factors, such as the stress of delivery. The picture of congenital hypothyroidism was only transient in some infants but remained unchanged in others (23).

The abnormalities of neonatal thyroid function were prevented by correcting iodine deficiency in mothers before or during pregnancy (123,126) (Fig. 11E.8). It has been suggested that permanent congenital hypothyroidism in severe iodine deficiency during the perinatal period causes myxedematous endemic cretinism and that transient hypothyroidism during the critical period of brain development is responsible for the endemic mental retardation frequently observed in clinically euthyroid children in severely affected areas (23) (see also Chapter 49).

A similar frequency of congenital hypothyroidism in association with severe endemic goiter has been reported from the Himalayas in northern India, Nepal, and Bhutan (127). Alterations of thyroid function in neonates have been subsequently reported from other less-severe endemic areas, even when thyroid function in adults was normal, and show a shift towards high serum TSH and lower T_4 values (128).

MILD-TO-MODERATE IODINE DEFICIENCY DISORDERS: THE SITUATION IN EUROPE

Epidemiology

Endemic goiter, occasionally complicated by endemic cretinism, was often reported in Europe up to the turn of the 20th century, especially from remote, isolated, mountainous areas in its central parts, including Switzerland, Austria, northern Italy, Bulgaria, and Poland (129,130). The problem of IDD has been entirely eliminated in Switzerland due to the implementation and monitoring of a program of salt iodization (131). Probably because of this remarkable program's impact on the medical world, IDD have not been considered a significant public health problem in Europe during the last 5 decades.

However, reevaluation of the problem in the late 1980s, under the sponsorship of the European Thyroid Association, clearly indicated that, with the exception of some of

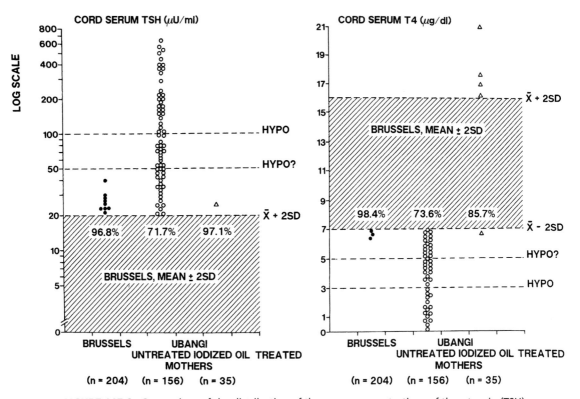

FIGURE 11E.8. Comparison of the distribution of the serum concentrations of thyrotropin (TSH) and thyroxine (T$_4$) in cord blood in Brussels and in newborns in the Ubangi endemic goiter area in the Democratic Republic of Congo born to untreated mothers or to mothers treated with one single injection of iodized oil during pregnancy. The number of newborns is shown in parentheses. The dotted lines correspond to the values considered as suggestive *(hypo?)* or characteristic *(hypo)* of permanent sporadic congenital hypothyroidism in the neonatal thyroid screening program of Brussels. (From Delange F, Thilly C, Bourdoux P, et al. Influence of dietary goitrogens during pregnancy in humans on thyroid function of the newborn. In: Delange F, Iteke FB, Ermans AM, eds. *Nutritional factors involved in the goitrogenic action of cassava.* Ottawa: International Development Research Centre, 1982:40, modified with permission.)

the Scandinavian countries, Austria, and Switzerland, most European countries, or at least certain areas of them, were still iodine deficient, especially in the south (132). Shortly thereafter, it was shown that differences in iodine intake among the adult populations of several countries or areas were accompanied by parallel differences in the iodine content of breast milk and of urine in neonates (133,134) (Table 11E.7). The status of iodine nutrition was reevaluated in 1992 in western and central Europe (135). Iodine deficiency was controlled in only five countries, namely Austria, Finland, Norway, Sweden, and Switzerland.

Programs aiming at the sustainable elimination of iodine deficiency were then reinforced or implemented in many European countries. A multicentre study conducted 5 years later in schoolchildren of 13 European countries, measuring thyroid volume by ultrasonography and urinary iodine, showed marked improvement in most (29).

Also, in 1997 the status of iodine nutrition was evaluated in the 26 countries of central and eastern Europe, the

Commonwealth of Independent States, and the Baltic States (136). This study indicated mild to severe iodine deficiency in many countries and a dramatic return of the deficiency within 5 to 7 years after the interruption of iodized salt programs, for example, in Russia.

Finally, the data on IDD and their prevention in all European countries have been reviewed again (137–140). Evidence of a marked improvement in the status of iodine nutrition was clearly shown, especially in central Europe. However, at least 18 countries still have inadequate iodine nutrition.

Public Health Consequences

The state of mild to severe iodine deficiency persisting in many countries or regions has important consequences for public health, including the intellectual development of infants and children. As an example, Table 11E.8 summarizes the situation in Belgium, where the consequences of mild

TABLE 11E.7. COMPARISON OF THE RESULTS OBTAINED IN EUROPEAN COUNTRIES FOR URINARY IODINE EXCRETION IN ADULTS, IODINE CONTENT OF BREAST MILK, AND URINE OF INFANTS ON DAY 5 OF LIFE

Country or Region (City)	Urinary Excretion of Iodine in Adults (µg/d)	Iodine Concentration (µg/dL)	
		Breast Milk (Mean ± SE) (n)	Urine from Infants on Day 5 (Median)
The Netherlands (Rotterdam)	88–140		16.2 (64)
Finland (Helsinki)	238–270		11.2 (39)
Sweden (Stockholm)	91–140	9.3 (60)	11.0 (52)
Sicily (nonendemic area) (Catania)	113		7.1 (14)
Switzerland (Zürich)	126–141		6.2 (62)
Spain (Madrid)	89	7.7 ± 0.9 (69)	
France (Paris)	55–126	8.2 ± 0.5 (68)	
(Lille)			5.8 (82)
Belgium (Brussels)	51	9.5 ± 0.6 (91)	4.8 (196)
Italy (Rome)	37		4.7 (114)
North Germany (Berlin)	35		2.8 (87)
South Germany (Freiburg)	20	2.5 (41)	1.2 (41)
(Iena)	16	1.2 ± 0.1 (55)	0.8 (54)
Sicily (endemic area) (San Angelo)	22	2.7 ± 0.3 (59)	

Adapted from Delange F, Heidemann P, Bourdoux P, et al. Regional variations of iodine nutrition and thyroid function during the neonatal period in Europe. *Biol Neonate* 1986;49:322; and Delange F, Bürgi H. Iodine deficiency disorders in Europe. *Bull World Health Organ* 1989;67:317, with permission.

IDD on the main target groups, that is, pregnant and lactating women, neonates, and young infants, have been extensively investigated. A recent national survey of iodine nutrition in Belgium has shown marked improvement (141).

More generally, the consequences of iodine deficiency in Europe can be summarized in the following sections.

Adults

The frequency of simple goiter is high in many countries and the cost of treating thyroid problems resulting from iodine deficiency in the adult population is enormous. For example, the diagnosis and treatment of goiter due to iodine deficiency in Germany cost an estimated US$1 billion per year (142), while prevention with iodized salt would cost only US$0.02 to $0.08 per person per year (143). Thyroidal uptake of radioiodine varies markedly from one European country to another and is inversely related to iodine intake (144). High thyroidal uptake due to iodine deficiency increases the risk of thyroid irradiation and development of thyroid cancer in case of a nuclear accident (145).

Thyroid function is usually normal in adults in Europe. In contrast, it is frequently altered in pregnant women. During pregnancy, three synergic effects stimulate the gland: direct stimulation by human chorionic gonadotropin, stimulation through the usual feedback mechanism via the increase in TBG and the lowering of free hormone concentrations, and additional loss of iodide through increased renal clearance and to the fetoplacental unit (146) (see Chapter 80). At least in conditions of borderline iodine intake, as seen in Belgium and southwestern France (146,147) (50 to 70 µg/day), pregnancy is accompanied by a progressive decrease of serum free T_4 and consequently by an increase in serum TSH. This state of chronic TSH hyperstimulation causes goiter in about 10% of the pregnant women and progressively increases the serum Tg concentration (146,147). Goiter can persist after pregnancy in some women (148). Pregnancy, especially under conditions of borderline iodine intake, at least partly explains the higher frequency of thyroid problems in women than in men. Marginal iodine deficiency during pregnancy in Belgium causes even higher serum levels of TSH and Tg in neonates than in the mothers, and slight enlargement of the neonatal thyroid gland. The causal role of iodine deficiency in these changes is demonstrated by their prevention with iodine supplementation of the mothers during pregnancy (149) and their absence in iodine-replete areas of Europe, such as some parts of the Netherlands (150).

Adolescents and Children

Euthyroid goiter is especially frequent in adolescents and occasionally requires therapy with T_4 and/or iodide.

TABLE 11E.8. FUNCTIONAL CONSEQUENCES OF MILD IODINE DEFICIENCY IN BELGIUM

Age Groups	Recommended Iodine Intake (µg/day)[a]	Recommended Urinary Iodine Concentration (µg/L)	Actual Urinary Iodine Concentration (µg/L)	Functional Consequences
Pregnant and Lactating Women	200	200–300	<100 in 90% of the cases	Increased thyroid stimulation; goiter Prevention of the anomalies by iodine supplementation Iodine content of breast milk: 98 ± 5 µg/L (mean ± SE) (normal: 140–180 µg/L)
Adults	150	100–200	51–60	High thyroidal uptake of radioiodine Increased risk of thyroid irradiation in case of nuclear accident
Adolescents	150	100–200	30–50	Goiter
Children (6–12 y)	120	100–200	55–80	Goiter
Infants (6–36 mo)	90	180–220	101	Risk for impaired intellectual development
Neonates	90	150	48–86	High cord serum TSH and Tg High serum TSH and risk of transient neonatal hypothyrodism

[a] Per World Health Organization/United Nations International Children's Emergency Fund/International Council for Control of Iodine Deficiency Disorders (WHO/UNICEF/ICCIDD. *Assessment of the iodine deficiency disorders and monitoring their elimination.* Geneva: World Health Organization; 2001. Publication WHO/NHD/01.1:1).
Adapted from Delange F. Iodine deficiency in Europe anno 2002. *Thyroid International* 2002;5:1, with permission.

Even in Europe, clinically euthyroid schoolchildren born and living in an iodine-deficient area have subtle or overt neuropsychointellectual deficits compared to iodine-sufficient children living in the same ethnic, demographic, nutritional and socioeconomic system (151–155) (Table 11E.9). These deficits are of the same nature, although less marked, as those found in schoolchildren in areas with severe iodine deficiency and endemic mental retardation. They could result, as demonstrated in severe endemic goiter, from transient thyroid failure occurring during fetal or early postnatal life, i.e., during the critical period of brain development (see Chapters 49 and 74).

Neonates

The most important and frequent alterations of thyroid function due to iodine deficiency in Europe occur in neonates and young infants.

TABLE 11E.9. NEUROPSYCHOINTELLECTUAL DEFICITS IN INFANTS AND SCHOOLCHILDREN IN CONDITIONS OF MILD TO MODERATE IODINE DEFICIENCY IN EUROPE

Regions	Tests	Findings	Reference no.
Spain	Locally adapted Bayley, McCarthy, Cattell	Lower psychomotor and mental development than controls	151
Italy Sicily	Bender-Gestalt	Low preceptual integrative motor ability Neuromuscular and neurosensorial abnormalities	152
Tuscany	Wechsler, Raven	Low verbal IQ, perception, motor, and attentive functions	153
Tuscany	Wechsler	Lower velocity of motor response to visual stimuli Slower reaction time	154,155

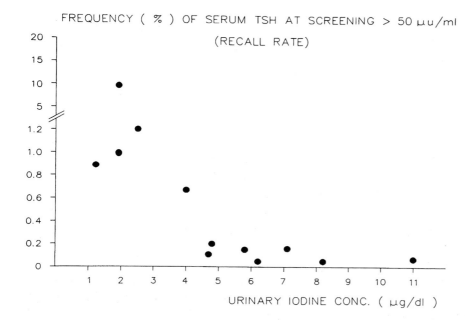

FREQUENCY (%) OF SERUM TSH AT SCREENING > 50 μu/ml
(RECALL RATE)

URINARY IODINE CONC. (μg/dl)

FIGURE 11E.9. Relationship between the urinary iodine concentration and the recall rate at the time of screening for congenital hypothyroidism in newborn populations in Europe. Each point results from the analysis of 50 to 200 urine samples and from 20,000 to 300,000 screening tests. (From Delange F. The disorders induced by iodine deficiency. *Thyroid* 1994; 4:107, with permission.)

The frequency of transient primary hypothyroidism is almost 8 times higher in Europe than in North America (156). The syndrome is characterized by postnatally acquired primary hypothyroidism lasting for a few weeks and requiring T$_4$ therapy (157). The risk of transient hypothyroidism in the neonate increases with the degree of prematurity (158). The specific role of iodine deficiency in the etiology of this hypothyroidism was demonstrated by its disappearance in Belgian preterm infants after they were systematically supplemented with 30 μg of potassium iodide per day.

As shown in Figure 11E.9, there is an inverse relationship between the urinary iodine concentration in newborn infants in Europe, used as an index of their status of iodine nutrition, and the frequency of serum TSH above 50 μU/mL at the time of screening for congenital hypothyroidism, that is, between iodine deficiency and the recall rate for suspected congenital hypothyroidism (19). Consequently, neonatal thyroid screening is a particularly sensitive indicator for the presence and action of environmental goitrogens, including iodine deficiency, and can be used as a monitoring tool in the evaluation of the effects of iodine prophylaxis on a population (159,160).

The reason for the particular sensitivity of the newborn, especially of the preterm infant, to the effects of iodine deficiency appears from the data summarized in Table 11E.10. In Toronto, where the iodine intake is high, the iodine content of the thyroid in full-term infants is 300 μg.

TABLE 11E.10. RELATIONSHIP BETWEEN THE IODINE CONTENT OF URINE IN ADULTS AND NEONATES, USED AS AN INDEX OF IODINE SUPPLY, AND THYROID WEIGHT, THYROID IODINE CONTENT, AND ESTIMATED TURNOVER RATE OF THYROIDAL IODINE IN NEONATES

	Adults	Neonates				
		Urine Iodine		Thyroid Gland		
City	Urinary Excretion of Iodine (μg/d)	Median Iodine Concentration (μg/L)[a,b]	Values <5 μg/L (%)	Weight (g)[a,b]	Iodine Content (μg)[a,b]	Estimated Turnover Rate (%/d)[c]
Toronto	600–800	148 (81)	11.9	1.00 ± 0.12 (13)	292 ± 47	17
Brussels	51	48 (196)[d]	53.2	0.76 ± 0.25 (4)	81 ± 9[e]	62
Leipzig	16	16 (70)[d]	97.2	3.27 ± 0.39 (10)[e]	43 ± 6[e]	125

[a]The number of patients is shown in parentheses.
[b]Results given as mean±SE.
[c]Based on a requirement of thyroxine 50 μg/day.
[d]Levels of significance as compared to Toronto, Canada *p*<0.001.
[e]Levels of significance as compared to Toronto, Canada *p*<0.01.
From Delange F. Screening for congenital hypothyroidism used as an indicator of IDD control. *Thyroid* 1998;8:1185–1192, with permission.

In Brussels, with a borderline iodine intake, the iodine content of the thyroid is 81 µg, and in Leipzig, which was severely iodine deficient, the content is only 43 µg. The table also shows that the turnover rate of intrathyroidal iodine is markedly accelerated in iodine-deficient neonates; therefore, thyroid failure is more likely to occur. These neonatal data contrast with those from adults, in whom thyroidal iodine stores are not affected by iodine deficiency unless it is severe (Fig. 11E.3).

TREATMENT AND PROPHYLAXIS OF IODINE DEFICIENCY DISORDERS

Prolonged administration of iodine or of thyroid hormones is highly effective in reducing the size of endemic goiters (161). Surgical treatment is often justified in large goiters with pressure symptoms. Nevertheless, such treatment is, in practice, impossible to apply to a general population in view of the extent of the problem and the general lack of adequate medical infrastructure in the most severely affected populations. The most logical approach is iodine prophylaxis. The public health features of iodine prophylaxis, including the planning and monitoring of prophylactic campaigns, the technical aspects of production and distribution of iodized salt, and the other methods of iodine delivery, as well as the cost-benefit evaluation of its effectiveness, are discussed in detail elsewhere (7,10,11,13,17, 22,143,162–166).

For almost 80 years, iodized salt has been used as the simplest and most effective way of providing extra iodine in the diet (162,163). Iodine can be added in the form of potassium iodide, but potassium iodate is preferred in humid regions, owing to its greater stability. The recommended levels for salt iodization vary widely. In the early phases of the programs, these levels varied from 1.9 to 100 parts iodine per million (ppm) of salt (131,163). The latest recommendation by WHO/UNICEF/ICCIDD (166) is that, in order to provide 150 µg/day of iodine via iodized salt, and considering the average salt intake and the loss of iodine from production to household and in cooking, the iodine concentration in salt at the site of production should be in the range of 20 to 40 mg iodine (or 34 to 66 mg iodate) per kilo of salt. These levels should be adjusted to ensure a median urinary iodine concentration of 100 to 200 µg/L in the population (5,166).

The first successful large-scale campaigns to prevent endemic goiter by iodized salt were carried out in the United States in 1917 (167) and in Switzerland in 1922 (131, 168). Subsequent pilot surveys confirmed the benefits of salt iodization, especially in Central and South America (7). In 1990, the World Summit for Children adopted the goal, endorsed by WHO and UNICEF, of virtual elimination of IDD by the year 2000 (5,11). Major programs of salt iodization were implemented, including in the most populated and affected parts of the world such as China (400 million at risk) and India. At the beginning of the 1990s, iodized salt reached probably <10% of consumers worldwide. In 1995, of 94 countries that were affected by IDD and had UNICEF programs, 58 had achieved the goal of iodization of 90% of all edible salt (169).

A world review of IDD control by iodized salt was performed by WHO/UNICEF/ICCIDD in late 1998 (Table 11E.11) (11); 130 countries with IDD had laws on iodization of all salt for human and animal nutrition and for the food industry, a strategy called universal salt iodization (USI). However, implementation of the regulations was achieved in only 94 of these countries, with a coverage by USI of >50% of the population in 63 countries and between 10% and 50% in the other 31. Monitoring the quality of iodized salt was reported in 98 countries, but iodine nutrition was monitored in only 79 of them. A further need is the systematic implementation of reliable monitoring of iodized salt from the site of production to the consumer.

Iodide has been used as a supplement in bread in the Netherlands and in Tasmania, but wide variations in con-

TABLE 11E.11. PROGRESS IN ELIMINATING IODINE DEFICIENCY DISORDERS (IDD) AS OF 1999

WHO Region	No. of Countries	No. With IDD Legislation	No. Monitoring Salt Quality	No. With Wide Access to Iodized Salt (%)	No. With Universal Salt Iodization (%)	Iodine Status Adequate (%)
Africa	46	44	34 (6)[a]	29	24	63
Americas	35	19	17	19	19	90
Southeast Asia	10	9	7 (1)	8	7	70
Eastern Mediterranean	22	17	14	14	10	66
Europe	51	32	20 (3)	17	13	27
Western Pacific	27	9	6 (2)	8	6	76
Total	191	130	98 (12)	95	79	68

[a]The figures in parentheses refers to the number of additional countries that have legislation in draft form.
From WHO/UNICEF/ICCIDD. *Progress towards the elimination of iodine deficiency disorders (IDD).* Geneva: World Health Organization; 1999. Publication WHO/NHD/99.4, with permission.

sumption make this a less than satisfactory technique (170). Iodization of water has been successfully used in some areas with adequate water supply and control of the iodization process (171–173). Iodized irrigation water has been successfully used in China (174) and decreased the mortality rate (175).

In many developing countries with severe iodine deficiency, iodization of salt, bread, or water had initially failed to prevent or eradicate the disease because various socioeconomic, climactic, or geographic conditions made systematic iodine supplementation difficult or impossible (162). In such conditions, prophylaxis and therapy could be achieved urgently by the administration of large quantities of iodine in the form of slowly resorbable iodized vegetable oil given intramuscularly or orally (176–178). The method is inexpensive and can be easily implemented through local health services using existing facilities or by small teams. The long-term effectiveness and safety of this procedure, including during pregnancy, have been extensively documented for at least 7 years in adults and for 2 to 3 years in young children after intramuscular injection and for 1 year after oral administration (179,180).

A United Nations Special Session in 2002 moved its previous deadline for IDD elimination from 2000 to 2005 (181). As already recounted in this chapter, the progress in the past 15 years has been enormous, but about half the world's countries still have significant iodine deficiency, and use of adequately iodized salt has leveled off at about 70% of households. The resistant pockets are predictably in areas that are economically poorest and most isolated. In addition, some countries that achieved iodine sufficiency are now in danger of backsliding because of inadequate monitoring and lack of effective governmental infrastructure and education. International agencies and many national governments have been vigorous in pursuing the goal of iodine sufficiency through universal salt iodization, but changes in personnel and new priorities pose real threats to sustaining the effort. Past history, especially in Latin America where salt iodization was widely introduced over 40 years ago only to be later neglected, shows that deficiency will recur if not constantly confronted (182).

SIDE EFFECTS OF IODINE SUPPLEMENTATION

As discussed so far in this chapter, iodine deficiency is associated with the development of thyroid function abnormalities. Similarly, iodine excess, including the overcorrection of a previous state of iodine deficiency, can also impair thyroid function. The effect of iodine on the thyroid gland is complex, with a U-shaped relationship between iodine intake and risk of thyroid diseases, as both low and high io-

dine intake are associated with an increased risk. Normal adults can tolerate up to about 1,000 µg iodine per day without any side effects (6,183). However this upper limit of normal is much lower in a population previously exposed to iodine deficiency. The optimal level of iodine intake to prevent any thyroid disease may be a relatively narrow range around the recommended daily adult intake of 150 µg (5,184).

Iodide Goiter and Iodine-Induced Hypothyroidism

The prevalences of both goiter and subclinical hypothyroidism are increased when iodine intake is chronically high, as for example in coastal areas of Japan (44) and China (45) (due to chronic intake of seaweeds rich in iodine such as laminaria) or in eastern China (because of the high iodine content of water from shallow wells (46)). The mechanisms behind this impairment of thyroid function are probably both iodine enhancement of thyroid autoimmunity and reversible inhibition of thyroid function by excess iodine (Wolff-Chaikoff effect) in susceptible subjects (see next section of this chapter). However, this type of thyroid failure has not been observed after correction of iodine deficiency, including in neonates after the administration of huge doses of iodized oil to their mothers during pregnancy (180).

Iodine-Induced Thyrotoxicosis

Iodine-induced thyrotoxicosis is the main complication of iodine prophylaxis. It has been reported in almost all iodine supplementation programs (15). The most extensively investigated outbreak occurred in Tasmania in the late 1960s following iodine supplementation simultaneously by tablets of iodide, iodized bread, and the use of iodophors in the milk industry (185). The incidence of thyrotoxicosis increased from 24 per 100,000 in 1963 to 125 per 100,000 in 1967. It occurred most frequently in individuals over 40 years of age with multinodular goiters. The most severe manifestations were cardiovascular and were occasionally lethal. The epidemic lasted for some 10 to 12 years, after which the incidence of thyrotoxicosis was somewhat below that existing prior to the epidemic.

Concern about this problem was recently renewed by reports from Zimbabwe that the introduction of iodized salt had sharply increased the incidence of thyrotoxicosis, from 3 per 100,000 to 7 per 100,000 over 18 months (186). A high risk of IIH was also reported from eastern Congo following the introduction of iodized salt (187). A multicenter study conducted in seven African countries, including Zimbabwe and Congo (188), showed that in the last two countries thyrotoxicosis stemmed from the sudden introduction of poorly monitored and excessively iodized salt in populations that had been severely iodine deficient for very long periods. The conclusion of the study was that the risk is related to a rapid increment of iodine intake resulting in acute iodine overload. However, a high frequency of thyrotoxicosis was not reported in populations that could adjust their thyroid function and its regulation to a chronically high iodine intake.

Iodine-induced thyrotoxicosis following iodine supplementation cannot be entirely avoided, even when the supplementation uses only physiological amounts of iodine. In a well-controlled longitudinal study in Switzerland the incidence increased by 27% during the year after the iodine supply was increased from 90 µg/day to the recommended value of 150 µg/day (189). Similarly, the introduction of salt iodization in a Chinese region with borderline deficiency (median urinary iodine of 86 µg/L) resulted in a slight but significant increase in the incidence of thyrotoxicosis (190).

Contrasting with these different reports, thyrotoxicosis was not reported in Iran following a single intramuscular injection of 1 mL iodized oil containing 480 mg iodine to 3,420 subjects with simple goiter in an area with moderate iodine deficiency (mean urinary iodine 35.8 µg/L). Follow-up by clinical and laboratory evaluation every 3 months for 1 year, and every 6 months for the next 4 years, revealed a 0.6% incidence, occurring mostly during the first 5 months after the injection. This figure is close to the incidence of spontaneous thyrotoxicosis in this population (0.4%) (191). Similarly, a clinical and biochemical 3-year survey of the effects of iodized oil injection found no case of iodine-induced thyrotoxicosis among 198 schoolchildren of Kiga, a village in a mountainous region of Iran, where the prevalence of visible goiter was 93% and the mean urinary iodine was 11.4 µg/g creatinine before intervention. Rather, serum T_4 increased from 5.0 to 9.5 µg/dL, TSH decreased from 20.3 to 2.2 mU/L, and Tg from 132.0 to 23.0 ng/mL, and the goiter prevalence lessened substantially (192).

Similarly reassuring results were obtained from long-term biochemical monitoring after oral administration of iodized oil to severely iodine-deficient schoolchildren in Romania (109).

The mechanism for the development of iodine-induced thyrotoxicosis has now been identified (193): iodine deficiency increases thyrocyte proliferation and mutation rates, which, in turn, trigger the development of multifocal autonomous growth with scattered cell clones harboring activating mutations of the TSH receptor. Measurement of intrathyroidal iodine by X-ray fluorescence scanning showed that some nodules retain their capacity to store iodine; these can become autonomous and cause thyrotoxicosis after iodine supplementation (194).

Thus, iodine-induced thyrotoxicosis appears to be largely unavoidable in the early phase of iodine supplementation. It affects principally the elderly with longstanding autonomous nodules. The incidence of thyrotoxicosis reverts to normal or even below normal after 1 to 10 years of iodine supplementation.

Iodine-Induced Thyroiditis

Another possible effect of iodine supplementation is the aggravation or even the induction of autoimmune thyroiditis. Under experimental conditions, excessive iodine intake can precipitate spontaneous thyroiditis in genetically predisposed strains of beagles, rats, or chickens (reviewed in reference 195). The mechanism may be that high dietary iodine triggers thyroid autoimmune reactivity by increasing the immunogenicity of Tg or by inducing damage to the thyroid and its cells by free radicals.

Attention was drawn to the possibility of iodine-induced thyroiditis in humans when an increased frequency of Hashimoto's thyroiditis was seen in goiters removed surgically in the United States after the implementation of salt iodization (196). Later studies reported the development of thyroid autoantibodies after the introduction of iodized oil in Greece (107). More recently, Kahaly et al (197) described the development of thyroid autoantibodies in 6 of 31 patients with endemic goiter treated for 6 months with a supraphysiological dose of 500 µg potassium iodide (KI) per day. The development of lymphocytic infiltration in the thyroids was noted as well. Cross-sectional studies of populations in Italy (198), Great Britain (199), and more recently Denmark and Iceland (16), each with different iodine intakes, showed that the frequencies of thyroid autoantibodies and hypothyroidism are higher in iodine-replete than in iodine-deficient populations. Similarly, the frequencies of thyroid antibodies (200) and of thyroiditis (201) are higher in the United States than in Europe, where the iodine intake is lower.

Acute massive iodine overload (daily consumption of at least 50 mg iodine daily) sharply increased thyroid peroxidase antibody values, serum TSH levels, and goiter prevalence, and all of these decreased after correcting iodine excess (202). However, although cross-sectional studies associated endemic goiter and the presence of thyroid autoantibodies, for example, in Sri Lanka (203), no large epidemiological, metabolic, or clinical surveys following iodine supplementation have uncovered significant iodine-induced thyroiditis with public health consequences (108, 109,191).

Thyroid Cancer

In animals, the chronic stimulation of the thyroid by TSH can produce thyroid tumors (204). There is a tendency toward higher incidence rates of thyroid cancer in autopsy material from endemic goiter areas, although the relationship between thyroid cancer and endemic goiter has often been debated without agreement being reached on many aspects, including causal relationship (114,161,205).

Iodine supplementation is accompanied by a change in the epidemiological pattern of thyroid cancer, with an increased prevalence of occult papillary cancer at autopsy (206,207). However, the prognosis of thyroid cancer is improved following iodine supplementation, due to a shift toward more differentiated forms that are diagnosed at earlier stages. Careful monitoring in Switzerland following iodine supplementation showed that the incidence of thyroid cancer steadily decreased from 2 to 3 per 100,000 in 1950 to 1 to 2 per 100,000 in 1988, during a period when iodine intake increased and reached an optimal value (208). In another example, fine-needle thyroid biopsies of 3,572 patients in Poland, where iodine deficiency was progressively corrected between 1985 and 1999, found that the frequency of neoplastic lesions significantly decreased over the period and the ratio of papillary to follicular carcinomas increased, as did the frequency of cytologically diagnosed chronic thyroiditis (from 1.5% to 5.7%) (209). Overall, correction of iodine deficiency appears to decrease the risk and morbidity of thyroid cancer.

In conclusion, the benefits of correcting iodine deficiency far outweigh its risks. Iodine-induced thyrotoxicosis and other adverse effects can be almost entirely avoided by adequate and sustained quality assurance and by monitoring of iodine supplementation, which should also confirm adequate iodine intake (182,195,210–212).

The progress toward correction of iodine deficiency globally in the past decade is a public health success unprecedented for a noninfectious disease (11,213) and its sustainable elimination is within reach.

REFERENCES

1. Hays M. Estimation of total body iodine content in normal young men. *Thyroid* 2001;11:671–675.
2. Koibuchi N, Chin WW. Thyroid hormone action and brain development. *Trends Endocrinol Metab* 2000;4:123–128.
3. Dobbing J, Sands J. Quantitative growth and development of human brain. *Arch Dis Child* 1973;48:757–767.
4. DeLong GR, Robbins J, Condliffe PG. *Iodine and the brain.* New York: Plenum Press, 1989:1–379.
5. WHO/UNICEF/ICCIDD. *Assessment of the iodine deficiency disorders and monitoring their elimination.* Geneva: World Health Organization; 2001. Publication WHO/NHD/01.1:1–107.
6. Thomson CD. Dietary recommendations of iodine around the world. *IDD Newsletter* 2002;18:38–42.
7. Stanbury JB, Hetzel B. *Endemic goiter and cretinism: iodine nutrition in health and disease.* New York: John Wiley and Sons, 1980:1–606.
8. Hetzel BS, Dunn JT, Stanbury JB. *The prevention and control of iodine deficiency disorders.* Amsterdam: Elsevier Science, 1987:1–354.
9. McMichael AJ, Potter JD, Hetzel BS. Iodine deficiency, thyroid function and reproductive failure. In: Stanbury JB, Hetzel BS eds. *Endemic goiter and endemic cretinism: Iodine nutrition in health and disease.* New York: John Wiley and Sons, 1980:445–460.
10. Hetzel BS. Iodine deficiency disorders (IDD) and their eradication. *Lancet* 1983;ii:1126–1129.
11. WHO/UNICEF/ICCIDD. *Progress towards the elimination of iodine deficiency disorders (IDD).* Geneva: World Health Organization; 1999. Publication WHO/NHD/99.4:1–33.
12. Koutras DA, Matovinovic J, Vought R. The ecology of iodine. In: Stanbury JB, Hetzel BS eds. *Endemic goiter and endemic cretinism.* New York: John Wiley and Sons, 1980:185–195.
13. WHO/UNICEF/ICCIDD. *Indicators for assessing iodine deficiency disorders and their control through salt iodization.* Geneva: World Health Organization; 1994. Publication WHO/NUT/94.6:1–55.
13a. http://www3.who.int/whosis/menu.cfm?path=mn (accessed August 23, 2004).
13b. http://www.icccidd.org (access August 23, 2004),
14. ICCIDD. Global iodine nutrition. *IDD Newsletter* 2003;19:24–25
15. Stanbury JB, Ermans AE, Bourdoux P, et al. Iodine-induced hyperthyroidism: occurrence and epidemiology. *Thyroid* 1998;8:83–100.
16. Laurberg P, Nohr SB, Pedersen KM, et al. Thyroid disorders in mild iodine deficiency. *Thyroid* 2000;10:951–963.
17. Boyages SC, Halpern JP. Endemic cretinism: toward a unifying hypothesis. *Thyroid* 1993;3:59–69.
18. Delange F. The disorders induced by iodine deficiency. *Thyroid* 1994;4:107–128.
19. Hetzel BS, Pandav CS. *S.O.S. for a billion: the conquest of iodine deficiency disorders,* 2nd ed. Dehli: Oxford University Press, 1996:1–466.
20. Hollowell JG, Hannon WH. Teratogen update: Iodine deficiency, a community teratogen. *Teratology* 1997;55:389–405.
21. Semba RD. Iodine deficiency disorders. In: Semba RD, Bloem MW, eds. *Nutrition and health in developing countries.* Totowa, NJ: Humana Press, 2001:343–363.
22. Delange F, Hetzel B. The iodine deficiency disorders. [Thyroid Disease Manager Web site]. Available at: http://http://www.thyroidmanager.org. Accessed August 22, 2004.
23. Delange F. Adaptation to iodine deficiency during growth: etiopathogenesis of endemic goiter and cretinism. In: Delange F, Fisher D, Malvaux P, eds. *Pediatric thyroidology.* Basel: S. Karger AG, 1985:295–326.
24. Delange F. Iodine nutrition and congenital hypothyroidism. In: Delange F, Fisher DA, Glinoer D, eds. *Research in congenital hypothyroidism.* New York: Plenum Press, 1989:173–185.
25. Gutekunst R, Teichert HM. Requirements for goiter surveys and the determination of thyroid size. In: Delange F, Dunn JT, Glinoer D, eds. *Iodine deficiency in Europe: a continuing concern.* New York: Plenum Press, 1993:109–118.
26. Vitti P, Martino E, Aghini-Lombardi F, et al. Thyroid volume measurement by ultrasound in children as a tool for the assessment of mild iodine deficiency. *J Clin Endocrinol Metab* 1994;79:600–603.
27. Zimmermann M, Saad A, Hess S, et al. Thyroid ultrasound compared with WHO 1960 and 1994 palpation criteria for determination of goiter prevalence in regions of mild and severe iodine deficiency. *Eur J Endocrinol* 2000;143:727–731.
28. WHO/ICCIDD. Recommended normative values for thyroid volume in children aged 6–15 years. *Bull World Health Organ* 1997;75:95–97.
29. Delange F, Benker G, Caron P, et al. Thyroid volume and urinary iodine in European schoolchildren: standardization of values for assessment of iodine deficiency. *Eur J Endocrinol* 1997;136:180–187.
30. Zimmermann MB, Molinari L, Spehl M, et al. Towards a consensus on reference values for thyroid volume in iodine replete schoolchildren: results of a workshop on interobserver and in-

terequipment variation in sonographic measurement of thyroid volume. *Eur J Endocrinol* 2001;144:213–220.

31. Zimmermann M, Hess S, Molinari L, et al. New reference values of thyroid volume by ultrasound in iodine-sufficient schoolchildren: a WHO/NHD Iodine Deficiency Study Group report. *Am J Clin Nutr* 2004;79:231.

32. Delange F. Endemic goitre and thyroid function in central Africa. *Monographs in pediatrics.* Basel: S. Karger AG, 1974:1–171.

33. Beckers C, Delange F. Etiology of endemic goiter. Iodine deficiency. In: Stanbury JB, Hetzel BS, eds. *Endemic goiter and endemic cretinism.* New York: John Wiley and Sons, 1980:199–217.

34. Gaitan E. *Environmental goitrogenesis.* Boca Raton: CRC Press, 1989:1–250.

35. Koutras DA, Papapetrou PD, Yataganas X, et al. Dietary sources of iodine in areas with and without iodine-deficiency goiter. *Am J Clin Nutr* 1970;23:870–874.

36. Follis RH. Patterns of urinary iodine excretion in goitrous and nongoitrous areas. *Am J Clin Nutr* 1964;14:253–268.

37. Jolin T, Escobar del Rey F. Evaluation of iodine/creatinine ratios of casual samples as indices of daily urinary iodine output during field studies. *J Clin Endocrinol* 1965;25:540–542.

38. Bourdoux P, Thilly C, Delange F, et al. A new look at old concepts in laboratory evaluation of endemic goiter. In: Dunn JT, Pretell E, Daza C, Viteri FE, eds. *Towards the eradication of endemic goiter, cretinism and iodine deficiency.* Washington, DC: Pan American Health Organization (PAHO); 1986. Scientific No. 502:115–129.

39. Hetzel BS, Potter BJ, Dulberg EM. The iodine deficiency disorders: nature, pathogenesis and epidemiology. *World Rev Nutr Diet* 1990;62:59–119.

40. Pandav CS, Rao AR. *Iodine deficiency disorders in livestock. Ecology and economics.* New Delhi: Oxford University Press, 1997:1–288.

41. Orts S, Dustin P, Delange F. Goitrous enzootic in the wild rat with a geographical distribution similar to endemic human goitre. *Acta Endocrinol (Copenh)* 1971;66:193–200.

42. Clements FW, Wishart JW. A thyroid-blocking agent in the etiology of endemic goiter. *Metabolism* 1956;5:623–639.

43. Peltola P, Virtanen A. Effect of the prophylactic use of iodine on the thyroid of cattle in the endemic goitre in Finland. *Ann Med Intern Fenn (Helsinki)* 1954;43:209–215.

44. Suzuki H, Higuchi T, Sawa K, et al. "Endemic coast goitre" in Hokkaido, Japan. *Acta Endocrinol (Copenh)* 1965;50:161–176.

45. Ma T, Zhi-Heng Y, Ti-Zhang L, et al. High-iodide endemic goiter. *Chin Med J (Engl)* 1982;95:692–696.

46. Zhao J, Wang P, Shang L, et al. Endemic goiter associated with high iodine intake. *Am J Public Health* 2000;90:1633–1635.

47. Choufoer JC, Van Rhijn M, Kassenaar AAH, et al. Endemic goiter in western New Guinea: iodine metabolism in goitrous and non-goitrous subjects. *J Clin Endocrinol Metab* 1963;23:1203–1217.

48. Delange F, Thilly C, Ermans AM. Iodine deficiency, a permissive condition in the development of endemic goiter. *J Clin Endocrinol Metab* 1968;28:114–116.

49. Roche M, Perinetti H, Barbeito A. Urinary excretion of stable iodine in a small group of isolated Venezuelan Indians. *J Clin Endocrinol Metab* 1961;21:1009–1012.

50. Ermans AM, Mbulamoko NM, Delange F, et al. *Role of cassava in the etiology of endemic goitre and cretinism.* Ottawa: International Development Research Centre, 1980:1–182.

51. Delange F, Iteke FB, Ermans AM. *Nutritional factors involved in the goitrogenic action of cassava.* Ottawa: International Development Research Centre, 1982:1–100.

52. Langer P, Greer MA. *Antithyroid substances and naturally occurring goitrogens.* Basel: S. Karger AG, 1977:1–178.

53. Podoba J, Langer P. *Naturally occurring goitrogens and thyroid function.* Bratislava: Publishing House of the Slovak Academy of Sciences, 1964:1–312.

54. Van Etten CH. Goitrogens. In: Liener IE, ed. *Toxic constituents of plant foodstuffs.* New York: Academic Press, 1969: 103–142.

55. Delange F, Ermans AM. Endemic goiter and cretinism. Naturally occurring goitrogens. *Pharmacol Ther* 1976;1:57–93.

56. Gmelin R, Virtanen AI. The enzymic formation of thiocyanate (SCN-) from a precursor(s) in Brassica species. *Acta Chem Scand* 1960;14:507–510.

57. Ermans AM, Bourdoux P. Antithyroid sulfurated compounds. In: Gaitan E, ed. *Environmental goitrogenesis.* Boca Raton, FL: CRC Press, 1989: 15–34.

58. Gibson HB, Howeler JF, Clements FW. Seasonal epidemics of endemic goitre in Tasmania. *Med J Aust* 1960;1:875–880.

59. Ermans AM, Kinthaert J, Van der Velden M, et al. Studies of the antithyroid effects of cassava and of thiocyanate in rats. In: Ermans AM, Mbulamoko NM, Delange F, Ahluwalia R, eds. *Role of cassava in the etiology of endemic goitre and cretinism.* Ottawa: International Development Research Centre, 1980:93–110.

60. Wolff J. Transport of iodide and other anions in the thyroid gland. *Physiol Rev* 1964;44:45–90.

61. Wollman SH. Inhibition by thiocyanate of accumulation of radioiodine by thyroid gland. *Am J Physiol* 1962;203:517–524.

62. Ekpechi OL. Pathogenesis of endemic goitre in eastern Nigeria. *Br J Nutr* 1967;21:537–545.

63. Delange F, Ermans AM. Role of a dietary goitrogen in the etiology of endemic goiter in Idjwi Island. *Am J Clin Nutr* 1971; 24:1354–1360.

64. Bourdoux P, Delange F, Gerard M, et al. Evidence that cassava ingestion increases thiocyanate formation: a possible etiology in endemic goiter. *J Clin Endocrinol Metab* 1978;216:613–621.

65. Maberly GF, Eastman CJ, Waite KV, et al. The role of cassava in endemic goitre in Sarawak, Malaysia. In: Ui N, Torizuka K, Nagataki S, Miayi K, eds. *Current problems in thyroid research.* Amsterdam: Excerpta Medica, 1983:341–344.

66. Gaitan E, Cooksey RC, Legan J, et al. Antithyroid effects in vivo and in vitro of babossu and manolioca: a staple food in goiter areas of Brazil. *Eur J Endocrinol* 1994;131:138–144.

67. Bourdoux P, Seghers P, Matufa M, et al. Cassava products: HCN content and detoxification processes. In: Delange F, Iteke FB, Ermans AM, eds. *Nutritional factors involved in the goitrogenic action of cassava.* Ottawa: International Development Research Centre, 1982:51–58.

68. Delange F, Vigneri R, Trimarchi F et al. Etiological factors of endemic goiter in north-eastern Sicily. *J Endocrinol Invest* 1978; 2:137–142.

69. Scranton JR, Nissen WM, Halmi NS. The kinetics of the inhibition of thyroidal iodine accumulation by thiocyanate: a reexamination. *Endocrinology* 1969;85:603–607.

70. Stanbury JB, Brownell GL, Riggs DS, et al. *Endemic goiter. The adaptation of man to iodine deficiency.* Cambridge, MA: Harvard University Press, 1954:1–209.

71. Studer H, Kohler H, Bürgi H. Iodine deficiency. In: Greer MA, Solomon DH, eds. *Handbook of physiology. Section 7. Endocrinology.* Washington, DC: American Physiological Society, 1974:303–328.

72. Dumont JE, Ermans AM, Maenhaut G, et al. Large goiter as a maladaptation to iodine deficiency. *Clin Endocrinol (Oxf)* 1995;43:1–10.

73. Chopra IJ, Sack J, Fisher DA. Circulating 3,3′,5′-triiodothyronine (reverse T3) in the human newborn. *J Clin Invest* 1975; 55:1137–1141.

74. Delange F, Hershman JM, Ermans AM. Relationship between the serum thyrotropin level, the prevalence of goiter and the pattern of iodine metabolism in Idjwi Island. *J Clin Endocrinol Metab* 1971;33:261–268.

75. Hennemann G, Djokomoeljanto R, Docter R, et al. The relationship between serum protein-bound iodine levels and urinary iodine excretion and serum thyrotropin concentrations in subjects from an endemic goitre area in central Java. *Acta Endocrinol (Copenh)* 1978;88:474–481.

76. Patel YC, Pharoah POD, Hornabrook RW, et al. Serum triiodothyronine, thyroxine and thyroid-stimulating hormone in endemic goiter: a comparison of goitrous and nongoitrous subjects in New Guinea. *J Clin Endocrinol Metab* 1973;37:783–789.

77. Pharoah POD, Lawton NF, Ellis SM, et al. The role of triiodothyronine (T3) in the maintenance of euthyroidism in endemic goitre. *Clin Endocrinol (Oxf)* 1973;2:193–199.

78. Dumont JE, Lamy F, Roger P, et al. Physiological and pathological regulation of thyroid cell proliferation and differentiation by thyrotropin and other factors. *Physiol Rev* 1992;72:667–697.

79. Wayne EJ, Koutras DA, Alexander WD. *Clinical aspects of iodine metabolism.* Oxford: Blackwell Science, 1964:1–303.

80. Spitzweg C, Morris JC. The sodium iodide symporter: its pathophysiological and therapeutic implications. *Clin Endocrinol (Oxf)* 2002;57:559–574.

81. Riggs DS. Quantitative aspects of iodine metabolism in man. *Pharmacol Rev* 1952;4:284.

82. Ermans AM, Dumont JE, Bastenie PA. Thyroid function in a goitrous endemic. II. Nonhormonal iodine escape from the goitrous gland. *J Clin Endocrinol Metab* 1963;23:550–560.

83. Schaefer AE. Status of salt iodization in PAHO member countries. In: Dunn JT, Medeiros-Neto GA, eds. *Endemic goiter and cretinism: continuing threats to world health.* Washington, DC: Pan American Health Organization (PAHO); 1974. Scientific No. 292:242–250.

84. Delange F, Bourdoux P, Chanoine JP, et al. Physiopathology of iodine nutrition during pregnancy, lactation and early postnatal life. In: Berger H, ed. *Vitamins and minerals in pregnancy and lactation.* New York: Raven Press, 1988:205–213.

85. Tovar E, Maisterrena JA, Chavez A. Iodine nutrition levels of schoolchildren in rural Mexico. In: Stanbury JB, ed. *Endemic goiter.* Washington, D.C.: Pan American Health Organization (PAHO); 1969. Scientific No. 193:411–415.

86. Oddie TH, Fisher DA, McConahey WM, et al. Iodine intake in the United States: a reassessment. *J Clin Endocrinol Metab* 1970;30:659–665.

87. Ermans AM. Etiopathogenesis of endemic goiter. In: Stanbury JB, Hetzel BS, eds. *Endemic goiter and endemic cretinism.* New York: John Wiley and Sons, 1980:287–301.

88. Ermans AM, Dumont J, Bastenie PA. Thyroid function in a goiter endemic. I. Impairment of hormone synthesis and secretion in the goitrous gland. *J Clin Endocrinol Metab* 1963;23:539–549.

89. Abrams GM, Larsen PR. Triiodothyronine and thyroxine in the serum and thyroid glands of iodine-deficient rats. *J Clin Invest* 1973;52:2522–2531.

90. Delange F, Ermans AM. Iodine deficiency. In: Braverman LE, Utiger RD, eds. *The thyroid: a fundamental and clinical text.* Philadelphia: JB Lippincott Co, 1991:368–390.

91. Delange F, Camus M, Ermans AM. Circulating thyroid hormones in endemic goiter. *J Clin Endocrinol Metab* 1972;4:891–895.

92. Kochupillai N, Karmakar MG, Weightman D, et al. Pituitary-thyroid axis in Himalayan endemic goitre. *Lancet* 1973;1:1021–1024.

93. Ermans AM, Kinthaert J, Delcroix C, et al. Metabolism of intrathyroidal iodine in nomal men. *J Clin Endocrinol Metab* 1968;28:169–180.

94. Dumont JE, Ermans AM, Bastenie PA. Thyroidal function in a goiter endemic. IV. Hypothyroidism and endemic cretinism. *J Clin Endocrinol Metab* 1963;23:325–335.

95. Camus M, Ermans AM, Bastenie PA. Alterations of iodine metabolism in asymptomatic thyroiditis. *Metabolism* 1968;17:1064–1072.

96. Greer MA, Grimm Y, Studer H. Qualitative changes in the secretion of thyroid hormones induced by iodine deficiency. *Endocrinology* 1968;83:1193–1198.

97. Medeiros-Neto GA, Imai Y, Kataoka K, et al. Thyroid function studies in endemic goiter and endemic cretinism. In: Robbins J, Braverman LE, eds. *Thyroid research.* Amsterdam: Excerpta Medica, 1976:497–500.

98. Evered DC, Ormston BJ, Smith PA, et al. Grades of hypothyroidism. *BMJ* 1973;i:657–662.

99. McDermott MT, Ridgway EC. Subclinical hypothyroidism is mild thyroid failure and should be treated. *J Clin Endocrinol Metab* 2001;86:4585–4590.

100. Silva JE, Dick TE, Larsen PR. The contribution of local tissue thyroxine monodeiodination to the nuclear 3,5,3′triiodothyronine in pituitary, liver and kidney of euthyroid rats. *Endocrinology* 1978;103:1196–1207.

101. Ingenbleek Y, Luypaert B, de Nayer P. Nutritional status and endemic goitre. *Lancet* 1980;i:388–392.

102. Van Herle AJ, Chopra IJ, Hershman JM, et al. Serum thyroglobulin in inhabitants of an endemic region of New Guinea. *J Clin Endocrinol Metab* 1976;43:512–516.

103. Pezzino V, Vigneri R, Squatrito S, et al. Increased serum thyroglobulin levels in patients with nontoxic goiter. *J Clin Endocrinol Metab* 1978;46:653–657.

104. Hershman JM, Due DT, Sharp B, et al. Endemic goiter in Vietnam. *J Clin Endocrinol Metab* 1983;57:243–249.

105. Fenzi GF, Ceccarelli C, Macchia E, et al. Reciprocal changes of serum thyroglobulin and TSH in residents of a moderate endemic goitre area. *Clin Endocrinol (Oxf)* 1985;23:115–122.

106. van den Briel T, West CE, Hautvast JGAJ, et al. Serum thyroglobulin and urinary iodine concentration are the most appropriate indicators of iodine status and thyroid function under conditions of increasing iodine supply. *J Nutr* 2001;131:2701–2706.

107. Boukis MA, Koutras DA, Souvatzoglou A, et al. Thyroid hormone and immunological studies in endemic goiter. *J Clin Endocr Metab* 1983;57:859–862.

108. Azizi F, Navai L, Fattahi F. Goiter prevalence, urinary iodine excretion, thyroid function and anti-thyroid antibodies after 12 years of salt iodization in Shahriar, Iran. *Int J Vitam Nutr Res* 2002;72:291–295.

109. Simescu M, Varciu M, Nicolaescu E, et al. Iodized oil as a complement to iodized salt in schoolchildren in endemic goiter in Romania. *Horm Res* 2002;58:78–82.

110. Correa P. Pathology of endemic goiter. In: Stanbury JB, Hetzel BS, eds. *Endemic goiter and endemic cretinism.* New York: John Wiley and Sons, 1980:303–332.

111. Studer H, Peter HJ, Gerber H. Natural heterogeneity of thyroid cells: the basis for understanding thyroid function and nodular goiter growth. *Endocr Rev* 1989;10:125–135.

112. Wahner HW, Cuell C, Correa P, et al. Thyroid carcinoma in an endemic goiter area, Cali, Colombia. *Am J Med* 1966;40:58–66.

113. Riccabona G. Thyroid cancer and endemic goiter. In: Stanbury JB, Hetzel BS, eds. *Endemic goiter and endemic cretinism.* New York: John Wiley and Sons, 1980:333–350.

114. Harach HR, Escalante DA, Onativia A, et al. Thyroid carcinoma and thyroiditis in an endemic goitre region before and after iodine prophylaxis. *Acta Endocrinol (Copenh)* 1985;108: 55–60.

115. De Visscher M, Beckers C, Van Den Schrieck HG, et al. Endemic goiter in the Uele region (Reic of Congo). I. General aspects and functional studies. *J Clin Endocrinol Metab* 1961;21: 175–188.

116. Maisterrena JA, Tovar E, Cancino A, et al. Nutrition and endemic goiter in Mexico. *J Clin Endocrinol Metab* 1964;24: 166–172.

117. Wahner HW, Gaitan E. Thyroid function in adolescents from the goiter endemic of the Cauca Valley, Columbia. In: Stanbury JB, ed. *Endemic goiter*. Washington, DC: Pan American Health Organization (PAHO); 1969. Scientific No. 193:291– 303.

118. Semiz S, Senol U, Bircan O, et al. Thyroid hormone profile in children with goiter in an endemic goiter area. *J Pediatr Endocrinol Metab* 2001;14:171–176.

119. Bourdoux P, Ermans AM. Factors influencing the levels of circulating T4, T3 and TSH in human beings submitted to severe iodine deficiency. *Ann Endocrinol (Paris)* 1981;42:40A.

120. Malvaux P. Thyroid function during the neonatal period, infancy and childhood. In: Delange F, Fisher DA, Malvaux P, eds. *Pediatric thyroidology*. Basel: S. Karger AG, 1985:33–43.

121. Bachtarzi H, Benmiloud M. TSH-regulation and goitrogenesis in severe iodine deficiency. *Acta Endocrinol (Copenh)* 1983;103: 21–27.

122. Delange F, Thilly C, Camus M, et al. Evidence for fetal hypothyroidism in severe endemic goiter. In: Robbins J, Braverman LE, eds. *Thyroid research*. Amsterdam: Excerpta Medica, 1976:493–496.

123. Thilly CH, Delange F, Lagasse R, et al. Fetal hypothyroidism and maternal thyroid status in severe endemic goiter. *J Clin Endocrinol Metab* 1978;47:354–360.

124. Delange F, Thilly C, Bourdoux P, et al. Influence of dietary goitrogens during pregnancy in humans on thyroid function of the newborn. In: Delange F, Iteke FB, Ermans AM, eds. *Nutritional factors involved in the goitrogenic action of cassava*. Ottawa: International Development Research Centre, 1982:40–50.

125. Courtois P, Delange F, Bourdoux P, et al. Significance of neonatal thyroid screening tests in severe endemic goiter. *Ann Endocrinol (Paris)* 1982;43:51A(abst).

126. Thilly CH, Vanderpas J, Bourdoux P, et al. Prevention of myxedematous cretinism with iodized oil during pregnancy. In: Ui N, Torizuka K, Nagataki S, Miyai K, eds. *Current problems in thyroid research*. Amsterdam: Excerpta Medica, 1983:386–389.

127. Kochupillai N, Pandav CS. Neonatal chemical hypothyroidism in iodine-deficient environments. In: Hetzel BS, Dunn JT, Stanbury JB, eds. *The prevention and control of iodine deficiency disorders*. Amsterdam: Elsevier Science, 1987:85–93.

128. Sava L, Delange F, Belfiore A, et al. Transient impairment of thyroid function in newborn from an area of endemic goiter. *J Clin Endocrinol Metab* 1984;59:90–95.

129. Merke F. *History and iconography of endemic goitre and cretinism*. Bern: Hans Huber, 1984:1–339.

130. König MP. *Die Kongenitale Hypothyreose und der Endemische Kretinismus*. Berlin: Springer-Verlag New York, 1968:1–175.

131. Bürgi H, Supersaxo Z, Selz B. Iodine deficiency diseases in Switzerland one hundred years after Theodor Kocher's survey: a historical review with some new goitre prevalence data. *Acta Endocrinol (Copenh)* 1990;123:577–590.

132. Gutekunst R, Scriba PC. Goiter and iodine deficiency in Europe: the European Thyroid Association report as updated in 1988. *J Endocrinol Invest* 1989;12:209–220.

133. Delange F, Heidemann P, Bourdoux P, et al. Regional variations of iodine nutrition and thyroid function during the neonatal period in Europe. *Biol Neonate* 1986;49:322–330.

134. Delange F, Bürgi H. Iodine deficiency disorders in Europe. *Bull World Health Organ* 1989;67:317–326.

135. Delange F, Dunn J, Glinoer D. *Iodine deficiency in Europe. A continuing concern*. New York: Plenum Press, 1993:1–491.

136. Delange F, Robertson A, McLoughney E, et al. *Elimination of iodine deficiency disorders (IDD) in central and eastern Europe, the Commonwealth of Independent States, and the Baltic States*. Geneva: World Health Organization; 1998. Publication WHO/ Euro/NUT/98.1:1–168.

137. Delange F. Iodine deficiency in Europe anno 2002. *Thyroid International* 2002;5:1–18.

138. Anonymous. West and central Europe assesses its iodine nutrition. *IDD Newsletter* 2002;18:51–55.

139. Vitti P, Delange F, Pinchera A, et al. Europe is iodine deficient. *Lancet* 2003;361.

140. Gerasimov G. IDD in eastern Europe and central Asia. *IDD Newsletter* 2002;18:33–37.

141. Delange F, Van Onderbergen A, Shabana W, et al. Silent iodine prophylaxis in western Europe only partly corrects iodine deficiency: the case of Belgium. *Eur J Endocrinol* 2000;143:189– 196.

142. Kahaly GJ, Dietlein M. Cost estimation of thyroid disorders in Germany. *Thyroid* 2002;12:909–914.

143. Mannar V. The iodization of salt for the elimination of iodine deficiency disorders. In: Hetzel BS, Pandav CS, eds. *S.O.S. for a billion: the conquest of iodine deficiency disorders*. New Delhi: Oxford University Press, 1996: 98–118.

144. Thilly CH, Vanderpas JB, Bebe N, et al. Iodine deficiency, other trace elements and goitrogenic factors in the etiopathogeny of iodine deficiency disorders (IDD). *Biol Trace Elem Res* 1992;32:229–243.

145. Malone J, Unger J, Delange F, et al. Thyroid consequences of Chernobyl accident in the countries of the European Community. *J Endocrinol Invest* 1991;14:707–717.

146. Glinoer D. Maternal and fetal impact of chronic iodine deficiency. *Clin Obstet Gynecol* 1997;40:102–116.

147. Caron P, Hoff M, Bazzi S, et al. Urinary iodine excretion during normal pregnancy in healthy women living in the Southwest of France: correlation with maternal thyroid parameters. *Thyroid* 1997;7:749–754.

148. Glinoer D, Lemone M, Bourdoux P, et al. Partial reversibility during late postpartum of thyroid abnormalities associated with pregnancy. *J Clin Endocrinol Metab* 1992;74:453–457.

149. Glinoer D, De Nayer P, Delange F, et al. A randomized trial for the treatment of excessive thyroid stimulation in pregnancy: maternal and neonatal effects. *J Clin Endocrinol Metab* 1995; 80:258–269.

150. Berghout A, Endert E, Ross A, et al. Thyroid function and thyroid size in normal pregnant women living in an iodine replete area. *Clin Endocrinol (Oxf)* 1994;41:375–379.

151. Bleichrodt N, Escobar del Rey F, Morreale de Escobar G, et al. Iodine deficiency: implications for mental and psychomotor development in children. In: DeLong GR, Robbins J, Condliffe PG, eds. *Iodine and the brain*. New York: Plenum Press, 1989:269–287.

152. Vermiglio F, Sidoti M, Finocchiaro MD, et al. Defective neuromotor and cognitive ability in iodine-deficient schoolchildren of an endemic goiter region in Sicily. *J Clin Endocrinol Metab* 1990;70:379–384.

153. Fenzi GF, Giusti LF, Aghini-Lombardi F, et al. Neuropsychological assessment in schoolchildren from an area of moderate iodine deficiency. *J Endocrinol Invest* 1990;13:427–431.

154. Vitti P, Aghini-Lombardi F, Antonangeli L, et al. Mild iodine deficiency in fetal/neonatal life and neuropsychological performances. *Acta Med Austriaca* 1992;19:57–59.

155. Aghini-Lombardi F, Pinchera A, Antonangeli L, et al. Mild iodine deficiency during fetal/ neonatal life and neuropsychological impairment in Tuscany. *J Endocrinol Invest* 1995; 18: 57–62.

156. Burrow GN, Dussault JH. *Neonatal thyroid screening.* New York: Raven Press, 1980:1–322.

157. Delange F, Dodion J, Wolter R, et al. Transient hypothyroidism in the newborn infant. *J Pediatr* 1978;92:974–976.

158. Delange F, Dalhem A, Bourdoux P, et al. Increased risk of primary hypothyroidism in preterm infants. *J Pediatr* 1984;105: 462–469.

159. Nordenberg D, Sullivan K, Maberly G, et al. Congenital hypothyroid screening programs and the sensitive thyrotropin assay: strategies for the surveillance of iodine deficiency disorders. In: Delange F, Dunn JT, Glinoer D, eds. *Iodine deficiency in Europe. A continuing concern.* New York: Plenum Press, 1993:211–218.

160. Delange F. Screening for congenital hypothyroidism used as an indicator of IDD control. *Thyroid* 1998;8:1185–1192.

161. Riccabona G. Treatment of the individual patient with endemic goiter. In: Stanbury JB, Hetzel BS, eds. *Endemic goiter and endemic cretinism.* New York: John Wiley and Sons, 1980: 351–394.

162. Stanbury JB, Ermans AM, Hetzel BS, et al. Endemic goitre and cretinism: public health significance and prevention. *WHO Chron* 1974;28:220–228.

163. Demaeyer EM, Lowenstein FW, Thilly CH. *The control of endemic goitre.* Geneva: World Health Organization, 1979:1–86.

164. Mannar VMG, Dunn JT. *Salt iodization for the elimination of iodine deficiency.* MI/ICCIDD/UNICEF/WHO; 1995:1–126.

165. Sullivan KM, Houston R, Gorstein J, et al. *Monitoring universal salt iodization programmes.* Wageningen: PAMM/MI/ICCIDD; 1995:1–101.

166. WHO/UNICEF/ICCIDD. *Recommended iodine levels in salt and guidelines for monitoring their adequacy and effectiveness.* Geneva: World Health Organization; 1996. WHO/NUT/ 96.13: 1–9.

167. Marine D, Kimball OP. Prevention of simple goiter in man. *Arch Intern Med* 1920;25:661–672.

168. Bürgi H. Iodine deficiency in Switzerland. In: Delange F, Robertson A, McLoughney E, Gerasimov G, eds. *Elimination of iodine deficiency disorders (IDD) in central and eastern Europe, the Commonwealth of Independent States, and the Baltic States.* Geneva: World Health Organization, 1998:15–20.

169. UNICEF. *The progress of nations.* New York: United Nations Children's Fund; 1995:1–54.

170. Clements W, Gibson HB, Coy JF. Goiter prophylaxis by addition of potassium iodate to bread. *Lancet* 1970;1:489–501.

171. Maberly GF, Eastman CJ, Corcoran JM. Effect of iodination of a village water-supply on goitre size and thyroid function. *Lancet* 1981;2:1270–1272.

172. Squatrito S, Vigneri R, Runello F, et al. Prevention and treatment of endemic iodine-deficient goiter by iodination of a municipal water supply. *J Clin Endocrinol Metab* 1986;63:368–375.

173. Fisch A, Pichard E, Prazuck T, et al. A new approach to combating iodine deficiency in developing countries: the controlled release of iodine in water by a silicone elastomer. *Am J Public Health* 1993;83:540–545.

174. Cao XY, Jian, XM, Kareem A, et al. Iodination of irrigation water as a method of supplying iodine to a severely iodine-deficient population in Xinjiang, China. *Lancet* 1994;344:107–110.

175. Delong GR, Leslie PW, Wang SH, et al. Effect on infant mortality of iodination of irrigation water in a severely iodine-deficient area of China. *Lancet* 1997;350:771–773.

176. Hetzel BS, Thilly CH, Fierro-Benitez R, et al. Iodized oil in the prevention of endemic goiter and cretinism. In: Stanbury JB, Hetzel BS, eds. *Endemic goiter and endemic cretinism.* New York: John Wiley and Sons, 1980:513–532.

177. Dunn JT. Iodized oil in the treatment and prophylaxis of IDD. In: Hetzel BS, Dunn JT, Stanbury JB, eds. *The prevention and control of iodine deficiency disorders.* Amsterdam: Elsevier Science, 1987:127–134.

178. Dunn JT. The use of iodized oil and other alternatives for the elimination of iodine deficiency disorders. In: Hetzel BS, Pandav CS, eds. *S.O.S. for a billion. The conquest of iodine deficiency disorders.* New Delhi: Oxford University Press, 1996: 119–128.

179. Benmiloud M, Chaouki M., Gutekunst R, et al. Oral iodized oil for correcting iodine deficiency: optimal dosing and outcome indicator selection. *J Clin Endocrinol Metab* 1994;19: 20–24.

180. Delange F. Administration of iodized oil during pregnancy: a summary of the published evidence. *Bull World Health Organ* 1996;74:101–108.

181. ICCIDD. UN General Assembly pledges sustainable elimination of iodine deficiency disorders by 2005. *IDD Newsletter* 2002;18:17–19.

182. Dunn JT. Complacency: the most dangerous enemy in the war against iodine deficiency. *Thyroid* 2000;10:681–683.

183. WHO. *Iodine and health. Eliminating iodine deficiency disorders safely through salt iodization.* Geneva: World Health Organization; 1994:1–7.

184. Knudsen N, Bülow I, Jorgensen T, et al. Comparative study of thyroid function and types of thyroid dysfunction in two areas in Denmark with slightly different iodine status. *Eur J Endocrinol* 2000;143:485–491.

185. Connolly RJ, Vidor GI, Stewart JC. Increase in thyrotoxicosis in endemic goitre area after iodation of bread. *Lancet* 1970;i: 500–502.

186. Todd CH, Allain T, Gomo ZAR, et al. Increase in thyrotoxicosis associated with iodine supplements in Zimbabwe. *Lancet* 1995;346:1563–1564.

187. Bourdoux P, Ermans AM, Mukalay AMW, et al. Iodine induced thyrotoxicosis in Kivu, Zaire. *Lancet* 1996;347:552–553.

188. Delange F, de Benoist B, Alnwick D. Risks of iodine-induced hyperthyroidism following correction of iodine deficiency by iodized salt. *Thyroid* 1999;9:545–556.

189. Baltisberger BL, Minde CE, Bürgi H. Decrease of incidence of toxic nodular goiter in a region of Switzerland after full correction of mild iodine deficiency. *Eur J Endocrinol* 1995;132: 546–549.

190. Yan F, Teng W, Shan Z, et al. Epidemiological survey on the relationship between different iodine intakes and the prevalence of hyperthyroidism. *Eur J Endocrinol* 2002;146:613–618.

191. Azizi F, Daftarian N. Side-effects of iodized oil administration in patients with simple goiter. *J Endocrinol Invest* 2001;24: 72–77.

192. Mirmiran P, Kimiagar M, Azizi F. Three-years survey of effects of iodized oil injection in schoolchildren with iodine deficiency disorders. *Exp Clin Endocrinol Diabetes* 2002;110:393–397.

193. Dremier S, Coppée F, Delange F, et al. Thyroid autonomy: mechanism and clinical effects. *J Clin Endocrinol Metab* 1996; 81:4187–4193.

194. Jonckheer MH, Velkeniers B, Van Haelst L. Further characterization of iodine-induced hyperthyroidism based on the direct

measurement of intrathyroidal iodine stores. *Nucl Med Commun* 1992;13:114–118.

195. Delange F, Lecomte P. Iodine supplementation: benefits outweigh risks. *Drug Saf* 2000;22:89–95.

196. McConahey WM, Keating FR, Beahr OH, et al. On the increasing occurrence of Hashimoto's thyroiditis. *J Clin Endocrinol Metab* 1962;22:542–544.

197. Kahaly GJ, Dienes HP, Beyer J, et al. Iodide induces thyroid autoimmunity in patients with endemic goiter: a randomised, double-blind, placebo-controlled trial. *Eur J Endocrinol* 1998;139:290–297.

198. Aghini-Lombardi F, Antonangeli L, Martino E, et al. The spectrum of thyroid disorders in an iodine-deficient community: the Pescoporgano survey. *J Clin Endocrinol Metab* 1999;84:561–566.

199. Vanderpump MPJ, Tunbridge WMG, French JM, et al. The incidence of thyroid disorders in the community: a twenty-year follow-up of the Wickham Survey. *Clin Endocrinol (Oxf)* 1995;43:55–68.

200. Hollowell JG, Staehling NW, Flanders WD, et al. Serum TSH, T4, and thyroid antibodies in the United States population (1988–1994): National Health and Nutrition Examination Survey (NHANES III). *J Clin Endocrinol Metab* 2002;87:489–499.

201. Braverman LE. Iodine and the thyroid: 33 years of study. *Thyroid* 1994;4:351–356.

202. Pearce EN, Gerber AR, Gootnick DB, et al. Effects of chronic iodine excess in a cohort of long-term American workers in West Africa. *J Clin Endocrinol Metab* 2002;87:5499–5502.

203. Premawardhana LDKE, Parkes AB, Smyth PPA, et al. Increased prevalence of thyroglobulin antibodies in Sri Lanka schoolgirls—is iodine the cause? *Eur J Endocrinol* 2000;143:185–188.

204. Money WL, Rawson RW. The experimental production of thyroid tumors in the rat exposed to prolonged treatment with thiouracil. *Cancer* 1950;3:321.

205. Pendergrast WJ, Milmore BK, Marcus SC. Thyroid cancer and thyrotoxicosis in the United States: their relation to endemic goiter. *J Chronic Dis* 1961;13:22–38.

206. Vigneri R, Pezzino V, Squatrito S, et al. Iodine deficiency and thyroid cancer. In: Delange F, Robertson A, McLoughney E, Gerasimov G, eds. *Elimination of iodine deficiency disorders (IDD) in central and eastern Europe, the Commonwealth of Independent States, and the Baltic States.* Geneva: World Health Organization; 1998.:67–72.

207. Williams ED. Dietary iodide and thyroid cancer. In: Hall R, Köbberling J, eds. *Thyroid disorders associated with iodine deficiency and excess.* New York: Raven Press, 1985: 201–207.

208. Levi F, Vecchia CL, Randriamiharisoa A. Cancer mortality in Switzerland, 1985–89. *Soz Praventivmed* 1991;36:112–126.

209. Slowinska-Klencka D, Klencki M, Sporny S, et al. Fine-needle aspiration biopsy of the thyroid in an area of endemic goitre: influence of restored sufficient iodine supplementation on the clinical significance of cytologic results. *Eur J Endocrinol* 2002;146:19–26.

210. Braverman LE. Adequate iodine intake-the good far outweights the bad. *Eur J Endocrinol* 1998;139:14–15.

211. Delange F. Risks and benefits of iodine supplementation. *Lancet* 1998;351:923–924.

212. Delange F, Bürgi H, Chen ZP, et al. World status of monitoring of iodine deficiency disorders control programs. *Thyroid* 2002;12:915–924.

213. Delange F, de Benoist B, Pretell E, et al. Iodine deficiency in the world: where do we stand at the turn of the century. *Thyroid* 2001;11:437–447.

11F   EFFECT OF EXCESS IODIDE: CLINICAL ASPECTS

ELIO ROTI
APOSTOLOS G. VAGENAKIS

An adequate supply of dietary iodide is essential for synthesis of the thyroid hormones. Iodide deficiency results in endemic goiter in many geographic areas, including continental western Europe; in many other regions, however, dietary iodide intake has increased, such as in the United States, Great Britain and Scandinavia. The National Health and Nutrition Examination Survey III 1988–1994 (NHANES III) found in the US population a median urinary iodide excretion rate of 145 µg/L. This value was significantly lower than that of 321 µg/L measured in the 1971 to 1974 period. Furthermore, urinary iodide concentrations were low (<50 µg/L) in 11.7% of the population, a 4.5-fold increase compared with that observed in 1971 to 1974. The proportion of women of childbearing age (15 to 47 years) and of pregnant women with low urinary iodide concentrations was 15% and 7%, 3.8 and 6.9 times the respective proportions in compared with the 1971 to 1974 survey (1). The decrement of iodide intake was probably due to the dairy industry's effort to reduce iodide in milk and a decrease in the use of iodide salts as the dough conditioner in commercial bread production (2). A recent survey of the iodide content in various brands of milk in Boston revealed a relatively high content of 116 µg iodide in 8 ounces of milk (2a). This trend in iodide consumption has also resulted in a decline in the percentage of the population with excessive iodide intake (>500 µg/L) from 27.8% in the 1971 to 1974 survey to 5.3% in the 1988 to 1994 survey. In a study in Denmark, urinary iodide excretion was extremely variable, dependent upon the iodide content in drinking water, which varied from <1.0 to 139 µg/L, and variable intake from day to day (3,4).

Strong evidence indicates that excess iodide can induce thyroid dysfunction, and these iodide-induced abnormalities in thyroid function are the subject of this subchapter.

NORMAL RESPONSE TO EXCESS IODIDE

In animals and humans, the thyroid gland has intrinsic autoregulatory mechanisms to effectively handle excess iodide intake, probably involving the iodide transporter (the sodium iodide (Na^+/I^-) symporter; NIS) recently cloned by Dal and colleagues (5).

The acute, transient inhibitory effect of iodide excess on thyroid iodide organification, the Wolff-Chaikoff effect, and the escape phenomenon are discussed in Chapter 4. It has been suggested that adaptation to or escape from the acute Wolff-Chaikoff effect is due to a decrease in NIS messenger RNA (mRNA) and protein (6) and to increased NIS protein turnover (7), thereby lowering intrathyroidal iodide and permitting normal hormone synthesis to resume (6). The well-known but less understood effect of iodide on the release of thyroxine (T_4) and triiodothyronine (T_3) from the thyroid has been studied prospectively in humans. When normal subjects were given approximately 40 to 150 mg iodide for 1 to 3 weeks, a small but significant decrease in the serum concentrations of T_4 and T_3 occurred, with a small but significant compensatory increase in the serum thyroid-stimulating hormone (thyrotropin, TSH) concentration and an increased TSH response to thyrotropin-releasing hormone (TRH) (8–10). These alterations were all within the normal range for each parameter. In another study, daily mouth rinsing with polyvinylpyrrolidone iodide for 6 months for gingivitis resulted in the absorption of about 3 mg iodide daily and in small but significant increases in the serum TSH concentration (11). After iodide withdrawal, all values returned to baseline levels. In contrast to these findings, an acute increase in serum iodide concentrations, approximately 90-fold above baseline values, following endoscopic retrograde cholangiopancreaticography with iopamidol, a nonionic contrast agent, was not followed by significant changes of serum TSH, free T_4, and free T_3 concentrations (12). This is in contrast with another study of 70 patients in whom there was a persistent decrease in serum TSH, especially in those with nodular goiters. The serum T_3 increased in all 70 patients and

serum free T_4 only in patients with nodular goiters. Symptoms of thyrotoxicosis were not present (13).

Smaller quantities of iodide (1,500 and 4,500 µg/day) administered to normal subjects who resided in iodide-replete areas resulted in significant decreases in serum T_4 and free T_4 but not in serum T_3 concentrations. Serum TSH concentrations increased, as did the serum TSH response to TRH. The smallest quantity of iodide that did not affect thyroid function was 500 µg/day (14). In another study, however, this small quantity of iodide enhanced the TSH response to TRH (15) and in a few patients also increased the basal serum TSH concentration above the normal range. Thus, iodide supplements of about 500 µg/day above the normal diet in iodide-sufficient areas might cause subtle changes in thyroid function (16).

These subtle changes in thyroid function during iodide administration are accompanied by a small increase of thyroid volume determined by echography (17) and by a decrement of thyroid blood flow evaluated by echo color Doppler (18). The latter finding, however, was not related to serum TSH changes.

SOURCES OF EXCESS IODIDE

Various drugs and food preservatives contain a large quantity of iodide that is either absorbed directly or released after metabolism of the drug. Many vitamin preparations are supplemented with about 150 µg iodide, a quantity that is considered to be the physiologic daily requirement. Iodophors contain large quantities of iodide and are used as udder antiseptics in the dairy industry, resulting in increased content of iodide in cow's milk from local contamination and increased secretion into milk from absorbed iodide. Iodide is concentrated by the mammary gland and secreted into the milk and, therefore, may influence thyroid function in the newborn fed cow's milk. Recent evidence in Boston suggests that human breast milk may contain insufficient quantities of iodide to maintain adequate iodide nutrition in breast fed neonates (E Pearce and L Braverman, unpublished data). Many iodide-rich products, such as kelp, kombu, and dolts, are available in natural food stores. In some areas of Japan, bread is made exclusively from seaweed, exposing the population to large quantities of iodide.

Iodides are present in high concentration in various proprietary and prescribed expectorants, including iodinated glycerol, although iodide has been removed from this latter medication in the United States. Another potential source of excess iodide is the use of contrast media in radiologic studies. Preparations used for computed tomography, arteriography, or pyelography are cleared from the plasma relatively quickly, but the iodide released during these procedures affects thyroid function. However, a dye commonly used for arteriography, meglumine ioxaglate, did not affect serum T_4, T_3, or free T_4 index up to 56 days after catheterization, but serum TSH was not measured (19). Coronary angiography performed in 788 unselected euthyroid patients, induced thyrotoxicosis in 2 patients within 12 weeks. The baseline serum TSH was normal and ultrasonography of the thyroid showed no abnormalities (20). Drugs used in the past for myelography, uterosalpingography, or bronchography were lipid soluble and cleared slowly, maintaining high plasma inorganic iodide concentrations for years. The newer water-soluble iodide-containing preparations,

such as metrizamide, have markedly reduced this problem. Occasionally drinking water may be a source of excess iodide intake, such as in some Chinese counties where the drinking water has an iodide concentration of 300 to 462 μg/L. The population residing in those areas has a urinary iodide excretion rate as high as 900 μg/L (21–24). Also, iodide-based water purification systems may cause chronic excessive iodide intake. A group of American volunteers working in west Africa had a median urinary iodide excretion of 5,048 μg/L, due to a faulty iodination system, and some developed goiter and subclinical hypothyroidism (25). A partial list of medications and other preparations containing large quantities of iodide is given in Table 11F.1.

TABLE 11F.1. COMMONLY USED IODIDE-CONTAINING DRUGS

Drugs	Iodide Content
Oral or Local	
Amiodarone	75 mg/tablet
Benziodarone[a]	49–100 mg/tablet
Calcium iodide (e.g., Calcidrine syrup)	26 mg/mL
Echothiophate iodide for ophthalmic solution (e.g., Phospholine)	5–41 mg/drop
Hydriodic acid syrup	13–15 mg/mL
Iodochlorhydroxyquin (e.g., Entero-Vioform)	104 mg/tablet
Iodide-containing vitamins	0.15 mg/tablet
Iodinated glycerol (e.g., Organidin,[b] Iophen)	15 mg/tablet, 25 mg/mL
Idoxuridine ophthalmic solution (e.g., Herplex)	18 mg/drop
Isopropamide iodide (e.g., Darbid, Combid)	1.8 mg/tablet
Kelp	0.15 mg/tablet
KI (e.g., Quadrinal)	145 mg/tablet, 24 mg/mL
Lugol's Solution	6.3 mg/drop
Niacinamide hydroiodide + KI (e.g., Iodo-Niacin)	115 mg/tablet
Ponaris nasal emollient	5 mg/0.8 mL
SSKI	38 mg/drop
Parenteral Preparations	
Sodium iodide, 10% solution	85 mg/mL
Topical Antiseptics	
Iodide tincture	40 mg/mL
Iodochlorhydroxyquin cream (e.g., Vioform)	12 mg/g
Iodoform gauze (e.g., NuGauze)	4.8 mg/ 100 mg gauze
Povidone iodide (e.g., Betadine)	10 mg/mL
Radiology Contrast Agents	
Diatrizoate meglumine sodium (e.g., Renografin-76)	370 mg/mL
Iodized oil	380 mg/mL
Iopanoic acid (e.g., Telepaque)	333 mg/tablet
Ipodate (e.g., Oragrafin)	308 mg/cap
Iothalamate (e.g., Angio-Conray)	480 mg/mL
Metrizamide (e.g., Amipaque)	483 mg/mL

KI, potassium iodide; SSKI, saturated solution of potassium iodide.
[a]Not U.S. Food and Drug Administration–approved.
[b]Iodide was removed from Organidin and Tuss Organidin in 1995.

IODIDE-INDUCED HYPOTHYROIDISM OR GOITER

In certain susceptible people, the thyroid cannot escape from the transient inhibitory effect of iodide on the organification mechanism. As a result, hypothyroidism may result after prolonged excess iodide administration. The hypothyroidism is usually transient, and thyroid function returns to normal after iodide withdrawal. Although the exact frequency of iodide goiter, hypothyroidism, or both, in subjects with apparently normal underlying thyroid function is not known, they are probably uncommon; in patients with underlying thyroid dysfunction, however, they are common (Table 11F.2). Iodide goiter may occur with or without hypothyroidism. Most patients who develop iodide goiter have received iodides for years. The mechanism by which the inhibitory effect of iodide is sustained in these susceptible people is not clear.

IODINE-INDUCED HYPOTHYROIDISM OR GOITER IN THE ABSENCE OF APPARENT THRYOID DISEASE

Normal Subjects

Iodide-induced goiter occurs in about 10% of the population of Hokkaido, a Japanese island. The inhabitants of this island, particularly the fishermen and their families, consume large quantities of an iodide-rich seaweed called kombu. The quantity of iodide ingested daily may exceed 200 mg. Despite goiter, hypothyroidism is rare. Endemic iodide-induced goiter has also been observed in 64% of children residing in a village in central China (21). These children drank water containing 462 mg iodide per liter. No increased prevalence of lymphocytic thyroiditis was found in these children. Thyroid autoantibodies as well as immunoglobulins that inhibited TSH binding were negative. Thyroid growth-stimulating immunoglobulins were found in 60% of goitrous children but were absent in children without goiter who resided in an

TABLE 11F.2. CAUSES OF IODIDE-INDUCED HYPOTHYROIDISM OR GOITER

In the case of underlying thyroid disease
    Fetus and neonate, mostly preterm
        Secondary to transplacental passage of iodide and exposure of newborn infants to topical
            or parenteral iodide-rich substances
    Infant
        Occasionally reported in infants drinking iodide-rich water (China) and after exposure to
            excess iodide
    Adult
        Frequently reported in Japanese subjects with high iodide intake (Hashimoto's thyroiditis
            has been excluded)
    Elderly
        Reported in elderly subjects with and without possible defective organification and
            autoimmune thyroiditis
    Chronic nonthyroidal illness
        Cystic fibrosis
        Chronic lung disease (Hashimoto's thyroiditis was not excluded)
        Chronic dialysis treatment
        Thalassemia major
        Anorexia nervosa
In the case of underlying thyroid disease
    Hashimoto's thyroiditis
    Euthyroid patients previously treated for Graves' disease by ^{131}I, thyroidectomy, or antithyroid
        drugs
    Subclinical hypothyroidism, especially in the elderly
    After transient postpartum thyroiditis
    After subacute, painful thyroiditis
    After hemithyroidectomy for benign nodules
    Euthyroid patients with a previous episode of amiodarone-induced destructive thyrotoxicosis
    Euthyroid patients with a previous episode of interferon-α-induced thyroid disorders
Iodide plus other potential goitrogens
    Sulfisoxazole: cystic fibrosis
    Lithium
    Sulfadiazine (?)

area with increased iodide concentrations in the drinking water (22). This finding has yet to be confirmed. In another study, goiter due to iodide-rich drinking water was observed in 10% of the subjects residing in 19 Chinese counties (23). In general, those subjects had normal thyroid function. Other Chinese subjects drinking iodide-rich water had a prevalence of clinical and subclinical hypothyroidism of 2% and 6%, respectively (24). In American workers drinking iodide-rich water serum TSH concentrations were above 4.2 mU/L in 29%. This value decreased to 5% after iodide removal (25). An increased prevalence of hypothyroidism (12%), defined by serum TSH concentrations >5 mU/L, was observed in thyroid autoantibody-negative Japanese subjects with an iodide concentration in morning urine samples greater than 75 mM (9.5 mg/L); in subjects with normal iodide excretion, the prevalence of hypothyroidism was only 2% (26). When the iodide intake was restricted, the increased serum TSH concentrations returned to normal in patients with negative antithyroid antibodies, but not in those with antibodies, suggesting that

excessive iodide intake should be considered a cause of hypothyroidism in addition to chronic thyroiditis in these areas (27). In an elderly Icelandic population, high urinary iodide excretion rates (median 150 μg/L, range 33 to 703 μg/L) were found to be accompanied by a high prevalence (18%) of serum TSH concentrations >4 mU/L. In subjects residing in Jutland with low urinary iodide excretion (median 38 μg/L, range 6 to 770 μg/L), serum TSH levels were low (<0.4 mU/L) in 10%. The incidence of positive thyroid antibodies was similar in both populations (28). In another study, the cumulative prevalence of overt and subclinical hypothyroidism progressively increased in respect to urinary iodide excretion, being 5%, 12%, and 32%, corresponding to a median urinary excretion of 72, 100, and 513 μg/g creatinine, respectively (29). The prevalence of positive antithyroid peroxidase (anti-TPO) and antithyroglobulin (anti-Tg) antibodies was similar in all three groups.

Treatment with povidone-iodide for 3 to 133 months resulted in subclinical hypothyroidism in 3 of 27 patients with neurologic diseases and negative antithyroid antibodies (30). These findings suggest that iodide-induced hypothyroidism might appear even in subjects with no underlying thyroid disease, and it is not strictly correlated with the presence of thyroid autoimmunity.

Histologic examination of the thyroid of patients with iodide-induced hypothyroidism revealed the presence of lymphocytic infiltration in only half the specimens examined. In the other specimens, hyperplastic changes in the follicles with papillary folding, cuboidal or columnar change of cells with clear and vesicular cytoplasm, and markedly reduced colloid in the distended follicles were seen. These changes were reversible after iodide withdrawal (31). In contrast to these findings, the administration of a single dose of 50 to 70 mg of potassium iodide (KI) to children for iodide prophylaxis following the Chernobyl reactor accident was not accompanied by an increment in serum TSH concentrations (32). Usually, serum T_4 and T_3 concentrations are low or low-normal and serum TSH is increased in patients with iodide-induced hypothyroidism. The thyroid radioactive iodide uptake would be expected to be very low in these patients; however, about 30% have a normal or high thyroid radioactive iodide uptake (33). Similar findings have been observed in European but not US patients who developed iodide-induced hypothyroidism after amiodarone administration (34,35).

Perinatal Period

Iodide readily crosses the placenta and is concentrated by the fetal thyroid. Large quantities of iodide administered to pregnant women resulted in goiter in the newborn, probably because the fetal thyroid is inordinately sensitive to the inhibitory effect of iodide on hormone synthesis (36). By ultrasonography and cordocentesis, goiter and hypothyroidism have been diagnosed in a fetus whose asthmatic mother consumed 2 to 3 spoonfuls per day of a syrup containing 130 mg/15 mL of iodide (37). Severe goitrous hypothyroidism was recently reported in a newborn infant with a history of iodide exposure in utero derived from an expectorant used by the mother (38). Whether the inhibitory effect was exerted on the organification mechanism or on the release of thyroid hormones, or both, is not clear. Studies in rats strongly suggest that the inhibitory effects are exerted in utero as well as in the late neonatal period, which corresponds to the last few weeks of human fetal life (39). Iodides are actively transported by breast tissue and secreted into the milk, and the administration of iodides to nursing mothers could result in iodide-induced hypothyroidism and goiter in their infants.

The thyroid of the fetus and newborn can be exposed to iodide from various routes. Vaginal douching with iodide-containing solutions in nonpregnant women results in a small increase in the serum TSH concentration (40). In contrast, in nonpregnant women vaginal disinfection with povidone-iodide vaginal pessaries and obstetric cream does not affect serum iodide concentrations and thyroid function (41,42). Transient hypothyroidism of the newborn, as indicated by an elevation of the serum TSH, has been reported to follow the application of vaginal solutions of povidone-iodide and in a few cases after povidone-iodide cream application (43) during the last trimester and during labor (36,43), or topical application of povidone-iodide to the skin of the newborns. The latter appears to be more common in premature, low-birthweight infants (44). Serum TSH concentrations above 20 mU/L occurred in 25% of the cases, promptly normalizing after the iodide-containing antiseptic was discontinued (45). The injection of small amounts of an iodinated contrast dye through nonradiopaque silastic catheters in premature infants induced hypothyroidism in some and thyrotoxicosis in others (44,46).

The administration of a single dose of 15 mg of KI to newborn infants for iodide prophylaxis after the Chernobyl nuclear reactor accident resulted in a transient increase of serum TSH concentrations in 0.4% of the 3,214 treated infants (32). In the same population, the exposure in utero to iodide due to maternal iodide prophylaxis did not result in an increase in congenital hypothyroidism (32).

Iodide contamination is the major cause of transient neonatal hypothyroidism (47), responsible for 3% of recalls at screening for congenital hypothyroidism (48). Because these reports emanate primarily from continental Europe, where mild iodide deficiency is present, it is possible that iodide deficiency might predispose the fetal and neonatal thyroid to the inhibitory effect of iodide. According to this hypothesis the supplementation of 150 µg iodide /day to pregnant women in Denmark, a mild to moderate iodide deficiency area, resulted in a significant increase of the percentage of cord serum TSH values above 10 mU/L, 41% in neonates whose mothers were supplemented with iodide and 31% in the control group (49). Brown et al reported that transient hypothyroidism is not a common sequela of routine skin cleansing with iodide in premature newborn infants in the United States, an iodide sufficient area (50). Furthermore, Momotani and colleagues (51) reported that only 2 of 35 newborns whose mothers had been treated with 6 to 40 mg iodide daily from 11 to 37 weeks of gestation for Graves' disease had elevated cord serum TSH concentrations. It is possible that the lack of fetal iodide-induced hypothyroidism in these newborns was due to the concomitant presence of autoimmune thyroid hyperfunction and the high ambient iodide intake in Japan.

Drugs containing iodide also may induce hypothyroidism in the fetus. Bartalena et al. (52) reviewed 64 cases of pregnant women treated with amiodarone. Hypothyroidism was detected in 17% of the progeny. All neonates had transient hypothyroidism.

Childhood

The administration of 40 to 65 mg iodide per day to euthyroid children residing in Greece resulted in serum TSH concentrations above 4.2 mU/L in 75% A similar finding was observed in euthyroid children who had transient neonatal hypothyroidism. In contrast, adult subjects did not have any increment in serum TSH concentrations (53). This finding suggests that in children, the autoregulatory mechanisms is immature and therefore the thyroid is susceptible to the inhibitory effects of excess iodide on hormone synthesis.

Chronic Nonthyroidal Illness

Patients with chronic nonthyroidal illness usually are not susceptible to the inhibitory effect of iodide despite the multiplicity of thyroid dysfunction. However, certain diseases may predispose the patient to iodide-induced thyroid dysfunction (54).

Iodide-induced hypothyroidism has been reported in patients with a variety of chronic lung diseases, including asthma, treated for a prolonged period with iodide-containing expectorants. However, underlying Hashimoto's thyroiditis predisposing these patients to the inhibitory effect of iodide was not ruled out (8,9).

Children with cystic fibrosis, especially those treated with sulfisoxazole, are particularly susceptible to iodide-induced hypothyroidism (55). No apparent thyroid dysfunction was found in these patients, although accumulation of lipofuscin has been observed in the thyroids of patients with cystic fibrosis. The significance of the latter finding is unclear because lipofuscin is found in the thyroid of mice fed large quantities of iodides.

In children and adults with thalassemia major and requiring chronic blood transfusions, iodide administration (60 mg/day) resulted in subclinical hypothyroidism (TSH >5 mU/L) in 60%. TSH returned to basal levels 2 to 3 weeks after iodide withdrawal. It appears that hemosiderosis renders the thyroid of these patients susceptible to the inhibitory effects of iodide (56).

Patients with chronic renal failure frequently have thyroid dysfunction, including thyroid enlargement and abnormal thyroid function tests. Some of these abnormalities are due to chronic disease, although iodides have been suspected as a potential pathogen because they are used as antiseptics in these patients. In one study, however, no relationship was found between thyroid abnormalities due to iodide and application of iodide-containing antiseptics (57). In another study, iodide-induced hypothyroidism was diagnosed in 3% of patients on chronic dialysis treatment (58). In these patients the thyroid was enlarged, thyroid radioactive uptake was normal or elevated, the iodide-perchlorate discharge test was positive, and no lymphocytic infiltration was present at cytologic examination. After re-

striction of iodide intake in 83% of patients with renal dysfunction and increased serum TSH concentrations, the thyroid function tests were normalized (59).

The use of mucolytic expectorants containing iodinated glycerol is particularly frequent in elderly subjects, although this problem may abate in the United States because iodide has been removed from the products. The occurrence of mild hypothyroidism after iodinated glycerol administration was observed in an elderly patient with a previous episode of severe hypothyroidism induced by KI administration, as well as in subjects without known thyroid disorders (60). In these subjects, the abnormalities of thyroid function resolved spontaneously after therapy was withdrawn.

Iodide-induced hypothyroidism has been reported in patients with anorexia nervosa (61,62). In one patient, excessive iodide intake resulting from kombu ingestion induced severe hypothyroidism despite negative antithyroid antibodies (62). After withdrawal of kombu, thyroid function returned to normal. Kombu is used in Japan as a low-calorie food, and one package contains approximately 13 mg of iodide.

In Japanese hypothyroid patients with negative thyroid antibodies, restriction of iodide intake resulted in a decrement of urinary iodide excretion from a median value of 834 μg I/g creatinine to 123 μg I/g creatinine a week later and a parallel decrement of serum TSH concentrations from 123 to 4 mU/L. Furthermore, during long-term follow-up these patients remained euthyroid, except for one subject, who resumed excessive iodide intake (63).

IODINE-INDUCED HYPOTHYROIDISM OR GOITER IN THE PRESENCE OF UNDERLYING THYROID DISEASE

Chronic Lymphocytic Thyroiditis

Patients with chronic lymphocytic (Hashimoto') thyroiditis often develop hypothyroidism due to thyroid destruction by the autoimmune process and the presence of TSH-blocking antibodies. In about 60% of patients, an abnormal iodide-perchlorate discharge test suggests a defect in the intrathyroidal organic binding of iodide. Administration of pharmacologic quantities of iodide (180 mg/day) resulted in hypothyroidism in more than 60% of the patients in one study. The iodide-perchlorate discharge test was positive in patients who developed iodide-hypothyroidism and negative in those who did not (8,9). The failure of the thyroid to escape from the inhibitory effect of iodide is probably due to a persistent Wolff-Chaikoff effect and not to inhibition of the release of T_4 and T_3 from the thyroid. Direct measurement of intrathyroidal thyroid hormone content, however, has not been performed. In Bio-Breeding/ Worcester (BB/Wor) rats, which are genetically susceptible to chronic lymphocytic thyroiditis, pharmacologic quantities of iodide surprisingly do not consistently induce hypothyroidism, and no demonstrable abnormality in intrathyroidal organification of iodide was found (64). In BB/Wor sublines with the most extensive lymphocytic thyroiditis, however, iodide administration does induce hypothyroidism (65). Contradictory results have been obtained when patients with Hashimoto's thyroiditis were exposed to a moderately increased iodide intake. The administration of 1.5 mg iodide daily for 3 months in patients with Hashimoto's thyroiditis did not induce hypothyroidism (66). A few Japanese patients with primary hypothyroidism due to lymphocytic thyroiditis and a high iodide intake became euthyroid when the iodide intake was restricted (67). This phenomenon has been confirmed in other studies (63,68). However, a large number of these patients had a relapse of hypothyroidism even in the presence of normal serum non-hormonal iodide concentrations (63).

Small quantities of iodide given chronically to four patients with Hashimoto's disease who resided in an area of sufficient iodide intake did not induce any changes in thyroid function (11). Of 40 patients, 8 with high TPO antibody levels residing in an area of mild iodide deficiency developed subclinical or overt hypothyroidism following the ingestion of only 250 μg KI/day for 4 months (69). These patients had serum TSH concentrations >3 mU/L before iodide supplementation. During iodide supplementation, the TPO antibody titer did not change. In another study conducted in patients with autoimmune thyroiditis also residing in an area of low iodide intake, small quantities of iodide caused a transient increase in serum T_4 and T_3 concentrations (70). Small quantities (150 μg/day) of iodide given to moderately iodide-deficient TPO-positive pregnant women did not induce or worsen post partum thyroid disease (71).

Graves' Disease

Before the discovery of antithyroid drugs, the sole medical treatment of Graves' thyrotoxicosis was the chronic administration of large quantities of iodide. Most patients were reasonably well controlled on this regimen, but thyrotoxicosis recurred in some patients, and a few patients developed reversible hypothyroidism. When patients with Graves' disease treated with iodide-131 (^{131}I) were given iodide (250 mg/day) 1 to 2 weeks after ^{131}I therapy, 60% developed transient hypothyroidism. Euthyroid patients treated years earlier either with ^{131}I or thyroidectomy also developed hypothyroidism during the administration of pharmacologic quantities of iodide. The hypothyroidism was transient, and thyroid function returned to normal after iodide withdrawal. All patients who developed hypothyroidism had a positive iodide-perchlorate discharge test (8,9).

In euthyroid subjects previously treated with antithyroid drugs for Graves' disease, the chronic administration of 10 drops of a saturated solution of potassium iodide

(SSKI) induced an increase in basal or TRH-stimulated serum TSH concentrations irrespective of iodide-perchlorate discharge test results (72). Basal and TRH-stimulated serum TSH concentrations returned to normal 60 days after SSKI withdrawal.

Postpartum Thyroiditis

Women euthyroid after a previous episode of postpartum thyroid dysfunction are prone to iodide-induced hypothyroidism. In 9 of 11 women, the administration of 300 mg iodide daily for 3 months induced hypothyroidism and, in some, goiter. As observed in patients with other thyroid diseases prone to develop iodide-induced hypothyroidism, a positive iodide-perchlorate discharge test was common (73). Two months after the iodide was withdrawn, thyroid function returned to normal (73). Consonant with those observations are findings suggesting that small doses of iodide administered to patients expected to develop postpartum thyroiditis may intensify rather than ameliorate the disease (74).

Post-subacute Thyroiditis

The chronic administration of large quantities of iodide (300 mg/day) to euthyroid patients long after an episode of painful subacute thyroiditis resulted in a significant increase in the serum TSH concentration in 10 of 18 subjects. Most of these patients had only a slight increase in serum TSH concentration, but two had values >50 mU/L and developed a goiter. A positive iodide-perchlorate discharge test was highly predictive of the occurrence of iodide-induced hypothyroidism (75). Persistent autoimmunity was found up to 39 months after the onset of subacute thyroiditis (76). The serum of these patients was negative for anti-Tg and antimicrosomal antibodies. The nature of the thyroid antigens reacting with serum antibodies in these patients has not been clearly defined, but the antigens were contained in the 2,000-g supernatant of crude thyroid extract. These findings may explain the subtle thyroid defects frequently observed in these patients and their sensitivity to iodide excess.

Post-hemithyroidectomy for Benign Nodules

Patients undergoing hemithyroidectomy for benign thyroid nodules are also susceptible to hypothyroidism when pharmacologic quantities of iodide are administered for a prolonged period (77). No underlying defect in thyroid hormone synthesis could be detected. Similar effects were observed in hemithyroidectomized BB/Wor rats prone to develop lymphocytic thyroiditis (78). This suggests that the hyperfunctioning thyroid remnant is unable to adapt to iodide excess.

After Thyroid Dysfunction Induced by Interferon-α

Treatment of patients with chronic active hepatitis with recombinant interferon-α (rIFN-α) is frequently complicated by the occurrence of autoimmune thyroiditis, thyrotoxicosis, or hypothyroidism (79,80) and a positive iodide-perchlorate discharge test (80). Pharmacologic quantities of iodide administered to euthyroid patients who had previously developed thyroid dysfunction during rIFN-α treatment resulted in subclinical thyroid dysfunction in some of the patients, independent of the presence of positive thyroid antibodies (81).

TABLE 11F.3. CAUSES OF IODIDE-INDUCED THYROTOXICOSIS

Iodide supplementation for endemic iodide-deficiency goiter
Iodide administration to patients with euthyroid Graves' disease, especially those in remission after antithyroid drug therapy
Nontoxic nodular goiter
Autonomously functioning adenoma
Nontoxic diffuse goiter
Iodide administration to patients with no underlying thyroid disease, especially in areas of mild-to-moderate iodide deficiency

SYNERGISM WITH OTHER DRUGS

Several drugs exert mild inhibitory effects on the intrathyroidal organification of iodide, although not when administered alone. When these drugs are administered with excess iodide, however, or when dietary iodide intake is greatly elevated, hypothyroidism or goiter may ensue.

Lithium is frequently used in the treatment of manic-depressive psychosis. It has multiple effects on thyroid function, including inhibition of thyroid hormone release and inhibition of organification of iodide, as judged by a positive iodide-perchlorate discharge test, and may induce goiter or hypothyroidism, especially in patients with Hashimoto's thyroiditis. Iodide-induced hypothyroidism has been reported in a patient receiving lithium.

The sulfonamides sulfadiazine and sulfisoxazole are mild inhibitors of thyroid hormone synthesis. Sulfisoxazole enhanced the inhibitory effects of iodide on hormone synthesis in patients with cystic fibrosis, resulting in goiter in many patients and mild hypothyroidism in others (55). The sulfonylurea hypoglycemic drugs, although potential goitrogens, had no significant inhibitory effect on iodide metabolism in patients, even when these drugs were administered with iodide-containing substances. Surprisingly, rIFN-α, which frequently induces different thyroid disorders, when administered with excess iodide does not potentiate the effect of iodide on thyroid function (82).

Iodide-Induced Thyrotoxicosis

Iodide-induced thyrotoxicosis is not a single etiologic entity. Since the initial description by Coindet in 1821 (83) and the subsequent definition by Breuer and Kocher in 1904, iodide-induced thyrotoxicosis has been reported in patients with a variety of underlying thyroid diseases. As shown in Table 11F.3, iodide-induced thyrotoxicosis may occur in patients with iodide-deficiency goiter, in euthyroid patients with Graves' disease after antithyroid drug therapy, in patients with multinodular goiters who reside in areas of iodide repletion or deficiency, and in people with no evidence of underlying thyroid disease (8,9,84,85). The pathogenesis and epidemiology of iodide-induced thyrotoxicosis have been thoroughly reviewed elsewhere (86, 87).

Iodide-Induced Thyrotoxicosis in Endemic Iodide-Deficient Areas

Widespread iodination of salt or administration of iodized oil has almost eliminated endemic goiter in many countries. The incidence of iodide-induced thyrotoxicosis in areas previously considered iodide deficient varied from 0% in Austria to 7% in Sweden after iodination programs. The incidence of iodide-induced thyrotoxicosis in one endemic goiter area has been estimated to be up to 2% (88). The natural course of the disease was mild, and it resolved spontaneously. Recently, in Denmark, a population with moderate iodide deficiency, the prevalence of thyrotoxicosis increased after iodide supplementation, which increased iodide intake, 50 μg/day (89).

Most patients (85%) who develop thyrotoxicosis have multinodular goiters, and they are elderly. Eight patients with iodide-induced thyrotoxicosis, diagnosed in Lucerne, Switzerland had a mean age of 61 years (90). Iodide-induced thyrotoxicosis occurs in 1.2% of all thyrotoxic patients with a mean age of 65 years (91). The risk of developing thyrotoxicosis is particularly high in these patients. Most are euthyroid before iodide administration, but they may have a nonsuppressible radioactive iodide uptake and low or undetectable serum TSH values. Approximately 20% of patients with multinodular goiters in Greece have either abnormal suppression of the radioactive iodide uptake or an undetectable serum TSH (A Vagenakis, unpublished observations). These patients are at risk to develop iodide-induced thyrotoxicosis. Similar results have been reported from central Europe (92). Single oral doses of 200, 400, and 800 mg iodide administered to goitrous adult subjects residing in Sudan induced four cases of thyrotoxicosis.

However, in the three groups of subjects, serum TSH concentrations <0.1 mU/L were present in 6% to 17% 12 months after iodide administration (93). Similar data have been reported 2 years after iodized salt distribution in Zaire. Among 190 adult subjects with nodular goiter, 14 (7%) developed severe thyrotoxicosis and 2 required antithyroid drug treatment (94). Thyroid-stimulating antibodies were absent in all patients. Surprisingly, these alterations lasted longer than 1 year (95). In Zimbabwe, following the iodination of salt at a level of 30 to 90 parts per million, a threefold increase of iodide-induced thyrotoxicosis was observed (96). Furthermore, there were more deaths in that population, mainly from cardiac complications. In contrast, Azizi et al (97) observed a prevalence of iodide-induced thyrotoxicosis of only 0.6% during an observation period of 4 years following the injection of 1 mL iodized oil containing 480 mg iodide.

It appears, therefore, that thyroid autonomy and thyrotoxicosis become evident when iodide repletion permits the autonomous tissue to synthesize and release excess quantities of thyroid hormone. The importance of thyroid autonomy for the development of iodide-induced thyrotoxicosis is strengthened by a report of iodide-induced thyrotoxicosis in a woman with a multinodular goiter treated with suppressive doses of T_4 and simultaneously exposed to high quantities of iodide (98). Attempts have been made to associate these events with thyroid autoimmunity, but the results are conflicting. Long-acting thyroid stimulator (LATS) or LATS protector was found in some patients but not in others (88). In another study, no change in the incidence of thyroid autoantibodies was found after oral iodized oil administration (99).

These observations suggest that the increased incidence of thyrotoxicosis in endemic areas after iodide exposure is due to an increased supply of iodide to patients with underlying macro- or micronodular disease with autonomous thyroid nodules or with underlying latent Graves' disease. This is consonant with studies from Belgium and Greece (100,101), in which the administration of small quantities of iodide (0.5 mg/day) to patients with autonomous nodules induced frank thyrotoxicosis. In Austria in 1990, salt iodination was doubled, from 10 to 20 mg KI/kg because urinary iodide excretion ranged from only 42 to 72 µg I/g creatinine (102). This increase was accompanied by an increase in the incidence of overt thyrotoxicosis from 30.5 to 41.7 cases per 100,000 in 1992 and a more marked increment of overt Graves' thyrotoxicosis from 10.4 to 20.9 cases per 100,000 in 1993.

It is interesting to note that among 147 patients reported in the literature who developed sporadic thyrotoxicosis without preexisting thyroid abnormality, 137 cases occurred in areas with urinary iodide excretion of 40 to 80 µg/day or iodide intake of <50 µg/day (84). It is evident, therefore, that the remarkably greater incidence of iodide-induced thyrotoxicosis in continental western Europe than in the United Kingdom, United States, and Japan is at least partially due to the iodide deficiency that occurs in Europe in contrast to the latter three countries, where iodide intake is sufficient.

It should be noted that notwithstanding the seriousness of iodide-induced thyrotoxicosis in the elderly in these areas, most observers agree that the risk should not undermine the benefits that iodide sufficiency in children and women, and should not prevent the proper correction of iodide deficiency in a community.

Iodide-Induced Thyrotoxicosis in Iodide-Sufficient Areas

In nonendemic euthyroid goiter areas, the incidence of iodide-induced thyrotoxicosis is low. The prevalence of goiter in the United States is about 3%, and it is surprising that only a few cases have been reported since the initial report from Boston (103), where four of eight patients with goiter developed severe iodide-induced thyrotoxicosis after administration of 180 mg iodide daily for several weeks. Although suppression scans or TRH stimulation tests were not performed, it is likely that the susceptible patients had nonsuppressible thyroid function. Many apparently euthyroid patients with a multinodular goiter who reside in iodide-replete areas may have abnormal suppression test results. Iodide-induced thyrotoxicosis also has been reported in other patients residing in the United States (84,104).

Iodide-induced thyrotoxicosis was identified in 13 of 60 hospitalized thyrotoxic elderly subjects in Australia (105, 106) and Germany (107) who had undergone nonionic contrast radiography. These subjects did not have TPO antibodies, and a thyroid scan revealed the presence of a multinodular goiter. In a prospective study in elderly subjects, frank thyrotoxicosis was uncommon following the administration of nonionic contrast agents, whereas subclinical thyrotoxicosis was observed (108). To reduce the incidence of iodide-induced thyrotoxicosis, the prophylactic use of methimazole or perchlorate given the day before and for 2 weeks after radiographic contrast agent administration to patients with thyroid autonomy has been suggested (109,110). However, the risk of iodide-induced thyrotoxicosis after coronary angiography was too low to recommend prophylactic therapy in unselected patients (111). Iodide-induced thyrotoxicosis also has been described in travelers (travelers' thyrotoxicosis) following the ingestion of iodinated preparations for water purification (112, 113). In all three cases, TPO antibodies were present at the time of the diagnosis of thyrotoxicosis. In a U.S. prospective study in eight normal subjects, the ingestion of four iodide purification tablets dissolved in water daily for 3 months markedly increased urine and serum iodide concentrations, and increased thyroid volume secondary to a small increase in TSH due to small decreases in serum T_4 and T_3 values (114).

The large difference in the rate of occurrence of iodide-induced thyrotoxicosis between iodide-deficient and iodide-replete areas is difficult to explain. It is possible that people with increased iodide intake are "resistant" to iodide-induced thyrotoxicosis because the sensitivity of the autoregulatory mechanism has changed, rendering the thyroid better able to handle the excessive quantities of iodide.

A characteristic of iodide-induced thyrotoxicosis in patients with multinodular goiter is its transient, although at times protracted, course. The thyrotoxicosis maneuver worsen after iodide withdrawal due to the abrupt release of preformed T_4 and T_3 from the thyroid. Serum T_4 is invariably increased, and serum T_3 is usually but not always elevated. Serum TSH is undetectable, and there is no response to TRH. Radioactive iodide uptake is usually low, but occasionally may be normal or increased. Due to the large store of preformed hormone in the thyroid, therapy is more difficult (see later section on amiodarone-induced thyroid disease).

Latent Graves' Disease

Antithyroid drug therapy for Graves' disease reduces thyroidal iodide content, and the thyroid is iodide depleted. Overt thyrotoxicosis can develop only if sufficient iodide is available. It has been reported that a small increase in dietary iodide from either iodide ingestion or thyroid hormone administration increases the frequency of recurrence of thyrotoxicosis after antithyroid drug therapy. The difference in remission rates between the United States and Europe and the preference of American thyroidologists to treat Graves' thyrotoxicosis with radioactive iodide instead of antithyroid drugs is attributed, at least in part, to the higher recurrence rate of Graves' disease in the United States due to adequate iodide intake (115). Administration of large quantities of iodide to patients with latent Graves' disease may result in thyrotoxicosis.

Consonant with this view are recent observations in Graves' disease patients treated with antithyroid drugs. In one study (116), simultaneous administration of methimazole and ipodate reduced the effectiveness of the antithyroid drug. In another study, iodide administration to patients rendered euthyroid after antithyroid drug therapy was accompanied by frank thyrotoxicosis in some and by an absent serum TSH response to TRH in others (72). Excess iodide administered to thyrotoxic patients with Graves' disease significantly increased TSH receptor antibody levels, suggesting that this phenomenon was responsible for iodide-induced thyrotoxicosis in these patients (117).

Unusual episodes of iodide-induced thyrotoxicosis have been observed in a few patients suffering from severe burns treated with povidone iodide (118) and in a patient who had metastatic thyroid carcinoma (119). In a patient with a TSH-producing pituitary tumor with mild thyrotoxicosis, accidental exposure to iodide resulted in severe thyrotoxicosis, which improved after iodide withdrawal (A Vagenakis, unpublished observation).

Amiodarone-Induced Thyroid Disease

Amiodarone, a benzofuranic derivative containing 75 mg iodide per 200-mg tablet, is widely used for the long-term treatment of cardiac arrhythmia. About 9 mg iodide is released daily during the metabolism of the drug (300-mg dose), which has a prolonged half-life of at least 100 days. Beyond its effects on the heart, amiodarone is a potent inhibitor of type I deiodinase, TSH secretion, and it is frequently associated with iodide-induced thyroid dysfunction. Amiodarone-induced thyrotoxicosis occurs in about 10% of patients residing in iodide-deficient areas (84,120,121). In the United States, amiodarone-induced hypothyroidism is more common, occurring in up to 20% of patients, whereas thyrotoxicosis is far less common. These differences are attributed to a higher ambient iodide intake in the United States (120,122).

The etiology of amiodarone-induced hypothyroidism can be partially explained by the excess iodide released during the metabolism of the drug. Measurements of intrathyroid iodide content by fluorescence imaging revealed increased iodide content in patients who developed hypothyroidism (70). Evidence for the essential role of iodide in the pathogenesis of amiodarone-associated hypothyroidism stems from the observation that administration of potassium perchlorate, which prevents thyroid iodide uptake and increases the release of inorganic iodide from the thyroid, restored euthyroidism in some patients. Perchlorate also can protect against inhibition of thyroid function and the resulting hypothyroidism caused by excess iodide, presumably by reducing the formation of an iodinated inhibitor (123,124). One study showed that hypothyroidism returned on withdrawal of potassium perchlorate (124). Iodide-induced hypothyroidism is also related to the presence of thyroid autoimmunity. Circulating antithyroid antibodies are common in patients who develop hypothyroidism during amiodarone treatment (120,122). Hypothyroidism is easy to diagnose because serum TSH is invariably high. T_4 treatment is indicated and does not require interruption of amiodarone therapy. However, in a single patient with amiodarone-induced hypothyroidism, continuation of amiodarone treatment induced destructive thyrotoxicosis (125).

Amiodarone-induced thyrotoxicosis results from two different mechanisms. The iodide released during the metabolism of the drug is responsible for the thyrotoxicosis in many cases. Predisposing factors include micro- and macronodular goiter, which are common in older patients who most often require amiodarone. Thyroid autoimmunity also has been incriminated as a predisposing factor, and antithyroid antibodies have been found in some patients (126) but not in others (127). In one study, the prevalence of serum thyroid-stimulating antibodies and TSH-binding inhibiting antibodies was similar to that in patients with spontaneous thyrotoxicosis (127). Amiodarone may also induce destructive thyroiditis, resulting in thyrotoxicosis, as suggested by clinical, histologic, and *in vitro* studies (128–130). The ultrastructural changes in the rat thyroid gland induced by amiodarone differ from those induced by excess iodide, and include disruption of subcellular organelles with a marked dilation of the endoplasmic reticulum (131). The clinical and laboratory characteristics of amiodarone-induced thyrotoxicosis are presented in Table 11F.4.

The evaluation of thyroid function is difficult in patients receiving amiodarone therapy. Serum T_4 may be elevated, serum T_3 decreased, and serum TSH slightly high in a euthyroid subject receiving the drug. Thyrotoxicosis is best confirmed by an elevation of serum T_3 and free T_3 concentrations as well as by an increase in sex hormone–binding globulin (132). The distinction between iodide-induced thyrotoxicosis (type I) and destructive thyrotoxicosis (type II) may be achieved by measurement of serum interleukin-6, which is elevated in some but not all cases of the destructive form (133), and by fine-needle biopsy, which yields cytologic findings consistent with thyroiditis (129). Color-flow Doppler sonography may show hypervascularity in type I amiodarone-induced thyrotoxicosis and hypovascularity in type II (134). The thyroid radioiodide uptake is always low in the destructive form and is most often low in the iodide-induced form, although may occasionally be normal or even elevated in Europe but not in the United States.

Distinction between the two forms is important for determining therapy. Amiodarone should almost always be discontinued. Large doses of antithyroid drugs are recommended for iodide-induced thyrotoxicosis. If this treatment fails, potassium perchlorate (250 mg three times daily) should be added (135,136). The latter drug blocks thyroid iodide uptake, thereby decreasing the intrathyroidal iodide content. If the thyroid radioiodide uptake is elevated, ^{131}I therapy is an alternative.

In patients with destructive thyrotoxicosis, administration of large doses of glucocorticoids is rapidly effective (129,137). Also, iopanoic acid has been successfully employed in the treatment of type II amiodarone-induced thyrotoxicosis (138,139). In a prospective and randomized study (139), both iopanoic acid and a glucocorticoid ameliorated the thyrotoxicosis. However, patients treated with the latter reached the euthyroid state more rapidly than those treated with iopanoic acid (139); normal serum T_3 concentrations were achieved after an average of 8 days. Relapses are frequent as the glucocorticoid dose is tapered (140). When the distinction between type I and type II amiodarone-induced thyrotoxicosis is not possible or when the two forms coexist in the same patient, a stepwise treatment approach is advisable, beginning with an antithyroid drug and potassium perchlorate. If after 1 month the patient is still thyrotoxic, potassium perchlorate can be discontinued and prednisone can be added, tapering the latter when the serum free T_4 concentrations are normalized. Lastly, the antithyroid drug can be reduced and discontinued when the urinary iodide excretion is <200 µg daily

TABLE 11F.4. FEATURES OF AMIODARONE-INDUCED THYROTOXICOSIS

	Iodide-induced thyrotoxicosis (type I)	Destructive thyrotoxicosis (type II)
Underlying thyroid abnormality	Yes	No
Thyroidal RAIU	Low, rarely normal or elevated	Low
Serum IL-6 concentrations	Slightly elevated	Occasionaly markedly elevated
Cytologic findings	?	Abundant colloid, hysticocytes
Pathogenic mechanism	Excessive thyroid hormone synthesis	Excessive thyroid hormone release (destructive thyroiditis) cells
Response to thionamides	Poor	No
Response to perchlorate	Yes	No
Response to glucocorticoids	?	Yes
Subsequent hypothyroidism	Unlikely	Possible
Effect of excess iodide following the thyrotoxic phase	Likely iodide-induced hypothyroidism	Possible recurrence of thyrotoxicosis
Color-flow Doppler sonography	Normal or increased blood flow	Decreased blood flow

?, not known; IL, interleukin; RAIU, radioiodide uptake.
From Bartalena L, Grasso L, Bragioni S, et al. Serum interleukin-6 in amiodarone-induced thyrotoxicosis. *J Clin Endocrinol Metab* 1994;78:423, modified with permission.

(141). Surgery has been successfully used for the treatment of amiodarone-induced thyrotoxicosis (142, 143) in patients with type I (144) and rarely type II (145). Patients with type I amiodarone-induced thyrotoxicosis can be treated with iopanoic acid prior to thyroidectomy (144).

After recovering from amiodarone-induced destructive thyrotoxicosis, patients may develop permanent hypothyroidism (125,129) as a result of fibrosis of the gland (146). The iodide-perchlorate discharge test result was positive in 60% of euthyroid patients who had recovered from amiodarone-induced destructive thyrotoxicosis (147). Chronic administration of 300 mg iodide daily to these patients induced a marked increase in basal and TRH-stimulated serum TSH concentrations, which returned to normal after iodide withdrawal.

In view of the high incidence of thyroid dysfunction, amiodarone should be administered with caution to patients with preexisting goiter or a history of thyroid disease. Adult patients with β-thalassemia have been shown to be particularly prone to develop both thyrotoxicosis and hypothyroidism during amiodarone therapy (148). Before beginning amiodarone treatment, a careful examination is required; serum TSH and TPO antibodies values must be obtained. During amiodarone treatment, measurement of serum TSH is required approximately every 6 months in order to detect the development of mild thyroid disorders.

Iodide as a Pathogen

Animal studies suggest that iodide administration has an important role in the development of autoimmune thyroid disease. Spontaneous lymphocytic infiltration of the thyroid has been observed in hamsters, beagles, nonobese diabetic mice, Buffalo rats, BB/Wor rats, and obese-strain chickens (149–152). Spontaneous lymphocytic thyroiditis occurs in about 30% of 90-day-old rats who also develop spontaneous insulin-dependent diabetes mellitus (BB/Wor rats) (64,150). The administration of iodide in their drinking water (0.05% sodium iodide) from 30 to 90 days strikingly increased the prevalence of lymphocytic thyroiditis to approximately 75% or more (64). Excess iodide administration to strains of rats that do not develop spontaneous thyroiditis does not induce histologic changes in the thyroid.

The mechanism by which iodide excess increases the occurrence of autoimmune thyroiditis may be due to the enhanced immunogenicity of iodide-rich Tg, as demonstrated in obese-strain chickens (153). Conversely, immunization of the BB/Wor rat with iodide-poor Tg did not induce thyroiditis (154). However, in obese-strain chickens, iodide excess induced thyroid infiltration only in predisposed animals (155), and the greatest effect was observed when iodide was given to the embryos (156). Furthermore, an essential requirement for the development of iodide-induced thyroiditis is the uptake and metabolism of iodide within the gland

(156). Other mechanisms for the development of iodide-induced thyroiditis, such as cellular damage due to elevated oxygen-free radicals, direct cytotoxic effects of iodide or autoregulation of major histocompatibility class I, and increased expression of intrathyroidal TNF-α have been proposed (155,157–159). In contrast to the present view that excess iodide increases the occurrence of autoimmune thyroiditis, iodide deficiency in Wistar rats led to goiter formation with signs of lymphocytic infiltration (160).

The relationship of iodide intake to the occurrence of Hashimoto's thyroiditis in humans is controversial. Some studies (161,162) have strongly suggested that increased iodide intake is associated with an increased incidence of Hashimoto's thyroiditis, especially when iodide is introduced into endemic goiter regions. In a randomized, double-blind, placebo-controlled study conducted in patients with endemic goiter, administration of 0.5 mg/day of KI for 6 months induced high serum anti-Tg antibody and antimicrosomal antibody levels in 19%. Fine-needle aspiration biopsy confirmed the presence of lymphocytic infiltration of the thyroid gland (163). These signs of thyroid autoimmunity disappeared after iodide withdrawal. The presence of lymphocytes in thyroid fine-needle aspiration specimens increased from 6% to 14% after the elimination of iodide deficiency in Greece (164). Also, the injection of 1 mL iodized oil intramuscularly in patients with nontoxic goiter living in Greece was accompanied by an increase in thyroid lymphocytic infiltration from 25% to 68% (165), and iodide prophylaxis has been followed by a threefold increase in the prevalence of autoimmune thyroiditis in schoolchildren (166). Similar results were reported by Markou et al in a study of iodide prophylaxis in Azerbaijan. The incidence of thyroid antibodies increased from 1% to 9% in 12 months in schoolchildren given 380 mg iodized oil orally (167). In elderly women residing in an area of adequate iodide intake, the prevalence of antimicrosomal antibodies was far higher than in those living in an area of mild iodide deficiency (149). In contrast, other studies did not find a relationship between iodide intake and the prevalence of thyroid autoimmunity (15,88). A lower prevalence of anti-TPO antibodies in children and adolescents following 5 years of iodide prophylaxis has been also reported (168). Possible explanations for these discrepant findings on the effect of iodide supplementation on thyroid autoimmunity are suggested by studies from Morocco and Sri Lanka (169–171). In these studies, following iodide prophylaxis the prevalence of thyroid antibodies increased, but decreased later to baseline or lower values. In a recent study iodide intake did not affect the pattern of epitope recognition by polyclonal TPO antibodies in elderly subjects (172).

The mechanism by which iodide interacts with the immune system is unknown. In the presence of iodide, the production of immunoglobulin G from human peripheral blood lymphocytes was increased after stimulation with

60. Drinka PJ, Nolten WE. Effects of iodinated glycerol on thyroid function: studies in elderly nursing home residents. *J Am Geriatr Soc* 1988;36:911.

61. Haraguchi K, Aida K, Akasu F, et al. Iodide-induced hypothyroidism in a patient with anorexia nervosa. *Endocrinol Jpn* 1986;33:61.

62. Matsubayashi S, Mukuta T, Watanabe H, et al. Iodide-induced hypothyroidism as a result of excessive intake of confectionery made with tangle weed, Kombu, used as a low calorie food during a bulimic period in a patient with anorexia nervosa. *Eating Weight Disord* 1998;3:50.

63. Sato K, Okamura K, Hirata T, et al. Immunological and chemical types of reversible hypothyroidism: clinical characteristics and long-term prognosis. *Clin Endocrinol (Oxf)* 1996; 45:519.

64. Allen EM, Appel MC, Braverman LE. The effect of iodide ingestion on the development of spontaneous lymphocytic thyroiditis in the diabetes-prone BB/W rat. *Endocrinology* 1986; 118:1977.

65. Rajatanavin R, Reinhardt W, Alex S, et al. Variable prevalence of lymphocytic thyroiditis among diabetes-prone sublines of BB/Wor rats. *Endocrinology* 1991;128:153.

66. Paul T, Reinhardt W, Meyers B, et al. Small increases in dietary iodide intake do not induce hypothyroidism in euthyroid patients with Hashimoto's thyroiditis. *Clin Res* 1987;35:400A.

67. Tajiri J, Higashi K, Morita M, et al. Studies of hypothyroidism in patients with high iodide intake. *J Clin Endocrinol Metab* 1986;63:412.

68. Takasu N, Yamada T, Takasu M, et al. Disappearance of thyrotropin-blocking antibodies and spontaneous recovery from hypothyroidism in autoimmune thyroiditis. *N Engl J Med* 1992;326:513.

69. Reinhardt W, Luster M, Rudorff KH, et al. Effect of small doses of iodide on thyroid function in patients with Hashimoto's thyroiditis residing in an area of mild iodide deficiency. *Eur J Endocrinol* 1998;139:23.

70. Fragu P, Schlumberger M, Tubiana M. Thyroid iodide content and serum thyroid hormone levels in autoimmune thyroiditis: effect of iodide supplementation. *J Nucl Med* 1985;26:133.

71. Nohr SB, Jorgensen A, Pedersen KM, et al. Postpartum thyroid dysfunction in pregnant thyroid peroxidase antibody-positive women living in an area with mild to moderate iodide deficiency: is iodide supplementation safe? *J Clin Endocrinol Metab* 2000;85:3191.

72. Roti E, Gardini E, Minelli R, et al. Effects of chronic iodide administration on thyroid status in euthyroid subjects previously treated with antithyroid drugs for Graves' thyrotoxicosis. *J Clin Endocrinol Metab* 1993;76:928.

73. Roti E, Minelli R, Gardini E, et al. Impaired intrathyroidal iodide organification and iodide-induced hypothyroidism in euthyroid women with a previous episode of postpartum thyroiditis. *J Clin Endocrinol Metab* 1991;73:958.

74. Kampe 0, Jansson R, Karlsson FA. Effects of L-thyroxine and iodide on the development of autoimmune post-partum thyroiditis. *J Clin Endocrinol Metab* 1990;70:1014.

75. Roti E, Minelli R. Gardini E, et al. Iodide induced hypothyroidism in euthyroid subjects with a previous episode of subacute thyroiditis. *J Clin Endocrinol Metab* 1990;70:1581.

76. Weetman AP, Smallridge RC, Nutman TB, et al. Persistent thyroid autoimmunity after subacute thyroiditis. *J Clin Lab Immunol* 1987;23:1.

77. Clark OH, Cavalieri RR, Moser C, et al. Iodide-induced hypothyroidism in patients after thyroid resection. *Eur J Clin Invest* 1990;20:573.

78. Allen EM, Appel MC, Braverman LE. Iodide-induced thyroiditis and hypothyroidism in the hemithyroidectomized BB/W rat. *Endocrinology* 1987;121:481.

79. Marcellin P, Pouteau M, Benhamou JP. Hepatitis C virus infection, alpha interferon therapy and thyroid dysfunction. *J Hepatol* 1995;22:364.

80. Roti E, Minelli R, Giuberti T, et al. Multiple changes in thyroid function in patients with chronic active HCV hepatitis treated with recombinant interferon-alpha. *Am J Med* 1996; 101:482.

81. Minelli R, Braverman LE, Giuberti T, et al. Effects of excess iodide administration on thyroid function induced by interferon-alpha treatment. *Clin Endocrinol (Oxf)* 1997;47:357.

82. Minelli R, Braverman LE, Valli MA, et al. Recombinant interferon a (rIFN-a) does not potentiate the effect of iodide excess on the development of thyroid abnormalities in patients with HCV chronic active hepatitis. *Clin Endocrinol (Oxf)* 1999;50:95.

83. Coindet JF. Nouvelles recherches sur les effects de l'iode, et sur les précautious à suivré dans le traitement de goitre par le nouveau remède. *Bibl Univ Sci Belles Lettres Arts* 1821;16: 140.

84. Fradkin JE, Wolff J. Iodide-induced thyrotoxicosis. *Medicine* (Baltimore) 1983;62:1.

85. McGregor AM, Weetman AP, Ratanachaiyavong S, et al. In: Hall R, Kobberling J, eds. *Thyroid disorders associated with iodide deficiency and excess.* Serono Symposia Series. New York: Raven Press, 1985:209.

86. Stanbury JB, Ermans AE, Bourdoux P, et al. Iodide-induced thyrotoxicosis: occurrence and epidemiology. *Thyroid* 1998; 8:83.

87. Roti E, Degli Uberti E. Iodide excess and thyrotoxicosis. *Thyroid* 2001;11:493.

88. Martins ML, Lima N, Knobel M, et al. Natural course of iodide-induced thyrotoxicosis (JodBasedow) in endemic goiter area: a 5 year follow up. *J Endocrinol Invest* 1989;12:329.

89. Bulow Pedersen I, Knudsen N, Jorgensen T et al. Large differences in incidences of overt hyper- and hypothyroidism associated with a small difference in iodide intake: a prospective comparative register-based population survey. *J Clin Endocrinol Metab* 2002;87:4462.

90. Henzen C, Buess M, Brander L. Iodide induced thyrotoxicosis (iodide-induced Basedow's disease): a current disease picture. *Schweiz Med Wochenschr* 1999;129:658.

91. Diez JJ. Thyrotoxicosis in patients older than 55 years: an analysis of the etiology and management. *Gerontology* 2003;49: 616.

92. Kutzin H, Modler C, Buschsieweke U. Iodide kinetics in facultative thyrotoxicosis. *J Mol Med* 1980;4:75.

93. Elnagar B, Eltom L, Karlsson FA, et al. The effects of different doses of oral iodized oil on goiter size, urinary iodide, and thyroid related hormones. *J Clin Endocrinol Metab* 1995;80: 891.

94. Ermans AM, Gullo D, Mugisho SG, et al. Iodide supplementation must be monitored at the population level in iodide deficient areas. *Thyroid* 1995;5[suppl 1]:37(Abstract).

95. Bourdoux P, Ermans AM, Mukalay WA, et al. Iodide induced thyrotoxicosis in Kiwu Zaire. *Lancet* 1996;347:552.

96. Todd CH, Allain T, Gomo ZAR, et al. Increase in thyrotoxicosis associated with iodide supplements in Zimbabwe. *Lancet* 1995;346:1563.

97. Azizi F, Daftarian N. Side-effects of iodized oil administration in patients with simple goiter. *J Endocrinol Invest* 2001; 24:72.

98. Reith PE, Granner DK. Iodide-induced thyrotoxicosis in a woman with a multinodular goiter taking levothyroxine. *Arch Intern Med* 1985;145:355.

99. Lazarus JH, Parkes AB, John R, et al. Endemic goitre in Senegal-thyroid function etiological factors and treatment with oral iodized oil. *Acta Endocrinol (Copenh)* 1992;126:149.

100. Ermans AM, Camus M. Modifications of thyroid function induced by chronic administration of iodide in the presence of "autonomous" thyroid tissue. *Acta Endocrinol (Copenh)* 1972; 70:463.

101. Livadas DP, Koutras PA, Souvatzoglou A, et al. The toxic effects of small iodide supplements in patients with autonomous thyroid nodules. *Clin Endocrinol (Oxf)* 1977;7:121.

102. Mostbeck A, Galvan G, Bauer P, et al. The incidence of thyrotoxicosis in Austria from 1987 to 1995 before and after an increase in salt iodization in 1990. *Eur J Nucl Med* 1998;25: 367.

103. Vagenakis AG, Wang CA, Burger A, et al. Iodide induced thyrotoxicosis in Boston. *N Engl J Med* 1972;287:523.

104. Rajatanavin R, Safran M, Stoller W, et al. Five patients with iodide-induced thyrotoxicosis. *Am J Med* 1984;77:378.

105. Martin FIR, Brian WT, Colman PG, et al. Iodide-induced thyrotoxicosis due to nonionic contrast radiography in the elderly. *Am J Med* 1993;95:78.

106. Martin FI, Deam DR. Thyrotoxicosis in elderly hospitalized patients. Clinical features and outcome. *Med J Aust* 1996;164: 200.

107. Steidle B. Iodide-induced thyrotoxicosis after contrast media. Animal experimental and clinical studies. In: Taenzer V, Wend S, eds. *Recent developments in non-ionic contrast media.* New York: Thieme Medical Publishers, 1989:6.

108. Conn JJ, Sebastian MJ, Deam D, et al. A prospective study of the effect of ionic media on thyroid function. *Thyroid* 1996;6: 107.

109. Nolte W, Müller R, Siggelkow H, et al. Prophylactic application of thyrostatic drugs during excessive iodide exposure in euthyroid patients with thyroid autonomy: a randomized study. *Eur J Endocrinol* 1996;134:337.

110. Lawrence JE, Lamm SH, Braverman LE. The use of perchlorate for the prevention of thyrotoxicosis in patients given iodide rich contrast agents. *J Endocrinol Invest* 1999;22:405.

111. Hinze G, Blombach O, Fink H, et al. Risk of iodide-induced thyrotoxicosis after coronary angiography: an investigation in 788 unselected subjects. *Eur J Endocrinol* 1999;140:264.

112. Liel Y, Alkan M. Transitory thyrotoxicosis induced by iodinated preparations for water purifications. *Arch Intern Med* 1996;156:807.

113. Mueller B, Diem P, Bürgi U. Travelers' thyrotoxicosis revisited. *Arch Intern Med* 1998;158:1723.

114. LeMar HJ, Georgitis WJ, McDermott MT. Thyroid adaptation to chronic tetraglycine hydroperiodide water purification tablet use. *J Clin Endocrinol Metab* 1995;80:220.

115. Solomon BL, Evanl JE, Burman KD, et al. Remission rates with antithyroid drug therapy: continuing influence of iodide uptake? *Arch Intern Med* 1987;107:510.

116. Roti E, Gardini E, Minelli R, et al. Sodium ipodate and methimazole in the long-term treatment of hyperthyroid Graves' disease. *Metabolism* 1993;42:403.

117. Wilson R, McKillop JH, Thomson JA. The effect of preoperative potassium iodide therapy on antibody production. *Acta Endocrinol (Copenh)* 1990;123:531.

118. Rath TH, Meissl G, Weissel M. Induction of thyrotoxicosis in burn patients treated topically with povidone-iodide. *Burns* 1988;14:320.

119. Yoshinari M, Tokuyama T, Okamura K, et al. Iodide-induced thyrotoxicosis in a thyroidectomized patient with metastatic thyroid carcinoma. *Cancer* 1988;61:1674.

120. Lombardi A, Martino E, Braverman LE. Amiodarone and the thyroid. *Thyroid Today* 1990;23:2.

121. Harjai KJ, Licata AA. Effects of amiodarone on thyroid function. *Ann Intern Med* 1997;126:63.

122. Martino E, Aghini-Lombardi F, Mariotti S, et al. Amiodarone iodide-induced hypothyroidism risk factors and follow-up in 28 cases. *Clin Endocrinol (Oxf)* 1987;26:227.

123. Wolff J. Perchlorate and the thyroid gland. *Pharmacol Rev* 1998;50:89.

124. Martino E, Mariotti S, Aghini-Lombardi F, et al. Short-term administration of potassium perchlorate restores euthyroidism in amiodarone iodide-induced hypothyroidism. *J Clin Endocrinol Metab* 1988;63:1233.

125. Minelli R, Gardini E, Bianconi L, et al. Subclinical hypothyroidism, overt thyrotoxicosis and subclinical hypothyroidism: the subsequent phases of thyroid function in a patient chronically treated with amiodarone. *J Endocrinol Invest* 1992;15:853.

126. Monteiro E, Galvao-Teles A, Santos ML, et al. Antithyroidal antibodies as an early marker for thyroid disease induced by amiodarone. *BMJ* 1986;292:227.

127. Safran M, Martino E, Aghini-Lombardi F, et al. Effect of amiodarone on circulating antithyroid antibodies. *BMJ* 1988;297: 456.

128. Chiovato L, Martino E, Tonacchera M, et al. Studies on the in vitro cytotoxic effect of amiodarone. *Endocrinology* 1994;134: 2277.

129. Roti E, Minelli R, Gardini E, et al. Thyrotoxicosis followed by hypothyroidism in patients treated with amiodarone. *Arch Intern Med* 1993;153:886.

130. Smyrk TC, Goellner JR, Brennan MD, et al. Pathology of the thyroid in amiodarone-associated thyrotoxicosis. *Am J Surg Pathol* 1987;11:197.

131. Pitsiavas V, Smerdely P, Li M, et al. Amiodarone induces a different pattern of ultrastructural change in the thyroid to iodide excess alone in both the BB/W rat and the Wistar rat. *Eur J Endocrinol* 1997;137:89.

132. Bambini G, Aghini-Lombardi F, Rosner W, et al. Sex hormone-binding globulin in amiodarone-treated patients: a marker for tissue thyrotoxicosis. *Arch Intern Med* 1987;147:1781.

133. Bartalena L, Grasso L, Brogioni S, et al. Serum interleukin-6 in amiodarone-induced thyrotoxicosis. *J Clin Endocrinol Metab* 1994;78:423.

134. Eaton SE, Euinton HA, Newman CM et al. Clinical experience of amiodarone-induced thyrotoxicosis over a 3-year period: role of colour-flow Doppler sonography. *Clin Endocrinol* 2002; 56:33.

135. Martino E, Aghini-Lombardi F, Mariotti S, et al. Treatment of amiodarone associated thyrotoxicosis by simultaneous administration of potassium perchlorate and methimazole. *J Endocrinol Invest* 1986;9:201.

136. Reichert LJ, Derooy HA. Treatment of amiodarone induced thyrotoxicosis with potassium perchlorate and methimazole during amiodarone treatment. *BMJ* 1989;298:1547.

137. Brousolle C, Ducotett X, Martin C, et al. Rapid effectiveness of prednisone and thionamides combined therapy in severe amiodarone iodide-induced thyrotoxicosis: comparison of two groups of patients with apparently normal thyroid glands. *J Endocrinol Invest* 1989;12:37.

138. Chopra IJ, Baber K. Use of oral cholecystographic agents in the treatment of amiodarone-induced thyrotoxicosis. *J Clin Endocrinol Metab* 2001;86:4707.

139. Bogazzi F, Bartalena L, Cosci C, et al. Treatment of type II amiodarone-induced thyrotoxicosis by either iopanoic acid or glucocorticoids: a prospective, randomized study. *J Clin Endocrinol Metab* 2003;88:1999.

140. Bartalena L, Brogioni S, Grasso L, et al. Treatment of amiodarone-induced thyrotoxicosis, a difficult challenge: results of a prospective study. *J Clin Endocrinol Metab* 1996;81:2930.

141. Erdogan MF, Gulec S, Tutar E, et al. A stepwise approach to the tratment of amiodarone-induced thyrotoxicosis. *Thyroid* 2003;13:205.

142. Farwell AP, Abend SL, Huang SK, et al. Thyroidectomy for amiodarone-induced thyrotoxicosis. *JAMA* 1990;263:1526.

143. Franzese CB, Stack BC Jr. Amiodarone-induced thyrotoxicosis: a case for surgical management. *Am J Otolaryngol* 2002; 23:358.

144. Bogazzi F, Aghini-Lombardi F, Cosci C,et al. Iopanoic acid rapidly controls type I amiodarone-induced thyrotoxicosis prior to thyroidectomy. *J Endocrinol Invest* 2002; 25: 176.

145. Claxton S, Sinha SN, Donovan S, et al. Refractory amiodarone-associated thyrotoxicosis: an indication for thyroidectomy. *Aust N Z J Surg* 2000;70:174.

146. Roti E, Bianconi L, De Chiara F, et al. Thyroid ultrasonography in patients with a previous episode of amiodarone induced thyrotoxicosis. *J Endocrinol Invest* 1994;17:259.

147. Roti E, Minelli R, Gardini E, et al. Iodide-induced subclinical hypothyroidism in euthyroid subjects with a previous episode of amiodarone-induced thyrotoxicosis. *J Clin Endocrinol Metab* 1992;75:1273.

148. Mariotti S, Loviselli A, Murenu S, et al. High prevalence of thyroid dysfunction in adult patients with beta-thalassemia major submitted to amiodarone treatment. *J Endocrinol Invest* 1999;22:55.

149. Safran M, Paul TL, Roti E, et al. Environmental factors affecting autoimmune thyroid disease. *Endocrinol Metab Clin North Am* 1987;16:32779.

150. Braverman LE, Paul T, Reinhardt W, et al. Effect of iodide intake and methimazole on lymphocytic thyroiditis in the BB/Wor rat. *Acta Endocrinol (Copenh)* 1987;281[suppl]:70.

151. Bagchi N, Brown TR, Urdanivia E. Induction of autoimmune thyroiditis in chickens by dietary iodide. *Science* 1985;230: 3258.

152. Allen EM, Braverman LE. The effect of iodide on lymphocytic thyroiditis in the thymectomized Buffalo rat. *Endocrinology* 1990;127:1613.

153. Sundick RS, Herdgen DM, Brown TR, et al. The incorporation of dietary iodide into thyroglobulin increases its immunogenicity. *Endocrinology* 1987;120:2078.

154. Ebner SA, Lueprasitsakul W, Alex S, et al. Iodide content of rat thyroglobulin affects its antigenicity in inducing lymphocytic thyroiditis in the BB/Wor rat. *Autoimmunity* 1992;13: 209.

155. Bagchi N, Brown TR, Anand P, et al. Early cellular events in the thyroid after exposure to iodide. *Thyroid* 1994;4[suppl 1]: S34.

156. Brown TR, Sundick RS, Dhar A, et al. Uptake and metabolism of iodide is crucial for the development of thyroiditis in obese strain chickens. *J Clin Invest* 1991;88:106.

157. Lit M, Boggiest SC. Iodide induced lymphocytic thyroiditis in the BOB/Worm rat: evidence of direct toxic effects of iodide on thyroid subcellular structure. *Autoimmunity* 1994;18:31.

158. Taniguchi SL, Giuliani C, Saji MS, et al. Transcriptional regulation of major histocompatibility (MHC) class I gene expression in thyroid cells by iodide involves enhancer A and transcription factor NF-KB. In: Program and abstracts of the 77th Annual Meeting of the Endocrine Society; Washington, DC 1995:77(Abstract).

159. Mori K, Mori M, Stone S, et al. Increased expression of tumor necrosis factor-alpha and decreased expression of thyroglobulin and thyroid peroxidase mRNA levels in the thyroids of iodide-treated BB/wor rats. *Eur J Endocrinol* 1998;139:539.

160. Mooij P, deWit HJ, Bloot AM, et al. Iodide deficiency induces thyroid autoimmune reactivity in Wistar rats. *Endocrinology* 1993;133:1197.

161. Boukis MA, Koutras DA, Souvatzoglou A, et al. Thyroid hormone and immunologic studies in endemic goiter. *J Clin Endocrinol Metab* 1983;57:4.

162. Harach HR, Escalante DA, Onativia A, et al. Thyroid carcinoma and thyroiditis in an endemic goiter region before and after iodide prophylaxis. *Acta Endocrinol (Copenh)* 1985; 108:55.

163. Kahaly GJ, Dienes HP, Beyer J, et al. Iodide induces thyroid autoimmunity in patients with endemic goitre: a randomised, double-blind, placebo-controlled trial. *Eur J Endocrinol* 1998; 139:290.

164. Doufas AG, Mastorakos G, Chatziioannou S, et al. The predominant form of non –toxic goiter in Greece is now autoimmune thyroiditis. *Eur J Endocrinol* 1999;140:505.

165. Papanastasiou L, Alevizaki M, Piperingos G et al. The effect of iodide administration on the development of thyroid autoimmunity in patients with nontoxic goiter. *Thyroid* 2000;10: 493.

166. Zois C, Stavrou I, Kalogera C, et al. High prevalence of autoimmune thyroiditis in schoolchildren after elimination of iodide deficiency in northwestern Greece. *Thyroid* 2003;13: 485.

167. Markou KB, Georgopoulos NA, Makri M, et al. Improvement of iodide deficiency after iodide supplementation in school children of Azarbaijan was accompanied by hypo and hyperthyrotropinemia and increase title of thyroid autoantibodies. *J Endocr Invest* 2003;26[Suppl]:43.

168. Kabelitz M, Liesenkotter KP, Stach B, et al. The prevalence of anti-thyroid peroxidase anibodies and autoimmune thyroiditis in children and adolescents in an iodide replete area. *Eur J Endocrinol* 2003;148:301.

169. Zimmermann MB, Moretti D, Chaouki N, et al. Introduction of iodised salt to severely iodide-deficient children does not provoke thyroid autoimmunity: a one-year prospective trial in Northern Morocco. *Thyroid* 2003;13:199.

170. Premawardhana LD, Parkes AB, Smyth PP, et al. Increased prevalence of thyroglobulin antibodies in Sri Lankan schoolchildren-is iodide the cause? *Eur J Endocrinol* 2000; 143:185.

171. Mazziotti G, Premawardhana LD, Parkes AB, et al. Evolution of thyroid autoimmunity during iodide prophylaxis. The Sri Lankan experience. *Eur J Endocrinol* 2003;149:103.

172. Czarnocka B, Szabolcs I, Pastuszko D, et al. In old age the majority of TPO thyroid peroxidase autoantibodies are directed to a single TPO domain irrespective of thyroid function and iodide intake. *Clin Endocrinol (Oxf)* 1998;48:803.

173. Grubeck-Loebenstein B, Buchan G, Sadegi R, et al. Transforming growth factor beta regulates thyroid growth: role in the pathogenesis of non toxic goiter. *J Clin Invest* 1989;83: 764.

174. Aeschimann S, Gerber H, Von Grunigen C, et al. The degree of inhibition of thyroid follicular cell proliferation by iodide is a highly individual characteristic of each cell and differs profoundly *in vitro* and in vivo. *Eur J Endocrinol* 1994;130: 595.

175. Philips DIW, Lazarus JH, Hall R. Iodide metabolism and the thyroid. *J Endocrinol* 1988;119:361.

176. Philips DIW, Nelson M, Barker DJP, et al. Iodide in milk and the incidence of thyrotoxicosis in England. *Clin Endocrinol (Oxf)* 1988;28:61.

177. Ford HC, Johnson LA, Feek CM, Newton JD. Iodide intake and seasonal incidence thyrotoxicosis in New Zealand. *Clin Endocrinol (Oxf)* 1991;34:179.

178. Azizi F. Environmental iodide intake affects the response to methimazole in patients with diffuse toxic goiter. *J Clin Endocrinol Metab* 1985;61:374.

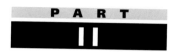

LABORATORY ASSESSMENT
OF THYROID FUNCTION

12

IN VIVO RADIONUCLIDE TESTS AND IMAGING

I. ROSS MCDOUGALL

The late Ralph Cavalieri was coauthor of this chapter for the sixth through eighth editions of *The Thyroid*. He is missed enormously. I hope he would have been in support of the additions, edits, and changes that have been made for this edition. The chapter covers the physical characteristics of radionuclides and radiopharmaceuticals that have a clinical role in nuclear imaging of the thyroid. Imaging instruments, including the gamma camera, rectilinear scanner, and positron emission tomographic camera (PET), are described briefly. The method for thyroid uptake measurement and routine scintigraphy for imaging the thyroid are discussed, and the scintigraphic findings in normal and disorders of the thyroid are presented. The role of diagnostic and posttreatment whole-body scintigraphy in patients with thyroid cancer is described. Controversies, including stunning and the role of radiopharmaceuticals for management of patients whose cancers do not trap iodine but secrete thyroglobulin (Tg) (iodine negative/Tg positive), are discussed.

RADIONUCLIDES FOR MEASUREMENT OF THYROID UPTAKE AND SCINTIGRAPHY

In regions with adequate dietary iodine, a normal thyroid traps about 10% to 35% of ingested radioiodine. The trapping mechanism is the sodium-iodide symporter (NIS) (1–3). The thyroidal NIS is regulated by thyrotropin (TSH). In contrast, NIS in other tissues such as salivary gland and breast is not under the control of TSH (3). The NIS cannot differentiate radioactive iodine from nonradioactive iodine (^{127}I). Therefore, tracers of radioactive iodine are trapped, organified, and incorporated into thyroid hormones like ^{127}I. There are more than 20 radionuclides of iodine, but only ^{123}I and ^{131}I are in widespread clinical use. ^{124}I and ^{125}I have physical properties that could be beneficial in selected situations, and they could become more important (4). The physical characteristics of these radionuclides are shown in Table 12.1. Because ^{123}I has a relatively short half-life and emits only γ photons, it is preferred for diagnostic testing. It has been used

for thyroid uptake and scanning and more recently for whole-body scans in patients with differentiated thyroid cancer. The 159 kev γ photon is almost ideal for scintigraphy with a gamma camera. ^{123}I is the radionuclide of choice for uptake measurements and for routine scintigraphy (5). In contrast, ^{131}I has a half-life of 8 days and emits β particles as well as high-energy γ photons. ^{131}I is therefore suited for therapy, but the γ photons can be imaged, and ^{131}I has a role in diagnostic and posttreatment whole-body scanning in patients with thyroid cancer. The use of ^{131}I for routine thyroid scintigraphy is discouraged because the radiation dose is about 100 times greater than that of ^{123}I, although it is legitimate to administer a 5 to 10 µCi tracer of ^{131}I to measure uptake prior to treatment of thyrotoxicosis. However, ^{123}I is preferred. Recently, there has been increasing interest in the use of ^{123}I for whole-body scintigraphy, as discussed in the section on cancer (6–8).

^{124}I is a positron emitter and, with the recent expansion in experience and availability of PET scanners, there will be increasing interest in this radionuclide. ^{124}I PET scanning, in addition to producing high-resolution images, can be used for volumetric and quantitative measurements (9). ^{125}I has primarily been used for *in vitro* testing because its low-energy emissions are not suited for imaging with a standard gamma camera. It has been used to treat thyrotoxicosis, and clearly the low energy Auger electron emissions can deliver sufficient radiation to kill cells (10). In theory, it could be used to treat small pulmonary metastases of functioning thyroid cancer by delivering the radiation at a subcellular level to the cancer cells, yet avoiding radiating the normal lung.

For testing and treatment, the radionuclides of iodine are administered by mouth, although they can be administered intravenously. In routine thyroid testing, uptake measurements are generally made after 24 hours; many physicians also obtain an early measurement after 4 to 6 hours. In patients with thyroid cancer, whole-body scans and uptakes are made after 24 hours when ^{123}I is given, although 48-hour measurements are possible when larger doses are given (185 to 370 MBq) (11,12). When ^{131}I is given, the scan and uptake are obtained after 48 to 72 hours.

TABLE 12.1. RADIONUCLIDES USED FOR *IN VIVO* THYROID STUDIES

Radionuclide	Half-life	Radioactive Emissions	Prescribed Dose, mCi (MBq)	Radiation toThyroid, Rads/mCi (cGy/MBq)	Clinical Uses
127I	Nonradioactive	None		None	Fluorescent scanning
123I	13.2 hr	γ159 kev	0.1–0.4 (3.7–14.8)	12 (0.32)	Routine thyroid scanning
			1–10 (37–370)		Whole-body scanning
131I	8.09 d	γ 364 kev (90%)	1–5 (37–185)	1,330 (36)	Whole-body scanning
		637 kev β	5–20 (185–740) 30–300 (1.1–11.1 GBq)		Therapy benign and malignant thyroid diseases
124I	4.2 d	β⁺ positron emitter		890 (24)	Whole-body scanning and dosimetry
125I	60 d	γ 25–35 kev Auger electrons	10–20 mCi (370–740)	790 (21)	In vitro Possibly therapy
		X-rays	Larger doses for cancer (has not been used but theoretically has a role)		
99mTcO4	6 hr	γ 140 kev	1–10 (37–370)	0.23 (0.006)	Widely available, used for routine imaging and uptake

aRadiation exposures, in centiGy (cGy) (= rads) per MBq administered, for radioiodines were calculated using the following assumptions: thyroid gland weight, 20 g (normal adult); maximum uptake, 25% of dose; half-time of uptake, 5 h; and biologic half-life in gland, 65 d. In children, the radiation exposure to the gland is threefold to fivefold higher than in adults. The value for 123I assumes no contamination with other radioiodines. The exposure calculations for radioiodines came from MIRD: Dose estimate report no. 5 (*J Nucl Med* 1975;16:857) and those for 99mTc from MIRD: Dose estimate report no. 8 (*J Nucl Med* 1977;17:74).

123I is not universally available, and many authorities recommend technetium pertechnetate (99mTcO4) for routine thyroid imaging. 99mTcO4 is trapped by the NIS, but it is not organified (13). 99mTcO4 is administered intravenously, and uptake and scan are obtained after 15 to 20 minutes. Some other differences between 99mTcO4 and 123I are discussed later in the chapter. Most nuclear medicine laboratories have 99mTcO4 available. Its availability, plus its low cost, makes it an attractive alternative to 123I.

OTHER RADIONUCLIDES AND RADIOPHARMACEUTICALS

Several noniodide radiopharmaceuticals are used for the evaluation of patients with thyroid disorders. These include thallium-201 (201Tl) (14,15), 99mTc-methoxyisobutylisonitrile (99mTc-sestamibi) (16,17), and 99mTc-tetrafosmin (18–20). These agents were introduced for imaging the myocardium, but they are also concentrated by follicular cells—especially cancer cells. 111In-pentreotide, an analogue of somatostatin, has a role in imaging medullary thyroid cancer and differentiated cancers that do not trap iodine (21,22). Pentavalent dimercaptosuccinate acid (99mTc-DMSA) is used in Europe for imaging medullary cancer, but this agent is not approved in the United States (23). One of the minor roles of these radiopharmaceuticals has been to differentiate benign from malignant thyroid nodules. They have also been used in the follow-up of patients who have had treatment for thyroid cancer. The benefits and shortcomings of the cancer-seeking radiopharmaceuticals in these situations are discussed later in this chapter. 18F-fluorodeoxyglucose (18F-FDG) is a positron (β⁺)-emitting radiopharmaceutical that has gained an important place in the staging and management of several cancers, including lymphoma, non–small-cell lung cancer, melanoma, head and neck cancer, colorectal cancer, and breast cancer (24–26). 18F-FDG is useful in patients whose thyroid cancers are unable to trap iodine and has recently been approved in the United States for this purpose (27).

INSTRUMENTS

The simplest instrument for measurement of thyroid uptake, which is discussed later in the chapter, is a probe with a single thallium-activated sodium-iodide crystal. For routine imaging, most nuclear medicine physicians recommend a gamma camera with a pin-hole collimator that has an aperture of <5 mm. The patient lies supine with the neck extended. The collimator should be at the same distance for all studies, except in the case of a large goiter, which cannot be imaged totally within the field of view. The gamma camera produces images of high quality with either ^{123}I or ^{99m}TcO$_4$, provided 30,000 to 50,000 counts are acquired for ^{123}I images and 100,000 to 200,000 counts are acquired for ^{99m}TcO$_4$ images, or replace imaging is continued for 10 minutes. The patient should be examined at the time of scintigraphy to ensure that a finding such as a nodule is correlated with the scintigraphic finding. A radioactive marker can be placed at the edges of a nodule and an image obtained of the marker superimposed on the thyroid image (Fig. 12.1). Markers can be used to identify anatomic sites such as the manubrium and thyroid cartilage. The gross anatomy can also be demonstrated by placing a source of radiation behind the patient; this produces a transmission scan (Fig. 12.2).

Some clinicians prefer the rectilinear scanner over the gamma camera for imaging the thyroid. The main reason is that the image is life size. However, the resolution of a rectilinear scanner is inferior to a modern gamma camera. In one comparative study the gamma camera had better sensitivity (97% vs. 69%), specificity (90% vs. 86%), and overall accuracy (94% vs. 77%) (28). It is impossible to obtain oblique images with a rectilinear scanner; oblique, or lateral, scintiscans can help define the presence of a nodule and determine its function (29). Tomographic scanning with a gamma camera is important in many aspects of nuclear medicine—for example, in evaluation of myocardial perfusion, cerebral function, and back pain. This technique is called single photon emission computed tomography (SPECT in the United States, or SPET in Europe). The camera head rotates around the patient 180 degrees to 360 degrees. The image is produced by back-projecting the data and using algorithms similar to those used for computed tomography (CT). Coronal, sagittal, and transaxial slices can be obtained. SPECT scanning improves resolu-

tion (30). It provides volumetric measurements that can help when the thyroid size is used for dosimetric calculations for treatment. One study found that the thyroid volume determined by SPECT was 108% of the actual size of the surgically removed glands (31). In another study of 25 patients with Graves' disease, planar imaging, SPECT, and ultrasound were compared with magnetic resonance imaging (MRI) in determining the volume of thyroid. MRI was considered to be the gold standard. Volumes calculated from planar images were quite inaccurate, giving an average of 35.2 mL compared with 25 mL by MRI. SPECT gave an average volume of 29.6 mL (32).

Gamma cameras capable of SPECT imaging have been equipped with a pinhole collimator. These instruments produce very high resolution and are able to identify nodules that could not be felt or identified on planar images (33). SPECT does not add information in patients with palpable nodules.

The low photon energies emitted from ^{125}I cannot be imaged by conventional gamma cameras. However, Beekman et al have recently designed a pinhole camera that can detect ^{125}I with a resolution of 0.2 mm for imaging small animals (34). Advances in instrumentation continue and will be translated into clinical use.

In patients with differentiated thyroid cancer who are candidates for ^{131}I treatment, a dual-headed gamma camera capable of whole-body scanning provides anterior and posterior whole-body scans after diagnostic doses of ^{123}I or ^{131}I, and after ^{131}I therapy. Whole-body scans are easier to interpret than multiple spot views. When the radionuclide is ^{131}I, a high-energy collimator is advised because the 364 kev photons of ^{131}I pass through the lead septa of a medium-energy collimator, resulting in images that are badly degraded.

With increased use of positron-emitting radiopharmaceuticals, including ^{18}F-FDG and ^{124}I, a dedicated PET camera provides better resolution than a hybrid PET/gamma camera (35). The reason is that positrons (positive electrons), when emitted from a source, travel a very short

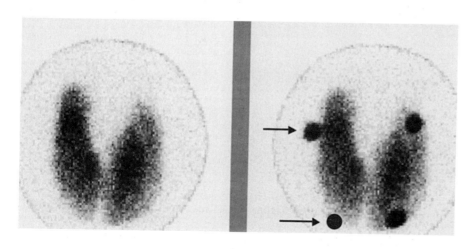

FIGURE 12.1. Left panel: Image of an enlarged thyroid obtained 24 hours after oral administration of 200 μCi (7.4 MBq) of ^{123}I. **Right panel:** Includes radioactive markers placed by the examiner at the upper and lower poles of the gland. This demonstrates that what is seen on the scintiscan corresponds with what is palpated.

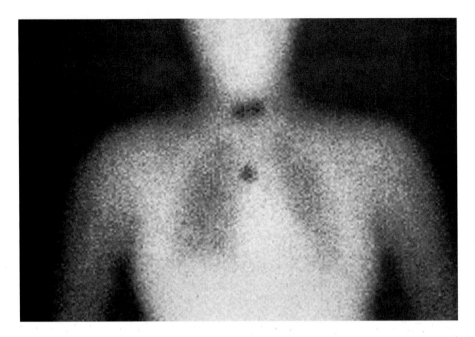

FIGURE 12.2. A transmission scan. The patient has had a thyroidectomy for thyroid cancer. The image is a diagnostic scan after 2 mCi (74 MBq) of [131]I. There are two small areas of uptake in the thyroid bed and one in the mediastinum. These would be difficult to position without some anatomic landmarks. This is achieved by putting a source of radiation behind the patient—in this case, a cobalt source used daily for obtaining quality-control images for each gamma camera.

distance and interact with electrons in the patient (negative charge). The positive and negative electrons of equal mass annihilate one another. The mass of the two electron particles is transmuted into two photons, each with 511 kev of energy. These photons travel at an angle of 180 degrees. Positron cameras usually have a ring of detectors surrounding the patient and electronics capable of identifying coincident photons, i.e., photons arriving at the same time and detected by opposing detectors. Modern PET scanners have an intrinsic resolution of <5 to 6 mm. A recent development has been the combination of a PET with a CT

scanner. The CT images are used for attenuation correction of the PET images. They also provide anatomic correlation for the functional PET scans (Fig. 12.3).

Miscellaneous instruments include handheld probes that can be used during surgery to identify focal sites of radioactivity. These instruments are used for sentinel node imaging after local injection of ^{99m}Tc sulfur colloid around the cancer. Sentinel node imaging is widely used for breast cancer and melanoma, and has been used in selected patients with thyroid cancer to identify the sentinel node, which, if it does not contain cancer, makes it likely that

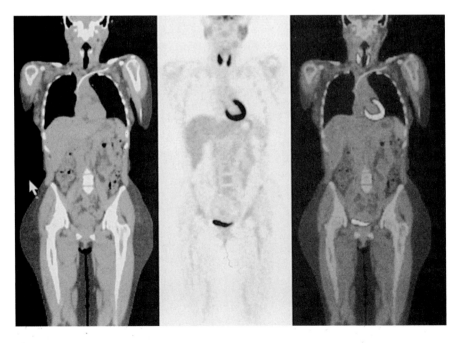

FIGURE 12.3. This figure shows the format of combined positron emission tomograpy/computed tomography (PET/CT) whole-body camera. The scan was used to evaluate the efficacy of chemotherapy for a nonthyroidal cancer. The central image is the PET scan, completed 1 hour after intravenous injection of 15 mCi (555 MBq) of ^{18}F-fluorodeoxyglucose. It shows physiological uptake in the myocardium, liver, urinary tract, and faintly in the muscles and skeleton. The intense uptake in the thyroid is characteristic of autoimmune thyroid disease, usually Hashimoto's thyroiditis. **Left panel:** CT which is used for attenuation correction of the PET images and for anatomic correlation. **Right panel:** Superimposition of the PET and CT images, combining function and anatomy.

secondary nodes are also free of cancer (36). Handheld detectors have also been used in patients who have been treated with ^{131}I, and that radionuclide is used as a road map for the surgeon as an aid to determine which tissue should be excised (37).

Fluorescent scanners detect nonradioactive iodine [127]I. The scanner has a source of radiation, usually americium ([241]Am), that emits photons with energies greater than the energy holding the K shell electrons of [127]I in their orbits (38). The photon energy of [241]Am of 59.6 kev ejects a K shell electron. The vacancy that results from the ejected electron is subsequently filled by an electron from the L shell. There is a difference in binding energy between the L and K electrons of 28.5 kev, and this energy is emitted as a fluorescent X-ray. The fluorescent scanner detects these x-rays and constructs an image that is representative of the quantity of [127]I in the gland (39).

THYROID UPTAKE: INDICATIONS AND PRINCIPLES

Measurements of thyroid uptake of radioiodine provide valuable information in the clinical situations listed in Table 12.2 (40). A known amount of tracer is administered orally, and the percentage accumulated at designated times is measured using either a probe or gamma camera. The fractional uptake is a function of the NIS, the rate of binding of iodine within the thyroid, and the rate of release of iodine from the thyroid. The uptake over the first hour reflects trapping. Measurements up to 6 to 8 hours reflect uptake, oxidation, and organification, and later measure-

TABLE 12.2. INDICATIONS FOR THYROID UPTAKE MEASUREMENT AND IMAGING

Indications for measuring thyroid uptake

To confirm the diagnosis of hyperthyroidism
To distinguish other causes of thyrotoxicosis from
  hyperthyroidism
To provide data for calculation of a therapeutic dose of [131]I
To detect intrathyroidal defects in organification

Indications for thyroid imaging

To compare structure and function of the thyroid
To differentiate different types of thyrotoxicosis
To determine whether a nodule is functioning
To determine whether a cervical or mediastinal mass contains
  functioning thyroid
To identify ectopic thyroid
To aid in the diagnosis of congenital hypothyroidism
To determine whether functioning metastases from thyroid
  carcinoma are present and amenable to ^{131}I therapy
To determine whether a patient with thyroid cancer has been
  treated successfully

ments depend on the balance of organification and release of radioiodine from the thyroid. In a hyperthyroid gland, the uptake can be higher at 4 to 6 hours than at 24 hours, but it is unusual to have an abnormal value early and a normal value at 24 hours. It is almost a universal procedure to obtain a 24-hour measurement, but the early 4- to 6-hour measurement allows the clinician to identify a thyroid with rapid turnover. Some authorities obtain only an early measurement and by extrapolation calculate the 24-hour value (41). The uptake is often used in the determination of therapy doses of ^{131}I to treat patients with Graves' thyrotoxicosis or toxic nodular goiter (42). A single early measurement allows for 1-day measurement of uptake and treatment. The author prefers the 24-hour value and finds the benefit of 1-day therapy is balanced by the opportunity to consult twice with the patient to ensure all clinical questions, follow-up arrangements, and legislative requirements related to radiation safety are answered.

TECHNIQUES AND RESULTS

When patients are referred for uptake and/or scan, it is important to ensure they are not taking thyroid hormone or an antithyroid medication. It is also important that they have not ingested an excess of iodine or been injected with radiographic contrast. It is very important to define that a woman is neither pregnant nor lactating. Please refer to the last paragraph in this chapter. The author prefers to administer the tracer in the morning with the patient fasting. When the patient has had prior studies, it is very helpful to have a copy for direct comparison. The uptake and scan should be interpreted in light of serum thyroid function tests.

For uptake alone, 50 to 100 μCi ^{123}I can be administered in a capsule. For patients who have difficulty swallowing, and children, ^{123}I can be given as a liquid. The dose to be administered is counted in a plastic phantom using the probe that is used for the uptake measurement in the patient. Correction for tissue background is made by counting over the midthigh and subtracting that count from the neck counts. Commercially available thyroid uptake units contain a dedicated computer that calculates the uptake from the standard and patient measurements. It is programmed to correct for the physical decay of [123]I. The formula for calculation by hand is

$$\text{Thyroid Uptake (\%)} = \frac{(\text{Net CPM Over Thyroid} - \text{Net CPM Over Thigh})}{\text{Net CPM Over Dose Standard} \times R \times F} \times 100$$

where CPM is counts per minute, R is the ratio of the dose administered to the dose of the standard, and F is the correction for physical decay.

UPTAKE OF ^{99m}TCO$_4$-PERTECHNETATE

Pertechnetate is trapped but not organified. The peak activity in a normal thyroid after intravenous injection occurs at about 15 to 30 minutes (13,43). The peak is earlier in hyperthyroid glands. The range of normal uptake is 0.25% to 3.0% of the injected dose. Therefore, the background activity is high. This has to be subtracted from thyroid counts. ^{99m}TcO$_4$ is trapped and secreted by salivary glands, and it is important to have the patient drink water to "clear" the esophagus before measuring uptake or scanning. When a probe is used for the uptake measurement, counts over the midthigh are used for this correction. When uptake is measured with a gamma camera, an area adjacent to the thyroid but avoiding the salivary glands can be used for background correction.

Some physicians use a neck-to-thigh ratio. This is rapid, and as little as 10 to 20 µCi ^{99m}Tc can be used, thus subjecting the patient and thyroid to very low doses of radiation. This is beneficial for children (44).

FACTORS INFLUENCING THYROID-UPTAKE TESTS

The function of the thyroid is only one of the factors that determine the uptake measurement. The uptake is generally increased in thyrotoxic patients with Graves' disease and toxic nodular goiter. Conversely, the uptake is generally decreased in subacute and silent thyroiditis and hypothyroidism. There are many other factors that influence this result (Table 12.3). The most important nonthyroidal influence is the serum inorganic iodine level, which is dependent on the intake of iodine.

STIMULATION AND SUPPRESSION TESTS

The use of recombinant human thyrotropin (rhTSH) to stimulate uptake of radioiodine in patients with thyroid cancer is described later in the chapter. There is no role for TSH stimulation in differentiating primary from secondary hypothyroidism. Similarly, there are no indications for triiodothyronine (T$_3$)- or thyroxine (T$_4$)-suppression tests. Historically, suppression tests were used to demonstrate that the uptake of the thyroid gland in patients with mild Graves' disease, or a autonomous hyperfunctioning nodule, was not suppressed after the administration of either T$_3$ or T$_4$. The tests were also used in an effort to predict whether a patient with Graves' disease was in remission. Remission was diagnosed when the thyroid uptake could be suppressed by exogenous T$_4$ or T$_3$. The following references are listed for those interested in the history and technical details (45,46). The differentiation of primary from secondary hypothyroidism and the diagnosis of mild thyrotoxicosis can be

TABLE 12.3. FACTORS THAT INFLUENCE THYROID RADIOIODINE UPTAKE

Causes of increased uptake

Hyperthyroidism
Iodine deficiency
Pregnancy (nuclear medicine tests should not be conducted in pregnant women)
Recovery phase of subacute, silent, or postpartum thyroiditis
Rebound after suppression of thyrotropin
Rebound after withdrawal of antithyroid medication
Lithium carbonate therapy
Some patients with Hashimoto's thyroiditis
Inborn errors of thyroid hormonogenesis apart from trapping defect

Causes of decreased uptake

Primary hypothyroidism
Destructive thyroiditis (subacute thyroiditis, silent thyroiditis, postpartum thyroiditis (ensure patient is not nursing)
After thyroidectomy, or ^{131}I treatment, or external neck radiation
Central hypothyroidism
Thyroid hormone
Excess iodine
Dietary variations
Dietary supplements
Radiological contrast
Amiodarone
Topical iodine
Medications other than those containing iodine
Antithyroid drugs
Perchlorate, thiocyanate
Sulphonamides, sulphonylurea
High-dose glucocorticosteroids

made by interpreting the scan along with serum thyroid function tests. A single test that can determine when a patient with Graves' disease is in permanent remission is not available.

THYROID SCINTIGRAPHY: NORMAL FINDINGS

The thyroid lies in the anterior cervical area and in adults weighs about 10 to 20 g. There are two lobes and an isthmus. In normal adults in the United States, the 24-hour uptake of oral radioiodine is in the range of 10% to 35% (Fig. 12.4). Therefore, about 1/5 to 1/3 of the administered dose is concentrated in a small superficial organ. This results in images of good quality. Nevertheless, the intrinsic resolution of the nuclear medicine instruments for ^{123}I is about 1 cm for planar images and 5 to 6 mm for tomographic images. Small lesions are not delineated. The pyramidal lobe is occasionally identified, in particular in patients with Graves' disease and less commonly in Hashimoto's thyroiditis (Fig. 12.5) (47).

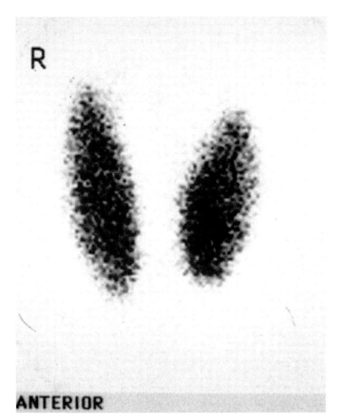

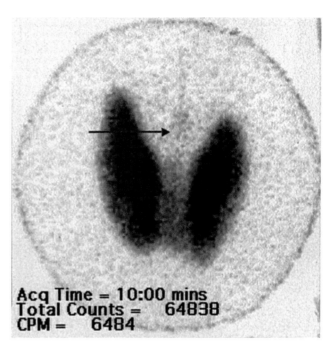

FIGURE 12.5. This image shows an enlarged thyroid with a faint pyramidal lobe is typical of Graves' hyperthyroidism. The early and 24-hour uptake values are usually above normal. This image was obtained at 24 hours after an oral dose of 200 µCi (7.4 MBq) of ^{123}I.

FIGURE 12.4. A normal thyroid scan obtained 24 hours after an oral dose of 200 µCi (7.4 MBq) of ^{123}I. The lobes are usually minimally asymmetric. The isthmus may not be imaged (as in this scan) when it is thin.

CONGENITAL DEFECTS

Congenital defects include anatomic and inherited disorders (48). Anatomic defects include agenesis and maldescent of the gland, which is positioned along the tract of the thyroglossal duct. Patients with agenesis are clinically and biochemically hypothyroid. Patients with a maldescended thyroid are usually hypothyroid. Imaging is valuable in defining agenesis of the thyroid. The thyroid is not identified, but there is uptake by salivary glands (49). Ectopic thyroid such as lingual thyroid can be identified on scintiscan. Anatomic defects such as hemiagenesis are infrequently identified because they are rare. They are usually identified only if the patient has some disorder such as thyrotoxicosis that results in the thyroid scan being ordered (50).

Pathophysiological defects resulting from inborn errors of synthesis of thyroid hormone can be diagnosed by correlating clinical findings, biochemical results, and uptake, and scintigraphy. Absent trapping due to mutations in NIS also show absence of the thyroid on scan, but in addition there is no trapping by the salivary glands. A defect in thyroid peroxidase can be identified by the combination of active trapping by the thyroid plus a positive perchlorate dis-

charge test. Defects in deiodination can be diagnosed by measuring radioactive monoiodotyrosine and diiodotyrosine in the urine.

THYROTOXICOSIS/HYPERTHYROIDISM

Thyrotoxicosis is the pathophysiological condition resulting from action of excess T_4 and T_3. Hyperthyroidism refers to an overactive gland, and patients with hyperthyroidism are thyrotoxic. However, not all thyrotoxic patients are hyperthyroid. Table 12.4 lists the more common conditions that result in excess thyroid hormones in the circulation (see Chapter 22 for a complete list). The important differentiation is whether the thyroid is actively trapping an excess of iodine or not. The common causes of hyperthyroidism are Graves' disease (Basedow's disease, diffuse toxic goiter), toxic multinodular goiter, and an autonomous hyperfunctioning nodule. The relative proportion of each varies significantly from country to country. Graves' disease is more common in countries with high intake of iodine, and toxic nodular goiters are more common in iodine-deficient countries. Figure 12.5 shows the typical appearance of Graves' disease on scan. Compared with a normal thyroid, the thyroid lobes are larger in all dimensions, the early and late uptakes are higher, there is less background activity, and the pyrami-

TABLE 12.4. CAUSES OF THYROTOXICOSIS, SEPARATED INTO THOSE WITH HIGH UPTAKE AND THOSE WITH LOW UPTAKE

Thyrotoxicosis with High Uptake	Thyrotoxicosis with Low Uptake
A. Autonomous gland	A. Thyroiditides
Graves' disease	Subacute thyroiditis
Toxic nodular goiter	Silent thyroiditis
Multinodular gland	Postpartum thyroiditis
Single autonomous nodule	
B. Gland-stimulated by excess	B. Exogenous thyroid
TSH or TSH-like hormone	hormone
TSH-secreting pituitary tumor	Factitious thyrotoxicosis
Placental tumors	Thyrotoxicosis medicamentosa
Hydatidiform mole	
Choriocarcinoma	Hamburger thyrotoxicosis
C. Ectopic source of hormone	C. Excess iodine exposure
secretion	
Widespread functioning	
thyroid cancer (usually	
follicular cancer)	
Struma ovarii	

TSH, thyrotropin.

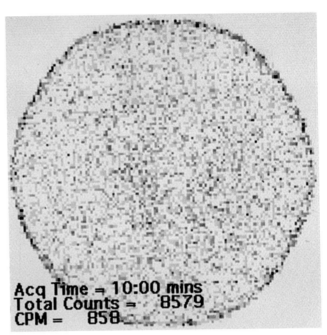

FIGURE 12.7. Thyroid scan of a patient with thyrotoxicosis due to inflammatory thyroiditis. There is no trapping of [123]I (200 μCi, 7.4 MBq). This appearance could be due to any of the disorders causing thyrotoxicosis with low uptake, as listed in Table 12.4.

dal lobe is often seen. Thyrotoxicosis as a result of a toxic nodular goiter shows the hyperfunctioning nodule(s), and normal tissue is usually suppressed because there is no TSH stimulation (Fig. 12.6). Figure 12.7 shows the scan of a patient with inflammatory thyroiditis, the uptake was <1%.

SOLITARY THYROID NODULE

Between 5% and 10% of solitary thyroid nodules are malignant; the main clinical question is whether the nodule is a cancer or not (51,52). Without question the best and most cost-effective test in a euthyroid patient is fine needle aspiration biopsy (53–56) (see Chap-

ter 73). Many primary care physicians continue to order a thyroid scintiscan to determine whether a nodule is malignant. This is not cost effective. Most cancers are nonfunctioning on scintiscan, and when they are large enough to be detected on scan, they are "cold." However, most nonfunctioning nodules are benign (57), and benign nodules are much more common than malignant nodules. Figure 12.8 shows a large cold nodule, which was histologically benign. If we accept that 5% of nodules are malignant and 95% are nonfunctioning, the a priori, chance of a nodule being cancerous is 1/20, and after the scan the a posteriori probability is 1/19. To add further confusion, there are occasional disparities when the same nodule is imaged with ^{123}I and [99m]TcO$_4$

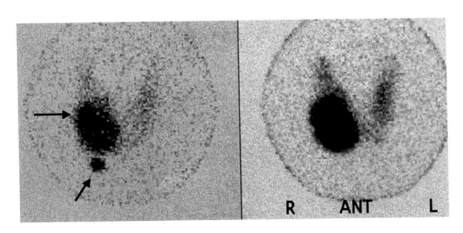

FIGURE 12.6. The image **on the right** shows a functioning nodule in the right lower pole with partial suppression of uptake in the remainder of the thyroid. The image **on the left** shows radioactive markers that were placed at the upper and lower edge of the palpable nodule. The patient had mild clinical and biochemical thyrotoxicosis. The images were obtained 24 hours after an oral dose of 200 μCi (7.4 MBq) of [123]I.

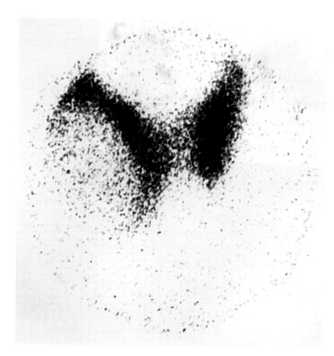

FIGURE 12.8. Thyroid scan administration of 24 hours after 200 μCi (7.4 MBq) of [123]I. There is a large nonfunctioning nodule in the right lobe. The patient, a teenager, had received external radiation therapy in childhood for cancer in the right neck. Because of the history and clinical and scintigraphic findings, the patient was referred for operation. The thyroid nodule was benign.

(58,59). A nodule that is hot on [99m]TcO$_4$ scan and cold on ^{123}I scan has an increased risk of being a cancer. In one study comparing ^{131}I and [99m]TcO$_4$ in 58 patients, 18 (31%) nodules had disparate results. Of the 18, 14 were malignant, with 12 being follicular and 2 being papillary cancers (59). A review of the literature suggests the disparity is less common than stated above. The difficulty is knowing which [99m]TcO$_4$ scan will be disparate by [123]I (or ^{131}I) imaging. As a result, those who recommend [99m]TcO$_4$ also recommend repeating the scan with ^{123}I in the case of a nodule that is hot on [99m]TcO$_4$ scan. Reverse disparity can occur, but rarely. The author prefers [123]I. In general, thyroid scintigraphy is not recommended as the first study in euthyroid patients with a solitary thyroid nodule. This is confirmed by the meta-analysis of Ashcraft and Van Herle (51). The positive predictive value of a cold nodule being malignant was 15%, and the specificity, that is, the likelihood that the scan will define the nodule as benign, was 6%.

There are exceptions to the dogma that fine needle aspiration (FNA) should be the first test. In regions of the world that are iodine deficient, there is a higher proportion of functioning nodules, and at a certain percentage it becomes more cost equivalent to obtain the scan. This is because the percentage of microfollicular lesions on biopsy increases with the increasing percentage of functioning

nodules. Second, when the patient has thyrotoxicosis, the probability of a functioning nodule increases, although occasionally patients with Graves' disease have a nonfunctioning nodule (60). That nonfunctioning nodule should be biopsied because thyroid cancer can occur in Graves' disease. Some authorities believe thyroid cancer in this setting behaves more aggressively (61,62).

There was hope that a cancer-seeking radiopharmaceutical could differentiate between a benign and malignant nodule. Relevant literature of results using ^{201}Tl, ^{99m}Tc-sestamibi, ^{99m}Tc-tetrafosmin, and ^{111}In-octreotide are presented later in the chapter. Previous investigators failed to differentiate benign from malignant nodules with [201]Tl. Mezosi et al evaluated 59 cold nodules with ^{99m}Tc-sestamibi (63). They concluded that it can differentiate degenerative from neoplastic nodules. However, it cannot differentiate adenoma from carcinoma. Demirel et al compared three methods of separating malignant from benign nodules (64). They imaged blood flow into the nodule immediately after injection of [99m]TcO$_4$ and ^{99m}Tc-sestamibi, and obtained delayed images with each agent. They also conducted Doppler ultrasound. They studied 43 patients who had cold nodules, and all went on to have histological proof of diagnosis. The authors accepted that a hypervascular nodule that demonstrated rapid washout of [99m]TcO$_4$ was malignant. When uptake of ^{99m}Tc-sestamibi in the nodule was 3+ on either an early or delayed scan, or both, the nodule was judged to be malignant. Radionuclide angiography diagnosed 8 of the 9 cancers and all 34 benign nodules (sensitivity 89%, specificity 100%). These results suggest that radionuclide angiography should be an important test. However, the technique has been available for more than 30 years, and one earlier report found the sensitivity to be 50% (65). ^{99m}Tc-sestamibi diagnosed 6 of 9 cancers and 31 of 34 benign nodules (sensitivity 67%, specificity 91%). In a similar study, ^{99m}Tc-sestamibi scans were compared with dynamic imaging with [99m]TcO$_4$, biopsy, and histology by Sathekge et al (66). They found a sensitivity of 91% and specificity of 77% for ^{99m}Tc-sestamibi. The specificity for radionuclide angiography was only 40%. ^{111}In-octreotide has not been shown to be of value in differentiating benign from malignant nodules (67).

Two reports describe the use of ^{18}F-FDG PET to differentiate benign from malignant thyroid nodules. In general, cancers showed high uptake, but there was considerable overlap with benign nodules. Autoimmune thyroid disorders also had high uptake of ^{18}F-FDG, as shown in Figure 12.3 (68,69).

There was then hope that the cancer-seeking radiopharmaceuticals could help in the management of patients with a nodule when biopsy results in indeterminate cytopathology. Lin et al used 10-minute and 3-hour ^{201}Tl images in 27 patients with indeterminate cytopathology and reported a sensitivity of 100% and specificity of 90% (70).

Chen et al concluded this would provide a considerable saving by reducing the number of patients referred for operation who have benign nodules. This was based on the estimated 17,000 to 29,000 indeterminate biopsies done annually in Taiwan (71).

In summary, cancer-seeking radiopharmaceuticals appear to have little role in the routine evaluation of solitary thyroid nodules. The tests are expensive and are not cost effective. The studies cited had an end point of excision of all nodules. The studies also had small numbers of patients and relatively high percentages of cancers. These results cannot be translated into clinical practice where very large numbers of patients are tested and the likelihood of cancer is low. There might be a limited role for imaging when biopsy is indeterminate in a patient who is reluctant to have surgery without compelling evidence the nodule is malignant. However, none of the radiopharmaceuticals are reliable at separating malignant from benign nodules. As a result, a clinician using one or other of these radiopharmaceuticals to determine which patient does not need surgery has to be responsible for follow-up to ensure a cancer is not overlooked. The role of these agents in patients with proven cancer is discussed later in the chapter.

SUBSTERNAL THYROID

When a goiter enlarges, the inferior aspect can enter the thoracic inlet. With time, a higher proportion of, or the entire, gland becomes substernal. This is usually detected on roentgenogram or CT scan done for some other clinical reason. The CT scan findings are occasionally typical and no additional tests are required (72). In many patients, it is not possible to exclude other diagnoses such as lymphoma. Thyroid scintigraphy with ^{123}I confirms that the intrathoracic mass contains functioning thyroid. ^{99m}TcO$_4$ is not recommended because uptake in the goiter is hard to differentiate from activity in the heart and great vessels.

HYPOTHYROIDISM

There is seldom an indication to measure uptake or obtain a scan in an adult with hypothyroidism. Their role in infants was discussed earlier in the chapter.

THYROID CANCER

Introduction

The role of scintigraphy in patients with thyroid cancer involves whole-body scintigraphy after the patient has undergone thyroidectomy. The patient has to have a high serum TSH concentration. In regions where the intake of dietary iodine is high, a low-iodine diet is recommended

for 2 weeks prior to imaging and therapy (73). A more detailed diet with recipes is available online at www. thyca.org. A diet for tube-fed patients has been published (74). The high serum TSH value can be obtained by stopping thyroid hormone, T$_4$ is stopped for 4 weeks, and T$_3$ for 2 weeks. Alternatively, thyroid hormone is not prescribed after thyroidectomy, and testing is undertaken after 4 weeks. There is no consensus as to how high the serum TSH value should be, but most accept a value above 25 mU/L. A high level of TSH can be achieved without withdrawing thyroid hormone by administering rhTSH by intramuscular injection (75,76). The most common regime is to inject rhTSH on a Monday and Tuesday, to administer the oral diagnostic dose of ^{131}I (or ^{123}I) on Wednesday, and do a whole-body scan on Friday (or Thursday in the case of ^{123}I). Two multinational trials reported on the value of rhTSH in comparison with standard diagnostic scans (75,77), and several authors have confirmed the value of rhTSH (78,79). The original trials suggested that about 10% of patients had mild transient nausea or headache after injection of rhTSH. In more than 170 studies, the author has found ~40% of patients to have one or the other symptom, but only 1 patient preferred the withdrawal protocol. Serum TSH values 24 hours after the second injection of TSH are in the range of 130 to 140 mU/L, and are inversely related to the mass of the patient.

The scan findings, whether obtained after injection of rhTSH or after withdrawal of thyroid hormone, have to be interpreted in relation to serum thyroglobulin (Tg) values. Knowledge of false positive radioiodine scan findings is important to ensure patients are not diagnosed and treated for nonexisting metastases.

A recent consensus report suggested that whole-body scanning following rhTSH is not necessary in low-risk patients previously treated with thyroidectomy and ^{131}I in whom the serum Tg after rhTSH does not rise to >2 ng/mL (79A).

There are several controversial aspects related to diagnostic whole-body scanning. First, should a diagnostic scan be obtained, or should the patient be treated with ^{131}I after thyroidectomy without obtaining the scan? Second, when a diagnostic scan is obtained, should ^{131}I be used, and if so, what dose should be given? When a decision has been made to give ^{123}I in place of ^{131}I, what is the appropriate dose? Lastly, what is the role of a posttherapy scan?

SHOULD A DIAGNOSTIC SCAN BE OBTAINED?

Some authorities recommend proceeding directly to ^{131}I therapy after surgery without a diagnostic scan. The diagnostic scan gives information about how much thyroid tissue is left and allows for demonstration of metastases once the surgeon has removed most or all of the normal thyroid. Therefore, it provides information on how much ^{131}I to prescribe. When dosimetric calculations are made, it is essential to have a diagnostic scan. The scan also demonstrates potential reasons for not proceeding to ^{131}I, for example, intense uptake in breast tissue in a young woman with good prognostic features.

WHICH RADIONUCLIDE IS BEST FOR WHOLE-BODY IMAGING?

[131]I, in doses of 1 to 2 mCi (37 to 74 MBq), has been used for diagnostic whole-body scans for several decades. Originally, ^{131}I was the only suitable radionuclide of iodine, and because it was also the radionuclide used for therapy, pretherapy diagnostic scans and uptake measurements were thought to reflect precisely the behavior of the larger therapy dose. It then became apparent that posttherapy scans could show more lesions and demonstrate known lesions better. Therefore, there was a trend to prescribe larger diagnostic doses of [131]I (80,81). They were increased to 5 and then 10 mCi (185 to 370 MBq). In contrast, this author found that 2mCi (74 MBq) of ^{131}I seldom underestimated the stage of disease, and other authors confirmed that finding (82). Nevertheless, the popularity of larger diagnostic doses increased, until Park et al described absent or reduced uptake on posttherapy scans in comparison with diagnostic scans (83). The implication was that the diagnostic dose of ^{131}I delivered sufficient radiation to thyroid cells that they were incapable of trapping the therapeutic dose. This has been called "stunning." Park et al described a linear increase in the frequency of stunning as the diagnostic dose of ^{131}I increased. As a result, some clinicians abandoned diagnostic scans, and others reverted to lower doses of ^{131}I, or changed to [123]I. Stunning has become a very controversial topic. Again, this author found it to be rare when 2 mCi (74 MBq) [131]I are prescribed (Fig. 12.9). Several other authors have found no evidence of stunning with larger doses of [131]I. Cholewinski et al did not encounter this in 122 patients after 5 mCi (185 MBq) (84). Morris et al compared the outcome of ^{131}I therapy in two groups of patients, one treated directly with ^{131}I and the second treated after a diagnostic scan (85). There was no difference in the percentage of patients with a successful outcome after radioiodine therapy. In contrast, several authors strongly support the concept of stunning. Leger et al found that 71% of patients who first had a diagnostic scan with ^{131}I were not successfully ablated, compared with 7% who had ^{123}I diagnostic scans (86). Lees et al also found fewer patients were successfully ablated when given 5 mCi (185 MBq) of [131]I (87). Many of these reports require careful evaluation to explain the different conclusions. One disparity is the difference in the diagnostic dose, larger doses being more likely to cause stunning. A second difference is the delay between the diagnostic scan and therapy. The longer the delay, the greater the radiation delivered and the more likely for stunning to occur.

The concern about stunning has prompted several authorities to administer ^{123}I instead of [131]I. However, this author has reported less uptake on posttherapy scans when ^{123}I was the tracer (88). This adds fuel to the concept that

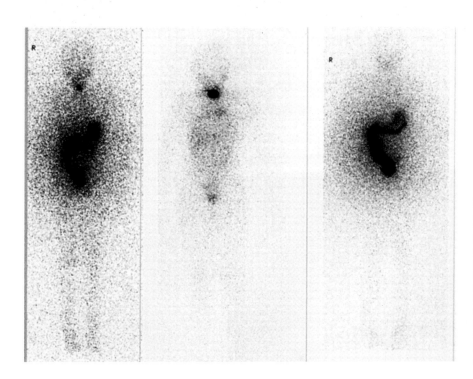

FIGURE 12.9. Whole-body images in a patient who had a thyroidectomy for differentiated thyroid cancer. The **left panel** shows a scan made 72 hours after 2 mCi (74 MBq) of [131]I. The **middle panel** is a posttherapy scan 1 week after 100 mCi (3.7 GBq) of [131]I. The **right panel** is follow-up scan after 1 year. The diagnostic and posttherapy scans show uptake in the thyroid bed and no evidence of "stunning" or additional lesions. The follow-up scan shows that residual thyroid was successfully ablated.

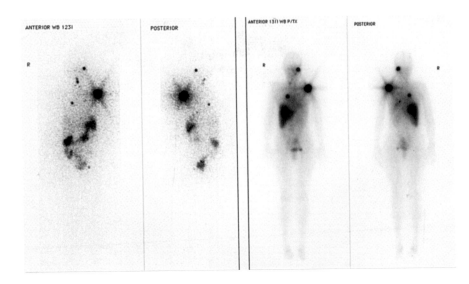

FIGURE 12.10. The scintiscans **on the left** are whole-body images made 24 hours after 2 mCi (74 MBq) of ¹²³I. The patient had undergone a thyroidectomy 6 years earlier. The pathology was a follicular adenoma (confirmed on review). She then presented with a mass in her left mandible that was metastatic follicular cancer. The whole-body scan shows lesions in the mandible, left shoulder, left groin and thorax. The images **on the right** are posttreatment scans acquired 7 days after 200 mCi (7.4 GBq) of ¹³¹I showing the same lesions; no additional metastases are recognized. The liver is easily identified on the posttreatment images.

the difference in timing of the posttreatment scan compared with the diagnostic scan must be considered. ¹²³I has also been used after stimulation with rhTSH (89).

POSTTHERAPY SCANNING

Posttreatment scans are the most sensitive imaging tests to determine the extent of functioning thyroid cancer. There are several reports of the posttreatment scan showing more lesions than diagnostic ¹³¹I scans (80,81). This led to the use of higher doses of ¹³¹I for diagnostic whole-body scans, which in turn resulted in the description of stunning. There are differences in when physicians order the posttreatment scan. Some obtain them at the time the patient is discharged from the hospital after treatment. Historically, that was when the retained dose of ¹³¹I was <30 mCi (<1.1 GBq). Others, including this author, have the patient return for the posttreatment scan after approximately 7 days. This timing also allows for a measurement of emitted radiation to determine whether the patient can be released from the restrictions of their activity intended to protect his or her family and the public. Lesions can be recognized with more certainty on a posttreatment scan in comparison with a diagnostic scan, but the stage of disease is increased in only 3% to 5% of patients (Fig. 12.10). This was confirmed in a study from the Mayo Clinic (90). Because the posttreatment scan can show more lesions, this altered the philosophy of management by some authorities who recommend treatment with ¹³¹I when a patient has a negative diagnostic whole-body scan but a high serum Tg level. They describe identification of the site of Tg production on the posttherapy scan (91,92). Alternative methods for finding the thyroid tissue are described later in the chapter.

FALSE-POSITIVE RADIOIODINE SCANS

Iodine is trapped not only by thyroid cells, but also by choroid plexus, salivary and mammary glands, and parietal cells. Iodine is also secreted by these glands, and it is cleared through the kidneys into urine. As a result, uptake in these tissues and in the urinary system can be misinterpreted as functioning metastases. There are many benign and malignant conditions that concentrate iodine and can therefore result in a false-positive radioiodine scan (93–95) (Table 12.5). It is important for the

TABLE 12.5. CAUSES OF A FALSE-POSITIVE WHOLE-BODY RADIOIODINE SCAN THAT CAN BE MISINTERPRETED AS METASTASIS

Physiologic	Pathologic
Salivary glands	Wig
Contamination with saliva	Meningioma
Nasopharynx	Artificial eye
Esophagus	Dacrocystitis
Thymus	Parotid tumor
Breast	Sinusitis
Stomach	Dental caries
Liver (posttherapy scan)	Tracheostomy
Gall bladder	Inflammatory lung disease
Intestine	Carcinoma of lung
Contamination with stool	Pleuropericardial cyst
Urinary tract	Struma cordis
Contamination with urine	Hiatal hernia
	Zenker's diverticulum
	Barrett's esophagus
	Adenocarcinoma of stomach
	Renal cyst
	Meckel's diverticulum
	Cystadenoma of ovary

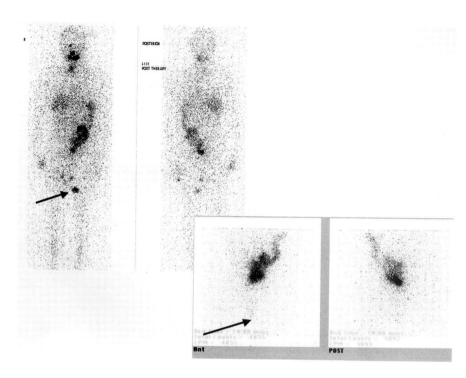

FIGURE 12.11. Whole-body images obtained 7 days after treatment of 100 mCi (3.7 GBq) of ^{131}I in a patient with thyroid cancer treated by surgery. There is uptake in the thyroid bed, salivary glands, liver, and intestine. There is also uptake in the left groin. The patient was not expected to have distant metastases. The pelvic "lesions" were cured by removing the patient's trousers and underwear.

clinician interpreting the radioiodine scan to determine whether abnormal concentration of radioiodine can reasonably be attributed to thyroid cancer. Knowledge of the natural history and pattern of spread of thyroid cancer is important. In addition, comparison of the scan findings with serum Tg measurements helps determine whether metastases are likely to be present. Figure 12.11 shows abnormal uptake in the left groin area due to contamination of underwear. Repeating the scan with the patient "gowned" demonstrated the uptake was a false-positive.

ALTERNATIVE CANCER-SEEKING RADIOPHARMACEUTICALS AND TECHNIQUES

The imaging methods discussed later in the chapter are employed in patients who have negative iodine scans and measurable serum Tg, or in whom the iodine scan is thought to underestimate the extent of disease. Management of patients with a measurable serum Tg value but a negative diagnostic scan with ^{131}I or ^{123}I is controversial. There is evidence that therapeutic doses of ^{131}I can demonstrate lesions and decrease serum Tg (91). Others find that lesions are seldom identified and that the serum Tg does not change (96). Each of the alternative radiopharmaceuticals is discussed briefly, but most authorities agree that PET using ^{18}F-FDG has replaced the other radiopharmaceuticals, including ^{201}Tl, ^{111}In-pentetreotide, ^{99m}Tc-sestamibi, and ^{99m}Tc-tetrafosmin.

Thallium

^{201}Tl atoms are substantially larger than K atoms. However, both are concentrated in cells through the potassium channel. ^{201}Tl is used for imaging the myocardium, parathyroid adenomas, and several nonthyroidal cancers. The photon emissions are of low energy, and the half-value (the length of tissue that attenuates 50% of the emitted photons) is about 4 cm. Two to four mCi (74 to 148 MBq) injected intravenously and imaging started within 10 to 15 minutes. Because ^{201}Tl can be trapped and washed out of cells at different rates, it is best to image early and after 2 to 3 hours. The quality of ^{201}Tl images is inferior to those of ^{99m}Tc compounds and to PET using ^{18}F-FDG. Most authorities no longer recommend this radionuclide for imaging thyroid cancer.

^{111}Indium-Pentetreotide

^{111}In-Pentetreotide is a radiolabeled somatostatin analogue that binds to somatostatin receptors 2, 3, and 5 (97). The radiopharmaceutical is valuable in imaging neuroendocrine cancers such as carcinoids, insulinomas, and some thyroid cancers. Five to six mCi (185 to 222 MBq) is injected intravenously and whole-body and tomographic images obtained at 4 and 24 hours. Most of the published series are of small numbers of patients. In one series of 48 patients, ^{111}In-pentetreotide images positive in 74% of patients (98). Sarlis et al compared this agent with ^{18}F-FDG PET and conventional radiologic studies, including whole-body CT and MRI, ultrasound of the neck, and skeletal surveys (99). The sensitivity of ^{111}In-pentetreotide was 49.5%, and for PET 67.6%; however, some lesions were only detected by the former.

[99m]Tc-Sestamibi and ^{99m}Tc-Tetrafosmin

These radiopharmaceuticals are discussed together because they are both technetium-labeled agents used primarily for evaluation of myocardial perfusion. They have also been used to identify parathyroid adenomas. ^{99m}Tc-radiopharmaceuticals give excellent resolution, radiation to the patient is low and thyroid hormone need not be withdrawn. Twenty to twenty-five mCi (740 to 925 MBq) are injected intravenously, and whole-body imaging started early, some recommend immediately. In an analysis of 110 patients, 22 of 24 patients with abnormal scans had high serum Tg values (17). Of the 86 who had normal serum Tg values, 83 had negative ^{99m}Tc-sestamibi scans. ^{99m}Tc-sestamibi has identified local recurrences and metastases in lymph nodes, lung, and skeleton. Not all of the reports have such good sensitivity and specificity. Clinical reports and reviews of ^{99m}Tc-tetrafosmin give similar results (100–102).

POSITRON EMISSION TOMOGRAPHY WITH ^{18}F-FLUORODEOXYGLUCOSE

This technology is based on the principle that cancers utilize more glucose than normal tissues. There is very little glucose uptake in normal thyroid tissue. Similarly, well-differentiated thyroid cancers trap little ^{18}F-FDG. However, these cancers concentrate radioiodine. When thyroid cancers lose the ability to trap iodine they are less well differentiated, in which case they may concentrate glucose and be imaged by PET scan after intravenous injection of ^{18}F-FDG. The images are made 1 hour after injection of 10 to 15 mCi ^{18}F-FDG (370 to 555 MBq). This technique finds the site of Tg production in 50% to 75% of patients (27,103–113). The scan is more likely to be positive when the serum Tg is higher. Figure 12.12 shows a PET scan in a patient with extensive papillary cancer, a high serum Tg value, and a negative ^{123}I whole-body scan. The author has experience with PET in 80 patients, several of whom have had two or more studies. The images are easy to interpret, the pathology of abnormal sites can be confirmed by directed biopsy, and proven lesions treated by operation or external radiation, depending on their accessibility. Lesions which are FDG avid are usually resistant to ^{131}I therapy.

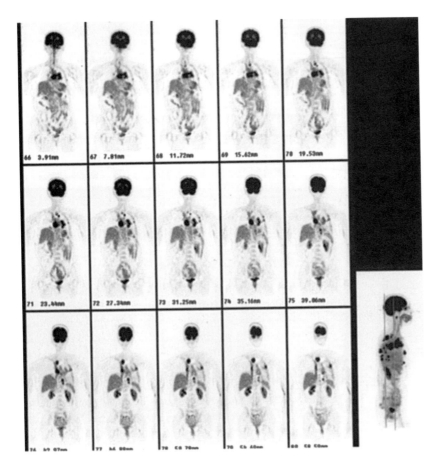

FIGURE 12.12. Coronal images of a positron emission tomograpy (PET) scan made 1 hour after injection of 15 mCi (555 MBq) of ^{18}F-fluorodeoxyglucose (^{18}F-FDG). The patient has had thyroid cancer with recurrences and progression for 50 years. Her serum thyroglobulin concentration is very high. A diagnostic scan showed no uptake of [123]I. The PET scan shows intense uptake of ^{18}F-FDG in the mediastinum, lung hila, spine, sternum, and lungs. There is physiological uptake in the brain, myocardium, liver, kidneys, and bladder.

PET has been used to follow the response of thyroid cancers to retinoid therapy (114). Most of the patients were studied when they were euthyroid or when TSH secretion was suppressed. Recent reports have shown a higher sensitivity for PET when serum TSH values are high (115). This raises the possibility that a negative PET scan in a euthyroid patient should be repeated after stimulation by TSH, either after withdrawal of thyroid hormone or after injection of rhTSH. ^{18}F-FDG scan has a high sensitivity in Hürthle-cell cancer. The author has used it in selected patients with anaplastic cancer to stage the extent of disease with a single imaging procedure. False-positive PET scans can result from inflammatory conditions such as tuberculosis and sarcoidosis. Active muscles use glucose for metabolism, and patients who are tense or shivering can have increased uptake of ^{18}F-FDG in neck muscles that could be misinterpreted as cervical nodal metastases. This can be avoided by reviewing the images on a computer terminal, and scrolling through the tomographic images and following the linear anatomy of muscles. Recently similar uptake of ^{18}F-FDG has been attributed to metabolism in brown fat, and combined PET/CT has confirmed this (Fig. 12.13).

INTRAOPERATIVE IMAGING

There are several different approaches to intraoperative imaging. One is to administer a tracer of [125]I 24 hours before the operation and use a handheld probe to identify tissue that concentrates the radionuclide. In a study of 64 patients undergoing total thyroidectomy, 43 patients had detectable activity, which could be completely excised in 33. This ensured the thyroidectomy was complete and could eliminate the need for ^{131}I ablation (116).

Schlumberger described a technique in which patients were scanned during surgery several days after a therapeutic dose of ^{131}I, to help the surgeon identify functioning metastases. Potential drawbacks from this approach are that the patient is hypothyroid and the surgeon is exposed to the radioactive patient. The question is whether it is necessary to operate, since ^{131}I alone is a very effective treatment.

Lastly, sentinel node imaging has been described. This is used routinely in patients with breast cancer and melanoma. There are a few reports on the use of sentinel node technique in thyroid carcinoma (36,117,118). Colloidal particles, usually [99c]Tc-sulfur colloid, is injected in or around the primary cancer. Four hundred to one thousand μCi (15 to 37 MBq) provides sufficient radiation to be detected by a gamma camera and later in the operating room by a handheld probe. There is also a report of this technique using ^{99m}Tc-sestamibi as the tracer (119). Whether sentinel node imaging in patients with thyroid cancer will become more widely employed is not certain, since the current approach with thyroidectomy and removal of clinically suspicious nodes produces excellent results.

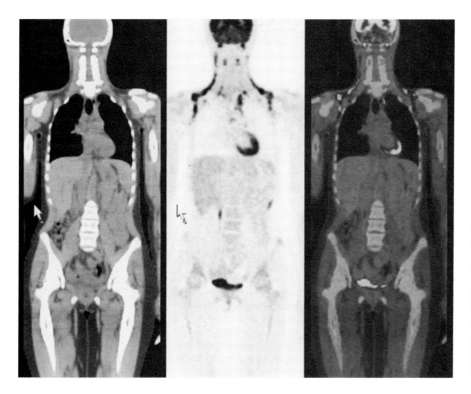

FIGURE 12.13. Coronal images of a positron emission tomograpy/computed tomography (PET/CT) scan made 1 hour after injection of 15 mCi (555 MBq) of ^{18}F-fluorodeoxyglucose (^{18}F-FDG). The patient was being scanned after treatment for Hodgkin's disease. The PET scan is **in the middle,** CT scan **on the left,** and fused images are **on the right.** There is uptake of ^{18}F-FDG in the lateral neck and upper mediastinum. This could be misinterpreted as nodal metastases, but is uptake in brown fat.

FLUORESCENT SCANNING

Fluorescent scanners are not widely available, and although they can quantitate the iodine content of the thyroid, they have not gained wide acceptance. The procedure has been used to measure the amount of iodine in the thyroid in different geographic regions. In the United States, the normal range is 5 to 15 mg. In France, the range is 2.5 to 7.5 mg (120). One study found the mean value in Graves' disease to be 36.5 mg, and the result is also high in patients who have received radiographic contrast or who take iodine-rich medications such as amiodarone (39). Because cancers trap less iodine than normal thyroid, it was hoped that fluorescent scanning could differentiate benign from malignant nodules. Unfortunately, the majority of benign nodules contain less iodine than normal thyroid, so the test has little discriminatory power (121).

IMAGING STUDIES FOR MEDULLARY THYROID CARCINOMA

Standard radioiodine scintigraphy is not helpful in patients with medullary thyroid cancer. The usual problem is to find the site of production of calcitonin measurable after total thyroidectomy. Standard radiological studies such as CT, ultrasonography, and MRI can be useful. Nuclear medicine techniques have the advantage of imaging the entire body. [201]Tl, ^{99m}Tc-sestamibi, and ^{99m}Tc-tetrafosmin have been used with some success, ranging from modest to disappointing (20,122). There are reports from Europe of the value of ^{99m}Tc-DMSA, but it is not approved in the United States (123). Adalet et al evaluated 34 known lesions with ^{99m}Tc-DMSA, ^{201}Tl, and ^{99m}Tc-tetrafosmin. ^{99m}Tc-DMSA readily detected 30 lesions, whereas 21 and 20 lesions were visualized very faintly with ^{201}Tl or ^{99m}Tc-tetrafosmin, respectively. Rhenium-labeled DMSA has been produced for targeted treatment of medullary thyroid cancer (124,125). [131]I- and ^{123}I-metaiodobenzylguanidine (MIBG) have been used to image medullary cancer, but the sensitivity is disappointing. ^{111}In-pentetreotide in one study correctly diagnosed 11 of 17 patients (67). In studies comparing ^{111}In-pentetreotide, ^{201}Tl, ^{99m}Tc-sestamibi, and ^{99m}Tc-DMSA, no single test identified all lesions (22, 23). Several investigators have found ^{18}F-FDG PET to be the most sensitive test for identifying medullary cancer (126–129). In a study comparing PET with ^{111}In-pentetreotide, each procedure found some lesions that were missed by the other (22). There are recent data on the benefit of combined PET/CT imaging (130). This author has had useful results with ^{18}F-FDG PET. However, the test is likely to be negative when the serum calcitonin is <100 pg/mL.

RADIOACTIVE IODINE AND PREGNANT OR NURSING WOMEN

Pregnant women should not be given radionuclides of iodine. Most patients with thyroid disorders are women of child-bearing potential, and it is important for nuclear medicine personnel to ensure that a pregnant or nursing woman does not receive radioiodine, in particular [131]I. This is even more important when larger doses are prescribed for therapy or for whole-body scintigraphy. In the case of patients receiving small tracer doses of ^{123}I, if there is any doubt about the possibility of pregnancy, a serum pregnancy test should be ordered. Because larger doses of ^{131}I can cause ablation of fetal thyroid, a U.S. court has determined that an oral declaration of nonpregnancy is not good enough (131). Urinary pregnancy tests are not sensitive in early pregnancy and do not exclude conception. Therefore, a serum pregnancy test should be obtained in all women who could bear children.

The lactating breast concentrates and secretes iodine. The nursing baby would therefore be exposed to radiation. Because of the small size and increased activity of the thyroid in the newborn, tracer doses of radioiodine given to the mother necessitate cessation of nursing. In the case of a tracer of ^{123}I, we advise complete cessation for 2 to 3 days, and afterward that the radioactivity in an aliquot of milk be measured, to determine whether it is safe to resume nursing. In the case of ^{131}I, because of its half-life and electron emissions, nursing should be stopped completely. There are limited references on this topic (132–134).

In the case of a pregnant or nursing patient, the following questions should be answered. Is the study essential? Are there alternative procedures that do not require administration of radionuclides? If not, which radiopharmaceutical will give the lowest radiation dose, and would it be possible to obtain the desired information with a lower dose?

REFERENCES

1. Dai G, Levy O, Carrasco N. Cloning and characterization of the thyroid iodide transporter. *Nature* 1996;379:458–460.
2. Dohan O, De La Vieja A, Paroder V, et al. The sodium/iodide symporter (NIS): characterization, regulation, and medical significance. *Endocr Rev* 2003;24:48–77.
3. De La Vieja A, Dohan O, Levy O, et al. Molecular analysis of the sodium/iodide symporter: impact on thyroid and extrathyroid pathophysiology. *Physiol Rev* 2000;80:1083–105.
4. Gorges R, Antoch G, Brandau W, et al. Combination PET/CT with 124I positron rays in metastatic follicular thyroid carcinoma. *Nuklearmedizin* 2002;41:N68–N71.
5. Solomon B, Glinoer D, Lagasse R, et al. Current trends in the management of Graves' disease. *J Clin Endocrinol Metab* 1990; 70:1518–1524.

6. Yaakob W, Gordon L, Spicer KM, et al. The usefulness of iodine-123 whole-body scans in evaluating thyroid carcinoma and metastases. *J Nucl Med Technol* 1999;27:279–281.
7. Violet J, Nutting C, Plowman PN, et al. 123I imaging in the follow-up of differentiated thyroid cancer. *Clin Oncol (R Coll Radiol)* 2001;13:313–314.
8. Kalinyak JE. 123I as a diagnostic tracer in the management of thyroid cancer. *Nucl Med Commun* 2002;23:509–511.
9. Pentlow KS, Graham MC, Lambrecht RM, et al. Quantitative imaging of iodine-124 with PET. *J Nucl Med* 1996;37:1557–1562.
10. McDougall I, Greig WR, Gillespie FC. Radioactive iodine-125 therapy for thyrotoxicosis: background and evaluation in 148 patients. *N Engl J Med* 1971;285:1099–1104.
11. Alzahrani AS, Bakheet S, Al Mandil M, et al. 123I isotope as a diagnostic agent in the follow-up of patients with differentiated thyroid cancer: comparison with post 131I therapy whole body scanning. *J Clin Endocrinol Metab* 2001;86:5294–5300.
12. Gerard SK, Cavalieri RR. I-123 diagnostic thyroid tumor whole-body scanning with imaging at 6, 24, and 48 hours. *Clin Nucl Med* 2002;27:1–8.
13. Atkins, HL. Technetium-99m pertechnetate uptake and scanning in the evaluation of thyroid function. *Semin Nucl Med* 1971;1:345–355.
14. Hoefnagel B, Delprat CC, Marcuse HR, et al. Role of thallium-201 total-body scintigraphy in follow-up of thyroid carcinoma. *J Nucl Med* 1986;27:1854–1857.
15. Iida Y, Hidaka A, Hatabu H, et al. Follow-up study of postoperative patients with thyroid cancer by thallium-201 scintigraphy and serum thyroglobulin measurement. *J Nucl Med* 1991;32:2098–2100.
16. Yen T-C, Lin H-D, Lee C-H, et al. The role of technetium-99m sestamibi whole-body scans in diagnosing metastatic Hurthle cell carcinoma of the thyroid gland after total thyroidectomy: a comparison with iodine-131 and thallium-201 whole-body scans. *J Nucl Med* 1994;21:980–983.
17. Almeida-Filho P, Ravizzini GC, Almeida C, et al. Whole-body Tc-99m sestamibi scintigraphy in the follow-up of differentiated thyroid carcinoma. *Clin Nucl Med* 2000;25:443–446.
18. Gallowitsch H, Mikosch P, Kresnik E, et al. Thyroglobulin and low-dose iodine-131 and technetium-99m-tetrofosmin whole-body scintigraphy in differentiated thyroid carcinoma. *J Nucl Med* 1998;39:870–875.
19. Gallowitsch HJ, Mikosch P, Kresnik E, et al. Comparison between 99mTc-tetrofosmin/pertechnetate subtraction scintigraphy and 99mTc-tetrofosmin SPECT for preoperative localization of parathyroid adenoma in an endemic goiter area. *Invest Radiol* 2000;35:453–459.
20. Adalet I, Demirkale P, Unal S, et al. Disappointing results with Tc-99m tetrofosmin for detecting medullary thyroid carcinoma metastases comparison with Tc-99m VDMSA and TI-201. *Clin Nucl Med* 1999;24:678–683.
21. Tenenbaum F, Lumbroso J, Schlumberger M, et al. Radiolabeled somatostatin analog scintigraphy in differentiated thyroid carcinoma. *J Nucl Med* 1995;36:807–810.
22. Adams S, Baum RP, Hertel A, et al. Comparison of metabolic and receptor imaging in recurrent medullary thyroid carcinoma with histopathological findings. *Eur J Nucl Med* 1998;25:1277–1283.
23. Ugur O, Kostaglu L, Guler N, et al. Comparison of 99mTc (V)-DMSA, 201Tl, and 99mTc-MIBI imaging in the follow-up of patients with medullary carcinoma of the thyroid. *Eur J Nucl Med* 1996. 23:1367–1381.
24. Huebner RH, Park KC, Shepherd JE, et al. A meta-analysis of the literature for whole-body FDG PET detection of recurrent colorectal cancer. *J Nucl Med* 2000;41:1177–1189.
25. Meta J, Seltzer M, Schiepers C, et al. Impact of 18F-FDG PET on managing patients with colorectal cancer: the referring physician's perspective. *J Nucl Med* 2001;42:586–590.
26. Schwimmer J, Essner R, Patel A, et al. A review of the literature for whole-body FDG PET in the management of patients with melanoma. *Q J Nucl Med* 2000. 44:153–167.
27. McDougall IR, Davidson J, Segall GM. Positron emission tomography of the thyroid, with an emphasis on thyroid cancer. *Nucl Med Commun* 2001;22:485–492.
28. Sostre S, Ashare AB, Quinones JD, et al. Thyroid scintigraphy: pinhole images versus rectilinear scan. *Radiology* 1978;129:759–762.
29. Smith ML, Wraight EP. Oblique views in thyroid imaging. *Clin Nucl Med* 1989;40:505–507.
30. Chen J, La France ND, Rippin R, et al. Iodine-123 SPECT of the thyroid in multinodular goiter. *J Nucl Med* 1988;29:110–113.
31. Webb S, Flower MA, Ott RJ, et al. Single photon emission computed tomography imaging and volume estimation of the thyroid using fan beam geometry. *Br J Radiol* 1986;59:951–955.
32. Van Isselt JW, de Klerk JM, van Rijk PP, et al. Comparison of methods for thyroid volume estimation in patients with Graves' disease. *Eur J Nucl Med Mol Imaging* 2003;30:525–531.
33. Krausz Y, Wil M, Saliman F. Role of high-resolution pinhole tomography in the evaluation of thyroid abnormalities. *Thyroid* 1997;7:847–852.
34. Beekman F, McElray DP, Berger F. Towards in vivo nuclear microscopy: iodine-125 imaging in mice using micro-pinholes. *Eur J Nucl Med* 2002;29:933–938.
35. Patton J. Turkington TG. Coincidence imaging with a dual-head scintillation camera. *J Nucl Med* 1999;40:432–441.
36. Catarci M, Zaraca F, Angeloni R, et al. Preoperative lymphoscintigraphy and sentinel lymph node biopsy in papillary thyroid cancer. A pilot study. *J Surg Oncol* 2001;77:21–24; [discussion] 25.
37. Schlumberger, MJ. Papillary and follicular thyroid carcinoma. *N Engl J Med* 1998;338:297–306.
38. Hoffer PB, Gottschalk A. Fluorescent thyroid scanning: scanning without radioisotopes. Initial clinical results. *Radiology* 1971;99:117–123.
39. Leger AF, Fragu P, Rougier P, et al. Thyroid iodine content measured by x-ray fluorescence in amiodarone-induced thyrotoxicosis: concise communication. *J Nucl Med* 1983;24:582–585.
40. Becker D. Charkes ND, Hurley JR. Society of Nuclear Medicine Procedure Guideline for thyroid scintigraphy. *J Nucl Med* 1996;37:1264–1266.
41. Morris LF, Waxman AD, Braunstein GD. Accuracy considerations when using early (four- or six-hour) radioactive iodine uptake to predict twenty-four-hour values for radioactive iodine dosage in the treatment of Graves' disease. *Thyroid* 2000;10:779–787.
42. Kalinyak JE, McDougall IR. How should the dose of iodine-13I be determined in the treatment of Graves' hyperthyroidism? *J Clin Endocrinol Metab* 2003;88:975–977.
43. Hays M, Wesselossky B. Simultaneous measurement of thyroid trapping (99mTcO4-) and binding (131I): clinical and experimental studies in man. *J Nucl Med* 1973;14:785–792.
44. Duck SC, Sty J. Technetium thyroid uptake ratios in pediatric Graves' disease. *J Pediatr* 1985;107:905–909.
45. Werner S. Response to triiodothyronine as an index of persistance of disease in the thyroid remnant of patients in remission from hyperthyroidism. *J Clin Invest* 1956;35:57.
46. Charkes N, Cantor RE, Goluboff B. A three day, double isotope, L-triiodothyronine suppression test of thyroid autonomy. *J Nucl Med* 1967;8:627.

47. Levy H, Sziklas JJ, Rosenber RJ, et al. Incidence of pyramidal lobe on thyroid scans. *Clin Nucl Med* 1987;12:560–561.

48. Knobel M, Medeiros-Neto G. An outline of inherited disorders of the thyroid hormone generating system. *Thyroid* 2003;13:771–801.

49. Verelst J, Chanoine J-P, Delange F. Radionuclide imaging in primary permanent congenital hypothyroidism. *Clin Nucl Med* 1991;16:652–655.

50. Matsumura L, Russo EMK, Dib SA, et al. Hemiagenesis of the thyroid gland and T3 hyperthyroidism. *Postgrad Med J* 1982;58: 244–246.

51. Ashcraft MW, Van Herle AJ. Management of thyroid nodules. Scanning techniques, thyroid suppressive therapy and fine needle aspiration. *Head Neck Surg* 1981;3:297–322.

52. Mazzaferri E. Management of a solitary thyroid nodule. *N Engl J Med* 1993;328:553–559.

53. McDougall I. Thyroid nodules. In: *Thyroid disease in clinical practice*. Oxford Press, London. 1992:193–206.

54. Ross DS. Evaluation of the thyroid nodule. *Nucl Med* 1991; 32:2181–2192.

55. Roman SA. Endocrine tumors: evaluation of the thyroid nodule. *Curr Opin Oncol* 2003.;15:66–70.

56. Weiss RE, Lado-Abeal J. Thyroid nodules: diagnosis and therapy. *Curr Opin Oncol* 2002;14:45–52.

57. Nagai GR, Pitts WC, Basso L, et al. Scintigraphically hot nodules and thyroid cancer. *Clin Nucl Med* 1987;6:123–127.

58. Kusic Z, Becker DV, Sanger EL, et al. Comparison of technetium-99m and iodine-123 imaging of thyroid nodules: comparison with pathological findings. *J Nucl Med* 1990;31:393–399.

59. Erjavec M, Morvin T, Auersperg M, et al. Comparative accumulation of 99m-Tc and 131-I in thyroid nodules: case report. *J Nucl Med* 1977;18:346–347.

60. Kraimps J, Bouin-Pineau MH, Mathonnet M, et al. Multicenter study of thyroid nodules in patients with Graves' disease. *Br J Surg* 2000;87:1111–1113.

61. Belfiori A, Garofalo MR, Giuffrida D, et al. Increased aggressiveness of thyroid cancer in patients with Graves' disease. *J Clin Endocrinol Metab* 1990;75:830–835.

62. Carnell N, Valente WA. Thyroid nodules in Graves' disease: classification, characterization, and response to treatment. *Thyroid* 1998;8:647–652.

63. Mezosi E, Bajnok L, Gyory F, et al. The role of technetium-99m methoxyisobutylisonitrile scintigraphy in the differential diagnosis of cold thyroid nodules. *Eur J Nucl Med* 1999;26:798–803.

64. Demiral K, Kapucu O, Yucel C, et al. A comparison of radionuclide thyroid angiography, 99mTc-MIBI scintigraphy and power Doppler ultrasonography in the differential diagnosis of solitary cold thyroid nodules. *Eur J Nucl Med Mol Imaging* 2003;30:642–650.

65. Moe RD, Franekl SF, Chacko AK, et al. Radionuclide thyroid angiography and surgical correlation. A five-year study. *Arch Otolaryngol Head Neck Surg* 1984;110:717–720.

66. Sathekge M, Mageza RB, Muthupheli MN, et al. Evaluation of thyroid nodules with technetium-99m MIBI and technetium-99m pertechnetate. *Head Neck* 1991;23:305–310.

67. Krenning E, Kwekkeboom DJ, Bakkar WH, et al. Somatostatin receptor scintigraphy with (111In-DTPA-D-Phe1)- and (123I-Tyr3)-octreotide: the Rotterdam experience with more than 1000 patients. *Eur J Nucl Med* 1993;20:716–731.

68. Bloom AD, Adler LP, Shuck JM. Determination of malignancy of thyroid nodules with positron emission tomography. *Surgery* 1993;114:728.

69. Yasuda S, Shohtsu A, Ide M, et al. Chronic thyroiditis: diffuse uptake of FDG at PET. *Radiology* 1998;207:775–778.

70. Lin C, Sun SS, Yang MD, et al. The use of 201Tl thyroid scan for equivocal fine-needle aspiration results in cold thyroid nodules. *Anticancer Res* 2001;21:2969–2972.

71. Chen Y, Wang WH, Chan T, et al. The cost effectiveness of dual phase 201Tl thyroid scan in detecting thyroid cancer for evaluating thyroid nodules with equivocal fine-needle aspiration results: the preliminary Taiwanese experience. *Neoplasma* 2002;49:129–132.

72. Bashist B, Ellis K, Gold RP. Computed tomography and intrathoracic goiter. *AJR Am J Roentgenol* 1983;140:455–460.

73. Lakshmanan M, Schaffer A, Robbins J, et al. A simplified low iodine diet in I-131 scanning and therapy of thyroid carcinoma. *Clin Nucl Med* 1988;13:866–868.

74. Ain K, Dewitt PA, Gardner TG, et al. Low-iodine tube-feeding diet for I-131 scanning and therapy. *Clin Nucl Med* 1994;19:504–507.

75. Ladenson P, Braverman LE, Mazzaferri EL, et al. Comparison of administration of recombinant human thyrotropin with withdrawal of thyroid hormone for radioactive iodine scanning in patients with thyroid carcinoma. *N Engl J Med* 1997;337:888–896.

76. Ladenson PW. Recombinant thyrotropin for detection of recurrent thyroid cancer. *Trans Am Clin Climatol Assoc* 2002;113:21–30.

77. Haugen BR, Pacini F, Reiners C, et al. A comparison of recombinant human thyrotropin and thyroid hormone withdrawal for the detection of thyroid remnant or cancer. *J Clin Endocrinol Metab* 1999;84:3877–3885.

78. McDougall I, Weigel RJ. Recombinant human thyrotropin in the management of thyroid cancer. *Curr Opin Oncol* 2001;13:39–43.

79. Mazzaferri EL, Kloos RT. Using recombinant human TSH in the management of well-differentiated thyroid cancer: current strategies and future directions. *Thyroid* 2000;10:767–778.

79A. Mazzaferri EL, Robbins RJ, Spencer CA, et al. A consensus report of the role of serum thyroglobulin as a monitoring method for low-risk patients with papillary thyroid carcinoma. *J Clin Endocrinol Metab* 2003;88:14333–1441.

80. Nemec J, Röhling S, Zamrazil V, et al. Comparison of the distribution of diagnostic and thyroablative I-131 in the evaluation of differentiated thyroid cancers. *J Nucl Med* 1979;20:92–97.

81. Pacini F, Lippi L, Formica M, et al. Therapeutic doses of iodine-131 reveal undiagnosed metastases in thyroid cancer patients with detectable serum-thyroglobulin levels. *J Nucl Med* 1987;28:1888–1891.

82. McDougall I. 74 MBq radioiodine 131I does not prevent uptake of therapeutic doses of 131I (i.e. it does not cause stunning) in differentiated thyroid cancer. *Nucl Med Commun* 1997;18:505–512.

83. Park H, Perkins OW, Edmondson JW, et al. Influence of diagnostic radioiodines on the uptake of ablative dose of iodine-131. *Thyroid* 1994;4:49–54.

84. Cholewinski SP, Yoo KS, Klieger PS, et al. Absence of thyroid stunning after diagnostic whole-body scanning with 185 MBq 131I. *J Nucl Med* 2000;41:1198–1202.

85. Morris LF, Waxman AD, Braunstein GD. The nonimpact of thyroid stunning: remnant ablation rates in 131I-scanned and nonscanned individuals. *J Clin Endocrinol Metab* 2001;86:3507–511.

86. Leger F, Izembart M, Dagousset F, et al. Decreased uptake of therapeutic doses of iodine-131 after 185-MBq iodine-131 diagnostic imaging for thyroid remnants in differentiated thyroid carcinoma. *Eur J Nucl Med* 1998;25:242–246.

87. Lees W, Mansberg R, Roberts J, et al. The clinical effects of thyroid stunning after diagnostic whole-body scanning with 185 MBq 131I. *Eur J Nucl Med* 2002;2002:1421–1427.

88. Cohen J, Kalinyak JE, McDougall IR. Clinical implications of the differences between diagnostic 123I and post-therapy 131I scans. *Nucl Med Commun* 2004;25:129.

89. Fish SA, Alavi A, Mandel SJ. I-123 imaging after recombinant human thyroid–stimulating hormone to diagnose metastatic disease in an intubated patient with papillary thyroid cancer. *Clin Nucl Med* 2002;27:895.

90. Fatourechi V, Hay ID, Mullan BP, et al. Are posttherapy radioiodine scans informative and do they influence subsequent therapy of patients with differentiated thyroid cancer? *Thyroid* 2000;10:573–577.

91. Pineda J, Lee T, Ain K, et al. Iodine-131 therapy for thyroid cancer patients with elevated thyroglobulin and negative diagnostic scan. *J Clin Endocrinol Metab* 1995;80:1488–1492.

92. Schlumberger M, Mancusi F, Baudin E, et al. 131I therapy for elevated thyroglobulin levels. 1997;7:273–276.

93. Carlisle M, Lu C, McDougall IR. The interpretation of 131I scans in the evaluation of thyroid cancer, with an emphasis on false positive findings. *Nucl Med Commun* 2003;24:715–735.

94. McDougall I. Whole-body scintigraphy with radioiodine-131. A comprehensive list of false positives with some examples. *Clin Nucl Med* 1995;20:869–875.

95. Bakheet S, Hammami MM. False-positive radioiodine whole-body scan in thyroid cancer patients with unrelated pathology. *Clin Nucl Med* 1994;19:325–329.

96. Fatourechi V, Hay ID. Treating the patient with differentiated thyroid cancer with thyroglobulin-positive iodine-131 diagnostic scan-negative metastases: including comments on the role of serum thyroglobulin monitoring in tumor surveillance. *Semin Nucl Med* 2000;30:107–114.

97. England RJ, Atkin SL. Somatostatins and their role in thyroid cancer. *Clin Otolaryngol* 2002;27:120–123.

98. Gorges R, Kahaly G, Muller-Brand J, et al. Radionuclide-labeled somatostatin analogues for diagnostic and therapeutic purposes in nonmedullary thyroid cancer. *Thyroid* 2001;11:647–659.

99. Sarlis NJ, Gourgiotis L, Guthrie LC, et al. In-111 DTPA-octreotide scintigraphy for disease detection in metastatic thyroid cancer: comparison with F-18 FDG positron emission tomography and extensive conventional radiographic imaging. *Clin Nucl Med* 2003;28:208–217.

100. Lind P, Gallowitsch HJ, Langsteger W, et al. Technetium-99m-tetrofosmin whole-body scintigraphy in the follow-up of differentiated thyroid carcinoma. *J Nucl Med* 1997;38:348–352.

101. Lind P, Gallowitsch HJ, Mikosch P, et al. Comparison of different tracers in the follow up of differentiated thyroid carcinoma. *Acta Med Austriaca* 1999;26:115–117.

102. Drac-Kaniewska J, Kozlowicz-Gudzinska I, Tomaszewicz-Kubasiki H, et al. 99mTc tetrofosmin in diagnosis of distant metastases from differentiated thyroid cancer. [in Polish]. *Wiad Lek* 2001;54[Suppl 1]:357–362.

103. Joensuu H, Ahonen A. Imaging of metastases of thyroid carcinoma with fluorine-18 fluorodeoxyglucose. *J Nucl Med* 1987; 28:910–914.

104. Alnafisi NS, Driedger AA, Coates G, et al. FDG PET of recurrent or metastatic 131I-negative papillary thyroid carcinoma. *J Nucl Med* 2000;41:1010–1015.

105. Fiene U. Fluoro-18-deoxyglucose positron emission tomography in differentiated thyroid carcinoma. *Eur J Endocrinol* 1998; 138:492–496.

106. Grunwald F, Kalicke T, Feine U, et al. Fluorine-18 fluorodeoxyglucose positron emission tomography in thyroid cancer: results of a multicentre study. *Eur J Nucl Med* 1999;26:1547–1552.

107. Wang W, Macapinlac H, Finn RD, et al. PET scanning with (18F) 2-fluoro-2 deoxy-D-glucose (FDG) can localize residual differentiated thyroid cancer in patients with negative (131I)-iodine whole-body scans. *J Clin Endocrinol Metab* 1999;84:2291–2302.

108. Wang W, Larson SM, Fazzari M, et al. Prognostic value of (18F) fluorodeoxyglucose positron emission tomographic scanning in patients with thyroid cancer. *J Clin Endocrinol Metab* 2000;85:1107–1113.

109. Chung JK, So Y, Lee JS, et al. Value of FDG PET in papillary thyroid carcinoma with negative 131I whole-body scan. *J Nucl Med* 1999;40:986–992.

110. Altenvoerde G, Lerch H, Kuwert T, et al. Positron emission tomography with F-18-deoxyglucose in patients with differentiated thyroid carcinoma, elevated thyroglobulin levels, and negative iodine scans. *Langenbecks Arch Surg* 1998;383:160–163.

111. Muros MA, Llamas-Elvira JM, Ramirez-Navarro A, et al. Utility of fluorine-18-fluorodeoxyglucose positron emission tomography in differentiated thyroid carcinoma with negative radioiodine scans and elevated serum thyroglobulin levels. *Am J Surg* 2000;179:457–461.

112. Huang T, Chieng PU, Chang CC, et al. Positron emission tomography for detecting iodine-131 nonvisualized metastasis of well-differentiated thyroid carcinoma: two case reports. *J Endocrinol Invest* 1998. 21:392–398.

113. van Tol KM, Jager PL, Dullaart RP, et al. Follow-up in patients with differentiated thyroid carcinoma with positive 18F-fluoro-2-deoxy-D-glucose-positron emission tomography results, elevated thyroglobulin levels, and negative high-dose 131I posttreatment whole body scans. *J Clin Endocrinol Metab* 2000;85:2082–2083.

114. Boerner AR, Petrich T, Weckesser E, et al. Monitoring isotretinoin therapy in thyroid cancer using 18F-FDG PET. *Eur J Nucl Med Mol Imaging* 2002;29:231–236.

115. Petrich T, Helmeke HJ, Meyer GJ, et al. Influence of rhTSH on (18)F fluorodeoxyglucose uptake by differentiated thyroid carcinoma. *Eur J Nucl Med Mol Imaging* 2002;29:641–647.

116. Lennquist S, Persliden J, Smeds S. The value of intraoperative scintigraphy as a routine procedure in thyroid carcinoma. *World J Surg* 1988;12:586–592.

117. Rettenbacher L, Sungler P, Gmeiner D, et al. Detecting the sentinel lymph node in patients with differentiated thyroid carcinoma. *Eur J Nucl Med* 2000;27:1399–1401.

118. Kelemen P, Van Herle AJ, Guiliano ARE. Sentinel lymphadenectomy in thyroid malignant neoplasms. *Arch Surg* 1998; 133:288–294.

119. Boz A, Arici C, Gungor F, et al. Gamma probe-guided resection and scanning with TC-99m MIBI of a local recurrence of follicular thyroid carcinoma. *Clin Nucl Med* 2001;26:820–822.

120. Meignan M, Galle P. Fluorescent thyroid scanning and intrathyroidal iodine quantification: study in 140 patients. [in French, author's translation] *Nouv Presse Med* 1978;7:13–19.

121. Patton JA, Hollifield JW, Brill AB, et al. Differentiation between malignant and benign solitary thyroid nodules by fluorescent scanning. *J Nucl Med* 1976;17:17–21.

122. Hoefnagel C, Delprat CC, Zanin D, et al. New radionuclide tracers for the diagnosis and therapy of medullary cancer. *Clin Nucl Med* 1988;13:159–165.

123. Shikare S, Bashir K, Menon PS, et al. Detection of medullary carcinoma of thyroid, with liver metastasis, using 99mTc DMSA(V) scintigraphy. *J Postgrad Med* 1995;41:12–13.

124. Bisunadan MM, Blower PJ, Clarke SE, et al. Synthesis and characterization of (186Re)rhenium(V)dimercaptosuccinic acid: a possible tumour radiotherapy agent. *Int J Rad Appl Instrum (A)* 1991;42:167–171.

125. Blower PJ, Lam AS, O'Doherty MJ, et al. Pentavalent rhenium-188 dimercaptosuccinic acid for targeted radiotherapy: synthesis and preliminary animal and human studies. *Eur J Nucl Med* 1998;25:613–621.

126. Brandt-Mainz K, Muller SP, Gorges R, et al. The value of fluorine-18 fluorodeoxyglucose PET in patients with medullary thyroid cancer. *Eur J Nucl Med* 2000;27:490–496.

127. Diehl M, Risse JH, Brandt-Mainz K, et al. Fluorine-18 fluorodeoxyglucose positron emission tomography in medullary thyroid cancer: results of a multicentre study. *Eur J Nucl Med* 2001;28:1671–1676.

128. Szakall S, Jr., Esik O, Bajzik G, et al. 18F-FDG PET detection of lymph node metastases in medullary thyroid carcinoma. *J Nucl Med* 2002;43(1):66–71.

129. Gourgiotis L, Sarlis NJ, Reynolds JC, et al. Localization of medullary thyroid carcinoma metastasis in a multiple endocrine neoplasia type 2A patient by 6-(18F)-fluorodopamine positron emission tomography. *J Clin Endocrinol Metab* 2003;88:637–641.

130. Bockisch A, Brandt-Mainz K, Gorges R, et al. Diagnosis in medullary thyroid cancer with (18F) FDG-PET and improvement using a combined PET/CT scanner. *Acta Med Austriaca* 2003;30:22–25.

131. Berlin L. Iodine-131 and the pregnant patient. *AJR Am J Roentgenol* 2001;176:869–871.

132. Romney B, Nickoloff EL, Esser PD, et al. Radionuclide administration to nursing mothers: mathematically derived guidelines. *Radiology* 1988;160:549–554.

133. Romney B, Nickoloff EL, Esser PD. Excretion of radioiodine in breast milk. *J Nucl Med* 1989;30:124–126.

134. Mountford PJ, Coakley AJ. A review of the secretion of radioactivity in human breast milk: data, quantitative analysis and recommendations. *Nucl Med Commun* 1989;10:15–27.

MEASURING SERUM THYROTROPIN AND THYROID HORMONE AND ASSESSING THYROID HORMONE TRANSPORT

ANTHONY D. TOFT
GEOFFREY J. BECKETT

This chapter reviews the various serum tests of thyroid function; outlines how these tests should be selected, performed, reported, and interpreted; and discusses how the pitfalls of the tests can be recognized or avoided. The United States National Academy of Clinical Biochemistry has published extensive guidelines concerning the Laboratory Support for the Diagnosis and Monitoring of Thyroid Disease, which are of relevance to both clinicians and laboratories (1). In general, measurements of serum thyrotropin (TSH) and the thyroid hormones thyroxine (T_4) and triiodothyronine (T_3) should be performed to determine thyroid status before embarking upon the tests necessary to determine the cause of the thyroid dysfunction or any treatment for it. Diagnosis of thyroid disorders relies heavily on the results of measurements of serum TSH and thyroid hormones, and it is essential that reliable assay systems be used for these measurements.

SERUM THYROTROPIN

Measurement of TSH in a basal serum sample by a sensitive immunometric assay is the single most sensitive, specific, and reliable test of thyroid status. In patients with primary (thyroidal) hypothyroidism, serum TSH concentrations are high, whereas in almost all patients with thyrotoxicosis, serum TSH concentrations are low, usually below 0.02 mU/L. However, measurement of serum TSH alone is not a reliable test for detecting thyroid dysfunction arising from hypothalamic-pituitary disease, or other specific instances, such as assay interference and end-organ resistance (2).

Evolution of Serum Thyrotropin Measurements

The introduction in the 1980s of sensitive and specific immunoassays for TSH revolutionized the way in which thyroid function testing is approached (3,4). Before then,

serum TSH was measured by relatively insensitive and nonspecific radioimmunoassays (5). These assays could only detect serum TSH concentrations as low as about 1 mU/L, and therefore serum TSH could not be detected in all normal subjects. The assays could detect the high serum TSH concentrations found in patients with primary hypothyroidism, but because of their limited sensitivity they were unable to distinguish reliably between normal subjects and patients with thyrotoxicosis or other conditions associated with decreased TSH secretion without recourse to thyrotropin-releasing hormone (TRH) stimulation.

Serum TSH is now measured by immunometric assays that use noncompetitive labeled-antibody methods. These assays use two highly specific monoclonal antibodies raised to epitopes on the alpha and beta subunits, respectively, of the TSH molecule. Nonisotopic labels are now preferred over radioactive labels, because they improve assay sensitivity and readily lend themselves to automation (Fig. 13.1). With immunometric assay methodologies it is now possible to detect serum TSH concentrations < 0.02 mU/L with a high degree of specificity (1,6). As a result of the improvements, serum TSH assays have become the most sensitive and specific method for assessing thyroid status (7).

Functional Sensitivity

The introduction of immunometric assays for serum TSH led to a problem regarding the nomenclature describing the assays. Manufacturers described their products with a variety of qualifying adjectives such as "sensitive," "supersensitive," and "ultrasensitive," terms that did not necessarily equate with the relative degree of sensitivity of the assays. Also, analytical sensitivity was frequently quoted. This is the lowest serum concentration of TSH that can be distinguished by statistical analysis from the zero standard within a single assay when multiple replicates are analyzed. This is an inappropriate and misleading way of estimating sensitivity because laboratories do not analyze multiple

Capture Antibody

Signal Antibody

**Gel / Resin Particle
Plastic Bead
Plastic tube
Microtitre Plate
Fibre Strip**

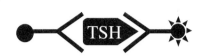

**^{125}I-Radiolabel
Fluorescent
Chemiluminescent
Enzyme**

FIGURE 13.1. Configurations of immunoradiometric assays (IRMAs). An IRMA usually consists of a capture antibody and a signal antibody. Both antibodies may be added together with the sample to form a sandwich, or the capture antibody and analyte may be added first, followed by a wash step, before the addition of signal antibody. The capture antibody is usually immobilized on an insoluble matrix. The signal antibody may be labeled with ^{125}I, but is more often labeled with a fluorescent or chemiluminescent chemical or an enzyme, usually horseradish peroxidase or alkaline phosphatase. These enzymes can be linked to substrates that give a colorimetric end point. Greater sensitivity can be achieved if the enzyme is linked to a substrate that produces fluorescence or chemiluminescence.

replicates of a sample routinely (1,6,8,9). Also, the sensitivity of a single assay does not represent the day-to-day variability that occurs in routine use. The key to identifying the sensitivity of an assay lies in constructing a precision profile. This is a plot of the coefficient of variation (CV) against serum TSH concentration, using results obtained over a long period of time with multiple batches of reagents (Fig. 13.2). The concentration of TSH at which the response in the assay has a CV of 20% is the "functional sensitivity" of the assay, and is the value that most accurately represents the performance of an assay when used routinely (1,6,8–10). The use of functional sensitivity gave rise to the "generation" nomenclature for TSH assays. The early assays with a functional sensitivity of 1.0 to 2.0

mU/L were termed first-generation assays, and those with a functional sensitivity of 0.1 to 0.2 mU/L and 0.01 to 0.02 mU/L were termed second- and third-generation assays, respectively (6). Fourth-generation assays, which have a sensitivity of 0.001 to 0.002 mU/L, have been developed for research purposes (11). These are arbitrary terms and should not be used; instead, serum TSH assays should simply be described in terms of their functional sensitivity in milliunits per liter.

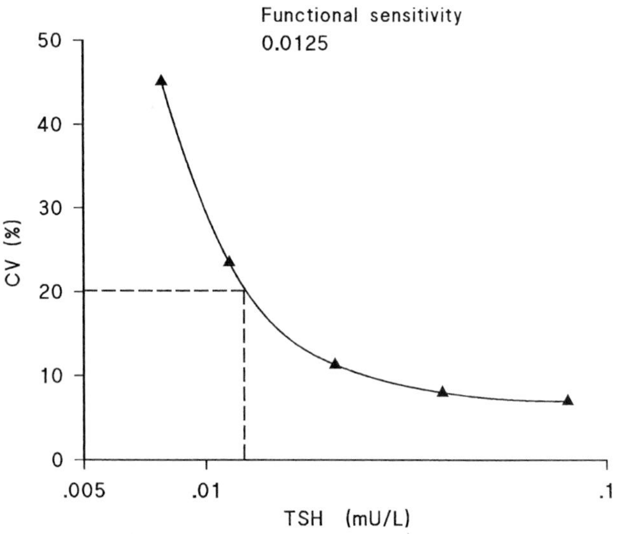

It is essential that serum TSH assays be sufficiently sensitive for clinical diagnostic purposes. To this end, the laboratories should use a method to measure serum TSH that has a functional sensitivity of ≤ 0.02 mU/L, and that functional sensitivity should be defined as briefly noted earlier as the 20% between-run CV determined by a protocol that allows for changes in operator and reagent batch, and is assessed in at least 10 different assay runs. Laboratories should also confirm the functional sensitivity quoted by the manufacturer and have quality-assurance procedures in place to ensure that the functional sensitivity of the assay is regularly monitored.

**Functional sensitivity
0.0125**

FIGURE 13.2. The precision profile and functional sensitivity of a serum thyrotropin (TSH) assay. The precision profile of an assay is derived from multiple assays using different batches of reagents. The quantity of TSH that can be measured with a coefficient of variation of 20% is the functional sensitivity of the assay. In this example the functional sensitivity is 0.0125 mU/L.

MEASUREMENTS OF SERUM THYROID HORMONES

Thyroid hormones are transported in serum almost entirely reversibly bound to protein (see Chapter 6). Most (70% to 80%) of the T_4 and T_3 in serum is bound to thyroxine-binding globulin (TBG), and the remainder is bound to transthyretin (also known as thyroxine-binding prealbumin) and albumin. Approximately 0.05% of the T_4 and 0.2% of the T_3 in serum are free (i.e., not bound to any protein). Most available evidence indicates that only the free hormone can cross the cell membrane and affect intracellular metabolism (12,13). Thus, patients with marked TBG deficiency have low serum total T_4 and T_3

concentrations, but they are euthyroid and have normal serum concentrations of TSH, free T_4, and free T_3. This does not necessarily mean that the complexes of T_4 or T_3 and binding protein have no biological role; binding proteins may be involved in targeting T_4 and T_3 to specific tissues. The reversible binding of T_4 and T_3 to these binding proteins also ensures that a relatively constant concentration of free hormone is supplied to tissues. The ability of T_4 and T_3 to dissociate from the binding proteins and maintain a constant free hormone concentration forms the basis of the methods used to measure free T_4 and free T_3 in serum.

MEASUREMENTS OF SERUM FREE THYROXINE AND FREE TRIIODOTHYRONINE

Theoretical Considerations

Serum free hormone measurements theoretically provide a more reliable means of diagnosing thyroid dysfunction than measurements of serum total hormone concentration, because the latter can be altered not only by thyroid dysfunction, but also by changes in the production of the binding proteins. Because the serum concentrations of free T_4 and free T_3 are extremely low, measuring them in the presence of the high concentrations of T_4 and T_3 that are protein-bound has proved challenging. Indeed, poor assay design has resulted in a mass of conflicting literature regarding the results of measurements of serum free T_4 and free T_3 in patients with nonthyroidal illness and those taking certain drugs (14,15). The theoretical basis on which reliable measurements of serum free T_4 and free T_3 should be designed has been reviewed recently in detail (16). In humans, the serum free T_4 (and free T_3) fraction is mostly affected by changes in the affinity and concentration of TBG, whereas changes in the affinity and concentration of albumin or transthyretin have little effect (16).

In essence, the serum free T_4 (and free T_3) concentration results from the equilibrium between the bound and free hormone.

$$TBG\text{-}T_4 \leftrightarrows TBG + T_4$$

The law of mass action dictates the proportion of T_4 that binds to TBG, i.e., the affinity of the binding protein (Keq) multiplied by its concentration. This is the "relative binding capacity." Thus, if the affinity or concentration of TBG decreases, the proportion of T_4 bound will also diminish, and the serum free T_4 concentration will increase. This illustrates the mechanism for the low serum total T_4 and high free T_4 concentrations found in patients with nonthyroidal illness who have a decrease in serum TBG-binding capacity.

Measurements of serum free T_4 (and T_3) involve sampling the fraction of T_4 in serum that is free (unbound).

This can be done using physical separation of free T_4 from bound T_4 [through equilibrium dialysis (ED) or ultrafiltration], or, alternatively, by adding an antibody that "captures" a proportion of the pool of free T_4. The removal of free T_4 from the original equilibrium will result in dissociation of T_4 from the binding protein to create a new equilibrium. A crucial requirement of any valid method for measurement of serum free T_4 is that there is minimal disruption of the original equilibrium during the assay process. If this principle is adhered to, then the measured serum free T_4 value will be a good estimate of the serum free T_4 concentration *in vivo*. The disruption of the equilibrium will be minimal if there is little dilution of the sample and only a small proportion of the T_4 pool is captured. Other factors that influence the affinity of binding proteins for T_4 and thus modify serum free T_4 concentrations include temperature, pH, and the ionic composition of any buffer used in the assay. These factors all need to be controlled in any assay for serum free T_4 (16). The inadequacies of many commercial assays have led to the suggestion that the term "free hormone estimate" be used for all serum free T_4 measurements used in clinical practice (1). However, this term fails to indicate that some assays are better than others, and it may also cause the clinician to have inappropriate lack of confidence in the result.

Methods for Measuring Serum Free Thyroxine and Triiodothyronine

Equilibrium Dialysis and Ultrafiltration

Equilibrium dialysis and ultrafiltration are widely regarded as reference methods for assays of serum free T_4 and free T_3, although neither is completely satisfactory (1,16–21). Both methods involve the initial separation of free hormone through a semipermeable membrane followed by quantification of the separated hormone by sensitive and specific immunoassay.

A typical dialysis apparatus comprises two compartments separated by a semipermeable membrane. Serum is added to one compartment and buffer to the other. The sample is then incubated with agitation, during which time small molecules like T_4 pass across the membrane into the opposite compartment. This process will proceed until equilibrium has been reached such that the concentration of the permeable molecules is equal on both sides of the membrane. The T_4 concentration in the buffer compartment at this new equilibrium should provide a good estimate of the free T_4 concentration in the original sample. Equilibrium is reached typically in 16 to 24 hours. This long incubation period can cause problems in certain samples (e.g., patients given heparin), because nonesterified fatty acids (NEFAs) may be released by the hydrolysis of endogenous triglyceride through the action of lipoprotein lipase, which is activated by heparin (19). When present in high concentrations, these fatty acids diminish the binding capacity of

TBG for T_4, thus increasing the free T_4 concentration during the dialysis period. A similar increase in free T_4 will occur if serum samples from patients given heparin are stored unfrozen before analysis. Ions from the buffer compartment can also move into the sample during dialysis and modify the pH and composition of the sample, thereby affecting binding of T_4 to TBG or other protein. It is also essential to minimize disruption of the original equilibrium by keeping both the sample dilution and ratio of the volume of buffer to volume of sample as low as possible. It can be predicted that, for serum samples with normal or high binding capacity, the free T_4 concentration will not change significantly, even when the sample is diluted more than 100-fold. Figure 13.3 illustrates this in serum samples from a normal subject, and in patients with thyrotoxicosis and hypothyroidism. In contrast, serum free T_4 values decline markedly when serum from a patient with low serum-binding capacity (e.g., renal failure or other severe illness) or serum rich in NEFAs is diluted (Fig. 13.3). In these sick patients, the low serum-binding capacity may result from the presence of drugs, fatty acids, or various compounds that accumulate when hepatic or renal function is impaired, or by the synthesis of modified TBG that has a low

affinity for T_4 (19,22–25). The effect of dilution on serum free T_4 concentrations has been advocated as a useful test to validate commercial assays for serum free T_4 (16,26–28).

Validity of Commercial Methods for Measurements of Serum Free Thyroxine and Triiodothyronine

Routine assays for serum free T_4 and free T_3 have been given a variety of names, depending on the methodology. The first widely available assays were the so-called analogue assays. These assays are based on a T_4 analogue that has similar immunoreactivity to T_4 but does not bind to the serum-binding proteins. If this is achieved, the analogue should equilibrate only with the free T_4 fraction, and therefore the results should accurately reflect the free T_4 content of the serum sample. However, while many of the early analogues did not bind to TBG, they did bind to albumin or transthyretin. As a consequence, the free serum T_4 results were dependent on the binding capacity of those proteins in the sample (29–32).

All assays for serum free T_4 now in wide use have the following steps in common: The serum sample is diluted, an anti-T_4 antibody is added to "capture" a proportion of the free T_4 pool, and the unoccupied T_4-binding sites on the antibody are then estimated by adding T_4 that has been labeled in some way. Sample dilution, temperature, and buffer composition can be controlled to some extent, but these assays have additional problems over those of equilibrium dialysis (16). T_4 binding to the antibody tends to disrupt the original equilibrium, an effect that is dependent on the T_4-binding capacity of the serum sample, and the affinity and concentration of the anti-T_4 antibody. Also, the binding capacity of the serum sample may be quite different from that used in the assay calibrators. The effect of this is that serum samples with low binding capacity (low serum TBG, e.g., nonthyroidal illness) tend to yield serum free T_4 values that are lower than the true value, whereas serum samples with high binding capacity (high serum TBG, e.g., pregnancy) tend to yield results that are higher than the true value. Many assays include albumin, added in an attempt to diminish nonspecific binding and nullify the effects of fatty acids on serum free T_4 concentrations (33,34). Unfortunately, albumin binds T_4 and, if present in sufficient concentrations, will disrupt the equilibrium (35). Serum samples with low binding capacity are more prone to this effect than are samples with normal or high binding capacity. These various effects explain why serum free T_4 concentrations may be low, normal, or high in a patient with nonthyroidal illness, depending on which assay was used. Figure 13.4 shows the correlation between the results of measurements of serum free T_4 by ED and two serum free T_4 assays currently on the market in several groups of patients. The labeled-antibody assay (left panel) contains no added bovine serum albumin, whereas the

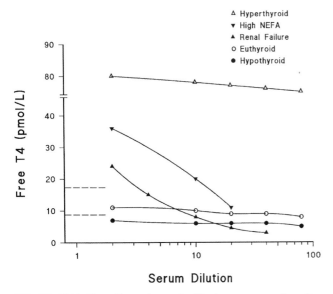

FIGURE 13.3. The effect of sample dilution on serum free thyroxine (T_4) concentrations measured by equilibrium dialysis. Serum samples from a normal subject (euthyroid) and patients with thyrotoxicosis (hyperthyroid), a high serum nonesterified fatty acid concentration (high NEFA), renal failure, and hypothyroidism were analyzed in dilutions, ranging from 1:2 to 1:80. The results of the measurements in the serum samples from the normal subject and the patients with thyroid dysfunction did not vary when the samples were diluted up to 80-fold. In contrast, the serum free T_4 concentrations decreased with dilution in the samples from a patient with renal failure or a patient who had a high serum nonesterified fatty acid concentration after heparin administration (i.e., low serum-binding capacity). The dashed horizontal lines denote the normal reference range. To convert serum free T_4 values to ng/dL, multiply by 0.078.

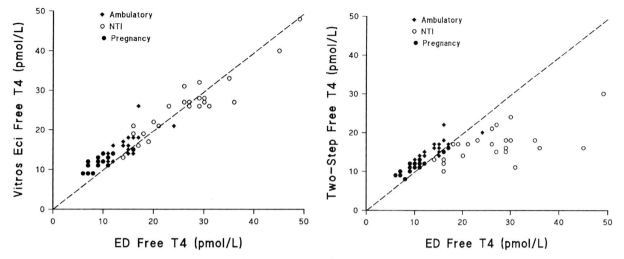

FIGURE 13.4. Relationship between measurements of serum free thyroxine (T$_4$) by equilibrium dialysis (ED) and by two commercial methods in ambulatory patients, patients with nonthyroidal illness, and pregnant women. **Left panel:** The results of measurements by equilibrium dialysis and the Vitros ECi–labeled antibody serum free T$_4$ assay (Ortho Clinical Diagnostics, High Wycombe, Bucks, UK), which has no bovine serum albumin included in the reagents, are similar. **Right panel:** The results of ED and the AxSYM two-step free T$_4$ assay (Abbott Diagnostics, North Chicago, IL, USA), which includes albumin, disagree markedly in patients with nonthyroidal illness. The ED was performed using the Nichols method (Nichols Institute Diagnostics, San Clemente, CA, USA). To convert serum free T$_4$ values to ng/dL, multiply by 0.078. (From Christofides ND, Wilkinson E, Stoddart M, et al. Serum thyroxine binding capacity-dependent bias in an auomated free thyroxine assay. *J Immunoassay* 1999;20:201; and Christofides ND, Wilkinson E, Stoddart M, et al. Assessment of serum thyroxine binding capacity-dependent biases in free thyroxine assays. *Clin Chem* 1999;45:520, with permission.)

two-step assay (right panel) has albumin included. The results from both methods agree with the results of equilibrium dialysis in serum samples from pregnant women (high serum TBG) and euthyroid ambulatory patients with normal serum binding capacity. However, the results of the labeled antibody assay (no added albumin)—not the results of the two-step assay (albumin added)—agree with those of dialysis in serum samples with low binding capacity from patients with nonthyroidal illness.

The validity of an assay can be assessed in two ways (16, 27,28). One is by comparison with a reference method. For any assay, the results should be similar to those obtained using a validated equilibrium dialysis or ultrafiltration method. This applies not only to patients with thyroid dysfunction, but also to patients with a wide range of serum-binding capacities. These should include pregnant women, women taking estrogen, patients with nonthyroidal illness, and patients taking drugs such as furosemide or salicylate that inhibit T$_4$ binding to TBG or other binding proteins. The second validation method is to document that the results are similar when serum samples, particularly those with normal or high binding capacity, are diluted. Because dilution itself may modify nonspecific effects, dilutions of no more than eightfold should be tested. Assays in which the measured serum free T$_4$ values fall substantially at these dilutions are likely to underestimate the true free T$_4$ values in patients with low serum-binding ca-

pacity. An example of this dilution test performed using two current assays is shown in Fig. 13.5. Many current assays for serum free T$_4$ fail these validation tests (27,36,37).

Nomenclature of Assays for Serum Free Thyroxine and Free Triiodothyronine

Serum free T$_4$ assays have been given a wide range of names, including one-step, analogue, two-step, back-titration, and labeled antibody. The principles of each of these assay have been reviewed in the literature (1,12,16,19,26). The names do not guarantee validity or performance. For example, clearly different serum free T$_4$ concentrations may be found in the same samples assayed using two different assays of the same type (Fig. 13.6).

Serum Free Triiodothyronine Assays

Serum free T$_3$ concentrations are lower than those of free T$_4$, and their measurement is much more problematic. Under normal circumstances, approximately 80% of the T$_3$ in serum is derived from the extrathyroidal deiodination of T$_4$ (see Chapter 7). In patients with nonthyroidal illness, tissue uptake and deiodination of T$_4$ are decreased, and therefore serum total T$_3$ concentrations fall (see section on nonthyroidal illness in Chapter 11). However, for

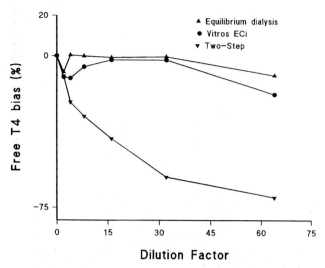

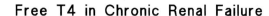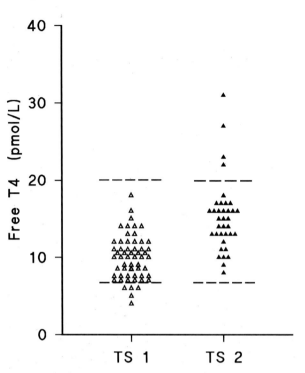

FIGURE 13.5. Dilution test used to assess the validity of serum free thyroxine (T_4) assay methods. This plot shows the effects of dilution of serum on the measured free T_4 concentration in a pool of serum samples from normal pregnant women, who have a high serum thyroxine-binding globulin concentration, as determined by equilibrium dialysis and the two commercial methods shown in Fig. 13.4. Dilution of serum did not alter the results as measured by equilibrium dialysis and the Vitro ECi method (Ortho Clinical Diagnostics, Hugh Wycombe, Bucks, UK), but resulted in underestimation of the serum free T_4 concentration (negative free T_4 bias) in the Abbott AxSYM two-step serum free T_4 assay (Abbot Diagnostics, North Chicago, IL, USA). (From Christofides ND, Wilkinson E, Stoddart M, et al. Serum thyroxine binding capacity-dependent bias in an automated free thyroxine assay. *J Immunoassay* 1999;20:201, and Christofides ND, Wilkinson E, Stoddart M, et al. Assessment of serum thyroxine binding capacity-dependent biases in free thyroxine assays. *Clin Chem* 1999;45:520, with permission.)

FIGURE 13.6. Serum free thyroxine (T_4) concentrations in patients with chronic renal failure measured by two commercial two-step methods (TS1, TS2). The reference ranges of the two assays were similar, but the results in the patients, who had decreased serum binding of T_4, were consistently lower in the TS1 assay. To convert serum free T_4 values to ng/dL, multiply by 0.078.

serum free T_3, other factors come into play, including modification of serum T_3-binding capacity, which tends to increase the free T_3 fraction (14,15). Although results from most commercial methods indicate that serum free T_3 concentrations are low in these patients, the concentrations as measured by ultrafiltration or some labeled antibody methods may be normal or occasionally even slightly high (38,39).

Serum Free Thyroxine and Free Triiodothyronine Indexes

Serum free T_4 and free T_3 can be estimated indirectly as the serum free T_4 index and the serum free T_3 index. These index methods require measurement of serum total T_4 or total T_3 (see later in the chapter) together with measurement of the thyroid hormone–binding ratio (THBR, also known as the T_3-resin uptake) (1). The THBR is an estimate of the number of unoccupied thyroid hormone–binding sites in a serum sample, as compared with the number in normal subjects. The THBR is usually measured by adding labeled T_3 (T_4 can be used instead) and an insoluble hormone-binding resin to the serum sample. The

proportion of labeled T_3 that binds to the resin (resin uptake) is then measured. The ratio of the resin uptake in the presence of the patient's serum, as compared with that in a pool of normal serum, is the THBR. In patients with thyrotoxicosis there are few unoccupied serum-binding sites, and proportionately more labeled T_3 binds to the resin, whereas in pregnant women, in whom there are many unoccupied binding sites, proportionately less labeled T_3 binds to the resin. The serum free hormone index is then calculated by multiplying the serum total hormone concentration by the THBR (1). In thyrotoxicosis, both the serum THBR and total T_4 values are high, giving an appropriately high serum free T_4 index. In pregnancy, although the serum total T_4 value is high, the THBR is low, and the serum free T_4 index is normal. Sometimes, the results are expressed as the percentage of labeled T_3 bound to the resin, and the serum free T_4 index is calculated as the product of the serum total T_4 concentration and the percentage T_3-resin uptake.

In a similar test, serum total T_4 and TBG are measured separately by immunoassays, and a serum T_4/TBG ratio is calculated. This ratio fails to take into account changes in the other thyroid hormone–binding proteins, although, as discussed earlier, even large changes in the concentration or affinity of transthyretin TTR or albumin have relatively little effect on the free T_4 (or free T_3) concentration in serum. More importantly, modifications in the binding capacity or affinity of TBG that may occur in patients taking certain drugs or those with nonthyroidal illness are not accounted for by the serum T_4/TBG ratio (23,40).

Furthermore, the ratio does not accurately describe the serum free T_4 concentration, because the calculation uses the serum total TBG concentration rather the concentration of unoccupied binding sites; the relationship between the serum T_4/TBG ratio and serum total T_4 concentrations is linear, whereas the relationship between serum free T_4 and total T_4 concentrations is curvilinear. At high serum total T_4 concentrations, there are few unoccupied T_4 binding sites on TBG, and thus the T_4/TBG ratio underestimates the serum free T_4 concentration. The converse is true when serum total T_4 concentrations are low (16). These indirect tests have largely been replaced by direct measurements of serum free T_4 and free T_3.

Introduction of a Method for Assay of Serum Free Thyroxine and Free Triiodothyronine

Clinicians should inform themselves on how well the serum free T_4 and free T_3 assays used by the laboratory perform in patients with thyroid disorders, pregnant women, patients with nonthyroidal illness, patients taking drugs that alter serum protein binding of T_4, or patients who have abnormalities in the production of one of the binding proteins (see section on effects of drugs and other substances on thyroid hormone synthesis and metabolism in Chapter 11). Laboratories should take appropriate action to minimize sample deterioration during storage, for example, by freezing samples that cannot be assayed within 24 hours of collection.

MEASUREMENT OF SERUM TOTAL THYROXINE AND TOTAL TRIIODOTHYRONINE

It is much easier to measure serum total T_4 and T_3 than free T_4 and T_3. To do this, T_4 or T_3 is displaced from the binding proteins using various chemical agents, and the released hormone is measured using a competitive immunoassay. The technical problems associated with measurements of serum total T_4 and total T_3 are limited to assay interference and calibration issues. The purity of the standard, the type of matrix (serum) used to prepare the calibrators, and the lack of an international reference method are important problems (1).

In clinical practice, most problems associated with measurements of serum total T_4 (and total T_3) arise in patients with abnormalities in serum hormone binding that may increase or decrease the serum total hormone concentration (41). Among these abnormalities, the most common is the increase in serum TBG concentrations, and therefore the increases in serum total T_4 and total T_3 concentrations, that occur in pregnant women and women taking any form of estrogen. The estrogen analogue tamoxifen has a small effect, and raloxifene has very little effect, on serum TBG concentrations. Genetic variants of TBG, transthyretin, and albumin have been described to have altered T_4-binding characteristics, which in turn alter serum total T_4 and total T_3 concentrations (see Chapter 6) (41). In patients with nonthyroidal illness, the TBG that is produced may have lower affinity for T_4 and T_3 than normal TBG. Many drugs may also lower the T_4-binding capacity of serum. Some patients produce autoantibodies to T_4 or T_3, which increase the hormone-binding capacity of serum and interfere with the assays for the respective hormone (42).

The use of serum total T_4 and total T_3 measurements is becoming less popular with the advent of more reliable methods for measurements of serum free T_4 and free T_3. However, the results of measurements of serum total T_4 are still considered to have a role in assessing thyroid status in some patients with nonthyroidal illness in whom serum free T_4 and TSH values do not concur (1).

EFFECTS OF DRUG TREATMENT

Drugs may modify secretion of TSH, or the production, secretion, transport and metabolism of T_4 and T_3 (Table 13.1) (43,44). Some drugs alter thyroid secretion, whereas others result in abnormal thyroid function test results in otherwise euthyroid subjects in other ways (see section on the effects of drugs and other substances on thyroid hormone synthesis and metabolism in Chapter 11).

In general, serum TSH concentrations are less affected by drugs than are serum T_4 and T_3 concentrations. High doses of glucocorticoids and dopaminergic drugs inhibit TSH release acutely, but do not cause hypothyroidism (45,46). High doses of propranolol and other β-adrenergic antagonist drugs (but not all of them), and glucocorticoids decrease serum T_3 concentrations slightly by inhibiting the extrathyroidal conversion of T_4 to T_3 (47).

Phenytoin, carbamazepine, and phenobarbital accelerate the clearance of T_4 and T_3, and may lower serum free T_4 and free T_3 concentrations slightly. High doses of furosemide, salicylates, and some other nonsteroidal antiinflammatory drugs competitively inhibit T_4 and T_3 binding to serum TBG and may transiently raise serum free T_4 and free T_3 concentrations (22,48–51). *In vivo* administration

TABLE 13.1. DRUGS THAT ALTER THYROID FUNCTION AND THE RESULTS OF THYROID FUNCTION TESTS

Decreased TSH Secretion	Decreased Thyroid Hormone Secretion	Increased Thyroid Hormone Secretion[a]	Decreased Thyroid Hormone Synthesis[a]
Dopamine	Iodide	Iodide	Methimazole
Glucocorticoids	Lithium	Lithium	Carbimazole
Octreotide	Amiodarone	Amiodarone	Propylthiouracil
	Thalidomide		Lithium
High Serum TBG, Total T$_4$, Total T$_3$[b]	**Low Serum TBG, Total T$_4$, Total T$_3$[b]**	**Displacement of T$_4$ from Serum Proteins**	**Increased Hepatic Metabolism of T$_4$[b]**
Estrogen	Androgen	Furosemide	Phenytoin
Tamoxifen	Anabolic steroids	Salicylates	Carbamazepine
Heroin	Glucocorticoids	Fenclofenac	Phenobarbital
Methadone		Mefenamic acid	Rifampin
Impaired T$_4$ to T$_3$ Conversion	**Impaired Absorption of T$_4$[c]**		
β-Adrenergic antagonists	Calcium carbonate		
	Cholestyramine		
Glucocorticoids	Colestipol		
Amiodarone	Aluminium hydroxide		
Propylthiouracil	Ferrous sulfate		
Iopanoic acid	Sucralfate		

[a]Modify thyroid hormone synthesis and thus may alter thyroid status.
[b]Modify the requirement for T$_4$ in patients with hypothyroidism.
[c]Interfere with T$_4$ absorption from the gastrointestinal tract. Patients taking T$_4$ should be advised against taking these drugs and T$_4$ at the same time.
T$_3$, triiodothyronine; T$_4$, thyroxine; TBG, thyroxine-binding globulin; TSH, thyrotropin.

of heparin liberates NEFAs, which may then displace T$_4$ and T$_3$ from the binding proteins, and therefore increase serum free T$_4$ and free T$_3$ concentrations; the effect of these drugs on measured serum free T$_4$ (and free T$_3$) concentrations is very method dependent (52–54).

Drugs that alter the serum concentration or binding capacity of the thyroid hormone–binding proteins (particularly TBG) will alter serum total T$_4$ and total T$_3$ concentrations, but not serum free T$_4$ and free T$_3$ concentrations if the hypothalamic-pituitary-thyroid axis is intact.

REFERENCE RANGES

By convention, a reference range usually comprises 95% of a reference population. Thus, whatever is being measured, 2.5% of "normal" subjects will have values above the reference range, and 2.5% will have values below the range. The distribution of serum total and free T$_4$ and total and free T$_3$ concentrations is normal in reference populations. In contrast, for serum TSH the distribution is log normal, even when subjects who have high serum antithyroid peroxidase antibody concentrations are excluded from the reference population (55). Serum TSH, but not serum free T$_4$ and free T$_3$, concentrations vary twofold at different times of the day, peak values occurring during the night (between

2300 and 0200 hours) and nadir values during the day (between 1000 and 1600 hours) (56). TSH secretion is also pulsatile, with about 8 to 12 small pulses per 24 hours. For serum TSH, reference ranges should be established using specimens collected between 0800 and 1800 hours and using 95% confidence limits from log-transformed data. The reference population should have no personal or family history of thyroid disease, have normal serum antithyroid peroxidase antibody concentrations, and should not be taking medications known to alter TSH or thyroid secretion or serum binding proteins (1). Clearly, method-related reference ranges need to be used for all thyroid function tests. Manufacturers' reference ranges should be confirmed locally in at least 120 normal subjects (1). Typical adult reference ranges are serum TSH, 0.3 to 4.0 mU/L; serum total T$_4$, 5 to 12 µg/dL (65 to 155 nmol/L); serum total T$_3$, 65 to 170 ng/dL (1.0 to 2.6 nmol/L); serum free T$_4$, 0.7 to 2.0 ng/dL (9 to 25 pmol/L); and serum free T$_3$, 0.2 to 0.5 ng/dL (3 to 8 pmol/L).

The results of all these measurements are higher in neonates, infants, and children, and therefore age-related reference ranges are needed (see Chapter 74) (1,57). Also, serum TSH and free and total T$_4$ and T$_3$ concentrations all change during pregnancy, and therefore trimester-related reference ranges should be available for each of these analytes (see Chapter 80) (58,59).

CHANGES IN THYROID FUNCTION TESTS

Knowledge of the analytical variability and estimates of the intra-individual and inter-individual variability allows estimation of the differences in thyroid tests that can be considered as clinically important when repeated measurements are made during thyroid hormone or antithyroid treatment (60,61). For serum TSH, total T_4, and total T_3, these are approximately 0.8 mU/L, 1.2 µg/dL (15 nmol/L), and 40 ng/dL (0.6 nmol/L), respectively. For serum free T_4 and free T_3, these values are probably about 0.5 ng/dL (6 pmol/L) for free T_4 and 0.1 ng/dL (1.5 pmol/L) for free T_3, but many of these results were determined using older assays, and these data may not be applicable to the newer assays.

ASSAY INTERFERENCE

All assays are prone to interference from a range of substances in serum, including human anti-animal (heterophil) antibodies, antithyroid antibodies, and rheumatoid factor. For example, if mouse monoclonal antibodies are used in an immunometric assay for measurements of serum TSH, then antimouse antibodies in a serum sample might bind to both the capture antibody and signal antibody and form a bridge between the antibodies in a similar manner to TSH, resulting in a spuriously high serum TSH value. Assay manufacturers try to minimize such interference by adding mouse immunoglobulins to the reagents in the hope that they will neutralize any antimouse antibodies and prevent bridging. Unfortunately, in some serum samples the concentration of these antimouse antibodies may be so high that interference still occurs (42,62–65). Laboratories should have protocols available to determine if results are analytically valid. Such protocols could include determining if the result shows linearity on dilution (not valid for free hormone measurements), testing for the presence of heterophil antibodies, antimouse antibodies, and antithyroid hormone antibodies, and confirmation by an alternative assay method (66).

THYROID HORMONE–BINDING PROTEINS

The thyroid hormone–binding proteins TBG, transthyretin, and albumin transport the hydrophobic thyroid hormones in serum and provide a buffer to stabilize free T_4 and free T_3 for cell uptake (41). TBG is a member of the serine protease inhibitor (serpin) family of proteins, and it may facilitate the transport of maternal T_4 to the fetus. Most structural variants of TBG have either normal or diminished affinity for T_4 and T_3 (see Chapter 6.) Genetic variants of albumin may have a markedly increased affinity

for T_4, but not T_3, giving rise to a disorder known as familial dysalbuminemic hyperthyroxinemia. Patients with this disorder have high serum total T_4 concentrations, but normal serum total T_3, free T_3, and TSH concentrations. Some analogue-based methods for measuring serum free T_4 give high values due to assay artefact, whereas serum free T_4 concentrations measured by equilibrium dialysis or two-step assays are normal (67). A much less common mutation in albumin has been described that results in an increased affinity for T_3 but not T_4 (68). Several mutations in transthyretin (TTR) have been described which result in high serum total T_4 concentrations (24,69,70).

Electrophoresis of serum after the addition of radiolabeled T_3 or T_4 allows the identification of abnormal proteins that have high affinity for either hormone. Incubation of serum with radiolabeled T_3 or T_4 and precipitation of the gammaglobulin fraction using 20% polyethylene glycol is a simple way to detect serum anti-T_3 and anti-T_4 antibodies (71).

INTERPRETATION OF THE RESULTS OF THYROID FUNCTION TESTS

Thyrotoxicosis

With the exception of the rare cases of thyrotoxicosis caused by a TSH-secreting pituitary tumor, serum TSH concentrations are low, usually <0.02 mU/L, in patients with thyrotoxicosis. Both serum total and free T_3 and T_4 concentrations are high in over 95% of these patients. Those patients with thyrotoxicosis caused by Graves' disease are usually more clinically thyrotoxic than those with nodular goiter, and this is reflected in higher serum total and free T_4 and T_3 concentrations. A typical patient with Graves' thyrotoxicosis has a serum free T_4 concentration of 3 to 4 ng/dL (40 to 52 pmol/L), a serum total T_4 concentration of 15 to 17 µg/dL (190 to 220 nmol/L), a serum free T_3 concentration of 0.8 to 1.0 ng/dL (12 to 15 pmol/L), and a serum total T_3 concentration of 350 to 450 ng/dL (5.4 to 7.0 nmol/L). The corresponding values in a patient with thyrotoxicosis caused by a nodular goiter are likely to be about 25% to 30% lower. In younger patients, there is a reasonably good correlation between serum free T_4 and free T_3 concentrations and symptoms and signs of thyrotoxicosis, but the correlation is weak in older patients.

Triiodothyronine Thyrotoxicosis

About 2% to 4% of patients with thyrotoxicosis have high serum T_3 concentrations, but their serum T_4 concentrations are within the reference range (usually the upper part of that range); they are said to have T_3-thyrotoxicosis. The incidence of T_3-thyrotoxicosis is higher when serum total rather than free T_4 is measured (72). It is most likely to be found in patients who live in areas of iodine deficiency and in patients with nodular goiter, those receiving antithyroid drug therapy, and those with recurrent thyrotoxicosis after subtotal thyroidectomy or antithyroid drug therapy.

Subclinical Thyrotoxicosis

The combination of a low serum TSH concentration and normal serum free T_4 and free T_3 concentrations is known as subclinical thyrotoxicosis. This condition reflects the sensitivity of the pituitary thyrotrophs to the inhibitory action of small increases in serum T_4 and T_3 concentrations (see section on regulation of thyrotropin secretion in Chapter 10) (73). An absence of symptoms was once part of the definition of subclinical thyrotoxicosis, but, in fact, subtle clinical features of thyrotoxicosis may be present (see Chapter 79). Also, subclinical thyrotoxicosis is a risk factor for atrial fibrillation (74,75) and low bone mineral density (76). These biochemical findings may also be present in patients with nonthyroidal illness or central hypothyroidism (Table 13.2) (77).

In the absence of clinical manifestations of thyroid disease, and even after additional studies such as measurements of thyroid radioiodine uptake or TSH-receptor antibodies, it may be difficult to decide whether patients with low serum TSH concentrations and normal serum free T_4 and T_3 concentrations have subclinical thyrotoxicosis or nonthyroidal illness. In such circumstances, thyroid function tests should be repeated several weeks later; a normal or high serum TSH concentration at this time suggests recovery from nonthyroidal illness or the hypothyroid phase of thyroiditis. If the pattern persists, the choices are a trial of antithyroid drug therapy or close clinical follow-up.

Factitious Thyrotoxicosis

In this condition, excessive quantities of thyroid hormone are taken without the knowledge of the physician, usually by women wishing to lose weight. In all cases, serum TSH concentrations are low. Serum concentrations of T_3 and T_4 vary, depending upon the thyroid hormone preparation being taken. Ingestion of T_4 alone results in a greater rise in serum total and free T_4 than in total and free T_3 concentrations, so that the serum T_4:T_3 ratio is higher in these patients than in those with spontaneously occurring thyrotoxicosis; for example, a patient might have a serum free T_4 concentration of 4.6 ng/dL (60 pmol/L) but a serum free T_3 concentration of 0.9 ng/dL (1.4 pmol/L). If T_3 is taken, serum total and free T_4 concentrations are low, whereas serum total and free T_3 concentrations are high (how high will depend on when the patient last took T_3). If thyroid extract is taken, the serum T_3 and T_4 concentrations will depend upon the relative proportions of the two thyroid hormones in the tablets, which may vary from batch to batch. If factitious thyrotoxicosis is suspected, serum thyroglobulin should be undetectable, in contrast to all other forms of thyrotoxicosis (see Chapters 14 and 29) (78).

Changes in Serum Thyroxine and Triiodothyronine Concentrations during Treatment of Thyrotoxicosis

In patients with thyrotoxicosis, serum T_4 and T_3 concentrations are usually normal within 6 to 8 weeks after iodine-131 therapy and in 3 to 4 weeks after initiation of antithyroid drug therapy (79). There is a delay, however, in the recovery of TSH secretion; as a result, serum TSH concentrations may remain low for several weeks or even a few months after serum T_4 and T_3 concentrations have fallen to within, or even below, their respective normal ranges (see Chapter 45) (80). It follows that measurements of serum free T_4 are a better indicator of the patient's clinical status than measurements of serum TSH during the first few months of any type of antithyroid therapy. After recovery

TABLE 13.2. CAUSES OF LOW SERUM THYROID-STIMULATING HORMONE CONCENTRATIONS

Condition or Factor	Serum Triiodothyronine		Serum Thyroxine	
	Free	Total	Free	Total
Endogenous subclinical thyrotoxicosis	High normal	High normal	High normal	High normal
Exogenous subclinical thyrotoxicosis (T_4 therapy)	Normal	Normal	High normal or high	High normal or high
Nonthyroidal illness	Normal, low, or high[a]	Normal or low	Normal, low, or high[b]	Normal, low, or high[c]
Central hypothyroidism	Normal or low	Normal or low	Low normal or low	Low normal or low

[a]In patients with nonthyroidal illness, serum free T_3 concentrations may be high if a particular commercial assay system (e.g., Vitros ECi, Ortho Clinical Diagnostics, High Wycombe, Bucks, UK) is used.
[b]The values depend on both the severity of the illness and the method of measurement used.
[c]The values depend on the type and severity of the illness.
Adapted from Toft AD. Subclinical hyperthyroidism. *N Engl J Med* 2001;345:512, with permission. Copyright 2001 Massachusetts Medical Society.

of TSH secretion, measurements of serum TSH are the best way to gauge the effect of treatment for thyrotoxicosis.

Predicting Relapse of Thyrotoxicosis

No single test of thyroid function is reliable in predicting relapse of thyrotoxicosis in patients with Graves' disease (see Chapter 45). On a group basis, antithyroid drug treatment can be expected to induce long-term remission in many patients with mild thyrotoxicosis [serum total T_3 concentration less than approximately 300 ng/dL (4.5 nmol/L)] and a small goiter, but not in patients with a large goiter and a higher serum T_3 concentration (81). Patients with Graves' thyrotoxicosis who have a serum T_3:T_4 ratio of > 20, calculated in nanograms per micrograms (> 0.024 calculated on a molar basis) that persists during antithyroid drug treatment are unlikely to have a remission (82).

Pregnancy

In normal pregnant women, serum TSH concentrations fall slightly during the first trimester; up to 20% of these women may have values below the normal reference range at that time (see Chapter 80) (83). Therefore, trimester-related reference values should be used (1). This decrease in serum TSH concentrations is due to the weak thyroid-stimulating activity of chorionic gonadotropin, which has structural homology with TSH (see section on chemistry and biosynthesis of thyrotropin in Chapter 10). In a few pregnant women, the resulting increase in serum free T_4 concentrations may be sufficient to cause clinical manifestations of thyrotoxicosis (gestational thyrotoxicosis). Gestational thyrotoxicosis is frequently associated with hyperemesis, in which serum chorionic gonadotropin concentrations tend to be high (see Chapter 26) (84,85). Serum chorionic gonadotropin concentrations also are higher in women with multiple pregnancies, as compared with those who have singleton pregnancies, and they are therefore more likely to have high serum free T_4 concentrations (and low serum TSH concentrations) during the first trimester.

While serum free T_4 and free T_3 concentrations rise slightly in response to the thyroid-stimulating action of chorionic gonadotropin during the first trimester, they then fall. As for serum TSH, it is wise, as noted earlier, to use trimester-related reference ranges in evaluating the results of these measurements, particularly in pregnant women with thyrotoxicosis (1,58,59). In the past, good control of thyrotoxicosis consisted of maintaining a normal serum TSH concentration in the mother; however, but there is now evidence that mothers with no thyroid disease and who have a serum free T_4 concentration in the lowest tenth percentile in the first trimester have children with lower scores on neurodevelopment tests, as compared with children of mothers who have higher serum free T_4 concentrations (see Chapter

74) (86). Pregnant women with thyrotoxicosis, therefore, should be given the lowest dose of antithyroid drug which results in a low normal serum TSH concentration and a serum free T_4 concentration in the upper part of the reference range throughout pregnancy.

Hypothyroidism

Serum TSH concentrations are usually in excess of 20 mU/L in patients with overt primary hypothyroidism, defined as high serum TSH and low T_4 concentrations, whereas most patients with serum TSH concentrations between 5 and 20 mU/L have normal serum T_4 concentrations, albeit in the lower part of reference range (subclinical hypothyroidism) (see Chapter 78). Markedly high serum TSH values of 500 mU/L and higher are usually found only in young patients who have severe, long-standing hypothyroidism. The increase in TSH secretion in these patients is accompanied by hypertrophy and hyperplasia of the thyrotrophs, which occasionally is sufficiently intense to cause enlargement of the pituitary (see Chapter 3). Otherwise, there is little relationship between serum TSH concentrations and clinical findings in patients with hypothyroidism (87). Patients with central hypothyroidism have normal or low serum TSH concentrations (see Chapter 51). Measurements of serum T_3 are not indicated in evaluating patients with hypothyroidism, because the values are normal in a substantial proportion of the patients.

Subclinical Hypothyroidism

Subclinical hypothyroidism is defined as high serum concentrations of TSH and normal serum concentrations of T_4 and T_3. The serum TSH concentrations are usually between 5 and 20 mU/L. Most patients are asymptomatic, but some have nonspecific symptoms compatible with hypothyroidism, such as tiredness and lack of energy (see Chapter 78). Subclinical hypothyroidism represents the mildest form of thyroid failure; whether these patients should be treated is debated. Those favoring therapy are most influenced by the knowledge that 25% to 50% feel better when taking T_4 and by the evidence that approximately 3 to 5% have progression to overt hypothyroidism each year. Progression is most likely in patients who have a high serum antithyroid peroxidase antibody concentration (88).

Changes in Serum Thyroxine and TSH Concentrations during Treatment of Hypothyroidism

After initiation of T_4 therapy in patients with hypothyroidism, serum TSH concentrations fall slowly as serum T_4 concentrations rise. For example, in hypothyroid patients with serum TSH concentrations of 100 to 200 mU/L, treatment with T_4 in a dose of 100 μg daily results in a fall in serum TSH concentrations to near normal only after 6 to 8 weeks, whereas serum T_4 concentrations increase to within the normal range in about 2 weeks (89). The appropriate dose of T_4 is that which restores the patient to the euthyroid state with a serum TSH concentration at the lower part of the reference range; when this is done, serum free T_4 concentrations are usually in the upper part of its reference range or slightly high, e.g., serum TSH 0.5 mU/L and serum free T_4 1.6 ng/dL (20 pmol/L) (see Chapter 67). Once the maintenance dose of T_4 is established, it remains relatively constant. However, some medications reduce the absorption of T_4 (Table 13.1). Patients should be advised not to take these medications within 4 hours after ingestion of T_4. Drugs such as phenytoin and carbamazepine, which increase hepatic metabolism of T_4, may result in the need for a higher dose of T_4 as well. Sertraline, by an unknown mechanism, may also increase the requirement for T_4 (90,91). The rise in serum TBG concentrations that occurs in pregnant women and those given estrogen results in the need for more T_4; conversely, the fall in serum TBG concentrations that occurs in patients given androgen results in the need for less T_4. A high serum TSH concentration in a patient taking T_4 who had been previously well controlled does not necessarily imply poor compliance; it should raise the suspicion of whether the patient is taking a new medication.

One biochemical combination that is very suggestive of poor compliance with T_4 therapy is a high serum free T_4 concentration and a high serum TSH concentration. These results indicate that the patient, having been erratic in tablet-taking, consumed high doses of T_4 in the few days before the clinic visit.

Many patients taking T_4 have a low serum TSH concentration and feel better than when the concentration is normal. There is little evidence that this exogenous form of subclinical thyrotoxicosis is detrimental, as long as the patient's serum T_3 concentration is normal (92).

Nonthyroidal Illness

Patients who have any of a wide range of acute or chronic nonthyroidal illnesses may have abnormalities in thyroid function tests, even though they are clinically euthyroid. The majority of these patients have normal serum TSH concentrations, and therefore this measurement provides the best guide to thyroid status in sick people, as it does in more healthy people. However, some acutely ill patients have low serum TSH concentrations, and then during recovery their concentrations may be slightly high (5 to 20 mU/L) for a few days (93,94). Serum total and free T_3 concentrations usually fall as a result of impaired tissue uptake of T_4 and conversion of T_4 to T_3 (15). However, serum free T_3 concentrations measured by ultrafiltration of undiluted serum (38) or some commercial assays may be normal or

high in these patients (39). The serum concentrations and binding capacity (or affinity) of thyroid hormone-binding proteins tend to be reduced in patients with nonthyroidal illness (95), which in turn tends to reduce serum total T_4 and T_3 concentrations and raise the free fraction of serum T_4 and T_3. The contribution of each of these mechanisms varies with the type, severity, and stage of the illness, and therefore the results of thyroid function tests may be extremely variable; they in fact may mimic the changes that occur in patients with thyroid dysfunction. In hospitalized patients, a low serum TSH value is at least twice as likely to be caused by nonthyroidal illness as thyrotoxicosis, whereas a high serum TSH concentration is as likely to be associated with recovery from illness as hypothyroidism (93). The poor predictive value of thyroid function tests in hospitalized patients indicates that these tests should be requested only in patients who have some clinical manifestations of thyroid dysfunction, such as unexplained atrial fibrillation or hypothermia. In such patients, low serum total or free T_3 concentrations strongly suggest nonthyroidal illness, and repeated measurements after the patients have recovered from the illness will determine whether the abnormal results were caused by the illness or by thyroid dysfunction (see section on nonthyroidal illness in Chapter 11) (96).

PHILOSOPHY OF THYROID FUNCTION TESTING

Measurement of serum TSH is the best single test of thyroid function (4). The sensitivity of this measurement is such that some organizations have recommended that all adults be screened for thyroid disease using TSH, beginning at age 35 years and every 5 years thereafter (97). However, the yield will be low (see Chapter 19). Furthermore, it is important to note that measurements of serum TSH as a first-line test may yield misleading information, for example, missing patients with central hypothyroidism in whom serum TSH concentrations may be normal or even high (98), and those admittedly rare patients with thyrotoxicosis caused by a TSH-secreting pituitary tumor or thyroid hormone resistance (see Chapter 24 and see Chapter 81) (Table 13.3). On the other hand, patients with low serum TSH concentrations as a result of nonthyroidal illness may be mistakenly diagnosed as having central hypothyroidism. Measurements of serum TSH are widely used for screening newborn infants for hypothyroidism (see section on neonatal screening in Chapter 75).

Isolated TSH deficiency is rare; impaired thyrotroph function is usually accompanied by growth hormone and gonadotropin deficiencies, although corticotropin secretion is less frequently affected. Clinical suspicion of pitu-

TABLE 13.3. CLINICAL SITUATIONS IN WHICH MEASUREMENTS OF SERUM THYROTROPIN ALONE MAY YIELD MISLEADING RESULTS

Condition	Serum TSH	Consequences of Clinical Action Based on Serum TSH Value Alone	Serum Free T_4 (If Measured)
Heterophil antibodies	Normal	Failure to diagnose thyrotoxicosis	High
Central hypothyroidism	Normal[a]	Failure to diagnose hypothyroidism and investigate hypothalamic-pituitary structure and function	Low
TSH-secreting pituitary adenoma	Normal[a]	Failure to diagnose thyrotoxicosis and investigate pituitary structure and function	High
Thyroid hormone resistance	Normal[a]	Failure to recognize the condition	High
Poor compliance with T_4 therapy	High	Inappropriate increase in dose of T_4	High
Delayed recovery of TSH secretion	Normal or low	Failure to diagnose impending hypothyroidism	Low

[a]Serum TSH concentrations may be high in these conditions, which should prompt measurements of serum free T_4 and further investigation.
T_4, thyroxine; TSH, thyrotropin.

itary or hypothalamic disease should override any misleading biochemical findings (99). However, such a policy not only gives undue weight to the clinical skills of a profession that is more reliant than ever before on biochemical tests, but also fails to appreciate that the majority of requests for thyroid function tests originate in primary care. Few primary care physicians have much experience in the diagnosis and treatment of central hypothyroidism, the symptoms of which are often nonspecific. In this respect, recent reports cast considerable doubt on the wisdom of adopting measurement of serum TSH alone as the first-line test of thyroid function (100,101). Together, these reports describe a series of 21 patients with pituitary or hypothalamic disease in whom hypothyroidism was manifested by low serum T_4 but normal serum TSH concentrations. Although some of the patients had clinical signs of pituitary disease, and almost 50% had a pituitary tumor, the diagnosis of hypopituitarism was unsuspected in the majority. The study from Liverpool, United Kingdom (101), concluded that the incidence of partial or complete hypopituitarism was 55 cases per million per year, severalfold higher than that recognized previously (102). If translated to the United Kingdom as a whole, there would be some 2500 new cases of central hypothyroidism each year, of which some 60% would not be detected by either clinical examination or measurement of serum TSH.

The main reason to measure serum TSH alone is to control laboratory expenditure. However, the issue of cost of thyroid function tests is complex and depends upon factors such as total laboratory workload, the costs of reagents for particular tests, discounts given by diagnostic laboratories, and degree of laboratory automation. Restricting assessment to measurements of serum TSH alone, rather than measurements of serum TSH and free T_4, is unlikely to result in the savings anticipated. Indeed, any savings realized by not measuring serum free T_4 at the initial stage are minor when set against the potential costs of misdiagnosis. If both serum TSH and free T_4 are measured at the outset

and interpreted correctly, it should be possible to detect all causes of thyroid dysfunction or prompt measurement of serum T_3 to identify nonthyroidal illness or assay interference (103).

REFERENCES

1. Baloch Z, Carayon P, Conte-Devolx B, et al. Laboratory medicine practice guidelines. Laboratory support for the diagnosis and monitoring of thyroid disease. *Thyroid* 2003;13:3.
2. Dayan CM. Interpretation of thyroid function tests. *Lancet* 2001;357:619.
3. Seth J, Kellett HA, Caldwell G, et al. A sensitive immunoradiometric assay for serum thyroid stimulating hormone: a replacement for the thyrotrophin releasing hormone test? *BMJ* 1984; 289:1334.
4. Caldwell G, Kellett HA, Gow SM, et al. A new strategy for thyroid function testing. *Lancet* 1985;i:1117.
5. Hall R. The need for more sensitive assays for the measurement of thyroid-stimulating hormone (TSH) and the long-acting thyroid stimulator (LATS). *Clin Endocrinol (Oxf)* 1974;3:361.
6. Spencer CA, Takeuchi M, Kazarosyan M. Current status and performance goals for serum thyrotropin (TSH) assays. *Clin Chem* 1996;42:140.
7. Nicoloff JT, Spencer CA. The use and misuse of the sensitive thyrotropin assays. *J Clin Endocrinol Metab* 1990;71:553.
8. Spencer CA, LoPresti JS, Patel A, et al. Applications of a new chemiluminometric thyrotropin assay to subnormal measurement. *J Clin Endocrinol Metab* 1990;70:453.
9. Spencer CA, Takeuchi M, Kazarosyan M, et al. Interlaboratory/intermethod differences in functional sensitivity of immunometric assays of thyrotropin (TSH) and impact on reliability of measurement of subnormal concentrations of TSH. *Clin Chem* 1995;41:367.
10. McConway MG, Chapman RS, Beastall GH, et al. How sensitive are immunometric assays for thyrotropin? *Clin Chem* 1989; 35:289.
11. Spencer CA, Schwarzbein D, Guttler RB, et al. Thyrotropin (TSH)-releasing hormone stimulation test responses employing third and fourth generation TSH assays. *J Clin Endocrinol Metab* 1993;76:494.
12. Ekins R. The free hormone hypothesis and measurement of free hormones. *Clin Chem* 1992;38:1289.

13. Ekins R. Measurement of free hormones in blood. *Endocr Rev* 1990;11:5.

14. Kaptein E. Nonthyroidal illness. In: Henneman G KE, ed. *Thyroid international.* Darmstadt: Merck KG, 1998.

15. Beckett GJ, Wilkinson E. Thyroid hormone metabolism in non-thyroidal illness. *CPD Bulletin of Clinical Biochemistry* 1998;1:9.

16. Christofides N. Free analyte immunoassay. In: Wild D, ed. *The immunoassay handbook.* 2nd ed. London: Nature Publishing Group, 2001:61.

17. Faber J, Waetjen I, Siersbaek-Nielsen K. Free thyroxine measured in undiluted serum by dialysis and ultrafiltration: effects of non-thyroidal illness, and an acute load of salicylate or heparin. *Clin Chim Acta* 1993;223:159.

18. Tikanoja S. Ultrafiltration devices tested for use in a free thyroxine assay validated by comparison with equilibrium dialysis. *Scand J Clin Lab Invest* 1990;50:663.

19. Stockigt J. Free thyroid hormone measurement. A critical appraisal. *Endocrinol Metab Clin North Am* 2001;30:265.

20. Nelson JC, Wilcox RB. Analytical performance of free and total thyroxine assays. *Clin Chem* 1996;42:146.

21. Holm SS, Andreasen L, Hansen SH, et al. Influence of adsorption and deproteination on potential free thyroxine reference methods. *Clin Chem* 2002;48:108.

22. Wang R, Nelson JC, Wilcox RB. Salsalate and salicylate binding to and their displacement of thyroxine from thyroxine-binding globulin, transthyrin, and albumin. *Thyroid* 1999;9:359.

23. Hennemann G, Everts ME, de Jong M, et al. The significance of plasma membrane transport in the bioavailability of thyroid hormone. *Clin Endocrinol (Oxf)* 1998;48:1.

24. Lim CF, Stockigt JR, Curtis AJ, et al. A naturally occurring furan fatty acid enhances drug inhibition of thyroxine binding in serum. *Metabolism* 1993;42:1468.

25. Lim CF, Stockigt JR. Influence of uremic toxins and nonesterified fatty acids on drug and thyroid hormone binding in serum. *Clin Chem* 1998;44:2380.

26. Ekins R. Analytic measurements of free thyroxine. *Clin Lab Med* 1993;13:599.

27. Christofides ND, Wilkinson E, Stoddart M, et al. Serum thyroxine binding capacity-dependent bias in an automated free thyroxine assay. *J Immunoassay* 1999;20:201.

28. Christofides ND, Wilkinson E, Stoddart M, et al. Assessment of serum thyroxine binding capacity-dependent biases in free thyroxine assays. *Clin Chem* 1999;45:520.

29. Bayer MF. Free thyroxine results are affected by albumin concentration and nonthyroidal illness. *Clin Chim Acta* 1983;130:391.

30. Csako G, Zweig MH, Benson C, et al. On the albumin dependence of measurements of free thyroxin. I. Technical performance of seven methods. *Clin Chem* 1986;32:108.

31. Csako G, Zweig MH, Benson C, et al. On the albumin-dependence of measurements of free thyroxin. II. Patients with non-thyroidal illness. *Clin Chem* 1987;33:87.

32. Csako G, Zweig MH, Glickman J, et al. Direct and indirect techniques for free thyroxin compared in patients with nonthyroidal illness. I. Effect of free fatty acids. *Clin Chem* 1989;35:102.

33. Wilkins TA. Albumin in analog FT4 assay reagents: the facts. *Clin Chem* 1987;33:1293.

34. Wilkins TA, Midgley JE. Albumin-dependence of free thyroxin in nonthyroidal illness. *Clin Chem* 1987;33:1494.

35. Ekins R. One-step, labeled-antibody assay for measuring free thyroxine. I. Assay development and validation. *Clin Chem* 1992;38:2355.

36. Sapin R. Serum thyroxine binding capacity-dependent bias in five free thyroxine immunoassays: assessment with serum dilu-

tion experiments and impact on diagnostic performance. *Clin Biochem* 2001;34:367.

37. Sapin R, d'Herbomez M. Free thyroxine measured by equilibrium dialysis and nine immunoassays in sera with various serum thyroxine-binding capacities. *Clin Chem* 2003;49:1531.

38. Faber J, Siersbaek-Nielsen K. Serum free 3,5,3'-triiodothyronine (T3) in non-thyroidal somatic illness, as measured by ultrafiltration and immunoextraction. *Clin Chim Acta* 1996;256:115.

39. Sapin R, Schlienger JL, Kaltenbach G, et al. Determination of free triiodothyronine by six different methods in patients with non-thyroidal illness and in patients treated with amiodarone. *Ann Clin Biochem* 1995;32:314.

40. Wiersinga WM. *Thyroid* hormone metabolism in non-thyroidal illness. *Curr Opin Endocrinol Diabetes* 1996;3:422.

41. Schussler GC. The thyroxine binding proteins. *Thyroid* 2000;10:141.

42. Despres N, Grant AM. Antibody interference in thyroid assays: a potential for clinical misinformation. *Clin Chem* 1998;44:440.

43. Surks MI, Sievert R. Drugs and thyroid function. *N Engl J Med* 1995;333:1688.

44. Kailajarvi M, Takala T, Gronroos P, et al. Reminders of drug effects on laboratory test results. *Clin Chem* 2000;46:1395.

45. Brabant A, Brabant G, Schuermeyer T, et al. The role of glucocorticoids in the regulation of thyrotropin. *Acta Endocrinol (Copenh)* 1989;121:95.

46. Kaptein EM, Spencer CA, Kamiel MB, et al. Prolonged dopamine administration and thyroid hormone economy in normal and critically ill subjects. *J Clin Endocrinol Metab* 1980;51:387.

47. Geffner DL, Hershman JM. Beta-adrenergic blockade for the treatment of hyperthyroidism. *Am J Med* 1992;93:61.

48. Hawkins RC. Furosemide interference in newer free thyroxine assays. *Clin Chem* 1998;44:2550.

49. Lim CF, Munro SL, Wynne KN, et al. Influence of nonesterified fatty acids and lysolecithins on thyroxine binding to thyroxine-binding globulin and transthyretin. *Thyroid* 1995;5:319.

50. Munro SL, Lim CF, Hall JG, et al. Drug competition for thyroxine binding to transthyretin (prealbumin): comparison with effects on thyroxine-binding globulin. *J Clin Endocrinol Metab* 1989;68:1141.

51. Surks MI, DeFesi CR. Normal serum free thyroid hormone concentrations in patients treated with phenytoin or carbamazepine. A paradox resolved. *JAMA* 1996;275:1495.

52. Beckett GJ, Ratcliffe WA, Chapman B, et al. Non-isotopic, two-step free thyroxine immunoassay: a better measure of free thyroxine than analogue radioimmunoassay. *Ann Clin Biochem* 1990;27:581.

53. Beckett GJ, Wilkinson E, Rae PW, et al. The clinical utility of a non-isotopic two-step assay (DELFIA) and an analogue radioimmunoassay (SimulTRAC) for free thyroxine compared. *Ann Clin Biochem* 1991;28:335.

54. Mendel CM, Frost PH, Kunitake ST, et al. Mechanism of the heparin-induced increase in the concentration of free thyroxine in plasma. *J Clin Endocrinol Metab* 1987;65:1259.

55. Hollowell JG, Staehling NW, Flanders WD, et al. Serum TSH, T4, and thyroid antibodies in the United States population (1988 to 1994): National Health and Nutrition Examination Survey (NHANES III). *J Clin Endocrinol Metab* 2002;87:489.

56. Brabant G, Prank K, Hoang-Vu C, et al. Hypothalamic regulation of pulsatile thyrotropin secretion. *J Clin Endocrinol Metab* 1991;72:145.

57. Elmlinger MW, Kuhnel W, Lambrecht HG, et al. Reference intervals from birth to adulthood for serum thyroxine (T4), tri-

iodothyronine (T3), free T3, free T4, thyroxine binding globulin (TBG) and thyrotropin (TSH). *Clin Chem Lab Med* 2001; 39:973.

58. Gow SM, Kellett HA, Seth J, et al. Limitations of new thyroid function tests in pregnancy. *Clin Chim Acta* 1985;152:325.

59. Price A, Obel O, Cresswell J, et al. Comparison of thyroid function in pregnant and non-pregnant Asian and western Caucasian women. *Clin Chim Acta* 2001;308:91.

60. Andersen S, Pedersen KM, Bruun NH, et al. Narrow individual variations in serum T4 and T3 in normal subjects: a clue to the understanding of subclinical thyroid disease. *J Clin Endocrinol Metab* 2002;87:1068.

61. Browning MC, Ford RP, Callaghan SJ, et al. Intra- and interindividual biological variation of five analytes used in assessing thyroid function: implications for necessary standards of performance and the interpretation of results. *Clin Chem* 1986;32:962.

62. Boscato LM, Stuart MC. Heterophilic antibodies: a problem for all immunoassays. *Clin Chem* 1988;34:27.

63. John R, Henley R. Antibody interference in free thyroxine assays. *Ann Clin Biochem* 1992;29:472.

64. John R, Othman S, Parkes AB, et al. Interference in thyroid-function tests in postpartum thyroiditis. *Clin Chem* 1991;37:1397.

65. Kricka LJ. Interferences in immunoassay—still a threat. *Clin Chem* 2000;46:1037.

66. Ismail AA, Walker PL, Cawood ML, et al. Interference in immunoassay is an underestimated problem. *Ann Clin Biochem* 2002;39:366.

67. Stockigt JR, DeGaris M, Barlow JW. "Unbound-analogue" methods for free T4: a note of caution. *N Engl J Med* 1982; 307:126.

68. Sunthornthepvarakul T, Likitmaskul S, Ngowngarmratana S, et al. Familial dysalbuminemic hypertriiodothyroninemia: a new, dominantly inherited albumin defect. *J Clin Endocrinol Metab* 1998;83:1448.

69. Curtis AJ, Scrimshaw BJ, Topliss DJ, et al. Thyroxine binding by human transthyretin variants: mutations at position 119, but not position 54, increase thyroxine binding affinity. *J Clin Endocrinol Metab* 1994;78:459.

70. Stockigt JR, Stevens V, White EL, et al. "Unbound analog" radioimmunoassays for free thyroxin measure the albumin-bound hormone fraction. *Clin Chem* 1983;29:1408.

71. Stockigt JR, Dyer SA, Mohr VS, et al. Specific methods to identify plasma binding abnormalities in euthyroid hyperthyroxinemia. *J Clin Endocrinol Metab* 1986;62:230.

72. Seth J, Beckett G. Diagnosis of hyperthyroidism: the newer biochemical tests. *Clin Endocrinol Metab* 1985;14:373.

73. Snyder PJ, Utiger RD. Inhibition of thyrotropin response to thyrotropin-releasing hormone by small quantities of thyroid hormones. *J Clin Invest* 1972;51:2077.

74. Forfar JC, Feek CM, Miller HC, et al. Atrial fibrillation and isolated suppression of the pituitary-thyroid axis: response to specific antithyroid therapy. *Int J Cardiol* 1981;1:43.

75. Sawin CT. Subclinical hyperthyroidism and atrial fibrillation. *Thyroid* 2002;12:501.

76. Faber J, Jensen IW, Petersen L, et al. Normalization of serum thyrotrophin by means of radioiodine treatment in subclinical hyperthyroidism: effect on bone loss in postmenopausal women. *Clin Endocrinol (Oxf)* 1998;48:285.

77. Toft AD. Subclinical hyperthyroidism. *N Engl J Med* 2001; 345:512.

78. Cohen JH, Ingbar SH, Braverman LE. Thyrotoxicosis due to ingestion of excess thyroid hormone. *Endocr Rev* 1989;10:113.

79. Page SR, Sheard CE, Herbert M, et al. A comparison of 20 or 40 mg per day of carbimazole in the initial treatment of hyperthyroidism. *Clin Endocrinol (Oxf)* 1996;45:511.

80. Toft AD, Irvine WJ, Hunter WM, et al. Anomalous plasma TSH levels in patients developing hypothyroidism in the early months after 131I therapy for thyrotoxicosis. *J Clin Endocrinol Metab* 1974;39:607.

81. Young ET, Steel NR, Taylor JJ, et al. Prediction of remission after antithyroid drug treatment in Graves' disease. *QJM* 1988; 66:175.

82. Takamatsu J, Kuma K, Mozai T. Serum triiodothyronine to thyroxine ratio: a newly recognized predictor of the outcome of hyperthyroidism due to Graves' disease. *J Clin Endocrinol Metab* 1986;62:980.

83. Panesar NS, Li CY, Rogers MS. Reference intervals for thyroid hormones in pregnant Chinese women. *Ann Clin Biochem* 2001;38:329.

84. Talbot JA, Lambert A, Anobile CJ, et al. The nature of human chorionic gonadotrophin glycoforms in gestational thyrotoxicosis. *Clin Endocrinol (Oxf)* 2001;55:33.

85. Hershman JM. Human chorionic gonadotropin and the thyroid: hyperemesis gravidarum and trophoblastic tumors. *Thyroid* 1999;9:653.

86. Pop VJ, Brouwers EP, Vader HL, et al. Maternal hypothyroxinaemia during early pregnancy and subsequent child development: a 3-year follow-up study. *Clin Endocrinol (Oxf)* 2003; 59:282.

87. Meier C, Trittibach P, Guglielmetti M, et al. Serum thyroid stimulating hormone in assessment of severity of tissue hypothyroidism in patients with overt primary thyroid failure: cross sectional survey. *BMJ* 2003;326:311.

88. Cooper DS. Subclinical hypothyroidism. *N Engl J Med* 2001; 345:260.

89. Cotton GE, Gorman CA, Mayberry WE. Suppression of thyrotropin (h-TSH) in serums of patients with myxedema of varying etiology treated with thyroid hormones. *N Engl J Med* 1971;285:529.

90. Sagud M, Pivac N, Muck-Seler D, et al. Effects of sertraline treatment on plasma cortisol, prolactin and thyroid hormones in female depressed patients. *Neuropsychobiology* 2002;45: 139.

91. Harel Z, Biro FM, Tedford WL. Effects of long term treatment with sertraline (Zoloft) simulating hypothyroidism in an adolescent. *J Adolesc Health* 1995;16:232.

92. Toft AD, Beckett GJ. Thyroid function tests and hypothyroidism. *BMJ* 2003;326:295.

93. Spencer C, Eigen A, Shen D, et al. Specificity of sensitive assays of thyrotropin (TSH) used to screen for thyroid disease in hospitalized patients. *Clin Chem* 1987;33:1391.

94. Hamblin PS, Dyer SA, Mohr VS, et al. Relationship between thyrotropin and thyroxine changes during recovery from severe hypothyroxinemia of critical illness. *J Clin Endocrinol Metab* 1986;62:717.

95. Wilcox RB, Nelson JC, Tomei RT. Heterogeneity in affinities of serum proteins for thyroxine among patients with non-thyroidal illness as indicated by the serum free thyroxine response to serum dilution. *Eur J Endocrinol* 1994;131:9.

96. Stockigt JR. Guidelines for diagnosis and monitoring of thyroid disease: nonthyroidal illness. *Clin Chem* 1996;42:188.

97. Ladenson PW, Singer PA, Ain KB, et al. American Thyroid Association guidelines for detection of thyroid dysfunction. *Arch Intern Med* 2000;160:1573.

98. Oliveira JH, Persani L, Beck-Peccoz P, et al. Investigating the paradox of hypothyroidism and increased serum thyrotropin (TSH) levels in Sheehan's syndrome: characterization of TSH carbohydrate content and bioactivity. *J Clin Endocrinol Metab* 2001;86:1694.

99. Price A, Weetman AP. Screening for central hypothyroidism is unjustified. *BMJ* 2001;322:798.

100. Waise A, Belchetz PE. Lesson of the week: unsuspected central hypothyroidism. *BMJ* 2000;321:1275.
101. Wardle CA, Fraser WD, Squire CR. Pitfalls in the use of thyrotropin concentration as a first-line thyroid-function test. *Lancet* 2001;357:1013.
102. Lamberts SW, de Herder WW, van der Lely AJ. Pituitary insufficiency. *Lancet* 1998;352:127.
103. Mitchell DR, Parvin CA, Gronowski AM. Rules-based detection of discrepancies between TSH and free T4 results. *Clin Chim Acta* 2003;332:89.

14

THYROGLOBULIN

CAROLE ANN SPENCER

Thyroglobulin (Tg), the scaffold protein within which the biologically active thyroid hormones thyroxine (T_4) and triiodothyronine (T_3) are synthesized, comprises up to 75% of the protein content of the thyroid gland. It contains not only T_4 and T_3, but also their precursors, diiodotyrosine (DIT) and monoiodotyrosine (MIT). Tg is also an autoantigen involved in thyroid autoimmunity. The tissue-specific origin of Tg has led to its use as a marker for differentiated (papillary and follicular) thyroid carcinoma (hereafter referred to as thyroid carcinoma) (1). Serum Tg concentrations vary in response to changes in thyroid volume, thyroid stimulation, and thyroid damage (2). This chapter will focus on the pathophysiology, methodology, and clinical utility of measurements of serum Tg.

BIOSYNTHESIS, SECRETION, AND METABOLIC CLEARANCE OF THYROGLOBULIN

Tg is a 19S (660 kDa) glycoprotein composed of two identical 12S (330 kDa) subunits produced only by thyroid follicular cells. Tg is encoded by a single-copy gene mapped to chromosome 8q24.2–8q24.3 (see Chapter 5) (3,4). Tg mutations can result in thyroid dyshormonogenesis (see Chapter 48) (5–7). There can also be within-individual Tg heterogeneity, as a result of variations in splicing of Tg transcripts (3,6,8). As shown schematically in Figure 14.1 (Part 1), Tg gene transcription is regulated by the thyroid-specific transcription factors (TTF-1, TTF-2) and Pax-8 (4,9,10). Hormones such as thyrotropin (TSH), TSH receptor–stimulating antibodies of Graves' disease, interleukin-1, insulin, and insulin-like growth factor-1 act synergistically through cyclic adenosine monophosphate to stimulate Tg gene expression (11–15). There is growing evidence that Tg, particularly poorly iodinated Tg, binds to asialoglycoprotein receptors in the apical membrane of thyroid follicular cells and autoregulates thyroid function by suppressing the expression of the genes for thyroid-specific transcription factors, vascular endothelial growth factor, and the sodium iodide symporter, and by increasing expression of the apical membrane iodide porter, pendrin (9,16–20). Other hormonal factors such as epidermal

growth factor, interferon-γ, tumor necrosis factor-α, and retinoic acid inhibit Tg gene expression (21–27).

The biosynthesis of the mature, iodinated Tg homodimer is a complex process that is orchestrated by multiple molecular chaperone molecules that transport newly synthesized Tg to the apical membrane (Fig. 14.1, Parts 3–5) (28–31). During this process, Tg is glycosylated and sulfated, and disulfide bonds are formed—steps necessary for appropriate conformational folding and, ultimately, thyroid hormonogenesis (see Chapter 5). Homodimerization to form mature 660 kDa Tg, which is the substrate for thyroid peroxidase/H_2O_2–mediated iodination, takes place in the follicular lumen. Thereafter, the MIT and DIT residues are coupled to form T_4 and T_3 within the protein backbone of Tg at specific hormonogenic sites (32,33). Mature hormone-rich Tg is stored as large multimers in the follicular lumen (34); the Tg concentration in the colloid that fills the lumen can be as high as 500 mg/mL (34,35). Liberation and secretion of T_4 and T_3 requires endocytosis of Tg [which involves asialoglycoprotein and megalin receptors in the apical membrane (Fig. 14.1, Part 6) (18,36–39)] into the thyroid follicular cells, and the subsequent proteolysis of Tg in lysosomes (40–43). Tg that is internalized by megalin may be protected from lysosomal proteolysis, and therefore intact Tg may reach the basolateral membrane of the cells (38,39). A small amount of Tg is secreted as such, and perhaps also as Tg-megalin complexes; antimegalin antibodies have been detected in the serum in some patients (38).

TSH regulates trafficking of Tg in thyroid follicular cells in two ways. It stimulates Tg endocytosis at the apical membrane and subsequent Tg proteolysis, and it stimulates receptor-mediated uptake of Tg from the circulation at the basolateral membrane (44,45). Tg is also taken up by nonthyroid cells such as macrophages in the liver and other tissues (46). The mechanisms responsible for Tg uptake by these tissues, which determines the rate of clearance of Tg from the circulation, are poorly understood. The plasma half-life of Tg in patients with benign thyroid disorders and those with thyroid carcinoma is similar (~4 days) (47,48). Tg clearance is influenced by its molecular size and sialic acid content, and thyroid status. The variations in the estimates of Tg half-life may be due to differences in the Tg preparations used in the studies; some were done by measuring the disappearance of exogenously administered

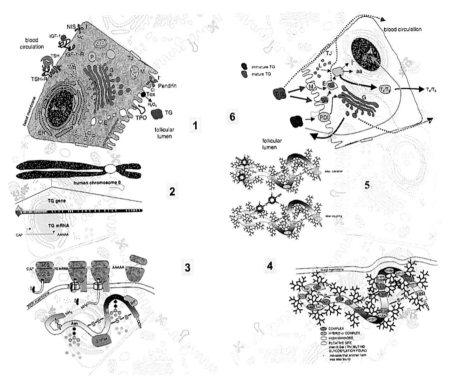

FIGURE 14.1. Schematic diagram of the biosynthesis, storage, and breakdown of thyroglobulin. **Part 1:** A thyroid follicular cell and its constituent organelles (E, endosome; ER, endoplasmic reticulum; G, Golgi apparatus; L, lysosome; M, mitochondrion; N, nucleus; P, peroxisome; R, bound and free ribosome) and proteins [IGF-1, insulin-like growth factor-1; IGF-1-R, receptor for IGF-1; NIS, sodium iodide symporter; Tg, thyroglobulin; TJ, tight function; Tox, thyroid oxidases; TPO, thyroid peroxidase; TSH, thyrotropin; TSH-R, receptor for TSH; 1, thyroid transcription factor-1 (TTF-1); 2, thyroid transcription factor-1 (TTF-2)]. **Part 2:** Human chromosome 8 expanded to show the thyroglobulin (Tg) *(TG)* gene and Tg messenger RNA (cell nucleus in background). **Part 3:** Transcription of Tg messenger RNA and maturation of newly synthesized thyroglobulin, showing chaperone molecules *(BIP, GRP94)*, formation of disulfide bonds *(-S-S-)*, and sites of glycosylation *(Asn)* (cytoplasm of cell in background). **Part 4:** Details of glycosylation of thyroglobulin showing sites of carbohydrate attachment (Golgi apparatus in background). **Part 5:** Mature thyroglobulin in follicular lumen after iodination of tyrosine residues and iodotyrosine coupling to form T_4 and T_3 (thyroid follicular cell and follicular lumen in background). **Part 6:** Thyroid follicular cell and follicular lumen showing luminal thyroglobulin and its resorption into the cell and subsequent breakdown in lysomones to form T_4, T_3, iodine, and amino acids. aa, amino acids; E, endosome; I⁻, iodine; G, Golgi apparatus; L, lysosomes; M, megalin; PDI, protein disulfide isomerase; TJ, tight junction; 1, thyroid transcription factor-1 (TTF-1); 2, thyroid transcription factor-1 (TTF-2). (Reproduced from van de Graaf SA, Ris-Stalpers C, Pauws E, et al. Up to date with human thyroglobulin. *J Endocrinol* 2001;170:307, with permission.)

Tg that had been purified from thyroid tissue, and others by measuring the disappearance of endogenous Tg after thyroidectomy (48). The high serum Tg concentrations found in some patients with acute and chronic liver diseases may be due to impaired hepatocyte clearance of Tg or increased Tg secretion secondary to a toxic effect of alcohol on the thyroid gland (49).

Physicochemical analysis of Tg extracted from normal and diseased thyroid tissue reveals differences in both Tg glycosylation and iodination (50–53). These differences may change the molecular conformation of Tg and thereby mask or expose epitopes that alter its immunoactivity (53–59). In fact, the Tg found in the serum of some patients with thyroid carcinoma differs immunologically from that of normal subjects (51,56,60,61). [These differ-

ences have led to the development of several thyroid carcinoma–specific monoclonal Tg antibodies, although none of these antibodies are currently used for diagnostic purposes (61).] The differences can have clinical consequences; in some patients with thyroid carcinoma, the iodine content of the Tg produced by the tumor is low, with the result that it reacts poorly in assays for serum Tg (55,57,58,60).

MEASUREMENT OF THYROGLOBULIN

Tg is most often measured in serum, but it can also be measured in cyst or pleural fluid and in fluid rinses of needles used for biopsy of neck masses. Its presence in cells or tissue sections can be detected by immunocytochemistry (62–64). These latter procedures can be helpful in determining whether a thyroid nodule is a thyroid epithelial carcinoma or a medullary thyroid carcinoma, and whether a neck or other mass is of thyroid or other origin.

Currently, serum Tg is measured by immunometric assay (IMA) or radioimmunoassay (RIA) techniques (2); among them, automated nonisotopic IMA methods are the most widely used. These IMA methods take little time, have a wide working range, and use reagents with a long shelf life (2,65). In contrast, RIA methods are manual, technically demanding, and take longer (2,65). The sensitivity of most current serum Tg assays is 0.5 to 1.0 µg/L (66–68). This level of sensitivity is not sufficient to allow reliable distinction between normal subjects and patients with no functioning thyroid tissue.

MEASUREMENTS OF SERUM THYROGLOBULIN IN THE ABSENCE OF THYROGLOBULIN ANTIBODIES

Measurement of serum Tg remains technically challenging, and current Tg assays have several serious limitations. One

limitation is the large between-method variation in results, a variation that persists despite the recent availability of an International Reference Preparation (CRM-457) (69,70). Between-method variations are greater than within-person variations (~30% vs. ~15%, respectively), and therefore the same assay should be used during long-term follow-up of patients with thyroid carcinoma (2,68,71,72). Between-method variations are likely to persist because serum Tg is immunologically heterogeneous, especially because many Tg epitopes are conformational (59,61,73,74). Current Tg IMA methods using monoclonal capture antibodies may not recognize well the different forms of Tg that circulate in different patients (75,76). Furthermore, the serum Tg of patients may differ from the Tg extracted from normal thyroid tissue that is used as the standard in different assays, a problem not eliminated by the availability of the reference standard (51,53,56). In addition, any Tg that circulates complexed with its endocytotic receptor, megalin, may not be detected (38,39).

The second limitation of serum Tg assays is suboptimal sensitivity, so that the limit of detection is a little lower than the lower limit of the normal reference range (Fig. 14.2, left panel). The most important consequence of this limitation is that basal (unstimulated) serum Tg measurements cannot be used for the early detection of

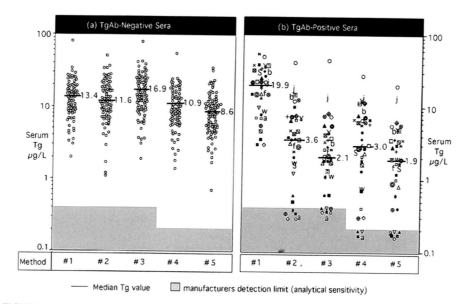

FIGURE 14.2. Serum thryoglobulin (Tg) concentrations in 88 normal subjects with no detectable serum anti-Tg antibodies **(left panel)** and 36 normal subjects with high serum anti-Tg antibody concentrations **(right panel)**, as determined by five different methods: (1) RIA, University of Southern California, Los Angeles, CA, USA; (2) Nichols Bead IMA, Nichols Institute Diagnostics, San Juan Capistrano, CA, USA; (3) Nichols Advantage IMA, Nichols Institute Diagnostics, San Juan Capistrano, CA, USA; (4) Access IMA, Beckman-Coulter Co., Fullerton, CA, USA; and (5) Immulite IMA, Diagnostic Products Corporation, Los Angeles, CA, USA. Note the logarithmic scale of the y-axis. The *shaded areas* indicate the analytical sensitivity of the respective assay. The *short bold horizontal lines* indicate the median values, with the actual median values shown beside these lines. The *symbols in the right panel* indicate the results in individual subjects in each of the assays. (Reproduced from Spencer CA. New insights for using serum thyroglobulin (Tg) measurement for managing patients with differentiated thyroid carcinomas. *Thyroid International* 2003;4:1, with permission.)

recurrent thyroid carcinoma (1,2,77). More sensitive assays are being developed (66,67). A 10- to 100-fold increase in sensitivity will likely allow detection of persistent and recurrent thyroid carcinoma without the need for stimulation testing with recombinant human TSH (1,66,67, 78).

MEASUREMENTS OF SERUM THYROGLOBULIN IN THE PRESENCE OF THYROGLOBULIN ANTIBODIES

The most serious limitation of all current methods for serum Tg assay is their susceptibility to interference by anti-Tg antibodies and, to a lesser extent, heterophile antibodies (2,79,80). Estimates of the prevalence of high serum anti-Tg antibody concentrations vary with the sensitivity and specificity of the detection method (79,81–83), but most studies suggest that approximately 10% of adults have high concentrations, and the frequency is twofold higher (~20%) in patients with thyroid carcinoma (see Chapter 15) (2,79,84). Given these results, anti-Tg antibodies should be measured in any serum sample in which Tg is to be measured, using immunoassay in preference to agglutination assays because of its greater sensitivity (2,79).

The presence, magnitude, and direction of the effect of anti-Tg antibodies on measurements of serum Tg measurement depend on the method of serum Tg assay (IMA or RIA), the specific reagents used, the assay conditions, and the characteristics of the serum anti-Tg antibodies (Fig. 14.2, right panel) (2,65,79,85,86). There appears to be no serum anti-Tg antibody concentration below which there is no interference (79,87). In IMA assays for serum Tg, the presence of anti-Tg antibodies in serum results is falsely low or undetectable serum Tg values (2,68), presumably because Tg complexed with anti-Tg antibodies in the serum sample cannot bind to the antibodies used in the IMA. In all of the IMA methods used to obtain the results shown in the right panel of Figure 14.2, some patients with serum anti-Tg antibodies had inappropriately low, and in some cases undetectable, serum Tg concentrations. In patients with thyroid carcinoma, a serum Tg value measured by IMA that is artifactually low because of the presence of anti-Tg antibodies can mask clinically important disease (2,79). IMA methods in which the presence of anti-Tg antibodies results in inappropriately low or undetectable serum Tg values are not suitable for monitoring patients with thyroid carcinoma, unless the presence of anti-Tg antibodies has been excluded by sensitive direct assays for anti-Tg antibodies (2).

One approach designed to overcome interference by anti-Tg antibodies in IMAs has been the use of monoclonal capture antibodies that selectively bind Tg epitopes not involved in thyroid autoimmune disease (88,89). [Epitope mapping of Tg has revealed Tg to have six different antigenic domains (regions 1 to VI), and the reactivity of serum anti-Tg antibodies in normal subjects and patients with thyroid disease with these different domains varies (90).] Unfortunately, anti-Tg antibodies still react in these modified IMAs, probably because of differences in epitope specificity and/or affinity of the anti-Tg antibodies in patients with thyroid carcinoma and those with other thyroid disorders (91,92). One reason for this variation is that the antigenicity of Tg relates to its iodine content (57,58,93); the anti-Tg antibodies produced by patients with nonneoplastic thyroid disorders often have specificity for epitopes close to the iodine (hormone)-rich regions of Tg (94), whereas the anti-Tg antibodies produced by patients with thyroid carcinoma lack this specificity because they are directed against Tg that is iodine-poor (95).

RIA methods for measuring serum Tg are less prone to interference by anti-Tg antibodies than IMA methods, but anti-Tg antibodies can cause falsely high or low serum Tg values in RIAs (79,85). In these assays, the magnitude and direction of the effects of anti-Tg antibodies are determined by the factors that affect the partitioning of Tg between the anti-Tg antibody used in the assay and the endogenous anti-Tg antibodies present in the serum (85). The usual effect of anti-Tg antibodies in serum Tg RIAs is to cause an artifactually high values. Discordance between serum Tg values measured by IMA and RIA, specifically low serum Tg values measured by IMA and high serum Tg values measured by RIA, is an indicator of the presence of serum anti-Tg antibodies (79).

Serum anti-Tg antibodies are usually measured directly by immunoassay, as noted above. They can also be measured indirectly, by determining the recovery of Tg added to the serum sample *in vitro* (if recovery is high, the serum sample presumably contains no anti-Tg antibodies, and vice versa). There is now consensus, however, that this is not an adequate test for serum anti-Tg antibodies, and that anti-Tg antibodies should be measured directly (2,79,87, 96). Not all anti-Tg antibodies are detected by the recovery test, and, in addition, serial measurements of serum anti-Tg antibodies can be used as a surrogate marker for thyroid carcinoma, high values indicating persistent carcinoma and disappearance of the antibodies indicating elimination of all thyroid tissue (79,87,96–98).

SERUM THYROGLOBULIN CONCENTRATIONS IN NORMAL ADULTS

All normal subjects should have Tg detected in their serum, since some Tg is always cosecreted with T_4 and T_3

(2). A measured serum Tg value is the result of three factors: the mass of thyroid tissue; the presence, if any, of thyroid damage caused by thyroiditis, surgery, hemorrhage, radiation injury, or chemicals or drugs; and the presence, or lack thereof, of TSH, chorionic gonadotropin, or TSH receptor–stimulating antibodies (11,78,99–107). Based on the result of twin studies, serum Tg concentrations are to some extent genetically determined, but the above factors are much more important (100,108). There is no diurnal or seasonal variation in serum Tg concentrations (71,100).

Serum Tg concentrations tend to be higher in women than in men (100); it is unclear whether this relates to the effects of estrogen or a higher prevalence of occult thyroid disorders in women (84,109,110). The difference is small, and therefore the same normal reference range is used for women and men (100,108). However, the reference ranges for different assays vary as a consequence of both pathophysiologic and methodologic factors (Fig. 14.2, left panel) (2).

There is a rise in serum Tg concentrations during the first trimester of pregnancy, caused by the high serum chorionic gonadotropin concentrations at that time; during the latter half of gestation, serum Tg concentrations return to pre-pregnancy values if iodine intake is adequate (see Chapter 80) (111–113). At delivery, maternal serum Tg concentrations are correlated with thyroid size as assessed by ultrasonography (111,113).

SERUM THYROGLOBULIN CONCENTRATIONS IN FETUSES, INFANTS, AND CHILDREN

Tg is present in the fetal thyroid by 8 weeks of gestation; iodine transport begins several weeks later. The appearance of Tg mRNA coincides with the appearance of the immature 12S Tg protein. Mature 19S Tg is detected later, coincident with iodination, which appears necessary for the aggregation of 12S to form 19S Tg (114). As gestation progresses, Tg iodination and intrathyroidal T_4 content increase and approach adult levels at term (see Chapters 74 and 80). Birth weight and gestational age correlate positively with the cord serum concentrations of T_4, T_3, and free T_4, but negatively with cord serum Tg and TSH concentrations (115,116). Cord serum Tg concentrations are higher than maternal serum Tg concentrations and are correlated positively with cord serum TSH concentrations (116,117).

In iodine-deficient areas, the deficient maternal iodine intake is associated with high cord serum TSH and Tg concentrations and increased thyroid volume (111,118), and cord serum Tg concentrations are negatively correlated with maternal urinary iodine excretion (111,116,119). Neonatal serum Tg concentrations are correlated with the

serum T_3/T_4 ratio, but not serum TSH concentrations, suggesting that iodine availability affects the degree of Tg iodination and is an independent determinant of serum Tg concentrations at birth (119). Thyroid size and cord serum Tg concentrations are increased in infants born to mothers who smoke (120–122). These changes are thought to be secondary to a goitrogenic effect of thiocyanate, because its concentrations are positively correlated with cord and maternal serum Tg concentrations (123).

In normal full-term infants, serum Tg concentrations increase in the first days after birth, presumably in response to the postnatal surge in TSH secretion (124). This increase is attenuated in sick or preterm infants (125). During the first few months of life, serum Tg concentrations decrease by approximately 50%, and they continue to decline slowly throughout childhood to reach adult levels after puberty (126).

SERUM THYROGLOBULIN CONCENTRATIONS IN THYROID DISEASES

Serum Tg concentrations are high in patients with many thyroid disorders, including patients with any type of thyroid enlargement, autonomy, injury, or stimulation. Serum Tg concentrations are low in patients in whom the thyroid did not develop (thyroid agenesis) and those in whom the gland is destroyed or removed, or its function is suppressed.

Goiter

Patients with simple goiter may have high serum Tg concentrations. The values are usually independent of the patients' serum TSH concentration and markers of autoimmunity, but are correlated inversely with iodine content and intrathyroidal iodine stores (127–132). In contrast, patients with a multinodular goiter often have high serum Tg concentrations, and the concentrations are inversely correlated with serum TSH concentrations and positively correlated with goiter size (133). After thyroidectomy, serial measurements of serum Tg can be used to monitor goiter regrowth in these patients (103).

Serum Tg concentrations are high in many patients with iodine deficiency, even those who do not have high serum TSH concentrations (see section on iodine deficiency in Chapter 11). Measurements of serum Tg can be used to monitor the iodine status of populations (100, 134–138).

Most patients with any type of goiter caused by an increase in TSH secretion, whether clinically euthyroid or hypothyroid, have high serum Tg concentrations. These patients include those with thyroid dyshormonogenesis secondary to molecular defects in thyroid hormone biosynthesis, except for those defects that result in defective thyroglobulin synthesis (see Chapter 48). They also include patients with goiter induced by drugs or environmental agents (see Chapter 50). The frequency of goiter is increased in patients with acromegaly. They also tend to have high serum Tg concentrations, and the concentrations are not correlated with serum TSH concentrations. In these patients, the goiter and high serum Tg concentrations are probably caused by insulin-like growth factor-1 (139).

Thyroid Nodular Disease

Patients with benign thyroid nodules, nonfunctioning and autonomously functioning thyroid adenomas, and multinodular goiter may have normal or high serum Tg concentrations (103,133,134,140). In all these patients, serum Tg concentrations are correlated with the number and size of nodules and their functional activity; the values therefore tend to be higher in those patients with an autonomously functioning thyroid adenoma or a toxic multinodular goiter (see Chapters 25 and 69) (133,140–145).

In patients with a solitary nodule, serum Tg concentrations decline when nodule volume shrinks in response to T_4 therapy (146,147). In patients at risk for thyroid nodules as a result of head or neck irradiation, a high serum Tg concentration is associated with an increased risk of a nodule during a 10-year follow-up period (142,148). Serum Tg concentrations correlate with the number, not the volume, of nodules present in these patients (142).

Thyrotoxicosis

Serum Tg concentrations are high in patients with thyrotoxicosis caused by excess secretion (hyperthyroidism) or release of T_4 and T_3, whether caused by Graves' disease, a TSH-secreting pituitary tumor, chorionic gonadotropin, a thyroid adenoma or multinodular goiter, or thyroid inflammation (101,149–156). However, serum Tg measurements in many (40% to 70%) patients with Graves' thyrotoxicosis are confounded by high serum anti-Tg antibody concentrations and their resulting effect in serum Tg assays (see above) (86,87,96,149,157). The only thyrotoxic condition in which serum Tg concentrations are low is that caused by exogenous thyroid hormone, whether iatrogenic or factitious (158,159).

Among patients with Graves' thyrotoxicosis, serum Tg concentrations usually decline in response to antithyroid drug treatment, probably as a consequence of a decrease in production of TSH receptor–stimulating antibodies and the resulting decrease in thyroid mass (149–151,160). The

concentrations tend to remain high in those patients with persistent thyrotoxicosis, even when their serum T_4 and T_3 concentrations fall to normal in response to the antithyroid drug (149,150). Although serum Tg concentrations seem to be correlated better with the status of Graves' disease than thyroid secretion in these patients, the prognostic value of serum Tg measurements as a marker of the activity of Graves' disease is not high, because serum Tg concentrations are influenced by other factors such as goiter size, an increase in TSH secretion in response to antithyroid drug therapy, and interference by serum anti-Tg antibodies (see Chapter 45) (87,151,152).

Surgical or radioiodine treatment of patients with thyrotoxicosis results in acute (1- to 2-day) and chronic (1- to 3-month) increases in serum Tg concentrations secondary to surgical trauma and radiation-induced thyroid destruction, respectively (101,149,161).

Hypothyroidism

Measurements of serum Tg have little clinical value in the diagnosis or treatment of adults with hypothyroidism.

Patients with the most common cause of hypothyroidism, chronic autoimmune thyroiditis, may have normal or high serum Tg concentrations. However, many of them have high serum anti-Tg antibody concentrations (see Chapter 15), so that serum Tg cannot usually be measured accurately (2,87,162). Indeed, the antigenicity of iodine-rich Tg has been implicated in the initiation of this disorder (see Chapter 47). Serum Tg concentrations are low in most patients who have hypothyroidism after thyroidectomy, radioiodine, or external radiation therapy, or any disorder that destroys thyroid tissue (and that is not mediated by autoimmunity) (163,164). In any of these situations, the serum Tg value will depend on the amount of thyroid tissue remaining and the degree of elevation of TSH secretion. Serum Tg concentrations tend to be low in patients with central hypothyroidism.

Measurements of serum Tg do have value in the evaluation of infants with congenital hypothyroidism, because the results can help to identify the cause of hypothyroidism. Infants with thyroid agenesis have undetectable serum Tg concentrations, and the concentrations are low or undetectable in infants with central hypothyroidism; those with inactivating mutations of the TSH receptor, thyroid transcription factor-1, and the molecular chaperone proteins involved in the maturation of Tg; and mutations in Tg itself (if the protein cannot be exported into the circulation) (5,165–168). Infants with other causes of hypothyroidism, such as thyroid dysgenesis and other defects in thyroid hormone biosynthesis, have normal or high concentrations (see Chapter 48 and see section on congenital hypothyroidism in Chapter 75).

Thyroiditis

High serum Tg concentrations are a sensitive indicator of thyroid injury caused by both acute and chronic thyroid inflammation. They are, therefore, high in patients with subacute granulomatous thyroiditis (de Quervain's thyroiditis) and in those with silent (painless) thyroiditis (including postpartum thyroiditis) (see Chapters 27 and 28). In all these patients, the concentrations are highest during the thyrotoxic phase of the thyroiditis, but they also may be high during the hypothyroid phase, as a result of TSH stimulation. While recovery is usually complete, some of these patients may have high serum Tg concentrations for a year or two (107,169–171). There is a growing list of therapeutic agents (amiodarone, interferon-α, interleukin-2, and lithium) that induce thyroiditis closely mimicking silent thyroiditis (see section on effects of drugs and other substances on thyroid hormone synthesis and metabolism, and section on the effect of excess iodide in Chapter 11) (172–176).

Patients with thyrotoxicosis caused by silent thyroiditis can be distinguished from those with thyrotoxicosis caused by exogenous thyroid hormone by measurements of serum Tg; the values are high in the former and low in the latter (158,177). However, patients with silent thyroiditis may have high serum anti-Tg antibody concentrations during their illness, and women with postpartum thyroiditis usually have high serum anti-Tg antibody concentrations before the onset of thyroiditis. The presence of high serum anti-Tg antibody concentrations may predispose patients to drug-induced thyroiditis.

Thyroid Carcinoma

Most differentiated thyroid carcinomas produce Tg, although their content of Tg messenger RNA (mRNA) transcripts tends to be lower that that of normal thyroid tissue (178–180). The content of Tg mRNA and Tg protein in thyroid carcinomas varies and correlates poorly with serum Tg concentrations (181–184). Rarely, medullary carcinomas express both calcitonin and Tg (185,186). Anaplastic thyroid carcinomas produce little Tg, and among differentiated carcinomas its production is correlated with the degree of differentiation of the tumor (179,187). As these carcinomas dedifferentiate, expression of sodium iodide symporters and TSH receptors disappears before expression of Tg, so that the patients have detectable serum Tg concentrations, but their tumors do not concentrate radioiodine (188–194).

Many patients with thyroid carcinoma, especially those with follicular carcinoma, have high serum Tg concentrations at the time of diagnosis (195–196). However, measurements of serum Tg do not aid in the diagnosis of thyroid carcinoma, because many patients with benign nodules also have high serum Tg concentrations (195). In patients with thyroid carcinoma, preoperative serum Tg concentrations are correlated with the degree of differentiation and extent of tumor (193,195–198); patients with metastases, especially bony metastases, have the highest (often > 1000 µg/L) serum Tg concentrations (199,200). A high serum Tg concentration at this time suggests not only that the tumor produces Tg, but also that postoperative measurements of serum Tg will be useful for monitoring changes in tumor burden (99,201). The difference between pre- and postoperative serum Tg values provides an indicator of the completeness of surgery, and patients with more extensive disease tend to have higher postoperative serum Tg concentrations (99,202,203).

After thyroidectomy and radioiodine therapy, patients are monitored indefinitely for recurrent disease using serial serum Tg measurements, in conjunction with a variety of imaging techniques (see section on radioiodine therapy and other treatments and outcomes in Chapter 70) (203–205). In this regard, measurements of serum Tg have proven very useful, and indeed their main value is in the follow-up of patients with thyroid carcinoma. The specificity of postoperative serum Tg monitoring for detection of recurrent carcinoma is highest in patients with no residual normal thyroid tissue (201,206). However, this monitoring is also valuable in patients who were treated with surgery and radioiodine but in whom the thyroid remnant was not destroyed (207,208).

In patients with thyroid carcinoma, postoperative serum Tg concentrations should be interpreted relative to the reference values of the assay used, the extent of surgery, whether radioiodine was given, and the patient's serum TSH concentration (Fig. 14.3) (2,202). In particular, serum Tg values cannot be interpreted without knowing the patients' serum TSH concentration and whether they were given TSH. In patients who have detectable serum Tg concentrations while receiving T_4 therapy, serum Tg concentrations increase from 3- to 100-fold in response to TSH administration (1,68,78,209–216).

Approximately 80% of patients with thyroid carcinoma have an undetectable postoperative serum Tg concentration (< 1 µg/L, using current Tg methodology) while being treated with T_4 (7). In approximately 20% of these patients, serum Tg will be detectable after T_4 is stopped or they are given TSH (1). These patients must be evaluated further, by ultrasonography of the neck and radioiodine and other imaging procedures, for possible recurrent carcinoma (1,217). Not all of them have recurrent carcinoma. In some, the rise in serum Tg concentration results from stimulation of normal thyroid tissue that was not destroyed by previous surgical and radioiodine therapy (206,218, 219). In others, ultrasonography and diagnostic radioiodine imaging studies reveal no evidence of recurrent carci-

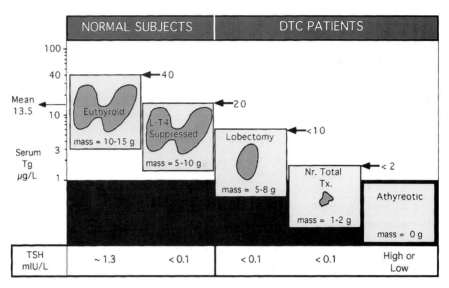

FIGURE 14.3. Expected serum thyroglobulin (Tg) concentrations as a function of thyroid mass and changes in serum TSH concentrations in normal subjects [mean (±SD) serum Tg concentration, 13.5 µg/L; range, 3 to 40 µg/L], normal subjects taking T_4 to inhibit TSH secretion (maximal serum Tg value, 20 µg/L), and patients with differentiated thyroid carcinoma (DTC) after thyroid lobectomy (maximal serum Tg value, <10 µg/L), after near-total thyroidectomy *(Nr. Total Tx.)* (maximal serum Tg value, <2 µg/L), and after thyroidectomy and radioiodine therapy (Athyreotic) (maximal serum Tg value, 1 µg/L). Normal thyroid mass, 10 to 15 g, i.e., 1 g normal thyroid tissue, produces ~1 µg Tg/L of serum when the serum TSH concentration is ~1.3 mU/L, and it produces ~0.5 µg Tg/L of serum when the TSH concentration is < 0.1 mU/L. (From Baloch Z, Carayon P, Conte-Devoix B, et al. Laboratory medicine practice guidelines: laboratory support for the diagnosis and monitoring of thyroid disease. *Thyroid* 2003;13:3, modified with permission.)

noma (1,220–223). Some of these patients have disease revealed by scanning after high-dose radioiodine therapy (221–225). False-negative radioiodine scans are characteristic of more poorly differentiated carcinomas that concentrate little if any iodine because of a loss of sodium iodide symporters and TSH receptors (188–194). These poorly differentiated carcinomas may be detected by positron emission tomography after administration of 18-F-fluorodeoxygluose (226,227).

Notwithstanding these inconsistencies between the results of serum Tg measurements and other tests for detecting recurrent thyroid carcinoma, the overall value of serum Tg measurements, particularly serum Tg measurements after endogenous or exogenous TSH stimulation, as a marker of thyroid carcinoma is high. Among over 1000 patients who had serum Tg concentrations < 1 µg/L while taking T_4, approximately 80% had no increase in serum Tg in response to TSH stimulation, and may be considered free of disease (Fig. 14.4). Among the approximately 20% who had a rise in serum Tg in response to TSH stimulation, less than half had evidence of recurrent carcinoma (8.7% of those with unstimulated serum TSH concentrations <1 µg/L) (1,211–217). In the future, more sensitive serum Tg assays are likely to make it unnecessary to stop T_4

therapy or administer TSH before measuring serum Tg during follow-up of patients with thyroid carcinoma.

MEASUREMENT OF THYROGLOBULIN MRNA IN PERIPHERAL BLOOD

Tg mRNA transcripts can be detected in peripheral blood by molecular biologic techniques, suggesting that measurements of Tg mRNA could be used as a tumor marker in patients with thyroid carcinoma in whom serum Tg cannot be measured because of the presence of anti-Tg antibodies (182,228). Tg mRNA has been measured by quantitative reverse transcriptase-polymerase chain reaction in both peripheral blood and cervical lymph node metastases using different Tg primers (229–231). The blood levels of Tg mRNA are TSH-dependent, but do not correlate with thyroid pathology (231,232). Tg mRNA is always detected in peripheral blood of normal subjects and in patients with an intact thyroid gland; patients with metastatic thyroid carcinoma may or may not have detectable levels (181,182, 229,231,233). The false-negative Tg mRNA results could be due production of fewer Tg transcripts or production of splice-variant forms of Tg mRNA (4,180). Conversely,

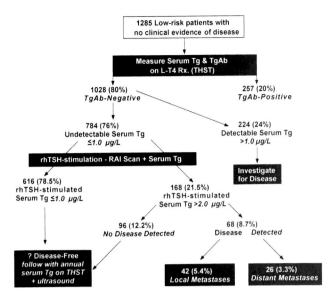

FIGURE 14.4. Diagram summarizing the results of measurements of serum thyroglobulin (Tg) and anti-Tg antibodies (TgAb) in 1285 patients (from eight studies) with thyroid carcinoma considered at low risk of recurrence after thyroidectomy and radioiodine therapy. All patients were receiving T$_4$ therapy *(L-T4 Rx.)* in doses sufficient to suppress TSH secretion to below normal *(THST)*. The patients who had undetectable serum Tg concentrations (< 1.0 μg/L) received recombinant human TSH *(rhTSH)* and then underwent radioiodine scanning *(RAI Scan)* and measurement of serum Tg. Further study was based on the results of these tests. (From Mazzaferri EL, Robbins RJ, Spencer CA, et al. A consensus report of the role of serum thyroglobulin as a monitoring method for low-risk patients with papillary thyroid carcinoma. *J Clin Endocrinol Metab* 2003;88:1433; Haugen BR, Pacini F, Reiners, C, et al. A comparison of recombinant human thyrotropin and thyroid hormone withdrawal for the detection of thyroid remnant or cancer. *J Clin Endocrinol Metab* 1999;84:3877; David A, Blotta A, Bondanelli M, et al. Serum thyroglobulin concentrations and (131)I whole-body scan results in patients with differentiated thyroid carcinoma after administration of recombinant human thyroid-stimulating hormone. *J Nucl Med* 2001;42:1470; Giovanni V, Arianna LG, Antonio C, et al. The use of recombinant human TSH in the follow-up of differentiated thyroid cancer: experience from a large patient cohort in a single centre. *Clin Endocrinol (Oxf)* 2002;56:247; Haugen BR, Ridgway EC, McLaughlin BA, et al. Clinical comparison of whole-body radioiodine scan and serum thyroglobulin after stimulation with recombinant human thyrotropin. *Thyroid* 2002; 12:37; Mazzaferri EL, Kloos RT. Is diagnostic iodine-131 scanning with recombinant human TSH useful in the follow-up of differentiated thyroid cancer after thyroid ablation? *J Clin Endocrinol Metab* 2002:87:1490; Pacini F, Molinaris E, Lippi F, et al. Prediction of disease status by recombinant human TSH-stimulated serum Tg in the postsurgical follow-up of differentiated thyroid carcinoma. *J Clin Endocrinol Metab* 2001;86:5686; Robbins RJ, Chon JT, Fleisher M, et al. Is the serum thyroglobulin response to recombinant human thyrotropin sufficient, by itself, to monitor for residual thyroid carcinoma? *J Clin Endocrinol Metab* 2002; 87:3242; and Wartofsky L. Management of low-risk well-differentiated thyroid cancer based only on thyroglobulin measurement after recombinant human thyrotropin. *Thyroid* 2002;12: 583, with permission.)

false-positive Tg mRNA results have been found in patients with no thyroid tissue, including patients with congenital athyreosis, raising the question of tissue specificity of the origin of Tg mRNA (181,233,234).

REFERENCES

1. Mazzaferri EL, Robbins RJ, Spencer CA, et al. A consensus report of the role of serum thyroglobulin as a monitoring method for low-risk patients with papillary thyroid carcinoma. *J Clin Endocrinol Metab* 2003; 88:1433.
2. Baloch Z, Carayon P, Conte-Devoix B, et al. Laboratory medicine practice guidelines: laboratory support for the diagnosis and monitoring of thyroid disease. *Thyroid* 2003;13:3.
3. Bertaux F, Noel M, Lasmoles F, et al. Identification of the exon structure and four alternative transcripts of the thyroglobulin-encoding gene. *Gene* 1995;156:297.
4. van de Graaf SA, Ris-Stalpers C, Pauws E, et al. Up to date with human thyroglobulin. *J Endocrinol* 2001;170:307.
5. Kim PS, Hossain SA, Park YN, et al. A single amino acid change in the acetylcholinesterase-like domain of thyroglobulin causes congenital goiter with hypothyroidism in the cog/cog mouse: a model of human endoplasmic reticulum storage diseases. *Proc Natl Acad Sci U S A* 1998;95:9909.
6. van de Graaf SA, Cammenga M, Ponne NJ, et al. The screening for mutations in the thyroglobulin cDNA from six patients with congenital hypothyroidism. *Biochimie* 1999;81:425.
7. van de Graaf SA, Ris-Stalpers C, Veenboer GJM, et al. A premature stop codon in thyroglobulin mRNA results in familial goiter and moderate hypothyroidism. *J Clin Endocrinol Metab* 1999;84:2537.
8. Hishinuma A, Takamatsu J, Ohyama Y, et al. Two novel cysteine substitutions (C1263R and C1995S) of thyroglobulin cause a defect in intracellular transport of thyroglobulin in patients with congenital goiter and the variant type of adenomatous goiter. *J Clin Endocrinol Metab* 1999;84:1438.
9. Suzuki K, Lavaroni S, Mori A, et al. Autoregulation of thyroid-specific gene transcription by thyroglobulin. *Proc Natl Acad Sci U S A* 1998;95:8251.
10. Damante G, Tell G, Di Lauro R. A unique combination of transcription factors controls differentiation of thyroid cells. *Prog Nucleic Acid Res Mol Biol* 2001;66:307.
11. Kung AW, Collison K, Banga JP, et al. Effect of Graves' IgG on gene transcription in human thyroid cell cultures. Thyroglobulin gene activation. *FEBS Lett* 1988;232:12.
12. Kung AW, Lau KS. Interleukin-1 beta modulates thyrotropin-induced thyroglobulin mRNA transcription through 3′,5′-cyclic adneosine monophosphate. *Endocrinology* 1990;127:1369.
13. Santisteban P, Acebron A, Schwarz MP, et al. Insulin and insulin-like growth factor 1 regulate a thyroid-specific nuclear protein that binds to the thyroglobulin promoter. *Mol Endocrinol* 1992;6:1310.
14. Ortiz L, Zannini M, Di Lauro R, et al. Transcriptional control of the forkhead thyroid transcription factor TTF-2 by thyrotropin, insulin, and insulin-like growth factor I. *J Biol Chem* 1997;272:23334.
15. Rasmussen AK, Bendtzen K, Feldt-Rasmussen U. Thyrocyte-interleukin-1 interactions. *Exp Clin Endocrinol Diabetes* 2000; 108:67.
16. Suzuki K, Mori A, Levaroni S, et al. In vivo expression of thyroid transcription factor-1 RNA and its relation to thyroid function and follicular heterogeneity; identification of follicu-

lar thyroglobulin as a feedback suppressor of thyroid transcription factor-1 RNA levels and thyroglobulin synthesis. *Thyroid* 1999; 9:319.

17. Suzuki K, Mori A, Saito J, et al. Follicular thyroglobulin suppresses iodide uptake by suppressing expression of the sodium/iodide symporter gene. *Endocrinology* 1999;140:5422.

18. Ulianich L, Suzuki K, Mori A, et al. Follicular thyroglobulin (TG) suppression of thyroid-restricted genes involves the apical membrane sialoglycoprotein receptor and TG phosphorylation. *J Biol Chem* 1999;274:25099.

19. Nakazato M, Chung HK, Ulianich L, et al. Thyroglobulin repression of thyroid transcription factor 1 (TTF-1) gene expression is mediated by decreased DNA binding of nuclear factor I proteins which control constitutive TTF-1 expression. *Mol Cell Biol* 2000;20:8499.

20. Kohn LD, Suzuki K, Nakazato M, et al. Effects of thyroglobulin and pendrin on iodide flux through the thyrocyte. *Trends Endocrinol Metab* 2001;12:10.

21. Pohl V, Roger PP, Christophe D, et al. Differentiation expression during proliferative activity induced through different pathways: in situ hybridization study of thyroglobulin gene expression in thyroid epithelial cells. *J Cell Biol* 1990;111: 663.

22. Namba H, Yamashita S, Morita S, et al. Retinoic acid inhibits human thyroid peroxidase and thyroglobulin gene expression. *J Endocrinol Invest* 1993;16:87.

23. Holting T, Siperstein AE, Clark OH, et al. Epidermal growth factor enhances proliferation, migration and invasion of follicular and papillary thyroid cancer in vitro and in vivo. *J Clin Endocrinol Metab* 1994;79:401.

24. Kung WQ, Lau KS. Gamma-interferon activates a nuclear protein that binds to gamma-interferon activation site of the thyroglobulin gene. *J Mol Endocrinol* 1998;20:293.

25. Tang KT, Braverman LE, DeVito WJ. Tumor necrosis factor-alpha and interferon-gamma modulate gene expression of type I 5'-deiodinase, thyroid peroxidase, and thyroglobulin in FRTL-5 rat thyroid cells. *Endocrinology* 1995;136:881.

26. Holting T, Zielke A, Siperstein AE, et al. Transforming growth factor beta-1 is a negative growth regulator for differentiated thyroid cancer: studies of growth, mitration, invasion, and adhesion of cultured follicular and papillary thyroid cancer cell lines. *J Clin Endocrinol Metab* 1994;79:806.

27. Rasmussen AK, Kayser L, Feldt-Rasmussen U, et al. Influence of tumour necrosis factor-alpha, tumour necrosis factor-beta and interferon-gamma, separately and added together with interleukin-1 beta, on the function of cultured human thyroid cells. *J Endocrinol* 1994;143:359.

28. Arvan P, Kim PS, Kuliawat R, et al. Intracellular protein transport to the thyrocyte plasma membrane: potential implications for thyroid physiology. *Thyroid* 1997;7:89.

29. Kim PS, Arvan P. Endocrinopathies in the family of endoplasmic reticulum (ER) storage diseases: disorders of protein trafficking and the role of ER molecular chaperones. *Endocr Rev* 1998;19:173.

30. Di Jeso B, Pereira R, Consiglio E, et al. Demonstration of a Ca2+ requirement for thyroglobulin dimerization and export to the golgi complex. *Eur J Biochem* 1998;252:583.

31. Di Jeso B, Ulianich L, Pacifico F, et al. Folding of thyroglobulin in the calnexin/calreticulin pathway and its alteration by loss of Ca2+ from the endoplasmic reticulum. *Biochem J* 2003;370: 449.

32. Lamas L, Anderson PC, Fox JW, et al. Consensus sequences for early iodination and hormonogenesis in human thyroglobulin. *J Biol Chem* 1989;264:13541.

33. de Vijlder JJM, Den Hartog MT. Anionic iodotyrosine residues are required for iodothyronine synthesis. *Eur J Endocrinol* 1998; 138:227.

34. Berndorfer U, Wilms H, Herzog V. Multimerization of thyroglobulin (TG) during extracellular storage: isolation of highly cross-linked TG from human thyroids. *J Clin Endocrinol Metab* 1996;81:1918.

35. Herzog V, Berndorfer U, Saber Y. Isolation of insoluble secretory product from bovine thyroid: extracellular storage of thyroglobulin in covalently cross-linked form. *J Cell Biol* 1992; 118:1071.

36. Zheng G, Marino M, Zhao J, et al. Megalin (gp330); a putative endocytic receptor for thyroglobulin. *Endocrinology* 1998;139: 1462.

37. Marino M, Lisi S, Pinchera A, et al. Targeting of thyroglobulin to transcytosis following megalin-mediated endocytosis: evidence for a preferential pH-independent pathway. *J Endocrinol Invest* 2003;26:222.

38. Marino M, Pinchera A, McCluskey RT, et al. Megalin in thyroid physiology and pathology. *Thyroid* 2001;11:47.

39. Marino M, Chiovato L, Mitsiades N, et al. Circulating thyroglobulin transcytosed by thyroid cells in complexed with secretory components of its endocytic receptor megalin. *J Clin Endocrinol Metab* 2000;85:3458.

40. Bernier-Valentin F, Kostrouch Z, Rabilloud R, et al. Analysis of the thyroglobulin internalization process using in vitro reconstituted thyroid follicles: evidence for a coated vesicle-dependent endocytic pathway. *Endocrinology* 1991;129:2194.

41. Kostrouch Z, Bernier-Valentin F, Munari-Silem Y, et al. Thyroglobulin molecules internalized by thyrocytes are sorted in early endosomes and partially recycled back to the follicular lumen. *Endocrinology* 1993;132:2645.

42. Dunn AD, Crutchfield HE, Dunn JT. Proteolytic processing of thyroglobulin by extracts of thyroid lysosomes. *Endocrinology* 1991;128:3073.

43. Brix K, Lemansky P, Herzog V. Evidence for extracellularly acting cathepsins mediating thyroid hormone liberation in thyroid epithelial cells. *Endocrinology* 1996;137:1963.

44. Gire V, Kostrouch Z, Bernier-Valentin F, et al. Endocytosis of albumin and thyroglobulin at the basolateral membrane of thyrocytes organized in follicles. *Endocrinology* 1996;137: 522.

45. Mezgrhani H, Mziaut H, Courageot J, et al. Identification of the membrane receptor binding domain of thyroglobulin. Insights into the quality control of thyroglobulin biosynthesis. *J Biol Chem* 1997;272:23340.

46. Giraud A, Siffroi S, Lanet J, et al. Binding and internalization of thyroglobulin: selectivity, pH dependence, and lack of tissue specificity. *Endocrinology* 1997;138:2325.

47. Hocevar M, Auersperg M, Stanovnik L. The dynamics of serum thyroglobulin elimination from the body after thyroid surgery. *Eur J Surg Oncol* 1997;23:208.

48. Izumi M, Kubo I, Taura M, et al. Kinetic study of immunoreactive human thyroglobulin. *J Clin Endocrinol Metab* 1986; 62:410.

49. Hegedus L, Reasmussen N, Kastrup RV, et al. Independent effects of liver disease and chronic alcoholism on thyroid function and size: the possibility of a toxic effect of alcohol on the thyroid gland. *Metabolism* 1988;37:229.

50. Gardas A, Domek H. Iodine induced alteration in immunological and biochemical properties of thyroglobulin. *Am J Physiol* 1993;265:237.

51. Maruyama M, Kato R, Kobayashi S, et al. A method to differentiate between thyroglobulin derived from normal thyroid tissue and from thyroid carcinoma based on analysis of reactivity to lectins. *Arch Pathol Lab Med* 1998;122:715.

52. Magro G, Perissinotto D, Schiappacassi M, et al. Proteomic and postproteomic characterization of keratan sulfate-glycanated isoforms of thyroglobulin and transferrin uniquely elabo-

rated by papillary thyroid carcinomas. *Am J Pathol* 2003;163:183.

53. Feldman A, Singh A, Diamond EJ, et al. Variability in production and immunoreactivity of in-vitro secreted human thyroglobulin. *Clin Endocrinol (Oxf)* 1987;27:691.

54. Fenouillet E, Fayet G, Hovsepian S, et al. Immunochemical evidence for a role of complex carbohydrate chains in thyroglobulin antigenicity. *J Biol Chem* 1986;261:15153.

55. Schulz R, Bethauser H, Stempka L, et al. Evidence for immunological differences between circulating and tissue-derived thyroglobulin in men. *Eur J Clin Invest* 1989;19:459.

56. Saboori AM, Rose NR, Kuppers RC, et al. Immunoreactivity of multiple molecular forms of human thyroglobulin. *Clin Immunol Immunopathol* 1994;72:121.

57. Saboori AM, Rose NR, Burek CL. Iodiation of human thyroglobulin (Tg) alters its immunoreactivity. II. Fine specificity of a monoclonal antibody that recognizes iodinated Tg. *Clin Exp Immunol* 1998;113:303.

58. Saboori AM, Rose NR, Bresler HS, et al. Iodiation of human thyroglobulin (Tg) alters its immunoreactivity. I. Iodiation alters multiple epitopes of human Tg. *Clin Exp Immunol* 1998;113:297.

59. Druetta L, Croizet K, Bornet H, et al. Analyses of the molecular forms of serum thyroglobulin from patients with Graves' disease, subacute thyroiditis or differentiated thyroid cancer by velocity sedimentation on sucrose gradient and Western blot. *Eur J Endocrinol* 1999;139:498.

60. Heilig B, Hufner M, Dorken B, et al. Increased heterogeneity of serum thyroglobulin in thyroid cancer patients as determined by monoclonal antibodies. *Klin Wochenschr* 1986;64:776.

61. Sugawa H, Smith E, Imura H, et al. A thyroid cancer specific monoclonal antibody which recognizes cryptic epitope(s) of human thyroglobulin. *Mol Cell Endocrinol* 1993;93:207.

62. Pacini F, Pinchera A. Serum and tissue thyroglobulin measurement: clinical applications in thyroid disease. *Biochimie* 1999;81:463.

63. Chang TC, Tung CC, Hsiao YL, et al. Immunoperoxidase staining in the differential diagnosis of parathyroid from thyroid origin in fine needle aspirates of suspected parathyroid lesions. *Acta Cytologica* 1998;42:619.

64. Pacini F, Fugazzola L, Lippi F, et al. Detection of thyroglobulin in fine needle aspirates of nonthyroidal neck masses: a clue to the diagnosis of metastatic differentiated thyroid cancer. *J Clin Endocrinol Metab* 1992;74:1401.

65. Spencer CA, Takeuchi M, Kazarosyan M. Current status and performance goals for serum thyroglobulin assays. *Clin Chem* 1996;42:164.

66. Fugazzola L, Mihalich A, Persani L, et al. Highly sensitive serum thyroglobulin and circulating thyroglobulin mRNA evaluations in the management of patients with differentiated thyroid cancer in apparent remission. *J Clin Endocrinol Metab* 2002;87:3201.

67. Zophel K, Wunderlich G, Smith BR. Serum thyroglobulin measurements with a high sensitivity enzyme-linked immunosorbent assay: is there a clinical benefit in patients with differentiated thyroid carcinoma? *Thyroid* 2003;13:861.

68. Spencer CA. New insights for using serum thyroglobulin (Tg) measurement for managing patients with differentiated thyroid carcinomas. *Thyroid International* 2003;4:1

69. Feldt-Rasmussen U, Profilis C, Colinet E, et al. Human thyroglobulin reference material (CRM 457). I. Assessment of homogeneity, stability and immunoreactivity. *Ann Biol Clin* 1996;54:337.

70. Feldt-Rasmussen U, Profilis C, Colinet E, et al. Human thyroglobulin reference material (CRM 457). II. Physicochemical characterization and certification. *Ann Biol Clin* 1996;54:343.

71. Feldt-Rasmussen U, Petersen PH, Blaabjerg O, et al. Long-term variability in serum thyroglobulin and thyroid related hormones in healthy subjects. *Acta Endocrinol (Copenh)* 1980;95:328.

72. Feldt-Rasmussen U, Schlumberger M. European interlaboratory comparison of serum thyroglobulin measurement. *J Endocrinol Invest* 1988;11:175.

73. Tomer Y. Anti-thyroglobulin autoantibodies in autoimmune thyroid diseases: cross-reactive or pathogenic? *Clin Immunol Immunopathol* 1997;82:3.

74. Erregragui K, Prato S, Miquelis R, et al. Antigenic mapping of human thyroglobulin—topographic relationship between antigenic regions and functional domains. *Eur J Biochem* 1997;244:801.

75. Saboori AM, Rose NR, Yuhasz SC, et al. Peptides of human thyroglobulin reactive with sera of patients with autoimmune thyroid disease. *J Immunol* 1999;163:6244.

76. Benvenga S, Burek CL, Talor M, et al. Heterogeneity of the thyroglobulin epitopes associated with circulating thyroid hormone autoantibodies in Hashimoto's thyroiditis and non-autoimmune thyroid diseases. *J Endocrinol Invest* 2002;25:977.

77. Wunderlich G, Zophel K, Crook L, et al. A high sensitivity enzyme-linked immunosorbent assay for serum thyroglobulin. *Thyroid* 2001;11:819.

78. Haugen BR, Pacini F, Reiners C, et al. A comparison of recombinant human thyrotropin and thyroid hormone withdrawal for the detection of thyroid remnant or cancer. *J Clin Endocrinol Metab* 1999;84:3877.

79. Spencer CA, Wang C, Fatemi S, et al. Serum thyroglobulin autoantibodies: prevalence, influence on serum thyroglobulin measurement and prognostic significance in patients with differentiated thyroid carcinoma. *J Clin Endocrinol Metab* 1998;83:1121.

80. Preissner CM, O'Kane DJ, Singh RJ, et al. Phantoms in the assay tube: heterophile antibody interferences in serum thyroglobulin assays. *J Clin Endocrinol Metab* 2003;88:3069.

81. Arai T, Kurashima C, Utsuyama M, et al. Measurement of anti-thyroglobulin and anti-thyroid peroxidase antibodies using highly sensitive radioimmunoassay: an effective method for detecting asymptomatic focal lymphocytic thyroiditis in the elderly. *Endocr J* 2000;47:575.

82. Tozzoli R, Bizzaro N, Tonutti E, et al. Immunoassay of anti-thyroid autoantibodies: high analytical variability in second generation methods. *Clin Chem Lab Med* 2002;40:568.

83. Cubero JM, Rodriguez-Espinosa J, Gelpi C, et al. Thyroglobulin autoantibody levels below the cut-off for positivity can interfere with thyroglobulin measurement. *Thyroid* 2003;13:659.

84. Hollowell JG, Staehling NW, Hannon WH, et al. Serum thyrotropin, thyroxine, and thyroid antibodies in the United States population (1988 to 1994): NHANES III. *J Clin Endocrinol Metab* 2002;87:489.

85. Schneider AB, Pervos R. Radioimmunoassay of human thyroglobulin: effect of antithyroglobulin autoantibodies. *J Clin Endocrinol Metab* 1978;47:126.

86. Mariotti S, Barbesino G, Caturegli P, et al. Assay of thyroglobulin in serum with thyroglobulin autoantibodies: an unobtainable goal? *J Clin Endocrinol Metab* 1995;80:468.

87. Massart C, Maugendre D. Importance of the detection method for thyroglobulin antibodies for the validity of thyroglobulin measurements in sera from patients with Graves' disease. *Clin Chem* 2002;48:102.

88. Marquet PY, Daver A, Sapin R, et al. Highly sensitive immunoradiometric assay for serum thyroglobulin with minimal interference from autoantibodies. *Clin Chem* 1996;42:258.

89. Erali M, Bigelow RB, Meikle AW. ELISA for thyroglobulin in serum: recovery studies to evaluate autoantibody interference and reliability of thyroglobulin values. *Clin Chem* 1996;42:766.

90. Estienne B, McIntosh RS, Ruf J, et al. Comparative mapping of cloned human and murine antithyroglobulin antibodies: recognition by human antibodies of an immunodominant region. *Thyroid* 1998;8:643.

91. Henry M, Malthiery Y, Zasnelli E, et al. Epitope mapping of human thyroglobulin: Heterogeneous recognition by thyroid pathologic sera. *J Immunol* 1990;145:3692.

92. Okosieme OE, Premawardhana LD, Jayasinghe A, et al. Thyroglobulin epitope recognition in a post iodine-supplemented Sri Lankan population. *Clin Endocrinol (Oxf)* 2003;59:190.

93. Rasooly L, Rose NR, Saboori AM, et al. Iodine is essential for human T cell recognition of human thyroglobulin. *Autoimmunity* 1998;27:213.

94. Erregragui K, Cheillan F, Defoort JP, et al. Autoantibodies to thyroid hormones: the role of thyroglobulin. *Clin Exp Immunol* 1996;105:140.

95. Schneider A, Ikekubo K, Kuma K. Iodine content of serum thyroglobulin in normal individuals and patients with thyroid tumors. *J Clin Endocrinol Metab* 1983;57:1251.

96. Sapin R, Schlienger JL. Thyroglobulin assay ambiguities. *Ann Biol Clin (Paris)* 1998;56:41.

97. Chung JK, Park YJ, Kim TY, et al. Clinical significance of elevated level of serum antithyroglobulin antibody in patients with differentiated thyroid cancer after thyroid ablation. *Clin Endocrinol (Oxf)* 2002;57:215.

98. Chiovato L, Latrofa F, Braverman LE, et al. Disappearance of humoral thyroid autoimmunity after complete removal of thyroid antigens. *Ann Intern Med* 2003;139:346.

99. Bachelot A, Cailleux AF, Klain M, et al. Relationship between tumor burden and serum thyroglobulin level in patients with papillary and follicular thyroid carcinoma. *Thyroid* 2002;12:707.

100. Knudsen N, Bulow I, Jorgensen T, et al. Serum Tg–a sensitive marker of thyroid abnormalities and iodine deficiency in epidemiological studies. *J Clin Endocrinol Metab* 2001;86:3599.

101. Feldt-Rasmussen U, Blichert-Toft M, Christiansen C, et al. Serum thyroglobulin and its autoantibody following subtotal thyroid resection of Graves' disease. *Eur J Clin Invest* 1982;12:203.

102. Nakazato N, Yoshida K, Mori K, et al. Antithyroid drugs inhibit radioiodine-induced increases in thyroid autoantibodies in hyperthyroid Graves' disease. *Thyroid* 1999;9:775.

103. Date J, Feldt-Rasmussen U, Blichert-Toft M, et al. Long-term observation of serum thyroglobulin after resection of nontoxic goiter and relation to ultrasonographically demonstrated relapse. *World J Surg* 1996;20:351.

104. Bayraktar M, Ergin M, Boyacioglu A, et al. A preliminary report of thyroglobulin release after fine needle aspiration biopsy of thyroid nodules. *J Int Med Res* 1990;18:253.

105. Muller E, Franke WG, Koch R. Thyroglobulin and violent asphyxia. *Forensic Sci Int* 1997;90:165.

106. Kawamura S, Kishino B, Tajima K, et al. Elevated serum thyroglobulin as a manifestation of acute haemorrhage into the thyroid gland. *Clin Endocrinol (Oxf)* 1984;20:213.

107. Smallridge RC, De Keyser FM, Van Herle AJ, et al. *Thyroid* iodine content and serum thyroglobulin: clues to the natural history of destruction-induced thyroiditis. *J Clin Endocrinol Metab* 1986;62:1213.

108. Premawardhana LD, Lo SS, Phillips DI, et al. Variability of serum thyroglobulin levels is determined by a major gene. *Clin Endocrinol (Oxf)* 1994;41:725.

109. Clark OH, Gerend PL, Davis M, et al. Estrogen and thyroid stimulating hormone (TSH) receptors in neoplastic and non-neoplastic human thyroid tissue. *J Surg Res* 1985;38:89.

110. Hoelting T, Siperstein AE, Duh QY, et al. Tamoxifen inhibits growth, migration, and invasion of human follicular and papillary thyroid cancer cells in vitro and in vivo. *J Clin Endocrinol Metab* 1995;80:308.

111. Glinoer D, De Nayer P, Delange F, et al. A randomized trial for the treatment of mild iodine deficiency during pregnancy: maternal and neonatal effects. *J Clin Endocrinol Metab* 1995;80:258.

112. Gonzalez-Jimenez A, Fernandez-Soto ML, Escobar-Jimenez F, et al. *Thyroid* function parameters and TSH-receptor antibodies in healthy subjects and Graves' disease patients: a sequential study before, during and after pregnancy. *Thyroidology* 1993;5:13.

113. Glinoer D, De Nayer P, Bourdoux P, et al. Regulation of maternal thyroid during pregnancy. *J Clin Endocrinol Metab* 1990;71:276.

114. Rodriguez M, Santisteban P, Acebron A, et al. Expression of thyroglobulin gene in maternal and fetal thyroid in rats. *Endocrinology* 1992;131:415.

115. Penny R, Spencer CA, Frasier SD, et al. Cord serum thyroid-stimulating hormone and thyroglobulin levels decline with increasing birth weight in newborns. *J Clin Endocrinol Metab* 1984;59:979.

116. Glinoer D. The regulation of thyroid function in pregnancy: pathways of endocrine adaptation from physiology to pathology. *Endocr Rev* 1997;18:404.

117. Glinoer D, Delange F, Laboureur I, et al. Maternal and neonatal thyroid function at birth in an area of marginally low iodine intake. *J Clin Endocrinol Metab* 1992;75:800.

118. Vulsma T, Gons MH, de Vijlder JJ. Maternal-fetal transfer of thyroxine in congenital hypothyroidism due to a total organification defect or thyroid agenesis. *N Engl J Med* 1989;321:13.

119. Nohr SB, Laurberg P. Opposite variations in maternal and neonatal thyroid function induced by iodine supplementation during pregnancy. *J Clin Endocrinol Metab* 2000;85:623.

120. Chanoine JP, Toppet V, Bourdoux P, et al. Smoking during pregnancy: a significant cause of neonatal thyroid enlargement. *Br J Obstet Gynaecol* 1991;98:65.

121. Gasparoni A, Autelli M, Ravagni-Probizer MF, et al. Effect of passive smoking on thyroid function in infants. *Eur J Endocrinol* 1998;138:379.

122. Klett M, Ohlig M, Manz F, et al. Effect of iodine supply on neonatal thyroid volume and TSH. *Acta Paediatr Suppl* 1999;88:18.

123. Fukayama H, Nasu M, Murakami S, et al. Examination of antithyroid effects of smoking products in cultured thyroid follicles: only thiocyanate is a potent antithyroid agent. *Acta Endocrinol (Copenh)* 1992;127:520.

124. Pezzino V, Filetti S, Belfiore A, et al. Serum thyroglobulin levels in the newborn. *J Clin Endocrinol Metab* 1981;52:364.

125. Black EG, Bodden SJ, Hulse JA, et al. Serum thyroglobulin in normal and hypothyroid neonates. *Clin Endocrinol (Oxf)* 1982;16:267.

126. Penny R, Spencer CA, Frasier SD, et al. *Thyroid*-stimulating hormone and thyroglobulin levels decrease with chronological age in children and adolescents. *J Clin Endocrinol Metab* 1983;56:177.

127. Feldt-Rasmussen U, Hegedus L, Hansen JM, et al. Relationship between thyroid volume and serum thyroglobulin during long-term suppression with triiodothyronine in patients with diffuse non-toxic goitre. *Acta Endocrinol (Copenh)* 1984;105:184.

128. Hershman JM, Due DT, Sharp B, et al. Endemic goiter in Vietnam. *J Clin Endocrinol Metab* 1983;57:243.

129. Unger J, De Maertelaer V, Golstein J, et al. Relationship between serum thyroglobulin and intrathyroidal stable iodine in human simple goiter. *Clin Endocrinol (Oxf)* 1985;23:1.

130. Fenzi GF, Ceccarelli C, Macchia E, et al. Reciprocal changes of serum thyroglobulin and TSH in residents of a moderate endemic goitre area. *Clin Endocrinol (Oxf)* 1985;23:115.

131. Fenzi GF, Giani C, Ceccarelli P, et al. Role of autoimmune and familial factors in goiter prevalence. Studies performed in a moderately endemic area. *J Endocrinol Invest* 1986;9:161.

132. Brix TH, Hegedus L. Genetic and environmental factors in the aetiology of simple goitre. *Ann Med* 2000;32:153.

133. Berghout A, Wiersinga WM, Smits NJ, et al. Interrelationships between age, thyroid volume, thyroid nodularity, and thyroid function in patients with sporadic nontoxic goiter. *Am J Med* 1990;89:602.

134. Missler U, Gutekunst R, Wood WG. Thyroglobulin is a more sensitive indicator of iodine deficiency than thyrotropin: development and evaluation of dry blood spot assays for thyrotropin and thyroglobulin in iodine-deficient geographical areas. *Eur J Clin Chem Clin Biochem* 1994;32:137.

135. Rasmussen LB, Ovesen L, Bulow I, et al. Relations between various measures of iodine intake and thyroid volume, thyroid nodularity, and serum thyroglobulin. *Am J Clin Nutr* 2002;76:1069.

136. van den Briel T, West CE, Hautvast JG, et al. Serum thyroglobulin and urinary iodine concentration are the most appropriate indicators of iodine status and thyroid function under conditions of increasing iodine supply in schoolchildren in Benin. *J Nutr* 2001;131:2701.

137. Simsek E, Safak A, Yavuz O, et al. Sensitivity of iodine deficiency indicators and iodine status in Turkey. *J Pediatr Endocrinol Metab* 2003;16:197.

138. Zimmermann MB, Moretti D, Chaouki N, et al. Development of a dried whole-blood spot thyroglobulin assay and its evaluation as an indicator of thyroid status in goitrous children receiving iodized salt. *Am J Clin Nutr* 2003;77:1453.

139. Miyakawa M, Saji M, Tsushima T, et al. *Thyroid* volume and serum thyroglobulin levels in patients with acromegaly: correlation with plasma insulin-like growth factor 1 levels. *J Clin Endocrinol Metab* 1988;67:973.

140. Madeddu G, Casu AR, Marrosu A, et al. Serum thyroglobulin in patients with autonomous thyroid nodules. *Clin Endocrinol (Oxf)* 1984;21:377.

141. Knudsen N, Bulow I, Laurberg P, et al. Low socio-economic status and familial occurrence of goitre are associated with a high prevalence of goitre. *Eur J Epidemiol* 2003;18:175.

142. Schneider AB, Bekerman C, Leland J, et al. *Thyroid* nodules in the follow-up of irradiated individuals: comparison of thyroid ultrasound with scanning and palpation. *J Clin Endocrinol Metab* 1997;82:4020.

143. Gebel F, Ramelli G, Burgi U, et al. The site of leakage of intrafollicular thyroglobulin into the blood stream in simple human goiter. *J Clin Endocrinol Metab* 1983;57:915.

144. Ongphiphadhanakul B, Rajatanavin R, Chiemchanya S, et al. Systematic inclusion of clinical and laboratory data improves diagnostic accuracy of fine-needle aspiration biopsy in solitary nodules. *Acta Endocrinol (Copenh)* 1992;126:233.

145. Mizokami T, Okamura K, Hirata T, et al. Acute spontaneous hemorrhagic degeneration of the thyroid nodule with subacute thyroiditis-like symptoms and laboratory findings. *Endocr J* 1995;42:683.

146. Kuo SW, Hu CA, Pei D, et al. Efficacy of thyroxine-suppressive therapy and its relation to serum thyroglobulin levels in solitary nontoxic thyroid nodules. *J Formos Med Assoc* 1993;92:55.

147. Koc M, Ersoz HO, Akpinar I, et al. Effect of low- and high-dose levothyroxine on thyroid nodule volume: a crossover placebo-controlled trial. *Clin Endocrinol (Oxf)* 2002;57:621.

148. Schneider AB, Bekerman C, Favus M, et al. Continuing occurrence of thyroid nodules after head and neck irradiation. Relation to plasma thyroglobulin concentration. *Ann Intern Med* 1981;94:176.

149. Uller RP, Van Herle AJ. Effect of therapy on serum thyroglobulin levels in patients with Graves' disease. *J Clin Endocrinol Metab* 1978;46:747.

150. Aizawa T, Ishihara M, Koizumi Y, et al. Serum thyroglobulin concentration as an indicator for assessing thyroid stimulation in patients with Graves' disease during antithyroid drug therapy. *Am J Med* 1990;89:175.

151. Yamaguchi Y, Inukai T, Iwashita A, et al. Changes in thyroid volume during antithyroid drug therapy for Graves' disease and its relationship to TSH receptor antibodies, TSH and thyroglobulin. *Acta Endocrinol (Copenh)* 1990;123:411.

152. Werner RS, Romaldini JH, Farah CS, et al. Serum thyroid-stimulating antibody, thyroglobulin levels, and thyroid suppressibility measurement as predictors of the outcome of combined methimazole and triiodothyronine therapy in Graves' disease. *Thyroid* 1991;1:293.

153. Chou FF, Wang PW, Chen SM. The presence of higher levels of thyroglobulin, but not thyroid autoantibodies, in the thyroid vein in Graves' disease. *J Endocrinol Invest* 1994;17:41.

154. Roti E, Uberti ED. Iodine excess and hyperthyroidism. *Thyroid* 2001;11:493.

155. Matsubara S, Inoh M, Tarumi Y, et al. An outbreak (159 cases) of transient thyrotoxicosis without hyperthyroidism in Japan. *Intern Med* 1995;34:514.

156. Daniels GH. Amiodarone-induced thyrotoxicosis. *J Clin Endocrinol Metab* 2001;86:3.

157. Takaichi Y, Tamai H, Honda K, et al. The significance of antithyroglobulin and antithyroidal microsomal antibodies in patients with hyperthyroidism due to Graves' disease treated with antithyroidal drugs. *J Clin Endocrinol Metab* 1989;68:1097.

158. Cohen JH, Ingbar SH, Braverman LE. Thyrotoxicosis due to ingestion of excess thyroid hormone. *Endocr Rev* 1989;10:113.

159. Meurisse M, Preudhomme L, Lamberty G, et al. Iatrogenic thyrotoxicosis. Causal circumstances, pathophysiology and principles of treatment. Review of the literature. *Acta Chir Belg* 2001;101:257.

160. Talbot JN, Duron F, Feron R, et al. Thyroglobulin, thyrotropin and thyrotropin binding inhibiting immunoglobulins assayed at the withdrawal of antithyroid drug therapy as predictors of relapse of Graves' disease within one year. *J Endocrinol Invest* 1989;12:589.

161. Feldt-Rasmussen U, Petersen PH, Date J, et al. Serum thyroglobulin in patients undergoing subtotal thyroidectomy for toxic and nontoxic goiter. *J Endocrinol Invest* 1982;5:161.

162. Kasagi K, Kousaka T, Higuchi K, et al. Clinical significance of measurements of antithyroid antibodies in the diagnosis of Hashimoto's thyroiditis: comparison with histological findings. *Thyroid* 1996;6:445.

163. Contempre B, Duale GL, Gervy C, et al. Hypothyroid patients showing shortened responsiveness to oral iodized oil have paradoxically low serum thyroglobulin and low thyroid reserve. Thyroglobulin/thyrotropin ratio as a measure of thyroid damage. *Eur J Endocrinol* 1996;134:342.

164. Markou K, Georgopoulos N, Kyriazopoulou V, et al. Iodine-induced hypothyroidism. *Thyroid* 2001;11:501.

165. Acebron A, Aza-Blanc P, Rossi DL, et al. Congenital human thyroglobulin defect due to low expression of the thyroid-

specific transcription factor TTF-1. *J Clin Invest* 1995;96: 781.

166. Medeiros-Neto G, Kim PS, Yoo SE, et al. Congenital hypothyroid goiter with deficient thyroglobulin. Identification of molecular chaperones. *J Clin Invest* 1996;98:2838.

167. Caron P, Moya CM, Malet D, et al. Compound heterozygous mutations in the thyroglobulin gene (1143delC and 6725G—>A [R2223H]) resulting in fetal goitrous hypothyroidism. *J Clin Endocrinol Metab* 2003;88:3546.

168. Czernichow P, Schlumberger M, Pomarede R, et al. Plasma thyroglobulin measurements help determine the type of thyroid defect in congenital hypothyroidism. *J Clin Endocrinol Metab* 1983;56:242.

169. Parkes AB, Black EG, Adams H, et al. Serum thyroglobulin: an early indicator of autoimmune post-partum thyroiditis. *Clin Endocrinol (Oxf)* 1994;41:9.

170. Fragu P, Rougier P, Schlumberger M, et al. Evolution of thyroid 127-I stores measured by X-ray fluorescence in subacute thyroiditis. *J Clin Endocrinol Metab* 1982;54:162.

171. Madeddu G, Casu AR, Costanza C, et al. Serum thyroglobulin levels in the diagnosis and follow-up of subacute 'painful' thyroiditis. *Arch Intern Med* 1985;145:243.

172. Prummel MF, Laurberg P. Interferon-alpha and autoimmune thyroid disease. *Thyroid* 2003;13:547.

173. Carella C, Mazziotti G, Morisco F, et al. Long-term outcome of interferon-alpha-induced thyroid autoimmunity and prognostic influence of thyroid autoantibody pattern at the end of treatment. *J Clin Endocrinol Metab* 2001;86:1925.

174. Martino E, Bartalena L, Bogazzi F, et al. The effects of amiodarone on the thyroid. *Endocr Rev* 2001;22:240.

175. Johnston AM, Eagles JM. Lithium-associated clinical hypothyroidism. Prevalence and risk factors. *Br J Psychiatry* 1999;175: 336.

176. Miller KK, Daniels GH. Association between lithium use and thyrotoxicosis caused by silent thyroiditis. *Clin Endocrinol (Oxf)* 2001;55:501.

177. Parmar MS, Sturge C. Recurrent hamburger thyrotoxicosis. *CMAJ* 2003;169:415.

178. Bejarano PA, Nikiforov YE, Swenson ES, et al. Thyroid transcription factor-1, thyroglobulin, cytokeratin 7, and cytokeratin 20 in thyroid neoplasms. *Appl Immunohistochem Mol Morphol* 2000;8:189.

179. Basolo F, Pisaturo F, Pollina LE, et al. N-ras mutation in poorly differentiated thyroid carcinomas: correlation with bone metastases and inverse correlation to thyroglobulin expression. *Thyroid* 2000;10:19.

180. Ringel MD, Anderson J, Souza SL, et al. Expression of the sodium iodide symporter and thyroglobulin genes are reduced in papillary thyroid cancer. *Mod Pathol* 2001;14:289.

181. Takano T, Miyauchi A, Yoshida H, et al. Quantitative measurement of thyroglobulin mRNA in peripheral blood of patients after total thyroidectomy. *Br J Cancer* 2001;85:102.

182. Ringel MD, Balducci-Silano PL, Anderson JS, et al. Quantitative reverse transcription-polymerase chain reaction of circulating thyroglobulin messenger ribonucleic acid for monitoring patients with thyroid carcinoma. *J Clin Endocrinol Metab* 1999;84:4037.

183. Biscolla RP, Cerutti JM, Maciel RM. Detection of recurrent thyroid cancer by sensitive nested reverse transcription-polymerase chain reaction of thyroglobulin and sodium/iodine symporter messenger ribonucleic acid transcripts in peripheral blood. *J Clin Endocrinol Metab* 2000;85:3623.

184. Eszlinger M, Neumann S, Otto L, et al. Thyroglobulin mRNA quantification in the peripheral blood is not a reliable marker for the follow-up of patients with differentiated thyroid cancer. *Eur J Endocrinol* 2002;147:575.

185. Noel M, Delehye MC, Segond N, et al. Study of calcitonin and thyroglobulin gene expression in human mixed follicular and medullary thyroid carcinoma. *Thyroid* 1991;1:249.

186. Shimizu M, Hirokawa M, LiVolsi VA, et al. Combined "mixed medullary-follicular" and "papillary" carcinoma of the thyroid with lymph node metastasis. *Endocr Pathol* 2000;11:353.

187. Ohta K, Endo T, Onaya T. The mRNA levels of thyrotropin receptor, thyroglobulin and thyroid peroxidase in neoplastic thyroid tissues. *Biochem Biophys Res Commun* 1991;174: 1148.

188. Caillou B, Troalen F, Baudin E, et al. Na+/I- symporter distribution in human thyroid tissues: an immunohistochemical study. *J Clin Endocrinol Metab* 1998;83:4102.

189. Lazar V, Bidart JM, Caillou B, et al. Expression of the Na+/I-symporter gene in human thyroid tumors: a comparison study with other thyroid-specific genes. *J Clin Endocrinol Metab* 1999;84:3228.

190. Gerard AC, Daumerie C, Mestdagh C, et al. Correlation between the loss of thyroglobulin iodination and the expression of thyroid-specific proteins involved in iodine metabolism in thyroid carcinomas. *J Clin Endocrinol Metab* 2003;88: 4977.

191. Arturi F, Russo D, Schlumberger M, et al. Iodide symporter gene expression in human thyroid tumors. *J Clin Endocrinol Metab* 1998;83:2493.

192. Tanaka K, Sonoo H, Yamamoto Y, et al. et al. Changes of expression level of the differentiation markers in papillary thyroid carcinoma under thyrotropin suppression therapy in vivo immunohistochemical detection of thyroglobulin, thyroid peroxidase, and thyrotropin receptor. *J Surg Oncol* 2000;75: 108.

193. Dralle H, Schwarzrock R, Lang W, et al. Comparison of histology and immunohistochemistry with thyroglobulin serum levels and radioiodine uptake in recurrences and metastases of differentiated thyroid carcinomas. *Acta Endocrinol (Copenh)* 1985; 108:504.

194. Filetti S, Bidart JM, Arturi F, et al. Sodium/iodide symporter: a key transport system in thyroid cancer cell metabolism. *Eur J Endocrinol* 1999;141:443.

195. Ericsson UB, Tegler L, Lennquist S, et al. Serum thyroglobulin in differentiated thyroid carcinoma. *Acta Chir Scand* 1984; 150:367.

196. Hrafnkelsson J, Tulinius H, Kjeld M, et al. Serum thyroglobulin as a risk factor for thyroid carcinoma. *Acta Oncol* 2000;39: 973.

197. Okamoto T, Kanbe M, Iihara M, et al. Measuring serum thyroglobulin in patients with follicular thyroid nodule: its diagnostic implications. *Endocr J* 1997;44:187.

198. Sharma AK, Sarda AK, Chattopadhyay TK, et al. The role of estimation of the ratio of preoperative serum thyroglobulin to the thyroid mass in predicting the behaviour of well differentiated thyroid cancers. *J Postgrad Med* 1996;42:39.

199. Shah DH, Dandekar SR, Jeevanram RK, et al. Serum thyroglobulin in differentiated thyroid carcinoma: histological and metastatic classification. *Acta Endocrinol (Copenh)* 1981; 98:222.

200. Edmonds CJ, Willis CL. Serum thyroglobulin in the investigation of patients presenting with metastases. *Br J Radiol* 1988; 61:317.

201. Ozata M, Suzuki S, Miyamoto T, et al. Serum thyroglobulin in the follow-up of patients with treated differentiated thyroid cancer. *J Clin Endocrinol Metab* 1994;79:98.

202. Ronga G, Filesi M, Ventroni G, et al. Value of the first serum thyroglobulin level after total thyroidectomy for the diagnosis of metastases from differentiated thyroid carcinoma. *Eur J Nucl Med* 1999;26:1448.

203. Lima N, Cavalieri H, Tomimori E, et al. Prognostic value of serial serum thyroglobulin determinations after total thyroidectomy for differentiated thyroid cancer. 2002;25:110.
204. Schlumberger MJ. Diagnostic follow-up of well-differentiated thyroid carcinoma: historical perspective and current status. *J Endocrinol Invest* 1999;22:3.
205. Baudin E, Do Cao C, Cailleux AF, et al. Positive predictive value of serum thyroglobulin levels, measured during the first year of follow-up after thyroid hormone withdrawal, in thyroid cancer patients. *J Clin Endocrinol Metab* 2003;88:1107.
206. Savelli G, Chiti A, Rodari M, et al. Predictive value of thyroglobulin changes for the efficacy of thyroid remnant ablation. *Tumori* 2001;87:42.
207. Lin JD, Huang MJ, Hsu BR, et al. Significance of postoperative serum thyroglobulin levels in patients with papillary and follicular thyroid carcinomas. *J Surg Oncol* 2002;80:45.
208. Fatemi S, Nicoloff J, LoPresti J, et al. Use of 2 year post-tx serum thyroglobulin (Tg) to assess risk of recurrent/persistent papillary thyroid cancer. *J Endocrinol Invest* 2001;24(Suppl 6).
209. Spencer CA, Lo Presti JS, Fatemi S, et al. Detection of residual and recurrent differentiated thyroid carcinoma (DTC) by serum thyroglobulin (Tg) measurement. *Thyroid* 1999;9:435.
210. David A, Blotta A, Bondanelli M, et al. Serum thyroglobulin concentrations and (131)I whole-body scan results in patients with differentiated thyroid carcinoma after administration of recombinant human thyroid-stimulating hormone. *J Nucl Med* 2001;42:1470.
211. Giovanni V, Arianna LG, Antonio C, et al. The use of recombinant human TSH in the follow-up of differentiated thyroid cancer: experience from a large patient cohort in a single centre. *Clin Endocrinol (Oxf)* 2002;56:247.
212. Haugen BR, Ridgway EC, McLaughlin BA, et al. Clinical comparison of whole-body radioiodine scan and serum thyroglobulin after stimulation with recombinant human thyrotropin. *Thyroid* 2002;12:37.
213. Mazzaferri EL, Kloos RT. Is diagnostic iodine-131 scanning with recombinant human TSH useful in the follow-up of differentiated thyroid cancer after thyroid ablation? *J Clin Endocrinol Metab* 2002;87:1490.
214. Pacini F, Molinaris E, Lippi F, et al. Prediction of disease status by recombinant human TSH-stimulated serum Tg in the postsurgical follow-up of differentiated thyroid carcinoma. *J Clin Endocrinol Metab* 2001:86;5686.
215. Robbins RJ, Chon JT, Fleisher M, et al. Is the serum thyroglobulin response to recombinant human thyrotropin sufficient, by itself, to monitor for residual thyroid carcinoma? *J Clin Endocrinol Metab* 2002;87:3242.
216. Wartofsky L. Management of low-risk well-differentiated thyroid cancer based only on thyroglobulin measurement after recombinant human thyrotropin. *Thyroid* 2002;12:583.
217. Pacini F, Molinaro E, Castagna MG, et al. Recombinant human thyrotropin-stimulated serum thyroglobulin combined with neck ultrasonography has the highest sensitivity in monitoring differentiated thyroid carcinoma. *J Clin Endocrinol Metab* 2003;88:3668.
218. Siddiqui AR, Edmondson J, Wellman HN, et al. Feasibility of low doses of I-131 for thyroid ablation in postsurgical patients with thyroid carcinoma. *Clin Nucl Med* 1981;6:158.
219. Arslan N, Ilgan S, Serdengecti M, et al. Post-surgical ablation of thyroid remnants with high-dose (131)I in patients with differentiated thyroid carcinoma. *Nucl Med Commun* 2001;22:1021.
220. Torlontano M, Crocetti U, D'Aloiso L, et al. Serum thyroglobulin and 131I whole body scan after recombinant human TSH stimulation in the follow-up of low-risk patients with differentiated thyroid cancer. *Eur J Endocrinol* 2003;148:19.
221. Schlumberger M, Baudin E. Serum thyroglobulin in the follow-up of patients with differentiated thyroid carcinoma. *Eur J Endocrinol* 1998;138:249.
222. Pachucki J, Burmeister LA. Evaluation and treatment of persistent thyroglobulinemia in patients with well-differentiated thyroid cancer. *Eur J Endocrinol* 1997;137:254.
223. van Tol KM, Jager PL, de Vries EG, et al. Outcome in patients with differentiated thyroid cancer with negative diagnostic whole-body scanning and detectable stimulated thyroglobulin. *Eur J Endocrinol* 2003;148:589.
224. Fatourechi V, Hay ID, Mullan BP, et al. Are posttherapy radioiodine scans informative and do they influence subsequent therapy of patients with differentiated thyroid cancer? *Thyroid* 2000;10:573.
225. Fatourechi V, Hay ID, Javedan H, et al. Lack of impact of radioiodine therapy in Tg-positive, diagnostic whole-body scan-negative patients with follicular cell-derived thyroid cancer. *J Clin Endocrinol Metab* 2002;87:1521.
226. Hung MC, Wu HS, Kao CH, et al. F18-fluorodeoxyglucose positron emission tomography in detecting metastatic papillary thyroid carcinoma with elevated human serum thyroglobulin levels but negative I-131 whole body scan. *Endocr Res* 2003;29:169.
227. Lowe VJ, Mullan BP, Hay ID, et al. 18F-FDG PET of patients with Hurthle cell carcinoma. *J Nucl Med* 2003;44:1402.
228. Ditkoff BA, Marvin MR, Yemul S, et al. Detection of circulating thyroid cells in peripheral blood. *Surgery* 1996;120:959.
229. Denizot A, Delfino C, Dutour-Meyer A, et al. Evaluation of quantitative measurement of thyroglobulin mRNA in the follow-up of differentiated thyroid cancer. *Thyroid* 2003;13:867.
230. Arturi F, Russo D, Giuffrida D, et al. Early diagnosis by genetic analysis of differentiated thyroid cancer metastases in small lymph nodes. *J Clin Endocrinol Metab* 1997;82:1638.
231. Savagner F, Rodien P, Reynier P, et al. Analysis of Tg transcripts by real-time RT-PCR in the blood of thyroid cancer patients. *J Clin Endocrinol Metab* 2002;87:635.
232. Fenton C, Anderson JS, Patel AD, et al. Thyroglobulin messenger ribonucleic acid levels in the peripheral blood of children with benign and malignant thyroid disease. *Pediatr Res* 2001;49:429.
233. Bellantone R, Lombardi CP, Bossola M, et al. Validity of thyroglobulin mRNA assay in peripheral blood of postoperative thyroid carcinoma patients in predicting tumor recurrence varies according to the histologic type: results of a prospective study. *Cancer* 2001;92:2273.
234. Bugalho MJ, Domingues RS, Pinto AC, et al. Detection of thyroglobulin mRNA transcripts in peripheral blood of individuals with and without thyroid glands: evidence for thyroglobulin expression by blood cells. *Eur J Endocrinol* 2001;145:409.

THYROID-DIRECTED ANTIBODIES

CLAUDIO MARCOCCI
MICHELE MARINÒ

Humoral and cellular immune responses are involved in the two main types of autoimmune thyroid disease (AITD), Graves' disease and chronic autoimmune thyroiditis. The humoral immune response is dominant in Graves' disease, as indicated by the fact that thyrotoxicosis in patients with the disease is caused by the action of antibodies that activate the thyrotropin receptor (TSHR). In contrast, the cellular immune response is dominant in chronic autoimmune thyroiditis. Although nearly all patients with chronic autoimmune thyroiditis have high serum concentrations of antibodies against several thyroid antigens, for the most part the disorder appears to be the consequence of tissue damage initiated by T cells (1). Whatever the pathophysiologic role of antibodies, in clinical practice measurements of serum antibodies against thyroid antigens are useful for the evaluation of patients suspected of having either Graves' thyrotoxicosis or chronic autoimmune thyroiditis (see section on Pathogenesis of Graves' Disease in Chapter 23 and Chapter 47).

The major thyroid antigens are thyroglobulin (Tg), thyroid peroxidase (TPO), and the TSHR (Table 15.1). Other thyroid antigens include the thyroid hormones thyroxine (T_4) and triiodothyronine (T_3), as components of Tg; the sodium iodide symporter (NIS); megalin (gp330); uncharacterized membrane antigens other than TPO and TSHR; and antigens cloned from the complementary DNA (cDNA) of human thyroid libraries.

ANTITHYROGLOBULIN ANTIBODIES

Structure and Forms of Thyroglobulin

Thyroid follicles, the functional units of the thyroid, are composed of a single layer of epithelial cells (thyrocytes) surrounding a lumen that contains a viscous substance known as colloid. Thyroglobulin, both the precursor and storage form of thyroid hormone, is the major protein component of colloid (see Chapter 5) (2). In its major, mature form, Tg is a large 660 kDa dimeric glycoprotein composed of two identical 330 kDa monomers (2).

Iodination of tyrosyl residues of Tg and coupling of iodotyrosyl residues within Tg at the cell-colloid interface result in the formation of T_4 and T_3 within the Tg molecule, a process catalyzed by TPO (2). The hormonal content of Tg depends on iodide availability, and, on average, a molecule of human Tg contains 2.3 molecules of T_4 and 0.3 molecule of T_3 (2). Thyroglobulin molecules within the colloid are heterogeneous in terms of hormone content, extent of glycosylation, and size (some are present as monomers, and others as polymers or proteolytic fragments) (2). Newly secreted Tg molecules adjacent to the apical surface of thyrocytes are readily available for reabsorption into thyrocytes and proteolysis, with release of T_4 and T_3 (3). Those Tg molecules that are not reabsorbed are stored in the colloid (4).

Thyroglobulin Recognition by Antibodies

The immune properties of Tg depend, at least in part, on its hormone content (5). Thus, formation of T_4 and T_3 within Tg changes its conformation so that certain epitopes are masked and others are unmasked (5,6). As a consequence, the binding ability of antibodies is variably affected by the hormonal content of Tg (5). Anti-Tg antibodies found in the serum of normal subjects usually recognize only highly conserved epitopes located in the hormone-containing regions of Tg, whereas among patients with AITD and mice with experimental thyroiditis the anti-Tg antibodies are less restricted (5–8). This implies some sort of epitopes spreading. In addition, the epitopes recognized by anti-Tg antibodies from patients with chronic autoimmune thyroiditis, Graves' disease, and differentiated thyroid carcinoma differ in some respects (5). In general, anti-Tg antibodies recognize conformational epitopes preferentially, and linear epitopes are less important (5), indicating that the immunogenic potential of intact Tg is greater than that of fragments of Tg that have lost the ability to form conformational epitopes.

Importance of the Presence of Thyroglobulin in the Circulation

Thyroglobulin is uniquely produced by thyroid cells, and most of it is stored within thyroid follicles, but small amounts are present in the circulation (9). In this regard, exposure of the immune system to Tg may be responsible

TABLE 15.1. THYROID ANTIGEN ANTIBODY SYSTEMS AND INDICATIONS FOR MEASUREMENTS OF SERUM ANTITHYROID ANTIBODIES

Antigen	Antibody	Indications for Measurement
Tg	Anti-Tg antibodies	Diagnosis of autoimmune thyroid disease in anti-TPO-negative cases when serum Tg is measured
TPO	Anti-TPO antibodies	Diagnosis of chronic autoimmune thyroiditis
	TSHR antibodies	
	TBII	Diagnosis of Graves' thyrotoxicosis and euthyroid ophthalmopathy
TSHR		Third trimester of pregnancy in women with Graves' disease or chronic autoimmune thyroiditis
	TSHR-SAb	
	TSHR-BAb)	
Tg + TPO	Tg-TPOAb	
CA2	CA2-Ab	
Megalin	Megalin-Ab	
Thyroid hormones	Anti-T$_3$ and anti-T$_4$ antibodies	
NIS	NIS-Ab	

Ab, antibody; CA2, second colloid antigen; NIS, sodium iodide symporter; Tg, thyroglobulin; TPO, thyroid peroxidase; TSH, thyrotropin; TSHR, TSH receptor; TSHR-BAb, TSH-blocking antibodies; TSHR-SAb, thyroid-stimulating antibodies.

for T-cell reactivity or antibody production. However, this does not seem to be crucial for the production of anti-Tg antibodies, because many patients with high serum Tg concentrations have no circulating anti-Tg antibodies (10,11). On the other hand, massive release of Tg after destruction of the thyroid can be followed by the appearance of anti-Tg antibodies in the serum (11). Indeed, exposure of the immune system to thyroid antigens is probably necessary for maintaining an autoimmune response. Thus, in patients with thyroid carcinoma, both anti-Tg antibodies and anti-TPO antibodies disappear from the circulation after the complete elimination of thyroid tissue by thyroidectomy and radioiodine treatment (12).

Thyroglobulin can reach the circulation by several mechanisms (9). One is transepithelial transport (transcytosis), by which Tg is internalized, in conjunction with the endocytic receptor megalin, at the apical surface of thyrocytes and transported through the thyrocyte to be released into the extracellular space (13). This is the main mechanism of Tg secretion under conditions in which thyroid follicular structure is intact (9,13). Another mechanism is leakage of Tg because of disruption of the thyroid follicles, as it occurs in destructive processes (14). Finally, Tg may be directly secreted by thyrocytes immediately after synthesis; this seems to be the cause of high serum Tg concentrations in thyroid carcinoma (13). Whether the mechanism of Tg release affects anti-Tg antibody production is not known.

Importance of Antithyroglobulin Antibodies in the Pathogenesis of Autoimmune Thyroid Disease

Most anti-Tg antibodies are IgG antibodies. They may be of any subclass, but in patients with AITD they are predominantly IgG 4 and IgG 2 (15). IgA and IgM anti-Tg antibod-

ies can also be found (15). Anti-Tg antibodies do not fix complement, probably because the immunodominant epitopes of Tg are widely spaced in the Tg molecule, thereby preventing IgG cross-linking (16). The lack of defined biological actions of anti-Tg antibodies implies that they have no pathogenic role. This is supported by the presence of high serum anti-Tg antibody concentrations in some otherwise healthy subjects (Fig. 15.1) (10) and in patients with monoclonal gammopathy (17), as well as the lack of correlation between serum anti-Tg antibody concentrations and disease activity in patients with chronic autoimmune thyroiditis and mice with experimental autoimmune thyroiditis (10,11,18).

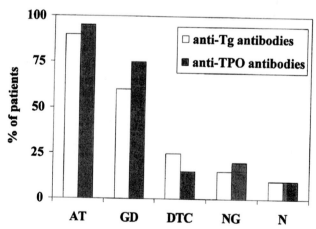

FIGURE 15.1. Frequency of high serum anti-Tg and anti-TPO antibody concentrations in patients with autoimmune thyroiditis *(AT)*, Graves' disease *(GD)*, differentiated thyroid cancer *(DTC)*, and nodular goiter *(NG)*, and in normal subjects *(N)*. (From Mariotti S, Pisani S, Russova A, et al. A new solid-phase immunoradiometric assay for anti-thyroglobulin autoantibody. *J Endocrinol Invest* 1982;5:227; and Mariotti S, Caturegli P, Piccolo P, et al. Antithyroid peroxidase autoantibodies in thyroid diseases. *J Clin Endocrinol Metab* 1990;71:661,with modifications.)

There is, however, some evidence for a role of anti-Tg antibodies in chronic autoimmune thyroiditis. Serum anti-Tg antibodies are oligoclonal in patients with chronic autoimmune thyroiditis, whereas they are polyclonal in normal subjects (15,19). There is deposition of Tg–anti-Tg immune complexes in kidney basal membranes in some patients with glomerulonephritis (20). Pregnant women who have high serum anti-Tg antibody concentrations are more likely to have postpartum thyroiditis than pregnant women who have normal serum anti-Tg antibody concentrations (21). Finally, passive transfer of anti-Tg antibodies can result in autoimmune thyroiditis in animals (22).

Serum Antithyroglobulin Antibody Concentrations in Various Conditions

Anti-Tg antibodies have been measured in serum using several techniques (11,23). Initially, they were measured by passive agglutination, and the results were reported simply as positive or negative or as the dilution of serum giving a positive response (titer). Subsequently, much more sensitive methods, including radioimmunoassays (RIAs), immunoradiometric assays (IRMAs), enzyme-linked immunosorbent assays (ELISAs), and chemiluminescence assays were developed. The latter methods are now used in clinical practice, and the results are usually reported quantitatively, in units per milliliter of serum.

Anti-Tg antibodies are rarely present in children without thyroid disease. Among normal adults, about 10% have high serum anti-Tg antibody concentrations, and among women age 60 years and older 15% may have high concentrations (Fig. 15.1) (10,11,24). Among patients with chronic autoimmune thyroiditis, 80% to 90% have high concentrations. The concentrations are high in 50% to 60% of patients with thyrotoxicosis caused by Graves' disease (20,21), and in an even higher percentage of patients with Graves' thyrotoxicosis who become hypothyroid after radioiodine treatment (25). They also are high in about 20% to 25% of patients with thyroid carcinoma (26,27), and in 10% to 20% of patients with nodular goiter (10,11), but are undetectable or present in low concentrations in patients with subacute thyroiditis (11). The presence of high serum anti-Tg antibody concentrations in patients with thyroid carcinoma limits the value of measurements of serum Tg as a tumor marker in these patients (see Chapter 14).

Among patients with chronic autoimmune thyroiditis, serum anti-Tg antibody concentrations are high less often than are serum anti-TPO antibody concentrations (Fig. 15.1) (10,11), and therefore serum anti-Tg antibodies should not be measured routinely in these patients. A few patients with this disorder, however, have normal serum anti-TPO antibody concentrations but high serum anti-Tg antibody concentrations (27,28).

ANTITHYROID PEROXIDASE ANTIBODIES

Structure and Functions of Thyroid Peroxidase

Thyroid peroxidase (TPO) is a poorly glycosylated membrane-bound enzyme that contains a heme group (29). The human TPO gene encodes an approximately 100 kDa protein composed of 933 amino acids (29). TPO is expressed on the apical membrane of thyrocytes, directly facing the colloid, where it catalyzes iodine oxidation and iodination of tyrosyl residues of Tg (see section on thyroid hormone synthesis in Chapter 4) (2,29).

Antibodies reacting with an antigen located in the cytoplasm and at the apical surface of thyrocytes were originally identified by immunofluorescence (29). The antigen was originally called the "microsomal antigen," based on the apparent subcellular localization of most of the staining. Subsequent studies revealed the antigen to be TPO, and the antibodies are measured now as TPO antibodies.

Immunodominant Epitopes of Thyroid Peroxidase

Anti-TPO antibodies have an IgG subclass distribution similar to that of anti-Tg antibodies (29,30). The major immunogenic region of TPO is located near the carboxyl-terminal end of the molecule. Most human anti-TPO antibodies bind to conformational epitopes in this region of TPO, although some react with linear epitopes (30–33). There are some differences in epitope recognition between the anti-TPO antibodies found in patients with AITD and those found in occasional normal subjects, suggesting that recognition of specific epitopes may have pathogenic importance (34). Unlike anti-Tg antibodies, anti-TPO antibodies do not display a high degree of epitope spreading (30).

Importance of Antithyroid Peroxidase Antibodies in the Pathogenesis of Autoimmune Thyroid Disease

There is little evidence that anti-TPO antibodies play a role in the pathogenesis of AITD, but they are more likely to be of pathogenic importance than anti-Tg antibodies, for several reasons. Serum anti-TPO antibody concentrations are correlated with the active phase of the disease in patients with chronic autoimmune thyroiditis (29,30). More patients with chronic autoimmune thyroiditis have high serum anti-TPO antibody concentrations than high anti-Tg antibody concentrations (Fig. 15.1) (10,11,27). Anti-TPO antibodies can fix complement, and they can bind to thyrocytes and kill them *in vitro*; if similarly active *in vivo*, they could contribute to the development of hypothyroidism (35–37). However, in one study there was no correlation between the level of cytotoxic activity and anti-TPO antibody concentration in serum (36).

Formation of immune complexes containing thyroid-directed antibodies may be involved in cell damage (38–40). Deposits of immune complexes have been found along the basal membrane of thyrocytes, both in Graves' disease and chronic autoimmune thyroiditis, and the complexes contained terminal components of complement, suggesting the formation of membrane attack complexes (38). Circulating soluble immune complexes containing small amounts of Tg and anti-Tg antibodies, but not TPO and anti-TPO antibodies, have been found in patients with AITD (38). These immune complexes could activate the killer T cells that mediate antibody-dependent cell-mediated cytotoxicity (38). Passive infusion of serum from patients with chronic autoimmune thyroiditis that contained high concentrations of complement-fixing anti-TPO antibodies into monkeys did not cause thyroid injury (41).

With respect to possible anti-TPO antibody-mediated inhibition of TPO activity, infants of mothers with chronic autoimmune thyroiditis and high serum anti-TPO antibody concentrations have normal thyroid function, despite transplacental transfer of the antibodies to the infants (42). Serum containing anti-TPO antibodies inhibited the enzymatic activity of TPO *in vitro* in some but not other studies (43–46). However, when present, the inhibition was not dose dependent and was unrelated to the thyroid function of the donors.

Serum Antithyroid Peroxidase Antibody Assay in Various Conditions

Several methods are available to measure anti-TPO antibodies in serum (47). Most early studies were done using immunofluorescence or passive agglutination, and, as for anti-Tg antibodies, the results were reported as positive or negative or as antibody titers. These methods have been replaced by RIA, IRMA, ELISA and chemiluminescence methods, with the results being reported quantitatively (usually as units per milliliter of serum) (47).

About 10% of normal adults have high serum anti-TPO antibody concentrations, and the prevalence increases to up to 30% in the elderly (Fig. 15.1) (see Chapter 19) (24,47,48). The concentrations are high in 10% to 20% of patients with nodular goiter or thyroid carcinoma, about 75% of patients with Graves' thyrotoxicosis, and nearly all (> 90%) patients with chronic autoimmune thyroiditis (47). Serum anti-TPO antibody concentrations are not correlated with thyroid function or type of thyroid disease; the concentrations can be similarly high in patients with chronic autoimmune thyroiditis and Graves' disease (47). The concentrations decrease during antithyroid drug therapy in patients with Graves' thyrotoxicosis,

but measurements are not helpful in predicting the outcome of thyrotoxicosis after withdrawal of antithyroid drug therapy (49). Serum anti-TPO antibody concentrations levels may decrease during T_4 therapy in patients with chronic autoimmune thyroiditis, especially in those with atrophic thyroiditis (see Chapter 47) (50). In contrast, the concentrations rise transiently in patients with thyrotoxicosis after radioiodine therapy, probably due to massive release of thyroid antigens (51). The presence of a high serum anti-TPO antibody concentration during the first trimester of pregnancy may predict the occurrence of postpartum thyroiditis, and the concentrations are high in women with postpartum thyroiditis (see Chapter 27).

Regardless of the assay used, high serum anti-TPO antibody concentrations are more commonly found than high serum anti-Tg antibody concentrations in patients with AITD (Fig. 15.1) (10,11,27). In addition, as mentioned earlier, some patients have high serum anti-TPO antibody concentrations but normal serum anti-Tg antibody concentrations, although the opposite is rare (27,28). Therefore, measurement of serum anti-TPO antibodies is a more sensitive test of thyroid autoimmunity, and it should be the main diagnostic tool for the identification of the autoimmune origin of thyroid disease (Table 15.1).

ANTIBODIES THAT REACT WITH BOTH THYROGLOBULIN AND THYROID PEROXIDASE

Some antibodies react with both Tg and TPO. In mice, these Tg-TPO antibodies can be induced by immunization with Tg, but not with TPO (52). In a large multicenter study, high serum Tg-TPO antibody concentrations were found in approximately 40% of patients with chronic autoimmune thyroiditis, 35% of patients with Graves' disease, 15% of those with postpartum thyroiditis, and 20% of patients with thyroid carcinoma (53). The proportions were slightly higher in another, smaller study (54). These antibodies may react with other unrelated antigens besides Tg and TPO, e.g., a Tg-TPO antibody cloned from an IgG gene combinatory library constructed from B cells infiltrating the thyroid of a patient with a high serum Tg-TPO antibody concentration bound Tg, TPO, and other unrelated thyroid antigens (55).

ANTIBODIES TO THE SECOND COLLOID ANTIGEN

Antibodies that bind to a colloid antigen other than Tg, known as the second colloid antigen (CA2), have been found in the serum of patients with AITD and occasionally other thyroid disorders (56). These antibodies were detected by immunofluorescence on sections of fixed thyroid tissue. The biochemical properties and function of this antigen have not been characterized.

ANTIBODIES TO CELL SURFACE ANTIGENS OTHER THAN THYROID PEROXIDASE AND THYROTROPIN RECEPTORS

Antibodies capable of binding to antigens on the surface of thyrocytes have been detected by immunofluorescence and by mixed hemadsorption using cultured thyrocytes (57). TPO antibodies and TSHR antibodies would be expected to be detected by these techniques, as would megalin, a recently identified thyroid protein (58).

Antibodies to Megalin

Megalin, also known as gp330, is a multiligand receptor expressed in several organs (9); in the thyroid it can be found on the apical surface of thyrocytes, where it functions as a receptor for Tg and is then responsible for Tg transcytosis across thyrocytes (59). Thyroglobulin that is carried across thyrocytes by megalin enters the circulation complexed with components of megalin (13). Thus, when transcytosis is increased, the immune system may be exposed to large amounts of megalin, which may induce antibody production. Indeed, the ability of megalin to induce antibodies in rats with Heymann nephritis prompted the search for megalin antibodies in the serum of patients with AITD (58). Using flow cytometry to measure binding of serum IgG to megalin expressed on cultured cells, antibodies to megalin were detected in 50% of patients with chronic autoimmune thyroiditis and in some patients with Graves' disease and thyroid carcinoma, but not in normal subjects. These IgGs also precipitated megalin extracted from cells. The pathogenic role or clinical importance of megalin antibodies is not known.

ANTIBODIES TO THYROID HORMONES

Antibodies reacting with T_4 and T_3 are present in the serum of some patients with chronic autoimmune thyroiditis and Graves' disease, and rarely in patients with other thyroid diseases (60,61). The appearance of these antibodies in the serum seems to be related to massive exposure of the immune system to the hormonogenic epitopes of Tg (62,63). Anti-T_4 and anti-T_3 antibodies can also be found in the serum of patients with non-organ-specific autoimmune diseases, including Sjögren's syndrome and rheumatoid arthritis, suggesting that cross-reacting epitopes are present in connective tissue (61).

Anti-T_4 and anti-T_3 antibodies are not commonly measured in the clinical practice, and their importance is related mainly to the fact that they can interfere with measurement of T_4 and T_3, thereby causing either falsely high or low values, depending on the method used for measurements of serum T_4 and T_3 (Table 15.1) (see Chapter 13).

ANTIBODIES TO THE SODIUM IODIDE SYMPORTER

The sodium iodide symporter (NIS) is a membrane protein belonging to the superfamily of ion transporters. It is expressed on the basolateral surface of thyrocytes, where it mediates entry of iodide ions into the cells (see section of thyroid iodine transport in Chapter 4) (64). Investigations on NIS as a thyroid autoantigen stemmed from findings suggesting that serum immunoglobulins inhibited iodide uptake by thyrocytes (64). However, subsequent studies indicated that the inhibition of iodide transport was not mediated by immunoglobulins (65,66).

Antibodies against the NIS protein have been detected in serum from patients with AITD using several techniques (64). The frequency of detection of these antibodies in the serum of patients with thyroid disease has varied, from approximately 5% to 25%, depending on the criteria used to define a positive test (67); when present, their epitope specificity is limited (68). Thus, anti-NIS antibodies seem to be rather rare and of little pathophysiologic importance.

OTHER ANTIBODIES

Antibodies to *Yersinia Enterocolitica*

Antibodies against constituents of *Yersinia enterocolitica* have been implicated in the pathogenesis of Graves' disease, based on similarities between the envelope of this organism and the TSHR (69). However, anti-*Yersinia* antibodies can be found not only in patients with Graves' disease, but also in patients with chronic autoimmune thyroiditis (69), and therefore they are not clearly related to TSHR antibodies. In addition, there is no evidence that Graves' disease or any other AITD is more common in patients with *Yersinia* infection, as compared with those with no evidence of *Yersinia* infection (69).

Antibodies to Antigens Shared by Thyroid and Orbital Tissue

Based on the hypothesis that the pathogenesis of Graves' ophthalmopathy is related to immunologic cross-reactivity against antigenic determinants shared by thyroid and orbital tissue (70), several investigators have attempted to identify and characterize the responsible antigens and the antibodies directed against these antigens. The search has led to the identification of several possible autoimmune targets in extraocular muscle and thyroid tissue, among which at least three have been characterized: a 67 kDa protein, the flavoprotein subunit of mitochondrial succinate dehydrogenase (71); a 55 kDa protein, G2s (72); and a 63 kDa protein, calsequestrin (73). Serum antibodies against these proteins have been detected in some patients with Graves' ophthalmopathy, patients with Graves' thyrotoxicosis but no ophthalmopathy, patients with chronic autoimmune thyroiditis, and normal subjects (71–73). These antibodies could be markers of muscle damage in patients with ophthalmopathy, but their prevalence in patients with ophthalmopathy is relatively low (30% to 70% in various studies), it is almost as high in patients with the other disorders listed in the preceding sentence, and it is as high as 15% of normal subjects and patients with unrelated diseases.

Antibodies to Thyrotropin

Serum antibodies against thyrotropin (TSH) have been detected in a few patients (74), usually in patients who had some type of AITD and in whom the measured serum TSH concentration was not the expected value.

THYROTROPIN RECEPTOR ANTIBODIES

TSHR antibodies have a direct pathogenic role in AITD. In patients with Graves' thyrotoxicosis, TSHR antibodies act as a TSH agonist and activate TSHRs in the same way TSH does. In a proportion of patients with chronic autoimmune thyroiditis, TSHR antibodies have a TSH antagonist action. As a result of these different properties, and variations in methods of detection, the nomenclature of TSHR antibodies is complex (Table 15.1). TSHR antibodies that are measured by their ability to inhibit the binding of TSH to TSH receptors *in vitro* are called TSH-binding inhibitory immunoglobulins (TBII). TSHR antibodies that are measured by their ability to stimulate cyclic adenosine monophosphate production (cyclic AMP) in cultured cells expressing TSHRs (either thyrocytes or other cell types transfected with TSHR cDNA) are called thyroid-stimulating antibodies (TSHR-SAb). TSHR antibodies that are measured by their ability to inhibit the action of TSH in cultured cells expressing TSH receptors are called thyroid-stimulating-blocking antibodies (TSHR-BAb).

Thyrotropin Receptor Structure and Functions

The TSH receptor is a member of the G-protein-coupled family of receptors, and, like other members of this family, its structure is characterized by seven transmembrane-spanning domains linked by three sets of alternating intracellular and extracellular loops, a relatively large amino-terminal extracellular tail, and a carboxyl-terminal cytoplasmic tail (75,76). The human TSHR gene is located on chromosome

14, and it encodes a 744-amino-acid molecule, with a molecular weight of 84 kDa, approximately 35 kDa of which is carbohydrate. The receptor is highly homologous among different species, which allows the use of TSH receptors from species other than humans for *in vitro* assays of TSHR antibodies (see section on the thyrotropin receptor in Chapter 10 and the section on pathogenesis of Graves' disease in Chapter 23) (75,76).

High-affinity TSH binding sites are located in the extracellular domain of the TSHR, whereas its transmembrane and intracellular regions are involved in signal transduction (75,76). Binding of TSH to the extracellular domain of the receptor at the basolateral surface of thyrocytes results in conformational modifications that lead to high-affinity interactions of the cytoplasmic tail with guanine nucleotide-binding (G) proteins, which ultimately triggers intracellular signaling (see section on biological actions of thyrotropin in Chapter 10) (75,76).

Thyrotropin Receptor Antibody Interactions with Thyrotropin Receptors

Proposed models of the TSHR suggest the existence of a TSH-binding pocket in the extracellular domain, which contains major conformational binding sites for both TSH and TSHR antibodies (75,76). Although the binding sites for TSHR antibodies and TSH overlap and encompass much of the extracellular domain of the receptor, they are not identical. Thus, the major functional epitopes for TSHR-SAb binding are located in the extreme amino-terminal portion of the extracellular domain of the receptor, whereas TSHR-BAb bind more to the carboxyl-terminal portion of the extracellular domain closer to the cell membrane (75–81). However, TSHR antibodies are heterogeneous in terms of epitope recognition, possibly due to epitope spreading during the immune response (75–82). Whether and to what extent glycosylation of the extracellular domain of the TSHR affects its recognition by antibodies is uncertain. Although glycosylation is certainly fundamental for correct folding of the receptor during biosynthesis, variations in oligosaccharide content of the receptor do not much alter the binding of TSHR-SAb from patients with Graves' thyrotoxicosis (83), but some glycosylation of the extracellular domain of the receptor is necessary for antibody recognition (84).

Shedding of the amino-terminal 310 amino-acid residues of the extracellular domain of the TSHR (the A subunit) may either initiate or amplify the immune response against the receptor, and epitopes recognized by TSHR-SAb are partially sterically hindered on the holoreceptor on the plasma membrane (85,86). Thus, TSHR-SAb from patients with Graves' thyrotoxicosis react to a greater extent with a chimeric A subunit-fusion protein, as compared with the wild type holoreceptor (both transfected in cultured cells), suggesting better recognition of the A subunit by TSHR-SAb when this portion of the receptor is not in its native conformation, as should occur after shedding (85). In addition, immunization of mice with the A subunit of the receptor results in a greater proportion of TSHR antibodies with stimulating activity, as compared with immunization with the wild type holoreceptor (86).

Biological Actions of Thyrotropin Receptor Antibodies

Thyrotropin Receptor–Stimulating Antibodies

TSHR-SAb are TSH agonists, and they are the cause of thyrotoxicosis and goiter in patients with Graves' disease. TSHR-SAb are oligoclonal or pauciclonal, based on isoelectric focusing studies, IgG1-subclass restriction, and light-chain restriction (75,76). Indeed, monoclonal TSHR-SAb have been reported to be produced by lymphocytes from patients with Graves' thyrotoxicosis (87), a human monoclonal TSHR-SAb has been purified and characterized (88), and several monoclonal TSHR-SAb have been produced in mice immunized with the TSHR or TSHR cDNA (89–91). TSHR-SAb that are IgG4 subclass also exist (92).

TSHR-SAb stimulate adenylyl cyclase activity, iodide uptake, TPO and Tg synthesis, and T_4 and T_3 release by thyrocytes, as well as growth, DNA accumulation, and mitotic activity in thyrocytes (93–96). Like TSH, TSHR-SAb exert most of their biological effects via the cyclic AMP pathway, and to a lesser extent via the phosphoinositol pathway (75,76).

Thyrotropin Receptor–Blocking Antibodies

TSHR-BAb bind to TSHRs and block the action of TSH. They contribute to the development of hypothyroidism in some patients with atrophic chronic autoimmune thyroiditis and occasional patients with goitrous chronic autoimmune thyroiditis (97). Unlike TSHR-SAb, TSHR-BAb are not subclass restricted and are therefore likely to have a polyclonal origin (98). TSHR-BAb act by blocking binding of TSH to TSHRs, thereby reducing the stimulating actions of TSH on thyroid cells, such as cyclic AMP production, iodine uptake and organification, and cell growth (75,76,99).

Serum Assays for Thyrotropin Receptor Antibodies in Various Conditions

As mentioned above, serum TSHR antibodies can be measured by two major types of assays, radioreceptor assays, by which it is not possible to distinguish whether the antibodies are stimulating or blocking antibodies, and *in vitro* bioassays, by which it is possible to determine the biologic activity (stimulating or blocking) of the antibodies.

Radioreceptor Assays

Radioreceptor assays measure the inhibition of binding of labeled TSH to TSHRs; as mentioned above, TSHR antibodies measured in this way are called TSHR-binding inhibitory antibodies (TBII). The assays for TBII are based on the ability or serum or the IgG fraction of serum to inhibit the binding of labeled TSH to porcine TSHRs, TSHRs purified from Chinese hamster ovary (CHO) cells transfected with recombinant human TSHR cDNA (100), or TSHRs expressed in leukemic cells transfected with human TSHR cDNA (101). With the latter assay, TBII can be detected in up to 99% of patients with untreated Graves' thyrotoxicosis, approximately 90% of patients with Graves' thyrotoxicosis treated with methimazole, 50% of patients with Graves' thyrotoxicosis who are in remission after cessation of methimazole therapy, 15% of patients with chronic autoimmune thyroiditis, and 0.5% of normal subjects (Fig. 15.2) (101). The prevalence of high values in patients with Graves' disease using the latter assay is clearly higher than that reported in studies in which older methods were used (99,102).

In Vitro *Bioassays for Thyrotropin Receptor Antibodies*

In vitro bioassays for TSHR antibodies are mainly based on measurements of cyclic AMP production in rat thyrocytes (FRTL5 cells) or in CHO cells transfected with human TSHR cDNA (103–105). Unlike assays for TBII, these assays are not widely available.

TSHR-SAb assays measure the ability of serum or serum IgG to increase cyclic AMP production by cultured cells (103–105). Using these assays TSHR-SAb can be detected in the serum of about 90% of patients with Graves' thyrotoxicosis at the time of diagnosis (103–105). Assays using CHO cells transfected with human TSHR cDNA are more sensitive than those using FRTL5 cells, probably because of the use of human rather than rat TSHRs (104). Using transfected CHO cells, TSHR-SAb can be detected in up to 95% of patients with Graves' thyrotoxicosis at the time of diagnosis; approximately 90% of patients with Graves' thyrotoxicosis treated with methimazole, but still thyrotoxic; 60% of patients with Graves' thyrotoxicosis who are taking methimazole and are euthyroid; and 35% of patients with Graves' thyrotoxicosis who remain euthyroid after cessation of methimazole (Fig. 15.2) (104).

In general, there is a good correlation between serum TBII and TSHR-SAb values in patients with Graves' thyrotoxicosis (106). The presence of TBII activity but not TSHR-SAb activity is indicative of atrophic chronic autoimmune thyroiditis, and many of these patients have high serum TSHR-BAb activity (107).

TSHR-BAb assays measure the ability of the whole serum or of serum IgG to inhibit the TSH-stimulated increase of cyclic AMP production in cultured cells express-

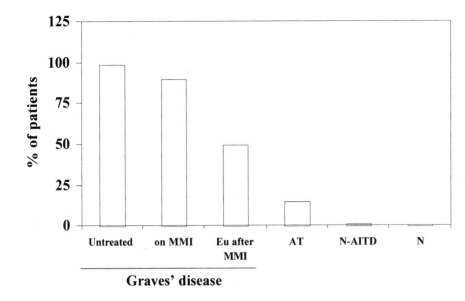

FIGURE 15.2. Frequency of high serum TSH-binding inhibitory immunoglobulin *(TBII)* activity in patients with Graves' thyrotoxicosis, autoimmune thyroiditis *(AT)*, non-autoimmune thyroid disease *(N-AITD)*, and in normal subjects *(N)*. On MMI, patients studied during methimazole therapy; Eu after MMI, patients remaining euthyroid after cessation of methimazole therapy. (From Costagliola S, Morgenthaler NG, Hoermann R, et al. Second generation assay for thyrotropin receptor antibodies has superior diagnostic sensitivity for Graves' disease. *J Clin Endocrinol Metab* 1999;84:90, with modifications.)

ing TSHRs (99,105). For TSHR-SAb assays, the cell types used are FRTL5 cells and CHO cells transfected with TSHR cDNA (99,105). In addition, primary cultures of human or porcine thyrocytes can be used. As for TSHR-SAb, the CHO cell-based system provides greater sensitivity (99). With this type of assay, TSHR-BAb can be detected in the serum of approximately 65% of patients with atrophic chronic autoimmune thyroiditis, 25% of patients with goitrous chronic autoimmune thyroiditis who have overt hypothyroidism, and 10% of patients with goitrous chronic autoimmune thyroiditis who have subclinical hypothyroidism, whereas they are undetectable in normal subjects (Fig. 15.2) (97).

Coexistence of Thyrotropin Receptor–Stimulating and –Blocking Antibodies

TSHR antibodies with stimulating and blocking activity have been found at the same or different times in some patients with AITD (107,108). These patients may have hypothyroidism, and high serum TSHR-BAb activity, at one time, and thyrotoxicosis, and high serum TSHR-SAb activity, at another time (107,108). In rare patients, most of whom have thyrotoxicosis, both activities can be detected at the same time. The coexistence of TSHR-SAb and TSHR-BAb is suggested by a biphasic dose-response curve in the TSHR-SAb assay.

Clinical Value of Measurements of Thyrotropin Receptor Antibodies

Most patients with Graves' thyrotoxicosis have positive serum tests for TBII and TSHR-SAb (Fig. 15.2 and Fig.

15.3) (99–106). Nevertheless, the diagnostic value of measurements of serum TSHR antibodies in serum is rather limited (Table 15.1). Thus, the presence of a diffuse goiter, and especially signs of Graves' ophthalmopathy, and measurements of serum TSH and free T_4 are sufficient to confirm a diagnosis of Graves' thyrotoxicosis in the majority of patients.

Serum assays for TBII may, however, be useful in certain patients, for example euthyroid patients with ophthalmopathy, patients with the nodular variant of Graves' disease, and pregnant women with either Graves' thyrotoxicosis of chronic autoimmune thyroiditis. In euthyroid patients with ophthalmopathy and in those with nodular goiter and thyrotoxicosis, the presence of TBII in the serum helps to demonstrate that the patient's ophthalmopathy or thyrotoxicosis is caused by Graves' disease (70). In pregnant women, transplacental passage of TSHR-SAb or TSHR-BAb can result in transient fetal and neonatal thyrotoxicosis or hypothyroidism (109–112); measurements of maternal serum TBII are helpful in assessing the likelihood of fetal or neonatal thyrotoxicosis in pregnant women with Graves' thyrotoxicosis (even if treated with thyroidectomy or radioiodine and taking T_4) and the likelihood of neonatal hypothyroidism in pregnant women with hypothyroidism and chronic autoimmune thyroiditis (see section on congenital hypothyroidism in Chapter 75 and Chapter 76). The tests should be done in the third trimester. If the maternal serum TBII value is high, serum TSHR-SAb or TSHR-BAb can be measured. The risk of neonatal thyrotoxicosis is very low unless maternal serum TBII and TSHR-SAb activity is very high (112).

Among postpartum women with thyrotoxicosis, measurements of serum TSHR antibodies may help to distinguish between Graves' thyrotoxicosis and postpartum thyroiditis as the cause of the thyrotoxicosis (see Chapter 27) (113). Women with postpartum thyroiditis may have high

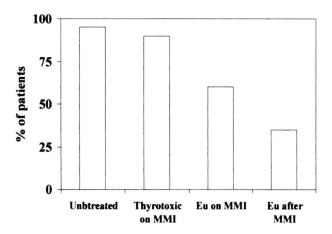

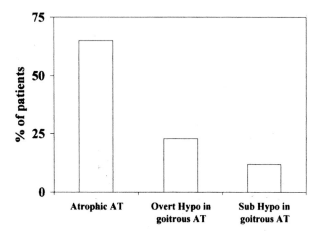

FIGURE 15.3. Frequency of high serum TSH receptor antibody activity in patients with Graves' thyrotoxicosis **(top)** and chronic autoimmune thyroiditis **(bottom)**. In the top panel, the antibodies were measured as TSH receptor–stimulating antibodies (TSHR-SAb). In the bottom panel, the antibodies were measured as TSH receptor–blocking antibodies (TSHR-BAb). AT, autoimmune thyroiditis; Eu, euthyroid; Hypo, hypothyroidism; MMI, methimazole; Sub Hypo, subclinical hypothyroidism. (From Chiovato L, Vitti P, Bendinelli G, et al. Detection of antibodies blocking thyrotropin effect using Chinese hamster ovary cells transfected with the cloned human TSH receptor. *J Endocrinol Invest* 1994;17:809, with modifications; and Costagliola S, Morgenthaler NG, Hoermann R, et al. Second generation assay for thyrotropin receptor antibodies has superior diagnostic sensitivity for Graves' disease. *J Clin Endocrinol Metab* 1999;84:90, with modifications.)

with Graves' thyrotoxicosis, serum TBII and TSHR-SAb activity decline during antithyroid drug therapy (116), and the decline is greater in patients who remain euthyroid after cessation of therapy. The risk of later recurrence of thyrotoxicosis may be lower in those patients in whom serum TBII or TSHR-SAb activity disappears, but the issue is debated (102,117–120). Overall, the presence of high levels of serum TSHR antibodies at the end of antithyroid drug therapy has a high positive predictive value (98%) and specificity (73% to 99%) for relapse of thyrotoxicosis, but a low negative predictive value (47%) and sensitivity (28% to 49%) (117,119). Whether measurements of serum TBII or TSHR-SAb activity at the start antithyroid drug therapy have predictive value is a matter of debate (102, 117,120,121).

Thyroid Growth–Promoting and –Blocking Antibodies

The extent of thyroid enlargement varies substantially among patients with Graves' disease and those with chronic autoimmune thyroiditis, and years ago some investigators obtained evidence for the presence of serum antibodies that stimulated thyroid growth or inhibited the growth-stimulating action of TSH, without affecting cyclic AMP production (122). However, subsequent studies have not confirmed the existence of thyroid growth-promoting or growth-blocking antibodies (96,122).

MEASUREMENT OF THYROID-DIRECTED ANTIBODIES IN CLINICAL PRACTICE

Measurements of thyroid-directed antibodies in serum can be clinically useful in the evaluation of some patients with chronic autoimmune thyroiditis or Graves' disease (Table 15.1). Measurements of serum anti-TPO antibodies are more useful in evaluating patients suspected to have chronic autoimmune thyroiditis than are measurements of serum anti-Tg antibodies, and the latter measurement is indicated only if suspicion of the disorder is high and the patient's serum anti-TPO antibody concentration is normal. Measurements of serum anti-TPO antibodies in pregnant women are useful in estimating the risk of postpartum thyroiditis, but it is debated whether it should be performed routinely. Serum anti-Tg antibodies should be measured whenever serum Tg is measured, especially in patients with thyroid carcinoma, because serum Tg cannot be measured reliably when anti-Tg antibodies are present (see Chapter 14).

Measurements of serum TBII can help to identify, or exclude, Graves' disease as a cause of thyrotoxicosis, but other clinical parameters serve the same purpose in most instances. However, these measurements may be helpful in confirming, or excluding, the presence of Graves' disease in

serum TSHR-BAb activity during the hypothyroid phase of the illness (113), but measurements of TBII or TSHR-BAb are rarely indicated.

The occasional presence of serum TSHR-SAb in euthyroid patients with diffuse goiter or a family history of AITD can forecast the development of Graves' thyrotoxicosis (114). Similarly, occasional patients with subclinical thyrotoxicosis have high levels of serum TBII or TSHR-SAb activity, indicating that the cause of the subclinical thyrotoxicosis is Graves' disease (115). Among patients

patients with a nodular goiter and euthyroid patients with ophthalmopathy, and for assessing the risk of fetal or neonatal thyrotoxicosis or hypothyroidism in pregnant women with Graves' disease or chronic autoimmune thyroiditis, respectively.

ACKNOWLEDGMENTS

We are grateful to Dr. Francesco Latrofa for his critical reading of the manuscript and helpful suggestions.

REFERENCES

1. Weetman AP, McGregor AM. Autoimmune thyroid disease: further developments in our understanding. *Endocr Rev* 1994; 15:788.
2. Dunn JT, Dunn AD. Thyroglobulin: chemistry, biosynthesis and proteolysis. In: Braverman LE, Utiger LD, eds. *Werner and Ingbar's The thyroid: a fundamental and clinical text*. 8th ed. Philadelphia: Lippincott Williams & Wilkins, 2000:91.
3. Schneider PB. Thyroidal iodine heterogeneity: "last come, first served" system of iodine turnover. *Endocrinology* 1964;74:973.
4. Berndorfer U, Wilms H, Herzog V. Multimerization of thyroglobulin (TG) during extracellular storage: isolation of highly cross-linked TG from human thyroids. *J Clin Endocrinol Metab* 1996;81:1918.
5. Rose NR, Burek CL. Autoantibodies to thyroglobulin in health and disease. *Appl Biochem Biotechnol* 2000;83:245.
6. Saboori AM, Rose NR, Bresler HS, et al. Iodination of human thyroglobulin (Tg) alters its immunoreactivity. I. Iodination alters multiple epitopes of human Tg. *Clin Exp Immunol* 1998; 113:297.
7. Tomer Y. Anti-thyroglobulin autoantibodies in autoimmune thyroid diseases: cross-reactive or pathogenic? *Clin Immunol Immunopathol* 1997;82:3.
8. Bresler HS, Burek CL, Hoffman WH, et al. Autoantigenic determinants on human thyroglobulin. II. Determinants recognized by autoantibodies from patients with autoimmune thyroiditis compared to autoantibodies from healthy subjects *Clin Immunol Immunopathol* 1990;54:76.
9. Marinò M, McCluskey RT. Role of thyroglobulin endocytic pathways in the control of thyroid hormone release. *Am J Physiol* 2000;279:C1295.
10. Mariotti S, Pisani S, Russova A, et al. A new solid-phase immunoradiometric assay for anti-thyroglobulin autoantibody. *J Endocrinol Invest* 1982;5:227.
11. Spencer CA. Thyroglobulin. In: Braverman LE, Utiger LD, eds. *Werner and Ingbar's The thyroid: a fundamental and clinical text*. 8th ed. Philadelphia: Lippincott Williams & Wilkins, 2000:402.
12. Chiovato L, Latrofa F, Braverman LE, et al. Disappearance of humoral thyroid autoimmunity after complete removal of thyroid antigens. *Ann Intern Med* 2003;139:346.
13. Marinò M, Chiovato L, Mitsiades N, et al. Circulating thyroglobulin derived from transcytosis is combined with a secretory component of its endocytic receptor megalin. *J Clin Endocrinol Metab* 2000;85:3458.
14. Druetta L, Bornet H, Sassolas G, et al. Identification of thyroid hormone residues on serum thyroglobulin: a clue to the source of circulating thyroglobulin in thyroid diseases. *Eur J Endocrinol* 1999;140:457.
15. Caturegli P, Kuppers RC, Mariotti S, al. IgG subclass distribution of thyroglobulin antibodies in patients with thyroid disease. *Clin Exp Immunol* 1994;98:464.
16. McIntosh RS, Weetman AP. Molecular analysis of the antibody response to thyroglobulin and thyroid peroxidase. *Thyroid* 1997;7:471.
17. Yativ N, Buskila D, Blank M et al. The detection of anti-thyroglobulin activity in human serum monoclonal immunoglobulins (monoclonal gammopathies). *Immunol Res* 1993;12:330.
18. Rose NR, Kong YM, Okayasu I, et al. T-cell regulation in autoimmune thyroiditis. *Immunol Rev* 1981;55:299.
19. Dietrich G, Kazatchkine MD. Normal immunoglobulin G (IgG) for therapeutic use (intravenous Ig) contain anti-idiotypic specificities against an immunodominant, disease associated, cross-reactive, idiotype of human anti-thyroglobulin autoantibodies. *J Clin Invest* 1990;85:620.
20. Jordan SC, Buckingham B, Sakai R, et al. Studies of immune-complex glomerulonephritis mediated by human thyroglobulin. *N Engl J Med* 1981;304:1212.
21. Lazarus JH, Hall R, Othman S, et al. The clinical spectrum of postpartum thyroid disease. *QJM* 1996;89:429.
22. Nakamura RM, Weigle WO. Transfer of experimental autoimmune thyroiditis by serum from thyroidectomized donors. *J Exp Med* 1969;130:263.
23. Feldt-Rasmussen U. Analytical and clinical preformance goals for testing autoantibodies to thyroperoxidase, thyroglobulin, and thyrotropin receptor. *Clin Chem* 1996;42:160.
24. Mariotti S, Sansoni P, Barbesino G, et al. Thyroid and other organ-specific autoantibodies in healthy centenarians. *Lancet* 1992;339:1506.
25. Marcocci C, Gianchecchi D, Masini I, et al. A reappraisal of the role of methimazole and other factors on the efficacy and outcome of radioiodine therapy of Graves' thyrotoxicosis. *J Endocrinol Invest* 1990;13:513.
26. Spencer CA, Takeuchi M, Kazarosyan M, et al. Serum thyroglobulin autoantibodies: prevalence, influence of serum thyroglobulin measurement, and prognostic significance in patients with differentiated thyroid carcinoma. *J Clin Endocrinol Metab* 1998;83:1121.
27. Mariotti S, Barbesino G, Caturegli P, et al. Assay of thyroglobulin in serum with thyroglobulin autoantibodies: an unobtainable goal? *J Clin Endocrinol Metab* 1995;80:468.
28. Mariotti S, Barbesino G, Caturegli P, et al. False negative results observed in anti-thyroid peroxidase autoantibody determination by competitive radioimmunoassays using monoclonal antibodies. *Eur J Endocrinol* 1994;130:552.
29. McLachlan SM, Rapoport B. The molecular biology of thyroid peroxidase: cloning, expression and role as autoantigen in autoimmune thyroid disease. *Endocr Rev* 1992;13:192.
30. McLachlan SM, Rapoport B. Autoimmune response to the thyroid in humans: thyroid peroxidase—the common autoantigenic denominator. *Int Rev Immunol* 2000;19:587.
31. Pichurin P, Guo J, Yan X, et al. Human monoclonal autoantibodies to B-cell epitopes outside the thyroid peroxidase autoantibody immunodominant region. *Thyroid* 2001;11:301.
32. Guo J, Wang Y, Jaume JC, et al. Rarity of autoantibodies to a major autoantigen, thyroid peroxidase, that interact with denatured antigen or with epitopes outside the immunodominant region. *Clin Exp Immunol* 1999;117:19.
33. Tonacchera M, Cetani F, Costagliola S, et al. Mapping thyroid peroxidase epitopes using recombinant protein fragments. *Eur J Endocrinol* 1995;132:53.
34. Grennan Jones F, Ziemnicka K, Sanders J, et al. Analysis of autoantibody epitopes on human thyroid peroxidase. *Autoimmunity* 1999;30:157.

35. Guo J, Jaume JC, Rapoport B, et al. Recombinant thyroid peroxidase-specific Fab converted to immunoglobulin G (IgG) molecules: evidence for thyroid cell damage by IgG1, but not IgG4, autoantibodies. *J Clin Endocrinol Metab* 1997;82:925.

36. Chiovato L, Bassi P, Santini F, et al. Antibodies producing complement-mediated thyroid cytotoxicity in patients with atrophic or goitrous autoimmune thyroiditis. *J Clin Endocrinol Metab* 1993;77:1700.

37. Khoury EL, Bottazzo GF, Roitt IM. The thyroid microsomal antibody revisited. Its paradoxical binding in vivo to the apical surface of the follicula epithelium. *J Exp Med* 1984;159:577.

38. Kalderon AE, Bogaars HA. Immune complex deposits in Graves' disease and Hashimoto's thyroiditis. *Am J Med* 1977; 63:729.

39. Rodien P, Madec AM, Ruf J, et al. Antibody-dependent cell-mediated cytotoxicity in autoimmune thyroid disease: relationship to antithyroperoxidase antibodies. *J Endocrinol Invest* 1996;81:2595.

40. Bogner U, Kotulla P, Peters H, et al. Thyroid peroxidase/microsomal antibodies are not identical with thyroid cytotoxic antibodies in autoimmune thyroiditis. *Acta Endocrinol (Copenh)* 1990;123:431.

41. Roitt IM, Doniach D. Human auto-immune thyroiditis: serological studies. *Lancet* 1958;2:1027.

42. Dussault JH, Letarte J, Guyda H, et al. Lack of influence of thyroid antibodies on thyroid function in the newborn infant and on a mass screening program for congenital hypothyroidism. *J Pediatr* 1980;96:385.

43. Okamoto Y, Hamada N, Saito H, et al. Thyroid peroxidase activity-inhibiting immunoglobulins in patients with autoimmune thyroid disease. *J Clin Endocrinol Metab* 1989;68:730.

44. Saller B, Hormann R, Mann K. Heterogeneity of autoantibodies against thyroid peroxidase in autoimmune thyroid disease: evidence against antibodies directly inhibiting peroxidase activity as regulatory factors in thyroid hormone metabolism. *J Clin Endocrinol Metab* 1991;72:188.

45. Nishikawa T, Jaume JC, McLachlan SM, et al. Human monoclonal autoantibodies against the immunodominant region on thyroid peroxidase: lack of cross-reactivity with related peroxidases or thyroglobulin and inability to inhibit thyroid peroxidase enzymatic activity. *J Clin Endocrinol Metab* 1995;80:1461.

46. Kohno Y, Naito N, Saito K, et al. Anti-thyroid peroxidase antibody activity in sera of patients with systemic lupus erythematosus. *Clin Exp Immunol* 1989;75:217.

47. Mariotti S, Caturegli P, Piccolo P, et al. Antithyroid peroxidase autoantibodies in thyroid diseases. *J Clin Endocrinol Metab* 1990;71:661.

48. Pedersen IB, Knudsen N, Jorgensen T, et al. Thyroid peroxidase and thyroglobulin autoantibodies in a large survey of populations with mild and moderate iodine deficiency. *Clin Endocrinol (Oxf)* 2003;58:36.

49. Marcocci C, Chiovato L, Mariotti S, et al. Changes of circulating thyroid autoantibody levels during and after therapy with methimazole in patients with Graves' disease. *J Endocrinol Invest* 1982;5:13.

50. Chiovato L, Marcocci C, Mariotti S, et al. L-Thyroxine therapy induces a fall of thyroid microsomal and thyroglobulin antibodies in idiopathic myxedema but not in euthyroid Hashimoto's thyroiditis. *J Endocrinol Invest* 1986;9:299.

51. Einhorn J, Fagraeus A, Jonsson J. Thyroid antibodies after 131-I treatment for hypethyroidism. *J Clin Endocrinol Metab* 1965; 25:1218.

52. Ruf J, Feldt-Rasmussen U, Hegedus L, et al. Bispecific thyroglobulin and thyroperoxidase autoantibodies in patients with various thyroid and autoimmune diseases. *J Clin Endocrinol Metab* 1994;79:1404.

53. Estienne V, Duthoit C, Costanzo VD, et al. Multicenter study on TGPO autoantibody prevalence in various thyroid and nonthyroid diseases; relationships with thyroglobulin and thyroperoxidase autoantibody parameters. *Eur J Endocrinol* 1999; 141:563.

54. Zophel K, Gruning T, Wunderlich G, et al. Clinical value of a bispecific antibody binding to thyroglobulin and thyroperoxidase (TGPO-aAb) in various thyroid diseases. *Autoimmunity* 1999;29:257.

55. Latrofa F, Pichurin P, Guo J, et al. Thyroglobulin-thyroperoxidase autoantibodies are polyreactive, not bispecific: analysis using human monoclonal autoantibodies. *J Clin Endocrinol Metab* 2003;88:371–378.

56. Doniach D, Roitt IM. In: Gell PGH, Coombs RA, Lachmann PJ, eds. *Clinical aspects of immunology.* Oxford: Blackwell Science, 1975:1355.

57. Fagraeus A, Jonsson J. Distribution of organ antigens over the surface of thyroid cells as examined by the immunofluorescence test. *Immunology* 1970;18:413.

58. Marino M, Chiovato L, Friedlander JA, et al. Serum antibodies against megalin (gp330) in patients with autoimmune thyroiditis. *J Clin Endocrinol Metab* 1999;84:2468.

59. Lisi S, Pinchera A, McCluskey RT, et al. Preferential megalin-mediated transcytosis of low hormonogenic thyroglobulin: a novel control mechanism for thyroid hormone release. *Proc Natl Acad Sci USA* 2003;100:148–158.

60. Sakata S, Nakamura S, Miura K. Autoantibodies against thyroid hormones or iodothyronines. *Ann Intern Med* 1985;103: 579.

61. Ruggeri RM, Galletti M, Mandolfino MG, et al. Thyroid hormone autoantibodies in primary Sjogren syndrome and rheumatoid arthritis are more prevalent than in autoimmune thyroid disease, becoming progressively more frequent in these diseases. *J Endocrinol Invest* 2002;25:447–454.

62. Benvenga S, Trimarchi F. Triggering of thyroid hormone autoantibodies. *J R Soc Med* 2003;96:50.

63. Benvenga S, Bartolone L, Squadrito S, et al. Thyroid hormone autoantibodies elicited by diagnostic fine needle biopsy. *J Clin Endocrinol Metab* 1997;82:4217.

64. Dohan O, De la Vieja A, Paroder V, et al. The sodium/iodide symporter (NIS): characterization, regulation, and medical significance. *Endocr Rev* 2003;24:48.

65. Chin HS, Chin DK, Morgenthaler NG, et al. Rarity of anti-Na+/I- symporter (NIS) antibody with iodide uptake inhibiting activity in autoimmune thyroid diseases (AITD). *J Clin Endocrinol Metab* 2000;85:3937.

66. Tonacchera M, Agretti P, Ceccarini G, et al. Autoantibodies from patients with autoimmune thyroid disease do not interfere with the activity of the human iodide symporter gene stably transfected in CHO cells. *Eur J Endocrinol* 2001;144:611.

67. Seissler J, Wagner S, Schott M, et al. Low frequency of autoantibodies to the human Na(+)/I(-) symporter in patients with autoimmune thyroid disease. *J Clin Endocrinol Metab* 2000; 85:4630.

68. Kemp EH, Waterman EA, Ajjan RA, et al. Identification of antigenic domains on the human sodium-iodide symporter which are recognized by autoantibodies from patients with autoimmune thyroid disease. *Clin Exp Immunol* 2001;124:377.

69. Corapcioglu D, Tonyukuk V, Kiyan M, et al. Relationship between thyroid autoimmunity and *Yersinia enterocolitica* antibodies. *Thyroid* 2002;12:613.

70. Prummel MF. Pathogenetic and clinical aspects of endocrine ophthalmopathy. *Exp Clin Endocrinol Diabetes* 1999;107 [Suppl 3]:S75.

71. Kemp EH, Ridgway JN, Smith KA, et al. Autoantibodies to the flavoprotein subunit of succinate dehydrogenase: analysis of

specificity in autoimmune thyroid disease. *Clin Endocrinol (Oxf)* 2000;53:291.

72. Gunji K, De Bellis A, Li AW, et al. Cloning and characterization of the novel thyroid and eye muscle shared protein G2s: autoantibodies against G2s are closely associated with ophthalmopathy in patients with Graves' hyperthyroidism. *J Clin Endocrinol Metab* 2000;85:1641.

73. Gunji K, Kubota S, Stolarski C, et al. A 63 kDa skeletal muscle protein associated with eye muscle inflammation in Graves' disease is identified as the calcium binding protein calsequestrin. *Autoimmunity* 1999;29:1.

74. Akamizu T, Mori T, Kasagi K, et al. Anti-TSH antibody with high specificity to human TSH in sera from patient with Graves' disease: its isolation from, and interaction with, TSH receptor antibodies. *Clin Endocrinol (Oxf)* 1987;26:311.

75. Rapoport B, Chazenbalk GD, Jaume JC, et al. The thyrotropin (TSH) receptor: interaction with TSH and autoantibodies. *Endocr Rev* 1998;19:673.

76. Graves PN, Davies TF. New insights into the thyroid-stimulating hormone receptor. The major antigen of Graves' disease. *Endocrinol Metab Clin North Am* 2000;29:267.

77. Chazenbalk GD, Wang Y, Guo J, et al. A mouse monoclonal antibody to a thyrotropin receptor ectodomain variant provides insight into the exquisite antigenic conformational requirement, epitopes and in vivo concentration of human autoantibodies. *J Clin Endocrinol Metab* 1999;84:702.

78. Chen CR, Tanaka K, Chazenbalk GD, et al. A full biological response to autoantibodies in Graves' disease requires a disulfide-bonded loop in the thyrotropin receptor N terminus homologous to a laminin epidermal growth factor-like domain. *J Biol Chem* 2001;276:14767.

79. Cundiff JG, Kaithamana S, Seetharamaiah GS, et al. Studies using recombinant fragments of human TSH receptor reveal apparent diversity in the binding specificities of antibodies that block TSH binding to its receptor or stimulate thyroid hormone production. *J Clin Endocrinol Metab* 2001;86:42540.

80. Tahara K, Ishikawa N, Yamamoto K, et al. Epitopes for thyroid stimulating and blocking autoantibodies on the extracellular domain of the human thyrotropin receptor. *Thyroid* 1997;7:867.

81. Akamizu T, Kohn LD, Hiratani H, et al. Hashimoto's thyroiditis with heterogeneous antithyrotropin receptor antibodies: unique epitopes may contribute to the regulation of thyroid function by the antibodies. *J Clin Endocrinol Metab* 2000;85:2116.

82. Schwarz-Lauer L, Chazenbalk GD, Mclachlan SM, et al. Evidence for a simplified view of autoantibody interactions with the thyrotropin receptor. *Thyroid* 2002;12:115.

83. Seetharamaiah GS, Dallas JS, Patibandla SA, et al. Requirement of glycosylation of the human thyrotropin receptor ectodomain for its reactivity with autoantibodies in patients' sera. *J Immunol* 1997;158:2798.

84. Nagayama Y, Namba H, Yokoyama N, et al. Role of asparagine-linked oligosaccharides in protein folding, membrane targeting, and thyrotropin and autoantibody binding of the human thyrotropin receptor. *J Biol Chem* 1998;273:33423.

85. Chazenbalk GD, Pichurin P, Chen CR, et al. Thyroid-stimulating autoantibodies in Graves disease preferentially recognize the free A subunit, not the thyrotropin holoreceptor. *J Clin Invest* 2002;110:209.

86. Chen CR, Pichurin P, Nagayama Y, et al. The thyrotropin receptor autoantigen in Graves' disease is the culprit as well as the victim. *J Clin Invest* 2003;111:1897.

87. Kohn LD, Suzuki K, Hoffman WH, et al. Characterization of monoclonal thyroid-stimulating and thyrotropin binding-inhibiting autoantibodies from a Hashimoto's patient whose children had intrauterine and neonatal thyroid disease. *J Clin Endocrinol Metab* 1997;82:3998.

88. Sanders J, Evans M, Premawardhana LD, et al. Human monoclonal thyroid stimulating autoantibody. *Lancet* 2003;362:126.

89. Costagliola S, Rodien P, Many MC, et al. Genetic immunization against the human thyrotropin receptor causes thyroiditis and allows production of monoclonal antibodies recognizing the native receptor. *J Immunol* 1998;160:1458.

90. Davies TF, Bobovnikova Y, Weiss M, et al. Development and characterization of monoclonal antibodies specific for the murine thyrotropin receptor. *Thyroid* 1998;8:693.

91. Ando T, Latif R, Pritsker A, et al. A monoclonal thyroid-stimulating antibody. *J Clin Invest* 2002;110:1667.

92. Latrofa F, Chazenbalk GD, Pichurin P, et al. Characterization of TSH receptor autoantibodies affinity-enriched to near purity from the serum of Graves patients. *Thyroid* 2003;13:734(abst).

93. Vitti P, Rotella CM, Valente WA, et al. Characterization of the optimal stimulatory effect of Graves' monoclonal and serum immunoglobulin G on adenosine 3',5'-monophosphate production in FRTL-5 thyroid cells: a potential clinical assay. *J Clin Endocrinol Metab* 1983;57:782.

94. Marcocci C, Valente WA, Pinchera A, et al. Graves' IgG stimulation of iodide uptake in FRTL-5 rat thyroid cells: a clinical assay complementing FRTL-5 assays measuring adenylate cyclase and growth-stimulating antibodies in autoimmune thyroid thyroid disease. *J Endocrinol Invest* 1983;6:463.

95. Chiovato L, Hammond LJ, Hanafusa T, et al. Detection of thyroid growth immunoglobulins (TGI) by 3H-thymidine incorporation in cultured rat thyroid follicles. *Clin Endocrinol (Oxf)* 1983;19:581.

96. Vitti P, Chiovato L, Tonacchera M, et al. Failure to detect thyroid growth-promoting activity in Immunoglobulin G of patients with endemic goiter. *J Clin Endocrinol Metab* 1994;78:1020.

97. Chiovato L, Vitti P, Bendinelli G, et al. Detection of antibodies blocking thyrotropin effect using Chinese hamster ovary cells transfected with the cloned human TSH receptor. *J Endocrinol Invest* 1994;17:809.

98. Tokuda Y, Kasagi K, Iida Y, et al. Inhibition of thyrotropin-stimulated iodide uptake in FRTL-5 thyroid cells by crude immunoglobulin fractions from patients with goitrous and atrophic autoimmune thyroiditis. *J Clin Endocrinol Metab* 1988;67:251.

99. Chiovato L, Vitti P, Santini F, et al. Incidence of antibodies blocking thyrotropin effect in vitro in patients with euthyroid or hypothyroid autoimmune thyroiditis. *J Clin Endocrinol Metab* 1990;71:40.

100. Filetti S, Foti D, Costante G, et al. Recombinant human thyrotropin (TSH) receptor in a radioreceptor assay for the measurement of TSH receptor autoantibodies. *J Clin Endocrinol Metab* 1991;72:1096.

101. Costagliola S, Morgenthaler NG, Hoermann R, et al. Second generation assay for thyrotropin receptor antibodies has superior diagnostic sensitivity for Graves' disease. *J Clin Endocrinol Metab* 1999;84:90.

102. Takasu N, Oshiro C, Akamine H, et al. Thyroid-stimulating antibody and TSH-binding inhibitor immunoglobulin in 277 Graves' patients and in 686 normal subjects. *J Endocrinol Invest* 1997;20:452.

103. Vitti P, Valente WA, Ambesi-Impiombato FS, et al. Graves' IgG stimulation of continuously cultured rat thyroid cells: a sensitive and potentially useful clinical assay. *J Endocrinol Invest* 1982;5:179.

104. Vitti P, Elisei R, Tonacchera M, et al. Detection of thyroid-stimulating antibody using Chinese hamster ovary cells transfected with cloned human thyrotropin receptor. *J Clin Endocrinol Metab* 1993;76:499.

105. Morgenthaler NG, Pampel I, Aust G, et al. Application of a bioassay with CHO cells for the routine detection of stimulating and blocking autoantibodies to the TSH-receptor. *Horm Metab Res* 1998;30:162.

106. Creagh FN, Teece M, Williams S, et al. An analysis of thyrotropin receptor binding and thyroid stimulating activities in a series of Graves' sera. *Clin Endocrinol (Oxf)* 1985;23:395.

107. Macchia E, Concetti R, Carone G, et al. Demonstration of blocking immunoglobulins G, having a heterogeneous behaviour, in sera of patients with Graves' disease: possible coexistence of different autoantibodies directed to the TSH receptor. *Clin Endocrinol (Oxf)* 1988;28:147.

108. Takasu N, Yamada T, Takasu M, et al. Disappearance of thyrotropin-blocking antibodies and spontaneous recovery from hypothyroidism in autoimmune thyroiditis. *N Engl J Med* 1992;326:513.

109. McKenzie JM, Zakarija M. Fetal and neonatal thyrotoxicosis and hypothyroidism due to maternal TSH receptor antibodies. *Thyroid* 1992;2:155.

110. Brown RS, Bellisario RL, Botero D, et al. Incidence of transient congenital hypothyroidism due to maternal thyrotropin receptor-blocking antibodies in over one million babies. *J Clin Endocrinol Metab* 1996;81:1147.

111. Zakarija M, McKenzie JM, Hoffman WH. Prediction and therapy of intrauterine and late onset neonatal thyrotoxicosis. *J Clin Endocrinol Metab* 1986;62:368.

112. McKenzie JM, Zakarija M. The clinical use of thyrotropin receptor antibody measurements. *J Clin Endocrinol Metab* 1989;72:1093.

113. Amino N, Tada H, Hidaka Y. Autoimmune thyroid disease and pregnancy. *J Endocrinol Invest* 1996;19:59.

114. Kasagi K, Tamai H, Morita T, et al. Role of thyrotropin receptor antibodies in the development of thyrotoxicosis: follow-up studies on nine patients with Graves' disease. *J Clin Endocrinol Metab* 1989;68:1189.

115. Kasagi K, Takeuchi R, Misaki T, et al. Subclinical Graves' disease as a cause of subnormal TSH levels in euthyroid subjects. *J Endocrinol Invest* 1997;20:183.

116. Fenzi GF, Hashizume K, Roudeboush CP, et al. Changes in thyroid-stimulating immunoglobulins during antithyroid therapy. *J Clin Endocrinol Metab* 1979;48:572.

117. Vitti P, Rago T, Chiovato L, et al. Clinical features of patients with Graves' disease undergoing remission after antithyroid drug treatment. *Thyroid* 1997;7:369.

118. Madec AM, Laurent MC, Lorcy Y, et al. Thyroid stimulating antibodies: an aid to the strategy of treatment of Graves' disease? *Clin Endocrinol (Oxf)* 1984;21:247.

119. Schleusener H, Schwander J, Holle R, et al. Prospective multicentre study on the prediction of relapse after anti-thyroid drug treatment in patients with Graves' disease. *Acta Endocrinol (Copenh)* 1989;120:689.

120. Zingrillo M, D'Aloiso L, Ghiggi MR, et al. Thyroid hypoechogenicity after methimazole withdrawal in Graves' disease: a useful index for predicting recurrence? *Clin Endocrinol (Oxf)* 1996;45:201.

121. Michelangeli V, Poon C, Taft J, et al. The prognostic value of thyrotropin receptor antibody measurement in the early stages of treatment of Graves' disease with antithyroid drugs. *Thyroid* 1998;8:119.

122. Brown RS. Immunoglobulins affecting thyroid growth: a continuing controversy. *J Clin Endocrinol Metab* 1995;80:1506.

16

NONISOTOPIC TECHNIQUES OF THYROID IMAGING

LASZLO HEGEDÜS
FINN NOE BENNEDBAEK

Imaging has revolutionized the evaluation of patients with thyroid disease during the past three decades. However, it is important to bear in mind that the use of thyroid imaging, fascinating as it may be, is in general not evidence-based, and there have been few cost-benefit evaluations of these procedures (1).

Clinical examination and biochemical evaluation of thyroid function are fundamental in the evaluation of patients with thyroid disorders, but there is wide observer variation in the assessment of clinical findings in these patients, particularly in relation to palpation of the thyroid gland (2). Therefore, it is not surprising that imaging of the thyroid is often performed. In most cases, it cannot distinguish between benign and malignant lesions, and its clinical value is generally thought to be limited (1,3). Nevertheless, in a recent survey of members of the European Thyroid Association, 88% said they would use imaging in an index case of a euthyroid patient with a solitary thyroid nodule and no clinical suspicion of carcinoma (4). In contrast, American endocrinologists place less value on this technology, which in many patients is considered superfluous (5).

The thyroid gland can be evaluated by several imaging techniques. One is radionuclide imaging, which is discussed in detail in Chapter 12 and will not be considered further here. The others are plain radiography, ultrasonography, computed tomography (CT), and magnetic resonance imaging (MRI). Each has advantages and limitations, and there is no absolute clinical indication for performing any of them in the majority of patients (3,6,7). The major limitation of all the techniques, in addition to expense, is their lack of specificity for tissue diagnosis. This chapter will focus on the clinical use of ultrasonography, CT, and MRI, and as far as possible compare their advantages and disadvantages (Table 16.1).

PLAIN RADIOGRAPHY

A routine chest radiograph is rarely indicated for evaluation of patients with thyroid disease. An X-ray taken for another purpose can disclose mediastinal extension of a goiter or deviation or compression of the trachea caused by a goiter in the neck or mediastinum (7) (Fig. 16.1).

ULTRASONOGRAPHY

Ultrasonographic examination of the neck is performed using high-frequency transducers (7 to 13 MHz) with the patient in the supine position and the neck hyperextended. The transducer is coupled to the skin with gel because the sound waves do not pass through air. Ultrasonography can detect thyroid lobes or lesions as small as 2 mm. It can distinguish solid nodules from simple and complex cysts. It allows accurate estimation of thyroid size, gives a rough estimate of tissue density (echogenicity), shows vascular flow and velocity (color-flow Doppler), and aids in the accurate placing of needles for diagnostic or therapeutic purposes (8,9). Finally, it allows in utero investigation of the fetal thyroid (10). The major limitations of ultrasonography are the high degree of observer dependency (11) and the inability to identify retrotracheal, retroclavicular, or intrathoracic extensions of the thyroid (7,9,12). Images are obtained in the transverse (axial) and longitudinal (sagittal) planes, and sometimes in the oblique planes. The procedure rarely takes more than 10 minutes.

Ultrasonography is based on the emission of high-frequency sound waves and their subsequent reflection as they pass through the tissue. The amplitude of the reflections of the sound waves varies according to differences in the acoustic impedance of the various tissues. Therefore, small calcifications of 1 mm with a high acoustic impedance may be seen, whereas a large thyroid nodule with acoustic characteristics similar to that of normal thyroid tissue may not be seen. High-frequency sound waves penetrate tissue less well than do low-frequency waves, but the structural resolution of the high-frequency waves is better. The frequency used to visualize the thyroid is a compromise between the need for depth of penetration and that for resolution. The use of real time allows differentiation hypoechogenicity, probably related to areas that are affected by the inflammatory process (34), and vascularity is decreased (35). With recovery, size decreases, but areas of hypoechogenicity may be detected for many months (34). Color-Doppler ultrasonography distinguishes patients with the multinodular variant of Graves' disease (extranodular diffuse hypoechogenicity with increased color Doppler signal and maximal peak systolic velocity) from those with nonautoimmune toxic multinodular goiter (normal extranodular vascularity) (36).

Multinodular Goiter

Multinodular goiters are usually larger than diffuse goiters, and 10% to 20% have a substernal or intrathoracic extension that cannot be visualized by ultrasonography because the bony thorax prevents penetration of sound waves (37). The echographic structure of multinodular goiters may be heterogeneous without well-defined nodules, or there may be multiple nodules interspersed throughout a normal-appearing gland. Areas of hemorrhage, necrosis, and calcifications are often seen. These goiters, as noted above, may be diffusely hypoechogenic and therefore difficult to distinguish from goitrous autoimmune thyroiditis.

The majority of patients evaluated for a solitary nodule have additional small thyroid nodules detected by ultrasonography (37). The echogenicity of the nodules varies from hyper- to iso- to hypoechoic, often even in the same patient. The presence of multiple nodules, as detected by ultrasonography or any other imaging procedure, does not exclude carcinoma, and indeed it is just as likely to be present in a multinodular goiter as in a solitary nodule (38,39). Therefore, especially in view of the increasing use of nonsurgical treatment for multinodular goiter (see Chapter 69) (37,40), fine-needle aspiration biopsy is usually indicated, especially in euthyroid patients with a dominant or a growing nodule. Ultrasound guidance is recommended because it facilitates sampling of nodular lesions and is associated with a lower rate of false-negative results (see Chapter 73) (41).

Thyroid Cysts

Thyroid cysts are well-defined areas with greatly reduced or no echogenicity (Fig. 16.4), but there may be a few echoes if the cyst contains debris or necrotic tissue. True simple cysts are rare (perhaps 1% of all nodules) and virtually always benign (37). More often, cysts are complex or mixed, with both cystic and solid components. A complex cyst is as likely to be a carcinoma as is a solid nodule (39,42), and the risk of initial nondiagnostic cytology is largely predicted by the presence of a cystic component of the nodule (43). After ultrasound-guided aspiration, the residual solid component should be examined via biopsy (Fig. 16.4). If the cytology is benign and the cyst recurs, as it does in approximately 50% of patients (44), ultrasound-guided treatment can be offered. Injection of tetracycline is not effective in preventing further recurrence (45), but injection of ethanol may be effective (46). The presence of only benign cells in the cystic component of a complex nodule cannot be taken as evidence that the solid component is not a carcinoma, nor can the color of the cyst fluid (42,47).

Benign Thyroid Nodules

Most benign thyroid nodules (thyroid adenomas, hyperplastic nodules) are hypoechoic relative to normal thyroid tissue, but so are thyroid carcinomas, and the two cannot be distinguished reliably on the basis of size, degree of echogenicity, or presence of a sonographic halo, calcifica-

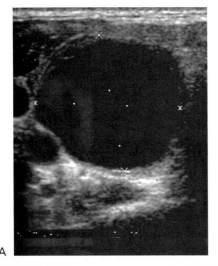 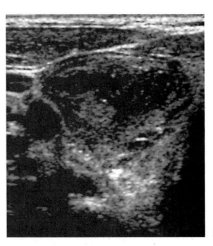

FIGURE 16.4. Transverse sonogram of a right thyroid nodule with a central cystic region before **(A)** and after aspiration of the cyst **(B)**. More solid tissue is seen after the aspiration, and it should be biopsied to reduce the likelihood of overlooking carcinoma.

tions, or vascularization (48–50). Therefore, it has been argued that the most cost-effective investigation of these patients is fine-needle aspiration biopsy guided by palpation, and this is the usual practice in many places (3). In Europe, however, most thyroidologists prefer ultrasound-guided biopsy (4), which slightly increases the likelihood of obtaining a sufficient sample (41).

The frequent detection of nonpalpaple nodules or incidentalomas raises the same concern about possible malignancy as when the nodule is palpable. The risk of carcinoma in a nonpalpable nodule found in patients who have not had head or neck irradiation varies from 0.13% to 0.45% (19). In case of suspicion of carcinoma, or if the nodule is at least 1 cm in diameter, fine-needle aspiration biopsy guided by ultrasonography is recommended (3,19, 41). Carcinoma is just as common in nonpalpable nodules that are at least 1 cm in diameter as it is in palpable nodules of this size (51).

Interventional ultrasonography is being increasingly used as a nonsurgical therapeutic tool for percutaneous ablation of symptomatic benign nodules, e.g. ethanol injection (52) or interstitial laser photocoagulation (Fig. 16.5) (53).

Thyroid Carcinomas

Most thyroid carcinomas are hypoechoic, as compared with normal thyroid tissue, and microcalcifications are often present, especially in papillary carcinomas (7,8,14). Excluding microcalcifications, there are no sonographic differences among the different types of thyroid carcinoma

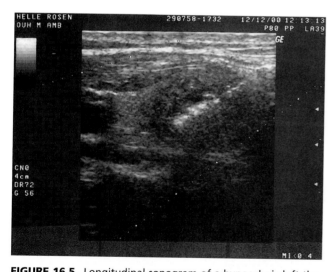

FIGURE 16.5. Longitudinal sonogram of a hypoechoic left thyroid nodule obtained during laser photocoagulation showing the needle tract and a roughly cylindrical hyperechoic area centrally in the nodule. A needle with a stylet is positioned centrally in the nodule, the stylet is removed, and a quartz laser fiber is inserted throught the needle into the nodule. Laser energy from an infrared laser power source is then delivered through the fiber to destroy the nodule.

or between thyroid carcinomas and benign thyroid nodules. Some vascular patterns recorded by color-Doppler or power-Doppler ultrasonography are suggestive of carcinoma, but the only ultrasound findings that are highly suggestive of carcinoma are invasion of adjacent structures and lymph node enlargement (14). The newly introduced contrast agents for ultrasonography may provide complementary information to differentiate benign from malignant nodules but cannot replace fine-needle aspiration biopsy (54).

Because nodules 2 to 3 mm in diameter can be detected, ultrasonography is increasingly used in the follow-up of patients treated for thyroid carcinoma or at risk for it because of previous irradiation (e.g., after the nuclear accident at Chernobyl). The presence of hypoechoic masses in the thyroid bed or adjacent tissues suggests recurrent carcinoma (see section on radioiodine and other treatments and outcomes in Chapter 70) (8).

COMPUTED TOMOGRAPHY

Computed tomography offers excellent anatomic resolution because of its ability to identify small differences in density between different tissues. Differences in density as small as 0.5% can be detected, as compared with 5% to 10% for conventional X-ray techniques. It is the ability to detect accurately the absorption of X-rays by tissues (attenuation) that enables individual tissues to be identified (6,7).

Computed tomography is highly sensitive for detecting thyroid nodules, but as with ultrasonography, benign nodules cannot be distinguished from carcinomas (7,55,56). It can distinguish solid from simple and complex cysts. Thyroid volume can be determined with an accuracy of approximately 88% (57). It is superior to ultrasonography in detecting thyroid tissue in the retrotracheal, retroclavicular, and intrathoracic regions (58), and it is not as observer dependent as is ultrasonography. The limitations of CT are cost, limited availability for studying patients with thyroid disease, length of the procedure, need for patient cooperation, artifacts caused by swallowing or breathing, and exposure to ionizing irradiation (1 to 4 rad) (7,55,56). The image is not dynamic and, although possible, CT-guided biopsy is more cumbersome than is ultrasound-guided biopsy (59). Patients with nodular goiter who are to undergo CT should not be given a radiographic contrast agent as part of the procedure because of the risk of iodine-induced thyrotoxicosis (Table 16.1) (60).

Computed tomography depends on the attenuation of an X-ray beam as it passes through tissues. The extent of attenuation depends on the constituents of the tissue, and the brightness of each portion (pixel) of the final image is proportional to the degree that it attenuates the X-rays passing through it. The image is usually depicted in shades of gray. Density values are expressed in CT numbers (Hounsfield units), which are related to the attenuation value of water. The thyroid is readily seen on CT because of its high iodine content, and the CT density of the thyroid is closely correlated with its iodine content and can be used to estimate it (61).

The Normal Thyroid Gland

The normal thyroid gland is easily seen on CT, and its density is always higher than that of the surrounding tissues. Differences in density reported from various countries are due to differences in iodine intake. There is no sex difference in density, but it decreases with age and as a consequence of T_4 treatment (62), and it increases after intravenous administration of a radiographic contrast agent.

Disease in the thyroid often leads to decreased ability to concentrate iodine or rapid iodine turnover; therefore, reduced density on CT is the hallmark of many thyroid diseases (7,55,56). Exact density measurements, however, have not proven useful in distinguishing between the different diseases. Thus, the CT image may be compatible with a certain diagnosis but is rarely specific for it (56).

Diffuse Thyroid Disease

Nonautoimmune nontoxic diffuse goiters appear as homogeneously enlarged thyroid glands with a varying degree of hypodensity. In patients with Graves' thyrotoxicosis, the density is decreased by 50% to 70% due to decreased iodine stores, and the tissue may be slightly inhomogeneous (63,64). In patients with goitrous autoimmune thyroiditis, the density is reduced in an inhomogeneous pattern and is lowest in patients with hypothyroidism, and increasing goiter size is characteristically associated with decreasing density (65,66). Asymmetric low-density areas should raise the suspicion of lymphoma or carcinoma (66,67).

Subacute thyroiditis is also characterized by focal or diffuse low density (68). In the initial phases acute suppurative thyroiditis has no characteristic CT image, but as infection progresses loculated hypodense abscesses may appear (68).

Multinodular Goiter

Multinodular goiters usually are seen as an enlarged asymmetric thyroid gland with multiple areas of low density of varying degrees of discreteness (Fig. 16.6) (63). The density increases after intravenous administration of a radiographic contrast agent, except in areas of hemorrhage or necrosis or in cysts (66). Calcifications are seen in up to 50% of these goiters. Compression of the trachea, esophagus, and great vessels is easily detected, and CT is ideal for estimating the extent of tracheal compression by a goiter and intrathoracic extension of a goiter (58). In a patient with an intrathoracic mass, CT showing anatomic continuity of the mass with the cervical thyroid and CT density greater than muscle provide evidence of the thyroidal origin of the mass. Mediastinal lymphomas, thymomas, or lymphadenopathy usually have markedly lower CT density (62).

Thyroid Cysts

Simple cysts are hypodense lesions, are smooth walled, and are surrounded by normal thyroid tissue. The density of cyst fluid is always less than muscle, and it does not increase after administration of a radiographic contrast agent. Complex cysts are easily distinguished from simple cysts (55,66).

Benign Thyroid Nodules and Carcinomas

Thyroid adenomas and other benign nodules are usually round or oval lesions of low density, and, as noted above, thyroid adenomas or other benign nodules cannot be distinguished from carcinomas using CT when the lesion is confined to the thyroid. Focal calcifications are seen in approximately 10% of benign nodules (7,55,66). Invasive growth into surrounding structures and metastases to cervical lymph nodes are indicative of carcinoma (69).

Papillary and follicular carcinomas are usually seen as irregular low-density masses, and punctate calcifications are present in approximately 60%. There may be slight enhancement after contrast injection. Medullary thyroid carcinomas characteristically appear as single or multiple low-density lesions of variable size in one or both lobes (55,66). Calcification is less often seen than in papillary carcinomas. Patients with C-cell hyperplasia have normal CT scans (70).

Large irregular masses of low attenuation with central cystic or necrotic areas are suggestive of anaplastic carcinoma, especially if many calcifications are seen, but some multinodular goiters have the same appearance. Invasion of the trachea, cricoid or thyroid cartilage, and growth

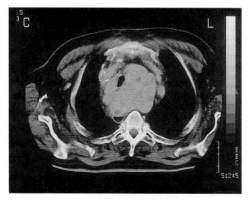

FIGURE 16.6. Computed tomography of a large intrathoracic goiter. Lateral dislocation and compression of the trachea are evident.

into the tracheal lumen are highly suggestive of anaplastic carcinoma. Both goitrous autoimmune thyroiditis and thyroid lymphoma appear as masses of low to intermediate density with little enhancement after contrast injection (71).

Computed tomography is of value in the follow-up of patients with thyroid carcinoma because of its sensitivity for detecting recurrent carcinoma in the neck and metastases elsewhere. Recurrent carcinoma appears as discrete low-density lesions within or outside the thyroid bed. Lymph node metastases typically have a regular rim and a core of central lucency and no enhancement after contrast injection (69). The ability of CT to detect recurrent thyroid carcinoma is not related to the ability of the tumor to take up radioiodine. Therefore, CT complements whole-body scintigraphy in the follow-up of these patients (see Chapter 12).

Developmental Abnormalities

Scintigraphy and not CT is the imaging procedure of choice when thyroid tissue is being sought anywhere (72). The exception is fetuses, in whom ultrasonography is the preferred procedure (10,73).

Ectopic thyroid tissue may be located anywhere from the foramen cecum at the base of the tongue to the anterior mediastinum. Although radioiodine or pertechnetate scintigraphy can uniquely identify tissue as being of thyroid origin, CT can aid in localization if radionuclide uptake is poor (74). Figure 16.7 shows a CT image of an unusual intratracheal location of ectopic thyroid tissue (74).

MAGNETIC RESONANCE IMAGING

MRI offers excellent anatomic resolution and generation of images in multiple planes. The technique is highly sensitive but just as nonspecific as ultrasonography and CT in differentiating benign thyroid nodules from carcinomas. It

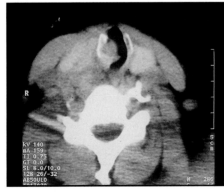

FIGURE 16.7. Computed tomography showing slightly enlarged thyroid lobes and ectopic thyroid tissue located within the trachea.

can distinguish solid from simple and complex cysts (7,55,56). Like CT it provides highly accurate estimates of thyroid volume and is useful especially in irregularly enlarged goiters. For this purpose, the observer variation of MR imaging is 2% to 4% (75,76). Like CT, and in contrast to ultrasonography, it can identify thyroid tissue in the retrotracheal, retroclavicular, and intrathoracic regions (77). The paramagnetic contrast agent gadolinium allows visualization of tumor vascularity (78). The limitations of MRI are its cost, limited availability for studying patients with thyroid disease, length of the procedure, need for patient cooperation (5% to 10% of patients cannot tolerate it due to claustrophobia, and some, especially children, need to be sedated) (79). Patient and tissue movement (e.g., swallowing) decreases image quality, and calcifications are better seen with CT (80,81). MRI cannot be used in patients with cardiac pacemakers, implantable defibrillators, CNS aneurysmal clips, cochlear implants, and ferromagnetic ocular fragments. Small metal objects, stainless steel surgical clips, and orthopedic devices decrease resolution and cause field inhomogeneity, but do not hinder MR imaging. Dental substances, if ferromagnetic, cause image distortion (Table 16.1).

Magnetic resonance images depend on the magnetic properties of certain atomic nuclei. Protons have a positive electrical charge and generate a magnetic field as they spin. The protons can be excited using a radiofrequency pulse, lifting some of the protons to a higher energy state. When radiofrequency is turned off, the protons realign themselves with the static external magnetic field through a process called relaxation. The resulting realignment results in protons returning to a lower energy state and the release of energy as a small voltage. This voltage is detected by the surface coil receiver, relayed to a computer, and reconstructed into an image. The MRI signal contains several variable components. The T1 relaxation time (longitudinal or spin-lattice relaxation time) reflects the time for protons to give up their energy to the surrounding environment (lattice) and return to their original alignment parallel to the magnetic field. The T2 relaxation time (transverse or spin-spin relaxation time) is the time needed for synchronous transverse spinning to decay after excitation. Adjustment of the pulse sequence can favor one or the other of these magnetic properties. As a rule, T1-weighted transverse images are initially obtained from cranial to caudal. Coronal scans allow the evaluation of substernal goiters (82,83). Subsequently, T2-weighted images are obtained. These require longer scan times and are more dependent on patient cooperation.

The Normal Thyroid Gland

On T1-weighted images the normal thyroid gland has a nearly homogeneous signal with an intensity similar to that of the adjacent neck muscles (Fig. 16.8A) (79–83). Air, blood, and vessels usually appear black. On T2-weighted

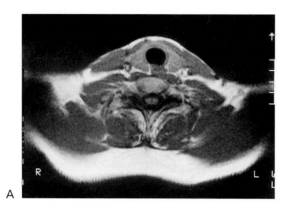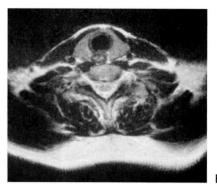

FIGURE 16.8. T1-weighted **(A)** and T2-weighted **(B)** MRIs of a normal thyroid gland.

images, the normal thyroid has a greater signal intensity than the adjacent muscles (Fig. 16.8B). Blood vessels, lymph nodes, fat, and muscle are clearly identified and distinguished from the thyroid. As with ultrasonography and CT, small solitary or multiple focal abnormalities of the thyroid are seen in up to nearly 50% of normal subjects (84). Normal parathyroid glands cannot be seen, but enlarged ones can (85). MRI, like ultrasonography and CT, detects parathyroid adenomas with a sensitivity of 60% to 80% (85,86).

Diffuse Thyroid Disease

In Graves' disease both T1- and T2-weighted images show a diffusely increased but slightly heterogeneous signal (87,88). There is a linear relationship between the thyroid:muscle signal ratio and serum T_4 concentrations and 24-hour thyroid radioiodine uptake values (87). After treatment with radioiodine, this signal ratio decreases, concomitant with the decrease in serum T_4 concentrations (87).

The thyroid in patients with goitrous autoimmune thyroiditis is heterogeneous on T1-weighted images and has a

diffusely increased signal on T2-weighted images, and there may be linear bands of increased intensity. These bands are thought to reflect areas of fibrosis (89). Infiltration of adjacent neck structures and hypointensity on T1- and T2-weighted images are suggestive of Riedel's thyroiditis (90).

Multinodular Goiter

MRI can detect nodules as small as 3 to 5 mm (55). Characteristically, multinodular goiters have various degrees of heterogeneity and low to increased signal intensity on T1-weighted images (Fig. 16.9) (82). Focal hemorrhage and cystic degeneration are characterized by high signal intensity (89). T2-weighted images show more pronounced heterogeneity and increased intensity (82). Nodules are better visualized on T2-weighted images (89). The MR characteristics of hypo- or hyperfunctioning nodules do not differ.

Thyroid Cysts

Simple cysts have a homogeneous high-intensity signal on both T1- and T2-weighted imaging (79). The intensity on T1-weighted images increases with increasing protein and lipid content.

Benign Thyroid Nodules and Carcinomas

Thyroid adenomas and other benign nodules appear round or oval with a heterogeneous signal equal to or greater than that of normal thyroid tissue (82,87). On T2-weighted images the nodules have increased signal intensity. No MRI characteristics accurately distinguish between benign nodules and carcinomas, although benign nodules characteristically have a smoother, more uniform, and thicker capsule than carcinomas. Thyroid carcinomas

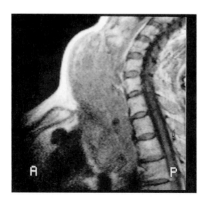

FIGURE 16.9. T1-weighted sagittal MRI of a large multinodular goiter extending into the thorax.

appear as focal or nonfocal lesions of variable size; they are isointense or slightly hyperintense on T1-weighted images and hyperintense on T2-weighted images. The imaging characteristics of all types of thyroid carcinomas including medullary carcinoma and lymphoma are similar (71,83, 89).

The extent of thyroid carcinoma can be determined preoperatively, which may be useful in planning surgery. Extension into adjacent structures (such as muscles, vessels, the larynx, and the trachea) is usually evident. MRI cannot distinguish metastatic from inflammatory adenopathy. An important application of MRI is for the detection of recurrent carcinoma. Although the thyroid remnant is usually seen as peritracheal tissue with low signal intensity on T1- and T2-weighted images, recurrent carcinoma and lymph node metastases have low to medium signal intensity on T1-weighted images and medium to high signal intensity on T2-weighted images (82). Features such as asymmetry, increased signal intensity in the thyroid bed, and invasion or displacement of adjacent tissue, as well as enlarged lymph nodes with increased signal intensity, thus suggest recurrent carcinoma (7,56,91). Gadolinium injection may be useful because metastatic nodes are enhanced centrally after gadolinium injection (78). Furthermore, recurrent carcinoma enhances with gadolinium, whereas scar tissue usually does not (78). However, in the differentiation between benign and malignant thyroid tumors the time-intensity curves after gadolinium injection overlap in benign and malignant nodules (92).

CONCLUSION

There is no absolute clinical indication for performing any of the imaging procedures described herein, and none of them accurately distinguish benign thyroid nodules from thyroid carcinomas. Nonetheless, these procedures, particularly ultrasonography, are being increasingly used (4,8). Ultrasonography is widely available, it costs relatively little, and many physicians have found it of value in patients with several different thyroid disorders (4,9,37,93). Even if it cannot reliably identify or exclude thyroid carcinoma, it provides superior morphologic detail, as compared with scintigraphy, and allows more accurate placing of needles for biopsy and therapy (9,37). Additionally, it provides far more accurate estimates of thyroid volume than does palpation, and some have found the information about echogenicity and vascularization provided by ultrasonography to be useful in the classification and follow-up of patients with thyroid disorders.

CT and MRI provide information similar to that provided by ultrasonography. Their greater expense and more limited availability argue against their use, with rare exceptions. CT is valuable in determining the extent of a substernal goiter or in the evaluation of a mediastinal mass. It can give valuable information in the evaluation of thyroid carcinoma and its spread. MRI is useful in the same clinical situations and may be superior to CT in the evaluation of patients suspected of having recurrent carcinoma, be it in the thyroid bed or in regional lymph nodes.

REFERENCES

1. Ortiz R, Hupart KH, DeFesi CR, et al. Effect of early referral to an endocrinologist on efficiency and cost of evaluation and development of treatment plan in patients with thyroid nodules. *J Clin Endocrinol Metab* 1998;83:3803.
2. Jarlov AE, Nygaard B, Hegedus L, et al. Observer variation in the clinical and laboratory evaluation of patients with thyroid dysfunction and goiter. *Thyroid* 1998;8:393.
3. Singer PA, Cooper DS, Daniels GH, et al. Treatment guidelines for patients with thyroid nodules and well-differentiated thyroid cancer. *Arch Intern Med* 1996;156:2165.
4. Bennedbaek FN, Perrild H, Hegedus L. Diagnosis and treatment of the solitary thyroid nodule. Results of a European survey. *Clin Endocrinol (Oxf)* 1999;50:357.
5. Bennedbaek FN, Hegedus L. Management of the solitary thyroid nodule: results of a North American survey. *J Clin Endocrinol Metab* 2000;85:2493.
6. Nusynowitz ML. Thyroid imaging. *Lippincott's Prim Care Pract* 1999;3:546.
7. Naik KS, Bury RF. Imaging the thyroid. *Clin Radiol* 1998;53: 630.
8. Solbiati L, Osti V, Cova L, et al. Ultrasound of thyroid, parathyroid glands and neck lymph nodes. *Eur Radiol* 2001;11: 2411.
9. Hegedus L. Thyroid ultrasound. *Endocrinol Metab Clin North Am* 2001;30:339.
10. Achiron R, Rotstein Z, Lipitz S, et al. The development of the foetal thyroid: in utero ultrasonographic measurements. *Clin Endocrinol (Oxf)* 1998;48:259.
11. Jarlov AE, Nygard B, Hegedus L, et al. Observer variation in ultrasound assessment of the thyroid gland. *Br J Radiol* 1993;66: 625.
12. Gotway MB, Higgins CB. MR imaging of the thyroid and parathyroid glands. *Magn Reson Imaging Clin N Am* 2000;8:163.
13. Gritzmann N, Koischwitz D, Rettenbacher T. Sonography of the thyroid and parathyroid glands. *Radiol Clin North Am* 2000; 38:1131.
14. Cerbone G, Spiezia S, Colao A, et al. Power Doppler improves the diagnostic accuracy of color Doppler ultrasonography in cold thyroid nodules: follow-up results. *Horm Res* 1999;52:19.
15. Correas JM, Bridal L, Lesavre A, et al. Ultrasound contrast agents: properties, principles of action, tolerance, and artifacts. *Eur Radiol* 2001;11:1316.
16. Maiorana R, Carta A, Floriddia G, et al. Thyroid hemiagenesis: prevalence in normal children and effect on thyroid function. *J Clin Endocrinol Metab* 2003;88:1534.
17. Gupta P, Maddalozzo J. Preoperative sonography in presumed thyroglossal duct cysts. *Arch Otolaryngol Head Neck Surg* 2001; 127:200.
18. Ying M, Brook F, Ahuja A, et al. The value of thyroid parenchymal echogenicity as an indicator of pathology using the sternomastoid muscle for comparison. *Ultrasound Med Biol* 1998; 24:1097.
19. Tan GH, Gharib H. Thyroid incidentalomas: management approaches to nonpalpable nodules discovered incidentally on thyroid imaging. *Ann Intern Med* 1997;126:226.

20. Knudsen N, Bulow I, Jorgensen T, et al. Goitre prevalence and thyroid abnormalities at ultrasonography: a comparative epidemiological study in two regions with slightly different iodine status. *Clin Endocrinol (Oxf)* 2000;53:479.

21. Brunn J, Block U, Ruf G, et al. Volumetric analysis of thyroid lobes by real-time ultrasound [author's transl]. *Dtsch Med Wochenschr* 1981;106:1338.

22. Hegedus L, Perrild H, Poulsen LR, et al. The determination of thyroid volume by ultrasound and its relationship to bodyweight, age, and sex in normal subjects. *J Clin Endocrinol Metab* 1983;56:260.

23. Schlogl S, Werner E, Lassmann M, et al. The use of three-dimensional ultrasound for thyroid volumetry. *Thyroid* 2001;11:569.

24. Hegedus L. Thyroid size determined by ultrasound. Influence of physiological factors and non-thyroidal disease. *Dan Med Bull* 1990;37:249.

25. Delange F, Benker G, Caron P, et al. Thyroid volume and urinary iodine in European schoolchildren: standardization of values for assessment of iodine deficiency. *Eur J Endocrinol* 1997;136:180.

26. Pedersen OM, Aardal NP, Larssen TB, et al. The value of ultrasonography in predicting autoimmune thyroid disease. *Thyroid* 2000;10:251.

27. Raber W, Gessl A, Nowotny P, et al. Thyroid ultrasound versus antithyroid peroxidase antibody determination: a cohort study of four hundred fifty-one subjects. *Thyroid* 2002;12:725.

28. Matsuzuka F, Miyauchi A, Katayama S, et al. Clinical aspects of primary thyroid lymphoma: diagnosis and treatment based on our experience of 119 cases. *Thyroid* 1993;3:93.

29. Vitti P, Rago T, Mancusi F, et al. Thyroid hypoechogenic pattern at ultrasonography as a tool for predicting recurrence of hyperthyroidism after medical treatment in patients with Graves' disease. *Acta Endocrinol (Copenh)* 1992;126:128.

30. Zingrillo M, D'Aloiso L, Ghiggi MR, et al. Thyroid hypoechogenicity after methimazole withdrawal in Graves' disease: a useful index for predicting recurrence? *Clin Endocrinol (Oxf)* 1996;45:201.

31. Baldini M, Castagnone D, Rivolta R, et al. Thyroid vascularization by color doppler ultrasonography in Graves' disease. Changes related to different phases and to the long-term outcome of the disease. *Thyroid* 1997;7:823.

32. Bogazzi F, Bartalena L, Vitti P, et al. Color flow Doppler sonography in thyrotoxicosis factitia. *J Endocrinol Invest* 1996;19:603.

33. Bogazzi F, Bartalena L, Brogioni S, et al. Color flow Doppler sonography rapidly differentiates type I and type II amiodarone-induced thyrotoxicosis. *Thyroid* 1997;7:541.

34. Bennedbaek FN, Hegedus L. The value of ultrasonography in the diagnosis and follow-up of subacute thyroiditis. *Thyroid* 1997;7:45.

35. Hiromatsu Y, Ishibashi M, Miyake I, et al. Color Doppler ultrasonography in patients with subacute thyroiditis. *Thyroid* 1999;9:1189.

36. Boi F, Loy M, Piga M, et al. The usefulness of conventional and echo colour Doppler sonography in the differential diagnosis of toxic multinodular goitres. *Eur J Endocrinol* 2000;143:339.

37. Hegedus L, Bonnema SJ, Bennedbaek FN. Management of simple nodular goiter: current status and future perspectives. *Endocr Rev* 2003;24:102.

38. Tollin SR, Mery GM, Jelveh N, et al. The use of fine-needle aspiration biopsy under ultrasound guidance to assess the risk of malignancy in patients with a multinodular goiter. *Thyroid* 2000;10:235.

39. Belfiore A, La Rosa GL, La Porta GA, et al. Cancer risk in patients with cold thyroid nodules: relevance of iodine intake, sex, age, and multinodularity. *Am J Med* 1992;93:363.

40. Hermus AR, Huysmans DA. Treatment of benign nodular thyroid disease. *N Engl J Med* 1998;338:1438.

41. Danese D, Sciacchitano S, Farsetti A, et al. Diagnostic accuracy of conventional versus sonography-guided fine-needle aspiration biopsy of thyroid nodules. *Thyroid* 1998;8:15.

42. Abbas G, Heller KS, Khoynezhad A, et al. The incidence of carcinoma in cytologically benign thyroid cysts. *Surgery* 2001;130:1035.

43. Alexander EK, Heering JP, Benson CB, et al. Assessment of nondiagnostic ultrasound-guided fine needle aspirations of thyroid nodules. *J Clin Endocrinol Metab* 2002;87:4924.

44. Monzani F, Lippi F, Goletti O, et al. Percutaneous aspiration and ethanol sclerotherapy for thyroid cysts. *J Clin Endocrinol Metab* 1994;78:800.

45. Hegedus L, Hansen JM, Karstrup S, et al. Tetracycline for sclerosis of thyroid cysts. A randomized study. *Arch Intern Med* 1988;148:1116.

46. Bennedbaek FN, Hegedus L. Treatment of recurrent thyroid cysts with ethanol: a randomized double-blind controlled trial. *J Clin Endocrinol Metab* 2003;88:5773.

47. McHenry CR, Slusarczyk SJ, Khiyami A. Recommendations for management of cystic thyroid disease. *Surgery* 1999;126:1167.

48. Giuffrida D, Gharib H. Controversies in the management of cold, hot, and occult thyroid nodules. *Am J Med* 1995;99:642.

49. Rago T, Vitti P, Chiovato L, et al. Role of conventional ultrasonography and color flow-Doppler sonography in predicting malignancy in 'cold' thyroid nodules. *Eur J Endocrinol* 1998;138:41.

50. Hegedus L, Karstrup S. Ultrasonography in the evaluation of cold thyroid nodules. *Eur J Endocrinol* 1998;138:30.

51. Hagag P, Strauss S, Weiss M. Role of ultrasound-guided fine-needle aspiration biopsy in evaluation of nonpalpable thyroid nodules. *Thyroid* 1998;8:989.

52. Bennedbaek FN, Karstrup S, Hegedus L. Percutaneous ethanol injection therapy in the treatment of thyroid and parathyroid diseases. *Eur J Endocrinol* 1997;136:240.

53. Dossing H, Bennedbaek FN, Karstrup S, et al. Benign solitary solid cold thyroid nodules: US-guided interstitial laser photocoagulation—initial experience. *Radiology* 2002;225:53.

54. Spiezia S, Farina R, Cerbone G, et al. Analysis of color Doppler signal intensity variation after levovist injection: a new approach to the diagnosis of thyroid nodules. *J Ultrasound Med* 2001;20:223.

55. Youserm DM, Huang T, Loevner LA, et al. Clinical and economic impact of incidental thyroid lesions found with CT and MR. *AJNR Am J Neuroradiol* 1997;18:1423.

56. Loevner LA. Imaging of the thyroid gland. *Semin Ultrasound CT MR* 1996;17:539.

57. Hermans R, Bouillon R, Laga K, et al. Estimation of thyroid gland volume by spiral computed tomography. *Eur Radiol* 1997;7:214.

58. Jennings A. Evaluation of substernal goiters using computed tomography and MR imaging. *Endocrinol Metab Clin North Am* 2001;30:401.

59. DelGaudio JM, Dillard DG, Albritton FD, et al. Computed tomography—guided needle biopsy of head and neck lesions. *Arch Otolaryngol Head Neck Surg* 2000;126:366.

60. Shimura H, Takazawa K, Endo T, et al. T4-thyroid storm after CT-scan with iodinated contrast medium. *J Endocrinol Invest* 1990;13:73.

61. Imanishi Y, Ehara N, Shinagawa T, et al. Correlation of CT values, iodine concentration, and histological changes in the thyroid. *J Comput Assist Tomogr* 2000;24:322.

62. Reede DL, Bergeron RT, McCauley DI. CT of the thyroid and of other thoracic inlet disorders. *J Otolaryngol* 1982;11:349.

63. Silverman PM, Newman GE, Korobkin M, et al. Computed tomography in the evaluation of thyroid disease. *AJR Am J Roentgenol* 1984;142:897.

64. Kamijo K. Clinical studies on thyroid CT number in Graves' disease and destructive thyrotoxicosis. *Endocr J* 1994;41:25.

65. Kamijo K. Clinical studies on thyroid CT number in chronic thyroiditis. *Endocr J* 1994;41:19.

66. Weber AL, Randolph G, Aksoy FG. The thyroid and parathyroid glands. CT and MR imaging and correlation with pathology and clinical findings. *Radiol Clin North Am* 2000;38:1105.

67. Kim HC, Han MH, Kim KH, et al. Primary thyroid lymphoma: CT findings. *Eur J Radiol* 2003;46:233.

68. Bernard PJ, Som PM, Urken ML, et al. The CT findings of acute thyroiditis and acute suppurative thyroiditis. *Otolaryngol Head Neck Surg* 1988;99:489.

69. Van den Brekel MW. Lymph node metastases: CT and MRI. *Eur J Radiol* 2000;33:230.

70. Wells SA Jr., Donis-Keller H. Current perspectives on the diagnosis and management of patients with multiple endocrine neoplasia type 2 syndromes. *Endocrinol Metab Clin North Am* 1994;23:215.

71. Takashima S, Nomura N, Noguchi Y, et al. Primary thyroid lymphoma: evaluation with US, CT, and MRI. *J Comput Assist Tomogr* 1995;19:282.

72. Meller J, Becker W. The continuing importance of thyroid scintigraphy in the era of high-resolution ultrasound. *Eur J Nucl Med Mol Imaging* 2002;29[Suppl 2]:S425.

73. Polk DH. Diagnosis and management of altered fetal thyroid status. *Clin Perinatol* 1994;21:647.

74. Dossing H, Jorgensen KE, Oster-Jorgensen E, et al. Recurrent pregnancy-related upper airway obstruction caused by intratracheal ectopic thyroid tissue. *Thyroid* 1999;9:955.

75. Bonnema SJ, Andersen PB, Knudsen DU, et al. MR imaging of large multinodular goiters: observer agreement on volume versus observer disagreement on dimensions of the involved trachea. *AJR Am J Roentgenol* 2002;179:259.

76. Huysmans DA, de Haas MM, van den Broek WJ, et al. Magnetic resonance imaging for volume estimation of large multinodular goitres: a comparison with scintigraphy. *Br J Radiol* 1994;67:519.

77. Newman E, Shaha AR. Substernal goiter. *J Surg Oncol* 1995;60:207.

78. Crawford SC, Harnsberger HR, Lufkin RB, et al. The role of gadolinium-DTPA in the evaluation of extracranial head and neck mass lesions. *Radiol Clin North Am* 1989;27:219.

79. Gefter WB, Spritzer CE, Eisenberg B, et al. Thyroid imaging with high-field-strength surface-coil MR. *Radiology* 1987;164:483.

80. Baker HL Jr, Berquist TH, Kispert DB, et al. Magnetic resonance imaging in a routine clinical setting. *Mayo Clin Proc* 1985;60:75.

81. Stark DD, Clark OH, Moss AA. Magnetic resonance imaging of the thyroid, thymus, and parathyroid glands. *Surgery* 1984;96:1083.

82. Higgins CB, McNamara MT, Fisher MR, et al. MR imaging of the thyroid. *AJR Am J Roentgenol* 1986;147:1255.

83. Higgins CB, Auffermann W. MR imaging of thyroid and parathyroid glands: a review of current status. *AJR Am J Roentgenol* 1988;151:1095.

84. Funari M, Campos Z, Gooding GA, et al. MRI and ultrasound detection of asymptomatic thyroid nodules in hyperparathyroidism. *J Comput Assist Tomogr* 1992;16:615.

85. Seelos KC, DeMarco R, Clark OH, et al. Persistent and recurrent hyperparathyroidism: assessment with gadopentetate dimeglumine-enhanced MR imaging. *Radiology* 1990;177:373.

86. Karstrup S. Ultrasonically guided localization, tissue verification, and percutaneous treatment of parathyroid tumours. Thesis. *Dan Med Bull* 1995;42:175.

87. Charkes ND, Maurer AH, Siegel JA, et al. MR imaging in thyroid disorders: correlation of signal intensity with Graves' disease activity. *Radiology* 1987;164:491.

88. Tezuka M, Murata Y, Ishida R, et al. MR imaging of the thyroid: correlation between apparent diffusion coefficient and thyroid gland scintigraphy. *J Magn Reson Imaging* 2003;17:163.

89. Noma S, Nishimura K, Togashi K, et al. Thyroid gland: MR imaging. *Radiology* 1987;164:495.

90. Perez Fontan FJ, Cordido CF, Pombo FF, et al. Riedel thyroiditis: US, CT, and MR evaluation. *J Comput Assist Tomogr* 1993;17:324.

91. Takashima S, Takayama F, Wang J, et al. Using MR imaging to predict invasion of the recurrent laryngeal nerve by thyroid carcinoma. *AJR Am J Roentgenol* 2003;180:837.

92. Kusunoki T, Murata K, Nishida S, et al. Histopathological findings of human thyroid tumors and dynamic MRI. *Auris Nasus Larynx* 2002;29:357.

93. Brennan MD, Miner KM, Rizza RA. Profiles of the Endocrine Clinic: the Mayo Clinic. *J Clin Endocrinol Metab* 1998;83:3427.

INTRODUCTION TO THYROID DISEASES

SURGICAL ANATOMY

ROBERT M. BEAZLEY

HISTORY

An understanding of the embryology and anatomy of the thyroid gland is important in both the medical and surgical management of thyroid diseases. In the former, it is critical to interpreting diagnostic studies especially ultrasound (US), nuclear, magnetic resonance image (MRI), and computed tomography scans (CT). In the latter case, the requirement is self-evident, with the best surgical results occurring in the hands of those individuals with an extensive and complete understanding and appreciation of the anatomy of the thyroid. Indeed, the great surgeon Halsted said "the extirpation of the thyroid gland for goiter typifies better than any operation the supreme triumph of the surgeon's art" (1).

Anatomical manifestations of the abnormal thyroid gland were recognized centuries before the gland itself was described. Goiters were first appreciated in China in 2700 B.C., while 300 years later the Romans recognized endemic goiters in the Alps. In the 7th century A.D., Paul of Aegina is reported to have been the first physician to describe a goiter, which he called a "bronchocele." Albucasis, the great Arabian physician, remarked on "the elephant of the throat" seen in women in the 11th century. Leonardo da Vinci sketched a bilobed structure he observed in the neck around 1500. Vesalius's great anatomical work *De Fabrica Humani Corporis* (1543) illustrates two "glandulae larynges," which he postulated functioned to lubricate the larynx. Although the Roman Bartholomaeus Eustachius (1520–1574), discoverer of the "adrenal glands," described a single glandulam thyroideum, with an isthmus connecting the lobes, his work was not published until the 18th century. Thomas Wharton (1614–1673) of London described the "glandula thyroidoeis," naming it because of its relationship to the thyroid cartilage. Frederick Ruysch of Leiden utilized the microscope in 1750 to reveal the vesicles in the thyroid gland.

Thyroid surgery did not come of age until the seventh decade of the 19th century, although sporadic attempts at surgical manipulation were recorded in Europe and America between 1596 and 1848, largely with disastrous results. Indeed, the evolution of thyroid surgery is the paradigm of modern surgery. Billroth (1829–1894) and Kocher (1841–1917) in Europe and Charles Mayo (1866–1939), William Halsted (1852–1922), and George Crile (1864–1943) in America were prominent contributors to the evolution of thyroid surgery. In his classic review "The Operative Story of Goiter," Halsted stated that the operation had become "essentially perfected in Switzerland, Germany and Austria by 1883" (1). Interestingly, the major technical details of thyroidectomy have changed very little in the last 125 years.

EMBRYOLOGY

Thyroid Gland

A thorough understanding of the embryologic development of the thyroid is the key to understanding surgical anatomy. Initial thyroid development is discernible around the third week with appearance, at the level of the second branchial arch, of a median anlage on the ventral pharyngeal wall. Invagination of this midline thickening evolves as a single or paired diverticulum, which migrates caudally toward the base of the neck to become the lateral thyroid lobes. In the developed fetus, the origin of the median anlage is recognized as the "foramen cecum." A stalk of degenerating follicular cells connects the invaginated median anlage to the foramen cecum, thus forming the thyroglossal duct. By the fifth week, the thyroglossal duct is markedly attenuated and begins to break into fragments, disappearing in most cases by the eighth week. Also, around the fifth week the lateral thyroid anlage, having developed from the ventral portion of the fourth pharyngeal pouch, originates and fuses to the posterior aspect of the lateral thyroid lobes, contributing up to 30% of thyroid weight. Neural crest derived cells are contributed by the abortive fifth branchial pouch. These neural crest cells of the ultimobranchial body ultimately migrate into the upper third of the thyroid lobes giving rise to the parafollicular cells or calcitonin-secreting "C-cells." In the developed thyroid, the point of fusion of this lateral thyroid anlage may be recognized as the "tubercle Zuckerkandl" located on the posterior surface of the thyroid lobe, an anatomical landmark useful in identifying the recurrent nerve (2). Recognizable thyroid follicles begin to appear around the second month, with most follicles having been formed by the fourth month. Iodine uptake occurs early and is present before mature follicles are identifiable.

The thyroglossal duct may completely disappear or remain intact, leaving an epithelial tube or cord—thus setting the stage for development of a thyroglossal duct cyst (3). These solitary cysts are generally smooth and well defined; most are midline and attached to the hyoid bone and can be seen to rise in the anterior neck when the tongue is protruded. Most cysts are recognized in childhood, but one third appear after the age of 30 years. A connection or potential connection to the foramen cecum predisposes to infection with oral flora. The resulting infection may cause spontaneous rupture with development of a thyroglossal sinus. The cysts are typically lined by either pseudostratified ciliated columnar epithelium, squamous epithelium, or both. In 20% of cases, the fibrous wall may contain heterotopic thyroid tissue in addition to chronic inflammatory infiltrate. It is said that approximately 1% of thyroglossal cysts will undergo malignant transformation, which is most commonly of the papillary variety, although squamous cell cancers are also seen.

A caudal midline thyroglossal remnant attached to the isthmus or adjacent thyroid lobe may become the pyramidal lobe. Present in about 50% of patients, the pyramidal lobe can extend cephalad, a variable distance toward the hyoid bone. Failure to recognize and remove this extension is a common cause of "incomplete total thyroidectomy." Occasionally, the pyramidal lobe is attached to the hyoid bone by a fibrous band—the obliterated thyroglossal duct. When muscle fibers are identified in this band or cord, it has been dubbed the "levator glandulae superioris."

Anomalous formation of the thyroid can lead to failure of descent and lingual thyroid or thyroid tissue in the submental area, hyoid bone region, or anywhere along the normal pathway of descent. Such abnormal positioning may be misinterpreted as a thyroglossal duct cyst. Thyrothymic thyroid rests, which are attached to the thyroid gland by connective tissue, are common. Occasionally, such nodules are recognized to descend into the anterior or posterior mediastinum, possibly giving rise to retrosternal goiters. Blood supply of these aberrant nodules usually arises from the inferior thyroid artery. In a recent study, Sackett et al studied 100 patients for thyrothymic rests, examining 180 sides of the neck in 90 individuals. Eighty-three separate sides (46%) revealed histologic thyroid rests. In those patients with recognized rests, 57% were bilateral, 30% right sided, and only 13% left sided. Eighty percent of rests were attached to the thyroid gland, 20% entirely separate, and 88% <1 cm in size (4). It has been speculated that thyrothymic rests that remain after thyroidectomy may account for the occasional failure of total thyroidectomy. Clearly, this is a finding that has not been recognized by thyroid surgeons in the past.

Our understanding of the genetics of the thyroid development and control of embryologic migration is evolving. Mouse chromosome 4 is the location of Ttf-2, which is expressed in the developing thyroid. Gene expression is down-regulated, as thyroid cell precursors complete migration. Ttf-2 null mutant mice exhibit only sublingual thyroid or a total agenesis of the thyroid gland. Heterozygous mutations in Pax-8 are associated with hemiagenesis (5). Murine HoxA3 disruption results in thyroid hypoplasia. However, the exact molecular mechanisms of thyroid development remain to be elucidated.

Recurrent Laryngeal Nerve

Embryologic formation of the recurrent laryngeal nerves is intimately associated with the sixth branchial arch. The vagus nerve primordia is recognizable by the fifth week of fetal life, with the recurrent nerve clearly discernible by the sixth to seventh week (6). The embryonic aortic arches initially lie cranial to the larynx, so the recurrent nerve passes directly to the larynx. However, with further development the larynx moves cranially, the neck lengthens, while the aortic arch remains in the thorax. The recurrent nerve descending laterally must course medially under the sixth arch to maintain intimate contact with the larynx. Thus a medial "looping pathway" for the recurrent nerve is established. On the right side the sixth arch disappears and the fifth is transitory, so the nerve ascends to loop around the proximal portion of the fourth arch, which ultimately becomes the subclavian artery. The sixth arch on the left becomes the ductus arteriosus, so one finds the recurrent nerve on the left coursing under and around this structure (ligamentum arteriosum).

The blood supply of the recurrent laryngeal nerve arises from the inferior thyroid artery. The nerve enters the neck from behind the clavicle and the subclavian vessel on the right and the aorta on the left, coursing cephalad in the tracheoesophageal groove. Frequently, the right nerve ascends slightly lateral to the groove, while the left tends to course more medially in the groove. Approximately 50% of the time a nerve branches along its course into ventral and dorsal branches, with the dorsal branch innervating the esophagus and the ventral branch the larynx. Occasionally, more than two branches may be observed. The nerve is intimately associated with the inferior thyroid, crossing it at an oblique angle. It may cross dorsally or ventrally or between branches of the artery. This unpredictable anatomical situation is a constant source of concern to the thyroid surgeon because of the potential of inadvertent injury.

The surgeon must be aware of anatomical anomalies of the recurrent nerve that may be encountered. The most common is the "nonrecurring" recurrent nerve on the right side (~1%). This anomaly occurs as a result of the absence of the proximal portion of the fourth arch, with the right subclavian artery arising from the distal aortic arch and passing behind the esophagus. As a result, the right recurrent nerve courses directly from the vagus in the neck and enters the cricothyroid membrane behind the inferior cornu of thyroid cartilage from the area of the upper pole of the thyroid. The nerve can approach the thyroid gland in a course parallel with the inferior thyroid artery and can thus be confused as a vascular structure. A right aortic arch with the ligamentum arteriosum, which in two thirds of cases is associated with a left retro esophageal subclavian artery, will set the anatomical stage for a "nonrecurring" left recurrent nerve. This is an exceedingly rare occurrence. Preoperative imaging studies, especially CT, may alert the surgeon to these recurrent nerve anomalies.

The superior laryngeal nerve is a second nerve related to thyroid anatomy. It arises from the caudal end of the nodose ganglia after the vagus nerve exits the jugular foramen. It passes caudally deep to the carotid artery and along the pharynx toward the superior cornu of the thyroid cartilage, where it divides into a large internal branch (sensory to the epiglottis, base of the tongue, and larynx) and a smaller external branch (motor to the cricothyroideus and the inferior phargeal constrictors, with some sensory fibers to the intralaryngeal mucous membrane) (7). The external branch of the superior laryngeal nerve chiefly tenses the vocal cord, resulting in the timbre of the voice. As the nerve approaches the cricothyroid muscle, it is in close relationship to the superior thyroid artery and thus may be injured during thyroid surgery, requiring ligation of the upper pole vascular pedicle. At the operating table, it is affectionately known as the "nerve of Amelita Galli-Curci," after the Italian coloratura soprano who lost the exquisite quality of her voice after goiter surgery (although speculated to have been the result of nerve injury) in 1930.

GROSS ANATOMY

The normal adult thyroid gland lies anterior to the upper trachea and consists of two lateral lobes connected by a midline isthmus. Each lobe is approximately 5 cm in length, 3 cm in width, and 2 cm in thickness. The superior pole of the lateral lobe is applied medially to the thyroid cartilage and cricothyroid muscle, posteriorly against the inferior pharyngeal constrictors and esophagus. Laterally, the lobe is adjacent to the carotid artery. The middle portion of the thyroid lobe is molded medially by the trachea, while laterally the gland abuts the carotid artery. The inferior pole lies laterally on the trachea at the level of the fourth and fifth tracheal ring. The average adult thyroid weighs between 20 and 30 g. The thyroid is covered by the sternohyoid muscle and most immediately by the sternothyroid muscle, which inserts into the thyroid cartilage

in an oblique fashion and affectively prevents the lateral thyroid lobes from encroaching medially (Fig. 17.1).

Blood Supply and Lymphatics

The arterial blood supply to the thyroid gland is derived from two main sources. The superior thyroid artery, first branch of the external carotid, descends parallel to the larynx to vascularize the upper pole. The inferior thyroid artery arises from the thyrocervical trunk and courses cephalad behind the carotid sheath to the level of the cricoid cartilage, turning medially and looping caudally to intersect the midportion of the thyroid gland. Near the capsule of the gland it divides into multiple terminal branches, one of which will generally supply the inferior parathyroid gland.

The thyroid gland is invested by the deep layer of cervical fascia, which forms a "filmy" capsule over the gland projecting into the thyroid substance, dividing the gland into irregularly shaped and sized lobules. Posteriorly, the fascia condenses forming the suspensory ligament of the thyroid (Berry's ligament), attaching the gland to the upper two or three tracheal rings. This dense attachment accounts for the up and down movement of the thyroid gland when the patient swallows. Additionally, the recurrent nerve often passes through Berry's ligament on its way to the cricothyroid membrane. The capsule provides a plane of surgical dissection between the gland, overlying sternohyoid, and sternothyroid muscles. Superficially, the thyroid surface is covered with multiple veins of varying size and a network of small lymphatic vessels. The veins for a plexus on the thyroid surface from which superior middle and inferior veins arise. The superior and middle vein empty into the jugular, while the inferior empties into the innominate vein.

The lymphatic drainage of the thyroid is profuse and flows in multiple directions. Intraglandular lymphatics communicate with capsular vessels, which may communicate diffusely across both lobes of the thyroid gland. The initial area of capsular drainage is felt to be the central or visceral compartment, defined as the space between the two common carotid arteries. Nodes in the visceral compartment may be divided into pretracheal, prelaryngeal, and paratracheoesophageal groups. Pretracheal nodes lie in anterior relationship to the isthmus and drain inferiorly into the mediastinal group, while the prelaryngeal nodes (delphian) drain cephalad toward the superior thyroid artery and into the lateral neck. Paratracheoesophageal nodes lie deep to the thyroid lobe, running in relationship to the recurrent nerve, and ultimately communicate with lymph nodes lateral to the carotid artery. Central and lower thyroid pole lymphatics normally drain toward the paratracheoesophageal nodes, while upper pole lymphatics follow the superior thyroid artery and thence to subdiagastric

Occlusion of the thoracic outlet by a large retrosternal goiter may occur when the arms are extended over the head. The "Pemberton's sign" results in the obstruction of venous return from the head and neck region, results in visible venous distension over the neck, plethoric changes in the color of the facial skin, and may be associated with difficulty breathing and/or rarely syncope (5,7).

There is no consensus as to the optimal position of the examiner to the patient when palpating the thyroid (1,5,7,20). Most agree that with practice and patience the normal thyroid gland can be readily palpated, and the ability to feel thyroid tissue does not automatically signify enlargement of the thyroid (1,3,5,10). The patient may be seated with the head tilted slightly posteriorly but avoiding extreme stretching to relieve tension on the overlying tissues. Bed-bound patients may be examined by the positioning of a pillow across the scapulae, allowing a backward head tilt and easier palpation of the thyroid in the supine position (1).

The author of this section in the previous edition favors thyroid palpation while facing the patient (1). The examiner identifies the cricoid cartilage and seeks the isthmus of the thyroid directly below this landmark (Fig. 1A). The presence of kyphosis and emphysema in the elderly may result in the cricoid being displaced behind the sternum, making thyroid palpation in such individuals extremely difficult (1). Palpation of the isthmus with the thumb is accomplished by moving the thumb over the isthmus and with the thumb stationary during swallowing. As outlined in the previous edition, the examiner approaches the patient from the right to examine the left lobe and from the left to examine the right lobe. From the right, the left lobe is palpated with two or three fingers of the right hand lateral to the trachea and medial to the SCM muscles, with the thumb placed right of the trachea (1) (Fig. 1B). Palpation starts above the expected location of the thyroid and moves downward in a circular, rubbing motion, applying gentle (but adequate) pressure as the lobe is examined. The fingers are kept stationary at various levels of interest, and the patient swallows, sliding the thyroid beneath the fingers. An alternative to examining from alternate sides of the patient is accomplished, i.e., from the right by using the right thumb to palpate the right lobe and the fingers to examine the left lobe, as described earlier.

Others recommend palpation with the examiner positioned behind the seated or standing patient (4,6,10,20). The examiner places the fingers of both hands on the patient's neck with the index fingers initially localizing the cricoid cartilage, then moving just below to palpate the isthmus. The head is tilted posteriorly enough to relieve tension of the overlying structures and allow the SCM muscles to displace somewhat laterally. With the tips of two or three fingers overlying the thyroid lobes (Fig. 1C), the examiner may slide the fingers over the thyroid, applying sufficient pressure to feel beneath the overlying struc-

TABLE 18.1. CLINICAL FINDINGS AND ASSOCIATION OF MALIGNANCY IN THYROID NODULES

Finding	Favors Benign	Favors Malignant (L.R.)
Pain, tenderness	X	—
Soft, smooth, mobile	X	—
Change in nodule size	↓	↑
Firm, hard, irregular nodule	—	X
Multinodular goiter	?	?
Dominant nodule	—	X
Vocal cord paralysis with		
Goiter	—	X (45.2)
Nodule	—	X (12.0)
Fixed to surroundings—		
Goiter	—	X (9.7)
Nodule	—	X (7.2)
Cervical lymph nodes with		
Goiter	—	X (13.4)
Nodule	—	X (7.4)

X, finding when present favors either benign or malignant diagnosis; ↓, decrease in nodule size; ↑, increase in nodule size; L.R., likelihood ratio of malignancy being present; ?, data inconsistent. From Boyle JA, Greig WR, Franklin DA, et al. Construction of a model for computer-assisted diagnosis: application to the problem of non-toxic goiter. *QJM* 1966;35:565–588; Hamming JF, Goslings BM, van Steenis GJ, et al. The value of fine needle aspiration biopsy in patients with nodular thyroid disease divided into groups of suspicious of malignant neoplasms on clinical grounds. *Arch Intern Med* 1990;150:113–116; Belfiore A, La Rosa GL, La Porta GA, et al. Cancer risk in patients with cold thyroid nodules: relevance of iodine intake, sex, age, and multinodularity. *Am J Med* 1992;93:363–369; Singer P, Cooper DS, Daniels GH, et al. Treatment guidelines for patients with thyroid nodules and well differentiated thyroid cancer. *Arch Intern Med* 1996;156:2165–2172; Feld S, Garcia M, Baskin HJ, et al. AACE clinical practice guidelines for the diagnosis and management of thyroid nodules. *Endocrine Practice* 1996;2:80–84; McGee S. The thyroid and its disorders. In: Fathman L, ed. *Evidence-based physical diagnosis.* Philadelphia: WB Saunders, 2001:271–303; and Blum M, Hussain MA. Evidence and thoughts about thyroid nodules that grow after they have been identified as benign by aspiration cytology. *Thyroid* 2003;13:637–641, with permission.

tures and outlining the borders of both lobes. With the finger tips then stationary over the thyroid (Fig. 1C), the patient swallows, moving the thyroid under the examiner's fingers.

If nodules are appreciated, the upper and lower borders may be trapped between two examining fingers so as to allow a gross determination of size in the caudo-cranial as well as lateral-medial dimension. A simple pocket ruler is used by many clinicians for this initial measurement. Alternatively the overlying skin may be marked and measured, or tape may be applied to the skin over the nodule, marked to outline the nodule, and adhered to a note in the patient's record to document size.

The normal isthmus has a felt-like consistency and is several millimeters in thickness (1). Extending from the isthmus upward and either left or right of midline, a pyramidal lobe may be palpable. The pyramidal lobe, a vestige of the embryonic thyroglossal duct, is present in up to 80% of thyroids examined at surgery (21). A pyramidal lobe

TABLE 18.2. CORRELATION OF CLINICAL STATUS WITH PHYSICAL FINDINGS SUGGESTS DIFFERENTIAL DIAGNOSIS

Clinical	Thyroid Palpation	Differential Diagnosis
Euthyroid	Normal size, no nodules	Thyroid disease unlikely[a]
	Diffuse enlargement	Nontoxic goiter, Graves' disease, Hashimoto's thyroiditis, iodine deficiency, silent and postpartum thyroiditis
	Nodule	Benign adenoma, thyroid cyst, thyroid carcinoma
	Right lobe enlarged	Hemiagenesis of left lobe
	Sudden painful enlargement	Hemorrhage; benign, carcinoma, subacute thyroiditis (focal)
	Midline mass	
	Moves with tongue extension	Thyroglossal duct cyst
	Moves with thyroid	Pyramidal lobe
Thyrotoxic	No palpable thyroid	Exogenous thyroid ingestion, ectopic thyroid hormone production
	Diffuse enlargement (+/- pyramidal lobe)	Graves' disease, nonautoimmune hyperthyroidism, silent and postpartum thyroiditis
	Nodular bilateral enlargement	Toxic multinodular goiter
	Nodule	Toxic nodule, Graves' with cold nodule, toxic nodular goiter with dominant cold nodule
Hypothyroid	No palpable thyroid	Atrophic thyroiditis, secondary hypothyroidism, S/P 131-I Rx for Graves' disease, S/P thyroidectomy
	Diffuse enlargement (+/- pyramidal lobe)	Hashimoto's thyroiditis, iodine deficiency, iodine organification defect, silent and postpartum thyroiditis
	Nodule	Thyroid carcinoma, Hashimoto's thyroiditis, thyroid cyst

S/P, status post; Rx, treatment.
[a]Does not rule out the presence of small nodules or nonhomogenous tissue consistency.

may be palpated in the presence of generalized thyroid enlargement, as seen in Hashimoto's thyroiditis or Graves' disease (21), and may be mistaken for an isthmus nodule or a pretracheal, "delphian" lymph node (5).

During palpation of the thyroid, a vascular thrill may be appreciated, suggesting significantly increased thyroidal blood flow (10,22). Auscultation of the thyroid is important when examining the thyrotoxic patient with goiter. Blood flow is enhanced in the hyperthyroid gland (i.e., Graves' disease), and pulsating murmurs (bruit) may be heard (4–6,11). Examination of the thyroid lobes should give the examiner a sense of the size, texture, consistency, and presence of nodules or tenderness. The right lobe may be somewhat larger than the left, and each is expected to be about 4 to 5 cm less in length and 2 to 3 cm in width (4). A thyroid that is both visibly enlarged with the head in the normal position and confirmed by an estimate of increased thyroid size by palpation is highly likely to correlate with increased gland volume on ultrasound and is designated a goiter. Each lobe is estimated to be about the size of the distal phalanx of the individual's thumb (5,6). Estimates of normal adult thyroid volume (weight) in iodine-replete areas of the world range from 10 to 20 g (10,20,23,24) and varies directly by body size, sex, and, to a lesser degree, age (23). The average-sized woman has a thyroid of about 15 g; if the estimate of diffusely hypertrophied lobes, when compared to the patient's thumb, is two or three times normal size, the estimated weight is 30 to 45 g. Correlation with

objective methods of thyroid volume measurement have shown this method to be imprecise. Smaller goiters may go undetected, and the size of larger goiters tend to be underestimated (25–27). Another method of documenting diffuse thyroidal enlargement is the use of a tape measure to document neck circumference. The tape is positioned at specific landmarks that can be duplicated for serial measurements (10). If the lower borders of the gland cannot be discerned, the goiter may extend retrosternally, and the full extent of the enlargement may be underestimated by the examiner.

The consistency of the normal thyroid tissue is described as rubbery (5). A patient with Graves' disease has a thyroid that feels softer than normal (5), often described as spongy and malleable, similar to the feel of uncooked sirloin steak (10). A spectrum of increasing firmness of the thyroid tissue has been described from the Graves' gland, to colloid goiter and early Hashimoto's thyroiditis. Adenomatous and multinodular goiters are said to be even firmer than those described earlier, and late Hashimoto's glands with extensive fibrosis tend to be very firm (5). Infiltrating primary malignancies and thyroid lymphomas have been described as "stony" hard (15). Fibrotic glands affected by Reidel's thyroiditis have been said to have a woody consistency (5).

The size, location, and consistency of nodular lesions palpated in the course of the thyroid exam should be noted. When an apparent solitary nodule is palpated, multiple occult nodules are likely to be present in about half of patients (11). Correlation of physical findings and high-resolution ultrasound document show that only about 6% of nodules < 0.5 cm in diameter are palpable; as size increases, more are palpable, but only about one half of the nodules > 2 cm are reliably detected by experienced examiners (28).

Pure cysts are more likely transilluminated by the beam of a penlight pressed against the side of the nodule when compared to absent transmission observed by the unaffected contralateral lobe (10). Readily palpable enlargement of a single (usually right) thyroid lobe and absence of the contralateral (left) lobe is characteristic of the rarely seen (0.05% prevalence) hemiagenesis of a thyroid lobe (29). Fluctuant nodules may be appreciated in acute suppurative thyroiditis (4), inflamed thyroglossal duct cysts (8), and infected branchial cleft cysts (9).

Pain in the thyroid may indicate the presence of thyroiditis. Subacute granulomatous (de Quervain's) thyroiditis (SAT) is usually associated with diffusely distributed severe pain potentially making palpation problematic. Rarely, this diffuse form of thyroidal pain has been observed in Hashimoto's thyroiditis. The pain associated with SAT may occasionally be localized to an isolated area of the gland (4) and then differentiated from other conditions such as acute hemorrhage within a nodule (4), the occasional case of painful malignant thyroid disease, and acute suppurative thyroiditis (10).

Examination requires a careful determination of the presence or absence of enlarged cervical lymph nodes (2,4, 7) (Fig. 1D). A palpable node in the central cricoid area anterior to the cricothyroid ligament and just above the isthmus is termed a delphian node and may be the earliest sign of metastatic papillary cancer. The delphian node is not specific to thyroid cancer, as it may also be enlarged in patients with laryngeal cancer (11), subacute granulomatous thyroiditis (4), Graves' disease, and, rarely, in individuals with Hashimoto's thyroiditis (5,10). A differential approach to evaluating the presence of malignancy in palpable thyroid nodules and goiters is outlined in the Table 8.1. Table 8.2 correlates the clinical context and characteristics of palpable thyroid nodules and goiters with differential diagnosis.

REFERENCES

1. Daniels GH. Physical examination of the thyroid. In: Braverman LE, Utiger RD, eds. *Werner & Ingbar's the thyroid: A fundamental and clinical text*. Philadelphia: Lippincott Williams & Wilkins, 2000: 462–466.
2. Singer P, Cooper DS, Daniels GH, et al. Treatment guidelines for patients with thyroid nodules and well differentiated thyroid cancer. *Arch Intern Med* 1996;156:2165–2172.
3. Feld S, Garcia M, Baskin HJ, et al. AACE clinical practice guidelines for the diagnosis and management of thyroid nodules. *Endocrine Practice* 1996;2:80–84.
4. Dillman WH. The thyroid. In: Goldman L, Bennett JC, eds. *Cecil textbook of medicine*. Philadelphia: WB Saunders, 2000: 1231–1249.
5. Larsen PR, Davies TF, Schlumberger M-J, et al. Thyroid physiology and diagnostic evaluation of patients with thyroid disorders. In: Larsen PR, Kronenberg HM, Melmed S, et al, eds. *Williams textbook of endocrinology*. Philadelphia: WB Saunders, 2003:364–365.
6. Bickley LS, Hoekelman RA. The head and neck. In: *Physical examination and history taking*. Philadelphia: Lippincott, 1999: 202–206, 211, 244.
7. Jameson JL, Weetman AP. Disorders of the thyroid gland. In: Braunwald E, Fauci AS, Kasper DL, et al, eds. *Harrison's principles of internal medicine*. New York: McGraw-Hill, 2001:2060–2048.
8. Leonhardt JM, Heymann WR. Thyroid disease and the skin. *Dermatol Clin* 2002;20:471–481.
9. Glosser JW, Pires CAS, Feinberg SE. Branchial cleft or crevical lymphoepithelial cysts: etiology and management. *J Am Dent Assoc* 2003;134:81–86.
10. Wartofsky L. Approach to the patient with thyroid disease. In: Becker KL, ed. *Principles and practice of endocrinology*. Philadelphia: Lippincott Williams & Wilkins, 2001:308–310.
11. McGee S. The thyroid and its disorders. In: Fathman L, ed. *Evidence-based physical diagnosis*. Philadelphia: WB Saunders, 2001: 271–303.
12. Stanbury JB, Ermans AM, Hetzel BS, et al. Endemic goiter and cretinism: public health significance and prevention. *World Health Organization Chronicle* 1974;28: 220–228.
13. Perez D, Scrimshaw NS, Munoz JA. Classification of goitre and technique of endemic goiter surveys. *Bull World Health Organ* 1958;18:217–232.
14. Siminoski K. Differential movement during swallowing as an aid in the detection of thyroid pseudonodules. *Head Neck* 1994; 16:21–24.
15. Ansell SM, Grant CS, Habermann TM. Primary thyroid lymphoma. *Semin Oncol* 1999;26:316–323.
16. Gwinup G. Morton E. The high lying thyroid: a cause of pseudogoiter. *J Clin Endocrinol Metab* 1975;40:37–42.
17. Leonidas J-R, Goldman JM, Wheeler MF. Cervical lipomas masquerading as thyroid nodules. *JAMA* 1985;253:1436–1437.
18. Mercer RD. Pseudo-goiter: the Modigliani syndrome. *Cleve Clin J Med* 1975;42:319–326.
19. Pribitkin EA, Freidman O. Papillary carcinoma in a thyroglossal duct remnant. *Arch Otolaryngol Head Neck Surg* 2002;128:461–462.
20. Siminoski K. The rational clinical examination: does this patient have a goiter? *JAMA* 1995;273:813–817.
21. Dumont JE, Corvilain B, Maenhaut C. The phylogeny, ontogeny, anatomy, and metabolic regulation of the thyroid. In: De Groot LJ, ed. *Thyroid manager*. Chicago: Endocrine Education Inc, 2002:1–6.
22. Saleh A, Cohnen M Furst, G., et al. Differential diagnosis of hyperthyroidism: Doppler sosgraphic quantification of thyroid blood flow distingues between Graves' disease and diffuse toxic goiter. *Exp Clin Endocrinol Diabetes* 2002;110:32–36.
23. Hegedus L, Perrild H, Poulsen LR, et al. The determination of thyroid volume by ultrasound and its relationship to body weight, age, and sex in normal subjects. *J Clin Endocrinol Metab* 1983;56:260–263.
24. Hegedus L, Karstrup S, Veirgang D, et al. High frequency of goitre in cigarette smokers. *Clin Endocrinol (Oxf)* 1985;22:287–292.
25. Berghout A, Wiersinga WM, Smits NJ, et al. The value of thyroid volume measured by ultrasonography in the diagnosis of goiter. *Clin Endocrinol (Oxf)* 1988;28:409–414.
26. Vitti P, Martino E, Aghini-Lombardi F, et al. Thyroid volume measurement by ultrasound in children as a tool for the assess-

ment of mild iodine deficiency. *J Clin Endocrinol Metab* 1994;79:600–603.

27. Smyth PP, Darke C, Parkes AB, et al. Assessment of goiter in an area of endemic iodine deficiency. *Thyroid* 1999;9:895–901.

28. Wiest PW, Hartshorne MF, Inskip PD, et al. Thyroid palpation versus high-resolution thyroid ultrasonography in the detection of nodules. *J Ultrasound Med* 1998;17:487–496.

29. Maiorana R, Carta A, Floriddia G, et al. Thyroid hemiagenisis: prevalence in normal children and effect on thyroid function. *J Clin Endocrinol Metab* 2003;88:1534–1536.

30. Boyle JA, Greig WR, Franklin DA, et al. Construction of a model for computer-assisted diagnosis: application to the problem of non-toxic goiter. *QJM* 1966;35:565–588.

31. Hamming JF, Goslings BM, van Steenis GJ, et al. The value of fine needle aspiration biopsy in patients with nodular thyroid disease divided into groups of suspicious of malignant neoplasms on clinical grounds. *Arch Intern Med* 1990;150:113–116.

32. Belfiore A, La Rosa GL, La Porta GA, et al. Cancer risk in patients with cold thyroid nodules: relevance of iodine intake, sex, age, and multinodularity. *Am J Med* 1992;93:363–369.

33. Blum M, Hussain MA. Evidence and thoughts about thyroid nodules that grow after they have been identified as benign by aspiration cytology. *Thyroid* 2003;13:637–641.

THE EPIDEMIOLOGY OF THYROID DISEASES

MARK P.J. VANDERPUMP

The most common cause of thyroid disorders worldwide is iodine deficiency, leading to goiter formation and hypothyroidism. In iodine-replete areas, most persons with thyroid disorders have autoimmune disease, ranging from thyrotoxicosis to hypothyroidism. The problems encountered in epidemiologic studies of thyroid disorders are those of definition (e.g., overt hypothyroidism and subclinical hypothyroidism), selection criteria, influence of age and sex, environmental factors, the use of different techniques for assessment of thyroid function, and the relative paucity of incidence data. Recent data from screening large population samples in the United States have revealed differences in the frequency of thyroid dysfunction and high serum antithyroid antibody concentrations in different ethnic groups, whereas studies from Europe have revealed the influence of dietary iodine intake on the epidemiology of thyroid dysfunction.

THYROTOXICOSIS

A decrease in serum thyrotropin (TSH) concentration is the earliest measure of thyroid overactivity (subclinical thyrotoxicosis), followed by an increase in serum thyroxine (T_4) and triiodothyronine (T_3) concentrations (overt thyrotoxicosis). The most common causes of thyrotoxicosis are Graves' disease, followed by toxic multinodular goiter; rarer causes include an autonomously functioning thyroid adenoma, thyroiditis, and excessive T_4 therapy. In epidemiologic studies, however, the etiology of thyrotoxicosis is rarely ascertained.

Prevalence of Thyrotoxicosis

The prevalence of thyrotoxicosis in women is between 0.5% and 2%, and it is 10 times more common in women than in men in iodine-replete communities [1]. A cross-sectional study of 2779 subjects in the 1970s, in the community of Whickham, a mixed urban and rural area in northeast England, first documented the prevalence of thyroid disorders [2]. The prevalence of undiagnosed thyrotoxicosis, based on clinical features and high serum T_4 concentrations and high serum-free T_4 index values was 4.7 per 1000 women. Thyrotoxicosis had been previously diagnosed and treated in 20 per 1000 women, increasing to 27 per 1000 women when possible, but unproven cases were included, as compared with 1.6 to 2.3 per 1000 men, in whom no new cases were found during the survey. Subsequent studies from Europe, Japan, and the United States confirmed these results [1]. A cross-sectional survey of 25,682 subjects aged over 18 years attending a health fair in Colorado found that overt thyrotoxicosis, defined as serum TSH concentration ≤0.01mU/L, was present in only 1 per 1000 of those not taking thyroid medication [3]. In the Third National Health and Nutrition Examination Survey (NHANES III) in the United States, serum TSH and total T_4 were measured in a representative sample of 16,533 subjects aged over 12 years [4]. In those subjects who were neither taking thyroid medication nor reporting histories of thyroid disease, 2 per 1000 had "clinically significant" thyrotoxicosis, defined as a serum TSH concentration <0.1 mU/L and a serum total T_4 concentration ≥13.0 µg/dL (170 nmol/L). In a survey of 1210 elderly persons over the age of 60 years in a single general practice in Birmingham, England, only 1 subject (sex not identified) was found to have thyrotoxicosis [5]. A recent U.S. cross-sectional study of 2799 healthy community-dwelling adults aged 70 to 79 years found evidence of thyrotoxicosis (defined biochemically as a serum TSH concentration ≤0.1m U/L and a serum free T_4 concentration >1.8 ng/dL (23 pmol/L) in only 5 subjects (1 man and 4 women) [6].

The prevalence of undiagnosed thyrotoxicosis in Pescopagano, Italy, an area of mild iodine deficiency (median urinary iodine excretion, 55 µg/L), was higher, at 2%, with a further 1% of adults there having a history of toxic nodular goiter [7]. Approximately one third had a diffuse goiter; the frequency in men and women was similar. In a population sample of 2656 from Copenhagen, another area of mild iodine deficiency (median urinary iodine excretion, 70 µg/L), newly diagnosed thyrotoxicosis was found in 1.2% of women and no men, and the prevalence of known thyrotoxicosis was 1.4% [8].

Subclinical Thyrotoxicosis

The introduction of assays for serum TSH that were sensitive enough to distinguish between normal and low concentrations allowed subjects with subclinical thyrotoxicosis to be identified. Subclinical thyrotoxicosis is defined as a low serum TSH concentration and normal serum T_4 and T_3 concentrations, in the absence of hypothalamic or pituitary disease, nonthyroidal illness, or ingestion of drugs that inhibit TSH secretion (see Chapter 79). The available studies differ in the definition of a low serum TSH concentration and whether the subjects included were receiving T_4 therapy.

The reported overall prevalence ranges from 0.5% to 6.3%, with men and women aged over 65 years having the highest prevalence, approximately half of whom were taking T_4 (3–5,9,10). Among these studies, the serum TSH cut-off value ranged from <0.1 to <0.5 mU/L; it is not clear how this difference affected the reported prevalence rates. In the Colorado study of 25,862 subjects (of whom 88% were white), and in which the serum TSH cut-off value was 0.3 mU/L, the overall prevalence of subclinical thyrotoxicosis was 2.1% (3). In contrast, the NHANES III study, defining subclinical thyrotoxicosis using a more stringent serum TSH cut-off value of 0.1 mU/L, reported an overall prevalence of 0.7% in the total population and 0.2% in the thyroid disease-free population ($n = 13,344$) (4). The rates were highest in those subjects aged 20 to 39 years and in those older than 79 years. In this study, the percentage of subjects with serum TSH concentrations <0.4 mU/L was significantly higher in women than men, and black subjects had significantly lower mean serum TSH concentrations, and therefore a higher prevalence of subclinical thyrotoxicosis (0.4%) than whites (0.1%) or Mexican Americans (0.3%).

At the 20-year follow-up of the Whickham survey cohort, 4% had serum TSH values <0.5 mU/L (normal, 0.5 to 5.2 mU/L), decreasing to 3% if those subjects were taking T_4; those with newly diagnosed overt thyrotoxicosis were excluded (9). When serum TSH was measured in the same subjects using a more sensitive TSH assay (detection limit of 0.01 mU/L, coefficient of variation of 10% at 0.08 mU/L, and a normal range of 0.17 to 2.89 mU/L), approximately 2% had subnormal serum TSH concentrations ($\geq$0.01 but <0.17 mU/L), and 1% had undetectable serum TSH concentrations (<0.01 mU/L). In subjects over 60 years of age in the Framingham Heart Study, 4% had a low serum TSH concentration (<0.1 mU/L), of whom half were taking T_4 (10).

Among subjects with subclinical thyrotoxicosis, those with low but detectable serum TSH values may recover spontaneously when retested. In the community survey in Birmingham, UK, 6% had low serum TSH concentrations, and 2% of women and 1% of men had undetectable values (<0.05 mU/L) (5). One year later, 88% of those with undetectable serum TSH values continued to have a

subnormal value, and 76% of those with a value of 0.05 to 0.5 mU/L had normal values.

The prevalence of subnormal serum TSH concentrations (detection limit 0.01 mU/L and excluding those subjects taking T_4) was higher in the iodine-deficient population of Pescopagano (6%), due to functional autonomy from a nodular goiter (7). In Jutland, an area of mild iodine deficiency in Denmark, 10% of a random sample of 423 subjects had low serum TSH concentrations, as compared with 1% of 100 subjects of similar age in iodine-rich Iceland (11). Subclinical thyrotoxicosis was not detected in a group of elderly nursing home residents in an iodine-rich region of Hungary (12).

Incidence of Overt Thyrotoxicosis

The annual incidence data available for overt thyrotoxicosis from large population studies are comparable, at 0.4 per 1000 women and 0.1 per 1000 men, but the age-specific incidence varies considerably (1). The peak age-specific incidence of Graves' disease was between 20 and 49 years in two studies (13,14), but increased with age in Iceland (15) and peaked at 60 to 69 years in Malmö, Sweden (16). The peak age-specific incidence of thyrotoxicosis caused by toxic nodular goiter and autonomously functioning thyroid adenomas in the Malmö study was over 80 years. The only available data in a black population, from Johannesburg, South Africa, also suggest a tenfold-lower annual incidence of thyrotoxicosis (0.09 per 1000 women and 0.007 per 1000 men) than in whites (17). In a prospective study of 12 towns in England and Wales, the annual incidence of thyrotoxicosis strongly correlated with the prevalence of endemic goiter among schoolchildren 60 years earlier (18). Subsequent to this survey, serum samples from 216 of the 290 cases identified were assayed for TSH receptor antibodies. The frequency of antibody-positive thyrotoxicosis, an indicator of Graves' disease, did not correlate with goiter in the past (19).

In a 20-year follow-up of the Whickham cohort, the mean annual incidence of thyrotoxicosis in women was 0.8 per 1000 survivors (95% confidence interval, 0.5 to 1.4) (9). The incidence rate was similar in the women who had died during the 20-year interval. No new cases were detected in men. An estimate of the probability of the development of thyrotoxicosis in women at a particular time averaged 1.4 per 1000 between the ages of 35 and 60 years (Fig. 19.1). Neither serum thyroid antibody status nor the presence of a goiter during the first survey was associated with the development of thyrotoxicosis at follow-up. Other cohort studies provide comparable incidence data, which suggests that many cases of thyrotoxicosis remain undiagnosed in the community unless routine testing is undertaken (1).

Data on the risk of progression of subclinical to overt thyrotoxicosis are limited. At the 1-year follow-up of the subjects over 60 years of age in Birmingham, of 50 who

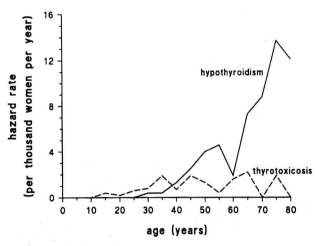

FIGURE 19.1. The age-specific hazard rates for the development of overt thyrotoxicosis (hyperthyroidism) and hypothyroidism in women followed for 20 years in the community survey in Whickham, England. (From Vanderpump MPJ, Tunbridge WMG, French JM, et al. The incidence of thyroid disorders in the community: a twenty-year follow-up of the Whickham Survey. *Clin Endocrinol (Oxf)* 1995;43:55–69, with permission.)

initially had serum TSH values below normal, only 1 subject developed overt thyrotoxicosis (5). In short follow-up studies, the incidence has been calculated at 5% per year (20).

CHRONIC AUTOIMMUNE THYROIDITIS

The presence of high serum concentrations of thyroid antibodies [antithyroid peroxidase (microsomal) and antithyroglobulin] correlates with the presence of focal thyroiditis in thyroid tissue obtained by biopsy and at autopsy from patients with no evidence of hypothyroidism during life (21). Patients with hypothyroidism caused by either atrophic or goitrous autoimmune thyroiditis usually have high serum concentrations of these same antibodies. High serum concentrations of these antibodies, especially thyroid peroxidase antibodies, also are often found in patients with Graves' disease and other thyroid diseases, but not as often, and the serum concentrations are usually lower (see Chapter 15).

In all the early studies, regardless of the methodology, a progressive increase in prevalence of positive serum tests for thyroid antibodies was found with age in women, as compared with a uniformly low prevalence and no age trend in men. In the Whickham survey, mean serum TSH concentrations were significantly higher in both men and women with positive serum antithyroid antibody tests, and 3% of the subjects (5% of women, 1% of men) had both positive antibody tests and a serum TSH value >6 mU/L (2). In the NHANES III survey, the percentage of subjects

with high serum antithyroid peroxidase and antithyroglobulin antibody concentrations increased with age in both men and women, and high concentrations were more prevalent in women than in men and less prevalent in blacks than in other ethnic groups (4). High serum antithyroglobulin antibody concentrations alone were not significantly associated with thyroid disease in this study.

At the 20-year follow-up of the Whickham survey, 19% of the survivors had high serum antithyroid peroxidase antibody concentrations and 5% had high serum antithyroglobulin antibody concentrations (9). Seventeen percent of women and 7% of men who initially had normal values now had high values, 9% of women and 2% of men had high values on both occasions, and 2% of women and 0.5% of men had high values initially but not at follow-up. Over 50% of the women in whom the serum antithyroid antibody concentrations changed from high to normal were receiving T_4 treatment for hypothyroidism. There was no evidence that a high serum antithyroid antibody concentration at the original survey was a risk factor for premature death in this cohort (22).

HYPOTHYROIDISM

The earliest biochemical abnormality in hypothyroidism is an increase in serum TSH concentration associated with normal serum T_4 and T_3 concentrations (subclinical hypothyroidism). This is followed by a decrease in serum T_4 concentration, at which stage most patients have symptoms and benefit from treatment (overt hypothyroidism). In persons living in iodine-replete areas, the cause is usually either chronic autoimmune thyroiditis (atrophic autoimmune thyroiditis or goitrous autoimmune thyroiditis [Hashimoto's thyroiditis]) (see Chapter 47) or destructive treatment for thyrotoxicosis, but the cause was not often determined in the large cohort studies.

Prevalence of Hypothyroidism

In iodine-replete communities, the prevalence of spontaneous hypothyroidism is between 1% and 2%, and it is more common in older women and about ten times more common in women than in men (23). In the Whickham survey, the prevalence of newly diagnosed overt hypothyroidism was 3 per 1000 women (2). The prevalence of previously diagnosed and treated hypothyroidism was 14 per 1000 women, increasing to 19 per 1000 women when possible, but unproven, cases were included. The overall prevalence in men was <1 case per 1000. One third had been previously treated by surgery or radioiodine for thyrotoxicosis. Excluding iatrogenic causes, the prevalence of hypothyroidism was 10 per 1000 women, increasing to 15 per 1000 when possible, but unproven, cases were included (Fig. 19.1). This is comparable with other studies, including the Colorado and NHANES III studies, in which the prevalence of newly diagnosed hypothyroidism was 4 per 1000 and 3 per 1000, respectively (3,4). In Pescopagano, the prevalence of newly diagnosed overt hypothyroidism was 0.3% of 573 women (chronic autoimmune thyroiditis confirmed as etiology) (there were no cases among 419 men), and no subject had been diagnosed and treated for hypothyroidism (7). In Copenhagen, 6 per 1000 of the women and 2 per 1000 men had overt but undiagnosed hypothyroidism, and 1% were taking T_4 (8).

Subclinical Hypothyroidism

In the original Whickham survey, 8% of women (10% of women over 55 years of age) and 3% of men had subclinical hypothyroidism (2). Serum TSH concentrations did not change as a function of age among adult men, but in women over 40 years of age the concentrations increased. If, however, women with high serum antithyroid antibody concentrations were excluded, there was no age-related increase (2). In the Colorado study, 9.4% of the subjects had a high serum TSH concentration, of whom 9.0% had subclinical hypothyroidism (3). Among those with a high serum TSH concentration, 74% had a value between 5.1 and 10 mU/L, and 26% had a value >10 mU/L. The percentage of subjects with a high serum TSH concentration was higher for women than men in each decade of age, and ranged from 4% to 21% in women and 3% to 16% in men (Fig. 19.2). In the NHANES III study, serum TSH concentrations increased with age in both men and women and were higher in whites than blacks, independent of serum antithyroid antibody concentrations (4).

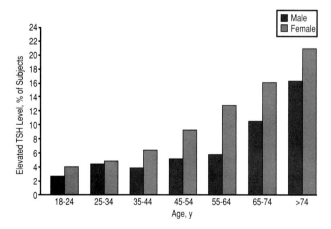

FIGURE 19.2. The percentage of 25,682 subjects with a high serum thyrotropin concentration, by sex and decade of age, in the Colorado Thyroid Study. (From Canaris GJ, Manowitz NR, Mayor G, et al. The Colorado Thyroid Disease Prevalence Study. *Arch Intern Med* 2000;160:526–534, with permission.)

Community studies of elderly persons have confirmed the high prevalence of subclinical hypothyroidism in this age group, with approximately 10% of subjects over the age of 60 years having serum TSH values above the normal range (5,24). Recent data from a cohort of people aged 70 to 79 years in the United States found that black subjects had a significantly lower prevalence of subclinical hypothyroidism (2% in men, 3% in women), as compared with white subjects (4% in men, 6% in women) (6). In iodine-deficient Pescopagano, there was a slightly lower prevalence of subclinical hypothyroidism (4% of women and 3% of men), but high serum antithyroid antibody concentrations were as prevalent, although lower, as in iodine-replete communities (7). In Copenhagen (mild iodine deficiency), only 0.7% of subjects had subclinical hypothyroidism, and 83% of them had serum antithyroid antibody concentrations >200 kU/L (8). Among elderly persons living in iodine-deficient areas, approximately 10% of subjects over age 60 years had serum TSH values above the normal range (10,11). Subclinical hypothyroidism is found at higher frequency (18% in Iceland and 24% in Hungary) in areas where iodine intake is high, but most cases are not of autoimmune origin (11,12).

Overt Hypothyroidism

After destructive treatment of thyrotoxicosis with either radioiodine or surgery, the incidence of overt hypothyroidism is greatest in the first year (25,26). In an audit of 813 consecutive patients treated for thyrotoxicosis in Birmingham, United Kingdom, there was an increase in the incidence of hypothyroidism at 1 year in those given higher doses of radioiodine (61% among those given 10 mCi (370 MBq) versus 41% among those given 5 mCi (185 MBq) (27). The incidence of hypothyroidism in patients with Graves' thyrotoxicosis was higher than that in patients with nodular goiter (55% vs. 32%). If the patient had subclinical hypothyroidism 1 year or more after radioiodine or surgical treatment, then the rate of progression to overt hypothyroidism was 2% to 6% per year (25,26).

The incidence of hypothyroidism after surgery, external radiation therapy of the neck, or both, in patients with head and neck cancer (including lymphoma) is as high as 50% within the first year after treatment, particularly in patients who underwent surgery and received high doses of radiation (28,29). The effect is dose dependent, the onset is gradual, and subclinical hypothyroidism can be present for many years before the development of overt hypothyroidism.

The 20-year follow-up of the Whickham cohort provided incidence data and allowed the determination of risk factors for spontaneous hypothyroidism in this period (9). The mean annual incidence of spontaneous hypothyroidism in the surviving women during the 20-year follow-up period was 3.5 per 1000 (95% confidence interval, 2.8 to 4.5), increasing to 4.1 per 1000 (95% confidence interval, 3.3 to 5.0) if all cases, including those who had received destructive treatment for thyrotoxicosis, were included. The hazard rate (i.e., the estimate of the probability of a woman developing hypothyroidism at a particular time) increased with age to 13.7 per 1000 in women 75 to 80 years of age (Fig 19.1). The mean annual incidence during the 20-year follow-up period in men (all spontaneous except for 1 case of lithium-induced hypothyroidism) was 0.6 per 1000 (95% confidence interval, 0.3 to 1.2). The risk of having developed hypothyroidism was examined with respect to risk factors identified in the first survey. In the surviving women, the annual risk of spontaneous overt hypothyroidism was 4% in those who had both high serum TSH and antithyroid antibody concentrations, 3% if only their serum TSH concentration was high, and 2% if only their serum thyroid antibody concentration was high; at the time of follow-up, the respective rates overall of hypothyroidism were 55%, 33%, and 27%. The probability of developing hypothyroidism was higher in those women who had serum TSH concentrations above 2.0 mU/L and high serum titers of antithyroid microsomal antibodies during the first survey (Fig. 19.3). Neither a positive family history of any thyroid disease, the presence of a goiter at either the first or the follow-up survey, nor parity at first survey was associated with an increased risk of hypothyroidism.

The other incidence data for hypothyroidism are from short (and often small) follow-up studies. In a follow-up study of 437 healthy women 40 to 60 years of age in the Netherlands, 24% of those who initially had a positive serum test for antithyroid microsomal antibodies and normal serum TSH concentrations had a high serum TSH concentration (>4.2 mU/L) 10 years later, as compared with 3% in the women who had a negative test for the antibodies (30). As in the 20-year follow-up of the Whickham cohort, serum TSH concentrations in the upper part of the normal range in this study also appeared to have a predictive value. In a 9-year follow-up of a cohort of 82 women with subclinical hypothyroidism, the cumulative incidence of overt hypothyroidism was 0% in those with serum TSH concentrations of 4 to 6 mU/L, 43% in those with serum TSH concentrations >6 to 12 mU/L, and 77% in those with serum TSH concentrations >12 mU/L (31).

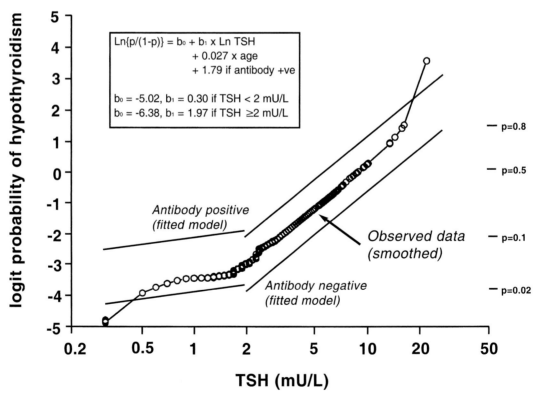

FIGURE 19.3. The probability of development of overt hypothyroidism in 20 years among 912 women of the original Whickham cohort, as a function of their serum thyrotropin values at baseline. (From Vanderpump MPJ, Tunbridge WMG, French JM, et al. The incidence of thyroid disorders in the community: a twenty-year follow-up of the Whickham Survey. *Clin Endocrinol (Oxf)* 1995;43:55–69, with permission.)

In this study, the incidence of overt hypothyroidism also was higher in those women with high serum antithyroid microsomal antibody concentrations at baseline (59% vs. 23%; $p = 0.03$), but a high serum antithyroid antibody concentration contributed much less to the risk of overt hypothyroidism than did a high baseline serum TSH concentration, in contrast to the Whickham data. All studies indicate that the higher the serum TSH value, the greater the likelihood of development of overt hypothyroidism in subjects with chronic autoimmune thyroiditis. High serum antithyroid antibody and TSH concentrations have prognostic importance in elderly subjects as well (5,32,33).

SPORADIC GOITER

The most common thyroid disease in the community is simple (diffuse) goiter. The clinical grading of thyroid size is subjective and imprecise (34,35). Ultrasonography has been used in epidemiologic studies to assess thyroid size (36–38), leading to much higher estimates of goiter prevalence than in studies in which goiter size was assessed by physical examination.

Considerable regional variations in the incidence of goiter exist, even in nonendemic goiter areas. In cross-sectional surveys, the prevalence of diffuse goiter declines with age, the greatest prevalence is in premenopausal women, and the ratio of women to men is at least 4:1 (2). This decline in frequency of goiter with age is in contrast to the age-related increase in frequency of thyroid nodules and high serum antithyroid antibody concentrations. In the Framingham study of subjects over 60 years of age, the prevalence of single thyroid nodules was 3% and that of multiple nodules was 1%, as assessed by palpation (39). In a survey of 101 women 49 to 58 years of age, thyroid nodules were detected by ultrasonography in 36%, of which less than one third were detected by palpation (40). Ultrasonography as a screening test is too sensitive and will result in the unnecessary pursuit of findings that are so common that they rarely have any pathologic importance (see Chapter 16). A higher prevalence of multinodular goiter is found in areas of iodine deficiency (41).

Longitudinal studies confirm the decreasing frequency of goiter with age. In the 20-year follow-up of the Whickham cohort, 10% of women and 2% of men had a goiter, as compared with 23% and 5%, respectively, at the first survey (9). The presence of a diffuse goiter was not predictive of any clinical or biochemical evidence of thyroid dysfunction. In women, an association was found between the development of a goiter and thyroid antibody status at follow-up, but not initially. In a 20-year follow-up study of 11- to 18-year-old subjects in southwestern United States, 60% of the 92 subjects who had a diffuse goiter initially had spontaneous regression by the age of 30 years (42).

Longitudinal data from Framingham suggests an annual incidence of thyroid nodules of 1 per 1000, and that, once formed, they tend to remain present for a long period of time; virtually all are benign (39).

SCREENING FOR THYROID DYSFUNCTION

Congenital hypothyroidism affects about one newborn in 3500 to 4500 births and is the most treatable cause of mental retardation. Iodine deficiency (intake below 25 μg/day), particularly in preterm infants, still accounts for many cases of congenital hypothyroidism in Europe, Asia, and Africa. Clinical diagnosis occurs in <5% of newborns with hypothyroidism because symptoms and signs are often minimal (43). The value of screening for congenital hypothyroidism in heel-prick blood specimens is unquestioned, and it is now done routinely in many countries (see section on neonatal screening in Chapter 75).

Certain groups of adults who should have an assessment of thyroid function (e.g. measurement of serum TSH) at least once to detect thyroid dysfunction include those with atrial fibrillation (44) or hyperlipidemia (45). There is a high frequency of asymptomatic thyroid dysfunction in unselected patients with diabetes mellitus, and annual assessment of thyroid function in patients with diabetes is cost-effective (46). There is no consensus on whether healthy women should be screened for postpartum thyroiditis (see Chapters 27 and 80). However, women with type 1 diabetes are three times more likely to develop postpartum thyroid dysfunction than are normal women, and therefore all such diabetic women should be tested (47). Any woman with a past history of postpartum thyroiditis should be offered annual assessment of thyroid function, in view of their increased long-term risk of permanent hypothyroidism. Similarly, in view of the high prevalence of hypothyroidism in patients with Down's syndrome (48) and Turner's syndrome (49), these patients should also have an annual assessment of thyroid function. Assessment of thyroid function is indicated every 6 months in patients receiving amiodarone and lithium and every 12 months in those treated with head and neck radiation (see section of effects of drugs and other substances on thyroid hormone synthesis and the section on effect of excess iodide in Chapters 11 and 50) (23).

All patients with thyrotoxicosis who receive destructive treatment for thyrotoxicosis should be followed indefinitely for the development of hypothyroidism; this follow-up should begin 4 to 8 weeks after treatment, then at 3-month intervals for 1 year, and then annually thereafter (see Chapter 45). Among patients hospitalized for acute illness, the occurrence of thyroid disease is no more common than in the general population. Therefore, testing should be limited but with a high index of clinical suspicion, particularly in elderly women, and with an awareness of the difficulties in interpreting thyroid function tests in the presence of acute illness (see section on nonthyroidal illness in Chapter 11) (50).

Controversy exists as to whether healthy adults living in an area of iodine sufficiency benefit from screening for thyroid disease. The prevalence of unsuspected overt thyroid disease is low, but as described above a substantial proportion of subjects tested will have evidence of thyroid dysfunction, usually subclinical hypothyroidism. In the absence of the confounding effects of nonthyroidal illness or drugs, a normal serum TSH concentration has a high predictive value in ruling out thyroid disease in healthy subjects. In unselected populations, measurement of serum TSH has a sensitivity of 89% to 95% and specificity of 90% to 96% for overt thyroid dysfunction, as compared with cases confirmed by history, examination, and additional testing. Normal serum TSH concentrations are found in some patients with hypothyroidism caused by pituitary or hypothalamic disease, but both these situations are rare (see Chapter 13). In nearly all studies serum TSH value >5 or 6 mU/L is accepted as being raised (51).

Various physician organizations have made different recommendations as to whether subclinical thyroid disease is of sufficient clinical importance to warrant screening and therapy (1,52–59). A cost-utility analysis using a computer decision model suggested that the cost-effectiveness of screening for subclinical hypothyroidism compared favorably with other preventive medical practices, such as screening for hypertension or breast cancer in women in the same age group, while providing a similar increase in quality-adjusted life years (60–61). Over one half of the presumed benefit in the latter was accounted for by preventing progression to overt hypothyroidism, 30% by improving associated mild symptoms, and 2% by preventing cardiovascular disease. The cost of detecting subclinical hypothyroidism was $9,223 for women and $22,595 for men per quality-of-life year gained, but this cost was heavily dependent on the cost of the serum TSH assay. The cost-benefit analysis did not allow for the extra costs of detecting, investigating, and potentially treating subclinical thyrotoxicosis.

This analysis led the American Thyroid Association to recommend population-based screening for thyroid dysfunction by measurement of serum TSH, beginning at age 35 years and every 5 years thereafter (62). Those organizations that assess screening programs, such as the U.S. Preventive Services Task Force, have not recommended regular assessment of thyroid function in adults (55). The reason is that there have been no trials to determine whether identification and treatment of subjects with thyroid dysfunction, which would mostly be subclinical hypothyroidism, results in any long-term benefit. The potential benefits in terms of decreased symptoms or other systemic effects are generally small and may not enhance quality of life (see Chapters 78 and 79). In a recent observational 10-year study, a low serum TSH concentration (<0.05 mU/L), but not a high serum TSH concentration, was associated with

an increase in all-cause mortality and cardiovascular mortality (63).

If screening is done, and a high serum TSH concentration is found, the measurement should be repeated 1 or 2 months later, along with measurement of serum-free T_4, after excluding nonthyroidal illness and drug interference. If the serum TSH concentration is high and the serum-free T_4 concentration is low, then the subject has overt hypothyroidism, and, even if asymptomatic on further questioning, should be treated with T_4. If the serum free T_4 concentration is normal, but the serum TSH concentration is >10 or 15 mU/L, then treatment with T_4 is reasonable, if only because of the likelihood of progression. If the serum TSH concentration is between 5 and 10 mU/L, then serum antithyroid peroxidase antibodies should be measured. If the serum antibody concentration is high, then serum TSH should be measured annually; T_4 therapy should be started if the serum TSH concentration rises above 10 mU/L. If the serum antibody concentration is normal, then repeat measurement of serum TSH every 3 to 5 years may be all that is required (1).

Few subjects screened will have overt thyrotoxicosis, but the consequences of finding subclinical thyrotoxicosis have to be addressed. If a subject has a low screening serum TSH value, the first step is to repeat the measurement of serum TSH and measure serum free T_4, to identify overt thyrotoxicosis (and also central hypothyroidism). Usually, subclinical thyrotoxicosis will be confirmed. In addition to the risk of overt thyrotoxicosis, the subject may be at risk for atrial fibrillation and osteoporosis (see Chapter 79) (64, 65). No consensus exists regarding the treatment of subclinical thyrotoxicosis, although therapy with an antithyroid drug or radioiodine may be indicated (66). Any potential benefits of therapy in subclinical thyrotoxicosis must be weighed against the substantial morbidity associated with the treatment of thyrotoxicosis (see Chapter 45). If treatment is not undertaken, serum TSH should be measured at least annually, with follow-up measurements of serum-free T_4 if the serum TSH value is low.

There is an urgent need for long-term studies of the effects of treatment of both subclinical hypothyroidism and subclinical thyrotoxicosis to determine if there is indeed benefit from screening for thyroid dysfunction in adults.

REFERENCES

1. Tunbridge WMG, Vanderpump MPJ. Population screening for autoimmune thyroid disease. *Endocrinol Metab Clin North Am* 2000;29:239–253.
2. Tunbridge WMG, Evered DC, Hall R, et al. The spectrum of thyroid disease in the community: The Whickham Survey. *Clin Endocrinol (Oxf)* 1977;7:481–491.
3. Canaris GJ, Manowitz NR, Mayor G, et al. The Colorado Thyroid Disease Prevalence Study. *Arch Intern Med* 2000; 160:526–534.

4. Hollowell JG, Staehling NW, Flanders D, et al. Serum TSH, T$_4$, and thyroid antibodies in the United States population (1988 to 1994): National Health and Nutrition Survey (NHANES III). *J Clin Endocrinol Metab* 2002;87:489–499.

5. Parle JV, Franklyn JA, Cross KW, et al. Prevalence and follow-up of abnormal thyrotrophin (TSH) concentrations in the elderly in the United Kingdom. *Clin Endocrinol (Oxf)* 1991;34:77–83.

6. Kanaya AM, Harris F, Volpato S, et al. Association between thyroid dysfunction and total cholesterol level in an older biracial population: The Health, Aging and Body Composition Study. *Arch Intern Med* 2002;162:773–779.

7. Aghini-Lombardi F, Antonangeli L, Martino E, et al. The spectrum of thyroid disorders in an iodine-deficient community: The Pescopagano Survey. *J Clin Endocrinol Metab* 1999;84:561–566.

8. Knudsen N, Jørgensen T, Rasmussen S, et al. The prevalence of thyroid dysfunction in a population with borderline iodine deficiency. *Clin Endocrinol (Oxf)* 1999;51:361–367.

9. Vanderpump MPJ, Tunbridge WMG, French JM, et al. The incidence of thyroid disorders in the community: a twenty-year follow-up of the Whickham Survey. *Clin Endocrinol (Oxf)* 1995;43:55–69.

10. Sawin CT, Geller A, Kaplan MM, et al. Low serum thyrotropin (thyroid-stimulating hormone) in older persons without hyperthyroidism. *Arch Intern Med* 1991;151:165–168.

11. Laurberg P, Pedersen KM, Hreidarsson A, et al. Iodine intake and the pattern of thyroid disorders: a comparative epidemiological study of thyroid abnormalities in the elderly in Iceland and in Jutland, Denmark. *J Clin Endocrinol Metab* 1998;83:765–769.

12. Szabolcs I, Padoba J, Feldkamp J, et al. Comparative screening for thyroid disorders in old age in areas of iodine deficiency, long-term iodine prophylaxis and abundant iodine intake. *Clin Endocrinol (Oxf)* 1997;47:87–92.

13. Furszyfer J, Kurland LT, McConahey WM, et al. Graves' disease in Olmsted County, Minnesota, 1935 through 1967. *Mayo Clin Proc* 1970;45:636–644.

14. Mogensen EF, Green A. The epidemiology of thyrotoxicosis in Denmark. Incidence and geographical variation in the Funen region 1972–1974. *Acta Med Scand* 1980;208:183–186.

15. Haraldsson A, Gudmundsson ST, Larusson G, et al. Thyrotoxicosis in Iceland 1980–1982. An epidemiological survey. *Acta Medica Scandinavica* 1985;217:253–258.

16. Berglund J, Christensen SB, Hallengren B. Total and age-specific incidence of Graves' thyrotoxicosis, toxic nodular goitre and solitary toxic adenoma in Malmö 1970–1974. *J Intern Med* 1990;227:137–141.

17. Kalk WJ, Kalk J. Incidence and causes of hyperthyroidism in blacks. *S Afr Med J* 1989;75:114–116.

18. Barker DJB, Phillips DIW. Current incidence of thyrotoxicosis and past prevalence of goiter in 12 British towns. *Lancet* 1984;2:567–570.

19. Phillips DIW, Barker DJ, Rees Smith B, et al. The geographical distribution of thyrotoxicosis in England according to the presence or absence of TSH-receptor antibodies. *Clin Endocrinol (Oxf)* 1985;23:283–287.

20. Wiersinga WM. Subclinical hypothyroidism and hyperthyroidism. I. Prevalence and clinical relevance. *Neth J Med* 1995;46:197–204.

21. Dayan CM, Daniels GH. Chronic autoimmune thyroiditis. *N Engl J Med* 1996;335:99–107.

22. Vanderpump MPJ, Tunbridge WMG, French JM, et al. The development of ischemic heart disease in relation to autoimmune thyroid disease in a 20-year follow-up of an English community. *Thyroid* 1996;6:155–160.

23. Vanderpump MPJ, Tunbridge WMG. Epidemiology and prevention of clinical and subclinical hypothyroidism. *Thyroid* 2002;12:839–847.

24. Sawin CT, Bigos ST, Land S, et al. The aging thyroid: relationship between elevated serum thyrotropin level and thyroid antibodies in elderly patients. *Am J Med* 1985;79:591–595.

25. Franklyn JA, Daykin J, Droic Z, et al. Long term follow-up of treatment of thyrotoxicosis by three different methods. *Clin Endocrinol (Oxf)* 1991;34:71–76.

26. Berglund J, Christensen SB, Dymling JF, et al. The incidence of recurrence and hypothyroidism following treatment with antithyroid drugs, surgery or radioiodine in all patients with thyrotoxicosis in Malmö during the period 1970–1974. *J Intern Med* 1991;229:435–442.

27. Allahabadia A, Daykin J, Sheppard MC, et al. Radioiodine treatment of hyperthyroidism—prognostic factors for outcome. *J Clin Endocrinol Metab* 2001;86:3611–3617.

28. Grande C. Hypothyroidism following radiotherapy for head and neck cancer: multivariate analysis of risk factors. *Radiother Oncol* 1992;25:31–36.

29. Tell R, Sjodin H, Lundell G, Lewin F, et al. Hypothyroidism after external radiotherapy for head and neck cancer. *Int J Radiat Oncol Biol Phys* 1997;39:303–308.

30. Geul KW, van Sluisveld ILL, Grobbee DE, et al. The importance of thyroid microsomal antibodies in the development of elevated serum TSH in middle-aged women: associations with serum lipids. *Clin Endocrinol (Oxf)* 1993;39:275–280.

31. Huber G, Staub J-J, Meier C, et al. Prospective study of the spontaneous course of subclinical hypothyroidism: Prognostic value of thytoropin, thyroid reserve, and thyroid antibodies. *J Clin Endocrinol Metab* 2002;87:3221–3226.

32. Sawin CT, Castelli WP, Hershman JM, et al. The aging thyroid: thyroid deficiency in the Framingham Study. *Arch Intern Med* 1985;145:1386–1388.

33. Rosenthal KJ, Hunt WC, Garry PJ, et al. Thyroid failure in the elderly: microsomal antibodies as discriminant for therapy. *JAMA* 1987;258:209–213.

34. Jarløv EA, Hegedüs L, Gjørup T, et al. Observer variation in the clinical assessment of the thyroid gland. *J Intern Med* 1991;229:159–161.

35. Jarløv EA, Hegedüs L, Gjørup T, et al. Inadequacy of the WHO classification of the thyroid gland. *Thyroidology* 1992;4:107–110.

36. Brander A, Viikinkoski P, Nickels J, et al. Thyroid gland: US screening in random adult population. *Radiology* 1991;181:683–687.

37. Hintze G, Windeler J, Baumert J, et al. Thyroid volume and goitre prevalence in the elderly as determined by ultrasound and their relationships to laboratory indices. *Acta Endocrinologica* 1991;124:12–18.

38. Nygaard B, Gideon P, Dige-Petersen H, et al. Thyroid volume and morphology and urinary iodine excretion in a Danish municipality. *Acta Endocrinologica* 1993;129:505–510.

39. Vander JB, Gaston EA, Dawber TR. The significance of nontoxic thyroid nodules: final report of a 15-year study of the incidence of malignancy. *Ann Intern Med* 1968;69:537.

40. Brander A, Viikinkoski P, Nickels J, et al. Thyroid gland: US screening in middle-aged women with no previous thyroid disease. *Radiology* 1989;173:507–510.

41. Smyth PPA, Darke C, Parkes AB, et al. Assessment of goitre in an area of endemic iodine deficiency. *Thyroid* 1999;9:895–901.

42. Rallison ML, Dobyns BM, Meikle AW, et al. Natural history of thyroid abnormalities: prevalence, incidence, and regression of thyroid diseases in adolescents and young adults. *Am J Med* 1991;91:363–370.

43. Anonymous. Newborn Screening for congenital hypothyroidism: recommended guidelines. *Pediatrics* 1993;91:1203–1209.

American Academy of Pediatrics AAP Section on Endocrinology and Committee on Genetics and American Thyroid Association on Public Health.

44. Woeber KA. Thyrotoxicosis and the heart. *N Eng J Med* 1992;327:94–98.

45. Pirich C, Mullner M, Sinzinger H. Prevalence and relevance of thyroid dysfunction in 1922 cholesterol screening participants. *J Clin Epidemiol* 2000;53:623–629.

46. Perros P, McCrimmon RJ, Shaw G, et al. Frequency of thyroid dysfunction in diabetic patients: value of annual screening. *Diabet Med* 1996;12:622–627.

47. Alvarez-Marfany M, Roman S, Drexler A, et al. Long-term prospective study of postpartum thyroid dysfunction in women with insulin-dependent diabetes mellitus. *J Clin Endocrinol Metab* 1994;79:10–16.

48. Karlsson B, Gustafsson J, Hedov G, et al. Thyroid dysfunction in Down's syndrome: relation to age and thyroid autoimmunity. *Arch Dis Child* 1998;79:242–245.

49. Chiovato L, Larizza D, Bendinelli G, et al. Autoimmune hypothyroidism and hyperthyroidism in patients with Turner's syndrome. *Eur J Endocrinol* 1996;134:568–575.

50. Attia J, Margetts P, Guyatt G. Diagnosis of thyroid disease in hospitalized patients: a systematic review. *Arch Intern Med* 1999;159:658–665.

51. Baloch Z, Carayon P, Conte-Devolx B, et al. Laboratory medicine practice guidelines: laboratory support for the diagnosis and monitoring of thyroid disease. *Thyroid* 2003;13:3–126.

52. Surks MI, Chopra IJ, Mariash CN, et al. American Thyroid Association guidelines for use of laboratory tests in thyroid disorders. *JAMA* 1990;263:1529–1532.

53. Singer PA, Cooper DS, Levy EG, et al. Treatment guidelines for patients with hyperthyroidism and hypothyroidism. *JAMA* 1995;273:808–812.

54. Glenn GC. Practice parameter on laboratory panel testing for screening and case finding in asymptomatic adults: the Laboratory Testing Strategy Task Force of the College of American Pathologists. *Arch Pathol Lab Med* 1996;120:929–943.

55. US Preventive Services Task Force. Screening for thyroid disease. In: *Guide to clinical preventive services.* 2nd ed. Baltimore: Williams & Wilkins, 1996:209–218.

56. Vanderpump MPJ, Ahlquist JAO, Franklyn JA, et al. Consensus statement for good practice and audit measures in the management of hypothyroidism and hyperthyroidism. *BMJ* 1996;313: 539–544.

57. Weetman AP. Hypothyroidism: screening and subclinical disease. *BMJ* 1997;314:1175–1178.

58. Helfand M, Redfern CC. Clinical guideline, part 2: Screening for thyroid disease: an update. *Ann Intern Med* 1998;129:144–158.

59. Buskin HJ. American Association of Clinical Endocrinologists Medical Guidelines for clinical practice for the evaluation and treatment of hyperthyroidism and hypothyroidism. *Endocr Pract* 2002; 8:458–467.

60. Danese MD, Powe NR, Sawin CT, et al. Screening for mild thyroid failure at the periodic health examination: a decision and cost-effectiveness analysis. *JAMA* 1996;276:285–292.

61. Powe NR, Danese MD, Ladenson PW. Decision analysis in endocrinology and metabolism. *Endocrinol Metab Clin North Am* 1997;26:89–111.

62. Ladenson PW, Singer PA, Ain KB, et al. American Thyroid Association Guidelines for detection of thyroid dysfunction. *Arch Intern Med* 2000;160:1573–1575.

63. Parle JV, Maisonneuve P, Sheppard MC, et al. Prediction of all-cause and cardiovascular mortality in elderly people from one thyrotropin result: a 10-year cohort study. *Lancet* 2001;358: 861–865.

64. Sawin CT, Geller A, Wolf PA, et al. Low serum thyrotropin concentrations as a risk factor for atrial fibrillation in older persons. *N Engl J Med* 1994;331:1249–1252.

65. Uzzan B, Campos J, Cucherat M, et al. Effects of bone mass of long-term treatment with thyroid hormones: a meta-analysis. *J Clin Endocrinol Metab* 1996;81:4278–4289.

66. Toft AD. Subclinical hyperthyroidism. *N Eng J Med* 2001; 345:512–516.

GENETIC FACTORS IN THYROID DISEASE

SIMON H.S. PEARCE
PAT KENDALL-TAYLOR

The spectrum of clinical thyroid disease that is strongly influenced by genetic factors runs from congenital hypothyroidism and thyroid agenesis, through transient gestational hyperthyroidism and autoimmune thyroid diseases (AITDs), to benign and malignant thyroid tumors. Indeed, a family history is a particularly frequent finding in patients with all forms of thyroid autoimmunity and for many types of goiter. This chapter reviews the inherited (germ line) basis for thyroid diseases, including those disorders with a strict monogenic (Mendelian) basis and those more common conditions that are inherited as complex multigenic traits. The pathogenesis of thyroid tumors and the role of somatic gene mutations in thyroid disease is covered in detail elsewhere (see section on oncogenes in Chapters 70 and 71).

MONOGENIC DISORDERS

Monogenic disorders of the thyroid axis frequently present as congenital or childhood hypothyroidism. They are usefully classified according to the level of the defect, i.e., pituitary thyrotrophs, thyroid development or hormonogenesis, hormone transport, and end-organ responsiveness (Table 20.1). Developmental problems of the thyroid account for the majority of infants with congenital hypothyroidism and are broadly referred to as thyroid dysgenesis, which includes thyroid agenesis, hemiagenesis, hypoplasia, and ectopic thyroid (i.e., abnormalities of both morphogenesis and migration) (1,2). Less than 15% of infants with thyroid dysgenesis are found to have one of the currently defined molecular defects (3–6). Of these gene abnormalities, only infants with a *PAX8* gene mutation appear to have a disorder that is manifest as thyroid dysgenesis alone (6). Interestingly, even in families with a characterized *PAX8* molecular abnormality, the morphology of the thyroid abnormality is not always consistent between patients (6,7). Defects in thyroid hormonogenesis account for only about 10% of congenital hypothyroidism, and often present with goiter as an additional feature (see Chapter 48). There undoubtedly are other single gene defects, and most likely some complex ones causing or modifying both thyroid dysgenesis and hormonogenesis, that await discovery.

Inherited disorders of thyroid hormone transport comprise abnormalities of both the serum-binding and transmembrane passage of thyroid hormones. Abnormalities of serum transport are due to altered quantity or binding affinity of the serum binding proteins, thyroxine-binding globulin (TBG), transthyretin, and albumin. Thyroxine-binding globulin is the major carrier protein, and abnormalities range from complete TBG deficiency, altered affinity for thyroid hormones, to excess production of TBG (27,28). The TBG gene is located on the X chromosome, and the biochemical manifestations of abnormal TBG production are more marked in males. Alleles encoding TBG isoforms with altered binding affinity are particularly prevalent in certain racial groups (29). Mutations in the albumin gene cause familial dysalbuminemic hyperthyroxinemia (30,31). Interestingly, a kindred with an albumin variant that has a high affinity for triiodothyronine (T_3) but not thyroxine (T_4) has been reported, demonstrating that the binding of T_4 and T_3 has different molecular specificities within the albumin molecule (32).

With the widespread use of serum thyrotropin (TSH) and free thyroid hormone assays, these familial states of euthyroid hypothyroxinemia and euthyroid hyperthyroxinemia, which are only apparent on assay of serum total hormone concentrations, rarely cause significant diagnostic confusion. These conditions of altered biochemistry are in marked contrast to the devastating disorder recently described in male children with abnormal transmembrane thyroid hormone transport (33). These children present with hypotonia, severe psychomotor retardation, failure of speech, nystagmus, and a low serum T_4 concentration in conjunction with a high serum T_3 concentration (33). Serum TSH values are normal at birth and become moderately elevated, but the developmental abnormalities are not reversed by T_4 treatment. Mutations in an X-chromosome membrane transporter, MCT8, are responsible for this disorder (33). The disorders of end-organ responsiveness to thyroid hormones are termed resistance to thyroid hormone (RTH) and are caused by a variety of dominantly in-

**TABLE 20.1. SINGLE GENE DEFECTS THAT CAUSE DISORDERS OF THE
HYPOTHALAMIC-PITUITARY-THYROID AXIS**

Disorder	Phenotype	Gene Defect (Inheritance)	OMIM No.[a]	Reference No.	Chapter
Hypothalamic-pituitary disorders					51
Insensitivity to TRH	Hypothyroidism, no response to TRH	TRH-R (AR)	188545	8	
Combined pituitary hormone deficiency	Hypothyroidism, serum TSH low to slightly high	Pit1 [POU1F1] (AR, AD)	173110	9	
	—	PROP1 (AR)	601538	10	
	-with rigid cervical spine	LHX3 (AR)	600577	11	
	-with septo-optic dysplasia	HESX1 (AR, AD)	601802	12	
Isolated TSH deficiency	Hypothyroidism	TSH-β (AR)	275100	13	
Thyroid development					75
Thyroid dysgenesis	Hypothyroidism, ectopic or hypoplastic thyroid	PAX8 (AD)	218700	6,7	
	Variable degree of hypothyroidism, pulmonary hypoplasia and choreoathetosis	TTF1 [NKX2–1] (haploinsufficient)	600635	4,5	
Thyroid agenesis	Hypothyroidism, with palatal clefts, spiky hair, choanal atresia [Bamforth-Lazarus syndrome]	TTF2 (AR)	241850	3	
Thyroid hormonogenesis[b]					48
Iodide transport defect	Hypothyroidism, goiter	NIS (AR)	274400	14	
Total organification defect	Hypothyroidism, goiter	TPO (AR)	274500	15	
	Hypothyroidism, goiter	THOX2 (AR)	606759	16	
Partial organification defect	Transient neonatal hypothyroidism	THOX2 (AD)	606759	16	
	Goiter, variable sensorineural deafness, [Pendred's syndrome]	PDS (AR)	274600	17	
Thyroglobulin defect	Variable hypothyroidism, goiter	Tg (AR)	188450	18	
	Simple goiter	Tg (AD)	188450	19	
TSH-receptor signaling					10,25
Complete TSH resistance	Hypothyroidism, thyroid hypoplasia	TSH-R (AR)	275200	20	
Partial TSH resistance	Euthyroid hyperthyrotropinemia	TSH-R (AR)	275200	21	
	Pseudohypoparathyroidism type 1a, parathyroid hormone resistance, osteodystrophy	GNAS1 (AD & paternal imprinting)	103580	22	
Familial gestational hyperthyroidism	Hyperthyroidism in pregnancy	TSH-R (AD) [K183R]	603373	23	
Hereditary toxic thyroid hyperplasia	Congenital hyperthyroidism and goiter	TSH-R activation (AD)	603373	24	
Toxic thyroid adenoma	Autonomous follicular adenoma	TSH-R activation (somatic)	603373	25	
	McCune-Albright syndrome, polyostotic fibrous dysplasia, precocious puberty	GNAS1 activation (mosaic)	174800	26	
Thyroid hormone transport					13
Euthyroid hypothyroxinemia	TBG deficiency (complete or partial)	TBG (XR)	314200	27	
Euthyroid, excess serum total thyroid hormones	TBG excess	TBG duplication (XR)	314200	28	
	Increased TTR affinity	TTR (AD)	176300	30	
	Familial dysalbuminemic hyperthyroxinemia	Alb (AD)	103600	31	
	Familial dysalbuminemic hypertriiodothyroninemia	Alb (AD)	103600	32	
Transmembrane defect	Low serum T_4, high serum T_3, psychomotor retardation, nystagmus	MCT8 (XR)		33, 33A	

(continued)

TABLE 20.1. SINGLE GENE DEFECTS THAT CAUSE DISORDERS OF THE HYPOTHALAMIC-PITUITARY-THYROID AXIS *(continued)*

Disorder	Phenotype	Gene Defect (Inheritance)	OMIM No.[a]	Reference No.	Chapter
End-organ response					81
Resistance to thyroid hormone	High serum T$_4$ and T$_3$, normal to high serum TSH, goiter	THRB (AD)	190160	34	
Thyroid tumorigenesis					70,71
Medullary carcinoma	Familial medullary carcinoma	RET (AD)	171400	35,36	
	MEN2a with pheochromocytoma	RET (AD)	171400	36	
	MEN2b with ganglioneuroma and pheochromocytoma	RET (AD)	162300	36,37	
Thyroid hamartoma/ carcinoma and thyroiditis	Breast adenoma/ carcinoma, skin hamartoma [Cowden's syndrome]	PTEN (AD)	158350	38	
Differentiated thyroid carcinoma	Short stature, cataract, skin changes, type 2 diabetes [Werner syndrome]	RECQL2 (AR)	277700	39	
Papillary carcinoma	with polyposis coli [Gardner's syndrome]	APC (AD)	175100	40	
Thyroid adenoma/ carcinoma	Pigmentary adrenal adenoma, cardiac myxoma, [Carney complex]	PRKAR1A (AD)	160980	41	
Thyroid autoimmunity					23,47
Autoimmune hypothyroidism	Hypoparathyroidism, hypoadrenalism, candidiasis [APECED syndrome, APS1]	AIRE (AR)	240300	42,43	
	Immune diabetes, autoimmune enteropathy [IPEX syndrome]	FOXP3 (XR)	304790	44	
Miscellaneous					
Cystinosis	Hypothyroidism, renal failure, corneal deposition	CTNS (AR)	219800	45	50
Thyrotoxic periodic paralysis	Muscle paralysis when hypokalemic	KCNE3 (AD)	188580	46	41

[a]OMIM no. refers to the catalog of "Online Mendelian Inheritance in Man," as found on www.ncbi.nlm.nih.gov/entrez/query.fcgi?db=OMIM.
[b]An additional form of dyshormonogenesis, dehalogenase deficiency, has been characterized at a biochemical, but not molecular, level.
Alb, albumin; APC, adenomatous polyposis coli; APECED, autoimmune polyendocrinopathy candidiasis and ectodermal dysplasia; APSI, autoimmune polyendocrinopathy syndrome type 1; CTNS, cystinosin; FOXP3, Forkhead box P3; GNAS1, Gs-alpha subunit gene; KCNE3, Voltage gated potassium channel-3; MCT8, Monocarboxylate transporter-8; NKX2-1, (no full form); PAX8, paired box gene-8; PDS, Pendrin; PRKAR1A, Regulatory c-AMP dependent protein kinase-1α; PTEN, Phosphatase and tensin homolog; RECQL2, RECQ-like2; RET, (no full form); THOX2, thyroid oxidase-2; THRB, Thyroid hormone receptor-β; TTF1, thyroid transcription factor-1; TTF2, thyroid transcription factor-2.

herited mutations of the thyroid hormone β receptor (34). RTH syndromes have a variable phenotype, which ranges from asymptomatic goiter or tachycardia to hyperactivity, learning difficulty, developmental delay, and retarded bone growth with short stature. The biochemical hallmarks of these conditions are high serum thyroid hormone and normal or slightly high serum TSH concentrations (see Chapter 81).

CHROMOSOMAL DISORDERS

Several chromosomal deletion or rearrangement syndromes are associated with thyroid disorders. The most common disorders in which thyroid dysfunction is a frequent accompaniment are listed in Table 20.2. Patients with Down's syndrome, with trisomy of chromosome 21, have a high prevalence of both autoimmune and congenital thyroid disease. Autoimmune hypothyroidism (chronic autoimmune thyroiditis) is the most common thyroid problem, affecting 15% to 20% of adults with Down's syndrome (47–49). Graves' disease occurs less frequently, with a prevalence of 1% to 2%, which may not be increased compared with the general population (47,48). Congenital hypothyroidism is found in about 2% of infants with Down's syndrome. Turner's syndrome, which is characterized by complete or partial loss of X-chromosome material in a phenotypic female, is also associated with autoimmune thyroid disease (AITD). About 15% of patients with Turner's syndrome have autoimmune hypothyroidism, with 30% to 40% having high serum antithyroid antibody concentrations (50–52). There is a correlation between cytogenetic abnormalities and AITD in patients with Turner's syndrome, with overt hypothyroidism being found in up to 40% of patients with an Xq isochromosome (deleted short arm and duplicated long arm) (52–54). The DiGeorge syndrome (cardiac outflow tract defects, thymic hypoplasia, hypoparathyroidism, and facial anomalies) and

TABLE 20.2. CHROMOSOMAL DISORDERS WITH THYROID DISEASE AS A COMPONENT

Disorder	Thyroid Phenotype	Other Features	Cytogenetic Abnormality	OMIM No.[a]	Reference No.
Down's syndrome	Autoimmune hypothyroidism	Mental retardation, cardiac anomalies, characteristic facies, others	Trisomy 21	190685	47–49
DiGeorge/CATCH22 syndrome	Graves' disease	Cardiac outflow tract anomalies, thymic hypoplasia, hypoparathyroidism	22q11del	188400	55–57
Turner's syndrome	Autoimmune hypothyroidism, Thyroid antibodies	Web neck, ovarian dysgenesis, short stature, renal and aortic root abnormalities	X0		50–52
Smith-Magenis syndrome	Hypothyroidism	Mental retardation, eye anomalies, self-injury	17p11del	182290	59,60
1p terminal deletion	Hypothyroidism	Mental retardation, microcephaly, large fontanelle, hearing loss, characteristic facies	1p36 del	607872	58

[a]OMIM no. refers to the catalog of "Online Mendelian Inheritance in Man," as found on www.ncbi.nlm.nih.gov/entrez/query.fcgi?db=OMIM.

the overlapping chromosome 22q11 deletion syndromes are associated with Graves' disease in up to 20% of cases (55–57). Two rarer chromosomal disorders, 1p terminal deletion and Smith-Magenis syndrome, are each associated with hypothyroidism in about one third of cases (Table 20.2). The pathogenesis of the hypothyroidism is ill defined, although it is likely to be developmental in nature.

COMPLEX DISORDERS

Complex disorders are determined by a combination of genetic and nongenetic factors (including environmental and other influences). Most common complex traits are thought to have a multigenic basis; i.e., in different individuals they are determined by a varying combination of susceptibility alleles in different genes (61). However, even for an apparently simple genetic trait, the phenotype may be dependent to some extent upon environmental influences. For instance, in mendelian forms of thyroid dyshormonogenesis the presence or severity of hypothyroidism and the rate of goiter development may be determined by dietary iodide availability. AITD is the most prevalent of the autoimmune conditions, with at least 2% of women being affected by overt thyroid dysfunction. Similarly, simple euthyroid goiter is a frequent finding in women, even in iodine-replete areas. Both these common disorders have a complex multigenic basis.

Simple (Euthyroid) Goiter

Simple goiter is defined as a diffuse or nodular enlargement of the thyroid that is not the result of neoplasia or inflammation in a subject who is euthyroid (62). It is a heterogeneous disorder that affects up to 15% of women and about 3% of men who live in iodine-sufficient regions (63,64). It is an important problem on a population level due to its prevalence, and also because some subjects with simple goiter may be predisposed to nonmedullary thyroid cancer (65–67). However, it is notable that in the majority of patients who have recurrent thyroid nodules after surgery for goiter the new nodules are polyclonal in nature, indicating that the condition is predominantly a hyperplastic rather than neoplastic process (68). Surprisingly, in iodine-deficient regions, goiter has a familial tendency (69), with a higher concordance in monozygotic than dizygotic twins (70). In the absence of iodine deficiency, simple goiter also has a strong genetic basis (71). In a large Danish cohort of female twins, the concordance rate in monozygotic twins was 42%, as compared with 13% in dizygotic twins (72), and data from this study suggested that about 80% of the susceptibility to simple goiter may be determined by genetic factors.

Heterozygous mutations in the thyroglobulin (Tg) molecule have been described in three kindreds with simple goiter, identified from 30 probands (19). In these families, about 50% of patients carrying the mutation had a goiter, with an increasing penetrance after the age of 25 years (19). Thus, at least 10% of cases of simple goiter may be due to mild defects in thyroid hormonogenesis (19,72). However, in contrast to the "dyshormonogenic" presentation as a recessive trait associated with hypothyroidism, these Tg mutations are manifest as euthyroid goiter in later life and are inherited in an autosomal-dominant fashion (19,72,73). In recent years, several large kindreds with dominantly inherited multinodular goiter have been identified, and genome-wide linkage studies have mapped novel susceptibility loci to chromosomes 14q32, Xp22, and 3q26 (designated MNG1 to MNG3) (74–76). Of these three loci, only MNG1 on 14q32 has been independently confirmed

(77). Of the three families in whom linkage was initially established, the phenotype of one kindred was distinct in having an onset of goiter in prepubertal children, rapid ^{123}I uptake, and high serum TSH concentrations in some subjects, suggesting that the MNG3 locus may encode another mild form of dyshormonogenesis (76). Reassuringly, these linkages appear distinct from those for familial non-medullary thyroid cancer (1p21, 2q21, 19p13) (78–80) (see section on oncogenes in Chapter 70). Thus, simple goiter is certainly a complex trait in terms of its molecular pathogenesis, with iodine availability as the major environmental component. Whether its inheritance is as a multiple monogenic trait comprising a series of different single gene disorders with a common phenotype, or is a truly complex trait with alleles at several genetic loci contributing to the disorder in each patient, is unknown. It will be interesting to determine whether the gene defects underlying MNG1 to MNG3 are subtle abnormalities of hormonogenesis or whether a proportion of cases will be due to inherited defects in the regulation of cell cycling or growth of thyroid follicular cells.

Autoimmune Thyroid Disease

AITD comprises a series of interrelated conditions including Graves' disease, Hashimoto's (goitrous) thyroiditis, atrophic autoimmune hypothyroidism, postpartum thyroiditis, and thyroid-associated ophthalmopathy. These different manifestations of AITD may occur sequentially, and sometimes synchronously, in the same patient. This clustering of different phenotypes of AITD within a patient suggests that these conditions have a common pathophysiologic basis (see section on pathogenesis of Graves' disease in Chapters 23 and 47). A widely accepted model for the pathogenesis of AITD suggests that each patient has a background inherited predisposition to autoimmunity, with additional environmental and hormonal factors that trigger or contribute to the development of disease. In support of this model, there is good evidence that both cigarette smoking and adverse psychosocial events are associated with the development of Graves' disease (81–83). Similarly, the female preponderance of AITD (63), the modulation of animal models of the disease with sex steroids (84), the amelioration of Graves' disease during pregnancy, and the occurrence of postpartum thyroiditis all support the important role of sex steroids in these disorders.

Genetic Epidemiology of Autoimmune Thyroid Disease

Twin studies show an increased concordance of Graves' disease and autoimmune hypothyroidism in monozygotic twins as compared to dizygotic twins (reviewed in reference

85). In a series of careful investigations of 8966 Danish twins, concordance for Graves' disease in monozygotic twins was 35% as compared with 3% in dizygotic twins (86). Similarly, there was 55% concordance of autoimmune hypothyroidism (combining both atrophic and goitrous forms of the disease) in monzygotic twins, but no concordance among dizygotic twins (87). A statistical model based on these data suggested that 79% of the predisposition to Graves' disease is due to genetic factors, with only 21% due to nongenetic (environmental and hormonal) factors (86), confirming the dominant role of heredity in the pathogenesis of the disease.

In addition to twin studies, a measure of the heritability of a disorder can be gained from the ratio of the risk to a relative of an affected proband compared with the background population prevalence (a value termed λs for siblings and λo for parents/offspring) (61). A study from Hungary found 5.3% of 435 probands with Graves' disease had siblings with the disease (21 sisters, 2 brothers), compared with a background population frequency of Graves' disease of 0.6% (88). This allows estimation of the λs for Graves' disease as 8.1 in this population. In a similar study carried out in England, the λs for Graves' disease was 9.9 (89). To put these values into context, the λs for type 1 diabetes mellitus is 15, and that for rheumatoid arthritis is 8 (90). An important message for patients with Graves' disease is that their female siblings and children have a 5% to 8% chance of also being affected by the disease, and an approximately similar risk of developing autoimmune hypothyroidism.

Heritability of Thyroid Antibodies

Soon after the first description of thyroid antibodies (91), their occurrence in 22 of 39 siblings (56%) of probands with AITD was noted, and a dominant pattern of inheritance was suggested (92). The finding of thyroid antibodies in 30% to 50% of first-degree female relatives has been confirmed using sensitive assays for serum anti-thyroglobulin (Tg) and antithyroid peroxidase (TPO) antibodies (93). The prevalence of these antibodies in male relatives is less (~10% to 30%); this pattern has been attributed to dominant inheritance with reduced penetrance in males (93). Naturally occurring TPO antibodies are not uniform in specificity, and tend to be directed against certain defined "immunodominant" epitopes of TPO. Interestingly, these patterns of TPO antibody response (epitopic fingerprints) can be inherited in a dominant fashion (94), and can persist for many years. It is striking that even in families in which several members have antibodies to TPO or Tg, clinically overt AITD is not the rule (95). This demonstrates that, although the generation of a B-cell immune response to thyroid antigens is one component of thyroid autoimmunity, it is not in itself sufficient to cause disease, and that other tissue-specific responses or immune system factors are also necessary.

Association of Autoimmune Thyroid Disease with Other Autoimmune Disorders

The occurrence of Hashimoto's thyroiditis in patients with type 1 diabetes mellitus, and in their family members, is well recognized. In large groups of families with type 1 diabetes in the United Kingdom and the United States, at least one case of AITD was reported in relatives of 22% and 40% of patients with type 1 diabetes, respectively (96,97). A higher-than-expected prevalence of AITD has been found in patients with other autoimmune disorders and in their families (98). In two studies of families with two or more rheumatoid arthritis cases, about 50% of the families had a patient with rheumatoid arthritis or a relative had AITD (99,100). Similarly, AITD is often found in patients with autoimmune Addison's disease, being present in 40% to 50% of patients with sporadic Addison's disease [i.e., those who do not have the autoimmune polyendocrinopathy, candidiasis, or ectodermal dysplasia (APECED) syndrome] (101,102). Other weaker associations exist between AITD and other autoimmune endocrinopathies (e.g., autoimmune premature ovarian failure) and nonendocrine autoimmune disorders (e.g., pernicious anemia, celiac disease, myasthenia gravis, multiple sclerosis) (103). This clustering of different autoimmune conditions suggests that several different autoimmune disorders are likely to have a disease susceptibility allele (or alleles) in common.

Monogenic Disorders with Autoimmune Thyroid Disease as a Component

AITD is a component of three monogenic syndromes. The most common of these rare disorders is the APECED (type 1 polyendocrinopathy) syndrome (Table 20.1). The cardinal features of this condition are autoimmune hypoparathyroidism, Addison's disease, and chronic mucocutaneous candidiasis, which begin in childhood or early adolescence (see reference 42 for a comprehensive review). Other autoimmune disorders such as type 1 diabetes, pernicious anemia, and hypogonadism occur in 15% to 30% of patients with the APECED syndrome, but autoimmune hypothyroidism is comparatively uncommon, affecting only about 5% of patients. The extreme rarity of Graves' disease in APECED is notable. APECED is an autosomal recessive syndrome caused by mutations in the autoimmune regulator (*AIRE*) gene on chromosome 21 (43). AIRE is a nuclear transcription factor that is expressed predominantly in dendritic antigen presenting cells in the thymus and peripheral lymphoid tissues. *AIRE* gene mutations lead to

defective negative selection of potentially autoreactive thymocytes and ineffective peripheral antigen presentation for some antigens (e.g., *Candida*). One large family has been described with dominantly inherited severe and persistent candidiasis and hypothyroidism with goiter, a condition that is distinct from APECED. Linkage studies found that the disorder mapped to chromosome 2p, but the causative gene has not been identified (104). A third, rarer disorder is the immune dysregulation, polyendocrinopathy, and enteropathy (X-linked) syndrome (IPEX). This is a devastating disorder of male infants with failure to thrive due to autoimmune enteropathy (44). Autoimmune hypothyroidism and type 1 diabetes develop in the first year of life in about 50% and 90% of affected males, respectively. IPEX is caused by mutations in the *FOXP3* gene on chromosome Xp11. FOXP3 is expressed in T lymphocytes and is critical to the development of regulatory T cells, without which inappropriate activation and proliferation of CD4 lymphocytes occurs (44). These monogenic syndromes point towards two cell types, namely the dendritic antigen-presenting cell and the CD4 lymphocyte, whose normal functioning is critical to the maintenance of immune tolerance to thyroid tissues.

Autoimmune Thyroid Diseases as Complex Genetic Traits

In contrast to the unusual monogenic forms of autoimmunity mentioned above, most cases of AITD, along with other common autoimmune disorders, are now thought to have a complex genetic basis; i.e., the genetic predisposition to the disease is determined by a series of interacting susceptibility alleles of several different genes (90). These various genetic loci may also have differing influences on the predisposition to AITD in different populations (locus heterogeneity), which makes the identification of disease susceptibility genes a more difficult task. There are two standard approaches for identifying disease genes for either monogenic or complex traits (61). First, candidate gene studies involve examining polymorphic markers within a particular gene, which has been selected because it is thought that disruption of its function may result in the phenotype. There has been some success in using this approach to identify susceptibility genes for AITD. A second approach is linkage scanning, in which widely spaced anonymous genetic markers (usually microsatellite repeat polymorphisms between genes) are used to detect chromosomal segments with evidence for linkage in affected families. Linkage analysis is more robust than association analysis, because it may detect genetic effects many millions of nucleotides away and does not rely on the same allele being linked to disease in each kindred. However, linkage studies may lack sensitivity to detect loci with small effects and are poor at localizing a disease allele. Several genetic tests now combine elements of familial linkage and association analysis (linkage in the presence of association), the most widely used analysis being the transmission disequilibrium test (105).

Luckily for investigators interested in AITD, linkage studies of type 1 diabetes have been prominent in the field of complex trait mapping. It is now clear from genomewide linkage studies encompassing more than 750 families with type 1 diabetes that there are seven loci where there is firm or suggestive evidence of genetic linkage (106,107). Of these loci, one is the major histocompatibility complex (MHC) on chromosome 6p21, another is the insulin gene region on chromosome 11p15, and a third is the cytotoxic T lymphocyte antigen-4 (*CTLA-4*) gene on chromosome 2q33 (see later in the chapter). The other four linked loci, and a further 12 putative type 1 diabetes loci, have all been defined on the basis of linkage to anonymous markers, and there is no defined allelic association. These studies of type 1 diabetes have advanced the field by demonstrating that a common autoimmune disorder has a complex (multigenic) genetic basis (90). Indeed, similar findings have subsequently been made for rheumatoid arthritis, multiple sclerosis, and systemic lupus erythematosus, albeit with smaller numbers of families (108,109). There is likely to be a similar number of genetic loci implicated in the pathogenesis of AITD, and because of the familial clustering of the disease with type 1 diabetes, some susceptibility alleles are likely to be shared by both disorders.

Genetic studies of AITD have proceeded in recent years with a series of linkage and association studies, and by fine-mapping studies. Although some progress has been made, there is still no detailed molecular view of the pathogenesis of AITD. The limiting factors for these genetic approaches have been small sample sizes, disease loci with small effects, and the expense and relatively slow speed of genotyping large numbers of people for multiple markers.

The Major Histocompatibility Complex

The MHC, which contains the human leukocyte antigen (HLA) genes, is located on chromosome 6p21. It is subdivided into three regions: the class I region, which encodes the HLA antigens A, B, and C; the class II region, which encodes HLA antigens DR, DQ, and DP, each with one or more α and β chains; and the class III region, encoding several immunoregulatory molecules including complement components, heat shock protein 70 (*HSP70*), and tumour necrosis factors (*TNF*) (Fig. 20.1). The class II region also contains the peptide transporters associated with antigen processing (*TAP*) and large multifunctional protease (*LMP*) genes. Tight linkage disequilibrium (i.e., conserved haplotypes) exists between the alleles of the MHC region. Major histocompatibility complex class II molecules play a critical part in the initiation of adaptive immune responses.

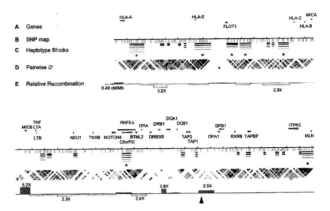

FIGURE 20.1. Linkage disequilibrium map of the human major histocompatility complex (MHC) region. A gene and single nucleotide polymorphism *(SNP)* map showing seven regions *(*)* with highly conserved haplotype blocks, the linkage disequilibrium measure *(D')*, and recombination rates across the MHC region. The terminal end of the 6p arm is to the left in the upper chain, and the centromere is to the right of the lower chain. The numerous genes in the MHC region can be seen, with some areas of particularly strong linkage disequilibrium. (From Walsh EC, Mather KA, Schaffner SF, et al. An integrated haplotype map of the human major histocompatibility complex. *Am J Hum Genet* 2003;73:580, with permission.)

Peptide antigens can only be recognized by T-cell antigen receptors when they are attached to the binding groove of an MHC molecule on the surface of an antigen-presenting cell.

The first recognition of an association between Graves' disease and alleles of MHC class I molecules was the finding of a higher frequency of the HLA-B8 allele in patients with Graves' disease (47%), as compared with normal subjects (21%) (110). Several studies in white populations confirmed this association (111,112). However, a stronger association of Graves' disease was found with the MHC class II allele, HLA-DR3, which is in strong linkage disequilibrium with HLA-B8 (113). Many case-control studies in white populations have since found Graves' disease to be associated with HLA-DR3, with relative risks between 2.5 and 5 (reviewed in references 85 and 114). More recently, this association of MHC with Graves' disease was confirmed in a study using the transmission disequilibrium test, which showed preferential transmission of the HLA DRB1*0304-DQB1*02-DQA1*0501 (DR3-DQ2) haplotype (115). Although there is no doubt about the association of Graves' disease with the HLA-DR3 haplotype in whites, the primary disease susceptibility allele in the region remains unknown. An association of Graves' disease, particularly in males, with the HLA-DQA1*0501 allele, which was stronger than, and independent of, the HLA-DR3 status, has also been reported (116). This independent association of HLA-DQA1*0501 with Graves' disease has been supported by some studies (115,117,118), but not by others (119–121). In other populations, Graves' disease has been found to be associated with several different HLA alleles. For example, it has been found to be associated with HLA-B35, -B46, -A2, and -DPB1*0501 in Japanese patients (122–124); HLA-A10, -B8, and -DQw2 in Indians (125); HLA-DR1 and -DR3 in South African blacks (126); the DRB3*020/DQA1*0501 haplotype in black Americans (127); and HLA-B46, -DR9, -DRB1*303, and -DQB1*0303 in Hong Kong Chinese (128). Furthermore, case-control studies have also shown an association of Graves' disease with alleles of several different non-HLA genes within the MHC complex, including the *HSP70, TNF, TAP,* and *LMP* genes (121,129–132). Thus, it is likely that other, non-HLA genes within the MHC locus contribute to susceptibility to AITD. Due to the strong linkage disequilibrium within this region (Fig. 20.1), it is difficult to determine the independent effect of a particular allele in disease susceptibility, and much larger association studies are needed to resolve these issues.

The results of HLA association studies in autoimmune thyroiditis have been less consistent. In whites, autoimmune hypothyroidism has been associated with HLA alleles that include HLA-B8, -DR3, -DR4, -DR5, -DQA1* 0201/*0301, and -DQB1*03 (121,133–137). Small sample sizes and phenotypic heterogeneity (for example, goitrous vs. atrophic autoimmune hypothyroidism) make it difficult to draw a firm conclusion from these studies, but they suggest a modest association of autoimmune hypothyroidism with HLA-DR3, -DR4, and -DR5. Postpartum thyroiditis has also been found to be associated with HLA-DR4 (135,138) and -DR5 (139,140), suggesting a close relationship between these two disorders.

Although case-control studies in whites have consistently demonstrated an association of Graves' disease with HLA alleles, the results of familial linkage studies of the HLA locus in the disease have been discrepant. Among early studies, several found excess sharing of HLA alleles in sibs affected with the disease, suggesting linkage (88,141), but linkage was not confirmed in other studies (reviewed in reference 89). However, all the studies were small, and there was phenotypic heterogeneity in the kindreds in some studies (e.g., inclusion of members with both Graves' disease and autoimmune hypothyroidism) (89). Based on a transmission disequilibrium test approach in a larger cohort of Graves' disease families, Graves' disease was linked to HLA (115). Linkage analysis in a cohort of sib-pairs with Graves' disease in the United Kingdom also found modest evidence to support linkage of the disease to the MHC region (142). However, three recent genome-wide scans in families with AITD have failed to detect linkage at chromosome 6p21 markers (143–145). Therefore, the contribution of genes in the MHC region to the genetic susceptibility to Graves' disease is comparatively small, perhaps accounting for 10% to 20% of the inherited susceptibility in certain populations (142). This is in marked contrast to type 1 diabetes, in which MHC is the dominant

locus, accounting for 30% to 40% of the total genetic susceptibility (106,107). In addition, most of the susceptibility to type 1 diabetes within the MHC locus is thought to be encoded by HLA-DQB and -DRB alleles, with lesser contributions from other adjacent genes (146,147). For AITD, it is likely that other, non-HLA genes within 6p21 determine a more substantial part of the inherited predisposition encoded by this region of the genome.

Cytotoxic T Lymphocyte Antigen-4

CTLA-4 is an immunoregulatory molecule that is expressed on the surface of activated T lymphocytes. Several lines of evidence support its role as a key negative regulator of T-cell activation. CTLA-4 knockout mice develop a rampant lymphoproliferative disorder resulting in splenomegaly, lymphadenopathy, and death from autoimmunity before 3 to 4 weeks of age (148). The administration of CTLA-4 blocking antibodies also precipitates or exacerbates autoimmunity in several murine models (149). Conversely, a soluble fusion protein of CTLA-4 and the immunoglobulin G1 Fc region (CTLA-4-Ig) ameliorates different experimental autoimmune disorders, including diabetes (150). Furthermore, the engagement of CTLA-4 with its ligands arrests the progression of activation-induced T-cell cycling (151), possibly by inducing apoptosis of activated T cells (152). This regulatory role of CTLA-4 in T-cell activation makes the CTLA-4 gene an attractive candidate locus for autoimmune disorders.

In 1995, Yanagawa and coworkers reported a significant association of Graves' disease with an allele of a microsatellite polymorphism (designated *CTLA-4[AT]$_n$*) within the 3′-untranslated region of the *CTLA-4* gene (153). Subsequently, the G allele of a single-nucleotide polymorphism that encoded a threonine to alanine change within the signal peptide of CTLA-4 (*CTLA-4[49]A/G*) was also found to be associated with Graves' disease (154). The association of these two *CTLA-4* polymorphisms with Graves' disease has been confirmed by subsequent studies in many different populations, with odds ratios between 1.4 and 3.2 (reviewed in reference 89). Of note, one study in Tunisians found the association with Graves' disease was with the A allele at *CTLA-4[49]A/G* (155), suggesting that despite the change in the coding sequence encoded by this polymorphism, it was probably not the disease allele. The G allele at the *CTLA-4[49]A/G* polymorphism was also found to be associated with autoimmune hypothyroidism in several different populations, although with less consistency than with Graves' disease (reviewed in reference 156). This is most likely to be due to the small size of some of the studies, and perhaps the phenotypic heterogeneity in ascertainment of autoimmune hypothyroidism.

Despite the clear finding of association of CTLA-4 alleles with Graves' disease and autoimmune hypothyroidism in many studies from different populations, initial family studies failed to detect linkage at *CTLA-4* (143,157). However, detailed analysis of the CTLA-4 locus in a cohort of sib pairs in the United Kingdom revealed strong evidence of linkage to *CTLA-4* (peak nonparametric linkage score 3.4), conferring up to one third of the total genetic susceptibility to Graves' disease in this population (142). Significant linkage of *CTLA-4* to thyroid autoantibody status was also subsequently reported (158), but genome-wide scans in Chinese families with Graves' disease and Japanese families with AITD did not show linkage at *CTLA-4* (144,145).

In order to identify the underlying susceptibility polymorphism within *CTLA-4*, a detailed fine-mapping study of the entire *CTLA-4* locus using markers for 108 single nucleotide polymorphisms was done (Fig. 20.2) (159). Using a regression model, the marker most highly associated with the disease (designated *CT60*) was located in the 3′ untranslated region of the gene, and the susceptibility allele had an odds ratio of about 1.5 for both Graves' disease and autoimmune hypothyroidism, but a lower contribution to type 1 diabetes (odds ratio ~1.2). The *CT60* polymorphism appears to regulate a splice variant of an upstream exon, which determines the expression of membrane-bound versus soluble forms of the mature *CTLA-4* molecule. It is hypothesized that under-expression of the mRNA for the soluble *CTLA-4* isoform (encoded by the

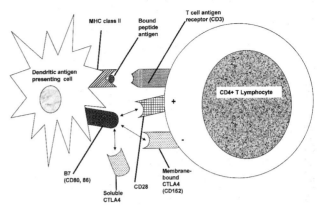

FIGURE 20.3. Schematic drawing of an antigen-presenting cell interacting with a T lymphocyte. The dendritic antigen-presenting cell presents a cleaved peptide antigen bound to the groove of the MHC class II molecule. This complex is recognized by a T lymphocyte with an antigen receptor (CD3 complex) with high affinity for the peptide-MHC complex. For the lymphocyte to become activated, a second signal must be delivered. This occurs when CD28 molecules on the T cell bind to B7 (CD80 and CD86) molecules on the antigen-presenting cell. This binding results in T-cell proliferation and activation. In contrast, T cells become quiescent or die when B7 molecules bind to *CTLA-4* molecules. Either membrane-bound or soluble *CTLA-4* may inhibit B7 binding to CD28, thereby stopping the costimulatory activation of the lymphocyte via the B7-CD28 interaction. Subjects with the susceptibility allele for autoimmune thyroid disease at *CTLA-4* produce relatively small amounts of soluble *CTLA-4* messenger RNA (159); if reflected at the protein level, this could allow a greater B7 binding to CD28, and therefore greater activation of T cells.

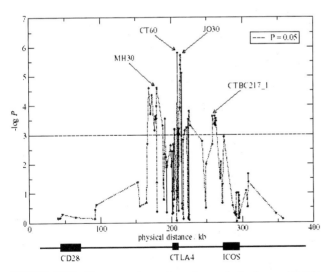

FIGURE 20.2. Fine-mapping of markers of single nucleotide polymorphisms markers at CTLA-4 and adjacent loci. A plot of −log P values in favor of association against the physical map of the markers in the adjacent transcripts CD28, CTLA-4, and ICOS on chromosome 2q33, each of which has a role in lymphocyte costimulation. The most evidence for association is found at the CT60 polymorphism within the 3′ untranslated region of CTLA-4. Alleles of this polymorphism were found to correlate with relative amounts of membrane-bound and soluble CTLA-4 production. (From Ueda H, Howson JM, Esposito L, et al. Association of the T-cell regulatory gene CTLA4 with susceptibility to autoimmune disease. *Nature* 2003;423:506, with permission.)

CT60 allele) leads to an imbalance in positive versus "negative" costimulatory signaling to activated T lymphocytes (Fig. 20.3). The CTLA-4 CT60 susceptibility allele has a high population prevalence (60% carrier rate in whites in the United Kingdom), and is likely to be a susceptibility allele not just for AITD and type 1 diabetes, but also for other autoimmune disorders. The high frequency of this low penetrance "disease" allele/haplotype in the normal population is the probable explanation as to why several linkage studies failed to identify the locus (160). A key question is whether this allele can be used to predict the outcome of treatment of Graves' disease, or the development of Graves' ophthalmopathy (161,162). Finally, the effect of nongenetic factors (e.g., smoking, pregnancy, sex hormones) on the expression of the soluble form of CTLA-4 are needed to understand better the interaction of the genetic predisposition and "environmental" factors.

Other Candidate Autoimmune Thyroid Disease Genes and Results of Linkage Scanning

Case-control studies of many other candidate immune system and thyroid-specific genes for AITD have not led to substantial advances in our understanding of pathogenesis. Immunoregulatory genes, including the immunoglobulin heavy-chain (Gm), T-cell receptor β-chain, interleukin-1 receptor antagonist, interleukin-4, interferon-γ, and Fas ligand genes have been studied, but no allele of any of these genes has been consistently associated with AITD (reviewed in references 89 and 163). Similarly, studies of the TSH receptor, the thyroid receptor-β and TPO genes have not yielded significant associations (89). Studies of the vitamin D receptor and the vitamin D–binding protein gene have suggested a possible role in Graves' disease (164,165) but await replication.

In recent years, four different cohorts of patients have been examined for genetic linkage to a large number of anonymous chromosomal markers by US, UK, Japanese, and Chinese investigators (142–145,157,158,166–168). The results of these studies need to be viewed in the context that with 102 families (US study), 82 sib-pairs (UK study), 123 sib-pairs (Japanese study), and 54 families (Chinese study), no individual study has been large enough to detect susceptibility loci with modest effects (169). Thus, only highly significant linkages, or those that are replicated in a second cohort of patients, are likely to stand the test of time. Despite this caution, several promising chromosomal loci have emerged (Table 20.3) (170). In

particular, loci for AITD on chromosomes 5q31–q33, 8q23, 18q21, and 20q13 have each been replicated to some degree by a second study (143–145,166–168,171), suggesting that novel disease susceptibility alleles are likely to be identified from at least some of these loci. Of particular interest, the chromosome 8 linkage appears to be strongest in patients with autoimmune hypothyroidism, and it overlaps the Tg locus, and in one study preliminary evidence for association within the Tg gene was found (172,173).

Summary of Autoimmune Thyroid Disease Genetics

AITD can be considered a complex trait with a predominant genetic component. Several gene loci determine susceptibility to the disease, with a major contribution from CTLA-4. Currently, there is moderate evidence that other loci are involved to a lesser degree, including one or more genes in the MHC region. As work progresses, it is likely that other disease genes and immune system pathways will be identified that predispose to the disease. The evaluation of gene-environment interaction at a molecular level is likely to cast further light on disease pathogenesis.

TABLE 20.3. LINKAGE OF AUTOIMMUNE THYROID DISEASE IN DIFFERENT POPULATIONS[a]

Chromosomal Loci[b]	U.S. Study (Reference Nos. 143,157,158,168)	Japanese Study (Reference No. 144)	Chinese Study (Reference No. 145)	UK Study (Newcastle) (Reference Nos. 142,161,166,167)	UK Study (Birmingham) (Reference Nos. 115,131)
1p33	−	−	+	ND	ND
1q42	−	−	+	ND	ND
2q33 (CTLA-4)	+++[c]	−	−	++	+TDT
5q31-q33	-	++	+++	ND	ND
6p21 (MHC)	++	−	−	+	++TDT
6p (AITD1)	++	−	−	−	ND
8q23-q24	+++	+++	−	ND	ND
10q22	+++	−	−	ND	ND
11p14	-	−	+	ND	ND
12q22 (HT2)	++	−	−	ND	ND
13q32 (HT1)	+	−	−	ND	ND
14q31 (GD1)	++	−	−	−	ND
15q21	-	−	+	ND	ND
18q21	-	+	−	++	ND
20q11 (GD2)	+++	−	−	+[d]	ND
Xp11	−	−	−	++	ND
Xq21 (GD3)	++	−	−	−	ND

AITD1, Autoimmune thyroid disease-susceptibility to 1; *CTLA-4*, cytotoxic T lymphocyte antigen-4; *GD1*, Graves' disease-susceptibility to 1; *GD2*, Graves' disease-susceptibility to 2; *GD3*, Graves' disease-susceptibility to 3; *HT1*, Hashimoto's thyroiditis-susceptibility to 1; *HT2*, Hashimoto's thyroiditis-susceptibility to 2; MHC, major histocompatibility complex; ND, not done; TDT, transmission disequilibrium test.
[a]Significance levels for linkage are designated according to the criteria of Lander and Kruglyak: —, no linkage; +, nominal linkage (LOD score >1.0); ++, suggestive linkage (LOD score >1.9); +++, significant linkage (LOD score >3.3). Equivalent nonparametric linkage scores are >1.2, >2.2, and >3.6 for nominal, suggestive and significant linkage, respectively (169).
[b]Loci found linked in more than one dataset are shown in bold.
[c]Linkage with thyroid autoantibody production (158).
[d]Evidence for linkage found *only* in the Graves' disease families with apparent dominant mode of transmission (a tentative finding).

THE FUTURE

In the last few years there have been unprecedented advances in knowledge about the sequence and organization of the human and murine genomes, such that there are now comprehensive gene maps of each chromosome, and tissue-specific expression profiles at both the mRNA and protein level are rapidly being developed. In time, these advances will more fully inform our knowledge of the physiology of normal thyroid function and its disturbance in many more disease states. Impressive progress in understanding both monogenic and complex thyroid disorders at a genomic level has been made in the last decade. The next decade holds the promise of allowing the integration of genetic and epidemiologic approaches to understanding disease, through a determination of the underlying molecular pathology.

REFERENCES

1. Kopp P. Perspective: genetic defects in the etiology of congenital hypothyroidism. *Endocrinology* 2002;143:2019.
2. Van Vliet G. Development of the thyroid gland: lessons from congenitally hypothyroid mice and men. *Clin Genet* 2003;63:445.
3. Clifton-Bligh RJ, Wentworth JM, Heinz P, et al. Mutation of the gene encoding human TTF-2 associated with thyroid agenesis, cleft palate and choanal atresia. *Nat Genet* 1998;19:399.
4. Krude H, Schutz B, Biebermann H, et al. Choreoathetosis, hypothyroidism, and pulmonary alterations due to human NKX2–1 haploinsufficiency. *J Clin Invest* 2002;109:475.
5. Pohlenz J, Dumitrescu A, Zundel D, et al. Partial deficiency of thyroid transcription factor 1 produces predominantly neurological defects in humans and mice. *J Clin Invest* 2002;109:469.
6. Macchia PE, Lapi P, Krude H, et al. PAX8 mutations associated with congenital hypothyroidism caused by thyroid dysgenesis. *Nat Genet* 1998;19:83.
7. Congdon T, Nguyen LQ, Nogueira CR, et al. A novel mutation (Q40P) in PAX8 associated with congenital hypothyroidism and thyroid hypoplasia: evidence for phenotypic variability in mother and child. *J Clin Endocrinol Metab* 2001;86:3962.
8. Collu R, Tang J Castagné J, et al. A novel mechanism for isolated central hypothyroidism: inactivating mutations in the thyrotropin-releasing hormone receptor. *J Clin Endocrinol Metab* 1997;82:1561.
9. Radovick S, Nations M, Du Y, et al. A mutation in the POU-specific domain of Pit1 and hypopituitarism without pituitary hypoplasia. *Science* 1992;257:1115.
10. Wu W, Cogan JD, Pfäffle RW, et al. Mutations in PROP1 cause familial combined pituitary hormone deficiency. *Nat Genet* 1998;18:147.
11. Netchine I, Soubrier M-L, Krude H, et al. Mutations in LHX3 result in a new syndrome revealed by combined pituitary hormone deficiency. *Nat Genet* 2000;25:182.
12. Dattani MT, Martinez-Barbera JP, Thomas PQ, et al. Mutations in the homeobox gene HESX1/hesx1 associated with septo-optic dysplasia in human and mouse. *Nat Genet* 1998;19:125.
13. Hayashiziki Y, Hinoka Y, Tatsumi K, et al. Deoxyribonucleic acid analysis of five families with familial inherited thyroid stimulating hormone deficiency. *J Clin Endocrinol Metab* 1990;71:792.
14. Fujiwara H, Tatsumi K, Miki K, et al. Congenital hypothyroidism caused by a mutation in the Na+/I- symporter. *Nat Genet* 1997;16:124.
15. Abramowicz M, Targovnik H, Varela V, et al. Identification of a mutation in the coding sequence of the human thyroid peroxidase gene causing congenital goiter. *J Clin Invest* 1992;90:1200.
16. Moreno JC, Bikker H, Kempers MJE, et al. Inactivating mutations in the gene for thyroid oxidase 2 (THOX2) and congenital hypothyroidism. *N Engl J Med* 2002;347:95.
17. Everett LA, Glaser B, Beck JC, et al. Pendred syndrome is caused by mutations in a putative sulphate transporter gene (PDS). *Nat Genet* 1997;17:411.
18. Ieiri T, Cochaux P, Targovnik H, et al. A 3′ spliced site mutation in the thyroglobulin gene responsible for congenital goiter with hypothyroidism. *J Clin Invest* 1991;88:1901.
19. Corral J, Martín C, Pérez R, et al. Thyroglobulin gene point mutation associated with non-endemic simple goitre. *Lancet* 1993;341:462.
20. Biebermann H, Schoneberg T, Krude H, et al. Mutations of the human thyrotropin receptor gene causing thyroid hypoplasia and persistent congenital hypothyroidism. *J Clin Endocrinol Metab* 1997;82:3471.
21. Sunthornthepvarakul T, Gottschalk ME, Hayashi Y, et al. Resistance to thyrotropin caused by mutations in the thyrotropin-receptor gene. *N Engl J Med* 1995;332:155.
22. Weinstein LS, Gejman PV, Friedman E, et al. Mutations of the Gs alpha-subunit gene in Albright hereditary osteodystrophy detected by denaturing gradient gel electrophoresis. *Proc Natl Acad Sci USA* 1990;87:8287.
23. Rodien P, Bremont C, Sanson ML, et al. Familial gestational hyperthyroidism caused by a mutant thyrotropin receptor hypersensitive to human chorionic gonadotropin. *N Engl J Med* 1998;339:1823.
24. Duprez L, Parma J, Van Sande J, et al. Germline mutations in the thyrotropin receptor gene cause non-autoimmune autosomal dominant hyperthyroidism. *Nat Genet* 1994;7:396.
25. Parma J, Duprez L, Van Sande J, et al. Somatic mutations in the thyrotropin receptor gene cause hyperfunctioning thyroid adenomas. *Nature* 1993;365:649.
26. Mastorakos G, Mitsiades NS, Doufas AG, et al. Hyperthyroidism in McCune-Albright syndrome with a review of thyroid abnormalities sixty years after the first report. *Thyroid* 1997;7:433.
27. Mori Y, Seino S, Takeda K, et al. A mutation causing reduced biological activity and stability of thyroxine-binding globulin probably as a result of abnormal glycosylation of the molecule. *Mol Endocrinol* 1989;3:575.
28. Mori Y, Miura Y, Takeuchi H, et al. Gene amplification as a cause of inherited thyroxine-binding globulin excess in two Japanese families. *J Clin Endocrinol Metab* 1995;80:3758.
29. Takeda K, Mori Y, Sobieszczyk S, et al. Sequence of the variant thyroxine-binding globulin of Australian aborigines. Only one of two amino acid replacements is responsible for its altered properties. *J Clin Invest* 1989;83:1344.
30. Moses AC, Rosen HN, Moller DE, et al. A point mutation in transthyretin increases affinity for thyroxine and produces euthyroid hyperthyroxinemia. *J Clin Invest* 1990;86:2025.
31. Sunthornthepvarakul T, Angkeow P, Weiss RE, et al. An identical missense mutation in the albumin gene results in familial dysalbuminemic hyperthyroxinemia in 8 unrelated families. *Biochem Biophys Res Commun* 1994;202:781.

32. Sunthornthepvarakul T, Likitmaskul S, Ngowngarmratana S, et al. Familial dysalbuminemic hypertriiodothyroninemia: a new, dominantly inherited albumin defect. *J Clin Endocrinol Metab* 1998;83:1448.

33. Friesema EC, Grueters A, Bierbermann H, et al. Severe X-linked psychomotor retardation caused by mutations in a thyroid hormone transporter. Lancet 2004 (in press).

33a. Dumitrescu AM, Liao XH, Best TB, et al. A novel syndrome combining thyroid and neurological abnormalities is associated with mutations in a monocarboxylate transporter gene. *Am J Hum Genet* 2004:74:168.

34. Weiss RE, Refetoff S. Resistance to thyroid hormone. *Reviews in Endocrine and Metabolic Disorders* 2000;1:97.

35. Mulligan LM, Kwok JB, Healey CS, et al. Germ-line mutations of the RET proto-oncogene in multiple endocrine neoplasia type 2A. *Nature* 1993;363:458.

36. Eng C, Clayton D, Schuffenecker I, et al. The relationship between specific RET proto-oncogene mutations and disease phenotype in multiple endocrine neoplasia type 2. *JAMA* 1996;276:1575.

37. Eng C, Smith DP, Mulligan LM, et al. Point mutation within the tyrosine kinase domain of the RET proto-oncogene in multiple endocrine neoplasia type 2B and related sporadic tumours. *Hum Mol Genet* 1994;3:237.

38. Marsh DJ, Coulon V, Lunetta KL, et al. Mutation spectrum and genotype-phenotype analyses in Cowden disease and Bannayan-Zonana syndrome, two hamartoma syndromes with germline PTEN mutation. *Hum Mol Genet* 1998;7:507.

39. Ishikawa Y, Sugano H, Matsumoto T, et al. Unusual features of thyroid carcinomas in Japanese patients with Werner syndrome and possible genotype-phenotype relations to cell type and race. *Cancer* 1999;85:1345.

40. Bell B, Mazzaferri EL. Familial adenomatous polyposis (Gardner's syndrome) and thyroid carcinoma. A case report and review of the literature. *Dig Dis Sci* 1993;38:185.

41. Kirschner LS, Carney JA, Pack SD, et al. Mutations of the gene encoding the protein kinase A type I-alpha regulatory subunit in patients with the Carney complex. *Nat Genet* 2000;26:89.

42. Perheentupa J. APS-I/APECED: the clinical disease and therapy. *Endocrinol Metab Clin North Am* 2002;31:295.

43. Bjorses P, Aaltonen J, Horelli-Kuitunen N, et al. Gene defect behind APECED: a new clue to autoimmunity. *Hum Mol Genet* 1998;7:1547.

44. Wildin RS, Smyk-Pearson S, Filipovich AH. Clinical and molecular features of the immunodysregulation, polyendocrinopathy, enteropathy, X linked (IPEX) syndrome. *J Med Genet* 2002;39:537.

45. Gahl WA, Thoene JG, Schneider JA. Cystinosis. *N Engl J Med* 2002;347:111.

46. Dias Da Silva MR, Cerutti JM, Arnaldi LA, et al. A mutation in the KCNE3 potassium channel gene is associated with susceptibility to thyrotoxic hypokalemic periodic paralysis. *J Clin Endocrinol Metab* 2002;87:4881.

47. Karlsson B, Gustafsson J, Hedov G, et al. Thyroid dysfunction in Down's syndrome: relation to age and thyroid autoimmunity. *Arch Dis Child* 1998;79:242.

48. Friedman DL, Kastner T, Pond WS, et al. Thyroid dysfunction in individuals with Down syndrome. *Arch Intern Med* 1989;149:1990.

49. Murdoch JC, Ratcliffe WA, McLarty DG, et al. Thyroid function in adults with Down's syndrome. *J Clin Endocrinol Metab* 1977;44:453.

50. Medeiros CC, Marini SH, Baptista MT, et al. Turner's syndrome and thyroid disease: a transverse study of pediatric patients in Brazil. *J Pediatr Endocrinol Metab* 2000;13:357.

51. Elsheikh M, Wass JA, Conway GS. Autoimmune thyroid syndrome in women with Turner's syndrome—the association with karyotype. *Clin Endocrinol (Oxf)* 2001;55:223.

52. Radetti G, Mazzanti L, Paganini C, et al. Frequency, clinical and laboratory features of thyroiditis in girls with Turner's syndrome. *Acta Paediatr* 1995;84:909.

53. de Kerdanet M, Lucas J, Lemee F, et al. Turner's syndrome with X-isochromosome and Hashimoto's thyroiditis. *Clin Endocrinol (Oxf)* 1994;41:673.

54. Sparkes RS, Motulsky AG. The Turner syndrome with isochromosome X and Hashimoto's thyroiditis. *Ann Intern Med* 1967;67:132.

55. Kawame H, Adachi M, Tachibana K, et al. Graves' disease in patients with 22q11.2 deletion. *J Pediatr* 2001;139:892.

56. Adachi M, Tachibana K, Masuno M, et al. Clinical characteristics of children with hypoparathyroidism due to 22q11.2 microdeletion. *Eur J Pediatr* 1998;157:34.

57. Kawamura T, Nimura I, Hanafusa M, et al. DiGeorge syndrome with Graves' disease: a case report. *Endocr J* 2000;47:91.

58. Heilstedt HA, Ballif BC, Howard LA, et al. Physical map of 1p36, placement of breakpoints in monosomy 1p36, and clinical characterization of the syndrome. *Am J Hum Genet* 2003;72:1200.

59. Greenberg F, Lewis RA, Potocki L, et al. Multi-disciplinary clinical study of Smith-Magenis syndrome (deletion 17p11.2). *Am J Med Genet* 1996;62:247.

60. Slager RE, Newton TL, Vlangos CN, et al. Mutations in RAI1 associated with Smith-Magenis syndrome. *Nat Genet* 2003;33:466.

61. Lander ES, Schork NJ. Genetic dissection of complex traits. *Science* 1994;265:2037.

62. Hegedüs L, Bonnema SJ, Bennedbæk FN. Management of simple nodular goiter: current status and future perspectives. *Endocr Rev* 2003;24:102.

63. Tunbridge WM, Evered DC, Hall R, et al. The spectrum of thyroid disease in a community; the Whickham survey. *Clin Endocrinol (Oxf)* 1977;7:481.

64. Knudsen N, Perrild H, Christiansen E, et al. Thyroid structure and size and two year follow up of solitary cold thyroid nodules in an unselected population with borderline iodine deficiency. *Eur J Endocrinol* 2000;142:224.

65. Ron E, Kleinerman RA, Boice JD, et al. A population-based case-control study of thyroid cancer. *J Nat Cancer Inst* 1987;79:1.

66. Preston-Martin S, Bernstein L, Pike MC, et al. Thyroid cancer among young women related to prior thyroid disease and pregnancy history. *Br J Cancer* 1987;55:191.

67. Lesueur F, Stark M, Tocco T, et al. Genetic heterogeneity in familial nonmedullary thyroid carcinoma: exclusion of linkage to RET, MNG1, and TCO in 56 families. *J Clin Endocrinol Metab* 1999;84:2157.

68. Harrer P, Broeker M, Zint A, et al. Thyroid nodules in recurrent multinodular goiters are predominantly polyclonal. *J Endocrinol Invest* 1998;21:380.

69. Hadjidakis SG, Koutras DA, Daikos GK. Endemic goitre in Greece: family studies. *J Med Genet* 1964;1:82.

70. Malamos B, Koutras DA, Kostamis P, et al. Endemic goitre in Greece: a study of 379 twin pairs. *J Med Genet* 1967;4:16.

71. Greig WR, Boyle JA, Duncan A, et al. Genetic and non-genetic factors in simple goitre formation: evidence from a twin study. *QJM* 1967;36:175.

72. Brix TH, Kyvik KO, Hegedus L. Major role of genes in the etiology of simple goiter in females: a population-based twin study. *J Clin Endocrinol Metab* 1999;84:3071.

73. González-Sarmiento R, Corral J, Mories MT, et al. Monoallelic deletion in the 5′ region of the thyroglobulin gene as a cause of sporadic nonendemic simple goiter. *Thyroid* 2001;8:789.

74. Bignell GR, Canzian F, Shayeghi M, et al. Familial nontoxic multinodular goiter locus maps to chromosome 14q but does not account for familial nonmedullary thyroid cancer. *Am J Hum Genet* 1997;61:1123.

75. Capon F, Tacconelli A, Giardina E, et al. Mapping a dominant form of multinodular goiter to chromosome Xp22. *Am J Hum Genet* 2000;67:1004.

76. Takahashi T, Nozaki J, Komatsu M, et al. A new locus for a dominant form of multinodular goiter on 3q26.1-q26.3. *Biochem Biophys Res Commun* 2001;284:650.

77. Neumann S, Willgerodt H, Ackermann F, et al. Linkage of familial euthyroid goiter to the multinodular goiter-1 locus and exclusion of the candidate genes thyroglobulin, thyroperoxidase and Na/I symporter. *J Clin Endocrinol Metab* 1999;84:3750.

78. Malchoff CD, Sarfarazi M, Tendler B, et al. Papillary thyroid carcinoma associated with papillary renal neoplasia: genetic linkage analysis of a distinct heritable tumor syndrome. *J Clin Endocrinol Metab* 2000;85:1758.

79. Canzian F, Amati P, Harach R, et al. A gene predisposing to familial thyroid tumors with cell oxyphilia maps to chromosome 19p13.2. *Am J Hum Genet* 1998;63:1743.

80. McKay JD, Lesueur F, Jonard L, et al. Localization of a susceptibility gene for familial nonmedullary thyroid carcinoma to chromosome 2q21. *Am J Hum Genet* 2001;69:440.

81. Vestergaard P. Smoking and thyroid disorders—a meta-analysis. *Eur J Endocrinol* 2002;146:153.

82. Winsa B, Adami HO, Bergstrom R, et al. Stressful life events and Graves' disease. *Lancet* 1991;338:1475.

83. Sonino N, Girelli ME, Boscaro M, et al. Life events in the pathogenesis of Graves' disease. A controlled study. *Acta Endocrinol* 1993;128:293.

84. Okayasu I, Kong YM, Rose NR. Effect of castration and sex hormones on experimental autoimmune thyroiditis. *Clin Immunol Immunopathol* 1981;20:240.

85. Brix TH, Kyvik KO, Hegedus L. What is the evidence of genetic factors in the etiology of Graves' disease? A brief review. *Thyroid* 1998;8:627.

86. Brix TH, Kyvik KO, Christensen K, et al. Evidence for a major role of heredity in Graves' disease: a population-based study of two Danish twin cohorts. *J Clin Endocrinol Metab* 2001;86:930.

87. Brix TH, Kyvik KO, Hegedus L. A population-based study of chronic autoimmune hypothyroidism in Danish twins. *J Clin Endocrinol Metab* 2000;85:536.

88. Stenszky V, Kozma L, Balazs C, et al. The genetics of Graves' disease: HLA and disease susceptibility. *J Clin Endocrinol Metab* 1985;61:735.

89. Vaidya B, Kendall-Taylor P, Pearce SHS. The genetics of autoimmune thyroid disease. *J Clin Endocrinol Metab* 2002; 87: 5385.

90. Wandstrat A, Wakeland E. The genetics of complex autoimmune diseases: non-MHC susceptibility genes. *Nature Immunol* 2001;2:802.

91. Roitt IM, Doniach D, Campbell PN, et al. Auto-antibodies in Hashimoto's disease (lymphadenoid goitre). *Lancet* 1956;ii:820.

92. Hall R, Owen SG, Smart GA. Evidence for a genetic predisposition to formation of thyroid autoantibodies. *Lancet* 1960;ii:187.

93. Phillips D, McLachlan S, Stephenson A, et al. Autosomal dominant transmission of autoantibodies to thyroglobulin and thyroid peroxidase. *J Clin Endocrinol Metab* 1990;70:742.

94. Jaume JC, Guo J, Pauls DL, et al. Evidence for genetic transmission of thyroid peroxidase autoantibody epitopic fragments. *J Clin Endocrinol Metab* 1999;84:1424.

95. Phillips D, Prentice L, Upadhyaya M, et al. Autosomal dominant inheritance of autoantibodies to thyroid peroxidase and thyroglobulin—studies in families not selected for autoimmune thyroid disease. *J Clin Endocrinol Metab* 1991;72:973.

96. Heward J, Gough SCL. Genetic susceptibility to the development of autoimmune disease. *Clin Sci* (London)1997;93:479.

97. Payami H, Joe S, Thomson G. Autoimmune thyroid disease in type 1 diabetic families. *Genet Epidemiol* 1989;6:137.

98. Torfs CP, King MC, Huey B, et al. Genetic interrelationship between insulin-dependent diabetes mellitus, the autoimmune thyroid diseases, and rheumatoid arthritis. *Am J Hum Genet* 1986;38:170.

99. Walker DJ, Griffiths M, Griffiths ID. Occurrence of autoimmune diseases and autoantibodies in multicase rheumatoid arthritis families. *Ann Rheum Dis* 1986;45:323.

100. Grennan DM, Dyer PA, Clague R, et al. Family studies in RA—the importance of HLA-DR4 and of genes for autoimmune thyroid disease. *J Rheumatol* 1983;10:584.

101. Nerup J. Addison's disease: clinical studies a report of 108 cases. *Acta Endocrinol* (Copenh) 1974;76:127.

102. Dittmar M, Kahaly GJ. Polyglandular autoimmune syndromes: immunogenetics and long-term follow-up. *J Clin Endocrinol Metab* 2003;88:2983.

103. Broadley SA, Deans J, Sawcer SJ, et al. Autoimmune disease in first-degree relatives of patients with multiple sclerosis. *Brain* 2000;123:1102.

104. Atkinson TP, Schäffer AA, Grimbacher B, et al. An immune defect causing dominant chronic mucocutaneous candidiasis and thyroid disease maps to chromosome 2p in a single family. *Am J Hum Genet* 2001;69:791.

105. Spielman RS, McGinnis RE, Ewens WJ. Transmission test for linkage disequilibrium: the insulin gene region and insulin-dependent diabetes mellitus (IDDM). *Am J Hum Genet* 1993; 52:506.

106. Davies JL, Kawaguchi Y, Bennett ST, et al. A genome-wide search for human type 1 diabetes susceptibility genes. *Nature* 1994;371:130.

107. Cox NJ, Wapelhorst B, Morrison VA, et al. Seven regions of the genome show evidence of linkage to type 1 diabetes in a consensus analysis of 767 multiplex families. *Am J Hum Genet* 2001;69:820.

108. Cornelis F, Faure S, Martinez M, et al. New susceptibility locus for rheumatoid arthritis suggested by a genome-wide linkage study. *Proc Natl Acad Sci USA* 1998;95:10746.

109. Shai R, Quismorio FP, Li L, et al. Genome-wide screen for systemic lupus erythematosus susceptibility genes in multiplex families. *Hum Mol Genet* 1999;8:639.

110. Grumet FC, Payne RO, Konishi J, et al. HL-A antigens as markers for disease susceptibility and autoimmunity in Graves' disease. *J Clin Endocrinol Metab* 1974;39:1115.

111. Seignalet J, Mirouze J, Jaffiol C, et al. HLA in Graves' disease and in diabetes mellitus insulin-dependent. *Tissue Antigens* 1975;6:272.

112. Bech K, Lumholtz B, Nerup J, et al. HLA antigens in Graves' disease. *Acta Endocrinol* (Copenh) 1977;86:510.

113. Farid NR, Sampson L, Noel EP, et al. A study of human leukocyte D locus related antigens in Graves' disease. *J Clin Invest* 1979;63:108.

114. Tomer Y, Davies TF. The genetic susceptibility to Graves' disease. *Baillieres Clin Endocrinol Metab* 1997;11:431.

115. Heward JM, Allahabadia A, Daykin J, et al. Linkage disequilibrium between the human leukocyte antigen class II region of the major histocompatibility complex and Graves' disease: replication using a population case control and family-based study. *J Clin Endocrinol Metab* 1998;83:3394.

116. Yanagawa T, Mangklabruks A, Chang Y, et al. Human histocompatability leukocyte antigen-DQA1*0501 allele associated with genetic susceptibility to Graves' disease in a Caucasian population. *J Clin Endocrinol Metab* 1993;76:1569.

117. Barlow AB, Wheatcroft N, Watson P, et al. Association of HLA-DQA1*0501 with Graves' disease in English Caucasian men and women. *Clin Endocrinol (Oxf)* 1996;44:73.

118. Maciel LM, Rodrigues SS, Dibbern RS, et al. Association of the HLA-DRB1*0301 and HLA-DQA1*0501 alleles with Graves' disease in a population representing the gene contribution from several ethnic backgrounds. *Thyroid* 2001;11:31.

119. Cuddihy RM, Bahn RS. Lack of an independent association between the human leukocyte antigen allele DQA1*0501 and Graves' disease. *J Clin Endocrinol Metab* 1996;81:847.

120. Philippou G, Krimitzas A, Kaltsas G, et al. HLA DQA1*0501 and DRB1*0301 antigens do not independently convey susceptibility to Graves' disease. *J Endocrinol Invest* 2001;24:88.

121. Hunt PJ, Marshall SE, Weetman AP, et al. Histocompatibility leucocyte antigens and closely linked immunomodulatory genes in autoimmune thyroid disease. *Clin Endocrinol (Oxf)* 2001;55:491.

122. Kawa A, Nakamura S, Nakazawa M, et al. HLA-BW35 and B5 in Japanese patients with Graves' disease. *Acta Endocrinol (Copenh)* 1977; 86:754.

123. Dong RP, Kimura A, Okubo R, et al. HLA-A and DPB1 loci confer susceptibility to Graves' disease. *Hum Immunol* 1992; 35:165.

124. Onuma H, Ota M, Sugenoya A, et al. Association of HLA-DPB1*0501 with early-onset Graves' disease in Japanese. *Hum Immunol* 1994;39:195.

125. Tandon N, Mehra NK, Taneja V, et al. HLA antigens in Asian Indian patients with Graves' disease. *Clin Endocrinol (Oxf)* 1990;33:21.

126. Omar MA, Hammond MG, Desai RK, et al. HLA class I and II antigens in South African blacks with Graves' disease. *Clin Immunol Immunopathol* 1990;54:98.

127. Chen QY, Nadell D, Zhang XY, et al. The human leukocyte antigen HLA DRB3*020/DQA1*0501 haplotype is associated with Graves' disease in African Americans. *J Clin Endocrinol Metab* 2000;85:1545.

128. Wong GW, Cheng SH, Dorman JS. The HLA-DQ associations with Graves' disease in Chinese children. *Clin Endocrinol (Oxf)* 1999;50:493.

129. Ratanachaiyavong S, Demaine AG, Campbell RD, et al. Heat shock protein 70 (HSP70) and complement C4 genotypes in patients with hyperthyroid Graves' disease. *Clin Exp Immunol* 1991;84:48.

130. Badenhoop K, Schwarz G, Schleusener H, et al. Tumor necrosis factor beta gene polymorphisms in Graves' disease. *J Clin Endocrinol Metab* 1992;74:287.

131. Heward JM, Allahabadia A, Sheppard MC, et al. Association of the large multifunctional proteasome (LMP2) gene with Graves' disease is a result of linkage disequilibrium with the HLA haplotype DRB1*0304-DQB1*02-DQA1*0501. *Clin Endocrinol (Oxf)* 1999;51:115.

132. Kamizono S, Hiromatsu Y, Seki N, et al. A polymorphism of the 5′ flanking region of tumour necrosis factor alpha gene is associated with thyroid-associated ophthalmopathy in Japanese. *Clin Endocrinol (Oxf)* 2000;52:759.

133. Moens H, Farid NR, Sampson L, et al. Hashimoto's thyroiditis is associated with HLA-DRw3. *N Engl J Med* 1978;299:133.

134. Tandon N, Zhang L, Weetman AP. HLA associations with Hashimoto's thyroiditis. *Clin Endocrinol (Oxf)* 1991;34:383.

135. Thompson C, Farid NR. Post-partum thyroiditis and goitrous (Hashimoto's) thyroiditis are associated with HLA-DR4. *Immunol Lett* 1985;11:301.

136. Bogner U, Badenhoop K, Peters H, et al. HLA-DR/DQ gene variation in nongoitrous autoimmune thyroiditis at the serological and molecular level. *Autoimmunity* 1992;14:155.

137. Badenhoop K, Schwarz G, Walfish PG, et al. Susceptibility to thyroid autoimmune disease: molecular analysis of HLA-D region genes identifies new markers for goitrous Hashimoto's thyroiditis. *J Clin Endocrinol Metab* 1990;71:1131.

138. Jansson R, Safwenberg J, Dahlberg PA. Influence of the HLA-DR4 antigen and iodine status on the development of autoimmune postpartum thyroiditis. *J Clin Endocrinol Metab* 1985; 60:168.

139. Vargas MT, Briones-Urbina R, Gladman D, et al. Antithyroid microsomal autoantibodies and HLA-DR5 are associated with postpartum thyroid dysfunction: evidence supporting an autoimmune pathogenesis. *J Clin Endocrinol Metab* 1988;67:327.

140. Parkes AB, Darke C, Othman S, et al. Major histocompatibility complex class II and complement polymorphisms in postpartum thyroiditis. *Eur J Endocrinol* 1996;134:449.

141. Uno H, Sasazuki T, Tamai H, et al. Two major genes, linked to HLA and Gm, control susceptibility to Graves' disease. *Nature* 1981;292:768.

142. Vaidya B, Imrie H, Perros P, et al. The cytotoxic T lymphocyte antigen-4 is a major Graves' disease locus. *Hum Mol Genet* 1999;8:1195.

143. Tomer Y, Barbesino G, Greenberg DA, et al. Mapping the major susceptibility loci for familial Graves' and Hashimoto's diseases: evidence for genetic heterogeneity and gene interactions. *J Clin Endocrinol Metab* 1999;84:4656.

144. Sakai K, Shirasawa S, Ishikawa N, et al. Identification of susceptibility loci for autoimmune thyroid disease to 5q31-q33 and Hashimoto's thyroiditis to 8q23-q24 by multipoint affected sib-pair linkage analysis in Japanese. *Hum Mol Genet* 2001;10:1379.

145. Jin Y, Teng W, Ben S, et al. Genome-wide scan of Graves' disease: evidence for linkage on chromosome 5q31 in Chinese Han pedigrees. *J Clin Endocrinol Metab* 2003;88:1798.

146. Zavattari P, Lampis R, Motzo C, et al. Conditional linkage disequilibrium analysis of a complex disease superlocus, IDDM1 in the HLA region, reveals the presence of independent modifying gene effects influencing the type 1 diabetes risk encoded by the major HLA-DQB1, -DRB1 disease loci. *Hum Mol Genet* 2001;10:881.

147. Johansson S, Lie BA, Todd JA, et al. Evidence of at least two type 1 diabetes susceptibility genes in the HLA complex distinct from HLA-DQB1, -DQA1 and -DRB1. *Genes Immun* 2003;4:46.

148. Waterhouse P, Penninger JM, Timms E, et al. Lymphoproliferative disorders with early lethality in mice deficient in CTLA-4. *Science* 1995;270:985.

149. Luhder F, Hoglund P, Allison JP, et al. Cytotoxic T lymphocyte-associated antigen 4 (CTLA-4) regulates the unfolding of autoimmune diabetes. *J Exp Med* 1998;187:427.

150. Lenschow DJ, Ho SC, Sattar H, et al. Differential effects of anti-B7–1 and anti-B7–2 monoclonal antibody treatment on the development of diabetes in the nonobese diabetic mouse. *J Exp Med* 1995;181:1145.

151. Krummel MF, Allison JP. CTLA-4 engagement inhibits IL-2 accumulation and cell cycle progression upon activation of resting T cells. *J Exp Med* 1996;183:2533.

152. Scheipers P, Reiser H. Fas-independent death of activated CD4(+) T lymphocytes induced by CTLA-4 crosslinking. *Proc Natl Acad Sci U S A* 1998;95:10083.

153. Yanagawa T, Hidaka Y, Guimaraes V, et al. CTLA-4 gene polymorphism associated with Graves' disease in a Caucasian population. *J Clin Endocrinol Metab* 1995;80:41.

154. Nisticò L, Buzzetti R, Pritchard LE, et al. The CTLA-4 gene region of chromosome 2q33 is linked to, and associated with, type 1 diabetes. *Hum Mol Genet* 1996;5:1075.

155. Hadj Kacem H, Bellassoued M, Bougacha-Elleuch N, et al. CTLA-4 gene polymorphisms in Tunisian patients with Graves' disease. *Clin Immunol* 2001;101:361.

156. Nithiyananthan R, Heward JM, Allahabadia A, et al. Polymorphism of the CTLA-4 gene is associated with autoimmune hypothyroidism in the United Kingdom. *Thyroid* 2002;12:3.

157. Barbesino G, Tomer Y, Concepcion E, et al. Linkage analysis of candidate genes in autoimmune thyroid disease. I. Selected immunoregulatory genes. *J Clin Endocrinol Metab* 1998;83:3290.

158. Tomer Y, Greenberg DA, Barbesino G, et al. CTLA-4 and not CD28 is a susceptibility gene for thyroid autoantibody production. *J Clin Endocrinol Metab* 2001;86:1687.

159. Ueda H, Howson JM, Esposito L, et al. Association of the T-cell regulatory gene CTLA4 with susceptibility to autoimmune disease. *Nature* 2003;423:506.

160. Risch N, Merikangas K. The future of genetic studies of complex human diseases. *Science* 1996;273:1516.

161. Vaidya B, Imrie H, Perros P, et al. Cytotoxic T lymphocyte antigen-4 (CTLA-4) gene polymorphism confers susceptibility to thyroid associated orbitopathy. *Lancet* 1999;354:743.

162. Allahabadia A, Heward JM, Nithiyananthan R, et al. MHC class II region, CTLA4 gene, and ophthalmopathy in patients with Graves' disease. *Lancet* 2001;358:984.

163. Stuck BJ, Pani MA, Besrour F, et al. Fas ligand gene polymorphisms are not associated with Hashimoto's thyroiditis and Graves' disease. *Hum Immunol* 2003;64:285.

164. Ban Y, Taniyama M, Ban Y. Vitamin D receptor gene polymorphism is associated with Graves' disease in the Japanese population. *J Clin Endocrinol Metab* 2000;85:4639.

165. Pani MA, Regulla K, Segni M, et al. A polymorphism within the vitamin D–binding protein gene is associated with Graves' disease but not with Hashimoto's thyroiditis. *J Clin Endocrinol Metab* 2002;87:2564.

166. Pearce SHS, Vaidya B, Imrie H, et al. Further evidence for a susceptibility locus on chromosome 20q13.11 in families with dominant transmission of Graves' disease. *Am J Hum Genet* 1999;65:1462.

167. Vaidya B, Imrie H, Perros P, et al. Evidence for a new Graves' disease susceptibility locus at chromosome 18q21. *Am J Hum Genet* 2000;66:1710.

168. Tomer Y, Ban Y, Concepcion E, et al. Common and unique susceptibility loci in Graves' and Hashimoto diseases: results of whole-genome screening in a data set of 102 multiplex families. *Am J Hum Genet* 2003;73:000.

169. Risch N. Linkage strategies for genetically complex traits. II. The power of affected relative pairs. *Am J Hum Genet* 1990;46:229.

170. Lander E, Kruglyak L. Genetic dissection of complex traits: guidelines for interpreting and reporting linkage results. *Nat Genet* 1995;11:241.

171. Akamizu T, Hiratani H, Ikegami S, et al. Association study of autoimmune thyroid disease at 5q23-q33 in Japanese patients. *J Hum Genet* 2003;48:236.

172. Ban Y, Greenberg DA, Concepcion E, et al. Amino acid substitutions in the thyroglobulin gene are associated with susceptibility to human and murine autoimmune thyroid disease. *Proc Natl Acad Sci USA* 2003;100:15119.

173. Gough S. The thyroglobulin gene: the third locus for autoimmune thyroid disease or a false dawn? *Trends Molecular Medicine* 2004;10:302.

21

PATHOLOGY

ZUBAIR WAHID BALOCH
VIRGINIA A. LIVOLSI

NORMAL THYROID

The normal thyroid gland is a bilobed structure, connected by an isthmus. The thyroid capsule is thin, does not strip easily, and contains sizable venous channels that become strikingly prominent when vascularity is increased. The normal gland is soft and yellowish-red; the colloid gives the cut surfaces a glistening, translucent appearance. Normal thyroid weights in the United States range from 10 to 20 g. The functional unit of the thyroid is the follicle, which averages about 20 μm in diameter (1). A thyroid lobule consists of 20 to 40 follicles bound together by a thin sheath of connective tissue and supplied by a lobular artery (2). The thyroid follicles are formed by a single layer of low cuboidal epithelium. The nucleus of the follicular cell is round to ovoid, sometimes irregular in shape, centrally placed, and uniform in size. The nucleolus is inconspicuous. A basal lamina envelops the entire follicle. Numerous capillaries and lymphatics surround the follicle. Considerable interstitial connective tissue and fat cells may be present (3). The follicular lumen is occupied by colloid, partly composed of thyroglobulin, which is evenly applied to the luminal cell borders. Calcium oxalate crystals are common in the colloid of adults (4,5).

Electron microscopy demonstrates that the normal flat to low-cuboidal follicular cells interdigitate and overlap one another, and that they are intimately related to the capillaries that surround the follicle; microvilli on the apical surface are numerous near the cellular margins (6–8).

C-cells are intrafollicular and lie next to the follicular cells and within the basal lamina that surrounds each follicle of the normal gland. C-cells are most numerous in the central portions of the middle and upper thirds of the thyroid lobes (9–12). They are believed to originate from the last branchial pouches (ultimobranchial bodies). C-cells are typically more numerous in infant thyroid than in adult glands (9,13).

Sizable C-cell aggregates have been observed in some adults without any known endocrinologic abnormality (10, 11,14). The C-cells are polygonal to spindle-shaped, have "light," or low-density cytoplasm, and contain numerous membrane-limited cytoplasmic granules, which contain calcitonin. A small number of C-cells (or cells similar to

them) contain somatostatin (15,16). Guyetant et al (17) define C-cell hyperplasia as consisting of >40 C-cells/cm² and the presence of at least three low-power microscopic fields containing >50 C-cells.

The tiny solid cell nests of ovoid to spindled epidermoid cells are also considered to be of ultimobranchial origin (18–21). Typically, the nests have about the same distribution in the thyroid lobes as the C-cells. Tiny cysts that contain fluid, and a few mucous cells, may lie within or accompany the solid cell nests. So-called mixed follicles (19) are lined by follicular cells and epidermoid cells (and sometimes C-cells) and contain both colloid and mucoid material. The ultimobranchial structures probably also contribute a small proportion of normal thyroid follicles (21–25).

Oxyphil cells (oncocytes, Askanazy cells, Hürthle cells) are altered follicular cells; they are enlarged, have granular eosinophilic cytoplasm, and have large, hyperchromatic, or bizarre nuclei (26,27). The cytoplasm is filled with swollen mitochondria. They are common in long-standing Graves' disease, autoimmune thyroiditis, thyroids damaged by adiation, tumors, and some adenomatous nodules (28).

Small clusters of lymphoid cells are so common in the thyroid stroma that they are essentially a normal finding (29). Also present in the interstitial tissue are antigen-presenting dendritic cells; these are sparse in the normal gland but increased in autoimmune thyroid disease (30).

DEVELOPMENTAL VARIATIONS

The thyroglossal tract extends in the midline from the foramen cecum at the base of the tongue to the isthmus of the normal gland (31). The tract consists of connective tissue, the thyroglossal duct, lymphoid tissue, and thyroid follicles; it is attached to and may extend through the center of the hyoid bone and is intimately related to the surrounding skeletal muscle. Thyroid tissue may persist at the base of the tongue, and in some patients may represent the only thyroid present (32). The thyroglossal duct typically is a tube lined by ciliated pseudostratified epithelium. If the duct is traumatized or infected, the epithelium may be transitional or squamous, or it may be partially or completely lost and replaced by fibrous tissue. Foreign-body reaction and chronic inflammation may be conspicuous. If fluid accumulates in part of the thyroglossal duct, a thyroglossal cyst may develop (31,33) (See Chapter 2).

Any type of diffuse thyroid disease can involve lingual thyroid (34) and the thyroid tissue along the tract.

Occasionally, segments of thyroglossal duct are included within the thyroid gland proper and, rarely, may serve as the origin of an intrathyroidal cyst (35). Parathyroid glands, thymic tissue, tiny masses of cartilage, and tiny glands lined by ciliated cells may be seen in normal thyroid glands, presumably related to anomalies of the development of the branchial pouches (36–38).

Because of the intimate relationship that exists in the embryo between the immature thyroid tissue and the adjacent developing skeletal muscle, strips of striated muscle are occasionally included within the thyroid (2,39,40). Conversely, thyroid tissue may be found in perithyroidal skeletal muscle. Such nodules of thyroid tissue are particularly prominent when the gland is hyperplastic, and they should not be confused with carcinoma.

Groups of thyroid follicles in lymph nodes nearly always represent metastatic carcinoma (papillary carcinoma). A few experienced pathologists state normal thyroid follicles rarely occur in cervical lymph nodes (41–43). Hence, normal thyroid tissue lying only within the capsule of a node, especially if the node is located in the midline, may represent an embryologic remnant and not metastatic cancer.

GOITER

Goiter is a diffuse or nodular enlargement of the thyroid gland, usually resulting from a benign process or a process of unknown origin.

When there is a deficiency of circulating thyroid hormone because of inborn errors of metabolism, iodine deficiency, or goitrogenic agents, and if the hypothalamic–pituitary axis is intact, production of thyroid-stimulating hormone (TSH, thyrotropin) is increased; consequently, cellular activity and increased glandular activity and glandular mass result in an attempt to restore the euthyroid state.

Worldwide, the most common cause of thyroid hormone deficiency is an inadequate amount of iodine in the diet, leading to iodine-deficiency goiter (44). Other causes include inborn errors of thyroidal metabolism (dyshormonogenetic goiter) (45,46), dietary goitrogens, and goitrogenic drugs and chemicals.

The pathologic changes of simple nontoxic goiter include one or more of the following: (a) hyperplasia, (b) colloid accumulation, or (c) nodularity (44,47,48).

Hyperplasia represents the response of the thyroid to TSH, other growth factors, or circulating stimulatory antibodies (49). The hyperplasia may compensate for thyroid hormonal deficiency, but in some patients, even severe hyperplasia does not produce sufficient hormonal output to avoid hypothyroidism.

If the deficiency of thyroid hormone occurs at birth or early in life, cretinism or juvenile myxedema may result, even though the gland is enlarged and hyperplastic; this is especially likely when an inborn error of thyroidal metabolism is present. A hyperplastic gland is hyperemic, diffusely enlarged, and not nodular.

The epithelium is tall and columnar; the follicles are collapsed and contain only scanty colloid. When the hyperplastic stage is extreme and prolonged, there may be confusion with carcinoma because of the degree of cellularity and the presence of enlarged cells. The nuclei are enlarged, hyperchromatic, and even bizarre. Because of follicular collapse and epithelial hyperplasia and hypertrophy, papillary changes can be seen (50). This pattern occurs most often in untreated dyshormonogenetic goiter (45, 46). Recognition of the benign nature of the process is possible because all the glandular tissue is abnormal, unlike carcinoma, in which the neoplastic masses constitute one or more localized groups of abnormal cells with a background of nonneoplastic parenchyma.

Thyroid follicles may not remain in a state of continuous hyperplasia, but instead undergo involution, with the hyperplastic follicles reaccumulating colloid. The epithelium becomes low cuboidal or flattened and resembles that of the normal gland. Some follicles become much larger than normal, contain excessive colloid, and are lined with flat epithelium (overinvolution; exhaustion atrophy). The gland is diffusely enlarged, soft, and has a glistening cut surface because of the excess of stored colloid. In addition to large follicles filled with colloid, there are foci in the gland where hyperplasia is still evident. This phase of nontoxic goiter is often termed colloid goiter.

Patients with long-standing thyroid deficiency typically develop nodular goiters that result from overdistention of some involuted follicles, and persistence of regions of epithelial hyperplasia. The new follicles form nodules and may be heterogeneous in their appearance, in their capacity for growth and function, and in their responsiveness to TSH. The vascular network is altered through the elongation and distortion of vessels, leading to hemorrhage, necrosis, inflammation, and fibrosis. These localized degenerative and reparative changes produce some nodules that are poorly circumscribed, and others that are well demarcated and resemble true adenomas (adenomatous goiter) (47,50,51). Because the nodules distort the vascular supply to some areas of the gland, some zones will contain larger-than-normal amounts of colloid and/or iodide, and others will have relative colloid and/or iodide deficiency. Growth of goiters therefore may be related to focally excessive stimulation by TSH, stimulation by growth factors, focally abnormal iodide concentration, growth-promoting thyroid antibodies, and poorly understood intrathyroidal factors.

Nodular goiter is essentially a process involving the entire gland, but the nodularity may be asymmetric, and individual nodules within the same gland may vary greatly in size. If one nodule is much larger or more prominent than the others, distinguishing it from a true neoplasm may not be possible. Several studies have shown that about 70% of dominant nodules in nodular goiter are indeed clonal proliferations (52–55). The formation of cysts, hemorrhage, fibrosis, and calcification further complicates the assessment of the gland.

The heterogeneity of the generations of replicating follicular cells in responsiveness to outside stimuli, functional capacity, and rate of growth, results in formation of groups of cells appear that are hyperfunctional or autonomous, or both. These form "hot" nodules that may cause thyrotoxicosis (Plummer's disease) (56).

Studies with radioactive iodine administered before operation have not always demonstrated correlations between the morphology of a nodule and its iodine metabolism (57) (see Chapter 68).

GRAVES' DISEASE

In this disorder, also termed diffuse toxic goiter, the thyroid is diffusely enlarged up to several times normal size.

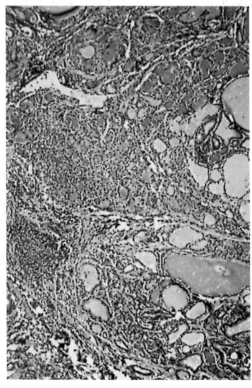

FIGURE 21.1. Diffuse hyperplasia of Graves' disease. Some colloid has accumulated **(right side)** because of preoperative antithyroid drug therapy.

The capsule is smooth, and the gland is hyperemic. The cut surfaces are fleshy and lack normal translucence because of loss of colloid. If the patient is untreated, treated briefly, or receives only propranolol, the microscopic appearance shows cellular hypertrophy and hyperplasia (Fig. 21.1) (6,9). There is almost no colloid. The cells are tall columnar, and are thrown into papillary folds that extend into the lumina of the follicles. Blood vessels are congested. At the ultrastructural level, microvilli are increased in number and elongated, the Golgi apparatus and endoplasmic reticulum are large, and mitochondria are numerous (6). Infiltrates of lymphocytes lie between the follicles, ranging from minimal to extensive. T-cells predominate among the epithelial cells (cytotoxic-suppressor cells) and in the interstitial tissue (helper-inducer cells), where there are no lymphoid follicles (58–60). B-cells are numerous in the lymphoid follicles. Class II major histocompatibility complex antigens are expressed on the epithelial cells, and these epithelial cells induce the proliferation of T-cells, helping to perpetuate the process (58,61,62).

Lymphoid hyperplasia may occur elsewhere in the body: thymus, lymph nodes, and spleen.

Because nearly all patients now receive antithyroid medication and then iodide before surgery, the glands have undergone varying degrees of involution (63). Some appear almost normal except for numerous large follicles filled with colloid. A few papillae may remain. The hyperemia is notably decreased, especially if there has been preoperative administration of iodide (63).

If hyperplasia continues for many years, oxyphilic metaplasia of the cells begins to occur, the amount of stroma increases in an irregular fashion, and nodularity develops, just as in diffuse euthyroid goiter. If the process subsides spontaneously or because of maintenance on antithyroid medication, the involution may be remarkably complete, it may be irregular (with some foci of hyperplasia evident), or the gland may be altered by chronic lymphocytic thyroiditis (64).

DYSHORMONOGENETIC GOITER

When an inborn error of thyroid metabolism exists, and sufficient amount of circulating thyroid hormone is not available, the normal physiologic response of the pituitary to increase TSH causes a larger, more active thyroid, which may or may not be able to produce enough hormone to reach a normal equilibrium. If TSH stimulation is marked and prolonged, the thyroid becomes large and nodular; microscopically enlargement of follicular cells, virtual absence of colloid, and increased stroma are seen (45,46).

Large follicular cells with bizarre, hyperchromatic nuclei may be numerous. The enlarged gland, the bizarre cells, and the cellular nodules have at times been mistaken for carcinoma. Cancer can occur in a dyshormonogenetic goiter, but it is very rare (65) (see Chapter 48).

IATROGENIC AND RELATED HYPERPLASIAS

Chronic ingestion of excess iodide, for whatever reason, occasionally leads to diffuse hyperplasia. Papillary formations and small nodules may be numerous. Infiltration of lymphocytes may occur.

About 3% of patients given lithium salts for a prolonged period develop goiter or hypothyroidism, or both. Patients so treated have been reported to have diffuse hyperplasia with considerable cellular and nuclear pleomorphism (66).

Bromide ingestion may lead to hypothyroidism because of loss of iodide from the gland. There are hyperplastic cells, foci of papillary proliferation, and loss of colloid (67).

AUTOIMMUNE THYROIDITIS

Common synonyms for autoimmune thyroiditis include Hashimoto's thyroiditis, lymphocytic thyroiditis, and struma lymphomatosa.

The disorder, most common in women, encompasses a spectrum of clinical and pathologic changes (44), ranging from an absence of symptoms to hypothyroidism and rarely, hyperthyroidism, from a large goiter to an atrophic gland, and from scattered clusters of infiltrating lymphocytes to extensive chronic inflammation and scarring with almost complete loss of follicular epithelium.

Various antithyroid antibodies and other immune phenomena occur, including in situ immune complex deposition and basement membrane changes in the gland, and expression of major histocompatibility complex antigens on the thyroid cells (58,59,68). Thyroiditis may be found in the same families in which idiopathic hypothyroidism and Graves' disease are common. It may follow typical Graves' disease (64).

The hyperthyroid variant of autoimmune thyroiditis is closely related to Graves' disease and may be almost identical in its gross and microscopic appearance to the latter condition (69), suggesting that this variant may indeed be Graves' disease. The presence of TSH-receptor antibodies in such patients would confirm the diagnosis of Graves' disease.

If the thyroiditis is slight and focal, then the thyroid is normal in size and contains scattered infiltrates of lymphocytes, predominantly T-cells. Some of the infiltrates contain lymphoid follicular centers, mostly B-cells. The thyroid follicles involved by the infiltrates appear atrophic; they have lost part or all of their colloid.

Small numbers of plasma cells (mostly immunoglobulin G (IgG)-positive) are mixed with lymphocytes (68). Glands

involved by this focal thyroiditis typically are asymptomatic; therefore, the thyroiditis is discovered when thyroid tissue is surgically removed for other reasons, or the process is found at autopsy. Focal lymphocytic thyroiditis probably represents the mild or early form of autoimmune thyroiditis (29). When focal lymphocytic thyroiditis is more than minimal and the foci of involvement are larger and more numerous, occasional follicular cells undergo metaplasia toward oxyphilic cells. Part of a lobe sometimes may be extensively involved by lymphocytic thyroiditis, with minor changes occurring elsewhere in the gland; hence nodularity may result (nodular Hashimoto's thyroiditis).

In more advanced cases of autoimmune thyroiditis, little or no normal parenchyma is visible. The gland on gross examination is enlarged, and its cut surfaces are fleshy and pale.

Microscopic examination shows that many follicles are small, the amount of colloid is decreased, and infiltrates of lymphocytes, plasma cells, and macrophages are extensive (Fig. 21.2) (70,71). Lymphoid follicular centers are numerous, and their antibody-producing B-cells are polyclonal; those containing IgG are the most numerous (59–61,68, 72). T-cells are most frequent among the epithelial cells and in the interstitial tissue away from lymphoid follicles. In-

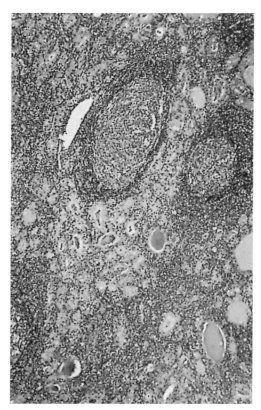

FIGURE 21.2. Autoimmune thyroiditis. Lymphoid follicles are conspicuous. Only a few colloid-filled thyroid follicles remain; most of these follicles are small and were formed by hyperplastic and metaplastic cells.

flammatory giant cells may be scattered through the damaged follicles; their presence should not lead the pathologist to mistake autoimmune thyroiditis for de Quervain's thyroiditis (71). The amount of connective tissue in the gland often increases. Some follicular cells appear atrophic or damaged; many are hyperplastic or metaplastic (oncocytic or Hürthle cells; squamous metaplasia) (73,74). The solid-cell nests have been suggested as the origin of the latter (21,74). Possibly related rare cystic lesions have also been noted (38,40,75,76).

Most cases of adult hypothyroidism not related to pituitary failure, radiation, or surgical removal, probably represent an atrophic form of autoimmune thyroiditis (see Chapter 47). These glands are fibrotic and usually small, with a few nests of abnormal epithelial cells; scattered small groups of lymphocytes and plasma cells are present.

SILENT THYROIDITIS

Some patients with autoimmune thyroiditis have one or more episodes of painless enlargement of the gland accompanied by transient thyrotoxicosis and reduced radioiodine uptake, followed by transient and less commonly permanent hypothyroidism (77–79). The episodes often occur postpartum (79). Biopsies have demonstrated that the thyroid may have diffuse or focal lymphocytic thyroiditis. The entities of "silent thyroiditis" or postpartum thyroiditis have been shown to fall into the spectrum of autoimmune thyroid disease (77,79) (see Chapter 27).

SPECIFIC INFECTIOUS THYROIDITIS

Acute suppurative thyroiditis results from infection by pyogenic organisms. Tuberculosis, syphilis, parasitic infestations, and fungal infections may occur (80,81). In children, suppurative thyroiditis may occur by direct extension of infection from the pyriform sinus (82). Pneumocystis carinii thyroiditis and cytomegalovirus infection have been identified in patients with acquired immunodeficiency syndrome (83,84). Thyroidal infections are usually associated with the presence of the organism elsewhere in the body and occur in patients who lack a normal immune system (transplant recipients, patients with acquired immune deficiency syndrome) or who are debilitated by a chronic disease.

GRANULOMATOUS THYROIDITIS

Synonyms for granulomatous thyroiditis are subacute thyroiditis and de Quervain's thyroiditis. This disorder, proba-

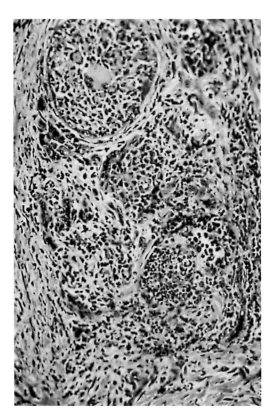

FIGURE 21.3. de Quervain's thyroiditis. The five follicles shown are distended by inflammatory cells.

bly of viral origin, is characteristically self-limiting, lasting 1 to 3 months. Grossly, the gland is slightly enlarged. The changes are usually bilateral but may be asymmetric or focal. The involved regions are firm, poorly defined, and resemble carcinoma grossly (85). Microscopic changes in the regions involved consist of disrupted follicles, with fragmentation of the colloid and many macrophages (Fig. 21.3) (85).

Microabscesses form, as some follicles are filled with polymorphonuclear leukocytes. Both follicular cells and colloid are destroyed focally. Giant cells of the foreign-body type arise from the fusion of macrophages, and they lie adjacent to or surround the disrupted colloid. Fibrous tissue proliferates around the damaged follicles, and lymphocytes infiltrate the connective tissue. Because the damaged foci contain necrotic cells, macrophages, and giant cells, and because they are surrounded by proliferative connective tissue that contains lymphocytes, there is a distinct resemblance to pathologic processes characterized by the formation of granulomas.

The thyroid tissue between the damaged regions appears normal. Healing occurs by fibrosis and by proliferation of remaining follicular cells; new follicles appear.

PALPATION THYROIDITIS

In many thyroid specimens, particularly surgically resected ones, an occasional follicle is disorganized, with breakdown of colloid, macrophages, and foreign-body giant cell reaction. This incidental microscopic finding is believed to be the result of palpation of the gland and hence is a post-traumatic thyroiditis (86).

AMIODARONE INJURY WITH THYROTOXICOSIS

Administration of amiodarone may cause thyrotoxicosis. Tissue changes are usually focal. Groups of follicles contain degenerated follicular cells (with granular or vacuolated cytoplasm), some follicles have lost follicular cells, and there is partial or complete loss of colloid. Zones of fibrosis are evident. The intervening thyroid tissue is normal (87,88).

RIEDEL'S STRUMA

Riedel's struma (Riedel's thyroiditis fibrosclerosis) invasive fibrous thyroiditis (89,90) is a very rare condition that represents one manifestation of a systemic collagenosis. It may include sclerosing mediastinitis, retroperitoneal fibrosis, pseudotumor of the orbit, and sclerosis of the biliary tract (90). The involvement of the thyroid seems to be incidental. Typically, a lobe of the thyroid and the adjacent skeletal muscle, nerves, blood vessels, and trachea are extensively replaced by dense, inflamed fibrous tissue. The mass formed is firm to hard, pale gray, and easily mistaken for cancer on clinical examination or by the surgeon at operation. Inflammatory cells, especially lymphocytes and plasma cells, are present in the dense connective tissue; angiitis usually involving veins may be conspicuous. There is no atypia of the fibroblasts or of the inflammatory cells; no oxyphilic metaplasia is found.

Carcinomas with extensive fibrosis and sclerosing lymphomas should be considered in the differential diagnosis; absence of cytological atypia is helpful in this distinction.

There does not appear to be any relation to other types of thyroiditis. Riedel's struma may be unilateral, and the portion of the gland not involved by the process is normal. In some cases, remnants of a nodule or adenoma are found.

COMBINED RIEDEL'S STRUMA AND FIBROSING HASHIMOTO'S THYROIDITIS

This rare condition shows simultaneous involvement of thyroid by Riedel's struma and Hashimoto's thyroiditis.

The patients usually present with goiter and the serologic profile of Hashimoto's thyroiditis; however, the microscopic picture is that of Riedel's struma. Most authors believe that this simultaneous occurrence is coincidental (91).

MISCELLANEOUS DISORDERS
Radiation Effects

Ionizing radiation delivered in small doses to the thyroid glands of infants, children, and adolescents causes a marked increase in the later incidence of benign and malignant neoplasms (92–95). The neoplasms begin to appear about 5 to 10 years later, but many occur decades later. Larger doses cause more numerous nodules; many of these nodules are particularly cellular, and some are atypical in their structure and cytologic features, suggesting premalignant characteristics (92). The cancers that develop after small doses of radiation are mostly papillary carcinomas, are often multicentric or bilateral, and are frequently small (94). In addition to the nodules and neoplasms that occur, other changes are believed to be more common as well, including focal epithelial hyperplasia, chronic lymphocytic thyroiditis, oxyphilic metaplasia of follicular cells, and slight fibrosis (95 (see Chapter 70).

Large doses of ionizing radiation (e.g., therapeutic radiation for head and neck cancer, or radioiodine therapy) initially cause injury to vessels, irregular necrosis and sloughing of the follicular epithelium, and breakdown of some follicles. Hemorrhage, edema, and small numbers of inflammatory cells appear. As the damage heals, sclerosis and dilatation of vessels occur, the fibrous stroma of the gland increases, and a mixture of atrophic, hyperplastic, and metaplastic changes take place in the follicular epithelium (96,97). In some cases, oxyphilic cells with bizarre nuclei line the follicles.

AMYLOIDOSIS

The thyroid may be involved in primary or secondary amyloidosis (98,99). The amyloid deposition may be sufficiently uneven to produce an amyloid tumor or mass. Such an accumulation must be differentiated from that occurring in some instances of medullary carcinoma.

BLACK THYROID

Prolonged therapy with tetracycline antibiotics, especially minocycline, may cause the accumulation of sufficient pigment in the follicular cells to produce a dark brown to black gland (100,101). Much of the pigment is lipofuscin, but part may be a metabolite of the drug. Rarely, there may be interference with thyroid function (100).

NEOPLASMS

Thyroid neoplasms demonstrate a variety of morphologic patterns that complicate their pathologic interpretation. All neoplasms that arise from thyroid epithelial cells may have some functional capacities. They may respond to TSH and may even produce excessive amounts of thyroid hormones (56,102–104) or, if medullary carcinoma, produce excessive amounts of calcitonin. Immunohistochemical evaluation has been of diagnostic value. Localization of thyroglobulin or calcitonin aids in the classification of unusual thyroidal tumors and in providing definite identification of metastatic thyroid carcinomas (105).

In general, evaluation of nuclear ploidy (27,106–109) has been of little use in assessing malignancy in thyroid tumors. Some apparently diploid tumors are malignant; some aneuploid tumors are benign (107,109–112). Measurements of steroid receptors (113), oncogenes (114), proliferation indices (115,116), particular antigens (117), and studies of the nucleolar organizing regions (118) have provided some limited diagnostic or prognostic data (see Chapter 70).

Changes that occur with moderate frequency in thyroid epithelial tumors are the appearance of clear cells (119) and oxyphilic cells (oncocytes, Hürthle cells, Askanazy cells) (120,121).

BENIGN NEOPLASMS

Adenomas and Adenomatous Nodules

Nearly all adenomas have follicular patterns. Those follicular adenomas with papillary hyperplasia (some of which are functional) should not be classified as papillary adenomas (56), but as papillary hyperplastic nodules. An adenoma is defined as a solitary, encapsulated lesion having a uniform internal architecture that is substantially different from the surrounding thyroidal parenchyma, and it compresses the surrounding parenchma (46,122).

On gross examination, adenomas and nodules are well circumscribed and are often sharply demarcated from the adjacent tissue. They vary in size from about 1 mm in diameter to several centimeters (Fig. 21.4). The typical nodule contains so much colloid that it appears translucent, whereas the classic adenoma is cellular, fleshy, and pale. Hemorrhage, fibrosis, and cystic change may be evident in both nodules and adenomas.

Microscopically, a typical adenomatous nodule has a varied pattern consisting of large and small follicles, usually with a large amount of colloid present (Figs. 21.5 and 21.6). Giant follicles (colloid cysts), often irregular in shape, are common. The cells range from flat to cuboidal or columnar, and their nuclei are small, rounded, uniform, and compact. The stroma often appears loose and edema-

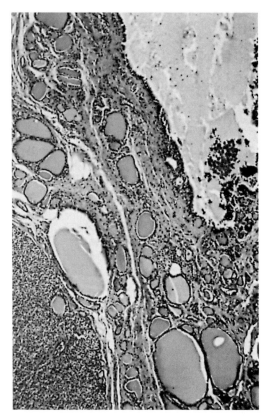

FIGURE 21.5. Adenomatous nodules. The lower left nodule is solid; the upper right nodule has undergone cystic degeneration.

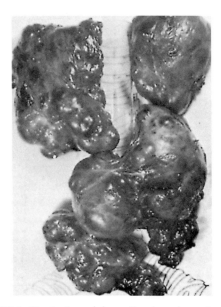

FIGURE 21.4. Nontoxic nodular goiter, largely mediastinal. The trachea and main-stem bronchi are represented diagrammatically.

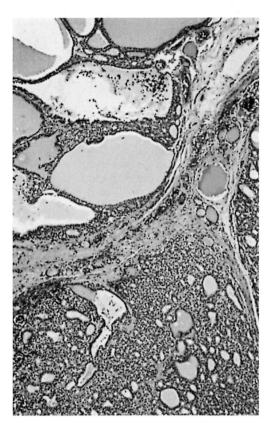

FIGURE 21.6. Adenomatous nodules. The nodule at the upper left contains large colloid-filled follicles.

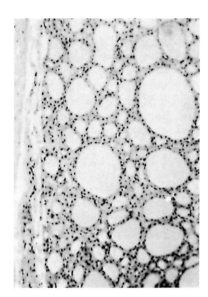

FIGURE 21.8. Follicular adenoma. The capsule is at the **left.**

Some, described as atypical adenomas, are hypercellular and may contain mitotic figures (44,122–125), therefore resembling well-encapsulated follicular carcinoma. Such a tumor requires careful study to avoid missing a carcinoma. Other atypical adenomas are also cellular but contain spin-

tous. Chronic inflammation, groups of macrophages, hemosiderin, fibrosis, and even calcification can be found.

The characteristic adenoma is encapsulated, cellular in comparison with the usual nodule, and relatively uniform in pattern (Figs. 21.7 and 21.8). It may present as a solid mass of cells with only a hint of follicular pattern, but, more often, adenomas are composed of relatively uniform follicles (Fig. 21.9). Adenomas sometimes have unusual patterns and cellular features (Fig. 21.10).

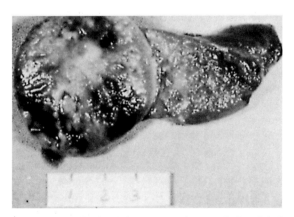

FIGURE 21.7. Follicular adenoma and normal thyroid tissue (gross). A capsule is visible, and the tumor contains central fibrosis and foci of hemorrhage.

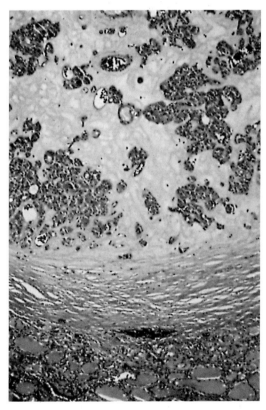

FIGURE 21.9. Follicular adenoma with a thick capsule. Extensive fibrous stroma is evident. Normal thyroid is at **bottom.**

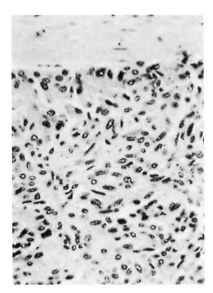

FIGURE 21.10. Atypical follicular adenoma. Many cells are elongated, some have large and irregular nuclei, and there is only a suggestion of follicle formation.

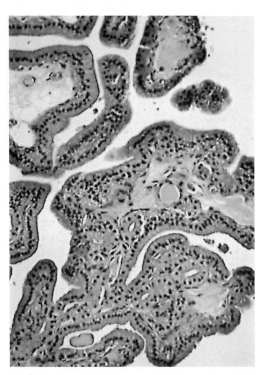

FIGURE 21.11. Adenoma or adenomatous nodule with papillae. The patient was 10 years old, and the nodule was hyperfunctional. The nuclei appear compact, regular, and round.

dle cells or polygonal cells with large and bizarre nuclei (125).

The so-called hyalinizing trabecular adenoma is a small, well-circumscribed tumor characterized by a trabecular and nesting pattern, with the nested, usually elongated cells surrounding hyaline connective tissue (126,127). Nuclei may contain cytoplasmic inclusions (126,127). Small psammoma bodies may occur. Gradations between typical follicular adenomas, trabecular adenomas, and the hyalinizing trabecular adenomas are seen (126,127). The differential diagnosis for these neoplasms is encapsulated medullary carcinoma; the adenomas contain thyroglobulin and no calcitonin. A majority of authors believe that hyalinizing trabecular adenoma is benign due to its clinical behavior. However, some authors have argued against the "benign" label of this tumor and believe that it is a form of papillary carcinoma. This is based on their similar cytologic characteristics, frequent coexistence, and similar immunoprofiles, and because some thyroid tumors with similar morphology have shown capsular and vascular invasion (128,129). We believe, until a conclusion is reached, that these tumors should be classified as hyalinizing trabecular neoplasm.

A rare variant of follicular adenoma is composed of vacuolated, signet-ring type cells (sometimes called mucinous), in which droplets of thyroglobulin and mucin-like material (possibly a carbohydrate or breakdown product of colloid) are present (130). An even more uncommon adenoma is the lipid-rich cell adenomas (131).

Cystic change is common, especially in adenomatous nodules, and almost all the typical architecture may disap-

pear, except for tiny remnants of the periphery. Cystic changes in nodules are frequently accompanied by the formation of papillae (Fig. 21.11).

Critical examination of adenomatous nodules shows that many of these lesions are not solitary, that encapsulation and compression are inconstant phenomena, and that their internal architecture is quite variable. Studies of clonality (52–55) suggest that they are true neoplasms. Most adenomas or nodules take up little or no radioiodine and are thus "cold" on scan.

A few of these benign lesions are hyperfunctional, or "hot"; usually this occurs with nodules of nodular goiter rather than with a classic adenoma (56). In adolescents and young women, many of the hot, or toxic, nodules contain numerous papillae, often sufficient in number to cause a pathologist to suggest a diagnosis of papillary carcinoma.

Teratomas of the thyroid and of the tissues adjacent to the thyroid occur predominantly in infants and are usually diagnosed at the time of birth (132). They may become large, sufficiently so to cause dystocia by hyperextension of the neck. They are often associated with polyhydramnios. These tumors are almost always benign. Teratomas of the thyroid and the perithyroidal region are rare in adults, but may be malignant (133). Microscopically, the teratoma is composed of multiple elements, often with a preponderance of neural components.

MALIGNANT NEOPLASMS

The most common malignant neoplasms that originate in the thyroid are the well-differentiated carcinomas of follicular epithelial origin: most are papillary carcinomas. These constitute about 80% of thyroid carcinomas.

In predicting the prognosis in thyroid cancer, one must include the patient's age and sex, the size of the primary tumor, the presence or absence of direct extension into the juxtathyroidal tissues, and the presence or absence of metastatic foci. In some neoplasms, features such as DNA content and the presence of certain cells and antigens must be considered (27,107,134–137).

Most nonneoplastic diseases of the thyroid do not seem to be precursors of malignant diseases, with the exception that autoimmune thyroiditis may predispose to malignant lymphoma. An occasional adenoma or adenomatous nodule may contain a focus of papillary carcinoma when removed at operation, but this is a rare occurrence.

Anaplastic carcinomas often have arisen in goitrous thyroids, and careful examination of the resected tissues has frequently demonstrated benign tumors or well-differentiated carcinomas in close association with the anaplastic carcinoma. Such findings have led to suggestions that the benign tumor or low-grade carcinoma has become "transformed" into the anaplastic carcinoma (125,138,139).

The characteristics of well-differentiated carcinomas can be appreciated only by careful microscopic examination of multiple, well-prepared sections. Frozen sections at times may be misleading (140), and the surgeon must accept this limitation.

PAPILLARY CARCINOMA

About 80% of thyroid carcinomas are papillary carcinomas. More common in women than in men and rarely familial (141), papillary carcinoma occurs most frequently in those parts of the world where ample iodine is present in the diet and the environment (142,143). The association of radiation, especially low-dose external radiation in childhood, with the development of adult papillary thyroid cancer, is well documented (144,145). Recent studies from the areas of the former Soviet Union near the Chernobyl nuclear plant indicate an "epidemic" of thyroid carcinoma in children and teenagers following the nuclear accident and release of radioactive iodine. Virtually all of these tumors are papillary carcinomas (146).

Grossly, papillary cancers are predominantly solid, although small cystic foci may be present. A distinctly cystic character is evident in some cases, with one or more cystic spaces occupying most of the neoplasm (125,147). Bits of calcified material and crystals may be present in the cyst fluid. Papillae protruding into the cysts may be seen and at

times are so numerous that portions of the cut surfaces appear granular.

Papillary carcinomas usually are infiltrative, and their margins often are poorly defined; however, about 10% to 20% of papillary cancers appear grossly encapsulated.

Fibrosis is common in and around papillary carcinomas (147–149), and it may be distributed in an extremely irregular fashion, grossly and microscopically (147–151). Occasionally, fibrosis is so extensive that almost no neoplastic cells can be found. Rarely, the stroma of the carcinomas is myxoid or similar to that of nodular fasciitis (152,153). Nonlamellated calcification is also common.

Small papillary carcinomas ("occult" carcinomas) are defined as being 1 cm in diameter or less and may be called minimal carcinomas or microcarcinomas (125,154–158). The incidence of these lesions ranges from 6% to 36% (125). When visible on gross examination, they present as small, irregular, firm scars, as soft foci of discoloration, or as tiny calcific lesions. Occasionally, such a tumor presents as a metastatic focus, usually as an enlarged cervical lymph node, rarely in a distant site (159–163). Microscopically, they contain neoplastic follicles or papillae, with the smallest ones showing a predominance of follicular pattern (159,162). They may be encapsulated or infiltrative.

Microscopic examination shows that most clinically evident papillary cancers contain papillae (Fig. 21.12); how-

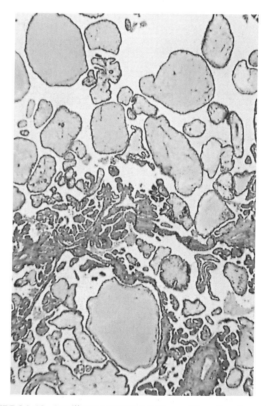

FIGURE 21.12. Papillary carcinoma with papillae of various sizes.

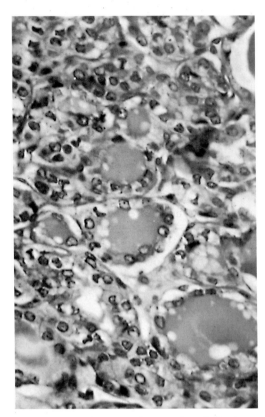

FIGURE 21.13. Papillary carcinoma with a follicular pattern. Nuclei vary in size and shape, and some have clear centers.

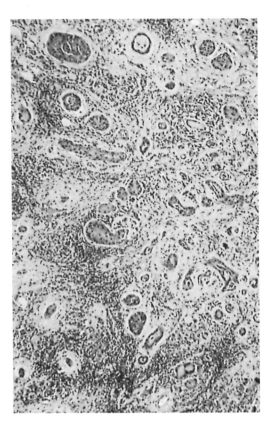

FIGURE 21.14. Papillary carcinoma with extensive fibrosis, chronic inflammation, and squamous metaplasia.

ever, papillae may constitute only a tiny part of the neoplasm. Papillary cancer may be solid, may be composed of follicles (Fig. 21.13), which is classified as follicular variant, or may be almost entirely papillary (125,148–151, 164,165). Trabecular (150,164), cribriform (150), and diffuse (125,151, 165–171), patterns occur (Fig. 21.14).

The most diagnostic single feature in papillary carcinoma is the epithelial cell, which is usually cuboidal to low columnar, and contains a distinctive nucleus (see Fig. 21.13) (125,147–151,172–174).

The nucleus is relatively large and irregular in shape, with folds, indentations, and cytoplasmic inclusions (147–151,172–174). The nucleolus is often inconspicuous because it lies near the nuclear membrane. The nuclear heterochromatin tends to be concentrated near the nuclear membrane, causing the central portion of the nucleus to appear relatively pale, empty, or like ground glass. When the cells form papillae or follicles, often most of the cytoplasm is concentrated in the apical or basal portions of the cells, thereby causing neighboring nuclei to appear to touch or overlap one another.

The papillae are distinctive, typically gnarled, with well-developed fibrovascular cores, and covered with a single layer of the characteristic cells (172). When papillae are crowded and close together, the cancer may appear almost solid. Many papillary carcinomas have a substantial num-

ber of follicles (indeed, they may predominate) (125,147–151). An occasional papillary carcinoma, however, is composed almost entirely of distended, colloid-filled follicles of moderately uniform size and shape, thereby closely resembling the pattern of an adenomatoid nodule (151). Rare papillae, an occasional focus of infiltration at the periphery, and the characteristic nuclei allow the diagnosis to be made.

Papillary carcinoma may be largely or exclusively solid. In young people, it is not known if this pattern affects prognosis (125,146,148), but in the middle-aged and elderly it may be associated with a loss of differentiation that suggests an aggressive neoplasm. Follicles or papillae may be rare or nonexistent in the primary focus, although they are more likely to be present in metastatic foci in lymph nodes.

The characteristic nuclei, the frequent presence of psammoma bodies, the tendency to focal metaplasia suggestive of squamous metaplasia, and the infiltration by lymphocytes in and around the neoplasm help distinguish this variant from medullary carcinoma, solid follicular carcinoma, and insular carcinoma (125). Immunoreactive thyroglobulin can be demonstrated focally in these variants; no calcitonin is present.

Rarely, papillary thyroid carcinoma appears as a diffuse involvement of all the lymphatic channels of one lobe or of the entire thyroid (125,148,166–171), accompanied by severe lymphocytic thyroiditis or interstitial fibrosis. Psammoma bodies are numerous. A primary mass lesion (epicenter) may not be found in the gland. This variant occurs more often in young people, is usually accompanied by lymph node metastases, and often pulmonary metastases.

The tall cell variant is an unusual type of papillary carcinoma that appears to be more aggressive than the usual variety (125,147,150,175,176). Some of these tumors are composed of cells with oncocytic cytoplasm, but the cells are narrow and elongated (at least twice as long as they are wide). These tumors often show extrathyroidal soft tissue extension and vascular invasion (20% to 25%). Most occur in older people, and the mortality rate is relatively high (176).

Rarely, a papillary carcinoma is composed of oxyphilic cells (oncocytes, Askanazy cells, Hürthle cells) (26,125, 151,177) that arise in a thyroid altered by lymphocytic thyroiditis. This lesion may show central cystic change and consists of papillary fronds infiltrated by a brisk lymphoplasmacytic infiltrate. Due to this peculiar morphology, which closely resembles Warthin's tumor of the salivary glands, this tumor is termed Warthin-like papillary carcinoma of thyroid (177). This variant appears to have the same spectrum of behavior as the common variety.

Encapsulation of the primary carcinoma is associated with a lower frequency of lymph node involvement, (125, 147–151,178,179).

About one third to one half of papillary carcinomas contain laminated calcific spherules, known as psammoma bodies (Fig. 21.15) (125,147–151,164,180). They measure 5 to 100 µm in diameter and probably begin in damaged or dying cells. Anytime a psammoma body is found in normal thyroid tissue, cervical lymph nodes, or juxtathyroidal soft tissue, a search of the resected tissues should be instituted for papillary carcinoma. Structures resembling psammoma bodies are occasionally found inside the follicles of adenomas or adenomatous nodules, especially those composed of oxyphilic cells, where they seem to arise from calcification of inspissated colloid.

Lymphocytic infiltration is often present within and around papillary carcinomas (148,149) (Fig. 21.16).

Lymphatic invasion accounts for the high frequency of multiple intrathyroidal foci of the tumor and metastasis to cervical lymph nodes (Fig. 21.17). Occasionally, cervical nodal enlargement due to metastatic papillary carcinoma is the presenting complaint. If a nodal metastasis is cystic, it must be differentiated from a branchial cleft cyst (125). If well-differentiated neoplastic follicles enlarge the node, it must not be mistaken for a sequestered thyroid nodule (40,181). The nuclear features of papillary carcinoma may

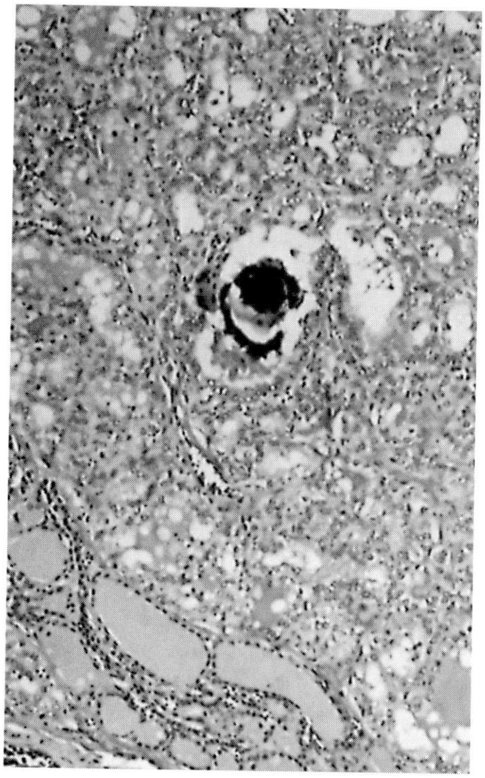

FIGURE 21.15. Papillary carcinoma containing a psammoma body. **Lower left:** Normal thyroid.

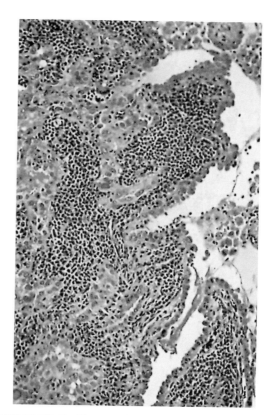

FIGURE 21.16. Papillary carcinoma with extensive infiltration by lymphocytes and plasma cells.

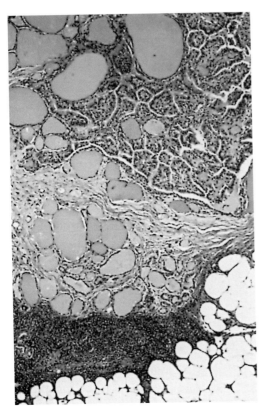

FIGURE 21.17. Papillary carcinoma in a lymph node. Half of it has a follicular pattern; half is composed of papillae.

not be present in these differentiated follicular-patterned metastases. Blood vessel invasion by papillary carcinoma is uncommon (125,147–151), and metastatic foci in distant sites are unusual, with the lungs most frequently involved (125,147–151,182,183).

The presence of many mitotic figures, enlarged or hyperchromatic nuclei, abnormal DNA content, deviation from the usual recognized histologic patterns, and regions of nondescript neoplastic cells not clearly recognizable as typical of papillary carcinoma (loss of differentiation) constitute characteristics believed to indicate that more aggressive behavior is likely (137,150,183). These features occur most often in older people and in large cancers.

FOLLICULAR CARCINOMA

Follicular carcinoma accounts for about 5% or less of all thyroid carcinomas in the United States, is more common in women than in men, and may occur at any age, but is more frequent with increasing age (especially after 30 years). The incidence is higher in regions of the world where iodine deficiency occurs (142,143).

Follicular carcinoma is an expansile neoplasm that is nearly always more or less encapsulated and has many sim-

ilarities to follicular adenoma (125,184–190). Grossly, it usually presents as a fleshy, solid, encapsulated mass, sometimes with focal fibrosis or calcification. The capsule is usually well developed, but if the tumor is aggressive, extensions beyond the capsule may be readily apparent. Sometimes invasion of sinusoids or veins is seen at the periphery of the neoplasm (125,184).

On microscopic examination, follicular carcinomas most often have a microfollicular pattern and resemble a cellular follicular adenoma. Trabecular or solid patterns are fairly common and often accompany the microfollicular pattern. Medium-sized to large follicles filled with colloid typically are a minor component or are absent; only rarely do they comprise most of the cancer (Fig. 21.18) (184). Thyroglobulin immunostaining may be used to detect colloid droplets, thereby demonstrating that some of the apparently solid neoplasms do contain microfollicles (191) and confirming the follicular derivation of the tumor.

The cells of follicular carcinoma are slightly to moderately larger than those present in most adenomas and adenomatous nodules, but otherwise they are similar. Mitotic figures range from rare to frequent.

Follicular carcinomas are divided into (a) localized, minimally invasive cancers and (b) more widely invasive cancers (125,184–190). Because follicular carcinomas are

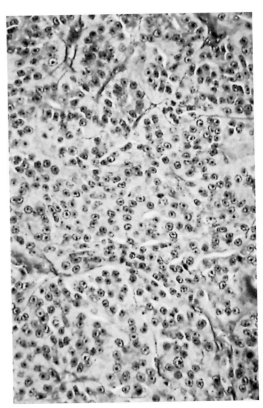

FIGURE 21.18. Follicular carcinoma with a mostly solid pattern. A few closed follicles are evident. Nucleoli are conspicuous.

nearly always encapsulated, the distinction between adenoma and minimally invasive carcinoma may be difficult. Carcinoma is recognized by its extension into vessels at its periphery, by its penetration into and through the capsule that surrounds it, and (occasionally) by the presence of distant metastasis (184,189). Even a minimally invasive carcinoma can present as a metastatic lesion (185,189). Many sections of the periphery of the neoplasm may need to be examined to find evidence of invasion, although most cancers will be diagnosed on examination of 10 sections (184,185,189).

A follicular carcinoma that invades only two or three small vessels may be termed "minimally invasive." A carcinoma that penetrates or invades its capsule to a limited extent but does not show vascular invasion is also termed "minimally invasive" (Figs. 21.19 and 21.20). The term invasive adenoma should be avoided; these are cancers.

The minimally invasive carcinomas rarely recur or spread to distant sites, so the outlook for most patients is good. However, since the literature contains numerous studies in which distributions between follicular variant of papillary carcinoma and true follicular carcinoma were not made (192,193), accurate data on long-term prognosis for minimally invasive follicular carcinoma are not available. Follicular carcinoma has little tendency to invade lym-

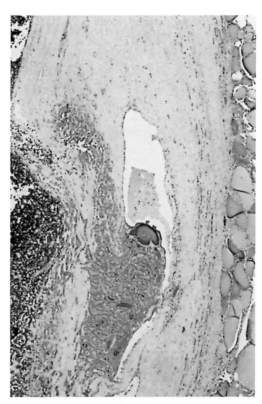

FIGURE 21.20. Follicular carcinoma (same as in Fig. 21.19). The cells protrude into a vessel in the capsule.

phatic vessels and spread to lymph nodes (184–190,192, 194).

Metastatic spread to the skeleton, lungs, brain, liver, and other tissues through the bloodstream may occur.

The follicular carcinomas that are not localized or minimally invasive have been grouped as "widely invasive"; these include examples in which multiple fingers of neoplastic cells extend into the surrounding thyroid or in which there is extensive replacement of the thyroid gland and soft tissue of the neck.

ONCOCYTIC (HÜRTHLE-CELL) TUMORS

Perhaps no thyroid neoplasm has elicited more confusion or debate than Hürthle-cell (or oncocytic) neoplasms. Clinicians and pathologists alike have considered that such tumors do not "follow the rules" for histopathologic diagnosis of malignancy (26–27,195–199).

Over the past decade, studies from numerous institutions throughout the world have shown that oncocytic or Hürthle-cell tumors can be divided into benign and malignant categories by careful adherence to strict pathologic criteria. More importantly, these pathologic distinctions predict clinical behavior (26,27,120,121,195,198,199).

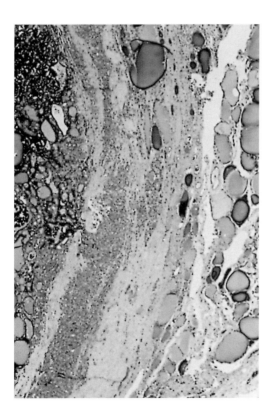

FIGURE 21.19. Follicular carcinoma that is small, hemorrhagic, and associated with skeletal metastases. Irregular infiltrates of tumor cells are visible in the capsule.

Most oncocytic neoplasms behave as follicular carcinomas, i.e., pathologically one must assess the capsule for invasion and/or vascular invasion (26,27,199). However, some papillary carcinomas show oncocytic cytology; these behave as usual papillary cancers and often arise in glands with chronic thyroiditis (177).

Hürthle-cell carcinomas should be separated as a category of thyroid neoplasms different from true follicular carcinomas. First, Hürthle-cell cancers can metastasize to regional lymph nodes as well as hematogenously (30); in addition, histologic evidence of invasive characteristics is found more commonly in oncocytic cancers (192).

Since approximately one third of oncocytic thyroid tumors show invasion (i.e., are cancers), as compared with 2% to 5% of nononcocytic follicular tumors, the finding of Hürthle-cell cytology in a fine-needle aspiration sample of a thyroid nodule should lead to surgical resection of the lesion to assess malignancy (26,199).

PATHOLOGIC DIAGNOSIS OF PAPILLARY AND FOLLICULAR CARCINOMA OF THYROID: CONTROVERSIES AND USE OF IMMUNOHISTOCHEMICAL MARKERS

The pathologic diagnosis of various thyroid lesions can be challenging. The two lesions that comprise a major portion of difficult cases in thyroid pathology are follicular variant of papillary thyroid carcinoma and follicular carcinoma (200,201)

Excluding classical papillary carcinoma, follicular variant of papillary thyroid carcinoma (FVPTC) is the most common variant of papillary carcinoma; it is characterized by follicular growth pattern and nuclear morphology characteristic of papillary carinomas. These lesions can be partially or completely encapsulated, and up to 15% can show capsular and vascular invasion (202–204). A majority of FVPTC are easily diagnosed by the characteristic nuclear morphology of papillary carcinoma; however, there exists a subset of cases in which the diagnosis of FVPTC can be challenging (200). This group consists of tumors, which arise in a background of nodular goiter, are completely encapsulated, lack capsular and/or vascular invasion, and shows multifocal rather than diffuse distribution of nuclear features of papillary carcinoma (204).

Controversy exists among experts about the diagnosis of such lesions. Some believe due to excellent clinical behavior and questionable morphology these tumors should be classified as "tumors of undetermined malignant potential" to avoid unnecessary therapy (205). Others believe that due to multifocal presence of nuclear features of papillary carcinoma the entire tumor should be classified as FVPTC for treatment and staging purposes (200). However, some authors have reported similar cases, which were classified as benign, atypical, or as "tumors of undetermined malignant

potential," that recurred as lymph node and even distant metastases (186,189,200).

Several studies have explored the role of various immunohistochemical and molecular markers as an aid to the histologic diagnosis of FVPTC (206–210). The markers studied include cytokeratin-19, HBME-1, galectin-3, and RET-PTC. None of these markers has been shown to be 100% specific; but when used in a panel, all these can prove to be helpful in the diagnosis of FVPTC (205–212).

As mentioned above, follicular carcinoma can be divided into so-called minimally invasive and widely invasive (163,183). In our practice we use a three-tiered classification: *minimally invasive, grossly encapsulated angioinvasive, and widely invasive* (200). There is much debate among pathologists regarding the criteria for the diagnosis of minimally invasive follicular carcinoma (185,188,192,200,213). Some believe that the diagnosis of follicular carcinoma should only be made in cases which demonstrate invasion of the capsular vessels with or without capsular invasion (189,192,205). Others believe that invasion is the key: thus invasion *of* the capsule, invasion *through* the capsule, and invasion *into* veins in or beyond the capsule represent the diagnostic criteria for carcinoma in a follicular thyroid neoplasm (200,212). Some have suggested the term "follicular tumor of undetermined malignant potential" for tumors which only show minimal capsular invasion, because a majority of these tumors will behave in a benign fashion (205). However, follow-up studies of some tumors diagnosed as follicular carcinoma on the basis of capsular invasion only have demonstrated distant metastases (188).

Are there any immunohistochemical markers available that can be helpful in the diagnosis of follicular carcinoma? Kroll et al reported that the chromosomal translocation t(2;3)(q13;25), that results in a fusion protein consisting of the DNA-binding domain of the thyroid transcription factor Pax-8 and the activation domain of peroxisome proliferator-activated receptor gamma (PPAR-gamma), was present in follicular carcinomas but not in papillary carcinomas, follicular adenomas, or multinodular goiter (214). However, follow-up studies have shown that while PPAR-gamma expression is seen in the majority of follicular carcinomas, it is also seen in other follicular-patterned lesions (follicular variant of papillary carcinoma and follicular adenoma) as well as in non-lesional surrounding thyroid tissue (215–217).

CLEAR-CELL TUMORS

Clear-cell change can be identified focally in many follicular-derived lesions in the thyroid—thyroiditis, nodules and neoplasms (118). Most clear-cell metaplasia is associated with oncocytic or Hürthle-cell change. Hence, distinction of proliferative or neoplastic nodules (and benign from malignant nodules) relies on adherence to accepted criteria for follicular lesions. Of greatest import is the differentiation of clear-cell change in follicular lesions from clear-cell renal cell carcinomas metastatic to the thyroid (118,129). Immunostaining for thyroglobulin may be helpful in sorting out this diagnostic problem.

POORLY DIFFERENTIATED CARCINOMA

Reviews of large numbers of thyroid carcinomas have often included examples of carcinomas that are recognizable as originating from follicular epithelium (often with evidence of coexistent papillary or follicular carcinoma), but that have moderate to high rates of mitotic activity, are composed of solid masses or trabeculae of relatively uniform epithelial cells, have tiny follicles present in varying numbers, may contain regions of acute necrosis, and are more aggressive than the usual well-differentiated carcinomas (218–226). Nishida et al in their study of poorly differentiated thyroid cancers noted that tumors with greater than 10% of "poorly differentiated" areas had a significantly worse prognosis than those tumors with small foci of poorly differentiated growth (220). Included among these lesions are insular carcinoma, columnar cell, tall cell and trabecular types of papillary cancer (219–226), and "poorly differentiated" carcinoma of Sakamoto (221). These tumors generally lack the usual histologic features and exceptional aggressiveness of anaplastic carcinomas, but they are neither typical follicular nor papillary carcinomas (220).

The role of oncogenes in thyroid carcinogenesis is not discussed in detail in this chapter (see section Oncogenes in Chapter 70). However, several investigators have reported results of immunostaining for p53, bcl-2, Ras oncogenes, and nM23 gene (113,227–234). Well-differentiated thyroid cancers are rarely positive for p53, whereas many anaplastic carcinoma are (40% to 60%) (233,234). Correspondingly, bcl-2 (related to the mechanism of apoptosis) oncogene is often expressed in well-differentiated cancers and rarely in undifferentiated cancers. Tumors in the poorly differentiated group (tall cell or columnar cell papillary cancer, and insular carcinoma) show intermediate patterns of expression of p53 (and of bcl 2 (231,232). Immunostaining for oncogene nM23 has not proven useful in thyroid tumors (114).

Evaluation for proliferative markers in thyroid neoplasms (immunostaining for PCNA or Ki67 antigen) has shown, as expected, low proliferation rates for well-differentiated tumors and high rates in poorly or undifferentiated lesions. The value of these tests is not evident in the clinical evaluation of affected patients (115,116).

ANAPLASTIC CARCINOMA

Fewer than 10% of thyroid carcinomas may be classified as anaplastic or undifferentiated (235). They are most com-mon in regions of the world where iodine is deficient (142, 143). Traditionally, these tumors include the rare small-cell carcinomas and the more common spindle cell and giant cell types. However, most lesions originally classified as small-cell anaplastic carcinomas represent medullary carcinoma, insular carcinoma or small cell malignant lymphoma (235–237). An oat-cell thyroid carcinoma, apparently separate from small-cell medullary carcinoma, has been described (236,237). The possibility of a metastatic carcinoma from another organ always has to be considered (237).

The following discussion will focus on spindle and giant-cell tumors. All are aggressive neoplasms that usually occur in elderly people, more often women. The patient may relate a history of a thyroid nodule that, after many years of stability, suddenly begins to grow rapidly. Some patients are known to have had low-grade thyroid carcinoma; some have low-grade thyroid carcinoma discovered at the time of diagnosis of the anaplastic tumor; and some have no history of thyroid disease (142,143,238).

Careful pathologic examination of thyroid glands that contain anaplastic carcinomas has demonstrated a high (50% to 70%) incidence of remnants of well-differentiated follicular or papillary carcinoma (138,139,217,237,238) or sometimes an adenoma or adenomatous nodules (238), confirming the clinical impression that anaplastic carcinomas arise out of low-grade tumors.

Gross examination demonstrates a hard, pale, infiltrative mass that may contain foci of necrosis and hemorrhage. These tumors invade the cervical soft tissues and involve the regional lymph nodes, often by direct extension. Microscopic examination reveals varied histologic patterns, many mitotic figures, and regions of acute necrosis.

Anaplastic carcinomas are usually pleomorphic (Fig. 21.21) and are composed of medium-sized to large cells with a vaguely epithelial appearance (138,139,237,238). There may be squamous cell differentiation (138,139) (or a tendency toward this pattern). Others appear sarcomatous (Fig. 21.22), especially resembling malignant fibrous histiocytoma, fibrosarcoma, or angiosarcoma (138,139, 237,238). Spindle cells may dominate. The giant-cell carcinomas often have malignant spindle cells. The most common type has bizarre giant cells, frequently multinucleated, and containing abnormal mitotic figures. Less commonly, some giant cells resemble osteoclasts (139,238,239).

Ultrastructural studies have demonstrated the presence of structures resembling tiny follicles, and junctions between the cells, supporting an epithelial phenotype (138, 139,237,238). Immunohistochemical evidence of thyroglobulin has been found in a few anaplastic carcinomas; it is likely that in most of these cases, the thyroglobulin staining represents diffusion of thyroglobulin from destroyed thyroid follicles (138,237); 50% to 100% of these tumors contain keratin (138,139,237,238). Carcinosarcoma of the thyroid (240) has been described.

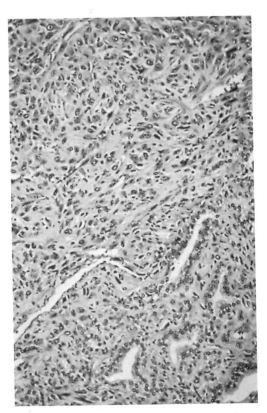

FIGURE 21.21. Anaplastic carcinoma. Remnants of neoplastic follicles are present in the lower portion.

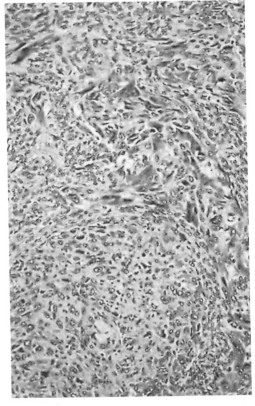

FIGURE 21.22. Anaplastic carcinoma with sarcomatous appearance.

SQUAMOUS CELL CARCINOMA, MUCOEPIDERMOID CARCINOMA, AND INTRATHYROIDAL THYMOMALIKE NEOPLASMS

Chronic inflammation and scarring in the thyroid may cause the affected epithelium to undergo benign squamous metaplasia (122,241). Squamous metaplasia may occur in papillary carcinoma (125,148) and in anaplastic carcinoma (138,139,237,238). Sometimes, typical squamous cell carcinoma occurs in association with papillary or anaplastic carcinoma (221,241,242). Occasionally, squamous cell carcinoma appears as an entity independent of any other form of thyroid cancer (243). Variants associated with leukocytosis and hypercalcemia have been described (244). The major differential diagnosis is metastatic squamous carcinoma, especially from the head and neck, lung, or esophagus. Primary squamous carcinoma of the thyroid is usually aggressive, with a poor prognosis (243).

Mucoepidermoid carcinoma of the thyroid is rare (245–252) and may originate from ultimobranchial remnants or follicular epithelium (252). Two distinct tumors have been described under this category: *mucoepidermoid carcinoma* and *sclerosing mucoepidermoid carcinoma with eosinophilia* (245–246,250,252). Mucoepidermoid carcinoma is more common in women and usually presents as solitary painless mass. These tumors consist of areas of squamous differentiation and mucin production. By immunohistochemisty these tumors are positive for thyroglobulin, which confirms their follicular origin (250,252). Sclerosing mucoepidermoid carcinoma with eosinophilia is similar in its clinical presentation and biologic behavior to mucoepidermoid carcinoma. This tumor is usually seen in glands affected by Hashimoto's thyroiditis and shows squamous and glandular differentiation. These tumors are negative for thyroglobulin and have immunoprofile similar to ultimobranchial body rest/solid cell nests (251,252).

Rare thyroid tumors composed of spindled epithelial cells arranged in nests, sometimes associated with mucous microcysts, and resembling thymomas *(SETTLE tumors — spindled and epithelial tumor with thymus like differentiation)* have been reported (250,253,254). A few examples of neoplasms resembling thymic carcinomas also have been described, *(CASTLE tumor-carcinoma with thymus-ike differentiation)* (254). These lesions may originate from branchial pouch remnants within and adjacent to the thyroid (250,253).

MEDULLARY CARCINOMA

C-cell proliferation has been reported in adults as a possible change with advancing age (12,15), as a familial disorder associated with medullary carcinoma with or without multiple endocrine neoplasia (254–256), as an association

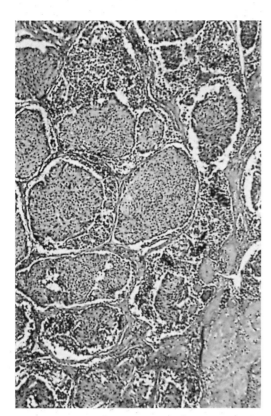

FIGURE 21.23. Medullary carcinoma with insular pattern. Amyloid is present at the lower right.

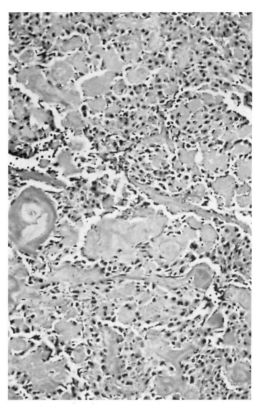

FIGURE 21.24. Medullary carcinoma with numerous small deposits of amyloid.

with hypercalcemia (13), in areas of thyroid-abutting follicular tumors (257), in chronic thyroiditis (258), and as an isolated event of unknown significance (11,18,257). Medullary carcinoma (259–261) constitutes about 5% of thyroid carcinomas, originates from C-cells (261), may be sporadic or familial, and may be associated with disorders of other endocrine glands (see Chapter 71).

On gross examination, most medullary carcinomas are found to be firm, white or yellow, and infiltrative. Some are well defined and even encapsulated; the latter have a better prognosis (106,262).

On light microscopic examination, the cells are rounded or polygonal or may be spindled (Figs. 21.23 and 21.24) (259–264). They appear as a diffuse solid mass, as islands separated by fibrous tissue (usually dense or hyalinized), as trabeculae or ribbons of cells, and (uncommonly) as glandular structures (Figs. 21.25 and 21.26) (261–263). Small vessels in the tumor may be conspicuous, with the cells oriented around them. Pseudopapillary formations (264) and even true papillary patterns (263–265) have been reported. The carcinomas may be composed of small cells (in the past confused with small-cell anaplastic carcinoma) (263, 265,266), may contain numerous giant cells (265–267), may have large cells with eosinophilic cytoplasm, resembling oncocytic follicular cells (268), and can form glandular structures (269). *Clear cell medullary carcinomas* have been reported (270). Cells producing mucus may be pres-

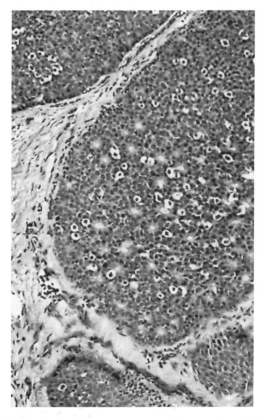

FIGURE 21.25. Medullary carcinoma with many tiny acini present in the islands of cells.

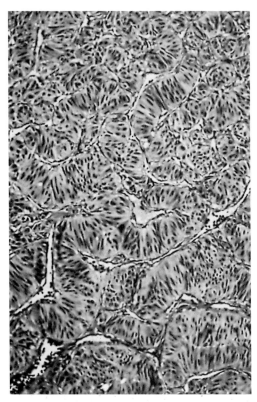

FIGURE 21.26. Medullary carcinoma with a trabecular pattern.

ent in varying numbers (271, 272). Rarely, these carcinomas produce melanin (273, 274).

The nuclei are rounded or elongated; occasionally nuclei are large and irregular. Cytoplasmic inclusions in nuclei may occur. Aneuploid DNA patterns indicate a less favorable prognosis (106,275).

Multiple small foci of necrosis sometimes are present, especially in the medullary carcinomas composed of small cells. *Anaplastic variants of medullary carcinoma* have been described, but these are extremely rare (138,237,263, 266).

Amyloid deposits formed by the secretory products of the neoplastic cells are frequently present, both in the primary tumor and in the metastatic foci. About 20% of medullary cancers lack amyloid (106,263). The presence of amyloid indicates a better prognosis (106). Tumor stroma and the amyloid may undergo calcification.

Medullary carcinomas nearly always produce calcitonin, although a few may lack this peptide (236,263). Other substances detected include chromogranin, calcitonin gene-related peptide, carcinoembryonic antigen, somatostatin, β-endorphin, adrenocorticotropin, serotonin, bombesin, chorionic gonadotropin, histaminase, and prostaglandins (276–279). The demonstration of only small amounts of calcitonin by immunostaining has been associated with a poor prognosis (280,281).

Invasion of lymphatic and blood vessels and metastases in cervical nodes are common. A few patients who develop widespread disease and die from the disease in 2 or 3 years. A few have very indolent tumors (usually misdiagnosed as adenoma initially) that persist for as long as 30 years. Some reports indicate familial medullary carcinomas (especially patients with Sipple's syndrome) have a better prognosis (280–282). Patients with multiple andocrine neoplasia type 28 have tumors that are particularly aggressive (281).

Most cases of medullary carcinoma are sporadic, particularly in patients over 40 years old, involve only one lobe, and are not associated with other endocrine lesions. A considerable number of cases are familial, however, especially in younger patients (254–256). Such cancers may be associated with bilateral pheochromocytomas or adrenal medullary hyperplasia and with parathyroid hyperplasia (Sipple's syndrome, multiple endocrine neoplasia type 2A).

Some patients have a variant syndrome, with mucosal and cutaneous neuromas (type 2B) (255). The familial medullary carcinomas are usually bilateral and multicentric. Other family members may have C-cell hyperplasia and medullary carcinomas of microscopic size, some of which may have already spread to lymph nodes. In this situation, the C-cell hyperplasia must be regarded as premalignant.

Recent evidence suggests that immunostaining for a component of the neural adhesion molecule can distinguish familial C-cell hyperplasia from secondary reactive states (283). However, with the advent of genetic testing for familial medullary carcinoma, the pathologist can be relieved of the burden of defining C-cell hyperplasia in glands removed for medullary carcinoma (284–286). C-cell adenoma ("medullary adenoma") has not been identified pathologically; lesions diagnosed as C-cell adenoma may be small and circumscribed, but they are cancers.

A few medullary carcinomas are discovered incidental to thyroid operations for other conditions (287), at autopsy (288,289), or because of high serum calcitonin (290). The so-called *micromedullary carcinomas* (equivalent to micropapillary carcinoma and defined as tumors of 1 cm or less) have an excellent prognosis if confined to the gland (291,292). Some of the micromedullary cancers arise in the background of chronic thyroiditis and may be associated with C-cell hyperplasia even in the absence of familial disease. Some of these patients have hypothyroidism and high serum TSH levels; animal studies have shown that TSH can stimulate growth of C-cells. Hence this type of C-cell hyperplasia and micromedullary carcinoma may represent a secondary "reactive" phenomenon leading to early neoplastic change (290–292). The nontumoral parenchyma should be examined for evidence of C-cell hyperplasia in a thyroid removed for a medullary carcinoma.

Occasionally, the gland contains moderate to severe autoimmune thyroiditis (258,287), adenomatoid nodules, or a follicular-derived thyroid cancer (257).

Some medullary carcinomas grow sufficiently slowly to allow them to trap thyroid follicles. A few neoplasms have been reported that appear to represent joint C-cell and follicular cell proliferations (293–296). These are rare and are classified as *mixed medullary and follicular carcinomas*; nodal metastases from these tumors also exhibit both follicular and medullary components.

Several hypotheses have been suggested regarding the origin of these tumors (293,294); some authors have proposed that they are collision tumors, where others believe that they develop from an uncommitted stem cell capable of producing both follicular and C-cell progeny (293–297). Volante et al microdissected the individual components of 12 mixed tumors and performed genetic analysis for the RET proto-oncogene and allelic losses of nine loci on chromosome 6, and studied the clonal composition of tumor cells in female patients. Their results showed that the follicular and medullary components of the mixed tumors are not derived from single stem cells. In addition, the follicular-patterned areas were oligo/polyclonal and most likely are hyperplastic rather than neoplastic (297).

LYMPHOMA

Secondary involvement of the thyroid by malignant lymphoma that first appeared elsewhere in the body has been reported in 20% of patients dying from generalized lymphoma (122).

Malignant lymphoma presenting as a primary neoplasm in the thyroid is uncommon (298–301). Its apparent rarity in the older literature reflects diagnosis of lymphoma as anaplastic carcinoma. Most patients have a history of diffuse goiter (probably the result of autoimmune thyroiditis) that suddenly increased in size.

Gross examination reveals firm, fleshy tissue that is usually pale. Evidence of previous lymphocytic thyroiditis is present in most cases in which some thyroid parenchyma still persists (298,300).

Most thyroid lymphomas are diffuse (Fig. 21.27). Virtually all examples are B-cell types (298,299,302–304); many may be extranodal lymphomas that arise in mucosa-associated lymphoid tissue (MALT) (298,302). Some patients have typical plasmacytomas (305,306); these have a good prognosis. Hodgkin's disease is extremely rare.

Invasion of lymphoma into and through the thyroid capsule, extension into the adjacent soft tissues, and involvement of regional lymph nodes occur fairly often and represent unfavorable prognostic factors. Some reports have suggested that gastrointestinal involvement is fairly

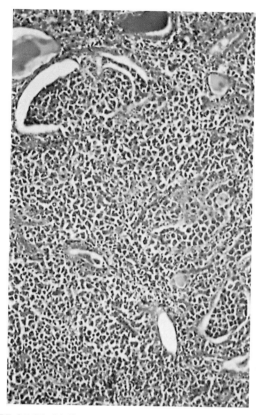

FIGURE 21.27. Malignant lymphoma. Several thyroid follicles are distended by the infiltrate; this is the so-called lymphoepithelial lesion.

common in patients with thyroid lymphoma, but experience varies in this regard (298).

Distinguishing lymphoma from small-cell carcinoma, either primary or metastatic, may be difficult; appropriate special procedures usually allow this to be done (307). Malignant lymphoma also has to be differentiated from advanced autoimmune thyroiditis; this distinction may require assessment of lymphocyte clonality by special studies (e.g., flow cytometry, gene rearrangement).

SARCOMA

Sarcomas of the thyroid are rare and comprise less than 1% of all thyroid malignancies. There is a tendency to overdiagnose sarcoma of the thyroid (308). In some cases follicular thyroid tumors may undergo extensive spindle cell metaplasia and can be mistaken for a sarcoma. In such instances immunostaining for thyroglobulin proves helpful (309). On complete, critical examination most proposed sarcomas prove to be anaplastic carcinomas. Reports of angiosarcoma (310–312) and leiomyosarcoma (313) have been published.

CARCINOMA IN ECTOPIC THYROID TISSUE

The tumors that arise in the thyroglossal tract have been mostly papillary carcinomas (314–318). In contrast with the thyroglossal carcinomas, tumors of sublingual and lingual ectopic thyroid tissue constitute the various types found in the main gland.

Carcinomas, usually papillary subtype (319), and lesions that resemble carcinoid tumors (320) have been reported in struma ovarii.

METASTATIC NEOPLASMS

Metastatic neoplasms in the thyroid that masquerade as primary tumors are rare. They have been reported to be most often carcinomas from the breast, lung, and kidney (321–323). Metastatic renal cell carcinoma probably is the secondary neoplasm that not only may appear clinically as a primary thyroid neoplasm but also may be mistaken as a thyroid tumor by the pathologist (119,322). Immunostaining for thyroglobulin is helpful in making the distinction. Sometimes the thyroid mass represents the initial manifestation of the renal neoplasm; on other occasion, it appears so long after nephrectomy that the possibility of a metastasis has been forgotten by the patient and the physician (321–323). In rare cases metastases may occur to a thyroid tumor, representing cases of tumor-to-tumor metatstasis (324).

REFERENCES

1. Toda S, Yonemitsu N, Hikichi Y, et al. Differentiation of human thyroid follicle cells from normal subjects and Basedow's disease in three dimensional collagen gel culture. *Pathol Res Pract* 1992;188:874.
2. Klinck GH. Structure of the thyroid. In: Hazard JB, Smith DE, eds. *The thyroid.* Baltimore: Williams & Wilkins, 1964:1.
3. Gnepp DR, Ogorzalek JM, Heffess CS. Fat-containing lesions of the thyroid gland. *Am J Surg Pathol* 1989;13:605.
4. MacMahon HE, Lee HY, Rivelis CF. Birefringent crystals in human thyroid. *Acta Endocrinol (Copenh)* 1968;58:172.
5. Reid JD, Choi CH, Oldroyd NO. Calcium oxalate crystals in the thyroid: their identification, prevalence origin and possible significance. *Am J Clin Pathol* 1987;87:443.
6. Heimann P. Ultrastructure of human thyroid: a study of normal thyroid, untreated and treated diffuse toxic goiter. *Acta Endocrinol (Copenh)* 1966;53[Suppl 110]:1.
7. Klinck GH, Oertel JE, Winship T. Ultrastructure of normal human thyroid. *Lab Invest* 1970;22:2.
8. Sobrinho-Simoes M, Johannessen JV. Scanning electron microscopy of the normal human thyroid. *J Submicrosc Cytol Pathol* 1981;13:209.
9. Gibson W, Croker B, Cox C. C cell populations in normal children and young adults. *Lab Invest* 1980;42:119.
10. Gibson WGH, Peng TC, Croker BP. C-cell nodules in adult human thyroid. A common autopsy finding. *Am J Clin Pathol* 1981;75:347.
11. Gibson WGH, Peng TC, Croker BP. Age-associated C-cell hyperplasia in the human thyroid. *Am J Pathol* 1982;106:388.
12. Wolfe HJ, Voelkel EF, Tashjian AH. Distribution of calcitonin-containing cells in the nromal adult human thyroid gland: a correlation of morphology with peptide content. *J Clin Endocrinol Metab* 1974;38:688.
13. Wolfe HJ, DeLellis RA, Voelkel EF, et al. Distribution of calcitonin-containing cells in neonatal human thyroid gland: a correlation of morphology with peptide content. *J Clin Endocrinol Metab* 1975;41:1076.
14. O'Toole K, Fenoglio-Preiser C, Pushparaj N. Endocrine changes associated with the human aging process. III. Effect of age on the number of calcitonin immunoreactive cells in the thyroid gland. *Hum Pathol* 1985:16:991.
15. Baschieri L, Castagna M, Fierabracci A, et al. Distribution of calcitonin-and somatostatin-containing cells in thyroid lymphoma and in Hashimoto's thyroiditis. *Appl Pathol* 1989;7:99.
16. Kameda Y, Oyama H, Endoh M, et al. Somatostatin immunoreactive C cells in thyroid glands from various mammalian species. *Anat Rec* 1982;204:161.
17. Guyetant S, Wion-Barbot N, Rousselet MC, et al. C-cell hyperplasia associated with chronic lymphocytic thyroiditis. *Hum Pathol* 1994;25:514.
18. Harach JR. Solid cell nests of the thyroid: an anatomical survey and immunohistochemical study for the presence of thyroglobulin. *Acta Anat (Basel)* 1985;122:249.
19. Harach JR. Mixed follicles of the human thyroid gland. *Acta Anat (Basel)* 1987;129:27.
20. Harach JR. Solid cell nests of the thyroid. *J Pathol* 1988;155:191.
21. Harach HR, Viyanic GM, Jasani B. Ultimobranchial body nest in human fetal thyroid: an autopsy histological and immunohistochemical study in relation to solid cell nests and mucoepidermoid carcinoma of the thyroid. *J Pathol* 1993;169:465.
22. Cameselle-Teijeero J, Valera-Duran J, Sambade C, et al. Solid cell nests of the thyroid. *Hum Pathol* 1994;25:684.
23. Mizukami Y, Nonomura A, Mishigishi T, et al. Solid cell nests of the thyroid. *Am J Clin Pathol* 1994;101:186.
24. Parham DM. Laterally situated neck cysts derived from the embryological remnants of thyroid development. *Histopathology* 1988;12:95.
25. Williams ED, Toyn CE, Harach HR. The ultimobranchial gland and congenital thyroid abnormalities in man. *J Pathol* 1989;159:135.
26. Bronner MP, LiVolsi VA. Oxyphilic (Askanazy/Hurthle cell) tumors of the thyroid: microscopic features predict biologic behavior. *Surg Pathol* 1988;1:137.
27. Flint A, Davenport RD, Lloyd RV, et al. Cytomorphometric measurements of Hurthle cell tumors of the thyroid gland: correlation with pathologic features and clinical behavior. *Cancer* 1988;61:110.
28. Friedman NB. Cellular involution in the thyroid gland: significance of Hürthle cells in myxedema, exhaustion atrophy, Hashimoto's disease and the reactions to irradiation, thiouracil therapy and subtotal resection. *J Clin Endocrinol* 1949; 9:874.
29. Mitchell JD, Kirkham N, Machin D. Focal lymphocytic thyroiditis in Southampton. *J Pathol* 1984;144:269.
30. Kabel PJ, Voorbij HAM, DeHaan M, et al. Intrathyroidal dendritic cells. *J Clin Endocrinol Metab* 1988;66:199.
31. Allard RHB. The thyroglossal cyst. *Head Neck Surg* 1982;5:134.
32. Neinas FW, Goman CA, Devine KD, et al. Lingual thyroid: clinical characteristics of 15 cases. *Ann Intern Med* 1973;79:205.

33. Pollock WF, Stevenson EO. Cysts and sinuses of the thyroglossal duct. *Am J Surg* 1966;112:225.
34. Sauk JJ. Ectopic lingual thyroid. *J Pathol* 1970;102:239.
35. Shareef DS, Salm R. Ectopic vestigial lesions of neck and shoulders. *J Clin Pathol* 1981;34:1155.
36. Apel RL, Asa SL, Chalvardjian A, et al. Intrathyroidal lymphoepithelial cysts of probable branchial origin. *Hum Pathol* 1994;25:1238.
37. Carpenter GR, Emery JL. Inclusions in the human thyroid. *J Anat* 1976;122:77.
38. LiVolsi VA. Branchial and thymic remnants in the thyroid and cervical region. An explanation for unusual tumors and microscopic curiosities. *Endocrine Pathol* 1993;4:115.
39. Gardiner WR. Unusual relationships between thyroid gland and skeletal muscle in infants: a review of the literature and four case reports. *Cancer* 1956;9:681.
40. Hathaway BM. Innocuous accessory thyroid nodules. *Arch Surg* 1965;90:222.
41. Gerard-Merchant R, Caillou B. Thyroid inclusions in cervical lymph nodes. *Clin Endocrinol Metab* 1981;10:337.
42. Meyer JS, Steinberg LS. Microscopically benign thyroid follicles in cervical lymph nodes:serial section study of lymph node inclusions and entire thyroid gland in 5 cases. *Cancer* 1969;24:302.
43. Roth LM. Inclusions of nonneoplastic thyroid tissue within cervical lymph nodes. *Cancer* 1965;18:105.
44. Doniach I. The thyroid gland. In: Symmers W StC, ed. *Systemic pathology*, 2nd ed. Edinburgh: Churchill Livingstone, 1978:1976.
45. Kennedy JS. The pathology of dyshormonogenetic goitre. *J Pathol* 1969;99:251.
46. Moore GH. The thyroid in sporadic goitrous cretinism: a report of three new cases, description of the pathologic anatomy of the thyroid glands and a review of the literature. *Arch Pathol* 1962;74:35.
47. Studer H, Ramelli F. Simple goiter and its variants; euthyroid and hyperthyroid multinodular goiters. *Endocr Rev* 1982;3:40.
48. Taylor S. The evolution of nodular goiter. *J Clin Endocrinol Metab* 1953;13:1232.
49. van der Gaag RD, Drexhage HA, Wiersinga WM, et al. Further studies on thryoid growth-stimulating immunoglobulins in euthyroid nonendemic goiter. *J Clin Endocrinol Metab* 1974;39:719.
50. Ramelli F, Studer H, Bruggisser D. Patholgenesis of thyroid nodules in multinodular goiter. *Am J Pathol* 1982;109:215.
51. Studer H, Gerber H, Zbaeren J, et al. Histomorphological and immunohistochemical evidence that nodular goiters grow by episodic replication of multiple clusters of thyroid follicular cells. *J Clin Endocrinol Metab* 1992;75:1151.
52. Aeschemann S, Kopp PA, Kemura ET, et al. Morphological and functional polymorphism within clonal thyroid nodules. *J Clin Invest* 1993;77:846.
53. Apel RL, Ezzat S, Bapat BV, et al. Clonality of thyroid nodules in sporadic goiter. *Diagn Mol Pathol* 1995;4:113.
54. Hicks DG, LiVolsi VA, Neidich JA, et al. Clonal analysis of solitary follicular nodules in the thyroid. *Am J Pathol* 1990;137:553.
55. Namba H, Matsuo K, Fagin JA. Clonal composition of benign and malignant thyroid tumors. *J Clin Invest* 1990;86:120.
56. Mizukami Y, Michigishi T, Nonomura A, et al. Autonomously functioning (hot) nodule of the thyroid gland: a clinical and histopathologic study of 17 cases. *Am J Clin Pathol* 1994;101:29.
57. Campbell WL, Santiago HE, Perzin KH, et al. The autonomous thyroid nodule: correlation of scan appearance and histopathology. *Radiology* 1973; 107:133.
58. DeGroot LJ, Quintans J. The causes of autoimmune thyroid disease. *Endocr Rev* 1989;10:537.
59. Wick MR, Sawyer MD. Antigenic alterations in autoimmune thyroid diseases: observations and hypotheses. *Arch Pathol Lab Med* 1989;113:77.
60. Derwahl M, Huber G, Studer H. Slow growth but intense hypertrophy of thyrocytes in longstanding Graves' goitres. *Acta Endocrinol (Copenh)* 1989;121:389.
61. Margolick JB, Hsu SM, Volkman DJ, et al. Immunohistochemical characterization of intrathyroid lymphocytes in Graves' disease: interstitial and intraepithelial populations. *Am J Med* 1984;76:815.
62. Matsunaga M, Eguchi K, Fukuda T, et al. Class II major histocompatibility complex antigen expression and cellular interactions in thyroid glands of Graves' disease. *J Clin Endocrinol Metab* 1986;62:723.
63. Eggen PC, Seljelid R. The histological appearance of hyperfunctioning thyroids following various preoperative treatments. *Acta Pathol Microbiol Immunol Scand (A)* 1973;71:1663.
64. Hirota Y, Tamai H, Hayashi Y, et al. Thyroid function and histology in forty-five patients with hyperthyroid Graves' disease in clinical remission more than ten years after thionamide drug treatment. *J Clin Endocrinol Metab* 1986;62:165.
65. Vickery AL. The diagnosis of malignancy in dyshormonogenetic goiter. *Clin Endocrinol Metab* 1985;2:90.
66. Fauerholdt L, Vendsborg P. Thyroid gland morphology after lithium treatment. *Acta Pathol Microbiol Immunol Scand (A)* 1981;89:339.
67. Mizukami Y, Funaki N, Hashimoto T, et al. Histologic features of thyroid gland in a patient with bromide induced hypothyroidism. *Am J Clin Pathol* 1988;89:802.
68. Aichinger G, Fill H, Wick G. *In situ* immune complexes, lymphocyte subpopulations, and HLA-DR-positive epithelial cells in Hashimoto's thyroiditis. *Lab Invest* 1985;52;132
69. Fatourechi V, McConahey WM, Woolner LB. Hyperthyroidism associated with histologic Hashimoto's thyroiditis. *Mayo Clin Proc* 1971;46:682.
70. LiVolsi VA. The pathology of autoimmune thyroid disease: a review. *Thyroid* 1994;4:333.
71. Mizukami Y, Michigishi T, Kawato M, et al. Chronic thyroiditis: thyroid function and histologic correlation in 601 cases. *Hum Pathol* 1992;23:980.
72. Ben-Ezra J, Wu A, Sheibani K. Hashimoto's thyroiditis lacks detectable clonal immunoglobulin and T cell receptor gene rearrangements. *Hum Pathol* 1988;19:1444.
73. LiVolsi VA, Merino MJ. Squamous cells in the human thyroid gland. *Am J Surg Pathol* 1978;2;133.
74. Vollenweider I, Hedinger C. Solid cell nests (SCN) in Hashimoto's thyroiditis. *Virchows Arch* 1988;412:357.
75. Carney JA. Thyroid cysts. *Am J Surg Pathol* 1989;13:1072.
76. Louis DN, Vickery AL, Rosai J, et al. Multiple branchial cleft-like cysts in Hashimoto's thyroiditis. *Am J Surg Pathol* 1989; 13:45.
77. Mizukami Y, Michigishi F, Hashimoto T, et al. Silent thyroiditis: a histologic and immunohistochemical study. *Hum Pathol* 1988;19:423.
78. Woolf PD. Transient painless thyroiditis with hyperthyroidism: a variant of lymphocytic thyroiditis? *Endocr Rev* 1980;1:411.
79. LiVolsi VA. Postpartum thyroiditis: the pathology slowly unravels. *Am J Clin Pathol* 1993;100:193.
80. deMent SH, Smith RRL, Karp JE, et al. Pulmonary, cardiac, and thyroid involvement in disseminated *Pseudoallescheria boydii. Arch Pathol Lab Med* 1984;108:859.
81. Loeb JM, Livermore BM, Wofsy D. Coccidioidomycosis of the thyroid. *Ann Intern Med* 1979;91:409.

82. Lucaya J, Bordon WE, Enriquez G, et al. Congenital pyriform sinus fistula: a cause of acute left-sided suppurative thyroiditis and neck abscess in children. *Pediatr Radiol* 1990;21:27.

83. Drucker DJ, Bailey D, Rotstein L. Thyroiditis as the presenting manifestation of disseminated extrapulmonary *Pneumocystis carinii* infection. *J Clin Endocrinol Metab* 1990;71:1663.

84. Frank TS, LiVolsi VA, Connor AM. Cytomegalovirus infection of the thyroid in immunocompromised adults. *Yale J Biol Med* 1987;60:1.

85. Lindsay S, Dailey ME. Granulomatous or giant cell thyroiditis. *Surg Gyn Obstet* 1954;98:197.

86. Carney JA, Moore SB, Northcutt RC, et al. Palpation thyroiditis (multifocal granulomatous folliculitis). *Am J Clin Pathol* 1975;64:639.

87. Leung WH, Lau CP, Wong CK, et al. Amiodarone induced thyroiditis. *Am Heart J* 1989;118:848.

88. Smyrk TC, Goellner JR, Brennan MD, et al. Pathology of the thyroid in amiodarone assoicated thyrotoxicosis. *Am J Surg Pathol* 1987;11:197.

89. Schwaegerle SM, Bauer TW, Esselstyn CB. Riedel's thyroiditis. *Am J Clin Pathol* 1988;90:715.

90. Comings DE, Skubi KB, Van Eyes J, et al. Familial multifocal fibrosclerosis: findings suggesting that retroperitoneal fibrosis, mediastinal fibrosis, sclerosing cholangitis, Riedel's thyroiditis and pseudotumor of the orbit may be different manifestations of a single disease. *Ann Intern Med* 1967;66:884.

91. Julie C, Vieillefond A, Desligneres S, et al. Hashimoto's thyroiditis associated with Riedel's thyroiditis and retroperitoneal fibrosis. *Pathol Res Pract* 1997;193:573.

92. Conrad RA, Dobyns BM, Sutow WW. Thyroid neoplasia as late effect of exposure to radioactive iodine in fallout. *JAMA* 1970;214:316.

93. Carr RF, LiVolsi VA. Morphologic changes in the thyroid after irradiation for Hodgkin's and non-Hodgkin's lymphoma. *Cancer* 1989;64:825.

94. Schneider AB, Pinsky S, Bekerman C, et al. Characteristics of 108 thyroid cancers detected by screening in a population with a history of head and neck irradiation. *Cancer* 1980;46:1218.

95. Spitalnick PF, Strauss FH. Patterns of human thyroid parenchymal reaction following low dose childhood irradiation. *Cancer* 1978;41:1098.

96. Curran RC, Eckert H, Wilson GM. The thyroid gland after treatment of hyperthyroidism by partial thyroidectomy or iodine 131. *J Pathol* 1958;76:541.

97. Dobyns, BM, Vickery Al, Maloof F, et al. Functional and histologic effects of therapeutic doses of radioactive iodine on the thyroid of man. *J Clin Endocrinol Metab* 1953;13:548.

98. Kanoh T, Shimada H, Uchino H, et al. Amyloid goiter with hypothyroidism. *Arch Pathol Lab Med* 1989;113:542.

99. Kennedy JS, Thomson JA, Buchanan WM. Amyloid in the thyroid. *QJM* 1974;43:127.

100. Alexander CB, Herrera GA, Jaffe K, et al. Black thyroid: clinical manifestations, ultrastructural findings, and possible mechanisms. *Hum Pathol* 1985;16:72

101. Landas SK, Schelper RL, Tio FO, Turner JW, Moore KC, Bennett-Gray J. Black thyroid syndrome: exaggeration of a normal process? *Am J Clin Pathol* 1986;85:411.

102. McConahey WM, Hay ID, Woolner LB, et al. Papillary thyroid cancer treated at the Mayo Clinic, 1946 through 1970: initial manifestations, pathological findings, therapy and outcome. *Mayo Clin Proc* 1986;61:978.

103. McConnon JK, Von Westarp C, Mitchell RI. Follicular carcinoma of the thyroid with functioning metastases and clinical hyperthyroidism. *Can Med Assoc J* 1975;112:724.

104. Panke TW, Croxson MS, Parker JW, et al. Triiodothyronine secreting (toxic) adenoma of the thyroid gland: light and electron microscopic characteristics. *Cancer* 1978;12:95.

105. Ryff-de Leche A, Staub JJ, Kohler-Faden R, et al. Thyroglobulin production by malignant thyroid tumors: an immunocytochemical and radioimmunassay study. *Cancer* 1986;57:1145.

106. Bergholm U, Adami HO, Auer G, et al. Histopathologic characterisics and nuclear DNA content as prognostic factors in medullary thyroid carcinomas: a nationwide study in Sweden. *Cancer* 1989;64:135.

107. Bronner MP, Clevenger CV, Edmonds PR, et al. Flow cytometric analysis of DNA content in Hürthle cell adenomas and carcinoma of the thyroid. *Am J Clin Pathol* 1988;89:764.

108. Joensuu H, Klemi PJ. Comparison of nuclear DNA content in primary and metastatic differentiated thyroid carcinoma. *Am J Clin Pathol* 1988;89:35.

109. Joensuu H, Klemi PJ, Eerola E. DNA aneuploidy in follicular adenomas of the thyroid gland. *Am J Pathol* 1986;124:373.

110. Fukunga M, Shinozaki N, Endo Y, et al. Atypical adenoma of the thyroid. *Acta Pathol Jpn* 1992;42:432.

111. Oyama T, Vickery AL, Preffer FI, et al. A comparative study of flow cytometry and histopathologic findings in thyroid follicular carcinomas and adenomas. *Hum Pathol* 1994;25:271.

112. Zedenius J, Auer G, Backdahl M, et al. Follicular tumors of the thyroid gland: diagnosis, clinical aspects and nuclear DNA analysis. *World J Surg* 1992;16:589.

113. van Hoeven KH, Menendez-Botel CJ, Strong EW, et al. Estrogen and progesterone receptor content in human thyroid disease. *Am J Clin Pathol* 1993;99:175.

114. Farley DR, Eberhardt NL, Grant CS, et al. Expression of a potential metastasis suppressor gene (nm23) in thyroid neoplasms. *World J Surg* 1993;17:615.

115. Shimizu T, Usuda N, Yamanda T, et al. Proliferative activity of human thyroid tumors evaluated by proliferating cell nuclear antigen/cyclin immunohistochemical studies. *Cancer* 1993;71:2807.

116. Tateyama H, Yang YP, Ermoto T, et al. Proliferative cell nuclear antigen expression in follicular tumors of the thyroid with special reference to oxyphilic cell lesions. *Virchows Arch* 1994;424:533.

117. Loy TS, Darkow GV, Spollen LE, et al. Immunostaining for Leu-7 in the diagnosis of thyroid carcinoma. *Arch Pathol Lab Med* 1994;118:172.

118. Nairn ER, Crocker J, McGovern J. Limited value of AgNOR enumeration in assessment of thyroid neoplasms. *J Clin Pathol* 1988;41:1136.

119. Carcangiu ML, Sibley RK, Rosai J. Clear cell change in primary thyroid tumors: a study of 38 cases. *Am J Surg Pathol* 1989;13:1041.

120. Arganini M, Behar R, Wu T-C, et al. Hürthle cell tumors: a twenty-five year experience. *Surgery* 1986;100:1108.

121. Bondeson L, Bondeson AG, Ljungberg O, et al. Oxyphil tumors of the thyroid: followup of 42 surgical cases. *Ann Surg* 1981;194:677.

122. Meissner WA, Warren S. Tumors of the thyroid gland. *Atlas of tumor pathology*, 2nd series, fascicle 4. Washington, D.C.: Armed Forces Institute of Pathology, 1969.

123. Hazard JB, Kenyon R. Atypical adenoma of the thyroid. *Arch Pathol* 1954;58:554.

124. Lang W, Georgii A, Stauch G, et al. The differentiation of atypical adenomas and encapsulated follicular carcinomas in the thyroid gland. *Virchows Arch* 1980;385:125.

125. Rosai J, Carcangiu ML, DeLellis RA. *Tumors of the thyroid gland*, 3rd series, fascicle 5. Washington, D.C.: Armed Forces Institute of Pathology, 1992.

126. Rothenberg HJ, Goellner JR, Carney JA. Hyalinizing adenoma of the thyroid gland: recognition and characterization of its yellow cytoplasmic body. *Am J Surg Pathol* 1999;23:118.

127. LiVolsi VA, Gupta PK. Thyroid fine needle aspiration-paraganglioma-like adenoma of the thyroid. *Diagn Cytopathol* 1992; 8:82.

128. Sambade C, Franssila K, Cameselle-Teijeiro J, et al. Hyalinizing trabecular adenoma: a misnomer for a peculiar tumor of the thyroid gland. *Endocr Pathol* 1991;2:83.

129. Fonseca E, Nesland JM, Sobrinho-Simoes. Expression of stratified epithelial-type cytokeratins in hyalinizing trabecular adenomas support their relationship with papillary carcinomas of the thyroid. *Histopathology* 1997;31:330.

130. Gherardi G. Signet ring cell "mucinous" thyroid adenomas: a follicle cell tumour with abnormal accumulation of thyroglobulin and a peculiar histochemical profile. *Histopathology* 1987; 11:317.

131. Toth K, Peter I, Kremmer T, et al. Lipid rich cell thyroid adenoma: histopathology and comparative lipid analysis. *Virchows Arch* 1990;417:273.

132. Bale GF. Teratoma of the neck in the region of the thyroid gland: a review of the literature and report of four cases. *Am J Pathol* 1950;26:565.

133. Kimler SC, Muth WF. Primary malignant teratoma of the thyroid: case report and literature review of cervical teratomas in adults. *Cancer* 1978;42:311.

134. Hrafnkelsson J, Stal O, Enestrom S, et al. Cellular DNA pattern, S-phase frequency and survival in papillary thyroid cancer. *Acta Oncol* 1988;27:329.

135. Schroder S, Schwarz W, Rehpenning W, et al. Prognostic significance of Leu-M1 immunostaining in papillary carcinomas of the thyroid gland. *Virchows Arch* 1987;411:435.

136. Schroder S, Schwarz W, Rehpenning W, et al. Dendritic/Langerhans cells and prognosis in patients with papillary thyroid carcinomas: immunohistochemical study of 106 thyroid neoplasms correlated with followup data. *Am J Clin Pathol* 1988;89:295.

137. Tennvall J, Biorklund A, Moller T, et al. Prognostic factors of papillary, follicular and medullary carcinomas of the thyroid gland: retrospective multivariate analysis of 216 patients with a median followup of 11 years. *Acta Radiol Oncol* 1985; 24:17.

138. LiVolsi VA, Brooks JJ, Arendash-Durand B. Anaplastic thyroid tumors: immunohistology. *Am J Clin Pathol* 1987;87:434.

139. Carcangiu ML, Steeper T, Zampi G, et al. Anaplastic thyroid carcinoma: a study of 70 cases. *Am J Clin Pathol* 1985;83:135.

140. Bronner MP, Hamilton R, LiVolsi VA. Utility of frozen section analysis on follicular lesions of the thyroid. *Endocr Pathol* 1994;5:154.

141. Lote K, Andersen K, Nordal E, et al. Familial occurrence of papillary thyroid carcinoma. *Cancer* 1980;46:1291.

142. Cuello C, Correa P, Eisenberg H. Geographic pathology of thyroid carcinoma. *Cancer* 1969;23:230.

143. Hofstadter F. Frequency and morphology of malignant tumours of the thyroid before and after the introduction of iodine prophylaxis. *Virchows Arch* 1980;385:263.

144. Samaan NA. Papillary carcinoma of the thyroid: hereditary or radiation induced? *Cancer Invest* 1989;7:399.

145. Kerber RA, Till JE, Simon SL, et al. A cohort study of thyroid disease in relation to fallout from nuclear weapons testing. *JAMA* 1993;270:2076.

146. Nikiforov Y, Grepp DR. Pediatric thyroid cancer after the Chernobyl disaster. *Cancer* 1994;74:748.

147. Hawk WA, Hazard JB. The many appearances of papillary carcinoma of the thyroid. *Cleve Clin Q* 1976;43:207.

148. Carcangiu ML, Zampi G, Pupi A, et al. Papillary carcinoma of the thyroid: a clinicopathologic study of 241 cases treated at the University of Florence, Italy. *Cancer* 1985;55:805.

149. Carcangiu ML, Zampi G, Rosai J. Papillary thyroid carcinoma: a study of its many morphologic expressions and clinical correlates. *Pathol Annu* 1985;20[Pt 1]:1.

150. Tscholl-Ducommun J, Hedinger CE. Papillary thyroid carcinomas: morphology and prognsois. *Virchows Arch* 1982; 396:19.

151. Vickery Al, Carcangiu ML, Johannessen JV, et al. Papillary carcinoma. *Semin Diagn Pathol* 1985;2:90.

152. Chan JKC, Rosai J. Papillary carcinoma of thyroid with exuberant nodular fasciitis like stroma: report of three cases. *Am J Clin Pathol* 1991;95:309.

153. Ostrowski MA, Asa SL, Chamberlain D, et al. Myxomatous change in papillary carcinoma of the thyroid. *Surg Pathol* 1989; 2:249.

154. Salvadori B, DelBo R, Pilotti S, et al. Occult papillary carcinoma of the thyroid: a questional entity. *Eur J Cancer* 1993; 13:1817.

155. Franssila KO, Harach HR. Occult papillary carcinoma of the thyroid in children and young adults: a systematic autopsy study in Finland. *Cancer* 1986;58:715.

156. Harach HR, Franssila KO, Wasenius VM. Occult papillary carcinoma of the thyroid: a "normal" finding in Finland: a systematic autopsy study. *Cancer* 1985;56:531.

157. Kasai N, Sakamoto A. New subgrouping of small thyroid carcinomas. *Cancer* 1987;60:1767.

158. Komorowski RA, Hanson GA. Occult thyroid pathology in the young adult: an autopsy study of 138 patients without clinical thyroid disease. *Hum Pathol* 1988;19:689.

159. Yamamoto Y, Maeda T, Izumi K, et al. Occult papillary carcinoma of the thyroid: a study of 408 autopsy cases. *Cancer* 1990;65:1173.

160. Harach HR, Franssila KO. Occult papillary carcinoma of the thyroid appearing as lung metastasis. *Arch Pathol Lab Med* 1984;108:529.

161. Patchefsky AS, Keller IB, Mansfield CM. Solitary vertebral column metastasis from occult sclerosing carcinoma of the thyroid gland. *Am J Clin Pathol* 1970;53:596.

162. Sampson RJ, Key CR, Buncher CR, et al. Smallest forms of papillary carcinoma of the thyroid: a study of 141 microcarcinomas less than 0.1 cm in greatest dimension. *Arch Pathol* 1971;91:334.

163. Strate SM, Lee EL, Childers JH. Occult papillary carcinoma of the thyroid with distant metastases. *Cancer* 1984;54:1093.

164. Hedinger CE, Williams ED, Sobin LH. *Histological typing of thyroid tumours*, 2nd ed. International Histological Classification of Tumours, no.11. Berlin: Springer-Verlag, 1988.

165. Lindsay S. Papillary thyroid carcinoma revisited. In: Hedinger CE, ed. *Thyroid cancer*. Berlin: Springer-Verlag, 1969.

166. Carcangiu ML, Bianchi S. Diffuse sclerosing variant of papillary thyroid carcinoma: clinicopathologic study of 15 cases. *Am J Surg Pathol* 1989;13:1041.

167. Fujimoto Y, Obara T, Ito Y, et al. Diffuse sclerosing variant of papillary carcinoma of the thyroid. *Cancer* 1990;66:2306.

168. Chan JKC, Tsui MS, Tse CH. Diffuse sclerosing variant of papillary carcinoma of the thyroid: a histological and immunohistochemical study of three cases. *Histopathology* 1987;11:191.

169. Schroder S, Bay V, Dumke K, et al. Diffuse sclerosing variant of papillary thyroid carcinoma: S-100 protein immunocytochemistry and prognosis. *Virchows Arch* 1990;416: 367.

170. Soares J, Limbert E, Sobrinho-Simoes M. Diffuse sclerosing variant of papillary thyroid carcinoma: a clinicopathologic study of 10 cases. *Pathol Res Pract* 1989;185:200.

171. Moreno-Egea A, Rodriguez-Gonzalez JM, Sola-Perez J, et al. Clinicopathological study of the diffuse sclerosing variety of papillary cancer of the thyroid. *Eur J Surg Oncol* 1994; 20:7.

172. Kini SR. *Guides to clinical aspiration biopsy: thyroid.* New York: Igaku-Shoin, 1987.

173. Gray A, Doniach I. Morphology of the nuclei of papillary carcinoma of the thyroid. *Br J Cancer* 1969;23:49.

174. Johannessen JV, Gould VE, Jao W. The fine structure of human thyroid cancer. *Hum Pathol* 1978;9:385.

175. Akslen LA, Varhaug JE. Thyroid carcinoma with mixed tall cell and columnar cell features. *Am J Clin Pathol* 1990;94: 442.

176. Johnson TL, Lloyd RV, Thompson NW, et al. Prognostic implications of the tall cell variant of papillary thyroid carcinoma. *Am J Surg Pathol* 1988;12:22.

177. LiVolsi VA, Apel RL, Asa SL. Papillary Hürthle cell carcinoma with lymphocytic stroma: "Warthin-like tumor" of the thyroid. *Am J Surg Pathol* 1995;19:810.

178. Evans HL. Encapsulated papillary neoplasms of the thyroid: a study of 14 cases followed for a minimum of 10 years. *Am J Surg Pathol* 1987;11:592.

179. Schroder S, Bocker W, Dralle H, et al. The encapsulated papillary carcinoma of the thyroid: a morphologic subtype of the papillary thyroid carcinoma. *Cancer* 1984;54:90.

180. Johannessen JV, Sobrinho-Simoes M. The origin and significance of thyroid psammoma bodies. *Lab Invest* 1980;43:287.

181. Sisson JC, Schmidt RW, Beierwaltes WH. Sequestered nodular goiter. *N Engl J Med* 1964;270:927.

182. Russell WO, Ibanez ML, Clark RL, et al. Thyroid carcinoma: classification, intraglandular dissemination and clinicopathological study based upon whole organ sections in 80 glands. *Cancer* 1963;16:1425.

183. Smith SA, Hay ID, Goellner JR, et al. Mortality from papillary thyroid carcinoma: a case control study of 56 lethal cases. *Cancer* 1988;62: 1381.

184. Franssila KO, Ackerman LV, Brown CL, et al. Follicular carcinoma. *Semin Diagn Pathol* 1985;2:101.

185. Yamashina M. Follicular neoplasms of the thyroid. *Am J Surg Pathol* 1992;16:392.

186. Kahn NF, Perzin KH. Follicular carcinoma of the thyroid. An evaluation of the histologic criteria used for diagnosis. *Pathol Annu* 1983;18[Pt 1]:221.

187. Lang W, Choritz H, Hundeshagen H. Risk factors in follicular thyroid carcinoma: a retrospective followup study covering a 14 year period with emphasis on morphologic findings. *Am J Surg Pathol* 1986;10:246.

188. Hazard JB, Kenyon R. Encapsulated angioinvasive carcinoma (angioinvasive adenoma) of thyroid gland. *Arch Pathol* 1954; 19:152.

189. Evans HL. Follicular neoplasms of the thyroid: a study of 44 cases followed for a minimum of 10 years with emphasis on differential diagnosis. *Cancer* 1984;54:535.

190. Schroder S, Pfannschmidt N, Dralle H, et al. The encapsulated follicular carcinoma of the thyroid: a clinicopathologic study of 35 cases. *Virchows Arch* 1984;402:259.

191. Harach HR, Franssila KO. Thyroglobulin immunostaining in follicular thyroid carcinoma: relationship to the degree of differentiation and cell type. *Histopathology* 1988;13:43.

192. LiVolsi VA, Asa SL. The demise of follicular carcinoma of the thyroid gland. *Thyroid* 1994;4:233.

193. van Heerden JA, Hay ID, Goellner JR, et al. Follicular thyroid carcinoma with capsular invasion alone: a nonthreatening malignancy. *Surgery* 1992;112:1130.

194. Franssila KO. Is the differentiation between papillary and follicular thyroid carcinoma valid? *Cancer* 1973;32:853.

195. Watson DG, Brennan MD, Goellner JR, et al. Invasive Hürthle cell carcinoma of the thyroid: natural history and management. *Mayo Clin Proc* 1984;59:851.

196. Gundry SR, Burney RE, Thompson NW, et al. Total thyroidectomy for Hürthle cell neoplasm of the thyroid. *Arch Surg* 1983;118:529.

197. Thompson NW, Dunn EL, Batsakis JG, et al. Hürthle cell lesions of the thyroid gland. *Surg Gynecol Obstet* 1974;139: 555.

198. Flint A, Lloyd RV. Hürthle cell neoplasms of the thyroid gland. *Pathol Annu* 1990;25[Pt 1]:37.

199. Tallini G, Carcangiu ML, Rosai J. Oncocytic neoplasms of the thyroid gland. *Acta Pathol Jpn* 1992;42:305.

200. Baloch ZW, Livolsi VA. Follicular-patterned lesions of the thyroid: the bane of the pathologist. *Am J Clin Pathol* 2002;117: 143.

201. Chan JK. Strict criteria should be applied in the diagnosis of encapsulated follicular variant of papillary thyroid carcinoma. *Am J Clin Pathol* 2002;117:16.

202. Chen KTC, Rosai J. Follicular variant of thyroid papillary carcinoma: a clinicopathologic study of six cases. *Am J Surg Pathol* 1977;1:123.

203. Tielens ET, Sherman SI, Hruban RH, et al. Follicular variant of papillary thyroid carcinoma: a clinicopathologic study. *Cancer* 1994;73:424.

204. Baloch ZW, Gupta PK, Yu GH, et al. Follicular variant of papillary carcinoma. Cytologic and histologic correlation. *Am J Clin Pathol* 1999;111:216.

205. Williams ED, Abrosimov A, Bogdanova TI, et al. Two proposals regarding the terminology of thyroid tumors. [Guest editorial.] *Int J Surg Pathol* 2000;8:181.

206. Baloch ZW, Abraham S, Roberts S, et al. Differential expression of cytokeratins in follicular variant of papillary carcinoma: an immunohistochemical study and its diagnostic utility. *Hum Pathol* 1999;30:1166.

207. Cheung CC, Ezzat S, Freeman JL, et al. Immunohistochemical diagnosis of papillary thyroid carcinoma. *Mod Pathol* 2001;14: 338.

208. Rigau V, Martel B, Evrard C, et al. Interet de l'HBME-1 en pathologie thyroidienne. *Annales de Pathologie* 2001;21:15.

209. Kawachi K, Matsushita Y, Yonezawa S, et al. Galectin-3 expression in various thyroid neoplasms and its possible role in metastasis formation. *Human Pathol* 2000;31:428.

210. Herrmann ME, LiVolsi VA, Pasha TL, et al. Immunohistochemical expression of galectin-3 in benign and malignant thyroid lesions. *Arch Pathol Lab Med* 2002;126:710.

211. Cerilli LA, Mills SE, Rumpel CA, et al. Interpretation of RET immunostaining in follicular lesions of the thyroid. *Am J Clin Pathol* 2002;118:186.

212. Baloch ZW, LiVolsi VA. The quest for a magic tumor marker: continuing saga in the diagnosis of the follicular lesions of thyroid. *Am J Clin Pathol* 2002;118:165.

213. Thompson LD, Wieneke JA, Paal E, et al. A clinicopathologic study of minimally invasive follicular carcinoma of the thyroid gland with a review of the English literature. *Cancer* 2001;91: 505.

214. Kroll TG, Sarraf P, Pecciarini L, et al. PAX8-PPARgamma 1 fusion in oncogene human thyroid carcinoma. *Science* 2000; 289:1357.

215. Marques AR, Espadinha C, Catarino AL, et al. Expression of PAX8-PPAR gamma 1 rearrangements in both follicular thyroid carcinomas and adenomas. *J Clin Endocrinol Metab* 2002; 87:3947.

216. Villanueva-Siles E, Tanaka K, Wenig BM. Peroxisome proliferator-activated receptor gamma 1 (PPAR-g) in benign and malignant thyroid lesions: an immunohistochemical study. *Mod Pathol* 2002;15:121A(abst).

217. Gustafson KG, LiVolsi VA, Furth EE, et al. Peroxisome prolif-erator-activated receptor-gamma expression in follicular-patterned thyroid lesions: caveats for the use of immunohisto-chemical studies. *Am J Clin Pathol* 2003;120:175.

218. Rosai J, Saxen EA, Woolner LB. Undifferentiated and poorly differentiated carcinoma. *Semin Diagn Pathol* 1985;2:123.

219. Carcangiu ML, Zampi G, Rosai J. Poorly differentiated ("insu-lar") thyroid carcinoma. *Am J Surg Pathol* 1984;8:655.

220. Nishida T, Katayama S, Tsujimoto M, et al. Clinicopathologi-cal significance of poorly differentiated thyroid carcinoma. *Am J Surg Pathol* 1999;23:205.

221. Sakamoto A, Kasai N, Sugano H. Poorly differentiated carci-noma of the thyroid: a clinicopathologic entity for a high risk group of papillary and follicular carcinomas. *Cancer* 1983;52:1849.

222. Evans HL. Columnar cell carcinoma of the thyroid: a report of two cases of an aggressive variant of thyroid carcinoma. *Am J Clin Pathol* 1986;85:77.

223. Mizukami Y, Nonomura A, Michigishi T, et al. Columnar cell carcinoma of the thyroid gland. *Hum Pathol* 1994;25:1098.

224. Robbins J, Merino MJ, Boice JD, et al. Thyroid cancer: a lethal endocrine neoplasm. *Ann Intern Med* 1991;115:133.

225. Sobrinho-Simoes M, Nesland JM, Johannessen JV. Columnar cell carcinoma. Another variant of poorly differentiated carci-noma of the thyroid. *Am J Clin Pathol* 1988;89:264.

226. Sobrinho-Simoes M, Sambade C, Nesland JM, et al. Tall cell papillary carcinoma. *Am J Surg Pathol* 1989;13:79.

227. Auguste LJ, Masood S, Westerband O, et al. Oncogene expres-sion in follicular neoplasms of the thyroid. *Am J Surg* 1992;164:592.

228. Dobashi Y, Sakamoto A, Sugimura H, et al. Over expression of p53 as a possible prognostic factor in human thyroid carcinoma. *Am J Surg Pathol* 1993;17:375.

229. Dobashi Y, Sugimura H, Sakamoto A, et al. Stepwise participa-tion of p 53 gene mutation during dedifferentiation of human thyroid carcinomas. *Diagn Mol Pathol* 1994;3:9–14.

230. Matias-Guiu X, Cuatrecasas M, Musulen E, et al. P 53 expres-sion in anaplastic carcinomas arising from papillary carcino-mas. *J Clin Pathol* 1994;47:337.

231. Pilotti S, Collini P, DelBo R, et al. A novel panel of antibodies that segregates immunocytochemically poorly differentiated carcinoma from undifferentiated carcinoma of the thyroid gland. *Am J Surg Pathol* 1994;18:1054.

232. Pilotti S, Collini P, Rilke F, et al. Bcl-2 protein expression in carcinomas originating from the follicular epithelium of the thyroid gland. *J Pathol* 1994;172:337.

233. Soares P, Cameselle-Teijeiro J, Sobrinho-Simoes M. Immuno-histochemical detection of p 53 in differentiated, poorly differ-entiated and undifferentiated carcinomas of the thyroid. *Histo-pathology* 1994;24:205.

234. Fagin JA, Matsuo K, Karmakar A, et al. High prevalence of mutations of the p 53 gene in poorly differentiated human thy-roid carcinomas. *J Clin Invest* 1993;91:179.

235. Mambo NC, Irwin SM. Anaplastic small cell neoplasms of the thyroid: an immunoperoxidase study. *Hum Pathol* 1984;15:55.

236. Eusebi V, Damiani S, Riva C, et al. Calcitonin free oat cell car-cinoma of the thyroid gland. *Virchows Arch* 1990;14:737.

237. Hurlimann J, Gardiol D, Scazziga B. Immunohistology of anaplastic thyroid carcinoma: a study of 43 cases. *Histopathol-ogy* 1987;11:567.

238. Venkatesh YSS, Ordonez NG, Schultz PN, et al. Anaplastic carcinoma of the thyroid: a clinicopathologic study of 121 cases. *Cancer* 1990;66:321.

239. Hashimoto H, Koga S, Watanabe H, et al. Undifferentiated carcinoma of the thryoid gland with osteoclast like giant cells. *Acta Pathol Jpn* 1980;30:323.

240. Donnell CA, Pollock WJ, Sybers WA. Thyroid carcinosarcoma. *Arch Pathol Lab Med* 1987;111:1169.

241. Katoh R, Sakamoto A, Kasai N, et al. Squamous differentiation in thyroid carcinoma: with special reference to histogenesis of squamous cell carcinoma of the thyroid. *Acta Pathol Jpn* 1989;39:306.

242. Mikukami Y, Matsubara F, Hashimoto T, et al. Primary mucin producing adenosquamous carcinoma of the thyroid gland. *Acta Pathol Jpn* 1987;37:1157.

243. Huang TY, Assor D. Primary squamous cell carcinoma of the thyroid gland: a report of four cases. *Am J Clin Pathol* 1971;11:567.

244. Riddle PE, Dinesoy HP. Primary squamous cell carcinoma of the thyroid associated with leukocytosis and hypercalcemia. *Arch Pathol Lab Med* 1987;111:373.

245. Chan JKC, Albores-Saavedra J, Battifora H, et al. Sclerosing mucoepidermoid thyroid carcinoma with eosinophilia. *Am J Surg Pathol* 1991;15:438.

246. Franssila KO, Harach HR, Wasenius VM. Mucoepidermoid carcinoma of the thyroid. *Histopathology* 1984;8:847.

247. Katoh R, Sugai T, Ono S, et al. Mucoepidermoid carcinoma of the thyroid gland. *Cancer* 1990;65:2020.

248. Mizukami Y, Matsubara F, Hashimoto T, et al. Primary mu-coepidermoid carcinoma in the thyroid gland: a case report in-cluding an ultrastructural and biochemical study. *Cancer* 1984;53:1741.

249. Rhatigan RM, Roque J, Bucker RL. Mucoepidermoid carci-noma of the thyroid gland. *Cancer* 1977;39:210.

250. Chan JKC, Rosai J. Tumors of the neck showing thymic or re-lated branchial pouch differentiation. *Hum Pathol* 1991;22:349.

251. Wenig BM, Adair CF, Heffess CS. Primary mucoepidermoid carcinoma of the thyroid gland: a report of six cases and a re-view of the literature of a follicular epithelial-derived tumor. *Hum Pathol* 1995;26:1099.

252. Baloch ZW, Solomon AC, LiVolsi VA. Primary mucoepider-moid carcinoma (MEC) and sclerosing mucoepidermoid carci-noma with eosinophilia (SMECE) of the thyroid: a report of nine cases. *Mod Pathol* 2000;13:802–807.

253. Miyauchi A, Kuma K, Matsuzuka F, et al. Intrathyroidal ep-ithelial thymoma: an entity distinct from squamous cell carci-noma of the thyroid. *World J Surg* 1985;9:128.

254. Bigner SH, Mendelsohn G, Wells SA, et al. Medullary carci-noma of the thyroid in the multiple endocrine neoplasia IIB syndrome. *Am J Surg Pathol* 1981;5:459.

255. Carney JA, Sizemore GW, Hayles AB. C cell disease of the thy-roid gland in multiple endocrine neoplsia type 2b. *Cancer* 1979;44:2173.

256. Melvin KEW, Tashjian AH, Miller HH. Studies in familial medullary thyroid carcinoma. *Recent Prog Horm Res* 1972;28:399.

257. Albores-Saavedra J, Montfonte H, Nadji M, et al. C-cell hyper-plasia in thyroid tissue adjacent to follicular cell tumors. *Hum Pathol* 1988;19:795.

258. Libbey NP, Nowakowski KJ, Tucci JR. C cell hyperplasia of the thyroid in a patient with goitrous hypothyroidism and Hashi-moto's thyroiditis. *Am J Surg Pathol* 1989;13:71.

259. Hazard JB, Hawk WA, Crile G. Medullary (solid) carcinoma of the thyroid: a clinicopathologic entity. *J Clin Endocrinol Metab* 1959;19:152.

260. Williams ED, Brown CL, Doniach I. Pathological and clinical findings in a series of 67 cases of medullary carcinoma of the thyroid. *J Clin Pathol* 1966;19:103.

261. Hazard JB. The C (parafollicular) cells of the thyroid gland and medullary thyroid carcinoma: a review. *Am J Pathol* 1977;88:214.

262. Huss LJ, Mendelsohn G. Medullary carcinoma of the thyroid gland: an encapsulated variant resembling the hyalinizing tra-

becular (paraganglioma-like) adenoma of thyroid. *Mod Pathol* 1990;3:581.

263. Albores-Saavedra J, LiVolsi VA, Williams ED. Medullary carcinoma. *Semin Diagn Pathol* 1985;2:137.

264. Kakudo K, Miyauchi A, Takai S, et al. C cell carcinoma of the thyroid: papillary type. *Acta Pathol Jpn* 1979;29:653.

265. Sambade C, Baldaque-Faria A, Cardoso-Oliveira M, et al. Follicular and papillary variants of medullary carcinoma of the thyroid. *Pathol Res Pract* 1989;184:98.

266. Nieuwenhuizen-Kruseman AC, Bosman FT, van Bergen-Henegouw JC, et al. Medullary differentiation of anaplastic thyroid carcinoma. *Am J Clin Pathol* 1992;77:541.

267. Kakudo K, Miyauchi A, Ogihara T, et al. Medullary carcinoma of the thyroid: giant cell type. *Arch Pathol Lab Med* 1978;102:445.

268. Harach HR, Bergholm U. Medullary (C cell) carcinoma of the thyroid with features of follicular oxyphilic cell tumours. *Histopathology* 1988;13:645.

269. Harach HR, Williams ED. Glandular (tubular and follicular) variants of medullary carcinoma of the thyroid. *Histopathology* 1983;7:83.

270. Landon G, Ordonez NG. Clear cell variant of medullary carcinoma of the thyroid. *Hum Pathol* 1985;16:844.

271. Martin-Lacave I, Gonzalez-Campora R, Moreno-Fernandez A, et al. Mucosubstances in medullary carcinoma of the thyroid. *Histopathology* 1988;13:55.

272. Zaatari GS, Saigo PE, Huvos AG. Mucin production in medullary carcinoma of the thyroid. *Arch Pathol Lab Med* 1983;107:70.

273. Beerman H, Rigaud C, Bogomoletz WV, et al. Melanin production in black medullary thyroid carcinoma (MTC). *Histopathology* 1990;16:227.

274. Marcus JN, Dise CA, LiVolsi VA. Melanin production in a medullary thyroid carcinoma. *Cancer* 1982;49:2518.

275. Schroder S, Bocker W, Baisch H, et al. Prognostic factors in medullary thyroid carcinoma: survival in relation to age, sex, stage, histology, immunocytochemistry and DNA content. *Cancer* 1988;61:806.

276. Capella C, Bordi C, Monga G, et al. Multiple endocrine cell types in thyroid medullary carcinoma: evidence for calcitonin, somatostatin, ACTH, 5HT and small granule cells. *Virchows Arch* 1978;377:111.

277. Dasovic-Knezevic M, Bormer O, Holm R, et al. Carcinoembryonic antigen in medullary thyroid carcinoma: an immunohistochemical study applying six novel monoclonal antibodies. *Mod Pathol* 1989;2:610.

278. Pacini F, Elisei R, Anelli S, et al. Somatostatin in medullary thyroid cancer: in vitro and in vivo studies. *Cancer* 1989;63:1189.

279. Lippman SM, Mendelsohn G, Trump DL, et al. The prognostic and biological significance of cellular heterogeneity in medullary thyroid carcinoma: a study of calcitonin, L-dopa decarboxylase, and histaminase. *J Clin Endocrinol Metab* 1982;54:233.

280. Saad MF, Ordonez NG, Rashid RK, et al. Medullary carcinoma of the thyroid: a study of the clinical features and prognostic factors in 161 patients. *Medicine (Baltimore)* 1984;63:319.

281. Samaan NA, Schultz PN, Hickey RC. Medullary thyroid carcinoma: prognosis of familial versus sporadic disease and the role of radiotherapy. *J Clin Endocrinol Metab* 1988;67:801.

282. Gharib H, McConahey WM, Tregs RD, et al. Medullary thyroid carcinoma: clinicopathologic features and longterm followup of 65 patients treated during 1946 through 1970. *Mayo Clin Proc* 1992;67:934.

283. Komminoth P, Roth J, Saramaslani P, et al. Polysialic acid of the neural adhesion molecule in the human thyroid: a marker for medullary thyroid carcinoma and primary C-cell hyperplasia. *Am J Surg Pathol* 1994;18:399.

284. Feldman GL, Kambouris M, Talpos GB, et al. Clinical value of direct DNA analysis of the RET proto-oncogene in families with multiple endocrine neoplasia type 2A. *Surgery* 1994;116:1042.

285. O'Riordain DS, O'Brien T, Weaver A, et al. Medullary thyroid carcinoma in multiple endocrine neoplasia types 2A and 2B. *Surgery* 1994;116:1017.

286. Utiger RD. Medullary thyroid carcinoma, genes and the prevention of cancer. *N Engl J Med* 1994;331:870.

287. Weiss LM, Weinberg DS, Warhol MJ. Medullary carcinoma arising in a thyroid with Hashimoto's thyroiditis. *Am J Clin Pathol* 1983;80:534.

288. Bondeson L, Ljungberg O. Occult thyroid carcinoma at autopsy in Malmo, Sweden. *Cancer* 1981;47:319.

289. Lang W, Borrusch H, Bauer L. Occult carcinoma of the thyroid: evaluation of 1020 consecutive autopsies. *Am J Clin Pathol* 1988;90:72.

290. White IL, Vimadalal SD, Catz B, et al. Occult medullary carcinoma of thyroid: an unusual clinical and pathological presentation. *Cancer* 1981;47:1364.

291. Krueger JE, Maitra A, Albores-Saavedra J. Inherited medullary microcarcinoma of the thyroid: a study of 11 cases. *Am J Surg Pathol* 2000;24:853.

292. Kaserer K, Scheuba C, Neuhold N, et al. Sporadic versus familial medullary thyroid microcarcinoma: a histopathologic study of 50 consecutive patients. *Am J Surg Pathol* 2001;25:1245.

293. Apel RL, Alpert LC, Rizzo A, et al. A metastasizing composite carcinoma of the thyroid with distinct medullary and papillary components. *Arch Pathol Lab Med* 1994;118:1143.

294. Holm R, Sobrinho-Simoes M, Nesland JM, et al. Medullary thyroid carcinoma with thyroglobulin immunoreactivity: a special entity? *Lab Invest* 1987;57:258.

295. Kovacs CS, Mase RM, Kovacs K, et al. Thyroid medullary carcinoma with thyroglobulin immunoreactivity in sporadic multiple endocrine neoplasia type 2B. *Cancer* 1994;74:928.

296. Lax SF, Beham A, Kronberger-Schonecker D, et al. Coexistence of papillary and medullary carcinoma of the thyroid gland-mixed or collision tumor? *Virchows Arch* 1994;424:441.

297. Volante M, Papotti M, Roth J, et al. Mixed medullary-follicular thyroid carcinoma. Molecular evidence for a dual origin of tumor components. *Am J Pathol* 1999;155:1499.

298. Anscombe AM, Wright DH. Primary malignant lymphoma of the thyroid—a tumor of mucosa-associated lymphoid tissue: review of seventy-six cases. *Histopathology* 1985;9:81

299. Aozasa K, Inoue A, Tajima K, et al. Malignant lymphomas of the thyroid gland. Analysis of 79 patients with emphasis on histologic prognostic factors. *Cancer* 1986;58:100

300. Compagno J, Oertel JE. Malignant lymphoma and other lymphoproliferative disorders of the thyroid gland: a clinicopathologic study of 245 cases. *Am J Clin Pathol* 1980;74:1.

301. Oertel JE, Heffess CS. Lymphoma of the thyroid and related disorders. *Semin Oncol* 1987;14:333.

302. Hyjek E, Isaacson PG. Primary B-cell lymphoma of the thyroid and its relationship to Hashimoto's thyroiditis. *Hum Pathol* 1988;19:1315.

303. Aozasa K, Inoue A, Yoshimura H, et al. Intermediate lymphocytic lymphoma of the thyroid. An immunologic and immunohistologic study. *Cancer* 1986;57:1762

304. Faure P, Chittal S, Woodman-Memeteau F, et al. Diagnostic features of primary malignat lymphomas of the thyroid with monoclonal antibodies. *Cancer* 1988;61:1852.

305. Aozasa K, Inoue A, Yoshimura H, et al. Plasmacytoma of the thyroid gland. *Cancer* 1986;58:105.

306. Kovacs CA, Mant MJ, Nguyen GK, et al. Plasma cell lesions of the thyroid. *Thyroid* 1994;4:65.

307. Burke JS. Histologic criteria for distinguishing between benign and malignant extranodal lymphoid infiltrates. *Semin Diagn Pathol* 1985;2:152.

308. Hedinger CE. Sarcomas of the thyroid gland. In: Hedinger CE, ed. *Thyroid cancer.* Berlin: Springer-Verlag, 1969:47.

309. Vergilio J, Baloch ZW, LiVolsi VA. Spindle cell metaplasia of the thyroid arising in association with papillary carcinoma and follicular adenoma. *Am J Clin Pathol* 2002;117:199–204.

310. Eusebi V, Carcangiu ML, Dina R, et al. Keratin positive epithelioid angiosarcoma of thyroid: a report of four cases. *Am J Surg Pathol* 1990;14:737.

311. Pfaltz M, Hedinger CE, Saremaslani P, et al. Malignant hemangioendothelioma of the thyroid and factor VIII-related antigen. *Virchows Arch* 1983;401:177.

312. Ruchti C, Gerber HA, Schaffner T. Factor VIII-related antigen in malignant hemangioendothelioma of the thyroid: additional evidence for the endothelial origin of this tumor. *Am J Clin Pathol* 1984;82:474.

313. Kawahara E, Nakanishi T, Terahata S, et al. Leiomyosarcoma of the thyroid gland: a case report with a comparative study of five cases of anaplastic carcinoma. *Cancer* 1988;62:2558.

314. Bhagavan BS, Govinda Rao DR, Weinberg T. Carcinoma of thyroglossal duct cyst: case reports and review of the literature. *Surgery* 1970;67:281.

315. Boswell WC, Zoller M, Williams JS, et al. Thyroglossal duct carcinoma. *Am Surg* 1994;60:650.

316. Heshmati HM, Fatourechi V, van Heerden JA, et al. Thyroglossal duct carcinoma: report of 12 cases. *Mayo Clin Proc* 1997;72:315.

317. LiVolsi VA, Perzin KH, Savetsky L. Carcinoma arising in median ectopic thyroid (including thyroglossal duct tissue). *Cancer* 1974;34:577.

318. Yang YJ, Haghir S, Wanamaker JR, et al. Diagnosis of papillary carcinoma in a thyroglossal duct cyst by fine-needle aspiration biopsy. *Arch Pathol Lab Med* 2000;124:139.

319. Devaney K, Snyder R, Norris HJ, et al. Proliferative struma ovarii and histologically malignant struma ovarii—a clinicopathologic study of 54 cases. *Int J Gynecol Pathol* 1993;12:333.

320. Snyder RR, Tavassoli FA. Ovarian strumal carcinoid: immunohistochemical, ultrastructural and clinicopathologic observations. *Int J Gynecol Pathol* 1986;5:187.

321. Czech JM, Lichtor TR, Carney JA, et al. Neoplasms metastatic to the thyroid gland. *Surg Gynecol Obstet* 1982;155:503.

322. Green LK, Ro JY, Mackay B, et al. Renal cell carcinoma metastatic to the thyroid. *Cancer* 1989;63:1810.

323. Lam KY, Lo CY. Metastatic tumors of the thyroid gland: a study of 79 cases in Chinese patients. *Arch Pathol Lab Med* 1998;122:37–41.

324. Baloch ZW, LiVolsi VA. Tumor-to-tumor metastasis to follicular variant of papillary carcinoma of thyroid. *Arch Pathol Lab Med* 1999;123:703.

THYROID DISEASES: THYROTOXICOSIS

INTRODUCTION

22

INTRODUCTION TO THYROTOXICOSIS

LEWIS E. BRAVERMAN
ROBERT D. UTIGER

This chapter introduces the section on thyrotoxicosis, a common and important thyroid disorder. It has multiple causes, and its recognition and treatment are important components of endocrine practice.

We use the term *thyrotoxicosis* to mean the clinical syndrome of hypermetabolism and hyperactivity that results when the serum concentrations of free thyroxine (T_4), free triiodothyronine (T_3), or both, are high. The term *hyperthyroidism* is used to mean sustained increases in thyroid hormone biosynthesis and secretion by the thyroid gland. Thus, the terms *thyrotoxicosis* and *hyperthyroidism* are not synonymous. While many patients with thyrotoxicosis have hyperthyroidism, others—for example, those in whom thyrotoxicosis is caused by thyroiditis or exogenous thyroid hormone administration—do not.

The clinical manifestations of thyrotoxicosis are, for the most part, independent of its cause. However, certain features of the illness often provide clues about the cause of thyrotoxicosis in an individual patient. These features include the duration of thyrotoxicosis, the size and shape of the thyroid gland, and the presence or absence of the extrathyroidal manifestations of Graves' disease. For example, at the time of diagnosis, patients with thyrotoxicosis caused by thyroiditis rarely have had symptoms for more than a few weeks, whereas those with Graves' disease have usually had symptoms for at least several months. An attempt should be made to determine the cause of thyrotoxicosis in all patients, because knowledge of the cause determines prognosis and guides therapy.

The causes of thyrotoxicosis can be subdivided into those disorders that are associated with hyperthyroidism and those that are not (Table 22.1). All these disorders are discussed in detail in the following chapters. Among the causes of spontaneously occurring thyrotoxicosis, Graves' disease is the most common; its frequency as the cause of thyrotoxicosis ranges from approximately 60% to 90% in different regions of the world. Most of the remaining cases are caused by toxic nodular goiter, autonomously functioning thyroid adenomas (toxic adenomas), or the several types of thyroiditis (1–3). Except for exogenous thyrotoxicosis, all the other causes of thyrotoxicosis are rare.

While many patients with thyrotoxicosis have overt clinical and biochemical disease, thyrotoxicosis may be subclinical. Subclinical thyrotoxicosis is defined as normal serum free T_4 and T_3 concentrations and low serum thyrotropin (TSH) concentrations; the patients may or may not have symptoms of thyrotoxicosis, but if present the symptoms are usually mild and nonspecific. The causes of overt and subclinical thyrotoxicosis are similar, but the most common cause of subclinical thyrotoxicosis is exogenous thyroid hormone administration rather than Graves' disease (4). Whether and how patients with endogenous subclinical thyrotoxicosis should be treated is controversial (see Chapter 79).

The underlying problem in patients with thyrotoxicosis is acceleration of many physiologic processes, and the clinical manifestations reflect that acceleration. The more common clinical manifestations are listed in Table 22.2,

TABLE 22.1. CAUSES OF THYROTOXICOSIS

Common Causes	
Type of Thyrotoxicosis	**Pathogenic Mechanism**
Thyrotoxicosis associated with hyperthyroidism[a]	
Production of abnormal thyroid stimulator (Graves' disease)	TSH receptor-stimulating antibody
Intrinsic thyroid autonomy	
Toxic adenoma	Benign tumor
Toxic multinodular goiter	Foci of functional autonomy
Thyrotoxicosis not associated with hyperthyroidism[b]	
Inflammatory disease	
Silent (painless) thyroiditis[d]	Release of stored hormones
Subacute thyroiditis	Release of stored hormones
Extrathyroidal source of hormone	
Exogenous thyroid hormone	Hormone in medication or rarely, food or nutritional supplements

Uncommon Causes	
Type of Thyrotoxicosis	**Pathogenic Mechanism**
Thyrotoxicosis associated with hyperthyroidism[a]	
Production of thyroid-stimulating hormones	
TSH hypersecretion	Thyrotroph adenoma
	Thyrotroph resistance to thyroid hormone
Trophoblastic tumor	Chorionic gonadotropin
Hyperemesis gravidarum	Chorionic gonadotropin
Gestational thyrotoxicosis	TSH-receptor mutation resulting in increased sensitivity to chorionic gonadotropin
Intrinsic thyroid autonomy	
Thyroid carcinoma	Foci of functional autonomy
Nonautoimmune autosomal-dominant hyperthyroidism	Constitutive activation of TSH receptors
Struma ovari	Toxic adenoma in a dermoid tumor of ovary
Drug-induced hyperthyroidism	
Iodine and iodine-containing drugs and radiographic contrast agents[c]	
Iodine excess plus thyroid autonomy	
Thyrotoxicosis not associated with hyperthyroidism[b]	
Inflammatory disease	
Drug-induced thyroiditis (amiodarone, interferon-α)	Release of stored thyroid hormone
Infarction of thyroid adenoma	Release of stored thyroid hormone
Radiation thyroiditis	Release of stored thyroid hormone

[a] Radioiodine uptake by thyroid gland (or abnormal or abnormally located thyroid tissue) high.
[b] Thyroid radioiodine uptake low.
[c] Thyroid radioiodine uptake usually low, but may be normal.
[d] Including postpartum thyroiditis.
TSH, thyrotropin.

and they are discussed in detail in the following chapters. None of the clinical manifestations are specific; it is usually the combination of several of them that brings to mind the possibility of the disorder in a patient. The frequency and severity of these symptoms and signs vary considerably among patients; some patients have only a few symptoms or signs and others many, and their severity varies widely; rarely thyrotoxicosis is life threatening (see Chapter 43).

Among the factors that determine the manifestations of thyrotoxicosis are the age of the patient (5,6) and the presence of concomitant disturbances in the function of one or another organ system, so that the impact of thyrotoxicosis is either exaggerated or diminished. For example, as com-

pared with younger patients, older patients have fewer symptoms and signs of sympathetic activation, such as anxiety, hyperactivity, and tremor, and more symptoms and signs of cardiovascular dysfunction, such as dyspnea and atrial fibrillation, and they are more likely to lose weight. The extent and severity of the clinical manifestations of thyrotoxicosis are not strongly correlated with its biochemical severity (7).

It is now easy to obtain biochemical confirmation of thyrotoxicosis by measurements of serum TSH and direct or indirect measurements of the serum free T_4, free T_3, or both (see Chapter 13). Other tests, such as measurements of radioiodine uptake, radioiodine and other imaging tests,

TABLE 22.2. COMMON CLINICAL MANIFESTATIONS OF THYROTOXICOSIS

Symptoms
  Nervousness
  Fatigue
  Weakness
  Increased perspiration
  Heat intolerance
  Tremor
  Hyperactivity
  Palpitation
  Appetite change (usually increase)
  Weight change (usually weight loss)
  Menstrual disturbances
Signs
  Hyperactivity
  Tachycardia or atrial arrhythmia
  Systolic hypertension
  Warm, moist, smooth skin
  Stare and eyelid retraction
  Tremor
  Hyperreflexia
  Muscle weakness

TABLE 22.3. CLINICAL MANIFESTATIONS OF SPECIFIC CAUSES OF THYROTOXICOSIS

Clinical Finding	Cause
Diffuse goiter	Graves' disease, silent thyroiditis
Uninodular goiter	Thyroid autonomy
Multinodular goiter	Thyroid autonomy
Impalpable thyroid gland	Exogenous thyroid hormone
Thyroid pain and tenderness	Subacute thyroiditis
Ophthalmopathy	Graves' disease
Localized dermopathy	Graves' disease
Thyroid acropachy	Graves' disease

and measurements of TSH-receptor antibodies, may be done to determine the cause of thyrotoxicosis. Fortunately, however, the cause can usually be determined by history and physical examination, and tests to determine the cause are not routinely necessary. Among these tests, measurement of thyroid radioiodine is the most useful, because it distinguishes between thyrotoxicosis caused by hyperthyroidism and that caused by thyroiditis or exogenous thyroid hormone administration.

Finally, the various antithyroid treatments available—antithyroid drugs, radioactive iodine, and thyroidectomy—effectively ameliorate hyperthyroidism and therefore thyrotoxicosis (see Chapter 45). However, none is ideal, because they do not address the fundamental abnormality that causes thyrotoxicosis in most patients, and preferences for them vary widely throughout the world (8,9).

REFERENCES

1. Brownlie BEW, Wells JE. The epidemiology of thyrotoxicosis in New Zealand: incidence and geographical distribution in North Canterbury, 1983–1985. *Clin Endocrinol (Oxf)* 1990;33:249.
2. Reinwein D, Benker G, Konig MP, et al. The different types of hyperthyroidism in Europe: results of a prospective study of 924 patients. *J Endocrinol Invest* 1988;11:193.
3. Williams I, Ankrett VO, Lazarus JH, et al. Aetiology of hyperthyroidism in Canada and Wales. *J Epidemiol Community Health* 1983;37:245.
4. Marqusse E, Haden S, Utiger RD. Subclinical thyrotoxicosis. *Endocrinol Metab Clin North Am* 1998;27:37.
5. Nordyke RA, Gilbert FI Jr, Harada ASM. Graves' disease: influence of age on clinical findings. *Arch Intern Med* 1988;148:626.
6. Trivalle C, Doucet J, Chassagne P, et al. Differences in the signs and symptoms of hyperthyroidism in older and younger patients. *J Am Geriatr Soc* 1996;44:50.
7. Trzepacz PT, Klein I, Robert M, et al. Graves' disease: an analysis of thyroid hormone levels and hyperthyroid signs and symptoms. *Am J Med* 1989;87:558.
8. Solomon B, Glinoer D, Lagasse R, et al. Current trends in the management of Graves' disease. *J Clin Endocrinol Metab* 1990;70:1518.
9. Romaldini JH. Case selection and restrictions recommended to patients with hyperthyroidism in South America. *Thyroid* 1997;7:225.

CAUSES OF HYPERTHYROIDISM

23

GRAVES' DISEASE

23A   THE PATHOGENESIS OF GRAVES' DISEASE

TERRY F. DAVIES

Graves' disease is a uniquely human autoimmune disease with an interesting immunopathogenesis, because unique stimulating autoantibodies to the thyrotropin (TSH) receptor are the major pathogenic feature of the disease. Unlike many autoimmune diseases, these antibodies are not just markers of the disease but are responsible for the hyperthyroidism that is the predominant feature of the disease. In most patients with Graves' disease, both B- and T-lymphocytes are directed at all three well-characterized thyroid autoantigens—thyroglobulin (Tg), thyroid peroxidase (TPO), and the TSH receptor (TSH-R)—as well as a variety of minor antigens such as the sodium iodide transporter (NIS). However, much evidence suggests that only the TSH-R is the primary autoantigen of Graves' disease, and that the other thyroid antigens are only secondarily involved (1).

AUTOIMMUNITY

Definition of an Autoantigen

There are a number of simple rules concerning the self-molecules (autoantigens) with which T cells and autoantibodies interact. Autoantigens are present from birth and do not just appear during later development. In fact, autoantigens are highly conserved structural proteins coded for by genes with low mutation rates. Hence, autoantigens are not abnormal molecules, but they may be coded for by polymorphic genes within the population. Such polymorphisms may cause structural and functional variations, which may be important such as reported for Tg (2). However, autoimmune diseases are thought primarily to involve defects in immune surveillance pathways. The molecular recognition sites (epitopes) for autoantibodies versus T cells usually differ, and immunization of animals with the appropriate purified antigen always induces antigen-specific T- and B-cell responses against both T- and B- cell-directed epitopes.

The Nature of T Cells

The T cells that survive both intrathymic deletion and peripheral deletion are a complex mixture of cells of different phenotypes. Both CD4+ and CD8+ cells consist of many subsets; therefore, a full discussion of them is not possible here. Furthermore, many such T cells are in transition between immature and mature forms, and this may occur within an autoimmune infiltrate. However, knowledge of biologic function is probably more important than phenotype. On the whole, CD4+ cells tend to be regulatory cells (especially the CD4+/CD25+ subset) (3), and CD8+ cells tend to be cytotoxic cells capable of lysing target cells. Many T cells exert their function by the secretion of cytokines, and studies of cytokine secretion in mice have provided useful criteria to help understand the way T cells initiate and control the immune response. The CD4+ T cells have been shown to be of two principal types, T helper 1 and T helper 2 (Th1 and Th2), which differ functionally in their pattern of cytokine secretion and differ phenotypically in their pattern of chemokine receptor expression (4,5). In fact, Th1 and Th2 cells represent two polarized forms of the T-cell response, while other T cells fall outside this pattern. Th1 cells secrete principally interleukin (IL)-2, interferon (IFN)-γ, and tumor necrosis factor (TNF)-β and induce target cell cytotoxicity, while Th2 cells secrete IL-4, IL-5, IL-10, and IL-13 and are particularly effective at inducing antibody secretion. In humans, this dichotomy is not as strict as in mice, and much cellular interchange has been shown. However, there is general agreement that human Th2 cells may be best defined as those that always secrete IL-4, while Th1 cells usually, but not always, secrete IFN-γ. This Th1/Th2 concept has been most helpful in understanding immunopathology.

Antibody and T-Cell Interactions with Antigen

Antibodies are immunoglobulins that may be present in the serum or expressed on the surface of B cells and are able to bind to their specific antigenic molecules directly. The strength of this binding is measured as the affinity of the antibody and is directly dependent, to a large degree, on the number of antigen-binding sites (Fig. 23A.1). Hence,

the binding energy is usually greater for conformational antigens with multiple binding sites than for the binding to a small linear antigen (6). Pathogenic antibodies of high affinity are therefore most likely to interact with conformational antigens (7), and this is an important concept in understanding Graves' disease where stimulating TSH-R antibodies (TSHR-Ab) only interact appropriately with the extracellular domain of TSH-Rs. In contrast to immunoglobulins, T cells recognize the complexity of antigen and major histocompatibility antigens (HLA) (Fig. 23A.2). The T-cell antigen receptor is also a member of the immunoglobulin family, but it has a transmembrane domain that anchors it within the cell surface. The CD8+ T cells recognize antigens complexed with HLA class I molecules (A, C, and B), and CD4+ T cells recognize antigens with HLA class II molecules (DR, DP, and DQ). T cells, through their T-cell antigen receptor, recognize small linear peptides complexed with an appropriate HLA molecule and therefore are termed HLA restricted. In thyroid autoimmunity, thyroid antigens are first engulfed by antigen-presenting cells (APCs) such as macrophages and dendritic cells, then digested by proteases within these cells. Antigen breakdown products (peptides) are then bound to intracellular HLA molecules, and the complexes are transported onto the cell surface by transporters associated with antigen processing (TAPs). Thyroid cells may act as APCs (see later in the chapter).

Second Signals

Both B cells and T cells rely on secondary signals once antigen has been identified in order to enter a proliferative and secretory state (8). A variety of cytokines secreted by T cells and APCs serve as second B-cell signals. In con-

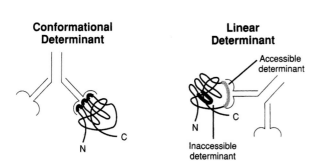

FIGURE 23A.1. Antigen-antibody interactions. **Left:** An immunoglobulin (Ig)G antibody interacts with a conformational (nonlinear) determinant involving noncontiguous parts of the antigen. **Right:** An IgG antibody reacts with a linear (accessible) determinant; an inaccessible determinant is buried within the antigen. (From Abbas AK, Lichtman AH, Pober JS. *Anonymous cellular and molecular immunology.* Philadelphia: WB Saunders, 1991, adapted with permission.)

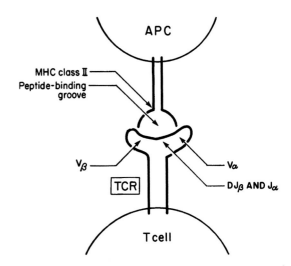

FIGURE 23A.2. Diagram of the mechanism of antigen presentation by an antigen-presenting cell to the T-cell antigen receptor of a T cell. APC, antigen-presenting cell.

**TABLE 23A.1. SECOND SIGNALS
FOR T-CELL ACTIVATION**

CD28/B7s
B7–1 > B7–2 (CD80) (e.g., dendritic cells)
B7h (GL50, ICOS-L) (e.g., fibroblasts)
PD-1/PD-1L (e.g., hematopoietic cells)
CD40/CD40L (e.g., B cells, fibroblasts, and thyroid cells)
ICAM/LFA-1 (e.g., thyroid cells)

trast, T-cell second signals are supplied by signal transduction from cell-surface molecules (such as the B7 family and CD40) (Table 23A.1), which are activated by ligands on the surface of the APCs (CD28 and CD40L). B cells and T cells that interact with specific antigen in the absence of a second signal become desensitized, a state referred to as anergy. Hence, anergy is one of the mechanisms that may be used for suppressing an immune response (9).

Criteria for an Autoimmune Disease

Three types of evidence can be marshaled to establish that a human disease is autoimmune in origin:

1. Direct evidence is provided if the disease, or manifestations of the disease, arise from transfer of pathogenic antibody or pathogenic T cells to humans or animals.
2. Indirect evidence may be based on studies in experimental animals by immunization with candidate antigens, and a disorder similar to the human disease ensues.
3. Circumstantial evidence may be obtained from clinical studies demonstrating, for example, an immune infiltrate at the site of disease or associated autoimmune diseases.

In Graves' disease, the antibody and cell-mediated thyroid antigen-specific immune responses are well defined, and there are now induced animal models of this uniquely human disease. Historically, the induction of thyroid hyperfunction by TSHR-Ab in normal subjects by the transfer of serum from patients with Graves' disease (10) was the first direct proof for an autoimmune origin of a human disease.

Restriction vs. Polyclonality

It is now possible to learn whether autoimmune reactions are multireactive and more likely to be representative of a secondary polyclonal immune response, or whether the immune response is much more focused, involving restricted sets of B cells and T cells (11). In an autoimmune disease, the immune system is where the abnormality is to be found and, therefore, the primary autoimmune re-

sponse at the onset of the disease should be oligoclonal. This has, indeed, proven to be the case for most of the human autoimmune diseases, including Graves' disease, as discussed later in the chapter.

THYROID IMMUNOLOGY

Intrathyroidal B cells

The B cells that accumulate within the thyroid gland of patients with Graves' disease have reduced proliferative responses to B-cell mitogens and greater basal immunoglobulin secretion than peripheral blood B cells, indicative of their activated state. B cells from Graves' thyroid tissue may also secrete thyroid autoantibodies spontaneously *in vitro*, again implying preactivation (12). Hence, the thyroid gland is a primary, but not exclusive, site of thyroid autoantibody secretion in autoimmune thyroid disease (AITD), perhaps best described by studies in mice with severe combined immunodeficiency (SCID) (Fig. 23A.3). Transplantation of Graves' thyroid tissue into T cell– and B cell–deficient mice resulted in the detection of human thyroid autoantibodies in the serum of the recipient mice (13). Additional direct evidence came from studies with

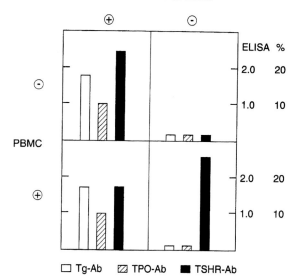

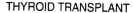

FIGURE 23A.3. Production of antibodies in mice with subacute combined immunodeficiency disease after thyroid tissue engraftment or intraperitoneal injection of peripheral blood mononuclear cells (PBMC) from a patient undergoing surgery for the treatment of Graves' disease. Thyroid antibodies were measured in mouse serum 4 to 6 weeks after transplantation. In the absence of thyroid tissue and PBMC, no thyroid antibodies were detectable **(upper right)**. In contrast, transplantation of thyroid tissue resulted in the production of thyroglobulin (Tg), thyroid peroxidase (TPo), and thyrotropin-receptor (TSH-R) antibodies (Ab) by the mice.

animal models of thyroiditis (see later in the chapter) and, indirectly, from the decline in thyroid autoantibodies after antithyroid drug treatment, thyroidectomy, and, in the long term, radioiodine therapy (14–16).

Autoantibodies to the Human Thyrotropin Receptor

Long-acting thyroid stimulator (LATS) was discovered by Adams and Purves almost 50 years ago during a search for thyroid-stimulating activity in the serum of patients with Graves' disease using a bioassay for pituitary TSH (17). The patients' serum stimulated radioiodine release from the prelabeled thyroid glands of guinea pigs for a much longer time period than did a pituitary TSH preparation (hence the term "long-acting"). This prolonged stimulating activity was then found to reside in the immunoglobulin (Ig)G fraction of serum. With the advent of biologically active radiolabeled TSH, it became possible to detect TSH-Rs on thyroid membranes, and subsequently this IgG activity in Graves' disease patients was found to compete with TSH for receptor occupancy, proving that it contained TSHR-Ab acting as TSH agonists (18). In patients with Graves' disease, the thyroid gland is no longer under the control of pituitary TSH but is continuously stimulated by circulating antibodies with TSH-like activity. Hence, it is not possible to put the thyroid to "sleep" using exogenous thyroxine suppression of any remaining endogenous TSH because of the presence of thyroid-stimulating antibodies.

Bioactivity of Thyrotropin-Receptor Antibodies

We now know that antibodies that bind to the TSH-R may or may not initiate an intracellular signal. Those that induce signal transduction are referred to as TSHR-stimulating, and those that do not are TSHR-blocking or TSHR-neutral antibodies (19). Further complicating this issue has been the observation of the simultaneous presence of TSHR-stimulating and TSHR-blocking antibodies in the same serum samples from patients with Graves' disease. The effective degree of thyroid stimulation under such circumstances is dependent on the relative concentration and bioactivities of the different antibodies (20). The original self-infusion of serum from patients with Graves' disease by Adams and colleagues and the resulting thyroid stimulation was the first direct evidence for the role of TSHR-Ab in the induction of hyperthyroidism in humans (10). Another early demonstration of the *in vivo* effects of TSHR-Ab came from studies demonstrating stimulation of the thyroid in neonates by transplacental passage of TSHR-Ab from their mothers (21).

Prevalence of Thyrotropin-Receptor Antibodies in Graves' Disease

TSHR-Ab are detectable only in patients with AITD. Such antibodies are therefore disease specific in great contrast to the high prevalence of Tg and TPO-antibodies in people with apparently normal thyroid function. Eighty to 100% of untreated patients with thyrotoxicosis caused by Graves' disease have detectable TSHR-Ab in their serum (22–24). The titers of TSHR-Ab may be reduced by treatment of thyrotoxicosis, and when they persist in higher concentrations they often predict a recurrence after withdrawal of antithyroid drug treatment (25–28) (Table 23A.2). TSHR-blocking antibodies may, in time, become the more prevalent antibody after treatment of thyrotoxic patients with Graves' disease, contributing to the development of later thyroid failure (29).

Immunologic Characteristics of Thyrotropin-Receptor Antibodies

TSHR-Ab are oligoclonal. Patients with Graves' disease have TSHR-Ab with light chain restriction, and the TSH agonist bioactivity is found mostly in the IgG1 subclass (30). However, this evidence of a pauciclonal B-cell response may not be typical of all patients with Graves' disease. For example, it is in contrast to the variable biologic nature of the antibodies when examined *in vitro*, and as discussed earlier in the chapter, with many patients having stimulating and blocking antibodies at the same time.

Thyrotropin Antibody Epitopes

The cloning of the TSH-R has permitted the initiation of detailed studies of its epitopes and structure-function relationships (31–33). The large extracellular domain of the TSH-R is the major immunogenic region, and TSHR-Ab bind to this domain of the receptor (Fig. 23A.4). The difference in functional activity of different TSHR-Ab may relate to molecular binding characteristics dependent on conformational changes and affinity. Many studies have now indicated that high affinity–stimulating antibodies to the TSH-R are dependent on the receptor being in its normal conformation (34,35) and interact with highest affin-

TABLE 23A.2. FACTORS INFLUENCING RECURRENCE OF GRAVES' DISEASE

High thyrotropin-receptor antibody concentration
Large iodine intake
Marked residual goiter
Short duration of antithyroid drug treatment
Previous recurrence
Failure to normalize low serum thyrotropin concentrations

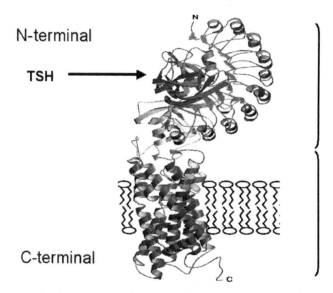

N-terminal

TSH →

C-terminal

FIGURE 23A.4. A model of the thyrotropin receptor (TSH-R). Note the α- and β-subunits of the receptor, which are disulfide linked and formed by protease cleavage of the intact molecule. The α-subunit is subsequently thought to be shed into the circulation, where it most likely contributes to the maintenance of tolerance to the TSH-R.

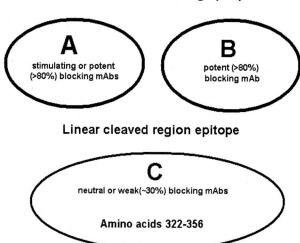

Conformational TSH binding epitopes

A
stimulating or potent (>80%) blocking mAbs

B
potent (>80%) blocking mAb

Linear cleaved region epitope

C
neutral or weak(~30%) blocking mAbs

Amino acids 322-356

FIGURE 23A.5. A scheme for thyrotropin (TSH)-receptor epitopes based on monoclonal antibody binding to the wild type receptor. Three major sites are illustrated. Monoclonal antibodies to one site do not bind to any of the other sites. (From Ando T, Latif R, Davies T. First identification of three binding sites for monoclonal antibodies to the native TSH receptor. *Thyroid* 2003; 13:734(abst), with permission.)

ity to the extracellular domain of the receptor alone (36). However, some TSHR-Ab recognize linear epitopes, but with low affinity, and many of these may be blocking or neutral in their activity. To date, there is suggestive evidence that stimulating antibodies bind to a restricted conformational epitope in the extracellular domain, but that blocking antibodies bind to more than one epitope. This conclusion is based on three primary conformational epitopes on the TSH-R identified using mouse monoclonal antibodies to the TSHR (37) (Fig. 23A.5). However, the location of such epitopes in the normally conformed TSH-R is uncertain.

Thyrotropin Receptor Regulation in Graves' Disease

Similar to TSH, TSHR-stimulating antibodies activate both cyclic adenosine monophosphate (cyclic AMP)-mediated signal transduction and the phosphoinositol cascade (38). The result is release of thyroid hormone and Tg, and stimulation of iodine uptake, protein synthesis, and thyroid cell growth. Although desensitization of the thyroidal cyclic AMP response by prolonged exposure to TSHR-Ab occurs *in vitro* and *in vivo*, this effect is highly concentration dependent. The low levels of antibody in patients therefore ensure that this does not occur to a great extent *in vivo* or they would not remain thyrotoxic (39,40). Resistance to desensitization by lower concentrations of TSH and of TSHR-Ab allows the hyperthyroid state to persist. In addition, although the TSH-R is not transcriptionally regulated,

at lower levels of stimulation there is evidence for positive regulation of the TSH-R by TSH, perhaps on the basis of messenger RNA stabilization (41,42).

Lessons from Monoclonal Thyrotropin-Receptor Antibodies with Stimulating Activity

For many years, attempts to induce Graves' disease in animals resulted in TSHR-Ab that blocked the TSH-R. Recently, several groups have isolated high-affinity TSHR-stimulating antibodies (43,44) (Fig. 23A.6), allowing new probes to be developed for the TSH-R. Such stimulating antibodies only interact with the natural, fully conformed receptor and appear to share the same conformational epitopes. Chronic treatment of mice with stimulating TSHR-Ab, however, did not produce severe thyrotoxicosis as expected, but a relatively mild degree of thyroid overactivity secondary to desensitization of the host thyroid (45). The low levels of TSHR-Ab in Graves' disease patients (46,47) may explain why the thyroid is able to continue to oversecrete thyroid hormone for many years.

Other Thyroid Antibodies in Graves' Disease

The majority of patients with Graves' disease have circulating antibodies to additional thyroid autoantigens, not just

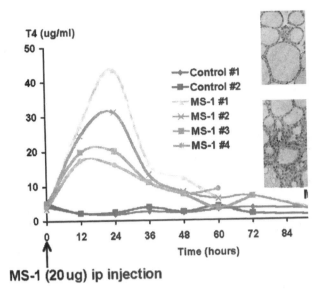

FIGURE 23A.6. *In vivo* thyroid stimulation by monoclonal thyroid-stimulating antibody. 20 μg of antibody (MS-1) was administered intraperitoneally, and the serum thyroid hormone response measured at the illustrated time intervals. The *insets* show the histologic response of the thyroid gland with thyroid cell hypertrophy and colloid droplet formation.

the TSH-R. In particular, Tg and TPO antibodies, sometimes in high titers, are found in the majority of such patients. Since these antibodies are polyclonal in nature, and the role of TSHR-Ab is so important in the disease, the Tg and TPO antibodies appear to reflect a coincidental but controlled autoimmune thyroiditis (48). Autoantibodies to the iodide transporter have also been demonstrated in pa-

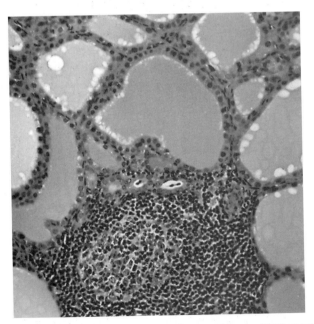

FIGURE 23A.7. Histologic section from a patient with Graves' disease showing mild thyroid hyperplasia and a patchy lymphocytic infiltrate, which is characteristic of the disease.

tients with Graves' disease, but are likely to be similar signs of coincidental thyroiditis (49). Hence, Graves' disease appears to develop on a background of or is coincidental with autoimmune thyroiditis. This explains why many patients not treated with destructive therapy become hypothyroid in time (29).

The Intrathyroidal Lymphocytic Infiltrate

Much of the early evidence that Graves' disease was an autoimmune disease was based on the discovery of TSHR-Ab by Adams and Kennedy (50). However, supporting evidence was in fact found much earlier within the thyroid gland itself. The thyroid in Graves' disease is characterized by a lymphocytic infiltration, that is nonhomogeneous, suggestive of differing degrees of antigenicity between follicles. Also suggestive of this explanation is thyroid follicular hyperplasia, which tends to be more extensive in areas of infiltration (51,52) (Fig. 23A.7). Antithyroid drug treatment may markedly reduce the degree of lymphocytic infiltration, which should be kept in mind when examining individual patient samples. Although the intrathyroidal lymphocyte population is mixed, immunohistologic staining and functional studies have shown that the majority of cells are T cells and that B-cell germinal centers are much less common than in chronic autoimmune thyroiditis (Hashimoto's disease) (53,54). Intra-epithelial T cells and plasma cells can be seen both adjacent to and within the thyroid follicles. Staining for cytokines has suggested the presence of both Th1 and Th2 T cells, sometimes with a predominance of Th2 (55). There is none of the follicular destruction seen in Hashimoto's disease, despite the lymphocytic infiltration (see Chapter 21). In fact, as mentioned earlier, thyroid follicular epithelial cell size has been correlated with the intensity of the local infiltrate, which suggests local thyroid cell stimulation by TSHR-Ab (52).

Functional Analysis of Intrathyroidal T Cells

As would be expected, activated B cells and T cells are more frequent in intrathyroidal lymphocyte cultures than peripheral blood cultures. T cells in patients with AITD are reactive to processed thyroid antigens (as peptides) (56). Such activated T cells enhance antibody (anti-Tg, anti-TPO, and TSHR-Ab) production and have helper and regulatory functions. About 10% of activated T cells infiltrating the thyroid gland in patients with AITD proliferate in response to thyroid cell antigens (57). In Graves' disease, intrathyroidal T-cell clones, when grown under appropriate conditions, are primarily Th2 with considerable T-cell helper activity (58,59) (Table 23A.3). This supports the concept that the functional role of T cells in Graves' disease is primarily a helper role rather than a suppressor or cytotoxic role.

TABLE 23A.3. CHARACTERISTICS OF INTRATHYROIDAL T-CELL CLONES

Source	n	CD4+	CD8+	MLR[a]	Thyroid	Cytotoxic
PBMC	21	100%	0	55%	0	ND
Graves' disease	21	75%	25%	50%	33%	0
Hashimoto's disease	36	41%	58%	55%	11%	14%

Data were expressed as % cells exhibiting autologous mixed lymphocyte reactions.
[a]Proliferation in response to crude thyroid antigen (thyroid), or lysis of autologous thyroid cells (cytotoxic).
MLR, mixed lymphocyte reaction; ND, not done; PBMC, peripheral blood mononuclear cells.
From Mackenzie WA, Schwartz AE, Friedman EW, et al. Intrathyroidal T-cell clones from patients with autoimmune thyroid disease. *J Clin Endocrinol Metab* 1987;64:818, with permission.

Apoptosis in Graves' Disease

It is now clear that deletion of T cells is achieved via apoptosis, and there are a number of pathways that signal this mechanism via T-cell surface molecules such as Fas antigen. Such signaling is initiated by binding of Fas ligand expressed, for example, by thymic epithelium; regulatory T cells, and even thyroid cells, may be involved in this pathway (see later in the chapter) (60). Autoimmune disease is a reflection of the failure to delete or anergize antigen-specific T cells, in other words, a failure to achieve tolerance of thyroid self. However, controversy has arisen over the importance of the role of thyroid cell apoptosis in autoimmune thyroiditis, and this will be dealt with elsewhere in this volume (see Chapter 47). There is, however, evidence that thyroid cells may become apoptosed even in hypertrophied Graves' thyroid glands (61), but this is a minor population of cells and may be the normal response to coincidental thyroiditis and dividing thyroid cells.

The Intrathyroidal T-Cell Receptor V Gene Repertoire

Most antigen receptors on the surface of T cells consist of two noncovalently linked chains (α and β), each with variable (V), diversity (D) (mainly β), and junctional (J) regions with common constant (Cα and Cβ) regions (62). Other T cells of less-certain function have γ/δ receptors. The V, D, and J genes code for recognition of the antigen-HLA complex by the T-cell receptor, affording antigen specificity. In addition to the many V (> 100) and J (> 50) genes present in the genome, random nucleotide (N) additions and deletions to the D region add immense complexity to the T-cell antigen receptor repertoire, causing this region, referred to as the third complementarity determining region (CDR3), to be of prime importance in antigen recognition (63). Most studies of intrathyroidal T cells have demonstrated bias in V gene utilization by T cells from within the thyroid as compared with peripheral blood from the same patient (11,64) (Fig. 23A.8). Evidence has also been sought for clonal expansion of T-cell populations within the thyroid gland of patients by direct sequencing of the CDR3 regions of the T-cell antigen receptors of in-

trathyroidal T cells generated by reverse transcription–polymerase chain reaction (RT-PCR). The most prominent V-gene families were indeed representative of clonally expanded T cells, based on the evidence of multiple identical sequences within the generated fragments (65). Such information once again supports the concept of pauciclonal intrathyroidal T-cells in Graves' disease and points to the importance of T-cells in disease etiology. Identical T-cell antigen receptors have also been shown to occur within the thyroid and retroorbital tissues of patients with Graves'

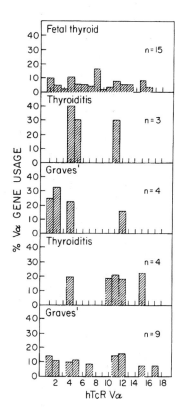

FIGURE 23A.8. Results of Southern blot analyses of thyroid tissue from a normal fetus, two patients with Graves' disease, and two patients with autoimmune thyroiditis. Results are shown as densitometric measurements of Vα gene fragments. Note the reduced V gene use in the tissue from the four patients as compared with the widespread use in the fetal thyroid. *n*, number of V-gene families detected.

thyroid and eye disease (64). A similar T-cell receptor bias has been observed in many other autoimmune diseases, including rheumatoid arthritis and multiple sclerosis (Fig. 23A.8). We, and others, have suggested that highly restricted T-cell responses occur early in autoimmune disease, but that, as the pathologic process progresses, the response is less restricted secondary to "determinant spreading" and bystander activation (see later in the chapter) (66–68).

Regulatory Effects of T Cells in Autoimmune Thyroid Disease

With the identification of the CD4+/CD25+ T-cell subset as a major regulatory cell population (3,69), these cells have been reported to be abnormal in some immune diseases, including experimental autoimmune thyroiditis (69). Their importance in human AITD is uncertain because other mechanisms are in place to maintain thyroid-specific tolerance. These include:

1. The secretion of inhibitory cytokines by immune cells.
2. The induction of anergized T cells because of the absence of second signals.
3. The induction of apoptosis leading to immune-cell deletion.

T-Cell Selection

Positive and negative selection of T cells and B cells occurs in the thymus and in the peripheral immune system (70,71). TSH-R and Tg have been shown to be expressed by thymic epithelial cells (72). Thyroid-reactive T cells should, in principal, therefore, be removed or anergized within the thymus, and if they escape deletion at that site, they should normally be deleted by peripheral mechanisms. Anergy occurs when T cells and B cells bind antigen in the absence of second signals, as discussed earlier. The resulting anergized T cells have potent suppressive actions and may act as regulatory cells (73), but are also subject to apoptosis. Early data demonstrated that certain HLA-DR haplotypes conferred a reduced nonspecific regulatory T-cell function. For example, normal subjects with HLA-DR3 had reduced suppressor T-cell activity as compared with non-DR3 subjects (74,75), associated with reduced IL-2 secretion and impaired lymphocyte apoptosis (76,77).

IMMUNE MECHANISMS IN THE PATHOGENESIS OF GRAVES' DISEASE

Several possible explanations for the onset of all autoimmune diseases, including Graves' disease, have been hypothesized on the basis of how the immune system works (Table 23A.3). However, only recently have clear experimental data been generated in the exploration of these hypotheses. Here we review just a few of these hypotheses and

the evidence for, or against, their involvement in Graves' disease.

Self-Antigen Expression

Viral infection may lead to the virus becoming a persistent endogenous antigen, or in theory may lead to overexposure of previously sequestered or unexposed antigens. For example, transgenic mice expressing lymphocytic chorismeningitis (LCM) virus antigens in pancreatic β cells, when challenged with LCM virus, developed lymphocytic infiltrates in their β cells and then diabetes mellitus (78). Expression of retroviral protein has been reported in thyroid tissue from patients with AITD, but confirmation has not been forthcoming (see later in the chapter).

Failure of Deletion

TSH-R and Tg are expressed in the thymus and lead to central deletion of autoreactive T cells. In autoimmune diabetes (type 1), variations in the thymic expression of insulin have been related to a failure to delete insulin-reactive T cells (79). However, this was not related to the insulin itself, but rather to transcriptional regulation of its expression. Similar phenomena may play a role in other autoimmune diseases. The autoimmune regulator gene (AIRE) has been shown to be a major regulator of intrathymic gene expression (80). However, this gene has not been linked to or associated with AITD.

Specificity Crossover (Molecular Mimicry)

Structural similarity between antigens encoded by different genes can lead to crossover of specificity (81). Antigenic similarity between infectious agents and host-cell proteins is common, and in one analysis of 600 monoclonal antibodies raised against a large variety of viruses, 4% crossreacted with host determinants expressed in uninfected tissues (82). Mice infected with reovirus type 1 develop an autoimmune polyendocrinopathy and generate antibodies directed against normal pancreas, pituitary, thyroid, and gastric mucosa, which suggests antigenic similarity between a retroviral antigen and a tissue antigen expressed in multiple endocrine tissues (83). Molecular mimicry has also been reported between *Yersinia enterocolitica* and the TSH-R, based on the crossreaction between *Y. enterocolitica* and serum from patients with Graves' disease. Similar observations have been made between retroviral sequences and the TSH-R (84). However, there is no evidence that either *Y. enterocolitica* or retroviral infection leads to Graves' disease.

Bystander Effects

A potential mechanism for inducing thyroid autoimmunity *in vivo* would be a local viral infection that would induce an inflammatory reaction and stimulate production of γ-interferon and/or other cytokines by nonthyroid-specific (bystander) immune cells infiltrating the thyroid gland. This activity would have an effect on any resident thyroid-specific T cells within the gland. Such activity within the gland would also induce expression of HLA class II molecules on thyroid epithelial cells. HLA class II expression would endow the thyroid cell with the potential ability to self-present its own autoantigens in a unique way (see later in the chapter) and would induce further activation of resident thyroid-specific autoreactive T cells and development of disease. This bystander hypothesis has experimental support in NOD mice, in which pancreatic inflammation induced with Coxsackie B4 virus (85) was followed by autoimmune diabetes. Of course, this explanation assumes there are thyroid-specific T cells standing by in the gland of susceptible individuals. There is evidence of the failure to lose thyroid-specific T cells from the Graves' thyroid gland (86), but there are no data analyzing the glands of susceptible individuals before the onset of disease. We have used a murine model of experimental autoimmune thyroiditis to examine bystander effects. When we transferred Tg-specific T cells, labeled with a green fluorescent tag into naive hosts, they accumulated in the host thyroids. However, the infiltrate was not just of green cells but also of host lymphocytes, indicating they had been attracted into the gland as a result of bystander activation (87).

Thyroid Cell Expression of Histocompatibility Antigen Molecules

Major histocompatibility complex (MHC) class II molecules (HLA-DR, DP, DQ in humans) are expressed on thyroid cells from patients with AITD but not on the thyroid cells from normal subjects (Fig. 23A.9) (88). Because T-cell derived cytokines, such as γ-interferon, are well known to be able to overexpress HLA class I molecules and to induce the expression of class II molecules on thyroid epithelial cells, this thyroid cell phenomenon has been considered to be a secondary response. For example, *in vivo* induction of MHC class II molecules on thyroid follicular cells by γ-interferon can induce autoimmune thyroiditis in susceptible mice (89). However, viruses may also be able to directly induce the expression of class II MHC molecules independently of cytokine secretion (90). Cultured rat thyroid cells infected with reovirus types 1 and 3 expressed MHC class II antigens in a dose-dependent manner in the absence of T cells (91). Cytomegalovirus infection of primary cultures of human thyroid cells also resulted in induction of HLA-DR expression on the cells (92). This approach would fit the original hypothesis of aberrant HLA expression of Bottazzo et al. (93). In support of this hypothesis is one of the mouse models of Graves' disease (94,95). The Shimojo model is dependent on the constitutive expression of MHC class II antigens on TSH-expressing L-fibroblast cells used as immunizing antigen. Such a model provides additional evidence for this potential mechanism of thyroid antigen presentation. Nevertheless, there are currently no data to support a direct induction of thyroid cell HLA expression as the initiator of human thyroid disease.

Evidence for Thyroid Cells as Antigen-Presenting Cells

In order for many of these hypotheses to be attractive, the thyroid antigen presentation to the immune system must occur within the gland itself. All cells that express HLA molecules have the potential to present antigen directly to T cells. Efficient APCs such as dendritic cells and B cells are plentiful in the Graves' thyroid gland (96,97). However, it is also possible that the thyroid epithelial cells

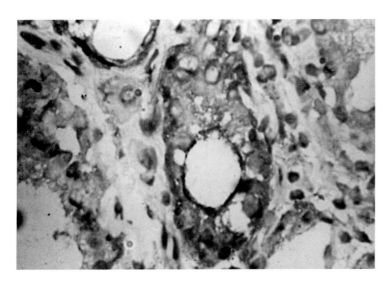

FIGURE 23A.9. HLA-DR expression (*dark immuno-per-oxidase-stained areas*) in thyroid tissue from a patient with Graves' disease (200× magnification).

TABLE 23A.4. SUMMARY OF EVIDENCE THAT THYROID CELLS MAY ACT AS ANTIGEN-PRESENTING CELLS

HLA-DR positive thyroid cells will stimulate an autologous mixed lymphocyte reaction with proliferation of helper T cells.

Coculture of thyroid cells and peripheral blood mononuclear cells from patients with Graves' disease leads to γ production and thyroid cell HLA-DR expression.

Human thyroid epithelial cells were able to present an influenza-specific peptide to a peptide-specific human T-cell clone a reaction that was blocked by HLA class II antibody. However, the thyroid cells were unable to process complex antigen (intact influenza virus) for presentation.

Thyroid epithelial cells were capable of phagocytosis but at a slower rate than macrophages. This function was inhibited by interleukin-1, methimazole, and dexamethasone, but enhanced by interleukin-2 and interferon-γ.

A cloned line of thyroid cells from Wistar rats was able to interact directly with cloned antigen-specific T cells in the absence of other antigen presenting cells.

Expression of CD40 antigen on thyroid epithelial cells.

HLA, histocompatibility antigens.
From Davies TF. Co-culture of human thyroid monolayer cells and autologous T cells: impact of HLA class II antigen expression. *J Clin Endocrinol Metab* 1985;61:418 (152); Eguchi K, Otsubo T, Kawabe K, et al. The remarkable proliferation of helper T cell subset in response to autologous thyrocytes and intrathyroidal T cells from patients with Graves' disease. *Isr J Med Sci* 1987;70:403 (153); Iwatani Y, Gerstein HC, Iitaka M, et al. Thyrocyte HLA-DR expression and gamma interferon production in autoimmune thyroid disease. *J Clin Endocrinol Metab* 1986;63:695 (154); Londei M, Lamb JR, Bottazzo GF, et al. Epithelial cells expressing aberrant MHC class II determinants can present antigen to cloned human T cells. *Nature* 1984;312:639; Matsunaga M. The effects of cytokines, antithyroidal drugs, and glucocorticoids on phagocytosis by thyroid cells. *Acta Endocrinol (Copenh)* 1988;119: 413 (155); Kimura H, Davies TF. Thyroid-specific T cells in the normal Wistar rat. II. T cell clones interact with cloned Wistar rat thyroid cells and provide direct evidence for autoantigen presentation by thyroid epithelial cells. *Clin Immunol Immunopathol* 1991;58:195; and Metcalfe RA, McIntosh RS, Marelli-Berg F, et al. Detection of CD40 on human thyroid follicular cells: analysis of expression and function. *J Clin Endocrinol Metab* 1998;83:1268, with permission.

themselves present thyroid antigen directly (see Fig. 23A.2; Table 23A.4). Thyroid follicular cells bearing HLA class II determinants can present preprocessed viral peptide antigens to cloned human T cells (98). In addition, thyroid antigen-specific T-cell clones react specifically with cloned autologous thyroid cells in the absence of conventional antigen-presenting cells, suggesting the presence of secondary signals as well as presentation (99). The observation of CD40 cofactor expression on thyroid cells also supports this potential property of human thyroid cells (100). However, as discussed earlier, HLA antigen expression in the absence of second signal would have the opposite effect, exerting a suppressive influence on the local immune response, and there is evidence of such protection in certain circumstances (101,102).

Lessons from Animal Models

Induced animal models of autoimmune disease rely on mechanisms that differ from the apparently spontaneous disease in patients, but have provided much of our basic understanding of disease mechanisms. Immunization of mice with recombinant TSH-R extracellular domain resulted in thyroid failure rather than thyroid overactivity (103). However, both Shimojo et al (94,95) and Costagliola et al (104) reported new approaches to the induction of Graves'

disease in mice, the former using fibroblasts expressing the human TSH-R, as discussed earlier in the chapter, and the latter using human TSH-R complementary DNA immunizations. More recently, a highly effective immunizing agent has been shown to be an adenovirus construct incorporating the full length TSH-R (46). The immunized mice became hyperthyroid and had many, but not all, of the features of Graves' disease, including thyroid-stimulating antibodies and markedly increased serum triiodothyronine and thyroxine levels, and weight loss and hyperactivity. Their thyroids had the histological features of thyroid hyperactivity, including thyroid cell hypertrophy and colloid droplet formation—all consistent with Graves' disease (Fig. 23A.10)—and some investigators have observed retroorbital tissue involvement. However, the only model to have an intrathyroidal lymphocytic infiltrate has been a hamster model—perhaps because of their outbred nature (105). Monoclonal antibodies to the TSH-R obtained in these models were discussed earlier. These results have demonstrated that immunization with human TSH-R expressed on mammalian cells, in the presence of MHC class II antigen, induced functional TSH-R autoantibodies that stimulated the host thyroid gland. Interestingly, some animals developed gross thyroid failure rather than hyperthyroidism, and both TSH-R-stimulating and -blocking antibodies were formed, again reminiscent of human Graves' disease.

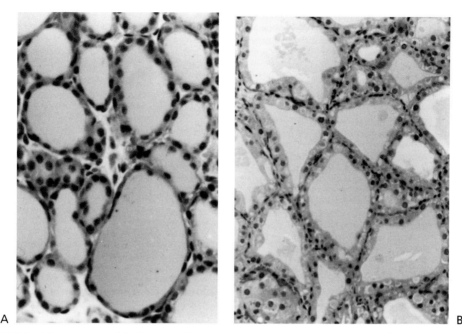

FIGURE 23A.10. A model of Graves' disease. A. Thyroid histology of a normal mouse. B. Thyroid histology of a mouse immunized with thyrotropin (TSH) receptors. (From Kita M, Ahmad L, Marians RC, et al. Regulation and transfer of a murine model of thyrotropin receptor mediated Graves' disease. *Endocrinology* 1999;140:1392, with permission.)

KNOWN RISK FACTORS FOR GRAVES' DISEASE

Susceptibility Genes and the Precipitation of Graves' Disease

The genetics of AITD are discussed at length in Chapter 20. Graves' disease is a complex genetic disease with several gene loci involved (Table 23A.5). However, it is important to note here that for Graves' disease to occur, the individual must be susceptible and that a large part of this susceptibility is inherited, as shown by a sibling recurrence risk (λs) of 11.6 for Graves' disease (106,107). Presumably, this inherited susceptibility is expressed via the presence of T cells and B cells, which induce AITD under appropriately abnormal conditions secondary to molecular mimicry or bystander stimulation. Only some of the factors likely to precipitate Graves' disease are known; these include infection, thyroid autoantibodies, trauma and injury, stress, sex steroids, pregnancy, iodine, and irradiation (Table 23A.5).

Infection

For infection to be defined as the cause of Graves' disease, an identifiable agent should, in theory, be present in the majority of patients and transfer of the agent should transfer the disease. As discussed earlier, some data have directly and indirectly implicated infectious agents in the possible immune mechanisms involved in the pathogenesis of Graves' disease (108). The disease has been associated with a variety of infectious agents (e.g., *Y. enterocolitica*; 109–111), but there is no evidence that such infections lead directly to it. Infection of the thyroid gland itself (e.g., subacute thyroiditis, congenital rubella) is associated with thyroid autoimmune phenomena, including thyroid autoantibody secretion and the development of AITD (for review, see reference 108), and, therefore, AITD may be the common endpoint of many different infections working via their bystander effect (see earlier in the chapter). However, the causative role of infectious agents in Graves' disease is unproven. Autoimmune thyroiditis can be induced in experimental animals by certain viral infections, but Graves' disease does not ensue. Reports of retroviral sequences in the thyroid glands of patients with Graves' disease have not been substantiated (112–116).

Thyroid Autoantibodies

The Whickham survey in the northeast of England followed a community for 20 years and confirmed that the presence of ant-TPO and anti-Tg antibodies more than doubled the risk of developing clinical AITD (117). There are also data that produce the propensity to produce thyroid autoantibodies is an autosomal dominant trait (118), and recent data have linked this propensity to the CTLA-4 gene, which codes for a modulator of the second signal for T-cell activation (119). Lastly, there is a large literature on the presence of TSHR-Ab as a predictor of recurrence of Graves' disease (27).

TABLE 23A.5. POTENTIAL PATHOGENIC MECHANISMS IN GRAVES' DISEASE

Immune mechanisms
  Self-antigen expression of a viral antigen or a previously
    hidden antigen
  Specificity crossover between self-antigens or an infectious
    agent
  Bystander activation
  Indirect or direct induction of thyroid cell HLA class II
    antigens
Risk factors
  External factors
    Infection
    Trauma
    Stress
    Iodine intake
    Irradiation
  Internal factors
    Thyroid autoantibodies
    Sex steroids
    Pregnancy (microchimerism, the postpartum period)
  Genetic susceptibility
    HLA
    CTLA-4
    CD40
    Thyroglobulin
    The X chromosome

HLA, histocompatibility antigens.

Tissue Damage

This may take the form of a direct insult to the thyroid by an infection or another external influence, including trauma (108,120). The mechanism for such initiation is most likely to be the activation and attraction of host immune cells and a potent bystander effect on thyroid-specific T cells. Clinical examples of this effect have been most impressive in pretibial myxedema in which recurrence is common after plastic surgery or injury (121).

Stress

The second case of thyrotoxicosis originally described by Parry in 1825 (122) was a 21-year-old woman who became symptomatic after she had fallen down the stairs in a wheelchair. Since that time, a major stress has often been associated with the onset of Graves' disease, including data on the high incidence of thyrotoxicosis among refugees from German concentration camps (123). Both acute and chronic stress induces an overall state of immune suppression by nonantigen-specific mechanisms, perhaps secondary to the effects of cortisol and corticotropin-releasing hormone at the level of the immune cell. In several studies, more patients with Graves' disease had a history of major stresses than control subjects (124–126), and women may be more susceptible to such stress (127). Acute stress-induced immune suppression may be followed by immune

system hyperactivity, which could precipitate AITD, as in the postpartum period (see later in the chapter).

Sex Steroids

Far more women than men have Graves' disease (~10:1), and some evidence suggests that sex steroids may contribute to this difference in susceptibility. Evidence in favor of such an influence includes the presentation of disease onset at the time of the menopause and the fact that Graves' disease is uncommon before puberty. Although estrogen may influence the immune system, particularly the B-cell repertoire, this influence of estrogen has been one of B-cell suppression rather than stimulation (128). Progesterone, however, favors the production of Th2-type cytokines, which would result in enhanced autoantibody production, an important component in the development of Graves' disease (129). In animals, androgen protected against estrogen enhanced thyroiditis after Tg immunization. These results provide evidence for an influence of sex steroids on the development of AITD. It remains unclear how important their influence is (130).

The X Chromosome

Women have two X chromosomes, thus potentially receiving a double dose of any susceptibility genes. Evidence suggesting a possible susceptibility gene locus on the X chromosome (131,132) has not been substantiated in larger studies (133). Interest in the role of X-chromosome inactivation in the etiology of autoimmune disease is also relevant to this discussion (134). Since women may use different X chromosomes in different tissues, it is possible that an immune response may occur from undeleted T cells interacting with antigens from a different X chromosome to the one they were tolerant to.

The Postpartum Period

The onset, or recurrence, of Graves' disease in the postpartum period offers a unique opportunity to identify those factors that herald its onset. Unfortunately, only data relating to autoantibodies are available, and the role of antigen-specific T cells has not been explored. Graves' disease sometimes appears to be aggravated in early pregnancy (135), but most patients show a falling level of TSHR-Ab at this time with a decreasing need for antithyroid drugs, in just the same way as TPO and Tg antibodies fall (135, 136). This decline in TSHR-Ab is clinically important because of the potential transfer of stimulating TSHR-Ab to the fetus (21,137). When the antibody level falls insufficiently, the fetus may be born with transient neonatal thyrotoxicosis. In addition, if the mother transfers TSHR-blocking antibodies, then transient neonatal hypothyroidism may ensue (20,138). Following delivery, and the end of the placental-driven immunosuppression, there is usually a rebound increase in the quantity of thyroid autoantibodies, including TSHR-Ab, in the serum of the mother with a peak 3 to 6 months later. The onset of new or recurrent thyrotoxicosis correlates with this rise in TSHR-Ab. Hence, the recurrence, or the new onset, of Graves' disease is seen with a similar timing as for postpartum thyroiditis and is caused by the rising levels of TSHR-Ab.

Maternal Microchimerism

During pregnancy, both T-cell and B-cell function is diminished, and the rebound from this immunosuppression is thought to contribute to the development of the postpartum thyroid syndromes. Fetal progenitor cells persist in some maternal circulations for 20 or more years after childbirth (139,140). Although it appears that this observation is not true after all pregnancies, as documented so well in experimental animals (141), when it does occur the maternal T cells may or may not have become tolerant to paternal alloantigens. Tolerance certainly appears to have occurred during a successful pregnancy but, presumably, may also be lost in the postpartum period in some women (142). However, the more different the paternal HLA class II genes (DR and DQ) when compared with the mother, and, therefore, the more different the haplotype of the fetus, the stronger the immune suppression in the resulting pregnancy. This causes a greater relief from autoimmune diseases, such as rheumatoid arthritis, during pregnancy (143). Could microchimerism explain these HLA data and contribute to the rebound and to the female preponderance in autoimmune disease, including that of the thyroid gland? Recent data from a number of groups have confirmed the presence of intrathyroidal microchimerism in patients and animals with AITD (144,145) (Fig. 23A.11). Their persistence in the postpartum period, when the immune suppression of pregnancy is no longer active, may cause them to be a major thyroid autoimmune stimulant unless a permanent state of tolerance is induced. Failure to develop such tolerance may have serious consequences. Support for this hypothesis comes from evidence that in some women these fetal cells may initiate an intradermal "graft versus host" reaction, leading to scleroderma and long-standing immune stimulation (146).

Iodine

As well as being a substrate for the production of thyroid hormones, there is evidence that iodine can act as an immune stimulant precipitating the onset of AITD and may also be directly toxic to the thyroid epithelial cell. There is strong support for increased iodination of Tg being involved in the onset of autoimmune thyroiditis (147), and polymorphisms in the Tg gene have been associated with AITD. Similarly, iodine-induced thyrotoxicosis becomes common when iodine-deficient individuals are supplemented with dietary iodide (148). This takes the form of

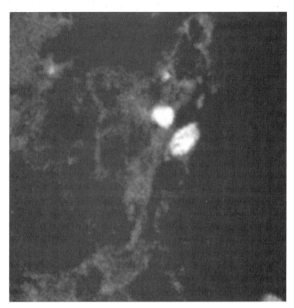

FIGURE 23A.11. Intrathyroidal fetal microchimerism in the gland of a mouse with experimental thyroiditis. By following the mating of a fluorescent green mouse with a normal female, it was possible to detect green fluorescent male fetal cells in the thyroid tissue of the pregnant female mouse who had been previously immunized with thyroglobulin and developed experimental autoimmune thyroiditis. Such observations confirmed the presence of not just male DNA within the thyroid gland but intact fetal cells, which may have pluripotential properties. Only mice with thyroiditis had significant accumulation of fetal cells within their thyroid glands. (From Ando T, Imaizumi M, Graves PN, et al. Intrathyroidal fetal microchimerism in Graves' disease. *J Clin Endocrinol Metab* 2002;87:3315–3320, with permission.)

either toxic nodular goiter or Graves' disease. In addition, patients with Graves' thyrotoxicosis become more difficult to control with antithyroid drugs if their dietary iodine intake is too high, probably because iodine increases the stores of preformed hormone. In areas of iodine sufficiency, dietary iodine probably has little influence on the onset of Graves' disease. Nevertheless, iodine-containing drugs, such as amiodarone, frequently precipitate Graves' disease in susceptible patients, particularly in iodine-deficient areas (149), while hypothyroidism is more common in iodine-replete parts of the world. This is due to the onset of either a direct toxic action on the thyroid cells or the precipitation of hypothyroidism in patients with autoimmune thyroiditis.

Irradiation

Irradiation has differential effects on T-cell subsets, setting the stage for immune dysregulation. The most impressive data for irradiation-induced thyroid autoimmunity has come from the areas downwind of the Chernobyl nuclear accident, where many of the children developed thyroid antibodies when compared with unexposed populations (150). However, there are no data yet on the precipitation of Graves' disease in these populations. Radioiodine treatment has been reported to exacerbate or precipitate ophthalmic Graves' disease, most likely by the same effects on different T-cell subsets in a susceptible population (151).

Conclusion

The intrathyroidal lymphocytic infiltrate is the initial abnormality in AITD and can be correlated with the levels of thyroid autoantibodies. In susceptible persons, mostly women, thyroid-specific T cells and B cells capable of developing Graves' disease become activated (152–155). The two major theories of autoimmune disease etiology at this time are molecular mimicry and bystander effects. Molecular mimicry relies on crossover specificity of an immune response (perhaps an extrathyroidal infection), with an intrathyroidal antigen leading to the presence of activated T cells in the gland. In the bystander hypothesis, an intrathyroidal insult such as a virus would coincidentally activate T cells present in the gland. These activated T cells would then induce the expression of HLA class I and class II antigens by the thyroid epithelial cells, which, together with their second signal potential and that of other APCs present, would provide an efficient means of clonally expanding locally infiltrated thyroid antigen-specific cells capable of initiating disease. Once activated, the thyroid-specific T cells would induce B-cell proliferation and secretion of TSHR-Ab, and hyperthyroidism would ensue.

REFERENCES

1. Davies TF, Larsen PR. Thyrotoxicosis. In: Wilson GM, Foster D, Kronenberg M, Larsen PR, eds. *Williams textbook of endocrinology.* Philadelphia: Saunders, 2002.
2. Ban Y, Greenberg DA, Concepcion E. Amino acid substitutions in the thyroglobulin gene are associated with susceptibility to human and murine autoimmune thyroid disease. *Proc Natl Acad Sci USA* 2003;100:15119–15124.
3. Shih FF, Mandik-Nayak L, Wipke BT. Massive thymic deletion results in systemic autoimmunity through elimination of CD4+ CD25+ T regulatory cells. *J Exp Med* 2004;199:323–335.
4. Romagnani S. An update on human Th1 and Th2 cells. *Int Arch Allergy Immunol* 1997;113:153–156.
5. Abbas AK, Murphy KM, Sher A, et al. Functional diversity of helper T lymphocytes. *Nature* 1996;383:787–793.
6. Tainer JA, Deal CD, Geysen HM, et al. Defining antibody-antigen recognition: towards engineered antibodies and epitopes. *Int Rev Immunol* 1991;7:165–188.
7. Weiss A. Structure and function of the T cell antigen receptor. *J Clin Invest* 1990;86:1015–1022.
8. Schwartz RH. T cell anergy. *Sci Am* 1993;269:66–71.
9. Arnold B, Schonrich G, Hammerling GJ. Multiple levels of peripheral tolerance. *Immunol Today* 1993;14:12–14.
10. Adams DD, Fastier FN, Howie JB, et al. Stimulation of the human thyroid by infusions of plasma containing LATS protector. *J Clin Endocrinol Metab* 1974;39:826–832.
11. Davies TF. T cell receptor gene expression in autoimmune thyroid disease. In: Davis MM, Buxbaum J, eds. *T cell receptor use in human autoimmune diseases,* vol. 756. New York: New York Academy of Sciences, 1995:331–344.
12. Ueki Y, Eguchi K, Otsubo T, et al. Abnormal B lymphocyte function in thyroid glands from patients with Graves' disease. *J Clin Endocrinol Metab* 1989;69:939–945.
13. Martin A, Valentine M, Unger P, et al. Engraftment of human lymphocytes and thyroid tissue into Scid and Rag2-deficient mice: absent progression of lymphocytic infiltration. *J Clin Endocrinol Metab* 1994;79:716–723.
14. McGregor AM, Petersen MM, McLachlan SM, et al. Carbimazole and the autoimmune response in Graves' disease. *N Engl J Med* 1980;303:302–304.
15. McGregor AM, Petersen MM, Capiferri R, et al. Effects of radioiodine on thyrotrophin binding inhibiting immunoglobulins in Graves' disease. *Clin Endocrinol (Oxf)* 1979;11:437–444.
16. Weetman AP. The immunomodulatory effects of antithyroid drugs. *Thyroid* 1994;4:145–146.
17. Adams DD, Purves HD. Abnormal responses in the assay of thyrotropin. *Proceedings of the University of Otago Medical School* 1956;34:11–12.
18. Rees Smith B, McLachlan SM, Furmaniak J. Autoantibodies to the thyrotropin receptor. *Endocr Rev* 1988;9:106–121.
19. Kraiem Z, Lahat N, Glaser B, et al. Thyrotropin receptor blocking antibodies: incidence, characterization and in-vitro synthesis. *Clin Endocrinol (Oxf)* 1987;27:409–421.
20. Zakarija M, McKenzie JM, Eidson MS. Transient neonatal hypothyroidism: characterization of maternal antibodies to the thyrotropin receptor. *J Clin Endocrinol Metab* 1990;70:1239–1246.
21. Zakarija M, McKenzie JM. Pregnancy-associated changes in thyroid-stimulating antibody of Graves' disease and the relationship to neonatal hyperthyroidism. *J Clin Endocrinol Metab* 1983;57:1036–1040.
22. Shewring G, Rees Smith B. An improved radioreceptor assay for TSH receptor antibodies. *Clin Endocrinol (Oxf)* 1982;17:409–411.
23. Costagliola S, Morgenthaler NG, Hoermann R, et al. Second generation assay for thyrotropin receptor antibodies has superior diagnostic sensitivity for Graves' disease. *J Clin Endocrinol Metab* 1999;84:90–97.
24. Bolton J, Sanders J, Oda Y, et al. Measurement of thyroid-stimulating hormone receptor autoantibodies by ELISA. *Clin Chem* 1999;45:2285–2287.
25. Weetman AP, McGregor AM, Hall R. Evidence for an effect of antithyroid drugs on the natural history of Graves' disease. *Clin Endocrinol (Oxf)* 1984;21:163–172.
26. Davies TF, Yeo PP, Evered DC, et al. Value of thyroid-stimulating-antibody determinations in predicting short-term thyrotoxic relapse in Graves' disease. *Lancet* 1977;1:1181–1182.
27. Davies TF. Thyroid-stimulating antibodies predict hyperthyroidism. *J Clin Endocrinol Metab* 1998;83:3777–3781.
28. Wilson R, McKillop JH, Henderson N, et al. The ability of the serum TSH receptor antibody index and HLA status to predict long-term remission of thyrotoxicosis following medical therapy for Graves' disease. *Clin Endocrinol (Oxf)* 1986;25:151–156.
29. Wood LC, Ingbar SH. Hypothyroidism as a late sequela in patients with Graves' disease treated with antithyroid agents. *J Clin Invest* 1979;64:1429–1436.
30. Weetman AP, Yateman ME, Ealey PA, et al. Thyroid-stimulating antibody activity between different immunoglobulin G subclasses. *J Clin Invest* 1990;86:723–727.
31. Libert F, Lefort A, Gerard C, et al. Cloning, sequencing and expression of the human TSH receptor: evidence for binding of autoantibodies. *Biochem Biophys Res Commun* 1989;165:1250–1255.

32. Nagayama Y, Kaufman KD, Seto P, et al. Molecular cloning, sequence and functional expression of the cDNA for the human thyrotropin receptor. *Biochem Biophys Res Commun* 1989;165:1184–1190.

33. Misrahi M, Loosfelt H, Atger M, et al. Cloning, sequencing, and expression of human TSH receptor. *Biochem Biophys Res Commun* 1990;166:394–403.

34. Sanders J, Evans M, Premawardhana LDKE, et al. Human monoclonal thyroid stimulating autoantibody. *Lancet* 2003;362:126–128.

35. Vlase H, Graves PN, Magnusson R, et al. Human autoantibodies to the TSH receptor: recognition of linear, folded and glycosylated recombinant extracellular domain. *J Clin Endocrinol Metab* 1995;80:46–53.

36. Chazenbalk GD, Pichurin P, Chen CR, et al. Thyroid-stimulating autoantibodies in Graves' disease preferentially recognize the free A subunit, not the thyrotropin holoreceptor. *J Clin Invest* 2002;110:209–217.

37. Ando T, Latif R, Davies T. First identification of three binding sites for monoclonal antibodies to the native TSH receptor. *Thyroid* 2003;13:734(abst).

38. Anderson MS, Venanzi ES, Klein L, et al. Projection of an immunological self shadow within the thymus by the aire protein. *Science* 2002;298:1395–1401.

39. Damante G, Foti D, Catalfamo R, et al. Desensitization of thyroid cyclic AMP response to thyroid stimulating immunoglobulin: comparison with TSH. *Metabolism* 1987;36:768–773.

40. Kraiem Z, Alkobi R, Sadeh O. Sensitization and desensitization of human thyroid cells in culture: effects of thyrotropin and thyroid-stimulating immunoglobulin. *J Endocrinol* 1988;119:341–349.

41. Davies TF. Positive regulation of the guinea pig thyrotropin receptor. *Endocrinology* 1985;117:201–207.

42. Huber G, Concepcion LE, Graves P, et al. Positive regulation of the human TSH receptor mRNA by recombinant human TSH is at the nuclear level. *Endocrinology* 1992;130:2858–2864.

43. Ando T, Latif R, Pritsker A, et al. A monoclonal thyroid-stimulating antibody. *J Clin Invest* 2002;110:1667–1674.

44. Sanders J, Jeffreys J, Depraetere H, et al. Thyroid-stimulating monoclonal antibodies. *Thyroid* 2002;12:1043–1050.

45. Ando T, Latif R, Davies TF. Concentration-dependent regulation of thyrotropin function by thyroid-stimulating antibody. *J Clin Invest* 2004;113:1589.

46. Nagayama Y, Kita-Furuyama M, Ando T, et al. A novel murine model of Graves' hyperthyroidism with intramuscular injection of adenovirus expressing the thyrotropin receptor. *J Immunol* 2002;168:2789–2794.

47. Jaume JC, Kakinuma A, Chazenbalk GD, et al. Thyrotropin receptor autoantibodies in serum are present at much lower levels than thyroid peroxidase autoantibodies: analysis by flow cytometry. *J Clin Endocrinol Metab* 1997;82:500–507.

48. McLachlan SM, Feldt-Rasmussen U, Young ET, et al. IgG subclass distribution of thyroid autoantibodies: a "fingerprint" of an individual's response to thyroglobulin and thyroid microsomal antigen. *Clin Endocrinol (Oxf)* 1987;26:335–346.

49. Klintschar M, Schwaiger P, Mannweiler S, et al. Evidence of fetal microchimerism in Hashimoto's thyroiditis. *J Clin Endocrinol Metab* 2001;86:2494–2498.

50. Adams DD, Kennedy TH. Occurrence in thyrotoxicosis of a gamma globulin which protects LATS from neutralization by an extract of thyroid gland. *J Clin Endocrinol Metab* 1967;27:173–177.

51. Livolsi VA. *Surgical pathology of the thyroid*. Philadelphia: Saunders, 1990.

52. Paschke R, Bruckner N, Eck T, et al. Regional stimulation of thyroid epithelial cells in Graves' disease by lymphocytic aggregates and plasma cells. *Acta Endocrinol* (Copenh) 1991;125:459–465.

53. Martin A, Goldsmith NK, Friedman EW, et al. Intrathyroidal accumulation of T cell phenotypes in autoimmune thyroid disease. *Autoimmunity* 1990;6:269–281.

54. Paschke R, Bruckner N, Schmeidl R, et al. Predominant intraepithelial localization of primed T cells and immunoglobulin-producing lymphocytes in Graves' disease. *Acta Endocrinol* (Copenh) 1991;124:630–636.

55. Srivatsa B, Srivatsa S, Johnson KL, et al. Microchimerism of presumed fetal origin in thyroid specimens from women: a case-control study. *Lancet* 2001;358:2034–2038.

56. Dayan CM, Londei M, Corcoran AE, et al. Autoantigen recognition by thyroid-infiltrating T cells in Graves' disease. *Proc Natl Acad Sci USA* 1991;88:7415–7419.

57. Mackenzie WA, Schwartz AE, Friedman EW, et al. Intrathyroidal T cell clones from patients with autoimmune thyroid disease. *J Clin Endocrinol Metab* 1987;64:818–824.

58. Martin A, Schwartz AE, Friedman EW, et al. Successful production of intrathyroidal human T cell hybridomas: evidence for intact helper T cell function in Graves' disease. *J Clin Endocrinol Metab* 1989;69:1104–1108.

59. Watson PF, Pickerill AP, Davies R, et al. Analysis of cytokine gene expression in Graves' disease and multinodular goiter. *J Clin Endocrinol Metab* 1994;79:355–360.

60. Arscott PL, Knapp J, Rymaszewsi M, et al. Fas (APO-1, CD95)-mediated apoptosis in thyroid cells is regulated by a labile protein inhibitor. *Endocrinology* 1997;138:5019.

61. Hiromatsu Y, Hoshino T, Yagita H, et al. Functional Fas ligand expression in thyrocytes from patients with Graves' disease. *J Clin Endocrinol Metab* 1999;84:2896–2902.

62. Malissen M, Minard K, Mjolsness S, et al. Mouse T cell antigen receptor: structure and organization of constant and joining gene segments encoding the beta polypeptide. *Cell* 1984;37:1101–1110.

63. Davis MM, Bjorkman PJ. T-cell antigen receptor genes and T-cell recognition. *Nature* 1988;334:395–402.

64. Heufelder AE, Herterich S, Ernst G, et al. Analysis of retroorbital T cell antigen receptor variable region gene usage in patients with Graves' opthalmopathy. *Eur J Endocrinol* 1995;132:266–277.

65. Nakashima M, Martin A, Davies TF. Intrathyroidal T cell accumulation in Graves' disease: delineation of mechanisms based on in situ T cell receptor analysis. *J Clin Endocrinol Metab* 1996;81:3346–3351.

66. Davies T, Concepcion E, Ben Nun A, et al. T-cell receptor V gene usage in autoimmune thyroid disease: direct assessment by thyroid aspiration. *J Clin Endocrinol Metab* 1993;76:660–666.

67. Matsuoka N, Martin A, Concepcion ES, et al. Preservation of functioning human thyroid organoids in the *scid* mouse. II. Biased use of intrathyroidal T cell receptor V genes. *J Clin Endocrinol Metab* 1993;77:311–315.

68. Lehmann PV, Sercarz EE, Forsthuber T, et al. Determinant spreading and the dynamics of the autoimmune repertoire. *Immunol Today* 1993;14:203–208.

69. Morris GP, Chen LP, Kong YCM. CD137 signaling interferes with activation and function of regulatory CD4(+)CD25(+) T cells in induced tolerance to experimental autoimmune thyroiditis (EAT). *FASEB J* 2003;17:C259.

70. Jenkins M. The role of cell division in the induction of clonal anergy. *Immunol Today* 1992;13:69–73.

71. Morahan G, Hoffmann M, Miller J. A nondeletional mechanism of peripheral tolerance in T-cell receptor transgenic mice. *Proc Natl Acad Sci USA* 1992;88:11421–11425.

72. Spitzweg C, Joba W, Heufelder AE. Expression of thyroid-related genes in human thymus. *Thyroid* 1999;9:133–141.

73. Lombardi G, Sidhu S, Batchelor R, et al. Anergic T cells as suppressor cells in vitro. *Science* 1994;264:1587–1589.

74. Ambinder JM, Chiorazzi N, Gibofsky A, et al. Special characteristics of cellular immune function in normal individuals of the HLA-DR3 type. *Clin Immunol Immunopathol* 1982;23:269–274.

75. Kallenberg CGM, Klaassen RJL, Beelen JM, et al. HLA-B8/DR3 phenotype and the primary immune response. *Clin Immunol Immunopathol* 1985;34:135–140.

76. Stassi G, Todaro M, De Maria R, et al. Defective expression of CD95 (FAS/APO-1) molecule suggests apoptosis impairment of T and B cells in HLA-B8, DR3-positive individuals. *Hum Immunol* 1997;55:39–45.

77. Candore G, Cigna D, Gervasi F, et al. In vitro cytokine production by HLA-B8,DR3 positive subjects. *Autoimmunity* 1994;18:121–132.

78. Oldstone MBA, Nerenberg M, Southern P, et al. Virus infection triggers insulin-dependent diabetes mellitus in a transgenic model: role of anti-self (virus) immune response. *Cell* 1991;65:319–331.

79. Puglise A, Zeller M, Fernandez Jr A, et al. The insulin gene is transcribed in the human thymus and transcription levels correlate with allelic variation at the INS VNTR-IDDM2 susceptibility locus for type 1 diabetes. *Nat Genet* 1997;15:293–297.

80. Pitkanen J, Peterson P. Autoimmune regulator: from loss of function to autoimmunity. *Genes Immun* 2003;4:12–21.

81. Oldstone MBA. Molecular mimicry and autoimmune diseases. *Cell* 1987;50:819–820.

82. Srinivasappa J, Saegusa J, Prabhakar BS, et al. Molecular mimicry: frequency of reactivity of monoclonal antiviral antibodies with normal tissues. *J Virol* 1986;57:397–401.

83. Haspel MV, Onodera T, Prabhakar BS, et al. Virus-induced autoimmunity: monoclonal antibodies that react with endocrine tissues. *Science* 1983;220:304–306.

84. Burch HB, Nagy EV, Lukes YG, et al. Nucleotide and amino acid homology between the human thyrotropin receptor and HIV-1 nef protein: identification and functional analysis. *Biochem Biophys Res Commun* 1991;181:498–505.

85. Horwitz MS, Bradley LM, Harbertson J, et al. Diabetes induced by Coxsackie virus: initiation by bystander damage and not molecular mimicry [see comments]. *Nat Med* 1998;4:781–785.

86. Valentine M, Martin A, Unger P, et al. Preservation of functioning human thyroid "organoids" in the *scid* mouse. III. Thyrotropin independence of thyroid follicle formation. *J Clin Endocrinol Metab* 1994;134:1225–1230.

87. Arata N, Ando T, Davies T. By-stander activation in autoimmune thyroiditis: studies on experimental autoimmune thyroiditis in the green fluorescent mouse. *Thyroid* 2003;13:707.

88. Hanafusa T, Pujol Borrell R, Chiovato L, et al. Aberrant expression of HLA-DR antigen on thyrocytes in Graves' disease: relevance for autoimmunity. *Lancet* 1983;2:1111–1115.

89. Kawakami Y, Kuzuya N, Watanabe T, et al. Induction of experimental thyroiditis in mice by recombinant interferon gamma administration. *Acta Endocrinol (Copenh)* 1990;122:41–48.

90. Massa PT, Dorries R, Meulen V. Viral particles induce Ia antigen expression on astrocytes. *Nature* 1986;320:543–546.

91. Neufeld DS, Platzer M, Davies TF. Reovirus induction of MHC class II antigen in rat thyroid cells. *Endocrinology* 1989;124:543–545.

92. Khoury E, Pereira L, Greenspan F. Induction of HLA-DR expression on thyroid follicular cells by cytomegalovirus infection in vitro. *Am J Pathol* 1991;138:1209–1223.

93. Bottazzo GF, Pujol Borrell R, Hanafusa T, et al. Role of aberrant HLA-DR expression and antigen presentation in induction of endocrine autoimmunity. *Lancet* 1983;2:1115–1119.

94. Shimojo N, Kohno Y, Yamaguchi K-I, et al. Induction of Graves'-like disease in mice by immunization with fibroblasts transfected with the thyrotropin receptor and a class II molecule. *Proc Natl Acad Sci U S A* 1996;93:11074–11079.

95. Kita M, Ahmad L, Marians RC, et al. Regulation and transfer of a murine model of thyrotropin receptor antibody mediated Graves' disease. *Endocrinology* 1999;140:1392–1398.

96. Kabel PJ, Voorbij HA, De Haan M, et al. Intrathyroidal dendritic cells. *J Clin Endocrinol Metab* 1988;66:199–207.

97. Hutchings P, Rayner DC, Champion BR, et al. High efficiency antigen presentation by thyroglobulin-primed murine spleen B cells. *European J Immunol* 1987;17:393–398.

98. Londei M, Lamb JR, Bottazzo GF, et al. Epithelial cells expressing aberrant MHC class II determinants can present antigen to cloned human T cells. *Nature* 1984;312:639–641.

99. Kimura H, Davies TF. Thyroid-specific T cells in the normal Wistar rat. II. T cell clones interact with cloned wistar rat thyroid cells and provide direct evidence for autoantigen presentation by thyroid epithelial cells. *Clin Immunol Immunopathol* 1991;58:195–206.

100. Metcalfe RA, McIntosh RS, Marelli-Berg F, et al. Detection of CD40 on human thyroid follicular cells: analysis of expression and function. *J Clin Endocrinol Metab* 1998;83:1268–1274.

101. Tang H, Sharp GC, Peterson KP, et al. IFN-gamma-deficient mice develop severe granulomatous experimental autoimmune thyroiditis with eosinophil infiltration in thyroids. *J Immunol* 1998;160:5105–5112.

102. Caturegli P, Hejazi M, Suzuki K, et al. Hypothyroidism in transgenic mice expressing IFN-gamma in the thyroid. *Proc Natl Acad Sci U S A* 2000;97:1719–1724.

103. Vlase H, Weiss M, Graves PN, et al. Characterization of the murine immune response to the murine TSH receptor ectodomain: induction of hypothyroidism and TSH receptor antibodies. *Clin Exp Immunol* 1998;113:111–118.

104. Costagliola S, Rodien P, Many MC, et al. Genetic immunization against the TSH receptor causes thyroiditis and allows production of monoclonal antibodies recognizing the native receptor. *J Immunol* 1998;160:1458–1465.

105. Ando T, Imaizumi M, Graves P, et al. Induction of thyroid-stimulating hormone receptor autoimmunity in hamsters. *Endocrinology* 2003;144:671–680.

106. Tomer Y, Davies TF. The genetic susceptibility to Graves' disease. *Bailliere's Clin Endocrinol Metab* 1997;11:431–450.

107. Villanueva R, Greenberg DA, Davies TF, et al. Sibling recurrence risk in autoimmune thyroid disease. *Thyroid* 2003;13:761–764.

108. Tomer Y, Davies TF. Infection, thyroid disease and autoimmunity. *Endocr Rev* 1993;14:107–120.

109. Lidman K, Eriksson U, Norberg R, et al. Indirect immunofluorescence staining of human thyroid by antibodies occurring in *Yersinia enterocolitica* infections. *Clin Exp Immunol* 1976;23:429–435.

110. Wenzel BE, Heeseman J, Wenzel KW, et al. Antibodies to plasmid-encoded proteins of enteropathogenic *Yersinia* in patients with autoimmune thyroid disease. *Lancet* 1988;1:56–59.

111. Toivanen P, Toivanen A. Does Yersinia induce autoimmunity? *Int Arch Allergy Immunol* 1994;104:107–111.

112. Ciampolillo A, Mirakian R, Schulz T, et al. Retrovirus-like sequences in Graves' disease: implications for human autoimmunity. *Lancet* 1989;1:1096–1099.

113. Wick G, Trieb K, Aguzzi A, et al. Possible role of human foamy virus in Graves' disease. *Intervirology (Basel)* 1993;35:101–107.

114. Lagaye S, Vexiau P, Morozov V, et al. Human spumaretrovirus-related sequences in the DNA of leukocytes from patients with

Graves' disease. *Proc Natl Acad Sci USA* 1992;89:10070–10074.

115. Humphrey M, Baker JR Jr, Carr FE, et al. Absence of retroviral sequences in Graves' disease. *Lancet* 1991;337:17–18.

116. Neumann-Haefelin D, Fleps U, Renne R, et al. Foamy viruses. *Intervirology (Basel)* 1993;35:196–207.

117. Vanderpump MPJ, Tunbridge WMG, French JM, et al. The incidence of thyroid disorders in the community: a twenty-year follow-up of the Whickham survey. *Clin Endocrinol (Oxf)* 1995;43:55–68.

118. Phillips D, Prentice L, Upadhyaya M, et al. Autosomal dominant inheritance of autoantibodies to thyroid peroxidase and thyroglobulin—studies in families not selected for autoimmune thyroid disease. *J Clin Endocrinol Metab* 1991;72:973–975.

119. Tomer Y, Greenberg DA, Barbesino G, et al. CTLA-4 and not CD28 is a susceptibility gene for thyroid autoantibody production. *J Clin Endocrinol Metab* 2001;86:1687–1693.

120. Davies TF. Trauma and pressure explain the clinical presentation of the Graves' disease triad. *Thyroid* 2000;10:629–630.

121. Rapoport B, Alsabeh R, Aftergood D, et al. Elephantiasic pretibial myxedema: insight into (and a hypothesis regarding) the pathogenesis of the extrathyroidal manifestations of Graves' disease. *Thyroid* 2000;10:685–692.

122. Parry CH. Disease of the heart. *Collections from the unpublished writings,* vol. 2. London: Underwoods, 1825:111–125.

123. Weisman SA. Incidence of thyrotoxicosis among refugees from Nazi prison camps. *J Clin Endocrinol Metab* 1958;48:747–752.

124. Leclere J, Weryha G. Stress and auto-immune endocrine diseases. *Horm Res* 1989;31:90.

125. Winsa B, Adami H-O, Bergstrom R, et al. Stressful life events and Graves' disease. *Lancet* 1991;338:1475–1479.

126. Sonino N, Girelli M, Boscaro M, et al. Life events in the pathogenesis of Graves' disease: a controlled study. *Acta Endocrinologica* 1993;128:293–296.

127. Gaillard RC, Spinedi E. Sex- and stress-steroids interactions and the immune system: evidence for a neuroendocrine-immunological sexual dimorphism. *Domest Anim Endocrinol* 1998;15:345–352.

128. Kincade PW, Medina KL, Smithson G, et al. Pregnancy: a clue to normal regulation of B lymphopoiesis. *Immunol Today* 1994;15:539–544.

129. Piccinini M-P, Giudizi M-G, Biagiotti R, et al. Progesterone favors the development of human T helper cells producing Th2-type cytokines and promotes both IL-4 production and membrane CD30 expression in established Th1 cell clones. *J Immunol* 1995;155:128–133.

130. Ansar AS, Young PR, Penhale WJ. Beneficial effect of testosterone in the treatment of chronic autoimmune thyroiditis in rats. *J Immunol* 1986;136:143–147.

131. Barbesino G, Tomer Y, Concepcion ES, et al. Role of the estrogen receptor gene and the X chromosome in the genetic susceptibility to AITD. *Thyroid* 1997;7[Suppl 1]:S103(abst).

132. Imrie H, Vaidya B, Perros P, et al. Evidence for a Graves' disease susceptibility locus at chromosome Xp11 in a United Kingdom population. *J Clin Endocrinol Metab* 2001;86:626–630.

133. Tomer Y, Ban Y, Concepcion E, et al. Common and unique susceptibility loci in Graves' and Hashimoto diseases: results of whole-genome screening in a data set of 102 multiplex families. *Am J Hum Genet* 2003;73:736–747.

134. Trejo V, Derom C, Vlietinck R, et al. X chromosome inactivation patterns correlate with fetal-placental anatomy in monozygotic twin pairs: implications for immune relatedness and concordance for autoimmunity. *Mol Med* 1994;1:62–70.

135. Amino N, Tanizawa O, Mori H, et al. Aggravation of thyrotoxicosis in early pregnancy and after delivery in Graves' disease. *J Clin Endocrinol Metab* 1982;55:108–111.

136. Tamaki H, Amino N, Aozasa M, et al. Serial changes in thyroid-stimulating antibody and thyroid binding inhibitor immunoglobublin at the time of postpartum occurrence of thyrotoxicosis in Graves' disease. *J Clin Endocrinol Metab* 1987;65:324–330.

137. Munro DS, Major PW. Thyroid stimulating activity in human sera. *J Endocrinol* 1960;2:19.

138. Arikawa K, Ichikawa Y, Yoshida T, et al. Blocking type antthyrotropin receptor antibody in patients with nongoitrous hypothyroidism: its incidence and characteristics of action. *J Clin Endocrinol Metab* 1985;60:953–959.

139. Hsieh T, Pao C, Hor J, et al. Presence of fetal cells in the maternal circulation. *Hum Gene* 1993;92:204–209.

140. Bianchi DW, Zickwolf GK, Weil GJ, et al. Male fetal progenitor cells persist in maternal blood for as long as 27 years postpartum. *Proc Natl Acad Sci U S A* 1996;93:705–708.

141. Bonney EA, Matzinger P. The maternal immune system's interaction with circulating fetal cells. *J Immunol* 1997;158:40–47.

142. Harris DT, Schumbacher MJ, LoCascio J, et al. Immunoreactivity of umbilical cord blood and post-partum maternal peripheral blood with regard to HLA-haploidentical transplantation. *Bone Marrow Transplant* 1994;14:63–68.

143. Nelson JL, Hughes KA, Smith AG, et al. Maternal-fetal disparity in HLA class II alloantigens and the pregnancy-induced amelioration of rheumatoid arthritis. *N Engl J Med* 1993;329:466–471.

144. Ando T, Imaizumi M, Graves PN, et al. Intrathyroidal fetal microchimerism in Graves' disease. *J Clin Endocrinol Metab* 2002;87:3315–3320.

145. Ando T, Davies TF. Postpartum autoimmune thyroid disease: the potential role of fetal microchimerism. *J Clin Endocrinol Metab* 2003;88:2965–2971.

146. Artlett CM. Identification of fetal DNA and cells in skin lesions from women with systemic sclerosis. *N Engl J Med* 1998;338:1186–1191.

147. Sundick RS, Herdegen DM, Brown T, et al. The incorporation of dietary iodine into thyroglobulin increases its immunogenicity. *Endocrinology* 1987;120:2078–22084.

148. Liel Y, Alkan M. 'Travelers' thyrotoxicosis': transitory thyrotoxicosis induced by iodinated preparations for water purification. *Arch Intern Med* 1996;156:807–810.

149. Bartalena L, Bogazzi F, Martino E. Amiodarone-induced thyrotoxicosis: a difficult diagnostic and therapeutic challenge. *Clin Endocrinol (Oxf)* 2002;56:23–24.

150. Pacini F, Vorontsova T, Molinaro E, et al. Prevalence of thyroid autoantibodies in children and adolescents from Belarus exposed to the Chernobyl radioactive fallout. *Lancet* 1998;352:763–766.

151. Bartalena L, Marcocci C, Bogazzi F, et al. Relation between therapy for hyperthyroidism and the course of Graves' ophthalmopathy. *N Engl J Med* 1998;338:73–78.

152. Davies TF. Co-culture of human thyroid monolayer cells and autologous T cells: impact of HLA class II antigen expression. *J Clin Endocrinol Metab* 1985;61:418–422.

153. Eguchi K, Otsubo T, Kawabe K, et al. The remarkable proliferation of helper T cell subset in response to autologous thyrocytes and intrathyroidal T cells from patients with Graves' disease. *Isr J Med Sci* 1987;70:403–410.

154. Iwatani Y, Gerstein HC, Iitaka M, et al. Thyrocyte HLA-DR expression and gamma interferon production in autoimmune thyroid disease. *J Clin Endocrinol Metab* 1986;63:695–708.

155. Matsunaga M. The effects of cytokines, antithyroidal drugs, and glucocorticoids on phagocytosis by thyroid cells. *Acta Endocrinologica (Copenh)* 1988;119:413–419.

23B OPHTHALMOPATHY

PETROS PERROS
A. JANE DICKINSON

Ophthalmic abnormalities, better known as ophthalmopathy, are the principal extrathyroidal manifestations of Graves' disease. The numerous synonyms for Graves' ophthalmopathy (orbitopathy, thyroid eye disease) reflect its multifaceted clinical expression and the uncertainties about its pathogenesis, natural history, and treatment.

EPIDEMIOLOGY

Graves' ophthalmopathy is clinically evident in about a third of patients with Graves' disease, although it can be demonstrated by orbital imaging in nearly all (1–3). Its incidence seems to have declined in recent years for reasons that are unclear (3). Most patients have mild eye disease not requiring specific treatment, while approximately 5% have severe potentially sight-threatening ophthalmopathy (2). The incidence of Graves' ophthalmopathy in the United States, based on a population study, was 16/100,000 per annum for women and 2.9/100,000 per annum for men (4). The age distribution at the time of presentation shows two peaks, one at 40 to 44 years and a later one at 60 to 64 years for women, and 65 to 69 years for men (1). The female to male ratio in patients attending specialist centers is approximately 2:1 (2).

PATHOGENESIS

Current evidence favors an autoimmune pathogenesis with important genetic and environmental influences, particularly smoking (5). Orbital muscle, connective tissue, and adipose tissue are infiltrated by lymphocytes and macrophages (2). The extracellular compartment of extraocular muscles and orbital fibroadipose tissue becomes edematous, secondary to deposition of hydrophilic glycosoaminoglycans, while the muscle cells themselves are unaffected (1,5).

Anatomic Considerations

The orbit resembles a rigid cone with its base open anteriorly, where it is bounded by the semidistensible anterior orbital septum. Edematous expansion of orbital tissue has predictable consequences: dysfunction of affected muscles, increased orbital pressure, and proptosis (exophthalmos,

forward displacement of the eye). The clinical expression relating to each of these factors depends on the site and severity of inflammation and the potential for forward displacement. Several extraocular muscles, including the levator palpebrae superioris, are usually affected, although with variable frequency (2,6,7). This leads to restriction of the eye (dysmotility), lid lag, and incomplete eyelid closure. The latter may provoke sight-threatening corneal exposure, often compounded by proptosis. The degree of proptosis is limited by the length of the rectus muscles and the tightness of the anterior orbital septum. If the muscles are unable to stretch and the septum is tight, proptosis is minimal, but orbital pressure and venous congestion increase, and the rectus muscles may then compress the optic nerve at the orbital apex, with resulting visual loss. Conversely, if the septum is lax and the muscles are able to stretch, then proptosis increases, occasionally allowing subluxation of the eyeball. Acute inflammation may also cause erythema and swelling of the conjunctivae and eyelids, compounded by venous and lymphatic congestion. Muscle inflammation gives way to fatty degeneration and scarring, sometimes with further tethering and restriction. Various stages of this process may coexist in one or more muscles.

Immunology

The expansion of orbital tissues is primarily due to the edema that results from deposition of the very hydrophilic glycosaminoglycans. Orbital fibroblasts appear to synthesize and secrete these glycosoaminoglycans in response to cytokines produced by infiltrating immune cells and macrophages and by the fibroblasts themselves (5). Cytokines also stimulate orbital fibroblasts, vascular endothelium, and macrophages to produce other immunomodulatory and inflammatory mediators. These in turn aid recruitment of T cells into the orbit and antigen recognition and presentation, and therefore perpetuate the local inflammatory response (5). A cell-mediated (Th1-type) immune response appears prominent early in the evolution of Graves' ophthalmopathy, whereas humoral immunity (Th2-type), or both, may be relevant later in the course of the disease (5,6).

Evidence of autoimmune responses to thyroid antigens is invariably present in patients with Graves' ophthalmopathy, including those with euthyroid Graves' ophthalmopathy (2). An autoantigen shared by thyroid and orbit would explain the specific targeting of the latter, and the close association between Graves' thyroid disease and Graves' eye disease. The most studied and promising candidate autoantigen is the thyrotropin (TSH) receptor. This is expressed in orbital connective tissue, orbital fat (5,8,9), and extraocular muscle fibers (10), but at higher levels in patients with Graves' ophthalmopathy than normal subjects (5). Orbital connective tissue contains adipocyte precursors (preadipocytes), which under appropriate conditions can differentiate into adipocytes (11). *In vitro*, expression of TSH receptors increases as fibroblasts differentiate to preadipocytes and adipocytes (12), and both differentiation and TSH-receptor expression are stimulated by cytokines (5). These are likely events in the evolution of Graves' ophthalmopathy, because there is often an increase in orbital fat content (11). A role for antibodies to the TSH receptor is also possible (13,14). Other candidate antigens shared between the thyroid and orbital tissue include a surface antigen known as G2s, thyroglobulin (5), and the insulin-like growth factor (IGF-1) receptor (15). Two animal models for Graves' ophthalmopathy have been described. Mice immunized with the cDNAs for TSHR or G2s and TSHR appear to develop orbital infiltration similar to Graves' ophthalmopathy (5).

Genetic and Other Influences

The genetic contribution to Graves' disease is substantial (see Chapter 20). The same risks and associations apply to Graves' ophthalmopathy (16). Several studies examining genes that may distinguish between patients with Graves' disease with and without eye disease have focused on associations between ophthalmopathy and alleles at the major histocompatibility complex (MHC), cytotoxic lymphocyte-associated antigen (CTLA)-4 (17), and other loci (18). These studies have yielded contradictory results, which may be partly due to differences in allelotyping methodology, disease definition, race/ethnicity of the study subjects, and small sample sizes (16). Other factors that are associated with severe eye disease include advanced age, male sex, smoking, and persistent thyroid dysfunction, particularly hypothyroidism (1,5).

NATURAL HISTORY

The onset of eye disease usually coincides with that of the thyrotoxicosis however, exceptions are not uncommon, and Graves' ophthalmopathy can precede or follow thyrotoxicosis by months or even years (Fig. 23B.1) (2). The severity of ophthalmopathy follows a phasic pattern: a phase of progressive deterioration lasting several months; a short period of peak severity; a phase of spontaneous improvement lasting up to a year or longer; and a quiescent phase when inflammatory signs disappear and clinical features stabilize, although they do not usually resolve completely. This pattern of change in severity over time was first de-

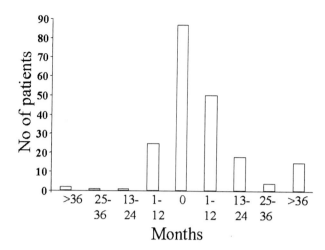

FIGURE 23B.1. Relationship between onset of Graves' ophthalmopathy and thyrotoxicosis. Most patients who ultimately have clinically important Graves' ophthalmopathy have some mild features of ophthalmopathy at the time of presentation with thyrotoxicosis (0 months). In a few patients ophthalmopathy precedes, in slightly more it follows the onset of thyrotoxicosis by 1 to 12 months, and in occasional patients the interval is much longer. (From Bartalena L, Pinchera A, Marcocci C. Management of Graves' ophthalmopathy: reality and perspectives. *Endocr Rev* 2000;21:168, with permission.)

scribed years ago (Fig. 23B.2) and has been confirmed by later studies (19). A related concept is disease activity, which relates to the presence of an acute inflammatory process within the orbit. Change in activity is implied by change in severity over time; its assessment is discussed later. Graves' ophthalmopathy rarely becomes active again once it has become quiescent, but the activity and course may vary in individual eyes (20).

CLINICAL PRESENTATION

Graves' ophthalmopathy is usually bilateral, but it may be asymmetric. The onset can be rapid or insidious. Typical

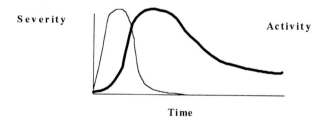

FIGURE 23B.2. The natural history of the changes in severity (*bold line*) and activity (*thin line*) of Graves' ophthalmopathy as a function of time. The phases of severity of ophthalmopathy are progressive deterioration, plateau, slow improvement, and, lastly, stability. The phases of activity of ophthalmopathy relate to changes in severity but are more prolonged. (From Rundle FF, Wilson CW. Development and course of exophthalmos and ophthalmoplegia in Graves' disease with special reference to the effect of thyroidectomy. *Clin Sci* 1945;5:177, with permission.)

TABLE 23B.1. EVALUATION OF SYMPTOMS OF GRAVES' OPHTHALMOPATHY

Patients are asked whether any of the following symptoms are present, whether the symptom has changed in the last 1 to 2 months, and its severity on a scale of 0 to 10.

Overall appearance of the eyes
  Normal
  Abnormal
Surface symptoms
  Grittiness
  Excessive watering
  Aversion to bright light
Swelling of the eyelids
Protrusion of the eyes
Pain or ache in or behind the eye
  Spontaneous orbital pain
  Pain only on gaze in a particular direction
Double vision
  Intermittent: apparent on waking but resolves, apparent only
    when tired, or apparent intermittently at other times.
  Inconstant: always present in certain directions of gaze
  Constantly present unless a particular head posture is
    adopted
  Constantly present regardless of head posture
Blurred vision
  Clears with blinking
  Clears on covering one eye
  Persistent blurring or awareness of gray areas in field of
    vision
Reduced color intensity or difference between eyes

initial symptoms relate most commonly to discomfort of the surfaces of the eyes and changes in appearance, particularly periorbital swelling (Table 23B.1). These symptoms usually develop gradually over weeks to months, and although itching is absent, misdiagnosis as allergy is common. Other common symptoms are retroorbital pain, pain provoked by gazing in particular directions, and diplopia (21). Some patients describe slight diplopia as "blurring"; however, the blurring clears with monocular occlusion (2,21). Significant dysmotility may be accompanied by a compensatory head tilt (Fig. 23B.3A). The myopathy of Graves' ophthalmopathy relates to failure of relaxation, thus impeding the action of ipsilateral antagonist muscles. Rectus muscle involvement is usually asymmetrical, with restriction most evident in the inferior and medial rectus muscles and rare in the lateral rectus muscles. Hence, upward gaze and abduction are commonly restricted. Although dysmotility affects up to 60% of patients with Graves' ophthalmopathy (2), many have no diplopia due to symmetric involvement of both orbits or amblyopia, or because the restriction affects extremes of gaze irrelevant to daily life. Optic neuropathy is uncommon, but such patients may notice blurred vision unaffected by blinking or closing one eye, reduced color appreciation, or an awareness of gray areas of field loss (2,21). Older men with diabetes and vascular disease are most at risk for optic neuropathy (21).

Most patients with ophthalmopathy develop thyroid dysfunction concurrently or several months before onset ophthalmopathy (Fig. 23B.1), but 6% to 10% have characteristic ophthalmopathy without discernible thyroid dysfunction, termed euthyroid Graves' ophthalmopathy or ophthalmic Graves' disease (2). Most of these patients have onset of thyrotoxicosis within 18 months. About 5% of patients with Graves' ophthalmopathy have primary hypothyroidism rather than thyrotoxicosis. Concealed proptosis (Fig. 23B.3) is a clinical variant in which ophthalmopathy is obscured by only minimal proptosis. It is not uncommon, and is important to recognize because of the high risk of optic neuropathy; these patients almost always have tense orbits and dysmotility, and often aching eye pain.

SEVERITY AND ACTIVITY OF EYE DISEASE

Severity is defined as the degree of functional or cosmetic deficit at any time point in the course of the disease (21). Thus, variations in periorbital edema, proptosis, diplopia, corneal integrity, and optic nerve function are measures of severity. In contrast, activity implies the presence of acute inflammation, and therefore potential for change either spontaneously or in response to medical treatment. Activity can be inferred directly when symptoms and signs of acute inflammation are present, or by demonstrating change in measures of severity via sequential assessments.

CLINICAL ASSESSMENT

The aim of initial assessment is to verify the diagnosis, ascertain severity, and determine the phase of the ophthalmopathy (Fig. 23B.2). A detailed assessment of symptoms (Table 23B.1) helps to highlight the patient's concerns and priorities, and informs mutual understanding and counselling. Ascertaining severity allows the clinician to determine the need for interventional treatment, while ascertaining activity and disease phase dictates the therapeutic options then available. Disease phase may be partly determined by a trend in symptoms, but reassessment in two to three months is sometimes required.

Diagnosis

Most signs of Graves' ophthalmopathy are nonspecific, reflecting inflammation or volume changes in extraocular muscles or other tissue within the confined retrobulbar

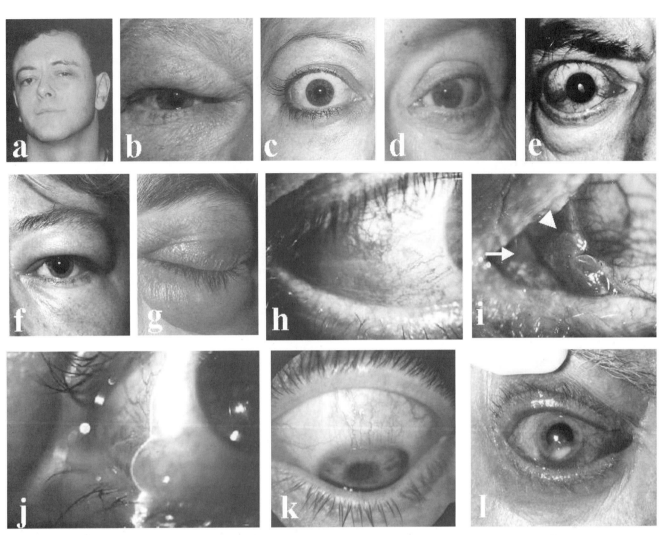

FIGURE 23B.3. Photographs of eyes of patients with Graves' ophthalmopathy. **A:** Extraocular muscle dysmotility associated with compensatory head tilt and chin-up position. **B:** Concealed proptosis (exophthalmos): acuity was 20/100 with loss of color vision. **C:** Lid retraction in a patient with inactive ophthalmopathy. **D:** Lateral flare of the contour of the upper eyelid. **E:** Proptosis and lid swelling caused by forward displacement of orbital fat in a patient with inactive ophthalmopathy. **F:** Lid swelling due to active ophthalmopathy. **G:** Eyelid festoons (marked edema of lids). **H:** Dilated superficial vessels over insertion of the lateral rectus muscle in a patient with active ophthalmopathy disease. **I:** Inflamed caruncle (*arrowhead*) and plica (*arrow*) in a patient with active ophthalmopathy. **J:** Chemosis in a patient with active ophthalmopathy (slit-lamp examination). **K:** Superior limbic keratoconjunctivitis. **L:** Corneal ulcer. (From Dickinson AJ, Perros P. Controversies in the clinical evaluation of active thyroid-associated orbitopathy: use of a detailed protocol with comparative photographs for objective assessment. *Clin Endocrinol (Oxf)* 2001;55:283, with permission; and Perros P, Dickinson AJ, Kendall-Taylor P. Clinical presentation and natural history of Graves' ophthalmopathy. In: Bahn RS, ed. *Thyroid eye disease.* Boston: Kluwer Academic Publishers, 2001:119, with permission.)

space; hence other causes of ophthalmopathy should be considered. These include myasthenia gravis, retroorbital tumors, carotid-cavernous fistula, and especially other inflammatory orbitopathies (2,22,23). Nevertheless, Graves' ophthalmopathy is the most common cause of not only bilateral but also unilateral proptosis (2,22). Typically, the combination of ophthalmic symptoms and signs plus the presence of thyrotoxicosis at that time or in the recent past will confirm the diagnosis without the need for supplementary studies (24). In patients with eyelid retraction (Fig. 23B.3C), Graves' ophthalmopathy is considered to be present if the patient has one of the following: abnormal thyroid function, proptosis, optic neuropathy, or restrictive myopathy. If eyelid retraction is absent, then thyroid dysfunction must be present together with proptosis, optic neuropathy, or restrictive myopathy to reach a confident diagnosis. Other signs that are highly suggestive of Graves' ophthalmopathy are lid lag and a change in the contour of the upper eyelid known as lateral flare (Fig. 23B.3D).

Evaluation of Disease Severity

Recommendations for objective assessment of Graves' ophthalmopathy have been proposed (25), but there is no agreement as to precisely what to score and how to define it (21). A more detailed protocol with a soft tissue atlas was published (21) and adopted by the European Group on Graves' ophthalmopathy (EUGOGO) (26); however, worldwide consensus remains elusive. Given the variable presentation of Graves' ophthalmopathy, summary descriptions are of little use, and each feature should be assessed individually. The NOSPECS scheme (Table 23B.2) provides a useful mnemonic to assist this, although as a scoring system it has been justifiably criticized for poor definitions and reproducibility, and for failing to record important change (2,21).

Assessment of Soft Tissue Changes

A complete examination protocol and photographic color atlas for assessment of the soft tissue changes that occur in patients with Graves' ophthalmopathy can be found at http://www.EUGOGO.org.

Eyelid and Periorbital Swelling

Orbital fat or lacrimal gland displacement can cause visible discrete eyelid swelling during any phase of ophthalmopathy (Fig. 23B.3E), whereas acute inflammation with subdermal fluid accumulation or tense skin thickening suggests active ophthalmopathy (Fig. 23B.3F). The edema of

TABLE 23B.2. NOSPECS CLASSIFICATION OF THE OCULAR CHANGES IN GRAVES' DISEASE

Classes	Grades	Ocular Symptoms and Signs
0		<u>N</u>o symptoms or signs
1		<u>O</u>nly (signs limited to upper lid retraction and stare, with or without lid lag and proptosis)
2		<u>S</u>oft tissue involvement (symptoms of excessive lacrimation, sandy sensation, retrobulbar discomfort, and photophobia, but not diplopia); objective signs as follows:
	0	Absent
	a	Minimal (edema of conjunctivae and lids, conjunctival injection, and fullness of lids, often with orbital fat extrusion, palpable lacrimal glands, or swollen extraocular muscle palpable beneath lower lids)
	b	Moderate (above plus chemosis, lagophthalmos lid fullness)
	c	Marked
3		<u>P</u>roptosis associated with classes 2 to 6 only (specify if inequality of 3 mm or more between eyes, or if progression of 3 mm or more under observation)
	0	Absent (20 mm or less)
	a	Minimal (21–23 mm)
	b	Moderate (24–27 mm)
	c	Marked (28 mm or more)
4		<u>E</u>xtraocular muscle involvement (usually with diplopia)
	0	Absent
	a	Minimal (limitation of motion, evident at extremes of gaze in one or more directions)
	b	Moderate (evident restriction of motion without fixation of position)
	c	Marked (fixation of position of a globe or globes)
5		<u>C</u>orneal involvement (primarily due to lagophthalmos)
	0	Absent
	a	Minimal (stippling or cornea)
	b	Moderate (ulceration)
	c	Marked (clouding, necrosis, perforation)
6		<u>S</u>ight loss (due to optic nerve involvement)
	0	Absent
	a	Minimal (disc pallor or choking, or visual field defect; vision 20/20 to 20/60)
	b	Moderate (disc pallor or choking, visual field defect, 20/70 to 20/200)
	c	Marked (blindness, i.e. failure to perceive light; vision less than 20/200)

From Werner SC. Modification of the classification of the eye changes of Graves' disease: recommendations of the Ad Hoc committee of the American Thyroid Association. *J Clin Endocrinol Metab* 1977; 44:203.

the eyelids, especially the lower lids, may be very marked (festoons) (Fig. 23B.3G), and it can persist long-term. Like many soft tissue features, lid swelling is best graded by photographic comparison to assess trend and treatment response (21).

Lid Erythema

Erythema of the eyelids implies active disease.

Conjunctival Erythema

Erythema of the bulbar conjunctivae is associated with active disease (21). Dilated superficial vessels overlying the insertion of the lateral rectus muscle (Fig. 23B.3H) may be especially prominent in patients with active ophthalmopathy (21).

Inflammation of the Caruncle or Plica

The caruncle is the triangular-shaped tissue inside the inner corner of the eyelids rich in sebaceous glands, while the plica is the vertical fold of conjunctiva just lateral to the caruncle. Inflammation in either of these structures suggests active ophthalmopathy (Fig. 23B.3I).

Chemosis

Chemosis denotes conjunctival edema (Fig. 23B.3J), which implies acute orbital congestion, a surrogate marker of retroorbital inflammation.

Superior Limbic Keratoconjunctivitis

This describes inflammation of the upper bulbar and eyelid conjunctiva where they move over one another. It occurs in about 3% of patients with active ophthalmopathy (Fig. 23B.3K) and is associated with upper lid retraction (27).

Palpebral Aperture

Widening of the palpebral fissure is usually due to retraction of both upper and lower eyelids, and is caused by multiple factors (2,21). For the upper lids these include contraction of both the levator and Müller's muscles, proptosis, scarring of the lacrimal fascia, and tightness of the inferior rectus muscle, while lower lid retraction correlates strongly with proptosis (Fig. 23B.3E). Standardized measurements require a consistent technique (distance fixation in a relaxed state, standardized head position, and, if vertical strabismus is present, occlusion of the contralateral eye). The width of the mid-pupil vertical fissure is measured, noting the distance between each lid and the adjacent limbus, plus the presence or absence of the upper lid contour abnormality known as lateral flare (Fig. 23B.3D).

Proptosis (Exophthalmos)

Proptosis is the forward displacement of the eyeball, measured clinically with an exophthalmometer. This is a measure of the position of the cornea relative to a fixed bony point, which is usually the lateral margin of the bony orbit. Normal values depend on race, age, sex, extent of myopia, and the instrument used (21). Accuracy to within two millimeters requires a consistent method with the same instrument and ideally by the same observer (21,28).

Motility

Motility can be assessed either subjectively or objectively (21). Those methods that compare the two eyes (Maddox rod test, Lancaster red-green test, prism cover test, and Hess Lees screen test) have limited use as outcome measures for patients with a bilateral disease such as Graves' ophthalmopathy, but the latter two still guide the use of prisms to improve vision and surgical management. The field of binocular single vision describes the area in which the patient has no double vision and is valuable for assessment, treatment monitoring, and surgical planning. In recent years, uniocular fields of fixation plotted by perimetry have been used as outcome measures (21,29), as they have proved the most reliable method for quantifying the excursion of each eye in different directions of gaze, thus permitting sequential analysis regardless of the muscles involved.

Cornea

Lid retraction causes relative corneal exposure, often with punctate epithelial breakdown that can be highlighted by fluorescein staining. Provided the eyelids can close to cover the cornea there is no real risk of ulceration, but if closure is incomplete, then ulceration and even perforation can occur. This usually happens when there is levator dysfunction with poor lid movement, and an absent Bell's phenomenon (no reflex upward eyeball rotation on attempted lid closure) caused by a tight inferior rectus muscle.

Intraocular Pressure

High intraocular pressure is caused by orbital venous congestion and globe compression by a tight inferior rectus, and increases further during upward gaze. This rarely progresses to true glaucoma.

Visual Function

Optic neuropathy is almost always caused by compression of the optic nerve at the apex of the orbit by grossly swollen muscles (21), but occasionally it is due to nerve stretching by extreme proptosis (30) or prolonged subluxation of the eyeball. Nearly all patients with optic neuropathy have associated dysmotility; the orbit is usually tense (assessed by palpation) and intraocular pressure is relatively high. Corrected visual acuity, color vision (blue discrimination is most sensitive), pupillary responses (swinging light test), and the appearance of the optic disc should be determined. Disc swelling is diagnostic of optic neuropathy in the absence of other causes, but other features are less reliable. Most patients with optic neuropathy have a visual acuity of 20/40 or better, 50% have normal discs, and 75% have bilateral compression with no afferent pupil defect (2,21). Perimetry, contrast sensitivity, and visual-evoked potential recordings help support the diagnosis, but the results of these tests should not be used as a basis for treatment decisions in the absence of clinical evidence of optic neuropathy (21). Perimetry is abnormal in 35% of patients with optic neuropathy, but the results are influenced by normal variations in test results and other pathology such as cataract or glaucoma, and are grossly unreliable if visual acuity is ≤20/80 (31). Confounding pathology such as cataract and age-related macular degeneration affect contrast sensitivity, while thyroid dysfunction and age affect visual-evoked potentials (21,32).

Clinical Evaluation of Disease Activity

The inflammatory soft-tissue changes that imply activity were described earlier. The Clinical Activity Score (CAS) provides a way to quantitate these changes. This score consists of two scores for pain, five for inflammatory features, and three for change in severity of proptosis, diplopia and, visual acuity over two months (Table 23B.3) (33,34). Although partly subjective, it is a simple, useful tool for

TABLE 23B.3. CLINICAL ACTIVITY SCORE

Pain
  Painful, oppressive feeling on or behind the globe
  Pain on attempted up-, side-, or down-gaze
Redness
  Redness of the eyelids
  Diffuse redness of the conjunctiva (Fig. 23.3H)
Swelling
  Chemosis (Fig. 23.3J)
  Swollen caruncle (Fig. 23.3I)
  Edema of the eyelid(s) (Fig. 23.3F,G)
  Increase in proptosis of 2 mm or more during 1- to 3-month
    period
Impaired Function
  Decrease in visual acuity of 1 or more lines on the Snellen
    chart (using a pinhole) during a 1- to 3-month period
  Decrease of eye movements in any direction equal to or more
    than 5 degrees during a 1- to 3-month period

One point is given for each sign present. The sum of the points defines the activity score. (From Mourits MP, Koornneef L, Wiersinga WM, et al. Clinical criteria for the assessment of disease activity in Graves' ophthalmopathy: a novel approach. *Br J Ophthalmol* 1989;73:63, with permission of the publisher.)

everyday patient management. A score of 4 or higher signifies active disease.

Quality of Life and Self-Assessment

Patients with newly diagnosed Graves' ophthalmopathy describe impairment in psychological health comparable to patients with other chronic diseases (35), and the impairment persists for several years (36). Approximately half of the patients describe anxiety and depression (37), which are strongly correlated with their altered facial appearance and visual dysfunction, particularly diplopia. A validated disease-specific quality of life questionnaire is available (38) and is an essential outcome measure for clinical therapeutic trials (25).

Diagnostic Imaging

Most patients with Graves' ophthalmopathy do not need to undergo orbital imaging, whether ultrasonography, computed tomography (CT), magnetic resonance imaging (MRI), or octreotide scintigraphy (39). The exceptions include diagnostic uncertainty, in which case CT or MRI is mandatory, particularly for excluding orbital tumors (2); further evaluation of disease activity (A-mode ultrasonography, MRI and octreotide scintigraphy) (34); identifying patients with only expansion of orbital adipose tissue (CT or MRI); planning of surgical decompression or orbital radiation (CT); and identifying patients at high risk for optic neuropathy, in whom either CT or MRI will show "apical crowding" (40). Apical crowding denotes swollen muscles effacing the optic nerve at the orbital apex. If orbital fat also prolapses through the superior orbital fissure, then these combined features are highly sensitive and specific for optic neuropathy (41).

Ultrasonography

B-mode ultrasonography is of limited value because of technical factors that limit its accuracy and also prevent any imaging of the posterior orbit (42). A-mode ultrasonography provides qualitative information, with high muscle reflectivity (hyperechogenicity) implying edema, and therefore active Graves' ophthalmopathy. However, this result does not predict the response to medical treatment, whereas low reflectivity (hypoechogenicity) predicts a poor response (42).

Computed Tomography

Computed tomography (CT) is widely used to evaluate ophthalmopathy in patients with Graves' disease. The large differences in contrast between bone, muscle, and fat allow recognition of proptosis, the dimensions of fat and especially muscle, and the risk of optic neuropathy (40). CT is ideal for bone and sinus imaging before decompression, but cannot reliably distinguish closely adjacent muscles, e.g., the levator and superior rectus muscles.

Magnetic Resonance Imaging

Magnetic resonance imaging (MRI) is expensive and less widely available than CT. The indications for this test are the same as those for CT, except that it is not appropriate for predecompression bony imaging. Its advantages include lack of radiation, improved detection of optic neuropathy, and the potential for more accurate measurements of retroorbital tissues for treatment monitoring (43). Additionally, more sophisticated tissue characterization allows the potential for qualitative tissue analysis, which may help identify active disease. T2 relaxation times (34,42) and STIR (Short Tau Inversion Recovery) sequences help to identify tissue edema and have some correlation with the Clinical Activity Score, but do not accurately predict the response to treatment (44).

Orbital Scintigraphy

Orbital scintigraphy using radiolabeled somatostatin analogs (45) may be helpful in identifying patients with active ophthalmopathy, however its place in routine management is uncertain.

Biochemistry and Immunology

No serum tests can confirm, refute, or predict Graves' ophthalmopathy. Biochemical assessment of thyroid function is mandatory in all newly presenting patients, and should be repeated regularly to ensure euthyroidism is rapidly achieved and maintained (see Chapter 13). Measurements of serum TSH-receptor antibodies confirm the presence of Graves' disease. Approximately 75% of patients with Graves' ophthalmopathy have high serum concentrations of antithyroid peroxidase antibodies (2).

TREATMENT OF GRAVES' OPHTHALMOPATHY

Choice of Treatment for Thyrotoxicosis

The effect of different treatments for thyrotoxicosis on the natural history of Graves' ophthalmopathy has been a subject of debate, with much of the debate focused on the question of whether radioiodine treatment results in onset or exacerbation of ophthalmopathy (see Chapter 45). In a randomized prospective study, the risk of onset or exacerbation of ophthalmopathy was higher in patients treated with radioiodine, as compared with either antithyroid drug therapy or subtotal thyroidectomy (46). Thyroxine therapy ini-

tiated two weeks after radioiodine was given, thus preventing hypothyroidism, reduced the appearance or worsening of ophthalmopathy (47). A further, larger randomized study compared antithyroid drug therapy with radioiodine therapy, with and without the addition of prednisone (48). Radioiodine was associated with a small but significantly higher risk of onset or worsening of ophthalmopathy, as compared with antithyroid drug therapy; there was no increase in risk in those patients treated with radioiodine and prednisone. In a prospective study of patients with thyrotoxicosis who had inactive Graves' ophthalmopathy, radioiodine therapy combined with early thyroxine therapy to prevent hypothyroidism was not associated with onset or exacerbation of ophthalmopathy (49). The adverse effect of radioiodine in patients with ophthalmopathy is probably at least partly due to radioiodine-induced hypothyroidism. However, it is likely that radioiodine therapy itself has a detrimental effect on the eyes during the active phase of the disease. Antithyroid drugs and thyroidectomy are neutral with regards to the course of Graves' ophthalmopathy (46,50), and therefore are the preferred therapy for patients who have active ophthalmopathy.

Indications for Referral to an Ophthalmologist or Specialist Clinic

Most patients who develop Graves' ophthalmopathy present initially to a primary care physician or endocrinologist. Most of them have mild ophthalmopathy, and referral to a specialist is usually unnecessary. A brief history and a basic ophthalmologic examination, which can be rapidly performed by any physician, should identify those patients who would benefit from referral (Table 23B.4).

Sequence and Planning of Treatment

The first priority in patients with active Graves' ophthalmopathy is to ensure that the patient's vision is not threatened because of optic neuropathy or corneal ulceration. The presence of either of these findings mandates urgent treatment, usually with glucocorticoids. For other patients with active ophthalmopathy, the indications for glucocorticoid therapy are less well defined, but may include orbital pain, marked soft tissue involvement, or dysmotility that substantially reduces the patient's quality of life. Once ophthalmopathy becomes inactive, rehabilitative reconstructive surgery should be considered (Table 23B.5).

Simple Treatments

The corneal exposure that results from lid retraction frequently induces surface-related symptoms, but responds

TABLE 23B.4. INDICATIONS FOR REFERRAL OF PATIENTS WITH GRAVES' OPHTHALMOPATHY TO AN OPHTHALMOLOGIST OR SPECIALIST CLINIC

Inability to close the eyelids (lagophthalmos), leaving the cornea visible*
Corneal ulceration or abscess* (Fig. 23.3I)
Diminished corrected visual acuity*
Awareness of diminished color vision*
Afferent pupillary defect*
Swollen optic disc*
Severe orbital pain
Symptomatic deterioration of preexisting Graves' ophthalmopathy
Troublesome diplopia, particularly affecting forward gaze or reading position or associated with compensatory head tilt (Fig. 23.2A)
Surface symptoms, unresolved after 1 to 2 weeks of regular use of topical lubricants
History of subluxation of the globe
Patients severely distressed by their appearance
Severe periorbital edema (Fig. 23.3B, F, G)
Severe proptosis (Fig. 23.3E)

*Urgent referral required if there is suspicion of optic neuropathy or corneal ulceration.

well to topical lubricants, although overuse of preservative-containing preparations should be avoided. Upper-lid retraction may be reduced by botulinum toxin injection (51). Use of sunglasses often helps photophobia and tearing. Sleeping semi-recumbent rather than flat may improve morning tissue congestion. Temporary (fresnel) prisms often relieve diplopia in patients with active ophthalmopathy and may be permanently incorporated into glasses when dysmotility stabilizes. Diplopia unrelieved by prisms requires monocular occlusion, which may en-

able the patient to continue to drive a car. Patients who have subluxation of the eyes should be taught how to reposition the globe while awaiting decompression surgery (52).

Major Treatments

Glucocorticoids

Glucocorticoids have multiple immunosuppressive actions, including inhibition of leukocyte chemotaxis and cytokine release, reduction in glycosaminoglycan synthesis by orbital fibroblasts, and down-regulation of adhesion molecules (53). Prospective randomized studies have demonstrated a beneficial effect of glucocorticoids, as compared with no treatment, in thyrotoxic patients with ophthalmopathy who were treated with radioiodine (48,54).

The benefit of glucocorticoids in other patients with ophthalmopathy is less well documented; overall, about 60% to 75% of patients treated with glucocorticoids have improved, but all the studies were uncontrolled (53). Glucocorticoids can be administered orally, intravenously, or by retrobulbar injection; the latter route has no advantage and has largely been abandoned. They are usually given orally in high doses (e.g. prednisone, 60 to 80 mg daily) for 2 to 4 weeks, then gradually reduced; disease exacerbation is common during dose reduction. High doses of intravenous glucocorticoids, for example, 500 mg of methylprednisolone given daily for 3 days, may be more effective than oral glucocorticoids, with reported response rates of 73% to 100% (20,55,56). In one study this type of therapy resulted in a favorable clinical response in 88% of patients, as compared with a response rate of 63% in patients given

TABLE 23B.5. PLANNING AND SEQUENCE OF TREATMENTS FOR PATIENTS WITH GRAVES' OPHTHALMOPATHY

Vision threatened by:	Action:
Optic nerve compression	Urgent medical or surgical decompression and/or orbital irradiation
Severe corneal exposure (eyelids cannot cover cornea)	Urgent immunosuppression to improve closure; may also need urgent surgical decompression or occasionally lid lengthening
Globe subluxation	Semi-urgent surgical decompression
Active disease of moderate or worse severity:	Action:
Soft tissue signs and/or dysmotility	Consider immunosuppressive treatment
Inactive eye disease with marked proptosis	Action:
	Consider surgical decompression
Inactive disease with important dysmotility	Action:
	Consider strabismus surgery
Inactive disease with important lid problems	Action:
	Consider lid surgery, but first ensure that lid problems will not be addressed by prior decompression or strabismus surgery

oral glucocorticoid therapy (56), and there were fewer side effects in the intravenous-therapy group than in the oral-therapy group, even though the total dose was higher in the intravenous-therapy group.

Overall, glucocorticoid therapy is most appropriate for patients with active ophthalmopathy in whom sight is threatened; those with substantial dysmotility, especially diplopia affecting primary gaze or reading position; and those with moderate to severe inflammatory features. Glucocorticoid therapy is unlikely to be beneficial in patients whose principal problem is proptosis, and the risk of side effects far outweighs their value in patients with mild ophthalmopathy. Whenever glucocorticoids are given, the duration of therapy should be as short as possible, but attempts to reduce or discontinue glucocorticoid therapy are often followed by exacerbation of ophthalmopathy, and therefore the need for higher doses or reinstitution of therapy. Thus, patients may develop Cushing's syndrome. Osteoporosis prophylaxis should be considered, although in one study repeated pulses of high-dose intravenous glucocorticoid therapy did not accelerate bone loss (56). This therapy, however, can induce rises in serum concentrations of hepatic enzymes, and three deaths from liver failure have been reported in approximately 800 patients with ophthalmopathy treated with high intravenous doses of glucocorticoids (56,57).

Orbital Radiation

Orbital radiation may be of benefit in patients with Graves' ophthalmopathy. The benefit is presumed to be due to a suppressive effect on activated intraorbital lymphocytes and fibroblasts, leading to a decrease in the production of cytokines and glycosaminoglycans by these cells (58). The standard protocol consists of 20 Gy, delivered in 10 fractions over 2 weeks using well-collimated beams generated by a supervoltage linear accelerator (58). Planning includes CT and preparing a plastic mold for head immobilization. A short course of glucocorticoids (10 to 20 mg of prednisone daily) is sometimes given concurrently to avoid transient conjunctivitis. An alternative regimen delivering the same radiation dose over 20 weeks yielded slightly better results (59), however, most efficacy and safety data derive from studies using the standard protocol. The efficacy of radiation was similar to that of glucocorticoids in uncontrolled studies (53), but with a slower onset and peak effect at about 6 months.

There have been two prospective randomized placebo-controlled studies of the efficacy of orbital radiation in patients with moderately severe Graves' ophthalmopathy. In one study, 60% of patients treated with radiation improved, as compared with 31% of those who received sham radiation; the main improvement was in increased motility, especially in upgaze (60). In the other study, patients were randomly assigned to receive radiation to one eye and sham

radiation to their other eye (61). There was no difference in the two eyes six months later. Patient selection may account for these discordant findings.

Given the safety of orbital radiation therapy, it should be considered in patients with active Graves' ophthalmopathy (62), particularly those in whom the ophthalmopathy is of recent onset and in whom dysmotility is a problem. The indications for glucocorticoid and radiation therapy are similar, and the two treatments should be viewed as complementary. Orbital radiation is appropriate as monotherapy in patients whose ophthalmopathy is not severe, and those in whom glucocorticoids are contraindicated. With modern equipment the radiation can be focused on the retroorbital tissues, and the radiation dose to surrounding tissues is very low. The estimated risk of fatal cancer following any radiation is 7 per 1000 (63), but no cases have ever been reported in patients with Graves' ophthalmopathy treated with orbital radiation. Nevertheless, it is not recommended for patients younger than 35 years of age, because few data are available for this group. Radiation-induced cataracts are rare in patients treated with radiation generated by a linear accelerator. So also is radiation-induced retinopathy; however, it is more likely in patients with retinal vascular disease or previous exposure to chemotherapeutic drugs (64–66).

Combined Therapy with Glucocorticoids and Orbital Radiotherapy

The combination of orbital radiation and glucocorticoids is more effective than either treatment alone (53), and in patients treated with both it may be possible to discontinue the glucocorticoid within three months.

Other Medical Treatments

Numerous other medical treatments have been described (2,53,67), but all should be considered experimental. The combination of cyclosporine and an oral glucocorticoid was marginally better than either alone, but cyclosporine therapy requires close monitoring. Intravenous immunoglobulin was reported to be as effective as glucocorticoids in one small study, but its expense and unknown long-term effects are strong arguments against its use. Octreotide appeared useful in a case-controlled study (68), but not in a randomized prospective study in patients with moderate Graves' ophthalmopathy (69). Plasmapheresis, often combined with a glucocorticoid, was effective in small uncontrolled studies. The combination of two antioxidants (allopurinol and nicotinamide) was beneficial in a small study (70). Pentoxifylline (71), colchicine, methotrexate, bromocriptine, metronidazole, chlorambucil, and cyclophosphamide have been thought to be beneficial in a few patients, but they have substantial side effects (53); given the variable natural history of Graves' ophthalmopathy, the benefit of any of these drugs may well have been due to chance alone.

Prognosis and Prediction of Response to Medical Treatment

Among patients with thyrotoxicosis caused by Graves' disease who do not have clinically evident ophthalmopathy at the time antithyroid treatment is initiated, the risk of developing ophthalmopathy is approximately 20% in the next 18 months but is negligible later (2). Patients most likely to develop ophthalmopathy are those who have severe thyrotoxicosis (46), a large goiter, high serum TSH-receptor antibody concentrations (1), or persistent thyroid dysfunction (2); those who are smokers (8); and possibly those treated with radioiodine (48,72). Similarly, these same risk factors are associated with severe ophthalmopathy and, by inference, with possible progression of mild ophthalmopathy. In addition, old age and male sex are adverse prognostic factors (5). Based only on clinical signs during a single assessment, progression of ophthalmopathy could be predicted accurately in 69% of eyes using a neural network (73), however, this approach has not been validated prospectively. The small risk of onset or exacerbation of ophthalmopathy associated with radioiodine therapy may be prevented by glucocorticoid therapy (48); there appears to be no risk of radioiodine therapy in patients with inactive ophthalmopathy (49). There is circumstantial evidence that cessation of smoking leads to improvement in ophthalmopathy (74). Additionally, non-smokers have less severe ophthalmopathy of shorter duration, and therapy is more effective, as compared with smokers (48,75). Therefore, smoking cessation should be considered for all patients with Graves' disease.

Glucocorticoid therapy or orbital radiation therapy are more effective in patients with ophthalmopathy of recent onset than in those with chronic ophthalmopathy (53); therefore, the prognosis is better in patients treated promptly. The Clinical Activity Score, measurements of cytokines in serum, ultrasonography, MRI, and octreotide scintigraphy have all been reported to predict response to medical treatment (34,44,45,53). Multivariate logistic regression analysis including clinical, biochemical, and imaging measures was only marginally better than the Clinical Activity Score for predicting response to medical treatment (76). At present, the duration of eye disease and clinical assessment of disease activity are the only practical guides to predicting outcome. In patients treated with high intravenous doses of glucocorticoids, reassessment within a week usually gives an accurate indication as to response, which even at this early stage is predictive of longer-term outcome (2).

Surgical Treatment

Surgical therapy for patients with Graves' ophthalmopathy has expanded in recent years (77), due to the development of safer surgical techniques coupled with higher patient expectations. Three types of surgery are available, orbital decompression, correction of strabismus, and eyelid adjustment. While few patients require all procedures, the order should virtually always be decompression, then strabismus surgery, and then lid surgery. Premorbid photographs and supportive counselling help determine the functional and cosmetic concerns of the patient, and should allow development of a realistic plan, which is especially important when the scope for improvement is limited. Despite this, surgery can contribute very significantly to an improved outcome in patients with Graves' ophthalmopathy.

Orbital Decompression

Orbital decompression entails expansion of the bony boundaries of the orbits, removal of orbital fat, or both, thereby reducing the effects of the expanded orbital fibroadipose and muscle tissue. In patients with active ophthalmopathy, decompression may be indicated urgently to prevent visual loss due to optic neuropathy or corneal exposure. It may also be indicated in patients with active or inactive ophthalmopathy who have subluxation of their eyes. In patients with inactive ophthalmopathy, it may be indicated to improve appearance if eyelid surgery alone is unlikely to result in a satisfactory result.

The choice of decompression procedure depends on the indications for surgery and the desired amount of proptosis reduction, balanced against the risks, particularly of induced dysmotility, which is the most frequent complication (78–81). Hence, the surgical team should offer a range of procedures differing in approach, and with clear objectives: which walls of the bony orbits are to be opened, and by how much; how much periorbital tissue should be disrupted; and how much retroorbital fat should be removed (79,82–84). Four bony surfaces are available for decompression: the medial wall adjacent to the ethmoid sinuses; the floor of the orbit, which is the roof of the maxillary sinus; the anterolateral wall of the orbit adjacent to the temporal fossa above and buccal fat below; and the deep lateral wall comprising most of the greater wing and part of the lesser wing of the sphenoid bone (85). Decompression of the roof of the orbit has little effect on proptosis, induces orbital pulsation, and is virtually obsolete. In patients with optic neuropathy the posteromedial wall should at least be removed (86,87), either by an external or endoscopic approach. For rehabilitation, however, there is controversy as to which walls to remove first (78,80,86), and this debate has been further hampered by the lack of standardized reporting of both pre- and postoperative dysmotility (81). Dysmotility occasionally improves after decompression, particularly in patients in whom muscle thickness is not increased but the muscles are stretched from proptosis. Fat decompression is often done in conjunction with bony decompression; performed alone, decompression of fibroadipose tissue rarely worsens dysmotility, but proptosis isn't reduced much (78,88). Other complications of decompression, in addition to dysmotility, include blindness, orbital cellulitis, cerebrospinal fluid leak, cerebral hematoma, cutaneous sensory loss, sinus obstruction, anosmia, nasolacrimal outflow obstruction, and lid malposition.

Surgery for Strabismus

Strabismus surgery should be performed only when the ocular alignment has been stable for 6 months, although it may be done earlier if the ophthalmopathy is inactive or as a sequel to decompression (89,90). The goal of strabismus surgery is to improve ocular alignment and eliminate any abnormal head posture, and thereby create an optimal binocular field for straight-ahead vision and reading. Preoperative planning should include assessment of occupation, driving status, and hobbies to determine goals for that patient, as it is seldom possible to achieve binocular vision in all directions or accurately correct tiny deviations (91). Strabismus surgery in patients with Graves' ophthalmopathy for the most part involves loosening tight muscles (20,91). Multiple operations may be required (20,92). Most patients achieve useful binocular vision, but 10% have to resort to monocular occlusion. Surgical complications include lid malposition and perforation of the globe.

Eyelid Surgery

Eyelid surgery is rarely indicated in patients with active ophthalmopathy, because decompression is usually sufficient to prevent corneal perforation or globe subluxation. Lid surgery is usually the final stage of rehabilitation. Several procedures may be needed. They include adjustment of upper and lower eyelid positions; cautious removal of excess skin; repositioning of a prolapsed lacrimal gland; and occasionally a small lateral tarsorrhaphy. The latter is obsolete as a stand-alone procedure, as the esthetic outcome is poor. Upper eyelid surgery addresses lid retraction and eyelid swelling, and often improves ocular comfort and tearing as well as appearance, but lid retraction due to a tight inferior rectus muscle should first be addressed by strabismus surgery. Upper lid lengthening techniques abound (93), but spacer material is not required. In contrast, lower eyelid lengthening does require spacer material, ideally autogenous. Cautious removal of excess skin may also be required but should never precede lid lengthening.

Organizational Aspects of Treating Patients with Ophthalmopathy

Multidisciplinary teams comprising physicians and surgeons who are interested and experienced in management of patients with Graves' ophthalmopathy achieve the best outcome. A critical mass of patient referrals is necessary to develop and maintain these skills. For a disease like Graves' ophthalmopathy with a low incidence (4), streamlining of referrals to a few centers with experience and expertise is imperative. The multidisciplinary team should ideally include an endocrinologist and an ophthalmologist, with access to expert orbital surgery, eye muscle surgery, oculoplastic surgery, and radiation therapy. The goals of the team include rapid achievement of euthyroidism and maintenance of the euthyroid state, and selection, timing, and delivery of most appropriate treatment for ophthalmopathy.

REFERENCES

1. Wiersinga WM, Prummel MF. Pathogenesis of Graves' ophthalmopathy-current understanding. *J Clin Endocrinol Metab* 2001; 86:501.
2. Burch HB, Wartofsky L. Graves' ophthalmopathy: current concepts regarding pathogenesis and management. *Endocr Rev* 1993; 14:747.
3. Kendall-Taylor P, Perros P. Clinical presentation of thyroid associated orbitopathy. *Thyroid* 1998;8:427.
4. Bartley GB, Fatourechi V, Kadrmas EF, et al. The incidence of Graves' ophthalmopathy in Olmsted County, Minnesota. *Am J Ophthalmol* 1995;120:511.
5. Bahn RS. Pathophysiology of Graves' ophthalmopathy: the cycle of disease. *J Clin Endocrinol Metab* 2003;88:1939.
6. Pappa A, Lawson JM, Calder V, et al. T cells and fibroblasts in affected extraocular muscles in early and late thyroid associated ophthalmopathy. *Br J Ophthalmol* 2000;84:517.
7. Cockerham KP, Hidayat AA, Brown HG, et al. Clinicopathologic evaluation of the Mueller muscle in thyroid-associated orbitopathy. *Ophthal Plast Reconstr Surg* 2002;18:11.
8. Wakelkamp IM, Bakker O, Baldeschi L, et al. TSH-R expression and cytokine profile in orbital tissue of active vs. inactive Graves' ophthalmopathy patients. *Clin Endocrinol (Oxf)* 2003; 58:280.
9. Agretti P, Chiovato L, De Marco G, et al. Real-time PCR provides evidence for thyrotropin receptor mRNA expression in orbital as well as in extraorbital tissues. *Eur J Endocrinol* 2002;147: 733.
10. Busuttil BE, Frauman AG. Extrathyroidal manifestations of Graves' disease: the thyrotropin receptor is expressed in extraocular, but not cardiac, muscle tissues. *J Clin Endocrinol Metab* 2001;86:2315.
11. Munsakul N, Bahn RS. Adipogenesis and TSH receptor expression. In: Bahn RS, ed. *Thyroid eye disease.* Boston: Kluwer Academic Publishers, 2001:37.
12. Starkey KJ, Janezic A, Jones G, et al. Adipose thyrotrophin receptor expression is elevated in Graves' and thyroid eye diseases ex vivo and indicates adipogenesis in progress in vivo. *J Mol Endocrinol* 2003;30:369.
13. Kaspar M, Archibald C, De BA, et al. Eye muscle antibodies and subtype of thyroid-associated ophthalmopathy. *Thyroid* 2002; 12:187.

14. Gerding MN, van der Meer JW, Broenink M, et al. Association of thyrotrophin receptor antibodies with the clinical features of Graves' ophthalmopathy. *Clin Endocrinol (Oxf)* 2000;52: 267.

15. Pritchard J, Han R, Horst N, et al. Immunoglobulin activation of T cell chemoattractant expression in fibroblasts from patients with Graves' disease is mediated through the insulin-like growth factor I receptor pathway. *J Immunol* 2003;170:6348.

16. Vaidya B, Kendall-Taylor P, Pearce SH. The genetics of autoimmune thyroid disease. *J Clin Endocrinol Metab* 2002;87:5385.

17. Bednarczuk T, Hiromatsu Y, Fukutani T, et al. Association of cytotoxic T-lymphocyte-associated antigen-4 (CTLA-4) gene polymorphism and non-genetic factors with Graves' ophthalmopathy in European and Japanese populations. *Eur J Endocrinol* 2003;148:13.

18. Kretowski A, Wawrusiewicz N, Mironczuk K, et al. Intercellular adhesion molecule 1 gene polymorphisms in Graves' disease. *J Clin Endocrinol Metab* 2003;88:4945-.

19. Perros P, Kendall-Taylor P. Natural history of thyroid eye disease. *Thyroid* 1998;8:423.

20. Kalman R, Mourits MP. Late recurrence of unilateral Graves' orbitopathy on the contralateral side. *Am J Ophthalmol* 2002;133: 727.

21. Dickinson AJ, Perros P. Controversies in the clinical evaluation of active thyroid-associated orbitopathy: use of a detailed protocol with comparative photographs for objective assessment. *Clin Endocrinol (Oxf)* 2001;55:283.

22. Rootman J, Chang W, Jones D. Distribution and differential diagnosis of orbital disease. In: Rootman J, ed. *Diseases of the orbit a multidisciplinary approach,* 2nd ed. Philadelphia: Lippincott Williams and Wilkins, 2003:53.

23. Lacey B, Chang W, Rootman J. Nonthyroid causes of extraocular muscle disease. *Surv Ophthalmol* 1999;44:187.

24. Bartley GB, Gorman CA. Diagnostic criteria for Graves' ophthalmopathy. *Am J Ophthalmol* 1995;119:792.

25. Pinchera A, Wiersinga W, Glinoer D, et al. Classification of eye changes of Graves' disease. *Thyroid* 1992;2:235.

26. Prummel MF, Bakker A, Wiersinga WM, et al. Multi-center study on the characteristics and treatment strategies of patients with Graves' orbitopathy: the first European Group on Graves' Orbitopathy experience. *Eur J Endocrinol* 2003;148:491.

27. Setty R, Varma D, O'Keeffe M, et al. Superior limbic keratoconjunctivitis (SLK) in Graves' orbitopathy (GO). In: Abstracts of the European Society of Ophthalmic Plastic and Reconstructive Surgery, 2003.

28. Sleep TJ, Manners RM. Interinstrument variability in Hertel type exophthalmometers. *Ophthal Plast Reconstr Surg* 2002;18: 254.

29. Haggerty H, Richardson S, Mitchell K, et al. A modified method for the reliable assessment of uniocular fields of fixation (UFOF). In: Proceedings of the European Strabismological Association, 2001.

30. Kazim M, Trokel SL, Acaroglu G, et al. Reversal of dysthyroid optic neuropathy following orbital fat decompression. *Br J Ophthalmol* 2000;84:600.

31. Henson DB, Chaudry S, Artes PH, et al. Response variability in the visual field: comparison of optic neuritis, glaucoma, ocular hypertension, and normal eyes. *Invest Ophthalmol Vis Sci* 2000; 41:417.

32. Tamburini G, Tacconi P, Ferrigno P, et al. Visual evoked potentials in hypothyroidism: a long-term evaluation. *Electromyogr Clin Neurophysiol* 1998;38:201.

33. Mourits MP, Koornneef L, Wiersinga WM, et al. Clinical criteria for the assessment of disease activity in Graves' ophthalmopathy: a novel approach. *Br J Ophthalmol* 1989;73:639.

34. Mourits MP. Assessment of disease activity. In: Bahn RS, ed. *Thyroid eye disease.* Boston: Kluwer Academic Publishers, 2001: 185.

35. Gerding MN, Terwee CB, Dekker FW, et al. Quality of life in patients with Graves' ophthalmopathy is markedly decreased: measurement by the Medical Outcomes Study instrument. *Thyroid* 1997;7:885.

36. Terwee C, Wakelkamp I, Tan S, et al. Long-term effects of Graves' ophthalmopathy on health-related quality of life. *Eur J Endocrinol* 2002;146:751.

37. Kahaly GJ, Hardt J, Petrak F, et al. Psychosocial factors in subjects with thyroid-associated ophthalmopathy. *Thyroid* 2002;12: 237.

38. Terwee CB, Gerding MN, Dekker FW, et al. Development of a disease specific quality of life questionnaire for patients with Graves' ophthalmopathy: the GO-QOL. *Br J Ophthalmol* 1998; 82:773.

39. Kahaly GJ. Imaging in thyroid-associated orbitopathy. *Eur J Endocrinol* 2001;145:107.

40. Giaconi JA, Kazim M, Rho T, et al. CT scan evidence of dysthyroid optic neuropathy. *Ophthal Plast Reconstr Surg* 2002;18:177.

41. Birchall D, Goodall KL, Noble JL, et al. Graves' ophthalmopathy: intracranial fat prolapse on CT images as an indicator of optic nerve compression. *Radiology* 1996;200:123.

42. Prummel M, Wiersinga W, Mourits MP. Assessment of disease activity in Graves' ophthalmopathy. In: Prummel M, ed. *Recent developments in Graves' ophthalmopathy.* London: Kluwer Academic Publishers, 2000:59.

43. Firbank MJ, Harrison RM, Williams ED, et al. Measuring extraocular muscle volume using dynamic contours. *Magn Reson Imaging Clin N Am* 2001;19:257.

44. Prummel, MF, Gerding MN, Zonneveld FW, et al. The usefulness of quantitative orbital magnetic resonance imaging in Graves' ophthalmopathy. *Clin Endocrinol (Oxf)* 2001;54:205.

45. Krassas GE. Octreoscan in thyroid-associated ophthalmopathy. *Thyroid* 2002;12:229.

46. Tallstedt L, Lundell G, Torring O, et al. Occurrence of ophthalmopathy after treatment for Graves' hyperthyroidism. *N Engl J Med* 1992;326:1733.

47. Tallstedt L, Lundell G, Blomgren H, et al. Does early administration of thyroxine reduce the development of Graves' ophthalmopathy after radioiodine treatment? *Eur J Endocrinol* 1994; 130:494.

48. Bartalena L, Marcocci C, Bogazzi F, et al. Relation between therapy for hyperthyroidism and the course of Graves' ophthalmopathy. *N Engl J Med* 1998;338:73.

49. Perros P, Neoh C, Frewin S, et al. Prophylactic steroids are unnecessary in patients with thyroid-associated ophthalmopathy receiving radioiodine therapy. *Endocrine Abstracts* 2003;5:OC36.

50. Marcocci C, Bruno-Bossio G, Manetti L, et al. The course of Graves' ophthalmopathy is not influenced by near total thyroidectomy: a case-control study. *Clin Endocrinol (Oxf)* 1999; 51:503.

51. Uddin JM, Davies PD. Treatment of upper eyelid retraction associated with thyroid eye disease with subconjunctival botulinum toxin injection. *Ophthalmology* 2002;109:1183.

52. Tse DT. A simple maneuver to reposit a subluxed globe. *Arch Ophthalmol* 2000;118:410.

53. Bartalena L, Pinchera A, Marcocci C. Management of Graves' ophthalmopathy: reality and perspectives. *Endocr Rev* 2000;21: 168.

54. Bartalena L, Marcocci C, Bogazzi F, et al. Use of corticosteroids to prevent progression of Graves' ophthalmopathy after radioiodine therapy for hyperthyroidism. *N Engl J Med* 1989;321: 1349.

55. Kauppinen-Makelin R, Karma A, Leinonen E, et al. High dose intravenous methylprednisolone pulse therapy versus oral prednisone for thyroid-associated ophthalmopathy. *Acta Ophthalmol Scand* 2002;80:316.

56. Marcocci C, Bartalena L, Tanda ML, et al. Comparison of the effectiveness and tolerability of intravenous or oral glucocorticoids associated with orbital radiotherapy in the management of severe Graves' ophthalmopathy: results of a prospective, single-blind, randomized study. *J Clin Endocrinol Metab* 2001;86:3562.

57. Marino M, Morabito E, Brunetto MR, et al. Acute and severe liver damage associated with intravenous glucocorticoid pulse therapy in patients with Graves' ophthalmopathy. *Thyroid* 2004; 14:203.

58. Kahaly GJ, Roesler HP, Kutzner J, et al. Radiotherapy for thyroid-associated orbitopathy. *Exp Clin Endocrinol Diabetes* 1999; 107[Suppl 5]:S201.

59. Kahaly GJ, Rosler HP, Pitz S, et al. Low- versus high-dose radiotherapy for Graves' ophthalmopathy: a randomized, single blind trial. *J Clin Endocrinol Metab* 2000;85:102.

60. Mourits MP, van Kempen-Harteveld ML, Garcia MB, et al. Radiotherapy for Graves' orbitopathy: randomised placebo-controlled study. *Lancet* 2000;355:1505.

61. Gorman CA, Garrity JA, Fatourechi V, et al. A prospective, randomized, double-blind, placebo-controlled study of orbital radiotherapy for Graves' ophthalmopathy. *Ophthalmology* 2001; 108:1523.

62. Bartalena L, Marcocci C, Gorman CA, et al. Orbital radiotherapy for Graves' ophthalmopathy: useful or useless? Safe or dangerous? *J Endocrinol Invest* 2003;26:5.

63. Akmansu M, Dirican B, Bora H, et al. The risk of radiation-induced carcinogenesis after external beam radiotherapy of Graves' orbitopathy. *Ophthalmic Res* 2003;35:150.

64. Kahaly GJ, Gorman CA, Kal HB, et al. Radiotherapy for Graves' ophthalmopathy. In: Prummel MF, ed. *Recent developments in Graves' ophthalmopathy.* Boston: Kluwer Academic Publishers, 2000:115.

65. Robertson DM, Buettner H, Gorman CA, et al. Retinal microvascular abnormalities in patients treated with external radiation for Graves' ophthalmopathy. *Arch Ophthalmol* 2003;121:652.

66. Marcocci C, Bartalena L, Rocchi R, et al. Long-term safety of orbital radiotherapy for Graves' ophthalmopathy. *J Clin Endocrinol Metab* 2003;88:3561.

67. Perros P, Kendall-Taylor P. Medical treatment for thyroid-associated ophthalmopathy. *Thyroid* 2002;12:241.

68. Krassas GE, Dumas A, Pontikides N, et al. Somatostatin receptor scintigraphy and octreotide treatment in patients with thyroid eye disease. *Clin Endocrinol (Oxf)* 1995;42:571.

69. Kendall-Taylor P, Dickinson AJ, Vaidya BJ et al. Double blind placebo controlled trial of octreotide LAR in thyroid-associated orbitopathy: clinical outcomes. *Thyroid* 2003;7:671.

70. Bouzas EA, Karadimas P, Mastorakos G, et al. Antioxidant agents in the treatment of Graves' ophthalmopathy. *Am J Ophthalmol* 2000;129:618.

71. Balazs C, Kiss E, Vamos A, et al. Beneficial effect of pentoxifylline on thyroid associated ophthalmopathy (TAO): a pilot study. *J Clin Endocrinol Metab* 1997;82:1999.

72. Bonnema SJ, Bartalena L, Toft AD, et al. Controversies in radioiodine therapy: relation to ophthalmopathy, the possible radioprotective effect of antithyroid drugs, and use in large goitres. *Eur J Endocrinol* 2002;147:1.

73. Salvi M, Dazzi D, Pellistri I, et al. Classification and prediction of the progression of thyroid-associated ophthalmopathy by an artificial neural network. *Ophthalmology* 2002;109:1703.

74. Wiersinga WM, Bartalena L. Epidemiology and prevention of Graves' ophthalmopathy. *Thyroid* 2002;12:855.

75. Eckstein A, Quadbeck B, Mueller G, et al. Impact of smoking on the response to treatment of thyroid associated ophthalmopathy. *Br J Ophthalmol* 2003;87:773.

76. Gerding MN, ed. *Assessment of disease activity in Graves' ophthalmopathy.* Amsterdam, NL: L. van der Velde BV, 1999.

77. Kalman R, Mourits MP, van der Pol JP, et al. Coronal approach for rehabilitative orbital decompression in Graves' ophthalmopathy. *Br J Ophthalmol* 1997;81;41.

78. Goldberg RA. The evolving paradigm of orbital decompression surgery. *Arch Ophthalmol* 1998;116:95.

79. Metson R. Reduction of diplopia following endoscopic orbital decompression: the orbital sling technique. *Laryngoscope* 2002; 112:1753.

80. Kacker A, Kazim M, Murphy M, et al. "Balanced" orbital decompression for severe Graves' orbitopathy: technique with treatment algorithm. *Otolaryngol Head Neck Surg* 2003;128: 228.

81. Paridaens D, Hans K, van Buitenen S, et al. The incidence of diplopia following coronal and translid orbital decompression in Graves' orbitopathy. *Eye* 1998;12:800.

82. Seiff SR, Tovilla JL, Carter SR et al. Modified orbital decompression for dysthyroid orbitopathy. *Ophthal Plast Reconstr Surg* 2000;16:62.

83. Abramoff MD, Kalman R, de Graaf MEL, et al. Rectus extraocular muscle paths and decompression surgery for Graves' orbitopathy: mechanism of motility disturbances. *Invest Ophthalmol Vis Sci* 2002;43:300.

84. Kikkawa DO, Pornpanich K, Cruz RC Jr, et al. Graded orbital decompression based on severity of proptosis. *Ophthalmology* 2002;109:1219.

85. Goldberg RA, Perry JD, Hortaleza V, et al. Strabismus after balanced medial plus lateral wall versus lateral wall only orbital decompression for dysthyroid orbitopathy. *Ophthal Plast Reconstr Surg* 2000;16:271.

86. Schaefer SD, Soliemanzadeh P, Della Rocca DA, et al. Endoscopic and transconjunctival orbital decompression for thyroid related orbital apex compression. *Laryngoscope* 2003;113:508.

87. Kazim M, Trokel SL, Acaroglu G, et al. Reversal of dysthyroid optic neuropathy following orbital fat decompression. *Br J Ophthalmol* 2000;84:600.

88. Olivari N. Thyroid-associated orbitopathy: transpalpebral decompression by removal of intraorbital fat. Experience with 1362 orbits in 697 patients over 13 years. *Exp Clin Endocrinol Diabetes* 1999;107[Suppl 5]:S208.

89. Yolar M, Oguz V, Pazarli H, et al. Early surgery for dysthyroid orbitomyopathy based on magnetic resonance imaging findings. *J Pediatr Ophthalmol Strabismus* 2002;39:336.

90. Bradley EA, Bartley GB, Garrity JA. Surgical management of Graves' ophthalmopathy. In: Bahn RS, ed. *Thyroid eye disease.* Boston: Kluwer Academic Publishers, 2001:219.

91. Esser J, Eckstein A. Ocular muscle and eyelid surgery in thyroid-associated orbitopathy. *Exp Clin Endocrinol Diabetes* 1999;107 [Suppl 5]:S214.

92. Prendiville P, Chopra M, Gauderman WJ, et al. The role of restricted motility in determining outcomes for vertical strabismus surgery in Graves' ophthalmology. *Ophthalmology* 2000;107: 545.

93. Mourits MP, Sasim IV. A single technique to correct various degrees of upper lid retraction in patients with Graves' orbitopathy. *Br J Ophthalmol* 1999;83:81.

23C LOCALIZED MYXEDEMA AND THYROID ACROPACHY

VAHAB FATOURECHI

Localized myxedema is an uncommon manifestation of autoimmune thyroiditis and in particular Graves' disease. It is almost always associated with Graves' ophthalmopathy (1–3). Although more than 91% of patients with localized myxedema have a history of thyrotoxicosis, it can occur in patients with ophthalmopathy who have never had thyrotoxicosis and also rarely in patients with chronic autoimmune thyroiditis with or without hypothyroidism (3–5). In a community-based epidemiologic study, 4% of patients with clinically evident ophthalmopathy had localized myxedema (6), and it occurs in 12% to 15% of patients with severe Graves' ophthalmopathy (2,4). The average age for females is 53 years and for males 54 years; patients younger than age 20 years rarely have the condition. The female-to-male ratio is 3.9:1 (3,5).

The characteristic abnormality of localized myxedema, skin thickening, usually is limited to the pretibial area. Thus, the disorder has been called pretibial myxedema. Because it can occur in other areas, however, localized myxedema, thyroid dermopathy, and dermopathy of Graves' disease are more appropriate terms. A subclinical form of the disorder can be identified by skin biopsy specimens that show deposition of glycosaminoglycans and activated fibroblasts in patients with Graves' disease without clinically evident skin changes (7,8), although no such abnormalities were seen in biopsy specimens of forearm skin from another group of patients with Graves' disease (9). Because most patients with localized myxedema have relatively severe ophthalmopathy (3,10) and high serum concentrations of thyrotropin (TSH) receptor–stimulating antibodies (11,12), localized myxedema most likely indicates more severe Graves' disease. When present, dermopathy is a marker for the existence or future development of severe ophthalmopathy and the likelihood of development of optic neuropathy, often requiring orbital decompression (10).

The lesions are characterized by an accumulation of glycosaminoglycans in the dermis and subcutaneous tissues (13–16). Although localized myxedema is uncommon, the histologic similarities between the fibroblast activation and glycosaminoglycan accumulation present in retroorbital tissue of patients with Graves' ophthalmopathy and in the dermal tissue of patients with localized myxedema suggest that insights into the pathogenesis of the latter would be helpful in the understanding and treatment of the more common and clinically important condition of ophthalmopathy (17).

CLINICAL MANIFESTATIONS

The lesions of localized myxedema occur not only in the pretibial area but almost as often on the feet and toes (2,3) (Fig. 23C.1). Isolated cases of involvement of the upper extremities, shoulders, upper back, pinnae, and nose have been reported (18–22). When the lesions occur in unusual sites, a history of trauma to the area is often present. A patient who carried heavy objects suspended from a stick balanced across his shoulders developed localized myxedema of the shoulders (Fig. 23C.2) (19). Lesions also may develop in burn and surgical scars (Fig. 23C.3) (22) and in smallpox vaccination sites (23).

Localized myxedema commonly begins with raised waxy lesions in the pretibial area. They are usually light-colored, but may be flesh-colored or yellowish brown (2, 3,24,25). Hyperpigmentation and hyperkeratosis may be present (2,3), as may hyperhidrosis (26,27). The latter may be caused by stimulation of sympathetic fibers by the surrounding mucin deposition (27). The lesions may be indurated and the hair follicles prominent, so that the lesions have an orange peel (peau d'orange) or pigskin appearance and texture. The lesions are usually asymptomatic and of only cosmetic importance, but they can impair function

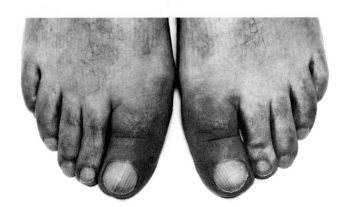

FIGURE 23C.1. Thyroid dermopathy involving the first toes.

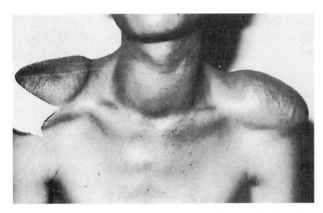

FIGURE 23C.2. Localized myxedema involving both shoulders. The patient had carried heavy objects suspended from a stick balanced across his shoulders. (From Noppakun N, Bancheun K, Chandraprasert S. Unusual locations of localized myxedema in Graves' disease: report of three cases. *Arch Dermatol* 1986;122: 85, with permission.)

(for example, causing difficulty wearing shoes) and rarely may be painful or pruritic. Nerve entrapment and reversible footdrop were reported in one patient (28). The lesions usually are aggravated by trauma, and exuberant recurrence may ensue if they are surgically excised (29).

Localized myxedema may appear in several distinct clinical forms (Fig. 23C.3): diffuse, nonpitting edema, the most common form (3,5); raised plaque lesions on a background of nonpitting edema; sharply circumscribed tubular or nodular lesions; and the rare elephantiasic form, consisting of nodular lesions mixed with lymphedema. Rarely, the lesions are polypoid or fungating. They usually do not ulcerate.

In a review of 178 consecutive patients with pretibial myxedema, 4 patients had no evidence of Graves' ophthalmopathy (10). Similar patients and patients with localized myxedema as the presenting symptom have been reported (30–33). The most common time of onset of ophthalmopathy was 0 to 12 months after diagnosis of thyrotoxicosis. For localized myxedema, the onset was 12 to 24 months after the diagnosis of thyrotoxicosis, but 12% of the patients developed localized myxedema 4 to 12 years after the diagnosis of thyrotoxicosis (Fig. 23C.4) (3).

BIOCHEMICAL NATURE AND HISTOPATHOLOGY

Light microscopy of biopsy specimens of lesions of localized myxedema shows large amounts of glycosaminoglycans (a mucin-like substance) in the reticular part of the dermis, but not usually in the papillary dermis. A few lymphocytes may be seen in the perivascular spaces, but extensive infiltration with lymphocytes is unusual. The number

of mast cells is moderately increased. Fragmentation and fraying of collagen fibers are seen when the tissue is stained with hematoxylin and eosin (Fig. 23C.5). Mucinous material with and without connective tissue separation is seen when the tissue is stained with Alcian blue and the periodic acid–Schiff stain. Collagen fibers are relatively reduced, and there is marked edema. Hyperkeratosis, acanthosis, and papillomatosis occasionally are seen (34).

Ultrastructural studies show dilated endoplasmic reticulum in fibroblasts, indicative of active glycosaminoglycan synthesis and secretion. The epidermis is usually normal except for widened intercellular spaces. Amorphous electron-dense material is seen close to the surface of the fibroblasts.

Overall, the structural changes of localized myxedema can be distinguished from hypothyroid myxedema by hyperkeratosis, a greater abundance of mucin, and mononuclear cell infiltration (34–37). The characteristics that distinguish localized myxedema from mucinosis associated with stasis dermatitis include preservation of a zone of normal-appearing collagen in the superficial papillary dermis, mucin deposition in the reticular dermis, lack of angioplasia, and relative absence of hemosiderin (37).

Quantitative lymphoscintigraphy and fluorescence microlymphography have shown that the deposited mucin promotes dermal edema by retention of fluid, which in turn causes compression or occlusion of small peripheral lymphatics and lymphedema (38). In one study, immunofluorescent staining of specimens from areas of localized myxedema showed evidence of immunoglobulin (Ig) A deposition in 75% of patients, IgG in 57%, and complement in 43% (39).

PATHOGENESIS

Graves' disease is a multigenic condition that develops as a result of susceptibility genes and environmental factors (40). However, no unique susceptibility genes specific to localized myxedema or Graves' ophthalmopathy have been identified (41). Graves' hyperthyroidism results from direct stimulation of thyroid follicular cells by TSH receptor–stimulating antibodies (see section on pathogenesis in this chapter). All patients with localized myxedema have high serum concentrations of TSH receptor–stimulating antibodies (2,5,11,12,42–44). Polymerase chain reaction techniques have shown RNA encoding the extracellular domain of the TSH receptor in cultured orbital, abdominal skin, and peripheral skin fibroblasts from patients with ophthalmopathy or localized myxedema as well as in skin from normal subjects (45,46). Pretibial myxedema tissue and normal skin express TSH receptor protein (46). TSH receptor immunoreactivity and transcripts have been identified in fibroblast cultures of orbital and pretibial myxedema and normal skin (47–49). Not all studies have

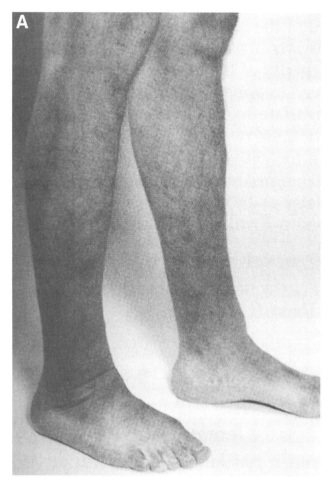

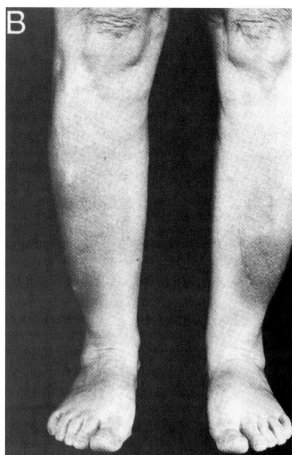

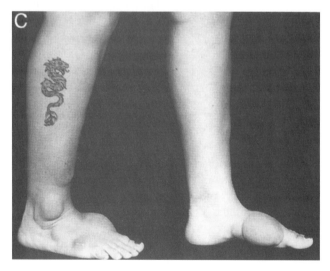

FIGURE 23C.3. Thyroid dermopathy (localized myxedema) in five patients. **A:** Nonpitting edema form in pretibial area. **B:** Plaque form in pretibial area. **C:** Nodular form in ankle and foot. **D:** Elephantiasic form. **E:** Occurrence of thyroid dermopathy in scar tissue. (From Schwartz KM, Fatourechi V, Ahmed DD, et al. Dermopathy of Graves' disease (pretibial myxedema): long-term outcome. *J Clin Endocrinol Metab* 2002;87:438, with permission.)

shown TSH receptor immunoreactivity in normal skin. In one study, TSH receptor immunoreactivity was demonstrated in pretibial hypodermis tissues of two patients with thyroid dermopathy but not in pretibial tissues of two control subjects. The immunoreactivity occurred in the cells resembling fibroblasts. It is not clear yet if this immunoreactivity is related to the receptor itself or to a crossreacting protein (50).

These results implicate TSH receptor–stimulating antibodies and TSH receptors in the pathogenesis of localized myxedema.

The serum of patients with localized myxedema may stimulate glycosaminoglycan production by fibroblasts *in vitro* (51,52). In other studies, however, serum IgG from patients with localized myxedema increased the synthesis of glycosaminoglycans, protein, and DNA by cultured

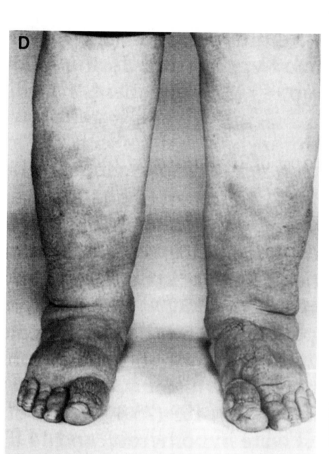

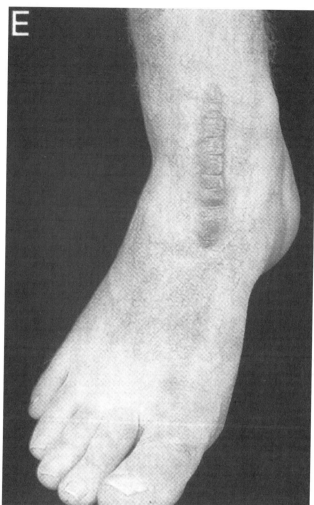

FIGURE 23C.3. *Continued*

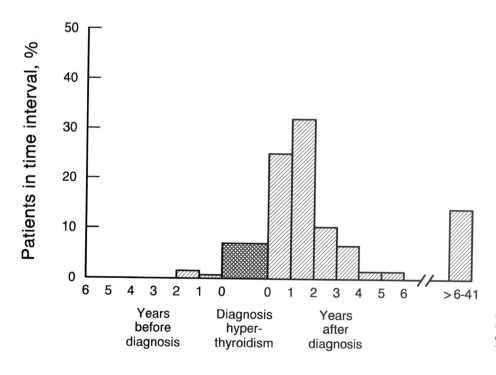

FIGURE 23C.4. Onset of localized myxedema in relation to time of diagnosis of thyrotoxicosis in 136 patients. *Cross-hatched bar*: Onset of localized myxedema within 3 months of diagnosis of thyrotoxicosis. (From Fatourechi V, Pajouhi M, Fransway AF. Dermopathy of Graves disease (pretibial myxedema): review of 150 cases. *Medicine (Baltimore)* 1994; 73:1, with permission.)

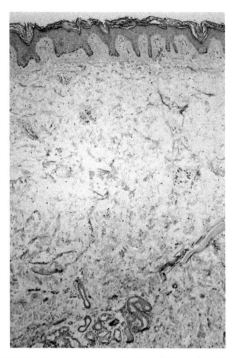

FIGURE 23C.5. Photomicrograph of skin biopsy specimen from patient with localized myxedema showing separation and fraying of connective tissue fibers and edema. The epidermis **(top)** is normal. (Hematoxylin and eosin, 340× original magnification.) (From Fatourechi V, Pajouhi M, Fransway AF. Dermopathy of Graves disease (pretibial myxedema): review of 150 cases. *Medicine (Baltimore)* 1994;73:1, with permission.)

FRTL-5 thyroid cells, but these IgGs and those of normal subjects were equally active in stimulating dermal fibroblasts (53).

If TSH receptors are expressed in normal skin, as shown by Rapoport et al (46), then how is it that the pretibial area is most commonly involved? There is a mechanical contribution to pathogenesis. Skin grafted to a lower extremity from areas that are not usually involved develops localized myxedema at the recipient site (46,54,55). Localized myxedema develops in areas exposed to repeated trauma (56), at the site of immunization (23), and after episodes of prolonged standing. Dependent edema because of a lower return of lymphatic fluid might reduce the clearance and increase the half-life of disease-related cytokines and chemokines within the affected tissue (46,57). This pooling of immune mediators increases the disease-producing effects. There is some evidence that trauma and injury may lead to activation of T cells and initiation of an antigen-specific response (58), in this case fibroblast activation and production of glycosaminoglycans.

Fibroblast activation in localized myxedema may occur indirectly, through sensitized T lymphocytes. T cells sensitized to antigens shared by thyroid follicular cells and fibroblasts, one candidate antigen being a portion of the TSH receptor, could infiltrate dermal tissue and release cy-

tokines, including interleukin 1α and transforming growth factor-β, which then stimulate synthesis of glycosaminoglycans and activate immunomodulatory proteins in dermal fibroblasts (17,59–61). There is evidence of accumulation of thyroid-specific T cells in the retroorbital and pretibial tissues in patients with Graves' ophthalmopathy and localized myxedema, respectively, and these T cells express a limited number of genes for T-cell antigen receptors, as is characteristic of antigen-sensitized T cells (62). Thus, in both extrathyroidal manifestations of Graves' disease, similar antigens may be responsible for recruitment and expansion of T cells.

Whatever the proximate cause of increased dermal production of glycosaminoglycans, the local accumulation of these substances leads to accumulation of fluid and expansion of dermal connective tissue and thus the characteristic skin changes (17). Secondarily, obstruction of the lymphatic microcirculation may aggravate the immune process and the lesions (38,46).

Some evidence for differences in the regulation of synthesis of glycosaminoglycans by fibroblasts from various anatomic sites has been presented (63,64), but the mechanical theory seems to apply better to localization of thyroid dermopathy in the lower extremity (65).

In summary, with the demonstration of TSH receptor transcripts and protein in fibroblasts, recognition of the role of various cytokines in stimulation of fibroblast activity, demonstration of high concentrations of TSH receptor–stimulating antibodies in the serum of patients with localized myxedema, and elucidation of the role of mechanical factors contributing to the pathogenesis of localized myxedema, the reasons for its (usual) location on the pretibial region have become better recognized.

DIFFERENTIAL DIAGNOSIS

The diagnosis of localized myxedema is usually obvious because of the typical pretibial lesions, the presence of Graves' ophthalmopathy, and a history of thyrotoxicosis. Biopsy may be necessary in some cases, however (3,5,37). Although dermopathy can be the initial presentation of Graves' disease in rare cases (10,30–33), the diagnosis of Graves' disease should be considered doubtful if Graves' ophthalmopathy is not present.

Skin changes somewhat similar to those of localized myxedema can occur in patients with simple edema as a result of fluid retention or venous insufficiency (66), generalized myxedema, chronic or lichenified dermatitis, hypertrophic lichen planus, and the urticarial phases of certain blistering eruptions, such as bullous pemphigoid. Cutaneous mucinoses, such as lichen myxedematosus (papular mucinosis), reticular erythematous mucinosis, and follicular mucinosis, are relatively rare dermatologic conditions in which accumulation of mucin in the dermis is a prominent feature (2,67). Most of these mucinoses involve the upper extremities, and thyroid dysfunction and ophthalmopathy are absent. Mucin deposition in recently recognized nephrogenic fibrosing dermopathy has some similarities with thyroid dermopathy, but the clinical picture and manifestations are different (68).

TREATMENT

Most patients require no therapy because the lesions are usually asymptomatic and not particularly unsightly, or they can be covered by clothing to the patient's satisfaction. Also, the lesions usually do not progress and may partially or completely regress with time (3). The natural course and long-term outcome of treated and untreated localized myxedema in a series of 178 patients were reported recently (5). Forty-six percent of these patients required no therapy for dermopathy.

When cosmetic concerns, functional impairment, or local discomfort necessitates treatment, topical application of a corticosteroid is the preferred therapy (5,69,70). The likelihood of therapeutic success decreases, however, as the extent of the lesions increases. The glucocorticoid is applied directly to the lesions, which for best results should be covered with a plastic film. In a group of 11 patients treated nightly or every other night by application of 0.2% midpotency corticosteroid fluocinolone acetonide cream to the lesions covered with occlusive plastic film dressings, all had substantial improvement (69). The improvement persisted after the frequency of treatment was gradually reduced to 2 to 4 times a month. A high-potency corticosteroid, such as clobetasol propionate, may also be used (71). Absorption of topical corticosteroid may be enhanced by hydrocolloid or plastic wrap occlusive dressing (71).

A trial of 4 to 10 weeks, followed by intermittent maintenance therapy (3,5), is usually needed. An occlusive dressing is kept in place for 12 hours. In the case of prolonged local therapy, skin should be watched for signs of adverse effects from the topical corticosteroid, such as atrophy, telangiectasia, and ecchymosis. Because of fluid accumulation, use of compressive bandages or an elastic stocking during the day offers additional benefit, especially in patients with the elephantiasic form of the disorder. Patients may require many months of therapy, the goal of which is to limit the degree of disfigurement, improve function, and avoid tissue breakdown and compressive complications. For patients with severe pretibial myxedema, such as the elephantiasic form, treatment similar to that used for patients with lymphedema may be required. In a recent report, complete decompressive physiotherapy resulted in sustained improvement in a patient with elephantiasic pretibial myxedema (72). This treatment, given by a certified physiotherapist, is a combination of manual lymphatic drainage and gentle massage, followed by the

application of multilayered low-stretch bandaging, exercise, and scrupulous skin care (73,74). Intradermal injections of a glucocorticoid (75) and hyaluronidase have been used, but these are not recommended because their efficacy is limited and they may cause irregular, lumpy skin. Local excision of pseudotumorous localized myxedema of the dorsum of the foot resistant to medical therapy has been reported, with apparent success (76). Surgical excision of nodules and skin grafting should be avoided, however, because of the possibility of exuberant recurrence of localized myxedema at the site of a surgical scar (29).

When ophthalmopathy overshadows the localized myxedema, as is often the case, systemic corticosteroid or other immunosuppressive therapy for the former may cause regression of the skin lesions (3,77). These drugs are rarely, if ever, indicated for localized myxedema alone. Other treatments that have been reported to be beneficial in a few patients include plasmapheresis, the somatostatin analogue octreotide, and high-dose intravenous immunoglobulin (78–82). The rationale for a beneficial effect of octreotide is the presence of somatostatin receptors in lymphocytes (83). However, a recent report showed no benefit from octreotide therapy in four patients with severe pretibial myxedema (84). Lack of benefit from high-dose intravenous immunoglobulin in a patient with elephantiasic pretibial myxedema also was reported recently (85). Evaluation of the effects of these therapies is difficult because of the small number of patients reported, short follow-up periods, and lack of controlled studies.

The long-term outcome for patients with localized myxedema varies. About half of patients with mild disease who receive no therapy have complete remission in 17 years. Severely affected patients who receive local corticosteroid and other therapies fare no better than patients with milder cases who receive no specific therapy. After 25 years of follow-up, 70% of untreated patients with milder myxedema and 58% of patients with severe forms who received local therapy achieved either partial or complete remission (Figs. 23C.6 and 23C.7) (5). Long-term remission appears to depend on the severity of initial disease rather than on the effect of therapy. Patients with milder cases without therapy have a better chance of complete remission than do patients with severe cases despite therapy. The present therapeutic modalities are palliative at best, and better and safer means of immune modulation are needed to treat this extrathyroidal manifestation of autoimmune thyroid disease.

THYROID ACROPACHY

Thyroid acropachy is the least common manifestation of Graves' disease. Similar to dermopathy, acropachy is a marker of a severe autoimmune process and a marker of severity of associated ophthalmopathy (10). A recently re-

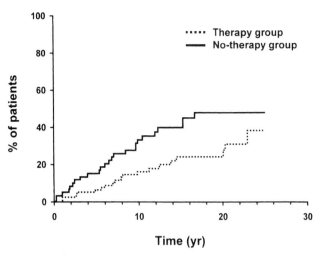

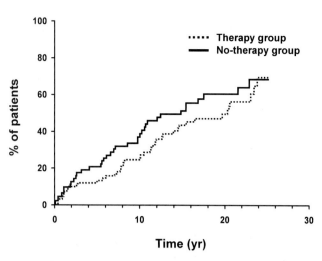

FIGURE 23C.6. Percentage of patients who had complete remission according to treatment group (Kaplan-Meier method). (From Schwartz KM, Fatourechi V, Ahmed DD, et al. Dermopathy of Graves' disease (pretibial myxedema): long-term outcome. *J Clin Endocrinol Metab* 2002;87:438, with permission.)

FIGURE 23C.7. Combined percentage of patients who had partial or complete remission according to treatment group (Kaplan-Meier method). (From Schwartz KM, Fatourechi V, Ahmed DD, et al. Dermopathy of Graves' disease (pretibial myxedema): long-term outcome. *J Clin Endocrinol Metab* 2002;87:438, with permission.)

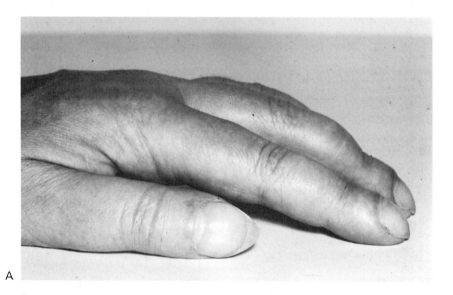

A

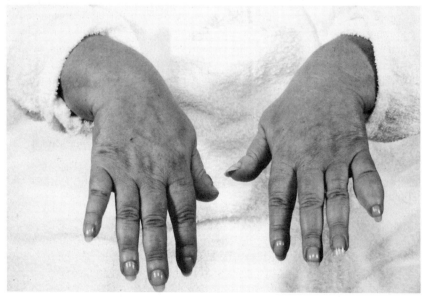

B

FIGURE 23C.8. A,B: Photographs of the hands in two patients with thyroid acropachy, showing clubbing of the fingertips and soft tissue swelling. **B:** Note the asymmetric involvement of the fingers.

ported series of patients with localized myxedema indicated that 22% of patients had thyroid acropachy (86). The most common form of acropachy is clubbing of the fingers and toes. Less commonly, swelling of digits and toes and periosteal reaction of distal extremity bones are seen. Previous reports had suggested a female-to-male ratio of 1:1 in this condition (87). However, in a recent report of 40 patients with acropachy, the female-to-male ratio was 3.4:1 (86). Acropachy almost always occurs in association with ophthalmopathy and localized myxedema, although an isolated case without either has been reported (88).

Typically, the process involves soft-tissue swelling of the hands and feet, usually in association with clubbing of the fingers and toes (Figs. 23C.8 and 23C.9). The skin is commonly pigmented and hyperkeratotic. Joints are not involved in thyroid acropachy, and the local warmth and increased blood flow characteristic of pulmonary osteoarthropathy are usually absent. The upper and lower ex-

tremities are equally involved (87,89). The process may be asymmetric, and involvement of a single digit has been reported (90). Acropachy is often painless, but some patients have pain and loss of function because of extreme swelling (86,91).

It is unusual for acropachy to occur before thyroid dysfunction, and in general the developmental chronology is thyroid dysfunction, ophthalmopathy, localized myxedema, and, lastly, acropachy (87,89). Although it can occur as late as 40 years after the onset of thyrotoxicosis, the median interval between diagnosis of the latter and acropachy is 2 to 3 years (87).

Radiography shows fusiform soft-tissue swelling of the digits and subperiosteal bone formation, usually involving the metacarpals, the proximal and middle phalanges of the fingers, and the metatarsal and proximal phalanges of the toes. The subperiosteal reaction is unusual in the long bones of the forearms or the legs, in contrast to pulmonary osteoarthropathy. Only one of 40 patients who had severe extremity pain had a periosteal reaction in the femur (Fig. 23C.10) (86). The periosteal new bone formation is most marked in the midportion of the diaphysis, and it characteristically appears spiculated, leathery, frothy, lacy, or bubbled (Fig. 23C.11) (87,89), quite different from the laminal periosteal proliferation of classic pulmonary osteoarthropathy. In the earlier stages of acropachy, when bone radiographs may appear normal, technetium (^{99m}Tc)-pyrophosphate bone scans show focal accumulation of the radionuclide in the affected areas (92). Most patients have a combination of skin changes, clubbing, bone changes, and radiographic changes, but patients in whom radiographic findings were the only manifestation of acropachy have been reported (89,93). Skin pathologic features are similar to those of localized myxedema (87,93). Little is known about the pathologic characteristics and pathogenesis of thyroid acropachy. One study of bone histology revealed nodular fibrosis of the periosteal area, subperiosteal bone formation, and fibrosis of the marrow space (94). One can speculate that the process involves autoimmune activation of periosteal fibroblasts.

Similar to patients with dermopathy and severe ophthalmopathy, a high percentage of patients with acropachy are current cigarette smokers. In a recent report, 81% of women and 75% of men were current smokers, respectively 3.7 and 2.6 times higher than the rate for the US general population (86). The association of acropachy with tobacco use, is also seen in patients with severe ophthalmopathy and dermopathy and is believed not to be related to pulmonary complications of tobacco use (86).

No specific treatment for thyroid acropachy is available. Systemic immunosuppressive therapy and local corticosteroid therapy are usually directed at associated ophthalmopathy and dermopathy. In most patients, clubbing is the only manifestation of acropachy, and it is asympto-

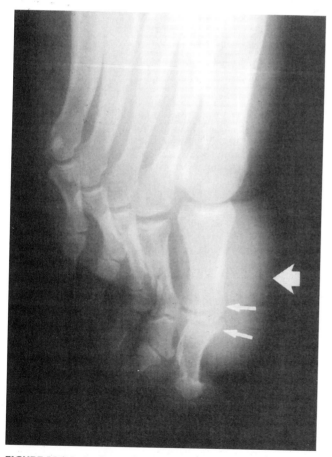

FIGURE 23C.9. Radiograph of the toes in a patient with thyroid acropachy. Note soft-tissue swelling (*arrowhead*) and mild, fluffy periosteal reaction of the first toe and distal end of the first metatarsal (*arrows*). (From Fatourechi V, Ahmed DD, Schwartz KM. Thyroid acropachy: report of 40 patients treated at a single institution in a 26-year period. *J Clin Endocrinol Metab* 2002;87:5435, with permission.)

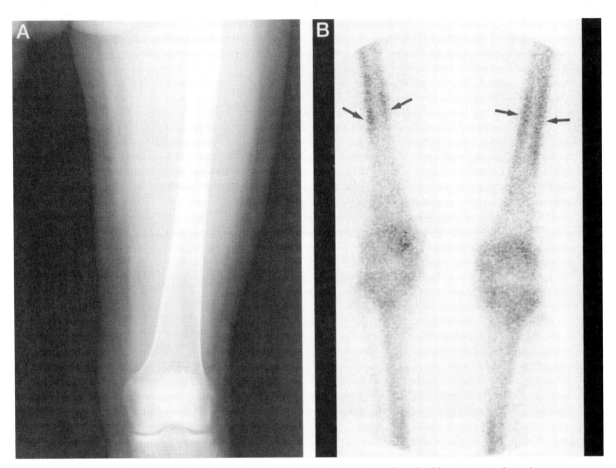

FIGURE 23C.10. Imaging of a patient with thyroid acropachy and marked lower extremity pain. **A:** Radiograph of the left femur is normal. **B:** Technetium-99m bone scan shows irregular increased uptake in the cortical area of both femurs (*arrows*) and tibae. (From Fatourechi V, Ahmed DD, Schwartz KM. Thyroid acropachy: report of 40 patients treated at a single institution in a 26-year period. *J Clin Endocrinol Metab* 2002;87:5435, with permission.)

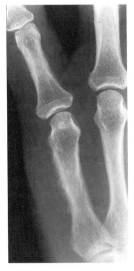

FIGURE 23C.11. Radiograph of fingers of a patient with thyroid acropachy. Note the asymmetric frothy appearance of subperiosteal bone formation in the midportion of the proximal phalanx on the **left**.

matic and requires no specific therapy. After long-term follow-up, remission of acropachy may occur. It is not clear from the reported cases how often remission of clubbing occurs. Long-term follow-up has shown that dermopathy and ophthalmopathy, not acropachy, are common sources of functional problems and the patient's chief complaints (86).

REFERENCES

1. Beierwaltes WH. Clinical correlation of pretibial myxedema with malignant exophthalmos. *Ann Intern Med* 1954;40:968–984.
2. Kriss JP. Pathogenesis and treatment of pretibial myxedema. *Endocrinol Metab Clin North Am* 1987;16:409–415.
3. Fatourechi V, Pajouhi M, Fransway AF. Dermopathy of Graves disease (pretibial myxedema): review of 150 cases. *Medicine (Baltimore)* 1994;73:1–7.
4. Fatourechi V, Garrity JA, Bartley GB, et al. Orbital decompression in Graves' ophthalmopathy associated with pretibial myxedema. *J Endocrinol Invest* 1993;16:433–437.

5. Schwartz KM, Fatourechi V, Ahmed DD, et al. Dermopathy of Graves' disease (pretibial myxedema): long-term outcome. *J Clin Endocrinol Metab* 2002;87:438–446.

6. Bartley GB, Fatourechi V, Kadrmas EF, et al. Clinical features of Graves' ophthalmopathy in an incidence cohort. *Am J Ophthalmol* 1996;121:284–290.

7. Wortsman J, Dietrich J, Traycoff RB, et al. Preradial myxedema in thyroid disease. *Arch Dermatol* 1981;117:635–638.

8. Salvi M, De Chiara F, Gardini E, et al. Echographic diagnosis of pretibial myxedema in patients with autoimmune thyroid disease. *Eur J Endocrinol* 1994;131:113–119.

9. Peacey SR, Flemming L, Messenger A, et al. Is Graves' dermopathy a generalized disorder? *Thyroid* 1996;6:41–45.

10. Fatourechi V, Bartley GB, Eghbali-Fatourechi GZ, et al. Graves' dermopathy and acropachy are markers of severe Graves' ophthalmopathy. *Thyroid* 2003;13:1141–1144.

11. Morris JC III, Hay ID, Nelson RE, et al. Clinical utility of thyrotropin-receptor antibody assays: comparison of radioreceptor and bioassay methods. *Mayo Clin Proc* 1988;63:707–717.

12. Schermer DR, Roenigk HH Jr, Schumacher OP, et al. Relationship of long-acting thyroid stimulator to pretibial myxedema. *Arch Dermatol* 1970;102:62–67.

13. Watson EM, Pearce RH. The mucopolysaccharide content of the skin in localized (pretibial) myxedema. *Am J Clin Pathol* 1947;17:507–512.

14. Sisson JC. Hyaluronic acid in localized myxedema. *J Clin Endocrinol Metab* 1968;28:433–436.

15. Smith TJ, Bahn RS, Gorman CA. Connective tissue, glycosaminoglycans, and diseases of the thyroid. *Endocr Rev* 1989;10:366–391.

16. Hanke CW, Bergfeld WF, Guirguis MN, et al. Hyaluronic acid synthesis in fibroblasts of pretibial myxedema. *Cleve Clin Q* 1983;50:129–132.

17. Bahn RS, Heufelder AE. Pathogenesis of Graves' ophthalmopathy. *N Engl J Med* 1993;329:1468–1475.

18. Cohen BD, Benua RS, Rawson RW. Localized myxedema involving the upper extremities. *Arch Intern Med* 1963;111:641–646.

19. Noppakun N, Bancheun K, Chandraprasert S. Unusual locations of localized myxedema in Graves' disease: report of three cases. *Arch Dermatol* 1986;122:85–88.

20. Akasu F, Takazawa K, Akasu R, et al. Localized myxedema on the nasal dorsum in a patient with Graves' disease: report of a case. *J Endocrinol Invest* 1989;12:717–721.

21. Slater DN. Cervical nodular localized myxoedema in a thyroidectomy scar: light and electron microscopy and histochemical findings. *Clin Exp Dermatol* 1987;12:216–219.

22. Wright AL, Buxton PK, Menzies D. Pretibial myxedema localized to scar tissue. *Int J Dermatol* 1990;29:54–55.

23. Pujol RM, Monmany J, Bague S, et al. Graves' disease presenting as localized myxoedematous infiltration in a smallpox vaccination scar. *Clin Exp Dermatol* 2000;25:132–134.

24. Frisch DR, Roth I. Pretibial myxedema: a review of the literature and case report. *J Am Podiatr Med Assoc* 1985;75:147–152.

25. Truhan AP. Pretibial myxedema. *Am Fam Physician* 1985;31:135–138.

26. Gitter DG, Sato K. Localized hyperhidrosis in pretibial myxedema. *J Am Acad Dermatol* 1990;23:250–254.

27. Kato N, Ueno H, Matsubara M. A case report of EMO syndrome showing localized hyperhidrosis in pretibial myxedema. *J Dermatol* 1991;18:598–604.

28. Siegler M, Refetoff S. Pretibial myxedema: a reversible cause of foot drop due to entrapment of the peroneal nerve. *N Engl J Med* 1976;294:1383–1384.

29. Chremos AN. Relentless localized myxedema, with exophthalmos, clubbing of the fingers and hypertrophic osteoarthropathy: observations on an unusual case. *Am J Med* 1965;38:954–961.

30. Georgala S, Katoulis AC, Georgala C, et al. Pretibial myxedema as the initial manifestation of Graves' disease. *J Eur Acad Dermatol Venereol* 2002;16:380–383.

31. Cho S, Choi JH, Sung KJ, et al. Graves' disease presenting as elephantiasic pretibial myxedema and nodules of the hands. *Int J Dermatol* 2001;40:276–277.

32. Jabbour SA, Miller JL. Endocrinopathies and the skin. *Int J Dermatol* 2000;39:88–99.

33. Omohundro C, Dijkstra JW, Camisa D, et al. Early onset pretibial myxedema in the absence of ophthalmopathy: a morphologic evolution. *Cutis* 1996;58:211–214.

34. Konrad K, Brenner W, Pehamberger H. Ultrastructural and immunological findings in Graves' disease with pretibial myxedema. *J Cutan Pathol* 1980;7:99–108.

35. Kobayasi T, Danielsen L, Asboe-Hansen G. Ultrastructure of localized myxedema. *Acta Derm Venereol* 1976;56:173–185.

36. Ishii M, Nakagawa K, Hamada T. An ultrastructural study of pretibial myxedema utilizing improved ruthenium red stain. *J Cutan Pathol* 1984;11:125–131.

37. Somach SC, Helm TN, Lawlor KB, et al. Pretibial mucin: histologic patterns and clinical correlation. *Arch Dermatol* 1993;129:1152–1156.

38. Bull RH, Coburn PR, Mortimer PS. Pretibial myxoedema: a manifestation of lymphoedema? *Lancet* 1993;341:403–404.

39. Antonelli A, Palla R, Casarosa L, et al. IgG, IgA and C3 deposits in the extra-thyroidal manifestations of autoimmune Graves' disease: their in vitro solubilization by intravenous immunoglobulin. *Clin Exp Rheumatol* 1996;14[Suppl 15]:S31–S35.

40. Tomer Y, Barbesino G, Greenberg DA, et al. Mapping the major susceptibility loci for familial Graves' and Hashimoto's diseases: evidence for genetic heterogeneity and gene interactions. *J Clin Endocrinol Metab* 1999;84:4656–4664.

41. Villanueva R, Inzerillo AM, Tomer Y, et al. Limited genetic susceptibility to severe Graves' ophthalmopathy: no role for CTLA-4 but evidence for an environmental etiology. *Thyroid* 2000;10:791–798.

42. Kriss JP, Pleshakov V, Chien JR. Isolation and identification of the long-acting thyroid stimulator and its relation to hyperthyroidism and circumscribed pretibial myxedema. *J Clin Endocrinol Metab* 1964;24:1005–1028.

43. Chang TC, Wu SL, Hsiao YL, et al. TSH and TSH receptor antibody-binding sites in fibroblasts of pretibial myxedema are related to the extracellular domain of entire TSH receptor. *Clin Immunol Immunopathol* 1994;71:113–120.

44. Tao TW, Leu SL, Kriss JP. Biological activity of autoantibodies associated with Graves' dermopathy. *J Clin Endocrinol Metab* 1989;69:90–99.

45. Heufelder AE, Dutton CM, Sarkar G, et al. Detection of TSH receptor RNA in cultured fibroblasts from patients with Graves' ophthalmopathy and pretibial dermopathy. *Thyroid* 1993;3:297–300.

46. Rapoport B, Alsabeh R, Aftergood D, et al. Elephantiasic pretibial myxedema: insight into a hypothesis regarding the pathogenesis of the extrathyroidal manifestations of Graves' disease. *Thyroid* 2000;10:685–692.

47. Spitzweg C, Joba W, Hunt N, et al. Analysis of human thyrotropin receptor gene expression and immunoreactivity in human orbital tissue. *Eur J Endocrinol* 1997;136:599–607.

48. Ludgate M, Crisp M, Lane C, et al. The thyrotropin receptor in thyroid eye disease. *Thyroid* 1998;8:411–413.

49. Wu SL, Chang TC, Chang TJ, et al. Cloning and sequencing of complete thyrotropin receptor transcripts in pretibial fibroblast culture cells. *J Endocrinol Invest* 1996;19:365–370.

50. Daumerie C, Ludgate M, Costagliola S, et al. Evidence for thyrotropin receptor immunoreactivity in pretibial connective tissue from patients with thyroid-associated dermopathy. *Eur J Endocrinol* 2002;146:35–38.

51. Cheung HS, Nicoloff JT, Kamiel MB, et al. Stimulation of fibroblast biosynthetic activity by serum of patients with pretibial myxedema. *J Invest Dermatol* 1978;71:12–17.

52. Shishiba Y, Imai Y, Odajima R, et al. Immunoglobulin G of patients with circumscribed pretibial myxedema of Graves' disease stimulates proteoglycan synthesis in human skin fibroblasts in culture. *Acta Endocrinol (Copenh)* 1992;127:44–51.

53. Metcalfe RA, Davies R, Weetman AP. Analysis of fibroblast-stimulating activity in IgG from patients with Graves' dermopathy. *Thyroid* 1993;3:207–212.

54. Schwartz KM, Ahmed DD, Ahmed I, et al. Development of localized myxedema in a skin graft. *Int J Dermatol* 2002;41:401–403.

55. Missner SC, Ramsay EW, Houck HE, et al. Graves' disease presenting as localized myxedema in a thigh donor graft site. *J Am Acad Dermatol* 1998;39:846–849.

56. Westphal SA. Extrathyroidal manifestations of Graves' disease: pretibial myxedema and thyroid acropachy. *Endocr Pract* 1995;1:116–122.

57. Bahn RS. Clinical review 157: pathophysiology of Graves' ophthalmopathy: the cycle of disease. *J Clin Endocrinol Metab* 2003;88:1939–1946.

58. Matzinger P. An innate sense of danger. *Semin Immunol* 1998;10:399–415.

59. Umetsu DT, Katzen D, Jabara HH, et al. Antigen presentation by human dermal fibroblasts: activation of resting T lymphocytes. *J Immunol* 1986;136:440–445.

60. Heufelder AE, Wenzel BE, Gorman CA, et al. Detection, cellular localization, and modulation of heat shock proteins in cultured fibroblasts from patients with extrathyroidal manifestations of Graves' disease. *J Clin Endocrinol Metab* 1991; 73:739–745.

61. Korducki JM, Loftus SJ, Bahn RS. Stimulation of glycosaminoglycan production in cultured human retroocular fibroblasts. *Invest Ophthalmol Vis Sci* 1992;33:2037–2042.

62. Heufelder AE. T-cell restriction in thyroid eye disease. *Thyroid* 1998;8:419–422.

63. Smith TJ, Bahn RS, Gorman CA. Hormonal regulation of hyaluronate synthesis in cultured human fibroblasts: evidence for differences between retroocular and dermal fibroblasts. *J Clin Endocrinol Metab* 1989;69:1019–1023.

64. Shishiba Y, Tanaka T, Ozawa Y, et al. Chemical characterization of high buoyant density proteoglycan accumulated in the affected skin of pretibial myxedema of Graves' disease. *Endocrinol Jpn* 1986;33:395–403.

65. Heufelder AE, Smith TJ, Gorman CA, et al. Increased induction of HLA-DR by interferon-gamma in cultured fibroblasts derived from patients with Graves' ophthalmopathy and pretibial dermopathy. *J Clin Endocrinol Metab* 1991;73:307–313.

66. Kim KJ, Kim HH, Chang SE, et al. A case of pretibial mucinosis without thyroid disease. *J Dermatol* 2002;29:383–385.

67. Truhan AP, Roenigk HH Jr. The cutaneous mucinoses. *J Am Acad Dermatol* 1986;14:1–18.

68. Mackay-Wiggan JM, Cohen DJ, Hardy MA, et al. Nephrogenic fibrosing dermopathy (scleromyxedema-like illness of renal disease). *J Am Acad Dermatol* 2003;48:55–60.

69. Kriss JP, Pleshakov V, Rosenblum A, et al. Therapy with occlusive dressings of pretibial myxedema with fluocinolone acetonide. *J Clin Endocrinol Metab* 1967;27:595–604.

70. Benoit FL, Greenspan FS. Corticoid therapy for pretibial myxedema: observations on the long-acting thyroid stimulator. *Ann Intern Med* 1967;66:711–720.

71. Volden G. Successful treatment of chronic skin diseases with clobetasol propionate and a hydrocolloid occlusive dressing. *Acta Derm Venereol* 1992;72:69–71.

72. Susser WS, Heermans AG, Chapman MS, et al. Elephantiasic pretibial myxedema: a novel treatment for an uncommon disorder. *J Am Acad Dermatol* 2002;46:723–726.

73. Connell M. Complete decongestive physiotherapy. *Innov Breast Cancer Care* 1998;3:93–96.

74. Smith JK. Oncology nursing in lymphedema management. *Innov Breast Cancer Care* 1998: 3:82–87.

75. Lang PG, Sisson JC, Lynch PJ. Intralesional triamcinolone therapy for pretibial myxedema. *Arch Dermatol* 1975;111:197–202.

76. Pingsmann A, Ockenfels HM, Patsalis T. Surgical excision of pseudotumorous pretibial myxedema. *Foot Ankle Int* 1996;17:107–110.

77. Koshiyama H, Mori S, Fujiwara K, et al. Successful treatment of hypothyroid Graves' disease with a combination of levothyroxine replacement, intravenous high-dose steroid and irradiation to the orbit. *Intern Med* 1993;32:421–423.

78. Kuzuya N, DeGroot LJ. Effect of plasmapheresis and steroid treatment on thyrotropin binding inhibitory immunoglobulins in a patient with exophthalmos and a patient with pretibial myxedema. *J Endocrinol Invest* 1982;5:373–378.

79. Noppen M, Velkeniers B, Steenssens L, et al. Beneficial effects of plasmapheresis followed by immunosuppressive therapy in pretibial myxedema. *Acta Clin Belg* 1988;43:381–383.

80. Chang TC, Kao SC, Huang KM. Octreotide and Graves' ophthalmopathy and pretibial myxoedema. *BMJ* 1992;304:158.

81. Priestley GC, Aldridge RD, Sime PJ, et al. Skin fibroblast activity in pretibial myxoedema and the effect of octreotide (Sandostatin) in vitro. *Br J Dermatol* 1994;131:52–56.

82. Antonelli A, Navarranne A, Palla R, et al. Pretibial myxedema and high-dose intravenous immunoglobulin treatment. *Thyroid* 1994;4:399–408.

83. Colao A, Lastoria S, Ferone D, et al. Orbital scintigraphy with [^{111}In-diethylenetriamine pentaacetic acid-D-phe^1]-octreotide predicts the clinical response to corticosteroid therapy in patients with Graves' ophthalmopathy. *J Clin Endocrinol Metab* 1998;83:3790–3794.

84. Rotman-Pikielny P, Brucker-Davis F, Turner ML, et al. Lack of effect of long-term octreotide therapy in severe thyroid-associated dermopathy. *Thyroid* 2003;13:465–470.

85. Terheyden P, Kahaly GJ, Zillikens D, et al. Lack of response of elephantiasic pretibial myxoedema to treatment with high-dose intravenous immunoglobulins. *Clin Exp Dermatol* 2003;28: 224–226.

86. Fatourechi V, Ahmed DD, Schwartz KM. Thyroid acropachy: report of 40 patients treated at a single institution in a 26-year period. *J Clin Endocrinol Metab* 2002;87:5435–5441.

87. Winkler A, Wilson D. Thyroid acropachy: case report and literature review. *Mol Med* 1985;82:756–761.

88. Goette DK. Thyroid acropachy. *Arch Dermatol* 1980;116:205–206.

89. Kinsella RA Jr, Back DK. Thyroid acropachy. *Med Clin North Am* 1968;52:393–398.

90. Chapman ME, Beggs I, Wu PS. Case report: thyroid acropachy in a single digit. *Clin Radiol* 1993;47:58–59.

91. Rothschild BM, Yoon BH. Thyroid acropachy complicated by lymphatic obstruction. *Arthritis Rheum* 1982;25:588–590.

92. Seigel RS, Thrall JH, Sisson JC. ^{99m}Tc-pyrophosphate scan and radiographic correlation in thyroid acropachy: case report. *J Nucl Med* 1976;17:791–793.

93. Parker LN, Wu SY, Lai MK, et al. The early diagnosis of atypical thyroid acropachy. *Arch Intern Med* 1982;142:1749–1751.

94. King LR, Braunstein H, Chambers D, et al. A case study of peculiar soft-tissue and bony changes in association with thyroid disease. *J Clin Endocrinol Metab* 1959;19:1323–1330.

THYROTROPIN-INDUCED THYROTOXICOSIS

PAOLO BECK-PECCOZ
LUCA PERSANI

Thyrotoxicosis results much more frequently from auto-antibody stimulation or primary disorders of the thyroid than from excessive secretion of thyrotropin (TSH). However, with the advent of ultrasensitive immunometric TSH assays, an increased number of patients with normal or high levels of TSH in the presence of high thyroid hormone concentrations have been recognized. In this situation, the negative feedback mechanism is clearly disrupted and TSH itself is responsible for the hyperstimulation of the thyroid gland and the consequent thyrotoxicosis. Therefore, it has been proposed this entity be termed central hyperthyroidism. Indeed, the old term, inappropriate secretion of TSH, which refers to the fact that TSH is not suppressed as expected, owing to the high thyroid hormone concentrations, appears inadequate, as it does not reflect the pathophysiological events underlying this unusual disorder.

Central hyperthyroidism is mainly due to an autonomous TSH hypersecretion from a TSH-secreting pituitary adenoma. However, signs and symptoms of thyrotoxicosis along with biochemical findings similar to those found in TSH-secreting tumors may be recorded in a minority of patients affected with resistance to thyroid hormones (RTH). This form of RTH is called pituitary RTH (PRTH), as the RTH action appears more severe at the pituitary than at the peripheral tissue level (see Chapter 81). The clinical importance of these rare entities is based on the diagnostic and therapeutical challenges they present. Failure to recognize these different disorders may result in dramatic consequences, such as improper thyroid ablation in patients with a TSH-secreting tumor or unnecessary pituitary surgery in patients with RTH. Conversely, early diagnosis and correct treatment of TSH-secreting tumor may prevent the occurrence of complications (visual defects by compression of the optic chiasm, hypopituitarism, etc.) and should improve the rate of cure. In this chapter, the salient clinical features of patients with a TSH-secreting tumor, as well as the diagnostic and therapeutic approaches and the prognostic criteria, will be discussed.

EPIDEMIOLOGY

TSH-secreting tumors are rare (1,2). The first patient was documented in 1960 by measuring serum TSH with a bioassay (3). These tumors account for about 0.5% to 1% of all pituitary adenomas, whose prevalence in the general population is about 0.02%. Thus, the prevalence of TSH-secreting tumors is about one case per million. However, this figure is probably underestimated, as the number of reported cases has tripled in the last decade. This trend is comparable to that observed in a large surgical series of pituitary tumors where an increased occurrence of TSH-secreting tumors (from <1% to 2.8% in the period 1989 to 1991) was documented (4). The increased number of reported cases principally results from the introduction of ultrasensitive immunometric assays for TSH as the first-line test for the evaluation of thyroid function. Based on the finding of measurable serum TSH levels in the presence of thyrotoxicosis, many patients previously thought to have Graves' disease can be correctly diagnosed as patients with TSH-secreting tumor or, alternatively, RTH (2,5,6).

The presence of a TSH-secreting tumor has been observed in patients of any age, from 8 to 84 years. However, most patients are diagnosed between the third and the sixth decade of life. Unlike the female predominance seen in the other common thyroid disorders, these tumors occur with equal frequency in men and women. Familial presentation has been reported only as part of the multiple endocrine neoplasia type 1 syndrome (MEN-1).

PATHOLOGICAL AND PATHOGENETIC ASPECTS

Almost all TSH-secreting tumors originate from pituitary thyrotrophs. Indeed, only two cases of ectopic nasopharynx adenoma overproducing TSH and causing thyrotoxicosis have been reported (7,8). These tumors are nearly always benign, and transformation into a TSH-secreting carcinoma with metastases has been reported in only one patient (9).

The great majority of TSH-secreting tumors are macroadenomas having a diameter of more than 10 mm at the time of diagnosis, while fewer than 15% are microadenomas. Extrasellar extension is present in more than two thirds of cases. Most of the tumors show localized or diffuse invasiveness into the surrounding structures, especially into the dura and bone. The occurrence of invasive macroadenomas is particularly frequent in patients with previous thyroid ablation by surgery or radioiodine, underlying the deleterious effects of incorrect diagnosis and treatment (Fig. 24.1). Such an aggressive transformation of the tumor resembles that occurring in Nelson's syndrome after adrenalectomy for Cushing's disease. By light microscopy, adenoma cells are often arranged in cords, usually with chromophobic appearance, though they occasionally stain with either basic or acid dyes. They appear large and polymorphous, with frequent nuclear atypia and mitoses, thus being often mistakenly recognized as a pituitary malignancy or metastasis from distant carcinomas (10). Electron microscopy demonstrates mostly monomorphous tumors, characterized by the presence of fusiform cells with long cytoplasmic processes, scanty rough endoplasmic reticulum, poorly developed Golgi apparatus, and a low number of small secretory granules (80–200 nm) mainly aligned under the plasma membrane (10,11).

About 75% of these tumors secrete TSH alone, which is often accompanied by an unbalanced hypersecretion of the α-subunit of glycoprotein hormones. Thus, cosecretion of other anterior pituitary hormones occurs in about 25% of patients. Hypersecretion of growth hormone (GH) and/or prolactin (PRL), resulting in acromegaly and/or amenorrhea/galactorrhea, are the most frequent associations. This may be due to the fact that GH and PRL share with TSH the common transcription factor Pit-1. The occurrence of a mixed adrenocorticotropic hormone (TSH)/

gonadotropin adenoma is rare, while no association with ACTH hypersecretion has been documented to date.

Immunostaining studies show the presence of TSH/β-subunit and/or α-subunit in the great majority of cases. By double immunostaining, the existence of mixed TSH/β-subunit adenomas composed of one cell type secreting α-subunit alone and another cosecreting α-subunit and TSH has been documented (11). In addition to α-subunit, TSH frequently colocalizes with other pituitary hormones in the same tumor cell. Nonetheless, immunopositivity for one or more pituitary hormones does not necessarily result in *in vivo* hypersecretion. Indeed, positive immunostaining for ACTH and gonadotropins generally occurs without evidence of hypersecretion of the corresponding hormone.

Due to the rarity of TSH-secreting tumors, *in vitro* hormone secretion from cultured tumors and its regulation by different agents have been investigated only rarely. Although some responses would be predicted from *in vivo* data, *in vitro* studies suggest that the majority of tumors express receptors for thyrotropin-releasing hormone (TRH) and somatostatin, while dopamine receptors seem to be variably present (12,13).

As for most pituitary tumors the pathogenesis of TSH-secreting tumors is largely unknown. Screening studies for genetic abnormalities resulting in transcriptional activation have yielded negative results (14). In particular, no activating mutations of putative protooncogenes, such as *ras, G-protein, TRH, and Pit-1,* or loss of genes with tumor suppressor activity, such as *p53* and *menin* gene, have been reported (14,15). Evidence for local overproduction of growth factors was provided in some tumors, in agreement with the constant presence of these substances in almost all pituitary adenomas. Recently, somatic mutations (16) and aberrant alternative splicing (17) of thyroid hormone receptor β have been reported, along with dysregulation of deiodinase expression and

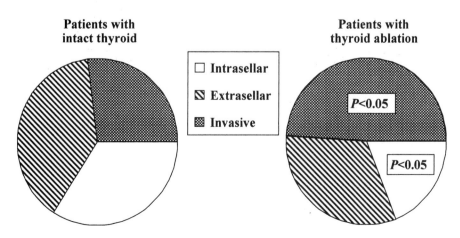

FIGURE 24.1. Effects of previous thyroid ablation on the size of TSH-producing adenomas. "Intrasellar" refers to both microadenomas and intrasellar macroadenomas, "extrasellar" to macroadenomas with suprasellar extension, and "invasive" to invasive macroadenomas. Data have been calculated from 264 reported patients (169 with an intact thyroid and 95 with thyroid ablation). Note the significant increase of invasive tumors in patients with thyroid ablation. Statistical analysis between the two groups was carried out by Fisher's exact test.

function (18,19). These findings may at least in part explain the defects in negative regulation of TSH by thyroid hormones in some tumors. Collectively, available data on a small number of tumors are too preliminary to draw definite conclusions on transcriptional and/or expression abnormalities in the tumors.

SIGNS AND SYMPTOMS

Patients with TSH-secreting tumor present with signs and symptoms of thyrotoxicosis that are frequently associated with those related to the pressure effects of the pituitary adenomas, causing loss of vision, visual field defects, and/or loss of other anterior pituitary functions (Table 24.1). Most patients have a long history of thyroid dysfunction, often misdiagnosed as Graves' disease, and about one third had an inappropriate thyroidectomy or radioiodine ablation (1,2,20,21). Clinical features of thyrotoxicosis are sometimes milder than expected on the basis of circulating thyroid hormone levels. In some acromegalic patients, signs and symptoms of thyrotoxicosis may be missed, as they are overshadowed by those of acromegaly. Contrary to what is observed in patients with primary thyroid disorders, atrial fibrillation and/or cardiac failure are rare events.

The presence of a goiter is the rule, even in patients with a previous thyroidectomy, since the remaining thyroid may regrow as a consequence of TSH hyperstimulation. Occurrence of uni- or multinodular goiter is frequent (about 72% of reported cases), whereas differentiated thyroid carcinoma was documented in a few cases (22,23). Progres-

sion toward functional autonomy seems to be infrequent (24). In contrast with Graves' disease, the occurrence of antithyroid autoantibodies is similar to that found in the general population, being about 8%. Bilateral exophthalmos occurred in a few patients who subsequently developed autoimmune thyroiditis, while unilateral exophthalmos due to orbital invasion by a pituitary tumor was reported in three patients (2).

Most patients with a TSH-secreting macroadenoma seek medical attention because of signs or symptoms of an expanding intracranial tumor. Indeed, as a consequence of tumor suprasellar extension or invasiveness, signs and symptoms of tumor mass prevail over those of thyroid hyperfunction in many patients. Visual field defects are present in about 40% and headache in 20% of patients (Table 24.1). Partial or total hypopituitarism occurs in about 25% of cases.

LABORATORY AND BIOCHEMICAL FEATURES

Serum Thyroid Hormone and Thyrotropin Levels

Serum TSH levels in untreated patients with TSH-secreting tumors may be high or in the normal range, whereas total and free thyroxine (T_4) and triiodothyronine (T_3) levels are definitely high (Table 24.2). Variations of the biological activity of secreted TSH molecules most likely account for the findings of normal TSH in the presence of high levels of free T_4 and free T_3, and goiter as well. Recent studies indicate that TSH molecules secreted by pituitary tumors may have normal, reduced, or increased biological activity relative to immunological activity, probably due to modification of glycosylation processes secondary to alterations of the posttranslational processing of the hormone within tumor cells (25,26).

In patients previously treated with thyroid ablation who still present with thyrotoxicosis serum, TSH levels are higher than in untreated patients, suggesting that tumoral thyrotroph cells may increase their TSH secretion in response to an even small reduction in thyroid hrmone levels (2,21). Therefore, while tumoral thyrotrophs are totally or partially resistant to the inhibitory action of high thyroid hormone levels, they have a preserved or even increased sensitivity to low serum thyroid hormone levels.

Particular clinical situations and possible laboratory artifacts may cause a biochemical profile similar to that characteristic of central thyrotoxicosis (2,5,6). Since these conditions are more common than are TSH-secreting tumors and RTH, they should be excluded before performing an extensive evaluation of the hypothalamic-pituitary-thyroid axis. Most of the other conditions may be recognized by measuring free, instead of total, thyroid

TABLE 24.1. CLINICAL CHARACTERISTICS OF PATIENTS WITH TSH-SECRETING TUMOR[a]

	Patients with a tumor *n*/total (%)[b]
Age range (years)	8–84
Female/male ratio	1.3
Previous thyroidectomy	95/301 (31.6)
Severe thyrotoxicosis	48/190 (25.2)
Goiter	177/194 (91.2)
Thyroid nodule(s)	47/65 (72.3)
Macroadenomas	229/264 (86.7)
Visual field defect	60/148 (40.5)
Headache	23/114 (20.2)
Menstrual disorders[c]	26/80 (32.5)
Galactorrhea[c]	11/36 (30.5)
Acromegaly	48/306 (15.7)

[a]Data from reports published through December 2003 and personal unpublished observations.
[b]*n*/total refers to the number of patients for whom the information was available.
[c]Data include women with or without associated prolactin hypersecretion.

TABLE 24.2. BIOCHEMICAL DATA OF PATIENTS WITH TSH-SECRETING TUMORS[a]

Serum parameter	Patients with intact thyroid	Patients with previous thyroidectomy	P
TSH (mU/L)[b]	9.3 ± 1.0 (125)	55.8 ± 10.2 (81)	<0.01
Normal TSH levels[c]	35.3% (60/170)	11.4% (9/79)	<0.01
α-subunit (mg/L)[b]	17.8 ± 5.4 (74)	14.5 ± 2.7 (46)	NS
α-subunit/TSH (m.r.)[b, d]	43.3 ± 15.5 (73)	3.7 ± 0.7 (46)	<0.03
High α-subunit levels[c]	66.6% (68/102)	72.9% (35/48)	NS
High α-subunit/TSH (m.r.)[c]	86.9% (86/99)	77.1% (37/48)	NS
TT_4 (nmol/L)[b]	239.8 ± 18.7 (33)	177.1 ± 9.8 (45)	<0.01
FT_4 (pmol/L)[b]	41.7 ± 2.3 (70)	28.7 ± 2.5 (30)	<0.01
TT_3 (nmol/L)[b]	4.9 ± 0.6 (33)	4.1 ± 0.3 (42)	NS
FT_3 (pmol/L)[b]	16.2 ± 0.8 (54)	10.5 ± 0.9 (20)	<0.01
High SHBG levels[c]	92.0% (23/25)	66.6% (6/9)	NS
Blunted TSH response to TRH test[c]	82.8% (116/140)	83.0% (58/70)	NS
Abnormal TSH response to T_3 suppression test[c, e]	100% (51/51)	100% (33/33)	NS

[a]Data from reports published through December 2003 and personal unpublished observations.
[b]Mean ± SE (n).
[c]% (n/total).
[d]To calculate α-subunit/TSH molar ratio divide α-subunit (µg/liter) by TSH (mU/liter) and multiply by 10.
[e]Lack of complete TSH inhibition after 8–10 days of T_3 administration (80–100 µg/day).

hormones (27). It is most important to measure serum free T_4 and T_3 by direct methods, not only to prevent possible misinterpretation due to variations in transport proteins, but also to assess true thyroid hormone production. Indeed, normal levels of total T_4 were reported in several patients, and only measurement free T_4 of led to the correct diagnosis (2,28).

Genetic alterations or treatment with certain drugs may cause quantitative/qualitative alterations of thyroxine-binding globulin, albumin, or transthyretin leading to increases in serum T_4 (see Chapter 6). Hyperthyroxinemia associated with measurable TSH may also be found in patients treated with the iodine-containing drug, amiodarone. In clinically ambiguous situations, the differential diagnosis rests on the recognition of the underlying disorder, as well as documenting normalization of thyroid function tests after drug withdrawal. Indeed, if patients with one of the above conditions were truly thyrotoxic, serum TSH levels should be undetectable.

Laboratory artifacts may cause falsely high levels of either thyroid hormones or TSH. Circulating anti-T_4 and/or anti-T_3 autoantibodies can interfere in the immunometric assay, leading to an overestimation of both total and free thyroid hormone levels (see Chapter 13). As far as the free T_4 and T_3 measurements are concerned, such overestimation is frequently observed when "one-step" analog methods are employed (29). The interference of the above autoantibodies may be counteracted by measuring free T_4 and free T_3 concentrations by equilibrium dialysis or by direct "two-step" methods, that is, methods able to avoid contact between serum proteins and tracer at the time of the assay. The more common factors interfering in TSH measurement are heterophilic antibodies directed against or cross-reacting with mouse IgG (30), and anti-TSH antibodies in patients previously treated with contaminated pituitary extracts. However, prevention of the formation of the "sandwich" anti-TSH antibodies usually leads to an underestimation of the actual levels of TSH and rarely to an overestimation.

Pituitary Glycoprotein Hormone α-Subunit

A helpful diagnostic tool for the diagnosis of a TSH-secreting tumor is the determination of the concentrations of the α-subunit common to each of the glycoprotein hormones, which are elevated in the majority of patients (Table 24.2) (1,2). Indeed, hypersecretion of the α-subunit is not unique to TSH-secreting tumors, being present in the majority of gonadotropinomas, in a subset of nonfunctioning pituitary adenomas, and in a low percentage of GH- or PRL-secreting tumors. TSH-secreting tumors commonly secrete excessive quantities of the free α-subunit, probably due to altered hormone synthesis within the tumoral cells. Secretion of the α-subunit by these tumors is in excess not only of the TSH β-subunit but also of the intact TSH molecule. This results in an α-subunit/TSH molar ratio, which usually is higher than 1.

Although previous studies have suggested that a ratio above 1 is indicative of the presence of a TSH-secreting tumor, similar values may be recorded in normal subjects, particularly postmenopausal women, indicating the need for appropriate control groups matched for TSH and gonadotropin levels (31).

Parameters of Peripheral Thyroid Hormone Action

Patients with central thyrotoxicosis may present with mild signs and symptoms of thyroid hormone overproduction. Therefore, the measurements of several parameters of peripheral thyroid hormone action both *in vivo* (basal metabolic rate, cardiac systolic time intervals, Achilles' reflex time) and *in vitro* (sex hormone–binding globulin: (SHBG), cholesterol, angiotensin–converting enzyme, osteocalcin, red–blood–cell sodium content, carboxyterminal cross-linked telopeptide of type I collagen, have been proposed to quantify the degree of thyrotoxicosis (2,5–7,21). Some of these parameters, and in particular SHBG, have been used to differentiate patients with TSH-secreting tumors from those with PRTH (Table 24.2). As occurs in the common forms of thyrotoxicosis, patients with TSH-secreting tumors have high SHBG levels, while they are in the normal range in patients with PRTH (32,33).

DIAGNOSTIC TESTING

In the past, several stimulatory and inhibitory tests have been proposed for the diagnosis of TSH-secreting tumors. None of these tests is of clear-cut diagnostic value, but the combination may increase their specificity and sensitivity. Classically, the T_3 suppression test has been used to assess the presence of a TSH-secreting tumor. From the analysis of different cases, complete inhibition of TSH secretion after T_3 administration (80 to 100 μg/day for 8 to 10 days) has never been recorded in patients with a TSH-secreting tumor (Table 24.2). In patients with previous thyroid ablation, T_3 suppression seems to be the most sensitive and specific test in assessing the presence of a TSH-secreting tumor (20,21). This test is contraindicated in elderly patients or those with coronary heart disease. The TRH test is another test that has been used to investigate the presence of a TSH-secreting tumor. In 83% of patients, TSH and α-subunit levels did not increase after TRH injection (34).

The majority of patients with a TSH-secreting tumor are sensitive to somatostatin or its analogs. Indeed, administration of native somatostatin or its analogs (octreotide and lanreotide) induces a reduction of TSH levels in the major-

ity of cases, and these tests may be predictive of the efficacy of long-term treatment (35).

IMAGING STUDIES AND LOCALIZATION

When considering the diagnosis of a TSH-oma, full imaging studies, particularly magnetic resonance imaging (MRI) or high-resolution computed tomography (CT), are mandatory. Nevertheless, since most TSH-omas are macroadenomas, in the majority of cases plain radiograms may reveal abnormalities of the sella turcica. Various degrees of suprasellar extension or sphenoidal sinus invasion are present in two thirds of cases.

Microadenomas are now reported with increasing frequency, accounting for about 15% of all recorded cases in both clinical and surgical series. Recently, pituitary scintigraphy with radiolabeled octreotide has been shown to successfully image TSH-omas (8,13,20,35). However, the specificity of these nuclear scans is very low, since pituitary tumors of different types, either secreting or nonsecreting, and even nonspecific pituitary lesions may have positive scans due to the presence of somatostatin receptors.

DIFFERENTIAL DIAGNOSIS

In a patient with signs and symptoms of hyperthyroidism, the presence of elevated TH and detectable TSH levels rules out primary hyperthyroidism. In patients receiving T_4 replacement therapy, the finding of measurable TSH in the presence of high TH levels may be due to poor compliance or to an incorrect high T_4 dose of T_4 ingested before blood sampling. In the case of euthyroid hyperthyroxinemia, it is mandatory to measure the concentrations of free, rather than total, thyroid hormones. If FT_4 and FT_3 concentrations are elevated in the presence of measurable TSH levels, it is important to exclude methodological interference due to the presence of circulating autoantibodies or heterophilic antibodies.

When the existence of central hyperthyroidism is confirmed, several diagnostic steps should be carried out to differentiate a TSH-oma from PRTH (2,5–7). Indeed, the possible presence of neurological signs and symptoms (visual defects, headache) or clinical features of concomitant hypersecretion of other pituitary hormones (acromegaly, galactorrhea, amenorrhea) points to the presence of a TSH-oma. The presence of alterations of pituitary content on MRI or CT scan strongly supports the diagnosis of TSH-oma. Nevertheless, the differential diagnosis may be difficult when the pituitary adenoma is undetectable by CT scan or MRI, or in the case of confusing lesions, such as empty sella or pituitary incidentalomas.

No significant differences in age, sex, previous thyroid ablation, TSH levels, or free thyroid hormone concentrations occur between patients with TSH-oma and those

TABLE 24.3. DIFFERENTIAL DIAGNOSIS BETWEEN TSH-SECRETING TUMORS AND RESISTANCE TO THYROID HORMONES (RTH)[a]

Parameter	TSH-omas	RTH	P
Female/male ratio	1.4	1.3	NS
Familial cases	0/18 (0%)	58/68 (85%)	<0.01
TSH (mU/L)	2.8 ± 0.6	2.0 ± 0.3	NS
FT$_4$ (pmol/L)	42.0 ± 4.5	28.5 ± 2.7	NS
FT$_3$ (pmol/L)	14.2 ± 1.5	11.9 ± 1.0	NS
SHBG (nmol/L)	117.0 ± 17.6	60.0 ± 4.1	<0.01
Lesions at CT or MRI	17/18 (95%)	1/54 (1.9%)	<0.01
High α-subunit levels	12/18 (66.7%)	1/60 (1.7%)	<0.01
High α-subunit/TSH m.r.	15/18 (83.3%)	1/60 (1.7%)	<0.01
Blunted TSH response to TRH	15/18 (83.3%)	3/68 (4.4%)	<0.01
Abnormal TSH response to T$_3$ suppression test[b]	17/17 (100%)	40/40 (100%)[c]	NS

[a]Only patients with intact thyroid are included. Data are obtained from patients followed at our Institute (18 TSH tumors and 68 RTH cases) and are expressed as mean ± SE.
[b] Werner's test (80–100 μg T$_3$ for 8–10 days). Quantitatively normal responses to T$_3$, i.e. complete inhibition of both basal and TRH-stimulated TSH levels, have never been recorded in either group of patients.
[c]Although abnormal in quantitative terms, TSH response to T$_3$ suppression test was qualitatively normal in all RTH patients.

with RTH (Table 24.3). However, in contrast with RTH patients, familial cases of TSH-secreting tumors have never been documented. Serum TSH levels within the normal range are more frequently found in RTH, while high α-subunit concentrations and/or high α-subunit/TSH molar ratio are typically present in patients with TSH-secreting tumors. Moreover, TSH unresponsiveness to TRH stimulation and/or to T$_3$ suppression favors the presence of a TSH-secreting tumor. Circulating SHBG levels are in the thyrotoxic range in patients with TSH-secreting tumors, while they are normal/low in RTH. Exceptions are the findings of normal SHBG levels in patients with mixed GH/TSH adenomas, due to the inhibitory action of GH on SHBG secretion, and of high SHBG in RTH patients treated with estrogen who have profound hypogonadism.

Finally, an apparent association between TSH-secreting tumor and RTH has been recently reported in a few patients (36,37), though genetic studies of possible mutations in the T$_3$-receptor β1 were not carried out in the Japanese case. Nonetheless, the occurrence of tumors in RTH patients is theoretically possible (37).

TREATMENT AND OUTCOME

Surgical resection is the recommended therapy for TSH-secreting pituitary tumors, with the aim of restoring normal pituitary/thyroid function. However, radical removal of large tumors, that still represent the majority of these tumors, is particularly difficult because of the marked fibrosis and the local invasion involving the cavernous sinus, internal carotid artery, or optic chiasm. Considering this high invasiveness, surgical removal or debulking of the tumor by transsphenoidal or subfrontal surgery, depending on the tumor volume and its suprasellar extension, should be undertaken as soon as possible. Particular attention should be paid to presurgical preparation of the patient: antithyroid drugs or octreotide along with propranolol should be given to restore the patient to euthyroidism. After surgery, partial or complete hypopituitarism may result. Evaluation of pituitary function, particularly ACTH secretion, should be undertaken soon after surgery and hormone replacement therapy initiated if needed.

If surgery is contraindicated or declined, as well as in the case of surgical failure, pituitary radiotherapy is mandatory. The recommended dose is no less than 45 Gy fractionated at 2 Gy/day or 10 to 25 Gy in a single dose if a stereotactic gamma unit is available. Experience with proton-beam and heavy particle radiotherapy in TSH-secreting tumors is lacking, though they have been successfully used in other pituitary tumors. Indeed, the radiosensitivity of these tumors has not been clearly evaluated.

Although earlier diagnosis has improved the surgical cure rate, some patients require medical therapy in order to control their thyrotoxicosis. Dopamine agonists, and particularly bromocriptine, have been given to some patients, with variable results, positive effects being mainly observed in some patients with a mixed PRL/TSH adenoma. Medical treatment depends upon long-acting somatostatin analogs, such as octreotide or lanreotide (35, 38–42). Treatment with these analogs leads to a reduction in TSH and α-subunit secretion in almost all cases, with restoration of the euthyroid state in the majority of them. In patients with a GH/TSH-producing adenoma such treatment not only restores euthyroidism, but also resolves acromegaly (Fig. 24.2). During octreotide therapy tumor shrinkage occurs in about a half of the patients and vision improvement in 75% (38). Resistance to oc-

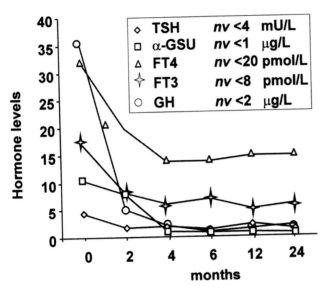

FIGURE 24.2. Treatment with long-acting somatostatin analogs (octreotide LAR, 20 mg every 28 days) of one acromegalic and thyrotoxic patient with a GH-/TSH-producing adenoma. α-GSU indicates the alpha subunit of pituitary glycoprotein hormones, whereas *nv* (normal values) indicates the upper limit of normal ranges for the various hormones. Note the normalization of GH, α-GSU, FT₃ and FT₄ levels along with the small decrement of TSH concentrations. Changes in the biological activity of secreted TSH may explain such a finding.

treotide treatment has been documented in only 4% of cases. Patients treated with somatostatin analogs should be carefully monitored, as untoward side effects, such as cholelithiasis and carbohydrate intolerance, may become manifest. The dose administered should be tailored for each patient, depending on therapeutic response and tolerance (including gastrointestinal side effects). Whether somatostatin analog treatment may be an alternative to surgery and irradiation in patients with TSH-secreting tumor remains to be established.

CRITERIA OF CURE AND FOLLOW-UP

The criteria of cure and follow-up of patients operated and/or irradiated for TSH-secreting tumors have not been clearly established, due to the rarity of the disease and the heterogeneity of parameters used. In particular, clinical remission of thyrotoxicosis, disappearance of neurological symptoms, resolution of neuroradiological alterations, and normalization of thyroid hormones, TSH, α-subunit, or the α-subunit/TSH molar ratio have been considered for evaluation of the efficacy of surgery or radiotherapy. It is obvious that previous thyroid ablation makes some of these criteria not applicable. In untreated patients, it is reasonable to assume that cure will result in clinical and biochemical reversal of thyroid hyperfunction. However,

the finding of normalization of serum free T₄ and free T₃ concentrations or indices of peripheral thyroid hormone action (SHBG, etc.) is not synonymous with complete removal or destruction of tumoral cells, since transient clinical remission accompanied by normalization of thyroid function tests has been observed (21). Disappearance of neurological signs and symptoms is a good prognostic event, but it may occur even after an incomplete debulking of the tumor. In our experience, undetectable TSH levels one week after surgery are likely to indicate complete adenomectomy, provided that presurgical treatments were stopped at least 10 days before surgery (21). The most sensitive and specific test to document the complete removal of the adenoma remains the T₃ suppression test. In fact, only patients in whom T₃ administration completely inhibits basal and TRH-stimulated TSH secretion, appear to be truly cured (21).

No data on recurrence rates of TSH-secreting tumors in patients judged cured after surgery or radiotherapy have been reported. However, recurrence of the adenoma does not appear to be frequent, at least in the first years after successful surgery (20,21). In general, the patient should be evaluated clinically and biochemically 2 or 3 times the first year postoperatively, and then every year. Pituitary imaging should be performed every 2 or 3 years, but should be done promptly whenever an increase in serum TSH and thyroid hormone levels or clinical symptoms occur. In the case of a persistent macroadenoma, close follow-up of visual fields is required, as visual function is threatened.

REFERENCES

1. Greenman Y, Melmed S. Thyrotropin-secreting pituitary tumors. In: Melmed S, ed. *The pituitary.* Boston: Blackwell Science, 1995: 546.
2. Beck-Peccoz P, Brucker-Davis F, Persani L, et al. Thyrotropin-secreting pituitary tumors. *Endocr Rev* 1996;17:610.
3. Jailer JW, Holub DA. Remission of Graves' disease following radiotherapy of a pituitary neoplasm. *Am J Med* 1960;28:497.
4. Mindermann T, Wilson CB. Thyrotropin-producing pituitary adenomas. *J Neurosurg* 1993;79:521–527.
5. Refetoff S, Weiss RE, Usala SJ. The syndromes of resistance to thyroid hormone. *Endocr Rev* 1993;14:348.
6. Beck-Peccoz P, Asteria C, Mannavola D. Resistance to thyroid hormone. In: Braverman LE, ed. *Contemporary endocrinology: diseases of the thyroid.* Totowa, NJ: Humana Press, 1997:199.
7. Cooper DS, Wenig BM. Hyperthyroidism caused by an ectopic TSH-secreting pituitary tumor. *Thyroid* 1996;6:337.
8. Pasquini E, Faustini-Fustini M, Sciarretta V, et al. Ectopic TSH-secreting pituitary adenoma of the vomerosphenoidal junction. *Eur J Endocrinol* 2003;148:253.
9. Mixson AJ, Friedman TC, Katz DA, et al. Thyrotropin-secreting pituitary carcinoma. *J Clin Endocrinol Metab* 1993; 76:529.
10. Bertholon-Grégoire M, Trouillas J, Guigard MP, et al. Mono- and plurihormonal thyrotropic pituitary adenomas: pathological, hormonal and clinical studies in 12 patients. *Eur J Endocrinol* 1999;140:519.

11. Terzolo M, Orlandi F, Bassetti M, et al. Hyperthyroidism due to a pituitary adenoma composed of two different cell types, one secreting alpha-subunit alone and another cosecreting alpha-subunit and thyrotropin. *J Clin Endocrinol Metab* 1991;72:415.

12. LeDafniet M, Brandi A-M, Kujas M, et al. Thyrotropin-releasing hormone (TRH) binding sites and thyrotropin response to TRH are regulated by thyroid hormones in human thyrotropic adenomas. *Eur J Endocrinol* 1994;130:559.

13. Bertherat J, Brue T, Enjalbert A, et al. Somatostatin receptors on thyrotropin-secreting pituitary adenomas: comparison with the inhibitory effects of octreotide upon *in vivo* and *in vitro* hormonal secretions. *J Clin Endocrinol Metab* 1992;75:540.

14. Boggild MD, Jenkinson S, Pistorello M, et al. Molecular genetics studies of sporadic pituitary tumors. *J Clin Endocrinol Metab* 1994;78:387.

15. Dong Q, Brucker-Davis F, Weintraub BD, et al. Screening of candidate oncogenes in human thyrotroph tumors: absence of activating mutations of the Ga$_q$, Ga$_{11}$, Ga$_s$, or thyrotropin-releasing hormone receptor genes. *J Clin Endocrinol Metab* 1996;81:1134.

16. Ando S, Sarlis NJ, Oldfield EH, et al. Somatic mutation of TR-beta can cause a defect in negative regulation of TSH in a TSH-secreting pituitary tumor. *J Clin Endocrinol Metab* 2001;86:5572.

17. Ando S, Sarlis NJ, Krishnan J, et al. Aberrant alternative splicing of thyroid hormone receptor in a TSH-secreting pituitary tumor is a mechanism for hormone resistance. *Mol Endocrinol* 2001;15:1529.

18. Tannahill LA, Visser TJ, McCabe CJ, et al. Dysregulation of iodothyronine deiodinase enzyme expression and function in human pituitary tumours. *Clin Endocrinol (Oxf)* 2002;56:735.

19. Baur A, Buchfelder M, Kohrle J. Expression of 5'-deiodinase enzymes in normal pituitaries and in various human pituitary adenomas. *Eur J Endocrinol* 2002 ;147:263.

20. Brucker-Davis F, Oldfield EH, Skarulis MC, et al. Thyrotropin-secreting pituitary tumors: diagnostic criteria, thyroid hormone sensitivity, and treatment outcome in 25 patients followed at the National Institutes of Health. *J Clin Endocrinol Metab* 1999;84:476.

21. Losa M, Giovanelli M, Persani L, et al. Criteria of cure and follow-up of central hyperthyroidism due to thyrotropin-secreting pituitary adenomas. *J Clin Endocrinol Metab* 1996;81:3084.

22. Gasparoni P, Rubello D, Persani L, et al. Unusual association between a thyrotropin-secreting pituitary adenoma and a papillary thyroid carcinoma. *Thyroid* 1998;8:181.

23. Ohta S, Nishizawa S, Oki Y, et al. Coexistence of thyrotropin-producing pituitary adenoma with papillary adenocarcinoma of the thyroid—a case report and surgical strategy. *Pituitary* 2001;4:271.

24. Abs R, Stevenaert A, Beckers A. Autonomously functioning thyroid nodules in a patient with a thyrotropin-secreting pituitary adenoma: possible cause-effect relationship. *Eur J Endocrinol* 1994;131:355.

25. Beck-Peccoz P, Persani L. Variable biological activity of thyroid-stimulating hormone. *Eur J Endocrinol* 1994;131:331.

26. Magner JA, Klibanski A, Fein H, et al. Ricin and lentil lectin affinity chromatography reveals oligosaccharide heterogeneity of thyrotropin secreted by 12 human pituitary tumors. *Metabolism* 1992;41:1009.

27. Ekins R. Measurement of free hormones in blood. *Endocr Rev* 1990;11:5.

28. Lind P, Langsteger W, Køltringer P, et al. Transient prealbumin-associated hyperthyroxinemia in a TSH-producing pituitary adenoma. *Nuklearmedizin* 1990;29:40.

29. Beck-Peccoz P, Piscitelli G, Cattaneo MG, et al. Evaluation of free thyroxine methods in the presence of iodothyronine binding autoantibodies. *J Clin Endocrinol Metab* 1984;58:736.

30. Zweig MH, Csako G, Spero M. Escape from blockade of interfering heterophile antibodies in a two-site immunoradiometric assay for thyrotropin. *Clin Chem* 1988;34:2589.

31. Beck-Peccoz P, Persani L, Faglia G. Glycoprotein hormone α-subunit in pituitary adenomas. *Trends Endocrinol Metab* 1992;3:41.

32. Beck-Peccoz P, Roncoroni R, Mariotti S, et al. Sex hormone-binding globulin measurement in patients with inappropriate secretion of thyrotropin (IST): evidence against selective pituitary thyroid hormone resistance in nonneoplastic IST. *J Clin Endocrinol Metab* 1990;71:19.

33. Persani L, Preziati D, Matthews CH, et al. Serum levels of carboxyterminal cross-linked telopeptide of type I collagen (ICTP) in the differential diagnosis of the syndromes of inappropriate secretion of TSH. *Clin Endocrinol (Oxf)* 1997;47:207.

34. Langlois M-F, Lamarche JB, Bellabarba D. Long-standing goiter and hypothyroidism: an unusual presentation of a TSH-secreting adenoma. *Thyroid* 1996;6:329.

35. Losa M, Magnani P, Mortini P, et al. Indium-111 pentetreotide single-photon emission tomography in patients with TSH-secreting pituitary adenomas: correlation with the effect of a single administration of octreotide on serum TSH levels. *Eur J Nucl Med* 1997;24:728.

36. Watanabe K, Kameya T, Yamauchi A, et al. Thyrotropin-producing adenoma associated with pituitary resistance to thyroid hormone. *J Clin Endocrinol Metab* 1993;76:1025.

37. Safer JD, Colan SD, Fraser LM, et al. A pituitary tumor in a patient with thyroid hormone resistance: a diagnostic dilemma. *Thyroid* 2001;11:281.

38. Chanson P, Weintraub BD, Harris AG. Octreotide therapy for thyroid stimulating-secreting pituitary adenomas. A follow-up of 52 patients. *Ann Intern Med* 1993;119:236.

39. Gancel A, Vuillermet P, Legrand A, et al. Effects of a slow-release formulation of the new somatostatin analogue lanreotide in TSH-secreting pituitary adenomas. *Clin Endocrinol (Oxf)* 1994;40:421.

40. Losa M, Mortini P, Franzin A, et al. Surgical management of thyrotropin-secreting pituitary adenomas. *Pituitary* 1999;2:127.

41. Kuhn JM, Arlot S, Lefebvre H, et al. Evaluation of the treatment of thyrotropin-secreting pituitary adenomas with a slow release formulation of the somatostatin analog lanreotide. *J Clin Endocrinol Metab* 2000;85:1487.

42. Caron P, Arlot S, Bauters C, et al. Efficacy of the long-acting octreotide formulation (octreotide-LAR) in patients with thyrotropin-secreting pituitary adenomas. *J Clin Endocrinol Metab.* 2001;86:2849.

65a. Krohn K, Maier J, van Steeg H. unpublished data, 2004.

66. Hermus AR, Huysmans DA. Treatment of benign nodular thyroid disease. *N Engl J Med* 1998;338:1438.

67. Ferrari C, Reschini E, Paracchi A. Treatment of the autonomous thyroid nodule: a review. *Eur J Endocrinol* 1996;135:383.

68. Gemsenjäger E. The surgical treatment of autonomous nodular goiter: prospective long-term study]. *Schweiz Med Wochenschr* 1992;122:687.

69. Thomusch O, Machens A, Sekulla C, et al. Multivariate analysis of risk factors for postoperative complications in benign goiter surgery: prospective multicenter study in Germany. *World J Surg* 2000;24:1335.

70. Miehle K, Paschke R. Therapy of thyrotoxicosis. *Exp Clin Endocrinol Diabetes* 2003;111:318.

71. Bogazzi F, Miccoli P, Berti P, et al. Preparation with opanoic acid rapidly controls thyrotoxicosis in patients with amiodaraone-induced thyrotoxicosis prior to thyroidectomy. *Surgery* 2002;132:1114.

72. Scholz GH, Hagemann E, Engelmann L, et al. Is there a place for thyroidectomy in older patients with thyrotoxic storm and cardiorespiratory failure? *Thyroid* 2003;13:933–940.

73. Reiners C, Schneider P. Radioiodine therapy of thyroid autonomy. *Eur J Nucl Med Mol Imaging* 2002;29[Suppl 2]:S471.

74. Marinelli LD, Quinby EH, Hine GJ. Dosage determination with radioactive isotopes. Practical considerations in therapy and protection. *Am J Roentgenol* 1948;59:281.

75. Holm LE, Hall P, Wiklund K, et al. Cancer risk after iodine-131 therapy for thyrotoxicosis. *J Natl Cancer Inst* 1991;83:1072.

76. Hall P, Boice JD Jr, Berg G, et al. Leukaemia incidence after iodine-131 exposure. *Lancet* 1992;340:1.

77. Franklyn JA, Maisonneuve P, Sheppard M, et al. Cancer incidence and mortality after radioiodine treatment for thyrotoxicosis: a population-based cohort study. *Lancet* 1999;353:2111.

78. Farahati J, Demidchik EP, Biko J, et al. Inverse association between age at the time of radiation exposure and extent of disease in cases of radiation-induced childhood thyroid carcinoma in Belarus. *Cancer* 2000;88:1470.

79. Lippi F, Ferrari C, Manetti L, et al. Treatment of solitary autonomous thyroid nodules by percutaneous ethanol injection: results of an Italian multicenter study: The Multicenter Study Group. *J Clin Endocrinol Metab* 1996;81:3261.

80. Zingrillo M, Modoni S, Conte M, et al. Percutaneous ethanol injection plus radioiodine versus radioiodine alone in the treatment of large toxic thyroid nodules. *J Nucl Med* 2003;44:207.

81. Miccoli P, Bendinelli C, Monzani F. Surgical aspects of thyroid nodules previously treated by ethanol injection. *Exp Clin Endocrinol Diabetes* 1998;106[Suppl 4]:S75.

82. Kahaly GJ, Dietlein M. Cost estimation of thyroid disorders in Germany. *Thyroid* 2002;12:909.

83. Vidal-Trecan GM, Stahl JE, Durand-Zaleski I. Managing toxic thyroid adenoma: a cost-effectiveness analysis. *Eur J Endocrinol* 2002;146:283.

84. Castro MR, Caraballo PJ, Morris JC. Effectiveness of thyroid hormone suppressive therapy in benign solitary thyroid nodules: a meta-analysis. *J Clin Endocrinol Metab* 2002;87:4154.

TROPHOBLASTIC TUMORS

JEROME M. HERSHMAN

Thyrotoxicosis occurs in patients with trophoblastic tumors, which are either hydatidiform moles or choriocarcinomas. Since the first report of thyrotoxicosis in women with a hydatidiform mole in 1955 (1), many additional cases have been reported (2–7). These reports revealed that the thyrotoxicosis disappeared rapidly after removal of the tumor, thus suggesting that the tumor produced a substance that caused the thyrotoxicosis. It is now clear that human chorionic gonadotropin (hCG) is the thyroid stimulator that causes thyrotoxicosis in patients with trophoblastic tumors.

In the United States, a hydatidiform mole occurs in about 1 in 1500 pregnancies, and is several times more common in Asian and Latin American countries. Choriocarcinoma occurs in 1 in 50,000 pregnancies in the United States and Europe; about one half of the cases occur in women with a previously diagnosed hydatidiform mole. Although thyrotoxicosis has been reported more often in women with a hydatidiform mole than in those with a choriocarcinoma, there have been many case reports of thyrotoxicosis in women with the latter (8–11), as well as in men with chorionic tumors of the testes (12–14).

The precise prevalence of thyrotoxicosis in patients with trophoblastic tumors is unknown. It was found in 5 of 20 women with trophoblastic tumors evaluated at a referral center in 1 year (15); 3 of these 5 women had a choriocarcinoma, and 2 had a hydatidiform mole. In another study, 30 of 52 women with gestational trophoblastic tumors were found to have thyrotoxicosis (2). In recent years, the routine use of ultrasonography during pregnancy has led to earlier diagnosis of hydatidiform moles when the tumor mass is smaller and thyrotoxicosis is less likely.

Hyperplacentosis, a rare nonneoplastic condition in which the placenta is enlarged and the serum hCG concentration is very high, may also cause thyrotoxicosis that remits promptly after delivery of the placenta (16).

GRADATIONS OF SEVERITY

In trophoblastic disease, the spectrum of alterations of thyroid function ranges from a small increase in serum free thyroxine (T_4) and triiodothyronine (T_3) concentrations, as evidenced by a low basal serum thyrotropin (TSH) con-
centration or a subnormal serum TSH response to thyrotropin-releasing hormone (TRH) (17), to moderate increases in serum free T_4 and T_3 concentrations with no symptoms of thyrotoxicosis, to marked increases with severe clinical thyrotoxicosis or even thyroid storm (4). The lack of clear clinical features of thyrotoxicosis in many patients with high serum free T_4 and T_3 concentrations may be attributable to the relatively brief duration of the increased thyroid function, so that there is insufficient time to develop overt clinical thyrotoxicosis (3,18). Also, the clinical manifestations of thyrotoxicosis may be overlooked because attention is focused on the toxemia that frequently accompanies the trophoblastic tumor. In addition, the toxemia may lower serum T_3 concentrations, as occurs in patients with nonthyroidal illness (see section on nonthyroidal illness in Chapter 11). Thyrotoxic patients with trophoblastic tumors have a lower serum T_3:T_4 ratio than do patients with thyrotoxicosis caused by Graves' disease.

CLINICAL FEATURES

Whereas many women with trophoblastic tumors have few symptoms and signs of thyrotoxicosis, despite having high serum free T_4 and T_3 concentrations, others do have the typical clinical findings, including weight loss, muscle weakness, fatigue, excessive perspiration, heat intolerance, tachycardia, nervousness, and tremor. The thyroid gland is either not enlarged or only minimally enlarged; only rarely is it more than twice normal size. Ophthalmopathy is absent, in contrast with Graves' disease. In addition, there are characteristic features of the trophoblastic tumor. Abnormal vaginal bleeding during pregnancy is the usual presentation; more than 95% of women with trophoblastic tumors have uterine bleeding between the 6th and 16th week of pregnancy, and the size of the uterus is large for the duration of the gestation. Nausea, vomiting, and toxemia of pregnancy occur commonly in molar pregnancy and may obscure the symptoms and signs of thyrotoxicosis.

Most women with choriocarcinoma present within 1 year of the preceding conception. Although the tumor may be confined to the uterus, it is usually widely metastatic, involving the pelvis, liver, lungs, and even the brain. The lung metastases may cause cough, dyspnea, hemoptysis, or pleuritic pain. Cerebral metastases may cause focal neurologic signs or seizures. The diagnosis of metastatic cancer is usually obvious. As in women with a hydatidiform mole, there may be laboratory evidence of increased thyroid function without clinically evident thyrotoxicosis. In men, choriocarcinoma nearly always arises in the testes, and is usually widely metastatic (12–14). Gynecomastia is a common complaint in men with choriocarcinoma, although gynecomastia can occur in any man with thyrotoxicosis (see Chapter 39) (2).

DIAGNOSIS

Chorionic gonadotropin is secreted by both hydatidiform moles and by choriocarcinomas. Therefore, hCG serves as a marker for the tumor. For diagnosis and follow-up of these patients, serum hCG should be measured by an immunoassay that detects all the main forms of the molecule and its β-subunits. Patients with trophoblastic tumors have high serum hCG concentrations and urinary hCG excretion, with values that greatly exceed those found in normal pregnant women. In patients with trophoblastic tumors, serum hCG concentrations always exceed 100 U/mL, the peak concentration that occurs in pregnant women at 10 to 12 weeks' gestation, and they usually exceed 200 U/mL (5,10,11). Not all patients with trophoblastic tumors with high serum hCG concentrations have thyrotoxicosis, however.

The diagnosis of thyrotoxicosis, or increased thyroid function, is established by finding high serum free T_4 and T_3 concentrations. Trophoblastic tumors secrete less estrogen than normal placental tissue, so that the increase of serum thyroxine-binding globulin (TBG) concentrations is less in women with a molar pregnancy than in normal pregnant women (2). Thyroid radioiodine uptake is increased (3). Even when serum T_4 and T_3 concentrations are only slightly high, both serum TSH concentrations and serum TSH responses to TRH are low (17). TSH-receptor antibodies are not detectable, excluding Graves' disease as the cause of thyrotoxicosis in women with trophoblastic tumors.

Ultrasonography of the uterus reveals a characteristic "snowstorm" pattern in women with a hydatidiform mole, and it also provides an accurate indication of tumor volume within the uterus. The definitive diagnosis of hydatidiform mole or choriocarcinoma is based on the histopathology of the tissue removed by curettage or surgery.

HYPEREMESIS GRAVIDARUM

Hyperemesis gravidarum is characterized by prolonged, severe nausea and vomiting in early pregnancy that lead to a loss of 5% of body weight, dehydration, and ketosis. It occurs in about 1.5% of pregnancies and is more common in Asian women than in white women. High serum free T_4 and T_3 concentrations are a common finding in women with hyperemesis gravidarum, having been reported in 25% to 75% of patients in various series (19–26). Women with hyperemesis and high serum free T_4 and T_3 concentrations have higher serum hCG concentrations than normal pregnant women (21,26). Their serum hCG concentrations correlate with the degree of elevation of serum free T_4 and T_3 concentrations and with serum thyroid-stimulating activity, as measured by bioassay. Vomiting is also more severe in women who have higher serum hCG concentrations, suggesting that another factor induced by hCG, perhaps estradiol, may be responsible for the vomiting (21). Although clinical features of thyrotoxicosis are usually absent, or overlooked, in women with hyperemesis gravidarum, some have clinically evident thyrotoxicosis, termed gestational thyrotoxicosis. Thyroid enlargement is rare. The thyrotoxicosis of hyperemesis gravidarum resolves spontaneously within several weeks as the vomiting disappears (19,25,27). Women with twin pregnancies have higher serum hCG concentrations than do women with singleton pregnancies, and are more likely to have hyperemesis gravidarum (28).

HUMAN CHORIONIC GONADOTROPIN

Human chorionic gonadotropin is composed of α- and β-subunits. The α-subunit is identical to the α-subunit of TSH, luteinizing hormone, and follicle-stimulating hormone. The β-subunit of hCG has considerable structural homology with the β-subunit of TSH, but it is larger because it contains a 21-amino-acid carboxy-terminal tail.

Material with thyroid-stimulating activity that has the characteristics of hCG can be extracted from hydatidiform moles and choriocarcinomas (9,29). The thyroid-stimulating activity of hCG has been demonstrated in mice, rats, chicks, and humans (29–31). Injection of large amounts of hCG (100,000 to 150,000 U) into normal men stimulates thyroid iodine release (30). In normal pregnant women, serum TSH concentrations decrease at 9 to 12 weeks of gestation when serum hCG concentrations are highest (see Chapter 80) (32–34), and 3% of pregnant women have transient subclinical thyrotoxicosis (low serum TSH and normal serum free T_4 and free T_3 concentrations) at that time (34). The high serum hCG concentrations correlate with increased thyroid-stimulating activity in a mouse bioassay (33). Serum thyroid-stimulating activity measured by a thyroid cell culture assay also is increased during the first trimester in normal pregnant women, and this activity was correlated with serum hCG and free T_4 concentrations (35). The thyroid-stimulating activity of purified hCG is equivalent to about 0.2 μU of bovine TSH per unit of hCG in a mouse bioassay (34) and 0.04 μU bovine TSH per unit of hCG in a rat thyroid-cell bioassay (Fig. 26.1), but is equivalent to only 0.0013 μU of human TSH per

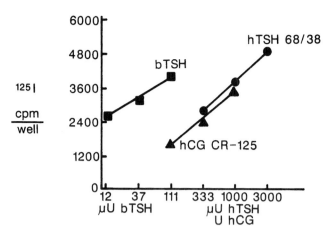

FIGURE 26.1. Comparison of the effects of bovine thyrotropin (TSH) and purified human chorionic gonadotropin (hCG) on iodide uptake in cultured rat thyroid (FRTL-5) cells. Relative potencies are 1 U hCG = 0.72 μU human TSH = 0.042 μU bovine TSH. (From Hershman JM, Lee H-Y, Sugawara M, et al. Human chorionic gonadotropin stimulates iodide uptake, adenylate cyclase, and deoxyribonucleic acid synthesis in cultured rat thyroid cells. *J Clin Endocrinol Metab* 1988;67:74, with permission.)

unit of hCG in a human thyroid-cell bioassay (36). Nevertheless, this thyroid-stimulating activity may be substantial in patients with trophoblastic tumors, in whom serum hCG concentrations may be as high as 2,000 U/mL. Serum hCG and T_3 concentrations were correlated in women with a hydatidiform mole (5), and in five women with trophoblastic thyrotoxicosis, serum hCG concentrations were correlated with serum T_4, free T_4, and T_3 concentrations (15). The high serum concentrations of hCG in early pregnancy may worsen the thyrotoxicosis of Graves' disease (37).

The thyroid-stimulating activity of hCG has been elucidated by a variety of studies. Human chorionic gonadotropin inhibits the binding of labeled TSH to its plasma membrane receptors on thyroid follicular cells (38,39), and activates adenylyl cyclase in rat thyroid cells and cells transfected with human TSH receptors (39,40). Human chorionic gonadotropin increases iodide uptake (37) by increasing the expression of the sodium/iodide transporter on thyroid cells (41).

The hCG extracted from hydatidiform moles has greatly increased thyroid-stimulating potency, as compared with hCG extracted from normal placentas (6,42). This material is enriched in the more basic forms of the molecule that contain less sialic acid than does normal hCG (6,42). Asialo-hCG purified from a patient with choriocarcinoma had potent thyroid-stimulating activity in a bioassay that used human thyroid follicles (36). Although asialo-hCG has much greater thyroid-stimulating activity *in vitro* than sialylated hCG, the lack of sialic acid greatly accelerates its clearance from plasma and thus reduces its physiologic action (43). Recombinant mutant hCG lacking the carboxy-terminal tail of the β-subunit stimulates the human TSH receptor about 10-fold more potently than does intact hCG (39). Presumably, the long carboxy-

terminal tail and the high sialic acid content reduce the ability of hCG to activate TSH receptors.

Although basic hCG that lacks sialic acid is more potent *in vitro*, women with hyperemesis gravidarum who have gestational thyrotoxicosis have high serum concentrations of acidic forms of hCG (44), and in them the acidic forms of hCG are correlated with the serum free T_4 and free T_3 concentrations (45). Human chorionic gonadotropin with increased sialic acid content has a longer serum half-life, which could increase its contribution to serum thyroid-stimulating activity.

MUTANT THYROID STIMULATING HORMONE–RECEPTOR

A woman with recurrent gestational thyrotoxicosis associated with hyperemesis gravidarum and a TSH-receptor mutation has been reported (46). Her mother had a similar history of hyperemesis and thyrotoxicosis during pregnancy. Study of the TSH receptor of the proband and her mother revealed an adenine to guanine substitution at codon 183 in exon 7 in one allele, resulting in substitution of arginine for lysine in the middle portion of the extracellular domain of the TSH receptor (see the section on the thyrotropin receptor in Chapter 10). The mutant TSH re-

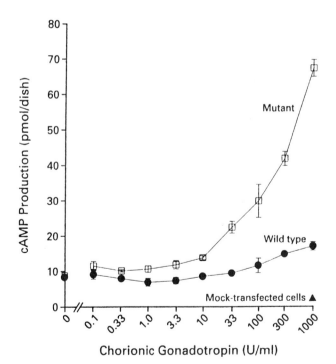

FIGURE 26.2. Functional characteristics of the mutant thyrotropin receptor in COS cells showing the effect of stimulation of cyclic adenosine monophosphate production by graded concentrations of chorionic gonadotropin in cells transfected with wild-type or mutant TSH receptor. (From Rodien P, Bremont C, Sanson M-LR, et al. Familial gestational hyperthyroidism caused by a mutant thyrotropin receptor hypersensitive to human chorionic gonadotropin. *N Engl J Med* 1998;339:1823.)

ceptor was transfected into COS cells, and the cells were incubated with hCG. These cells were more sensitive to hCG than cells transfected with wild-type receptors, as measured by the cyclic adenosine monophosphate responses to hCG (Fig. 26.2). Thus, the gestational thyrotoxicosis in these two women was due to an exaggerated thyroid-stimulating action of hCG. No other family with a TSH receptor mutation of this type has been reported. Substitution of methionine, asparagine, or glutamine for the lysine at position 183 in the TSH receptor also increases its affinity for hCG (47).

THERAPY

Surgical removal of the hydatidiform mole rapidly cures the thyrotoxicosis, as shown in Figure 26.3, and should be carried out as soon as possible. Other treatment of the thyrotoxicosis should be based on anticipation of the benefit of surgery. Propylthiouracil and methimazole can be given, but will have little immediate effect (see Chapter 45). Therapy with potassium iodide given orally will rapidly lower serum T_4 and T_3 concentrations (5). Propranolol and other β-adrenergic antagonist drugs are useful in controlling tachycardia and other symptoms of sympa-

thetic activation, and other supportive measures such as fluid and electrolyte replacement should be administered as needed.

Treatment of choriocarcinoma requires appropriate chemotherapy, which is best given in a specialized referral center. Cure of gestational choriocarcinoma cures the thyrotoxicosis (8,9,15). Unfortunately, patients with choriocarcinomas who have thyrotoxicosis usually have a large tumor mass, as indicated by high serum hCG concentrations, and therefore are less likely to be cured than the usual woman with choriocarcinoma, in whom the cure rate is greater than 90%. Nevertheless, several women with metastatic choriocarcinoma and thyrotoxicosis have achieved complete remission with chemotherapy. The prognosis for men with testicular choriocarcinoma and related hCG-secreting testicular tumors, however, is poor (13).

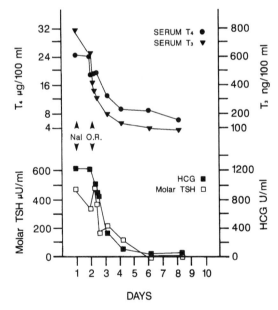

FIGURE 26.3. Serum thyroxine (T_4), triiodothyronine (T_3), thyrotropin (TSH), and human chorionic gonadotropin (hCG) concentrations in a 40-year-old woman with moderately severe thyrotoxicosis at 16 weeks gestation with a hydatidiform mole. She was given 1 g sodium iodide intravenously (*NaI*), and the hydatidiform mole was removed operatively (*O.R.*). There was a parallel fall in the serum hCG concentration, measured by radioimmunoassay, and in the serum molar TSH concentration, which was measured by a mouse bioassay. The patient's serum T_4 and T_3 concentrations also fell rapidly after removal of the mole. (From Higgins HP, Hershman JM, Kenimer JG, et al. The thyrotoxicosis of hydatidiform mole. *Ann Intern Med* 1975;83:307.)

REFERENCES

1. Tisne L, Barzelatto J, Stevenson C. Study of thyroid function during pregnancy and the post-partum period with radioactive iodine (Span). *Bol Soc Chil Obstet Ginecol* 1955;20:246.
2. Desai RK, Norman RJ, Jialal I, et al. Spectrum of thyroid function abnormalities in gestational trophoblastic neoplasia. *Clin Endocrinol (Oxf)* 1988;29:583.
3. Galton VA, Ingbar SH, Jimenez-Fonseca J, et al. Alterations in thyroid hormone economy in patients with hydatidiform mole. *J Clin Invest* 1971;50:1345.
4. Hershman JM, Higgins HP. Hydatidiform mole: a cause of clinical hyperthyroidism. *N Engl J Med* 1971;284:573.
5. Higgins HP, Hershman JM, Kenimer JG, et al. The thyrotoxicosis of hydatidiform mole. *Ann Intern Med* 1975;83:307.
6. Pekary AE, Jackson IMD, Goodwin TM, et al. Increased in vitro thyrotropic activity of partially sialated human chorionic gonadotropin extracted from hydatidiform moles of patients with hyperthyroidism. *J Clin Endocrinol Metab* 1993;76:70.
7. Sanchez JC, Sanchez JE. Pathological case of the month. *Arch Pediatr Adolesc Med* 1998;152:827.
8. Cohen JD, Utiger RD. Metastatic choriocarcinoma associated with hyperthyroidism. *J Clin Endocrinol Metab* 1970;30:423.
9. Cave WT Jr, Dunn JT. Choriocarcinoma with hyperthyroidism: probable identity of the thyrotropin with human chorionic gonadotropin. *Ann Intern Med* 1976;85:60.
10. Morley JE, Jacobson RJ, Melamed J, et al. Choriocarcinoma as a cause of thyrotoxicosis. *Am J Med* 1976;60:1036.
11. Nisula BC, Taliadouros GS. Thyroid function in gestational trophoblastic neoplasia: evidence that the thyrotropic activity of chorionic gonadotropin mediates the thyrotoxicosis of choriocarcinoma. *Am J Obstet Gynecol* 1980;138:77.
12. Karp PJ, Hershman JM, Richmond S, et al. Thyrotoxicosis from molar thyrotropin. *Arch Intern Med* 1973;132:432.
13. Giralt SA, Dexeus F, Amato R, et al. Hyperthyroidism in men with germ cell tumors and high levels of beta-human chorionic gonadotropin. *Cancer* 1992;69:1286.
14. Goodarzi MO, Van Herle AJ. Thyrotoxicosis in a male patient associated with excess human chorionic gonadotropin production by germ cell tumor. *Thyroid* 2000;10:611.
15. Rajatanavin R, Chailurkit LO, Srisupandit S, et al. Trophoblastic hyperthyroidism: clinical and biochemical features of five cases. *Am J Med* 1988;85:237.

16. Ginsberg J, Lewanczuk RZ, Honore LH. Hyperplacentosis: a novel cause of hyperthyroidism. *Thyroid* 2001;11:393.

17. Miyai K, Tanizawa O, Yamamoto T, et al. Pituitary-thyroid function in trophoblastic disease. *J Clin Endocrinol Metab* 1976; 42:254.

18. Nagataki S, Mizuno M, Sakamoto S, et al. Thyroid function in molar pregnancy. *J Clin Endocrinol Metab* 1977;44:254.

19. Goodwin TM, Montoro M, Mestman JH. Transient hyperthyroidism and hyperemesis gravidarum: clinical aspects. *Am J Obstet Gynecol* 1992;167:648.

20. Swaminathan R, Chin RK, Lao TTH, et al. Thyroid function in hyperemesis gravidarum. *Acta Endocrinol (Copenh)* 1989;120:155.

21. Goodwin TM, Montoro M, Mestman JH, et al. The role of chorionic gonadotropin in transient hyperthyroidism of hyperemesis gravidarum. *J Clin Endocrinol Metab* 1992;75:1333.

22. Bouillon R, Naesens M, Van Assche FA, et al. Thyroid function in patients with hyperemesis gravidarum. *Am J Obstet Gynecol* 1982;143:922.

23. Bober SA, McGill AC, Tunbridge WM. Thyroid function in hyperemesis gravidarum. *Acta Endocrinol (Copenh)* 1986;111:11404.

24. Shulman A, Shapiro MS, Behary C, et al. Abnormal thyroid function in hyperemesis gravidarum. *Acta Obstet Gynecol Scand* 1989;68:533.

25. Tan JYL, Loh KC, Yeo GSH, Chee YC. Transient hyperthyroidism of hyperemesis gravidarum. *Br J Obstet Gynaecol* 2002; 109:683.

26. Al-Yatama M, Diejomaoh M, Nandakumaran M, et al. Hormone profile of Kuwaiti women with hyperemesis gravidarum. *Arch Gynecol Obstet* 2002;266:218.

27. Kimura M, Amino N, Tamaki H, et al. Gestational thyrotoxicosis and hyperemesis gravidarum: possible role of hCG with higher stimulating activity. *Clin Endocrinol (Oxf)* 1993;38:345.

28. Grun JP, Meuris S, De Nayer P, et al. The thyrotrophic role of human chorionic gonadotrophin (hCG) in the early stages of twins (versus single) pregnancies. *Clin Endocrinol (Oxf)* 1997; 46:719.

29. Kenimer JG, Hershman JM, Higgins HP. The thyrotropin in hydatidiform moles is human chorionic gonadotropin. *J Clin Endocrinol Metab* 1975;40:482.

30. Sowers JR, Hershman JM, Carlson HE, et al. Effect of human chorionic gonadotropin on thyroid function in euthyroid men. *J Clin Endocrinol Metab* 1978;47:898.

31. Pekary AE, Azukizawa M, Hershman JM. Thyroidal responses to human chorionic gonadotropin in the chick and rat. *Horm Res* 1983;7:36.

32. Braunstein GD, Hershman JM. Comparison of serum pituitary thyrotropin and chorionic gonadotropin concentrations throughout pregnancy. *J Clin Endocrinol Metab* 1976;42:1123.

33. Harada A, Hershman JM, Reed AW, et al. Comparisons of thyroid stimulators and thyroid hormone concentrations in the sera of pregnant women. *J Clin Endocrinol Metab* 1979;48:793.

34. Glinoer D. The regulation of thyroid function in pregnancy: pathways of endocrine adaptation from physiology to pathology. *Endocr Rev* 1997;18:404.

35. Yoshikawa N, Nishikawa M, Horimoto M, et al. Thyroid-stimulating activity in sera of normal pregnant women. *J Clin Endocrinol Metab* 1989;69:891.

36. Yamazaki K, Sato K, Shizume K, et al. Potent thyrotropic activity of human chorionic gonadotropin variants in terms of 125I incorporation and de novo-synthesized thyroid hormone release in human thyroid follicles. *J Clin Endocrinol Metab* 1995;80:473.

37. Tamaki H, Itoh E, Kaneda T, et al. Crucial role of serum human chorionic gonadotropin for the aggravation of thyrotoxicosis in early pregnancy in Graves' disease. *Thyroid* 1993;3;189.

38. Azukizawa M, Kurtzman G, Pekary AE, et al. Comparison of the binding characteristics of bovine thyrotropin and human chorionic gonadotropin to thyroid plasma membranes. *Endocrinology* 1977;202:1880.

39. Yoshimura M, Hershman JM, Pang X-P, et al. Activation of the thyrotropin (TSH) receptor by human chorionic gonadotropin and luteinizing hormone in Chinese hamster ovary cells expressing functional human TSH receptors. *J Clin Endocrinol Metab* 1993;77:1009.

40. Hershman JM, Lee H-Y, Sugawara M, et al. Human chorionic gonadotropin stimulates iodide uptake, adenylate cyclase, and deoxyribonucleic acid synthesis in cultured rat thyroid cells. *J Clin Endocrinol Metab* 1988;67:74.

41. Arturi F, Presta I, Scarpelli D, et al. Stimulation of iodide uptake by human chorionic gonadotropin in FRTL-5 cells: effects on sodium/iodide symporter gene and protein expression. *Eur J Endocrinol* 2002; 147:655.

42. Yoshimura M, Pekary AE, Pang X-P, et al. Thyrotropic activity of basic isoelectric forms of human chorionic gonadotropin extracted from hydatidiform mole tissues. *J Clin Endocrinol Metab* 1994;78:862.

43. Hoermann R, Kubota K, Amir SM. Role of subunit sialic acid in hepatic binding, plasma survival rate, and in vivo thyrotropic activity of human chorionic gonadotropin. *Thyroid* 1993;3:41.

44. Jordan V, Grebe SK, Cooke RR, et al. Acidic isoforms of chorionic gonadotrophin in European and Samoan women are associated with hyperemesis gravidarum and may be thyrotrophic. *Clin Endocrinol (Oxf)* 1999; 50:619.

45. Talbot JA, Lambert A, Anobile CJ, et al. The nature of human chorionic gonadotrophin glycoforms in gestational thyrotoxicosis. *Clin Endocrinol (Oxf)* 2001; 55:33.

46. Rodien P, Bremont C, Sanson ML, et al. Familial gestational hyperthyroidism caused by a mutant thyrotropin receptor hypersensitive to human chorionic gonadotropin. *N Engl J Med* 1998; 339:1823.

47. Smits G, Govaerts C, Nubourgh I, et al. Lysine 183 and glutamic acid 157 of the TSH receptor: two interacting residues with a key role in determining specificity toward TSH and human CG. *Mol Endocrinol* 2002;16:722.

SPORADIC AND POSTPARTUM THYROIDITIS

JOHN H. LAZARUS

Sporadic thyroiditis, also known as silent thyroiditis, and postpartum thyroiditis are important causes of transient thyrotoxicosis as well as transient hypothyroidism. Pathologically, both conditions are characterized by chronic lymphocytic infiltration, and the term "destructive thyroiditis" is commonly used to describe the inflammation resulting in thyroid dysfunction (1). The thyrotoxicosis is caused by rapidly progressive tissue injury, followed by the release of large amounts of thyroid hormone into the circulation. While thyroid pain and tenderness are characteristic features of subacute thyroiditis, they are rare in sporadic or postpartum thyroiditis. The clinical hallmarks of destruction-induced thyrotoxicosis are abrupt onset of thyrotoxic symptoms, sometimes accompanied by the development of a goiter or enlargement of a preexisting goiter. Laboratory features, in addition to those that are diagnostic of thyrotoxicosis, include a low thyroid radioactive iodine uptake and high serum thyroglobulin (Tg) concentrations. Both these conditions are associated with the presence of thyroid antibodies, usually against thyroid peroxidase, and hypothyroidism, due to continuing immune activity, often follows the thyrotoxic phase. Because the destructive process is focal or self-limited, recovery to euthyroidism usually occurs. However, both sporadic and postpartum thyroiditis may evolve into permanent hypothyroidism either at the end of the acute episode or after years of slowly declining thyroid function.

SPORADIC (SILENT) THYROIDITIS

Sporadic (painless) thyroiditis associated with transient thyrotoxicosis was identified with increasing frequency some 25 years ago but now seems to be waning in frequency. The terms "silent thyroiditis" and "painless thyroiditis" (1–6) are most often used to describe this syndrome, although other terms have been used (7). Silent thyroiditis was initially described as a painless form of subacute thyroiditis (a disorder dominated by thyroid pain and tenderness) because of its similar clinical course (5,6); thyroid biopsy has shown it to be a form of lymphocytic thyroiditis (8–10), similar to, although usually less extensive than, that found in chronic autoimmune thyroiditis and indistinguishable from postpartum thyroiditis. The term "sporadic thyroiditis" is used to define this form of lymphocytic thyroiditis seen outside of the postpartum period. The condition follows a self-limited course of a few weeks to several months, and transient hypothyroidism often occurs during recovery. Multiple episodes may occur in the same person (10).

INCIDENCE

Silent thyroiditis has been reported in the United States, Europe, Canada, India, and Japan. Its recognition increased in the 1970s such that in some areas (e.g., Wisconsin) it accounted for as many as 23% of all cases of thyrotoxicosis (10). This high relative frequency of silent thyroiditis as a cause of thyrotoxicosis has not been reported in other parts of the United States and Europe, and may have been due in part to ingestion of ground beef contaminated with thyroid tissue, a form of iatrogenic thyrotoxicosis (see later in the chapter). Silent thyroiditis accounted for 6% of 100 consecutively referred thyrotoxic patients in Toronto but no cases in a similar population in Cardiff (11), and comprised less than 5% of all cases of thyrotoxicosis in Philadelphia (12), New York (13), and coastal Virginia (6) but 15% in Texas (6). The condition was a rare finding on the East and West Coasts of the United States, as well as in Europe and Argentina, but common around the Great Lakes in the United States and Canada (14). An occasional cluster of cases has been reported, for example, in association with subacute thyroiditis in Connecticut (15). The variable incidence may be due to variation in ascertainment rate as well as the fact that the transient and painless nature of the illness and its symptoms may be attributed to a "flu-like" illness by those unfamiliar with the disease. Some asymptomatic patients are also found to have silent thyroiditis by routine testing. Two epidemics of thyrotoxicosis in the Midwest believed to be due to silent thyroiditis proved to be due to the contamination of ground beef with thyroid tissue (16,17).

The affected patients are usually white or Asian. Women predominate in a ratio of 1.5 to 2:1, which is a much lower ratio than reported for almost all other types of thyroid disease, for which the ratios range from 3 to 10:1. Most patients are in the third through sixth decade of life, but patients as young as 5 years and as old as 93 years have been reported (10).

ETIOLOGY

Multiple reports describing only lymphocytic thyroiditis in biopsy specimens (8–10) disprove suggestions that the condition is a silent form of subacute thyroiditis. A search for antibodies to influenza viruses A and B, parainfluenza viruses types 1, 2, and 3, adenovirus, respiratory syncytial virus, mumps virus, measles virus, and coxsackie viruses types 1 through 6 in 18 patients with silent thyroiditis revealed only 1 patient with a significant rise in antibody titer during the course of the disease (10). No positive cultures for viruses or bacteria or electron microscopic evidence of viral inclusion bodies have been reported. A history of an illness such as an upper respiratory infection is unusual, although infection with rubella virus was implicated in one case (18), and an unidentified antecedent infection or exposure to antigen causing a transient increase in serum IgM concentration was reported in another (19). A seasonal cluster in summer and late autumn, the simultaneous occurrence of subacute thyroiditis and silent thyroiditis in a wife and husband (20), and the occurrence, in a short period of time, in five nursery school coworkers (21) suggest an infectious agent. However, viral serologic studies of acute and convalescent serum in the last group were negative.

Although most patients have a partial or complete remission, follow-up study for 1 to 10 years has shown the persistence of or later development of thyroid autoantibodies, thyroid enlargement, or permanent hypothyroidism in about half of the patients.

A substantial percentage of patients who have silent thyroiditis have personal or family histories of autoimmune thyroid disease. Histocompatibility antigen (HLA) haplotype studies show an increased frequency of HLA-DR3 and DR5 in patients with silent thyroiditis (22,23). Intrathyroidal T-cell phenotypes are similar in silent thyroiditis and chronic lymphocytic thyroiditis (24). Taken together, these facts suggest that silent thyroiditis is an early and unusual presentation of chronic lymphocytic thyroiditis, with an unknown factor causing the onset or exacerbation of the destructive process. Variant or atypical forms characterized by thyroid pain or tenderness similar to subacute thyroiditis are recognized only when biopsies are done (25,26).

TABLE 27.1. ETIOLOGICAL AND/OR INITIATING FACTORS IN SPORADIC THYROIDITIS

Infection	Rarely confirmed
Drugs	Amiodarone (27)
	Lithium (28–30a)
	Interleukin-2 (31,32)
	Interferon alpha (33–37)
	Granulocyte colony-stimulating factor (38)
	Leuprolide acetate (39)
Association with Other Autoimmune Diseases	Rheumatoid arthritis (40)
	Systemic lupus erythematosus (41)
	Graves' disease (42,43)
	Systemic sclerosis (44)
	Thymoma (45)
Local Factors	Palpation thyroiditis (46)
	Following parathyroid surgery (47)

Several factors have been suggested to be the initiating event in silent thyroiditis (Table 27.1). An increase in serum interleukin-6, an inflammatory mediator, has been found in patients with amiodarone-induced destructive thyroiditis with thyrotoxicosis (27). Thyroid iodine content has been found to be normal or slightly decreased during the thyrotoxic phase of silent thyroiditis (48), and urinary iodide excretion is increased during this phase but is decreased during recovery (10). This increase in urinary iodide reflects release of iodide and iodinated compounds from the damaged thyroid. Iodine-induced thyrotoxicosis and silent thyroiditis are sometimes indistinguishable, but the few patients with the former who have had thyroid biopsies have not had lymphocytic thyroiditis. Excessive iodine intake has been proposed as an aggravating or inciting factor because of its effects on lymphocytic thyroiditis in animals and on human thyroid disease. Other possible associated initiating factors include drugs, such as lithium (29), and immune disorders. Interestingly, in patients with hepatitis B treated with interferon-γ, no thyroid dysfunction or thyroid autoimmunity was observed (49). In contrast, patients with chronic active hepatitis C treated with interferon-α may develop thyrotoxicosis secondary to silent thyroiditis (29). Simple palpation has been reported to cause a multifocal granulomatous folliculitis without serum thyroid hormone concentration abnormalities (46). The thyrotoxicosis and thyroiditis noted in patients recovering from parathyroid surgery for parathyroid adenoma may be due to trauma to the thyroid gland during neck exploration for parathyroid surgery (47). Thyrotropin (TSH) receptor–stimulating antibodies (50,51) and TSH receptor–blocking antibodies may occur in patients with silent thyroiditis (52). Furthermore, there is evidence that antithyroid peroxidase antibodies are associated with the development of the hypothyroid phase (53) and also that both types of TSH-receptor antibodies are associated with transient hypothyroidism in this disease (54).

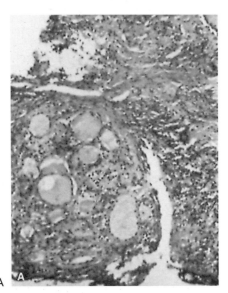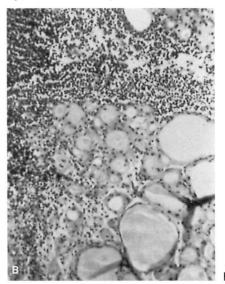

FIGURE 27.1. Histopathalogic findings in silent thyroiditis. **A:** Focal lymphocytic infiltration with partially or completely collapsed thyroid follicles. The thyroid follicular cells appear normal. **B:** Extensive lymphocytic infiltration with collapsed thyroid follicles and follicles containing mononuclear cells (Hematoxylin and eosin, 100× magnification).

The presence of these antibodies may be related to more severe immunological damage in the thyroid resulting in hypothyroidism.

PATHOLOGY

Thyroid tissue (Fig. 27.1) obtained by needle biopsy or surgery during the thyrotoxic phase of silent thyroiditis shows focal or diffuse lymphocytic infiltration (9,10,24) consistent with lymphocytic thyroiditis. Some thyroid follicles are disrupted or collapsed and contain intrafollicular macrophages, while adjacent follicles may be normal. Fibrosis is usually minimal but may be extensive. Lymphoid follicles are found in about half of patients, whereas Hürthle cells are sparse or absent. A few multinucleated giant cells within and around disrupted thyroid follicles may be seen in the biopsy specimens of some patients with painless thyroiditis. The pathologic changes of silent thyroiditis compared to those of chronic lymphocytic thyroiditis cannot be distinguished when unidentified biopsy specimens from patients with either disease are compared (10). While there is more extensive follicular disruption in silent thyroiditis, the pathological features are usually more extensive in chronic lymphocytic thyroiditis. Fine-needle aspiration biopsies are similar in the two conditions, the specimens containing lymphoid cells, thyroid follicular cells with Hürthle-cell changes, and a few multinucleated giant cells (31).

Thyroid tissue obtained during the hypothyroid or early recovery phase of silent thyroiditis usually shows mild lymphocytic thyroiditis and regenerating thyroid follicles that contain little colloid. Thyroid biopsies done after 6 months

to 3 years showed persistent mild lymphocytic thyroiditis in some patients and were normal in others (24).

CLINICAL FEATURES

The onset and severity of silent thyroiditis are variable. In one series, about 8% of patients were asymptomatic and were found by routine thyroid function testing (10). Thyrotoxicosis is usually mild, resulting in little if any disability. The symptoms and signs are those of thyrotoxicosis in general (including nervousness, fatigue, and tachycardia, all occurring in more than 80%) (10) but may include atrial fibrillation, diffuse myalgia, and periodic paralysis (8).

Exophthalmos, localized myxedema, and thyroid acropathy do not occur, although lid lag and lid retraction (signs of increased sympathetic tone) are frequently present. The thyroid is enlarged in 50% to 60% of patients (6), is usually symmetrical, and is rarely more than 2 to 3 times normal. It is usually described as being firmer than normal, and the surface may be slightly irregular. The disease has been found in single nodules and in ectopic thyroid tissue (10). Thyroid pain or tenderness is rare and when present is mild. Fever has been described (55).

COURSE

A schematic representation of the course of silent thyroiditis is shown in Figure 27.2. Most patients present in the thyrotoxic phase, but a few are in the euthyroid or hypothyroid phase. Most patients have had symptoms of thy-

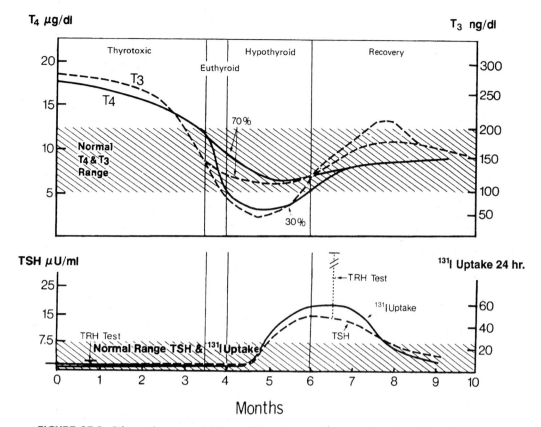

FIGURE 27.2. Schematic representation of the changes in serum thyroxine (T$_4$), triiodothyronine (T$_3$), and thyrotropin (TSH) concentrations, and 24-hour thyroid ^{131}I uptake during the course of silent thyroiditis and subacute thyroiditis. The *hatched areas* represent the normal ranges. The serum T$_4$ and T$_3$ lines separate during the early part of the euthyroid phase to show that only about 30% of patients subsequently develop hypothyroidism. In the recovery phase, the serum T$_3$ line separates to show that about 15% of patients have transient elevations in serum T$_3$ concentrations during this phase. To convert serum T$_4$ values to nmol/L, multiply by 12.87; to convert serum T$_3$ values to nmol/L, multiply by 0.015. (From Woolf PD. Transient painless thyroiditis with hyperthyroidism: a variant of lymphocytic thyroiditis? *Endocr Rev* 1980;1: 411, and The Endocrine Society, modified with permission.)

rotoxicosis for 1 to 4 weeks when the disease is discovered, and these symptoms persist for about 1 to 5 weeks after discovery. About 40% then have a hypothyroid phase, which usually lasts between 4 to 16 weeks but occasionally persists indefinitely.

LABORATORY FINDINGS

Thyroid function tests vary substantially, depending on the stage of the disease (6,10,52), and relate directly to the pathologic state of the thyroid gland.

THYROTOXIC PHASE

With inflammation and damage to the thyroid follicles, Tg proteolysis is activated, and its products leak into the circulation, resulting in high serum total and free T$_4$ and T$_3$ con-

centrations. The T$_4$ to T$_3$ ratio is higher than in Graves' thyrotoxicosis. Serum TSH is low and does not increase in response to thyrotropin-releasing hormone (TRH). Other iodinated materials, such as Tg and iodinated albumin, are found in the serum in increased quantities; the concentrations of the former may be as high as 400 ng/mL. As a result of both thyroid follicular cell damage and decreased TSH secretion, the thyroid follicular cells are unable to transport iodine, so that the thyroid radioiodine uptake falls to low values. Serum inorganic iodide concentrations are slightly increased and urinary iodide excretion is increased two- to fivefold because of the leakage of iodide from the damaged thyroid (6). Anti–thyroid peroxidase (anti-TPO) antibodies are high in about 60% and anti-Tg antibodies in 25% of patients, but TSH receptor antibodies are rarely found.

The erythrocyte sedimentation rate, total and differential white blood cell counts, and serum protein concentrations are high in about half of patients. Serum interleukin-12 concentrations are high, suggesting that a T helper 1

(Th1) type immune response occurs in this condition (56).

HYPOTHYROID AND RECOVERY PHASES

As the thyrotoxic phase abates, the serum T_4 and T_3 concentrations fall into the normal range and either remain there or, after 1 to 6 weeks in about 40% of patients, fall to subnormal concentrations (Fig. 27.2). In the interval when the serum T_4 and T_3 are normal, serum TSH concentrations and thyroid ^{131}I radioiodine uptake values remain low. After 2 to 4 weeks, if the patient remains euthyroid, or toward the end of the hypothyroid phase, these latter two tests become normal or elevated. Within another 1 to 3 weeks, serum T_4 and T_3 concentrations return to normal if hypothyroidism had occurred earlier. The hypothyroid interval lasts 4 to 10 weeks, occasionally longer. Permanent hypothyroidism occurs in less than 5% of patients. Antithyroid antibody titers usually reach their highest levels during the hypothyroid phase, then decrease and disappear in about half of patients (10). In the other half, the antibody titers fall but remain measurable for many years. The intrathyroidal iodine content is decreased by 50% to 70% 1 to 3 months after the onset of thyroiditis and still decreased by 20% to 30% at 10 to 12 months (48). Serum Tg concentrations gradually fall during the recovery phase but are often still slightly elevated one to two years later, indicating persistent thyroid inflammation (48). Urinary iodide excretion decreases markedly during the recovery phase because the thyroid is relatively depleted of its iodine and thyroid hormone stores (10).

DIAGNOSIS

The main features are a mild to moderate degree of thyrotoxicosis with corresponding elevation in serum T_4 and T_3 concentrations, a low thyroid ^{123}I uptake, slight thyroid enlargement (in 50% to 60% of patients), no thyroid tenderness, and no history of therapy with thyroid hormone. A fine-needle or core-needle biopsy of the thyroid gland showing lymphocytic thyroiditis confirms the diagnosis, but is rarely needed. As many patients are thought to have Graves' thyrotoxicosis, TSH-receptor antibody measurement will further differentiate the two conditions in most but possibly not every case, because a few patients with silent thyroiditis have those antibodies in their serum (52,57). A normal red blood cell zinc concentration has been claimed also to differentiate accurately silent thyroiditis from Graves' disease (58). Although a low thyroid radioiodine uptake value is most useful in identifying silent thyroiditis, it is important to rule out iodine con-

tamination due to any cause resulting in the suppressed uptake.

Iodine-induced thyrotoxicosis can easily be confused with silent thyroiditis. It has been recognized in patients with numerous preexisting thyroid diseases, such as a solitary nodule or nontoxic diffuse or multinodular goiter, as well as in patients without any history of thyroid disease. The thyroid ^{123}I uptake in such patients is usually low. Rare diseases that cause thyrotoxicosis with low thyroid radioiodine uptake values are struma ovarii (if the struma is a thyroid adenoma), differentiated carcinoma of the thyroid, and thyrotoxicosis factitia. The most difficult entity to recognize is thyrotoxicosis factitia. Surreptitious intake of thyroid hormone should always be suspected in a patient with thyrotoxicosis with low radioiodine uptake and no goiter. It may be differentiated from silent thyroiditis by history, if of long duration; patient behavior, often histrionic or denial; the absence of thyroid antibodies; and low serum Tg concentrations.

Ultrasonography usually reveals a slight increase in thyroid volume with decreased echogenicity. This study may be useful in diagnosis and further monitoring of these patients (4).

TREATMENT

Patients with silent thyroiditis may receive inappropriate treatment, such as an antithyroid drug, because of failure to recognize the disorder. Most often, the thyrotoxicosis is mild and not particularly bothersome, so patients need only be counseled about the disease and reassured that their symptoms will subside in a few weeks. They should be reminded that a short period of hypothyroidism may occur during recovery and that about 10% will have recurrent episodes in the future. When symptoms of thyrotoxicosis are troublesome, the patient may be given β-adrenergic antagonist, sedative, or tranquilizer therapy. Therapy with thionamide antithyroid drugs is inappropriate because increased thyroid hormone biosynthesis is not the cause of thyrotoxicosis in painless thyroiditis. Indeed, propylthiouracil administration does not change the course or severity of thyrotoxicosis in patients with silent thyroiditis (59). The few patients in whom thyrotoxicosis is more disabling may benefit from antiinflammatory therapy before the illness runs it natural course. Prednisone reduces the inflammatory process, causing decreases in both thyroid size and serum T_4 and T_3 concentrations, which may decline to the normal range within 7 to 10 days (59). The optimal starting dose of prednisone or duration of therapy has not been established, but therapy similar to that used successfully for many years in subacute thyroiditis works well. Initial therapy with 40 to 60 mg/day in single or divided doses and gradual reduction of the daily dose by 7.5 to 15 mg/week for a 4-week course is usually adequate.

Ipodate therapy, which also rapidly reduces serum T_3 concentrations is also an effective therapy in extremely severe cases of thyrotoxicosis (60). In rare patients who have been disabled from recurring episodes of silent thyroiditis, subtotal thyroidectomy has been beneficial (9,59). Ablation of the thyroid with ^{131}I could also be used in these instances, but one must wait until the thyroid ^{131}I uptake has recovered before this therapy can be given.

When hypothyroidism develops in silent thyroiditis, it is usually mild, and the patient can be advised that it will disappear within 4 to 10 weeks. If the symptoms of hypothyroidism are bothersome, sufficient T_4 should be given to relieve the hypothyroid symptoms but not so much as to decrease serum TSH to below normal, since continued TSH secretion may hasten recovery. The therapy can then be slowly withdrawn. In the occasional patient who develops permanent hypothyroidism, the serum T_4 concentration falls and the serum TSH concentration rises when T_4 therapy is withdrawn. If hypothyroidism lasts for longer than 6 months, it is probably permanent, and no further attempts at withdrawal need be undertaken. All patients should be followed at 1- to 2-year intervals for evidence of goiter or hypothyroidism, because up to half of patients who have an episode of silent thyroiditis eventually develop permanent thyroid disease (61).

POSTPARTUM THYROIDITIS

In 1948 H.E.W. Roberton, a general practitioner in New Zealand, described the occurrence of lassitude and other symptoms of hypothyroidism during the postpartum period (62). These complaints were treated successfully with thyroid extract. The syndrome remained generally unrecognized until the 1970s, when reports from Japan (63) and Canada (64) rediscovered the existence of postpartum thyroiditis (PPT) and recognized the immune nature of the condition (see reviews 65–68). Postpartum thyroiditis is essentially sporadic thyroiditis in the postpartum period. Several types of thyroid dysfunction that may arise following delivery (Fig. 27.3). The term "postpartum thyroiditis" relates to destructive thyroiditis occurring during the first 12 months postpartum and not to Graves' disease, although the two conditions may occur concurrently.

INCIDENCE

A variable incidence (from 3% to 17%) has been reported worldwide (70) because of wide variations in the number of women studied, the frequency of thyroid assessment, diagnostic criteria employed, and differences in hormone assay methodology. However, there is a general consensus that the disease occurs in 5% to 9% of unselected postpartum women (71–75). Recent studies have confirmed that the incidence and general characteristics of PPT are similar in different areas, e.g., Brazil (75), Iran (76), and Turkey (77). Women with type 1 diabetes have a threefold incidence of PPT compared to nondiabetic women (78). PPT is also more likely to occur in a woman who has had a previous episode (vide infra).

ETIOLOGY

There is abundant evidence that PPT is an immunologically related disease (79). Biopsy of the thyroid shows lymphocytic infiltration similar to that seen in Hashimoto's thyroiditis (80). Immunogenetic studies have demonstrated associations with haplotypes consistent with autoimmune thyroid disease. A higher incidence of HLA-A26, -BW46, and -BW67, together with a significantly lower frequency of HLA-BW62 and -CW7, as well as an increased incidence of HLA-A1 and -B8 in women with this condition, has been noted (81,82). HLA class II antigen associations with autoimmune thyroid disease have shown an association between HLA-DR3, -DR4, and -DR5 and PPT (83–86). The class III area of the major histocompatibility complex contains the coding for several proteins that are important in the pathogenesis of the autoimmune diseases (viz. tumor necrosis factor, heat shock

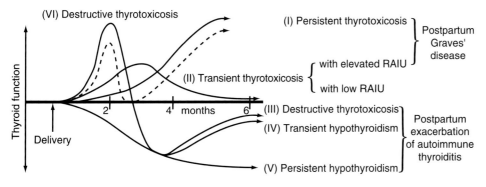

FIGURE 27.3. Development of thyroid dysfunction in the postpartum period. (From Amino N, Tada H, Hidaka Y. Thyroid disease after pregnancy: post-partum thyroiditis. In: Wass JAH, Shalet, SM, eds. *Oxford textbook of endocrinology and diabetes.* Oxford: Oxford University Press, 2002:527–532, adapted with permission.)

protein 70, complement). The frequency of the three complement proteins Bf, C4A, and C4B is significantly different in PPT compared with normal (86). Taken together, the immunogenetic findings suggest that PPT may well be similar to Hashimoto's disease.

Gestation and the postpartum period are characterized by fluctuations in the immune response, and PPT is accompanied by a significant elevation of circulating thyroid antibodies. This rapid perturbation of the immune system in the postpartum year contrasts with the relatively stable situation in chronic Hashimoto's thyroiditis (87). Although the antibody response is dramatic, its precise role in the immunopathogenesis of the condition remains to be determined; probably the antibody titer is merely a marker of disease, and the immunological damage is mediated by lymphocyte and complement associated mechanisms. Studies on antibody functional affinity (88) and IgG subclass distribution (89) of the TPO antibodies in PPT suggest that, as in other autoimmune diseases, activation of the complement system may have a role in pathogenesis. Quantitative analysis of the classical complement pathway activation has shown that not only is there activation of the complement system by thyroid-directed autoantibodies (90), but complement activation is related to the extent of the thyroiditis (42) and correlates with the severity of the thyroid dysfunction (91).

During pregnancy, maternal immune reactions are regulated to prevent rejection of the fetal allograft such that the cytokine profile is a T helper 2 (Th2) pattern, which switches back to the Th1 state postpartum (92).

Early postpartum (within 3 months) changes in T-cell subsets have been described similar to those seen in Hashimoto's disease (93). The peripheral T-lymphocyte subset ratio (CD4/CD8) has been shown to be higher in TPO antibody–positive women who developed postpartum thyroid dysfunction compared with similar antibody-positive women who did not (94). Study of lymphocyte populations during and after pregnancy has shown a generalized activation of immune activity at 36-weeks gestation in TPO antibody–positive women who went on to develop postpartum thyroid dysfunction, compared with those who did not; furthermore, the former group had lower serum cortisol concentrations predelivery (95).

Thus, both humoral and cellular immune reactions are involved in the development of postpartum thyroid disease, but the influence of the immunological changes in late gestation and the early postpartum period, which suggest a failure of continuing immunosuppression in late pregnancy, requires further clarification. Recent interest has focused on fetal microchimerism (defined as the presence of fetal cells in maternal tissues during and after pregnancy) as a potential immunomodulatory factor in the development of PPT (96); loss of placental immune suppression postpartum may allow activation of intrathyroidal fetal immune cells. Subsequent immune stimulation would initiate or exacerbate autoimmune thyroid disease, including PPT.

CLINICAL SPECTRUM

PPT with thyroid dysfunction (i.e., postpartum thyroid dysfunction, PPTD) is characterized by an episode of transient thyrotoxicosis followed by transient hypothyroidism. The former presents at about 14 weeks postpartum, followed by transient hypothyroidism at a median of 19 weeks (97). Very occasionally the hypothyroid state is seen first. Not all women manifest both thyroid states, and the thyrotoxic episode may escape detection as it may be of short duration. PPTD is almost always associated with the presence of antithyroid antibodies, usually anti-TPO antibodies that rise in titer after 6-weeks postpartum. Anti-Tg antibodies occur in about 15% and is the sole antibody in less than 5% of cases. However, postpartum thyroid dysfunction has been described in small numbers of women who do not have circulating thyroid antibodies (65,98). There is no evidence that variations in ambient iodine concentrations cause the condition (99).

The clinical course of PPTD is illustrated in Figure 27.4, which also shows the postpartum rise in anti-TPO titer associated with this condition. The thyroid dysfunction that occurs in up to 50% of the antibody-positive women comprises 19% with thyrotoxicosis alone, 49% hypothyroidism alone, and the remaining 32% with both (i.e., biphasic). Although the clinical manifestations of the thyrotoxicosis state are not usually severe, lack of energy and irritability are particularly prominent even in thyroid antibody–positive women who do not develop thyroid dysfunction. In contrast, the symptomatology of the hypothyroid phase may be profound. Many classic hypothyroid symptoms occur before the onset of overt hyperthyroidism and persist even after recovery is seen in hormone levels. The most frequent symptoms are lack of energy, aches and pains, poor memory, dry skin, and cold intolerance. Postpartum thyroiditis can also occur in women receiving T_4 therapy before pregnancy (100). Early accounts of noted an anecdotal association of depression with thyroid dysfunction in the postpartum period. Quantitative evaluation of depressive symptomatology shows an increase of mild to moderate depression in thyroid-antibody–positive women even when they remain euthyroid during the postpartum period, and this may present as early as 6-weeks postpartum (101,101a), although other smaller studies did not confirm these findings (102,103).

Postpartum Thyroid Function

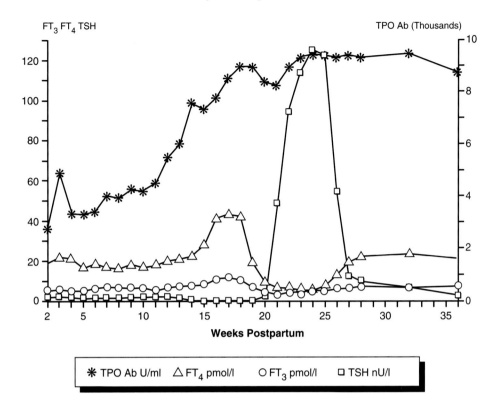

FIGURE 27.4. Emergence of transient thyrotoxicosis and hypothyroidism postpartum. The patient was found to have antithyroid peroxidase antibodies at 16-weeks gestation and was studied weekly postpartum for 36 weeks.

DIAGNOSIS

Thyrotoxicosis in the postpartum period may be due to a recurrence or the development of new Graves' disease or to the thyrotoxicosis phase of PPT. Despite the strong association between thyroid autoantibodies and the development of PPT (68), only some 50% of TPO Ab-positive women develop PPTD. Nevertheless, inspection of Table 27.2 shows that the presence of TPO-Ab measured at various times during gestation or postpartum has a useful predictive value for thyroid dysfunction (104–110). The occurrence of PPTD in TPO-Ab-negative women in most studies may relate to ethnic variability in the predilection for PPTD, the sensitivity of TPO-Ab assay used and the timing of TPO-Ab sampling (effects of immune modulation of pregnancy and the postpartum period may affect detection rates of TPO-Ab). A variety of screening strategies was used with screening done at variable times (antenatal, delivery, and postpartum). Screening for microsomal antibodies was the method used in earlier studies, but TPO-Ab was used in later studies. Sensitivity of TPO-Ab measurement in previous studies was relatively low compared with the present, although specificity was higher.

As PPTD is a destructive process, thyroidal radioiodine uptake will be very low at early and late times after isotope administration. TSH receptor antibodies are not seen in PPTD unless there is coexisting Graves' disease. Thyrotoxicosis due to PPT is diagnosed by a low serum TSH together with an elevated free T_4 or T_3, with either set of criteria occurring on more that one occasion. Thyroid hormone concentrations should be normal in the postpartum period. Antibodies to T_4 and T_3 may cause confusion in diagnosis, but they are infrequent (68).

Postpartum hypothyroidism may be defined as either a serum TSH concentration >3.6 mU/L (i.e., lower than the usual upper limit of the normal reference range) together with a free T_4 <0.6 ngldl (8 pmol/L) or a TSH 10 mU/L or more on one or more occasions. Thyroid ultrasonography has demonstrated diffuse or multifocal echogenicity, reflecting the abnormal thyroid morphology and consistent with the known lymphocytic infiltration of the thyroid (68). When anti-TPO antibodies are borderline during pregnancy, structural and echogenic changes might be of predictive value for the development of PPTD (75). The destructive nature of the thyroiditis is also shown by the increase in urinary iodine excretion in the thyrotoxic phase of the syndrome (68), as well as by an early rise in serum Tg (68). Despite active thyroiditis, there is no rise in interleukin-6 or C-reactive protein in PPTD (110a), but the inflammation may be responsible for a decrease in total transforming growth factor (TGF)-β1 and a concurrent increase in active TGF-β1 (111).

TABLE 27.2. ANALYSIS OF PREDICTIVE VALUE OF THYROID ANTIBODIES IN RELATION TO OCCURRENCE OF POSTPARTUM THYROID DYSFUNCTION[a]

Ab	Ab + ve Subjects	Sampling Time – pp (months)	Sensitivity	Specificity	PPV	Reference
Micro	44 (7)	2–5	0.77	0.95	0.52	104
Micro	62 (1)	3	0.89	0.92	0.4	105
Micro	38 (3)	3	0.87	0.97	0.53	106
Micro	41 (*)	Delivery	0.45	0.95	0.63	85
Micro	54 (11)	2–4	0.76	0.91	0.65	85
Micro	69 (8)	5–7	0.86	0.9	0.68	85
Micro	15 (6)	Trimester 3	0.71	0.92	0.52	107
TPO	31 (5)	Trimesters 1/3	0.67	0.93	0.31	108
TPO	55 (31)	6	0.64	0.95	0.64	103
Micro	40 (46)	6	0.46	0.98	0.78	103
Micro Tg	50 (65)	Early pregnancy	1/12pp 0.14 3/12pp 0.37	1/12pp 0.88 3/12pp 0.90	1/12pp 0.07 3/12pp 0.21	98
Micro	55 (*)	Delivery			0.73	109
TPO	66 (*)	Trimester 1	-	-	0.55	99
TPO	308 (0)	Ealy pregnancy	1.00	0.62	0.48	110

[a]Note the variable times at which antibody measurements were performed.
Key: Ab, thyroid antibody; micro, microsomal antibody; pp, postpartum; PPV, positive predictive value; Tg, thyroglobulin antibody; TPO, thyroid peroxidase antibody; ( ), number of PPTD subjects with negative antibodies; (*), unknown or not included.

MANAGEMENT

The thyrotoxic phase is relatively asymptomatic, although tachycardia and palpitations may be noted. These will respond to β-adrenoreceptor blocker therapy. Thionamide antithyroid drugs are contraindicated because of the destructive nature of the condition. While the thyrotoxicosis of PPTD always resolves, several long-term studies of the hypothyroid phase have documented persistence of hypothyroidism in 20% to 30% of cases (65). If postpartum hypothyroidism is diagnosed, the patient will respond to an initial dose of 100 μg of T_4 and should be subsequently managed as for primary hypothyroidism. It is impossible at this stage to determine which patients will have transient hypothyroidism (and therefore require only short-term T_4 treatment) or develop permanent disease. A pragmatic strategy is to treat all postpartum hypothyroid women for 1 year, then to stop T_4 and reevaluate thyroid function (112).

Women who have developed transient postpartum hypothyroidism and who have recovered spontaneously or have stopped T_4 therapy should have thyroid function checked annually, as a 50% rate of permanent hypothyroidism rate has been noted after 7 years' follow-up. In contrast, thyroid antibody–positive women who remain euthyroid during the first postpartum year require less frequent assessment; their rate of hypothyroidism at 7 years is only 5% (113). Recurrence of transient PPTD was observed in up to 30% to 40% in an early series (114), but in a larger number of women studied there was a 70% chance

of recurrent PPTD after a first attack and a 25% risk even if the woman was only anti-TPO-positive without thyroid dysfunction during the first postpartum period. From the foregoing discussion, it is apparent that PPTD occurs in 50% of the 10% of women who may be found to be anti-TPO–positive in early pregnancy. In addition, 30% of all anti-TPO–positive women postpartum will develop depressive symptomatology (independent of thyroid function) compared with about 20% of antibody-negative women. The incidence and morbidity of the thyroid dysfunction and depressive symptomatology suggest that screening for PPTD may be justified. For example, a strategy involving measurement of thyroid antibodies in early gestation at the time of "booking" may alert the clinician to the risk of postpartum problems and encourage early treatment (115).

REFERENCES

1. Dorfman SG, Cooperman MT, Nelson RS, et al. Painless thyroiditis and transient hyperthyroidism without goiter. *Ann Intern Med* 1977;86:24–28.
2. Gordon M. "Silent" thyroiditis with symptomatic hyperthyroidism in an elderly patient. *J Am Geriatr Soc* 1978;26:375–377.
3. Hofeldt FD, Weled BJ, Brown JE, et al. "Silent thyroiditis" versus thyrotoxicosis factitia. *Minn Med* 1976;59:380–382.
4. Miyakawa M, Tsushima T, Onoda N, et al. Thyroid ultrasonography related to clinical and laboratory findings in patients with silent thyroiditis. *J Endocrinol Invest* 1992;15:289–295.

5. Papapetrou PD, Jackson IMD. Thyrotoxicosis due to "silent" thyroiditis. *Lancet* 1975;1:361–363.

6. Woolf PD. Transient painless thyroiditis with hyperthyroidism: a variant of lymphocytic thyroiditis? *Endocr Rev* 1980;4:411–420.

7. Lazarus JH. Silent thyroiditis and subacute thyroiditis. In: *Werner & Ingbar's, The thyroid.* 7th ed. Philadelphia: JB Lippincott, 1996:577–591.

8. Gluck FB, Nusynowitz MD, Plymate S. Chronic lymphocytic thyroiditis, thyrotoxicosis, and low radioactive iodine uptake. Report of four cases. *N Engl J Med* 1975;293:624–628.

9. Gorman CA, Duick DS, Woolner LB, et al. Transient hyperthyroidism in patients with lymphocytic thyroiditis. *Mayo Clin Proc* 1978;53:359–365.

10. Nikolai TF, Brosseau J, Kettrick MA, et al. Lymphocytic thyroiditis with spontaneously resolving hyperthyroidism (silent thyroiditis). *Arch Intern Med* 1980;140:478–482.

11. Williams I, Ankrett VO, Lazarus JH, et al. Aetiology of hyperthyroidism in Canada and Wales. *J Epidemiol Community Health* 1983;37:245–248.

12. Schorr AB, Miller JL, Shtasel P, et al. Low incidence of painless thyroiditis in the Philadelphia area. *Clin Nucl Med* 1986;11:379–380.

13. Vitug AC, Goldman JM. Silent (painless) thyroiditis: evidence of a geographic variation in frequency. *Arch Intern Med* 1985;145:473–475.

14. Schneeberg NG. Silent thyroiditis. *Arch Intern Med* 1983;143:2214.

15. Dulipsingh L, Ikram Z, Malchoff CD, et al. A cluster of cases of subacute and silent thyroiditis in the northern Connecticut, Greater Hartford area. *Conn Med* 1998;62:395–397.

16. Hedberg CW, Fishbein DB, Janssen RS, et al. An outbreak of thyrotoxicosis caused by the consumption of bovine thyroid gland in ground beef. *N Engl J Med* 1987;316:993–998.

17. Kinney JS, Hurwitz ES, Fishbein DB, et al. Community outbreak of thyrotoxicosis: epidemiology, immunogenetic characteristics, and long-term outcome. *Am J Med* 1988;84:10–18.

18. Nakamura S, Kosaka J, Sugimoto M, et al. Silent thyroiditis following rubella. *Endocrinol Jpn* 1990;37:79–85.

19. Masuno M, Kosaka J, Makamura S. Silent thyroiditis in an eleven-year-old girl, associated with transient increase in serum IgM and thyroid hormone. *Endocrinol Jpn* 1991;38:219–222.

20. Morriston J, Caplan RH. Typical and atypical ("silent") subacute thyroiditis in a wife and husband. *Arch Intern Med* 1978;138:45–48.

21. Ogura T, Hirakawa S, Suzuki S, et al. Five patients with painless thyroiditis simultaneously developed in a nursery school. *Endocrinol Jpn* 1980;35:225–230.

22. Farid NR, Hawe BS, Walfish PG. Increased frequency of HLA-DR3 and 5 in the syndromes of painless thyroiditis with transient thyrotoxicosis: evidence for an autoimmune aetiology. *Clin Endocrinol (Oxf)* 1983;19:699–704.

23. Fein HG, Metz S. Nikolai TF, et al. HLA antigens in thyroiditis: differences between silent and postpartum lymphocytic forms, and comparison with subacute and goitrous autoimmune thyroiditis. In: Walfish PG, Wall J, Volpe R, eds. *Autoimmunity and the thyroid.* Orlando, FL: Academic Press, 1985:373–375.

24. Mizukami Y, Michigishi T, Hashimoto T, et al. Silent thyroiditis: a histologic and immunohistochemical study. *Hum Pathol* 1988;19:423–431.

25. Ishihara T, Mori T, Waseda N, et al. Histological, clinical and laboratory findings of acute exacerbation of Hashimoto's thyroiditis—comparison with those of subacute granulomatous thyroiditis. *Endocrinol Jpn* 1987;34:831–841.

26. Shigemasa C, Ueta Y, Mitani Y, et al. Chronic thyroiditis with painful tender thyroid enlargement and transient thyrotoxicosis. *J Clin Endocrinol Metab* 1990;70:385–390.

27. Bartalena L, Grasso L, Brogioni S, et al. Serum interleukin-6 in amiodarone-induced thyrotoxicosis. *J Clin Endocrinol Metab* 1994;78:423–427.

28. Chow CC, Lee S, Shek CC, et al. Lithium-associated transient thyrotoxicosis in 4 Chinese women with autoimmune thyroiditis. *Aust N Z J Psychiatry* 1993;27:246–253.

29. Miller KK, Daniels GH. Association between lithium use and thyrotoxicosis caused by silent thyroiditis. *Clin Endocrinol (Oxf)* 2001;55:501–508.

30. Dang AH, Hershman JM. Lithium-associated thyroiditis. *Endocr Pract* 2002;8:232–236.

30a. Shimizu M, Hirokawa M, Manabe T, et al. Lithium associated autoimmune thyroiditis. *J Clin Pathol* 1997;50: 172–174.

31. Vassilopoulou-Sellin R, Sella A, Dexeus FH, et al. Acute thyroid dysfunction (thyroiditis) after therapy with interleukin-2. *Horm Metab Res* 1992;24:434–438.

32. Reid I, Sharpe I, McDevitt J, et al. Thyroid dysfunction can predict response to immunotherapy with interleukin-2 and interferon-2 alpha. *Br J Cancer* 1991;64:915–918.

33. Lisker-Melman M, Di Biscelglie AM, Usala SJ et al. Development of thyroid disease during therapy of chronic viral hepatitis with interferon alfa. *Gastroenterology* 1992;102:2155–2160.

34. Kamikubo K, Takami R, Suwa T, et al. Silent thyroiditis developed during alpha-interferon therapy. *Am J Med* Sci 1993;306:174–176.

35. Kodama T, Katabami S, Kamijo K, et al. Development of transient thyroid disease and reaction during treatment of chronic hepatitis-C with interferon. *J Gastroenterol* 1994;29:289–292.

36. Roti E, Minelli R, Guiberti T, et al. Multiple changes in thyroid function in patients with chronic active HCV hepatitis treated with recombinant interferon-alpha. *Am J Med* 1996;101:482–487.

37. Mazziotti G, Sorvillo F, Stomaiuolo G, et al. Temporal relationship between the appearance of thyroid autoantibodies and development of destructive thyroiditis in patients undergoing treatment with two different type-1 interferons for HCV-related chronic hepatitis: a prospective study. *J Endocrinol Invest* 2002;25:624–630.

38. Hoekman K, Von Blomberg-Van der Flier BME, Wagstaff J, et al. Reversible thyroid dysfunction during treatment with GM-CSF. *Lancet* 1991;338: 541–542.

39. Kasayama S, Miyake S, Samejima Y. Transient thyrotoxicosis and hypothyroidism following administration of the GnRH agonist leuprolide acetate. *Endocr J.* 2000;47:783–785.

40. Sakata S, Nagai K, Shibata T, et al. A case of rheumatoid arthritis associated with silent thyroiditis. *J Endocrinol Invest* 1992;15:377–380.

41. Magaro M, Zoli A, Altomonte L, et al. The association of silent thyroiditis with active systemic lupus erythematosus. *Clin Exp Rheumatol* 1992;10:67–70.

42. Iitaka M, Ishii J, Ishikawa N, et al. A case of Graves' disease with false hyperthyrotropinemia who developed silent thyroiditis. *Endocrinol Jpn* 1991;38:667–671.

43. Ho SC, Eng PH, Fok AC, et al. Thyrotoxicosis due to the simultaneous occurrence of silent thyroiditis and Graves' disease. *Thyroid* 1999;9:1127–1132.

44. Yamamoto M, Fuwa Y, Chimori K, et al. A case of progressive systemic sclerosis (PSS) with silent thyroiditis and anti-bovine thyrotropin antibodies. *Endocrinol Jpn* 1991;38:265–270.

45. Murao S, Yoshinouchi T, Sato M, et al. Silent thyroiditis after excision of a thymoma. *Intern Med* 1998;37:604–605.

46. Carney AG, Moore SB, Northcutt RC, et al. Palpation thyroiditis (multifocal granulomatous folliculitis). *Am J Clin Pathol* 1975;64:639–647.

47. Walfish PG, Caplan D, Rosen IB. Postparathyroidectomy transient thyrotoxicosis. *J Clin Endocrinol Metab* 1992;75:224–227.

48. Smallridge RC, De Keyser FM, Van Herle AJ, et al. Thyroid iodine content and serum thyroglobulin: clues to the natural history of destruction-induced thyroiditis. *J Clin Endocrinol Metab* 1986;62:1213–1219.

48a. Wong V, Fu AX, George J, et al. Thyrotoxicosis induced by alpha-interferon therapy in chronic viral hepatitis. *Clin Endocrinol (Oxf)* 2002;56:793–798.

49. Kung AWC, Jones BM, Lai CL. Effects of interferon-γ therapy on thyroid function, T-lymphocyte subpopulations and induction of autoantibodies. *J Clin Endocrinol Metab* 1990;71:1230–1234.

50. Mitani Y, Shigesmasa C, Kouchi T, et al. Detection of thyroid stimulating antibody in patients with inflammatory thyrotoxicosis. *Horm Res* 1992;37:196–201.

51. Nakamura S, Sugimoto M, Kosaka J, et al. Silent thyroiditis with thyroid-stimulation-blocking antibodies (TSBAb). *Japanese Journal of Medicine* 1990;29:623–627.

52. Sarlis NJ, Brucker-Davis F, Swift JP, et al. Graves' disease following thyrotoxic painless thyroiditis. Analysis of antibody activities against the thyrotropin receptor in two cases. *Thyroid* 1997;7:829–836.

53. Yamamoto M, Sakurada T, Yoshida K, et al. Thyroid function and antimicrosomal antibody during the course of silent thyroiditis. *Endocrinol Jpn* 1987;34:357–363.

54. Nikolai TF, Coombs GJ, McKenzie AK, et al. Treatment of lymphocytic thyroiditis with spontaneously resolving hyperthyroidism (silent thyroiditis). *Arch Intern Med* 1982;142:2281–2283.

55. Baytner-Zamir H, Zelikovsky L, Jarchowsky J. Prolonged fever in painless subacute thyroiditis diagnosis by gallium scan. *Harefuah* 1996;130;453–455, 504.

56. Hidaka Y, Okumura M, Fukata S, et al. Increased serum concentration of interleukin-12 in patients with silent thyroiditis and Graves' disease. *Thyroid* 1999;2:149–153.

57. Ho SC, Eng PH, Fok AC, et al. Thyrotoxicosis due to the simultaneous occurrence of silent thyroiditis and Graves' disease. *Thyroid* 1999;9:1127–1132.

58. Sayama N, Yoshida K, Mori K, et al. Measurement of red blood cell zinc concentration with Zn-test kit: discrimination between hyperthyroid Graves' disease and transient thyrotoxicosis. *Endocr J* 1998;45:767–772.

59. Nikolai TF, Coombs GJ, McKenzie AK, et al. Treatment of lymphocytic thyroiditis with spontaneously resolving hyperthyroidism (silent thyroiditis). *Arch Intern Med* 1982;142:2281–2283.

60. Arem R, Munipalli B. Ipodate therapy in patients with severe destruction-induced thyrotoxicosis. *Arch Intern Med.* 1996;156:1752–1757.

61. Nikolai TF, Coombs GJ, McKenzie AK. Lymphocytic thyroiditis with spontaneously resolving hyperthyroidism and subacute thyroiditis: long-term follow-up. *Arch Intern Med* 1981;141:1455–1458.

62. Roberton HEW. Lassitude, coldness, and hair changes following pregnancy, and their response to treatment with thyroid extract. *BMJ* 1948;2:93–94.

63. Amino N, Miyai KJ, Onishi T, et al. Transient hypothyroidism after delivery in autoimmune thyroiditis. *J Clin Endocinol Metab* 1976;42:296–301.

64. Ginsberg J, Walfish PG. Postpartum transient thyrotoxicosis with painless thyroiditis. *Lancet* 1977;1:1125–1128.

65. Muller AF, Drexhage HA, Berghout A. Postpartum thyroiditis and autoimmune thyroiditis in women of childbearing age: recent insights and consequences for antenatal and postnatal care. *Endocr Rev* 2001;22:605–630.

66. Roti E, Uberti E. Post-partum thyroiditis—a clinical update. *Eur J Endocrinol* 2002;146:275–279.

67. Stagnaro-Green A. Clinical review 152: postpartum thyroiditis. *J Clin Endocrinol Metab* 2002;87:4042–4047.

68. Lazarus JH, Premawardhana LDKE, Parkes AB. Postpartum thyroiditis. *Autoimmunity* 2002;35:169–173.

69. Amino N, Tada H, Hidaka Y. Thyroid disease after pregnancy: post-partum thyroiditis. In: Wass JAH, Shalet, SM, eds. *Oxford textbook of endocrinology and diabetes.* Oxford: Oxford University Press, 2002:527–532.

70. Lazarus JH, Premawardhana LDKE, Parkes AB. Postpartum thyroiditis. In: Weetman AP, ed. *Immunology & medicine series: endocrine autoimmunity and associated conditions.* London: Kluwer Academic Publishers, 1998;27:83–97.

71. Nikolai TF, Turney SL, Roberts RC. Postpartum lymphocytic thyroiditis. *Arch Intern Med* 1987;47;221–224.

72. Fung HYM, Kologlu M, Collison K, et al. Postpartum thyroid dysfunction in mid Glamorgan. *BMJ* 1998;296:241–244.

73. Gerstein HC. How common is postpartum thyroiditis? *Arch Intern Med* 1990;150:1397–1400.

74. Walfish PG, Meyerson J, Provias JP, et al. Prevalence and characteristics of past-partum thyroid dysfunction: results of a survey from Toronto, Canada. *J Endocrinol Invest* 1992;15:265–272.

75. Barca MF, Knobel M, Tominori E, et al. Prevalence and characteristics of postpartum dysfunction in São Paulo, Brazil. *Clin Endocrinol (Oxf)* 2000;53:21–31.

76. Shahbazian HB, Sarvghadi F, Azizi F. Prevalence and characteristics of postpartum thyroid dysfunction in Tehran. *Eur J Endocrinol* 2001;145:397–401.

77. Bagis T, Gokcel A, Saygili ES. Autoimmune thyroid disease in pregnancy and postpartum period: relationship to spontaneous abortion. *Thyroid* 2001;11:1049–1053.

78. Gallas PRJ, Stolk, RP, Bakker K, et al. Thyroid dysfunction during pregnancy and in the first postpartum year in women with diabetes mellitus type 1. *Eur J Endocrinol* 2002;147:443–451.

79. Weetman AP, McGregor AM. Autoimmune thyroid disease: further developments in our understanding. *Endocr Rev* 1994;15:788–830.

80. Mizukami Y, Michigishi T, Nonomura A, et al. Postpartum thyroiditis—a clinical, histologic and immunologic study of 15 cases. *Am J Clin Pathol* 1993;100:200–205.

81. Tachi J, Amino N, Tamaki H, et al. Long term follow-up and HLA association in patients with postpartum hypothyroidism. *J Clin Endocrinol Metab* 1988;66:480–484.

82. Kologlu M, Fung H, Darke C, et al. Postpartum thyroid dysfunction and HLA status. *Eur J Clin Invest* 1990;20:56–60.

83. Farid NR, Haw BS, Walfish PG. Increased frequency of HLA-DR3 and 5 in the syndromes of painless thyroiditis with transient thyrotoxicosis: evidence for an autoimmune etiology. *Clin Endocrinol (Oxf)* 1983;19:699–704.

84. Jansson R, Safwenberg J, Dahlberg PA. Influence of the HLA-DR4 antigen and iodine status on the development of autoimmune postpartum thyroiditis. *J Clin Endocrinol Metab* 1985;60:168–173.

85. Vargas Mt, Briones-Urbina R, Gladman D, et al. Antithyroid microsomal autoantibodies and HLA-DR5 are associated with postpartum thyroid dysfunction: evidence supporting an autoimmune pathogenesis. *J Clin Endocrinol Metab* 1988;67:327–333.

86. Parkes AB, Darke C, Othman S, et al. MHC class II and complement polymorphism in postpartum thyroiditis. *Eur J Endocrinol* 1996;134:449–453.

87. Davies TF. The thyroid immunology of the postpartum period. *Thyroid* 1999;9;675–684.

88. Weetman AP, Fung HYM, Richards CJ, et al. IgG subclass distribution and relative functional affinity of thyroid microsomal antibodies in postpartum thyroiditis. *Eur J Clin Invest* 1990;20:133–136.

89. Briones-Urbina R, Parkes AB, Bogner U, et al. Increase in antimicrosomal antibody related IgG1, IgG2 and IgG3 and titres of antithyroid peroxidase antibodies, but not antibody dependent cell mediated cytotoxicity in post-partum thyroiditis with transient hyperthyroidism. *J Endocrinol Invest* 1990;13:879–876.

90. Parkes AB, Othman S, Hall R, et al. The role of complement in the pathogenesis of postpartum thyroiditis. *J Clin Endocrinol Metab* 1994;79:395–400.

91. Parkes AB, Adams H, Othman S, et al. The role of complement in the pathogenesis of postpartum thyroiditis: ultrasound echogenicity and the degree of complement induced thyroid damage. *Thyroid* 1996;6:169–174.

92. Wegmann TG, Lin H, Guilbert L, et al. Bidirectional cytokine interactions in the maternal-fetal relationship: is successful pregnancy a T_H2 phenomenon? *Immunol Today* 1993;14:353–356.

93. Watanabe M, Iwatani Y, Kaneda T, et al. Changes in T, B, and NK lymphocyte subsets during and after normal pregnancy. *J Reprod Immunol* 1997;37:368–377.

94. Stagnaro-Green A, Roman H, Cobin RH, et al. Prospective study of lymphocyte-initiated immunosuppression in normal pregnancy: evidence of a T-cell etiology for postpartum thyroid dysfunction. *J Clin Endocrinol Metab* 1992;74:645–653.

95. Kokandi AA, Parkes AB, Premawardhana LDKE, et al. Association of postpartum thyroid dysfunction with antepartum hormonal and immunological changes. *J Clin Endocrinol Metab* 2003;88:1126–1132.

96. Ando T, Davies TF. Postpartum autoimmune thyroid disease: The potential role of fetal microchimerism. *J Clin Endocrinol Metab* 2003;88:2965–2971.

97. Lazarus JH, Hall R, Othman S, et al. The clinical spectrum of postpartum thyroid disease. *QJM* 1996;89:429–435.

98. Sakaihara M, Yamada H, Kato EH, et al. Postpartum thyroid dysfunction in women with normal thyroid function during pregnancy. *Clin Endocrinol (Oxf)* 2000;53:487–492.

99. Nohr SB, Jorgensen A, Pedersen KM, et al. Postpartum thyroid dysfunction in pregnant thyroid peroxidase antibody-positive women living in an area with mild to moderate iodine deficiency: is iodine supplementation safe? *J Clin Endocrinol Metab* 2000;85:3191–3198.

100. Caixas A, Albareda M, Garcia-Patterson A, et al. Postpartum thyroiditis in women with hypothyroidism antedating pregnancy? *J Clin Endocrinol Metab* 1999;84:4000–4005.

101. Harris B, Othman S, Davies J, et al. Association between postpartum thyroid dysfunction and thyroid antibodies and depression. *BMJ* 1992;305:152–156.

101a. Kuijpens JL, Vader HL, Drexhage HA, et al. Thyroid peroxidase antibodies during gestation are a marker for subsequent depression postpartum. *Eur J Endocrinol* 2001;145:579–584.

102. Lucas A, Pizarro E, Granada ML, et al. Postpartum thyroid dysfunction and postpartum depression: are they two linked disorders? *Clin Endocrinol (Oxf)* 2001;55:809–814.

103. Kent GN, Stuckey AG, Allen JR, et al. Postpartum thyroid dysfunction; clinical assessment and relationship to psychiatric affective morbidity. *Clin Endocrinol (Oxf)* 1999;51:429–438.

104. Jansson R, Bernander S, Karlsson A, et al. Autoimmune thyroid dysfunction in the postpartum period. *J Clin Endocrinol Metab* 1984;58:681–687.

105. Amino N, Mori H, Iwatani Y, et al. High prevalence of transient postpartum thyrotoxicosis and hypothyroidism. *N Engl J Med* 1982;306:849–852.

106. Lervang HH, Pryds O, Ostergaard Kristensen HP. Thyroid dysfunction after delivery: incidence and clinical course. *Acta Med Scand* 1987;222:369–374.

107. Pop VJM, de Rooy HA, Vader HL, et al. Microsomal antibodies during gestation in relation to postpartum thyroid dysfunction and depression. *Acta Endocrinol* (Copenh) 1993;129:26–30.

108. Kuijpens JL, De Haan-Meulman M, Vader HL, et al. Cell-Mediated immunity and postpartum thyroid dysfunction: a possibility for the prediction of disease. *J Clin Endocrinol Metab* 1998;83:1959–1966.

109. Solomon BL, Fein HG, Smallridge RC. Usefulness of antimicrosomal antibody titres in the diagnosis of postpartum thyroiditis. *J Fam Pract* 1993;36:177–182.

110. Premawardhana LD, Parkes AB, John R, et al. Thyroid peroxidase antibodies in early pregnancy: utility for prediction of postpartum thyroid dysfunction and implications for screening. *Thyroid* 2004;14:610–615.

110a. Pearce EN, Bogazzi F, Martino E, et al. The prevalence of elevated serum C-reactive protein levels in inflammatory and noninflammatory thyroid disease. *Thyroid* 2003;13:643–648.

111. Oliveri A, De Angelis S, Vaccari V, et al. Postpartum thyroiditis is associated with fluctuations in transforming growth factor-β serum levels. *J Clin Endocrinol Metab* 2003;88:1280–1284.

112. Owen PJD, Lazarus JH. The treatment of post-partum thyroid disease. *J Endocrinol Invest* 2003;26:290–291.

113. Premawardhana LD, Parkes AB, Ammari F. Postpartum thyroiditis and long-term thyroid status: prognostic influence of thyroid peroxidase antibodies and ultrasound echogenicity. *J Clin Endocrinol Metab* 2000;85:71–75.

114. Dahlberg PA, Jansson R. Different aetiologies in post-partum thyroiditis. *Acta Endocrinol* (Copenh) 1983;104:195–200.

115. Lazarus JH, Ammari F, Oretti R, et al. Clinical aspects of recurrent postpartum thyroiditis. *Br J Gen Pract* 1997;47:305–308

SUBACUTE THYROIDITIS AND ACUTE INFECTIOUS THYROIDITIS

ALAN P. FARWELL

Subacute thyroiditis and acute infectious thyroiditis are two important causes of thyroid pain. The former is the most common cause of thyroid pain, while the latter is rare, but potentially life-threatening. Despite the common presentation of pain, two distinct clinical pictures evolve. Subacute thyroiditis is a relatively common disorder that has been attributed to a viral infection, although the evidence for a viral etiology is mostly circumstantial. In addition to pain, subacute thyroiditis causes transient thyrotoxicosis, followed by transient hypothyroidism and usually euthyroidism, and therapy is directed at thyroidal pain and dysfunction. In contrast, an infectious etiology is usually clear in the rare cases of acute infectious thyroiditis. Bacterial, fungal, and parasitic organisms all have been documented as etiologic agents, and therapy in acute thyroiditis is directed against the offending organism. In addition, acute thyroiditis is potentially life-threatening, and the prognosis is often dependent on the prompt recognition and treatment of this disorder.

DIFFERENTIAL DIAGNOSIS OF THE PAINFUL THYROID

In the patient who presents with neck pain, subacute and acute infectious thyroiditis must be differentiated from the other causes of anterior neck pain (Table 28.1). Essentially all of the nonthyroidal causes of neck pain are infectious in origin and present as discrete painful masses (1). Hemorrhage into either a thyroid cyst or a nodule usually presents with the sudden onset of unilateral neck pain associated with a marked increase in the size of a preexisting nodule. The pain associated with a rapidly enlarging carcinoma, usually anaplastic, is often more chronic in nature (2), as is painful Hashimoto's thyroiditis, which usually involves the entire gland, and antibodies directed against thyroglobulin (Tg) and thyroid peroxidase (TPO) are usually present in high titer (3). Radiation thyroiditis occurs in the setting of radioactive iodine treatment for hyperthyroidism or following supravoltage external radiation of the anterior neck for thyroid cancer or lymphoma. Amiodarone may cause thyroiditis, which may occasionally be painful (4,5).

Globus hystericus, an anxiety reaction that is characterized by a constrictive feeling in the throat, is a diagnosis of exclusion.

Because of the clinical presentation, frequency of occurrence, and differing etiology, subacute and acute infectious thyroiditis will be discussed separately.

SUBACUTE THYROIDITIS

Subacute thyroiditis is a spontaneous remitting inflammatory disorder of the thyroid that may last for weeks to months (6–9). This disorder has a number of eponyms, including de Quervain's thyroiditis, giant-cell thyroiditis, pseudogranulomatous thyroiditis, subacute painful thyroiditis, and subacute granulomatous thyroiditis (6). The first description of subacute thyroiditis was in 1895 by Mygind, who reported 18 cases of "thyroiditis akuta simplex" (10). The pathology of subacute thyroiditis was first described in 1904 by de Quervain, whose name is associated with the disorder, when he showed giant cells and granulomatous-type changes in the thyroids of affected patients (7). Subacute thyroiditis is the most common cause of the painful thyroid and may account for up to 5% of clinical thyroid abnormalities. As with other thyroid disorders, women are more frequently affected than men, with a peak incidence in the fourth and fifth decades (Table 28.2) (7–9). This disorder is rare in children (11) and the elderly (10).

Etiology

A viral etiology has most often been implicated in subacute thyroiditis (12–15). However, the evidence supporting this association is largely indirect. Only mumps virus (12) and an unidentified cytopathic virus (13) have been directly isolated from affected thyroids, while electron microscopy, an electromagnetic imaging study, demonstrated viral particles in thyroid tissue from a single patient with subacute thyroiditis (16).

Subacute thyroiditis often follows an upper respiratory tract infection and occasionally includes a prodromal phase of muscular aches and pains, fever, and malaise (10). In-

TABLE 28.1. DIFFERENTIAL DIAGNOSIS OF THE PAINFUL ANTERIOR NECK MASS

Thyroidal
  Subacute thyroiditis
  Acute infectious thyroiditis
  Hemorrhage into a cyst
  Hemorrhage into a benign or malignant nodule
  Rapidly enlarging thyroid carcinoma
  Painful Hashimoto's thyroiditis
  Radiation thyroiditis
  Painful amiodarone-induced thyroiditis
Nonthyroidal
  Infected thyroglossal duct cyst
  Infected branchial cleft cyst
  Infected cystic hygroma
  Cervical adenitis
  Cellulitis of the anterior neck
Other
  Globus hystericus

From Farwell AP, Braverman LE. Inflammatory thyroid disorders. *Otolaryngol Clin North Am* 1996;29:541–556, with permission.

deed, cases of subacute thyroiditis tend to be seasonal and geographical, coinciding with seasonal enterovirus infections (9). Subacute thyroiditis has been associated with infections by adenovirus, coxsackie, Epstein-Barr, and influenza viruses (10,13), and has been reported after hepatitis B vaccination (17) and during both interferon (18,19) and combination interferon and ribavirin therapy (20) for chronic hepatitis C. In 1967, Volpe et al (14) reported rising antibody titers to mumps virus, echovirus, adenovirus, and enterovirus in convalescent serum of 32 patients with subacute thyroiditis (Fig. 28.1). However, an additional 26 patients had viral antibody titers that did not change (14),

and in another study, serum, stool, and fine-needle thyroid aspirations in 27 consecutive patients with subacute thyroiditis revealed no evidence of enteroviral infection (21). A single report has described a fourfold rise in serum coxsackie antibody titers after a documented case of subacute thyroiditis (22). Recently, 10 patients presented with postviral thyroiditis that followed a similar course to subacute thyroiditis but was painless (23). In addition, there have been reports of painless subacute thyroiditis diagnosed by fine-needle aspiration biopsy.

Thyroid autoimmunity may be present during the acute phase of the disease, as indicated by the presence of antibodies against TPO, Tg, and the thyrotropin (TSH) receptor (6,26) and by sensitization of T lymphocytes against thyroid antigen (27). However, this is often transient and is most likely due to release of antigen during inflammation rather than a primary event. Several reports have suggested that subacute thyroiditis may trigger the production of TSH receptor antibodies (28), contributing to a prolonged hypothyroid phase (29) and occasionally leading to the development of Graves' disease (30), although this was not observed in the most recent epidemiological survey (9).

There is an apparent genetic predisposition to subacute thyroiditis, with histocompatibility antigen (HLA)–Bw35 reported in all ethnic groups (10), including approximately two-thirds of Caucasian and Chinese patients (31). The relative risk of HLA-Bw35 in subacute thyroiditis is high, ranging from 8.0 to 56.6 (10). Additional evidence for genetic susceptibility is the simultaneous development of subacute thyroiditis in identical twins heterozygous for the HLA-Bw35 haplotype (32). However, an epidemic of "atypical" subacute thyroiditis was described in a town in

TABLE 28.2. COMPARISON BETWEEN SUBACUTE AND ACUTE INFECTIOUS THYROIDITIS

	Subacute Thyroiditis	Acute Infectious Thyroiditis
Age of onset (yr)	20–60 (80% 40–50)	Adolescence, 20–40
Sex ratio (F:M)	5:1	1:1
Infectious agent	Possibly viral	Bacterial, fungal, parasitic, mycobacterial organisms
Genetic predisposition	Moderate, HLA Bw-35	Pyriform sinus fistula
Pathology	Giant cells, granulomas	Suppuration, offending organism
Culture	Negative	Positive for offending organism
Prodrome	Viral illness	Upper respiratory illness
Goiter	Painful, transient	Painful, transient
Fever and malaise	Yes	Yes
Thyroid function	Thyrotoxicosis, hypothyroidism, or both	Euthyroid
Thyroid peroxidase antibodies	Low titer/absent, transient	Low titer/absent, transient
Viral antibodies	Yes	No
ESR/C-reactive protein	High	High
24-h RAIU	<5%	Normal
Relapse	Rare	Common if patent pyriform sinus fistula
Permanent hypothyroidism	5%–15%	Rare

ESR, erythrocyte sedimentation rate; HLA, histocompatibility antigen; RAIU, radioactive iodine uptake.
Farwell AP, Braverman LE. Inflammatory thyroid disorders. *Otolaryngol Clin North Am* 1996;29:541–556; Pearce EN, Farwell AP, Braverman LE. Thyroiditis. *N Engl J Med* 2003;348:2646–2655; and Fatourechi V, Aniszewski JP, Fatourechi GZ, et al. Clinical features and outcome of subacute thyroiditis in an incidence cohort: Olmsted County, Minnesota, study. *J Clin Endocrinol Metab* 2003;88:2100–2105, with permission.

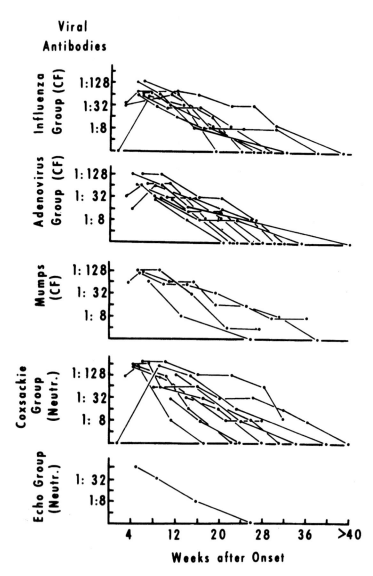

FIGURE 28.1. Viral antibody titers in subacute thyroiditis. A survey of 72 patients with subacute thyroiditis identified 32 with antibodies to common viruses that changed sufficiently in titer to suggest that they may play an etiologic role in the disorder. (From Volpe R, Row VV, Ezrin C. Circulating viral and thyroid antibodies in subacute thyroiditis. *J Clin Endocrinol Metab* 1967;27:1275–1284, with permission.)

the Netherlands in which a painful goiter was present in only 2 of 12 patients (33). HLA-B15/62 was found in 5 of 11 patients tested, while only 1 patient tested positive for HLA-Bw35. Lastly, a weak association of subacute thyroiditis with HLA-DRw8 has been reported in Japanese patients (34).

Pathology

The primary events in the pathology of subacute thyroiditis are destruction of the follicular epithelium and loss of follicular integrity; however, the histopathological changes are distinct from those found with Hashimoto's thyroiditis (35,36). Although the evaluation of subacute thyroiditis rarely requires histological examination, the diagnosis has been made on the basis of FNAB (37). The lesions are patchy in distribution and are of varying stages of development, with infiltration of mononuclear cells in affected re-

gions and partial or complete loss of colloid and fragmentation and duplication of the basement membrane (Fig. 28.2) (10). The characteristic follicular lesion is a central core of colloid surrounded by multinucleate giant cells (35,38). These follicular lesions progress to form granulomas. Carcinoembryonic antigen has been reported at the center of granulomas in acute-stage subacute thyroiditis, while carcinoma antigen 19–9 expression has been reported in the lesions in the later stages of the disease, suggesting a histiocytic or follicular cell origin for the giant cells (39). Caseation, hemorrhage, and calcification do not occur, and the pathological changes revert to normal, with minimal residual fibrosis, once the disease subsides.

Clinical Manifestations

The characteristic feature of subacute thyroiditis is pain in the region of the thyroid, either gradual or sudden in onset

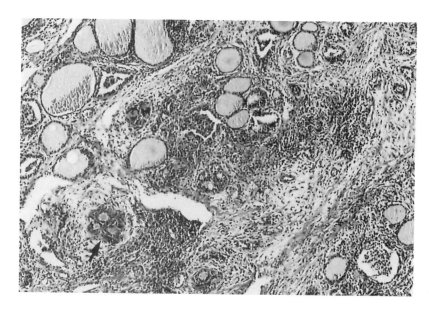

FIGURE 28.2. Histopathologic findings in subacute thyroiditis. Thyroid follicles are destroyed, and there is a mixed inflammatory infiltrate, desquamated thyroid epithelial cells, edema, and colloid undergoing phagocytosis by histiocytes (foreign body–type giant cells, *arrow*). (Hematoxylin and eosin, 40× magnification.) (From Lazarus JH. Silent thyroiditis and subacute thyroiditis. In: Braverman LE, Utiger RD, eds. *The thyroid*. Philadelphia: Lippincott-Raven Publishers, 1996:577–591, with permission.)

(Table 28.3) (7). The pain is usually constant and often severe, involving the entire thyroid in many patients. Occasionally, one side is initially affected and is followed in days to weeks by involvement of the contralateral side. The pain is often aggravated by turning the head or swallowing and may radiate to the jaw, ear, or occiput on the ipsilateral side. Rarely, subacute thyroiditis may present as a nontender solitary nodule. In these cases, the diagnosis has been made after FNAB (37).

Patients may report a viral prodrome, including myalgia, low-grade fever, lassitude (which may be debilitating), pharyngitis, and dysphagia. Symptoms of thyrotoxicosis are present in the majority of patients (6,9), due to follicular destruction and leakage of preformed hormone from the gland. Rarely, subacute thyroiditis may mimic temporal arteritis (40).

Palpation usually reveals an exquisitely tender, hard, ill-defined nodular thyroid (Table 28.3). The tender region may encompass an entire lobe, and mild tenderness may be present in the contralateral lobe. The overlying skin is occasionally warm and erythematous. Cervical lymphadenopathy is rarely present. While the vast majority of patients are only mildly to moderately ill, subacute thyroiditis may have a dramatic presentation, with marked fever, severe thyrotoxicosis, and obstructive symptoms due to pronounced thyroid inflammation and edema.

Laboratory Findings

During the active phase of subacute thyroiditis, the erythrocyte sedimentation rate (ESR) is usually markedly ele-

TABLE 28.3. COMMON CLINICAL FEATURES OF SUBACUTE THYROIDITIS[a]

Symptoms	Signs	Laboratory Findings
Pain in neck or thyroid	Tender, firm thyroid	High ESR
Constant, dull pain	Fever	High serum thyroid hormones
Fever	Acutely ill	High serum thyroglobulin
Dysphagia	Clinical thyrotoxicosis	High C-reactive protein
Malaise		24-h RAIU <5%
Fatigue		
Anxiety		
Sweats		

ESR, erythrocyte sedimentation rate; RAIU, radioactive iodine uptake.
[a]The clinical features have been reported in <50% of patients with subacute thyroiditis.
From Fatourechi V, Aniszewski JP, Fatourechi GZ, et al. Clinical features and outcome of subacute thyroiditis in an incidence cohort: Olmsted County, Minnesota, study. *J Clin Endocrinol Metab* 2003;88: 2100–2105; Lazarus JH. Silent thyroiditis and subacute thyroiditis. In: Braverman LE, Utiger RD, eds. *The thyroid*. Philadelphia: Lippincott-Raven Publishers, 1996:577–591; Pearce EN, Bogazzi F, Martino E, et al. The prevalence of elevated serum C-reactive protein levels in inflammatory and noninflammatory thyroid disease. *Thyroid* 2003;13:643–648; and Szabo SM, Allen DB. Thyroiditis: differentiation of acute suppurative and subacute thyroiditis. Case report and review of the literature [review]. *Clin Pediatr (Phila)* 1989;28:171–174, with permission.

vated (Table 28.3) (7). In fact, a normal ESR essentially rules out subacute thyroiditis as a tenable diagnosis. C-reactive protein is another inflammatory marker that appears to be selectively elevated in subacute thyroiditis (41). The white blood count is normal to mildly increased, and there is often a normochromic, normocytic anemia.

Biochemical thyrotoxicosis is present in approximately 50% of patients in the acute phase of subacute thyroiditis (6,9). The serum thyroxine (T_4) concentration is disproportionately elevated relative to the serum triiedothyronine T_3 concentration, reflecting the intrathyroidal T_4-to-T_3 ratio (42). In addition, the acute illness decreases the peripheral deiodination of T_4 to T_3, resulting in lower T_3 concentrations than expected (43). Serum TSH concentrations are low to undetectable. Consistent with follicular destruction, serum Tg concentrations are elevated (44,45). Antibodies directed against Tg and TPO are either absent or present in low titer.

The radioactive iodine uptake (RAIU) is low, most often <2% at 24 hours. Thus, subacute thyroiditis falls into the category of "low RAIU thyrotoxicosis" (46). As with the ESR discussed earlier, a normal RAIU essentially rules out subacute thyroiditis as a tenable diagnosis. Similarly, low uptake has been reported with technetium (Tc^{99}) pertechnetate, while Tc^{99}-sestamibi uptake may be elevated early in subacute thyroiditis (47). Ultrasound has been suggested as playing a useful supporting role in the diagnosis of subacute thyroiditis (48), particularly color-flow Doppler ultrasonography, in which the gland appears hypoechoic with low to normal vascularity (49). There has been a single report of increased radiogallium uptake in the thyroid in a patient with subacute thyroiditis (50).

Management

Salicylates and other nonsteroidal anti-inflammatory drugs are often adequate to decrease thyroidal pain in mild to moderate cases (6,9). In more severe cases, oral glucocorticoids (prednisone up to 40 mg/day) may provide dramatic relief of pain and swelling, often within a few hours of administration and in most cases within 24 to 48 hours (6,7). In fact, if thyroidal/neck pain fails to improve after 72 hours of prednisone corticosteroid therapy, the diagnosis of subacute thyroiditis should be questioned. Despite the clinical response, the underlying inflammatory process may persist, and symptoms may recur if the dose is tapered too rapidly. Up to 20% of patients will have a recurrence of thyroidal pain upon discontinuation of prednisone, which responds to restarting treatment (9,10,51,52). In general, full-doses prednisone are given for a week, followed by tapering the dose over 2 to 4 weeks. The use of steroid prednisone appears to have no effect on the development of transient hypothyroidism, but may be associated with a higher incidence of permanent hypothyroidism (9).

There appears to be no predictive differences between patients who have recurrent pain when prednisone is tapered and those whose pain has resolved (52). However, determination of the RAIU before discontinuing prednisone may be helpful in identifying those patients at the highest risk for early relapse (7). If the RAIU is still low, the inflammatory process is ongoing, and therapy should not be discontinued.

Patients with recurrent prednisone symptoms after withdrawal of corticosteroids usually respond to reinstitution or continuation of therapy for an additional month (10). While subacute thyroiditis is a self-limited disease and the vast majority of patients respond to the measures discussed above, there are occasional patients who suffer from repeated exacerbations of pain and inflammation (6). In these patients, therapy with T_4 has been helpful in preventing exacerbations, suggesting that endogenous TSH may contribute to their occurrence (6,10). Rarely, thyroidectomy or thyroid ablation with radioactive iodine when the uptake is normal may be indicated for management of patients with protracted courses of severe neck pain and malaise (6,10).

If clinical thyrotoxicosis is present, beta-adrenergic blocking drugs such as propranolol are useful. Antithyroid drugs have no role in the therapy of subacute thyroiditis, as the gland is not hyperfunctioning (46). The oral cholecystographic agents sodium iopanoate (1,000 mg daily) and sodium ipodate (500 mg daily) have been utilized to achieve rapid control of severe thyrotoxicosis in patients with subacute thyroiditis (53,54); however, both drugs are no longer available in the United States.

Clinical Course

The clinical course of subacute thyroiditis is self-limited, comprising four phases (Fig. 28.3) (6–8). The acute phase, consisting of thyroidal pain and thyrotoxicosis, usually lasts 3 to 6 weeks, but may last longer. A period of transient asymptomatic euthyroidism follows. Transient hypothyroidism occurs after several more weeks in 30% to 50% of patients (9,55) and may last for several months. The final recovery phase follows, when all aspects of thyroid function return to normal in 4 to 6 months, including morphology (48). While permanent hypothyroidism has been reported to be relatively rare, occurring in up to 5% of patients (55), recent studies suggest this incidence may be higher. A small study from France reported an incidence of permanent hypothyroidism of 31% (56), while a larger series from the Mayo Clinic reported an incidence of 15% (9).

Relapse of subacute thyroiditis is rare, occurring in up to 4% of patients (9,57). However, some patients with a history of subacute thyroiditis were found to be particularly sensitive to the inhibitory effects of exogenously administered iodide, suggesting a persistent thyroid abnor-

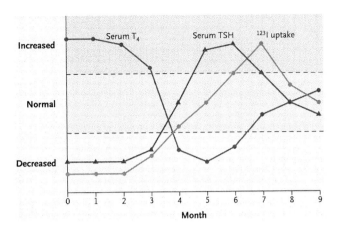

FIGURE 28.3. Clinical course of subacute thyroiditis. (From Pearce EV, Farwell AP, Braverman LE. Thyroiditis. *N Engl J Med* 2003;348:2646–55, with permission.)

mality (58). In addition, there have been case reports of Graves' disease occurring after subacute thyroiditis (30, 59). Thus, long-term follow-up of patients after an episode of subacute thyroiditis is suggested.

ACUTE INFECTIOUS THYROIDITIS

Acute infectious thyroiditis, also known as acute suppurative thyroiditis, infectious thyroiditis, bacterial thyroiditis, and pyogenic thyroiditis, is a rare disorder, with ~300 cases having been reported in the adult literature (15,60–62) and ~100 cases reported in the pediatric literature (63,64). However, bacterial infections of the thyroid are potentially life-threatening, often with an explosive onset, and the prognosis is often dependent on the prompt recognition and treatment. Immunosuppressed patients, such as those with human immunodeficiency virus (HIV) infection and acquired immunodeficiency syndrome (AIDS), as well as organ-transplant patients on pharmacologic immunosuppression, are particularly at risk for infectious thyroiditis. In these cases, opportunistic infections of the thyroid are more often chronic and insidious in onset.

Pathogenesis

In contrast to most other organs in the body, the thyroid gland is remarkably resistant to infection. Protective mechanisms contributing to the relative resistance of the thyroid to infection include (a) the rich blood supply to and lymphatic drainage from the thyroid; (b) the high glandular content of iodine, which may be bactericidal; and (c) the separation of the thyroid from other structures of the neck by fascial planes and the complete, protective fibrous capsule surrounding the gland. Indeed, experimental models

of infectious thyroiditis are difficult to develop, as shown by the observation that direct injection of either staphylococci or streptococci into the carotid arteries of dogs rarely resulted in thyroidal infection (65). Thyroidal infections are most commonly bacterial in origin, with fungi, parasitic organisms, and mycobacteria being isolated much less frequently (Table 28.4) (15,60–64). The most common predisposing factor to infections of the thyroid appears to be preexisting thyroid disease; simple goiter, nodular goiter, Hashimoto's thyroiditis, or thyroid carcinoma has been present in up to two thirds of women and one half of men with infectious thyroiditis (60,66–68).

The thyroid appears relatively resistant to direct inoculation of bacteria. Only one case of infectious thyroiditis has been reported as a complication of thyroid surgery (67), despite an incidence of wound infections of 0.5% to 1% (69). While the route of infection was rarely documented in the early literature, it is now apparent that transmission of infective organisms via a pyriform sinus fistula is the most common route of thyroidal infection, especially in children (Fig. 28.4). The first cases of infectious thyroiditis due to a fistula originating from the left pyriform sinus were reported in 1979 (70). Additional reports identified infected embryonic cysts of the third and fourth branchial pouches as routes of thyroidal infection (71–76). Subsequently, studies of over 100 patients with infectious thyroiditis have identified pyriform sinus fistulae, primarily left-sided, in up to 90% of these patients, especially in those with recurrent episodes (63,64,67,74,77–79). Infectious thyroiditis is often preceded by an upper respiratory infection, which may induce inflammation of the fistula and promote the transmission of pathogens to the thyroid. Consistent with these observations, infectious thyroiditis is more common in the late fall and late spring months (63,67,77).

Infectious thyroiditis has also been reported to occur as a result of direct spread of pathogenic organisms via patent thyroglossal duct fistulae (80). Infections of the retropharyngeal space (pharyngitis and tonsillitis) or the lateral

TABLE 28.4. PATHOGENESIS OF INFECTIOUS THYROIDITIS, 1900–1980

Organism	Frequency (%)
Bacterial	68
Fungal	15
Mycobacterial	9
Parasitic	5
Syphilitic	3

From Farwell AP, Braverman LE. Inflammatory thyroid disorders. *Otolaryngol Clin North Am* 1996;29:541–556; and Berger SA, Zonszein J, Villamena P, et al. Infectious diseases of the thyroid gland [Review]. *Rev Infect Dis* 1983;5:108–122, with permission.

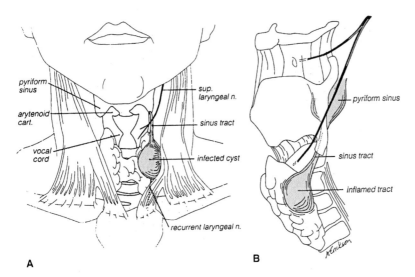

FIGURE 28.4. Thyroid abscess due to pyriform sinus fistula (*shaded*). Fistulous tract extends from apex of the left pyriform sinus to the abscess either adjacent to or within the left lobe of the thyroid. **A:** Frontal view. **B:** Lateral view. (From Har-el G, Sasaki CT, Prager D, Krespi YP. Acute suppurative thyroiditis and the branchial apparatus. *Am J Otolaryngol* 1991;12:6–11, with permission.)

pharyngeal spaces (pharyngitis, tonsillitis, parotitis, otitis, and mastoiditis) may rarely spread down posterior and lateral fascial planes into the neck and communicate with the structures in the pretracheal space (1). Infection may also arise directly from the pretracheal space through perforations in the esophagus (60).

As with any organ, infective organisms may reach the thyroid via spread from a distant focus through the bloodstream or lymphatics. Case reports of hematogenous spread from infections of the skin (81), lower respiratory tract, urinary tract, and gastrointestinal tract have been described

(60). This occurs more often in adults than children, usually in the presence of other underlying illnesses (68,82, 83), and acute suppurative thyroiditis has been reported in association with aggressive treatment of acute myelogenous leukemia in children (84).

Clinical Manifestations

Over 90% of patients with acute bacterial thyroiditis present with thyroidal pain, tenderness, fever, and local compression, resulting in dysphagia and dysphonia (Table 28.5) (68,77). The pain may radiate to the ear or mandible on the side of the infection (85). Signs and symptoms of systemic toxicity may be present. The thyroid is tender to palpation, with unilateral or bilateral lobar enlargement, and is associated with erythema and warmth of the skin. Abscess formation is indicated by fluctuance; a firm nodule may progress to fluctuance in the course of 1 to 3 days, so repeated physical examinations may be necessary. Cervical lymphadenopathy may be present but is not a prominent feature unless there is a predisposing pharyngitis.

Laboratory Findings

The laboratory evaluation of the painful thyroid should include determination of serum TSH as a reasonable initial thyroid function test. Normal thyroid function tests are seen in over two thirds of patients with acute suppurative thyroiditis (60,63,77), although thyrotoxicosis and hypothyroidism have been reported (77,86,87). Leukocytosis and an elevated ESR and C-reactive protein level are commonly observed in both subacute thyroiditis and infectious thyroiditis; thus these tests are not discriminatory. Radionuclide imaging, preferably with radioiodine, is useful in the case of a solitary painful nodule, and the RAIU will provide information on the overall function of the

TABLE 28.5. SIGNS AND SYMPTOMS OF ACUTE BACTERIAL THYROIDITIS

	Frequency (%)
Pain	89–100
Tenderness	89–100
Fever	91–100
High ESR/C-reactive protein	80–100
Antecedent upper respiratory illness	88–90
Left lobe involvement	85–89
Dysphonia	83
Leukocytosis	80
Erythema	70–82
Cough	73
Local warmth	63–70
Pharyngitis	69–90
Dysphagia/sore throat	40–91

ESR, erythrocyte sedimentation rate.
From Berger SA, Zonszein J, Villamena P, et al. Infectious diseases of the thyroid gland [review]. *Rev Infect Dis* 1983;5:108–122; Rich EJ, Mendelman PM. Acute suppurative thyroiditis in pediatric patients [review]. *Pediatr Infect Dis J* 1987;6:936–940; Chi H, Lee YJ, Chiu NC, et al. Acute suppurative thyroiditis in children. *Pediatr Infect Dis J* 2002;21:384–387; and Szabo SM, Allen DB. Thyroiditis. Differentiation of acute suppurative and subacute thyroiditis. Case report and review of the literature [review]. *Clin Pediatr (Phila)* 1989;28:171–174, with permission.

gland, which should be normal (88). The presence of soft-tissue gas on radiograph of the neck indicates infection with anaerobic, gas-forming organisms. Magnetic resonance imaging (MRI), ultrasonography, and computed tomography (CT) are most helpful in the identification of pyriform sinus fistulae or parathyroidal abscesses (89–94). These imaging studies, as well as other radionuclide studies, are best reserved for patients in whom the diagnosis is unclear (80,95).

FNAB is the best single laboratory test in the evaluation of infectious thyroiditis and will be diagnostic in most cases (15,60–64,96,97), especially when the tenderness is limited to a solitary nodule or a localized area and subacute thyroiditis has been ruled out. In addition to obtaining samples for cytology and gram stain and culture, provision should be made to obtain samples for special studies in the appropriate setting, such as Gomori's silver methenamine stain to identify *Pneumocystis carinii* in an immunocompromised patient (98,99).

Management

Bacterial Infections

Acute infectious thyroiditis is usually bacterial in origin (Table 28.4) (15,60–64,77). In adults, *Staphylococcus aureus* and *Streptococcus pyogenes* are the offending pathogens in >80% of patients and are the sole pathogen in over 70% of cases (Table 28.6) (60). In children, alpha- and beta-hemolytic *Streptococcus* and a variety of anaerobes account for 70% of cases, while mixed pathogens are identified in over 50% of cases (Table 28.6) (15,63,64). Other bacterial pathogens that have been shown to cause infectious thyroiditis include *Salmonella typhii, brandenberg,* and *enteriditis* (60,100–102), *Actinomyces naeslundi* (60), *Actinobacillus actinomycetemcomitans* (60), *Brucella melitensis* (103,104), *Clostridium septicum* (60), *Eikenella corrodens* (63,105), *Enterobacter* (63), *Escherichia coli, Haemophilus influenzae* (60), *Klebsiella* sp. (63), *Pseudomonas aeruginosa* (60), *Serratia marcescens* (106), and *Staphylococcus nonaureus* (60,63).

TABLE 28.6. CULTURE RESULTS IN ACUTE BACTERIAL THYROIDITIS

	Frequency (%)	
	Adults	Children
Pure cultures	72.9	35.5
Mixed cultures	18.8	56.5
Sterile cultures	8.2	8.1

From Berger SA, Zonszein J, Villamena P, et al. Infectious diseases of the thyroid gland [Review]. *Rev Infect Dis* 1983;5:108–122; and Rich EJ, Mendelman PM. Acute suppurative thyroiditis in pediatric patients [Review]. *Pediatr Infect Dis J* 1987;6:936–940, with permission.

Treatment of acute bacterial thyroiditis requires admission to the hospital, drainage of any abscess, and parenteral antimicrobial therapy aimed at the causative agent. Gram stain and culture of the fine-needle aspirate will reveal the causative organism in over 90% of cases. If no organisms are seen on the gram stain, nafcillin and gentamycin, or a third-generation cephalosporin, are appropriate initial therapy in adults, while a second-generation cephalosporin or clindamycin is reasonable in children. Since a pyriform sinus fistula is the most common route of infection in bacterial thyroiditis (63,67,74), a barium swallow (73), CT (90,91,94), or MRI (93) of the neck should be performed to look for a communicating fistula in most patients with the first episode and all patients with recurrent episodes. Such fistulae must be surgically excised for definitive cure and prevention of recurrent infection (67,74,76,78,107,108).

Mortality from acute bacterial thyroiditis has markedly improved from the 20% to 25% reported in the early 1900s, with the extensive review by Berger et al estimating an overall mortality of 8.6% (60). However, more recent reviews, including over than 100 patients, failed to list mortality as a complication of acute bacterial thyroiditis, possibly due to a higher index of suspicion and earlier therapy (63,64,67,68). Mortality still may occur if the diagnosis is delayed and antimicrobial therapy is not initiated (60). In survivors, complete recovery is the rule, although there have been reports of transient hypothyroidism, vocal cord paralysis (which may also be transient) (67,109), and recurrence of infection as sequelae of acute bacterial thyroiditis (60,63,67,68,110).

Fungal Infections

Fungal infection of the thyroid, while rare, is the second most common cause of infectious thyroiditis (Table 28.4). Over 30 cases of fungal thyroiditis have been reported in the world's literature, with at least 26 cases caused by *Aspergillus* species (60,111,112). Virtually all of the affected patients were immunocompromised, with the most common underlying conditions being glucocorticoid therapy, leukemia, and lymphoma. Disseminated aspergillosis was present, and most of the diagnoses were made postmortem. The pathology was consistent with hematogenous spread, with focal abscesses, hemorrhagic lesions surrounding blood vessels, or diffuse necrotizing thyroiditis. In one patient with disseminated aspergillosis, suppurative thyroiditis was suspected on an In-111 white-blood-cell scan and confirmed by biopsy (95). Case reports of fungal infections of the thyroid have included *Coccidioides immitis* (113) and *Histoplasma capsulatum* (114,115) in endemic regions and *Candida albicans* (116), *Allescheria boydii* (117), and *Nocardia asteroides* (118) as sporadic infections.

Mycobacterial Infections

The true incidence of infection of the thyroid with *Mycobacterium tuberculosis* is difficult to determine, as the pathology of lymphocytic infiltration and granuloma formation is nonspecific in the absence of demonstrable acid-fast bacilli. Using strict pathological criteria, only 19 cases have been reported in the literature (60). Thyroidal tuberculosis is associated with disseminated or miliary disease, and symptoms are usually present for months (119–121). Pain, tenderness, and fever are much less common than in cases of bacterial thyroiditis. While at least three of the reported patients with tuberculous thyroiditis died (60), resolution without sequelae usually follows appropriate antituberculous therapy. However, recurrent laryngeal nerve paralysis has been described (122).

Infections with atypical mycobacteria, including *M. chelonei* and *M. intracellulare*, have also been described (60). Thyroidal infection with *M. avian-intracellulare* has been reported in patients with AIDS in the setting of widely disseminated disease (123). While acid-fast organisms have been found in the thyroid of individuals with disseminated *M. leprae* (124), symptomatic thyroid infection has not been described.

Parasitic Infections

Parasitic thyroidal infection is extremely rare. Only nine reports of echinococcal (tapeworm) thyroiditis have been reported in the United States, located in sheep- and cattle-farming regions (60). Symptoms, primarily in the form of a goiter, are usually present for years, and the diagnosis is often made at the time of surgery. If echinococcal infection is suspected, biopsy of the lesion is contraindicated due to risk of spillage and rupture of the cyst contents. Surgical removal is the preferred mode of treatment, with antiparasitic agents useful as adjunctive therapy and for inoperable cases.

Strongyloides stercoralis, or roundworm, is widely disseminated in tropical climates, including the southeastern United States. Involvement of the thyroid has been described only in the setting of disseminated disease in immunocompromised patients (125). Therapy is aimed at the disseminated infection, with thiabendazole an effective drug. Mortality with disseminated *Strongyloides* infection is high due to both the infection and the immunocompromised status of the patient. A single patient with cysticercosis of the thyroid, acquired from ingestion of the eggs of the pork tapeworm *Taenia solium*, has been described (126).

Syphilitic Infections

Only seven cases of syphilitic infection of the thyroid have been reported in the world's literature (60). These infections most often presented as painless nodules. Other symptoms included local compression and occasionally hypothyroidism and ulceration of the skin.

Thyroidal Infections in Immunocompromised Patients

With the increasing incidence of infection by HIV leading to AIDS, as well as the increased use of immunosuppressive agents, several novel opportunistic pathogens have involved the thyroid. The most common infectious organism found in the thyroid at postmortem examination in patients with AIDS is cytomegalovirus (CMV), occurring in the setting of disseminated CMV infection (127,128). However, symptomatic thyroidal infection with CMV has not been reported. As mentioned above, thyroidal involvement with *M. avian-intracellulare* has been reported in the setting of widely disseminated disease (123).

The thyroid is a site of extrapulmonary infection with *Pneumocystis carinii*, a fungal organism based on RNA sequencing (129). In fact, asymptomatic infection of the thyroid was found in up to 20% of patients with disseminated *Pneumocystis* infection at autopsy (127). Extrapulmonary *Pneumocystis* infection occurs most often in patients receiving prophylaxis with aerosolized pentamidine. Symptomatic thyroidal infection, presenting as a painless nodule, was first reported in 1988 (130), followed by numerous other case reports. The diagnosis of *Pneumocystis carinii* infection is made by performing Gomori's silver methenamine stain on specimens obtained by biopsy. Since this is not a routine staining procedure, it must be requested when performing a biopsy on immunocompromised patients. Treatment with parenteral trimethoprim-sulfamethoxazole followed by prolonged oral administration (up to 2 months) is curative and may result in the restoration of normal thyroid function in regions that were previously "cold" by radioiodine scanning (98).

REFERENCES

1. Brook I. The swollen neck. Cervical lymphadenitis, parotitis, thyroiditis, and infected cysts [Review]. *Infect Dis Clin North Am* 1988;2:221–236.
2. van der Sluis RF, Wobbes T, Schoots FJ. Thyroid cancer mimicking thyroiditis. *J Surg Oncol* 1986;33:66–68.
3. Leung AK, Hegde K. Hashimoto's thyroiditis simulating De Quervain's thyroiditis. *J Adolesc Health Care* 1988;9:434–435.
4. Roti E, Minelli R, Gardini E, et al. Thyrotoxicosis followed by hypothyroidism in patients treated with amiodarone. *Arch Intern Med* 1993;153:886–892.
5. Bartalena L, Brogioni S, Grasso L, et al. Increased serum interleukin-6 concentration in patients with subacute thyroiditis: relationship with concomitant changes in serum T4-binding globulin concentration. *J Endocrinol Invest* 1993;16:213–218.
6. Volpe R. The management of subacute (de Quervain's) thyroiditis [Review]. *Thyroid* 1993;3:253–255.

7. Farwell AP, Braverman LE. Inflammatory thyroid disorders. *Otolaryngol Clin North Am* 1996;29:541–556.

8. Pearce EN, Farwell AP, Braverman LE. Thyroiditis. *N Engl J Med* 2003;348:2646–2655.

9. Fatourechi V, Aniszewski JP, Fatourechi GZ, et al. Clinical features and outcome of subacute thyroiditis in an incidence cohort: Olmsted County, Minnesota, study. *J Clin Endocrinol Metab* 2003;88:2100–2105.

10. Lazarus JH. Silent thyroiditis and subacute thyroiditis. In: Braverman LE, Utiger RD, eds. *The thyroid*. Philadelphia: Lippincott-Raven Publishers, 1996:577–591.

11. Ogawa E, Katsushima Y, Fujiwara I, et al. Subacute thyroiditis in children: patient report and review of the literature. *J Pediatr Endocrinol Metab* 2003;16:897–900.

12. Eylan E, Zmucky R, Sheba C. Mumps virus and subacute thyroiditis: evidence of a causal association. *Lancet* 1957;1:1062–1063.

13. Stancek D, Stanceková-Gressnerová M, Janotka M, et al. Isolation and some serological and epidemiological data on the viruses recovered from patients with subacute thyroiditis de Quervain. *Med Microbiol Immunol (Berl)* 1975;161:133–144.

14. Volpe R, Row VV, Ezrin C. Circulating viral and thyroid antibodies in subacute thyroiditis. *J Clin Endocrinol Metab* 1967;27:1275–1284.

15. Brook I. Microbiology and management of acute suppurative thyroiditis in children. *Int J Pediatr Otorhinolaryngol* 2003;67:447–451.

16. Sato M. Virus-like particles in the follicular epithelium of the thyroid from a patient with subacute thyroiditis (de Quervain). *Acta Pathol Jpn* 1975;25:499–501.

17. Toft J, Larsen S, Toft H. Subacute thyroiditis after hepatitis B vaccination [letter]. *Endocr J* 1998;45:135.

18. Falaschi P, Martocchia A, DqUrso R, et al. Subacute thyroiditis during interferon-alpha therapy for chronic hepatitis C. *J Endocrinol Invest* 1997;20:24–28.

19. Omur O, Daglyoz G, Akarca U, et al. Subacute thyroiditis during interferon therapy for chronic hepatitis B infection. *Clin Nucl Med* 2003;28:864–865.

20. Parana R, Cruz M, Lyra L, et al. Subacute thyroiditis during treatment with combination therapy (interferon plus ribavirin) for hepatitis C virus. *J Viral Hepat* 2000;7:393–395.

21. Luotola K, Hyoty H, Salmi J, et al. Evaluation of infectious etiology in subacute thyroiditis—lack of association with coxsackievirus infection. *APMIS* 1998;106:500–504.

22. Brouqui P, Raoult D, Conte-Devolx B. Coxsackie thyroiditis [Letter]. *Ann Intern Med* 1991;114:1063–1064.

23. Daniels GH. Atypical subacute thyroiditis: preliminary observations. *Thyroid* 2001;11:691–695.

24. Sanders LR, Moreno AJ, Pittman DL, et al. Painless giant cell thyroiditis diagnosed by fine needle aspiration and associated with intense thyroidal uptake of gallium. *Am J Med* 1986;80:971–975.

25. Piazza I, Girardi A. Painless giant cell thyroiditis. *Postgrad Med J* 1989;65:580–581.

26. Wall JR, Strackosch CR, Bandy P, et al. Nature of thyrotropin displacement activity in subacute thyroiditis. *J Clin Endocrinol Metab* 1982;54:587–593.

27. Wall JR, Fang SL, Ingbar SH, et al. Lymphocytic transformation in response to human thyroid extract in patients with subacute thyroiditis. *J Clin Endocrinol Metab* 1976;43:587–590.

28. Iitaka M, Momotani N, Hisaoka T, et al. TSH receptor antibody-associated thyroid dysfunction following subacute thyroiditis. *Clin Endocrinol (Oxf)* 1998;48:445–453.

29. Tamai H, Nozaki T, Mukuta T, et al. The incidence of thyroid stimulating blocking antibodies during the hypothyroid phase in patients with subacute thyroiditis. *J Clin Endocrinol Metab* 1991;73:245–250.

30. Bartalena L, Bogazzi F, Pecori F, et al. Graves' disease occurring after subacute thyroiditis: report of a case and review of the literature. *Thyroid* 1996;6:345–348.

31. Nyulassy S, Hnilica P, Buc M, et al. Subacute (de Quervain) thyroiditis: association with HLA-B35 antigen and abnormalities of the complement system immunoglobulins and other serum proteins. *J Clin Endocrinol Metab* 1977;45:270–274.

32. Rubin RA, Guay AT. Susceptibility to subacute thyroiditis is genetically influenced: familial occurrence in identical twins. *Thyroid* 1991;1:157–161

33. de Bruin TW, Riekhoff FP, de Boer JJ. An outbreak of thyrotoxicosis due to atypical subacute thyroiditis. *J Clin Endocrinol Metab* 1990;70:396–402.

34. Goto H, Uno H, Tamai H, et al. Genetic analysis of subacute (de Quervain's) thyroiditis. *Tissue Antigens* 1985;26:110–113.

35. Mizukami Y, Michigishi T, Kawato M, et al. Immunohistochemical and ultrastructural study of subacute thyroiditis, with special reference to multinucleated giant cells. *Hum Pathol* 1987;18:929–935.

36. Ofner C, Hittmair A, Kroll I, et al. Fine needle aspiration cytodiagnosis of subacute (de Quervain's) thyroiditis in an endemic goitre area. *Cytopathology* 1994;5:33–40.

37. Garcia Solano J, Gimenez Bascunana A, Sola Perez J, et al. Fine-needle aspiration of subacute granulomatous thyroiditis (de Quervain's thyroiditis): a clinico-cytologic review of 36 cases. *Diagn Cytopathol* 1997;16:214–220.

38. Kojima M, Nakamura S, Oyama T, et al. Cellular composition of subacute thyroiditis. an immunohistochemical study of six cases. *Pathol Res Pract* 2002;198:833–837.

39. Schmid KW, Ofner C, Ramsauer T, et al. CA 19–9 expression in subacute (de Quervain's) thyroiditis: an immunohistochemical study. *Mod Pathol* 1992;5:268–272.

40. Rosenstein ED, Kramer N. Occult subacute thyroiditis mimicking classic giant cell arteritis. *Arthritis Rheum* 1994;37:1618–1620.

41. Pearce EN, Bogazzi F, Martino E, et al. The prevalence of elevated serum C-reactive protein levels in inflammatory and noninflammatory thyroid disease. *Thyroid* 2003;13:643–648.

42. Amino N, Yabu Y, Miki T, et al. Serum ratio of triiodothyronine to thyroxine, and thyroxine-binding globulin and calcitonin concentrations in Graves' disease and destruction-induced thyrotoxicosis. *J Clin Endocrinol Metab* 1981;53:113–116.

43. Farwell AP. Sick euthyroid syndrome. *J Intensive Care Med* 1997;12:249–260.

44. Madeddu G, Casu AR, Costanza C, et al. Serum thyroglobulin levels in the diagnosis and follow-up of subacute 'painful' thyroiditis: a sequential study. *Arch Intern Med* 1985;145:243–247.

45. Smallridge RC, De Keyser FM, Van Herle AJ, et al. Thyroid iodine content and serum thyroglobulin: cues to the natural history of destruction-induced thyroiditis. *J Clin Endocrinol Metab* 1986;62:1213–1219.

46. Ross DS. Syndromes of thyrotoxicosis with low radioactive iodine uptake. *Endocrinol Metab Clin North Am* 1998;27:169–185.

47. Hiromatsu Y, Ishibashi M, Nishida H, et al. Technetium-99 m sestamibi imaging in patients with subacute thyroiditis. *Endocr J* 2003;50:239–244.

48. Bennedbaek FN, Hegedus L. The value of ultrasonography in the diagnosis and follow-up of subacute thyroiditis. *Thyroid* 1997;7:45–50.

49. Hiromatsu Y, Ishibashi M, Miyake I, et al. Color Doppler ultrasonography in patients with subacute thyroiditis. *Thyroid* 1999;9:1189–1193.

50. Miyake H, Tanaka R, Takeoka H, et al. Unsuspected painless subacute thyroiditis detected by radiogallium scintigraphy. *Jap J Nucl Med* 1992;29:1475–1478.

51. Nikolai TF, Coombs GJ, McKenzie AK. Lymphocytic thyroiditis with spontaneously resolving hyperthyroidism and and subacute thyroiditis. *Arch Intern Med* 1981;141:145.

52. Mizukoshi T, Noguchi S, Murakami T, et al. Evaluation of recurrence in 36 subacute thyroiditis patients managed with prednisolone. *Intern Med* 2001;40:292–295.

53. Arem R, Munipalli B. Ipodate therapy in patients with severe destruction-induced thyrotoxicosis. *Arch Intern Med* 1996;156:1752–1757.

54. Martinez DS, Chopra IJ. Use of oral cholecystography agents in the treatment of hyperthyroidism of subacute thyroiditis. *Panminerva Med* 2003;45:53–57.

55. Lio S, Pontecorvi A, Caruso M, et al. Transitory subclinical and permanent hypothyroidism in the course of subacute thyroiditis (de Quervain). *Acta Endocrinol* 1984;106:67–70.

56. Cordray JP, Nys P, Merceron RE, et al. Frequency of hypothyroidism after de Quervain thyroiditis and contribution of ultrasonographic thyroid volume measurement [in French]. *Ann Med Interne (Paris)* 2001;152:84–88.

57. Iitaka M, Momotani N, Ishii J, et al. Incidence of subacute thyroiditis recurrences after a prolonged latency: 24-year survey. *J Clin Endocrinol Metab* 1996;81:466–469.

58. Roti E, Minelli R, Gardini E, et al. Iodine-induced hypothyroidism in euthyroid subjects with a previous episode of subacute thyroiditis. *J Clin Endocrinol Metab* 1990;70:1581–1585.

59. Bennedbaek FN, Gram J, Hegedus L. The transition of subacute thyroiditis to Graves' disease as evidenced by diagnostic imaging. *Thyroid* 1996;6:457–459.

60. Berger SA, Zonszein J, Villamena P, et al. Infectious diseases of the thyroid gland [Review]. *Rev Infect Dis* 1983;5:108–122.

61. Shah SS, Baum SG. Diagnosis and management of infectious thyroiditis. *Curr Infect Dis Rep* 2000;2:147–153.

62. Farwell AP. Infectious thyroiditis. In: Braverman LE, Utiger RD, eds. *The thyroid*. Philadelphia: Lippincott Williams & Wilkins, 2000:1044–1050.

63. Rich EJ, Mendelman PM. Acute suppurative thyroiditis in pediatric patients [Review]. *Pediatr Infect Dis J* 1987;6:936–940.

64. Chi H, Lee YJ, Chiu NC, et al. Acute suppurative thyroiditis in children. *Pediatr Infect Dis J* 2002;21:384–387.

65. Womack NA. Thyroiditis. *Surgery* 1944;16:770–782.

66. Altemeier WA. Acute pyogenic thyroiditis. *Arch Surg* 1950;61:76–85.

67. Miyauchi A, Matsuzuka F, Kuma K, et al. Piriform sinus fistula: an underlying abnormality common in patients with acute suppurative thyroiditis. *World J Surg* 1990;14:400–405.

68. Jeng LB, Lin JD, Chen MF. Acute suppurative thyroiditis: a ten-year review in a Taiwanese hospital. *Scand J Infect Dis* 1994;26:297–300.

69. Foster RS. Morbidity and mortality after thyroidectomy. *Surg Gyn Ob* 1978;146:423–429.

70. Takai S-I, Miyauchi A, Matsuzuka F, et al. Internal fistula as a route of infection in acute suppurative thyroiditis. *Lancet* 1979;1:751–752.

71. Katz R, Bar-Ziv J, Preminger-Shapiro R, et al. Pyogenic thyroiditis due to branchial pouch sinus. *Isr J Med Sci* 1989;25:641–644.

72. Tovi F, Gatot A, Bar-Ziv J, et al. Recurrent suppurative thyroiditis due to fourth branchial pouch sinus. *Int J Ped Otorhinolaryngol* 1985;9:89–96.

73. Ueda J, Kobayashi Y, Hara K, et al. Routes of infection of acute suppurative thyroiditis diagnosed by barium examination. *Acta Radiol* 1986;27:209–211.

74. Har-el G, Sasaki CT, Prager D, et al. Acute suppurative thyroiditis and the branchial apparatus. *Am J Otolaryngol* 1991;12:6–11.

75. Yamashita J, Ogawa M, Yamashita S, et al. Acute suppurative thyroiditis in an asymptomatic woman: an atypical presentation simulating thyroid carcinoma. *Clin Endocrinol (Oxf)* 1994;40:145–149.

76. Ozaki O, Sugimoto T, Suzuki A, et al. Cervical thymic cyst as a cause of acute suppurative thyroiditis. *Jap J Surg* 1990;20:593–596.

77. Szabo SM, Allen DB. Thyroiditis. Differentiation of acute suppurative and subacute thyroiditis: case report and review of the literature [review]. *Clin Pediatr (Phila)* 1989;28:171–174.

78. DeLozier HL, Sofferman RA. Pyriform sinus fistula: an unusual cause of recurrent retropharyngeal abscess and cellulitis. *Ann Otol Rhinol Laryngol* 1986;95:377–382.

79. Lucaya J, Berdon WE, Enriquez G, et al. Congenital pyriform sinus fistula: a cause of acute left-sided suppurative thyroiditis and neck abscess in children [see comments]. *Pediatr Radiol* 1990;21:27–29.

80. Kawanaka M, Sugimoto Y, Suehiro M, et al. Thyroid imaging in a typical case of acute suppurative thyroiditis with abscess formation due to infection from a persistent thyroglossal duct. *Ann Nucl Med* 1994;8:159–162.

81. Agarwal A, Mishra SK, Sharma AK. Acute suppurative thyroiditis with demonstrable distant primary focus: a report of two cases. *Thyroid* 1998;8:399–401.

82. Li CC, Wang CH, Tsan KW. Graves' disease and diabetes mellitus associated with acute suppurative thyroiditis: a case report. *Chung Hua I Hsueh Tsa Chih (Taipei)* 1997;59:59–64.

83. Poelman M, Benoit Y, Laureys G, et al. Acute suppurative thyroiditis complicating second allogeneic transplant for juvenile CMML. *Bone Marrow Transplant* 1992;10:547–548.

84. Imai C, Kakihara T, Watanabe A, et al. Acute suppurative thyroiditis as a rare complication of aggressive chemotherapy in children with acute myelogeneous leukemia. *Pediatr Hematol Oncol* 2002;19:247–253.

85. Stevenson J. Acute bacterial thyroiditis presenting as otalgia. *J Laryngol Otol* 1991;105:788–789.

86. Walsh CH, Dunne C. Hyperthyroidism associated with acute suppurative thyroiditis. *Ir J Med Sci* 1992;161:137.

87. Fukata S, Miyauchi A, Kuma K, et al. Acute suppurative thyroiditis caused by an infected piriform sinus fistula with thyrotoxicosis. *Thyroid* 2002;12:175–178.

88. DiRusso G, Kern KA. Comparative analysis of complications from I-131 radioablation for well-differentiated thyroid cancer. *Surgery* 1994;116:1024–1030.

89. Ahuja AT, Griffiths JF, Roebuck DJ, et al. The role of ultrasound and oesophagography in the management of acute suppurative thyroiditis in children associated with congenital pyriform fossa sinus. *Clin Radiol* 1998;53:209–211.

90. Bar-Ziv J, Slasky BS, Sichel JY, et al. Branchial pouch sinus tract from the piriform fossa causing acute suppurative thyroiditis, neck abscess, or both: CT appearance and the use of air as a contrast agent. *American Journal of Roentgenology* 1996;167:1569–1572.

91. Bernard PJ, Som PM, Urken ML, et al. The CT findings of acute thyroiditis and acute suppurative thyroiditis. *Otolaryngol Head Neck Surg* 1988;99:489–493.

92. Hatabu H, Kasagi K, Yamamoto K, et al. Acute suppurative thyroiditis associated with piriform sinus fistula: sonographic findings. *American Journal of Roentgenology* 1990;155:845–847.

93. Hatakenaka M, Murakami J, Murayama S, et al. Acute suppurative perithyroiditis: MR findings. *Pediatr Radiol* 1997;27:353–355.

94. Kinoshita T, Ishii K, Naganuma H, et al. Acute suppurative thyroiditis arising from a piriform sinus fistula: CT diagnosis. *Radiat Med* 1998;16:217–219.

95. Pounds TR, Hattner RS. Surprise struma. Suppurative thyroiditis found by In-111 WBC imaging. *Clin Nucl Med* 1993; 18:1089.

96. Lin JD, Huang BY, Huang HS, et al. Ultrasonography and fine needle aspiration cytology of acute suppurative thyroiditis. *Chang Gung Med J* 1993;16:93–98.

97. Singh SK, Agrawal JK, Kumar M, et al. Fine needle aspiration cytology in the management of acute suppurative thyroiditis. *ENT J* 1994;73:415–417.

98. Battan R, Mariuz P, Raviglione MC, et al. *Pneumocystis carinii* infection of the thyroid in a hypothyroid patient with AIDS: diagnosis by fine needle aspiration biopsy. *J Clin Endocrinol Metab* 1991;72:724–726.

99. Guttler R, Singer PA, Axline SG, et al. *Pneumocystis carinii* thyroiditis: report of three cases and review of the literature [published erratum appears in *Arch Intern Med* 1993 Apr 26; 153(8):1002] [Review]. *Arch Intern Med* 1993;153:393–396.

100. Chiovato L, Canale G, Maccherini D, et al. Salmonella brandenburg: a novel cause of acute suppurative thyroiditis. *Acta Endocrinol* 1993;128:439–442.

101. Dai MS, Chang H, Peng MY, et al. Suppurative salmonella thyroiditis in a patient with chronic lymphocytic leukemia. *Ann Hematol* 2003;82:646–648.

102. Suskovic T, Vucicevic Z. Acute suppurative thyroiditis caused by Salmonella enteritidis. *Infection* 1995;23:180–181.

103. Mousa AR, al-Mudallal DS, Marafie A. Brucella thyroiditis [Letter]. *J Infect* 1989;19:287–288

104. von Graevenitz A, Colla F. Thyroiditis due to *Brucella melitensis*—report of two cases. *Infection* 1990;18:179–180.

105. Queen JS, Clegg HW, Council JC, et al. Acute suppurative thyroiditis caused by *Eikenella corrodens*. *J Pediatr Surg* 1988; 23:359–361.

106. Reichling JJ, Rose DN, Mendelson MH, et al. Acute suppurative thyroiditis caused by *Serratia marcescens*. *J Infect Dis* 1984; 149:281.

107. Rossiter JL, Topf P. Acute suppurative thyroiditis with bilateral piriform sinus fistulae. *Otolaryngol Head Neck Surg* 1991;105: 625–628.

108. Nonomura N, Ikarashi F, Fujisaki T, et al. Surgical approach to pyriform sinus fistula. *Am J Otolaryngol* 1993;14:111–115.

109. Boyd CM, Esclamado RM, Telian SA. Impaired vocal cord mobility in the setting of acute suppurative thyroiditis. *Head Neck* 1997;19:235–237.

110. Collazo-Clavell ML, Gharib H, Maragos NE. Relationship between vocal cord paralysis and benign thyroid disease. *Head Neck* 1995;17:24–30.

111. Winzelberg GG, Gore J, Yu D, et al. *Aspergillus flavis* as a cause of thyroiditis in an immunosuppressed host. *Johns Hopkins Med J* 1979;144:90–93.

112. Halazun JF, Anast CS, Lukens JN. Thyrotoxicosis associated with *Aspergillus* thyroiditis in chronic granulomatous disease. *J Pediatr* 1972;80:106–108.

113. Loeb JM, Levermore BM, Wofsy D. Coccidioidomycosis of the thyroid. *Ann Intern Med* 1979;91:409–411.

114. Goodwin RA, Shapiro JL, Thurman GH, et al. Disseminated histoplasmosis: clinical and pathological correlations. *Medicine (Baltimore)* 1980;59:1–33.

115. Goldani LZ, Klock C, Diehl A, et al. Histoplasmosis of the thyroid. *J Clin Microbiol* 2000;38:3890–3891.

116. Fernandez JF, Anaissie EJ, Vassilopoulou-Sellin R, et al. Acute fungal thyroiditis in a patient with acute myelogenous leukaemia. *J Int Med* 1991;230:539–541.

117. Rosen F, Deck JHN, Rewcastle NB. *Allescheria boydii*—unique systemic dissemination to thyroid and brain. *Can Med Assoc J* 1965;93:1125–1127.

118. Lewin SR, Street AC, Snider J. Suppurative thyroiditis due to *Nocardia asteroides* [Letter; Comment]. *J Infect* 1993;26:339–340.

119. Das DK, Pant CS, Chachra KL, et al. Fine needle aspiration cytology diagnosis of tuberculous thyroiditis: a report of eight cases. *Acta Cytol* 1992;36:517–522.

120. Hizawa K, Okamura K, Sato K, et al. Tuberculous thyroiditis and miliary tuberculosis manifested postpartum in a patient with thyroid carcinoma. *Endocrinol Jap* 1990;37:571–576.

121. Nieuwland Y, Tan KY, Elte JW. Miliary tuberculosis presenting with thyrotoxicosis. *Postgrad Med J* 1992;68:677–679.

122. Emery P. Tuberculous abscess of the thyroid with recurrent laryngeal nerve palsy: a case report and review of the literature. *J Laryngol Otol* 1980;94:553–558.

123. Horsburgh CR. *Mycobacterium avium* complex infection in the acquired immunodeficiency syndrome. *N Engl J Med* 1991; 324:1332–1338.

124. Hastings RC, Gillis TP, Krahenbuhl JL, et al. Leprosy. *Clin Microbiol Rev* 1988;1:330.

125. Scowden EB, Schaffner W, Stone WJ. Overwelming strongyloidias: an unappreciated opportunistic infection. *Medicine (Baltimore)* 1978;57:527–544.

126. Leelachaikul P, Chuahirun S. Cysticercosis of the thyroid gland in severe cerebral cysticercosis: report of a case. *J Med Assoc Thai* 1977;60:405.

127. Reichert CM, O'Leary TJ, Levens DL, et al. Autopsy pathology in the acquired immunodeficiency syndrome. *Am J Pathol* 1983;112:357–382.

128. Frank TS, LiVolsi VA, Connor AM. Cytomegalovirus infection of the thyroid in immunocompromised adults. *Yale J Biol Med* 1987;60:1–8.

129. Edman JC, Kovacs JA, Masur H, et al. Ribosomal RNA sequence shows *Pneumocystis carinii* to be a member of the fungi. *Nature* 1988;334:519–522.

130. Gallant JE, Enriquez RE, Cohen KL, et al. *Pneumocystis carinii* thyroiditis. *Am J Med* 1988;84:303–306.

29

THYROTOXICOSIS OF
EXTRATHYROID ORIGIN

ELIZABETH N. PEARCE

Extrathyroidal causes of thyrotoxicosis can be difficult to diagnose. The most common extrathyroidal cause of thyrotoxicosis is thyrotoxicosis factitia. The other causes, functional metastatic thyroid carcinoma and struma ovarii, are extremely rare.

THYROTOXICOSIS FACTITIA

Causes

Thyrotoxicosis due to the ingestion of exogenous thyroid hormone is most frequently iatrogenic—either intentionally [as when thyroid-stimulating hormone (TSH)–suppressive doses of sodium thyroxine (T_4) are prescribed in order to suppress tumor growth in thyroid cancer patients, or in an attempt to decrease goiter size] or unintentionally (as when overly vigorous T_4 therapy is prescribed for hypothyroidism).

Thyrotoxicosis factitia may also result from patients' surreptitious use of thyroid hormones. This usually occurs in the setting of psychiatric illness. Surreptitious thyroid hormone ingestion is more common in those working in medicine-related fields (who have more readily available access to thyroid hormone-containing medications) (1), and may occur at any age (2). Large doses of thyroid hormone may be ingested as a suicide attempt. In addition, some patients may ingest excessive doses of thyroid hormones, sometimes at the advice of their physicians, in an effort to lose weight, or to treat depression, menstrual disorders, or infertility (3).

Patients may also develop thyrotoxicosis from the unintentional ingestion of thyroid hormone. Accidental overdose of thyroid hormone most frequently occurs in children. Several community outbreaks of thyrotoxicosis from exogenous thyroid hormone ingestion have been reported. For example, 121 cases of thyrotoxicosis with low radioactive iodine uptake were documented in southwestern Minnesota and adjacent areas between 1984 and 1985. Subsequent investigations revealed the presence of bovine thyroid material in ground beef processed at a single local slaughtering plant (4). Beef-slaughtering techniques were also likely responsible for a similar community outbreak in Nebraska in 1984 (5). This type of community-wide thyrotoxicosis has been referred to as "hamburger thyroiditis" (3). Inadvertent exposure to thyroid hormone resulting in thyrotoxicosis has also been reported from occupational exposure to cosmetic creams containing iodine and thyroid hormones (6) and from accidental dosing with veterinary T_4 preparations (7).

Clinical Presentation and Diagnosis

Diagnosis of thyrotoxicosis resulting from exogenous thyroid hormone ingestion can be difficult and requires a high degree of clinical suspicion, as symptoms, initial laboratory values, and imaging studies are often indistinguishable from those of painless sporadic thyroiditis or other types of thyroiditis associated with low radioactive iodine uptakes. Serum TSH values will be low. Serum triiodothyronine (T_3) and T_4 levels are variably elevated, depending on the thyroid hormone preparation that has been ingested. T_3 poisoning may result in more severe and acute symptoms of thyrotoxicosis than poisoning with other forms of thyroid hormone (8). Because of the TSH suppression, the thyroid gland is small in patients without underlying thyroid disease. Exopthalmos is not present. Radioactive iodine uptake is low to undetectable. A serum thyroglobulin (Tg) measurement is frequently helpful, as serum Tg values are low to undetectable in thyrotoxicosis factitia, but are elevated in all other causes of thyrotoxicosis, such as Graves' disease, toxic nodular goiter, painless sporadic thyroiditis, and subacute thyroiditis (9). If antibodies to Tg are present in the serum, however, serum Tg measurements cannot reliably be used to differentiate thyrotoxicosis factitia from other causes of thyrotoxicosis. Fecal T_4 measurements may be used instead in such patients. Fecal T_4 measurements are approximately 1 nmol/g in normal healthy subjects, are mildly increased in Graves' disease (about 2 nmol/g), and are markedly elevated in individuals with thyrotoxicosis factitia (over 12 nmol/g) (10). Finally, color-flow Doppler sonography has been used to distinguish Graves' disease or toxic nodular goiter, in which the thyroid is hypervascular, two of their seven patients with thyrotoxicosis had decreased vital capacity (VC). Using only clinical signs and symptoms as markers of congestive heart failure (CHF), however, Lemon and Moersch (39) found that a decreased VC correlated only with "cardiac decompensation" and not with either the basal metabolic rate (BMR) or the severity of the thyrotoxic symptoms. Other early studies found an inverse correlation between the VC and the BMR (40). Despite several studies of the lung volumes in the subsequent 80 years, little more is known.

Because pulmonary function testing included analysis of the subdivisions of lung volume, one older study noted that one quarter of patients had decreased residual volume (RV), VC, and total lung capacity (TLC), with normal arterial blood gas (ABG) results and diffusing capacity for carbon monoxide (41). In 12 patients and 12 normal subjects, no differences were found in the mean baseline VC, TLC, RV, static compliance, or pressure-volume curves; but after treatment, the VC and TLC increased significantly in eight patients. Airway resistance and flow rates were normal in all studies (42). Studies of the subdivisions of lung volumes present a confusing picture (42–47), with frequent decreases of VC that increases in response to treatment, but inconsistent changes in the other lung volumes. These heterogeneous findings may reflect the presence of other underlying lung diseases in some patients; a more likely alternative is that thyrotoxicosis causes several types of changes in the lungs, all of which do not occur in the same patient. For example, respiratory muscle weakness resulting from chronic thyrotoxic myopathy probably occurs only in some patients.

ABG partial pressures and the oxygen and carbon dioxide–hemoglobin dissociation curves usually are normal (43). Mixed venous oxygen saturation typically increases because the elevation in cardiac output is greater than the increased oxygen consumption. Although the total amount of oxygen extracted by the peripheral tissues is increased, the efficiency of oxygen extraction is decreased. Diffusing capacity of the lung for carbon dioxide (DLCO) at rest may be normal (42,43,47) or low (48), but usually it is lower than expected for the high cardiac output. With exercise, the DLCO usually increases, but to a lesser extent than normal—or it may even decline. The reason for this decreased efficiency of gas exchange with exercise is not clear, but there may be disturbances in the alveolar capillary wall or in the recruitment of reserve capillaries.

LUNG COMPLIANCE AND RESPIRATORY MUSCLE WEAKNESS

Airway resistance, lung compliance, and respiratory muscle function determine the volumes of gas moved into or out of the lung. Airway resistance is normal in thyrotoxic patients. Some patients presumably have chronic thyrotoxic myopa-

thy that involves the diaphragm, but simultaneous changes in intrinsic lung compliance also may occur. Lung compliance could be altered by changes in the elastic properties (connective tissue) or by vascular engorgement. Compliance usually is determined from the static pressure–volume curve of the lung, with measurement of intrathoracic pressure using an esophageal balloon manometer. The maximal inspiratory pressure (Pi_{max}) at RV, maximal expiratory pressure (Pe_{max}) at TLC, maximal transdiaphragmatic pressure, and maximal voluntary minute ventilation (MVV) yield information about maximal respiratory muscle power. Even with these techniques, it is difficult to separate patients with pure respiratory muscle weakness from patients who have only decreased lung compliance. For example, almost all of 13 thyrotoxic patients had decreased lung compliance and decreased Pi_{max} and Pe_{max}, and in all of them, these parameters improved significantly after therapy (41). These findings have been confirmed in some studies (46), but not in others (47). Most patients whose lung compliance improved with treatment also had increases in VC, but TLC did not increase as expected if muscle function had improved.

Most thyrotoxic patients who complain of exertional dyspnea have diminished proximal muscle strength (48). In half the patients with proximal muscle weakness, Pi_{max} improved significantly after 6 weeks of therapy. The mean values of Pi_{max} and Pe_{max} were decreased in many thyrotoxic patients (42,43,45,47,49,50). Static lung compliance and elastic recoil were normal and did not improve with treatment. In the only study that directly measured transdiaphragmatic pressures of thyrotoxic patients with proximal muscle weakness and decreased Pi_{max} and Pe_{max}, transdiaphragmatic pressure was decreased in only one of the four patients, but all four patients had significantly increased transdiaphragmatic pressure after treatment that correlated with improvements in Pi_{max}, Pe_{max}, VC, and proximal muscle strength (49). In another study, the Pi_{max} and Pe_{max} were decreased in 5 and 8 of 14 patients, respectively (44). Significant increases in both values after correction of the thyrotoxicosis were typical. Structural and functional changes in the costal and crural parts of the diaphragm occurred in thyrotoxic dogs, evidenced by decreased transdiaphragmatic pressures and twitch shortening accompanied by vacuolization and loss of diaphragm muscle fibers (51).

The biochemical basis of these changes in respiratory muscle function is not understood. The thyrotoxic rat diaphragm has depressed glycolytic, tricarboxylic acid cycle, and fatty acid oxidative activity (50). The change in lung compliance could be due to altered lung extracellular matrix, but vascular engorgement is an unlikely cause because the DLCO is not increased as in other high cardiac output or capillary engorgement conditions, such as asthma or mild CHF.

In summary, chronic thyrotoxic myopathy affects the diaphragm and other respiratory muscles in up to half of

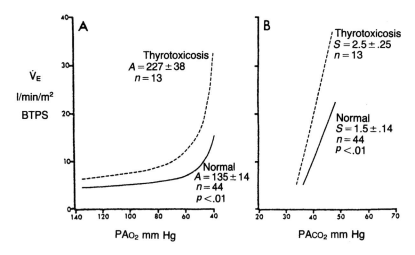

FIGURE 32.1. Mean ventilatory responses (*dotted lines*) to hypoxia (**A**) and hypercapnia (**B**) of 13 thyrotoxic patients are contrasted to the mean responses of 44 normal persons (*solid lines*). Both the hypoxic and the hypercapnic responses are significantly greater in the thyrotoxic group. (From Zwillich CW, Matthay M, Potts DE, et al. Thyrotoxicosis: comparison of the effects of thyroid ablation and beta adrenergic blockage on metabolic rate and ventilatory control. *J Clin Endocrinol Metab* 1978;46:495, with permission.)

thyrotoxic patients, causing loss of maximal respiratory muscle power. Involvement of the diaphragm must be inferred from physiologic tests because of the lack of specific pathologic or electromyographic hallmarks of chronic thyrotoxic myopathy. Easy fatigue also may cause exertional dyspnea. Whether chronic thyrotoxic myopathy of the diaphragm also predisposes to fatigue is unknown, and a shift in the high-low-power spectrum of the diaphragmatic electromyogram should be examined in future studies. Rarely, myasthenia gravis associated with thyrotoxicosis causes respiratory muscle weakness and easy fatigue.

VENTILATORY CONTROL

The increased oxygen consumption and carbon dioxide production of thyrotoxicosis lead to a homeostatic increase in minute ventilation. Thyrotoxicosis may affect the central regulatory response to a blood gas perturbation. Ventilatory response or drive is measured as the increase of minute ventilation, transdiaphragmatic pressure (Pdi), or mouth occlusion pressure (P0.1) while breathing either hyperoxic hypercapnic (HCVR) or hypoxic isocapnic (HVR) gas mixtures (52). The Pdi and P0.1 more directly reflect

neural output and are not as confounded by the presence of other lung disease.

Using a carbon dioxide rebreathing method of assessing HCVR, two studies of a total of 27 patients showed increased responses to carbon dioxide (53,54) (Fig. 32.1), although this was not true in another study (52). The effect of thyrotoxicosis on the HCVR was not mediated by catecholamines, since it was unaffected by propranolol (54) (Fig. 32.2). Hypoxic ventilatory response normally increases with exercise and fever in proportion to the elevation of the metabolism (55). Zwillich and co-workers found a significant increase of the HVR in 13 thyrotoxic patients, correlated with the increase in BMR (54) (Figs. 32.1 and 32.2) and unaffected by propranolol. A study using P0.1 as the output confirmed the increases in HVR and HCVR in 15 hyperthyroid patients (56).

In summary, both the HCVR and the HVR are increased in most thyrotoxic patients, likely contributing to dyspnea. This effect is independent of the β-adrenergic effects of catecholamines. It is not clear whether thyroid hormones affect the peripheral chemoreceptors or the medullary respiratory center. When superimposed on underlying lung disease, thyrotoxicosis can worsen dyspnea and might cause frank respiratory failure.

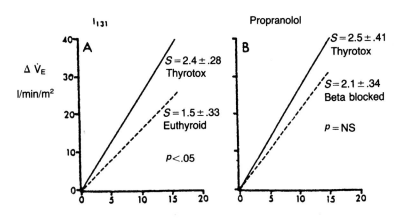

FIGURE 32.2. Effects of treatment with iodine-131 (**A**) and propranolol (**B**) on the mean ventilatory response to hypercapnia of 13 patients with thyrotoxicosis. Pretreatment responses (*solid lines*) and posttreatment responses (*dotted lines*) to hypercapnia. Radioactive iodine, but not propranolol, significantly diminished the hypercapnic ventilatory response. (From Zwillich CW, Matthay M, Potts DE, et al. Thyrotoxicosis: comparision of effects of thyroid ablation and beta adrenergic blockage on metabolic rate and ventilatory control. *J Clin Endocrinol Metab* 1978;46:496, with permission.)

EXERCISE

Thyrotoxicosis typically increases the resting heart rate, cardiac output, respiratory rate, and minute ventilation (57). The normal increases in these variables during exercise are magnified in thyrotoxic patients (41,43,45,47,58). The amount of oxygen consumed to perform any workload is increased. Although the rate of the increase in oxygen consumption with increasing work is normal (59) (Fig. 32.3), both the minute ventilation and the cardiac output for a given level of oxygen consumption are elevated at all levels of oxygen consumption (Fig. 32.4). The efficiency of oxygen extraction and utilization are decreased (60). The minute ventilation and P0.1 may be elevated disproportionately for the carbon dioxide production rate (42), possibly because of a rapid, shallow breathing pattern with more wasted dead space ventilation (61) and consistent with a more than compensatory increase in ventilatory drive. Ventilatory drive, expressed as the ratio of P0.1 to $PaCO_2$, increased proportionally with the T_3 level, and β-blockade decreased the ventilatory drive in the individuals with the highest T_3 levels. In one study, the anaerobic threshold was lower than predicted, but it was not clear whether this was due to poorer oxygen extraction by the peripheral tissues, greater lactate production, or both.

Thyrotoxic patients may be limited predominantly by their cardiac (62,63) or pulmonary systems. None of 15 patients achieved 80% of their predicted maximal oxygen uptake, and only 7 patients exceeded 80% of their predicted maximal heart rates (42). Because both organ systems are affected, cardiac limitation probably predomi-

nates in the absence of other lung disease or severe respiratory muscle weakness (63). With treatment, the maximal work performed usually increased significantly; surprisingly, however, the subjective sense of dyspnea and maximal oxygen uptake achieved during exercise testing did not improve in two studies (42,47), even with increases in maximal respiratory muscle pressures.

Pulmonary artery pressures of thyrotoxic patients may increase more than usual with exercise (58), but how often this occurs is uncertain. Exercise normally decreases the mixed venous oxygen saturation and the dead space:tidal volume ratio (61) the converse occurs in thyrotoxicosis (40). The DLCO of some patients decreases with exercise, especially at higher workloads (48). The elevated cardiac output may shorten capillary transit times and prevent complete gas equilibration. However, oxygen desaturation with exercise has not been reported. The normal respiratory exchange ratio suggests that oxidative phosphorylation is not uncoupled.

EFFECTS OF CARDIAC CHANGES ON THE LUNGS

The lungs may be affected by the cardiac consequences of thyrotoxicosis in two ways (see Chapter 31): high-output cardiac failure or pulmonary artery dilatation, possibly accompanied by pulmonary hypertension. The pulmonary capillary wedge pressure has been normal in most patients studied to date.

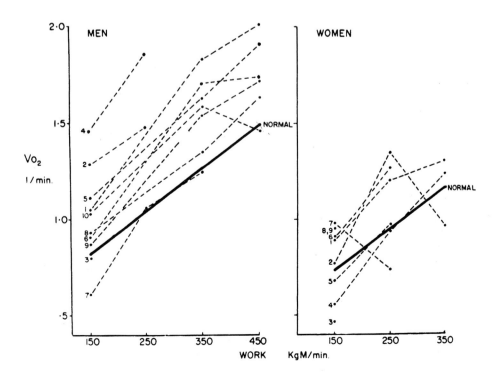

FIGURE 32.3. Oxygen consumption of 19 thyrotoxic patients at increasing workloads of bicycle exercise is shown. Most of the men (left panel) and women (right panel) had increased oxygen consumption at all workloads; the slope of the increase, however, was the same in the thyrotoxic patients as in the normal subjects. (From Massey DG, Becklake MR, McKenzie JM, et al. Circulatory and ventilatory response to exercise in thyrotoxicosis. *N Engl J Med* 1967; 276:1107, with permission.)

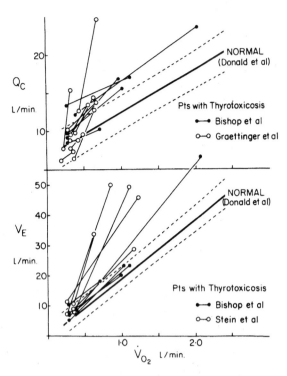

FIGURE 32.4. Cardiac output and minute ventilation responses to increasing oxygen consumption during exercise for patients with thyrotoxicosis. These are contrasted with the normal responses (*heavy lines*). The 95% confidence interval for the normal response is shown by the *broken lines*. (Data for cardiac output response are from Bishop JM, Donald KW, Wade OL. Circulatory dynamics at rest and on exercise in the hyperkinetic states. *Clin Sci* 1956;14:329; data for the minute ventilation response are from Bishop et al. and Stein M, Kimbel P, Johnson RL. Pulmonary function in hyperthyroidism. *J Clin Invest* 1961; 40348.) Both the cardiac output and the minute ventilation are higher than normal at all levels of oxygen consumption. (From data synthesized and plotted by Massey DG, Becklake MR, McKenzie J, Bates DV. Circulatory and ventilatory response to exercise in thyrotoxicosis. *N Engl J Med* 1967;276:1106.)

The pulmonary artery may appear dilated on plain chest radiography. Physical findings of an accentuated pulmonic second heart sound and a right ventricular heave suggest pulmonary hypertension. Elevation of resting pulmonary artery pressure are common with thyrotoxicosis, and the pressure frequently increases significantly during exercise (58). Most patients reported have had mild pulmonary hypertension, but the elevation may be moderate (64). Resting right ventricular stroke work often is elevated because an increased volume of blood is pumped against a somewhat increased pulmonary vascular resistance. The incidence of severe pulmonary hypertension attributable solely to thyrotoxicosis is not clear. Means-Lerman sign, a scratchy, coarse systolic ejection rub or murmur that is heard best along the left sternal border at the base of the heart, has been attributed either to rubbing of the di-

lated aorta or pulmonary artery against some other mediastinal structure or to turbulent pulmonary artery blood flow.

OTHER INTERACTIONS OF THE RESPIRATORY SYSTEM AND THYROID GLAND

Systemic processes may affect both the thyroid gland and the respiratory system. Alternatively, abnormalities of one system may affect the actual or apparent function of the other. Table 32.2 outlines these situations.

PULMONARY DISORDERS THAT INFLUENCE THE THYROID

Pulmonary diseases, such as chronic obstructive pulmonary disease (COPD), tuberculosis, and lung cancer, or critical illness can cause several patterns of change in thyroid function tests (see section on nonthyroidal illness in Chapter 11). In one study of patients in the intensive care unit, the degree of suppression of serum TSH responses to TRH correlated with outcome (65). In rats with sepsis, T_3 levels decreased markedly over 20 to 30 hours (66). Treatment with exogenous T_3 increased their ventilatory drive and lung mechanics, but it did not affect mortality or gas

TABLE 32.2. OTHER INTERACTIONS OF THE RESPIRATORY SYSTEM AND THYROID GLAND

Pulmonary disorders that influence the thyroid
  Hypercalcitonemia due to bronchogenic carcinoma
  Lung cancer metastatic to the thyroid
  Primary pulmonary hypertension
Thyroid disorders that influence the respiratory system
  Thyroid carcinoma with lung metastases
  Compression of trachea or superior vena cava due to
    enlarged thyroid
  Mediastinal goiter
  Chronic cough due to thyroiditis
  ? Increased airway reactivity in asthma
  Increased serum angiotensin-converting enzyme in
    hyperthyroidism
  Propylthiouracil-induced pleuritis or pneumonitis
Systemic conditions that affect both the lung and the thyroid
  Cystic fibrosis
  Cigarette smoking
  Acute respiratory distress after surgery or molar pregnancy
  Associated autoimmune disorders: systemic lupus
    erythematosus, Sjögren's syndrome, myasthenia gravis
  Infections: *Pneumocystis carinii* or *Aspergillus*
  Langerhans' cell histiocytosis

exchange. A controversial, untested suggestion is that TRH be used to treat endocrine disorders associated with critical illness (67).

Medullary carcinoma of the thyroid (MCT) can cause high elevated basal serum levels of calcitonin that increase markedly after pentagastrin administration. Hypercalcitonemia may occur in all pathologic types of bronchogenic carcinoma (68), but it occurs most commonly in small cell carcinoma. Some bronchogenic-carcinoma patients with normal basal calcitonin levels have a supranormal response to pentagastrin stimulation, but to a lesser degree than in MCT. The calcitonin can be produced ectopically by the tumor itself, or it may come from the thyroid gland owing to the presence of a factor secreted by the tumor.

Lung cancer can metastasize to the thyroid gland. Over 25 years at the Mayo Clinic, 5 of 30 cases of metastatic thyroid involvement were from a primary lung cancer (69). Typically, patients presented with a painful, tender thyroid mass, and a lung lesion was found either concurrently or later. Fine-needle aspiration biopsy of the thyroid has demonstrated small cell and squamous cell carcinomas metastatic from the lung (70).

Primary pulmonary hypertension seems to be associated with an increased frequency of thyrotoxicosis (71). This association does not seem to be due to drug therapy with prostacyclin. In some patients treatment of their hyperthyroidism has improved their pulmonary hypertension.

THYROID DISORDERS THAT INFLUENCE THE RESPIRATORY SYSTEM

Thyroid Cancer Metastatic to the Lung

Thyroid diseases other than thyrotoxicosis can affect the respiratory system. Thyroid cancer metastasizes to the lungs in 5% to 20% of cases (72,73), most commonly papillary carcinoma. In patients who die of thyroid cancer, more than 50% have lung metastases (74). The pulmonary metastases usually are asymptomatic, but they may cause dyspnea on exertion. Rarely, these patients present with hemoptysis from airway involvement, Pancoast's syndrome, or polycythemia from hypoxemia attributed to small arteriovenous shunts in the tumor. The chest radiograph may be normal or reveal diffuse miliary opacities that may have stippled calcification because of aggregation of psammoma bodies in the tumor. Less commonly, a smaller number of large nodules are present bilaterally on the chest radiograph. Airway involvement with thyroid carcinoma may be visualized with bronchoscopy, but biopsy usually is needed for diagnosis (75). Bronchial lavage and cytologic examination of the fluid may also reveal metastatic thyroid cancer (75a).

Pulmonary metastases most commonly occur in younger patients and usually present within 1 to 2 years of diagnosis rather than as a late complication. The metastases may or may not take up iodine, but rarely synthesize thyroid hormone (76). Patients with functioning metastases have a better prognosis than nonfunctioning metastases, especially if the chest radiograph is normal. Radioiodine scans are most likely to reveal pulmonary involvement after surgical removal of the primary tumor and thyroid gland. In some series, half the patients with lung metastases had normal chest radiographic films and diffuse uptake on radioiodine scans (76). Rarely, primary lung tumors, such as adenocarcinoma, or other conditions, such as bronchiectasis, concentrate iodine and are confused with metastatic thyroid cancer. Indium 111-DTPA scanning has moderate sensitivity for detecting thyroid cancer metastases and may be positive even when conventional imaging is normal (77).

The presence of pulmonary metastases does not necessarily mean a poor clinical course. Even without treatment, densities in the chest radiograph may persist without progression for many years (78). Many reports suggest that functional lung metastases disappear in half the patients treated with ^{131}I, but other reports showed lesser responses (79,80). A sudden increase in pulmonary involvement after a long period of stability suggests that the tumor may have undergone an anaplastic change. Documentation by biopsy and more aggressive treatment may be necessary.

Thyroid cancer in the neck or mediastinum can obstruct the trachea by compression or displacement, or it can erode into the trachea or esophagus, causing luminal obstruction or bleeding. Rarely, thyroid carcinomas originate in ectopic thyroid tissue located in the trachea (81). Thyroid carcinoma involves the upper airway in 1% to 6% of cases and causes hemoptysis and vocal cord paralysis more often than does benign thyroid disease (82). Airway invasion may be more common in older men. Lymphoma, in particular, infiltrates the tracheal wall, obstructing the lymphatics and causing laryngeal and subglottic edema. Compression or infiltration of the tracheal wall is more common than intraluminal tumor growth. Only 18 of 2,000 cases of thyroid carcinoma seen at the Mayo Clinic had intraluminal growth of tumor (83). Rarely, thyroid carcinoma develops in substernal or intrathoracic goiters, causing rapid enlargement and compressive symptoms.

Surgical treatment of thyroid carcinoma with laryngotracheal involvement may be complex (84–89). The tumor tends to grow along the trachea rather than causing early luminal obstruction. Resection often requires airway reconstruction, such as sleeve tracheal resection, tracheal and cricoid cartilage resection, or more complex procedures. Of 34 patients at Massachusetts General Hospital undergoing resection, three died postoperatively, but only two patients had airway recurrence (86). Patients who cannot be completely resected have a high mortality rate, whereas patients with total resection and external beam irradiation often do well (87). The 5-year prognosis for patients who undergo surgery may be significantly lower only if the tumor involved or expanded the tracheal mucosa as a nodule or ulcerated mass (90). Shave excision of thyroid carcinoma is dangerous because of the high likelihood of recurrence. Massive invasion prohibiting reconstruction, innominate artery invasion, and deep invasion into the mediastinum are considered major contraindications to resection.

Nonmalignant Upper Airway Compression

Enlargement of the thyroid resulting from a variety of non-malignant conditions, most commonly multinodular goiter, can compress or displace the surrounding structures (Fig. 32.5). Intrathoracic goiters have an incidence of 1 in 5,000 persons and up to 1 in 2,000 in women over age 45 years (91). The vast majority arise in the cervical thyroid and retain an anatomic connection to it and a similar blood supply. Of 144 patients with goiter, airway obstruction on flow volume loops occurred in 31% and was especially common in men (92).

The consequences of thyroid enlargement depend on the location of the enlarged thyroid tissue. In the neck, it can obstruct the trachea or esophagus or compress the superior vena cava or the recurrent laryngeal or cervical sympathetic nerves, resulting in exertional dyspnea, dysphagia, hoarseness, dysphonia, wheezing, stridor, or cough that may be positional (93). Bilateral vocal cord paralysis also can cause respiratory distress and stridor, which may be mistaken for asthma (94), but this occurs much more commonly in malignant thyroid disease. About 15% to 20% of patients are asymptomatic. Sudden onset of stridor occurs in 2% to 3% of these patients, usually because of sponta-

neous or traumatic hemorrhage within a multinodular goiter. Stridor also may occur immediately after extubation. In some cases, including subacute thyroiditis, it may be difficult to recognize that a thyroid abnormality is causing chronic cough because of a lack of marked thyroid enlargement (95). A markedly enlarged substernal or mediastinal thyroid is one of the rare benign causes of superior vena cava syndrome (96). In toxic multinodular goiter, propylthiouracil (PTU) may increase the size of the goiter and precipitate or worsen superior vena cava obstruction (97). Unilateral or bilateral Horner's sign also may occur with a large intrathoracic goiter that disrupts the cervical sympathetic nerves.

If the thyroid enlargement is at the level of the narrow thoracic inlet, compression of the trachea or esophagus is particularly likely, even with relatively small goiters. Elevating the arms or flexing the neck may raise the retroclavicular goiter into the inlet and aggravate the compression, which has been termed the "thyroid cork" (98). Thoracic inlet compression results in decreased venous return, increased jugular venous pressure, facial plethora, dysphonia, hoarseness, dizziness, and shortness of breath. Precipitation of these findings by raising the arms is defined as Pemberton's sign (99). In contrast to the superior vena cava syndrome, there is no venous dilatation over the chest wall because the obstruction is not central.

Tracheal obstruction can have severe consequences, such as difficulty with intubation or rapid airway obstruction after extubation. Stridor and recognizable upper airway obstruction occur only with loss of 75% or more of the trachea's cross-sectional area. Tracheomalacia may result from

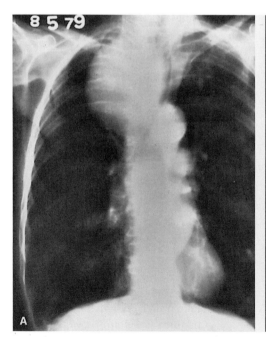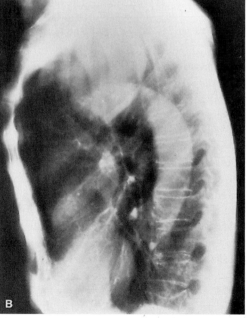

FIGURE 32.5. Posteroanterior **(A)** and lateral **(B)** chest radiographs showing a large substernal goiter, which is causing compression and anterolateral displacement of the trachea toward the left chest.

long-standing pressure on the trachea and may worsen after surgical tracheotomy. A sudden increase in the size of the thyroid mass, as with hemorrhage, can acutely obstruct the trachea, causing respiratory arrest (100).

Forty-three of 269 patients (16%) with enlarged thyroid glands had symptoms of obstruction to breathing or swallowing (101). Of the 5% of these patients with exertional dyspnea, most had tracheal deviation and hoarseness, but the degree of tracheal displacement was independent of the degree of compression (102). Intraluminal involvement, vocal cord paralysis, or hemoptysis did not always indicate malignant disease. Although the goiters frequently extended into the superior mediastinum and were visible on chest radiographs as a superior mediastinal mass, sternotomy usually was not required for surgical removal. In another series, 45 of 300 patients (15%) undergoing thyroidectomy had tracheal compression from benign thyroid disease (103). Four patients presented with acute upper airway obstruction requiring intubation, and four patients developed life-threatening obstruction while hospitalized. About half of 20 consecutive nonsurgical patients with euthyroid benign goiters, on careful questioning, had exertional dyspnea, and 80% had abnormalities of pulmonary function tests or tracheal tomography (104).

With airway obstruction, the peaks of the flow volume loop are cut off and flattened. Extrathoracic obstruction primarily diminishes inspiratory airflow, whereas intrathoracic obstruction predominantly affects expiratory airflow (105). Spirometric changes indicative of upper airway obstruction include decreased peak flow rates, a forced inspiratory flow measured at 50% of VC that is less than 100 L per minute, a ratio of forced inspiratory to forced expiratory flow rates measured at 50% of VC that is greater than 1, and a ratio of forced expiratory volume in 1 second to peak expiratory flow that is greater than 10 L/min. The inspiratory–expiratory flow volume loop is probably the most sensitive test, particularly if the test is performed with the patient in the supine position (106). A neural network algorithm based on the flow volume loop was 88% sensitive and 94% specific in detecting airway obstruction from goiter and was more accurate than specialist interpretation (107). Although chest radiography and ultrasonography predict retrosternal extension of goiter, they do not predict upper airway obstruction.

Tracheal tomography and computed tomography (CT) delineate the extent of luminal narrowing and may help plan airway and surgical management. A barium swallow can determine whether the esophagus also is compressed or deviated, as is true in up to one third of patients. Fluoroscopy can identify a pulsatile mass, indicating the presence of an aortic aneurysm rather than thyroid tissue. A radioactive iodine scan can confirm that a mediastinal mass takes up iodine and is likely to be thyroid tissue; a negative scan does not exclude the possibility that it is nonfunctioning thyroid tissue, but it must be done before CT scanning with iodinated contrast. Bronchoscopy or esophagoscopy may be necessary to ensure that primary cancer of one of these organs is not coexisting with a goiter.

About 10% of anterior mediastinal masses are mediastinal thyroid tissue. Overall, 5% of mediastinal tumors prove to be intrathoracic goiters. Suggestive CT features include anatomic continuity with the cervical thyroid, focal calcifications, high CT number (>70 HU), and a prolonged increase in CT number after iodinated intravenous contrast material (>100 HU) (108). Less commonly, mediastinal goiters occur in other parts of the mediastinum. Radionuclide scanning after administration of ^{123}I or ^{131}I may confirm this diagnosis.

Surgical treatment of a large substernal goiter with airway compression can be difficult (72,100). Most intrathoracic goiters should be removed because of the risk for sudden enlargement, unless the patient is in a high-risk group for surgical complications. Such goiters usually can be removed using a standard cervical collar incision, but sometimes a sternotomy or a thoracotomy is required. A combined surgical approach often is necessary for posterior mediastinal goiters. Tracheostomy should be avoided, if possible, unless laryngeal edema is present. Intubation should be attempted only in life-threatening situations or at the time of definitive surgery, after the diagnostic workup is otherwise complete. Surgery usually is recommended for goiters that cause peak inspiratory flow rates of 1.5 L per second or less. Peak and midinspiratory flow rates often double after removal of large goiters with significant tracheal obstruction. Two patients with hypercapnia preoperatively became normocapnic after removal of the goiter. Substernal goiters can recur in as many as 20% of postoperative patients. Until recently, there was reluctance to treat patients with large multinodular goiters and compressive symptoms with ^{131}I, but one study of 21 patients demonstrated objective improvement in tracheal luminal size and tracheal deviation (109).

Thyrotoxicosis and Asthma

Thyrotoxicosis has been said to worsen airway hyperreactivity in patients with asthma, based on several case reports and a study of five patients with severe intractable asthma who became responsive to therapy after several days of antithyroid treatment with PTU (110–113). In a small study, exogenous T_3 given chronically to asthmatics decreased their symptoms and increased their peak flow rates (114); however, peak flow measurement is highly variable and significantly effort dependent. In contrast, normal subjects who were made thyrotoxic with exogenous T_3 and challenged with methacholine inhalation did not increase their airway resistance (115). Nonasthmatic thyrotoxic patients did not have bronchoconstriction after histamine challenge or a change in response after becoming euthyroid (116). Mild asthmatics with T_3-induced thyrotoxicosis also did not have a change in methacholine-induced bronchospasm, pulmonary function tests, or exercise capacity (117). To confuse the subject further, thyrotoxicosis decreased bronchial reactivity to carbachol provocation in 8 of 11 patients studied before and after treatment (118). Acute hypothyroidism caused by thyroidectomy for cancer was associated with increased bronchial reactivity to carbachol in 11 patients without pulmonary disease (119).

In summary, most data do not support a consistent relationship between thyroid function and bronchial reactivity. It remains unclear whether or not hyperthyroidism and asthma are associated more frequently than expected based on their individual prevalence.

MISCELLANEOUS INTERACTIONS

Airway obstruction (asthma or COPD) and thyrotoxicosis interact in other ways. For example, β-blockers may worsen airway obstruction. Theophylline metabolism can be accelerated up to fourfold in patients with thyrotoxicosis because of increased hepatic metabolism by the cytochrome P450 system (120,121). Theophylline can increase serum T_4 concentrations, at least transiently, in adults and children (122).

Serum angiotensin-converting enzyme activity, once considered a diagnostic test for sarcoidosis, may be elevated in many granulomatous diseases, diabetes mellitus, and thyrotoxicosis (123). PTU can cause eosinophilic pleuritis or diffuse interstitial pneumonitis (124,125). The latter was documented by lung biopsies of two patients with dyspnea, a productive cough, and restrictive pulmonary function tests within 1 to 3 months after beginning PTU therapy. The pulmonary findings resolved rapidly after discontinuation of PTU. Antineutrophilic cytoplasmic antibody (ANCA) may occur in patients taking PTU (rarely methimazole) and occasionally results in ANCA-vasculitis, including alveolar hemorrhage (125a). Finally, Hashimoto's thyroiditis may be associated with an increase in the frequency of bronchogenic carcinoma, especially adenocarcinoma (126).

SYSTEMIC CONDITIONS THAT AFFECT BOTH LUNG AND THYROID

A variety of systemic conditions can affect both the lung and the thyroid. In the past, children with cystic fibrosis (CF) often were treated with potassium iodide as an expectorant. The goitrogenic effects of chronic iodide therapy led to a high incidence of goiter and hypothyroidism (127,128). In older studies, children with CF had lower than normal serum T_4 levels and high T_3/T_4 ratios with an increased serum TSH response to TRH (129), suggesting subclinical hypothyroidism, but these studies did not control for the effects of malnutrition or exocrine pancreatic deficiency.

Iodinated glycerol previously was used to increase clearance of mucus and for symptomatic treatment of COPD,

and may cause thyrotoxicosis or hypothyroidism (130, 131); consequently, iodine was removed from this medication. Chronic iodine therapy can cause pulmonary edema (132).

Cigarette smoking can alter thyroid function tests subtly; however, the changes are not clinically important in most people. Discontinuation of smoking may lead to decreases in serum T_4 and rT_3 levels, a small increase in the serum TSH level, and no change in the serum T_3 level (133). In contrast, in another study, heavy smokers had lower serum T_4 and T_3 levels compared with light smokers and control subjects (134). Other measures of thyroid function did not differ among the three groups. The pyridine components of cigarette smoke or higher serum thiocyanate concentrations in smokers may have a mild antithyroid effect. Smoking also is associated with a higher prevalence of ophthalmopathy in patients with Graves' disease (135–137) and nontoxic goiter, and it may increase the serum TSH further in subclinical hypothyroidism or impair the peripheral action of thyroid hormone (138). Nicotine per se is probably not the cause of the smoking-induced changes in thyroid function (139).

Systemic autoimmune disorders may involve the lung and often are associated with thyroid disease. Examples include Sjögren's syndrome, systemic lupus erythematosus, and rheumatoid arthritis. Myasthenia gravis occurs in 0.1% of patients with Graves' disease, which is a 30-fold increase over the prevalence in the general population. Pulmonary manifestations can include thymoma, aspiration resulting from bulbar involvement, and respiratory muscle weakness leading to respiratory failure.

Other systemic diseases can involve both the lung and thyroid. *Pneumocystis carinii* infection of the thyroid has been found in acquired immunodeficiency syndrome (AIDS) patients with enlarged thyroid glands, most of whom were receiving aerosolized pentamidine prophylaxis against *P. carinii* pneumonia (140). The goiters may or may not be tender, and patients have been thyrotoxic or hypothyroid. Radioactive iodine uptake usually is decreased in the affected region. *Aspergillus* also may infect the lungs and thyroid. Langerhans' cell granulomatosis may occur in the thyroid gland of patients with or without pulmonary involvement (141,142).

REFERENCES

1. Hitchcock KR, Reichlin S. Thyroid hormones in the adult rat lung. *Am Rev Respir Dis* 1978;117:807.
2. Obregon MJ, Deescobar M, Escobar Del Rey F. Concentrations of triiodo-L-thyronine in the plasma and tissue of normal rats, as determined by radioimmunoassay. *Endocrinology* 1979; 103:2145.
3. Escobar-Morreale JF, Obregon J, del Rey FE, et al. Replacement therapy for hypothyroidism with thyroxine alone does not ensure euthyroidism in all tissues, as studied in thyroidectomized rats. *J Clin Invest* 1995;96:2828.
4. Chopra IJ. A study of extrathyroidal conversion of thyroxine to 3,5,3′ triiodo-L-thyronine in the rat. *J Clin Invest* 1977;50:1124.

5. McCann UD, Shaw EA. Iodothyronine deiodination reaction types in several rat tissues: effects of age, thyroid status, and glucocorticoid treatment. *Endocrinology* 1984;114:1513.

6. Gonzales LW, Ballard PL. Identification and characterization of nuclear T$_3$-binding sites in fetal human lung. *J Clin Endocrinol Metab* 1981;53:21.

7. Gonzales LW, Ballard PL. Nuclear 3′,5′-tri-iodothyronine receptors in rabbit lung: characterization and developmental changes. *Endocrinology* 1982;111:542.

8. Morishige WK, Geurnsey DL. Triiodothyronine receptors in rat lung. *Endocrinology* 1978;102:1628.

9. Lindenberg JA, Brehier A, Ballard PL. Tri-iodothyronine nuclear binding in fetal and adult rabbit lung and cultured lung cells. *Endocrinology* 1979;103:1725.

10. Wilson M, Hitchcock KR, Douglas WJ, et al. Hormones and the lung. III: immunohistochemical localization of thyroid hormone binding in type II pulmonary epithelial cells clonally derived from adult rat lung. *Anat Rec* 1979;195:611.

11. Smith DM, Hitchcock KR. Thyroid hormone binding to adult rat alveolar type II cells. *Exp Lung Res* 1983;5:141.

12. Redding RA, Douglas WHJ, Stein M. Thyroid hormone influence on lung surfactant metabolism. *Science* 1972;175:994.

13. Hitchcock KR. Hormones and the lung. I. Thyroid hormones and glucocorticoids in lung development. *Anat Rec* 1979;194:15.

14. Holt, J, Canavan, JP, Goldspink, DF. The influence of thyroid hormones on the growth of the lungs in perinatal rats. *Int J Dev Biol* 1993;37:467.

15. Liggins GC. Thyrotrophin-releasing hormone and lung maturation. *Reprod Fertil Dev* 1995;7:443.

16. DeMello DE, Heyman S, Govindrajan R, et al. Delayed ultrastructural lung maturation in the fetal and newborn hypothyroid (hyt/hyt) mouse. *Pediatr Res* 1994;36:380.

17. Devaskar UP, Govindrajan R, Heyman S, et al. Fetal mouse lung ultrastructural maturation is accelerated by maternal thyrotropin-releasing hormone treatment. *Biol Neonate* 1996;70:101.

18. Ansari MA, Demello DE, Polk DH, et al. Thyrotropin-releasing hormone accelerates fetal mouse lung ultrastructural maturation via stimulation of extra thyroidal pathway. *Pediatr Res* 1997;42:709.

19. Chan L, Miller TF, Yuxin J, et al. Antenatal triiodothyronine improves neonatal pulmonary function in preterm lambs. *J Soc Gynecol Invest* 1998;5:122.

20. Moreno B, Rodriguez-Manzaneque JC, Perez-Castillo A, et al. Thyroid hormone controls the expression of insulin-like growth factor I receptor gene at different levels in lung and heart of developing and adult rats. *Endocrinology* 1997;138:1194.

21. Moraga FA, Riquelme RA, Lopez AA, et al. Maternal administration of glucocorticoid and thyrotropin-releasing hormone enhances fetal lung maturation in undisturbed preterm lambs. *Am J Obstet Gynecol* 1994;171:729.

22. Polk DH, Ikegami M, Newnham J, et al. Fetus-placenta-newborn: postnatal lung function in preterm lambs: effects of a single exposure to betamethasone and thyroid hormones. *Am J Obstet Gynecol* 1995;172:872.

23. Whitsett JA, Darovec-Beckerman C, Adams K, et al. Thyroid dependent maturation of beta-adrenergic receptors in the rat lung. *Biochem Biophys Res Commun* 1980;97:913.

24. Scarpace PJ, Abrass IB. Thyroid hormone regulation of rat heart, lymphocyte, and lung beta-adrenergic receptors. *Endocrinology* 1981;108:1007.

25. Folkesson H. Dexamethasone and thyroid pretreatment upregulate alveolar epithelial fluid clearance in adult rats. *J Appl Physiol* 2000;88:416–424.

26. Lei J, Nowbar S, Mariash CN, Ingbar DH. Thyroid hormone stimulates Na-K-ATPase activity and its plasma membrane insertion in rat alveolar epithelial cells. *Am J Physiol (Lung)* 2003;285:L762.

27. Lazzaro D, Price M, De Felice M, et al. The transcription factor TTF-1 is expressed at the onset of thyroid and lung morphogenesis and in restricted regions of the foetal brain. *Development* 1991;113:1093.

28. Bohinski RJ, Di Lauro R, Whitsett JA. The lung-specific surfactant protein B gene promoter is a target for thyroid transcription factor 1 and hepatocyte nuclear factor 3, indicating common factors for organ-specific gene expression along the foregut axis. *Mol Cell Biol* 1994;14:5671.

29. Minoo P, Hamdan H, Bu D, et al. TTF-1 regulates lung epithelial morphogenesis. *Dev Biol* 1995;172:694–698.

30. Kimura S, Hara Y, Pineau T, et al. The T/ebp null mouse: thyroid-specific enhancer-binding protein is essential for the organogenesis of the thyroid, lung, ventral forebrain and pituitary. *Genes Dev* 1996;10:60.

31. Bingle CD. Thyroid transcription factor-1. *Int J Biochem Cell Biol* 1997;29:1471.

32. Stahlman MT, Gray ME, Whitsett JA. Expression of thyroid transcription factor-1 in fetal and neonatal human lung. *J Histochem Cytochem* 1996;44:673.

33. Minoo P, Su G, Drum H, Bringas P, Kimura S. Defects in tracheoesophageal and lung morphogenesis in kx2.1 −/− mouse embryos. *Dev Biol* 1999;209:60–71.

34. Devriendt K, Vanhole C, Matthijs G, et al. Deletion of thyroid transcription factor-1 gene in an infant with neonatal thyroid dysfunction and respiratory failure [Letter]. *N Engl J Med* 1998;338:1317.

35. Sakiyama J, Yamagishi A, Kuroiwa A. Tbx4-Fgf10 system controls lung bud formation during chicken embryogenesis. *Development* 2003;130:1225–1234.

36. Matthay MA, Folkesson HG, Clerici C. Lung epithelial fluid transport and the resolution of pulmonary edema. *Physiol Rev* 2002;83:569–600.

37. Smith TJ, Murata Y, Horwitz AL, et al. Regulation of glycosaminoglycan synthesis by thyroid hormone in vitro. *J Clin Invest* 1982;70:1066.

38. Peabody FW, Wentworth JA. Clinical studies of the respiration. IV: the vital capacity of the lungs and its relation to dyspnea. *Arch Intern Med* 1917;20:443.

39. Lemon WS, Moersch JH. Basal metabolism and vital capacity. *Arch Intern Med* 1924;33:130.

40. Rabinowitch IM. The vital capacity in hyperthyroidism with a study of the influence of posture. *Arch Intern Med* 1923;31:910.

41. Stein M, Kimbel P, Johnson RL. Pulmonary function in hyperthyroidism. *J Clin Invest* 1961;40:348.

42. McElvaney GN, Wilcox PG, Fairbarn MS, et al. Respiratory muscle weakness and dyspnea in thyrotoxic patients. *Am Rev Respir Dis* 1990;141:1221.

43. Davies HW, Meakins J, Sands J. The influence of circulatory disturbances on the gaseous exchange of blood. V. blood gases and circulation rate in hyperthyroidism. *Heart* 1924;11:299.

44. Kendrick AH, O'Reilly JR, Laszlo G. Lung function and exercise performance in hyperthyroidism before and after treatment. *Q J Med* 1988;68:615.

45. Bates DM, Macklem PT, Christie RV. *Respiratory function in disease.* Philadelphia: WB Saunders, 1971:430.

46. Freedman S. Lung volumes and distensibility and maximum respiratory pressures in thyroid disease before and after treatment. *Thorax* 1978;33:785.

47. Massey DG, Becklake MR, McKenzie JM, et al. Circulatory and ventilatory response to exercise in thyrotoxicosis. *N Engl J Med* 1967;276:1104.

48. Ayres J, Clark TH, Maisey MN. Thyrotoxicosis and dyspnea. *Clin Endocrinol (Oxf)* 1982;164:645.

49. Mier A, Brophy C, Wass JAH, et al. Reversible respiratory muscle weakness in hyperthyroidism. *Am Rev Respir Dis* 1989; 139:529.

50. Ianuzzo CD, Chen V, O'Brien P, et al. Effect of experimental dysthyroidism on the enzymatic character of the diaphragm. *J Appl Physiol* 1984;56:117.

51. Miyashita A, Suzuki S, Suzuki M, et al. Effect of thyroid hormone on *in vivo* contractility of the canine diaphragm. *Am Rev Respir Dis* 1992;145:1456.

52. Valtin H, Tenney SM. Respiratory adaptations to hyperthyroidism. *J Appl Physiol* 1960;15:1107.

53. Engel LA, Ritchie B. Ventilatory response to inhaled carbon dioxide in hyperthyroidism. *J Appl Physiol* 1971;30:173.

54. Zwillich CW, Matthay M, Potts DE, et al. Thyrotoxicosis: comparison of effects of thyroid ablation and beta-adrenergic blockade on metabolic rate and ventilatory control. *J Clin Endocrinol Metab* 1978;46:491.

55. Stockley RA, Bishop JM. Effect of thyrotoxicosis on the reflex hypoxic respiratory drive. *Clin Sci* 1977;53:93.

56. Pino-Garcia JM, Garcia-Rio F, Diez JJ, et al. Regulation of breathing in hyperthyroidism: relationship to hormonal and metabolic changes. *Eur Respir J* 1998;12:400.

57. Kahaly GJ, Kampmann C, Mohr-Kahaly S. Cardiovascular hemodynamics and exercise tolerance in thyroid disease. *Thyroid* 2002;12:473–481

58. Bishop JM, Donald KW, Wade OL. Circulatory dynamics at rest and on exercise in the hyperkinetic states. *Clin Sci* 1956; 14:329.

59. McIlroy MD, Elridge FL, Stone RW. The mechanical properties of the lungs in anoxia, anaemia, and thyrotoxicosis. *Clin Sci* 1955;15:353.

60. Kimura H, Kawagoe Y, Kaneko N, et al. Low efficiency of oxygen utilization during exercise in hyperthyroidism. *Chest* 1996; 110:1264.

61. Small D, Gillons W, Levy RD, et al. Exertional dyspnea and ventilation in hyperthyroidism. *Chest* 1992;101:1268.

62. Forfar JC, Muir AL, Sawers, et al. Abnormal left ventricular function in hyperthyroidism. *N Engl J Med* 1982;307:1165.

63. Kahaly G, Hellermann J, Mohr-Kahaly S, et al. Impaired cardiopulmonary exercise capacity in patients with hyperthyroidism. *Chest* 1996;109:57.

64. Thurnheer R, Jenni TR, Russi EW, et al. Hyperthyroidism and pulmonary hypertension. J Intern Med 1997;242:185–188.

65. Sumita S, Ujike Y, Namiki A, et al. Suppression of the thyrotropin response to thyrotropin-releasing hormone and its association with severity of critical illness. *Crit Care Med* 1994; 22:1603.

66. Dulchavesky SA, Kennedy PR, Geller ER, et al. T_3 preserves respiratory function in sepsis. *J Trauma* 1991;31:753.

67. Van den Berghe G, de Zegher F, Vlasselaers D, et al. Thyrotropin-releasing hormone in critical illness. *Crit Care Med* 1996;24:590.

68. Samaan NA, Castillo S, Schultz PN, et al. Serum calcitonin after pentagastrin stimulation in patients with bronchogenic carcinoma and breast cancer compared to that in patients with medullary thyroid carcinoma. *J Clin Endocrinol Metab* 1980; 51:237.

69. Ivey HK. Cancer metastatic to the thyroid: a diagnostic problem. *Mayo Clin Proc* 1984;59:856.

70. Smith SA, Gharib H, Goellner JR. Fine-needle aspiration: usefulness for diagnosis and management of metastatic carcinoma to the thyroid. *Arch Intern Med* 1987;147:311.

71. Arroliga AC, Dweik RA, Rafanen AL. Primary pulmonary hypertension and thyroid disease. *Chest* 2000;118:1224–1225.

72. Worm AM, Holten I, Teaning E. Nuclear imaging of pulmonary metastases in thyroid carcinoma. *Acta Radiol Oncol Radiat Phys Biol* 1960;19:410.

73. Vassilopoulou-Sellin R, Klein MJ, Smith TH, et al. Pulmonary metastases in children and young adults with differentiated thyroid cancer. *Cancer* 1993;71:1348.

74. Kobayahi T, Asakawa H, Tamaki Y, et al. Fatal differentiated thyroid cancer. *J Surg Oncol* 1996;62:123.

75. Diaz G, Jimenez D, Dominguez-Reboiras S, et al. Yield of bronchoscopy in the diagnosis of neoplasm metastatic to the lung. *Respir Med* 2003;97:27–29.

75a. Mello CJ, Veronikis IE, Fraire AE, et al. Metastatic papillary thyroid carcinoma to lung diagnosed by bronchoalveolar lavage. *J Clin Endocrinol Metab* 1996;42:239.

76. Casara D, Rubello D, Saladini G, et al. Different features of pulmonary metastases in differentiated thyroid cancer: natural history and multivariate statistical analysis of prognostic variables. *J Nucl Med* 1993;34:809.

77. Sarlis NJ, Gourgiotis L, Guthrie LC, et al. In-111 DTPA-octreotide scintigraphy for disease detection in metastatic thyroid cancer. *Clin Nucl Med* 2003;28:208–217.

78. Maruyama M, Sugenoya A, Kobayashi S, et al. A case of papillary carcinoma of the thyroid with more than 30 years long-term asymptomatic pulmonary metastases. *Clin Endocrinol (Oxf)* 1993;38:331.

79. Sisson JC, Giordano TJ, Jamadar DA, et al. 131-I treatment of micronodular pulmonary metastases from papillary thyroid carcinoma. *Cancer* 1996;78:2184.

80. Schlumberger M, Challeton C, De Vathaire F, et al. Radioactive iodine treatment and external radiotherapy for lung and bone metastases from thyroid carcinoma. *J Nucl Med* 1996; 37:598.

81. Rotenberg D, Lawson VG, Van Nostrand AWP. Thyroid carcinoma presenting as a tracheal tumor: case report and literature review with reflections on pathogenesis. *J Otolaryngol* 1979; 8:4601.

82. Lawson V. The management of airway involvement in thyroid tumors. *Arch Otolaryngol* 1983;109:86.

83. Djalilian M, Bealirs OH, Devine KC, et al. Intraluminal involvement of the larynx and trachea by thyroid cancer. *Am J Surg* 1974;128:500.

84. Friedman M. Surgical management of thyroid carcinoma with laryngotracheal invasion. *Otolaryngol Clin North Am* 1990;23: 495.

85. Melliere DJM, Yashia NEB, Becquemin JP, et al. Thyroid carcinoma with tracheal or esophageal involvement: limited or maximal surgery? *Surgery* 1993;113:166.

86. Grillo HC, Suen HC, Mathisen DJ, et al. Resectional management of thyroid carcinoma invading the airway. *Ann Thorac Surg* 1992;54:3.

87. Lydiatt DD, Markin RS, Ogren FP. Tracheal invasion by thyroid carcinoma. *Ear Nose Throat J* 1990;69:145.

88. Nomori H, Kobayashi K, Ishihara T, et al. Thyroid carcinoma infiltrating the trachea: clinical, histologic, and morphometric analyses. *J Surg Oncol* 1990;44:78.

89. Hammoud AT, Mathisen DJ. Surgical management of the thyroid carcinoma invading the trachea. *Chest Surg Clin North Am* 2003;13:359–367.

90. Shin DH, Mark EJ, Suen HC, et al. Pathologic staging of papillary carcinoma of the thyroid with airway invasion based on the anatomic manner of extension to the trachea. *Hum Pathol* 1993;24:866.

91. Katlic MR, Wang CA, Grillo HC. Substernal goiter. *Ann Thorac Surg* 1985;39:391.

92. Miller MR, Pincock AC, Oates GD, et al. Upper airway obstruction due to goitre: detection, prevalence and results of surgical management. *Q J M* 1990;74:177.

93. Shambaugh GE, Seed R, Korn A. Airway obstruction in substernal goiters: clinical and therapeutic implications. *J Chron Dis* 1973;26:737.

94. Godwin JE, Miller KS, Goang KG, et al. Benign thyroid hyperplasia presenting as bilateral vocal cord paralysis: complete remission following surgery. *Chest* 1991;99:1029.

95. Irwin RS, Pratter MR, Hamolsky MW. Chronic persistent cough: an uncommon presenting complaint of thyroiditis. *Chest* 1982;81:386.

96. Siderys H, Rowe GA. Superior vena caval syndrome caused by intrathoracic goiter. *Am Surg* 1970;36:446.

97. Hershey CO, McVeigh RC, Miller RP. Transient superior vena cava syndrome due to propylthiouracil therapy in intrathoracic goiter. *Chest* 1981;79:356.

98. Blum M, Biller BJ, Bergman DA. The thyroid cork: obstruction of the thoracic inlet due to retroclavicular goiter. *JAMA* 1974;227:189.

99. Wallace C, Siminoski K. The Pemberton sign. *Ann Intern Med* 1996;125:568.

100. Torres A, Arroyo J, Kastanos N, et al. Acute respiratory failure and tracheal obstruction in patients with intrathoracic goiter. *Crit Care Med* 1983;11:265.

101. Calcaterra TC, Macari DR. Aerodigestive dysfunction secondary to thyroid tumors. *Laryngoscope* 1981;91:701.

102. Hassard AO, Holland JG. Benign thyroid disease and upper airway obstruction. *J Otolaryngol* 1982;11:77.

103. Alfonso A, Christoudias G, Amarruin Q, et al. Tracheal or esophageal compression due to benign thyroid disease. *Am J Surg* 1981;142:350.

104. Jaregui R, Liker ES, Bayley A. Upper airway obstruction in euthyroid goiter. *JAMA* 1977;238:2163.

105. Karbowitz SR, Edelman LB, Nath S, et al. Spectrum of advanced upper airway obstruction due to goiters. *Chest* 1985;87:18.

106. Meysman M, Noppen M, Vincken W. Effect of posture on the flow-volume loop in two patients with euthyroid goiter. *Chest* 1996;110:1615.

107. Bright P, Miller MR, Franklyn, JA, et al. The use of a neural network to detect upper airway obstruction caused by goiter. *Am J Respir Crit Care Med* 1998;157:1885.

108. Glazer GM, Axel L, Moss AA. CT diagnosis of mediastinal thyroid. *AJR* 1982;138:495.

109. Huysmans DAKC, Hermus ARMM, Corstens FHM, et al. Large, compressive goiters treated with radioiodine. *Ann Intern Med* 1994;121:757.

110. Settipane GA, Schoenfeld E, Hamolsky MW. Asthma and hyperthyroidism. *J Allergy Clin Immunol* 1972;49:348.

111. Shaha AR. Surgery for benign thyroid disease causing tracheoesophageal compression. *Otolaryngol Clin North Am* 1990;23:391.

112. Cockroft DW, Silverberg JDH, Dosman JA. Decrease in nonspecific bronchial reactivity in an asthmatic following treatment of hyperthyroidism. *Ann Allergy* 1978;41:163.

113. White NW, Raine RI, Bateman ED. Asthma and hyperthyroidism. *South Afr Med J* 1990;78:750.

114. Ismail AA, Shaleby E, Gadalla. Effect of tri-iodothyronine on bronchial asthma (part 2). *J Asthma Res* 1977;14:111.

115. Irwin RS, Pratter MR, Stivers DH, et al. Airway reactivity and lung function in triiodothyronine-induced thyrotoxicosis. *J Appl Physiol* 1985;58:1485.

116. Roberts JA, McLellan AR, Alexander WD. Effect of hyperthyroidism on bronchial reactivity in nonasthmatic patients. *Thorax* 1989;445:603.

117. Hollingsworth HM, Pratter MR, Dubois JM, et al. Effect of triiodothyronine-induced thyrotoxicosis on airway hyperresponsiveness. *J Appl Physiol* 1991;71:438.

118. Israel RH, Poe RH, Cave WT, et al. Hyperthyroidism protects against carbachol-induced bronchospasm. *Chest* 1987;91:243.

119. Wieshammer S, Keck FS, Shauffelen AC, et al. Effects of hypothyroidism on bronchial reactivity in non-asthmatic subjects. *Thorax* 1990;45:947.

120. Pokrajac M, Simic D, Varagic VM. Pharmacokinetics of theophylline in hyperthyroid and hypothyroid patients with chronic obstructive pulmonary disease. *Eur J Clin Pharmacol* 1987;33:483.

121. Bauman JH, Teichman S, Wible DA. Increased theophylline clearance in a patient with hyperthyroidism. *Ann Allergy* 1984;52:94.

122. Hiratani M, Muto K, Oshida Y, et al. Effect of sustained-release theophylline administration on pituitary-thyroid axis. *J Allergy Clin Immunol* 1982;70:481.

123. Yotsumoto H, Imai Y, Kuzuya N. Increased levels of serum angiotensin-converting enzyme activity in hyperthyroidism. *Ann Intern Med* 1982;96:326.

124. Miyazono K, Okazaki T, Uchida S, et al. Propylthiouracil-induced diffuse interstitial pneumonitis. *Arch Intern Med* 1984;144:1764.

125. Middleton KL, Santella R, Couser JI. Eosinophilic pleuritis due to propylthiouracil. *Chest* 1993;103:955.

125a. Dhillon SS, Lingh D, Doe N., et al. Diffuse alveolar hemorrhage and pulmonary capillaritis due to propylthiouracil. *Chest* 1999;116:1485.

126. Yamashita N, Maruchi N, Mori W. Hashimoto's thyroiditis: a possible risk factor for lung cancer among Japanese women. *Cancer Lett* 1979;7:9.

127. Dolan TF, Gibson LE. Complications of iodide therapy in patients with cystic fibrosis. *J Pediatr* 1971;79:684.

128. Segall-Blank M, Vagenakis AG, Schwachman H, et al. Thyroid gland function and pituitary TSH reserve in patients with cystic fibrosis. *J Pediatr* 1981;98:218.

129. De Luca F, Trimarchi F, Sferlazzas C, et al. Thyroid function in children with cystic fibrosis. *Eur J Pediatr* 1982;138:327.

130. Huseby JS, Benett SW, Hagensee ME. Hyperthyroidism induced by iodinated glycerol. *Am Rev Respir Dis* 1991;144:1403.

131. Becker CB, Gordon JM. Iodinated glycerol and thyroid dysfunction; four cases and a review of the literature. *Chest* 1993;103:188.

132. Geurian K, Branam C. Iodine poisoning secondary to long-term iodinated glycerol therapy. *Arch Intern Med* 1994;154:1153.

133. Melander A, Nordenskjold E, Lundh B, et al. Influence of smoking on thyroid activity. *Acta Med Scand* 1981;2049:441.

134. Sepkovic DW, Haley NJ, Wyner EL. Thyroid activity in cigarette smokers. *Arch Intern Med* 1984;144:501.

135. Bertelsen JB, Hegedüs L. Cigarette smoking and the thyroid. *Thyroid* 1994;4:327.

136. Bartalena L, Marcocci C, Tanda ML, et al. Cigarette smoking and therapeutic outcomes in Graves ophthalmopathy. *Ann Intern Med* 1998;129:632.

137. Bartalena L, Bogazzi F, Tanda ML. Cigarette smoking and the thyroid. *Eur J Endocrinol* 1995;133:507.

138. Miller B, Zulewski H, Huber P, et al. Impaired action of thyroid hormone associated with smoking in women with hypothyroidism. *N Engl J Med* 1995;333:964.

139. Colzani R, Fang SL, Alex S, et al. The effect of nicotine on thyroid function in rats. *Metabolism* 1998;47:154.

140. Guttler R, Singer PA. *Pneumocystis carinii* thyroiditis. *Arch Intern Med* 1993;153:393.

141. Tsang WYW, Lau MF, Chan JKC. Incidental Langerhans' cell histiocytosis of the thyroid. *Histopathology* 1994;24:397.

142. Maurea S, Lastoria S, Klain M, et al. Diagnostic evaluation of thyroid involvement by histiocytosis X. *J Nucl Med* 1994;35:263.

THE KIDNEYS AND ELECTROLYTE METABOLISM IN THYROTOXICOSIS

ELAINE M. KAPTEIN

Thyrotoxicosis, particularly severe thyrotoxicosis, is associated with multiple alterations in cardiovascular function, renal hemodynamics, and renal tubular reabsorptive function. Renal function is altered due to a combination of direct and indirect effects of thyroid hormone excess on the kidney (Fig. 33.1). The indirect effects include changes in cardiovascular hemodynamics and the renin–angiotensin-aldosterone system. Reversible alterations in sodium and water metabolism, calcium, phosphate, vitamin D, and uric acid homeostasis also occur.

HEMODYNAMIC CHANGES

Thyrotoxicosis results in a hyperkinetic circulation with increased heart rate and cardiac output, decreased peripheral vascular resistance, and increased blood flow to most organs, including the kidneys (see Chapter 31) (1). The decrease in peripheral vascular resistance may be due to relaxation of vascular smooth muscle cells, increased β-adrenergic receptor activity, and an increase in effective blood volume (2) (Fig. 33.1).

Nitric oxide is an important factor in regulating vascular tone, renal sodium excretion, and the renal pressure diuresis-natriuresis response, and therefore arterial blood pressure (3). Nitric oxide synthase activity is increased in the left ventricle, aorta and vena cava, and renal cortex and medulla of thyrotoxic rats (3). In thyrotoxic humans, decreased vascular resistance is largely due to increased endothelial production of nitric oxide and increased vascular sensitivity to acetylcholine, the endothelial-dependent vasodilator (4). Furthermore, the vasoconstrictor response to norepinephrine is increased, whereas plasma catecholamine concentrations are low (see Chapter 38) (4). These vascular abnormalities are corrected by correction of thyrotoxicosis (4). In addition, serum concentrations of the endothelial vasodilatory hormone adrenomedullin are high in patients with thyrotoxicosis (2). Thus, an increase in basal endothelial cell function and endothelial hyperresponsiveness to vasodilating stimuli provide an explanation for the decrease in peripheral vascular resistance and maintenance of a hyperkinetic state in patients with thyrotoxicosis (4). Activation of the renin–an-

giotensin–aldosterone system may play a causative role in development of cardiac hypertrophy in thyrotoxicosis (5,6).

HYPERTENSION

Systolic hypertension occurs in up to one third of patients with thyrotoxicosis (7). In one study, the mean systolic blood pressure was 10 mm Hg higher and diastolic blood pressure was 5 mm Hg lower during thyrotoxicosis than after euthyroidism was attained (1). Systolic blood pressure correlated with cardiac output, whereas diastolic blood pressure was related to systemic vascular resistance (1).

Thyrotoxicosis increases nitric oxide synthase activity, which as noted above regulates vascular tone, renal sodium excretion, and blood pressure (6). Thyrotoxicosis also results in activation of the renin–angiotensin system, the effects of which are blocked by angiotensin-converting enzyme inhibitors (6). In normal subjects, there is a functional balance between angiotensin II and nitric oxide production. In thyrotoxic rats, thyroxine (T_4) administration increased blood pressure and plasma concentrations of angiotensin II and nitrates/nitrites (6). Simultaneous administration of T_4 and subpressor doses of an inhibitor of nitric oxide synthesis caused a marked increase in blood pressure, which was attenuated by losartan, an angiotensin receptor–blocking drug (6). Plasma angiotensin II and nitric oxide concentrations were increased by T_4, whereas both were reduced in the rats given T_4 and the nitric oxide inhibitor (6). Impaired synthesis of nitric oxide results in increased sensitivity to the pressor effect of T_4, and the latter is attenuated by losartan. Thus, increased nitric oxide synthase activity may play a protective homeostatic role in ameliorating the prohypertensive effects of T_4 in thyrotoxicosis, as well as antagonizing the pressor actions of angiotensin II (6).

RENAL GLOMERULAR AND TUBULAR FUNCTION

In humans with thyrotoxicosis and animals treated with excess T_4, renal plasma flow and glomerular filtration rate

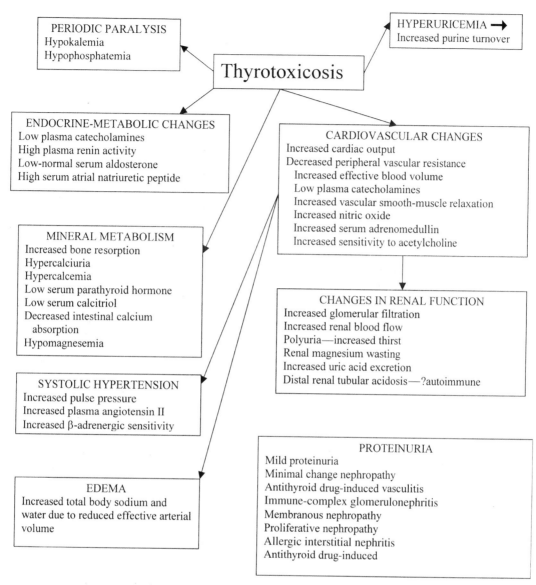

FIGURE 33.1. Diagram of the cardiovascular and other changes affecting renal function in patients with thyrotoxicosis.

are increased, probably because of the increase in cardiac output and decrease in peripheral resistance (8,9). Intrarenal vasodilatation also occurs (8). The renal content of the endogenous vasoconstrictor substance endothelin is lower in thyrotoxic rats, which may contribute to renal vasodilatation (10).

The glomerular filtration rate, as measured by inulin clearance, and renal blood flow, as measured by paraaminohippurate clearance, are increased by 12% to 20% in patients with thyrotoxicosis and normalize during antithyroid treatment (9,11) (Fig. 33.1). Serum creatinine concentrations tend to be low in patients with thyrotoxicosis and increase during antithyroid treatment (11). Normal subjects given large doses of thyroid hormone have a decrease in serum creatinine concentrations before substantial muscle

wasting occurs. Mean 24-hour urine creatinine excretion is significantly lower in patients with thyrotoxicosis due to loss of muscle mass, and it occurs despite an increase in the renal tubular secretion of creatinine (12–14).

Thyrotoxicosis induces both hypertrophy and hyperplasia of renal tubular epithelial cells. The increases are proportional to the increases in glomerular filtration rate and renal plasma flow. Intrarenal renin and angiotensin production are increased, as a result of increased renal renin messenger RNA expression, which leads to an increase in plasma renin activity and plasma angiotensin II concentrations and renal hypertrophy (15). The renal hypertrophy can be prevented by the angiotensin II antagonist losartan, indicating that it is dependent on intrarenal renin–angiotensin activation (15). Thyroid hormone also stimulates renal production of epidermal growth factor and renal growth in young animals (16), independent of protein intake and pituitary activity (8).

The functional and morphologic changes in renal tubules that occur in thyrotoxicosis are accompanied by an increase in renal tubular capacity for active transport. For example, transepithelial voltage and Na^+,K^+-adenosine triphosphatase (ATPase) activity are increased, with consequent increases in sodium transport. T_4 also stimulates sodium-dependent phosphate transport in cultured renal tubular cells (17), without changing sodium-dependent transport of sulfate, glucose, or proline (18,19). In thyrotoxic rats, proximal tubular sodium-proton exchange is increased (19); in particular, the predominant isoform (NHE_3) of the exchanger in proximal tubules is increased (20). These changes are not associated with clinically important increases in reabsorption of phosphate or bicarbonate.

WATER AND ELECTROLYTE METABOLISM

Patients with thyrotoxicosis rarely have discernible abnormalities in water metabolism. Serum electrolyte concentrations are usually normal. Occasional patients have polydipsia and polyuria, with 24-hour urine volumes as high as 3 or 4 L (21), associated at times with slightly hypotonic plasma. Some thyrotoxic patients have mild impairment in urinary concentrating ability (22), but this is not clinically important (23), and release of vasopressin in response to osmotic stimuli is normal (24). The polyuria is due to increased thirst, an explanation supported by observations in thyrotoxic animals (25,26). In patients with thyrotoxicosis, the sensation of thirst is initiated at a lower serum osmolality than when they are euthyroid (24). This increase in thirst may be secondary to the thirst-stimulating effect of high plasma angiotensin II concentrations (27). The increased thirst (polydipsia) and polyuria revert to normal after treatment of thyrotoxicosis.

Patients with thyrotoxicosis have high plasma renin activity and serum atrial natriuretic peptide concentrations (2,28–30). A higher cardiac preload in thyrotoxicosis may initiate secretion of atrial natriuretic peptide (2). The increase in plasma renin activity and serum atrial natriuretic peptide concentrations may also be due to a direct effect of T_4 on gene expression (2). The high serum atrial natriuretic peptide concentrations may contribute to the decrease in peripheral vascular resistance in thyrotoxicosis (2).

Thyrotoxic patients have normal or low serum aldosterone concentrations, particularly in relation to their plasma renin activity (2,30). Urinary excretion of sodium and potassium is normal when patients consume usual amounts of those ions. Whereas total body exchangeable potassium is decreased in thyrotoxicosis, as a result of a decrease in total muscle mass (31), total exchangeable sodium is often increased. Thyrotoxicosis in rats reduces sodium retention (6), which may be caused by increased renal perfusion and perhaps high serum atrial natriuretic peptide concentrations.

EDEMA

Thyrotoxic patients may have pitting edema involving the ankles, legs, and sacrum (32). Periorbital edema is usually a manifestation of Graves' ophthalmopathy rather than of thyrotoxicosis. Edema in thyrotoxic patients results from renal salt and water retention in response to a reduction in effective arterial volume, and the sodium retention contributes to an increase in blood volume and venous pressure. The edema that develops under these circumstances does not imply the presence of congestive heart failure. In support of this concept, exercise testing in thyrotoxic patients with edema usually results in a substantial increase in cardiac output with little or no increase in right atrial or pulmonary artery pressure. If the additional circulatory load imposed by high cardiac output overwhelms myocardial reserve, or if myocardial function is impaired by organic heart disease or by the thyrotoxicosis itself, congestive failure ensues (see Chapter 31). Severe thyrotoxicosis also may be associated with protein-calorie malnutrition and hypoalbuminemia, an additional cause of plasma volume expansion and edema.

MINERAL METABOLISM

Thyrotoxicosis causes increased bone resorption, as evidenced by low bone density and an increase in markers of bone resorption, such as urinary excretion of hydroxyproline, pyridinoline and deoxypyridinoline cross-links, and N-telopeptide of type I collagen (33). There is a compensatory increase in bone formation, as evidenced by increased serum osteocalcin and bone-specific alkaline phosphatase concentrations (see Chapter 40) (33). The increase in bone resorption is greater than that of bone formation (33); the result is osteopenia, and in some patients osteoporosis. These changes in mineral metabolism result in an increase in serum calcium concentrations and occasionally in hypercalcemia. The increase in serum calcium concentrations inhibits parathyroid hormone secretion, resulting in hypercalciuria and decreased renal 1α-hydroxylation of 25-hydroxyvitamin D, and therefore decreased intestinal calcium absorption. Occasional patients have renal calculi, nephrocalcinosis, and reversible renal insufficiency (34).

All these changes, including osteoporosis, are reversible with treatment of thyrotoxicosis.

Thyrotoxicosis may result in magnesium deficiency, with decreased serum total and ionized magnesium concentrations, due to renal magnesium wasting (33). Low serum magnesium concentrations may contribute to the low serum parathyroid hormone concentrations in thyrotoxicosis.

URIC ACID METABOLISM

Patients with long-standing thyrotoxicosis may have high serum uric acid concentrations (11,35). In one study, 28% of patients with toxic nodular goiter and 39% of those with thyrotoxicosis caused by Graves' disease had hyperuricemia, as compared with 2% to 10% of normal subjects (11). Renal clearance of uric acid was increased in proportion to the increase in glomerular filtration rate, and therefore the fractional excretion of uric acid was normal (11). The occurrence of high serum uric acid concentrations in the presence of increased urinary clearance of uric acid indicates that production of uric acid is increased more than is renal uric acid clearance (11). The increase in uric acid production is most likely due to increased purine turnover. There are no reports of an increase in gout in thyrotoxic patients.

THYROTOXIC PERIODIC PARALYSIS

Thyrotoxic periodic paralysis is characterized by localized or generalized attacks of muscle weakness, even flaccid paralysis, that last for a few hours to several days. Most patients are men, with the male to female ratio being 20:1; Asian men are particularly susceptible to the disorder, but it has been described in many ethnic/racial groups (36–39). The episodes of muscle weakness are associated with a decrease in serum potassium concentrations, although the concentration is not always subnormal (40), and may be accompanied by hypophosphatemia and hypomagnesemia (41). Hypophosphatemia may be caused by cellular uptake of phosphate in conjunction with the cellular uptake of potassium. Total body potassium content is normal; the hypokalemia results from the shift of potassium into cells, and is associated with low urinary potassium excretion and a low transtubular potassium concentration gradient (41, 42).

Thyrotoxicosis increases Na^+, K^+-ATPase activity in kidney, liver, and other tissues, and the activity of the enzyme increases in response to adrenergic stimulation (43–45). An increase in activity of this enzyme could explain the shift in potassium, but its periodic activation is unexplained. Na^+,K^+-ATPase-independent activation of potassium uptake may be more important (46). The epidemiol-

ogy, clinical manifestations, and treatment of this unusual manifestation of thyrotoxicosis are discussed in more detail in Chapter 41.

RENAL TUBULAR ACIDOSIS

Occasional patients with thyrotoxicosis have renal tubular acidosis, which has been characterized as distal because there is failure to achieve maximal urinary acidification. Renal bicarbonate wasting (proximal renal tubular acidosis) has not been described; in fact, expression of the proximal tubular sodium proton exchanger is increased in patients with thyrotoxicosis (20,47). Hypokalemia, a common feature of distal renal tubular acidosis, may exacerbate a tendency to periodic paralysis. Renal tubular acidosis rarely results from hypercalcemia and hypercalciuria, which can cause nephrocalcinosis, tubular damage, and impairment of urinary acidification (34,48). Renal tubular acidosis also may occur in association with thyrotoxicosis caused by Graves' disease in the absence of nephrocalcinosis, and may persist after resolution of the thyrotoxicosis (49). The renal tubular acidosis in these patients may have an autoimmune basis; antibodies to renal tubular cells were demonstrated in the serum of one patient with Graves' thyrotoxicosis and renal tubular acidosis (50). Urine pH, serum bicarbonate concentrations, and urine calcium excretion should be measured in the occasional thyrotoxic patient who has nephrolithiasis (49). Some patients with autoimmune thyroid disease and renal tubular acidosis also have Sjögren's syndrome, and this syndrome by itself may be associated with renal tubular acidosis (51).

PROTEINURIA AND IMMUNE COMPLEX GLOMERULONEPHRITIS

Some patients with autoimmune thyroid disease (Graves' disease or chronic autoimmune thyroiditis) have proteinuria, which is usually mild; it was found in 36% of patients in one study, most of whom were euthyroid (52,53) (Fig. 33.1). Administration of T_4 induces proteinuria in rats, which is unaffected by partial blockade of nitric oxide synthase or losartan. Thus, proteinuria may be the result of a direct effect of T_4 excess on glomerular permeability (6). Minimal change nephropathy has been reported in patients with autoimmune thyroid disease, including one patient who had multiple simultaneous relapses of Graves' thyrotoxicosis and the nephrotic syndrome (53,54).

Immune complex glomerulonephritis has been described in a few patients with thyrotoxicosis, with immune complexes containing thyroglobulin and antithyroglobulin antibodies implicated as a cause of the renal disease (55–57). The most common renal lesion was membranous glomerulonephritis, although proliferative changes also have been described (55–58). Similar patterns of immune complex deposition have been reported in patients with chronic autoimmune thyroiditis and hypothyroidism (59). The relative rarity of this entity contrasts with the frequency of circulating immune complexes in thyroid disease, estimated to be as high as 17% in thyrotoxicosis and higher in chronic autoimmune thyroiditis (60).

Proteinuria and even the nephrotic syndrome have been reported in rare patients with Graves' thyrotoxicosis after treatment with radioiodine (52,61). Biopsy findings have included membranous nephropathy, and immunofluorescence microscopy in several patients revealed thyroglobulin and thyroid peroxidase in the glomerular basement membrane and the mesangium (61). These changes could occur as a result of autoimmunization caused by radiation-induced release of thyroid antigens, but more likely are simply related to the autoimmune thyroid disease.

RENAL COMPLICATIONS OF ANTITHYROID DRUG THERAPY

Renal complications of antithyroid drug therapy are rare. Proteinuria has been reported in patients taking propylthiouracil or, rarely, methimazole, usually in patients with a drug-induced vasculitis (62–64) or lupuslike reaction (65). The full syndrome of lupus erythematosus with diffuse proliferative lupus nephritis was reported in one patient treated with propylthiouracil (66). Antineutrophil cytoplasmic antibody (ANCA)–positive vasculitis is an uncommon but well-recognized complication of therapy with propylthiouracil (see Chapter 45). Both C-ANCA (cytoplasmic) and P-ANCA (perinuclear) related disease has been described. Nephritis with or without systemic involvement is present in about two thirds of ANCA-positive patients (67–70). The duration of propylthiouracil therapy in these patients before onset of nephritis varied from weeks to years, more often the latter. Cessation of therapy may result in remission of the renal disease, but because of persistent renal disease, some patients have been treated with a glucocorticoid or cyclophosphamide, and a few patients have had permanent renal disease (70).

Two patients with thyrotoxicosis who developed severe allergic interstitial nephritis causing acute renal failure soon after initiation of propylthiouracil therapy have been reported. Both patients had a generalized rash, eosinophilia, and fever; both required hemodialysis and improved with glucocorticoid therapy (71,72). Another patient with amiodarone-induced thyrotoxicosis developed acute renal failure due to acute interstitial nephritis

and fatal Stevens-Johnson syndrome while receiving propylthiouracil (73).

REFERENCES

1. Marcisz C, Jonderko G, Kucharz E. Changes of arterial pressure in patients with hyperthyroidism during therapy. *Med Sci Monit* 2002;8:CR502.
2. Diekman MJ, Harms MP, Endert E, et al. Endocrine factors related to changes in total peripheral vascular resistance after treatment of thyrotoxic and hypothyroid patients. *Eur J Endocrinol* 2001;144:339.
3. Quesada A, Sainz J, Wangensteen R, et al. Nitric oxide synthase activity in hyperthyroid and hypothyroid rats. *Eur J Endocrinol* 2002;147:117.
4. Napoli R, Biondi B, Guardasole V, et al. Impact of hyperthyroidism and its correction on vascular reactivity in humans. *Circulation* 2001;104:3076.
5. Basset A, Blanc J, Messas E, et al. Renin-angiotensin system contribution to cardiac hypertrophy in experimental hyperthyroidism: an echocardiographic study. *J Cardiovasc Pharmacol* 2001;37:163.
6. Rodriguez-Gomez I, Sainz J, Wangensteen R, et al. Increased pressor sensitivity to chronic nitric oxide deficiency in hyperthyroid rats. *Hypertension* 2003;42:220.
7. Marcisz C, Jonderko G, Kucharz EJ. Influence of short-time application of a low sodium diet on blood pressure in patients with hyperthyroidism or hypothyroidism during therapy. *Am J Hypertens* 2001;14:995.
8. Bradley SE, Stephan F, Coelho JB, et al. The thyroid and the kidney. *Kidney Int* 1974;6:346.
9. Hlad CJ, Bricker NS. Renal function and I131 clearance in hyperthyroidism and myxedema. *J Clin Endocrinol Metab* 1954;14:1539.
10. Singh G, Sharma AC, Thompson EB, et al. Renal endothelin mechanism in altered thyroid states. *Life Sci* 1994;54:1901.
11. Sato A, Shirota T, Shinoda T, et al. Hyperuricemia in patients with hyperthyroidism due to Graves' disease. *Metabolism* 1995;44:207.
12. Shirota T, Shinoda T, Yamada T, et al. Alteration of renal function in hyperthyroidism: increased tubular secretion of creatinine and decreased distal tubular delivery of chloride. *Metabolism* 1992;41:402.
13. Adlerberth A, Angeras U, Jagenburg R, et al. Urinary excretion of 3-methylhistidine and creatinine and serum concentrations of amino acids in hyperthyroid patients following preoperative treatment with antithyroid drug or β-blocking agents: results from a prospective, randomized study. *Metabolism* 1987;36:637.
14. Ford HC, Lim WC, Chisnall WN, et al. Renal function and electrolyte levels in hyperthyroidism: urinary protein excretion and the plasma concentrations of urea, creatinine, urine acid, hydrogen ion and electrolytes. *Clin Endocrinol (Oxf)* 1989;30:293.
15. Kobori H, Ichihara A, Miyashita Y, et al. Mechanism of hyperthyroidism-induced renal hypertrophy in rats. *J Endocrinol* 1998;159:9.
16. Tang MJ, Lin YJ, Huang JJ. Thyroid hormone upregulates gene expression, synthesis and release of pro-epidermal growth factor in adult rat kidney. *Life Sci* 1995;57:1477.
17. Noronha-Blob L, Lowe V, Sacktor B. Stimulation by thyroid hormone of phosphate transport in primary cultured renal cells. *J Cell Physiol* 1988;137:95.

18. Beers KW, Dousa TP. Thyroid hormone stimulates the Na$^+$-PO$_4$ symporter but not the Na$^+$-SO$_4$ symporter in renal brush border. *Am J Physiol* 1993;265:F323.

19. Kinsella J, Sacktor B. Thyroid hormones increase Na$^+$/K$^+$ exchange activity in renal brush border membranes. *Proc Natl Acad Sci U S A* 1985;82:3606.

20. Azuma KK, Balkovetz DF, Magyar CE, et al. Renal Na$^+$/H$^+$ exchanger isoforms and their regulation by thyroid hormone. *Am J Physiol* 1996;270:C585.

21. Evered DC, Hayter CJ, Surveyor I. Primary polydipsia in thyrotoxicosis. *Metabolism* 1972;21:393.

22. Cutler RE, Glatte H, Dowling JT. Effect of hyperthyroidism on the renal concentrating mechanism in humans. *J Clin Endocrinol* 1967;27:453.

23. Katz AI, Emmanouel DS, Lindheimer MD. Thyroid hormone and the kidney. *Nephron* 1975;15:223.

24. Harvey JN, Nagi DK, Baylis PH, et al. Disturbance of osmoregulated thirst and vasopressin secretion in thyrotoxicosis. *Clin Endocrinol (Oxf)* 1991;35:29.

25. Thoday KL, Monney CT. Historical, clinical and laboratory features of 126 hyperthyroid cats. *Vet Record* 1992;131:257.

26. Hoey A, Page A, Brown L, et al. Cardiac changes in experimental hyperthyroidism in dogs. *Aust Vet J* 1991;68:352.

27. Phillips PA, Rolls BJ, Ledingham GG, et al. Angiotensin II–induced thirst and vasopressin release in man. *Clin Sci* 1985;68:669.

28. Rolandi E, Santaniello B, Bagnasco M, et al. Thyroid hormones and atrial natriuretic hormone secretion: study in hyper- and hypothyroid patients. *Acta Endocrinol (Copenh)* 1992;127:23.

29. Tajiri J, Noguchi S, Naomi S, et al. Plasma atrial natriuretic peptide in patients with Graves' disease. *Endocrinol Jpn* 1990;37:665.

30. Shigimatsu S, Iwasaki T, Aizawa T, et al. Plasma atrial natriuretic peptide, plasma renin activity and aldosterone during treatment of hyperthyroidism due to Graves' disease. *Horm Metab Res* 1989;21:514.

31. Aikawa JK. Isotopic studies of the body potassium content in thyrotoxicosis. *Proc Soc Exp Biol Med* 1953;84:594.

32. Klatsky SA, Manson PN. Thyroid disorders masquerading as aging changes. *Ann Plastic Surg* 1992;28:420.

33. Pantazi H, Papapetrou PD. Changes in parameters of bone and mineral metabolism during therapy for hyperthyroidism. *J Clin Endocrinol Metab* 2000;85:1099.

34. Epstein FH, Freedman LR, Levitan H. Hypercalcemia, nephrocalcinosis and reversible renal insufficiency associated with hyperthyroidism. *N Engl J Med* 1958;258:782.

35. Giordano N, Santacroce C, Mattii G, et al. Hyperuricemia and gout in thyroid endocrine disorders. *Clin Exp Rheumatol* 2001;19:661.

36. Ahlawat SK, Sachdev A. Hypokalaemic paralysis. *Postgrad Med J* 1999;75:193.

37. Shulkin D, Olson BR, Levey GS. Thyrotoxic periodic paralysis in a Latin-American taking acetazolamide. *Am J Med Sci* 1989;297:337.

38. Mellgren G, Bleskestad IH, Aanderud S, et al. Thyrotoxicosis and paraparesis in a young woman: case report and review of the literature. *Thyroid* 2002;12:77.

39. Ober KP. Thyrotoxic periodic paralysis in the United States: report of 7 cases and review of the literature. *Medicine* 1992;71:109.

40. Yeo PP, O'Neill WC. Thyrotoxicosis and periodic paralysis. *Med Grand Rounds* 1984;3:10.

41. Lin SH, Davids MR, Halperin ML. Hypokalaemia and paralysis. *Q J Med* 2003;96:161.

42. Shizume K, Shishiba Y, Sakuma M, et al. Studies on electrolyte metabolism in idiopathic and thyrotoxic periodic paralysis. II: total exchangeable sodium and potassium. *Metabolism* 1966;15:145.

43. Kubota K, Ingbar SH. Influences of thyroid states and sympathoadrenal system on extrarenal potassium disposal. *Am J Physiol* 1990;258:E428.

44. Chan A, Shinde R, Chow CC, et al. *In vivo* and *in vitro* sodium pump activity in subjects with thyrotoxic periodic paralysis. *BMJ* 1991;303:1096.

45. Sterns RH, Spital A. Disorders of internal potassium balance. *Semin Nephrol* 1987;7:399.

46. Oh VMS, Taylor EA, Yeo SH, et al. Cation transport across lymphocytic plasma membranes in euthyroid and thyrotoxic men with and without hypokalaemic periodic paralysis. *Clin Sci* 1990;78:199.

47. Baum M, Dwarakanath V, Alpern RJ, et al. Effects of thyroid hormone on the neonatal renal cortical Na$^+$/H$^+$ antiporter. *Kidney Int* 1998;53:1254.

48. Dash SC, Jain S, Khanna KN, et al. Thyrotoxicosis, renal tubular acidosis and renal stone. *J Assoc Phys India* 1980;28:323.

49. Jaeger P, Portmann L, Wauters JP, et al. Report of 1 case without nephrocalcinosis. *Am J Nephrol* 1985;5:116.

50. Konishi K, Hayashi M, Saruta T. Renal tubular acidosis with autoantibody directed to renal collecting-duct cells. *N Engl J Med* 1994;331:1593.

51. Mason A, Golding PL. Renal tubular acidosis and autoimmune thyroid disease. *Lancet* 1970;2:1104.

52. Weetman AP, Tomlinson K, Amos N, et al. Proteinuria in autoimmune thyroid disease. *Acta Endocrinol (Copenh)* 1985;109:341.

53. Holt S, Kingdon E, Morganstein D, et al. Simultaneous relapse of Graves' disease and minimal change glomerular disease. *Nephrol Dial Transplant* 2002;17:666.

54. Tanwani LK, Lohano V, Broadstone VL, et al. Minimal change nephropathy and Graves' disease: report of a case and review of the literature. *Endocr Pract* 2002;8:40.

55. Jordan SC, Buckingham B, Sakai R, et al. Studies of immune complex glomerulonephritis mediated by human thyroglobulin. *N Engl J Med* 1981;304:121.

56. O'Regan S, Fong JS, Kaplan BS, et al. Thyroid antigen-antibody nephritis. *Clin Immunol Immunopathol* 1976;6:341.

57. Matsuura M, Kikkawa Y, Akashi K, et al. Thyroid antigen-antibody nephritis: possible involvement of fucosyl-GMI as the antigen. *Endocrinol Jpn* 1987;34:587.

58. Horvath F, Teague P, Gaffney EF, et al. Thyroid antigen associated immune complex glomerulonephritis in Graves' disease. *Am J Med* 1979;67:901.

59. Jordan SC, Johnston WH, Bergstein JM. Immune complex glomerulonephritis mediated by thyroid antigens. *Arch Pathol Lab Med* 1978;102:530.

60. Calder EA, Penhale WJ, Barnes EW, et al. Evidence for circulating immune complexes in thyroid disease. *BMJ* 1974;2:30.

61. Becker BA, Fenves AZ, Breslau NA. Membranous glomerulonephritis associated with Graves' disease. *Am J Kidney Dis* 1999;33:369.

62. Griswold WR, Mendoza SA, Johnston W, et al. Vasculitis associated with propylthiouracil: evidence for immune complex pathogenesis and response to therapy. *West J Med* 1978;128:543.

63. McCormick RV. Periarteritis occurring during propylthiouracil therapy. *JAMA* 1950;144:1453.

64. Cassorla FG, Finegold DN, Parks JS, et al. Vasculitis, pulmonary cavitation, and anemia during antithyroid drug therapy. *Am J Dis Child* 1983;137:118.

65. Amrhein JA, Kenny FM, Ross D. Granulocytopenia, lupus-like syndrome, and other complications of propylthiouracil therapy. *J Pediatr* 1970;76:54.

66. Prasad GV, Bastacky S, Johnson JP. Propylthiouracil-induced diffuse proliferative lupus nephritis: review of immunological complications. *J Am Soc Nephrol* 1997;8:1205.

67. D'Cruz D, Chesser AM, Lightowler C, et al. Antineutrophil cytoplasmic antibody-positive crescentic glomerulonephritis associated with anti-thyroid drug treatment. *Br J Rheumatol* 1995; 34:1090.

68. Dolman KM, Gans RO, Vervaat TJ, et al. Vasculitis and antineutrophil cytoplasmic autoantibodies associated with propylthiouracil therapy. *Lancet* 1993;342:651.

69. Reynolds LR, Bhathena D. Nephrotic syndrome associated with methimazole therapy. *Arch Intern Med* 1979;139:236.

70. Winters MJ, Hurley RM, Lirenman DS. ANCA-positive glomerulonephritis and IgA nephropathy in a patient on propylthiouracil. *Pediatr Nephrol* 2002;17:257.

71. Reinhart SC, Moses AM, Cleary L, et al. Acute interstitial nephritis with renal failure associated with propylthiouracil therapy. *Am J Kidney Dis* 1994;24:575.

72. Fang JT, Huang CC. Propylthiouracil-induced acute interstitial nephritis with acute renal failure requiring haemodialysis: successful therapy with steroids. *Nephrol Dial Transplant* 1998;13: 757.

73. Dysseleer A, Buysschaert M, Fonck C, et al. Acute interstitial nephritis and fatal Stevens-Johnson syndrome after propylthiouracil therapy. *Thyroid* 2000;10:713.

THE GASTROINTESTINAL TRACT AND LIVER IN THYROTOXICOSIS

SANJEEV M. WASAN
JOSEPH H. SELLIN
RENA VASSILOPOULOU-SELLIN

The classic gastrointestinal (GI) manifestations of thyrotoxicosis are rapid intestinal transit, increased frequency of semi-formed stools, and weight loss from increased caloric requirement or malabsorption. This classic scenario is not necessarily common, and a caveat is in order. Although there are definite GI manifestations of thyrotoxicosis, their lack of specificity is such that they cannot serve as reliable diagnostic clues to the diagnosis. One may find, instead, a paradoxic weight gain despite the hypermetabolic state. The absence of constipation in the elderly patient occasionally has pointed the astute clinician to the diagnosis of thyrotoxicosis. Thyrotoxicosis has been associated with a multiplicity of liver-function abnormalities; however, the interpretation of these derangements may be clouded by the coexistence of congestive heart failure, malnutrition, or autoimmune liver disease. The clinical importance of a direct effect of thyrotoxicosis on the liver, through increased metabolic demand and a relative hypoxia, remains controversial. Because the diagnosis of thyrotoxicosis now can be made easily, more accurately, and earlier, and because effective treatment can promptly correct the symptoms and metabolic consequences of this disorder, prominent GI symptoms usually are confined to cases of diagnostic oversight.

The findings of GI dysfunction associated with thyrotoxicosis suggest that an excess of thyroid hormone disrupts the normal homeostatic mechanisms of the gut. Additionally, they point to a possible role for thyroid hormone in the physiology of the GI tract and liver and serve as a basis for further investigation into the peripheral effects of thyroid hormone.

THYROTOXICOSIS AND GUT MOTILITY

Frequent bowel movements (more than two a day) are significantly more common in patients with thyrotoxicosis than in normal subjects (1). Most thyrotoxic patients, however, have one bowel movement daily. Although constipation is rare, 3% of thyrotoxic patients take laxatives, about the same as in the general population, thus limiting the value of stool frequency as a clue toward the clinical diagnosis of thyrotoxicosis in an individual patient.

The increased stool frequency is generally ascribed to "hypermotility" of the intestine; however, the physiologic correlates of hypermotility are poorly defined, and the interrelationships between myoelectric activity (propulsive events and transit time) (2–4) and contractile force (5) need to be delineated more clearly.

Thyrotoxicosis may cause myopathy, leading to altered function of pharyngeal and upper esophageal muscles. As a result, patients may complain of dysphagia, which is reversed with correction of the thyroid excess. The esophagus has an increased rate of peristaltic propagation (6).

Studies of gastric emptying have yielded variable results. Despite expectations that gastric emptying might be accelerated, in clinical studies emptying was either normal or delayed (7–9). No specific relationship between dyspepsia and thyrotoxicosis has been demonstrated. Vomiting associated with thyrotoxicosis has been ascribed to either thyroid stimulation of a chemoreceptor trigger zone in the central nervous system (10) or to gastric stasis (11). Recent studies using electrogastrography (EGG) to measure gastric myoelectrical activity, revealed gastric dysrhythmia in both hypothyroid and thyrotoxic patients (12).

In thyrotoxicosis, the mouth-to-cecum transit time is approximately 40% of normal, and small and large intestinal transit is accelerated (13,14). These changes are reversible after correction of the thyrotoxicosis. Christensen and associates (15) demonstrated that the basic electric rhythm of slow-wave activity of the intestine is increased in thyrotoxicosis, indicating that the intestine is capable of more frequent contractions. In a study examining contractile rather than myoelectric activity, thyrotoxicosis induced changes in both the fasted and fed states, including an increase in contraction frequency during phase 2 of the migrating motor complex during digestion (5), and occasional giant migrating complexes were observed. By using a noninvasive measure of orocecal transit time, the lactulose–hydrogen breath test, investigators have demonstrated a shortened transit time in thyrotoxic patients that normalizes with treatment, with disappearance of gastrointestinal symptoms such as diarrhea and steatorrhea (14,16,17). Abnormalities of anal manometry and rectal sensation also exist in patients with altered thyroid function, with lower threshold sensation in thyrotoxic patients (18).

The clinical and experimental data on the effects of thyrotoxicosis on gut motility provide some evidence that thyroid excess affects the orderly propulsion of ingested materials through the GI tract. Significant gaps exist, however, in our knowledge of the thyrotoxic effects on intestinal motility.

GASTRIC FUNCTION IN THYROTOXICOSIS

The association between thyrotoxicosis and pernicious anemia was first described by Neuser (19) in 1899; since then, a strong clinical impression has prevailed that spontaneous thyroid disease and autoimmune gastritis coincide more frequently than expected by statistical probability. Pernicious anemia has been reported in 2% to 5% of thyrotoxic patients (3,20). The frequency of parietal cell or intrinsic factor antibodies as well as low serum vitamin B_{12} or intrinsic factor levels, however, has been on the order of 20% to 30% of patients (21,22). Atrophic gastritis, decreased acid secretion, and histamine-fast hypochlorhydria or achlorhydria have been found in thyrotoxic patients, even without overt pernicious anemia (23). Approximately one third of patients with autoimmune thyroid disease have atrophic gastritis (24). Hypergastrinemia also is found occasionally. The incidence of peptic ulcer disease is not increased; therefore, the hypergastrinemia is most probably secondary to decreased acid secretion. It is likely that the frequently coexisting abnormalities of thyroid and gastric function reflect the association of autoimmune hyperthyroid disease with other autoimmune diseases.

ABSORPTION AND INTESTINAL FUNCTION

Steatorrhea can occur in patients with thyrotoxicosis (23, 25,26), with daily fecal fat excretion as high as 20 g (normal, <7 g daily assuming a daily intake of 100 g fat). This cannot be ascribed exclusively to fat hyperphagia; an element of malabsorption appears to exist, although the cause remains obscure. Pancreatic exocrine function, as measured by standard secretion tests, is normal.

Small bowel biopsies in thyrotoxic patients have not demonstrated any alteration in the normal villous architecture, although minor increases in lymphocytic infiltration and edema have been observed. Small bowel radiographs have noted occasional dilatation and thickening of the circular folds (27). Intestinal absorption of D-xylose is normal. Decreased calcium absorption was demonstrated in clinical

and animal studies (28,29), perhaps due to deficient parathyroid-mediated synthesis of $1,25(OH)_2$ vitamin D.

Rapid intestinal transit is the generally accepted explanation for the steatorrhea of thyrotoxicosis. Analogous to postgastrectomy states, inadequate mixing of food and pancreatic secretions occurs as the intestinal chyme precedes the digestive enzymes through the length of the small bowel; maldigestion results because dietary fat, protein, and carbohydrates are not adequately broken down into components that a normal intestinal mucosa can absorb. An alternative explanation may involve thyroid down-regulation of intestinal brush-border enzymes, such as lactase, inducing selective carbohydrate malabsorption or steatorrhea (30). Propranolol therapy decreases both stool frequency and the amount of steatorrhea, suggesting that some of the intestinal findings are mediated by the sympathetic nervous system (31).

A significant association exists between autoimmune thyroid disorders and intestinal diseases with significant immune components. Careful surveys of patients with autoimmune thyroid disease demonstrated an approximate 5% incidence of celiac sprue; as for the converse, surveys in patients with sprue have revealed a 5% to 15% incidence of thyroid disease (32–35). Subclinical hypothyroidism is a frequent finding in celiac disease that is often normalized with strict gluten withdrawal (36). A study indicated that as many as 43% of patients with Hashimoto's thyroiditis had an increased density of the $\gamma\delta$ T-cell receptor–bearing intraepithelial lymphocytes and signs of mucosal T-cell activation, both features of celiac disease (37). Up to 4% of patients with ulcerative colitis have thyroid disorders (38,39). Thyrotoxicosis may exacerbate ulcerative colitis. The thyroid disease often appears before the colitis, but may occur simultaneously and impair the response to therapy. A hypermetabolic state may make the intestine more susceptible to damage from inflammation, related to autoantibodies or circulating immune complexes (40); a similar picture may occur in the liver (41). Treatment of the intestinal disorder is simplified after therapy for thyrotoxicosis. Secretory diarrhea may rarely occur (42).

THE LIVER IN THYROID DISEASE

The association between the liver and thyroid diseases has been a subject of investigation for over 50 years, but the exact nature of the relationship remains elusive. Possible thyroid–liver interactions include (a) liver damage secondary to the systemic effects of thyroid excess, (b) direct toxic effects of thyroid hormone on the liver, (c) association of intrinsic liver disease with intrinsic thyroid disease through autoimmune mechanisms, (d) alterations of thyroid hormone metabolism secondary to intrinsic liver disease, and (e) subclinical physiologic effects of thyroid hormone on liver function.

Early autopsy reports emphasized the severity of liver disease in patients dying of thyrotoxicosis (43) and described marked hepatic inflammation, steatosis, necrosis, and cirrhosis. It is not clear whether these were a direct effect of thyrotoxicosis or were caused by associated conditions (congestive heart failure, infection, or malnutrition) that can, in themselves, lead to hepatic dysfunction. Hepatic changes seen on light microscopy include vacuolization of hepatocytes, balloon degeneration, nuclear glycogen, and mild portal infiltration of mononuclear cells; electron microscopy reveals subtle ultrastructural changes, including hyperplasia of the smooth endoplasmic reticulum, a paucity of glycogen, and mitochondrial abnormalities (44). These are all nonspecific signs of liver injury. Abnormal liver function tests can often occur in thyrotoxic patients, especially with mild elevations of serum alkaline phosphatase or aminotransferases, with prevalence varying from 15% to 76%; these abnormalities are reversible with correction of the thyrotoxicosis (45–47). In patients receiving antithyroid drug therapy, it is important to consider that liver function abnormalities may be drug induced. Propylthiouracil therapy can result in mild elevation in liver enzymes, which is often transient and subclinical (48). Therapy is continued unless fulminant hepatotoxicity develops, which has been reported in a few cases (49). Methimazole therapy may rarely cause cholestasis and fulminant hepatic failure if the drug is continued (49a). Liver test abnormalities and hepatotoxicity occur more frequently in women, and tend to occur 3 to 4 months after therapy is begun. Baseline hepatic function tests are usually not performed before the initiation of propylthiouracil, so the true incidence of hepatotoxicity is not known (50).

Within the context of the generalized hypermetabolic state of thyrotoxicosis, resting metabolic rate and hepatic oxygen consumption increase (51), probably secondary to increased Na^+,K^+-ATPase activity. Increased hepatic oxygen uptake also has been described, despite normal fructose-6-phosphate and pentose cycling (52). The metabolic impact of thyroid hormone on the liver appears multifactorial, mediated by alterations of insulin-like growth factor homeostasis (53), cytochrome P450 regulation (54), and changes in fatty acid and lipid synthesis (55). Although mitochondrial metabolism is stimulated by thyroid hormone, it has been difficult to establish a clear-cut relationship between mitochondrial metabolism and thyroid function (56,57). Because hepatic blood flow is not increased (58), a combination of relative anoxia and increased metabolic demands develops that may lead to the centrizonal necrosis occasionally seen in severe thyrotoxicosis. A hypermetabolic state may make the liver more susceptible to injury. This has been observed in several experimental and clinical conditions, including ischemia-reperfusion and cold storage (59), drug-induced liver failure (60), and alcoholic hepatitis (61–63). Although propylthiouracil has been used clinically in the treatment of alcoholic hepatitis with possible

benefit, it has not achieved widespread acceptance as standard therapy among hepatologists.

No firm evidence has been found that thyroid hormone is directly toxic to the liver. Therefore, the thyrotoxic patients who present with liver dysfunction require careful investigation for nonthyroidal illness; this investigation frequently results in the detection of an autoimmune disorder because multisystem autoimmune diseases may affect both the liver and the thyroid (64). Perhaps the strongest association exists between lymphocytic thyroiditis and primary biliary cirrhosis (65,66). In a survey of 95 patients with primary biliary cirrhosis, Crowe and colleagues (67) found that 26% had thyroid microsomal antibodies, 16% had thyroglobulin antibodies, and 16% had either clinical or biochemical evidence of hypothyroidism.

THYROID FUNCTION IN LIVER DISEASE

The interpretation of concomitant thyroid and liver function abnormalities must take into account the fact that thyroid hormone metabolism is abnormal in severe liver disease. Both the production of thyroxine (T_4)-binding globulin (TBG) and the peripheral conversion of T_4 to triiodothyronine (T_3) may be decreased in patients with chronic liver disease. Conversely, serum TBG concentrations increase in patients with hepatitis, probably due to decreased clearance of TBG secondary to its increased sialic acid content (68). Despite the increased energy expenditure found in cirrhosis (69), most patients with cirrhosis are clinically euthyroid. In patients with chronic hepatitis C, therapeutic administration of interferon-α may precipitate clinical thyroid dysfunction, especially if antithyroid antibodies were present before treatment (70).

Several investigators have systematically examined thyroid function in patients with hepatitis and cirrhosis (usually alcohol-related). Despite considerable variability in serum total T_4 concentrations, serum free T_4 index values are usually normal or mildly increased, serum T_3 concentrations are usually decreased, and thyrotropin reverse T_3 concentrations are high (71–73). In cirrhosis, basal serum (TSH) concentrations may be high, and the TSH response to thyrotropin-releasing hormone is not different from that of normal subjects (73,74). Overall, this picture is most consistent with the changes that occur in systemic nonthyroidal illness (see section on nonthyroidal illness in Chapter 11).

THYROID HORMONE EFFECTS ON PHYSIOLOGIC FUNCTION OF GUT AND LIVER

The liver handles thyroid hormone similarly to the way it handles several organic anions. T_4 and T_3 are glucuronidated and sulfated, secreted into the biliary canaliccli, and concentrated in bile. The daily biliary excretion of T_4

(20 mmol) is miniscule compared with that of other organic anions (e.g., 600 mol bilirubin). Thyroid hormone has profound effects on hepatic organic anion transport and biliary excretion. Although bilirubin glucuronide formation is not changed *in vitro,* extrahepatic factors result in abnormal bilirubin metabolism *in vivo* (75,76). In experimental animals, thyrotoxicosis is associated with an increased bilirubin output in bile, which may result from increased degradation of hepatic heme (77). Thyroid-induced alterations in hepatic metabolism of bilirubin, specifically a decrease in glucuronyl transferase, may be responsible for the clinical occurrence of unconjugated hyperbilirubinemia, possibly by unmasking previously unrecognized Gilbert's syndrome (77).

Thyroid hormone decreases bile acid production and total bile acid pool size (78). Clinically, duodenal bile salt concentration in thyrotoxic patients appears to be normal (79). The clinical import of thyroid-induced alterations in organic anion excretion, bile flow, and microsomal enzyme activity requires further investigation but points to the important effects of thyroid hormone in normal liver function.

THYROID DISEASE AND CANCER

Medullary carcinoma of the thyroid (MCT) is a calcitonin-producing tumor of the thyroid gland. Calcitonin and calcitonin gene–related peptide (CGRP) are primary markers of MCT (80). One third of patients with this carcinoma develop a watery diarrhea, which is thought to be due to the high serum concentrations of calcitonin or CGRP. Initial studies suggested that calcitonin induces small intestinal fluid secretion; however, decreased colonic water absorption secondary to a motor disturbance may be the main mechanism of diarrhea in these patients (81,82).

Many patients with gastric cancer have been found to have antithyroid antibodies, as many as 25% in one study, but the presence of these antibodies did not necessarily indicate thyroid dysfunction (83).

Thyroid carcinomas can invade the aerodigestive tract, including the larynx, pharynx, and esophagus. A retrospective study found that papillary thyroid carcinoma, when invasive, involved the esophagus in 21% of cases (84). When thyroid carcinoma does invade the aerodigestive tract, complete resection offers prolonged palliation and best opportunity for cure (85). An association also appears to exist between carcinomas of the esophagus and the thyroid, albeit infrequent. Metachronous or synchronous esophageal cancer has been identified in patients with head and neck cancer and in other locations of the gastrointestinal tract, but cases also include the thyroid (86). Other primary gastrointestinal carcinomas also rarely metastasize to the thyroid gland.

Patients with familial adenomatous polyposis (FAP) have an increased incidence of extracolonic cancer, including thyroid cancer (87). Papillary thyroid cancer is the most common type and tends to occur in women with FAP more than in men. It is usually solitary and unilateral. Thyroid cancer tends to cluster in specific families with FAP. It may be that the mutation of the Adenomatous Polyposis Coli (APC) tumor-suppressor gene responsible for FAP is involved in the pathogenesis of thyroid cancer, but this is speculative (88).

SUMMARY

Thyroid hormones play an important role in the normal physiology of GI function; when present in excess, they may result most notably in hypermotility and malabsorption. Patients with thyrotoxicosis may have associated hepatic or gastric dysfunction because of underlying autoimmune disease. Overall, early detection and effective treatment have changed the clinical presentation of thyrotoxicosis so that GI symptoms have become clinically subtle in most patients.

REFERENCES

1. Baker JT, Harvey RF. Bowel habits in thyrotoxicosis and hyperthyroidism. *BMJ* 1971;1:322.
2. Nepotent MI, Spesivtseva VG. Motor function of gastrointestinal tract before and after I131 therapy in patients with thyrotoxicosis. *Fed Proc* 1963;22:T1177.
3. Schiller KRFR, Spray GH, Wangel AG, et al. Clinical and precursory forms of pernicious anaemia in hyperthyroidism. *Q J Med* 1968;174:451.
4. Wegener M, Wedmann B, Langhoff T, et al. Effect of hyperthyroidism on the transit of a caloric solid-liquid meal through the stomach, the small intestine, and the colon in man. *J Clin Endocrinol Metab* 1992;75:745.
5. Karaus M, Wienbeck M, Grussendorf M, et al. Intestinal motor activity in experimental hyperthyroidism in conscious dogs. *Gastroenterology* 1989;97:911.
6. Meshkinpour H, Afrasiabi MA, Valenta LJ. Esophageal motor function in Graves' disease. *Dig Dis Sci* 1979;24:159.
7. Jonderko K, Jonderko G, Marcisz C, Golab T. Gastric emptying in hyperthyroidism. *Am J Gastroenterol* 1997;92:835.
8. Barczynski M, Thor P. Reversible autonomic dysfunction in hyperthyroid patients affects gastric myoelectrical activity and emptying. *Clin Auton Res* 2001;11:243.
9. Pfaffenbach B, Adamek RJ, Hagelman D, et al. Effect of hyperthyroidism on antral myoelectric activity, gastric emptying and dyspepsia in man. *Hepatogastroenterology* 1997;44:1500.
10. Rosenthal DG, Jones C, Lewis SI. Thyrotoxic vomiting. *BMJ* 1976;2:209.
11. Parkin AJ, Bishop N, Nisbet AP. Vomiting due to gastric stasis as the presenting feature in thyrotoxicosis. *Postgrad Med J* 1982;57:405.
12. Gunsar F, et al. Effect of hypo- and hyperthyroidism on gastric myoelectrical activity. *Dig Dis Sci.* 2003;48:706.
13. Wegener M, et al. Effect of hyperthyroidism on the transit of a caloric solid-liquid meal through the stomach, the small intestine, and the colon in man. *J Clin Endocrinol Metab* 1992; 75: 745.
14. Shafer RB, Prentiss R, Bond JH. Gastrointestinal transit in thyroid disease. *Gastroenterology* 1984;86:852.

15. Christensen J, Schedl HP, Clifton JA. The basic electrical rhythm of the duodenum in normal human subjects and in patients with thyroid disease. *J Clin Invest* 1964;43:1659.
16. Tobin MV, Fisken RA, Diggory RT, et al. Orocaecal transit time in health and in thyroid disease. *Gut* 1989;30:26.
17. Papa A, et al. Effects of propylthiouracil on intestinal transit time and symptoms in hyperthyroid patients. *Hepatogastroenterology* 1997;44:426.
18. Deen KI, et al. Anorectal physiology and transit in patients with disorders of thyroid metabolism. *J Gastroenterol Hepatol* 1999; 14:384.
19. Neuser E. Anemia. *Wein Klin Wschr* 1899;122:288.
20. Furszyfer J, McConahey WM, Kurland LT, et al. On the increased association of Graves' disease with pernicious anemia. *Mayo Clin Proc* 1971;46:37.
21. Doniach D, Roitt IM, Taylor KP. Autoimmune phenomena in pernicious anema: serological overlap with thyroiditis, thyrotoxicosis, and systemic lupus erythematosus. *BMJ* 1963;1:1374.
22. Burman P, Kampe O, Kraaz W, et al. A study of autoimmune gastritis in the postpartum period and at a 5-year follow-up. *Gastroenterology* 1992;103:934.
23. Siurala M, Julkunen H, Lamberg BA. Gastrointestinal tract in hyperthyroidism before and after treatment. *Lancet* 1966;1:79.
24. Centanni M, et al. Atrophic body gastritis in patients with autoimmune thyroid disease: an underdiagnosed association. *Arch Intern Med* 1999;159:1726.
25. Goswani R, et al. Prevalence and significance of steatorrhea in patients with active Graves' disease. *Am J Gastroenterol* 1998;93: 1122.
26. Thomas FB, Caldwell JH, Greenberger NJ. Steatorrhea thyrotoxicosis: relation to hypermotility and excessive dietary fat. *Ann Intern Med* 1973;78:669.
27. Hellesen C, Friis Th, Larson S, et al. Small intestinal histology, radiology and absorption in hyperthyroidism. *Scand J Gastroenterol* 1968;4:169.
28. Noble HM, Matty AJ. The effect of thyroxine on the movement of calcium and inorganic phosphate through the small intestine of the rat. *J Endocrinol* 1967;37:111.
29. Peerenboom H, et al. The defect of intestinal calcium transport in hyperthyroidism and its response to therapy. *J Clin Endocrinol Metab* 1984;59:936.
30. Szilagy A, Lerman A, Barr RG, et al. Reversible lactose malabsorption and intolerance in Graves' disease. *Clin Invest* 1992;14:188.
31. Bricker LA, et al. Intractable diarrhea in hyperthyroidism: management with beta-adrenergic blockade. *Endocr Pract* 2001;7:28.
32. Volta U, Ravaglia G, et al. Coeliac disease in patients with autoimmune thyroiditis. *Digestion* 2001;64:61.
33. Counsell CE, Taha A, Ruddell S. Coeliac disease and autoimmune thyroid disease. *Gut* 1994;35:844.
34. Collin P, Kaukinen K, et al. Endocrinological disorders and celiac disease. *Endocr Rev* 2002;23:464.
35. Cuoco L, et al. Prevalence and early diagnosis of coeliac disease in autoimmune thyroid disorders. *Ital J Gastroenterol Hepatol* 1999;31:283.
36. Sategna-Guidetti C, et al. Prevalence of thyroid disorders in untreated adult celiac disease patients and effect of gluten withdrawal: an Italian multicenter study. *Am J Gastroenterol* 2001;96:751.
37. Valentino R, et al. Markers of potential coeliac disease in patients with Hashimoto's thyroiditis. *Eur J Endocrinol* 2002;146(4):479.
38. Modebe O. Autoimmune thyroid disease with ulcerative colitis. *Postgrad Med J* 1986;62:475.
39. Jarnerot G, et al. The thyroid in ulcerative colitis and Crohn's disease. II. Thyroid enlargement and hyperthyroidism in ulcerative colitis. *Acta Med Scand* 1975;197:83.
40. Bonapace ES, et al. Simultaneous occurrence of inflammatory bowel disease and thyroid disease. *Am J Gastroenterol* 2001;96: 1925.

41. Oren R, Maaravi Y, Karmel F, et al. Anti-thyroid drugs decrease mucosal damage in a rat model of experimental colitis. *Aliment Pharmacol Ther* 1997;11:341.
42. Culp KS, Piziak VK. Thyrotoxicosis presenting with secretory diarrhea. *Ann Intern Med* 1986;105:216.
43. Weller CV. Hepatic pathology in exophthalmic goiter. *Ann Intern Med* 1933;7:687.
44. Klion FM, Segal R, Schaffner F. The effect of altered thyroid function on the ultrastructure of the human liver. *Am J Med* 1971;50:317.
45. Huang MJ, Liaw YF. Clinical associations between thyroid and liver diseases. *J Gastro Hepatol* 1995;10:344.
46. Bicoveanu M, Hasinski, S. Abnormal results of liver function tests in patients with Graves' disease. *Endocr Pract* 2000;6: 367.
47. Gurlek A, Cobankara V, et al. Liver tests in hyperthyroidism: effect of antithyroid therapy. *J Clin Gastroenterol* 1997;24:180.
48. Liaw YF, Huang MJ, Fan KD, et al. Hepatic injury during propylthiouracil therapy in patients with hyperthyroidism: a cohort study. *Ann Intern Med* 1993;118:424.
49. Ruiz, J, et al. Fulminant hepatic failure associated with propylthiouracil. *Ann Pharm* 2003;37:224–228.
49a. Woeber KA. Methimazole-induced hepatotoxicity. *Endocr Pract* 2002;8:222–224.
50. Williams KV, et al. Fifty years of experience with propylthiouracil-associated hepatotoxicity: what have we learned? *J Clin Endocr Metab* 1997;82:1727.
51. Iossa S, Liverini G, Barletta A. Relationship between the resting metabolic rate and hepatic metabolism in rats: effect of hyperthyroidism and fasting for 24 hours. *J Endocrinol* 1992; 135:45.
52. Magnusson I, Wennlund A, Chandramouli V, et al. Fructose-6-phosphate cycling and the pentose cycle in hyperthyroidism. *J Clin Endocrinol Metab* 1990;70:461.
53. Angervo M, Tiihonen M, Leinonen P, et al. Thyroxine treatment increases circulating levels of insulin-like growth factor binding protein-1: a placebo-controlled study. *Clin Endocrinol (Oxf)* 1993;38:547.
54. Ram PA, Waxman DJ. Thyroid hormone stimulation of NADPH P450 reductase expression in liver and extrahepatic tissues. *J Biol Chem* 1992;267:3294.
55. Castellani LW, Wilcox HC, Heimberg M. Relationships between fatty acid synthesis and lipid secretion in the isolated perfused rat liver: effects of hyperthyroidism, glucose and oleate. *Biochim Biophys Acta* 1991;1086:197.
56. Lanni A, Moreno LM, Cioffi M, et al. Effect of 3,3′-di-iodothyronine and 3,5-di-iodothyronine on liver mitochondria. *J Endocrinol* 1993;136:59.
57. Soboll B, Horst C, Hummerich H, et al. Mitochondrial metabolism in different thyroid states. *Biochem J* 1992;281:171.
58. Myers JD, Brannon ES, Holland BC. A correlative study of the cardiac output and the hepatic circulation in hyperthyroidism. *J Clin Invest* 1950;29:1069.
59. Imberti R, Vairetti M, Gualea MR, et al. The effect of thyroid hormone modulation on rat liver injury associated with ischemia reperfusion and cold storage. *Anesth Anal* 1998;86:1187.
60. Bruck R, Oren R, Shirin H, et al. Hypothyroidism minimizes liver damage and improves survival in rats with thioacetamide induced fulminant hepatic failure. *Hepatology* 1998;27:1013.
61. Halle P, Pare P, Kaptern E, et al. Double-blind controlled trial of propylthiouracil in patients with severe acute alcoholic hepatitis. *Gastroenterology* 1982;82:925.
62. Kaplowitz N. Propylthiouracil treatment for alcoholic hepatitis: should it and does it work? *Gastroenterology* 1982;82:1468.
63. Orrego H, Blake JE, Blendis LM, et al. Long-term treatment of alcoholic liver disease with propylthiouracil. *N Engl J Med* 1987; 317;1421.

64. Doniach D, Roitt IM, Walker JG, et al. Tissue autoantibodies in primary biliary cirrhosis, active chronic hepatitis, cryptogenic cirrhosis. *Clin Exp Immunol Immunopathol* 1966;237:262.

65. Culp KS, Fleming CR, Duffy J, et al. Autoimmune associations in primary biliary cirrhosis. *Mayo Clin Proc* 1983;57:365.

66. Schussler GC, Schaffner F, Korn F. Increased serum thyroid hormone binding and decreased free hormone in chronic active liver disease. *N Engl J Med* 1978;299:510.

67. Crowe JP, Christensen E, Butler J, et al. Primary biliary cirrhosis: prevalence of hypothyroidism and its relationship to thyroid antibodies. *Gastroenterology* 1980;78:1437.

68. Ain KB, Refetoff S. Relationship of oligosaccharide modification to the cause of serum thyroxine-binding globulin excess. *J Clin Endocrinol Metab* 1988;66:1037.

69. Schneeweiss B, Graninger W, Ferenci P, et al. Energy metabolism in patients with acute and chronic liver disease. *Hepatology* 1990;11:387.

70. Watanabe U, Hashimoto E, Hisamitsu T, et al. The risk factor for development of thyroid disease during interferon-α therapy for chronic hepatitis C. *Am J Gastroenterol* 1994;89:399.

71. Chopra IJ. An assessment of daily production and significance of thyroidal secretion of reverse T₃ in man. *J Clin Invest* 1976;58:32.

72. Faber J, Thomsen JF, Lumholtz IB, et al. Kinetic studies of thyroxine, 3,5,3′-triiodothyronine, 3,3′,3′-triiodothyronine, 3′,5′-diiodothyronine, 3,3′-diiodothyronine, and 3′-monoiodothyronine in patients with liver cirrhosis. *J Clin Endocrinol Metab* 1981;53:1978.

73. Nomura S, Pittman CS, Chambers JB Jr, et al. Reduced peripheral conversion of thyroxine to triiodothyronine in patients with hepatic cirrhosis. *J Clin Invest* 1975;56:643.

74. Van Thiel DH, Smith WI, Wight B, et al. Elevated basal and abnormal thyrotropin-releasing-hormone induced thyroid-stimulating hormone secretion in chronic alcoholic men with liver disease. *Alcohol Clin Exp Res* 1979;3:302.

75. Gartner LM, Arias IM. Hormonal control of hepatic bilirubin transport and conjugation. *Am J Physiol* 1972;222;1091.

76. Reyes H, Levi J, Gatmaitan Z, et al. Studies of Y and Z, two hepatic cytoplasmic organic anion-binding proteins: effect of drugs, chemicals, hormones, and cholestasis. *J Clin Invest* 1971; 50:2242.

77. Van Steenbergen W, Fevery J, DeGroote J. Thyroid hormones and the hepatic handling of bilirubin: effects of hypothyroidism and hyperthyroidism on the apparent maximal biliary secretion of bilirubin in the Wistar rat. *J Hepatol* 1988;7:229.

78. Lin TH, Rubinstein R, Holmes WL. A study of the effect of d- and l-triiodothyronine on bile acid excretion of rats. *J Lipid Res* 1963;4:63.

79. Wiley ZD, Lavigne ME, Liu KM, et al. The effect of hyperthyroidism on gastric emptying rates and pancreatic exocrine and biliary secretion in man. *Am J Dig Dis* 1978;23:1003.

80. Hanna FW, et al. Regulatory peptides and other neuroendocrine markers in medullary carcinoma of the thyroid. *J Endocrinol* 1997;152:275.

81. Cox TM, et al. Role of calcitonin in diarrhoea associated with medullary carcinoma of the thyroid. *Gut* 1979;20:629.

82. Rambaud JC, et al. Pathophysiological study of diarrhoea in a patient with medullary thyroid carcinoma: evidence against a secretory mechanism and for the role of shortened colonic transit time. *Gut* 1988;29:537.

83. Syrigos KN, et al. Thyroid autoantibodies and thyroid function in patients with gastric cancer. *Acta Oncol* 1994;33:905.

84. McCaffrey TV, et al. Locally invasive papillary thyroid carcinoma: 1940–1990. *Head Neck* 1994;16:165.

85. Bayles SW, et al. Management of thyroid carcinoma invading the aerodigestive tract. *Laryngoscope* 1998;108:1402.

86. Naomoto Y, et al. Multiple primary cancers of the esophagus and the thyroid gland. *Jpn J Clin Oncol* 1999;29:349.

87. Lynch H, et al. Familial adenomatous polyposis and extracolonic cancer. *Dig Dis Sci* 2001;46:2325.

88. Perrier N, et al. Thyroid cancer in patients with familial adenomatous polyposis. *World J Surg* 1998;22:738.

THE BLOOD IN THYROTOXICOSIS

STEPHANIE A. FISH
SUSAN J. MANDEL

Thyrotoxicosis affects hematopoiesis in several ways, although clinically important abnormalities are rare. This chapter discusses the effects of thyrotoxicosis on erythrocytes, leukocytes, platelets, and coagulation factors.

ERYTHROCYTES

Thyrotoxicosis stimulates erythropoiesis both indirectly and directly. Serum erythropoietin concentrations are higher in thyrotoxic patients as compared with normal subjects, probably as a result of the increase in metabolic activity and the concomitant increase in need for peripheral oxygen delivery (1–4). Thyroid hormone may also stimulate mononuclear cells to release tissue-specific erythroid stimulatory factors (5) and directly stimulate the formation of erythroid progenitor cells and the synthesis of the globin chains of hemoglobin in those cells (3,5). The result is erythroid hyperplasia (2).

Despite the stimulatory effect of thyroid hormone on erythropoiesis, most patients with thyrotoxicosis have normal hemoglobin concentrations and hematocrit values (1,2,6,7). This may be explained in part by an increase in plasma volume, which is a frequent finding, as well as shortened red blood cell survival (2,5). Red cell morphology is usually normal, but the cells tend to be slightly smaller than normal (7). Some patients seem to have ineffective erythropoiesis, based on increased numbers of sideroblasts and increased amounts of hemosiderin in their marrow (8). However, other patients have low marrow iron stores (2). Serum iron concentrations are usually normal, those of transferrin tend to be low, and those of ferritin high (9).

Pernicious anemia occurs in 1% to 3% of patients with thyrotoxicosis, and 15% to 20% have high serum concentrations of parietal cell antibodies (6,10). These abnormalities are linked with Graves' thyrotoxicosis, not other types of thyrotoxicosis, and probably reflect the patients' vulnerability to autoimmune disorders rather than some interaction between thyroid hormone and vitamin B_{12} metabolism. In fact, patients with both type 1 diabetes mellitus and Graves' disease may be at even higher risk for the development of pernicious anemia (11). In addition to immunologic mechanisms, patients with thyrotoxicosis may have increased requirements for vitamin B_{12} and folate

(3,10). Serum vitamin B_{12} concentrations in patients with thyrotoxicosis who do not have pernicious anemia are lower than in normal subjects and increase after successful antithyroid therapy (12). Serum folate concentrations are high or normal in patients with thyrotoxicosis (2,3,12).

Thyroid hormone also exerts effects within erythrocytes. Thyrotoxic patients have high red blood cell 2,3-diphosphoglycerate concentrations, which shifts the oxyhemoglobin curve to the right (1,3,5). This change, like the stimulation of erythropoiesis, augments oxygen delivery to peripheral tissues. Red cell Na^+,K^+-ATPase activity is low in thyrotoxicosis, due to a decrease in the number of pump units per cell; therefore, the red cell sodium concentration is increased. In contrast, Na^+,K^+-ATPase activity is increased in most other tissues, including leukocytes, and indeed the increase is thought to contribute importantly to the increases in oxygen consumption and substrate utilization that are characteristic of thyrotoxicosis (see Chapter 38).

Red blood cell zinc concentrations are low in patients with thyrotoxicosis, as are the red cell concentrations of the zinc-containing enzyme carbonic anhydrase (13). In a study of patients with thyrotoxicosis before and during treatment, red cell zinc concentration and serum thyroxine (T_4) and triiodothyronine (T_3) concentrations were inversely correlated, but during treatment red cell zinc concentrations increased more slowly than serum T_4 and T_3 concentrations decreased, suggesting that red cell zinc concentrations reflect mean serum T_4 and T_3 concentrations over time, and therefore that measurements of red cell zinc could serve as a marker of time-integrated serum T_4 and T_3 concentrations (13).

In summary, erythropoiesis is increased in patients with thyrotoxicosis, largely to meet the need to increase oxygen delivery to peripheral tissues. Nevertheless, 10% to 25% of patients have anemia, which may be normocytic, microcytic, or macrocytic, but it is rarely severe (1,3,5–7). Among patients who are anemic, the causes include ineffective erythropoiesis, iron deficiency, vitamin B_{12} deficiency, and folate deficiency; among these causes only ineffective erythropoiesis is likely to be a direct effect of thyrotoxicosis.

Leukocytes

Most patients with thyrotoxicosis have normal leukocyte counts, normal or slightly low granulocyte counts, and normal or slightly increased lymphocyte counts (7,14–18). Furthermore, a few thyrotoxic patients have lymphoid enlargement and splenomegaly, and rare patients have thymic enlargement; these changes seem to occur mostly in patients with Graves' thyrotoxicosis, implying they are in some way related to immune activation rather than to thyrotoxicosis. No consistent abnormalities in the proportions of circulating B and T lymphocytes have been found in patients with Graves' thyrotoxicosis (19), but lymphocyte function may be abnormal, in that the cytotoxic activity of natural killer cells is lower in these patients than in normal subjects or patients with toxic nodular goiter (15).

Most patients with thyrotoxicosis caused by Graves' disease have normal granulocyte counts, but some have granulocytopenia (5,14,17). The cause is unknown. In a study of 17 patients with Graves' thyrotoxicosis, 8 had reduced bone marrow reserves of granulocytes, although only 1 had granulocytopenia (16). Although antineutrophil antibodies may be detected in up to 50% of patients with Graves' thyrotoxicosis, the contribution of the antibodies to the observed granulocytopenia is unclear (20). In a study of 63 patients with thyrotoxicosis, 17 (27%) had a granulocyte count less than 2,000/mm^3, 36 (57%) had a count of 2,000 to 4,000/mm^3 (2 to 4×10^9/L), and 10 (16%) had a count of greater than 4,000/mm^3 (4×10^9/L) (16); the patients' mean granulocyte count was 3,100/mm^3 (3.1×10^9/L), as compared with 3,600/mm^3 (3.6×10^9/ L) in normal subjects (17). In the patients the granulocyte counts were correlated positively with serum concentrations of granulocyte colony-stimulating factor (G-CSF), which on average slightly higher than in normal subjects, but not with their serum free T$_4$ concentrations. In patients with granulocyte counts of less than 2,000/mm^3 (2×10^9/L), the counts tended to increase after initiation of methimazole therapy. The three patients whose granulocyte counts declined transiently during methimazole therapy (none had agranulocytosis) had no change in serum G-CSF concentrations.

In another study of 37 patients treated with carbimazole in doses of 25 or 100 mg/day, granulocyte counts increased during the first 2 weeks of therapy in the former group and decreased in the latter group; however, there were no differences between the groups subsequently (18). Thus, the granulocyte count can increase during antithyroid drug treatment, even in patients with granulocytopenia (see Chapter 45).

HEMOSTASIS

Platelets

An occasional patient with thyrotoxicosis, nearly always caused by Graves' disease, has clinically important thrombocytopenia [platelet count <100,000/mm^3 (100×10^9/L)],

and many [42% in one study (21)] have platelet counts of less than 150,000/mm^3 (150×10^9/L) (22). Only rare patients, however, have clinical manifestations of thrombocytopenia or other disturbances in coagulation.

The thrombocytopenia has several causes (23). First, some patients with Graves' thyrotoxicosis have antiplatelet antibodies; they thus can be said to have autoimmune thrombocytopenia purpura (24). Its incidence may be increased in patients with Graves' disease (25), and it may precede the onset of thyrotoxicosis (26). In a study of 25 patients with Graves' thyrotoxicosis, 11 (44%) had high serum levels of platelet-bound immunoglobulin G (IgG) (24). Among the 11 patients, most had easy bruising or bleeding, and 3 had thrombocytopenia. Because of this association between autoimmune thrombocytopenia and Graves' disease, screening for hyperthyroidism should be considered in patients with unexplained thrombocytopenia (27). Another possible explanation for thrombocytopenia in patients with Graves' thyrotoxicosis is binding of thyrotropin (TSH) receptor–stimulating or other thyroid antibodies to truncated actin-binding protein on platelets, which links both the glycoprotein and the high-affinity Fc receptor for immunoglobulin G on the platelet membrane to the cytoskeleton of platelets, providing a mechanism whereby the antibodies could bind to platelets and accelerate their destruction (23).

Other factors that may contribute to thrombocytopenia in these patients are the thyrotoxicosis itself, which may increase the phagocytic activity of the reticuloendothelial system, including the spleen, and splenomegaly. Either would accelerate the clearance of platelets, whether sensitized or not (21,22,28).

All these effects are to some extent counterbalanced by increased production of platelets. The number of megakaryocytes in the bone marrow may be increased (29). The number of reticulated (young) platelets in the circulation is increased. These platelets are larger than more mature ones, and thus mean platelet volume is increased (28,30).

Platelet counts usually increase, platelet size decreases, and the amount of platelet-associated immunoglobulin G (IgG) decreases during antithyroid therapy (22,31). Patients with severe thrombocytopenia have been given concomitant glucocorticoid therapy (26), as would be done for thrombocytopenia alone. Antithyroid drugs may have immunosuppressive as well as antithyroid actions (see Chapter 45), which may reduce the production of IgG capable of binding to platelets.

Thyrotoxicosis may also alter platelet function; platelet aggregation in response to adenosine diphosphate (ADP), collagen, and ristocetin is decreased (32,33). These changes in platelet function may be due to inhibition of myosin light chain kinase, an enzyme that stimulates platelet contractile proteins (34). These abnormalities also improve during antithyroid therapy (32,33).

Clotting Factors and Warfarin Therapy

In thyrotoxicosis, the rate of clearance of most if not all coagulation factors is increased (35). However, the plasma concentrations of most of these factors are normal, except for small decreases in factor II concentrations and increases in factor VIII concentrations (36–38). Some thyrotoxic patients have shortened partial thromboplastin times, perhaps resulting from the increase in plasma factor VIII concentrations (36,38). Factor VIII deficiency due to an acquired circulating antibody that inhibited factor VIII coagulant activity was reported in two patients with Graves' thyrotoxicosis who presented with spontaneous bleeding (39,40). Serum concentrations of thrombomodulin, an endothelial surface glycoprotein that serves as a thrombin receptor, are high in patients with thyrotoxicosis (41).

The sensitivity of thyrotoxic patients to the anticoagulant effects of warfarin is increased. In one study in which thyrotoxic patients were given a single dose of warfarin, the decrease in both factors II and VII was greater and the increase in prothrombin time was greater before than after antithyroid treatment, but the responses of factors IX and X were similar (36). The explanation for the increased effect of warfarin in thyrotoxicosis is multifactorial, probably involving both more rapid clearance of clotting factors and reduced plasma protein binding of the drug. However, the results of pharmacokinetic studies of warfarin in thyrotoxic patients have been conflicting. In one study, the single-dose warfarin plasma half-life, plasma clearance, and volume of distribution were similar in patients studied when they were thyrotoxic and again when they were euthyroid (36); on the other hand, in a thyrotoxic patient receiving chronic warfarin therapy (5 mg/day), the plasma free warfarin concentration was high (37), consistent with decreased plasma protein binding of the drug (42). In addition, patients with thyrotoxicosis may be relatively resistant to reversal of warfarin-induced hypoprothrombinemia by vitamin K. Therefore, patients with thyrotoxicosis treated with warfarin may require lower doses.

Anticardiolipin Antibodies

Anticardiolipin antibodies have been found in the serum of patients with Graves' thyrotoxicosis, especially those with coexisting ophthalmopathy (43,44). These antibodies, especially those belonging to the immunoglobulin G isotype, may be associated with hypercoagulable states. With antithyroid therapy, the antibody concentrations decreased (44). Fortunately, thromboembolic events, the primary antiphospholipid syndrome, and recurrent abortions are rare occurrences in patients with Graves' thyrotoxicosis, and the presence of these antibodies may be a nonspecific marker of immune system activation (45).

REFERENCES

1. Lee GR. The anemias associated with renal disease, liver disease, endocrine disease and pregnancy. In: Lee GR, Foerster J, Lukens J, et al. *Wintrobe's clinical hematology.* Baltimore: Williams & Wilkins, 1999:1497.
2. Das KC, Mukherjee M, Sarkar TK, et al. Erythropoiesis and erythropoietin in hypo- and hyperthyroidism. *J Clin Endocrinol Metab* 1975;40:211.
3. Fein HG, Rivlin RS. Anemia in thyroid diseases. *Med Clin North Am* 1975;59:1133.
4. Donati RM, Gallagher NI. Hematologic alteration associated with endocrine disease. *Med Clin North Am* 1968;52:231.
5. Ford HC, Carter JM. The haematology of hyperthyroidism: abnormalities of erythrocytes, leucocytes, thrombocytes and haemostasis. *Postgrad Med J* 1988;64:735.
6. Nightingale S, Vitek PJ, Himsworth RL. The haematology of hyperthyroidism. *Q J Med* 1978;185:35.
7. Reddy J, Brownlie BEW, Heaton DC, et al. The peripheral blood picture in thyrotoxicosis. *N Z Med J* 1981;93:143.
8. Lahtinen R. Sideroblasts and haemosiderin in thyrotoxicosis. *Scand J Haematol* 1980;25:237.
9. Kubota K, Tamura J, Kurabayashi H, et al. Evaluation of increased serum ferritin levels in patients with hyperthyroidism. *Clin Invest* 1993;72:26.
10. Alperin JB, Haggard ME, Haynie TP. A study of vitamin B_{12} requirements in a patient with pernicious anemia and thyrotoxicosis: evidence of an increased need for vitamin B_{12} in the presence of hyperthyroidism. *Blood* 1970;36:632.
11. Perros P, Singh R K, Ludlam CA, et al. Prevalence of pernicious anaemia in patients with type 1 diabetes mellitus and autoimmune thyroid disease. *Diabetic Med* 2000;17:749.
12. Ford HC, Carter JM, Rendle MA. Serum and red cell folate and serum vitamin B_{12} levels in hyperthyroidism. *Am J Hematol* 1989;31:233.
13. Yoshida K, Kiso Y, Watanabe T, et al. Erythrocyte zinc in hyperthyroidism: reflection of integrated thyroid hormone levels over the previous few months. *Metabolism* 1990;39:182.
14. Irvine WJ, Wu FCW, Urbaniak SJ, et al. Peripheral blood leucocytes in thyrotoxicosis (Graves' disease) as studied by conventional light microscopy. *Clin Exp Immunol* 1977;27:216.
15. Marazuela M, Vargas JA, Alvarez-Mon M, et al. Impaired natural killer cytotoxicity in peripheral blood monomuclear cells in Graves' disease. *Eur J Endocrinol* 1995;132:175.
16. Ponassi A, Morra L, Caristo G, et al. Disorders of granulopoiesis in patients with untreated Graves' disease. *Acta Haematol* 1983;70:19.
17. Iitaka M, Noh JY, Kitahama S, et al. Elevated serum granulocyte colony-stimulating factor levels in patients with Graves' disease. *Clin Endocrinol (Oxf)* 1998;48:275.
18. Grebe S, Feek CM, Ford HC, et al. A randomized trial of short-term treatment of Graves' disease with high-dose carbimazole plus thyroxine versus low-dose carbimazole. *Clin Endocrinol (Oxf)* 1998;48:585.
19. Weetman AP, McGregor AM: Autoimmune thyroid disease: further developments in our understanding. *Endocr Rev* 15:788, 1994.
20. Weitzman SA, Stossel TP, Harmon DC, et al. Antineutrophil autoantibodies in Graves' disease. *J Clin Invest* 1985;75:119.
21. Adrouny A, Sandler RM, Carmel R. Variable presentation of thrombocytopenia in Graves' disease. *Arch Intern Med* 1982;142:1460.
22. Kurata Y, Nishioeda Y, Tsubakio T, et al. Thrombocytopenia in Graves' disease: effect of T_3 on platelet kinetics. *Acta Haematol* 1980;63:158.

23. Hofbauer LC, Heufelder AE. Coagulation disorders in thyroid diseases. *Eur J Endocrinol* 1997;136:1.

24. Hymes K, Blum M, Lackner H, et al. Easy bruising, thrombocytopenia, and elevated platelet immunoglobulin G in Graves' disease and Hashimoto's thyroiditis. *Ann Intern Med* 1981;94:27.

25. Marshall JS, Weisberger AS, Levy RP, et al. Coexistent idiopathic thrombocytopenic purpura and hyperthyroidism. *Ann Intern Med* 1967;67:411.

26. Hofbauer LC, Spitzweg C, Schmauss S, et al. Graves' disease associated with autoimmune thrombocytopenic purpura. *Arch Intern Med* 1997;157:1033.

27. Aggarwal A, Doolittle G. Autoimmune thrombocytopenic purpura associated with hyperthyroidism in a single individual. *South Med J* 1997;90:933.

28. Panzer S, Haubenstock A, Minar E. Platelets in hyperthyroidism: studies on platelet counts, mean platelet volume, 111-indium-labeled platelet kinetics, and platelet-associated immunoglobulins G and M. *J Clin Endocrinol Metab* 1990;70:491.

29. Axelrod AR, Berman L. The bone marrow in hyperthyroidism and hypothyroidism. *Blood* 1951;6:436.

30. Ford HC, Toomath RJ, Carter JM, et al. Mean platelet volume is increased in hyperthyroidism. *Am J Hematol* 1988;27:190.

31. Stiegler G, Stohlawetz P, Brugger S, et al. Elevated numbers of reticulated platelets in hyperthyroidism: direct evidence for an increase of thrombopoiesis. *Br J Haematol* 1998;101:656.

32. Myrup B, Bregengard C, Faber J. Primary haemostasis in thyroid disease. *J Intern Med* 1995;238:59.

33. Masunaga R, Nagasaka A, Nakai A, et al. Alteration of platelet aggregation in patients with thyroid disorders. *Metabolism* 1997;46:1128.

34. Mamiya S, Hagiwara M, Inoue S, et al. Thyroid hormones inhibit platelet function and myosin light chain kinase. *J Biol Chem* 1989;264:8575.

35. Loeliger EA, vanderEsch B, Mattern MJ, et al. The biological disappearance rate of prothrombin, factors VII, IX and X from plasma in hypothyroidism, hyperthyroidism and during fever. *Thromb Diath Hemorrh* 1964;10:267.

36. Kellett HA, Sawers JSA, Boulton FE, et al. Problems of anticoagulation with warfarin in hyperthyroidism. *Q J Med* 1986;58:43.

37. Chute JP, Tyan CP, Sladek G, et al. Exacerbation of warfarin-induced anticoagulation by hyperthyroidism. *Endocr Pract* 1997;3:77.

38. Simone JV, Abildgaard CF, Schulman I. Blood coagulation in thyroid dysfunction. *N Eng J Med* 1965;237:1057.

39. Sievert R, Goldstein ML, Surks MI. Graves' disease and autoimmune factor VIII deficiency. *Thyroid* 1996;6:245.

40. Marongiu F, Cauli C, Mameli G, et al. Apathetic Graves' disease and acquired hemophilia due to factor VIIIc antibody. *J Endocr Invest* 2002;25:246.

41. Morikawa Y, Morikawa A, Makino I. Relationship of thyroid states and serum thrombomodulin (TM) levels in patients with Graves' disease: TM, a possible new marker of the peripheral activity of thyroid hormones. *J Clin Endocrinol Metab* 1993;76:609.

42. O'Connor P, Feely J Clinical pharmacokinetics and endocrine disorders: therapeutic implications. *Clin Pharmacokinet* 1987;13:345.

43. Marongiu F, Conti M, Murtas ML, et al. Anticardiolipin antibodies in Graves' disease: relationship with thrombin activity *in vivo*. *Thromb Res* 1991;64:745.

44. Paggi A, Caccavo D, Ferri GM, et al. Anti-cardiolipin antibodies in autoimmune thyroid diseases. *Clin Endocrinol (Oxf)* 1994;40:329.

45. Hofbauer LC, Spitzweg C, Heufelder AE. Graves' disease associated with the primary antiphospholipid syndrome. *J Rheumatol* 1996;23:1435.

36

THE PITUITARY IN THYROTOXICOSIS

PETER J. SNYDER

Thyrotoxicosis affects the secretion of most pituitary hormones, but because the clinical consequences are not so great as are those in hypothyroidism, the abnormalities of pituitary hormone secretion have not been studied as well as those in hypothyroidism. The effects of thyrotoxicosis on the secretion of growth hormone (GH) and prolactin are discussed in this chapter; the effects on the secretion of vasopressin, corticotropin, and follicle-stimulating hormone and luteinizing hormone are discussed elsewhere (see Chapters 33, 37, and 39, respectively).

GROWTH HORMONE

Clinical Manifestations

Children with thyrotoxicosis may grow more rapidly than normal children. In one study of five children studied before and during antithyroid treatment, the height ages were all more than 3 standard deviations (SD) above the mean for normal children (1). The children's bone ages also were accelerated and to a similar degree; the relationship of bone age to height age remained normal. Consequently, when the children were treated, it appeared that their final heights would be normal.

Hormonal Abnormalities

Growth acceleration in children with thyrotoxicosis suggests that their GH secretion might be greater than normal. In one study of adults, both the production rate and metabolic clearance rate of GH were higher in thyrotoxic patients and lower in hypothyroid patients than in normal subjects (2). In eight patients with thyrotoxicosis, the mean (± SD) GH production rate was 529±242 ng/min, as compared with 347±173 ng/min in 22 normal subjects and 160±69 ng/min in six patients with hypothyroidism. Serum GH concentrations, however, are lower in thyrotoxic patients than in normal subjects. This decrease is not due to a lower serum concentration of GH-binding protein, because the concentrations were similar in 15 thyrotoxic patients and 19 normal subjects (3). Serum GH concentrations increase in response to deep sleep to a lesser degree in thyrotoxic children and adolescents than in normal subjects and increase when patients are treated with propylthiouracil (4) (Fig. 36.1). Likewise, the increase in serum GH concentrations in response to insulin-induced hypoglycemia is less in thyrotoxic children and adults than in normal subjects (5–7), especially in those with severe thyrotoxicosis (6). The serum GH response to growth hormone releasing hormone (GH-RH) also is less than normal in thyrotoxic patients, and it increases during antithyroid treatment (8,9), suggesting that the increased GH production rate is not due to increased stimulation by GH-RH.

The low serum GH concentrations, despite the increased production rate, are probably the result of the increased metabolic clearance rate (2). In fact, studies of GH secretion in seven thyrotoxic patients, based on measurements of serum GH concentrations at 10-minute intervals for 24 hours and deconvolution analysis (which removes the effect of metabolic clearance mathematically), revealed more frequent GH secretory bursts, a larger mass of GH released per burst, and a fourfold higher GH production rate than in seven normal subjects (10). Because GH secretion is greater than normal in thyrotoxicosis, the increase in linear growth in thyrotoxic children could be a GH effect. Thyroid hormone appears to act directly on somatotroph cells to stimulate GH secretion. In rats, triiodothyronine (T_3) activates the promoter region of the GH gene (11), an action that requires the expression of the transcription factor *Pit-1* (12).

The finding of higher than normal serum insulin-like growth factor-1 concentrations in thyrotoxic patients [mean (±SD) 259±34 µg/L] and a decrease to normal (189±15 µg/L) during antithyroid drug treatment (13) suggests that there is a greater than normal effect of GH in thyrotoxicosis. These results do not, however, exclude the possibility that increased linear growth in thyrotoxicosis could be due at least partly to a direct effect of thyroid hormone on bone.

PROLACTIN

Clinical Manifestations

Galactorrhea is a manifestation of hypothyroidism, and therefore one might expect that difficulty in lactation

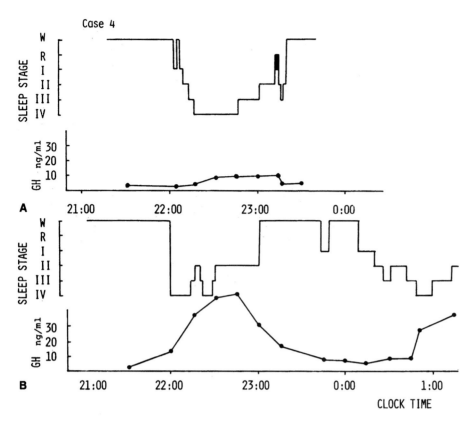

FIGURE 36.1. Serum GH concentrations during stages III and IV of sleep in a patient when thyrotoxic (**A**) and later after treatment when euthyroid (**B**). (From Sasaki N, Tsuyusaki T, Nakamura H, et al. Sleep-related growth hormone release in thyrotoxic patients before and during propylthiouracil therapy. *Endocrinol Jpn* 1985;32:39, with permission.)

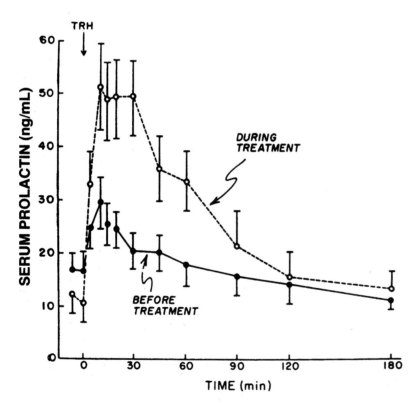

FIGURE 36.2. Mean (±5E) serum prolactin responses to thyrotropin-releasing hormone (TRH) in 10 patients when they were thyrotoxic (●, before treatment) and when they were euthyroid (○, during treatment). (From Snyder PJ, Jacobs LS, Utiger RD, Daughaday WH. Thyroid hormone inhibition of the prolactin response to thyrotropin-releasing hormone. *J Clin Invest* 1973;52:2324, with permission.)

would occur in postpartum women with thyrotoxicosis who attempt to nurse; however, this has not been reported, and it seems likely that prolactin secretion and serum prolactin concentrations in women with thyrotoxicosis are sufficient for normal lactation. In addition, postpartum thyroiditis, the most common cause of thyrotoxicosis at this time, usually begins several months after delivery and is mild and transient (see Chapter 27). Women with thyrotoxicosis who need antithyroid drug treatment can nurse their infants safely (see Chapter 45).

Hormonal Abnormalities

Secretion of prolactin in thyrotoxicosis is similar to that of GH in that the production rate and metabolic clearance rate are somewhat greater than normal, but serum prolactin concentrations are less than normal. In one study, the mean (±SD) production rate of prolactin in six patients with thyrotoxicosis was 504±91 µg/day and in six normal subjects was 367±144 µg/day (14). Not only are basal serum prolactin concentrations slightly lower in thyrotoxic patients, but so too are their serum prolactin responses to thyrotropin-releasing hormone (Fig. 36.2). Both basal and stimulated serum prolactin concentrations return to normal when the patients are treated (15) (Fig. 36.2). The serum prolactin response to arginine is also decreased in both women and men with thyrotoxicosis (16). The mechanism by which thyroid hormone suppresses prolactin secretion may involve an interaction with the activating response element and an inhibitory element on the promoter region of the human prolactin gene (17). So far, no physiologic or clinical consequences of these abnormalities are known.

REFERENCES

1. Schlesinger S, MacGillivray MH, Munschauer RW. Acceleration of growth and bone maturation in childhood thyrotoxicosis. *Pediatrics* 1973;83:233.
2. Taylor AL, Finster JL, Mintz DH. Metabolic clearance and production rates of human growth hormone. *J Clin Invest* 1969; 48:2349.
3. Amit T, Hertz P, Ish-Shalom S, et al. Effects of hypo- or hyperthyroidism on growth hormone-binding protein. *Clin Endocrinol (Oxf)* 1991;35:159.
4. Sasaki N, Tsuyusaki T, Nakamura H, et al. Sleep-related growth hormone release in thyrotoxic patients before and during propylthiouracil therapy. *Endocrinol Jpn* 1985;32:39.
5. Burgess JA, Smith BR, Merimee TJ. Growth hormone in thyrotoxicosis: effect of insulin-induced hypoglycemia. *J Clin Endocrinol* 1966;26:1257.
6. Giustina G, Reschini E, Valentini F, et al. Growth hormone and cortisol responses to insulin-induced hypoglycemia in thyrotoxicosis. *J Clin Endocrinol* 1971;32:571.
7. Katz HP, Youlton R, Kaplan SL, et al. Growth and growth hormone. III. Growth hormone release in children with primary hypothyroidism and thyrotoxicosis. *J Clin Endocrinol* 1969;29:346.
8. Valcalvi R, Dieguez C, Zini M, et al. Influence of hyperthyroidism on growth hormone secretion. *Clin Endocrinol (Oxf)* 1993;38:515.
9. Ramos-Dias JC, Lengyal A-MJ, Iopanoic acid–induced decrease of circulating T$_3$ causes a significant increase in GH responsiveness to GH-releasing hormone in thyrotoxic patients. *Clin Endocrinol (Oxf)* 1999;51:461.
10. Iranmanesh A, Lizarralde G, Johnson ML, et al. Nature of altered growth hormone secretion in hyperthyroidism. *J Clin Endocrinol Metab* 1991;72:108.
11. Brent GA, Harney JW, Moore DD, et al. Multihormonal regulation of the human, rat, and bovine growth hormone promoters: differential effects of 3'5'-cyclic adenosine monophosphate, thyroid hormone, and glucocorticoids. *Mol Endocrinol* 1988;2:792.
12. Palamino T, Barettino D, Aranda A. Role of GHF-1 in the regulation of the rat growth hormone gene promoter by thyroid hormone and retinoic acid receptors. *J Biol Chem* 1998;273:27541.
13. Miell JP, Taylor AM, Zini M, et al. Effects of hypothyroidism and hyperthyroidism on insulin-like growth factors (IGFs) and growth hormone- and IGF-proteins. *J Clin Endocrinol Metab* 1993;76:950.
14. Cooper DS, Ridgway EC, Kliman B, et al. Metabolic clearance and production rates of prolactin in man. *J Clin Invest* 1979;64:1669.
15. Snyder PJ, Jacobs LS, Utiger RD, et al. Thyroid hormone inhibition of the prolactin response to thyrotropin-releasing hormone. *J Clin Invest* 1973;52:2324.
16. Ciccarelli D, Zini M, Grottoli S, et al. Impaired prolactin response to arginine in patients with hyperthyroidism. *Clin Endocrinol* 1994;41:371.
17. Pernasetti F, Cacavelli L, Van der Weerdt C, et al. Thyroid hormone inhibits the human prolactin gene promoter by interfering with activating protein-1 and estrogen stimulations. *Mol Endocrinol* 1997;11:986.

THE ADRENAL CORTEX IN THYROTOXICOSIS

ROBERT G. DLUHY

Thyrotoxicosis has several effects on adrenocortical function and the metabolism of adrenocortical hormones, serving especially to accelerate the latter. Patients with thyrotoxicosis therefore have more rapid cortisol clearance than do normal subjects (Figs. 37.1 and 37.2). The function of the hypothalamic–pituitary–adrenal axis is normal; corticotropin (ACTH) and cortisol secretion increase to meet the need for more cortisol resulting from the increased clearance rate. Therefore, patients with thyrotoxicosis have normal serum ACTH and cortisol concentrations. If hypothalamic, pituitary, or adrenal function is impaired, however, the patient's serum cortisol concentrations are low.

Conversely, glucocorticoids affect a variety of thyroid functions, such as thyrotropin (TSH) secretion, the production and clearance of thyroxine (T_4), peripheral conversion of T_4 to triiodothyronine (T_3), renal clearance of iodide, and the production or clearance of serum thyroid hormone–binding proteins.

Finally, thyroid and adrenal function may be altered by concurrent disease processes, particularly autoimmune diseases, beyond the aforementioned hormonal interactions. Additional potential interactions include those resulting from the alterations in both adrenal and thyroid function that occur during acute and chronic illness (see section on nonthyroidal illness in Chapter 11).

THYROID-GLUCOCORTICOID INTERACTIONS IN PERIPHERAL TISSUES

In vitro, glucocorticoids act synergistically with T_3 to increase growth hormone (GH) production by pituitary tumor cells. The affinity of the T_3 nuclear receptors for T_3 in these cells is reduced by 50% in the absence of cortisol (1). Other interactions between thyroid hormones and glucocorticoids, for example, effects on the messenger RNAs (mRNAs) for the receptors for the two hormones and on GH gene expression, also have been reported (2–4). Thyroid hormone and glucocorticoid receptors are encoded by genes that are members of a single family, and the two

types of receptors have some structural similarity. In one study of GH_3 cells (a pituitary tumor cell line), T_3 increased glucocorticoid action by increasing glucocorticoid receptor mRNA concentrations (4). A reciprocal action of glucocorticoids on T_3 receptor mRNA was not found, even though T_3 action in GH_3 cells is augmented by glucocorticoids. In contrast to these interactions of glucocorticoids and thyroid hormone on GH secretion, there is no evidence for interactions in pituitary thyrotrophs or corticotrophs or in other tissues. In addition, some negative findings have emerged. For example, patients with either primary cortisol resistance (due to inactivating mutations of the glucocorticoid receptor) or the cortisol hyperreactive syndrome have normal serum TSH and thyroid hormone concentrations, and the responsiveness of their tissues to T_4 and T_3 is normal (5,6).

THYROID-ADRENOCORTICAL INTERACTIONS IN THE CENTRAL NERVOUS SYSTEM AND ANTERIOR PITUITARY

Neither ACTH nor cortisol is a major regulator of pituitary TSH secretion (7), and the release of ACTH and TSH is governed by separate hypothalamic signals (8,9). Thus, under physiologic conditions in humans, there is no functionally important feedback of cortisol on circadian TSH secretion, even though serum cortisol concentrations are lowest when serum TSH concentrations are highest in the late evening. On the other hand, moderate to high doses of glucocorticoids inhibit thyrotropin-releasing hormone (TRH)-induced TSH secretion and reduce mean 24-hour serum TSH concentrations and the nocturnal surge in TSH secretion. Patients with Cushing's syndrome have similar changes in TSH secretion (10). These changes are caused by a decrease in TSH pulse amplitude. TSH secretion returns to normal after the glucocorticoid is discontinued or Cushing's syndrome is treated; however, TSH secretion partially escapes from suppression during long-term glucocorticoid exposure so that hypothyroidism does not occur (11). The actions of glucocorticoids that affect TSH

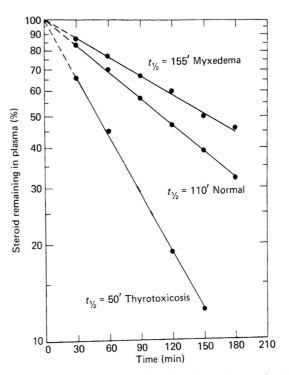

NORMAL

$$SC = \frac{SR}{MCR}$$

THYROTOXICOSIS

$$SC = \frac{\uparrow SR}{*\uparrow MCR}$$

* initiating event

FIGURE 37.1. The relationship between the serum concentrations and the secretion and clearance rates of cortisol in normal subjects and in patients with thyrotoxicosis. In normal subjects, the serum concentration (*SC*) of cortisol reflects its secretion at the time of measurement. The SC is dependent on two factors: the cortisol secretion rate (*SR*) and the rate at which cortisol is metabolized, that is, the metabolic clearance rate (*MCR*) of cortisol. In patients with thyrotoxicosis, the hepatic clearance of cortisol is accelerated due to augmentation of Δ4,5-reductase activity (see Fig. 37.3). If normal feedback relationships are preserved, the endogenous cortisol secretion rate increases and serum cortisol concentrations are normal.

secretion occur at the level of both the hypothalamus and the pituitary (11,12).

THYROTOXICOSIS AND ADRENOCORTICAL FUNCTION

In animals, thyrotoxicosis causes adrenocortical enlargement, but it does not occur in hypophysectomized animals given thyroid hormone, indicating that the effect of thyroid hormone is indirect. In early studies of patients with thyrotoxicosis, urinary 17-ketosteroid excretion was usually low and 17-hydroxycorticosteroid excretion was slightly high; both were low in patients in patients with hypothyroidism. Subsequent studies revealed that the metabolism of cortisol and other steroids is accelerated in thyrotoxicosis and slowed in hypothyroidism (13). These metabolic abnormalities are discussed in the next section with respect to the C_{21} steroids cortisol and aldosterone.

EFFECTS OF THYROTOXICOSIS ON CORTISOL SECRETION AND METABOLISM

Infused cortisol is cleared from the circulation at an accelerated rate in thyrotoxicosis, but not in other hypermetabolic states (13) (Fig. 37.2). The miscible pool of cortisol is normal, whereas the fractional turnover rate of the pool per unit time (metabolic clearance rate) and the secretion rate are increased (14); the latter occurs as a result of an increase in the number of cortisol secretory episodes. The raised cortisol secretion rate accounts for the increase in urinary 17-hydroxycorticoid excretion. These abnormalities are corrected after restoration of a euthyroid state by appropriate treatment (13). In hypothyroidism, the opposite changes occur, again with a normal cortisol pool size (Fig. 37.2); the reduced

FIGURE 37.2. Disappearance of cortisol from plasma after its intravenous administration to a single normal subject, a patient with hypothyroidism (myxedema), and a patient with thyrotoxicosis. The slowing and acceleration, respectively, of the plasma half-life ($t_{1/2}$) of cortisol are evident. In this study, the results were similar after infusion of tracer doses of ^{14}C-cortisol. (From Peterson RE. The influence of the thyroid on adrenal cortical function. *J Clin Invest* 1958;37:736, with permission.)

cortisol secretion rate is concordant with low urinary 17-hydroxycorticoid excretion, and treatment with thyroid hormone restores cortisol metabolism to normal (13).

In thyrotoxicosis, the normal pool of cortisol may be regarded as concordant with the normal serum cortisol concentrations. Serum corticosteroid-binding globulin concentrations are also normal, indicating that serum free cortisol concentrations should be normal. The latter is confirmed by the finding of normal urinary cortisol excretion. Therefore, thyrotoxicosis is not associated with abnormal adrenocortical function from the point of view of the peripheral tissues (13).

Thyrotoxicosis accelerates the disposal rate of endogenous or exogenous cortisol by accelerating reduction of ring A of the steroid molecule, chiefly by stimulating Δ4,5-steroid reductase activity in hepatic microsomes; this is the rate-limiting step in hepatic degradation of glucocorticoids (Fig. 37.3). The clearance of one of these metabolites, tetrahydrocortisone, in patients with thyrotoxicosis is normal. This finding indicates that the next step in the disposal of tetrahydrocortisone (and other ring A–reduced cortisol metabolites), which is conjugation with glucuronic acid, is normal (13).

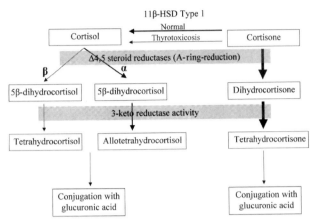

FIGURE 37.3. Alterations in hepatic metabolism of cortisol in thyrotoxicosis. Cortisol is inactivated primarily by reduction of the α,β-unsaturated ketone region in ring A, yielding 5α- and 5β-dihydrocortisol, which are inactive. These reactions are catalyzed by hepatic Δ4,5-steroid reductases. Subsequently 3-keto reduction of dihydrocortisol yields the tetrahydrohydroxy metabolites. Thyroid hormone increases the activity of these reductases. As a result, in thyrotoxicosis there is an overall increase in the metabolic clearance of cortisol, as well as a qualitative alteration in the pattern of metabolites produced, with a small increase in the fraction of cortisol metabolized to tetrahydrocortisone, a small increase in the allotetrahydrocortisol fraction, and a decrease in the fraction of tetrahydrocortisol. There are two isoforms of 11β-hydroxysteroid dehydrogenase (11β-HSD): type 1, which is located in the liver and acts as a reductase, thereby converting cortisone to cortisol; and type 2, which is located in the kidneys and acts as a dehydrogenase, converting cortisol to cortisone. Thyrotoxicosis results in a decrease in the reductase activity of 11β-HSD type 1 and therefore a decrease in hepatic conversion of cortisone to cortisol. The result is an accumulation of cortisone, which is biologically inactive. Thyrotoxicosis does not alter the conjugation of cortisol metabolites with glucuronic acid in the liver.
The larger and smaller arrows indicate changes in cortisol metabolism, as compared with normal.

Thyrotoxicosis not only influences the overall rate of cortisol degradation but also affects its metabolism qualitatively (Fig. 37.3). It increases the fraction of cortisol metabolized to 11-keto as opposed to 11β-hydroxy compounds; the quantities of tetrahydrocortisone and cortolones rise, whereas those of tetrahydrocortisol and cortols decline (13). T_4 also regulates hepatic 11β-hydroxysteroid dehydrogenase type 1 (11β-HSD1) mRNA and activity levels (15), although variable results have been reported in different species (16). In humans, thyrotoxicosis decreases the conversion of cortisone to cortisol (17), leading to accumulation of cortisone, which is biologically inactive (13). As a result, the ratio of tetrahydrocortisone to tetrahydrocortisol in urine is increased. Because these urinary cortisol metabolites provide an assessment of peripheral thyroid hormone action, a low or normal ratio in patients with high serum T_4 concentrations has been used as a marker of thyroid hormone resistance (17) (see Chapter 81). Cortisone, like cortisol, is also disposed of at an accelerated rate in thyrotoxicosis, as are corticosterone, deoxycorticosterone, aldosterone (see the next section), and most other steroids.

EFFECTS OF THYROTOXICOSIS ON THE PITUITARY-ADRENAL AXIS AND COUNTERREGULATORY HORMONES

In patients with thyrotoxicosis, basal serum cortisol concentrations and the responses to ACTH and insulin-induced hypoglycemia are usually normal. However, in patients with severe long-standing thyrotoxicosis, low-dose ACTH testing revealed significantly lower mean increments in serum cortisol concentrations, as compared with the increments when the patients were euthyroid (18). This effect of sustained thyrotoxicosis to diminish adrenocortical reserve is unlikely to be of clinical importance. Nevertheless, in patients with thyrotoxic crisis who have hypotension, treatment with hydrocortisone is the standard of practice because of the possibility of diminished adrenal reserve (relative adrenal insufficiency) or undiagnosed concomitant Addison's disease (see Chapter 43).

The responses of counterregulatory hormones to insulin-induced hypoglycemia in thyrotoxicosis are variable; serum glucagon responses are increased, ACTH responses are slightly increased, and GH responses are blunted. Serum glucose concentrations increase more rapidly after hypoglycemia in patients with thyrotoxicosis, as compared with normal subjects, most likely due to the heightened glucagon response (19).

Basal plasma epinephrine and norepinephrine concentrations are normal or slightly reduced, respectively, in patients with thyrotoxicosis (20) (see Chapter 38). The plasma epinephrine response to insulin-induced hypoglycemia is normal, whereas that of norepinephrine is reduced, consistent with a selective action of thyroid hormones on the sympathoadrenal system (20).

EFFECTS OF THYROTOXICOSIS ON THE RENIN–ANGIOTENSIN– ALDOSTERONE SYSTEM

In patients with thyrotoxicosis, the metabolic clearance rate of aldosterone is slightly increased, resulting in a compensatory increase in aldosterone secretion; serum concentrations of aldosterone are usually normal (13,21,22). In addition to increasing the hepatic degradation of aldosterone, thyrotoxicosis is associated with other alterations in the function of the renin–angiotensin–aldosterone system (Table 37.1). Plasma renin activity basally and in response to upright posture is increased, probably caused by increased activity of the β-adrenergic nervous system (22, 23). Serum angiotensin-converting enzyme concentrations are increased (24). Finally, serum angiotensinogen concentrations are increased (25), probably as a result of increased transcription of the angiotensinogen gene or increased stability of its mRNA (26). As a result of the increase in serum angiotensinogen, the generation of angiotensin peptides is

TABLE 37.1. EFFECTS OF THYROTOXICOSIS ON THE RENIN–ANGIOTENSIN–ALDOSTERONE SYSTEM

Hepatic clearance of aldosterone: increased
Plasma renin activity: high
Serum angiotensin-converting enzyme activity: increased
Serum aldosterone concentrations: normal[a]
Serum angiotensinogen concentrations: high

[a]Serum aldosterone concentrations: variable, probably due to varying states of sodium and potassium balance and the severity of thyrotoxicosis.

increased, because the serum concentration of angiotensinogen is near the Michaelis constant (K_m) of the proteolytic activity of renin. The actions of thyroid hormone on the production of angiotensinogen may contribute to the increased plasma renin activity in thyrotoxicosis. None of these changes is of clinical importance, nor do the changes underlie the cardiovascular manifestations of thyrotoxicosis, which are dominated by heightened adrenergic activity (see Chapter 31).

Thus, the regulation of aldosterone secretion in patients with thyrotoxicosis reflects thyroid hormone–induced alterations in hepatic steroid metabolism, and to a lesser extent independent actions on the renin–angiotensin–aldosterone system. In addition, patients with thyrotoxicosis may have low total-body potassium stores as a result of the kaliuretic effects of thyroid hormone; potassium depletion independently results in increased plasma renin activity and decreased production of aldosterone (27,28). These variables, as well as overall sodium balance and the severity of thyrotoxicosis, mean that the results of studies of the renin–angiotensin–aldosterone system are variable in patients with thyrotoxicosis. In general, plasma renin activity is increased (22,23), whereas basal serum aldosterone concentrations are normal, but they may be high or low (22,29,30). The serum aldosterone response to exogenous ACTH is normal (22, 29), but the response to exogenous angiotensin II is blunted (29). The altered relationship between plasma renin activity and aldosterone secretion may reflect potassium depletion; in one study, oral potassium loading corrected the abnormalities (22). Despite these alterations, the overall function of the renin–angiotensin–aldosterone system is preserved in thyrotoxicosis, so blood pressure regulation and sodium homeostasis are nearly always normal.

ANDROGENS AND ESTROGENS

Men with thyrotoxicosis have high serum estradiol concentrations, as a result of increased extraglandular conversion of androstenedione to estradiol, and some have gynecomastia (see Chapter 39). In addition, serum sex hormone–binding globulin concentrations are high, leading to increases in serum total testosterone and estradiol concentrations and concomitant decreases in the clearance rate of both

steroids (31). In human hepatoma cells, the mRNA for sex hormone–binding globulin is increased by T_3, suggesting that it increases expression of the gene for the binding protein (32).

The increase in hepatic $\Delta 4,5$-steroid reductase activity that occurs in thyrotoxicosis described above extends to androgens (Fig. 37.3). The result is a shift in the pattern of testosterone and androstenedione metabolism; the formation and urinary excretion of androsterone are increased, and those of etiocholanolone are decreased (13).

REFERENCES

1. DeNayer P, Dozin B, Vandeput Y, et al. Altered interaction between triiodothyronine and its nuclear receptors in absence of cortisol: a proposed mechanism for increased thyrotropin secretion in corticosteroid deficiency states. *Eur J Clin Invest* 1987; 17:106.
2. Brent GA, Harney JW, Moore DD, et al. Multihormonal regulation of the human, rat, and bovine growth hormone promoters: differential effects of 3′,5′-cyclic adenosine monophosphate, thyroid hormone, and glucocorticoids. *Mol Endocrinol* 1988;2: 792.
3. Brent GA. The molecular basis of thyroid hormone action. *N Engl J Med* 1994;331:847.
4. Williams GR, Franklyn JA, Sheppard MC. Thyroid hormone and glucocorticoid regulation of receptor and target gene mRNAs in pituitary GH3 cells. *Mol Cell Endocrinol* 1991;80:127.
5. Malchoff CD, Javier EC, Malchoff DM, et al. Primary cortisol resistance presenting as isosexual precocity. *J Clin Endocrinol Metab* 1990;70:503.
6. Iida S, Nakamura Y, Fujii H, et al. A patient with hypocortisolism and Cushing's syndrome-like manifestations: cortisol hyperreactive syndrome. *J Clin Endocrinol Metab* 1990;70:729.
7. Brabant A, Brabant G, Schuermeyer T, et al. The role of glucocorticoids in the regulation of thyrotropin. *Acta Endocrinol (Copenh)* 1989;121:95.
8. Alford FP, Baker HWG, Burger HG, et al. Temporal patterns of integrated plasma hormone levels during sleep and wakefulness. I: Thyroid-stimulating hormone, growth hormone and cortisol. *J Clin Endocrinol Metab* 1973;37:841.
9. Van Cauter E, Leclercq R, Vanhaelst L, et al. Simultaneous study of cortisol and TSH daily variations in normal subjects and patients with hyperadrenalcorticism. *J Clin Endocrinol Metab* 1974;39:645.
10. Adriaanse R, Brabant G, Endert E, et al. Pulsatile thyrotropin secretion in patients with Cushing's syndrome. *Metabolism* 1994; 43:782.
11. Nicoloff JT, Fisher DA, Appleman MD. The role of glucocorticoids in the regulation of thyroid function in man. *J Clin Invest* 1970;49:1922.
12. Wilber JF, Utiger RD. The effect of glucocorticoids on thyrotropin secretion. *J Clin Invest* 1969;48:2096.
13. Peterson RE. Metabolism of adrenal cortical steroids. In: Christy NP, ed. *The human adrenal cortex.* New York: Harper & Row, 1971:137.
14. Gallagher TF, Hellman L, Finkelstein J, et al. Hyperthyroidism and cortisol secretion in man. *J Clin Endocrinol Metab* 1972;34: 919.
15. Whorwood CB, Sheppard MC, Stewart PM. Tissue specific effects of thyroid hormone on 11β-hydroxysteroid dehydrogenase gene expression. *J Steroid Biochem Molec Biol* 1993;46(5): 539.

16. Ricketts ML, Shoesmith KJ, Hewison M, et al. Regulation of 11β-hydroxysteroid dehydrogenase type 1 in primary culture of rat and human hepatocytes. *J Endocrinol* 1998;156:159.

17. Taniyama M, Honma K, Ban Y. Urinary cortisol metabolites in the assessment of peripheral thyroid hormone action: application for diagnosis of resistance to thyroid hormone. *Thyroid* 1993;3:229.

18. Tsatsoulis A, Johnson EO, Kalogera CH, et al. The effect of thyrotoxicosis on adrenocortical reserve. *Eur J Endocrinol* 2000;142:231.

19. Moghetti P, Castello R, Tosi F, et al. Glucose counterregulatory response to acute hypoglycemia in hyperthyroid human subjects. *J Clin Endocrinol Metab* 1994;78:169.

20. Coulombe P, Dussault JH, Walker P. Catecholamine metabolism in thyroid diseases. II. Norepinephrine secretion rate in hyperthyroidism and hypothyroidism. *J Clin Endocrinol Metab* 1977;44:1185.

21. Luetscher JA Jr, Camargo CA, Cohen AP, et al. Observations on metabolism of aldosterone in man. *Ann Intern Med* 1963; 59:1.

22. Cain JP, Dluhy RG, Williams GH, et al. Control of aldosterone secretion in hyperthyroidism. *J Clin Endocrinol Metab* 1973;36:365.

23. Resnick LM, Laragh JH. Plasma renin activity in syndromes of thyroid hormone excess and deficiency. *Life Sci* 1982;30:585.

24. Brent GA, Hershman JM, Reed AW, et al. Serum angiotensin-converting enzyme in severe nonthyroidal illnesses associated with low serum thyroxine concentration. *Ann Intern Med* 1984; 100:680.

25. Dzau VJ, Hermann HC. Hormonal regulation of angiotensinogen synthesis. *Life Sci* 1982;30:577.

26. Deschepper CF, Hong-Brown LQ. Hormonal regulation of the angiotensinogen gene in liver and other tissues. In: Raizada MK, Phillips MI, Sumners C. eds. *Cellular and molecular biology of renin-angiotensin system.* Boca Raton, FL: CRC Press, 1993:152.

27. Dluhy RG, Underwood RH, Williams GH. Influence of dietary potassium on plasma renin activity in normal man. *J Appl Physiol* 1970;28:299.

28. Dluhy RG, Axelrod L, Underwood RH, et al. Studies of the control of plasma aldosterone concentration in normal man. II. Effect of dietary potassium and acute potassium infusion. *J Clin Invest* 1972;51:1950.

29. Kigoshi T, Kaneko M, Nakano S, et al. Aldosterone response to various stimuli in hyperthyroidism: *in vivo* and *in vitro* studies. *Folia Endocrinol Jpn* 1993;69:609.

30. Shigematsu S, Iwasaki T, Aizawa T, et al. Plasma atrial natriuretic peptide, plasma renin activity and aldosterone during treatment of hyperthyroidism due to Graves' disease. *Horm Metab Res* 1989;21:514.

31. Ridgway EC, Longcope C, Maloof F. Metabolic clearance and blood production rates of estradiol in hyperthyroidism. *J Clin Endocrinol Metab* 1975;41:491.

32. Barlow JW, Crowe TC, Cowen NL, et al. Stimulation of sex hormone-binding globulin mRNA and attenuation of corticosteroid-binding globulin mRNA by triiodothyronine in human hepatoma cells. *Eur J Endocrinol* 1994;130:166.

THERMOGENESIS AND THE SYMPATHOADRENAL SYSTEM IN THYROTOXICOSIS

J. ENRIQUE SILVA

OVERVIEW OF THERMOGENESIS

Living organisms are open systems wherein multiple energy transformations take place. Heat is constantly generated simply by virtue of the fundamental laws of thermodynamics. The energy contained in food is captured largely in the form of adenosine triphosphate (ATP), and this is used to sustain other biochemical processes, as well as physical processes such as movement or creation of ion or chemical gradients. In all these energy transformations, a fraction is lost as heat. Heat production or thermogenesis is thus the obligatory consequence of the multiple energy transformations that occur in living cells. Homeothermic species, however, must produce more heat than poikilothermic species because they must maintain the core temperature in environments usually colder than the body. To produce sufficient heat, homeothermic species (mammals and birds) had to increase the energy cost of living. Metabolic rate, as judged by oxygen consumption (QO_2), is clearly greater in mammals than in reptiles, whether measured in the whole animal or individual tissues (1). In addition to sustaining more energy transactions, the homeothermic machine has a lower thermodynamic efficiency; that is, for any given amount of work (chemical, mechanical), a larger amount of energy is dissipated as heat (2). The sum of the heat resulting from the minimal energy cost of living plus this extra thermogenesis derived from the vital process traditionally has been called obligatory thermogenesis, although it is probably more accurate to call it basal thermogenesis, because a fraction of it is not obligatory and can be reduced (Table 38.1). Indeed, most, if not all, this reducible fraction is thyroid hormone (TH) dependent and subject to regulation. In addition, homeothermic species can produce extra heat in response to cold or to dissipate energy when overfed. This is the so-called facultative or adaptive thermogenesis. This is activated when obligatory thermogenesis is not sufficient to maintain body temperature in colder environments. In such a situation, the body defends its temperature by reducing heat dissipation (vasoconstriction, piloerection) and by recruiting facultative thermogenesis in the form of shivering and increased metabolic heat. Shivering is the most acute response and is rapidly replaced by the production of metabolic heat. In small mammals, including the human newborn and infant, the main site of nonshivering facultative thermogenesis is the brown adipose tissue (BAT). In birds and larger mammals, including probably the adult human, skeletal muscle may be an important site of facultative thermogenesis (3–5). Not only is vasoconstriction a way to reduce heat dissipation, but it also constitutes a signal to activate thermogenic mechanisms. The reduction of blood flow to the skin in a cold environment makes it become rapidly colder, and temperature sensors bring this information to the hypothalamus, which coordinates the homeostatic responses.

The cold and heat intolerance of patients with hypothyroidism and thyrotoxicosis are well known even to the layperson. TH is present in all vertebrates, in which it plays an important developmental function and regulates the operation of specific genetic programs, but only in homeothermic species (birds and mammals) does TH stimulate obligatory thermogenesis. I have recently reviewed this topic (6). How TH acquired this new function with the advent of homeothermy is simply a matter of speculation.

In considering the thermogenic effects of TH, it is important to distinguish those that directly generate the heat from those that play an ancillary role to provide the fuel for thermogenesis. Even today we are not sure what biochemical mechanisms are used by TH to produce heat. In general, TH induces heat production by increasing ATP turnover and by reducing the thermodynamic efficiency of the biologic machine. This is schematically illustrated in Figure 38.1. This view has experimental support. For example, the ATP cost to produce a given amount of glycogen from gluconeogenic precursors is greater in euthyroid rat hepatocytes than in the hypothyroid counterpart (7); also, for any amount of mechanical work, the amount of energy dissipated as heat is greater in the euthyroid than in the hypothyroid skeletal muscle (8). In terms of thermogenesis, increased energy transformations and reduced thermodynamic efficiency is exactly what differentiates the homeothermic from the poikilothermic species. One may thus consider TH as essential to realize such differences.

**TABLE 38.1. THERMOGENESIS
IN HOMEOTHERMIC SPECIES**

Obligatory or basal thermogenesis
1. Heat derived from the minimal energy cost of living
2. Additional heat produced from
   a. Higher number of energy transactions (more active, more complex metabolism)
   b. Reduced fuel efficiency of at least some functions
Facultative or adaptive thermogenesis
1. Shivering thermogenesis
2. Nonshivering facultative thermogenesis

Basal metabolic rate could decrease 30% or more in severe hypothyroidism, indicating that heat production is reduced by the same amount, or probably more, because TH normally reduces fuel efficiency. Observations made in hepatocytes from hypothyroid, euthyroid, and thyrotoxic rats support this view. The difference in QO_2 between hypo-

and euthyroid hepatocytes was greater than the difference in ATP turnover (9), meaning that a larger fraction of the energy contained in the fuel oxidized was dissipated as heat in the euthyroid than in the hypothyroid condition.

Thermogenesis obviously increases energy needs. Essential to support TH thermogenesis is the provision of extra energy. It makes teleologic sense, therefore, that TH also stimulates food intake and lipogenesis (see references 6 and 10, and references therein). The former provides additional energy; the latter, a mechanism to store it in a high caloric density form, fat. Hepatic *de novo* synthesis of fatty acids and of triacylglycerols (triglycerides) is increased (11), and these are rapidly mobilized to white adipose tissue and muscle, where TH stimulates lipoprotein lipase (12,13). In addition, TH enhances the lipolytic responses to catecholamines in white adipose tissue (14–16). Increased thermogenesis also demands additional oxygen supply to tissues, and TH clearly stimulates cardiac function, increasing car-

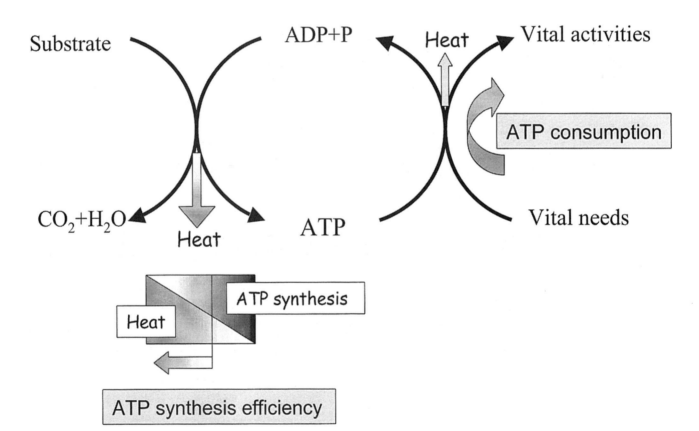

FIGURE 38.1. Schematic representation of energy transformations and heat generation in aerobic living cells. The energy contained in substrates is largely released in the mitochondria, where a fraction is captured in form of adenosine triphosphate (ATP) and a fraction is lost as heat. The energy contained in ATP is then used to sustain vital functions. Although a fraction of energy is also dissipated as heat when ATP is utilized, it is estimated that it is less than that dissipated in ATP synthesis and probably not subject to homeostatic regulation. Thermogenesis can increase by augmenting ATP demands, hence synthesis and utilization, as well as by lowering the efficiency of ATP synthesis. Thyroid hormone utilizes both types of mechanisms to augment obligatory thermogenesis. Facultative thermogenesis in brown adipose tissue largely results from uncoupling phosphorylation. This is stimulated by the sympathetic nervous system and amplified by thyroid hormone. (Adapted from Silva JE. The thermogenic effect of thyroid hormone and its clinical implications. *Ann Intern Med* 2003;139:205–213, with permission.)

diac performance and output as well as the capacity of blood to transport oxygen (17). Such an increase in myocardial efficiency and cardiac output would not be necessary if TH did not increase metabolic rate and heat production.

In many of these actions, but particularly those involving fuel and oxygen delivery, TH interacts with the sympathoadrenal system. Such interaction is also particularly important in facultative thermogenesis. TH is essential for BAT to express all its thermogenic potential, as discussed later. Such synergistic interaction takes place at several levels, namely potentiation of the norepinephrine signal at various steps, increase in enzyme activities needed for the thermogenic function, and a synergism with cyclic adenosine monophosphate (cAMP) at the gene expression level (18). On the other hand, sympathetic stimulation of BAT is affected by the thyroid status. By affecting basal thermogenesis, TH changes the need of facultative thermogenesis to maintain body temperature, hence sympathetic stimulation of BAT.

OVERVIEW OF THE SYMPATHOADRENAL SYSTEM

The sympathoadrenal system includes the sympathetic nervous system (SNS) and the adrenal medulla, the activity of which is centrally controlled at the level of the hypothalamus and brainstem. Both limbs of the sympathoadrenal system may be activated together, as in severe cold exposure and strenuous exertion, or independently, as in hypoglycemia, in which the adrenal medulla is stimulated and the activity of the SNS is suppressed. Norepinephrine, the main SNS neurotransmitter, is synthesized and stored in peripheral sympathetic nerve endings and released in response to coordinated nerve impulses targeted to specific tissues or organs. Epinephrine, in contrast, is a hormone secreted by the adrenal medulla in response to impulses carried in the splanchnic nerves and which influences processes throughout the body.

Catecholamines initiate their effects by interacting with cell surface receptors. Early pharmacologic and physiologic studies distinguished several types and subtypes of adrenergic receptors (19). With modern molecular cloning approaches, we have learned that this functional variability reflects the existence of different genes and variations in posttranscriptional processing (19–21). The α-adrenergic receptors mediate effects such as vasoconstriction, inhibition of insulin secretion (22), and stimulation of BAT type II thyroxine 5′deiodinase (23). The β-adrenergic receptors, on the other hand, mediate a variety of other processes, including cardiac stimulation, lipolysis, bronchodilation, vasodilation, and the production of metabolic heat. Both α_2- and β-adrenergic receptors are coupled to adenylyl cyclase by means of guanosine phosphate–binding proteins (G proteins). Whereas β-adrenergic receptors stimulate the production of cAMP by interacting with stimulatory G proteins (G_s), α_2 receptors interact with inhibitory G proteins (G_i) to inhibit adenylyl cyclase. Cyclic AMP activates protein kinases, generically called protein kinase A (PKA), which phosphorylates a wide variety of proteins, ultimately leading to end effects. The α_1-adrenergic receptor second messengers are inositol triphosphate (IP_3) and diacyl glycerol, both released from the hydrolysis of phosphatidylinositol. Diacyl glycerol directly stimulates protein kinase C (PKC), which in turn phosphorylates several proteins mediating a variety of end effects, and IP_3 elevates cytosolic Ca^{2+}, which influences cellular processes either directly or indirectly through the activation of Ca^{2+}-calmodulin-dependent protein kinases.

INTERACTIONS BETWEEN THYROID HORMONES AND THE SYMPATHOADRENAL SYSTEM: AN OVERVIEW

The sympathoadrenal system and TH normally interact in a coordinated manner in a number of responses to the environment. Whereas the adaptive role of the sympathoadrenal system is more readily evident, providing the means for rapid adjustments, TH increases the capacity of the cells to respond to most actions of catecholamines and maintains a metabolic rate appropriate for the availability and mobilization of substrates essential to ensure vigorous adrenergic responses. On the other hand, catecholamines increase thyroxine (T_4) to triiodothyronine (T_3) conversion in selected tissues and may increase the retention of the TH receptor in the nucleus or the recognition of DNA sequences through PKA-mediated phosphorylation of the T_3 receptor (24–26), the significance of which is yet to be defined. The synergistic interaction of both systems is essential, for example, in the response to cold exposure, when they interact to increase heat production. In general, a synergistic interaction is needed in states when the delivery of substrate or release of energy is required, such as during cold adaptation or overeating. In opposite situations, for example, starvation, both systems are turned down independently, at separate levels: sympathetic outflow decreases (27), and thyroidal secretion as well as T_4 to T_3 conversion are reduced (see Chapters 4B and 7).

In thyrotoxicosis and hypothyroidism, the interactions between the two systems are dominated by the fixation of one of them, the thyroid, at an abnormally high or low level. For example, in thyrotoxicosis, both obligatory thermogenesis and the responsiveness to catecholamines are increased, whereas the opposite occurs in hypothyroidism. The main response to these situations consists of a reduction or an increase, respectively, of sympathetic activity, as measured by norepinephrine turnover, in organs or tissues such as the heart and BAT (28–30). In patients with thyrotoxicosis, plasma and urinary levels of norepinephrine have been reported as either normal or diminished (31,32), whereas in hypothyroid patients urinary norepinephrine excretion is increased and plasma norepinephrine levels are significantly elevated (32,33), reflecting proportional increases in production rate (34,35) (see Chapter 60). As discussed later, the type II 5′deiodinase (D2) is stimulated by norepinephrine and inhibited by T_4. In thyrotoxicosis, therefore, the activity of D2 in BAT will be reduced and so will the generation of T_3 in this tissue, limiting heat generation. Studies in animals show that in T_4-induced thyrotoxicosis, the activity and the responses of BAT to cold are reduced (36,37). The opposite will occur in hypothyroidism, which enhances the activation of TH in BAT and helps to maintain its thermogenic function even in the presence of reduced plasma T_4 (38).

It follows from the preceding that the sympathomimetic features of thyrotoxicosis cannot be explained by increased sympathetic activity or epinephrine secretion, nor can the bradycardia or impaired thermogenesis of hypothyroidism be accounted for by reduced sympathetic activity. It is the exaggerated or the reduced response to catecholamines that explains these manifestations of thyrotoxicosis or hypothyroidism. In addition, some effects of TH are similar to those of sympathoadrenal activation, particularly in the cardiovascular and central nervous systems.

EFFECTS OF THYROID HORMONE ON PHYSIOLOGIC RESPONSES TO CATECHOLAMINES

TH clearly enhances the β-adrenergic receptor–mediated effects of catecholamines, and this action is important both physiologically and medically. Regarding the α-adrenergic signaling pathways, the effect of TH is neither as clear nor (seemingly) as physiologically important as on the β-adrenergic pathways. In part, this may result from TH acting at different levels downstream of the α-adrenergic receptor, often in the opposite direction. For example, T_3 reduces the expression of these receptors in liver and other organs (39) and enhances Ca^{2+}-mediated processes, but not PKC-mediated processes, whereas it directly stimulates gluconeogenesis and glycogenolysis and has a net stimulating effect on liver respiration (40).

MECHANISMS WHEREBY THYROID HORMONE ENHANCES β-ADRENERGIC RECEPTOR–MEDIATED RESPONSES TO CATECHOLAMINES

The mechanisms whereby TH enhances the β-adrenergic effects are varied both qualitatively and quantitatively, in

a tissue- and species-specific manner. They can be grouped into those whereby T_3 increases the accumulation of cAMP in response to adrenergic stimulation and those in which T_3 potentiates or enhances the effects of cAMP.

Amplification of the cAMP Response to β-Adrenergic Receptor Stimulation

TH can indeed markedly increase cAMP production. Plasma levels of cAMP are reduced in hypothyroid patients and are increased in hyperthyroid patients (41,42). In the latter group, the increase was diminished by the β-receptor antagonist, propranolol, whereas the infusion of epinephrine markedly increased urinary cAMP excretion in these patients (43). An increase of the number of β-adrenergic receptors, as well as a reduction in the number of α-adrenergic receptors by TH, has been documented in a number of tissues and cell systems from several species (see reference 39 for a review). For example, TH augments the density of β-adrenergic receptors in the heart (39,44), brown fat (45), and white adipose tissue (39) of rats. In humans, T_3 administration increases the density of β-receptors on circulating monocytes (46), and thyrotoxicosis is associated with about doubling the density of $β_2$-adrenergic receptors in white adipocytes (15). In general, the gain in receptor number in the transition from hypothyroidism to thyrotoxicosis is modest, rarely more than twofold, and additional mechanisms have to be invoked to explain the much larger increase in cAMP and some responses to catecholamines (15,16,47).

Thyroid hormones increase adenylyl cyclase activity in the rat epididymal fat pad (48) and brown adipocytes (47) and potentiate cAMP accumulation in response to catecholamines in isolated adipocytes from thyrotoxic human subjects or T_3-treated rats (16,49). In addition, TH affects the expression of adenylyl cyclase isoforms (50–52). Probably the most important postreceptor mechanism whereby thyroid hormones enhance cAMP responses is by decreasing the level of certain G-protein subunits. Several studies, using different systems, indicate that T_3 down-regulates some species of $G_{\alpha i}$ and G_β subunits (53–56). The former leads to less G_i-mediated inhibition of adenylyl cyclase, whereas the latter makes more $G_{\alpha S}$ subunits available to mediate stimulation of the cyclase. There is also evidence that TH may limit cAMP degradation by down-regulating some phosphodiesterases in adipose tissue (57). By other mechanisms less well characterized, such as an increase in cytosolic Ca^{2+}, thyroid hormones could contribute to amplifying cAMP accumulation in response to catecholamines (40).

Enhancement of cAMP Effects by Thyroid Hormone

In addition to increasing the availability of cAMP, TH may enhance the effects of cAMP. Examples of this level of action of TH are the gluconeogenic enzyme phosphoenolpyruvate carboxykinase (PEPCK) and BAT uncoupling protein 1 (UCP1). Given the growing list of genes regulated by cAMP (58), some of them also regulated by TH, this novel mechanism may well turn out to be common.

The enzyme PEPCK is a rate-limiting enzyme in gluconeogenesis. PEPCK gene transcription is stimulated by cAMP (produced in response to glucagon or epinephrine) through cAMP response elements (CREs) identified and characterized in the gene sequence (59). TH stimulates gluconeogenesis and the activity of PEPCK (60) interacting in a synergistic manner with cAMP at the gene level through a thyroid hormone response element (TRE) (61).

BAT is an important site of facultative thermogenesis regulated by catecholamines, a unique heat-producing organ in mammals (62,63). This tissue plays an important role in temperature regulation and diet-induced thermogenesis in small animals and during the newborn period in larger species, including humans (62,63). UCP1 is the key molecule in BAT thermogenesis. Norepinephrine (via cAMP) and T_3 synergistically stimulate the expression of the *UCP1* gene; each separately induces a twofold to threefold increase in gene expression, whereas together the induction is about 20-fold (64). The synergistic interaction also takes place at the gene level. Two TREs have been found high upstream in a critical enhancer element. Of the two, the downstream TRE and an adjacent downstream sequence seem essential for the synergism between cAMP and T_3, both of which interact with an additional, less well-defined downstream cAMP response sequence located near the minimal promoter of the gene (see reference 18 and references therein).

EFFECTS OF CATECHOLAMINES ON EXTRATHYROIDAL T₄ CONVERSION TO T₃

Catecholamines stimulate T_4 5'deiodination to T_3. Because T_3 is intrinsically 10 or more times more potent than T_4, this is a mechanism whereby catecholamines enhance the potency of thyroidal secretion. Interestingly, this activation may occur in a tissue-specific manner.

Biochemical and physiologic studies of T_4 to T_3 conversion have defined the existence of two pathways for the generation of T_3 (65,66). These two pathways correspond to two separate selenoproteins with iodothyronine 5'-deiodinating activity, type I (D1) and type II (D2) deiodinases encoded by two separate genes (comprehensively reviewed in reference 67) (see also Chapter 7B). D1 is largely present in the liver, kidney, and thyroid, and it is believed to be the main source of extrathyroidally generated plasma T_3, whereas D2 has been demonstrated in pituitary, central nervous system, placenta, and BAT, and, following its

cloning, in human skeletal muscle and heart (68). The D2 is believed to provide, predominantly, a local source of T_3 that is subject to tissue-specific regulation (69–71).

Catecholamines and D1

The possibility of a significant effect of catecholamines on peripheral conversion of T_4 to T_3 was raised by studies demonstrating that β-adrenergic blockade, both in hyperthyroid and in hypothyroid patients maintained on a fixed dose of T_4, decreased the circulating level of T_3 (see reference 72 for review). Nevertheless, subsequent work suggests, without excluding a minor *in vivo* stimulatory effect of catecholamines on D1, that inhibition by β-adrenergic antagonists is largely the result of a direct effect of these agents on D1. Thus, β-adrenergic blocking agents can actively block T_4 to T_3 conversion in crude homogenates of the liver, and catecholamines do not stimulate T_3 formation in whole-cell preparations. D- and L-propranolol are equally potent for inhibiting D1, and the inhibitory potency of various other compounds correlates better with the lipid solubility and membrane stabilizing properties than with their β-blocking potency (73,74).

Catecholamines and D2

In the BAT of rats (23,69) and other species (75,76), D2 can be vigorously stimulated by catecholamines. The α_1-receptor agonists suffice to stimulate D2 *in vivo*, and the stimulation by norepinephrine, a nonselective agonist, can be obliterated by prazosin, a specific α_1-receptor antagonist (23,77). However, experiments in isolated brown adipocytes show the need for both the α_1-pathway and cAMP for full stimulation (78) and suggest that the α_1-pathway somehow amplifies a cAMP-dependent signal. The brain is another tissue in which the local D2 is the major source of T_3 (71). An old report showing that the injection of epinephrine significantly increased the amount of tracer T_3 in the brains of mice after the injection of radiolabeled T_4 without detectable radiolabeled T_3 in the serum (79) indicated that catecholamines could stimulate the D2 in the brain. It was found later that this enzyme can be activated by cAMP, at least in astrocytes (80), and a CRE was identified on the 5'-flanking sequence of the D2 gene (81,82).

In the rat, acute or sustained adrenergic stimulation of BAT results in a striking increase in local T_3 generation, which can nearly saturate the T_3 receptors of this tissue (83) as well as contribute to the plasma pool of T_3 (77). The increase in local T_3 and the high level of nuclear T_3 occupancy have proved essential for a full response of uncoupling protein, α-glycerophosphate dehydrogenase, and other enzymes to adrenergic stimulation (70,84), which now has the support of observations in transgenic D2-deficient mice (85). This level of T_3 receptor occupancy in the absence of T_4 is possible only with more than a 10-fold elevation of the plasma T_3 levels (84). As mentioned earlier, in addition to its responsiveness to norepinephrine and cAMP, D2 activity is increased in hypothyroxinemia and is promptly and powerfully inhibited by T_4 (69,86), by virtue of which this enzyme plays a key role in coordinating the synergism between norepinephrine and T_3 in brown fat and possibly other tissues.

Early investigations suggested that a significant fraction of plasma T_3 in humans could derive from the activity of D2 (87). The recent finding of D2 messenger RNA (mRNA) and activity in human skeletal muscle (88) lends further support to this possibility. Furthermore, even though normal thyroid largely contains D1, the hyperactive thyroid gland of Graves' disease contains large amounts of D2 (89); however, because this enzyme is so sensitive to T_4 inhibition (69,86), it is not yet clear to what extent D2 could contribute to the extrathyroidal T_3 pool in thyrotoxicosis.

PHYSIOLOGIC AND CLINICAL CONSEQUENCES OF CATECHOLAMINE-THYROID HORMONE INTERACTIONS IN THYROTOXICOSIS

Cardiovascular Responses

The fact that the β-receptor blockade ameliorates some of the cardiovascular manifestations of thyrotoxicosis suggests that catecholamines play a role in their genesis. Because levels of catecholamines are not elevated and there is a reduction in the sympathetic input to the heart (90), the sympathetic component of the cardiovascular manifestations of thyrotoxicosis largely reflects an enhanced heart sensitivity, responsiveness, or both to catecholamines by virtue of mechanisms discussed previously. In humans, most studies [with a few exceptions (91,92)] demonstrated exaggerated heart rate responses to catecholamines in thyrotoxicosis (93). It is likely that the extent of participation of the SNS in the hyperdynamic cardiovascular state of thyrotoxicosis varies, depending on the physiologic status and the extent to which the sympathetic outflow in thyrotoxicosis is reduced (29). Even if lower than normal, the adrenergic stimulation of the heart, such as in stressful situations or exercise, will result in exaggerated cardiovascular responses. This exaggerated responsiveness of the thyrotoxic heart to adrenergic stimulation, on the other hand, may be advantageous at high load rates, as suggested by the negative effect of β-adrenergic blockade in the left ventricular ejection fraction during exercise in hyperthyroid persons (94).

It is important to emphasize that T_3 directly affects biochemical changes in the myocardium, leading to tachycardia, increased contractility, and accelerated relaxation

(95,96) (see also Chapter 31). The problem of the extent to which enhanced catecholamine responsiveness and sensitivity participate in the generation of hemodynamic changes in thyrotoxicosis, namely, the direct effects of TH, has been approached by studying the hemodynamic effects of β-blockers in thyrotoxicosis (see reference 17 for review). In general, results show that β-adrenergic blockade reduces, but does not normalize, heart rate and cardiac output. Most researchers agree that β-blockade does not significantly decrease the enhanced contractility characteristic of the thyrotoxic heart, in agreement with the observation that the reduction in cardiac output obtained with β-blockers is proportional to the drop in heart rate.

An important factor in the elevated cardiac output and hyperdynamic circulation of thyrotoxicosis is the reduction in peripheral vascular resistance (17). This reduction is thought to be mediated by a globally reduced sympathetic tone to skeletal muscle (29), along with decreased responses to contractile stimuli mediated by α_1-adrenergic receptors and enhanced responsiveness to β_2-adrenergic receptor–mediated dilatation (97,98). Indeed the contribution of β_2-adrenergic receptor in vascular peripheral resistance, particularly at the skeletal muscle level, has become more evident in recent times, and seems to be important in hyperthyroidism (17,99,100). Actually, β-adrenergic antagonists have been reported to increase peripheral vascular resistance (see references 93 and 101 and references therein), and this should be a reason to be cautious in the use of β-blockers in certain patients with severe hyperthyroidism (102), as discussed later.

Metabolic Responses

Lipolysis

TH accentuates the lipolytic effect of catecholamines in experimental animals and humans. T_3 not only enhances the strength of the norepinephrine signal by a variety of mechanisms, but it also may stimulate lipolysis by other, post–adenylyl cyclase mechanisms that as yet are not well defined. Increased sensitivity, responsiveness, or both to catecholamines in thyrotoxicosis has been documented *in vivo* and *in vitro*, in adipose tissue or adipocytes of several species, including humans (15,16,103). The mechanisms that strengthen the norepinephrine signal vary with the species. In rats, for example, it has been convincingly documented that TH inhibits the expression of G_b subunit (104) and G_i subunits (105,106). These proteins are underexpressed in adipocytes exposed to excess TH, whereas they are overexpressed in hypothyroidism. Recent studies in human white adipocytes from patients with hyperthyroidism, before and after treatment, as well as from euthyroid controls, suggest that an increase in β_2-adrenergic receptors occurs. This is associated with increased responsiveness to β_2, but not β_1 or α_2, agonists, as well as increased response to cAMP analogues or direct stimulation of adenylyl cyclase, suggesting a dual mechanism operating at both the receptor and postreceptor levels (15). The up- and down-regulation of several genes relevant to the lipolytic response has been documented in primary cultures of human subcutaneous adipocytes (107). There is indeed a coordinated increase in agonistic and decrease in antagonistic genes, such as α_2-adrenergic receptors, G_i protein, and phosphodiesterase, resulting in enhanced responses to norepinephrine via the β_2-adrenergic receptor. These observations are consistent with a much greater increase in lipolytic responses to norepinephrine (>10-fold) than in the number of β_2-adrenergic receptors (by twofold to threefold) in adipocytes from thyrotoxic persons. Pharmacologic approaches in the past, though, failed to support a major role for α_2-adrenergic receptors, which inhibit adenylyl cyclase through G_i proteins in the increased lipolytic responses (15,108). Lastly, TH also directly stimulates lipogenesis and fatty acid oxidation (109), contributing to accelerated fatty acid turnover.

Thermogenesis

As explained earlier, TH plays a critical role in thermogenesis. At least 30% of the heat produced from basal metabolic rate, so-called obligatory or basal thermogenesis (Table 38.1), is TH-dependent, and TH is essential for full facultative or adaptive thermogenesis responses. The relationship between catecholamines and thyroid hormones in the regulation of metabolic heat production in mammalian organisms is complex. Both thyroid hormones and the SNS participate in thermogenesis (reviewed in references 6 and 110). The SNS is concerned chiefly with rapid adjustments in heat production above basal rates in response to low environmental temperature or dietary intake (111) (facultative thermogenesis), whereas TH has the double role of being the main controller of basal thermogenesis and potentiating catecholamine-induced facultative thermogenesis.

TH increases basal thermogenesis, seemingly by a dual mechanism: by increasing ATP demands and by reducing the thermodynamic efficiency of ATP synthesis (Fig. 38.1). There is normally a fraction of energy dissipated as heat in the process of ATP synthesis as well as in the utilization in vital processes of the energy stored in ATP. Simply by increasing ATP demands and hence turnover, TH augments heat production, but this mechanism accounts for only a fraction, roughly 50%, of the increase in energy expenditure resulting from TH action (see reference 6 and references therein). The other part is probably the result of a decrease in the energy efficiency of vital processes, particularly in the synthesis of ATP. The fraction of energy dissipated as heat in ATP synthesis is greater than that lost in

the utilization of ATP and is subject to regulation. The concept that TH could reduce the efficiency of ATP synthesis is quite old but remained dormant for many years, and it was only recently revived (112) as a result of the analysis of the oxygen consumption as a function of the proton gradient across the inner mitochondrial membrane. Harper et al. have demonstrated that TH treatment of animals or cells results in increased proton leak in the mitochondria (9,113). Based on studies in rat hepatocytes, this mechanism is more important in the transition from hypothyroidism to euthyroidism than in thyrotoxicosis (9). These results support the concept that sustaining thermogenesis is a primary physiologic role of TH, rather than the mere consequence of increasing metabolic rate. While still significant in thyrotoxicosis, this mechanism is less important than increased ATP turnover as source of heat. The mechanism of the proton leak remains speculative. The novel uncoupling proteins UCP2 and UCP3 (see reference 114 for review) have the potential to account for the proton leak. It was recognized early on that UCP3 was stimulated by TH and adrenergic receptor activation (115). The major problem derives from the observation that transgenic UCP3 knockout mice do not respond differently from the cognate controls to T_3 (116), and neither this model nor the UCP2 knockout mice shows evidence of a thermogenic defect (116–118). Although this evidence is compelling, it is not definitive. TH can possibly utilize other thermogenic mechanisms that may be recruited as the level of TH increases, and the doses of T_3 injected in those experiments (116) were many times the daily production rate of this hormone.

Looking for alternative thermogenic mechanisms, we have investigated the mitochondrial glycerol-3-phosphate dehydrogenase (mGPD; EC 1.1.99.5), because this enzyme has long been known to be stimulated by TH (119). Moreover, mGPD is stimulated by TH only in tissues and species where TH increases thermogenesis (119–121). mGPD is the rate-limiting enzyme in the glycerol-3-phosphate (G3P) shuttle. This and the malate-aspartate shuttle transfer reducing equivalents (H^+, e^-) from cytoplasm to mitochondria to produce H_2O and capture the energy released as ATP. These shuttles are present in most cells, but their activity in absolute and relative terms varies substantially. For example, the G3P shuttle is very active in skeletal muscle, whereas the malate-aspartate shuttle is of minor importance (122). The other enzyme in the G3P shuttle is the cytoplasm glycerol-3-phosphate dehydrogenase (cGPD; EC 1.1.1.8). This enzyme reduces dihydroxyacetone-3-phosphate (DHAP) to G3P that can be used for lipid synthesis or reoxidized to DHAP by mGPD, which then transfers the reducing equivalents to the complex III of the mitochondrial respiratory chain. Depending on the tissues and prevailing conditions, the G3P shuttle can thus generate ATP or store energy as fat. Because the electrons enter the respiratory chain in complex III, only two ATPs are generated per pair of electrons or per atom of oxygen, as opposed to three ATPs when the electrons enter in complex I, as occurs with the use of the malate-aspartate shuttle. The G3P shuttle then allows for the rapid generation of ATP but with less efficiency. The G3P shuttle is, not surprisingly, quite active in cells that require rapid ATP generation such as flight muscle of insects, pancreatic islets, β cells, sperm cells, and muscle. Interestingly, mGPD is also abundant in BAT (123), although its role in this tissue has not been defined.

For the reasons briefly outlined, we have been investigating the phenotype of a mouse with targeted disruption of the mGPD gene (124). Mice with deletion of both alleles (mGPD−/−) had lower energy expenditure as judged by oxygen consumption and food intake (125). A compensated thermogenic defect was evident by the signs of chronic BAT stimulation and elevation of the plasma T_4 and T_3 concentrations. The elimination of these two responses made evident the thermogenic defect of mGPD−/− mice (125). They also have a twofold increase in UCP3 mRNA level in muscle, but the compensatory value of this change awaits confirmation. These results indicate that mGPD plays a role in the physiologic stimulation of obligatory thermogenesis by TH. Indeed, the increase in oxygen consumption caused by high doses of T_3 was not different between the mGPD−/− mice and the littermates of wild-type genotype.

It has been mentioned that BAT is an important site of facultative thermogenesis, where the synergism between the SNS and TH is essential to the realization of BAT thermogenic potential and where D2 plays a pivotal role. In thyrotoxicosis, the mechanisms regulating this deiodinase may serve the function of preventing an unwanted thermogenic synergism between TH and catecholamines because this enzyme is highly sensitive to inhibition by elevated plasma T_4 levels (69,86) and very dependent on continued adrenergic stimulation (64). Indeed, it has been found that brown-fat responses to cold are blunted in rats with T_4-induced thyrotoxicosis (36,37). Another locus of coordinated interaction between SNS and TH is the β_3-adrenergic receptor. These receptors are expressed predominantly in BAT and white adipose tissue of several species, including humans (see reference 126 for review). They are G protein–coupled receptors mediating metabolic responses, such as thermogenesis and lipolysis. Interestingly, the expression of β_3-adrenergic receptors is increased in hypothyroid BAT and is rapidly reversed by an injection of T_3, whereas the opposite occurs in white fat (127). This powerful effect of T_3 over BAT β_3-adrenergic receptors may be yet another mechanism for curbing facultative thermogenesis in thyrotoxicosis (127).

Skeletal muscle is likely an important site of facultative thermogenesis in adult humans (128) and in birds (see references 96 and 129 and references therein), who have little or no BAT. Muscle facultative thermogenesis is di-

rectly or indirectly (e.g., through fatty acids) stimulated by catecholamines (5) in a TH-dependent manner (8). It is conceivable that facultative thermogenesis in these sites also is reduced in human thyrotoxicosis and, furthermore, that the hyperthermia of thyroid storm represents the failure of the body to suppress the sympathetic activity in such sites. This view is supported by observations that thyroid storm may be triggered by stressful situations or by sympathomimetic agents (130). Moreover, propranolol has a beneficial effect on thyroid storm hyperthermia, but it does not reduce resting energy expenditure in uncomplicated thyrotoxicosis (131), in agreement with a suppressed adrenergic contribution to thermogenesis in this state.

Other Metabolic Responses

Muscle-protein loss (see Chapter 41) associated with thyrotoxicosis is not likely to be mediated by catecholamines because muscle sympathetic activity is frequently reduced in thyrotoxicosis (29), and β-blocking agents have no effects on protein degradation in thyrotoxicosis in either rats or humans, as judged by 3-methylhistidine excretion (132, 133).

Thyrotoxicosis also appears to modify the effect of catecholamines on insulin secretion in rats and in human subjects (134–136). Depending on the circumstances, catecholamines may either suppress or stimulate insulin secretion; suppression is mediated by an α-adrenergic mechanism (22), and stimulation involves the β-adrenergic receptor (137). In both experimental and clinical thyrotoxicosis, β-receptor-mediated stimulation of insulin secretion is enhanced (134).

Catecholamines are known to increase calcium mobilization from the skeleton (138), which is believed to be mediated by β-adrenergic receptors, as recently described in human and rat osteoblasts (139). That the stimulation of calcium release from bone in thyrotoxicosis may be mediated at least in part by catecholamines finds support in the observation that β-blockers may significantly reduce serum calcium in hypercalcemic but not in normocalcemic thyrotoxic patients or in normal subjects (140,141).

ADRENERGIC BLOCKADE IN HYPERTHYROIDISM

It follows from the foregoing discussion that, in view of the enhanced tissue responses to catecholamines, it may be beneficial in thyrotoxicosis to protect the body against residual sympathetic activity or during the derepression of SNS that may follow stimuli such as emotion, stress, and exercise. Reserpine, guanethidine, and propranolol all reverse some of the alterations that accompany the thyrotoxic state (101). Because most of the catecholamine effects enhanced by TH are mediated by β-adrenergic receptors, β-adrenergic antagonists probably represent the most specific way to accomplish the sympathetic blockade. The efficacy of propranolol in the symptomatic management of thyrotoxicosis was demonstrated in several studies (101). β-adrenergic blockade does not reduce thyroidal secretion, and although several β-blockers induce a modest decrease in plasma T_3 levels (72), these actions of β-blockers are believed to play a minor role in the beneficial effects of sympathetic blockade. Studies on the levels of cAMP (42) suggest that most of the clinical effect, particularly in lower doses, is due to β-adrenergic receptor blockade. Even though some reports comparing D- and L-propranolol (142) suggest that part of the beneficial effects of this drug may be independent from β-adrenergic antagonism, such a mechanism does not seem clinically important.

Clinical and Physiologic Effects of Adrenergic Blockade

The most dramatic effects of adrenergic blockade in uncomplicated thyrotoxicosis are symptoms derived from exaggerated responses to catecholamines and the hemodynamic changes associated with thyrotoxicosis. The hemodynamic effects of adrenergic blockade in experimental and spontaneous thyrotoxicosis have been the subject of repeated studies. Heart rate, cardiac output, systolic blood pressure, and pulse pressure are decreased, whereas circulation time is prolonged and peripheral vascular resistance is increased (17,93,101,143) by adrenergic blockade. This latter effect is probably due to the cancellation of β$_2$-adrenergic receptor activity, which is thought to mediate the peripheral vasodilatation of thyrotoxicosis, particularly in muscle (99). As mentioned earlier, the reduction in cardiac output following sympathetic blockade in hyperthyroidism closely corresponds to the decrease in heart rate with little or no effect on myocardial contractility (92,144,145), supporting the idea that most of the enhanced contractility reflects a direct action of T_3 on the myocardial Ca^{2+}-dependent- and myosin heavy-chain ATPases (95,144). It is important to recall that in exercise, in conditions of overload, or in impending congestive failure, the SNS contributes significantly to maintain cardiac output; in such conditions, the indiscriminate use of adrenergic blocking agents is likely to be detrimental (94,146,147). In such cases it is preferable to use selective β$_1$-adrenergic receptor blocking if β-adrenergic receptors are deemed necessary to reduce heart rate and restlessness.

Lid lag, lid retraction, widened palpebral fissure, as well as tremor and hyperreflexia, all expressions of increased adrenergic responses, are correspondingly reduced by sympathetic blockade (148–151). Interestingly, the tremor is a β$_2$-mediated effect, as may be the hypokalemia seen in a few patients (24). Nervousness and irritability also are diminished (152). Some of the more unusual but dramatic neurologic manifestations of thyrotoxicosis also are ameliorated by β-adrenergic blockade. Thyrotoxic periodic paralysis (24–153), choreoathetosis (154), and upper motor neuron weakness and spasticity (155) have been reported to improve with β-receptor blocking agents. Beta-adrenergic blockade also has been reported to reduce the hypercalcemia associated with hyperthyroidism (141,156,157).

Adrenergic blockade may reduce weight loss in hyperthyroid subjects at high doses (158), but it does not restore weight to normal (101,159). The reported improvement in nitrogen balance induced by β-blockers (159) probably is the result of a reduction in intestinal hypermotility and improved absorption (160) rather than from blocking catabolic effects of catecholamines. Although the clinical correlates of increased metabolic rate, heat intolerance, and sweating are ameliorated by β-blockade (101,161), β-blockade does not seem to reduce hypermetabolism to a clinically significant extent (131), except probably in thyroid storm, as discussed earlier.

Clinical Usefulness of Adrenergic Blockade in the Treatment of Thyrotoxicosis

Beta-blockers have significantly improved the management of the symptomatic thyrotoxic patient. In mild to moderate thyrotoxicosis, subjective symptomatic improvement often can be achieved with 40 to 80 mg of propranolol per day. Although thyrotoxicosis increases plasma clearance of propranolol (158,162,163), clinical goals can be attained with relatively low doses empirically determined. A reduction in pulse rate, particularly after mild exercise in the office, such as a few squattings, often provides a useful guide. In my experience, 40 mg of nadolol, a non-β-selective antagonist, at bedtime is an easy, effective way to obtain symptomatic relief.

Probably because of direct, unrestrained participation of the SNS, the effect of these agents in the thyroid storm is often dramatic (101). In these patients, doses of propranolol in excess of 160 mg per day may be necessary. A sensible approach is to control the acute manifestations with up to 5 to 10 mg of intravenous propranolol, at 1 mg per minute, followed by oral maintenance doses commenced 4 to 6 hours later and titrated to maintain reasonable control of the symptoms and tachycardia. When congestive failure, pressure, or volume overload is an issue, it is better to use short-acting β-blockers (102) and preferably β$_1$-adrenergic receptor selective agonists because blocking β$_2$-adrenergic receptors may be associated with increases in vascular peripheral resistance (99).

β-adrenergic blockade is also useful in thyrotoxic patients undergoing emergency surgery. Severely thyrotoxic patients undergoing surgery frequently have tachycardia and high temperature in the postoperative period, probably reflecting the sympathetic activation in response to the surgical stress (164). Propranolol, with or without concomitant inorganic iodides (164–166), or even with dexamethasone (167), has been used safely in hyperthyroid patients in preparation for thyroidal or nonthyroidal emergency surgery. Even though the metabolic and endocrine responses to surgical stress appear to be diminished by propranolol (168,169), β-blockers do not significantly antagonize the catabolic effects of the excess thyroid hormones or their direct thermogenic effects (159,170–173), as described in reports of failure of propranolol to prevent thyroid storm (174,175). In cases of untoward effects of thionamides, there is consensus that it is safer to include iodides to reduce thyroidal secretion (166,168) or dexamethasone (167) to counteract some effects of TH by inhibiting conversion of T_4 to T_3. Also, the higher doses of β-blocker used in these patients will eliminate completely the sympathetic stimulation of the heart, which may precipitate congestive heart failure in patients with limited reserve resulting from preexisting heart problems or pressure or volume overloads (94,146).

Propranolol also has been used in the treatment of thyrotoxicosis during pregnancy (176,177) and in the preoperative preparation of pregnant women for thyroidectomy (178). Although propranolol is effective for controlling the symptoms of thyrotoxicosis in the mother, it has potential adverse effects on the fetus and on the course of labor. Neonatal apnea, bradycardia, hypoglycemia, polycythemia, hyperbilirubinemia, and premature labor all have been described (176,179). Congestive heart failure in the newborn is a dreaded potential complication (180). In the thyrotoxic patient who is pregnant and in parturition or in need of cesarean section, propranolol may be life saving, but potential adverse effects on the fetus should be anticipated and call for an expectant attitude. Propranolol actually may play an important role in the management of neonatal thyrotoxicosis (181–183), but, as is the case of the transplacental passage route, it also may cause severe side effects (184) and should be used with extreme care.

Sympathetic blockade, particularly β-adrenergic blockade, certainly has an important place in the management of thyrotoxicosis. This approach should be used judiciously, however, and with the best possible understanding of the pathophysiology of the individual patient. It cannot be overemphasized that β-adrenergic blockade represents a palliative aspect in the preparation for surgery and to treat or ameliorate the manifestations of thyroid storm. Therefore, it must be used in conjunction with other measures that reduce TH secretion (large doses of iodine) and T_4 to T_3 conversion (propylthiouracil, iopanoic acid, and glucocorticoids) and that antagonize some end effects of T_3 (glucocorticoids).

REFERENCES

1. Else PL, Hulbert AJ. Comparison of the "mammal machine" and the "reptile machine": energy production. *Am Physiol* 1981;240:R3–R9.
2. Woledge RC. Energy transformations in living muscle. In: Wieser W, Gnaiger E, eds. *Energy transformations in cells and organisms.* New York: Georg Thieme Verlag, 1989:36–45.
3. Astrup A, Simonsen L, Bulow J, et al. Epinephrine mediates facultative carbohydrate-induced thermogenesis in human skeletal muscle. *Am J Physiol* 1989;257:E340–E345.
4. Astrup A, Bulow J, Christensen NJ, et al. Facultative thermogenesis induced by carbohydrate: a skeletal muscle component mediated by epinephrine. *Am J Physiol* 1986;250:E226–E229.
5. Block BA. Thermogenesis in muscle. *Annu Rev Physiol* 1994;56:535–577.
6. Silva JE. The thermogenic effect of thyroid hormone and its clinical implications. *Ann Intern Med* 2003;139:205–213.
7. Berry MN, Gregory RB, Grivell AR, et al. The thermodynamic regulation of cellular metabolism and heat production. In: Wieser W, Gnaiger E, eds. *Energy transformations in cells and organisms.* New York: Georg Thieme Verlag, 1989:18–27.
8. Leijendekker WJ, van Hardeveld C, Elzinga G. Heat production during contraction in skeletal muscle of hypothyroid mice. *Am Physiol* 1987;253(part 1):E214–E220.
9. Harper ME, Brand MD. The quantitative contributions of mitochondrial proton leak and ATP turnover reactions to the changed respiration rates of hepatocytes from rats of different thyroid status. *J Biol Chem* 1993;268:14850–14860.
10. Silva JE. The multiple contributions of thyroid hormone to heat production. *J Clin Invest* 2001;108:35–37.
11. Freake HC, Schwartz HL, Oppenheimer JH. The regulation of lipogenesis by thyroid hormone and its contribution to thermogenesis. *Endocrinology* 1989;125:2868–2874.
12. Ong JM, Simsolo RB, Saghizadeh M, et al. Expression of lipoprotein lipase in rat muscle: regulation by feeding and hypothyroidism. *J Lipid Res* 1994;35:1542–1551.
13. Saffari B, Ong JM, Kern PA. Regulation of adipose tissue lipoprotein lipase gene expression by thyroid hormone in rats. *J Lipid Res* 1992;33:241–249.
14. Riis AL, Gravholt CH, Djurhuus CB, et al. Elevated regional lipolysis in hyperthyroidism. *J Clin Endocrinol Metab* 2002;87:4747–4753.
15. Hellstrom L, Wahrenberg H, Reynisdottir S, et al. Catecholamine-induced adipocyte lipolysis in human hyperthyroidism. *J Clin Endocrinol Metab* 1997;82:159–166.
16. Wahrenberg H, Wennlund A, Arner P. Adrenergic regulation of lipolysis in fat cells from hyperthyroid and hypothyroid patients. *J Clin Endocrinol Metab* 1994;78:898–903.
17. Kahaly GJ, Kampmann C, Mohr-Kahaly S. Cardiovascular hemodynamics and exercise tolerance in thyroid disease. *Thyroid* 2002;12:473–481.
18. Silva JE, Rabelo R. Regulation of the uncoupling protein gene expression. *Eur J Endocrinol* 1997;136:251–264.
19. Goldstein DS. Catecholamine receptors and signal transduction: overview. *Adv Pharmacol* 1998;42:379–390.
20. Iyengar R. Molecular and functional diversity of mammalian Gs-stimulated adenylyl cyclases [Review]. *FASEB J* 1993;7:768–775.

21. Strasser RH, Ihl-Vahl R, Marquetant R. Molecular biology of adrenergic receptors. *J Hypertens* 1992;10:501–506.
22. Chan SL. Role of alpha 2-adrenoceptors and imidazoline-binding sites in the control of insulin secretion [Review]. *Clin Sci* 1993;85:671–677.
23. Silva JE, Larsen PR. Adrenergic activation of triiodothyronine production in brown adipose tissue. *Nature* 1983;305:712–713.
24. Tesfamariam B, Waldron T, Seymour AA. Quantitation of tremor in response to beta-adrenergic receptor stimulation in primates: relationship with hypokalemia. *J Pharmacol Toxicol Methods* 1998;40:201–205.
25. Nicoll JB, Gwinn BL, Iwig JS, et al. Compartment-specific phosphorylation of rat thyroid hormone receptor alpha1 regulates nuclear localization and retention. *Mol Cell Endocrinol* 2003;205:65–77.
26. Tzagarakis-Foster C, Privalsky ML. Phosphorylation of thyroid hormone receptors by protein kinase A regulates DNA recognition by specific inhibition of receptor monomer binding. *J Biol Chem* 1998;273:10926–10932.
27. Young JB, Saville E, Rothwell NJ, et al. Effect of diet and cold exposure on norepinephrine turnover in brown adipose tissue of the rat. *J Clin Invest* 1982;69:1061–1071.
28. Landsberg L, Axelrod J. Influence of pituitary, thyroid and adrenal hormones on norepinephrine turnover and metabolism in the rat heart. *Circ Res* 1968;22:559–571.
29. Matsukawa T, Mano T, Gotoh E, et al. Altered muscle sympathetic nerve activity in hyperthyroidism and hypothyroidism. *J Auton Nerv Syst* 1993;42:171–175.
30. Tu T, Nash CW. The influence of prolonged hyper- and hypothyroid states on the noradrenaline content of rat tissues and on the accumulation and efflux rates of tritiated noradrenaline. *Can J Physiol Pharmacol* 1975;53:74–80.
31. Bayliss RIS, Edwards OM. Urinary secretion of free catecholamines in Graves' disease. *Endocrinology* 1971;49:167.
32. Coulombe P, Dussault JH, Walker P. Plasma catecholamine concentrations in hyperthyroidism and hypothyroidism. *Metabolism* 1976;25:973–979.
33. Christensen NJ. Increased levels of plasma noradrenaline in hypothyroidism. *J Clin Endocrinol Metab* 1972;35:359.
34. Polikar R, Kennedy B, Ziegler M, et al. Plasma norepinephrine kinetics, dopamine-beta-hydroxylase, and chromogranin-A, in hypothyroid patients before and following replacement therapy. *J Clin Endocrinol Metab* 1990;70:277–281.
35. Coulombe P, and Dussault JH. Catecholamine metabolism in thyroid disease. II. Norepinephrine secretion rate in hyperthyroidism and hypothyroidism. *J Clin Endocrinol Metab* 1977;44:1185–1189.
36. Sundin U. GDP binding to rat brown fat mitochondria: effects of thyroxine at different ambient temperature. *Am J Physiol* 1981;241:C134–C139.
37. Triandafillou J, Gwilliam C, Himms-Hagen J. Role of thyroid hormone in cold-induced changes in rat brown adipose tissue mitochondria. *Can J Biochem* 1982;60:530–537.
38. Carvalho SD, Kimura ET, Bianco AC, et al. Central role of brown adipose tissue thyroxine 5'deiodinase on thyroid hormone-dependent thermogenic response to cold. *Endocrinology* 1991;128:2149–2159.
39. Bilezikian JP, Loeb JN. The influence of hyperthyroidism and hyperthyroidism on α- and β-adrenergic receptor systems and adrenergic responsiveness. *Endocr Rev* 1983;4:378–388.
40. Daza FJ, Parrilla R, Martin-Requero A. Influence of thyroid status on hepatic alpha 1-adrenoreceptor responsiveness. *Am J Physiol* 1997;273:E1065–E1072.
41. Karlberg BE, Henriksson KG, Andersson RG. Cyclic adenosine 3',5'-monophosphate concentration in plasma, adipose tissue

and skeletal muscle in normal subjects and in patients with hyper- and hypothyroidism. *J Clin Endocrinol Metab* 1974;39:96.
42. Guttler RB, Croxson MS, DeQuattro VL, et al. Effects of thyroid hormone on plasma adenosine 3',5'- monophosphate production in man. *Metabolism* 1977;26:1155–1162.
43. Guttler RG, Shaw JW, Otis CL, et al. Epinephrine-induced alterations in urinary cyclic AMP in hyper- and hypothyroidism. *J Clin Endocrinol Metab* 1975;41:707.
44. Crozatier B, Su JB, Corsin A, et al. Species differences in myocardial beta-adrenergic receptor regulation in response to hyperthyroidism. *Circ Res* 1991;69:1234–1243.
45. Rothwell NJ, Stock MJ, Sudera DK. Changes in adrenoreceptor density in brown adipose tissue from hyperthyroid rats. *Eur J Pharmacol* 1985;114:227–229.
46. Ginsberg AM, Clutter WE, Shah SD, et al. Triiodothyronine-induced thyrotoxicosis increases mononuclear leukocyte β-adrenergic receptor density in man. *J Clin Invest* 1981;67:1785.
47. Sundin U, Mills I, Fain JN. Thyroid-catecholamine interactions in isolated brown adipocytes. *Metabolism* 1984;33:1028–1033.
48. Bumgarner JR, Ramkumar V, Stiles GL. Altered thyroid status regulates the adipocyte A1 adenosine receptor-adenylate cyclase system. *Life Sci* 1989;44:1705–1712.
49. Mills I, Garcia-Sainz JA, Fain JN. Pertussis toxin effects on adenylate cyclase activity, cyclic AMP accumulation and lipolysis in adipocytes from hypothyroid, euthyroid and hyperthyroid rats. *Biochim Biophys Acta* 1986;876:619–630.
50. Pracyk JB, Slotkin TA. Thyroid hormone regulates ontogeny of beta adrenergic receptors and adenylate cyclase in rat heart and kidney: effects of propylthiouracil-induced perinatal hypothyroidism. *J Pharmacol Exp Ther* 1992;261:951–958.
51. Carvalho SD, Bianco AC, Silva JE. Effects of hypothyroidism on brown adipose tissue adenylyl cyclase activity. *Endocrinology* 1996;137:5519–5529.
52. Chaudhry A, Granneman JG. Effect of hypothyroidism on adenylyl cyclase activity and subtype gene expression in brown adipose tissue. *Am J Physiol* 1997;273:R762–R767.
53. Michel-Reher MB, Gross G, Jasper JR, et al. Tissue- and subunit-specific regulation of G-protein expression by hypo- and hyperthyroidism. *Biochem Pharmacol* 1993;45:1417–1423.
54. Orford MR, Leung FCL, Milligan G, et al. Treatment with triiodothyronine decreases the abundance of the α-subunits of Gi1 and Gi2 in the cerebral cortex. *J Neurol Sci* 1992;112:34–37.
55. Levine MA, Feldman AM, Robishaw JD, et al. Influence of thyroid hormone status on expression of genes encoding G proteins subunits in rat heart. *J Biol Chem* 1990;265:3553–3560.
56. Rapiejko PJ, Watkins DC, Ros M, et al. 1989. Thyroid hormones regulate G-protein β-subunit mRNA expression *in vivo*. *J Biol Chem* 1989;264:16183–16189.
57. Goswami A, Rosenberg IN. Effects of thyroid status on membrane-bound low Km cyclic nucleotide phosphodiesterase activities in rat adipocytes. *J Biol Chem* 1985;260:82–85.
58. Sassone-Corsi P. Transcription factors responsive to cAMP [Review]. *Annu Rev Cell Dev Biol* 1995;11:355–377.
59. Liu J, Park EA, Gurney AL, et al. Cyclic AMP induction of phosphoenolpyruvate carboxykinase (GTP) gene transcription is mediated by multiple promoter elements. *J Biol Chem* 1991;266:19095–19102.
60. Hoppner W, Sussmuth W, Seitz HJ. Effect of thyroid state on cyclic AMP-mediated induction of hepatic phosphoenolpyruvate carboxykinase. *Biochem J* 1985;226:67–73.
61. Giralt M, Park EA, Gurney AL, et al. Identification of a thyroid hormone response element in the phosphoenolpyruvate carboxykinase (GTP) gene: evidence for synergistic interaction be-

tween thyroid hormone and cAMP cis-regulatory elements. *J Biol Chem* 1991;266:21991–21996.

62. Himms-Hagen J. Brown adipose tissue metabolism and thermogenesis. *Annu Rev Nutr* 1985;5:69–94.

63. Cannon B, Nedergaard J. The biochemistry of an inefficient tissue: brown adipose tissue. *Essays Biochem* 1985;2:110–164.

64. Bianco AC, Sheng X, Silva JE. Triiodothyronine amplifies norepinephrine stimulation of uncoupling protein gene transcription by a mechanism not requiring protein synthesis. *J Biol Chem* 1988;263:18168–18175.

65. Visser TJ, Leonard JL, Kaplan MM, et al. Kinetic evidence suggesting two mechanisms for iodothyronine 5′-deiodination in rat cerebral cortex. *Proc Natl Acad Sci U S A* 1982;79:5080–5084.

66. Silva JE, Leonard JL, Crantz FR, et al. Evidence for two tissue-specific pathways for in vivo thyroxine 5′-deiodination in the rat. *J Clin Invest* 1982;69:1176–1184.

67. Bianco AC, Salvatore D, Gereben B, et al. Biochemistry, cellular and molecular biology, and physiological roles of the iodothyronine selenodeiodinases. *Endocr Rev* 2002;23:38–89.

68. Salvatore D, Low CS, Berry MJ, et al. Type 3 iodothyronine deiodinase: cloning, in vitro expression, and functional analysis of the placental selenoenzyme. *J Clin Invest* 1995;96:2421–2430.

69. Silva JE, Larsen PR. Hormonal regulation of iodothyronine 5′-deiodinase in rat brown adipose tissue. *Am J Physiol* 1986;251:E639–E643.

70. Bianco AC, Silva JE. Intracellular conversion of thyroxine to triiodothyronine is required for the optimal thermogenic function of brown adipose tissue. *J Clin Invest* 1987;79:295–300.

71. Silva JE, Matthews PS. Production rates and turnover of triiodothyronine in rat-developing-cerebral cortex and cerebellum: responses to hypothyroidism. *J Clin Invest* 1984;74:1035–1049.

72. Wiersinga WM. Propranolol and thyroid hormone metabolism. *Thyroid* 1991;1:273–277.

73. Shulkin BL, Peele ME, Utiger RD. Beta-adrenergic antagonist inhibition of hepatic 3,5,3′- triiodothyronine production. *Endocrinology* 1984;115:858–861.

74. Heyma P, Larkins RG, Campbell DG. Inhibition by propranolol of 3,5,3′-triiodothyronine formation from thyroxine in isolated rat renal tubules: an effect independent of β-adrenergic blockade. *Endocrinology* 1980;106:1437.

75. Kopecky J, Sigurdson L, Park IRA, et al. Thyroxine 5′-deiodinase in hamster and rat brown adipose tissue: effect of cold and diet. *Am J Physiol* 1986;251:E1–E7.

76. Kates A-L, Zaror-Behrens G, Himms-Hagen J. Adrenergic effects of thyroxine 5′-deiodinase in brown adipose tissue of lean and ob/ob mice. *Am J Physiol* 1990;258:R430–R435.

77. Silva JE, Larsen PR. Potential of brown adipose tissue type II thyroxine 5′-deiodinase as a local and systemic source of triiodothyronine in rats. *J Clin Invest* 1985;76:2296–2305.

78. Raasmaja A, Larsen PR. α1- and β-adrenergic agents cause synergistic stimulation of the iodothyronine deiodinase in rat brown adipocytes. *Endocrinology* 1989;125:2502–2509.

79. Grinberg R. Effect of epinephrine on metabolism of thyroxine by pituitary and brain. *Proc Soc Exp Biol Med* 1963;116:35.

80. Pallud S, Lennon AM, Ramauge M, et al. Expression of the type II iodothyronine deiodinase in cultured rat astrocytes is selenium-dependent. *J Biol Chem* 1997;272:18104–18110.

81. Song S, Adachi K, Katsuyama M, et al. Isolation and characterization of the 5′-upstream and untranslated regions of the mouse type II iodothyronine deiodinase gene. *Mol Cell Endocrinol* 2000;165:189–198.

82. Canettieri G, Celi FS, Baccheschi G, et al. Isolation of human type 2 deiodinase gene promoter and characterization of a functional cyclic adenosine monophosphate response element. *Endocrinology* 2000;141:1804–1813.

83. Bianco AC, Silva JE. Cold exposure rapidly produces virtual saturation of brown adipose tissue nuclear T$_3$ receptors. *Am J Physiol* 1988;255:E496–E508.

84. Bianco AC, Silva JE. Optimal response of key enzymes and uncoupling protein to cold in brown adipose tissue depends on local T$_3$ generation. *Am J Physiol* 1987;253:E255–E263.

85. de Jesus LA, Carvalho SD, Ribeiro MO, et al. The type 2 iodothyronine deiodinase is essential for adaptive thermogenesis in brown adipose tissue. *J Clin Invest* 2001;108:1379–1385.

86. Silva JE, Leonard JL. Regulation of rat cerebrocortical and adenohypophyseal type II 5′deiodinase by thyroxine, triiodothyronine and reverse triiodothyronine. *Endocrinology* 1985;116:1627–1635.

87. Lum SCM, Nicoloff JT, Spencer CA, et al. Peripheral tissue mechanism for maintenance of serum triiodothyronine values in a thyroxine-deficient state in man. *J Clin Invest* 1984;73:570–575.

88. Salvatore D, Bartha T, Harney JW, et al. Molecular biological and biochemical characterization of the human type 2 selenodeiodinase. *Endocrinology* 1996;137:3308–3315.

89. Salvatore D, Tu H, Harney JW, et al. Type 2 iodothyronine deiodinase is highly expressed in human thyroid. *J Clin Invest* 1996;98:962–968.

90. Gross G, Lues I. Thyroid-dependent alterations of myocardial adrenoceptors and adrenoceptor-mediated responses in the rat. *Naunyn Schmiedebergs Arch Pharmacol* 1985;329:427–439.

91. Aoki VS, Wilson WR, Thellen EO. Studies of the reputed augmentation of the cardiovascular effects of catecholamines in patients with spontaneous hyperthyroidism. *J Pharmacol Exp Ther* 1972;181:362.

92. Forfar JC, Stewart J, Sawers A, et al. Cardiovascular responses in hyperthyroidism before and during β-adrenoreceptor blockade: Evidence against adrenergic hypersensitivity. *Clin Endocrinol (Oxf)* 1982;16:441–452.

93. Levey GS, Klein I. Catecholamine-thyroid hormone interactions and the cardiovascular manifestations of hyperthyroidism [see comments]. *Am J Med* 1990;88:642–646.

94. Forfar JC, Muir AL, Sawers SA, et al. Abnormal left ventricular function in hyperthyroidism: evidence for a possible reversible cardiomyopathy. *N Engl J Med* 1982;307:1165.

95. Dillmann WH. Biochemical basis of thyroid hormone action in the heart. *Am J Med* 1990;88:626–630.

96. Hoit BD, Khoury SF, Shao Y, et al. Effects of thyroid hormone on cardiac beta-adrenergic responsiveness in conscious baboons. *Circulation* 1997;96:592–598.

97. McAllister RM, Grossenburg VD, Delp MD, et al. Effects of hyperthyroidism on vascular contractile and relaxation responses. *Am J Physiol* 1998;274:E946–E953.

98. Zwaveling J, Pfaffendorf M, van Zwieten PA. The influence of hyperthyroidism on vasoconstrictor and vasodilator responses in isolated coronary and renal resistance arteries. *Pharmacology* 1997;55:117–125.

99. Knuepfer MM. Muscarinic cholinergic and beta-adrenergic contribution to hindquarters vasodilation and cardiac responses to cocaine. *J Pharmacol Exp Ther* 2003;306:515–522.

100. Hoit BD, Suresh DP, Craft L, et al. Beta2-adrenergic receptor polymorphisms at amino acid 16 differentially influence agonist-stimulated blood pressure and peripheral blood flow in normal individuals. *Am Heart J* 2000;139:537–542.

101. Geffner DL, Hershman JM. Beta-adrenergic blockade for the treatment of hyperthyroidism [Review]. *Am J Med* 1992;93:61–68.

102. Fraser T, Green D. Weathering the storm: beta-blockade and the potential for disaster in severe hyperthyroidism. *Emerg Med (Fremantle)* 2001;13:376–380.

103. Elks ML, Manganiello VC. Effects of thyroid hormone on regulation of lipolysis and adenosine 3′,5′-monophosphate metabolism in 3T$_3$-L1 adipocytes. *Endocrinology* 1985;117:947–953.

104. Port JD, Hadcock JR, Malbon CC. Cross-regulation between G-protein-mediated pathways: acute activation of the inhibitory pathway of adenylylcyclase reduces β2-adrenergic receptor phosphorylation and increases β-adrenergic responsiveness. *J Biol Chem* 1992;267:8468–8472.

105. Milligan G, Spiegel AM, Unson CG, et al. Chemically induced hypothyroidism produces elevated amounts of the α subunit of the inhibitory guanine nucleotide binding protein (Gi) and the β subunit common to all G-proteins. *Biochem J* 1987;247: 223–227.

106. Milligan G, Saggerson ED. Concurrent up-regulation of guanine-nucleotide-binding proteins Gi1 alpha, Gi2 alpha and Gi3 alpha in adipocytes of hypothyroid rats. *Biochem J* 1990; 270:765–769.

107. Viguerie N, Millet L, Avizou S, et al. Regulation of human adipocyte gene expression by thyroid hormone. *J Clin Endocrinol Metab* 2002;87:630–634.

108. Del Rio G, Zizzo G, Marrama P, et al. Alpha 2-adrenergic activity is normal in patients with thyroid disease. *Clin Endocrinol (Oxf)* 1994;40:235–239.

109. Oppenheimer JH, Schwartz HL, Lane JT, et al. Functional relationship of thyroid hormone-induced lipogenesis, lipolysis and thermogenesis in the rat. *J Clin Invest* 1991;87:125–132.

110. Silva JE. Thyroid hormone control of thermogenesis and energy balance. *Thyroid* 1995;5:481–492.

111. Landsberg L, Saville ME, Young JB. The sympathoadrenal system and regulation of thermogenesis. *Am J Physiol* 1984;247: E181.

112. Brand MD, Steverding D, Kadenbach B, et al. The mechanism of the increase in mitochondrial proton permeability induced by thyroid hormones. *Eur J Biochem* 1992;206:775–781.

113. Harper ME, Ballantyne JS, Leach M, et al. Effects of thyroid hormones on oxidative phosphorylation [Review]. *Biochem Soc Trans* 1993;21:785–792.

114. Bouillaud F, Couplan E, Pecqueur C, et al. Homologues of the uncoupling protein from brown adipose tissue (UCP1): UCP2, UCP3, BMCP1 and UCP4. *Biochim Biophys Acta* 2001;1504: 107–119.

115. Gong DW, He YF, Karas M, et al. Uncoupling protein-3 is a mediator of thermogenesis regulated by thyroid hormone, β3-adrenergic agonists, and leptin. *J Biol Chem* 1997;272:24129–24132.

116. Gong DW, Monemdjou S, Gavrilova O, et al. Lack of obesity and normal response to fasting and thyroid hormone in mice lacking uncoupling protein-3. *J Biol Chem* 2000;275:16251–16257.

117. Vidal-Puig AJ, Grujic D, Zhang CY, et al. Energy metabolism in uncoupling protein 3 gene knockout mice. *J Biol Chem* 2000;275:16258–16266.

118. Arsenijevic D, Onuma H, Pecqueur C, et al. Disruption of the uncoupling protein-2 gene in mice reveals a role in immunity and reactive oxygen species production. *Nat Genet* 2000;26: 435–439.

119. Lee YP, Lardy HA. Influence of thyroid hormones on l-α-glycerophosphate dehydrogenases and other dehydrogenases in various organs of the rat. *J Biol Chem* 1965;240:1427–1436.

120. Barker SB, Klitgaard HM. Metabolism of tissues excised from thyroxine-injected rats. *J Physiol (Lond)* 1952;170:81–86.

121. Weirich RT, Schwartz HL, Oppenheimer JH. An analysis of the interrelationship of nuclear and plasma triiodothyronine in the sea lamprey, lake trout, and rat: evolutionary considerations. *Endocrinology* 1987;120:664–677.

122. Lehninger AL, Nelson DL, Cox MM. *Principles of biochemistry.* New York: Worth Publishers, 1993.

123. Ohkawa KI, Vogt MT, Farber E. Unusually high mitochondrial alpha glycerophosphate dehydrogenase activity in rat brown adipose tissue. *J Cell Biol* 1969;41:441–449.

124. Eto K, Tsubamoto Y, Terauchi Y, et al. Role of NADH shuttle system in glucose-induced activation of mitochondrial metabolism and insulin secretion. *Science* 1999;283:981–985.

125. DosSantos RA, Alfadda A, Eto K, et al. Evidence for a compensated thermogenic defect in transgenic mice lacking the mitochondrial glycerol 3-phosphate dehydrogenase gene. *Endocrinology* 2003;144:5469–5479.

126. Lowell BB, Flier JS. Brown adipose tissue, beta 3-adrenergic receptors, and obesity [Review]. *Annu Rev Med* 1997;48:307–316.

127. Rubio A, Raasmaja A, Silva JE. Effects of thyroid hormone on norepinephrine signalling in brown adipose tissue. II. Differential effects of thyroid hormone on β3-adrenergic receptors in brown and white adipose tissue. *Endocrinology* 1995;136: 3277–3284.

128. Astrup A, Bulow J, Madsen J, et al. Contribution of BAT and skeletal muscle to thermogenesis induced by efedrine in man. *Am J Physiol* 1985;248:E507–E515.

129. Duchamp C, Barré H. Skeletal muscle as the major site of nonshivering thermogenesis in cold-adapted ducklings. *Am J Physiol Reg Integ Comp Physiol* 1993;265:R1076–R1083.

130. Wilson BE, Hobbs WN. Case report: pseudoephedrine-associated thyroid storm: thyroid hormone-catecholamine interactions. *Am J Med Sci* 1993;306:317–319.

131. Moller N, Nielsen S, Nyholm B, et al. Glucose turnover, fuel oxidation and forearm substrate exchange in patients with thyrotoxicosis before and after medical treatment. *Clin Endocrinol (Oxf)* 1996;44:453–459.

132. Angeras U, Jagenburg R, Lindstedt G, et al. Effects of betablocking agents on urinary excretion of 3-methylhistidine during experimental hyperthyroidism in rats. *Eur Surg Res* 1987; 19:23–30.

133. Adlerberth A, Angeras U, Jagenburg R, et al. Urinary excretion of 3-methylhistidine and creatinine and plasma concentrations of amino acids in hyperthyroid patients following preoperative treatment with antithyroid drug or beta-blocking agent: results from a prospective, randomized study. *Metabolism* 1987;36: 637–642.

134. Wajchenberg BL, Cesar FP, Leme CE, et al. Effects of adrenergic stimulating and blocking agents on glucose-induced insulin responses in human thyrotoxicosis. *Metabolism* 1978;27:1715–1720.

135. Casla A, Arrieta F, Grant C, et al. Effect of short- and long-term experimental hyperthyroidism on plasma glucose level and insulin secretion during an intravenous glucose load and on insulin binding, insulin receptor kinase activity, and insulin action in adipose tissue. *Metabolism* 1993;42:814–821.

136. O'Meara NM, Blackman JD, Sturis J, et al. Alterations in the kinetics of C-peptide and insulin secretion in hyperthyroidism. *J Clin Endocrinol Metab* 1993;76:79–84.

137. Young JB, Landsberg L. Catecholamines and the regulation of hormone secretion [Review]. *Clin Endocrinol Metab* 1977;6: 657–695.

138. Skrabanek P. Catecholamines cause the hypercalciuria and hypercalcaemia in phaeochromocytoma and in hyperthyroidism [Review]. *Med Hypotheses* 1977;3:59–62.

139. Moore RE, Smith CK 2nd, Bailey CS, et al. Characterization of beta-adrenergic receptors on rat and human osteoblast-like cells and demonstration that beta-receptor agonists can stimulate

bone resorption in organ culture. *Bone Miner* 1993;23:301–315.

140. Hayes JR, Ritchie CM. Hypercalcaemia due to thyrotoxicosis. *Ir J Med Sci* 1983;152:422–423.

141. Feely J. Propranolol and the hypercalcaemia of thyrotoxicosis. *Acta Endocrinol (Copenh)* 1981;98:528–532.

142. Eber O, Buchinger W, Lindner W, et al. The effect of D- versus L-propranolol in the treatment of hyperthyroidism. *Clin Endocrinol (Oxf)* 1990;32:363–372.

143. Faber J, Wiinberg N, Schifter S, et al. Haemodynamic changes following treatment of subclinical and overt hyperthyroidism. *Eur J Endocrinol* 2001;145:391–396.

144. Morkin E, Flink IL, Goldman S. Biochemical and physiological effects of thyroid hormone on cardiac performance. *Metabolism* 1983;25:435–464.

145. Valensi P, Simon A, Pithois-Merli I, et al. Non-beta-adrenergic-mediated peripheral circulatory hyperkinesia in hyperthyroidism. *Angiology* 1992;43:996–1007.

146. Ikram H. Haemodynamic effects of beta-adrenergic blockade in hyperthyroid patients with and without heart failure. *BMJ* 1977;1:1505–1507.

147. Tulea E, Schneider F, Lungu G, et al. Functional response of the hyperthyroid patients with beta adrenoreceptor blockade to exercise. *Physiologie* 1985;22:263–267.

148. Henderson JM, Portmann L, Van Melle G, et al. Propranolol as an adjunct therapy for hyperthyroid tremor. *Eur Neurol* 1997;37:182–185.

149. Sneddon JM, Turner P. Adrenergic blockade and the eye signs of thyrotoxicosis. *Lancet* 1966;2:525–527.

150. Marsden CD, Gimlette TM, McAllister RG, et al. Effect of beta-adrenergic blockade on finger tremor and Achilles reflex time in anxious and thyrotoxic patients. *Acta Endocrinol (Copenh)* 1968;57:353–362.

151. Abila B, Lazarus JH, Kingswood JC, et al. Tremor: an alternative approach for investigating adrenergic mechanisms in thyrotoxicosis? *Clin Sci (Colch)* 1985;69:459–463.

152. Trzepacz PT, McCue M, Klein I, et al. Psychiatric and neuropsychological response to propranolol in Graves' disease. *Biol Psychiatry* 1988;23:678–688.

153. Shayne P, Hart A. Thyrotoxic periodic paralysis terminated with intravenous propranolol. *Ann Emerg Med* 1994;24:736–740.

154. Shahar E, Shapiro MS, Shenkman L. Hyperthyroid-induced chorea: case report and review of the literature [Review]. *Isr J Med Sci* 1988;24:264–266.

155. Rothberg MP, Shebert RT, Levey GS, et al. Propranolol and hyperthyroidism: reversal of upper motor neuron signs. *JAMA* 1974;230:1017.

156. Shahshahani MN, Palmieri GM. Oral propranolol in hypercalcemia associated with apathetic thyrotoxicosis. *Am J Med Sci* 1978;275:199–202.

157. Rude RK, Oldham SB, Singer FR, et al. Treatment of thyrotoxic hypercalcemia with propranolol. *N Engl J Med* 1976;294:431–433.

158. Feely J, Forrest A, Gunn A, et al. Propranolol dosage in thyrotoxicosis. *J Clin Endocrinol Metab* 1980;51:658.

159. Georges LP, Santangelo RP, Mackin JF, et al. Metabolic effects of propranolol in thyrotoxicosis. I. Nitrogen, calcium, and hydroxyproline. *Metabolism* 1975;24:11.

160. Bozzani A, Camboni MG, Tidone L, et al. Gastrointestinal transit in hyperthyroid patients before and after propranolol treatment. *Am J Gastroenterol* 1985;80:550–552.

161. Allen JA, Lowe DC, Roddie IC, et al. Studies on sweating in clinical and experimental thyrotoxicosis. *Clin Sci Mol Med* 1973;45:765–773.

162. Feely J, Stevenson IH, Crooks J. Propranolol dynamics in thyrotoxicosis. *Clin Pharmacol Ther* 1980;28:40.

163. Wells PG, Feely J, Wilkinson GR, et al. Effect of thyrotoxicosis on liver blood flow and propranolol disposition after long-term dosing. *Clin Pharmacol Ther* 1983;33:603–608.

164. Feely J, Crooks J, Forrest AL, et al. Propranolol in the surgical treatment of hyperthyroidism, including severely thyrotoxic patients. *Br J Surg* 1981;68:865.

165. Lennquist S, Jortso E, Anderberg B, et al. Betablockers compared with antithyroid drugs as preoperative treatment in hyperthyroidism: drug tolerance, complications, and postoperative thyroid function. *Surgery* 1985;98:1141–1147.

166. Lee KS, Kim K, Hur KB, et al. The role of propranolol in the preoperative preparation of patients with Graves' disease. *Surg Gynecol Obstet* 1986;162:365–369.

167. Baeza A, Aguayo J, Barria M, et al. Rapid preoperative preparation in hyperthyroidism. *Clin Endocrinol (Oxf)* 1991;35:439–442.

168. Peden NR, Browning MC, Feely J, et al. The clinical and metabolic responses to early surgical treatment for hyperthyroid Graves' disease: a comparison of three pre-operative treatment regimens. *QJM* 1985;56:579–591.

169. Feely J, Crooks J, Forrest AL, et al. Altered endocrine response to partial thyroidectomy in propranolol-prepared hyperthyroid patients. *Clin Endocrinol (Oxf)* 1981;14:597–604.

170. Angeras U, Hasselgren PO. Protein degradation in skeletal muscle during experimental hyperthyroidism in rats and the effect of beta-blocking agents. *Endocrinology* 1987;120:1417–1421.

171. Morrison WL, Gibson JN, Jung RT, et al. Skeletal muscle and whole body protein turnover in thyroid disease. *Eur J Clin Invest* 1988;18:62–68.

172. Martin WH III, Korte E, Tolley TK, et al. Skeletal muscle β-adrenoceptor distribution and responses to isoproterenol in hyperthyroidism. *Am J Physiol Endocrinol Metab* 1992;262:E504–E510.

173. Hasselgren PO, Adlerberth A, Angeras U, et al. Protein metabolism in skeletal muscle tissue from hyperthyroid patients after preoperative treatment with antithyroid drug or selective beta-blocking agent: results from a prospective, randomized study. *J Clin Endocrinol Metab* 1984;59:835–839.

174. Eriksson M, Rubenfeld S, Garber AJ, et al. Propranolol does not prevent thyroid storm. *N Engl J Med* 1977;296:263–264.

175. Strube PJ. Thyroid storm during beta blockade. *Anaesthesia* 1984;39:343–346.

176. Sherif IH, Oyan WT, Bosairi S, et al. Treatment of hyperthyroidism in pregnancy. *Acta Obstet Gynecol Scand* 1991;70:461–463.

177. Pruyn SC, Phelan JP, Buchanan GC. Long-term propranolol therapy in pregnancy: maternal and fetal outcome. *Am J Obstet Gynecol* 1979;135:485–489.

178. Levy CA, Waite JH, Dickey R. Thyrotoxicosis and pregnancy: use of preoperative propranolol for thyroidectomy. *Am J Surg* 1977;133:319–321.

179. Bullock JL, Harris RE, Young R. Treatment of thyrotoxicosis during pregnancy with propranolol. *Am J Obstet Gynecol* 1975;121:242–245.

180. Lightner ES, Allen HD, Loughlin G. Neonatal hyperthyroidism and heart failure: a differential approach. *Am J Dis Child* 1977;131:68–70.

181. Smith CS, Howard NJ. Propranolol in treatment of neonatal thyrotoxicosis. *J Pediatr* 1973;83:1046–1048.

182. Pemberton PJ, McConnell B, Shanks RG. Neonatal thyrotoxicosis treated with propranolol. *Arch Dis Child* 1974;49:813–815.

183. Orbeck H. Neonatal hyperthyroidism. *Acta Paediatr Scand* 1973;62:313–316.

184. Gardner LI. Is propranolol alone really beneficial in neonatal thyrotoxicosis? Bradycardia and hypoglycemia evoke the doctrine of primum non nocere. *Am J Dis Child* 1980;134:819–820.

THE MALE AND FEMALE REPRODUCTIVE SYSTEM IN THYROTOXICOSIS

GERASIMOS E. KRASSAS

The reproductive system has been suggested to be relatively resistant to the effects of thyroid dysfunctions. This view has been challenged by recent evidence, although most of the consequences are minor and reversible. However, the reproductive sequelae of thyroid disease are by no means trivial, particularly because the prevalence of thyroid dysfunction is high in the general population (1). The incidence of thyroid disease including thyrotoxicosis is far more common in women than in men. Whether this is directly or indirectly related to the hormonal status of women remains uncertain.

REPRODUCTIVE EFFECTS OF THYROTOXICOSIS IN THE FEMALE

For a better understanding of the effect of thyrotoxicosis on the female reproductive system, a brief review of the normal development and physiology of the female reproductive system follows.

Fetal and Neonatal Periods

In human fetuses, gonadotropin-releasing hormone (GnRH) cells are found in the olfactory placode in embryonic week 5.5, although a majority of GnRH cells originate in the olfactory pit at embryonic week 6.0 to 6.5. GnRH cells enter the forebrain through the terminal nerve by embryonic week 6.5, and they migrate into the hypothalamus by embryonic week 9.0 (2).

Follicle-stimulating hormone (FSH) and luteinizing hormone (LH) are detectable in the human pituitary by embryonic week 10, and their content increases until embryonic weeks 25 to 29. The pituitary starts to release gonadotropins (Gns) into the general circulation by embryonic weeks 11 to 12. Circulating Gns reach peak levels at midgestation, and subsequently both LH and FSH levels decline during late gestation (3). This peak in Gn levels may be causally related to the maximal development of follicles. The gonadotropes in human fetuses respond to GnRH by releasing LH and FSH both *in vivo* and *in vitro* (4). A sex difference in Gn levels is seen during midgestation. Pituitary content and circulating concentrations of LH and FSH in female fetuses are higher than those in male fetuses (5). Because circulating testosterone levels are higher in male fetuses as compared with circulating estrogen levels in female fetuses during midgestation, both the sex difference in Gn levels and the decrease in Gn levels toward late gestation in fetuses are attributed to the development of the negative feedback mechanism by the gonadal steroid hormones from the fetal gonads as well as from the placenta (6).

In female neonates, LH levels are only slightly elevated during the first few months of life, but FSH levels are high for the first 5 months (7). After the first 6 months of life, circulating levels of FSH, LH, and gonadal steroids are all low, and the hypothalamo-pituitary-gonadal system enters a quiescent stage until the time of puberty.

The Period at the Onset of and During Puberty

Puberty is defined as the transient period between childhood and adulthood during which reproductive function is reached. During this period the secondary sexual characteristics appear, the adolescent growth spurt occurs, the gonads start to produce mature gametes (sperm or oocytes) capable of fertilization, and major psychological changes occur.

Low levels of Gns during the childhood years are thought to result from exquisite sensitivity of the hypothalamic–pituitary axis (the so-called gonadostat), which remains suppressed despite extremely low levels of circulating gonadal steroids. The prepubertal gonadostat is 6 to 15 times more sensitive to estrogen than is the adult feedback mechanism (8). In addition to the gonadal steroid-dependent highly sensitive negative feedback system, a steroid-independent mechanism for inhibitory control of central nervous system responses is also operative, because Gn levels also decline in the absence of a gonad and in children with Turner's syndrome (8). Although the pineal gland has been proposed to be an inhibitor of Gn secretion in the human, neither the pineal gland nor melatonin has a major inhibitory effect on the gonadostat (8). GnRH is critical for the initiation of puberty. Grumbach and Styne (6) suggest that a gonadal steroid-dependent GnRH increase also occurs at the onset of puberty, since smaller amounts of gonadal steroids are effective in suppressing FSH and LH levels in prepubertal children than in adults. It is possible during the juvenile period in humans that a small amount of GnRH released from the hypothalamus is capable of maintaining the minimum levels of Gn secretion, which is susceptible to the negative feedback effect of steroid hormones. Before the onset of puberty, LH and FSH levels are low, but a highly sensitive assay indicates that circulating LH and FSH levels in prepubertal children are pulsatile, with slightly higher values at night than morning (9). In both boys and girls, preceding the physical signs of puberty, LH and FSH levels become elevated, pulsatility of these hormones becomes more pronounced, and the nocturnal increase in Gn release is enhanced (9,10). Both pulse frequency and amplitude of LH release increase at this stage as well (9). FSH increases early in puberty, with LH following (11). Before puberty the plasma FSH/LH ratio is greater than 1, whereas at the end of puberty the ratio is reversed. At menopause the FSH/LH ratio again becomes greater than 1 (12). During puberty the pituitary becomes more sensitive to infusions of GnRH, and the LH and FSH responses to GnRH increase in age-dependent increments (13). Three major developments characterize the approach of puberty: (a) adrenarche, the onset of adrenal androgen secretion; (b) decreased sensitivity of the gonadostat to feedback control by gonadal steroids, leading to activation or disinhibition of the GnRH neurosecretory neurons in the medial basal hypothalamus, with a consequent increase in pituitary Gn release; and (c) gonadarche, the enhancement of estrogen secretion by the ovary and the onset of ovulatory cycles.

An increase in secretion of adrenal androgens (adrenarche) occurs before maturation of Gn secretion. A variety of hormones have been proposed for the initiation of adrenarche, but evidence for the role of a hormone other than corticotropin remains elusive (14). As a consequence of increased FSH, the plasma level of 17-β-estradiol (E_2) increases progressively throughout puberty (11). Serum inhibin levels increase in parallel with FSH levels during puberty in girls (15). When inhibin levels reach those of adults, the inhibin-FSH negative feedback relationship is established. The factors that regulate the onset of gonadarche are thought to be initiated by a decreased sensitivity of the gonadostat to circulating levels of steroid hormones. Another hypothesis for the initiation of puberty involves loss of neuronal inhibition or enhanced neuronal stimulation (6).

Animal Studies

There are few data on the effects of excess thyroid hormone on the fetal development of the female reproductive tract. It has been shown that small doses of thyroid hormone given to young female mice resulted in the early attainment of sexual maturity with an early opening of the vagina and onset of estrous cycles (16). The ovaries of these mice revealed multiple corpora lutea and follicles. In contrast, the administration of large doses of thyroxine (T_4) to the neonatal rat resulted in a delay in vaginal opening and first estrous (17). Due to the short period of administration (5 days), which was followed by a period of hypothyroidism, it is uncertain whether the excess T_4 or the subsequent hypothyroidism caused the delay in sexual maturation. In the adult female rat, administration of T_4 in high doses resulted in long periods of diestrus with few mature follicles or corpora lutea (18). Moreover, the administration of excess thyroid hormone has been reported to produce an increase or no change in pituitary LH and a decrease in serum LH (19). A synergistic effect of thyroid hormone with FSH to stimulate differentiation of porcine granulosa cells has also been found (20).

Thyroid hormone receptors have been found in the uterus (21). Thus, changes in the uterus would be expected to occur after administration of thyroid hormone. Excess thyroid hormone given to mice produces thickened endometria. Moreover, administration of T_4 decreased estradiol uptake and retention by the rat uterus (22). Finally, a reduced uterine response to estrogen in thyrotoxic rats was reported (23).

In pregnancy it was shown that excess thyroid hormone is deleterious to pregnancy and could cause abortion and neonatal death, perhaps through a direct effect on trophoblastic function (24). However, mild thyrotoxicosis was found to help in the maintenance of implantation of delayed blastocysts and an increase in litter size (23).

Human Studies

Hormonal Changes

Thyrotoxicosis results in increased levels of sex hormone–binding globulin (SHBG) synthesized in the liver. Also, plasma estrogen levels may be two- or threefold higher in hyperthyroid than in normal women during all phases of the menstrual cycle (25). Whether the increase in plasma estrogens is entirely attributable to the elevated SHBG or whether there is an actual increase in unbound estrogen, as in the case of hyperthyroid men, remains to be determined. The metabolic clearance rate of E_2 is decreased in hyperthyroidism and is thought to be largely due to increased binding of E_2 to SHBG (26).

Changes also occur in circulating androgen metabolism in hyperthyroid women. Mean plasma levels of testosterone and androstenedione increase (27). The production rate of testosterone and androstenedione are significantly elevated in hyperthyroid women in comparison with normal females. The conversion ratio of androstenedione to estrone, as well as testosterone to E_2, is increased in hyperthyroid women (28).

Akande and Hockaday (29) found that the mean LH levels in both the follicular and luteal phases of the menstrual cycle are significantly higher in hyperthyroid women than in normal women. We found similar results when we studied women in the middle of the luteal phase of the cycle (30). Zahringer et al. (31) studied seven women with Graves' disease and six controls, sampling blood every 10 minutes for an 8-hour period. This was done in the early follicular phase of the menstrual cycle. They found that LH secretion was increased. Pulsatile characteristics of LH and FSH secretion (frequency, peak, shape) did not differ in patients when compared with controls (31). However, LH peaks may be absent in patients with amenorrhea. Serum LH levels decrease to normal after a few weeks of treatment with antithyroid drugs (32). Baseline FSH levels may be increased, although data on this are limited (30,33); however, some reports claim that FSH levels are normal in thyrotoxic women (31,34). The mechanism for the increase in serum LH and FSH in hyperthyroid women is unclear. Tanaka et al. (33) reported that hyperthyroxinemia results in an augmented Gn response to GnRH. Others, however, have been unable to confirm this finding (34).

We investigated 37 thyrotoxic women, all of reproductive age with normal periods and the same number of age- and weight-matched euthyroid controls. In all patients and controls, LH, FSH, and prolactin (PRL) levels were measured before and 30 and 60 minutes after a combined administration of thyrotropin-releasing hormone (TRH) and GnRH. In all patients, the same procedure was repeated 4 months after the initiation of antithyroid drugs, while the patients were euthyroid. We found that the Gn response was increased before treatment and remained slightly increased 4 months after treatment in comparison with controls (30). Moreover, no significant change in PRL secretion has been found (30,31). Usually, all these biochemical abnormalities are corrected after treatment.

Clinical Signs and Symptoms of the Reproductive System in Thyrotoxicosis

Children born with neonatal Graves' disease have no defects in the reproductive system that can be related to the pathologic entity. Hyperthyroidism occurring before puberty has been reported to delay sexual maturation and the onset of menses. However, others have reported no significant effect of hyperthyroidism on the age of menarche. Saxena et al. (35) found that in hyperthyroid girls the mean age of menarche was slightly advanced over that of their control population without thyroid disease.

Amenorrhea was one of the earlier of the known clinical changes associated with hyperthyroidism, as reported by von Basedow in 1840 (36). Since then, amenorrhea has been frequently reported, as well as a number of other changes in the menstrual cycle, including oligomenorrhea, hypomenorrhea, and anovulation. Biochemical and hormonal abnormalities, nutritional disturbances, and emotional upheavals associated with hyperthyroidism may, individually or in combination, be the cause of the menstrual disturbances.

Much confusion exists among physicians about the definition of different terms used to characterize menstrual abnormalities. It should be remembered that oligomenorrhea, polymenorrhea, and amenorrhea define the duration of the menstrual cycle, whereas hypomenorrhea, hypermenorrhea, and menorrhagia define the amount of menstrual flow. Thus, oligomenorrhea was identified when the interval between two periods was more than 35 days, polymenorrhea less than 21 days, and amenorrhea in women with previously normal periods when there was no menstruation for more than 3 months (37,38). Hypomenorrhea was arbitrarily defined when there was more than a 20% decrease in menstrual flow, hypermenorrhea when there was more than a 20% increase in menstrual flow in comparison with the previous periods, and menorrhagia as heavy menstrual bleeding (1).

The frequency of menstrual abnormalities in more recent studies is not the same as in earlier series. Thus, Benson and Dailey (39) found that of 221 hyperthyroid patients, 58% had oligomenorrhea or amenorrhea, and 5% had polymenorrhea. This is in general agreement with findings in older studies, such as those of Goldsmith et al. (40). Tanaka et al. (33) found that 8 of 41 thyrotoxic patients had amenorrhea and 15 had hypomenorrhea. More recently, Joshi et al. (41) found menstrual irregularities in 64.7% of hyperthyroid women in India, compared with 17.2% among healthy controls. These irregularities sometimes preceded identified thyroid dysfunction. We found irregular cycles in only 46 (21.5%) of 214 thyrotoxic patients. Twenty-four of them had hypo-, 15 poly-, 5 oligo-, and 2 hypermenorrhea. None had amenorrhea. From a similar number of normal controls, 18 (8.4%) had irregular periods, and of these 12 had oligomenorrhea. Although these findings indicate that menstrual disturbances in thyrotoxicosis are 2.5 times more frequent than in the normal population, they are still lower than has previously been described and support our notion that due to better medical care and public awareness, thyroid disturbances are diagnosed much earlier when the symptoms are still mild (42).

We also found that smoking aggravates the development of menstrual disturbances in thyrotoxicosis. Fifty percent of the thyrotoxic patients with abnormal menstruation were smokers, compared with 19% of the thyrotoxic patients with normal periods. We also found that patients with menstrual disturbances had higher total T_4 levels and that the levels were higher in smokers with abnormal periods. Thus, total T_4 levels appear to be an important factor related to the development of menstrual abnormalities in thyrotoxicosis, in contrast with total triiodothyronine, for which no such correlation was found (42).

Thyrotoxicosis in women has been linked with reduced fertility, although most thyrotoxic women remain ovulatory according to the results of endometrial biopsies (40). Joshi et al. (41) found that 3 (5.8%) of 52 thyrotoxic women had primary or secondary infertility. We measured progesterone levels, a fertility parameter, in the middle of the luteal phase of the cycle in 74 women of reproductive age, 37 of whom had Graves' disease and 37 of whom were euthyroid controls matched for age and weight. All patients and controls had normal periods. We remeasured progesterone levels at the same phase of the cycle, 4 months after the initiation of therapy with antithyroid when they were euthyroid. We found that progesterone levels were decreased before treatment in comparison with controls and were not restored 4 months after carbimazole therapy (43). Because endometrial biopsies were not performed, however, we are unable to reach final conclusions.

Thyrotoxicosis during and after pregnancy is discussed in detail in Chapters 27 and 80.

In summary, thyrotoxicosis occurring in prepubertal girls may result in slightly delayed menarche. In adult women, the effects of thyrotoxicosis on the reproductive system are present at the hypothalamic pituitary level with alterations in Gn release and in the circulating levels of SHBG, which result in alterations in sex steroid metabolism or their biologic activity. The variable clinical symptoms seen in women with thyrotoxicosis are the consequence of these alterations.

REPRODUCTIVE EFFECTS OF THYROTOXICOSIS IN THE MALE

Although the effects of hyper- and hypothyroidism on female gonadal function are well established (1), controversies exist regarding the impact of these diseases on male reproduction. This is due mainly to the clinical irrelevance of signs and symptoms related to male gonadal function, as compared with the systemic effects of hyper- and hypothyroidism, which results in the lack of well-controlled clinical studies. For a better understanding of the effect of thyrotoxicosis on the male reproductive system, a brief review of the normal physiology is followed.

The Male Reproductive System from Fetal to Adult Life

Male gonadal differentiation begins at 7 week of gestation, with organization of the gonadal blastema into interstitium and germ cell–containing testicular cords. Primitive Sertoli's cells and spermatogonia become visible within the cords, while the epithelium differentiates to form the tunica albuginea (44). Leydig's cells derived from the undifferentiated interstitium are visible by the end of the eighth week of gestation and are capable of androgen synthesis at this time. By 14 weeks of gestation these cells make up as much as 50% of the cell mass, but as the tubules develop they account for a smaller percentage of the tissue. The fetal testes grow from approximately 20 mg at 14 weeks of gestation to 800 mg at birth; at 5 to 6 months they descend into the inguinal canal in association with the epididymis and the ductus deferens (44). Testicular secretion of testosterone in the fetus reaches a peak late in the first trimester and then declines until parturition (45). The fetal testis also produces antimüllerian hormone, which causes dedifferentiation of the müllerian duct system in the male fetus (46). In the first year of life, there is a transient increase in testosterone, after which the testis remains relatively quiescent until the onset of puberty. The pulsatile secretion of GnRH causes pulsatile secretion of Gns. Plasma levels of LH and FSH in the fetus increase after the establishment of the hypothalamic–pituitary portal system until midgestation and then decrease toward term as inhibitory control begins to function; mean levels of fetal plasma FSH are higher in females than in males (47). During the first two years after birth, plasma levels of LH and FSH increase intermittently to adult values and occasionally higher, and then they remain low until puberty.

In the adult male, GnRH and the Gns are secreted in discrete pulses. The secretory pulses of LH occur at a frequency of 8 to 14 pulses per 24 hours and vary in magnitude (48). Pulsatile secretion of FSH is temporally coupled to that of LH but is lower in amplitude (49). The secretion of LH is controlled by the negative feedback action of gonadal steroids on the hypothalamus and the pituitary. Both testosterone and E_2 can effect this inhibition. Testosterone can be converted to E_2 in the brain and the pituitary, but on the basis of the results of many studies the two hormones are thought to act independently (50,51). LH stimulates the Leydig's cells to secrete testosterone and, to a minor extend, E_2 (52). Also, LH appears to govern testicular aromatization in the Leydig's cells. In the normal adult male, testosterone, dihydrotestosterone (DHT), and to some extend E_2 circulate in the plasma bound in part to SHBG, which synthesized in the liver (53). Thyroxine increases serum SHBG levels (53,54). Sex hormones bound to SHBG are inactive and appear not to be readily metabolized (53). The unbound sex hormones or those bound to albumin are biologically active. The testosterone concentration in the testes is maintained at a high concentration relative to serum by androgen-binding protein secreted by the Sertoli's cells under the influence of FSH. The high intratesticular concentration of testosterone may be necessary for normal Sertoli's cell function or may play a role in spermatogenesis or sperm transport (55). In certain tissues, especially the prostate, circulating testosterone enters the cell and is metabolized to more active products, especially DHT, through the action of the enzyme 5α-reductase II. In other tissues, 5α-reductase I is the major isoenzyme (56). Although DHT is the active androgen in some areas, testosterone itself is an active androgen in some tissues that lack the enzyme, like muscle. There is a decline in testicular function due to age (57), although the interplay of lifestyle and disease processes probably plays a role (58).

Although the testicular secretion of E_2 is important, the major source of circulating hormone derives from aromatization of testosterone in peripheral tissues, including adipose tissue, muscle, and skin; however, little aromatization appears to occur in the liver (59). These formed estrogens are further metabolized, primarily in the liver, to estriol and the catechol estrogens (60). The hypothalamus and pituitary can aromatize androgens, so it is uncertain whether testosterone itself or the estrogens formed locally from testosterone are the main negative feedback mechanisms for LH release (61). However, there is good evidence that one of the major factors controlling LH release is testosterone itself. Inhibin is a major factor in the control of FSH secretion (62).

Therefore, masculinization in men depends on the actions of both testosterone and DHT. The exact role of E_2 is uncertain, but it appears in some processes, like bone formation, to play an important role.

Animal Studies

Studies on the effects of alterations in thyroid hormone levels on the reproductive system have been performed extensively in animals (63). Changes from normal have generally resulted in a decrease in fertility and sexual activity. However, the mechanism is not constant throughout all species studied, and the results from different studies disagree. In intact rats, the administration of T_4 resulted in a decrease in serum Gn levels (64). In male mice the administration of T_4 doses, slightly greater than physiologic, resulted in shortening the time of development and with a tendency toward early maturation (63). However, large doses of thyroid hormone resulted in a decrease in the weights of the testes and seminal vesicles in mice and rabbits (63). In ram lambs, the administration of testosterone resulted in a decrease in testis volume and in an impairment of sexual development, in part due to alteration in LH pulse frequency (65). Studies on the effect of T_4 directly on the testes have indicated that there is a minimal change in oxygen consumption when T_4 is present in testicular slice incubations (66). Total lipids, cholesterol, and phospholipids in the testes are decreased after administration of excess T_4 to mature male rats (67). Testes from rats made thyrotoxic by T_4 administration synthesized increased amounts of testosterone (64). There are conflicting data on the effect of T_4 on spermatogenesis; it would appear that T_4 does not exert a direct effect on spermatogenesis in mature rats or rams (68).

Human Studies

Hormonal Changes in Male Thyrotoxicosis

An increase in SHBG is a consistent feature associated with thyrotoxicosis (69) and leads to an increase in circulating levels of total testosterone (69) and reduction in the metabolic clearance rate of testosterone (70). However, the plasma level of free testosterone is usually maintained within the normal range (71), which is in keeping with the lack of clinical consequences of the markedly elevated levels of total testosterone found in thyrotoxicosis. Circulating E_2 levels are increased in many men with thyrotoxicosis (72), which is partly due to increased bound E_2 to SHBG (72). However, an increase in the production rates of estrogens is also observed in some men with thyrotoxicosis, although it is unclear whether this is due to increased production of adrenal androgen precursors (specifically androstenedione) or to other mechanisms (73).

Thyrotoxicosis influences the metabolism of androgens and estrogens, leading to an increase in the excretion of 5α-reduced metabolites and an increase in the α:β ratio (74), although the mechanism for this is uncertain. Peripheral conversion of androgen to estrogen is enhanced in thyrotoxicosis, probably due to changes in peripheral blood flow (73) rather than a direct effect of T_4 on the aromatase complex. Furthermore, serum progesterone was reported to be higher in hyperthyroid than in euthyroid men (75), whereas mean basal testosterone bioactivity was lower in thyrotoxic patients when compared with controls (76). The hyperthyroid state also affects estrogen metabolism, and is associated with a marked increase in the excretion of the 2-hydroxyestrogens and a decrease in the excretion of 16α-hydroxyestrogens (77). Thyrotoxic males often present with clinical features that are compatible with exposure to increased estrogen bioactivity (gynecomastia, spider angiomas, and a decrease in libido) (78). Whether this results from alterations in estrogen metabolism, or is a direct effect of hyperthyroxinemia, is unknown.

Basal serum Gn concentrations are usually normal. In one study LH and FSH responses to exogenous GnRH were significantly greater in thyrotoxic patients in comparison with patients who were rendered euthyroid (79). A direct effect of thyroid hormone on Gn sensitivity to GnRH has been postulated (79). Other studies have observed an increase in basal serum levels of LH and FSH (31) and hyperresponsiveness to GnRH stimulation (76,80). It has been suggested that the LH elevation could be secondary to changes in sex steroid binding and peripheral metabolism, alterations in the hypothalamic–pituitary feedback, or due to the direct effect of thyroid hormones per se at this level.

All the above changes are fully reversible with restoration of the euthyroid state, and require no other specific treatment.

Spermatogenesis, Fertility, and Thyrotoxicosis

The effect of hyperthyroidism on semen quality has been the subject of only a few studies. Clyde et al. (81) investigated three young men and found that two had marked oligospermia with decreased motility. The third patient had a borderline low sperm count and decreased motility. Kidd et al. (71) studied five patients and found that all had total sperm counts of less than $40 \times 10^6/$ mL. In 1992 Hudson and Edwards (82) assessed testicular function in 16 thyrotoxic men. They found that although the mean sperm densities were low, they did not differ significantly from controls. However, the forward progressive sperm motility of thyrotoxic patients was significantly lower than that of normal men. In a more recent study, Abalovich et al. (76) investigated the effect of hyperthyroidism on spermatogenesis in 21 patients; 9 patients (43%) had a low total sperm count, 18 (85.7%) had "grade A" lineal motility defects, and 13 (61.9%) displayed "progressive motility" problems.

In a very recent study (78), 23 thyrotoxic men and 15 healthy controls were studied prospectively. Two semen analyses were obtained for examination before and about 5 months after achievement of euthyroidism either by methimazole alone (14 patients) or iodine 131 plus methimazole (9 patients). Total fructose, zinc, and magnesium concentrations were also measured in seminal plasma of 16 patients. Results in the patients represent the average of the values of the two measurements, whereas in the control group semen analysis was performed only once. Mean semen volume was within the normal range for both patients and controls. Mean sperm density was lower in patients, although the difference compared with controls did not reach statistical significance. Similar observations were made with regard to sperm morphology. However, mean sperm motility was lower in thyrotoxic men than in controls. Following treatment of the thyrotoxicosis, sperm density and motility improved, but sperm morphology did not change. The type of treatment administered for control of thyrotoxicosis (methimazole alone or ^{131}I plus methimazole) had no impact on sperm counts or morphology. Mean values for semen concentrations of fructose, zinc, and magnesium did not differ between patients and controls, either before or after achievement of euthyroidism, and did not correlate with sperm parameters or with pretreatment thyroid hormone levels (78).

In summary, most of the studies conducted so far have shown that men with thyrotoxicosis have abnormalities in seminal parameters, mainly sperm motility. These abnormalities improve or normalize when patients become euthyroid. Mechanisms that may explain these observations include alterations in sex steroid and Gn concentrations, direct effects of thyroid hormones, effects of thyroid-stimulating immunoglobulins on the testes, or other autoimmune mechanisms associated with Graves' disease.

Radioiodine Treatment for Hyperthyroidism and Reproduction

Radioiodine (^{131}I) is used widely in the diagnosis and treatment of thyroid diseases (83). The notion that radiation is mutagenic and may affect the gonads has raised concern in younger patients regarding its effect on reproductive function. Because the germinal epithelium and particularly the spermatogonia within it are very sensitive to radiation, there is concern that the radiation absorbed by the testes following large doses of radioiodine could result in azoospermia and permanent infertility (84). So far, several studies have reported normal reproductive performance in both male and female juvenile and adult patients with thyrotoxicosis after ^{131}I therapy (85). Many clinicians therefore justifiably use ^{131}I therapy as a first-line treatment for thyrotoxicosis for adults of all ages (1,86). However, given the considerable increase in the risk for thyroid cancer in young children exposed to external radiation, it has been hypothesized that there may be a small increase in the risk for thyroid cancer in young children treated with radioiodine therapy. This theoretic risk is probably highest in children before the age of 5 years and progressively lower in those treated at 5 to 10 and 10 to 20 years of age (87). Until safety long-term data are available for young children, radioiodine treatment in this age group should be administered with caution (88).

REFERENCES

1. Krassas GE. Thyroid disease and female reproduction. *Fertil Steril* 2000;74:1063.
2. Schwanzel-Fukuda M, Crossin KL, Pfaff DW, et al. Migration of luteinizing hormone-releasing hormone (LHRH) neurons in early human embryos. *J Comp Neurol* 1996;366:547.
3. Clements JA, Reyes FI, Winter JS, et al. Studies on human sexual development. III. Fetal pituitary and serum, and amniotic fluid concentrations of LH, CG, and FSH. *J Clin Endocrinol Metab* 1976;42:9.
4. Mueller PL, Sklar CA, Gluckman PD, et al. Hormone ontogeny in the ovine fetus. IX. Luteinizing hormone and follicle-stimulating hormone response to luteinizing hormone-releasing factor in mid- and late gestation and in the neonate. *Endocrinology* 1981;108:881.
5. Castillo RH, Matteri RL, Dumesic DA. Luteinizing hormone synthesis in cultured fetal human pituitary cells exposed to gonadotropin-releasing hormone. *J Clin Endocrinol Metab* 1992;75:318.
6. Grumbach MM, Styne DM. Puberty: ontogeny, neuroendocrinology, physiology, and disorders. In: Wilson JD, Foster DW, Kronenberg HM, et al., eds. *Williams textbook of endocrinology.* Philadelphia: WB Saunders, 1998:1509.
7. Winter JS, Faiman C, Hobson WC, et al. Pituitary-gonadal relations in infancy. I. Patterns of serum gonadotropin concentrations from birth to four years of age in man and chimpanzee. *J Clin Endocrinol Metab* 1975;40:545.
8. Styne DM, Grumbach MM. Disorders of puberty in the male and female. In: Yen SSC, Jaffe RB, eds. *Reproductive endocrinology: physiology, pathophysiology and clinical management,* 3rd ed. Philadelphia: WB Saunders, 1991:511.

9. Wu FC, Butler GE, Kelnar CJ, et al. Patterns of pulsatile luteinizing hormone and follicle-stimulating hormone secretion in prepubertal (midchildhood) boys and girls and patients with idiopathic hypogonadotropic hypogonadism (Kallmann's syndrome): a study using an ultrasensitive time-resolved immunofluorometric assay. *J Clin Endocrinol Metab* 1991;72:1229.

10. Wennink JM, Delemarre-van de Waal HA, Schoemaker R, et al. Luteinizing hormone and follicle stimulating hormone secretion patterns in boys throughout puberty measured using highly sensitive immunoradiometric assays. *Clin Endocrinol (Oxf)* 1989;31:551.

11. Winter JS, Faiman C, Reyes FI, et al. Gonadotrophins and steroid hormones in the blood and urine of prepubertal girls and other primates. *Clin Endocrinol Metab* 1978;7:513.

12. Carr BR. Disorders of the ovaries and female reproductive tract. In: Wilson JD, Foster DW, Kronenberg HM, et al., eds. *Williams textbook of endocrinology*, 9th ed. Philadelphia: WB Saunders, 1998:751.

13. Grumbach MM, Roth JC, Kaplan SL, et al. Hypothalamic-pituitary regulation of puberty in man: evidence and concepts derived from clinical research. In: Grumbach MM, Grave GD, Mayer FE, eds. *Control of the onset of puberty.* New York: Wiley & Sons, 1974:115.

14. Parker LN, Odell WD. Control of adrenal androgen secretion. *Endocr Rev* 1980;1:392.

15. Burger HG, McLachlan RI, Bangah M, et al. Serum inhibin concentrations rise throughout normal male and female puberty. *J Clin Endocrinol Metab* 1988;67:689.

16. Atalla F, Reineke FP. Influence of environmental temperature and thyroid status on reproductive organs of young female mice. *Fed Proc* 1951;10:1.

17. Gellert RJ, Bakke JL, Lawrence NL. Delayed vaginal opening in the rat following pharmacologic doses of T_4 administered during the neonatal period. *J Lab Clin Med* 1971;77:410.

18. Leathem JH. Nutritional effects on endocrine secretions. In: Young WC, ed. *Sex and internal secretions*, 3rd ed. Baltimore: Williams & Wilkins, 1961:666.

19. Howland BE, Ibrahim EA. Hyperthyroidism and gonadotropin secretion in male and female rats. *Experientia* 1973;29:1398.

20. Maruo T, Hiramatsu S, Otani T, et al. Increase in the expression of thyroid hormone receptors in porcine granulosa cells early in follicular maturation. *Acta Endocrinol (Copenh)* 1992;127:152.

21. Evans RW, Farwell AP, Braverman LE. Nuclear thyroid hormone receptor in the rat uterus. *Endocrinology* 1983;113:1459.

22. Ruh MF, Ruh TS, Klitgaard HM. Uptake and retention of estrogens by uteri from rats in various thyroid states. *Proc Soc Exp Biol Med* 1970;134:558.

23. Schultze AB, Noonan J. Thyroxine administration and reproduction in rats. *J Anim Sci* 1970;30:774–776.

24. Maruo T, Matsuo H, Mochizuki M. Thyroid hormone as a biological amplifier of differentiated trophoblast function in early pregnancy. *Acta Endocrinol (Copenh)* 1991;125:58.

25. Akande EO, Hockaday TDR. Plasma oestrogen and luteinizing hormone concentrations in thyrotoxic menstrual disturbance. *Proc R Soc Med* 1972;65:789.

26. Ridgway EC, Longcope C, Maloof F. Metabolic clearance and blood production rates of estradiol in hyperthyroidism. *J Clin Endocrinol Metab* 1975;4:491.

27. Southren AL, Olivo J, Gordon GG, et al. The conversion of androgens to estrogens in hyperthyroidism. *J Clin Endocrinol Metab* 1974;38:207.

28. Burrow GN. The thyroid gland and reproduction. In: Yen SSC, Jaffe RB, eds. *Reproductive endocrinology.* Philadelphia: WB Saunders, 1986:424.

29. Akande EO, Hockaday TDR. Plasma luteinizing hormone levels in women with thyrotoxicosis. *J Endocrinol* 1972;53:173.

30. Pontikides N, Kaltsas Th, Krassas GE. The hypothalamic–pituitary–gonadal axis in hyperthyroid female patients before and after treatment [Abstract 210]. *J Endocrinol Invest* 1990;13 (suppl 2):203.

31. Zahringer S, Tomova A, von Werder K, et al. The influence of hyperthyroidism on the hypothalamic-pituitary-gonadal axis. *Exp Clin Endocrinol Diabetes* 2000;108:282.

32. Akande EO. The effect of oestrogen on plasma levels of luteinizing hormone in euthyroid and thyrotoxic postmenopausal women. *J Obstet Gynecol* 1974;81:795.

33. Tanaka T, Tamai H, Kuma K, et al. Gonadotropin response to luteinizing hormone releasing hormone in hyperthyroid patients with menstrual disturbances. *Metabolism* 1981;30:323.

34. Distiller LA, Sagel J, Morley JE. Assessment of pituitary gonadotropin reserve using luteinizing hormone–releasing hormone (LRH) in states of altered thyroid function. *J Clin Endocrinol Metab* 1975;40:512.

35. Saxena KM, Crawford JD, Talbot NB. Childhood thyrotoxicosis: a long-term prospective. *BMJ* 1964;2:1153.

36. Von Basedow CA. Exophthalmos durch Hypertrophie des Zellgewebes in der Augenhohl. *Wochenschr Heilkunde* 1840;6:197.

37. Speroff L, Glass RH, Kase NG. Amenorrhoea. In: Speroff L, Glass RH, Kase NG, eds. *Clinical gynecologic endocrinology and infertility.* Baltimore:Williams & Wilkins, 1983:141.

38. Warren MP. Evaluation of secondary amenorrhoea. *J Clin Endocrinol Metab* 1996;81:437.

39. Benson RC, Dailey ME. Menstrual pattern in hyperthyroidism and subsequent post-therapy hypothyroidism. *Surg Gynaecol Obstet* 1955;100:19.

40. Goldsmith RE, Sturgis SH, Lerman J, et al. The menstrual pattern in thyroid disease. *J Clin Endocrinol Metab* 1952;12:846.

41. Joshi JV, Bhandakar SD, Chadha M, et al. Menstrual irregularities and lactation failure may precede thyroid dysfunction or goitre. *J Postgrad Med* 1993;39:137.

42. Krassas GE, Pontikides N, Kaltsas Th, et al. Menstrual disturbances in thyrotoxicosis. *Clin Endocrinol (Oxf)* 1994;40:641.

43. Pontikides N, Kaltsas Th, Krassas GE. The LH, FSH, PRL and progesterone levels in thyrotoxic female patients before and after treatment [Abstract 133]. *J Endocrinol Invest* 1990;13(suppl 2):164.

44. Pellimiemi LJ, Dym M. The fetal gonad and sexual differentiation. In: Tulchinsky D, Little AB, eds. *Maternal-fetal endocrinology,* 2nd ed. Philadelphia: WB Saunders, 1994:298.

45. George FW, Wilson JD. Sex determination and differentiation. In: Knobil E, Neill JD, eds. *The physiology of reproduction,* 2nd ed. New York: Raven, 1994:3.

46. Josso N. Antimüllerian hormone: new perspectives for a sexist molecule. *Endocr Rev* 1986;7:421.

47. Grumbach MM, Gluckman PD. The human fetal hypothalamus and pituitary gland: the maturation of neuroendocrine mechanisms controlling the secretion of fetal pituitary growth hormone, prolactin, gonadotropin, andrenocorticotropin-related peptides and thyrototropin. In: Tulchinsky D, Little AB, eds. *Maternal-fetal endocrinology,* 2nd ed. Philadelphia: WB Saunders, 1994:193.

48. Hayes FJ, Crowley WF Jr. Gonadotropin pulsations across development. *Horm Res* 1998;49:163.

49. Veldhuis JD, King JC, Urban RJ, et al. Operating characteristics of the male hypothalamo-pituitary-gonadal axis: pulsatile release of testosterone and follicle-stimulating hormone and their temporal coupling with luteinizing hormone. *J Clin Endocrinol Metab* 1987;65:929.

50. Winters SJ, Troen P. Evidence for a role of endogenous estrogen in the hypothalamic control of gonadotropin secretion in men. *J Clin Endocrinol Metab* 1985;61:842.

51. Morishima A, Grumbach MM, Simpson ER, et al. Aromatase deficiency in male and female siblings caused by a novel mutation and the physiological role of estrogens. *J Clin Endocrinol Metab* 1995;80:3689.

52. Weinstein RL, Kelch RP, Jenner MR, et al. Secretion of unconjugated androgens and estrogens by the normal and abnormal human testis before and after human chorionic gonadotropin. *J Clin Invest* 1974;53:1.

53. Rosner W. The functions of corticosteroid-binding globulin and sex hormone-binding globulin: recent advances. *Endocr Rev* 1990;11:80.

54. Yosha S, Fay M, Longcope C, et al. Effect of D-thyroxine on serum sex hormone binding globulin (SHBG), testosterone, and pituitary-thyroid function in euthyroid subjects. *J Endocrinol Invest* 1984;7:489.

55. Sharpe RM. regulation of spermatogenesis. In: Knobil E, Neill JD, eds. *The physiology of reproduction*, 2nd ed. New York: Raven, 1994:1363.

56. Jenkins EP, Andersson S, Imperato-McGinley J, et al. Genetic and pharmacological evidence for more than one human steroid 5 alpha-reductase. *J Clin Invest* 1992;89:293.

57. Kaufman JM, Vermeulen A. Declining gonadal function in elderly men. *Baillieres Clin Endocrinol Metab* 1997;11:289.

58. Gray A, Feldman HA, McKinlay JB, et al. Age, disease, and changing sex hormone levels in middle-aged men: results of the Massachusetts Male Aging Study. *J Clin Endocrinol Metab* 1991; 73:1016.

59. Longcope C, Sato K, McKay C, et al. Aromatization by splanchnic tissue in men. *J Clin Endocrinol Metab* 1984;58:1089.

60. Bolt HM. Metabolism of estrogens—natural and synthetic. *Pharmacol Ther* 1979;4:155.

61. Sheckter CB, Matsumoto AM, Bremner WJ. Testosterone administration inhibits gonadotropin secretion by an effect directly on the human pituitary. *J Clin Endocrinol Metab* 1989; 68:397.

62. Vale W, Bilezikjian LM, Rivier C. Reproductive and other roles of inhibins and activins. In: Knobil E, Neill JD, eds. *The physiology of reproduction*, 2nd ed. New York: Raven, 1994:1861.

63. Gomes WR. Metabolic and regulatory hormones influencing testis function. In: Johnson AD, Gomes WR, Vandemark NL, eds. *The testis*. Vol. III: *Influencing factors*. New York: Academic, 1970:67.

64. Schneider G, Kopach K, Ohanian H, et al. The hypothalamic-pituitary-gonadal axis during hyperthyroidism in the rat. *Endocrinology* 1979;105:674.

65. Chandrasekhar Y, D'Occhio MJ, Holland MK, et al. Activity of the hypothalamo-pituitary axis and testicular development in prepubertal ram lambs with induced hypothyroidism or hyperthyroidism. *Endocrinology* 1985;117:1645.

66. Massie ED, Gomes WR, Vandemark NL. Effects of thyroidectomy or thyroxine on testicular tissue metabolism. *J Reprod Fertil* 1969;18:173.

67. Aruldhas MM, Valivullah HM, Srinivasan N, et al. Role of thyroid on testicular lipids in prepubertal, pubertal and adult rats. I. Hyperthyroidism. *Biochim Biophys Acta* 1986;881:462.

68. Chandrasekhar Y, Holland MK, D'Occhio MJ, et al. Spermatogenesis, seminal characteristics and reproductive hormone levels in mature rams with induced hypothyroidism and hyperthyroidism. *J Endocrinol* 1985;105:39.

69. Ruder H, Corvol P, Mahoudeau JA, et al. Effects of induced hyperthyroidism on steroid metabolism in man. *J Clin Endocrinol Metab* 1971;33:382.

70. Vermeulen A, Verdonck L, Van Der Straeten M, et al. Capacity of the testosterone-binding globulin in human plasma and influence of specific binding to testosterone on its metabolic clearance rate. *J Clin Endocrinol Metab* 1969;29:1470.

71. Kidd GS, Glass AR, Vigersky RA. The hypothalamic-pituitary-testicular axis in thyrotoxicosis. *J Clin Endocrinol Metab* 1979; 48:798.

72. Chopra IJ, Tulchinsky D. Status of estrogen-androgen balance in hyperthyroid men with Graves' disease. *J Clin Endocrinol Metab* 1974;38:269.

73. Ridgway EC, Maloof F, Longcope C. Androgen and oestrogen dynamics in hyperthyroidism. *J Endocrinol* 1982;95:105.

74. Gallagher TF, Fukushima DK, Noguchi S, et al. Recent studies in steroid hormone metabolism in man. *Rec Prog Horm Res* 1966;22:283.

75. Nomura K, Suzuki H, Saji M, et al. High serum progesterone in hyperthyroid men with Graves' disease. *J Clin Endocrinol Metab* 1988;66:230.

76. Abalovich M, Levalle O, Hermes R, et al. Hypothalamic-pituitary-testicular axis and seminal parameters in hyperthyroid males. *Thyroid* 1999;9:857.

77. Michnovicz JJ, Galbraith RA. Effects of exogenous thyroxine on C-2 and C-16 alpha hydroxylations of estradiol in humans. *Steroids* 1990;55:22.

78. Krassas GE, Pontikides N, Deligianni V, et al. A prospective controlled study of the impact of hyperthyroidism on reproductive function in males. *J Clin Endocrinol Metab* 2002;87:3667.

79. Rojdmark S, Berg A, Kallner G. Hypothalamic-pituitary-testicular axis in patients with hyperthyroidism. *Horm Res* 1988;29: 185.

80. Velazquez EM, Bellabarba Arata G. Effects of thyroid status on pituitary gonadotropin and testicular reserve in men. *Arch Androl* 1997;38:85.

81. Clyde HR, Walsh PC, English RW. Elevated plasma testosterone and gonadotropin levels in infertile males with hyperthyroidism. *Fertil Steril* 1976;27:662.

82. Hudson RW, Edwards AL. Testicular function in hyperthyroidism. *J Androl* 1992;13:117.

83. Kaplan MM, Meier DA, Dworkin HJ. Treatment of hyperthyroidism with radioactive iodine. *Endocrinol Metab Clin North Am* 1998;27:205.

84. Hyer S, Vini L, O'Connell M, et al. Testicular dose and fertility in men following ^{131}I therapy for thyroid cancer. *Clin Endocrinol (Oxf)* 2002;56:755.

85. Safa AM, Schumacher OP, Rodriguez-Antunez A. Long-term follow-up results in children and adolescents treated with radioactive iodine (131-I) for hyperthyroidism. *N Engl J Med* 1975;292:167.

86. Krassas GE, Perros P. Thyroid disease and male reproductive function. *J Endocrinol Invest* 2003;26:372.

87. Rivkees SA, Sklar C, Freemark M. Clinical review 99: The management of Graves' disease in children, with special emphasis on radioiodine treatment. *J Clin Endocrinol Metab* 1998;83:3767.

88. Krassas GE. Treatment of juvenile Graves' disease and its ophthalmic complication: the "European way." *Eur J Endocrinol* 2004;150:407.

THE SKELETAL SYSTEM
IN THYROTOXICOSIS

MICHAEL C. SHEPPARD
NEIL J.L. GITTOES

Over a century ago a young woman who died from thyrotoxicosis was noted to have bones that looked "worm-eaten." The first systematic study of the clinical effects of thyrotoxicosis on the skeleton was published in 1972 (1). Among 187 patients with thyrotoxicosis, 15 (8%) had skeletal symptoms, and of these 80% were over 50 years old, and two thirds had a fracture or severe bone pain. Radiographic studies demonstrated generalized osteoporosis, and vertebral compression fractures were common. Since then, symptomatic osteoporosis and fractures resulting from thyrotoxicosis have become rare, as a result of earlier diagnosis and the widespread availability of effective treatments for thyrotoxicosis.

Although there is general acceptance that thyrotoxicosis increases bone turnover in general and bone resorption in particular, leading to osteopenia and osteoporosis, considerable controversy remains surrounding the relationship between thyrotoxicosis and bone, particularly in terms of fracture risk (Table 40.1).

THYROID HORMONE ACTIONS ON THE SKELETON

The skeleton is a metabolically active tissue in which mineralized bone is continuously remodeled by the coordinated recruitment of osteoclasts and osteoblasts that respectively resorb and form new bone. These processes are regulated by autocrine, paracrine, and endocrine pathways. Steroid hormones, particularly glucocorticoids (2), estrogens (3), androgens (3), and vitamin D (4), are particularly important regulators of bone metabolism. The effects of thyroid hormone on bone metabolism are perhaps less well characterized than are those of other hormones, but it is clear that perturbations in thyroid status have important effects on skeletal development, linear growth, and maintenance of normal bone mass.

BONE REMODELING IN THYROTOXICOSIS

In adults, the mechanical integrity of the skeleton is maintained by bone remodeling. Normally, recruitment and activation of osteoclasts and osteoblasts are tightly coupled (Fig. 40.1), resulting in maintenance of bone mass and strength. Osteoclasts initiate excavation of an area of bone; osteoblasts then invade the site to lay down new matrix that in turn is mineralized to form new bone. The activation-resorption-formation sequence occurs in discrete bone-remodeling units. In thyrotoxicosis, the processes of bone resorption, matrix deposition, and mineralization are accelerated and the activation frequency (rate at which sites undergo remodeling) is increased. Studies *in vitro* have demonstrated that thyroid hormone can stimulate bone resorption within a few days (5). Osteoclast and osteoblast activities are both increased (albeit disproportionately), and the duration of the remodeling cycle is reduced by approximately 50%. The uncoupling of osteoclast-osteoblast activation leads to an increase in the ratio of bone surface undergoing resorption to that undergoing formation. The net result is loss of bone, amounting to approximately 10% of mineralized bone per cycle in severe thyrotoxicosis (6–9).

In keeping with increased activity of both osteoclasts and osteoblasts, serum and urinary biochemical markers of bone turnover are high in thyrotoxicosis. They include markers of both bone formation (serum alkaline phosphatase and osteocalcin) and bone resorption (urinary excretion of pyridinoline and deoxypyridinoline cross-links and hydroxyproline), and the values are correlated with disease severity (10–13).

In addition to its direct effects on osteoclast-osteoblast cell function, thyrotoxicosis results in a negative calcium balance. Urinary calcium excretion is increased. Intestinal calcium absorption is decreased, and therefore fecal calcium excretion is increased. The increase in bone resorption raises serum calcium concentrations, sometimes enough to cause hypercalcemia. Years ago hypercalcemia was reported in up to 20% of patients with thyrotoxicosis, but the frequency is much lower now. Any increase in serum calcium concentration inhibits parathyroid hormone secretion, thus accounting, at least in part, for the increase in urinary calcium excretion. Another consequence of decreased parathyroid hormone secretion is reduced renal conversion of 25-hydroxyvitamin D (calcidiol) to 1,25-

TABLE 40.1. EFFECTS OF THYROID HORMONE EXCESS ON THE SKELETON

Endogenous thyrotoxicosis
   Decreased bone mineral density (osteopenia and
      osteoporosis)
   Increased risk of hip and vertebral fractures
   Increased mortality due to hip fracture
Exogenous thyroid hormone therapy
   No increase in fracture risk with thyroid hormone therapy
      per se
   TSH-suppressive therapy with thyroid hormone is associated
      with reduced bone mineral density in postmenopausal
      women
   TSH suppressive therapy is associated with an increased risk
      of hip and vertebral fracture

TSH, thyrotropin.

dihydroxyvitamin D (calcitriol). Reduced activation of vitamin D is exacerbated by increased metabolic clearance of vitamin D and its metabolites. Normal calcium homeostasis and parathyroid hormone secretion are restored after treatment for thyrotoxicosis. Administration of thyroid hormone to normal subjects results in similar changes in calcium homeostasis, with a prompt increase in both urinary and fecal calcium excretion.

The skeletal changes differ somewhat in children with thyrotoxicosis. In them, linear growth and bone age tend to be accelerated, and premature closure of growth plates and cranial sutures can occur in children with severe thyrotoxicosis (see Chapter 76).

MECHANISMS OF THYROID HORMONE ACTION IN BONE

Understanding of the cellular and molecular mechanisms of thyroid hormone action in bone is incomplete; what is known has been recently and comprehensively reviewed (14). Thyroid hormone receptor (TR) expression and function have been characterized in bone cells; the α_1, α_2, and β_1 isoforms of the receptor are present in osteoblasts (15–20) and some chondrocytes (21,22) (see Chapter 8). However, the results of studies of thyroid hormone effects in osteoblasts are conflicting, seemingly dependent on variables such as species, cell line/primary culture, and state of differentiation. Overall, thyroid hormone appears to stimulate osteoblast differentiation and activity, and increase synthesis of type 1 collagen, alkaline phosphatase (23), osteocalcin (24–26), and receptor activator of nuclear factor κB ligand (RANKL, a key molecule in osteoclast function) (27). Furthermore, thyroid hormone potentiates osteoblast responses to parathyroid hormone by increasing the expression of parathyroid hormone receptors (28). These effects of thyroid hormone appear to be mediated both directly and indirectly via other signaling pathways, such as fibroblast growth factor receptor-1 (29). Some of the effects of thyroid hormone on bone are extremely rapid and involve mobilization of intracellular calcium stores, suggesting that the hormone has nongenomic, TR-independent actions (30).

Although thyroid hormone stimulates osteoclastic bone resorption (the predominant mechanism responsible for

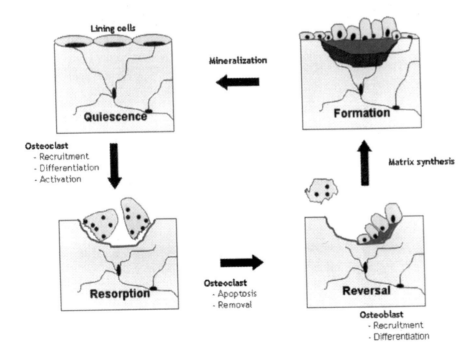

FIGURE 40.1. Schematic representation of the phases of bone remodeling.

reduced bone mineral density in patients with thyrotoxicosis), this effect is mediated indirectly via thyroid hormone–responsive osteoblasts (31,32); isolated osteoclasts alone cannot resorb bone (33). Osteoblast-derived signals, such as interleukin-6, prostaglandins, and RANKL (27), induce recruitment and differentiation of osteoclast progenitor cells or increase the activity of mature osteoclasts to effect osteoclastic bone resorption.

An important determinant of thyroid hormone action is prereceptor regulation of ligand availability (i.e., iodothyronine deiodinase function), although this is a poorly understood phenomenon in bone (27,34) (see Chapter 7). Type 2 iodothyronine deiodinase (D2) has been identified in osteoblasts (27), and D2 knockout mice have a mild transient period of growth retardation that curiously occurs only in males (35). D3 knockout mice develop severe progressive growth restriction soon after birth (36). It is likely that deiodinase function plays a critical role in determining the availability of triiodothyronine (T_3) and therefore its action in bone.

Autocrine effects mediated by thyroid hormone are also likely to be involved in regulation of bone turnover. Thyroid hormone stimulates the production of insulin-like growth factor-1 (IGF-1) in rat osteoblasts *in vitro* (37) and increases IGF-1 messenger RNA (mRNA) in mouse osteoblasts (38). IGF-1 in turn increases bone formation (39). Thyroid hormone increases IGF-1 mRNA in cultured vertebral, but not femoral, bone marrow cells (40), suggesting skeletal site-dependent differences in the *in vitro* responses of cells of osteoblastic lineage to thyroid hormone. Furthermore, thyroid hormone stimulates the production of interleukins in human bone marrow cultures (41,42); these cytokines may be additional mediators of thyroid hormone–induced bone loss.

BONE MINERAL DENSITY, FRACTURES, AND THYROTOXICOSIS

Many studies have reported reduced bone mineral density in patients with thyrotoxicosis. In addition, in some studies thyrotoxicosis was associated with an increase in risk for hip and spine fracture (43–48). A 2003 meta-analysis examined changes in bone mineral density and fracture risk after treatment for thyrotoxicosis (49). Using the terms *hyperthyroidism, bone mineral density,* and *fracture,* 289 references were retrieved; 20 references describing bone mineral density (902 patients) and 5 describing fracture risk (62,830 patients and control subjects) were included in the analysis. The bone mineral density of the spine and hip were significantly lower than normal in patients with thyrotoxicosis before treatment. After treatment, bone mineral density increased significantly, and it was normal in those patients studied more than 1 year after diagnosis and initi-

ation of therapy. Hip fracture risk in patients with previous thyrotoxicosis increased significantly with age, as compared with normal subjects (pooled risk estimate risk for hip fracture after diagnosis 1.6). A direct comparison of bone mineral density in patients treated with an antithyroid drug and those treated with radioiodine revealed no difference between the groups, but the groups differed in age and time after treatment. The hip fracture risk after diagnosis predicted from studies of bone mineral density was close to that observed in clinical studies comparing fracture risk in patients with thyrotoxicosis with normal subjects.

In sum, this analysis demonstrated that bone mineral density is decreased and fracture risk is increased in untreated patients with thyrotoxicosis. Antithyroid treatment alone, in the absence of any antiosteoporosis treatment, results in restoration of normal bone density. The increasing risk with age indicates that thyrotoxicosis augments age-related bone loss. These observations are consistent with previous reports that bone loss is greater in postmenopausal than premenopausal women with thyrotoxicosis (50,51).

With respect to fracture risk, a case control study of 116 postmenopausal women with hip fracture and 402 postmenopausal control women in Germany reported an odds ratio for thyrotoxicosis (present and past) among the women with hip fracture of 2.5 (48). Although screening for thyroid disease in elderly patients is not recommended by most authorities, the approximate 20% prevalence of thyroid disorders in this sample suggests the need for a high index of suspicion for thyroid disease in women who have fractures. In this study thyroxine (T_4) therapy was not a risk for hip fracture (odds ratio 0.67).

In another study, potential risk factors for hip fracture were assessed in 9,516 white women 65 years of age or older; 12% were taking thyroid hormone, and 9% had a history of thyrotoxicosis (43). These women were then followed for an average of 4.1 years to determine the frequency of hip fracture, validated by review of x-ray films. During the follow-up period 192 women had a first hip fracture not due to motor vehicle accidents. Independent risk factors for hip fracture included previous thyrotoxicosis, a maternal history of hip fracture, previous fractures of any type after the age of 50 years, and treatment with long-acting benzodiazepine or anticonvulsant drugs. A history of thyrotoxicosis independently increased the risk for hip fracture (relative risk 1.8), even after adjusting for femoral neck bone density. In this study, reduced bone mass did not account for the strong association between previous thyrotoxicosis and the risk for hip fracture, suggesting that thyrotoxicosis may cause long-lasting impairment of bone strength not detected by densitometry, or long-lasting muscle weakness that increases susceptibility to falls. Women taking thyroid hormone also appeared to have an increased risk for fracture; current thyroid hormone therapy was significantly associated with hip fracture (relative risk 1.6). However, current thyroid hormone therapy was not associated with the risk for hip fracture after adjustment for a history of thyrotoxicosis, which was reported by 36% of those women who were taking thyroid hormone.

In contrast, in a study of 300 postmenopausal white women, there was no difference in the frequency of a history of hip, vertebral, or forearm fracture in the 160 women who had a history of thyroid disease and the 140 women with no history of thyroid disease (52). In this cohort, 37 women (23%) with thyroid disease and 45 women (32%) without thyroid disease had a history of fracture. There were no differences between these groups in the number or type of fractures. Also, the duration of thyroid disease or therapy or dose of thyroid hormone did not affect fracture occurrence, although women with a history of thyrotoxicosis had their first fracture slightly earlier than women without thyroid disease.

A major study from Denmark reinforced these observations and clarified the risks. The study subjects consisted of 617 consecutive patients with toxic nodular goiter or diffuse toxic goiter (Graves' disease) treated between 1991 and 1997 (46). For each patient, an age- and sex-matched control subject was drawn from a random sample of the general population. Within the 5 years before the diagnosis of thyrotoxicosis there was no increase in fracture among the patients as compared with the controls. After diagnosis there was a significantly increased risk for fracture (relative risk 1.7), especially in patients over 50 years of age (relative risk 2.2). The sites of increased fracture were the spine and forearm, but not the femur, including the femoral neck. The fracture rates were similar in the patients with diffuse toxic goiter and those with toxic nodular goiter. There was no association between baseline serum T_4 or T_3 concentrations and subsequent fracture risk, suggesting that it may be the duration rather than the severity of the thyrotoxicosis that determines the detrimental effect on bone. Where this study conflicts with others is the absence of an increased frequency of hip fracture. Because the fracture rates in the control subjects and among the patients before the diagnosis of thyrotoxicosis were similar to the rate in the general population in Denmark, it seems unlikely that overreporting of fractures biased the results.

An unexpected finding of this study (46) was that an increase in fracture occurred only in patients who had been treated with radioiodine alone, but not those treated with radioiodine and methimazole or those treated with methimazole alone. The observation of an increase in fracture after radioiodine therapy, even after adjustment for age and other risk factors, agrees with the findings of a study published over 30 years ago (44). In the latter study, there was an increase in fracture in patients treated with radioiodine, but not those treated with either an antithyroid drug or thyroidectomy. It seems unlikely that radioiodine itself has an adverse skeletal effect. More likely, the difference was due to the older age of patients treated with radioiodine or slower correction of thyrotoxicosis by this treatment.

A contrasting study was reported from Malmo, Sweden (53). In this study of 333 patients who were treated for thyrotoxicosis for the first time during the 5-year period 1970 to 1974 and 618 age- and sex-matched control subjects, there was no difference in the 20-year frequency of fracture in the two groups. The size and design of this study did not allow, however, for analysis of the effect of duration of thyrotoxicosis or type of antithyroid treatment.

The close relationship between observed fracture risk and fracture risk based on the results of bone densitometry in patients with thyrotoxicosis, particularly as identified in the meta-analysis (49), leads to the conclusion that most of the changes in fracture risk are related to changes in bone mineral density. This conclusion is supported by the clear evidence that the decreased bone density associated with thyrotoxicosis is reversible after effective treatment (49,54–59) (Fig. 40.2). However, it is important to remember that fracture risk may also be increased as a result of decreased muscle strength (myopathy) and hyperactivity that occur in some patients with thyrotoxicosis (46).

MORTALITY AND FRACTURES

The relationship between thyrotoxicosis and mortality was examined in a population-based study in the United King-

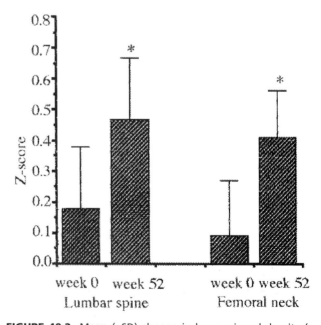

FIGURE 40.2. Mean (±SD) change in bone mineral density (z-score) in the lumbar spine and femoral neck before (week 0) and 1 year (week 52) after initiation of treatment in 17 patients with thyrotoxicosis. *$p < 0.01$, as compared with week 0. (From Siddiqi A, Burrin JM, Noonan K, et al. A longitudinal study of markers of bone turnover in Graves' disease and their value in predicting bone mineral density. *J Clin Endocrinol Metab* 1997; 82:753, with permission.)

dom with a long follow-up period (60). Among 7,299 patients with thyrotoxicosis treated with radioiodine between 1950 and 1989, there was an increase in all-cause mortality, particularly due to cardiovascular and cerebrovascular disease, as compared with the general population (see Chapter 77). In addition, there was an increase in mortality due to fractures of the femur (26 excess deaths; standardized mortality ratio 2.9). The risk for death due to fracture of the femur was limited to patients at least 59 years of age at the time of treatment, but it was not significantly associated with time after treatment. The influence of postradioiodine hypothyroidism or its treatment with T_4 on mortality in this cohort is not known.

EFFECTS OF EXOGENOUS THYROID HORMONE ON BONE MINERAL DENSITY AND FRACTURE RATES

While overt thyrotoxicosis is associated with osteopenia and sometimes osteoporosis, the effect of subclinical thyrotoxicosis [low serum thyrotropin (TSH) but normal serum T_4 and T_3 concentrations] on the skeleton is less clear (see Chapters 77 and 79). This is most often caused by T_4 therapy, even when it is prescribed as replacement therapy (61,62). In some, but not all, studies, patients taking T_4 in doses sufficient to cause subclinical thyrotoxicosis have had low bone density.

In the late 1980s and early 1990s, several studies revealed low bone density at multiple sites in patients, mostly women, receiving prolonged T_4 therapy who had low serum TSH concentrations (63–70). These studies were confounded by the inclusion of women who had previously had thyrotoxicosis and women of varying age and menopausal status. The results of subsequent cross-sectional and prospective studies of premenopausal women who had never had thyrotoxicosis and were taking TSH-suppressive doses of T_4 were contradictory; some revealed low bone density at one or more sites (64,65,71–73), whereas others did not (13,70,74–78). Similarly, in postmenopausal women, TSH-suppressive doses of T_4 have been reported to decrease (63–66,69,70,78) or have no effect (74,77,79,80) on bone mineral density. Many of these studies involved small numbers of women, most were cross-sectional, and there were variations in the doses of T_4 (and therefore the degree of TSH suppression), the extent to which TSH secretion was suppressed during the sometimes long follow-up period, and the extent to which the patients were matched with control subjects.

In a meta-analysis of 13 cross-sectional studies in which bone mineral density was measured in the distal forearm, femoral neck, or lumbar spine in T_4-treated women with low serum TSH concentrations and control women, there was no difference in bone density in the T_4-treated and

control premenopausal women, but among postmenopausal women those taking T_4 had lower bone density (81). The rate of excess bone loss in these women was estimated to be approximately 1% per year after 10 years ($p < 0.007$). The observed changes were distributed equally throughout the skeleton. The researchers concluded that suppressive T_4 thyroxine therapy caused significant bone loss in postmenopausal women, but not in premenopausal women.

A further meta-analysis of all published controlled cross-sectional studies between 1982 and 1984 (41 studies including approximately 1,250 patients) was performed concerning the impact of thyroid hormone therapy on bone mineral density (82). Women who were receiving estrogen therapy or who had a history of thyrotoxicosis were excluded, as were those with postoperative hypoparathyroidism. T_4 suppressive therapy was associated with significant bone loss at all sites, including lumbar spine and femoral neck, in postmenopausal women (but not in premenopausal women). Somewhat surprisingly, T_4 replacement therapy was associated with bone loss in premenopausal women (spine and hip), but not in postmenopausal women. The authors of this meta-analysis came to the same conclusion as above, namely that overtreatment with T_4 probably contributes to the development of osteoporosis in postmenopausal women.

In a study of 1,180 patients receiving T_4 replacement therapy in the United Kingdom, the rates of hip fracture were similar in patients with low serum TSH concentrations, as compared with those with normal serum TSH concentrations and with the general population (83). There was a trend toward an increased overall fracture rate in patients over 65 years of age with low serum TSH values (2.5% vs. 0.9%). However, the risk of hospitalization for fracture was approximately two times greater in persons over 65 years of age with low serum TSH concentrations.

The Study of Osteoporotic Fractures in the United States has provided important data relating to the risk for bone loss and fractures in older women with low serum TSH concentrations, many of whom were receiving T_4 (79). After adjustment for age, weight, previous thyrotoxicosis, and estrogen therapy, bone loss over 4 to 6 years was similar in women with low (<0.1 mU/L), normal (0.1–5 to 5 mU/L), and high (>5 mU/L) serum TSH values. At baseline, there were no differences in bone density of the calcaneus, spine, or femoral neck, but total hip density was 6% lower ($p = 0.01$) in the women with low serum TSH values. This was the first large prospective study of thyroid function and bone loss in a population-based group of postmenopausal women.

A subsequent study of the Study of Osteoporotic Fractures cohort examined the association between low serum TSH concentrations at baseline and subsequent fracture in 695 women over 65 years of age (84). During a mean follow-up period of 3.7 years, 148 women had a hip fracture, 149 women had a vertebral fracture, and 398 women had no fractures. The women with baseline serum TSH concentrations less than 0.1 mU/L, most of whom were taking thyroid hormone, had a greater than threefold increased risk for hip fracture and a fourfold increased risk for vertebral fracture, as compared with women who had normal serum TSH concentrations (0.5–5.5 mU/L).

In a similar but much larger study, the United Kingdom General Practice Research database was used to investigate the frequency of hip fracture in a large cohort of patients taking T_4 (84). Among 23,183 patients (88% women) who had taken T_4 for at least 1 year, 1.6% had a hip fracture, as compared with 1.4% of 92,732 control subjects ($p = 0.06$). Prescription of T_4 did not predict fracture occurrence in women but was an independent predictor in men. Serum TSH was not measured, so whether T_4 therapy was excessive is not known.

In summary, supraphysiologic doses of T_4 may decrease bone density and increase fracture risk, but the effects are small and most likely to occur only in postmenopausal women and those taking sufficient T_4 to decrease serum TSH concentrations to well below the normal range. In patients in whom high doses of T_4 are indicated, for example, those with recurrent thyroid carcinoma, a bisphosphonate or estrogen can be given to inhibit the detrimental effects of T_4 on the skeleton (85–88).

REFERENCES

1. Meunier PJ, Bianchi GGS, Eduoard CM, et al. Bony manifestations of thyrotoxicosis. *Orthop Clin North Am* 1972;3:745.
2. Canalis E, Giustina A. Glucocorticoid-induced osteoporosis: summary of a workshop. *J Clin Endocrinol Metab* 2001;86:5681.
3. Riggs BL, Khosla S, Melton LJ 3rd. Sex steroids and the construction and conservation of the adult skeleton. *Endocr Rev* 2002;23:279.
4. Lips P. Vitamin D deficiency and secondary hyperparathyroidism in the elderly: consequences for bone loss and fractures and therapeutic implications. *Endocr Rev* 2001;22:477.
5. Mundy GR, Shapiro JL, Bandelin JG, et al. Direct stimulation of bone resorption by thyroid hormones. *J Clin Invest* 1976;58:529.
6. Eriksen EF, Mosekilde L, Melsen F. Trabecular bone remodeling and bone balance in hyperthyroidism. *Bone* 1985;6:421.
7. Hasling C, Eriksen EF, Charles P, et al. Exogenous triiodothyronine activates bone remodeling. *Bone* 1987;8:65.
8. High WB, Capen CC, Black HE. Effects of thyroxine on cortical bone remodeling in adult dogs: a histomorphometric study. *Am J Pathol* 1981;102:438.
9. Mosekilde L, Melsen F. A tetracycline-based histomorphometric evaluation of bone resorption and bone turnover in hyperthyroidism and hyperparathyroidism. *Acta Med Scand* 1978;204:97.
10. Garnero P, Vassy V, Bertholin A, et al. Markers of bone turnover in hyperthyroidism and the effects of treatment. *J Clin Endocrinol Metab* 1994;78:955.
11. Harvey RD, McHardy KC, Reid IW, et al. Measurement of bone collagen degradation in hyperthyroidism and during thyroxine replacement therapy using pyridinium cross-links as specific urinary markers. *J Clin Endocrinol Metab* 1991;72:1189.
12. Guo CY, Weetman AP, Eastell R. Longitudinal changes of bone mineral density and bone turnover in postmenopausal women on thyroxine. *Clin Endocrinol (Oxf)* 1997;46:301.
13. Toivonen J, Tahtela R, Laitinen K, et al. Markers of bone turnover in patients with differentiated thyroid cancer with and following withdrawal of thyroxine suppressive therapy. *Eur J Endocrinol* 1998;138:667.
14. Duncan Bassett JH, Williams GR. The molecular actions of thyroid hormone in bone. *Trends Endocrinol Metab* 2003;14:356.
15. Williams GR, Bland R, Sheppard MC. Characterization of thyroid hormone (T_3) receptors in three osteosarcoma cell lines of distinct osteoblast phenotype: interactions among T_3, vitamin D3, and retinoid signaling. *Endocrinology* 1994;135:2375.
16. Rizzoli R, Poser J, Burgi U. Nuclear thyroid hormone receptors in cultured bone cells. *Metabolism* 1986;35:71.
17. Kasono K, Sato K, Han DC, et al. Stimulation of alkaline phosphatase activity by thyroid hormone in mouse osteoblast-like cells (MC3T3-E1): a possible mechanism of hyperalkaline phosphatasia in hyperthyroidism. *Bone Miner* 1988;4:355.
18. LeBron BA, Pekary AE, Mirell C, et al. Thyroid hormone 5'-deiodinase activity, nuclear binding, and effects on mitogenesis in UMR-106 osteoblastic osteosarcoma cells. *J Bone Miner Res* 1989;4:173.
19. Sato K, Han DC, Fujii Y, et al. Thyroid hormone stimulates alkaline phosphatase activity in cultured rat osteoblastic cells (ROS 17/2.8) through 3,5,3'-triiodo-L-thyronine nuclear receptors. *Endocrinology* 1987;120:1873.
20. Abu EO, Bord S, Horner A, et al. The expression of thyroid hormone receptors in human bone. *Bone* 1997;21:137.
21. Robson H, Siebler T, Stevens DA, et al. Thyroid hormone acts directly on growth plate chondrocytes to promote hypertrophic differentiation and inhibit clonal expansion and cell proliferation. *Endocrinology* 2000;141:3887.
22. Stevens DA, Hasserjian RP, Robson H, et al. Thyroid hormones regulate hypertrophic chondrocyte differentiation and expression of parathyroid hormone-related peptide and its receptor during endochondral bone formation. *J Bone Miner Res* 2000;15:2431.
23. Cooper DS, Kaplan MM, Ridgway EC, et al. Alkaline phosphatase isoenzyme patterns in hyperthyroidism. *Ann Intern Med* 1979;90:164.
24. Faber J, Perrild H, Johansen JS. Bone Gla protein and sex hormone-binding globulin in nontoxic goiter: parameters for metabolic status at the tissue level. *J Clin Endocrinol Metab* 1990;70:49.
25. Garrel DR, Delmas PD, Malaval L, et al. Serum bone Gla protein: a marker of bone turnover in hyperthyroidism. *J Clin Endocrinol Metab* 1986;62:1052.
26. Lukert BP, Higgins JC, Stoskopf MM. Serum osteocalcin is increased in patients with hyperthyroidism and decreased in patients receiving glucocorticoids. *J Clin Endocrinol Metab* 1986;62:1056.
27. Miura M, Tanaka K, Komatsu Y, et al. A novel interaction between thyroid hormones and 1,25(OH)(2)D(3) in osteoclast formation. *Biochem Biophys Res Commun* 2002;291:987.
28. Gu WX, Stern PH, Madison LD, et al. Mutual up-regulation of thyroid hormone and parathyroid hormone receptors in rat osteoblastic osteosarcoma 17/2.8 cells. *Endocrinology* 2001;142:157.
29. Stevens DA, Harvey CB, Scott AJ, et al. Thyroid hormone activates fibroblast growth factor receptor-1 in bone. *Mol Endocrinol* 2003;17:1751.
30. Lakatos P, Stern PH. Evidence for direct non-genomic effects of triiodothyronine on bone rudiments in rats: stimulation of the inositol phosphate second messenger system. *Acta Endocrinol (Copenh)* 1991;125:603.
31. Burger EH, van der Meer JW, Nijweide PJ. Osteoclast formation from mononuclear phagocytes: role of bone-forming cells. *J Cell Biol* 1984;99:1901.

32. Britto JM, Fenton AJ, Holloway WR, et al. Osteoblasts mediate thyroid hormone stimulation of osteoclastic bone resorption. *Endocrinology* 1994;134:169.

33. Zambonin Zallone A, Teti A, Primavera MV. Resorption of vital or devitalized bone by isolated osteoclasts in vitro: the role of lining cells. *Cell Tissue Res* 1984;235:561.

34. Miura M, Tanaka K, Komatsu Y, et al. Thyroid hormones promote chondrocyte differentiation in mouse ATDC5 cells and stimulate endochondral ossification in fetal mouse tibias through iodothyronine deiodinases in the growth plate. *J Bone Miner Res* 2002;17:443.

35. Schneider MJ, Fiering SN, Pallud SE, et al. Targeted disruption of the type 2 selenodeiodinase gene (DIO2) results in a phenotype of pituitary resistance to T_4. *Mol Endocrinol* 2001;15:2137.

36. Hernandez A, Fiering S, Martinez E, et al. The gene locus encoding iodothyronine deiodinase type 3 (Dio3) is imprinted in the fetus and expresses antisense transcripts. *Endocrinology* 2002;143:4483.

37. Schmid C, Schlapfer I, Futo E, et al. Triiodothyronine (T_3) stimulates insulin-like growth factor (IGF)-1 and IGF binding protein (IGFBP)-2 production by rat osteoblasts *in vitro*. *Acta Endocrinol (Copenh)* 1992;126:467.

38. Varga F, Rumpler M, Klaushofer K. Thyroid hormones increase insulin-like growth factor mRNA levels in the clonal osteoblastic cell line MC3T3-E1. *FEBS Lett* 1994;345:67.

39. Canalis E, Centrella M, Burch W, et al. Insulin-like growth factor I mediates selective anabolic effects of parathyroid hormone in bone cultures. *J Clin Invest* 1989;83:60.

40. Milne M, Kang MI, Quail JM, et al. Thyroid hormone excess increases insulin-like growth factor I transcripts in bone marrow cell cultures: divergent effects on vertebral and femoral cell cultures. *Endocrinology* 1998;139:2527.

41. Siddiqi A, Burrin JM, Wood DF, et al. Tri-iodothyronine regulates the production of interleukin-6 and interleukin-8 in human bone marrow stromal and osteoblast-like cells. *J Endocrinol* 1998;157:453.

42. Kim CH, Kim HK, Shong YK, et al. Thyroid hormone stimulates basal and interleukin (IL)-1-induced IL-6 production in human bone marrow stromal cells: a possible mediator of thyroid hormone-induced bone loss. *J Endocrinol* 1999;160:97.

43. Cummings SR, Nevitt MC, Browner WS, et al. Risk factors for hip fracture in white women: Study of Osteoporotic Fractures Research Group. *N Engl J Med* 1995;332:767.

44. Fraser SA, Anderson JB, Smith DA, et al. Osteoporosis and fractures following thyrotoxicosis. *Lancet* 1971;1:981.

45. Kelepouris N, Harper KD, Gannon F, et al. Severe osteoporosis in men. *Ann Intern Med* 1995;123:452.

46. Vestergaard P, Rejnmark L, Weeke J, et al. Fracture risk in patients treated for hyperthyroidism. *Thyroid* 2000;10:341.

47. Vestergaard P, Mosekilde L. Fractures in patients with hyperthyroidism and hypothyroidism: a nationwide follow-up study in 16,249 patients. *Thyroid* 2002;12:411.

48. Wejda B, Hintze G, Katschinski B, et al. Hip fractures and the thyroid: a case-control study. *J Intern Med* 1995;237:241.

49. Vestergaard P, Mosekilde L. Hyperthyroidism, bone mineral, and fracture risk—a meta-analysis. *Thyroid* 2003;13:585.

50. Campos-Pastor MM, Munoz-Torres M, Escobar-Jimenez F, et al. Bone mass in females with different thyroid disorders: influence of menopausal status. *Bone Miner* 1993;21:1.

51. Serraclara A, Jodar E, Sarabia F, et al. Bone mass after long-term euthyroidism in former hyperthyroid women treated with (131)I influence of menopausal status. *J Clin Densitom* 2001;4:249.

52. Solomon BL, Wartofsky L, Burman KD. Prevalence of fractures in postmenopausal women with thyroid disease. *Thyroid* 1993;3:17.

53. Hallengren B, Elmstahl B, Berglund J, et al. No increase in fracture incidence in patients treated for thyrotoxicosis in Malmo during 1970–74: a 20-year population-based follow-up. *J Intern Med* 1999;246:139.

54. Siddiqi A, Burrin JM, Noonan K, et al. A longitudinal study of markers of bone turnover in Graves' disease and their value in predicting bone mineral density. *J Clin Endocrinol Metab* 1997;82:753.

55. Arata N, Momotani N, Maruyama H, et al. Bone mineral density after surgical treatment for Graves' disease. *Thyroid* 1997;7:547.

56. Diamond T, Vine J, Smart R, et al. Thyrotoxic bone disease in women: a potentially reversible disorder. *Ann Intern Med* 1994;120:8.

57. Mudde AH, Houben AJ, Nieuwenhuijzen Kruseman AC. Bone metabolism during anti-thyroid drug treatment of endogenous subclinical hyperthyroidism. *Clin Endocrinol (Oxf)* 1994;41:421.

58. Rosen CJ, Adler RA. Longitudinal changes in lumbar bone density among thyrotoxic patients after attainment of euthyroidism. *J Clin Endocrinol Metab* 1992;75:1531.

59. Wakasugi M, Wakao R, Tawata M, et al. Change in bone mineral density in patients with hyperthyroidism after attainment of euthyroidism by dual energy x-ray absorptiometry. *Thyroid* 1994;4:179.

60. Franklyn JA, Maisonneuve P, Sheppard MC, et al. P. Mortality after the treatment of hyperthyroidism with radioactive iodine. *N Engl J Med* 1998;338:712.

61. Parle JV, Franklyn JA, Cross KW, et al. Prevalence and follow-up of abnormal thyrotrophin (TSH) concentrations in the elderly in the United Kingdom. *Clin Endocrinol (Oxf)* 1991;34:77.

62. Ross DS, Ardisson LJ, Meskell MJ. Measurement of thyrotropin in clinical and subclinical hyperthyroidism using a new chemiluminescent assay. *J Clin Endocrinol Metab* 1989;69:684.

63. Adlin EV, Maurer AH, Marks AD, et al. Bone mineral density in postmenopausal women treated with L-thyroxine. *Am J Med* 1991;90:360.

64. Diamond T, Nery L, Hales I. A therapeutic dilemma: suppressive doses of thyroxine significantly reduce bone mineral measurements in both premenopausal and postmenopausal women with thyroid carcinoma. *J Clin Endocrinol Metab* 1991;72:1184.

65. Greenspan SL, Greenspan FS, Resnick NM, et al. Skeletal integrity in premenopausal and postmenopausal women receiving long-term L-thyroxine therapy. *Am J Med* 1991;91:5.

66. Lehmke J, Bogner U, Felsenberg D, et al. Determination of bone mineral density by quantitative computed tomography and single photon absorptiometry in subclinical hyperthyroidism: a risk of early osteopaenia in post-menopausal women. *Clin Endocrinol (Oxf)* 1992;36:511.

67. Paul TL, Kerrigan J, Kelly AM, et al. Long-term L-thyroxine therapy is associated with decreased hip bone density in premenopausal women. *JAMA* 1988;259:3137.

68. Ross DS, Neer RM, Ridgway EC, et al. Subclinical hyperthyroidism and reduced bone density as a possible result of prolonged suppression of the pituitary-thyroid axis with L-thyroxine. *Am J Med* 1987;82:1167.

69. Stall GM, Harris S, Sokoll LJ, et al. Accelerated bone loss in hypothyroid patients overtreated with L-thyroxine. *Ann Intern Med* 1990;113:265.

70. Taelman P, Kaufman JM, Janssens X, et al. A. Reduced forearm bone mineral content and biochemical evidence of increased bone turnover in women with euthyroid goitre treated with thyroid hormone. *Clinical Endocrinology* 1990;33:107.

71. Pioli G, Pedrazzoni M, Palummeri E, et al. Longitudinal study of bone loss after thyroidectomy and suppressive thyroxine therapy in premenopausal women. *Acta Endocrinol (Copenh)* 1992;126:238.

72. De Rosa G, Testa A, Giacomini D, et al. Prospective study of bone loss in pre- and post-menopausal women on L-thyroxine

therapy for non-toxic goitre. *Clin Endocrinol (Oxf)* 1997;47: 529.

73. Jodar E, Begona Lopez M, Garcia L, et al. Bone changes in pre- and postmenopausal women with thyroid cancer on levothyroxine therapy: evolution of axial and appendicular bone mass. *Osteoporos Int* 1998;8:311.

74. Franklyn JA, Betteridge J, Daykin J, et al. Long-term thyroxine treatment and bone mineral density. *Lancet* 1992;340:9.

75. Goerres G, Theiler R, Muller-Brand J. Interfemur variation of bone mineral density in patients receiving high-dose thyroxin therapy. *Calcif Tissue Int* 1998;63:98.

76. Marcocci C, Golia F, Vignali E, et al. A. Skeletal integrity in men chronically treated with suppressive doses of L-thyroxine. *J Bone Miner Res* 1997;12:72.

77. Ribot C, Tremollieres F, Pouilles JM, et al. Bone mineral density and thyroid hormone therapy. *Clin Endocrinol (Oxf)* 1990;33: 143.

78. Stepan JJ, Limanova Z. Biochemical assessment of bone loss in patients on long-term thyroid hormone treatment. *Bone Miner* 1992;17:377.

79. Bauer DC, Nevitt MC, Ettinger B, et al. Low thyrotropin levels are not associated with bone loss in older women: a prospective study. *J Clin Endocrinol Metab* 1997;82:2931.

80. Gam AN, Jensen GF, Hasselstrom K, et al. Effect of thyroxine therapy on bone metabolism in substituted hypothyroid patients with normal or suppressed levels of TSH. *J Endocrinol Invest* 1991;14:451.

81. Faber J, Galloe AM. Changes in bone mass during prolonged subclinical hyperthyroidism due to L-thyroxine treatment: a meta-analysis. *Eur J Endocrinol* 1994;130:350.

82. Uzzan B, Campos J, Cucherat M, et al. Effects on bone mass of long term treatment with thyroid hormones: a meta-analysis. *J Clin Endocrinol Metab* 1996;81:4278.

83. Leese GP, Jung RT, Guthrie C, et al. Morbidity in patients on L-thyroxine: a comparison of those with a normal TSH to those with a suppressed TSH. *Clin Endocrinol (Oxf)* 1992;37:500.

84. Bauer DC, Ettinger B, Nevitt MC, et al. Risk for fracture in women with low serum levels of thyroid-stimulating hormone. *Ann Intern Med* 2001;134:561.

85. Ongphiphadhanakul B, Jenis LG, Braverman LE, et al. Etidronate inhibits the thyroid hormone-induced bone loss in rats assessed by bone mineral density and messenger ribonucleic acid markers of osteoblast and osteoclast function. *Endocrinology* 1993;133:2502.

86. Rosen HN, Sullivan EK, Middlebrooks VL, et al. Parenteral pamidronate prevents thyroid hormone-induced bone loss in rats. *J Bone Miner Res* 1993;8:1255.

87. Yamamoto M, Markatos A, Seedor JG, et al. The effects of the aminobisphosphonate alendronate on thyroid hormone-induced osteopenia in rats. *Calcif Tissue Int* 1993;53:278.

88. Rosen HN, Middlebrooks VL, Sullivan EK, et al. Subregion analysis of the rat femur: a sensitive indicator of changes in bone density following treatment with thyroid hormone or bisphosphonates. *Calcif Tissue Int* 1994;55:173.

THE NEUROMUSCULAR SYSTEM
AND BRAIN IN THYROTOXICOSIS

DAVID F. GARDNER

The earliest reports of thyrotoxicosis by Graves (1) and von Basedow (2) recognized muscle weakness as an important presenting complaint, and neuromuscular symptoms continue to be prominent clinical findings in patients with thyrotoxicosis. The frequency and severity of the abnormalities that have been described in these patients have varied considerably, undoubtedly due to variations in the severity of the thyrotoxicosis and in the ways that the diagnosis was established. Most patients with thyrotoxicosis who have abnormalities in neuromuscular function have Graves' disease, but the abnormalities occur in patients with thyrotoxicosis of any cause. This chapter focuses primarily on the direct effects of thyrotoxicosis on muscle and the central nervous system, but it also addresses primary neuromuscular disorders associated with thyrotoxicosis, specifically myasthenia gravis and thyrotoxic periodic paralysis.

MUSCLE DISORDERS

Myopathy

Symptoms or signs of muscle weakness occur in a high percentage of patients with thyrotoxicosis. In 54 consecutive patients evaluated by Ramsey, 50% gave a history of muscle weakness, and 63% had objective evidence of weakness or proximal muscle wasting (3). Similar data have been reported in numerous subsequent studies, with some variability in terms of the percentage of patients with subjective versus objective findings (4–7). A recent prospective study documented similar findings, with 67% of patients reporting weakness and 81% having decreased strength in at least one muscle group (8). In 36% of the patients in that study, muscle symptoms were the main reason for consulting a physician. Weakness is primarily proximal and often out of proportion to the degree of objective muscle wasting (3,9). Typical symptoms are similar to those in patients with other proximal myopathies and include difficulty arising from a sitting or supine position and raising the arms over the head, as well as generalized muscle aching. Distal muscle weakness is usually less prominent

than proximal (3) and tends to occur later in the course of the illness (4). Myopathic symptoms usually appear after the onset of the more typical clinical symptoms of thyrotoxicosis (3,10), although muscle weakness may be the presenting complaint (5,8,9). The degree of muscle weakness correlates more with the duration of the thyrotoxicosis than its biochemical severity (4,10), and weakness appears to be more common in men with thyrotoxicosis than women (9,10).

Less commonly, patients may have bulbar and esophagopharyngeal muscle weakness (11–13), with dysphonia, dysphagia, and dysarthria. Reversible diaphragmatic muscle weakness has been well documented and may contribute to the common complaint of dyspnea in patients with thyrotoxicosis (14–16). Substantial improvement in diaphragmatic movement and muscle strength was recently demonstrated in a study of 20 patients with thyrotoxicosis caused by Graves' disease studied before and after restoration of euthyroidism with carbimazole (14).

On physical examination, objective weakness is typically out of proportion to the degree of muscle atrophy, although some patients with long-standing thyrotoxicosis may have significant loss of muscle mass, particularly in the proximal musculature of the shoulders and the pelvic girdle. Distal weakness may be evident in the wrist flexors and extensors as well as the interosseous muscles (3). A minority of patients have muscle fasciculations, but they are usually overshadowed by the fine tremor of the hands and feet that is so characteristic of thyrotoxicosis. Signs of bulbar dysfunction may include dysphagia, dysphonia, and evidence of aspiration. Sphincter function is usually maintained (4). Deep tendon reflexes may be normal or hyperactive, but there is typically shortening of the relaxation phase (17,18).

An acute thyrotoxic myopathy has been described, with a predominance of bulbar symptoms and generalized weakness, usually in patients with preexisting thyrotoxicosis (4,19). It is likely that many of these patients had myasthenia gravis in addition to thyrotoxicosis, because of the predominance of bulbar symptoms and responsiveness to neostigmine. Rhabdomyolysis with acute renal failure has been reported in a single patient with thyroid storm (20).

The pathophysiology of muscle disease in thyrotoxicosis is probably multifactorial. That excess thyroid hormone has catabolic effects on muscle has been known for many years, with negative nitrogen balance being a consistent finding in virtually all studies (21) (see Chapter 38). Although protein synthesis is increased in thyrotoxic patients, protein degradation is accelerated to a greater degree, resulting in a net loss of muscle protein. This loss of muscle mass provides a ready explanation for both the subjective and objective muscle weakness that is so common in patients with thyrotoxicosis. Even mild degrees of thyrotoxicosis induced by exogenous administration of thyroid hormone result in negative nitrogen balance and sustained loss of muscle mass (22). Additional adverse effects of excess thyroid hormone may be related to the hormone's effects on the transcription of genes controlling calcium regulatory proteins and myosin heavy chain synthesis in muscle (23,24). Evidence that β-adrenergic antagonist drugs ameliorate muscle weakness in patients with thyrotoxicosis suggests that β-adrenergic stimulation and perhaps also cyclic adenosine monophosphate activation of muscle contribute to clinical myopathy (23,25). Finally, the multiple effects of thyroid hormone on the metabolism of muscle cells may contribute to the myopathy (4,10, 26–28). In thyrotoxicosis, glucose uptake and utilization by muscle are increased, as is glycogenolysis, and glycogen depletion is seen in muscle biopsy samples. In addition, mitochondrial oxidation is increased, with an associated increase in muscle heat production. Lipid oxidation, protein catabolism, and purine catabolism are also accelerated, and intracellular adenosine triphosphate (ATP) concentrations are low. In sum, in muscle, substrate uptake and utilization are increased, but the latter is less efficient than normal. Therefore, ATP generation and muscle contractility are decreased. The specific metabolic perturbations and exactly how they cause myopathy are not known.

Laboratory studies relating to muscle function and integrity are usually not revealing. Serum creatine kinase and myoglobin concentrations are usually normal (4,29), and a high serum concentration of either in a patient with thyrotoxicosis should raise the suspicion of a superimposed condition such as rhabdomyolysis (20) or an inflammatory myopathy (30).

Light microscopic findings on muscle biopsy may be normal or reveal mild, nonspecific changes. These include fiber atrophy (both type 1 and type 2), varying degrees of fatty infiltration, variability in the size of muscle fibers, occasional fiber necrosis, glycogen depletion, and lymphocytic infiltration (3,4,7,9,26). Electron microscopic studies usually show elongated mitochondria, an overall decrease in the number of mitochondria, swelling of transverse tubules, subsarcolemmal glycogen deposition, and papillary projections from the sarcolemma (4,31–33). None of these light microscopic or electron microscopic changes is specific for thyrotoxicosis.

Numerous electromyographic and nerve conduction studies have been performed on thyrotoxic patients with myopathy over the past 40 years (5,6,8,10,34,35). Motor and sensory nerve conduction is typically normal. Consistent findings on electromyography include short duration motor unit potentials and increased frequency of polyphasic potentials. Spontaneous electrical activity including fasciculations and fibrillations is uncommon. These findings are not specific for thyrotoxic myopathy, and some patients with clinical myopathy have normal electromyographic findings and others with normal strength have abnormal findings. The prevalence of electrical abnormalities is higher when the proximal rather than the distal musculature is evaluated. In older studies, a majority of patients with thyrotoxicosis had electromyographic abnormalities indicative of myopathy, but in a 2000 study only 2 of 21 patients (10%) had these abnormalities (67% complained of weakness, and 81% had objective weakness of at least one muscle group) (8). This same study found "neuropathic" changes in 24% of the patients, considerably higher than older studies.

There is no specific treatment for thyrotoxic myopathy, other than correction of the thyrotoxicosis, although some patients feel stronger when treated with a β-adrenergic antagonist drug alone (25). In the vast majority of patients with uncomplicated thyrotoxicosis, the clinical signs of myopathy and electromyographic abnormalities resolve completely within 3 to 6 months after restoration of normal thyroid function (3,6,8,36).

Myasthenia Gravis

Graves' disease and myasthenia gravis, disorders characterized by autoimmunity against the thyrotropin (TSH) and acetylcholine receptors, respectively, have been linked epidemiologically. The presence of thymic enlargement (17, 21), an association with HLA-B8 and -DR3 haplotypes, and the presence of antireceptor antibodies in both disorders suggest a common autoimmune pathophysiology. The prevalence of Graves' thyrotoxicosis in patients with myasthenia gravis ranges from 3% to 10% (37–40). The prevalence of all forms of autoimmune thyroid disease in patients with myasthenia is considerably higher, ranging from 25% to 30% (41,42). In an older autopsy study of 32 patients with myasthenia gravis, 19% had histologic evidence of thyroiditis, as compared with only 0.9% of a large control group (43). On the contrary, the prevalence of myasthenia gravis in patients with autoimmune thyroid disease was less than 1% in most studies (9,19,44–46). In a small series of patients with Graves' ophthalmopathy, 8% had acetylcholine receptor antibodies, but none had any symptoms or signs of myasthenia during a follow-up period of 4½ years (47). Thyrotoxicosis typically develops before or simultaneously with the myasthenia gravis, but it can occur later. Both thyrotoxicosis and hypothyroidism appear to exacerbate the clinical course of myasthenia gravis (4,19).

A study of 129 patients with myasthenia gravis in Italy found an interesting association between milder forms of myasthenia, specifically ocular myasthenia, and autoimmune thyroid disease (41). In patients with both disorders, the myasthenia was clinically milder, with a particular preference for ocular involvement, and the frequency of acetylcholine receptor antibodies and thymic disease was lower, as compared with patients with myasthenia alone. In these 129 patients, the overall prevalence of autoimmune thyroid disease was 62% in patients with ocular myasthenia, and only 29% in patients with generalized myasthenia (40). Similar findings were previously reported (48).

In occasional patients, the combination of bulbar symptoms, ocular symptoms, particularly ptosis and diplopia, respiratory muscle weakness, and severe generalized muscle weakness may make the distinction between thyrotoxic myopathy and myasthenia gravis difficult (49). The diagnosis of myasthenia gravis is based on the absence of infiltrative eye signs (periorbital and conjunctival edema, proptosis, extraocular muscle enlargement), a positive response to edrophonium (Tensilon), the characteristic decrement in response to repetitive nerve stimulation, and amelioration of symptoms with anticholinesterase drug therapy.

Thyrotoxic Periodic Paralysis

Familial periodic paralysis is an autosomal-dominant disorder characterized by acute generalized muscle weakness and hypokalemia, which usually presents in adolescence and rarely after the age of 30 years (50). Thyrotoxic periodic paralysis is the most common acquired form of periodic paralysis and typically presents in men of Asian descent, although it can occur in other ethnic groups as well (51–53). The reported incidence of periodic paralysis in Asian men with thyrotoxicosis ranges from 2% to 24%; a reasonable estimate of the overall incidence in this ethnic group is 5% to 10%. The incidence of thyrotoxic periodic paralysis in non-Asian North Americans has been estimated to be 0.1% to 0.2% (54). The disorder is rare in women (55), with an estimated male:female ratio of 20:1 (50). Thyrotoxic periodic paralysis typically presents between the ages of 20 and 40 years, reflecting the usual age of onset of Graves' thyrotoxicosis (55,56).

The typical clinical presentation of thyrotoxic periodic paralysis is similar to that of familial periodic paralysis. The patients have recurrent episodes of muscle weakness lasting minutes to days. The weakness is symmetric and may be local or generalized. Respiratory, sphincter, and cranial muscles are usually spared, but respiratory failure has been reported (50,57). The weakness characteristically begins in the legs, but it usually spreads, and it may progress to a generalized flaccid paralysis. Proximal musculature is more severely affected than distal, and lower extremity weakness tends to be more profound than upper extremity weakness (54,56). Sensation is normal, as is the sensorium. On examination, findings are usually limited to muscle weakness, diminished deep tendon reflexes, and evidence of coexisting thyrotoxicosis. However, the clinical manifestations of thyrotoxicosis may be subtle, so much so that serum TSH should be measured in any patient with periodic paralysis.

Patients often report prodromal symptoms of muscle pain, stiffness, and cramping. Precipitating factors include a carbohydrate challenge, insulin administration, cold exposure, and rest after vigorous exercise. Many attacks occur during sleep, with patients awakening in the morning with profound weakness, including the inability to walk (51, 54). Episodes rarely occur during ongoing physical activity; in fact, mild exercise may abort an attack. Attacks of thyrotoxic periodic paralysis cease when thyrotoxicosis is treated.

The most consistent laboratory abnormality during an acute attack is a low serum potassium concentration, with values as low as 1.1 mM (56); in a small series of patients, the mean serum potassium concentration was 1.69 mM (54). Serum potassium concentrations are consistently nomal between attacks, and occasional patients may be normokalemic during an attack. Some patients have high serum creatine kinase concentrations; the enzyme is entirely of skeletal muscle origin (56). Serum creatine kinase and myoglobin concentrations may increase during the recovery phase after an acute attack (58). An electrocardiogram obtained during an attack shows typical features of hypokalemia but no evidence of cardiac muscle injury or other abnormalities.

Treatment of acute episodes is straightforward, with potassium repletion by the oral route being the mainstay of therapy. Intravenous potassium should be reserved for the rare patients with nausea or vomiting or with bulbar muscle dysfunction. Intravenous glucose should be avoided because it may exacerbate hypokalemia by shifting potassium intracellularly. The hypokalemia in this disorder does not reflect a total body potassium deficit, but rather shift of potassium from the extracellular to the intracellular space, and rebound hyperkalemia during recovery has been reported (56). Thus, serum potassium should be measured and electrocardiograms done periodically during potassium therapy. In most patients, symptoms improve within 2 to 4 hours after potassium therapy is begun, and the weakness resolves completely within 24 to 36 hours.

Pending restoration of normal thyroid function, the likelihood of recurrent attacks can be minimized by avoidance of high-carbohydrate meals, vigorous exercise, prolonged cold exposure, and alcohol. Nonselective β-adrenergic antagonist drugs prevent attacks of thyrotoxic periodic paralysis while thyrotoxicosis is being corrected (51,59). The role of these drugs in the immediate treatment of weakness, however, is less clear. Several case reports suggest that the drugs have a beneficial effect (60–63); in two of these reports the patients improved rapidly after intravenous propranolol administration (61,62).

The pathophysiology of thyrotoxic periodic paralysis is not clear, although it is almost certainly a form of muscle ion-channel dysfunction or "channelopathy" (64). The intracellular potassium shifts associated with acute episodes result in progressive depolarization of the resting potential in the sarcolemma, precluding electrical excitability, and resulting in the clinical finding of muscle paralysis. Familial hypokalemic periodic paralysis has been attributed to mutations in the genes coding for calcium, sodium, and potassium channels (65). Recently, a mutation in the KCNE3 potassium channel gene was reported in a single patient with thyrotoxic periodic paralysis from Brazil (66). How thyrotoxicosis might affect the activity of the channel is not known.

NEUROLOGIC DISORDERS

With the exception of neuropsychiatric problems (see Chapter 42) and tremor, clinically important neurologic disorders are far less common in thyrotoxicosis than the muscle disorders reviewed above. In fact, it is unclear whether some of the neurologic syndromes discussed below are truly related to thyrotoxicosis, or simply coincidental findings.

Movement Disorders

The most prominent movement abnormality in thyrotoxicosis is a persistent fine tremor, both at rest and with movement. It most commonly affects the hands, but may also involve the feet, chin, lips, and tongue. In a prospective cohort study, 42 of 50 patients under 50 years of age (84%) with thyrotoxicosis had a tremor, as compared with 15 of 34 patients over 70 years of age (44%) (67). The latter value was not significantly different from the prevalence of tremor in elderly euthyroid subjects. However, there was no age-related decline in the prevalence of tremor in a group of 880 patients with thyrotoxicosis, with the rate in all age groups being approximately 70% (68).

Many patients note the tremor much of the time, but others recognize it only indirectly, for example, by deterioration in their ability to perform fine motor tasks, resulting in impaired handwriting, difficulty threading a needle, or difficulty performing other movements requiring fine muscular control. From a diagnostic perspective, the tremor caused by thyrotoxicosis is similar both clinically and electromyographically to that caused by generalized anxiety (69,70). β-adrenergic mechanisms are implicated in the

pathophysiology of the tremor, on the basis of the similarity of the tremor to that in patients with catecholamine excess syndromes and emotional stress, and the often dramatic improvement in tremor with β-adrenergic blocking agents (71,72). Tremor resolves in virtually all patients with correction of thyrotoxicosis.

The other reversible movement disorder reported in association with thyrotoxicosis is choreoathetosis. This is a rare complication of thyrotoxicosis, and most reports have described only one or two patients (73–76). Common findings in these cases include development of chorea after the onset of thyrotoxicosis, age less than 40 years, response of chorea to β-adrenergic antagonist drugs, and complete resolution of the choreiform movements with correction of the thyrotoxicosis.

Corticospinal Tract Disease

Rare patients with thyrotoxicosis present with symptoms and signs suggestive of corticospinal tract disease, including weakness, spasticity, hyperreflexia, a positive Babinski's sign, and bladder spasticity (77–80). Fasciculations are usually absent, and results of electromyographic studies are normal. As with choreoathetosis, neurologic signs resolve in most patients with correction of the thyrotoxicosis. The pathophysiology of this association has not been determined.

Neuropathy

Generalized peripheral neuropathy is also rare in patients with thyrotoxicosis. However, an acute neuropathy associated with paraplegia or quadriplegia has been described (10). This presentation has been referred to as Basedow's paraplegia, and it bears a close resemblance to the Guillain-Barré syndrome, in terms of its clinical presentation with profound lower extremity weakness and areflexia. Electrophysiologic studies in these patients reveal a mixed axonal and demyelinating sensorimotor neuropathy, and electromyographic findings are consistent with denervation (81,82). Symptoms and signs usually resolve with correction of thyrotoxicosis.

A recent prospective study of 21 patients with thyrotoxicosis found signs of a peripheral neuropathy, including depressed deep tendon reflexes and symmetric distal sensory disturbances, in a few (19%) of the patients (8). Electrophysiologic studies confirmed evidence of a peripheral neuropathy in 24% of these patients. There are a few reports of carpal tunnel syndrome in association with thyrotoxicosis that resolved with antithyroid therapy (83,84).

Seizures

Seizures are a rare complication of thyrotoxicosis. However, a report of three thyrotoxic patients presenting with seizures in a 2-year period at a single institution suggested that thyrotoxic seizures were more common than generally appreciated (85). The researchers estimated that thyrotoxicosis was the cause of an initial seizure in 1.2% of all patients admitted for seizures, and that 9% of patients admitted for thyrotoxicosis had seizures. The true prevalence of seizures in patients with thyrotoxicosis is certainly much lower than these figures suggest, because the study did not address the prevalence of seizures in nonhospitalized thyrotoxic patients. A causal relationship between thyrotoxicosis and seizures is suggested in several case reports documenting resolution of seizures and electroencephalographic abnormalities with correction of thyrotoxicosis, and relapse when thyrotoxicosis recurred (85–87). Reported electroencephalographic abnormalities have included diffuse bilateral slowing, alpha waves, the presence of triphasic waves suggestive of a diffuse encephalopathy, high voltage, and scattered sharp waves (85–88).

Central Nervous System Manifestations

The most common mental changes in patients with thyrotoxicosis are anxiety, irritability, emotional lability, apprehension, and difficulty concentrating. Cognitive abnormalities typically include a shortened attention span, distractibility, and occasionally impaired short-term memory. Psychosis is rare, but thyrotoxic patients may present with a frank psychosis associated with paranoia and delusions (89). An increased incidence of depression has also been reported (90,91). A detailed review of the neuropsychiatric manifestations of thyrotoxicosis is found in Chapter 42. A true encephalopathy can be observed in patients with thyroid storm. These patients typically present with agitation and delirium, associated with high fever, atrial fibrillation, congestive heart failure, vomiting, and diarrhea. Coma, sometimes associated with seizures, has also been reported (79,92,93). Central nervous symptoms and signs resolve with appropriate management of thyrotoxicosis. The clinical features of thyroid storm are covered in greater detail in Chapter 43.

The observation that elderly thyrotoxic patients may present in dramatically different fashion from younger patients was first reported many years ago (94). Rather than demonstrating hyperactivity and anxiety, these patients may present with a more "apathetic" clinical picture, including depression, lethargy, and pseudodementia. Weight loss, myopathy, atrial fibrillation, and congestive heart failure often dominate the clinical presentation (95–97). This atypical presentation has also been described in younger patients (98,99).

From the above summary of the neuropsychiatric manifestations of thyrotoxicosis, it follows that clinicians should have a low threshold for assessing thyroid function in patients with a wide spectrum of mental disorders.

REFERENCES

1. Graves RJ. Clinical lectures. *Lond Med Surg J* 1835;7:516.
2. von Basedow CA. Exophthalmos durch hypertrophie des Zellgewebes in der Augshole. *Wissenche Ann Ges Heilk Berl* 1840; 6:197.
3. Ramsay ID. Muscle dysfunction in hyperthyroidism. *Lancet* 1966;2:931.
4. Kaminski HJ, Ruff RL. Endocrine myopathies (hyper- and hypofunction of adrenal, thyroid, pituitary, and parathyroid glands and iatrogenic corticosteroid myopathy). In: Engel AG, Franzini-Armstrong C, eds. *Myology: basic and clinical,* 2nd ed, vol 2. New York: McGraw-Hill, 1994:1726.
5. Puvanendran K, Cheah JS, Naganathan N, et al. Thyrotoxic myopathy: a clinical and quantitative analytic electromyographic study. *J Neurol Sci* 1979;42:441.
6. Havard CWH, Campbell EDR, Ross HB, et al. Electromyographic and histological findings in the muscles of patients with thyrotoxicosis. *QJM* 1963;32:145.
7. Sayotoshi E, Murakami K, Kowa H, et al. Myopathy in thyrotoxicosis: with special emphasis on an effect of potassium ingestion on serum and urinary creatine. *Neurology* 1963;13:645.
8. Duyff RF, Van den Bosch J, Laman DM, et al. Neuromuscular findings in thyroid dysfunction: a prospective clinical and electrodiagnostic study. *J Neurol Neurosurg Psychiatry* 2000;68: 750.
9. Engel AG. Neuromuscular manifestations of Graves' disease. *Mayo Clin Proc* 1972;47:919.
10. Amato AA. Endocrine myopathies and toxic myopathies. In: Brown WF, Bolton CF, Aminoff MJ, eds. *Neuromuscular function and disease: basic, clinical, and electrodiagnostic aspects.* Vol. 2. Philadelphia: WB Saunders, 2002:1399.
11. Kammer GM, Hamilton CR. Acute bulbar muscle dysfunction and hyperthyroidism: a study of four cases and review of the literature. *Am J Med* 1974;56:464.
12. Marks P, Anderson J, Vincent R. Thyrotoxic myopathy presenting as dysphagia. *Postgrad Med J* 1980;56:669.
13. Sweatman MC, Chambers L. Disordered oesophageal motility in thyrotoxic myopathy. *Postgrad Med J* 1985;61:619.
14. Goswami R, Guleria R, Gupta AK, et al. Prevalence of diaphragmatic muscle weakness and dyspnoea in Graves' disease and their reversibility with carbimazole therapy. *Eur J Endocrinol* 2002; 147:299.
15. Mier A, Brophy C, Wass JA, et al. Reversible respiratory muscle weakness in hyperthyroidism. *Am Rev Respir Dis* 1989;139: 529.
16. McElvaney GN, Wilcox PG, Fairbarn MS, et al. Respiratory muscle weakness and dyspnea in thyrotoxic patients. *Am Rev Respir Dis* 1990;141:1221.
17. Reinfrank RF, Kaufman RP, Wetstone HJ, et al. Observations of the Achilles reflex test. *JAMA* 1967;199:1.
18. Lambert EH, Underdahl LO, Beckett S, et al. A study of the ankle jerk in myxedema. *J Clin Endocrinol* 1951;11:1186.
19. Swanson JW, Kelly JJ, McConahey WM. Neurologic aspects of thyroid dysfunction. *Mayo Clin Proc* 1981;56:504.
20. Bennett WR, Huston DP. Rhabdomyolysis in thyroid storm. *Am J Med* 1984;77:733.
21. Martin WH, Spina RJ, Kortte E, et al. Mechanisms of impaired exercise capacity in short duration experimental hyperthyroidism. *J Clin Invest* 1991;88:2047.
22. Lovejoy JC, Smith SR, Bray GA, et al. A paradigm of experimentally induced mild hyperthyroidism: effects on nitrogen balance, body composition, and energy expenditure in healthy young men. *J Clin Endocrinol Metab* 1997;82:765.
23. Klein I, Ojamaa K. Thyroid (neuro)myopathy. *Lancet* 2000;356: 614.

sixth decades of life, patients with a family history of autoimmune thyroid disease, and those with certain other disorders with an autoimmune pathogenesis (e.g., pernicious anemia, autoimmune diabetes mellitus, and myasthenia gravis). Patients who smoke cigarettes (5), are receiving the immunomodulatory agents interferon-α and interleukin-2 (6), or have a history of previous high-dose neck irradiation (7) are also at increased risk for developing Graves' disease.

Clinical features also may identify patients with less common forms of thyrotoxicosis. Patients with thyrotoxicosis caused by subacute (de Quervain's) thyroiditis have thyroid pain and tenderness and constitutional complaints, including fever, night sweats, and malaise. Those with toxic nodular goiter are usually older, and their thyrotoxicosis may have been provoked by recent exposure to iodine-containing medications (e.g., radiographic contrast agents). Detection of a thyroid nodule or multinodular goiter warrants screening for overt or subclinical thyrotoxicosis. The iodine-containing antiarrhythmic agent amiodarone can also provoke iodine-induced hyperthyroidism in patients without thyroid nodules as well as a painless thyroiditis that can cause transient thyrotoxicosis. Silent (painless, postpartum, or lymphocytic) thyroiditis most often affects women 2 to 8 months postpartum (see Chapter 27) but can occur after abortion. Rarely, it can occur in women who have not been pregnant and in men. Factitious thyrotoxicosis is most likely to occur in health-care workers or persons with access to thyroid hormone preparations, for example, those with a family member or canine pet taking thyroid hormone.

CLUES FROM ROUTINE LABORATORY TESTS

Certain abnormalities detected by routine biochemical screening also may suggest the presence of thyrotoxicosis. These include hypercalcemia, an elevated serum alkaline phosphatase concentration, and a serum cholesterol concentration that is either low or lower than previously determined. The concentrations of certain less commonly measured substances, including ferritin and angiotensin-converting enzyme, are also increased in thyrotoxicosis. The presence of thyrotoxicosis should be considered when atrial arrhythmias are detected by electrocardiography.

LABORATORY TESTING

Biochemical confirmation of thyrotoxicosis has traditionally been based on detection of elevated serum total and free thyroxine (T_4) and triiodothyronine (T_3) concentrations (8). Most patients have high serum concentrations of both hormones, but some have isolated increases of either T_4 or T_3. Although serum thyroid hormone measurements are useful for detecting thyrotoxicosis and monitoring treatment of it, they have two limitations. First, there are other causes of high serum T_4 or T_3 concentrations. Second, some thyrotoxic patients have serum T_4 and T_3 concentrations within the upper portion of the normal range. The development of sensitive assays for serum TSH has greatly simplified the diagnostic approach to thyrotoxicosis. TSH assays also have expanded the spectrum of thyrotoxicosis to include mild or subclinical thyrotoxicosis (see Chapter 79), in which suppression of the serum TSH to less than 0.1 mU/L occurs despite normal serum T_4 and T_3 levels.

SERUM THYROXINE DETERMINATIONS

The serum total T_4 concentration can be measured accurately by competitive protein-binding assays using either anti-T_4 antibodies or serum thyroid hormone–binding proteins. Most (99.97%) of the T_4 in serum is bound to thyroxine-binding globulin (TBG), transthyretin (TTR, or thyroxine-binding prealbumin), or albumin. An increase in the concentration or thyroid hormone-binding of any of these serum proteins, especially TBG, can cause a high serum total T_4 concentration (hyperthyroxinemia), which can be misconstrued as thyrotoxicosis (Table 44.1). Conversely, decreased T_4 binding by serum proteins may mask excess thyroid hormone production.

Determining the serum free T_4 concentration resolves most potential pitfalls associated with increased serum protein binding of T_4. Although equilibrium dialysis and ultrafiltration are the most accurate techniques for serum free

TABLE 44.1. CAUSES OF ELEVATED SERUM THYROXINE CONCENTRATIONS

Thyrotoxicosis
Increased serum protein binding
  Increased serum thyroxine-binding globulin concentrations
    Inherited
    Estrogen: pregnancy, exogenous, tumoral production
    Hepatitis, hepatoma
    HIV infection
    Drugs: methadone, heroin, clofibrate, 5-fluorouracil
  Familial dysalbuminemic hyperthyroxinemia
  Increased serum transthyretin binding or concentrations
    Inherited
    Carcinoma of pancreas, hepatoma
Psychiatric and medical illness
Drugs
  Propranolol (high doses)
  Amiodarone
  Radiographic contrast agents used for cholecystography
Anti-T_4 immunoglobulins

T_4 measurement, serum free T_4 immunoassays and the serum free T_4 index readily differentiate thyrotoxicosis from the most common cause of hyperthyroxinemia, which is TBG excess. Furthermore, free T_4 immunoassays and the serum free T_4 index are simpler, quicker, and less costly. Most serum free T_4 immunoassays employ an analogue of T_4 that does not bind to thyroid hormone–binding proteins. The free T_4 index is the product of the serum total T_4 and the thyroid hormone–binding ratio (THBR; also known as the T_3 or T_4 uptake) (9). These assays are discussed in detail in Chapter 13.

Other conditions that cause euthyroid hyperthyroxinemia may be more difficult to differentiate from thyrotoxicosis. Patients with familial dysalbuminemic hyperthyroxinemia have a mutated form of albumin that binds T_4 with increased affinity, increasing the serum total serum T_4 concentration (10,11). Because the mutated albumin usually binds T_3 poorly, the THBR value is typically normal, and therefore the serum free T_4 index value is deceptively high. Serum free T_4 analogue immunoassay methods also may yield falsely elevated values in this condition. Similarly, increased TTR binding of T_4, which occurs as both an inherited trait (12) and in patients with carcinoma of the pancreas or liver (13), causes an increased serum total T_4 concentration. Thyroid hormone–binding antibodies, which may be present in patients with chronic autoimmune thyroiditis or other autoimmune disorders, may cause spurious elevations in serum T_4 or T_3 concentrations (14).

Hyperthyroxinemia also may occur as a result of disorders that transiently increase the secretion of TSH (or chorionic gonadotropin) or disorders and medications that reduce T_4 clearance. For example, in one study of patients admitted to an inpatient medical service, modest elevations in serum total T_4 and free T_4 index values were found in 4% and 12%, respectively (15). Two disorders—acute psychosis (16,17) and hyperemesis gravidarum (18)—have been associated with a substantial prevalence of euthyroid hyperthyroxinemia. Propranolol, when given in high dosages [>160 mg/day (19)], and amiodarone (20) impair T_4 clearance, causing euthyroid hyperthyroxinemia (see section on Effects of Pharmacologic Agents on Thyroid Hormone Metabolism in Chapter 11). Even though they have no clinical evidence of thyrotoxicosis, some patients receiving T_4 therapy have modest hyperthyroxinemia. Finally, patients with generalized thyroid hormone resistance typically have elevated serum total and free T_4 and T_3 concentrations and normal or slightly increased TSH concentrations (21) (see Chapter 81).

Therefore, hyperthyroxinemia is not a pathognomonic manifestation of thyrotoxicosis. Differentiating thyrotoxicosis from euthyroid hyperthyroxinemia is often straightforward, based on clinical information (i.e., symptoms and signs of thyrotoxicosis or the other conditions associated with hyperthyroxinemia). Serum TSH measurement is in-valuable in distinguishing euthyroid hyperthyroxinemia, in which serum TSH usually is normal, from all common forms of thyrotoxicosis, in which serum TSH is low.

SERUM TRIIODOTHYRONINE DETERMINATIONS

Serum total and free T_3 concentrations are high in most patients with thyrotoxicosis. This is attributable to both increased thyroidal T_3 production and increased extrathyroidal conversion of T_4 to T_3. About 2% of thyrotoxic patients in the United States have T_3 thyrotoxicosis; that is, they have high serum T_3 but normal T_4 concentrations. The diagnostic sensitivity of serum T_3 determinations alone is limited because some thyrotoxic patients have T_4 thyrotoxicosis (22). T_4 toxicosis occurs primarily in patients with iodine-induced hyperthyroidism, inflammatory forms of thyroiditis, and intercurrent severe nonthyroidal illness in which extrathyroidal T_3 production from T_4 is inhibited. Although serum T_3 concentrations are high in patients who have elevated serum TBG concentrations, the lower affinity of TBG for T_3 leads to a lesser increase in serum T_3 than T_4. Serum T_3 concentrations may be spuriously elevated in rare patients with T_3-binding antibodies (14). A kindred has been reported with familial dysalbuminemic hypertriiodothyroninemia, in which a mutant albumin bound T_3, but not T_4 with higher affinity (23). Consequently, an elevated serum total T_3 concentration is only relatively specific for thyrotoxicosis. With the availability of sensitive serum TSH assays, the diagnostic utility of serum T_3 measurements—never great—has declined further. However, they are occasionally useful in monitoring treatment in patients with thyrotoxicosis, in whom antithyroid drug or radioactive iodine therapy may have discordant effects on serum T_4 and T_3 concentrations; for example, the serum T_3 concentration may remain elevated despite a normal or low serum T_4 (24).

SERUM THYROTROPIN DETERMINATIONS

The sensitivity of TSH secretion to inhibition by thyroid hormone makes serum TSH measurement a remarkably accurate test for diagnosis of all common forms of thyrotoxicosis. TSH assays with detection limits of 0.1 mU/L or lower readily differentiate between these patients and normal subjects (25). The recent authoritative National Association of Clinical Biochemistry guideline for laboratory diagnosis of thyroid disease specifies that TSH assay methods should have functional sensitivity of less than 0.02 mU/L, as defined by the assay's 20% between-run coefficient of variation (25a). These assays have rendered thyrotropin-releasing hormone (TRH) stimulation tests obsolete, except possibly in the investigation of very sick hospitalized patients, who may have very low serum TSH concentrations (26,27) (see the section on Nonthyroidal Illness in Chapter 11). Although a sensitive indicator of thyrotoxicosis in general, serum TSH concentrations are normal or even elevated in the rare patients with TSH-induced thyrotoxicosis due to TSH-secreting pituitary adenoma (28) or isolated pituitary resistance to thyroid hormone (see Chapters 24 and 81). Spurious elevation of the measured TSH level, potentially masking thyrotoxicosis, also may be the result of rare analytical problems, such as the presence of circulating anti-TSH immunoglobulins or human antimouse monoclonal immunoglobulins when these antibodies are used as an assay reagent (29).

SCREENING, CASE FINDING, AND DIAGNOSIS

Based on the infrequency of thyrotoxicosis, and the relative ease with which it can be recognized clinically, biochemical screening for thyrotoxicosis among healthy persons is unjustified. Case finding, that is, the identification of thyrotoxicosis in patients with vague symptoms or signs that could indicate the presence of thyrotoxicosis or in persons with special risk of thyrotoxicosis (e.g., amiodarone-treated patients), can best be done by measurement of the serum TSH concentration (30).

Virtually all patients with thyrotoxicosis have low or undetectable serum TSH concentrations; only the rare patient with TSH-induced thyrotoxicosis will be missed by this approach. Therefore, a normal serum TSH concentration is strong evidence that the patient is euthyroid. However, low (i.e., 0.1–0.5 mU/L) or even very low (0.1 mU/L or less) serum TSH values are not pathognomonic of thyrotoxicosis. Other causes of a low serum TSH concentration are subclinical thyrotoxicosis, nonthyroidal illness, central hypothyroidism, and early pregnancy. Among older outpatients, a low TSH level is common, occurring in about 5% (31–33) (see Chapter 79). Patients with nonthyroidal illness who have low serum TSH values are usually acutely ill and in the hospital (27,34) (see section on Nonthyroidal Illness in Chapter 11). Central hypothyroidism is unlikely to be encountered in case finding for thyrotoxicosis because it is rare, and most patients have clinical manifestations of hypothalamic or pituitary disease that are distinct from those of thyrotoxicosis. During the first trimester of pregnancy, particularly when complicated by hyperemesis gravidarum, the serum TSH concentration may be suppressed due to the relatively weak thyroid stimulatory effects of human chorionic gonadotropin, which circulates in high concentration at this time (35).

Alternatively, the serum free T_4 by immunoassay or free thyroxine index can be used, particularly if the level for excluding the diagnosis is arbitrarily set at a value somewhat below the upper limit of the normal reference range; for example, a free T_4 concentration of 1.4 ng/dL for an assay with a normal range of 0.6 to 1.6 ng/dL. Using this approach, only thyrotoxic patients with small increases in serum T_3 concentrations would be overlooked. Falsely elevated serum free T_4 index values may be encountered in patients with familial dysalbuminemic hyperthyroxinemia and those with certain nonthyroidal illnesses or in those receiving several drugs, as noted previously.

Whether TSH or free thyroxine testing is conducted for case finding, any patient having an abnormal result should have the other test performed before any conclusion is drawn or any sustained intervention is undertaken.

Among patients with substantial clinical suspicion of thyrotoxicosis, serum TSH and free T_4 should both be measured (Fig. 44.1). If the serum TSH value is low and the serum free T_4 value is high, the diagnosis is confirmed. If the serum TSH value is low and the serum free T_4 value is normal, the patient has either T_3 thyrotoxicosis, subclinical thyrotoxicosis, pregnancy, or nonthyroidal illness. Patients in the first three groups tend to have serum free T_4 values in the upper portion of the normal range and can be distinguished biochemically from one another by measurement of the serum T_3 concentration. If the serum TSH value is normal or high and the serum free T_4 value is high, then the patient should be evaluated for TSH-induced thyrotoxicosis. Other explanations for these results are generalized resistance to thyroid hormone, or, if serum free T_4 was determined by an analogue free T_4 assay or THBR method, familial dysalbuminemic hyperthyroxinemia. Patients with severe nonthyroidal illness often have low-normal or low serum free T_4 values and also can usually be identified by the context in which they are encountered.

DIAGNOSIS OF THE CAUSE OF THYROTOXICOSIS

Because the various causes of thyrotoxicosis require different therapies, it is essential that diagnosis of thyroid hormone excess be followed by definition of the underlying cause. In many patients, the history and physical examination alone are sufficient. Examples include the thyrotoxic woman with diffuse goiter and exophthalmos, indicating Graves' disease, or a thyrotoxic patient with neck pain and tenderness, suggesting subacute thyroiditis. In other patients, additional laboratory or *in vivo* radionuclide studies may be needed to establish the cause and guide therapeutic decision making. For example, a woman with postpartum thyrotoxicosis could have painless (postpartum) thyroiditis, Graves' disease, or even factitious thyrotoxicosis.

The relative elevations of serum T_3 and T_4 concentrations may provide a clue to the cause of thyrotoxicosis. Exuberant T_3 production is common in Graves' hyperthyroidism and toxic nodular goiter [i.e., a serum $T_3{:}T_4$ (ng/dL:µg/dL) ratio of >20]. T_4-predominant thyrotoxico-

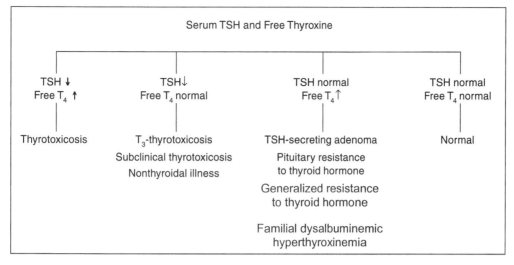

FIGURE 44.1. Diagnostic scheme for evaluating patients suspected of having thyrotoxicosis subdivided according to combinations of normal or low serum thyroid-stimulating hormone (TSH) concentrations and normal or high serum free thyroxine (T_4) values. Serum free T_4 can be measured either directly or indirectly as the serum free T_4 index (only the serum free T_4 index is high in patients with familial dysalbuminemic hyperthyroxinemia).

sis (i.e., a serum T_3:T_4 ratio of <15) suggests that thyroiditis (subacute or silent), iodine-induced thyrotoxicosis, or exogenous T_4 ingestion may be the cause. Measurements of thyroidal uptake of radioactive iodine or pertechnetate and thyroid imaging are only needed for differential diagnosis in some patients (Table 44.2). Thyrotoxicosis caused by excessive thyroid hormone synthesis and secretion is typically accompanied by increased uptake in functioning tissue, whereas thyroid inflammation and exogenous T_4 ingestion are associated with low thyroidal uptake (36). Radionuclide imaging often permits differentiation of Graves' disease from toxic nodular goiter, which have homogeneous and focal patterns of tracer distribution, respectively.

The clinical utility of assays for antibodies directed against the TSH receptor in Graves' disease is limited (37). These assays measure the ability of the patient's serum (or immunoglobulin fraction) either to inhibit the binding of TSH to its receptor (TSH receptor-binding inhibitory immunoglobulins) or to stimulate thyroid tissue in some way [e.g., adenylyl cyclase activity (thyroid-stimulating immunoglobulins)] (see Chapter 15). Tests for these antibodies may be used to diagnose Graves' disease in clinically and biochemically euthyroid patients with ophthalmopathy, and in unusual cases when differentiation of Graves' disease from toxic multinodular goiter is otherwise difficult and therapeutically important. In pregnant women with current or previously treated Graves' disease, the presence and level of thyroid-stimulating immunoglobulin activity can help predict the occurrence of fetal and neonatal thyrotoxicosis (37a).

Certain tests are useful in the diagnosis of other forms of thyrotoxicosis. Most patients with subacute thyroiditis

TABLE 44.2. THYROIDAL RADIOIODINE UPTAKE AND IMAGING IN THE DIFFERENTIAL DIAGNOSIS OF CAUSES OF THYROTOXICOSIS

Cause of Thyrotoxicosis	Fractional Uptake in 24 Hours (%)	Pattern of Distribution of Radionuclide in Thyroid
Graves' disease	35–95	Homogeneous
Toxic nodular goiter (uni- or multinodular)	20–60	Restricted to regions of autonomy
Subacute thyroiditis	0–2	Little or no uptake
Silent thyroiditis	0–2	Little or no uptake
Iodine-induced thyrotoxicosis	0–2	Little or no uptake
Factitious or iatrogenic thyrotoxicosis	0–2	Little or no uptake
Struma ovarii[a]	0–2	Uptake in ovary
Follicular carcinoma	0–5	Uptake in tumor metastases
TSH-induced thyrotoxicosis	30–80	Homogeneous

[a]Autonomously functioning thyroid tissue in an ovarian teratoma.

have an elevated erythrocyte sedimentation rate and C-reactive protein (37b), but those with silent thyroiditis do not. Serum thyroglobulin concentrations are high in patients with thyrotoxicosis caused by thyroid hypersecretion or inflammation, but not in those with factitious or iatrogenic thyrotoxicosis. Measurements of the serum glycoprotein hormone α subunit concentration may be of value in confirming a diagnosis of TSH-secreting pituitary adenoma (see Chapter 24).

REFERENCES

1. Bartalena L, Robbins J. Variations in thyroid hormone transport proteins and their clinical implications. *Thyroid* 1992;2:237.
2. Crooks J, Murray IPC, Wayne EL. Statistical methods applied to the clinical diagnosis of thyrotoxicosis. *Q J Med* 1959;28:211.
3. Trzepacz PT, Klein I, Roberts M, et al. Graves' disease: an analysis of thyroid hormone levels and hyperthyroid signs and symptoms. *Am J Med* 1989;87:558.
4. Nordyke RA, Gilbert FI Jr, Harada AS. Graves' disease: influence of age on clinical findings. *Arch Intern Med* 1988;248:626.
5. Prummel MF, Wiersinga WM. Smoking and risk of Graves' disease. *JAMA* 199327;269:479.
6. Koh LK, Greenspan FS, Yeo PP. Interferon-alpha induced thyroid dysfunction: three clinical presentations and a review of the literature. *Thyroid* 1997;7:891.
7. Hancock SL, Cox RS, McDougall IR. Thyroid diseases after treatment of Hodgkin's disease. *N Engl J Med* 1991;325:599.
8. Surks MI, Chopra IJ, Mariash CN, et al. American Thyroid Association guidelines for use of laboratory tests in thyroid disorders. *JAMA* 1990;263:1529.
9. Larsen PR, Alexander NM, Chopra IJ, et al. Revised nomenclature for tests of thyroid hormones and thyroid-related proteins in serum. *J Clin Endocrinol Metab* 1987;64:1089.
10. Heufelder AE, Klee GG, Wynne AG, et al. Familial dysalbuminemic hyperthyroxinemia: cumulative experience in 29 consecutive patients. *Endocr Pract* 1995;1:4.
11. Rushbrook JI, Becker E, Schussler GC, et al. Identification of a human serum albumin species associated with familial dysalbuminemic hyperthyroxinemia. *J Clin Endocrinol Metab* 1995; 80:461.
12. Moses AC, Rosen HN, Moller DE, et al. A point mutation in transthyretin increases affinity for thyroxine and produces euthyroid hyperthyroxinemia. *J Clin Invest* 1990;86:2025.
13. Rajatanavin R, Liberman C, Lawrence GD, et al. Euthyroid hyperthyroxinemia and thyroxine-binding prealbumin excess in islet cell carcinoma. *J Clin Endocrinol Metab* 1985;61:17.
14. Sakata S. Autoimmunity against thyroid hormones. *Crit Rev Immunol* 1994;14:157.
15. Gooch BR, Isley WL, Utiger RD. Abnormalities in thyroid function tests in patients admitted to a medical service. *Arch Intern Med* 1982;142:1801.
16. Spratt DI, Pont A, Miller MB, et al. Hyperthyroxinemia in patients with acute psychiatric disorders. *Am J Med* 1982;73:41.
17. Chopra IJ, Solomon DH, Huang T-S. Serum thyrotropin in hospitalized psychiatric patients: evidence for hyperthyrotropinemia as measured by an ultrasensitive thyrotropin assay. *Metabolism* 1990;39:538.
18. Goodwin TM, Montoro M, Mestman JH, et al. The role of chorionic gonadotropin in transient hyperthyroidism of hyperemesis gravidarum. *J Clin Endocrinol Metab* 1992;75:1333.
19. Cooper DS, Daniels GH, Ladenson PW, et al. Hyperthyroxinemia in patients with high-dose propranolol. *Am J Med* 1982;73:867.
20. Figge HL, Figge J. The effect of amiodarone on thyroid hormone function: a review of physiology and clinical manifestations. *J Clin Pharmacol* 1990;30:588.
21. Refetoff S, Usala SJ. The syndromes of resistance to thyroid hormones. *Endocr Rev* 1993;14:348.
22. Caplan RH, Pagliara AS, Wickus G. Thyroxine toxicosis: a common variant of hyperthyroidism. *JAMA* 1980;244:1934.
23. Sunthornthepvarakul T, Likitmaskul S, Ngowngarmratana S, et al. Familial dysalbuminemic hypertriiodothyroninemia: a new, dominantly inherited albumin defect. *J Clin Endocrinol Metab* 1998;83:1448.
24. Chen JJ, Ladenson PW. Discordant hypothyroxinemia and hypertriiodothyroninemia in treated patients with hyperthyroid Graves' disease. *J Clin Endocrinol Metab* 1986;63:102.
25. Klee GG, Hay ID. Assessment of sensitive thyrotropin assays for an expanded role in thyroid function testing: proposed criteria for analytic performance and clinical utility. *J Clin Endocrinol Metab* 1987;64:461.
25a. Baloch Z, Carayon P, Conte-Devolx B, et al., Guidelines Committee, National Academy of Clinical Biochemistry. Laboratory medicine practice guidelines: laboratory support for the diagnosis and monitoring of thyroid disease. *Thyroid* 2003;13:3–126.
26. Spencer CA, LoPresti JS, Patel A, et al. Applications of a new chemiluminescent thyrotropin assay to subnormal measurement. *J Clin Endocrinol Metab* 1990;70:453.
27. Franklyn JA, Black EG, Betteridge J, et al. Comparison of second and third generation methods for measurement of serum thyrotropin in patients with overt hyperthyroidism, patients receiving thyroxine therapy, and those with nonthyroidal illness. *J Clin Endocrinol Metab* 1994;78:1368.
28. McDermott MT, Ridgway EC. Central hyperthyroidism. *Endocrinol Metab Clin North Am* 1998;27:187.
29. Frost SJ, Hine KR, Firth GB, et al. Falsely lowered FT_4 and raised TSH concentrations in a patient with hyperthyroidism and human anti-mouse monoclonal antibodies. *Ann Clin Biochem* 1998;35(part 2):317.
30. de los Santos ET, Stanch GH, Mazzaferri EL. Sensitivity, specificity and cost-effectiveness of the sensitive thyrotropin assay in the diagnosis of thyroid disease in ambulatory patients. *Arch Intern Med* 1989;149:526.
31. Sawin CT, Geller A, Kaplan MM, et al. Low serum thyrotropin (thyroid-stimulating hormone) in older persons without hyperthyroidism. *Arch Intern Med* 1991;151:165.
32. Parle JV, Franklyn JA, Cross KW, et al. Prevalence and follow-up of abnormal thyrotrophin (TSH) concentrations in the elderly in the United Kingdom. *Clin Endocrinol* 1991;34:77.
33. Sawin CT, Geller A, Wolf PA, et al. Low serum thyrotropin concentrations as a risk factor for atrial fibrillation in older persons. *N Engl J Med* 1994;331:1249.
34. Eggertsen R, Petersen K, Lundberg P-A, et al. Screening for thyroid disease in a primary care unit with a thyroid stimulating hormone assay with a low detection limit. *BMJ* 1988;297:1586.
35. Glinoer D. Thyroid hyperfunction during pregnancy. *Thyroid* 1998;8:859–864.
36. Ross DS. Syndromes of thyrotoxicosis with low radioactive iodine uptake. *Endocrinol Metab Clin North Am* 1998;27:169.
37. Davies TF, Roti E, Braverman LE, et al. Thyroid controversy—stimulating antibodies. *J Clin Endocrinol Metab* 1998;83:3777.
37a. Peleg D, Cada S, Peleg A, Ben-Ami M. The relationship between maternal serum thyroid-stimulating immunoglobulin and fetal and neonatal thyrotoxicosis. *Obstet Gynecol* 2002;99:1040–1043.
37b. Pearce EN, Bogazzi F, Martino E, et al. The prevalence of elevated serum C–reactive protein levels in inflammatory and noninflammatory thyroid disease. *Thyroid* 2003;13:643.

TREATMENT OF THYROTOXICOSIS

DAVID S. COOPER

The ideal treatment of thyrotoxicosis would be directed at its cause. This is possible in only a few patients, for example, those with exogenous thyrotoxicosis or thyrotropin (TSH)-secreting pituitary adenomas. In patients with thyrotoxicosis due to its more common causes, especially Graves' disease, an autonomously functioning thyroid adenoma (toxic adenoma), and multinodular goiter, the fundamental causes are not known. Therapy is therefore directed at inhibiting thyroidal thyroxine (T_4) and triiodothyronine (T_3) synthesis and release or destroying thyroid tissue. Ancillary treatment involves ameliorating the effects of T_4 and T_3 on peripheral tissues. There are several means of accomplishing these goals, and their efficacy depends to some extent on the cause of the thyrotoxicosis. Because this is so, an attempt should be made to determine the cause; this usually can be achieved by history and physical examination, aided by selected tests such as measurement of thyroid radioiodine uptake and thyroid radionuclide imaging (see Chapter 12, and Chapters 23 through 29, in which the different causes of thyrotoxicosis are discussed).

This chapter considers the three forms of treatment of thyrotoxicosis—antithyroid drugs, radioactive iodine (radioiodine), and thyroidectomy—that are in wide use now. The emphasis is on treatment of the thyroid hyperactivity (hyperthyroidism) caused by Graves' disease, because it is the most common cause of thyrotoxicosis, and it is the disorder in which the relative merits of different treatments are most vigorously debated. When appropriate, the treatment of some of the other causes of thyrotoxicosis and of special patients (e.g., children, pregnant women, and patients with thyrotoxic storm) are mentioned. Information about treatment of some of the less-common causes of the disorder can be found in the chapters addressing those disorders.

THYROTOXICOSIS CAUSED BY GRAVES' DISEASE

Graves' disease is an autoimmune disease characterized by thyrotoxicosis caused by hypersecretion of the thyroid gland, thyroid hyperplasia, infiltrative ophthalmopathy, and localized myxedema. The thyroid hypersecretion and hyperplasia are caused by TSH receptor–stimulating antibodies (TSHR-Abs), which are antibodies against the TSH receptor on the cell membrane of thyroid follicular cells that mimic the effects of TSH (see section on pathogenesis of Graves' disease in Chapter 23) (1).

Autoimmune diseases tend to wax and wane over time, and Graves' disease is no exception. Although spontaneous remissions occur in patients who are not treated, Graves' disease—or rather the thyrotoxicosis that results from it—is virtually always treated because spontaneous remissions in untreated patients are uncommon and because the resulting thyrotoxicosis can have deleterious effects on multiple organ systems. In addition, there are several safe and effective therapies from which to choose, although each has certain drawbacks. Which therapy is best is a matter of debate, and opinions vary from country to country and from continent to continent (2,3). There is no "best" treatment, and the choice depends on several factors. Among the most important are the physician's experience and the patient's preferences. In some situations (e.g., in pregnant women and elderly patients), the therapeutic choices are more limited.

The chief therapeutic objective is to alleviate the patient's thyrotoxicosis. Antithyroid drugs act by decreasing thyroid hormone production. Whether the remissions that sometimes occur during or after antithyroid drug therapy are spontaneous, are due to amelioration of thyrotoxicosis, or are due to drug effects on the immune system is a matter of debate and is discussed later in detail. In contrast, surgery and radioiodine reduce the mass of thyroid tissue, but are not thought to alter the underlying Graves' disease, except possibly by removing intrathyroidal lymphocytes, a source of TSHR-Ab. Hypothyroidism usually follows the latter two treatments, but also may occur during or after drug therapy (4,5), possibly because of autoimmune destruction of the thyroid gland (6,7). Thus, the end result may be the same, regardless of the form of therapy.

DRUG THERAPY OF THYROTOXICOSIS CAUSED BY GRAVES' DISEASE

Antithyroid Drugs

Antithyroid drugs have been a mainstay of treatment of patients with Graves' thyrotoxicosis for almost 60 years (8,9). They can be given to patients with other forms of thyrotoxicosis (e.g., toxic nodular goiter), but they are not usually the primary mode of therapy for these conditions. These drugs inhibit the synthesis of T_4 and T_3, leading to gradual reduction in their serum concentrations. After several weeks or a few months, the dosage usually can be reduced; in some patients the drug can be discontinued, and the patient may remain euthyroid for months or years. A remission of Graves' disease, usually defined as being euthyroid for at least 1 year after treatment was stopped, occurs in about one half the patients. Thereafter, some patients have recurrent thyrotoxicosis (10), but others never do (11) (Fig. 45.1).

The antithyroid drugs to be considered here are heterocyclic compounds known as thioamides that contain a thioureylene group (Fig. 45.2). Three drugs of this type are available: methimazole [1-methyl 2-mercaptoimidazole; MMI (Tapazole)], carbimazole (1-methyl-2-thio-3 carbethoxy-imidazole), and propylthiouracil (6-propyl-2-thiouracil; PTU). MMI and PTU are used in the United States and South America, MMI in Europe and Japan, and carbimazole mainly in the United Kingdom. Carbimazole is rapidly metabolized to MMI (12) and has no properties not shared by MMI; therefore, these two drugs can be considered as one.

The origin of antithyroid drugs dates back to the early 1940s, with the serendipitous observations of two groups working independently at the Johns Hopkins Medical School. Richter and Clisby, who were studying taste preferences in laboratory animals, noted that the bitter substance phenylthiocarbamide caused goiter in rats (13). The MacKenzies, who were studying the gut flora of guinea pigs, recognized that the nonabsorbable antibiotic sulfaguanidine also caused goiter (14). They (15) and Astwood (16) subsequently determined that the cause of the goiter was stimulation of the thyroid by the pituitary gland, con-

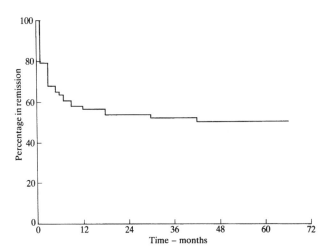

FIGURE 45.1. Kaplan-Meier plot showing the percentage of 72 patients with Graves' thyrotoxicosis remaining in remission after discontinuation of antithyroid drug therapy. Therapy was stopped at time 0. (From Young ET, Steel NR, Taylor JJ, et al. Prediction of remission after antithyroid drug treatment in Graves' disease. *QJM* 1988;250:175, with permission.)

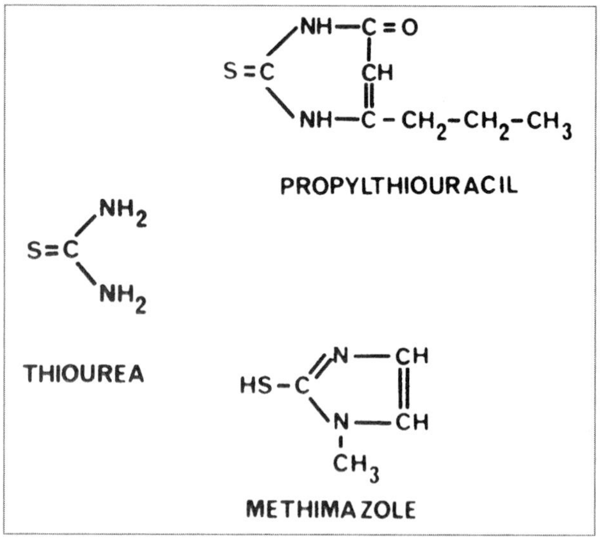

FIGURE 45.2. The structure of thiourea and two antithyroid drugs, propylthiouracil and methimazole, used clinically.

sequent to pharmacologic inhibition of thyroid hormone production. Within 18 months after the observations that sulfaguanidine and thiourea caused goiter, Astwood proposed that goitrogens could be used to treat thyrotoxicosis, screened many potentially useful compounds using a bioassay system, and conducted clinical studies with thiourea and thiouracil. Indeed, he coined the term "antithyroid drug" (17).

Mechanism of Action

The antithyroid drugs have intrathyroidal and extrathyroidal actions. The chief intrathyroidal actions are inhibition of iodine oxidation and organification, inhibition of iodotyrosine coupling, possible alteration of the structure of thyroglobulin, and possible inhibition of thyroglobulin biosynthesis. The main extrathyroidal action is inhibition of conversion of T_4 to T_3 (by PTU, but not MMI). The drugs' immunosuppressive actions, if they exist, could be at either or both sites.

Intrathyroidal Actions

Detailed descriptions of antithyroid drug pharmacology can be found in Chapter 4 and in the section on effects of drugs and other substances on thyroid hormone synthesis and metabolism in Chapter 11. Antithyroid drugs are actively transported into the thyroid gland (18–20), by a mechanism that is similar but probably not identical to the iodide transport system (21). They do not inhibit iodide transport or block the release of stored T_4 and T_3. Their most important actions are to interfere with thyroid peroxidase–mediated iodide oxidation, organification of iodine, and iodotyrosine coupling. With respect to the organification of iodine, the drugs compete with tyrosyl residues in thyroglobulin for oxidized iodine (22,23). As a result, the active iodine species is diverted away from tyrosyl residues in thyroglobulin, so that fewer are iodinated. The drugs themselves ultimately are oxidized and degraded. Antithyroid drugs also interfere with the peroxidase-catalyzed coupling process by which iodotyrosyl residues are coupled to form T_4 and T_3; the drug concentrations required to inhibit coupling are less than those required to inhibit iodine organification (24).

In addition to reducing iodine organification and iodotyrosyl coupling, the drugs may bind to thyroglobulin after they have been oxidized (25). Such binding could change the conformation of the thyroglobulin molecule, perhaps rendering it more resistant to subsequent iodination or hydrolysis. In addition, the drugs may inhibit the biosynthesis of thyroglobulin (26), although the concentrations required are probably higher (10^{-3} mol/L) than are achieved *in vivo* (27). They also may inhibit the growth of thyroid follicular cells (28,29).

Extrathyroidal Actions

Propylthiouracil, but not MMI, blocks the conversion of T_4 to T_3 in peripheral tissues (and the thyroid) by inhibiting the activity of type 1 T_4-deiodinase (see Chapter 7.) The mechanism is uncertain but may involve competition between the drug and cofactors for the reaction, which include reduced sulfhydryl groups (30). In addition, PTU may bind covalently to the enzyme via a selenosulfide bond (31), thereby inactivating it (32). MMI is not an inhibitor of this reaction, but other imidazole derivatives do inhibit T_4 conversion to T_3 *in vitro* (33). The clinical importance of the ability of PTU to block this conversion is discussed later.

Effects on the Immune System

Methimazole and PTU may have immunosuppressive as well as antithyroid actions (34–36). Although for the purpose of classification these putative effects are extrathyroidal, they probably involve actions on intrathyroidal immune function as well. The central question is whether the effects are caused by the action of the drugs on the immune system, or whether the abatement of autoimmune phenomena is simply the result of the decline in thyroid secretion induced by the drugs. In studies *in vitro*, the observed activity can be directly ascribed to the drug, but in studies *in vivo* the distinction between direct and indirect effects is ambiguous.

Despite some negative results (37), numerous *in vitro* studies have documented an effect of antithyroid drugs on various arms of the immune system. The drugs inhibit

lymphocyte transformation (38), and they may have other inhibitory (39–41) [as well as stimulatory (39–41)] effects on lymphocyte, monocyte (39), and neutrophil (39,42) function and on formation of soluble mediators such as interleukin-2 (IL-2) (43). The formation of free radicals, which may be important in T-cell responsiveness and in complement-mediated thyroid-cell injury, may be inhibited by MMI (44). In addition, the drugs may reduce expression of major histocompatibility complex (MHC) class II (HLA-DR) molecules on thyroid cells, which may be important for the initiation or maintenance of Graves' disease (45). Antithyroid drugs may reduce HLA-DR expression directly (46) or by inhibiting secretion of interferon-γ, which induces class II molecules (47). MMI reduces MHC class I messenger RNA concentrations in cultured thyroid cells (FRTL-5 cells) (48). Finally, antithyroid drugs may influence the immune system by inducing expression of Fas ligand (FasL) on thyroid cells, which could lead to activation of Fas on lymphocytes and consequently Fas-induced apoptosis of these cells (49).

There is also strong *in vivo* evidence, albeit circumstantial, for an immunologic effect of antithyroid drugs. The thyroid glands of patients with hyperthyroidism who were treated with an antithyroid drug before thyroidectomy were depleted of lymphocytes, as compared with patients who had received only the β-adrenergic receptor antagonist propranolol (50). In addition, the serum concentrations of TSHR-Ab, whether measured by bioassay or receptor assay, and other antithyroid antibodies decline during antithyroid drug therapy (51,52). The effects appear to be specific for thyroid-related antibodies, because the serum concentrations of antiparietal cell antibodies did not change in patients with coexisting autoimmune gastritis (53). Serum concentrations of the immunomodulator intercellular adhesion molecule-1 (ICAM-1) (54), and of some cytokines and soluble cytokine receptors, also decrease in response to antithyroid drug therapy, including those of IL-1β (55), soluble IL-2 receptors (55,56), and soluble IL-6 receptors (57). A study of thyroid aspirates from treated versus untreated patients suggested that thyrocyte HLA-DR expression is reduced by thioamide therapy (58). Furthermore, antithyroid drug treatment results in changes in cell-mediated immunity in patients with Graves' disease. For example, an increase (normalization) in suppressor T-cell number during treatment was found in several (59–61), but not all (62), studies, and helper T-cell (60) and natural killer cell activity decrease (63). Also, MMI decreases the number of activated T cells within the thyroid itself, as compared with the pretreatment number (60).

Despite the evidence for an immunomodulatory effect of antithyroid drugs, several caveats are necessary. With regard to the *in vitro* data, the effective doses have varied from 10^{-4} to 10^{-5} mol/L, whereas intrathyroidal concentrations *in vivo* are unlikely to exceed 5×10^{-5} mol/L (27,64), thus casting some doubt on the pharmacologic relevance of the observed effects. The changes in serum autoantibody concentrations and in T-cell subsets do not occur in all patients, and the changes that do occur are variable. The reasons for this are unclear, but they must relate to the question of whether remissions of Graves' disease are spontaneous, or whether they are induced by the antithyroid drug (see later discussion). Finally, any changes in immune response markers that may be induced by antithyroid drugs inevitably occur when thyroid secretion is declining and thyrotoxicosis is improving (34). Thus, if the thyrotoxic state were responsible for perpetuation of the altered immunity, then its correction should reduce the alterations. Therapy for Graves' thyrotoxicosis with potassium perchlorate leads to a decline in serum TSHR-Ab concentrations in a manner similar to that which occurs during antithyroid drug treatment (65), but since perchlorate also may have immunosuppressive effects (66), the matter remains unresolved.

Despite these reservations, additional *in vivo* data indicate an immunosuppressive effect of antithyroid drugs. First, administration of MMI causes serologic and histologic attenuation of experimental autoimmune thyroiditis in rats (67–69). Second, in one study of euthyroid patients with chronic autoimmune (Hashimoto's) thyroiditis, administration of carbimazole caused a decline in serum antithyroid peroxidase antibody concentrations (52), a result not confirmed, however, by two other studies (70,71). Finally, MMI, but not glucocorticoids, blocked the increase in serum TSHR-Ab concentrations that occurred in patients with Graves' disease treated with radioiodine (see later discussion), suggesting that an organ-specific effect, rather than generalized immunosuppression, is of primary importance (72). In another study, patients treated with either PTU or carbimazole had identical decrements in serum thyroid hormone concentrations, but the carbimazole-treated patients had greater decreases in serum TSHR-Ab concentrations and increases in the number of suppressor T cells, suggesting, indirectly, an effect on the immune system independent of thyroid function (73).

To summarize, antithyroid drugs can inhibit immune function *in vitro*, but the concentrations of drug required may be higher than are attained within the thyroid gland during treatment. Changes in serum concentrations of antithyroid antibodies and TSHR-Ab and in T-cell subsets occur in patients receiving chronic antithyroid drug therapy, but changes in thyroid function occur concomitantly, making it impossible to distinguish cause and effect satisfactorily.

CLINICAL PHARMACOLOGY OF THE ANTITHYROID DRUGS

Methimazole

MMI is almost completely absorbed from the gastrointestinal tract (74,75). Peak serum concentrations occur 1 to 2 hours after ingestion and are in the range of 300 ng/mL (2.6 mmol/L) after a 15-mg oral dose (Table 45.1) (75). The serum concentrations are dose related and correlate with effects on iodine organification (76). Carbimazole is rapidly converted to MMI in serum: 10 mg of carbimazole yields about 6 mg MMI (12). The serum half-life of MMI is 4 to 6 hours, but little is bound to serum proteins (75,77). The serum half-life is similar in patients with thyrotoxicosis (75,77), but it may be shorter in patients who do not respond to the drug (78). Drug clearance is unchanged in patients with renal disease (74) but is slowed in those with hepatic disease (77).

Intrathyroidal MMI concentrations are about 500 to 2000 ng/g (about 5×10^{-5} mol/L) (27,64). The intrathyroidal turnover of MMI is slow, the concentrations 17 to 20 hours after ingestion being similar to those 3 to 6 hours after ingestion (27), which may account for the longer duration of action of MMI as compared with PTU. The effects of MMI dissipate within 24 hours in one study (79), but other studies suggest a longer duration of action (80). Little MMI is excreted in the urine, and neither the products of metabolism nor their fate is known (81). Because it is not protein bound (77) and is lipid soluble, MMI freely crosses membranes [e.g., placenta (82) and breast epithelium (77)]. Given its relatively long serum (and intrathyroidal) half-life and its long duration of action, MMI is effective when given as a single daily dose (83–86).

Although the potency of MMI is commonly regarded as being about 10 times that of PTU, it is almost surely

TABLE 45.1. SELECTED PHARMACOLOGIC FEATURES OF ANTITHYROID DRUGS

	Propylthiouracil	Methimazole
Serum protein binding	~75%	Nil
Serum half-life	~1–2 h	~4–6 h
Volume of distribution	~20 L	~40 L
Metabolism of drug during illness		
Severe liver disease	Normal	Decreased
Severe kidney disease	Normal	Normal
Transplacental passage	Low	Higher
Concentrations in breast milk	Low	Higher

From Cooper DS, Bode HH, Nath B, et al. Methimazole pharmacology in man: studies using a newly developed radioimmunoassay for methimazole. *J Clin Endocrinol Metab* 1984;58:473; Cooper DS, Saxe VC, Meskell M, et al. Acute effects of propylthiouracil (PTU) on thyroidal iodine organification and peripheral iodothyronine deiodination: correlation with serum PTU levels measured by radioimmunoassay. *J Clin Endocrinol Metab* 1982;54:101; Cooper DS, Steigerwalt S, Migdal S. Pharmacology of propylthiouracil in thyrotoxicosis and chronic renal failure. *Arch Intern Med* 1987;147:785; Kampmann JP, Hansen JEM. Serum protein binding of propylthiouracil. *Br J Clin Pharmacol* 1983;16:549; Zaton A, Martinez A, DeGandarias JM. The binding of thioureylene compounds to human serum albumin. *Biochem Pharmacol* 1988;37:3127; and Kampmann JP, Hansen IM, Johansen K, et al. Propylthiouracil in human milk. *Lancet* 1980;2:736, with permission.

greater, and it may be up to 50 times more potent (76). Indeed, thyrotoxicosis can be controlled in most patients with doses of MMI that are less, for example, 10 to 15 mg daily, than those traditionally thought to be necessary (85,86). The difference in potency between MMI and PTU is probably not due to an actual difference at the biochemical level, but rather to differences in uptake into and metabolism within the thyroid gland, because *in vitro* MMI is not a significantly more potent inhibitor of thyroid peroxidase-catalyzed reactions (23). One study found an increase in prednisolone clearance in patients taking MMI, possibly related to hepatic enzyme induction (87). Therefore, patients requiring glucocorticoid therapy for Graves' ophthalmopathy may need higher doses if they are also taking MMI.

Propylthiouracil

Orally administered PTU is almost completely absorbed. Peak serum concentrations occur about 1 hour after ingestion and are dose dependent, with peak concentrations of about 3 mg/mL (18 mmol/L) after a 150-mg oral dose (88) (Table 45.1). Serum PTU concentrations correlate with the drug's effects on iodine oxidation and organification and with inhibition of T_4-deiodinase activity (84). There is little information about intrathyroidal concentrations, which are most relevant to efficacy and duration of action (20). The serum half-life of PTU is in the range of 1 to 2 hours, and it is not altered in patients with thyrotoxicosis (85) or hepatic (89) or renal failure (90), in children (91) or in elderly patients (92). PTU is strongly (80% to 90%) protein bound (93), largely to serum albumin (94), and is ionized at physiologic pH (95). This has implications for PTU therapy in pregnant and lactating women (see later discussion), because free (i.e., unbound) drug concentrations are low and ionized drug may not freely cross membranes. Most of an ingested dose of PTU is excreted in the urine, after conjugation with glucuronide in the liver (19).

The duration of action of PTU is about 12 to 24 hours (80,96). This rate probably depends on several factors, including the rates at which the drug is concentrated and degraded within the thyroid. Clearly, the duration of action is longer than the serum half-life. Although PTU can sometimes be given satisfactorily as a single daily dose (97), it usually is given every 6 to 8 hours (98), at least when therapy is initiated. With time, the frequency and total daily dose often can be decreased (96).

Clinical Considerations in the Use of Antithyroid Drugs

The thioamide antithyroid drugs are chiefly used for the long-term treatment of patients with thyrotoxicosis caused by Graves' disease, with the expectation—or at least the hope—that a remission of Graves' disease will occur. In

surveys of thyroidologists in the United States over a decade ago, radioiodine, not an antithyroid drug, was the preferred treatment for most patients, the exceptions being children, adolescents, and young adults (2,3). In contrast, an antithyroid drug is the treatment of choice in much of the rest of the world, including Europe, Japan, and South America (2).

The clinical factors that influence the choice of therapy and the likelihood of remission are discussed later. Antithyroid drugs rather than surgery are preferred for pregnant women, which is discussed separately, and for children and adolescents (also discussed later). They are often given before surgery and sometimes before radioiodine therapy, and they are standard therapy for neonates with Graves' disease, which is a transient condition.

Both MMI and PTU are very (at least 90%) effective in controlling thyrotoxicosis due to Graves' disease, and to some extent the choice between the two drugs is a matter of personal preference. Given the advantages of MMI (see later in the chapter), it is hard to understand why PTU remains rather widely used. Only PTU inhibits extrathyroidal T_4 conversion to T_3, and although serum T_3 concentrations do initially decline more rapidly after the initiation of PTU therapy, there is no evidence that the more rapid decline is clinically important, except possibly in patients with severe or life-threatening thyrotoxicosis (thyrotoxic storm) (99,100). In fact, MMI therapy results in more rapid normalization of serum T_4 and T_3 concentrations than does PTU therapy (101,102), probably related to the greater potency or the longer duration of action of MMI, as discussed earlier.

Generic MMI is available in either 5-, 10-, or 20 mg tablets (Tapazole® is only available as 5- and 10 mg tablets), and PTU in 50 mg tablets, a difference in formulation that means that fewer tablets of MMI need be given each day. The usual starting dose of MMI has been 20 to 30 mg daily, often in divided doses, but once-daily dosing—and lower doses—are adequate for most patients (103). In a prospective multicenter trial in Europe, 10 mg daily was nearly as effective as 40 mg daily (104); serum T_4 and T_3 concentrations were normal in 6 weeks in 85% of the patients given 10 mg daily and 92% of those given 40 mg daily. Patients living in areas of relative iodine deficiency had a more rapid response, an effect noted previously (105). There is little additional benefit of even higher doses (106). The usual starting dose of PTU is 100 mg three times daily.

One study found that baseline thyroid function is an important predictor of the required starting dosage. If the initial serum T_4 concentration was above 20 μg/dl (260 nmol/L), a daily carbimazole dose of 20 mg (equal to about 15 mg MMI) was inadequate for many patients; in contrast, if the initial serum T_4 concentration was lower, a starting dose of 40 mg per day (equivalent to 30 mg MMI), caused hypothyroidism in a substantial number of patients

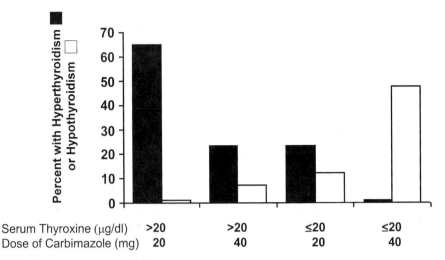

FIGURE 45.3. Percentages of patients with thyrotoxicosis who had persistent thyrotoxicosis or hypothyroidism 4 weeks after initiation of treatment with 20 mg/day or 40 mg/day of carbimazole, subdivided according to baseline serum thyroxine concentration ≤20 μg/dL or >21 μg/dL (260 nmol/L). Thirty-four patients were treated with 20 mg/day and 30 patients with 40 mg/day. (From Cooper DS. Antithyroid drugs in the management of patients with Graves' disease: an evidence-based approach to therapeutic controversies. *J Clin Endocrinol Metab* 2003; 88:3473, *copyright 2003, The Endocrine Society*, modified with permission; and from Page SR, Sheard CE, Herbert M, et al. A comparison of 20 or 40 mg per day of carbimazole in the initial treatment of hyperthyroidism. *Clin Endocrinol (Oxf)*1996;45:511, with permission.)

(Fig. 45.3) (107). Clearly, the dose should be increased if thyroid secretion does not decrease within 4 to 6 weeks. Doses of PTU as high as 2000 mg daily have been given to patients thought to be resistant to the drug, but in most instances the problem was poor compliance (108). In seriously ill patients who do not respond to high doses of antithyroid drugs, the addition of glucocorticoid therapy may provide additional benefit (109).

As thyroid secretion decreases during the first several weeks or months after antithyroid therapy is initiated, the dose of drug should be decreased, for example, to 5 or even 2.5 mg MMI or 100 or 50 mg PTU daily, or hypothyroidism may supervene. Other factors that determine the speed of recovery include disease activity, the initial degree of thyroid hypersecretion, and the intrathyroidal stores of T_4 and T_3. The ability to reduce the dose without exacerbation of thyrotoxicosis reflects not only waning of disease activity, possibly reflected by a decline in TSHR-Ab production, but also because the goal of therapy changes, from relatively complete to partial inhibition of T_4 and T_3 synthesis.

If high doses of drug are required for control of thyrotoxicosis, remission is unlikely, and ablative therapy usually is selected. Some authors have argued that continuous high-dose antithyroid drug therapy is preferable to reducing the dose to maintain thyroid function within normal limits, because rates of remission may be higher as a result of greater putative immunosuppressive effects. However, high-dose therapy has not been widely used because this theory is unproven, it requires concomitant T_4 therapy to prevent iatrogenic hypothyroidism, and because the fre-

quency of serious side effects is higher with high doses of antithyroid drug (104,110,111).

The choice of antithyroid drug is an individual matter, based mainly on the physician's personal preferences and experience, but there are many reasons to prefer MMI (112). First, the likelihood of compliance is higher because MMI can be given once daily and fewer tablets per day are needed; once-daily dosing of PTU is less effective (97,98). Second, patients treated with MMI become euthyroid sooner (101,102,113,114). The costs of MMI and PTU are comparable when doses of MMI in the 10 to 20 mg/day range are given; at higher doses, MMI is more expensive than PTU. Finally, MMI may be safer than PTU (115), at least in terms of the most important side effect of these drugs, which is agranulocytosis (see later discussion). In some special circumstances—pregnancy and thyrotoxic storm—PTU may be preferable.

Side Effects of Antithyroid Drugs

Antithyroid drugs have multiple potential side effects (Table 45.2). Most are considered to be allergic reactions. Fever, urticaria or other rashes, and arthralgia occur in 1% to 5% of patients (115,116), usually within the first several weeks or months after initiation of therapy, and are more common in patients treated with higher doses (104,116–118). In one study, serum aminotransferase concentrations increased slightly in one third of patients within 2 months after starting PTU therapy (119). The results of baseline

TABLE 45.2. SIDE EFFECTS OF ANTITHYROID DRUGS

Minor

Common (1%–5%)
  Urticaria or other rash
  Arthralgia
  Fever
  Transient granulocytopenia
Uncommon (<1%)
  Gastrointestinal
  Abnormalities of taste and smell
  Arthritis

Major

Rare (0.2%–0.5%)
  Agranulocytosis
Very rare (<1%)
  Aplastic anemia
  Thrombocytopenia
  Toxic hepatitis (PTU)
  Cholestatic hepatitis (MMI)
  Vasculitis, systemic lupus-like syndrome
  Hypoprothrombinemia (PTU)
  Hypoglycemia (due to anti-insulin antibodies) (MMI)

MMI, methimazole; PTU, propylthiouracil.

liver function tests, which are often abnormal in hyperthyroidism (120,121), were not predictive of this change in PTU-treated patients (119), and the high serum aminotransferase values resolved without discontinuation of therapy. Similar changes have not been reported for MMI. Serum alkaline phosphatase concentrations also may increase transiently during antithyroid drug therapy, not because of hepatobiliary dysfunction, but rather because of an increase in bone formation (121). Routine monitoring of liver function is not indicated.

The more serious and rarer toxic reactions (major side effects) are agranulocytosis, aplastic anemia, hepatitis [with PTU (122)] and cholestasis [with MMI (122)], polyarthritis (123), and a lupus-like syndrome or vasculitis (124, 125), all of which, with the possible exception of agranulocytosis, are more common in patients treated with PTU. Agranulocytosis, the most feared problem, probably occurs with equal frequency with both drugs (about 0.2% to 0.5%); the other severe reactions are less common. Fulminant PTU-induced hepatitis may be more common in children; deaths have been reported, and several other patients required liver transplantation (126). A few PTU-treated patients with isolated hypoprothrombinemia have been reported (127). MMI also can cause liver disease, usually cholestatic hepatitis; it may be severe (122,128,129). Patients should be warned about the potential for hepatotoxicity, and to discontinue the drug if they have malaise, jaundice, or dark urine. Patients with the lupus-like syndrome or vasculitis associated with PTU (and rarely MMI)

may have skin involvement, glomerulonephritis, or pulmonary hemorrhage, and often have high serum concentrations of antineutrophil cytoplasmic antibodies (ANCA) (124,125,130). Reports of ANCA-related vasculitis, mostly with PTU, are predominantly from Asian countries; some patients were ANCA positive before treatment was started (131,132), and many develop ANCA but do not have vasculitis (132,133). In most cases, the antibody is myeloperoxidase-ANCA (MPO-ANCA) (131,133,134).

Like the minor side effects, these major side effects usually occur within the first several weeks or months after the initiation of therapy, when drug dosage is higher. However, they can occur during prolonged treatment (110) and may be more common when the drug is resumed than when it was first given (45).

The cause of MMI- or PTU-induced agranulocytosis is not known, but it may be an immunologic phenomenon. Some patients have evidence of lymphocyte sensitization (135), an association with certain HLA class II haplotypes has been reported (136), and some patients have antibodies to granulocytes and granulocytic progenitor cells (137).

Agranulocytosis, which is often defined as a granulocyte count less than 250 cells/mm³ (0.25×10^9/L), usually develops so suddenly that routine monitoring of the leukocyte count has been thought to be of little value. Elderly patients may be more susceptible to agranulocytosis (115,138). However, in one study granulocytopenia [granulocyte count less than 500/mm³ (0.5×10^9/L)] was detected by routine monitoring of leukocyte counts before agranulocytosis occurred, suggesting the onset may be gradual (138). In the patients who had granulocytopenia, prompt discontinuation of therapy led to an increase in leukocyte count. If this observation is confirmed, periodic leukocyte counts would be reasonable, at least during the first few months of therapy, when most reported cases of agranulocytosis have occurred. However, due to the low frequency of this side effect, the cost effectiveness of routine monitoring must be questioned.

Patients with agranulocytosis typically present with fever and evidence of infection, usually of the oropharynx. All patients should be warned of the possible symptoms, and given written instructions that the drug should be discontinued and a physician contacted immediately if they have any symptoms of infection. Agranulocytosis must be distinguished from the transient, mild granulocytopenia [granulocyte count <1500/mm³ (1.5×10^9/L)] that occurs in up to 10% of antithyroid drug–treated patients, as well as that occasionally present in patients with thyrotoxicosis before therapy or in normal black subjects. As a practical matter, complete leukocyte counts should be obtained before initiation of therapy; if the baseline granulocyte count is normal but a subsequent count is <1500/mm³ (1.5×10^9/L), the drug should be discontinued. If the drug is not discontinued, the leukocyte count should be repeated weekly until it is stable or increasing. It may be possible to distinguish those patients with granulocytopenia during therapy who will recover rapidly from those who are likely to have agranulocytosis. In one study, 25 of 28 patients (89%) with moderate granulocytopenia [granulocyte count 500 to 1000/mm³ [0.5 to 1.0 × 10⁹/L)] and 4 of 6 patients (67%) with more severe granulocytopenia [granulocyte count 100 to 500/mm³ [0.1 to 0.5 × 10⁹/L)] had a normal granulocyte count 4 hours after a single injection of 75 mg of granulocyte colony stimulating factor (G-CSF) and subsequently recovered fully, whereas those patients who did not have a normal granulocyte count after G-CSF injection had progressive decreases in granulocyte counts (139). Thus, testing with G-CSF may allow recognition of those patients who will recover from those who will require additional care.

In addition to prompt discontinuation of the antithyroid drug, treatment of agranulocytosis typically involves the administration of broad-spectrum antibiotics and appropriate supportive measures; hospitalization should be avoided if possible, but is essential if the patient is febrile. The granulocyte count usually begins to increase within several days, but may not be normal for 10 to 14 days. G-CSF therapy has proven variably effective. Retrospective data suggest modest efficacy (140) in shortening the recovery time, but in a randomized trial of 24 patients, the combination of G-CSF (100 to 250 mg) and antibiotic therapy did not shorten the duration of agranulocytosis, as compared with antibiotic therapy alone (141). However, G-CSF may accelerate recovery in patients in whom the ratio of granulocytes to erythrocytes in the bone marrow is 0.5 or higher (142). Glucocorticoid therapy is probably ineffective (142).

In the case of minor drug-related side effects such as fever or rash, the side effect may subside in several days despite continuation of therapy, with or without a short course of antihistamine therapy. If the effect persists, the other antithyroid drug can be substituted, with reasonable probability that the side effect will subside. Substitution should not be attempted in the case of agranulocytosis or the other major side effects because cross-reactivity has been reported.

Patients with major side effects in whom antithyroid drug therapy is discontinued usually become thyrotoxic soon thereafter, if they were not thyrotoxic when the drug was discontinued. In them, antithyroid drug therapy is no longer an option. They should be treated with a β-adrenergic antagonist drug and inorganic iodine, an iodinated radiographic contrast agent, or lithium if the thyrotoxicosis is severe. If it is not, radioiodine therapy should be given as soon as practicable.

Other rare side effects of MMI are pancreatitis (143); hypoglycemia, caused by anti-insulin antibodies (the "insulin-autoimmune syndrome"), typically in Japanese patients (144,145); and myalgia and high serum creatine kinase concentrations (146). MMI can cause a decreased sense of taste (116), whereas PTU may cause a bitter or metallic taste.

Follow-up of Patients Taking an Antithyroid Drug for Graves' Disease

Once MMI or PTU therapy has been initiated, patients should be seen every 4 to 6 weeks until they are clinically and biochemically euthyroid. This usually occurs within 4 to 6 weeks with MMI, but it may take up to 12 weeks with PTU (101,113). As the thyrotoxicosis comes under control, the dose of antithyroid drug should be progressively reduced. Hypothyroidism, thyroid enlargement, or both may occur in patients if the dosage of drug is not decreased. Later, the frequency of follow-up visits can be decreased to every 2 to 3 months and then every 6 months.

The usual biochemical tests of thyroid function may be misleading early in the course of antithyroid drug therapy. TSH secretion is strongly inhibited by thyrotoxicosis, and therefore serum TSH concentrations may remain low for several months despite normalization of serum T_4 and T_3 concentrations. Some patients remain thyrotoxic despite having normal or even low serum T_4 concentrations; they have persistently high serum T_3 concentrations, indicating the need for an increase, rather than a decrease, in antithyroid drug dosage (147,148). This syndrome of so-called T_3-predominant thyrotoxicosis is due to incomplete inhibition of thyroid hormone synthesis and may be associated with a low likelihood of remission (149). Although an enlarging thyroid gland may indicate that hypothyroidism has developed, it also may be indicative of persistent or increasing TSHR-Ab production and a low likelihood of remission.

Remissions and Antithyroid Drug Therapy

The primary goal of antithyroid drug therapy is to render the patient euthyroid. However, this form of treatment is usually chosen in anticipation that the patient will eventually have a remission of Graves' disease, and therefore will not need destructive therapy. Unfortunately, the ability to predict which patients are likely to have a remission is poor (150), and there have been only a few large studies of the possible clinical, biochemical, and pharmacologic features that correlate with remission or relapse (151–153). One way of organizing the often-conflicting information concerning the factors that might be related to remission is to distinguish the clinical or patient-related factors from the drug-related factors, for example, type or dose of drug or duration of therapy. The goal is to identify those patients in whom remission is unlikely, so that they are not given treatment destined to fail.

PRETREATMENT CLINICAL FACTORS RELATING TO REMISSION OF GRAVES' DISEASE

Certain pretreatment clinical characteristics seem to be associated with a low likelihood of long-term remission (i.e.,

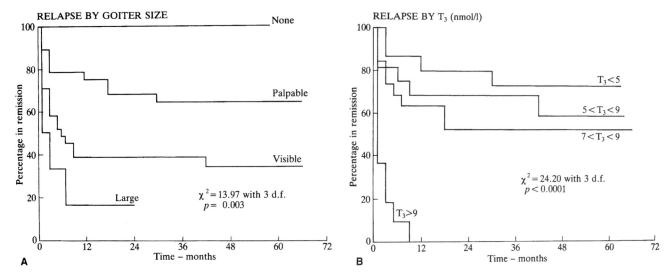

FIGURE 45.4. Likelihood of remission of Graves' thyrotoxicosis after discontinuation of antithyroid drug therapy in 72 patients as a function of **(A)** goiter size and **(B)** serum triiodothyronine (T_3) concentration at the beginning of therapy. Therapy was discontinued at time 0. To convert serum T_3 values to ng/dL, multiply by 65.1. (From Young ET, Steel NR, Taylor JJ, et al. Prediction of remission after antithyroid drug treatment in Graves' disease. *QJM* 1988;20:175, with permission.)

the patient remains euthyroid for at least 1 year after antithyroid drug therapy is discontinued). They include a large goiter and more severe biochemical thyrotoxicosis, in both adults (Fig. 45.4) (151–154) and children (155). Another may be a high ratio of T_3 to T_4 in serum [T_3 (ng/dL): T_4 (µg/dL) >20] before (and during) therapy (149), but this is disputed (156). High baseline serum concentrations of TSHR-Ab may (152,157) or may not (151) be predictive of eventual relapse, but an undetectable serum TSHR-Ab concentration at the time of diagnosis is associated with a very high (90%) rate of remission (158). Patients with certain HLA haplotypes (especially HLA-DR3) may be less likely (159), whereas those who are HLA-DR4 positive may be more likely, to have a remission (160); others have not found HLA typing to be useful (154–161). Likewise, a negative family history of Graves' disease may (162) or may not (161) be associated with an increased likelihood of remission. Patients with allergic diseases (e.g., atopy, allergic rhinitis, asthma), and high serum IgE concentrations may be less likely to have a remission (163).

Factors not consistently related to the likelihood of remission are the sex of the patient (164), smoking (165, 166), the presence of ophthalmopathy, or the duration of symptoms before the initiation of therapy. The remission rate may be higher in older patients, possibly due to milder thyrotoxicosis (167), but no relationship with age was found in another study (151). One study found that certain personality traits (e.g., hypochondriasis, depression, paranoia), as well as a higher prevalence of "daily hassles," were more common in those who relapsed versus those who remained euthyroid (168). Unfortunately, the low predictive value of any clinical finding makes it difficult to know *a priori* which patients are likely to have a remission and which are not.

Therapy Factors Relating to Remission of Graves' Disease

Duration of Therapy

Although many patients are treated with an antithyroid drug for 1 to 2 years before it is discontinued (2), some patients have a remission within weeks or months after treatment is begun (169,170). Longer courses of therapy intuitively seem preferable, and there are convincing retrospective data (171), particularly in children (172), that the longer the drug is given, the more likely the patient is to have a remission. However, recent prospective randomized studies on this point are conflicting (Fig. 45.5). In a French study of 114 patients, 62% of those treated with MMI for 6 months relapsed, as compared with 42% of those treated for 18 months (173). However, in two other similarly designed studies, the relapse rates were similar among patients treated for 12 months and 24 months (174), and among patients treated for 18 and 42 months (175). Furthermore, among 100 patients given a "block-replace" regimen of carbimazole plus T_4, the 1-year relapse rates were 41% in those treated for 6 months and 35% in those treated for 1 year (176). Given these results, treatment for 12 to 24 months seems reasonable, at which time treatment should be discontinued and the patient followed periodically.

Drug Dose

The possibility that high-dose antithyroid drug therapy might increase the likelihood of remission is based on the suggestion that the drugs have immunosuppressive effects, as discussed earlier. One study did find that the remission rate was higher (75% vs. 42%) with high-dose therapy

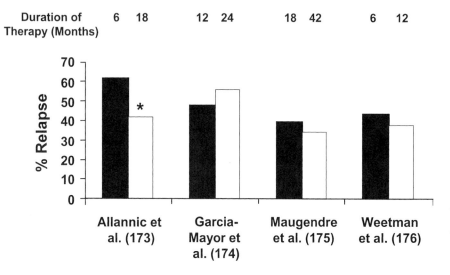

FIGURE 45.5. The rates of relapse of thyrotoxicosis caused by Graves' disease as a function of duration of antithyroid drug therapy in four prospective studies. The numbers overlying the bars are the number of months of in each treatment arm in each study. The rate of relapse was significantly lower in the patients treated longer in only one study (*$p<0.05$, for the comparison between the two groups). (From Cooper DS. Antithyroid drugs in the management of patients with Graves' disease: an evidence-based approach to therapeutic controversies. *J Clin Endocrinol Metab* 2003;88:3473, copyright 2003, The Endocrine Society).

(mean MMI dose 60 mg/day or PTU dose 700 mg/day), as compared with lower doses, but the study was confounded by the fact that the high-dose therapy group also received T_3 (177). In a subsequent study by the same group in which the patients given both high and low doses of antithyroid drug were given T_3, the rates of remission were similar (178), and they were similar in other prospective randomized studies in which high and low doses were compared (153,179–181).

Additional research casts doubt on the efficacy of high-dose regimens to improve the likelihood of remission. In one study there was no correlation between the MMI concentration in thyroid tissue obtained surgically and lymphocyte counts and numbers of activated T cells and antigen-presenting cells (182). In another, serum concentrations of β_2-microglobulin, soluble HLA class I antigen, and soluble IL-2 receptor were high in patients with Graves' thyrotoxicosis initially and decreased similarly whether the patients received high- or low-dose antithyroid drug therapy (56). Given the lack of evidence that high-dose therapy is more likely to be followed by remission and the higher likelihood of side effects (104,177,179,181), high-dose therapy cannot be recommended.

Combination Antithyroid Drug and Thyroxine Therapy

The possibility that the combination of an antithyroid drug and T_4 might improve the remission rate compared with an antithyroid drug alone is based on the hypothesis that T_4, by maintaining lower serum TSH concentrations, would decrease the expression of antigens (e.g., the TSH receptor) that are responsible for perpetuating the production of TSHR-Ab. In a study of 109 Japanese patients, 97% of those treated with MMI and T_4 for 18 months fol-

lowed by T_4 alone for 3 years remained in remission during the 3-year T_4 treatment period, as compared with 62% in patients given MMI for 18 months (183). Multiple attempts to replicate these remarkable results have been unsuccessful. In one study in the United Kingdom, for example, in which patients were treated for 17 months with carbimazole or carbimazole plus T_4, followed by T_4 or no therapy for 18 months, the proportion who remained in remission was similar (184). Similar negative results have been reported from Canada and several other European countries (185–190). Differences in ethnicity or iodine intake may be partly responsible but are unlikely to be the sole explanations for the difference. Furthermore, another group of Japanese investigators found no difference in serum TSHR-Ab concentrations in patients treated with MMI alone as compared with patients treated with MMI and T_4 (191).

Responses during Therapy Relating to Remission

Features during therapy that suggest that a patient may be entering remission include a decrease in goiter size (192), the ability to control the thyrotoxicosis with decreasing doses of drug, and normalization of the ratio of T_4 to T_3 in serum (148). Conversely, continuing thyroid enlargement, a requirement for a high dose of antithyroid drug, and persistence of high serum T_3 concentrations are evidence of continuing Graves' disease. Numerous other tests have been proposed to determine whether a patient's Graves' disease may be in remission so that antithyroid drug therapy can be discontinued with a low likelihood of relapse, but none has the requisite sensitivity and specificity to be useful in individual patients (151,193). The best studied of these tests is measurement of serum TSHR-Ab (194). Serum TSHR-Ab concentrations tend to decrease during antithyroid drug therapy because amelioration of thyrotoxicosis, an immunosuppressive effect of the drug, spontaneous remission, or a combination of these factors. The failure of serum TSHR-Ab to become undetectable during antithyroid drug therapy signifies almost certain relapse after discontinuation of therapy (154,195). If the antibodies disappear, however, there is still a 30% to 50% chance of relapse (152,157,166,194). Thus, detectable serum TSHR-Ab activity, but not its absence, has predictive value.

Other tests proposed as predictors of relapse or remission in patients treated with an antithyroid drug include T_3 suppression testing (196), thyrotropin-releasing hormone (TRH) testing (197), and measurements of serum thyroglobulin (198) and antithyroid peroxidase antibodies (199). These tests, if abnormal, indirectly indicate continuing production of TSHR-Ab, and therefore that remission has not occurred. Although each test has its proponents, in a large multicenter study of 451 patients (151) none of these tests had value in individual patients.

Discontinuation of Antithyroid Drug Therapy

In practice, it is most appropriate simply to reduce gradually and then discontinue the antithyroid drug after treatment for 12 to 24 months and follow the patient clinically and with serial measurements of serum TSH. Characteristically, as thyrotoxicosis recurs, serum TSH concentrations decrease, then serum T_3 concentrations increase, and then serum T_4 concentrations increase. However, a decrease in serum TSH concentration does not always mean recurrent thyrotoxicosis is imminent; some patients have low serum TSH concentrations but normal serum T_3 and T_4 concentrations (subclinical thyrotoxicosis) for prolonged periods (see Chapter 79). These latter patients provide evidence that Graves' disease can be subclinical (e.g., a patient can have Graves' thyroid disease without being overtly thyrotoxic), and they have a higher rate of relapse compared with patients who have normal serum TSH concentrations at discontinuation of therapy (200).

Most relapses of thyrotoxicosis occur within 3 to 6 months after antithyroid drug therapy is discontinued (152) (Fig. 45.1); relapses within this interval probably reflect persistent Graves' disease, rather than remission and recurrence of the disease. Thereafter, the rate of relapse gradually declines to near zero. In the older literature, about 60% of patients were still in remission after 4 years (192), but this was before our current ability to assess thyroid function accurately. More recent studies suggest that the rate of recurrent thyrotoxicosis plateaus at about 50% at 5 years (10,11,154,201). Relapse may be particularly likely in the postpartum period; in one study, almost 50% of women who were in remission before becoming pregnant developed recurrent thyrotoxicosis after delivery (202). A controlled trial suggested that this high rate of re-

lapse might be lowered by administration of T_4 during pregnancy (203), but these data have not been confirmed. Because relapses can occur at any time in a patient's life, and hypothyroidism can occur many years after antithyroid drug therapy, lifelong follow-up is recommended for all patients with Graves' disease.

The physician should have in mind a treatment strategy that can be implemented if and when a relapse occurs. In children, a second course of antithyroid drug therapy usually is advised. In young adults, either a second course of antithyroid drug therapy or radioiodine therapy is acceptable, although the likelihood of remission during another course of antithyroid drug therapy may be low. For older adults, radioiodine therapy is usually recommended. Very long-term administration of an antithyroid drug is safe, and some patients may prefer to take a low daily dose of either MMI or PTU for decades rather than receive destructive therapy (204).

In summary, primary antithyroid drug therapy is a reasonable choice in children and younger adults who have mild to moderate thyrotoxicosis caused by Graves' disease and who are likely to be compliant with therapy, in patients who have a bias against radioiodine, and in those with severe ophthalmopathy (see later in the chapter). It is a less reasonable choice as primary therapy for patients with severe biochemical thyrotoxicosis [serum T_3 concentration >600 ng/dL (9.2 nmol/L)] or a large goiter.

OTHER DRUGS USED IN THE TREATMENT OF THYROTOXICOSIS CAUSED BY GRAVES' DISEASE

Inorganic Iodide

The effects of iodide on thyroid function are complex and are discussed in detail in the section on the effect of excess iodide in Chapter 11. The major actions of iodide are to decrease T_4 and T_3 synthesis by inhibiting iodine oxidation and organification (the Wolff-Chaikoff effect), (205) and to block the release of T_4 and T_3 from the thyroid by inhibiting thyroglobulin proteolysis; the latter is the more rapid and prominent action in thyrotoxic patients.

Patients treated with inorganic iodide alone improve quickly, and their serum T_4 and T_3 concentrations decrease substantially, but not usually to within the normal range, in 7 to 14 days (206,207). Subsequently, many patients escape from its inhibitory effects, and their symptoms worsen as their serum T_4 and T_3 concentrations increase. However, in occasional patients with mild thyrotoxicosis, the disease can be controlled for prolonged periods with potassium iodide, given as Lugol's solution (8 mg iodide per drop) or as a saturated solution of potassium iodide (SSKI, 35 to 50 mg iodide per drop) (208). Typical dosages for this and other indications are three to five drops of Lugol's solution three times a day or one drop of SSKI three times a day.

These dosages were empirically derived, and doses in the range of 5 to 10 mg/day would probably suffice.

The three major uses of iodide today are for preparation of patients for surgery, treatment of thyrotoxic storm, and after radioiodine therapy. Preoperative iodide therapy was introduced when iodide was the only available antithyroid drug; in addition to reducing thyroid secretion, it was thought to reduce the vascularity of the thyroid gland. It is primarily for that reason that it is given today (209), usually for 10 days before surgery in patients who have already received antithyroid drug therapy. However, in a controlled study, iodide was not more effective than placebo in reducing operative blood loss or making thyroid gland manipulation easier (210). In patients previously treated only with a β-adrenergic antagonist drug, iodide does reduce thyroid function and blood flow; patients treated with both may have fewer perioperative complications, as compared with patients treated with a β-adrenergic antagonist drug alone (211). Thyroid surgery as therapy for thyrotoxicosis is discussed in detail later.

Patients with severe thyrotoxicosis are sometimes treated with iodide because of its ability to block thyroid hormone release acutely (see Chapter 43). Finally, iodide has been given with mixed success after radioiodine therapy alone (212–214) and rarely in combination with an antithyroid drug (215) to reduce thyroid secretion quickly. However, the combination of iodide and MMI does not result in more rapid lowering of serum T_4 and T_3 concentrations than MMI alone (216). Potassium iodide should be started 1 week after administration of the radioiodine so as not to interfere with thyroid uptake of the radioiodine. Close follow-up is important because hypothyroidism can develop quickly (212), although another study found no effect of iodine versus no therapy after radioiodine treatment (214). Patients treated with radioiodine or surgery are less likely to escape from the inhibitory effects of iodide on iodine oxidation and organification (217), and therefore are more likely to have a sustained antithyroid response (see section on effect of excess iodide in Chapter 11). Thus, iodide can be given as a single agent to patients with recurrent thyrotoxicosis after surgery or after radioiodine therapy.

Iodide cannot be given with impunity. In patients with toxic nodular goiter it can increase serum T_4 and T_3 concentrations and worsen symptoms, especially if the patient's iodine intake was marginal. In addition, although rare, sensitivity to iodine can occur in the form of acneform eruptions (iodism), sialoadenitis, and vasculitis.

Iodinated Radiographic Contrast Agents

Orally administered iodinated radiographic contrast agents used for cholecystography [e.g., sodium iopanoate [Telepaque] and sodium ipodate (Oragrafin)] are iodinated triiodoaniline derivatives that inhibit T_4-deiodinase activity, thereby acutely lowering serum T_3 concentrations (218, 219, and reviewed in 220 and 221). Additionally, the inorganic iodide formed as these compounds are deiodinated *in vivo* inhibits T_4 and T_3 release from the thyroid, and the iodide and perhaps also the compounds themselves inhibit synthesis of T_4 and T_3 (222). In normal subjects, serum T_4 concentrations increase slightly, probably as a result of a decrease in T_4 clearance and perhaps also a decrease in cellular T_4 uptake (223) (see section on effect of drugs and other substances on thyroid hormone synthesis and metabolism in Chapter 11). Although early reports suggested that these agents might be useful as primary therapy for Graves' thyrotoxicosis (224), they have limited value in long-term therapy (225,226), because of escape from the inhibitory effect of iodide on T_4 and T_3 synthesis. In addition, their administration may make subsequent control with an antithyroid drug more difficult, presumably because of the large iodine load (226). Subsequent radioiodine therapy also has to be delayed, because radioiodine uptake remains low for several months (227).

Because it rapidly lowers serum T_3 concentrations, ipodate has been used in conjunction with PTU (228) to decrease thyroid function in patients who required rapid control of thyrotoxicosis (e.g., in preparation for thyroidectomy) (229). In one study, MMI plus ipodate lowered serum T_3 concentrations and pulse rate more rapidly than MMI alone or MMI plus SSKI (216). The results were similar in another study in which ipodate, PTU, and PTU and propranolol were compared (228). These drugs have also been given to lower serum T_3 concentrations in patients with massive T_4 overdose (poisoning) (230), thyrotoxicosis from subacute thyroiditis (231), and amiodarone-induced thyrotoxicosis (232), and in severe neonatal thyrotoxicosis (233). The usual dose is 1 g daily. These agents have few side effects (renal failure with high doses, one reported case of thrombocytopenia), and they have potential benefits in patients with thyrotoxic storm, T_4 poisoning, and other conditions in which both rapid inhibition of thyroid secretion and inhibition of extrathyroidal T_3 production might be beneficial. Iopanoate (Telepaque) and ipodate (Oragrafin) are no longer available in the United States.

The water-soluble radiographic contrast agents given intravenously for angiography, pyelography, and computed tomography also contain large amounts of iodine. They are deiodinated, and the iodide has its expected antithyroid action, but it is short-lived because the agents are very rapidly excreted. The contrast agents themselves have no effects on thyroid hormone secretion or metabolism in normal subjects.

Potassium Perchlorate

The perchlorate anion (ClO_4^-) is a competitive inhibitor of thyroid iodide transport (234). It was used in the past as therapy for thyrotoxicosis but was abandoned because of its side effects (aplastic anemia, gastric ulceration) and because of the advent of MMI and PTU. In doses of 400 to 600 mg/day, it has proven effective (65) and safe. It also has proven effective in combination with an antithyroid drug in patients with iodine-induced thyrotoxicosis. Blockade of iodine transport by perchlorate would seem to be a reasonable adjunct in these patients, who often are resistant to therapy with an antithyroid drug alone (235).

Lithium Carbonate

Lithium is well known to have antithyroid actions, but its mechanism(s) of action is still not understood. It is concentrated by the thyroid (236), probably by active transport. Its primary action is to inhibit T_4 and T_3 release, a process that is stimulated by TSH and mediated by cyclic adenosine monophosphate (237–239). It also may inhibit T_4 and T_3 synthesis (240,241). As with iodide, there is a tendency for the thyroid gland to escape from the inhibitory actions of lithium; therefore, lithium has limited value for long-term treatment of patients with thyrotoxicosis. Lithium has little advantage over MMI (241), and it has many side effects. In practice, it should not be given as primary treatment for thyrotoxicosis, but it is an option for patients with severe thyrotoxicosis who are allergic to iodide, and it may have an adjunctive role in patients treated with radioiodine (see later in the chapter) and in those with amiodarone-induced thyrotoxicosis (242). The dose of lithium is 300 to 450 mg orally every 8 hours, the goal being to maintain serum lithium concentrations in the range of 1 mEq/L.

Beta-Adrenergic Antagonist Drugs

Beta-adrenergic antagonist drugs are useful adjuncts in the treatment of patients with thyrotoxicosis (243). Many of the manifestations of thyrotoxicosis mimic a hyperadrenergic state (244), and blockade of adrenergic receptors provides patients with considerable relief from some symptoms of thyrotoxicosis, notably anxiety, palpitations, tremor, and heat intolerance. Although the clinical benefit is not due to changes in thyroid function, these drugs cause small, clinically unimportant decrements in serum T_3 concentrations because of inhibition of extrathyroidal conversion of T_4 to T_3 (245).

Although these drugs improve the negative nitrogen balance (246) and decrease heart rate (247), cardiac output (248), and oxygen consumption (249) in patients with thyrotoxicosis, these measurements seldom become normal (250). Hence, these drugs are useful as primary therapy only in patients with transient thyrotoxicosis (e.g., the various forms of thyroiditis). On the other hand, they are useful as adjunctive therapy in alleviating symptoms during diagnostic evaluation or while awaiting the results of primary therapy.

Propranolol was the drug of this class originally given to patients with thyrotoxicosis, and it is still used widely, but some newer drugs of this class have a longer duration of action (long-acting propranolol, atenolol, metoprolol, and nadolol) or are more cardioselective (atenolol and metoprolol). The usual starting dose of propranolol is in the range of 80 mg/day; 50 mg/day of atenolol or metoprolol and 40 mg/day of nadolol have similar effects. High doses (e.g., 240 to 360 mg/day of propranolol) are occasionally needed to control symptoms and slow the heart rate (251). Propranolol and the cardioselective drug esmolol can be given intravenously to patients who are acutely ill.

In general, β-adrenergic antagonist drugs are well tolerated. The main side effects are nausea, headache, fatigue, insomnia, and depression; rare side effects are rash, fever, agranulocytosis, and thrombocytopenia. Complications related to the β-adrenergic antagonist actions are more common. Patients with a history of asthma should not be given these drugs, although a patient with mild asthma and, for example, marked tachycardia and palpitations could be given a cardioselective drug. Patients with a history of congestive heart failure also should not be given the drugs, except when the heart failure is clearly rate related or caused by atrial fibrillation (252). Even then, the drug should be given cautiously, preferably with digoxin. These drugs also are contraindicated in patients with bradyarrhythmias or Raynaud's phenomenon, and in patients being treated with a monoamine oxidase inhibitor.

Several studies have examined the potential usefulness of calcium channel–blocking drugs in thyrotoxicosis. In one study, diltiazem reduced resting heart rate by 17%, comparable with what can be achieved with a β-adrenergic antagonist drug (253). Calcium channel blockers have not been widely used in patients with thyrotoxicosis, but they should be considered for patients in whom β-adrenergic drugs are contraindicated.

RADIOACTIVE IODINE THERAPY FOR THYROTOXICOSIS

Since its introduction in the mid-1940s (254), radioiodine therapy has widely used for adults with thyrotoxicosis caused by Graves' disease (2). Although it is less rapidly effective than antithyroid drug therapy, it is in many other ways an ideal form of therapy; it is effective, safe, and relatively inexpensive. ^{131}I is the isotope of choice; other isotopes of iodine (e.g., ^{125}I-iodine) offer no clinical advantage. It is administered orally as a single dose in a capsule or in water, is rapidly and completely absorbed, and is quickly concentrated, oxidized, and organified by thyroid follicular cells. Although ^{131}I emits both β and γ radiation, it is the ionizing effects of the β particles, which have a path length of 1 to 2 mm, that destroy thyroid follicular cells. Because this distance exceeds the diameter of a thyroid cell, adjacent cells are irradiated even if they do not concentrate iodine.

Initially, radioiodine causes cellular necrosis that provokes an inflammatory response (255). Indeed, some patients have mild thyroid tenderness a few days after treatment; others have transient worsening of their thyrotoxicosis, due to leakage of stored T_4 and T_3 from disrupted follicles into the circulation (256). Histologically, cellular necrosis and inflammation are seen, as are bizarre nuclear changes reminiscent of carcinoma (257); the latter can persist for years and can cause confusion in the interpretation of thyroid cytology. Therefore, if a patient has a nodule that warrants biopsy, this should be done before radioiodine is given (258). Over time, chronic inflammation and fibrosis result in a substantial decrease in the size of the thyroid gland, ultimately and perhaps inevitably resulting in hypothyroidism. Some patients have relatively normal thyroid function for years or even decades, but they are in the minority.

Practical Therapeutic Considerations

Although worldwide experience in the use of radioiodine is vast, no unanimity of opinion exists concerning the optimal radioiodine dose or the most satisfactory method of dose calculation. In general, a dose that will deliver about 50 to 150 Gy (5000 to 15,000 rad) to the thyroid reduces thyroid hormone secretion to normal or below normal in patients with Graves' disease, but higher doses are required in patients with toxic nodular goiter. To achieve doses in this range, various factors must be considered, including the size of the thyroid, its avidity for iodine (i.e., the 6- or 24-hour radioiodine uptake), the turnover of radioiodine within the gland, the physical half-life of the isotope (8 days in the case of ^{131}I), and prior or planned antithyroid drug therapy, which may necessitate higher doses (see later discussion). When an antithyroid drug is given before radioiodine therapy, it should be discontinued for at least 3 days, lest it interfere with radioiodine organification or possibly act as a free radical scavenger (259), thereby diminishing the radiation effect.

Although estimations of gland size by physical examination are unreliable, the use of measurements of gland volume by ultrasonography for dose calculation does not improve outcome (260). Calculation of the biologic half-life of radioiodine is laborious but may be useful (261). Several less quantitative methods for determining radioiodine dosage have been proposed, including giving all patients the same fixed dosage (262,263). One common approach

(264) is to use the following formula, in which the administered dose is (in millicuries):

$$\frac{80\text{--}120 \ \mu Ci \ ^{131}I/g \ of \ thyroid \times estimated \ thyroid \ gland \ weight(g)}{24\text{-}h \ radioiodine \ uptake}$$

Using this formula, typical doses are in the range of 5 to 15 mCi (185 to 555 MBq), yielding a radiation dose of 50 to 100 Gy (5000 to 10,000 rad). The choice of microcuries per gram of thyroid tissue is empiric; higher doses should be given to patients with a relatively low 24-hour radioiodine uptake (<50%), a large goiter, those with severe thyrotoxicosis (associated with more rapid intrathyroidal iodine turnover), and those with a toxic nodular goiter. The dose should also be increased by 25% in patients treated with an antithyroid drug before and those who will be treated with one after radioiodine administration (265) (see later in the chapter). In a recent retrospective analysis the patients who failed to respond to therapy were young and had a large thyroid gland, more severe thyrotoxicosis, prior exposure to an antithyroid drug, or a higher radioiodine uptake value, as compared with those in whom treatment was successful (266). The authors recommended a dose that would deliver 11 mCi (407 MBq) of radioiodine for such patients, compared with a dose of 8 mCi (296 MBq) for the majority of patients. It also seems sensible to give higher doses to patients who require a second dose of radioiodine and to those patients in whom the risk of persistent disease should be minimized, such as the elderly or those with cardiac disease.

Some have suggested that large doses should be given to most patients and that hypothyroidism should be accepted as a desired consequence, rather than as a side effect, of therapy (267,268). Most patients become euthyroid, regardless of how the dose is determined (269), and ultimately develop hypothyroidism; lowering the likelihood of hypothyroidism by lowering the dose simply results in delay or failure to cure the thyrotoxicosis (270), necessitates additional therapy, and only delays hypothyroidism (271,272). Giving a fixed dose of radioiodine may simplify and reduce the cost of therapy, because radioiodine uptake need not be measured, and in randomized trials the outcome was similar in patients given calculated doses and those given fixed doses (262,263).

Thyroid secretion declines gradually within weeks to months after radioiodine treatment. Symptoms can be controlled during this interval with a β-adrenergic antagonist drug, if necessary; occasional patients may benefit from antithyroid drug or potassium iodide therapy, as discussed earlier. If either is given, it should be discontinued after several months to determine the efficacy of the radioiodine. The rate at which improvement occurs depends on factors that are poorly understood, but almost certainly include the initial level of thyroid function, the size of the thyroid, and the

rate of intrathyroidal radioiodine turnover, as well as the dose of radioiodine. Although no relationship between serum TSHR-Ab values and outcome was found in several studies (273,274), an inverse correlation between serum TSHR-Ab concentrations at baseline and the response to radioiodine was found in other studies (275,276). Serum TSHR-Ab concentrations tend to increase during the first year after radioiodine therapy, and then decline (273). This may be the cause of the post-radioiodine exacerbations that occasionally occur several months after therapy (277).

In general, 50% to 75% of patients have normal thyroid function and some shrinkage of goiter within 6 to 8 weeks after radioiodine therapy (278). Overall, over 80% to 90% of patients become euthyroid or hypothyroid after one dose of radioiodine (given according to the formula discussed earlier), 10% to 20% require a second dose, and a rare patient needs a third dose (278). The figures vary when other treatment philosophies are used. Because radioiodine sometimes acts slowly, an additional dose should not be given for 6 to 12 months.

Complications and Potential Risks of Radioiodine Therapy

Hypothyroidism

Hypothyroidism is an inevitable consequence of radioiodine therapy (279). In the past several decades its frequency has increased, and it has appeared sooner after radioiodine administration (280–282), probably because of the use of higher doses as well as the increased ease of detection of hypothyroidism using serum TSH determinations. Hypothyroidism develops in as many as 90% of patients within the first year after therapy (280), with a continuing rate of 2% to 3% per year thereafter. The rapidity with which hypothyroidism develops may relate to not only the dose of radioiodine but also immunologic factors; for example, hypothyroidism is particularly common in patients who have high serum antithyroid peroxidase antibody concentrations (283). Therapy with an antithyroid drug, given before or soon after radioiodine treatment, may lessen the rate of hypothyroidism and increase the risk of persistent thyrotoxicosis (284,285); one retrospective study suggested that these changes in the efficacy of radioiodine therapy were more frequent with PTU than MMI (286). In contrast, two prospective randomized trials found no effect of MMI pretreatment on the outcome of radioiodine therapy (287,288). In another prospective study the frequency of hypothyroidism 1 year later was higher in patients given MMI 4 days after radioiodine therapy as compared with patients treated with radioiodine alone (289).

In addition to permanent hypothyroidism, some patients have transient hypothyroidism (290–293), possibly due to transient thyroid injury, persistent TSH suppression, or both. Transient hypothyroidism usually occurs about 2 months after therapy and lasts for 1 to 4 months; serum TSH concentrations are often low, indicative of persistent suppression of TSH secretion. If hypothyroidism develops in the first 2 months after radioiodine therapy, particularly if there is persistence of goiter (293), therapy with T_4 may be withheld for 1 to 2 months unless the patient is unacceptably symptomatic.

Thyroid and Other Tumors

Despite the advantages of radioiodine therapy, it continues to be a controversial form of treatment, particularly for children and young adults (294). The major concern has been the possible carcinogenic effects of ionizing radiation, particularly late effects that might not be detected for decades. It is clear that external head and neck irradiation is associated with an increased rate of thyroid carcinoma (see section on pathogenesis of thyroid carcinoma in Chapter 70). However, notwithstanding a few case reports (295), there is little evidence that radioiodine therapy for thyrotoxicosis is a risk factor for thyroid carcinoma (296–302). With the exception of small bowel cancer in one study (303), there is no evidence for increased mortality from any other form of cancer (298–301), including leukemia (301,304).

Long-term follow-up data on radioiodine therapy in children and adolescents are sparse. In one study (296), thyroid adenomas appeared to be more frequent in patients who received radioiodine therapy as children or adolescents. In the largest studies dealing exclusively with children (305–307), the longest of which had a 14-year follow-up, the incidence of thyroid carcinoma, leukemia, or other cancers was not increased, nor was there evidence of abnormal reproductive histories in women. In a smaller study, 3 of 18 children treated with radioiodine developed thyroid nodules, one of which was a low-grade follicular carcinoma (308). Thus, because extensive long-term follow-up data are not available for children, most are treated with an antithyroid drug. Radioiodine has gained increasing acceptability as a first-choice therapy in adolescents (294). A more complete discussion of the treatment of thyrotoxicosis in children can be found at the end of this section and in Chapter 76.

Teratogenicity and Chromosomal Damage

Pregnancy, or the possibility of pregnancy, is an absolute contraindication to radioiodine therapy. Thus, a history of recent menses or a pregnancy test must be obtained in all sexually active women before the administration of radioiodine. In those rare women given radioiodine inadvertently before the 10th week of pregnancy (before the fetal thyroid can concentrate iodine), the outcome was normal

(309). If the radioiodine is given later, the fetal thyroid may be damaged, with consequent fetal hypothyroidism. Candid discussion with the parents is required in this unfortunate circumstance. Management options include fetal blood sampling for measurement of serum TSH, maternal or intraamniotic T_4 therapy, and careful follow-up with immediate evaluation at the time of birth. Among them the latter is most appropriate, given that infants with spontaneously occurring congenital hypothyroidism are normal at birth (see Chapter 75).

A more far-reaching question is that of possible genetic damage from radioiodine, with consequent deleterious health effects on the offspring of treated patients. Several studies have documented leukocyte chromosomal abnormalities in patients who received therapeutic doses of radioiodine (310,311), and minor abnormalities in those who received as little as 20 mCi (740 MBq) (312), but the clinical importance of these findings is uncertain. The whole body is exposed to radiation after radioiodine therapy, with gonadal radiation of particular concern because of γ irradiation from radioiodine in the urinary bladder. The estimates of the gonadal (ovarian) radiation dose after radioiodine therapy have varied by more than tenfold (313). A rough estimate of the dose is about 0.2 rad/mCi (0.054 Gy/Bq) of administered radioiodine (313), so that the dose to the ovaries would be 1 to 3 rad (0.01 to 0.03 Gy) for a woman receiving a usual therapeutic dose of 10 mCi (370 MBq). This dose is similar to that from several commonly performed radiologic procedures (e.g., barium enema and intravenous pyelography). The genetic risk of radioiodine therapy is less than the spontaneous rate of genetic abnormalities (0.003% or less vs. 0.8%), estimates that are borne out by the negative clinical data that are available (305, 306,314). Thus, Safa and colleagues (306) found no increase in congenital abnormalities in 86 children of 43 women who received radioiodine therapy as children. In a related study, none of 33 children of women who received radioiodine had cytogenetic abnormalities (315). In summary, there is no evidence that radioiodine therapy for thyrotoxicosis has adverse effects on the health of the offspring of treated patients. It seems prudent, however, to advise that pregnancy be avoided for at least 6 months after radioiodine therapy and until thyroid function is normal (316).

Despite these reassuring data, unnecessary exposure to radioiodine by family members, particularly children, should be minimized (317). It is almost impossible to avoid minor exposure as a result of environmental contamination (318). Because most of the radioactivity is excreted in the urine, patients should be instructed to use appropriate hygienic measures. Small amounts of radioiodine appear in the saliva, so that recently treated patients should not share food or drink with others and should avoid kissing them for several days after therapy. Because the thyroid is a source of γ radiation, parents are usually instructed not to hug their children for several days, and close contact with pregnant women should be avoided for a similar time period (318). Intimate physical contact should be avoided for several days. Lactation is also an absolute contraindication to radioiodine therapy because iodine is secreted into milk.

Miscellaneous Side Effects

There are no allergic reactions to radioiodine, even among people who are sensitive to iodide or iodinated contrast agents, because the mass of iodine in a typical radioiodine dose is only 1 mg (279). Persons who are allergic to radiographic contrast agents and seafood (allergic to proteins in the meat, not iodine) can safely be treated with radioiodine. Occasional patients note nausea, possibly caused by radiation gastritis. Mild anterior neck pain, caused by radiation thyroiditis, occurs rarely and is easily treated with a nonsteroidal antiinflammatory drug. Other rare associations with radioiodine therapy, not necessarily complications, are hypoparathyroidism, hyperparathyroidism, and vocal cord palsy (279).

Postradioiodine Worsening of Thyroid Function

Occasional transient exacerbation of thyrotoxicosis (256), possibly more frequent in patients with a toxic multinodular goiter (319), and very rare instances of thyrotoxic storm (320,321) have been reported as a result of release of T_4 and T_3 from the damaged thyroid follicles, but the transient increase in serum hormone concentrations usually is clinically silent, particularly in patients treated with a β-adrenergic antagonist drug.

Because MMI and PTU block the synthesis but not the release of T_4 and T_3, they deplete hormonal stores within the thyroid. In patients with severe thyrotoxicosis, elderly patients, and patients with cardiac disease, pretreatment with one of these drugs is prudent, not only because thyroid secretion is normalized sooner, but also because pretreatment may minimize the risk of aggravation of thyrotoxicosis after radioiodine therapy. Pretreatment is not necessary in most young patients with thyrotoxicosis. While pretreatment may not prevent worsening of thyroid function after radioiodine, the occasional biochemical exacerbations are less severe because the post-therapy level of thyroid function is reduced due to the pretreatment (322,323). Thyroid function may worsen in the few days between discontinuation of an antithyroid drug and administration of radioiodine, but the change is small and of little clinical importance (323,324). However, if that is a concern clinically, lithium given on the day of antithyroid drug withdrawal prevents any deterioration of thyroid function caused by antithyroid drug withdrawal (325).

Lithium therapy after radioiodine treatment may also prevent post-therapy worsening of thyroid function (326).

Radioiodine Therapy and Graves' Ophthalmopathy

The relationship between radioiodine therapy and the subsequent development or worsening of Graves' ophthalmopathy is an area of continuing controversy (327,328). Two large retrospective studies failed to document a relationship between the type of therapy for Graves' thyrotoxicosis (an antithyroid drug, radioiodine, or surgery) and subsequent changes in the eyes (329,330). Some other studies found that radioiodine therapy may lead to the development or worsening of ophthalmopathy (331–334), possibly because of the release of thyroid antigens and an increase in serum TSHR-Ab concentrations after therapy (273,335,336).

This question was examined in three prospective controlled studies of different antithyroid treatments. In the first, of 114 patients randomly assigned to treatment with MMI, surgery, or radioiodine, ophthalmopathy developed or worsened in 10%, 16%, and 33% of patients, respectively, during a 2-year follow-up period (333). The patients who received radioiodine became hypothyroid for a few weeks before T$_4$ therapy was initiated, whereas the drug and surgery groups were not hypothyroid at any time. Since other data suggest that post-therapy hypothyroidism may be related to worsening ophthalmopathy (337), there is the possibility that it was the posttherapy hypothyroidism rather than the radioiodine therapy *per se* that was responsible for the increased risk of ophthalmopathy in this study.

In the second prospective study, 40 patients with Graves' disease were randomly assigned to be treated with radioiodine or surgery. The likelihood of worsening after therapy was similar in the two groups (45% vs. 35%) (338). In the third study, 3% of 148 patients treated with MMI had the onset or worsening of eye disease, as compared with 15% of 150 patients treated with radioiodine, during a 1-year follow-up period (Fig. 45.6) (334). Among the radioiodine-treated patients, ophthalmopathy developed or worsened in 6% of nonsmokers as compared with 23% of smokers, suggesting that smoking may be an additional risk factor for radioiodine-related worsening of eye disease (339). The post-radioiodine therapy development or worsening of ophthalmopathy may be preventable by glucocorticoid therapy (0.4 to 0.5 mg/kg prednisone/day) for 3 months beginning immediately after radioiodine administration (331,334).

Based on these results, patients with Graves' thyrotoxicosis should be counseled that eye disease is more likely to occur or worsen after radioiodine therapy than antithyroid drug (or surgical) therapy. They should also be counseled

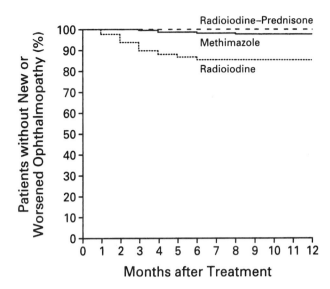

FIGURE 45.6. Kaplan-Meier plot showing the percentages of patients with Graves' thyrotoxicosis treated with radioiodine, radioiodine plus prednisone, or methimazole (MMI) who developed or had progression of ophthalmopathy during or after therapy. At 12 months there were 145 (of 145) patients in the radioiodine-prednisone group, 144 (of 148) patients in the MMI group, and 127 (of 150) patients in the radioiodine group. (From Bartalena L, Marcocci C, Bogazzi F, et al. Relation between therapy for hyperthyroidism and the course of Graves' ophthalmopathy. *N Engl J Med* 1998;338:73, with permission.)

about the risks and benefits of adjunctive glucocorticoid therapy.

Indications for Radioiodine Therapy

The indications for radioiodine therapy remain somewhat controversial. Although children and adolescents are being treated with radioiodine with increasing frequency (294), an antithyroid drug is usually preferred in these age groups (2). Others believe that all patients with thyrotoxicosis caused by Graves' disease should be given a trial of antithyroid drug therapy, in the hope that a remission will occur. However, remissions are uncommon in patients with moderate or severe thyrotoxicosis. For them, therefore, radioiodine is the most appropriate and perhaps cost-effective therapy, because it permanently ameliorates thyrotoxicosis quickly and safely.

SURGICAL THERAPY FOR THYROTOXICOSIS

Subtotal thyroidectomy is the oldest form of therapy for thyrotoxicosis. Although surgery was the only available therapy for many decades, it is presently performed in the United States only under special circumstances: in children, adolescents, and pregnant women who are allergic to or noncompliant with antithyroid drugs; in patients with large goiters or severe ophthalmopathy (340); and in patients who prefer destructive therapy but are apprehensive about radioiodine therapy (341).

Subtotal thyroidectomy usually is defined as removal of most of the thyroid gland, leaving a few grams of the posterior portion of each lobe (see Chapter 17) (342). Many surgeons now recommend total or near total thyroidectomy rather than subtotal thyroidectomy because of the possibility of recurrent thyrotoxicosis due to thyroid regrowth with the latter procedure (343). Although the mortality of subtotal or total thyroidectomy now is close to zero (342–345), two worrisome complications of surgery can occur, albeit rarely (1% to 2%), even in the most expert hands: recurrent laryngeal nerve damage and hypoparathyroidism. Other complications are transient hypocalcemia, postoperative bleeding, wound infection, and formation of keloids or otherwise unsightly scars. Although the skill of the surgeon is of paramount importance in avoiding perioperative morbidity (346), the number of surgeons experienced in performing thyroidectomy has decreased as other therapies increasingly dominate the treatment of thyrotoxicosis.

In a recent meta-analysis of thyroid surgery for Graves' disease, 100% of patients who underwent a total thyroidectomy were hypothyroid and remained so after follow-up periods ranging from 4 to 12 years (343). In contrast, after subtotal thyroidectomy, hypothyroidism occurs in the first postoperative year in 12% to 80% of patients (341, 347,348), with late-onset hypothyroidism in an additional 1% to 3% per year (347), possibly reflecting the natural history of Graves' disease. The development of hypothyroidism depends on several factors, most importantly the size of the thyroid remnant, but also the presence of antithyroid antibodies, perhaps reflecting autoimmune destruction of the remnant (349), and the duration of follow-up. In addition, 5% to 15% of patients have recurrent thyrotoxicosis (342–344,350,351). It is more common in patients who before treatment have high serum TSHR-Ab concentrations (352) and severe ophthalmopathy (353); these patients should have a total rather than a subtotal thyroidectomy. The recurrences may develop many years after surgery; in one study, 43% developed more than 5 years after surgery (354). Radioiodine is the treatment of choice for patients who have recurrent thyrotoxicosis after subtotal thyroidectomy.

Preoperative treatment has changed in recent years. Although an antithyroid drug in combination with inorganic iodide was standard therapy for several decades, many now recommend a β-adrenergic antagonist drug, with or without iodide (211,348,355). The latter regimen allows surgery to be performed sooner rather than later, because it has been customary to give the antithyroid drug until the patient is euthyroid, which may take 4 to 6 weeks, and then give iodide for 10 to 14 more days before surgery. The

propranolol (or similar drug) regimens consist of treatment for several weeks with doses sufficient to lower the resting pulse rate to <80 beats/min, with or without potassium iodide, for 10 to 14 days before surgery. Patients treated with propranolol are not clinically or biochemically euthyroid when they undergo surgery, even if they are also treated with iodide (356), and may still have high serum T_4 concentrations and require continued propranolol therapy postoperatively. Furthermore, patients treated in this way have more postoperative problems (e.g., fever and tachycardia), especially those with severe thyrotoxicosis (355–357). Therefore, unless surgery must be performed quickly for some reason, it seems wiser to treat patients who are to undergo surgery in the traditional manner with an antithyroid drug and then iodide. If surgery must be performed urgently, preparation for several days with a β-adrenergic antagonist drug (propranolol 40 mg every 6 hours), high doses of a glucocorticoid and dexamethasone should be safe and effective (229).

The addition of iodide (one to three drops of SSKI daily) to the traditional antithyroid drug regimen 10 days before surgery is controversial because of the lack of convincing evidence that it decreases blood loss during surgery (210), despite studies demonstrating a decrease in thyroid blood flow (209,358). Nevertheless, it is a commonly recommended practice (342). Even if it does not affect blood loss, its antithyroid action is helpful.

SPECIAL CONSIDERATIONS IN THE TREATMENT OF THYROTOXICOSIS

Treatment of Children and Adolescents

Children and adolescents can be treated with radioiodine (294), but an antithyroid drug is preferable, if only for the reason that most of the patients and their parents prefer to avoid destructive therapy and what it entails (see Chapter 76) (2,3). MMI is the drug of choice because of the ease of once-a-day administration. If antithyroid drugs are unsatisfactory or not tolerated, either radioiodine therapy or surgery is appropriate. Although radioiodine has obvious advantages over surgery, not the least being cost, surgery is still as acceptable alternative because of lingering doubts about radioiodine-induced carcinogenesis and genetic damage (359).

Children and adolescents with Graves' thyrotoxicosis are usually treated for many months or even many years; therefore, data on remission rates as a function of duration of treatment are available (172,360). These data suggest that longer periods of therapy are associated with more frequent remission; in one study (172), >75% of patients were in remission after treatment for about 11 years. On the other hand, some children and adolescents ultimately require radioiodine because of drug side effects (which may be more common in children and adolescents), poor compliance with drug therapy, or failure to achieve long-term remission (361–363).

Treatment of Elderly Patients

Elderly patients respond well to antithyroid drug therapy, and they are probably more likely to have a remission than are younger patients (167). Nevertheless, in the United States most are treated with radioiodine (2). They are more often pretreated with an antithyroid drug to reduce the risk of exacerbation of thyrotoxicosis after radioiodine therapy, which seems prudent (364). Antithyroid drug therapy may be resumed after radioiodine administration to ensure continuing euthyroidism while the radioiodine is taking effect (365). In patients with mild thyrotoxicosis, a β-adrenergic antagonist drug can be given as sole adjunctive therapy, both before and after radioiodine, with the usual caveats about these drugs in patients with underlying cardiac or pulmonary disease. With regard to the radioiodine dose, it should be high enough to ensure prompt resolution of the thyrotoxicosis, with a minimum chance for recurrence.

Most elderly patients in the United States with thyrotoxicosis probably have Graves' disease (366), but the frequency of solitary toxic adenoma and toxic multinodular goiter as the cause increases sharply with age (see later discussion). Patients with thyroid nodular disease usually require higher doses of radioiodine, because the goiters may be large and the radioiodine uptake relatively low (367). Hospitalization is required is some states in the United States if more than 30 mCi (1110 MBq) of radioiodine is given, and in some countries hospitalization is required even if very low doses are to be given. Patients with a toxic multinodular goiter should not be given iodide after radioiodine therapy or in preparation for surgery, for fear of exacerbating the thyrotoxicosis (368).

Thyrotoxicosis in Pregnant Women and during Lactation

Pregnancy

A full discussion of this topic is beyond the scope of this chapter; additional information can be found in Chapter 80 and in recent reviews (369). An antithyroid drug is the treatment of choice for pregnant women with thyrotoxicosis. In North America, PTU has usually been preferred because it has been thought that its fractional transfer to the fetus was less than that of MMI (82). However, this may not be the case (370). MMI is an acceptable alternative to PTU (371,372), and in fact it is the first-line drug in pregnant women in many parts of the world. A minor birth de-

fect (aplasia cutis) and more severe birth defects (MMI "embryopathy") have been rarely associated with MMI, and the latter anomaly even more rarely with PTU (373–375). This embryopathy includes choanal atresia and/or esophageal atresia.

Except for the very rare congenital abnormalities described above, antithyroid drugs are not teratogenic (376), but neonatal thyroid function can be affected by their transplacental passage. Fetal wastage and maternal morbidity are important problems in pregnant women with untreated or inadequately treated thyrotoxicosis (377), but to minimize fetal exposure to the antithyroid drug the dose should be just adequate, keeping the serum free T_4 value in the upper part of the normal range or slightly high (371, 378). Fortunately, thyrotoxicosis, which in pregnant women is nearly always caused by Graves' disease, often spontaneously improves in the later months of pregnancy, permitting the dose of drug to be lowered or even discontinued (378). Doses of PTU <150 mg/day are seldom associated with fetal thyroid dysfunction (379). If affected, neonatal thyroid function usually is only slightly depressed (380), it recovers quickly after delivery, and children exposed to an antithyroid drug in utero have no developmental or intellectual deficits (381,382). Combined antithyroid drug and T_4 therapy is not recommended because it does not prevent neonatal hypothyroidism and because it may result in the administration of higher doses of the antithyroid drug than are necessary. After delivery, there often is an exacerbation of mild thyrotoxicosis in the mother (202).

Other drugs may be given to pregnant women with thyrotoxicosis. A β-adrenergic antagonist drug can be given to alleviate bothersome symptoms and usually is considered to be safe in pregnancy (369). However, long-term treatment was associated with spontaneous abortion in one report (383). One of these drugs also can be given for preoperative therapy, should that become necessary because the patient is allergic to or noncompliant with antithyroid drug therapy. Potassium iodide also could be given preoperatively. Long-term iodide therapy was thought to be contraindicated in pregnant women because of the risk of development of fetal goiter, but in a Japanese study of pregnant women with mild thyrotoxicosis treated with 6 to 40 mg/day of potassium iodide alone, starting as early as 11 weeks of gestation, no fetal or neonatal abnormalities were noted (384).

Lactation

Antithyroid drug therapy is probably safe in nursing mothers, based not only on measurements of drug in milk but also clinical studies of breastfed infants. Although the concentration of MMI in milk is higher than that of PTU, neither drug has deleterious effects on thyroid function in newborn infants (95,385–388). It seems reasonable to permit breast feeding in women who desire to do so. The American Academy of Pediatrics has judged both PTU and MMI to be compatible with safe breast feeding (389).

THYROTOXIC STORM

Thyrotoxic storm is a rare condition characterized by uncompensated thyrotoxicosis, with fever, tachycardia or tachyarrhythmia, and altered mental status (99). It is almost always precipitated by an event such as infection, surgery, or trauma in a previously untreated or poorly controlled patient. Thyrotoxic storm is considered in detail in Chapter 43 and elsewhere in this book.

THYROTOXICOSIS DUE TO TOXIC ADENOMA AND MULTINODULAR GOITER

Toxic adenoma and multinodular goiter are unusual causes of thyrotoxicosis in young adults, but are more common among older adults (390,391). Treatment is rather straightforward; because the problem is intrinsic thyroid autonomy rather than external stimulation, spontaneous remissions do not occur. Therefore, an antithyroid drug is rarely the treatment of choice, except as preparation for therapy with radioiodine or surgery (392–395). In most patients with a toxic adenoma, the hyperthyroidism can be cured with radioiodine; posttreatment hypothyroidism is less common than in Graves' disease because the radioiodine is not concentrated by the suppressed, normal paranodular tissue (396–398). Even after a euthyroid state has been achieved however, the nodule may not disappear (399).

Theoretical arguments have been presented suggesting that the paranodular tissue receives potentially carcinogenic doses of γ radiation from the large doses of radioiodine sometimes required to treat these patients (400), but carcinoma is so rare that it is likely coincidental (295). Large doses of radioiodine may be needed to treat patients with a toxic adenoma, but 90% of patients were cured with a mean radioiodine dose of 10 mCi (370 MBq) in one study (396). On the other hand, surgery would be reasonable in a young patient with a large (>5 cm) adenoma. Ethanol injections have been used successfully for treatment of thyroid adenomas in Europe (401), but multiple injections that are often painful are needed, and therefore the procedure has not gained wide acceptance.

Most patients with toxic multinodular goiters are over 50 years old, and they often have other illnesses. Particular care must be taken to eliminate thyrotoxicosis in these patients. They may require large and often multiple doses of radioiodine (402), although a study from the United Kingdom found a higher cure rate at 6 months in patients with toxic nodular goiter than in patients with Graves' disease (403). Most patients should be treated initially with an antithyroid drug to reduce thyroid function quickly and to minimize the risk of exacerbation after radioiodine administration. Even if the thyrotoxicosis is cured, there may be little change in thyroid size because the goiters often contain many poorly or nonfunctioning nodules as well as the hyperfunctioning ones. Thus, surgery may be a better option in patients with a very large goiter, especially if there is evidence of tracheal narrowing or substernal extension; functional airway compromise from a goiter, substernal or otherwise, is an indication for surgery.

REFERENCES

1. McIver B, Morris JC. The pathogenesis of Graves' disease. *Endocrinol Metab Clin North Am* 1998;27:73.
2. Solomon B, Glinoer D, Lagasse R, et al. Current trends in the management of Graves' disease. *J Clin Endocrinol Metab* 1990; 70:1518.
3. Wartofsky L, Glinoer D, Solomon B, et al. Differences and similarities in the diagnosis and treatment of Graves' disease in Europe, Japan, and the United States. *Thyroid* 1991;1:129.
4. Hirota Y, Tamai H, Hayashi Y, et al. Thyroid function and histology in forty-five patients with hyperthyroid Graves' disease in clinical remission more than ten years after thionamide drug treatment. *J Clin Endocrinol Metab* 1986;62:165.
5. Wood LC, Ingbar SH. Hypothyroidism as a late sequela in patients with Graves' disease treated with antithyroid agents. *J Clin Invest* 1979;64:1429.
6. Tamai H, Hirota Y, Kasagi K, et al. The mechanism of spontaneous hypothyroidism in patients with Graves' disease after antithyroid drug treatment. *J Clin Endocrinol Metab* 1987;64: 718.
7. Tamai H, Kasagi K, Takaichi Y, et al. Development of spontaneous hypothyroidism in patients with Graves' disease treated with antithyroidal drugs: clinical, immunological, and histological findings in 26 patients. *J Clin Endocrinol Metab* 1989;69: 49.
8. Astwood EB. Treatment of hyperthyroidism with thiourea and thiouracil. *JAMA* 1943;122:78.
9. Astwood EB. Chemotherapy of hyperthyroidism. *Harvey Lect* 1944;40:195.
10. Sugrue D, McEvoy M, Feely J, et al. Hyperthyroidism in the land of Graves: results of treatment by surgery, radio-iodine and carbimazole in 837 cases. *QJM* 1980;49:51.
11. Hedley AJ, Young RE, Jones SJ, et al. Antithyroid drugs in the treatment of hyperthyroidism of Graves' disease: long-term follow-up of 434 patients. *Clin Endocrinol (Oxf)* 1989;31:209.
12. Jansson R, Dahlberg PA, Lindstrom B. Comparative bioavailability of carbimazole and methimazole. *Int J Clin Pharm Ther Toxicol* 1983;21:505.
13. Richter CR, Clisby KH. Toxic effects of the bitter tasting phenylthiocarbamide. *Arch Pathol* 1942;33:46.
14. MacKenzie JB, MacKenzie CG, McCollum EV. The effect of sulfanilylguanidine on the thyroid of the rat. *Science* 1941;94: 518.
15. MacKenzie CG, MacKenzie JB. Effect of sulfonamides and thioureas on the thyroid gland and basal metabolism. *Endocrinology* 1943;32:185.
16. Astwood EB, Sullivan J, Bissell A, et al. Action of certain sulfonamides and of thiourea upon the function of the thyroid gland of the rat. *Endocrinology* 1943;32:210.

17. Vanderlaan WP. Antithyroid drugs in hyperthyroidism. In: Van Middlesworth L, ed. *The thyroid gland.* Chicago: Year Book Medical Publishers, 1986:333.

18. Lazarus JH, Marchant B, Alexander WD, et al. 35S-antithyroid drug concentration and organic binding of iodine in the human thyroid. *Clin Endocrinol (Oxf)* 1975;4:609.

19. Marchant B, Alexander WD. The thyroid accumulation, oxidation and metabolic rate of 35S-methimazole in the rat. *Endocrinology* 1972;91:747.

20. Marchant B, Alexander WD, Robertson JWK, et al. Concentration of 35S-propylthiouracil by the thyroid gland and its relationship to anion trapping mechanism. *Metabolism* 1971; 20:989.

21. Connell JMC, Ferguson MM, Chang DSC, Alexander WD. Influence of sodium perchlorate on thioureylene antithyroid drug accumulation in mice. *J Endocrinol* 1983;98:183.

22. Davidson B, Soodak M, Neary JT, et al. The irreversible inactivation of thyroid peroxidase by methylmercaptoimidazole, thiouracil, and propylthiouracil in vitro and its relationship to in vivo findings. *Endocrinology* 1978;103:871.

23. Taurog A, Dorris M. A reexamination of the proposed inactivation of thyroid peroxidase in the rat thyroid by propylthiouracil. *Endocrinology* 1989;124:3038.

24. Engler H, Taurog A, Dorris ML. Preferential inhibition of thyroxine and 3,5,3′-triiodothyronine formation by propylthiouracil and methylmercaptoimidazole in thyroid peroxidase-catalyzed iodination of thyroglobulin. *Endocrinology* 1982;110:190.

25. Papapetrou PD, Mothon S, Alexander WD. Binding of the 35-S of 35S-propylthiouracil by follicular thyroglobulin in vivo and in vitro. *Acta Endocrinol* 1975;79:248.

26. Monaco F, Santolamazza C, DeRos I, et al. Effects of propylthiouracil and methylmercaptoimidazole on thyroglobulin synthesis. *Acta Endocrinol* 1980;93:32.

27. Jansson R, Dahlberg PA, Johansson H, et al. Intrathyroidal concentrations of methimazole in patients with Graves' disease. *J Clin Endocrinol Metab* 1983;57:129.

28. Taniguchi S, Yoshida A, Mashiba H. Direct effect of methimazole on rat thyroidal cell growth induced by thyrotropin and insulin-like growth factor I. *Endocrinology* 1989;124:2046.

29. Korytkowski M, Cooper D. Antithyroid drug effects on function and growth of FRTL-5 cells. *Thyroid* 1992;2:345.

30. Leonard JL, Rosenberg IN. Thyroxine 5′-deiodinase activity of rat kidney: observations on activation by thiols and inhibition by propylthiouracil. *Endocrinology* 1978;103:2137.

31. Berry MJ, Kieffer JD, Harney JW, et al. Selenocysteine confers the biochemical properties characteristic of the type I iodothyronine deiodinase. *J Biol Chem* 1991;266:14155.

32. Visser TJ, Overmeeren EV. Binding of radioiodinated propylthiouracil to rat liver microsomal fractions. *Biochem J* 1979; 183:167.

33. Visser TJ, Overmeeren E, Fekkes D, et al. Inhibition of iodothyronine 5′-deiodinase by thioureylenes: structure-activity relationship. *FEBS Lett* 1979;103:314.

34. Volpe R. Evidence that the immunosuppressive effects of antithyroid drug are mediated through actions on the thyroid cell, modulating thyrocyte-immunocyte signaling. *Thyroid* 1994;4: 217.

35. Wartofsky L. Has the use of antithyroid drugs of Graves' disease become obsolete? *Thyroid* 1993;3:335.

36. Weetman AP, McGregor AM, Hall R. Evidence for an effect of antithyroid drugs on the natural history of Graves' disease. *Clin Endocrinol (Oxf)* 1984;24:163.

37. Bagnasco M, Venuti D, Ciprandi G, et al. The effect of methimazole on the immune system is unlikely to operate directly on T lymphocytes. *J Endocrinol Invest* 1990;13:493.

38. Wall JR, Manwar GL, Greenwood DM, et al. The in vitro suppression of lectin induced 3H-thymidine incorporation into DNA of peripheral blood lymphocytes after the addition of propylthiouracil. *J Clin Endocrinol Metab* 1976;43: 1406.

39. Balazs C, Kiss E, Leovey A, et al. The immunosuppressive effect of methimazole on cell-mediated immunity is mediated by its capacity to inhibit peroxidase and to scavenge free oxygen radicals. *Clin Endocrinol (Oxf)* 1986;25:7.

40. Hallengren B, Forsgren A, Melander A. Effects of antithyroid drugs on lymphocyte function in vitro. *J Clin Endocrinol Metab* 1980;51:298.

41. Weiss I, Davies TF. Inhibition of immunoglobulin secreting cells by antithyroid drugs. *J Clin Endocrinol Metab* 1981;53: 1223.

42. Imamura M, Aoki N, Saito T, et al. Inhibitory effects of antithyroid drugs on oxygen radical formation in human neutrophils. *Acta Endocrinol* 1986;112:210.

43. Weetman AP. Effect of the anti-thyroid drug methimazole on interleukin-1 and interleukin-2 levels in vitro. *Clin Endocrinol (Oxf)* 1986;25:133.

44. Weetman AP, Tandon N, Morgan BP. Antithyroid drugs and release of inflammatory mediators by complement-attacked thyroid cells. *Lancet* 1992;340:633.

45. Volpe R. Graves' disease. In: Burrow GN, Oppenheimer JH, Volpe R, eds. *Thyroid function and disease.* Philadelphia: WB Saunders, 1989:214.

46. Bodolay E, Suranyi P, Juhasz F, et al. Methimazole blocks Graves' IgG but not interferon-HLA-DR expression by thyroid cells. *Immunol Lett* 1988;18:167.

47. Davies TF, Yang C, Platzer M. The influence of antithyroid drugs and iodine on thyroid cell MHC class II antigen expression. *Clin Endocrinol (Oxf)* 1989;31:125.

48. Saji M, Moriarty J, Ban T, et al. Major histocompatibility complex class I gene expression in rat thyroid cell is regulated by hormones, methimazole, and iodide as well as interferon. *J Clin Endocrinol Metab* 1992;75:871.

49. Mitsiades N, Poulaki V, Tseleni-Balafouta S, et al. Fas ligand expression in thyroid follicular cells from patients with thionamide-treated Graves' disease. *Thyroid.* 2000;10:527.

50. Beck JS, Young RJ, Simpson JG, et al. Lymphoid tissue in the thyroid gland and thymus of patients with primary thyrotoxicosis. *Br J Surg* 1973;60:769.

51. Hardisty CA, Fowles J, Munro DS. The effect of radioiodine and thyroid drugs on serum long acting thyroid stimulator protector (LATS-P): a three year prospective study. *Clin Endocrinol (Oxf)* 1984;20:547.

52. McGregor AM, Petersen MM, McLachlan SM, et al. Carbimazole and the autoimmune response in Graves' disease. *N Engl J Med* 1980;303:302.

53. McGregor AM, Rees-Smith B, Hall R, et al. Specificity of the immunosuppressive action of carbimazole in Graves' disease. *BMJ* 1982;284:1750.

54. Sonnet E, Massart C, Gibassier J, et al. Longitudinal study of soluble intercellular adhesion molecule-1 (ICAM-1) in sera of patients with Graves' disease. *J Endocrinol Invest* 1999;22: 430.

55. Tsatsoulis A, Vlachoyiannopoulos PG, Dalekos GN, et al. HM. Increased serum interleukin-1 beta during treatment of hyperthyroidism with antithyroid drugs. *Eur J Clin Invest* 1995; 25:654.

56. Escobar-Morreale H, Serrano-Gotarredona J, Villar L, et al. Methimazole has no dose-related effect on the serum concentrations of soluble class I major histocompatibility complex antigens, soluble interleukin-2 receptor, and beta 2-microglobulin in patients with Graves' disease. *Thyroid* 1996;6:29.

57. Salvi M, Girasole G, Pedrazzoni M, et al. Increased serum concentrations of interleukin-6 (IL-6) and soluble IL-6 receptor in patients with Graves' disease. *J Clin Endocrinol Metab* 1996; 81:2976.

58. Zantut-Wittmann DE, Tambascia MA, da Silva Trevisan MA, et al. Antithyroid drugs inhibit in vivo HLA-DR expression in thyroid follicular cells in Graves' disease. *Thyroid* 2001;11:575.

59. Madec AM, Allannic H, Genetet N, et al. T lymphocyte subsets at various stages of hyperthyroid Graves' disease: effect of carbimazole treatment and relationship with thyroid-stimulating antibody levels or HLA status. *J Clin Endocrinol Metab* 1986;62:117.

60. Totterman TH, Karlsson FA, Bengtsson M, et al. I. Induction of circulating activated suppressor-like T cells by methimazole therapy for Graves' disease. *N Engl J Med* 1987;316:15.

61. Ohashi H, Okugawa T, Itoh M. Circulating active T cell subsets in autoimmune thyroid diseases: differences between untreated and treated patients. *Acta Endocrinol* 1991;125:502.

62. Charreire J, Karsenty G, Bouchard P, et al. Effect of carbimazole treatment on specific and nonspecific immunological parameters in patients with Graves' disease. *Clin Exp Immunol* 1984;57:633.

63. Wang PW, Luo SF, Huang BY, et al. Depressed natural killer in Graves' disease and during antithyroid medication. *Clin Endocrinol (Oxf)* 1988;28:205.

64. Okuno A, Yano K, Inyaku F, et al. Pharmakokinetics of methimazole in children and adolescents with Graves' disease. *Acta Endocrinol* 1987;115:112.

65. Wenzel KW, Lente JR. Similar effects of antithyroid drugs and perchlorate on thyroid stimulating immunoglobulins in Graves' disease: evidence against an immunosuppressive effect of antithyroid drugs. *J Clin Endocrinol Metab* 1984;58:62.

66. Weetman AP, Gunn C, Hall R, et al. Immunosuppression by perchlorate. *Lancet* 1984;1:906.

67. Davies TF, Weiss I, Gerber M. Influence of methimazole on murine thyroiditis. *J Clin Invest* 1984;73:397.

68. Rennie DP, McGregor AM, Keast D, et al. The influence of methimazole on thyroglobulin-induced autoimmune thyroiditis in the rat. *Endocrinology* 1983;112:326.

69. Reinhardt W, Appel MC, Alex S, et al. The inhibitory effect of large doses of methimazole on iodine induced lymphocytic thyroiditis and serum anti-thyroglobulin antibody titers in BB/Wor rats. *J Endocrinol Invest* 1989;12:559.

70. Jansson R, Karlsson A, Dahlberg PA. Thyroxine, methimazole, and thyroid microsomal autoantibody titres in hypothyroid Hashimoto's thyroiditis. *BMJ* 1985;290:11.

71. Romaldini JH, Werner MC, Rodriques HF, et al. Graves' disease and Hashimoto's thyroiditis: effects of high doses of antithyroid drugs on thyroid autoantibody levels. *J Endocrinol Invest* 1986;9:233.

72. Gamstedt A, Wadman B, Karlsson A. Methimazole, but not betamethasone, prevents ^{131}I treatment-induced rises in thyrotropin receptor autoantibodies in hyperthyroid Graves' disease. *J Clin Endocrinol Metab* 1986;62:773.

73. Wilson R, McKillop JH, Pearson C, et al. Differential immunosuppressive action of carbimazole and propylthiouracil. *Clin Exp Immunol* 1988;73:312.

74. Jansson R, Lindstrom B, Dahlberg PA. Pharmacokinetic properties and bioavailability of methimazole. *Clin Pharmacokinet* 1985;10:443.

75. Okamura Y, Shigemasa C, Tatsuhara T. Pharmacokinetics of methimazole in normal subjects and hyperthyroid patients. *Endocrinol Jpn* 1986;33:605.

76. Low LCK, McCruden DC, Alexander WD. Intrathyroidal iodide binding rates and plasma methimazole concentrations in hyperthyroid patients on small doses of carbimazole. *Br J Clin Pharmacol* 1981;12:315.

77. Cooper DS, Bode HH, Nath B, et al. Methimazole pharmacology in man: studies using a newly developed radioimmunoassay for methimazole. *J Clin Endocrinol Metab* 1984;58:473.

78. Syrenicz A, Gawronska-Szklarz B, Wojcicki J, et al. Pharmacokinetic parameters of thiamazole in hyperthyroid patients responding rapidly and slowly to the treatment. *Pol J Pharmacol Pharm* 1991;43:207.

79. McCruden DC, Hilditch TE, Connell JMC, et al. Duration of antithyroid action of methimazole estimated with an intravenous perchlorate discharge test. *Clin Endocrinol (Oxf)* 1987;26:33.

80. Wartofsky L, Ingbar SH. A method for assessing the latency, potency and duration of action of antithyroid agents in man. In: Fellinger K, Hofer R, eds. *Further advances in thyroid research.* Wien: Verlag der Wiener Medizinischen Akademia, 1971;121.

81. Taurog A, Dorris ML. Propylthiouracil and methimazole display contrasting pathways of peripheral metabolism in both rat and human. *Endocrinology* 1988;122:592.

82. Marchant B, Brownlie BEW, Hart DM, et al. The placental transfer of propylthiouracil, methimazole and carbimazole. *J Clin Endocrinol Metab* 1977;45:1187.

83. MacFarlane IA, Davies D, Longson D, et al. Single daily dose short term carbimazole therapy for hyperthyroid Graves' disease. *Clin Endocrinol (Oxf)* 1983;18:557.

84. Messina M, Milani P, Gentile L, et al. Initial treatment of thyrotoxic Graves' disease with methimazole: a randomized trial comparing different dosages. *J Endocrinol Invest* 1987;10:291.

85. Roti E, Gardini E, Minelli R, et al. Methimazole and serum thyroid hormone concentrations in hyperthyroid patients: effects of single and multiple daily doses. *Ann Intern Med* 1989;111:181.

86. Shiroozu A, Okamura K, Ikenoue H, et al. Treatment of hyperthyroidism with a small single daily dose of methimazole. *J Clin Endocrinol Metab* 1986;63:125.

87. Legler UF. Impairment of prednisolone disposition in patients with Graves' disease taking methimazole. *J Clin Endocrinol Metab* 1988;66:221.

88. Cooper DS, Saxe VC, Meskell M, et al. Acute effects of propylthiouracil (PTU) on thyroidal iodine organification and peripheral iodothyronine deiodination: correlation with serum PTU levels measured by radioimmunoassay. *J Clin Endocrinol Metab* 1982;54:101.

89. Giles HG, Roberts EA, Orrego H, et al. Determination of free propylthiouracil clearance and single sample prediction of steady state. *J Pharm Pharmacol* 1982;34:62.

90. Cooper DS, Steigerwalt S, Migdal S. Pharmacology of propylthiouracil in thyrotoxicosis and chronic renal failure. *Arch Intern Med* 1987;147:785.

91. Hoffman WH, Miceli JN. Pharmacokinetics of propylthiouracil in children and .adolescents with Graves' disease in the hyperthyroid and euthyroid states. *Dev Pharmacol Ther* 1988;11:73.

92. Kampmann JP, Mortenson HB, Back D, et al. Kinetics of propylthiouracil in the elderly. *Acta Med Scand* 1979;624:93.

93. Kampmann JP, Hansen JEM. Serum protein binding of propylthiouracil. *Br J Clin Pharmacol* 1983;16:549.

94. Zaton A, Martinez A, DeGandarias JM. The binding of thioureylene compounds to human serum albumin. *Biochem Pharmacol* 1988;37:3127.

95. Kampmann JP, Hansen IM, Johansen K, et al. Propylthiouracil in human milk. *Lancet* 1980;2:736.

96. Barnes HV, Bledsoe T. A simple test for selecting the thioamide schedule in thyrotoxicosis. *J Clin Endocrinol Metab* 1972; 35: 250.

97. Greer MA, Meihoff WC, Studer H. Treatment of hyperthyroidism with a single daily dose of propylthiouracil. *N Engl J Med* 1965;272:888.

98. Gwinup G. Prospective randomized comparison of propylthiouracil. *JAMA* 78;239:2457.

99. Burch HB, Wartofsky L. Life-threatening thyrotoxicosis. *Endocrinol Metab Clin North Am* 1993;22:263.

100. Nicoloff JT. Thyroid storm and myxedema coma. *Med Clin North Am* 1985;69:1005.

101. Okamura K, Ikenoue H, Shiroozu A, et al. Reevaluation of the effects of methylmercaptoimidazole and propylthiouracil in patients with Graves' hyperthyroidism. *J Clin Endocrinol Metab* 1987;65:719.

102. Nicholas WC, Fischer RG, Stevenson RA, et al. Single daily dose of methimazole compared to every 8 hours propylthiouracil in the treatment of hyperthyroidism. *South Med J* 1995;88:973.

103. Mashio Y, Beniko M, Ikota A, et al. Treatment of hyperthyroidism with a small single daily dose of methimazole. *Acta Endocrinol* 1988;119:139.

104. Reinwein D, Benker G, Lazarus JH, et al. A prospective randomized trial of antithyroid drug dose in Graves' disease therapy. *J Clin Endocrinol Metab* 1993;76:1516.

105. Azizi F. Environmental iodine intake affects the response to methimazole in patients with diffuse toxic goiter. *J Clin Endocrinol Metab* 1985;61:374.

106. O'Malley BP, Rosenthal FD, Northover BJ, et al. Higher than conventional doses of carbimazole in the treatment of thyrotoxicosis. *Clin Endocrinol (Oxf)* 1988;29:281.

107. Page SR, Sheard CE, Herbert M, et al. A comparison of 20 or 40 mg per day of carbimazole in the initial treatment of hyperthyroidism. *Clin Endocrinol (Oxf)* 1996;45:511.

108. Cooper DS. Propylthiouracil levels in hyperthyroid patients unresponsive to large doses. *Ann Intern Med* 1985;102:328.

109. Jude EB, Dale J, Kumar S, et al. Treatment of thyrotoxicosis resistant to carbimazole with corticosteroids. *Postgrad Med J* 1996;72:439.

110. Cooper DS. Antithyroid drugs. *N Engl J Med* 1984;311:1353.

111. Werner MC, Romaldini JH, Bromberg N, et al. Adverse effects related to thionamide drugs and their dose regimen. *Am J Med Sci* 1989;297:216.

112. Cooper DS. Which antithyroid drug? *Am J Med* 1986;80:1165.

113. Kallner G, Vitols S, Ljunggren JG. Comparison of standardized initial doses of two antithyroid drugs in the treatment of Graves' disease. *J Intern Med* 1996;239:525.

114. Homsanit M, Sriussadaporn S, Vannasaeng S, et al. Efficacy of single daily dosage of methimazole vs. propylthiouracil in the induction of euthyroidism. *Clin Endocrinol (Oxf)* 2000;54:385.

115. Cooper DS, Goldminz D, Levin AA, et al. Agranulocytosis associated with antithyroid drugs. *Ann Intern Med* 1983;98:26.

116. Cooper DS. The side effects of antithyroid drugs. *The Endocrinologist* 1999;9:457.

117. Ducornet B, Duprey J. Effects secondaires des antithyroidiens de synthese. *Ann Med Interne* 1988;139:410.

118. Meyer-Gessner M, Benker G, Olbricht T, et al. Nebenwirkungen der antithyreoidalen therapie der hyperthyreose. *Dtsch Med Wochenschr* 1989;114:166.

119. Liaw Y-F, Huang M-J, Fan K-D, et al. Hepatic injury during propylthiouracil therapy in patients with hyperthyroidism. *Ann Intern Med* 1993;118:424.

120. Gurlek A, Cobaukara V, Bayraktar M. Liver tests in hyperthyroidism: effect of antithyroid therapy. *J Clin Gastroenterol* 1997;24:180.

121. Huang MJ, Li KL, Wei JS, et al. Sequential liver and bone biochemical changes in hyperthyroidism: prospective controlled follow-up study. *Am J Gastroenterol* 1994;89:1071.

122. Vitug AC, Goldman JM. Hepatotoxicity from antithyroid drugs. *Horm Res* 1985;21:229.

123. Bajaj S, Bell MJ, Shumak S, et al. Antithyroid arthritis. *J Rheumatol* 1998;25:1235.

124. Dolman KM, Gans RO, Vervaat TJ, et al. Vasculitis and antineutrophil cytoplasmic autoantibodies associated with propylthiouracil therapy. *Lancet* 1993;342:651.

125. Gunton JE, Stiel J, Caterson RJ, et al. Anti-thyroid drugs and antineutrophil cytoplasmic antibody positive vasculitis: a case report and review of the literature. *J Clin Endocrinol Metab* 1999;84:13.

126. Williams K, Nayak SU, Becker D, et al. Fifty years of experience with propylthiouracil-associated hepatotoxicity: what have we learned? *J Clin Endocrinol Metab* 1997;82:1727.

127. Gotta A, Sullivan CA, Seaman J, et al. Prolonged intraoperative bleeding caused by propylthiouracil-induced hypoprothrombinemia. *Anesthesiology* 1972;37:562.

128. Woeber KA. Methimazole-induced hepatotoxicity. *Endocr Pract* 2002;8:222.

129. Arab DM, Malatjalian DA, Rittmaster RS. Severe cholestatic jaundice in uncomplicated hyperthyroidism treated with methimazole. *J Clin Endocrinol Metab* 1995;80:1083.

130. Kitahara T, Hiromura K, Maezawa A, et al. Case of propylthiouracil-induced vasculitis associated with anti-neutrophil cytoplasmic antibody (ANCA): review of literature. *Clin Nephrol* 1997;47:336.

131. Sato H, Hattori M, Fujieda M, et al. High prevalence of antineutrophil cytoplasmic antibody positivity in childhood onset Graves' disease treated with propylthiouracil. *J Clin Endocrinol Metab* 2000;85:4270.

132. Guma M, Salinas I, Reverter JL, et al. Frequency of antineutrophil cytoplasmic antibody in Graves' disease patients treated with methimazole. *J Clin Endocrinol Metab* 2003;88:2141.

133. Sera N, Ashizawa K, Ando T, et al. Treatment with propylthiouracil is associated with appearance of antineutrophil cytoplasmic antibodies in some patients with Graves' disease. *Thyroid* 2000;10:595.

134. Noh JY, Asari T, Hamada N, et al. Frequency of appearance of myeloperoxidase-antineutrophil cytoplasmic antibody (MPO-ANCA) in Graves' disease patients treated with propylthiouracil and the relationship between MPO-ANCA and clinical manifestations. *Clin Endocrinol (Oxf)* 2001;54:651.

135. Wall JR, Fang SL, Kuroki T, et al. In vitro immunoreactivity to propylthiouracil, methimazole, and carbimazole in patients with Graves' disease: a possible cause of antithyroid drug-induced agranulocytosis. *J Clin Endocrinol Metab* 1984;58:868.

136. Tamai H, Sudo T, Kimura A, et al. Association between the DRB1*08032 histocompatibility antigen and methimazole-induced agranulocytosis in Japanese patients with Graves' disease. *Ann Intern Med* 1996;124:490.

137. Fibbe WE, Claas FHJ, Star-Dijkstra WVD, et al. Agranulocytosis induced by propylthiouracil: evidence of a drug dependent antibody reacting with granulocytes, monocytes and haematopoietic progenitor cells. *Br J Haematol* 1986;64:363.

138. Tajiri J, Noguehi S, Murakami T, et al. Antithyroid drug-induced agranulocytosis. *Arch Intern Med* 1990;150:621.

139. Tajiri J, Noguchi S, Murakami N. Usefulness of granulocyte count measurement four hours after injection of granulocyte colony-stimulating factor for detecting recovery from antithyroid drug-induced granulocytopenia. *Thyroid* 1997;7:575.

140. Andres E, Kurtz JE, Perrin AE, et al. Haematopoietic growth factor in antithyroid-drug-induced agranulocytosis. *QJM* 2001;94:423.

141. Fukata S, Kuma K, Sugawara M. Granulocyte colony-stimulating factor (G-CSF) does not improve recovery from antithyroid drug-induced agranulocytosis: a prospective study. *Thyroid* 1999; 9:29.

142. Tamai H, Mukuta T, Matsubayashi S, et al. Treatment of methimazole-induced agranulocytosis using recombinant human granulocyte colony stimulating factor (rhG-CSF). *J Clin Endocrinol Metab* 193;77:1356.

143. Taguchi M, Yokota M, Koyano H, et al. Acute pancreatitis and parotitis induced by methimazole in a patient with Graves' disease. *Clin Endocrinol (Oxf)* 1999;51:667.

144. Hakamata M, Itoh M, Sudo Y, et al. Insulin autoimmune syndrome after third therapy with methimazole. *Intern Med* 1995;34:410.

145. Uchigata Y, Hirata Y. Insulin autoimmune syndrome (IAS, Hirata disease). *Ann Med Interne (Paris)* 1999;150:245.

146. Suzuki S, Ichikawa K, Nagai M, et al. Elevation of serum creatine kinase during treatment with antithyroid drugs in patients with hyperthyroidism due to Graves' disease. *Arch Intern Med* 1997;157:693.

147. Hegedüs L, Hansen JM, Bech K, et al. Thyroid stimulating immunoglobulins in Graves' disease with goitre growth, low thyroxine and increasing triiodothyronine during PTU treatment. *Acta Endocrinol* 1984;107:482.

148. Wenzel KW, Lente JR. Syndrome of persisting thyroid stimulating immunoglobulins and growth promotion of goiter combined with low thyroxine and high triiodothyronine serum levels in drug treated Graves' disease. *J Endocrinol Invest* 1983;6:389.

149. Takamatsu J, Sugawara M, Kuma K, et al. Ratio of serum triiodothyronine to thyroxine and the prognosis of triiodothyronine-predominant Graves' disease. *Ann Intern Med* 1984;100:372.

150. Cooper DS. Antithyroid drugs for the treatment of hyperthyroidism caused by Graves' disease. *Endocrinol Metab Clin North Am* 1998;27:225.

151. Schleusener H, Schwander J, Fischer C, et al. Prospective multicentre study on the prediction of relapse after antithyroid drug treatment in patients with Graves' disease. *Acta Endocrinol* (Copenh) 1989;120:689.

152. Vitti P, Rago T, Chiovato L, et al. Clinical features of patients with Graves' disease undergoing remission after antithyroid drug treatment. *Thyroid* 1997;7:369.

153. Benker G, Rienwein D, Kahaly G, et al. Is there a methimazole dose effect on remission rate in Graves' disease? Results from a long-term prospective study. *Clin Endocrinol (Oxf)* 1998;49:451.

154. Young ET, Steel NR, Talor JJ, et al. Prediction of remission after antithyroid drug treatment in Graves' disease. *QJM* 1988;250:175.

155. Glaser NS, Styne DM. Predictors of early remission of hyperthyroidism in children. *J Clin Endocrinol Metab* 1997;82:1719.

156. Torring O, Tallstedt L, Wallin G, et al. Graves' hyperthyroidism: treatment with antithyroid drugs, surgery, or radioiodine—a prospective randomized study. *J Clin Endocrinol Metab* 1996;81:2986.

157. Michelangeli V, Poon C, Taft J, et al. The prognostic value of thyrotropin receptor antibody measurement in the early stages of treatment of Graves' disease with antithyroid drugs. *Thyroid* 1998;8:119.

158. Kawai K, Tamai H, Matsubayashi S, et al. A study of untreated Graves' patients with undetectable TSH binding inhibitor immunoglobulins and the effect of antithyroid drugs. *Clin Endocrinol(Oxf)* 1995;43:551.

159. McGregor AM, Smith BR, Hall R, et al. Prediction of relapse in hyperthyroid Graves' disease. *Lancet* 1980;1:1101.

160. DeBruin TWA, Bolk JH, Bussemaker JK, et al. Graves' disease: immunological and immunogenetic indicators of relapse. *BMJ* 1988;296:1292.

161. Allannic H, Fauchet R, Lorcy Y, et al. A prospective study of the relationship between relapse of hyperthyroid Graves' disease after antithyroid drugs and HLA haplotype. *J Clin Endocrinol Metab* 1983;57:719.

162. Eshoj O, Kvetny J, Mogensen EF, et al. Prediction of the course of Graves' disease after medical antithyroid treatment. *Acta Med Scand* 1985;217:225.

163. Komiya I, Yamada T, Sato A, Kouki T, Nishimori T, Takasu N. Remission and recurrence of hyperthyroid Graves' disease during and after methimazole treatment when assessed by IgE and interleukin 13. *J Clin Endocrinol Metab* 2001;86:3540.

164. Allahabadia A, Daykin J, Holder RL, et al. Age and gender predict the outcome of treatment for Graves' hyperthyroidism. *J Clin Endocrinol Metab* 2000;85:1038.

165. Kimball LE, Kulinskaya E, Brown B, et al. Does smoking increase relapse rates in Graves' disease? *J Endocrinol Invest* 2002;25:152.

166. Nedrebo BG, Holm PI, Uhlving S, et al. Predictors of outcome and comparison of different drug regimens for the prevention of relapse in patients with Graves' disease. *Eur J Endocrinol* 2002;147:583.

167. Yamada T, Aizawa T, Koizumi Y, et al. Age-related therapeutic response to antithyroid drug in patients with hyperthyroid Graves' disease. *J Am Geriatr Soc* 1994;42:513.

168. Fukao A, Takamatsu J, Murakami Y, et al. The relationship of psychological factors to the prognosis of hyperthyroidism in antithyroid drug-treated patients with Graves' disease. *Clin Endocrinol (Oxf)* 2003;58:550.

169. Bing RF, Rosenthal FD. Early remission in thyrotoxicosis produced by short courses of treatment. *Acta Endocrinol* (Copenh) 1982; 100:221.

170. Greer MA, Kammer H, Bouma DJ. Short-term antithyroid drug therapy for the thyrotoxicosis of Graves' disease. *N Engl J Med* 1977;297:173.

171. Tamai H, Nakagawa T, Fukino O, et al. Thionamide therapy in Graves' disease: relation of relapse rate to duration of therapy. *Ann Intern Med* 1980;92:488.

172. Lippe BM, Landaw EM, Kaplan SA. Hyperthyroidism in children treated with long term medical therapy: twenty-five percent remission every two years. *J Clin Endocrinol Metab* 1987;64:1241.

173. Allannic H, Fauchet R, Orgiazzi J, et al. Antithyroid drugs and Graves' disease: a prospective randomized evaluation of the efficacy of treatment duration. *J Clin Endocrinol Metab* 1990;70:675.

174. Garcia-Mayor RVG, Paramo C, Luna-Cano R, et al. Antithyroid drug and Graves' hyperthyroidism. Significance of treatment duration and TRAb determination on lasting remission. *J Endocrinol Invest* 1992;15:815.

175. Maugendre D, Gatel A, Campoin L, et al. Antithyroid drugs and Graves' disease—prospective randomized assessment of long-term teratment. *Clin Endocrinol (Oxf)* 1999;50:127.

176. Weetman AP, Pickerill AP, Watson P, et al. Treatment of Graves' disease with the block-replace regimen of antithyroid drugs: the effect of treatment duration and immunogenetic susceptibility on relapse. *QJM* 1994;87:337.

177. Romaldini JH, Bromberg N, Werner MC, et al. Comparison of effects of high and low dosage regimens of antithyroid drugs in the management of Graves' disease. *J Clin Endocrinol Metab* 1983;57:563.

178. Werner R, Romaldini J, Farah C, et al. Serum thyroid stimulating antibody, thyroglobulin levels, and thyroid suppressibility measurement as predictors of the outcome of combined methimazole and triiodothyronine therapy in Graves' disease. *Thyroid* 1991;1:293.

179. Jorde R, Ytre-Arne K, Stormer J, et al. Short-term treatment of Graves' disease with methimazole in high versus low doses. *J Intern Med* 1995;238:161.

180. Wilson R, Buchanan L, Fraser W, et al. Do higher doses of carbimazole improve remission in Graves' disease? *QJM* 1996;89:381.

181. Grebe SKG, Feek CM, Ford HC, et al. A randomized trial of short-term treatment of Graves' disease with high-dose carbimazole plus thyroxine versus low-dose carbimazole. *Clin Endocrinol (Oxf)* 1998;48:585.

182. Paschke R, Vogg M, Kristoferitsch R, et al. Methimazole has no dose-related effect on the intensity of the intrathyroidal au-

toimmune process in relapsing Graves' disease. *J Clin En-docrinol Metab* 1995;80:2470.

183. Hashizume K, Ichikawa I, Sakurai A, et al. Administration of thyroxine in treated Graves' disease. *N Engl J Med* 1991;324: 947.

184. McIver B, Rae P, Beckett G, et al. Lack of effect of thyroxine in patients with Graves' hyperthyroidism who are treated with an antithyroid drug. *N Engl J Med* 1996;334:220.

185. Rittmaster RS, Zwicker H, Abbott EC, et al. Effect of methimazole with or without exogenous l-thyroxine on serum concentrations of thyrotropin (TSH) receptor antibodies in patients with Graves' disease. *J Clin Endocrinol Metab* 1996;81:3283.

186. Pfeilschifter J, Zeigler R. Suppression of serum thyrotropin with thyroxine in patients with Graves' disease: effects on recurrence hyperthyroidism and thyroid volume. *Eur J Endocrinol* 1997;136:81.

187. Lucas A, Salinas I, Rius F, et al. Medical therapy of Graves' disease: does thyroxine prevent recurrence of hyperthyroidism? *J Clin Endocrinol Metab* 1997;82:2410.

188. Pujol P, Osman A, Grabar S, et al. TSH suppression combined with carbimazole for Graves' disease: effect on remission and relapse rates. *Clin Endocrinol (Oxf)* 1998;48:635.

189. Raber W, Kmen E, Waldhausl W, et al. Medical therapy of Graves' disease: effect on remission rates of methimazole alone and in combination with triiodothyronine. *Eur J Endocrinol* 2000;142:117.

190. Glinoer D, de Nayer P, Bex M. Effects of l-thyroxine administration, TSH-receptor antibodies and smoking on the risk of recurrence in Graves' hyperthyroidism treated with antithyroid drugs: a double-blind prospective randomized study. *Eur J Endocrinol* 2001;144:475.

191. Tamai H, Hayaki I, Kawai K, et al. Lack of effect of thyroxine administration on elevated thyroid stimulating receptor antibody levels in treated Graves' disease patients. *J Clin Endocrinol Metab* 1995;80:1481.

192. Hershman JM, Givens JR, Cassidy CE, et al. Long-term outcome of hyperthyroidism treated with antithyroid drugs. *J Clin Endocrinol Metab* 1966;26:803.

193. Benker G, Esser J, Kahaly G, et al. New therapeutic approaches in thyroidal autoimmune diseases. *Klin Wochenschr* 1990;68: 44.

194. Feldt-Rasmussen U, Schleusener H, Carayon P. Meta-analysis evaluation of the impact of thyrotropin receptor antibodies on long-term remission after medical therapy of Graves' disease. *J Clin Endocrinol Metab* 1994;78:98.

195. Teng CS, Yeung RTT. Changes in thyroid-stimulating antibody activity in Graves' disease treated with antithyroid drug and its relationship to relapse: a prospective study. *J Clin Endocrinol Metab* 1980;50:144.

196. Yamada T, Koizumi Y, Sato A, et al. Reappraisal of the 3,5,3'-triiodothyronine suppression test in the prediction of long-term outcome of antithyroid drug therapy in patients with hyperthyroid Graves' disease. *J Clin Endocrinol Metab* 1984;58:676.

197. Dahlberg PA, Karlsson FA, Jansson R, et al. Thyrotropin-releasing hormone testing during antithyroid drug treatment of Graves' disease as an indicator of remission. *J Clin Endocrinol Metab* 1985;61:1100.

198. Aizawa T, Ishiham M, Koizumi Y, et al. Serum thyroglobulin concentration as an indicator for assessing thyroid stimulation in patients with Graves' disease during antithyroid drug therapy. *Am J Med* 1990;89:175.

199. Hamada N, Ito K, Mimura T, et al. Retrospective evaluation of the significance of thyroid microsomal antibody in the treatment of Graves' disease. *Acta Endocrinol* (Copenh) 1987;114:328.

200. Cho BY, Shong MH, Yi KH, et al. Evaluation of serum basal thyrotrophin levels and thyrotrophin receptor antibody activi-

ties as prognostic markers for discontinuation of antithyroid drug treatment in patients with Graves' disease. *Clin Endocrinol (Oxf)* 1992;36:585.

201. Berglund J, Christensen SB, Dymling JF, et al. The incidence of recurrence and hypothyroidism following treatment with antithyroid drugs, surgery or radioiodine in all patients with thyrotoxicosis in Malmö during the period 1970–1974. *J Intern Med* 1991;229:435.

202. Amino N, Tanizawa O, Mori H, et al. Aggravation of thyrotoxicosis in early pregnancy and after delivery in Graves' disease. *J Clin Endocrinol Metab* 1982;55:108.

203. Hashizume K, Ichikawa K, Nishii Y, et al. Effect of administration of thyroxine on the risk of postpartum recurrence of hyperthyroid Graves' disease. *J Clin Endocrinol Metab* 1992;75:6.

204. Slingerland DW, Burrows BA. Long-term antithyroid treatment in hyperthyroidism. *JAMA* 1979;242:2408.

205. Burman KD, Wartofsky L. Iodine effects on the thyroid gland: biochemical and clinical aspects. *Rev Endocr Metab Disord* 2000;1:19.

206. Emerson CH, Anderson AJ, Howard WJ, et al. Serum thyroxine and triiodothyronine concentrations during iodide treatment of hyperthyroidism. *J Clin Endocrinol Metab* 1975;40:33.

207. Philippou G, Koutras DA, Piperingos G, et al. The effect of iodide on serum thyroid hormone levels in normal persons, in hyperthyroid patients, and in hypothyroid patients on thyroxine replacement. *Clin Endocrinol (Oxf)* 1992;36:573.

208. Thompson WO, Thompson PK, Brailey AG, et al. Prolonged treatment of exophthalmic goiter by iodine alone. *Arch Intern Med* 1930;45:481.

209. Chang DCS, Wheeler MH, Woodcock JP, et al. The effect of preoperative Lugol's iodine on thyroid blood flow in patients with Graves' hyperthyroidism. *Surgery* 1987;102:1055.

210. Coyle PJ, Mitchell JE. Thyroidectomy: is Lugol's iodine necessary? *Ann R Coll Surg Engl* 1982;64:334.

211. Peden NR, Gunn A, Browning MCK, et al. Nadolol and potassium iodide in the surgical treatment of thyrotoxicosis. *Br J Surg* 1982;69:638.

212. Ross DS, Daniels GH, DeStefano P, et al. Use of adjunctive potassium iodide after radioactive iodine (131I) treatment of Graves' hyperthyroidism. *J Clin Endocrinol Metab* 1983;57: 250.

213. Schimmel M, Utiger RD. Acute effect of inorganic iodide after 131I therapy for hyperthyroidism. *Clin Endocrinol (Oxf)* 1977; 6:329.

214. Bazzi MN, Bagchi N. Adjunctive treatment with propylthiouracil or iodine following radioiodine therapy for Graves' disease. *Thyroid* 1993;3:269.

215. Kasai K, Suzuki H, Shimoda SI. Effects of propylthiouracil and relatively small doses of iodide on early phase treatment of hyperthyroidism. *Acta Endocrinol (Copenh)* 1980;93:315.

216. Roti E, Robuschi G, Gardini E, et al. Comparison of methimazole, methimazole and sodium ipodate, and methimazole and saturated solution of potassium iodide in the early treatment of hyperthyroid Graves' disease. *Clin Endocrinol (Oxf)* 1988;28: 305.

217. Braverman LE, Woeber KA, Ingbar SH. Induction of myxedema by iodide in patients euthyroid after radioiodine or surgical treatment of diffuse toxic goiter. *N Engl J Med* 1969;281:816.

218. Burgi H, Wimpfheimer C, Burger A, et al. Changes of circulating thyroxine, triiodothyronine and reverse triiodothyronine after radiographic contrast agents. *J Clin Endocrinol Metab* 1976;43:1203.

219. Wu SY, Chopra IJ, Solomon DH, et al. Changes in circulating iodothyronines in euthyroid and hyperthyroid subjects given ipodate (Oragrafin), an agent for oral cholecystography. *J Clin Endocrinol Metab* 1978;46:691.

220. Braga M, Cooper DS. Oral cholecystographic agents and the thyroid. *J Clin Endocrinol Metab* 2001;86:1853.

221. Fontanilla JC, Schneider AB, Sarne DH. The use of oral radiographic contrast agents in the management of hyperthyroidism. *Thyroid* 2001;11:561.

222. Laurberg P. Multisite inhibition by ipodate of iodothyronine secretion from perfused dog thyroid lobes. *Endocrinology* 1985;117:1639.

223. Fellicetta JV, Green WL, Nelp WB. Inhibition of hepatic binding of thyroxine by cholecystographic agents. *J Clin Endocrinol Metab* 1980;65:1032.

224. Wu SY, Shyh TP, Chopra IJ, et al. Comparison of sodium ipodate (Oragrafin) and propylthiouracil in early treatment of hyperthyroidism. *J Clin Endocrinol Metab* 1982;54:630.

225. Martino E, Balzano S, Bartalena L, et al. Therapy of Graves' disease with sodium ipodate is associated with a high recurrence rate of hyperthyroidism. *J Endocrinol Invest* 1991;14:847.

226. Roti E, Gardini E, Minelli R, et al. Sodium ipodate and methimazole in the long-term treatment of hyperthyroid Graves' disease. *Metabolism* 1993;42:403.

227. Shen DC, Wu SY, Chopra IJ, et al. Long term treatment of Graves' hyperthyroidism with sodium ipodate. *J Clin Endocrinol Metab* 1985;61:723.

228. Sharp B, Reed AW, Tamagna EI, et al. Treatment of hyperthyroidism with sodium ipodate (Oragrafin) in addition to propylthiouracil and propranolol. *J Clin Endocrinol Metab* 1981;53:622.

229. Baeza A, Aguayo M, Barria M, et al. Rapid preoperative preparation in hyperthyroidism. *Clin Endocrinol (Oxf)* 1991;35:439.

230. Brown RS, Cohen JH 3rd, Braverman LE. Successful treatment of massive acute thyroid hormone poisoning with iopanoic acid. *J Pediatr* 1998;132:903.

231. Chopra IJ, van Herle AJ, Korenman SG, et al. Use of sodium ipodate in management of hyperthyroidism in subacute thyroiditis. *J Clin Endocrinol Metab* 1995 ;80:2178.

232. Chopra IJ, Baber K. Use of oral cholecystographic agents in the treatment of amiodarone-induced hyperthyroidism. *J Clin Endocrinol Metab* 2001;86:4707.

233. Transue D, Chan J, Kaplan M. Management of neonatal Graves disease with iopanoic acid. *J Pediatr* 1992;121:472.

234. Soldin OP, Braverman LE, Lamm SH. Perchlorate clinical pharmacology and human health: a review. *Ther Drug Monit* 2001;23:316.

235. Martino E, Lombardi-Aghini F, Mariotti S, et al. Treatment of amiodarone associated thyrotoxicosis by simultaneous administration of potassium perchlorate and methimazole. *J Endocrinol Invest* 1986;9:201.

236. Berens SC, Wolff J, Murphy DL. Lithium concentration by the thyroid. *Endocrinology* 1970;87:1085.

237. Berens SC, Bernstein RS, Robbins J, et al. Antithyroid effects of lithium. *J Clin Invest* 1970;49:1357.

238. Burrow G, Burke WR, Himmelhoch JM, et al. Effect of lithium on thyroid function. *J Clin Endocrinol Metab* 1971;32:647.

239. Williams JA, Berens SC, Wolff J. Thyroid secretion in vitro: inhibition of TSH and dibutyryl cyclic-AMP stimulated ^{131}I release by Li. *Endocrinology* 1971;88:1385.

240. Kristenson O, Andersen HH, Pallisgaard G. Lithium carbonate in the treatment of thyrotoxicosis. *Lancet* 1976;1:603.

241. Turner JG, Brownlie BEW, Sadler WA, et al. An evaluation of lithium as an adjunct to carbimazole treatment in acute thyrotoxicosis. *Acta Endocrinol* 1976;83:86.

242. Dickstein G, Shechner C, Adawi F, et al. Lithium treatment in amiodarone-induced thyrotoxicosis. *Am J Med* 1997;102:454.

243. Geffner DL, Hershman JM. Beta-adrenergic blockade for the treatment of hyperthyroidism. *Am J Med* 1992;93:61.

244. Ginsberg AM, Clutter WE, Shah SD, et al. Triiodothyronine-induced thyrotoxicosis increases mononuclear leukocyte beta-adrenergic receptor density in man. *J Clin Invest* 1981;67:1785.

245. Cooper DS, Daniels GH, Ladenson PW, et al. Hyperthyroxinemia in patients treated with high-dose propranolol. *Am J Med* 1982;73:867.

246. Georges LP, Santangelo RP, Mackin JF, et al. Metabolic effects of propranolol in thyrotoxicosis. I. Nitrogen, calcium and hydroxyproline. *Metabolism* 1975;24:11.

247. Valcavi R, Menozzi C, Roti E, et al. Sinus node function in hyperthyroid patients. *J Clin Endocrinol Metab* 1992;75:239.

248. Grossman W, Robin NI, Johnson LW, et al. Effects of beta blockade on the peripheral manifestations of thyrotoxicosis. *Ann Intern Med* 1971;74:875.

249. Saunders J, Hall SEH, Crowther A, et al. The effect of propranolol on thyroid hormones and oxygen consumption in thyrotoxicosis. *Clin Endocrinol (Oxf)* 1978;9:67.

250. O'Malley BP, Abbott RJ, Barnett DB, et al. Propranolol versus carbimazole as the sole treatment for thyrotoxicosis. A consideration of circulating thyroid hormone levels and tissue thyroid function. *Clin Endocrinol (Oxf)* 1982;16:545.

251. Feely J, Stevenson IH, Crooks J. Increased clearance of propranolol in thyrotoxicosis. *Ann Intern Med* 1981;94:472.

252. Klein I, Ojamaa K. Thyrotoxicosis and the heart. *Endocrinol Clin North Am* 1998;27:51.

253. Roti E, Montermini M, Roti S, et al. The effect of diltiazem, a calcium channel-blocking drug, on cardiac rate and rhythm in hyperthyroid patients. *Arch Intern Med* 1988;148:1919.

254. Becker DV, Sawin CT. Radioiodine and thyroid disease: the beginning. *Semin Nucl Med* 1996;26:155.

255. Jones BM, Kwok CC, Kung AW. Effect of radioactive iodine therapy on cytokine production in Graves' disease: transient increases in interleukin-4 (IL-4), IL-6, IL-10, and tumor necrosis factor-alpha, with longer term increases in interferon-gamma production. *J Clin Endocrinol Metab* 1999;84:4106.

256. Tamagna E, Levine GA, Hershman JM. Thyroid hormone concentrations after radioiodine therapy for hyperthyroidism. *J Nucl Med* 1979;20:387.

257. Dobyns BM, Vickery AL, Maloof F, et al. Functional and histologic effects of therapeutic doses of radioactive iodine on the thyroid of man. *J Clin Endocrinol Metab* 1953;13:548.

258. Centeno BA, Szyfelbein WM, Daniels GH, et al. Fine needle aspiration biopsy of the thyroid gland in patients with prior Graves' disease treated with radioactive iodine. Morphologic findings and practical pitfalls. *Acta Cytol* 1996;40:1189.

259. Sabri O, Zimny M, Schulz G, et al. Success rate of radioiodine therapy in Graves' disease: the influence of thyrostatic medication. *J Clin Endocrinol Metab* 1999;84:1229.

260. Tsuruta M, Nagayama Y, Yokoyama N, et al. Long-term follow-up studies on iodine-131 treatment of hyperthyroid Graves' disease based on the measurement of thyroid gland volume by ultrasonography. *Ann Nucl Med* 1993;7:193.

261. Berg G, Michanek A, Holmberg E, et al. Clinical outcome of radioiodine treatment of hyperthyroidism: a follow-up study. *J Intern Med* 1996;239:165.

262. Peters H, Fischer C, Bogner U, et al. Radioiodine therapy of Graves' hyperthyroidism: standard vs. calculated ^{131}I activity. Results from a prospective, randomized, multicentre study. *Eur J Clin Invest* 1995;25:186.

263. Leslie WD, Ward L, Salamon EA, et al. A randomized comparison of radioiodine doses in Graves' hyperthyroidism. *J Clin Endocrinol Metab* 2003;88:978.

264. Beierwaltes WH. The treatment of hyperthyroidism with iodine-131. *Semin Nucl Med* 1978;8:95.

265. Crooks J, Buchanan WW, Wayne EJ, et al. Effect of pretreatment with methylthiouracil on results of 131-I therapy. *BMJ* 1960;1:151.

266. Alexander EK, Larsen PR. High dose of (131)I therapy for the treatment of hyperthyroidism caused by Graves' disease. *J Clin Endocrinol Metab* 2002;87:1073.

267. Erikson E, Erikson K, Wahlberg P. Treatment of hyperthyroidism with standard doses of radioiodine aiming at ablation. *Acta Med Scand* 1985;214:55.

268. Safa AM, Skillern PG. Treatment of hyperthyroidism with a large initial dose of sodium iodide I^{131}. *Arch Intern Med* 1975; 135:673.

269. Franklyn JA, Daykin J, Droic Z, et al. Long-term follow-up of treatment of thyrotoxicosis by three different methods. *Clin Endocrinol (Oxf)* 1991;34:71.

270. Nordyke RA, Gilbert FI. Optimal iodine-131 dose for eliminating hyperthyroidism in Graves' disease. *J Nucl Med* 1991; 32:411.

271. Cevallos JL, Hagen GA, Maloof F, et al. Low-dose ^{131}I therapy of thyrotoxicosis (diffuse goiter). *N Engl J Med* 1974;290:141.

272. Sridama V, McCormick M, Kaplan EL, et al. Long-term follow-up study of compensated low-dose ^{131}I therapy for Graves' disease. *N Engl J Med* 1984;311:426.

273. Teng CS, Yeung RTT, Khoo RKK, et al. A prospective study of the changes in thyrotropin binding inhibitory immunoglobulins in Graves' disease treated by subtotal thyroidectomy or radioactive iodine. *J Clin Endocrinol Metab* 1980;50:1005.

274. Davies TF, Platzer M, Farid NR. Prediction of therapeutic response to radioiodine in Graves' disease using TSH-receptor antibodies and HLA-status. *Clin Endocrinol (Oxf)* 1982;16: 183.

275. Murakami Y, Takamatsu J, Sakane S, et al. Changes in thyroid volume in response to radioactive iodine for Graves' hyperthyroidism correlated with activity of thyroid-stimulating antibody and treatment outcome. *J Clin Endocrinol Metab* 1996; 81:3257.

276. Chiovato L, Fiore E, Vitti P, et al. Outcome of thyroid function in Graves' patients treated with radioiodine: role of thyroid-stimulating and thyrotropin-blocking antibodies and of radioiodine-induced thyroid damage. *J Clin Endocrinol Metab* 1998;83:40.

277. Stensvold AD, Jorde R, Sundsfjord J. Late and transient increases in free T4 after radioiodine treatment for Graves' disease. *J Endocrinol Invest* 1997;20:580.

278. Holm LE, Lundell G, Dahlqvist I, et al. Cure rate after ^{131}I therapy for hyperthyroidism. *Acta Radiol* 1981;20:161.

279. Graham GD, Burman KD. Radioiodine treatment of Graves' disease. *Ann Intern Med* 1986;105:900.

280. Cunnien AJ, Hay ID, Gorman CA, et al. Radioiodine-induced hypothyroidism in Graves' disease: factors associated with the increasing incidence. *J Nucl Med* 1982;23:978.

281. Holm LE. Changing annual incidence of hypothyroidism after iodine-131 therapy for hyperthyroidism, 1951–1975. *J Nucl Med* 1982;23:108.

282. Peden NR, Hart IR. The early development of transient and permanent hypothyroidism following radioiodine therapy for hyperthyroid Graves' disease. *Can Med Assoc J* 1984;130:1141.

283. Ahmad AM, Ahmad M, Young ET. Objective estimates of the probability of developing hypothyroidism following radioactive iodine treatment of thyrotoxicosis. *Eur J Endocrinol.* 2002; 146:767.

284. Marcocci C, Gianchecchi D, Masini I, et al. A reappraisal of the role of methimazole and other factors on the efficacy and outcome of radioiodine therapy of Graves' hyperthyroidism. *J Endocrinol Invest* 1990;13:513.

285. Tuttle RM, Patience T, Budd S. Treatment with propylthiouracil before radioactive iodine therapy is associated with a higher treatment failure rate than radioiodine therapy alone in Graves' disease. *Thyroid* 1995;5:243.

286. Imseis RE, VanMiddlesworth L, Massie JD, et al. Pretreatment with propylthiouracil but not methimazole reduces the therapeutic efficacy of iodine-131 in hyperthyroidism. *J Clin Endocrinol Metab* 1998;83:685.

287. Andrade VA, Gross JL, Maia AL. Effect of methimazole pretreatment on the efficacy of radioactive iodine therapy in Graves' hyperthyroidism: one-year follow-up of a prospective randomized study. *J Clin Endocrinol Metab* 2001;86:3488.

288. Braga M, Walpert N, Burch HB, et al. The effect of methimazole on cure rates after radioiodine treatment for Graves' hyperthyroidism: a randomized clinical trial. *Thyroid* 2002;12:135.

289. Kung AW, Yau CC, Cheng AC. The action of methimazole and L-thyroxine in radioiodine therapy: a prospective study on the incidence of hypothyroidism. *Thyroid* 1995;5:7.

290. Uy HL, Reasner CA, Samuels MH. Pattern of recovery of the hypothalamic–pituitary–thyroid axis following radioactive iodine therapy in patients with Graves' disease. *Am J Med* 1995;99:173.

291. Gomez N, Gomez JM, Ortiz A, et al. Transient hypothyroidism after iodine-131 therapy for Graves' disease. *J Nucl Med* 1995;36:1539.

292. Aizawa Y, Yoshida K, Kaise N, et al. The development of transient hypothyroidism after iodine-131 treatment in hyperthyroid patients with Graves' disease: prevalence, mechanism, and prognosis. *Clin Endocrinol (Oxf)* 1997;46:1.

293. Sawers JSA, Toft AD, Irvine WJ, et al. Transient hypothyroidism after iodine-131 treatment of thyrotoxicosis. *J Clin Endocrinol Metab* 1980;50:226.

294. Rivkees SA, Sklar C, Freemark M. The management of Graves' disease in children, with special emphasis on radioiodine treatment. *J Clin Endocrinol Metab* 1998;83:3767.

295. Wiener JD, Thijs LG, Meijer S. Thyroid carcinoma after ^{131}I treatment for hyperthyroidism. *Acta Med Scand* 1975;198:329.

296. Dobyns BM, Sheline GE, Workman JB, et al. Malignant and benign neoplasms of the thyroid in patients treated for hyperthyroidism: a report of the cooperative thyrotoxicosis therapy follow-up study. *J Clin Endocrinol Metab* 1974;38:976.

297. Holm LE, Dahlqvist I, Israelsson A, et al. Malignant thyroid tumors after iodine-131 therapy. *N Engl J Med* 1980;303:188.

298. Hoffman DA, McConahey WM, Diamond EL, et al. Mortality in women treated with hyperthyroidism. *Am J Epidemiol* 1982; 115:243.

299. Goldman MB, Maloof F, Monson RR, et al. Radioactive iodine therapy and breast cancer. *Am J Epidemiol* 1988;127:969.

300. Hall P, Lundell G, Holm LE. Mortality in patients treated for hyperthyroidism with iodine-131. *Acta Endocrinol* 1993;128:230.

301. Ron E, Doody MM, Becker DV, et al. Cancer mortality following treatment for adult hyperthyroidism. *JAMA* 1998;280:347.

302. Angusti T, Codegone A, Pellerito R, et al. Thyroid cancer prevalence after radioiodine treatment of hyperthyroidism. *J Nucl Med* 2000;41:1006.

303. Franklyn JA, Maisonneuve P, Sheppard M, et al. Cancer incidence and mortality after radioiodine treatment for hyperthyroidism: a population-based cohort study. *Lancet* 1999;353: 2111.

304. Hall P, Boice JD Jr, Berg G, et al. Leukaemia incidence after iodine-131 exposure. *Lancet* 1992;340:1.

305. Hayek A, Chapman EM, Crawford JD. Long-term results of treatment of thyrotoxicosis in children and adolescents with radioactive iodine. *N Engl J Med* 1970;283:949.

306. Safa AM, Schumacher OP, Rodriguez-Antunez A. Long-term follow-up results in children and adolescents treated with radioactive iodine (^{131}I) for hyperthyroidism. *N Engl J Med* 1975;292:167.

307. Freitas JE, Swanson DP, Gross MD, et al. Iodine-131: optimal therapy for hyperthyroidism in children and adolescents? *J Nucl Med* 1979;20:847.

308. Sheline GE, Lindsay S, Bell HG. Occurrence of thyroid nodules in children following therapy with radioiodine for hyperthyroidism. *J Clin Endocrinol Metab* 1959;19:127.

309. Stoffer SS, Hamburger JI. Inadvertent ^{131}I therapy for hyperthyroidism in the first trimester of pregnancy. *J Nucl Med* 1976;17:146.

310. Cantolino SJ, Schmickel RD, Ba UM, et al. Persistent chromosomal aberrations following radioiodine therapy for thyrotoxicosis. *N Engl J Med* 1966;275:739.

311. Nofal MM, Beierwaltes WH. Persistent chromosomal aberrations following radioiodine therapy. *J Nucl Med* 1964;5:840.

312. Vormittag W, Ring F, Kunze-Muhl E, et al. Structural chromosomal aberrations before and after administration of 20 mCi iodine-131. *Mutat Res* 1982;105:333.

313. Robertson JS, Gorman CA. Gonadal radiation dose and its genetic significance in radioiodine therapy of hyperthyroidism. *J Nucl Med* 1976;17:826.

314. Sarkar SD, Beierwaltes WH, Gill SP, et al. Subsequent fertility and birth histories of children and adolescents treated with 131I for thyroid cancer. *J Nucl Med* 1976;17:460.

315. Einhorn J, Hulten M, Lindsten J, et al. Clinical and cytogenetic investigation in children of parents treated with radioiodine. *Acta Radiol* 1972:11:193.

316. Gorman CA. Radioiodine and pregnancy. *Thyroid* 1999;9:721.

317. Kaplan MM, Meier DA, Dworkin HJ. Treatment of hyperthyroidism with radioactive iodine. *Endocrinol Metab Clin North Am* 1998;27:205.

318. Culver C, Dworkin HJ. Radiation safety considerations for post–iodine-131 hyperthyroid therapy. *J Nucl Med* 1991;32:169.

319. Koornstra JJ, Kerstens MN, Hoving J, et al. Clinical and biochemical changes following 131I therapy for hyperthyroidism in patients not pretreated with antithyroid drugs. *Neth J Med* 1999;55:215.

320. McDermott MT, Kidd GS, Dodson LE, et al. Radioiodine-induced thyroid storm. *Am J Med* 1983;75:353.

321. Kadmon PM, Noto RB, Boney CM, et al. Thyroid storm in a child following radioactive iodine (RAI) therapy: a consequence of RAI versus withdrawal of antithyroid medication. *J Clin Endocrinol Metab* 2001;86:1865.

322. Andrade VA, Gross JL, Maia AL. Effect of methimazole pretreatment on serum thyroid hormone levels after radioiodine treatment in Graves' hyperthyroidism. *J Clin Endocrinol Metab* 1999;84:4012.

323. Burch HB, Solomon BL, Cooper DS, et al. The effect of antithyroid drug pretreatment on acute changes in thyroid hormone levels after (131)I ablation for Graves' disease. *J Clin Endocrinol Metab* 2001;86:3016.

324. Cooper DS. Antithyroid drugs and radioiodine therapy: a grain of (iodized) salt. *Ann Intern Med* 1994;121:612.

325. Bogazzi F, Bartalena L, Campomori A, et al. Treatment with lithium prevents serum thyroid hormone increase after thionamide withdrawal and radioiodine therapy in patients with Graves' disease. *J Clin Endocrinol Metab* 2002;87:4490.

326. Bogazzi F, Bartalena L, Brogioni S, et al. Comparison of radioiodine with radioiodine plus lithium in the treatment of Graves' hyperthyroidism. *J Clin Endocrinol Metab* 1999;84:499.

327. Marcocci C, Bartalena L, Bogazzi F, et al. Relationship between Graves' ophthalmopathy and type of treatment of Graves' hyperthyroidism. *Thyroid* 1992;2:171.

328. Tallstedt L, Lundell G. Radioiodine treatment, ablation, and ophthalmopathy: a balanced perspective. *Thyroid* 1997;7:241.

329. Gwinup G, Elias AN, Ascher MS. Effect on exophthalmos of various methods of treatment of Graves' disease. *JAMA* 1982;247:2135.

330. Sridama V, DeGroot LJ. Treatment of Graves' disease and the course of ophthalmopathy. *Am J Med* 1989;87:70.

331. Bartalena L, Marcocci C, Bogazzi F, et al. Use of corticosteroids to prevent progression of Graves' ophthalmopathy after radioiodine therapy for hyperthyroidism. *N Engl J Med* 1989;321:1349.

332. Vestergaard H, Laurberg P. Radioiodine and aggravation of Graves' ophthalmopathy. *Lancet* 1989;1:47.

333. Tallstedt L, Lundell G, Torring O, et al. Occurrence of ophthalmopathy after treatment for Graves' hyperthyroidism. *N Engl J Med* 1992;326:1733.

334. Bartalena L, Marcocci C, Bogazzi F, et al. Relation between therapy for hyperthyroidism and the course of Graves' ophthalmopathy. *N Engl J Med* 1998;338:73.

335. Atkinson S, McGregor AM, Kendall-Taylor P, et al. Effect of radioiodine on stimulatory activity of Graves' immunoglobulins. *Clin Endocrinol (Oxf)* 1982;16:537.

336. Kung WC, Yau CC, Cheng A. The incidence of ophthalmopathy after radioiodine therapy for Graves' disease: prognostic factors and the role of methimazole. *J Clin Endocrinol Metab* 1994;79:542.

337. Tallstedt L, Lundell G, Blomgren H, et al. Does early administration of thyroxine reduce the development of Graves' ophthalmopathy after radioiodine treatment? *Eur J Endocrinol* 1994;130:494.

338. Vazquez-Chavez C, Nishimura Meguro E, Espinosa Said L, et al. Effect of the treatment of hyperthyroidism on the course of exophthalmos. *Rev Invest Clin* 1992;44:241.

339. Bartalena L, Marcocci C, Tanda ML, et al. Cigarette smoking and treatment outcomes in Graves ophthalmopathy. *Ann Intern Med* 1998;129:632.

340. Winsa B, Rastad J, Larsson E, et al. Total thyroidectomy in therapy-resistant Graves' disease. *Surgery* 1994;116:1068.

341. Parwardhan NA, Moront M, Rao S, et al. Surgery still has a role in Graves' hyperthyroidism. *Surgery* 1993;114:1108.

342. Klementschitsch P, Shen K, Kaplan EL. Reemergence of thyroidectomy as treatment for Graves' disease. *Surg Clin North Am* 1979;59:35.

343. Palit TK, Miller CC III, Miltenburg DM. The efficacy of thyroidectomy for Graves' disease: a meta-analysis. *J Surg Res* 2000;90:161.

344. Maier WP, Derrick BM, Marks AD, et al. Long-term follow-up of patients with Graves' disease treated by subtotal thyroidectomy. *Am J Surg* 1984;147:267.

345. Sugino K, Mimura T, Ozaki O, et al. Management of recurrent hyperthyroidism in patients with Graves' disease treated by subtotal thyroidectomy. *J Endocrinol Invest* 1995;18:415.

346. Sosa JA, Bowman HM, Tielsch JM, et al. The importance of surgeon experience for clinical and economic outcomes from thyroidectomy. *Ann Surg* 1998;228:320.

347. Hedley AJ, Bewsher PD, Jones SJ, et al. Late onset hypothyroidism after subtotal thyroidectomy for hyperthyroidism: implications for long term follow-up. *Br J Surg* 1983;70:740.

348. Lee TC, Coffey RJ, Currier BM, et al. Propranolol and thyroidectomy in the treatment of thyrotoxicosis. *Ann Surg* 1982;195:766.

349. Reid DJ. Hyperthyroidism and hypothyroidism complicating the treatment of thyrotoxicosis. *Br J Surg* 1987;74:1060.

350. Sugrue D, Drury MI, McEvoy M, et al. Long term follow-up of hyperthyroid patients treated by subtotal thyroidectomy. *Br J Surg* 1983;70:408.

351. Harada T, Shimaoka K, Arita S, et al. Follow up evaluation of thyroid function after thyroidectomy for thyrotoxicosis. *World J Surg* 1984;8:444.

352. Sugino K, Mimura T, Ozaki O, et al. Early recurrence of hyperthyroidism in patients with Graves' disease treated by subtotal thyroidectomy. *World J Surg* 1995;19:648.

353. Winsa B, Rastad J, Akerstrom G, et al. Retrospective evaluation of subtotal and total thyroidectomy in Graves' disease with and without endocrine ophthalmopathy. *Eur J Endocrinol* 1995;132:406.

354. Kalk WJ, Durbach D, Kantor S, et al. Postthyroidectomy thyrotoxicosis. *Lancet* 1978;1:2911.

355. Lennquist S, Jortso E, Anderberg BO, et al. Beta blockers compared with antithyroid drugs as preoperative treatment in hyperthyroidism: drug tolerance, complications, and postoperative thyroid function. *Surgery* 1985;98:1141.

356. Peden NR, Browning MCK, Feely J, et al. The clinical and metabolic responses to early surgical treatment for hyperthyroid Graves' disease: a comparison of three preoperative treatment regimens. *QJM* 1985;221:579.

357. Feely J, Crooks J, Forrest AL, et al. Propranolol in the surgical treatment of hyperthyroidism, including severely thyrotoxic patients. *Br J Surg* 1981;68:865.

358. Marigold JH, Morgan AK, Earle DJ, et al. Lugol's iodine: its effect on thyroid blood flow in patients with thyrotoxicosis. *Br J Surg* 1985;72:45.

359. Rudberg C, Johansson H, Akerstrom G, et al. Graves' disease in children and adolescents. Late results of surgical treatment. *Eur J Endocrinol* 1996;134:710.

360. Buckingham BA, Costin G, Roe TF, et al. Hyperthyroidism in children. *Am J Dis Child* 1981;135:112.

361. Hamburger JI. Management of hyperthyroidism in children and adolescents. *J Clin Endocrinol Metab* 1985;60:1019.

362. Glaser NS, Styne DM. Predictors of early remission of hyperthyroidism in children. *J Clin Endocrinol Metab* 1997;82:1719.

363. Zimmerman D, Lteif AN. Thyrotoxicosis in children. *Endocrinol Metab Clin North Am* 1998;27:109.

364. Cooper DS. Antithyroid drugs in the management of patients with Graves' disease: an evidence-based approach to therapeutic controversies. *J Clin Endocrinol Metab* 2003;88:3474.

365. Aro A, Huttunen JK, Lamberg B-A, et al. Comparison of propranolol and carbimazole as adjuncts to iodine-131 therapy of hyperthyroidism. *Acta Endocrinol* 1981;96:321.

366. Tibaldi JM, Barzel US, Albin J, et al. Thyrotoxicosis in the very old. *Am J Med* 1986;81:619.

367. Hamburger JI, Paul S. When and how to use higher ^{131}I doses for hyperthyroidism. *N Engl J Med* 1968;279:1361.

368. Roti E, Uberti ED. Iodine excess and hyperthyroidism. *Thyroid* 2001;11:493.

369. Masiukiewicz US, Burrow GN. Hyperthyroidism in pregnancy: diagnosis and treatment. *Thyroid* 1999;9:647.

370. Mortimer RH, Cannell GR, Addison RS, et al. Methimazole and propylthiouracil equally cross the perfused human term placental lobule. *J Clin Endocrinol Metab* 1997;82:3099.

371. Momotani N, Noh JY, Ishikawa N, et al. Effects of propylthiouracil and methimazole on fetal thyroid status in mothers with Graves' hyperthyroidism. *J Clin Endocrinol Metab* 1997;82:3633.

372. Wing DA, Millar LK, Koonings PP, et al. A comparison of propylthiouracil and methimazole in the treatment of hyperthyroidism in pregnancy. *Am J Obstet Gynecol* 1994;170:90.

373. Di Gianantonio E, Schaefer C, Mastroiacovo PP, et al. Adverse effects of prenatal methimazole exposure. *Teratology* 2001;64:262.

374. Mandel SJ, Brent GA, Larsen PR. Review of antithyroid drug use during pregnancy and report of a case of aplasia cutis. *Thyroid* 1994;4:129.

375. Mandel SJ, Cooper DS. The use of antithyroid drugs in pregnancy and lactation. *J Clin Endocrinol Metab* 2001;86:2354.

376. Momotani N, Ito K, Hamada N, et al. Maternal hyperthyroidism and congenital malformation in the offspring. *Clin Endocrinol (Oxf)* 1984;20:695.

377. Davis LE, Lucas MJ, Hankins GDV, et al. Thyrotoxicosis complicating pregnancy. *Am J Obstet Gynecol* 1989;160:63.

378. Momotani N, Noh J, Oyanagi H, et al. Antithyroid drug therapy for Graves' disease during pregnancy. *N Engl J Med* 1986;315:24.

379. Gardner DF, Cruikshank DP, Hays PM, et al. Pharmacology of propylthiouracil (PTU) in pregnant hyperthyroid women: correlation of maternal PTU concentrations with cord serum thyroid function tests. *J Clin Endocrinol Metab* 1986;62:277.

380. Cheron RG, Kaplan MM, Larsen PR, et al. Neonatal thyroid function after propylthiouracil therapy for maternal Graves' disease. *N Engl J Med* 1981;304:525.

381. Messer PM, Hauffa BP, Olbricht T, et al. Antithyroid drug treatment of Graves' disease in pregnancy: long-term effects on somatic growth, intellectual development and thyroid function of the offspring. *Acta Endocrinol* 1990;123:311.

382. Eisenstein Z, Weiss M, Katz Y, et al. Intellectual capacity of subjects exposed to methimazole or propylthiouracil in utero. *Eur J Pediatr* 1992;151:558.

383. Sherif IH, Oyan WT, Bosairi S, et al. Treatment of hyperthyroidism in pregnancy. *Acta Obstet Gynecol Scand* 1991;70:461.

384. Momotani N, Hisaokat, Noh J, et al. Effects of iodine on thyroid status of fetus versus mother in treatment of Graves' disease complicated by pregnancy. *J Clin Endocrinol Metab* 1992;75:738.

385. Lamberg BA, Ikonen E, Osterlung K, et al. Antithyroid treatment of maternal hyperthyroidism during lactation. *Clin Endocrinol (Oxf)* 1984;21:81.

386. Cooper DS. Antithyroid drugs: to breast-feed or not to breast-feed. *Am J Obstet Gynecol* 1987;157:234.

387. Momotani N, Yamashita R, Makino F, et al. Thyroid function in wholly breast-feeding infants whose mothers take high doses of propylthiouracil. *Clin Endocrinol (Oxf)* 2000;53:177.

388. Azizi F, Hedayati M. Thyroid function in breast-fed infants whose mothers take high doses of methimazole. *J Endocrinol Invest* 2002;25:493.

389. American Academy of Pediatrics, Committee on Drugs. Transfer of drugs and other chemicals into human milk. *Pediatrics* 2001;108:776.

390. Siegel RD, Lee SL. Toxic nodular goiter. *Endocrinol Metab Clin North Am* 1998;27:151.

391. Diez JJ. Hyperthyroidism in patients older than 55 years: an analysis of the etiology and management. *Gerontology* 2003;49:316.

392. Cooke ST, Ratcliffe G, Fogelman I, et al. Prevalence of inappropriate drug treatment in patients with hyperthyroidism. *BMJ* 1985;291:1491.

393. Van Soestbergen MJM, Van der Vijver JCM, Graafland AD. Recurrence of hyperthyroidism in multinodular goiter after long-term drug therapy: a comparison with Graves' disease. *J Endocrinol Invest* 1992;15:797.

394. Franklyn JA. The management of hyperthyroidism. *N Engl J Med* 1994;330:1731.

395. Ferrari C, Reschini E, Paracchi A. Treatment of the autonomous thyroid nodule: a review. *Eur J Endocrinol* 1996;135:383.

396. Ross DS, Ridgway EC, Daniels GH. Successful treatment of solitary toxic thyroid nodules with relatively low-dose iodine-131, with low prevalence of hypothyroidism. *Ann Intern Med* 1984;101:488.

397. Huysmans DA, Corstens FH, Kloppenborg PW. Long-term follow-up in toxic solitary autonomous thyroid nodules treated with radioactive iodine. *J Nucl Med* 1991;32:27.

398. Burch HB, Shakir F, Fitzsimmons TR, et al. Diagnosis and management of the autonomously functioning thyroid nodule: the Walter Reed Army Medical Center experience, 1975–1996. *Thyroid* 1998; 8:871.

399. Goldstein R, Hart IA. Follow-up of solitary autonomous thyroid nodules treated with [131]I. *N Engl J Med* 1983;309:1473.

400. Gorman CA, Robertson JS. Radiation dose in the selection of 131I or surgical treatment for toxic thyroid adenoma. *Ann Intern Med* 1978;89:85.

401. Zingrillo M, Torlontano M, Ghiggi MR, et al. Radioiodine and percutaneous ethanol injection in the treatment of large toxic thyroid nodule: a long-term study. *Thyroid* 2000;10:985.

402. Hamburger JI, Hamburger SW. Diagnosis and management of large toxic multinodular goiters. *J Nucl Med* 1985;26:888.

403. Franklyn JA, Daykin J, Holder R, et al. Radioiodine therapy compared in patients with toxic nodular or Graves' hyperthyroidism. *QJM* 1995;88:175.

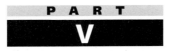
THYROID DISEASES: HYPOTHYROIDISM

SECTION A

INTRODUCTION

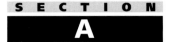

INTRODUCTION TO HYPOTHYROIDISM

LEWIS E. BRAVERMAN
ROBERT D. UTIGER

Hypothyroidism is the most common clinical disorder of thyroid function. It is most often caused by some disorder of the thyroid gland that leads to a decrease in thyroidal production and secretion of thyroxine (T_4) and triiodothyronine (T_3), in which case it is referred to as primary or thyroidal hypothyroidism. Primary hypothyroidism is invariably accompanied by increased thyrotropin (TSH) secretion. Much less often hypothyroidism is caused by decreased thyroidal stimulation by TSH, which is referred to as central, secondary, or hypothyrotropic hypothyroidism. Central hypothyroidism may be caused by pituitary or hypothalamic disease, the latter causing deficiency of thyrotropin-releasing hormone (TRH). It is usually accompanied by low or inappropriately normal serum TSH concentrations, but a few patients have high serum TSH concentrations because they secrete TSH that is immunoreactive but biologically inactive. Although most of the daily production of T_3 occurs in extrathyroidal tissue, and extrathyroidal T_3 production is decreased and serum T_3 concentrations are low in patients with nonthyroidal illness, the decrease in T_3 production in these patients is accompanied by few if any clinical manifestations of hypothyroidism (see section on Nonthyroidal Illness in Chapter 11). The rare patients with generalized resistance to thyroid hormone may have some residual signs of past hypothyroidism, but usually there are few if any symptoms or signs of hypothyroidism when the condition is recognized (see Chapter 81).

Hypothyroidism is sometimes referred to as myxedema, but the two terms are not interchangeable. Myxedema is the nonpitting edema caused by the accumulation of glycosaminoglycans in subcutaneous and other interstitial tissue that occurs in hypothyroid patients. It is most often present in long-standing or severe primary hypothyroidism (and is rarely seen today).

Primary hypothyroidism may result from diseases or treatments that destroy thyroid tissue or interfere with thyroid hormone biosynthesis (Table 46.1). Worldwide, iodine deficiency is the most common cause of hypothyroidism. In areas where iodine intake is adequate, the most common causes are chronic autoimmune thyroiditis, which occurs in both goitrous and atrophic forms, and radiation-induced hypothyroidism. The latter may be caused by radioactive iodine treatment of hyperthyroidism or external radiation therapy directed to the neck in patients with lymphoma or head and neck cancer. Although central hypothyroidism is rare, some of its causes (e.g., pituitary or hypothalamic tumors) may have disabling and even potentially fatal effects independent of the thyroid deficiency. For this reason, and because primary hypothyroidism may not be due to permanent thyroid destruction, an attempt should always be made to determine the cause of hypothyroidism in an individual patient.

The clinical manifestations of hypothyroidism are largely independent of its cause. It affects persons of all ages and both sexes, although the majority of patients are

TABLE 46.1. CAUSES OF HYPOTHYROIDISM

Primary hypothyroidism
  Destruction of thyroid tissue
    Chronic autoimmune thyroiditis—atrophic and goitrous
      forms
    Radiation—[131]I therapy for thyrotoxicosis, external
      radiotherapy to the head and neck for nonthyroid
      malignant disease
    Subtotal and total thyroidectomy
    Infiltrative diseases of the thyroid (amyloidosis,
      scleroderma)
  Defective thyroid hormone biosynthesis
    Iodine deficiency
    Drugs with antithyroid actions—lithium, iodine, and
      iodine-containing drugs and radiographic contrast
      agents
    Congenital defects in thyroid hormone biosynthesis
  Thyroid dysgenesis
Central hypothyroidism
  Pituitary disease
  Hypothalamic disease
Transient hypothyroidism
  Silent (painless) thyroiditis[a]
  Subacute thyroiditis
  After withdrawal of thyroid hormone therapy in euthyroid
    patients

[a]Including postpartum thyroiditis.

TABLE 46.2. CLINICAL MANIFESTATIONS OF HYPOTHYROIDISM

Symptoms
  Fatigue
  Lethargy
  Sleepiness
  Mental impairment
  Depression
  Cold intolerance
  Hoarseness
  Dry skin
  Decreased perspiration
  Weight gain
  Decreased appetite
  Constipation
  Menstrual disturbances
  Arthralgia
  Paresthesia
Signs
  Slow movements
  Slow speech
  Hoarseness
  Bradycardia
  Dry skin
  Nonpitting edema (myxedema)
  Hyporeflexia
  Delayed relaxation of reflexes

women, whatever the cause of the hypothyroidism. It may be overt or subclinical. The former is defined as high serum TSH concentrations and low serum free T_4 concentrations, and the latter as high serum TSH and normal serum free T_4 concentrations. Many but not all patients with overt hypothyroidism have some symptoms and signs of hypothyroidism, but the spectrum is broad; at one extreme are those patients who have no or very few symptoms and signs of hypothyroidism, and at the other extreme are those with myxedema coma (see Chapter 65) (1). Patients with subclinical hypothyroidism have few or no symptoms or signs of hypothyroidism (see Chapter 78).

The underlying problem in hypothyroidism is slowing of many physiologic processes, and the clinical manifestations reflect that slowing. Some of the more common symptoms and signs of hypothyroidism are listed in Tables 46.2 and 46.3 (2–4). These and other symptoms and signs are discussed in more detail in the chapters on the effects of hypothyroidism on different organ systems (see Chapters 52–64). None of them is a very sensitive or specific indicator of the presence of hypothyroidism (4,5). Indeed, the frequency of any individual symptom is not much higher in patients with overt hypothyroidism than in normal subjects (6). What is more important than the presence or absence of any particular symptom is the presence of multiple symptoms, particularly if of recent onset.

From the clinical perspective, therefore, hypothyroidism is a syndrome manifested by a collection of symptoms and signs. They are influenced by the age of the patient (7), the rate at which the hypothyroidism developed, and the presence of other disorders. In very young infants, hypothyroidism can result in irreversible mental and physical retardation, unless treatment is initiated within weeks after birth, whereas in children and adults its effects, while they may be profound, are reversible. Older patients tend to have fewer symptoms and signs of hypothyroidism, and those that they do have tend to be less specific (8). In general, patients who develop hypothyroidism rapidly have more symptoms than those in whom it develops slowly. In some patients, particularly those with chronic autoimmune thyroiditis, hypothyroidism may remain subclinical for many years, probably even decades, before becoming overt, testimony both to the indolent nature of the underlying process and the ability of the compensatory increase in

TABLE 46.3. CLINICAL MANIFESTATIONS OF SPECIFIC CAUSES OF HYPOTHYROIDISM

Finding	Cause of Hypothyroidism
Diffuse or nodular goiter	Chronic autoimmune thyroiditis, Ingestion of antithyroid substances Iodine deficiency or excess
Headache	Pituitary or hypothalamic tumor
Visual impairment	Pituitary or hypothalamic tumor
Deficiency or excess of pituitary hormones other than TSH	Pituitary or hypothalamic tumor

TSH secretion that occurs in all patients with any reduction in thyroid secretion to maintain near-normal thyroid hormone secretion if the thyroid gland is not seriously damaged.

We now have excellent tools to confirm the presence of hypothyroidism and to determine whether it is caused by thyroid or hypothalamic-pituitary disease in an individual patient (see Chapter 13). Determining its cause is less easy, but it is usually possible on the basis of history, physical examination, and measurements of thyroid autoantibodies in serum. T_4, the major product of the thyroid, can be easily replaced, but it is important to understand that, as shown in Table 46.1, hypothyroidism is not always due to thyroid destruction, and that in such patients the proper treatment is not to provide T_4 but to remedy the underlying disorder that led to decreased thyroid hormone synthesis, such as iodine deficiency or excess.

REFERENCES

1. Staub J-J, Althaus BU, Engler H, et al. Spectrum of subclinical and overt hypothyroidism: effect on thyrotropin, prolactin, and thyroid reserve, and metabolic impact on peripheral tissues. *Am J Med* 1992;92:621.
2. Billewicz WZ, Chapman RS, Crooks J, et al. Statistical methods applied to the diagnosis of hypothyroidism. *Q J Med* 1969;38:255.
3. Oddie TH, Boyd CM, Fisher DA, et al. Incidence of signs and symptoms in thyroid disease. *Med J Aust* 1972;2:981.
4. Zulewski H, Muller B, Exer P, et al. Estimation of tissue hypothyroidism by a new clinical score: evaluation of patients with various grades of hypothyroidism and controls. *J Clin Endocrinol Metab* 1997;82:771.
5. Bemben DA, Hamm RM, Morgan L, et al: Thyroid disease in the elderly. Part 2. Predictability of subclinical hypothyroidism. *J Fam Pract* 1994;38:583.
6. Canaris GJ, Steiner JF, Ridgway EC. Do traditional symptoms of hypothyroidism correlate with biochemical disease. *J Gen Intern Med* 1997;12:544.
7. Griffin JE. Hypothyroidism in the elderly. *Am J Med Sci* 1990;299:334.
8. Doucet J, Trivalle C, Chassagne P, et al. Does age play a role in clinical presentation of hypothyroidism? *J Am Geriatr Soc* 1994;42:984.

CAUSES OF HYPOTHYROIDISM

47

CHRONIC AUTOIMMUNE THYROIDITIS

ANTHONY P. WEETMAN

Chronic autoimmune thyroiditis is the original paradigm for autoimmune diseases in general. Only foreign proteins were considered to be antigens until Witebsky and Rose demonstrated that rabbits immunized with a saline extract of homologous thyroid tissue and Freund's adjuvant produced thyroid antibodies and had lymphocytic infiltration in the thyroid gland (1). In the same year, 1956, Doniach and Roitt reported that many patients with chronic goitrous (Hashimoto's) thyroiditis had high serum concentrations of antithyroglobulin antibodies (2). A year later, a second autoantigen was identified in the microsomal fraction of thyroid homogenates; it proved to be thyroid peroxidase (TPO) (3). We know now that other components of thyroid tissue, including the thyrotropin (TSH) receptor and, rarely, the sodium/iodide cotransporter, can serve as autoantigens.

The term *autoimmune thyroiditis* encompasses several different entities whose interrelationships remain unclear (Table 47.1). The most important are chronic goitrous thyroiditis and chronic atrophic thyroiditis. The pathology of these disorders, considered in detail in Chapter 21, consists of varying degrees of lymphocytic infiltration, fibrosis, and loss of follicular epithelium; occasionally some follicular hyperplasia is seen if the thyroid gland is enlarged. Repeat biopsies, performed at intervals of up to 20 years, reveal little alteration in thyroid histology, even in patients treated with thyroxine (T_4) (4). There is no good evidence that goitrous thyroiditis precedes atrophic thyroiditis. Among patients with hypothyroidism, the severity of fibrosis correlates with age (5). The atrophic and goitrous variants share

many clinical and biochemical, as well as pathologic, features, suggesting that their pathogenesis overlaps.

EXPERIMENTAL AUTOIMMUNE THYROIDITIS

Studies of various types of experimental autoimmune thyroiditis have provided major insights into the etiology and pathogenesis of autoimmune thyroiditis, although it is not completely satisfactory as a model of chronic autoimmune thyroiditis in humans. Immunization of mice with thyroglobulin (Tg) and an adjuvant causes transient thyroiditis, but its severity correlates only moderately well with Tg antibody production (6), and there is little change in thyroid function. Genetic susceptibility is determined predominantly but not exclusively by class I and II major histocompatibility complex (MHC) genes (6). A critical T-cell epitope in Tg includes conserved hormonogenic sites, and iodination of these may increase the antigenicity of Tg (7).

Experimental autoimmune thyroiditis can be transferred by T cells but not by serum, and both CD4 and CD8 T cells are required for optimal effects. However, a subpopulation of CD4 T cells has an important regulatory role in maintaining tolerance to Tg under normal circumstances (8). Cytotoxic CD8 T cells are important mediators of thyroid-cell damage in this type of experimental thyroiditis (9). A variation of experimental autoimmune thyroiditis is that which occurs in mice carrying human leukocyte antigen (HLA)-DR3 transgenes. These mice are susceptible to

TABLE 47.1. TYPES OF AUTOIMMUNE THYROIDITIS

	Course	Features
Goitrous (Hashimoto's) thyroiditis	Chronic	Goiter, lymphocytic infiltration, fibrosis, thyroid cell hyperplasia
Atrophic thyroiditis (primary myxedema)	Chronic	Atrophy, fibrosis
Juvenile thyroiditis	Chronic	Usually lymphocytic infiltration
Postpartum thyroiditis	Transient; may progress to chronic thyroiditis	Small goiter, some lymphocytic infiltration
Silent (painless) thyroiditis	Transient	Small goiter, some lymphocytic infiltration
Focal thyroiditis	Progressive in some patients	Present in the thyroid gland of 20% of people at autopsy

the induction of thyroiditis when immunized with Tg, unlike HLA-DR2 transgenic mice, thus confirming a role for the HLA haplotype in determining susceptibility to autoimmune thyroiditis (10).

Changes in the T-cell repertoire of mice or rats, as, for example, induced by thymectomy with or without sublethal irradiation, causes many organ-specific, genetically determined autoimmune diseases, including autoimmune thyroiditis (11). It can be transferred by CD4 cells, like when it is immunization induced, but a subfraction of normal CD4 cells prevents it, either directly or by inducing regulatory (suppressor) T cells. At least two explanations are offered for the etiology of this type of thyroiditis, related to different mechanisms for maintaining self-tolerance (Table 47.2). One is that autoreactive T cells escape tolerance because they do not encounter thyroid autoantigen in the appropriate setting in the athymic animals. However, intrathymic tolerance is never complete, and other mechanisms are required to prevent autoimmunity, such as T cell–mediated immune regulation. Thymectomy can therefore induce experimental autoimmune thyroiditis if performed at a stage of T-cell development when autoreactive, effector T cells have left the thymus for the periphery but the regulatory T cells have not. There has been intense recent interest in these regulatory T cells, one distinct population of which expresses CD4 and high levels of CD25 and may sample self antigens presented by dendritic cells in the thymus (12).

TABLE 47.2. T-CELL MECHANISMS INVOLVED IN IMMUNOLOGIC SELF-TOLERANCE

Intrathymic (central) deletion of autoreactive T cells
Intrathymic (central) anergy due to autoantigen presentation to CD4 cells in the absence of a costimulatory signal
Peripheral tolerance, usually by anergy, but deletion may occur
Active suppression of T-helper cells by several possible pathways, including cytokines and regulatory T cells
Sequestration of autoantigen, particularly by means of tissue expression of Fas ligand (immunologic privilege): autoreactive T cells expressing Fas undergo apoptosis
Absence of the activated CD4 cells required for expansion of CD8 cells or antigen sequestered by an anatomic barrier (immunologic ignorance)

Chronic thyroiditis occurs spontaneously in several animal species. A low proportion of female Buffalo strain rats develops chronic thyroiditis and high serum anti-Tg antibody concentrations, and the proportion can be increased by thymectomy or administration of methylcholanthrene (13). About 50% of diabetes-prone Biobreeding (BB) rats develop Tg antibodies and have lymphocytic infiltration of thyroid tissue, particularly when fed diets containing large amounts of iodide, but thyroid follicular destruction does not occur. The incidence of chronic thyroiditis and high serum antithyroid antibody concentrations is even higher in nonobese diabetic (NOD) mice (14).

Chronic thyroiditis in Obese strain (OS) chickens is perhaps the most like chronic goitrous thyroiditis, because these animals develop overt hypothyroidism as well as appropriate immunologic abnormalities (15). The MHC contributes slightly in determining susceptibility, but the major contribution is from uncharacterized immunoregulatory genes outside the MHC that affect T-cell responsiveness and control Tg antibody production. Additional genes increase the susceptibility of the thyroid to autoimmune damage, although no analogous genetic influence is apparent in other forms of experimental autoimmune thyroiditis.

Environmental factors are also important in the pathogenesis of autoimmune thyroiditis (16). The best characterized of these factors is iodide, which can cause thyroid injury through the generation of reactive oxygen intermediates and which may also increase the immunogenicity of Tg and directly stimulate the immune system, particularly dendritic cell function.

PREDISPOSITION TO CHRONIC AUTOIMMUNE THYROIDITIS

Autoimmune diseases usually occur when there is a failure of T-cell tolerance as a result of a combination of genetic and nongenetic factors (Table 47.3). The detailed genetics of chronic goitrous and chronic atrophic thyroiditis are considered in Chapter 20. Nongenetic factors may be endogenous or exogenous. The high prevalence of chronic autoimmune thyroiditis in women is partly related to the effects of sex hormones, and is best demonstrated by ma-

TABLE 47.3. ROLES OF GENETIC AND NONGENETIC FACTORS IN AUTOIMMUNITY

Factor	Effect
Major histocompatibility complex (MHC) class II genes	Encode products that delete autoreactive T cells, select for presentation of autoantigenic peptides, or activate suppressor T cells
Other MHC genes	Potential effects on antigen presentation; the cytokine tumor necrosis factor and some complement components also encoded in the MHC
Cytotoxic T-lymphocyte antigen-4 (CTLA-4) gene	CTLA-4 is important in terminating T-cell activation; polymorphic variants may fail to control autoreactive T cells fully
Cytokine genes	Control cytokine production
T-cell antigen receptor and immunoglobulin genes	Uncertain—some reports of association with autoimmunity
Infectious agents	May release autoantigens, alter expression of surface molecules, directly affect the immune system, or contain immunogenic sequences (epitopes) that mimic autoantigens
Dietary factors	Diverse potential effects; e.g., iodide may enhance the immunogenicity of thyroglobulin, alter thyroid cell function, or form toxic metabolites with oxygen
Toxins, pollutants	Diverse potential effects; e.g., methylcholanthrene enhances thyroiditis in Buffalo strain rats and toxins in cigarette smoke affect cytokine production
Hormones	Diverse potential effects; estrogens enhance most immune responses, whereas glucocorticoids and androgens suppress the responses
Stress	May alter neuroendocrine interactions with the immune system
Drugs	Diverse potential effects on the immune system; e.g., lithium, interferon-α, and some other cytokines exacerbate autoimmune thyroiditis

nipulation of estrogen and androgen concentrations in experimental autoimmune thyroiditis and other animal models of autoimmune disease (6), but a role for a gene on the long arm of the X chromosome is suggested by the high frequency of autoimmune thyroid disease in women with Turner's syndrome (17). Postpartum thyroiditis (see Chapter 27) also may result from hormonal effects on the immune system and is an important predictor of subsequent hypothyroidism. An alternative explanation for the effect of pregnancy in thyroid autoimmunity is the occurrence of intrathyroidal fetal microchimerism, demonstrated in both animals with experimental autoimmune thyroiditis during pregnancy and in women with Hashimoto's thyroiditis (18,19). Fetal cells may provoke an intrathyroidal alloimmune reaction that would be especially pronounced in those with preexisting subclinical autoimmune thyroiditis.

A role for stress is not apparent in chronic autoimmune thyroiditis, possibly because the disease evolves over such a long period, but stress-related variations in cortisol secretion could affect susceptibility, as suggested by observations in OS chickens (15). Low birth weight increases the prevalence of high serum antithyroid antibody concentrations in monozygotic twins discordant for birth size (20), demonstrating the potential effect of early nutritional and hormonal factors.

Despite the plausibility of the hypothesis that infectious agents cause autoimmunity via tissue damage or molecular mimicry, there is no evidence that infection plays a role in chronic autoimmune thyroiditis; this may be due to the difficulty in proving the influence of any environmental agent that may operate only at the beginning of what is a long preclinical course of disease (21). Normal gut microflora are required for the appearance of experimental autoimmune thyroiditis after thymectomy and irradiation in rats, although the mechanism is unclear (22). Polyclonal activation and molecular mimicry are both possible. There is an increase in autoimmune thyroid disease in patients with the congenital rubella syndrome (23), and hepatitis C virus infection has been associated with chronic goitrous thyroiditis in some but not other studies (24); on the other hand, chronic autoimmune thyroiditis is not a sequel of subacute granulomatous thyroiditis, which is presumed to be caused by a viral infection.

Observations in animals provide the most compelling evidence that a high dietary iodine intake can exacerbate thyroid autoimmunity. A high iodine intake increases the frequency of spontaneous thyroiditis in rats and OS chickens, as does a normal amount given after a period of iodine restriction (16). The effects of iodine supplementation on thyroid autoimmunity in humans are contradictory, probably due to the existence of immunoregulatory mechanisms that render any effects transient, and also genetic and environmental differences. Nonetheless, iodine administration can increase the frequency of high serum antithyroid antibody concentrations and lymphocytic thyroiditis in patients with goiter (25).

In patients with cancer or chronic hepatitis who have subclinical chronic autoimmune thyroiditis, treatment with interferon-α (IFN-α), interleukin-2 (IL-2), or granulocyte-macrophage colony-stimulating factor worsens the autoimmune process and may cause transient thyrotoxicosis, hypothyroidism, or both, and sometimes permanent hypothyroidism (26–28). The frequency of chronic autoimmune thyroiditis was increased in atomic bomb survivors in Japan and in children exposed to fallout after the Chernobyl nuclear reactor accident in the Ukraine (29,30).

GENETIC DEFECTS CAUSING HYPOTHYROIDISM

THOMAS VULSMA
JAN J.M. DE VIJLDER

Congenital hypothyroidism is the term applied to hypothyroidism that is present at birth. It is usually caused by defects in the development of the thyroid gland, which may be genetic, or genetic defects in the synthesis and secretion of thyroxine (T_4), the main product of the thyroid. Other, rarer causes include defects in the secretion and action of thyrotropin (TSH), the secretion and action of thyrotropin-releasing hormone (TRH), and the action of triiodothyronine (T_3), the biologically active thyroid hormone.

Congenital hypothyroidism thus includes a heterogeneous group of defects. Most cases of genetic origin are due to disorders of the thyroid gland, and for a long time the inherited disorders of thyroid hormone biosynthesis were the only ones that had been characterized in detail, based on abnormalities in iodine metabolism. During the past two decades the discovery of genes involved in thyroid development and thyroid hormone synthesis or action has expanded the spectrum of genetic disorders of the thyroid.

The clinical expression and long-term consequences of these genetic defects are dependent on the severity of the hypothyroidism, the age of onset, and the presence of associated malformations or disabilities. Congenital hypothyroidism of any cause is difficult to recognize at birth or very soon thereafter, in part because it is mitigated to some extent *in utero* by maternal-fetal transfer of T_4 (1,2). If therapy is not initiated very soon after birth, the result is irreversible damage to the developing brain (3,4). The difficulty in recognizing congenital hypothyroidism and the serious consequences of delayed therapy have led to the introduction of mass screening programs for newborn infants in many developed countries (see sections Neonatal Screening and Congenital Hypothyroidism in Chapter 75).

Approximately 70% to 80% of newborn infants with congenital hypothyroidism have an abnormality in thyroid development (thyroid dysgenesis) and 10% to 15% have an abnormality in one of the steps of thyroid hormone synthesis (thyroid dyshormonogenesis), they are said to have thyroidal congenital hypothyroidism. Most of the remainder have a hypothalamic or pituitary defect (central congenital hypothyroidism) (5,6). Disorders that affect the transport or metabolic action of thyroid hormone (peripheral hypothyroidism) are rare (see Chapter 81).

Early detection, made possible by neonatal screening, has increased the need for etiologic classification and DNA diagnosis, for adequate treatment of the affected infant and genetic counseling of the family. In this way, later progeny can be treated immediately after birth, or even prenatally. To obtain a good clinicopathologic classification (Table 48.1), sensitive immuno- and bioassays and imaging techniques are required, if necessary combined with in vivo radioiodine (^{123}I) studies, evaluation of iodine metabolism, and analysis of the iodinated compounds excreted in the urine. The results provide information about the type of congenital hypothyroidism, the proteins or factors that might be involved, and point to candidate genes that may harbor the causal gene mutations. The contribution of molecular biology to the diagnosis of genetic types of congenital hypothyroidism is increasing, and analysis of DNA is gradually replacing *in vitro* studies of tissues (7–9). Still, the molecular basis for the disorder in most infants is not known.

CENTRAL CONGENITAL HYPOTHYROIDISM

To detect central congenital hypothyroidism by neonatal screening, it is necessary to measure T_4 as well as TSH in the filter paper blood samples used for screening (see section Neonatal Screening in Chapter 75). In the Netherlands, where both T_4 and TSH are measured, the incidence of central hypothyroidism is about 1:20,000 newborn infants, substantially higher than usually assumed (5,10–12).

Central congenital hypothyroidism is a heterogeneous group of conditions. Although most cases are sporadic, they presumably originate from genetic defects. It is more common in males than females (11), for unknown reasons, but only a small percentage of cases can be ascribed to mutated genes located on the X chromosome.

Many infants with central congenital hypothyroidism, especially those with multiple pituitary hormone deficiencies, have a characteristic developmental abnormality of the infundibulum, also known as ectopic posterior lobe of the pituitary (posterior pituitary ectopia). This entity presents a distinctive appearance on T_1-weighted magnetic resonance imaging (MRI), with the hyperintense posterior lobe characteristically seen at the median eminence below the floor of the third ventricle.

Defects in Ontogeny of Hypothalamus and Pituitary Gland

The hypothalamus develops from the infundibulum, a region of the ventral diencephalons (see Chapter 2). It contains several nuclei that produce releasing and inhibiting hormones to regulate the synthesis and secretion of the various pituitary hormones. Defective neural migration in the developing infundibulum, resulting in posterior pituitary ectopia, is often accompanied by other malformations in the brain (e.g., periventricular heterotopia) (13) or elsewhere, and the functional problem may vary from isolated growth hormone deficiency to panhypopituitarism. The less visible the pituitary stalk by MRI, the more severe the anterior lobe hypoplasia and hormonal deficiencies (14). The etiology of the developmental defects is unknown. Almost all cases appear to be sporadic, with a strong male predominance. To date, *HESX1* is the only gene (rarely) associated with posterior pituitary ectopia (13,15).

The pituitary gland develops from two distinct ectoderm-derived structures, the infundibulum (a region of the ventral diencephalon) and Rathke's pouch (a derivative of the oral ectoderm). The posterior lobe develops from the infundibulum, and the intermediate and anterior lobes derive from Rathke's pouch (see Chapter 2). In the absence of the infundibulum the pituitary gland does not develop properly. Once the pituitary is developed, its secretory functions are controlled by hypothalamic neurons from the same region in the ventral diencephalon.

Mutations in several homeobox genes, including *HESX1, LHX3, LHX4, PHF6, PROP1,* and *POU1F1,* may cause central congenital hypothyroidism. In mice, the first four genes code for transcription factors that are required for the development of the forebrain, eyes, and other anterior structures, such as the hypothalamus, the pituitary gland, and the olfactory bulbs. The latter two genes code for pituitary-specific transcription factors.

Defects in *HESX1* in mice cause disorders that are comparable with septooptic dysplasia in humans (16). This entity is characterized by optic nerve hypoplasia, various forebrain defects, and multiple pituitary hormone deficiencies, including TSH deficiency. In a study of 38 patients with septooptic dysplasia, two siblings with agenesis of the corpus callosum, optic nerve hypoplasia, and panhypopituitarism were homozygous for an Arg53Cys mutation in the *HESX1* gene, resulting in a gene product incapable of binding to DNA (16). The affected siblings had consanguineous parents; heterozygous family members were normal. *HESX1* mutations have been described in other patients with congenital pituitary defects; the patients have had varying hormonal deficiencies, and some have had

optic nerve hypoplasia or abnormalities of the corpus callosum and septum pellucidum (17,18).

Homozygous mutations in the *LHX3* gene have been described in two unrelated consanguineous families. The patients had severe deficiency of all anterior pituitary hormones, except corticotropin, and a rigid cervical spine that limited head rotation. One missense mutation (Tyr116Cys) in LHX3 inhibits transcription of target genes but does not prevent DNA binding and interaction of LHX3 with partner proteins. Another mutation, an intragenic deletion, causes loss of the entire homeodomain, preventing binding of LHX3 to DNA (19).

In a family with short stature, pituitary and cerebellar defects, a poorly developed sella turcica, and multiple pituitary hormone deficiencies, including TSH deficiency, an intronic mutation in the LHX4 gene was identified that abolishes normal splicing of the LIM-homeobox transcription factor LHX4 (15). The inheritance was autosomal dominant.

The Börjeson-Forssman-Lehmann syndrome is a rare X-linked condition, characterized by early onset of multiple pituitary hormone deficiencies (most affected males are short and have hypogonadism), optic nerve hypoplasia, mild to moderate intellectual handicap, epilepsy, and the gradual development of coarse facial features. The heterozygous females are variably affected (20,21). This syndrome has been ascribed to mutations [Lys8Stop, Arg342Stop (22), and Asp333del (23)] in the *PHF6* gene. The function of the gene product is unknown, but the clinical features suggest that it plays an important role in midline neurodevelopment, including that of the hypothalamus and pituitary gland. There is a case report of a boy with a Börjeson-Forssman-Lehmann-like syndrome who had a duplication in chromosome Xq26.3-q28 (24).

Some cases of X-linked-recessive hypopituitarism have been explained by chromosomal duplication, leading to increased dosage of a still unknown gene that must be critical for pituitary development. The duplicated region, mapped to chromosome Xq26.1-q27.3, spans 9 Mb (25,26). Surviving patients had mild to moderate mental retardation.

The transcription factor POU1F1 acts as one of the main stimulators of TSH, growth hormone, and prolactin synthesis. Heterozygous, compound heterozygous, and homozygous POU1F1 deletions, and missense and nonsense mutations have been reported (27); the phenotype varies even between siblings with the same mutation (28–32). A heterozygous Arg271Try mutation exerts a dominant-negative effect (33). Hypothyroidism may be present at birth and has been detected in the screening program for congenital hypothyroidism in the Netherlands.

Mutations in *PROP1* account for the majority of cases of familial multiple pituitary hormone deficiencies. The disorder is recessively inherited; families with homozygosity or compound heterozygosity for inactivating point mutations and deletions in the PROP1 gene have been described (34). These mutations are responsible for subtypes of a multiple pituitary hormone deficiency syndrome that

TABLE 48.1. ETIOLOGIC CLASSIFICATION OF GENETIC DEFECTS CAUSING HYPOTHYROIDISM

Diagnostic Determinant vs. Etiologic Entity	Serum Free T$_4$ Concentration[a]	Serum TSH Concentration	Serum Tg Concentration	Urinary Iodopeptide Excretion	Thyroid Location and Size[b]	Thyroid Radioiodide Uptake[c]	Radioiodide Release after NaClO4[d]	Mode of Inheritance[e]
Congenital hypothyroidism of central origin								
Hypothalamic/pituitary dysgenesis	Low	Low to high	Low	Not indicated	Normal or hypoplastic	Not indicated	Not indicated	Autosomal recessive or dominant in a few cases
Hypothalamic/pituitary dyshormonogenesis								
TRH hypo-responsiveness	Low	Low	Low	Not indicated	Normal or hypoplastic	Not indicated	Not indicated	Autosomal recessive
TSH synthesis defect	Low	Low	Low	Not indicated	Normal or hypoplastic	Not indicated	Not indicated	Autosomal recessive
TSH hypoactivity	Low or normal	Normal or high	Low or normal	Not known	Not known	Low or normal	Absent	Autosomal recessive
Congenital hypothyroidism of thyroidal origin								
Thyroid dysgenesis								
Agenesis	Low or normal	Very high	Absent	Absent	Absent	Absent	Absent	Autosomal recessive or dominant in a few cases
Cryptic remnant	Low or normal	Very high	Low or normal	Absent	Absent	Absent	Absent	
Dystopic remnant	Low or normal	High	Low to high	Absent or low	(Sub-)lingual	Low or normal	Absent	
Eutopic remnant	Low or normal	High	Not known	Absent or low	Hypoplastic	Low or normal	Absent	
Thyroid dyshormonogenesis								
TSHR deficiency	Low or normal	High	Low or normal	Not known	Normal or hyperplastic	Low	Absent	Autosomal recessive
Gsa deficiency	Low or normal	Normal or high	Low or normal	Absent	Normal	Low	Absent	Autosomal dominant
Total sodium-iodide symporter defect	(Very) low	Very high	Very high	Absent	Normal or hyperplastic	Absent[f]	Absent	Autosomal recessive
Pendred's syndrome[g]	Low or normal	Normal or high	Normal or high	Absent	Normal or hyperplastic	Normal or high	Partial	Autosomal recessive
Total iodide organification defect	Low	Very high	Very high	Absent	Normal or hyperplastic	Rapid and high	Total	Autosomal recessive
Partial iodide organification defect	Low or normal	High	(Very) high	Absent or low	Normal or hyperplastic	High	Partial	Autosomal recessive
Thyroglobulin-synthesis defect	Low or normal	Normal or high	Low or normal	High	Normal or hyperplastic	Rapid and high	Absent	Autosomal recessive

Congenital hypothyroidism due to defects in peripheral tissues

Thyroidal and/or peripheral genetic defects	Serum T4	Serum T3	Serum TSH	Presence of MIT and DIT	Thyroid gland	Radioiodide uptake	Discharge	Inheritance
Iodide recycling defect (dehalogenase defect)	Low or normal	High	Very high		Normal or hyperplastic	High	Absent	Autosomal recessive
T4/T3 transmembrane transporter defect	Low	Very high T3	Not known Low reverse-T3	Not indicated	Normal or hyperplastic	Not known	Not indicated	X-linked
Thyroid hormone hyporesponsiveness	High	Normal or high	Normal or high	Not indicated	Normal or hyperplastic	High	Not indicated	Autosomal dominant
Excessive loss of thyroid hormone	Normal or low	Normal or high	Not known	Not indicated	Normal or hyperplastic	Not known	Not indicated	Depends on etiology

[a] In newborn infants who cannot produce any T_4, maternal-fetal transfer results in cord serum T_4 concentrations of 2.7–5.4 μg/dL (35–70 nmol/L) and comparable cord serum free T_4 concentrations, which decline with a half-life of 2.7–5.3 days.

[b] The thyroid's location in the neck region and its size is preferably examined by ultrasound imaging, or by radioiodide ($Na^{123}I$) imaging.

[c] $Na^{123}I$ is administered intravenously [27 μCi (1 MBq) for infants younger than 1 year and 54 μCi (2 MBq) for older children]. In general, the radioiodide uptake is a function of the amount of thyroid tissue and the degree of stimulation by TSH.

[d] Sodiumperchlorate is administered intravenously 2 hours after $Na^{123}I$ (10 mg/kg body mass, maximum 400 mg). Discharge of thyroidal radioiodide after 1 hour: <10% is normal; 10%–20% is borderline; >20% is abnormal.

[e] When the full-blown disease has an autosomal-recessive pattern of inheritance, some heterozygous relatives have mild abnormalities in the relevant tests.

[f] The most characteristic abnormality in patients with a total sodium-iodide symporter defect is a (very) low saliva/serum ratio of radioiodide: for neonates >10 is normal, 3–10 is borderline, <3 is abnormal. The saliva/blood ratio is 1.17 times the saliva/serum ratio (95% confidence interval 1.15–1.19). Partial iodide transport defect is an ill-defined condition; if it exists, the diagnostic test results depend entirely on the iodine intake, which varies greatly worldwide.

[g] The most important determinant of Pendred's syndrome is the sensorineural hearing defect.

DIT, diiodotyrosine; MIT, monoiodotyrosine; T_3, triiodothyronine; T_4, thyroxine; Tg, thyroglobulin; TSH, thyrotropin.

include TSH, growth hormone, prolactin, gonadotropin, and corticotropin deficiencies. The mutation is often a 2-bp deletion in an AG-rich region in exon 2 of the gene, resulting in a premature stop codon; another mutation (149delGA) resulting in the same stop codon has been described (see reference 34 for review).

The clinical abnormalities in patients with inactivating mutations in PROP1 differ from those of patients with inactivating POU1F1 mutations. The hormonal deficiencies emerge in a typical order, rather than being present at birth. Neonatal features of hypothyroidism such as prolonged jaundice have been described only once, and growth appears to be normal during infancy (35,36). Growth hormone deficiency becomes evident before TSH deficiency in 80% of patients, and gonadotropin deficiency comes later, although most patients fail to enter puberty spontaneously. Corticotropin deficiency is the last manifestation, often occurring several decades after birth. The degree of prolactin deficiency is variable. Although all untreated patients end up extremely short and sexually immature, their intelligence is normal, indicating that they were euthyroid during the first few years after birth. Central hypothyroidism caused by deficiency of PROP1 deficiencies has not been detected in the Dutch neonatal screening program for hypothyroidism.

Pituitary morphology in patients with PROP1 deficiency varies from hypoplastic to hyperplastic, without involvement of the surrounding tissues. The distinct MRI characteristics of pituitary enlargement may originate from the intermediate lobe (37).

Developmental defects such as solitary maxillary central incisor, nasal pyriform aperture stenosis, and variants of holoprosencephaly can be clues to the presence of deficiencies of one or more pituitary hormones (38). These entities have been associated with inactivating mutations in the *SHH* and *SIX3* genes; loss of one SHH allele is sufficient to cause holoprosencephaly (39). There are no case reports of isolated central hypothyroidism in patients with SHH or SIX3 mutations.

Defects in Thyrotropin-Releasing Hormone

Thyrotropin-releasing hormone (TRH), the tripeptide pyroglutamyl-histidyl-prolineamide, is the major hypothalamic mediator of the synthesis and secretion of TSH. It is present throughout the brain, but is found in highest concentrations in the paraventricular nuclei and median eminence of the hypothalamus (see section Regulation of Thyrotropin Secretion in Chapter 10). Hypothyroidism occurs in mice in which the TRH gene is deleted (40). However, no patient with a mutation in the gene for the precursor of TRH (preproTRH) or the gene for the enzymes that cleave prepro-TRH to its component TRH molecules has been described.

Central congenital hypothyroidism with complete absence of increases in serum TSH and prolactin concentrations in response to exogenous TRH has been described (41). The affected patient was compound heterozygous for two mutations in the TRH receptor. Both mutations resulted in production of receptors unable to bind TRH. The patient had mild hypothyroidism, short stature, and markedly delayed bone maturation. The parents and eldest brother, who were heterozygous for one of the mutations, were normal.

Defects in Synthesis of Thyrotropin

Thyrotropin is a heterodimer composed of noncovalently linked α- and β-subunits. It shares the α-subunit with follicle-stimulating hormone, luteinizing hormone, and chorionic gonadotropin; each has a different β-subunit (see section Chemistry and Biosynthesis Of Thyrotropin in Chapter 10). TSH stimulates the growth and function of the thyroid via interaction with its specific plasma membrane receptor.

Genetic disorders of TSH synthesis are rare. They include patients whose TSH has decreased bioactivity, resulting in mild hypothyroidism and high serum concentrations of immunoreactive TSH (42), as well as patients with totally inactive TSH and severe congenital hypothyroidism (43).

A variety of inactivating mutations has been described in the gene for the β-subunit of TSH. A nonsense mutation (Glu12X) was found in two Greek families (44). Three Japanese families had a Gly29Arg mutation in the [Cys-Ala-Gly-Tyr-Cys] region of the gene, which results in synthesis of β-subunits that cannot combine with α subunits (45). Other mutations include a Glu49X mutation that resulted in a truncated inactive TSH (46,47), a Cys85Arg mutation (48), and a defect in the donor splice site of intron 2 (G → A + 5) (49). The most frequent mutation is a single-base deletion in codon 105 in exon 3, resulting in a frame shift and a premature stop codon (Cys105FS114X). A disulfide bond between Cys19 and Cys105 in the β-subunit is predicted to form the "buckle" of a "seat-belt" that surrounds the subunit and maintains the conformation and bioactivity of the hormone (50–56). Another mutation, 313deltaT, is recognized as a founder effect in several German families (57).

Most patients with defects in TSH had severe hypothyroidism when discovered, mostly after the neonatal period. They are not identified by screening programs that measure only blood-spot TSH concentrations (56) (see section Neonatal Screening in Chapter 75).

THYROIDAL CONGENITAL HYPOTHYROIDISM

The overall incidence of thyroidal congenital hypothyroidism is on average 1:4,000, but varies considerably in different countries and among different racial and ethnic groups (5) (see section Neonatal Screening in Chapter 75).

The majority of patients with thyroidal congenital hypothyroidism have abnormal thyroid development (thyroid dysgenesis). Therefore, diagnostic evaluation should include an imaging procedure. If the infant has a normally shaped and located thyroid gland, irrespective of its size, and a high serum TSH concentration, further studies with radioiodide will provide information about thyroidal iodide metabolism. Measurements of serum thyroglobulin and low-molecular-weight iodopeptides in the urine help to discriminate between the various types of defects, and measurement of urinary iodide excretion helps to differentiate genetic defects from iodine deficiency or excess (Fig. 48.1 and Table 48.1). Because it is essential to treat newborn infants with congenital hypothyroidism immediately, blood and urine samples must be obtained immediately after referral. Radioiodide studies can be conducted a few days after T_4 therapy is started, before the infant's serum TSH concentration decreases to normal. Alternatively, these studies can be performed at 3 to 4 years of age, when T_4 therapy can be interrupted safely for several weeks.

Defects in Ontogeny of the Thyroid Gland

The development of the thyroid gland starts with an invagination of the ventral endoderm of the future oral cavity (median anlage). This invagination develops into a bilobar structure, and subsequently each lobe fuses with an ultimobranchial body (lateral anlage) derived from the fourth pharyngeal pouches while migrating to the distal part of the neck (see Chapter 2). Thyroid follicles appear at 10 weeks of gestation, indicating that the thyroid follicular cells can synthesize thyroglobulin. At the same time, iodine accumulates in the fetal thyroid, indicating that thyroid oxidase and peroxidase are active. By mid-gestation the thyroid is able to secrete substantial amounts of T_4. Serum free T_4 concentrations gradually increase until adult values are reached at about 36 weeks of gestation (see Chapter 74).

Thyroid dysgenesis, the most common cause of congenital hypothyroidism in iodine-sufficient areas), is easy to recognize, but its cause is not known. The great majority of cases are sporadic (5), but multiple cases occur in a few families (8), and up to 5% of patients have other congenital, mainly cardiac malformations (58). Some observations point to genetic defects. Thyroid dysgenesis is more prevalent among people of European origin than African or Asian origin, and the patients are predominantly (~70%) female (5,58). A peculiar phenomenon is the striking discordance of monozygotic twins for thyroid dysgenesis (5,59), a major argument against an exogenous (maternal) factor as its primary cause. Among the rare descriptions of

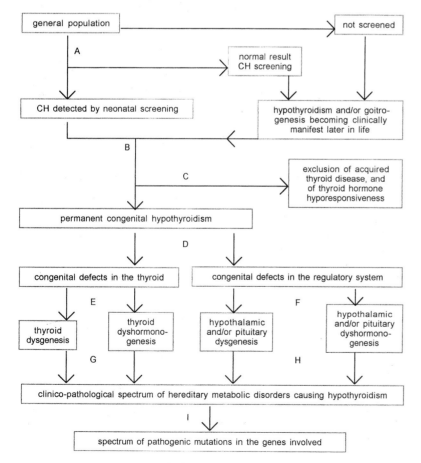

FIGURE 48.1. Flow chart for etiologic classification of disorders causing congenital hypothyroidism (*CH*). **A:** Neonatal screening by measurements of thyroxine (T_4) and thyrotropin (TSH) in dried blood samples on filter paper. **B:** Confirmation by measurement of serum TSH and serum free T_4. **C:** If the serum free T_4 concentration is inappropriately high in relation to the serum TSH concentration, clinical evaluation of the infant and measurement of maternal TSH receptor–stimulating antibodies and urinary iodine excretion are indicated. **D:** Decide whether the serum free T_4 and TSH values indicate the presence of thyroidal or central congenital hypothyroidism. **E:** Perform thyroid radionuclide imaging or ultrasonography to distinguish between thyroid dysgenesis or thyroid dyshormonogenesis. **F:** Perform magnetic resonance imaging of the hypothalamus and pituitary. **G:** Measure serum thyroglobulin and thyroid radioiodide uptake (including discharge after perchlorate), and test urine for iodopeptides or iodotyrosines. **H:** Evaluate other components of hypothalamic-pituitary function. **I:** Perform mutation analysis to identify the specific defect.

monozygotic twins concordant for thyroid dysgenesis, the rudiments of thyroid tissue were concordant or discordant (5,60).

The clinical consequences are highly variable, from severe hypothyroidism due to thyroid agenesis to moderate hypothyroidism due to ectopic (usually sublingual) thyroid rudiments to subclinical hypothyroidism (high serum TSH but normal serum free T_4 concentrations) in patients with thyroid hemiagenesis.

In mice, the transcription factors Nkx2.1 (Ttf1), FoxE1 (Ttf2; Fkhl15), Pax8, and Shh are essential for thyroid development (61–64), whereas thyroid development is normal in the absence of TSH or TSH receptors (65). Few humans with thyroid dysgenesis have had mutations in the human homologues NKX2.1 (TTF1), FOXE1 (TTF2, FKHL15), or PAX8. The thyroid phenotype is highly variable, including agenesis, hypoplastic eutopic or ectopic rudiments, and an (apparently) normally developed thyroid gland (8). Mutations in the human homologue of Shh causing thyroid dysgenesis have not been described.

Several infants with both neonatal thyroid dysfunction and respiratory failure who had a deletion of chromosome 14q12–13.3 containing the homeobox gene *NKX2.1* have been described (66,67). Other patients with congenital hypothyroidism caused by mutations in the NKX2.1 gene had a variable degree of hypothyroidism, as well as mental retardation, choreoathetosis, hypotonia, pulmonary problems, and hypothalamic abnormalities (68,69).

A homozygous missense mutation in FOXE1 (Ala65Val, within the forkhead-binding domain) was found in two siblings with the Bamforth-Lazarus syndrome (cleft palate, choanal atresia, and thyroid dysgenesis). The defect resulted in impaired DNA binding and loss of transcriptional function (70). Another biallelic Ser57Asn mutation in the DNA-binding domain was found in patients with thyroid agenesis and cleft palate, but no choanal atresia (71). The less severe phenotype in the latter patients suggests partial function of the mutated *FOXE1* gene.

In a study of 145 patients with congenital hyperthyroidism, several were found to have mutations in one allele of the *PAX8* gene (72). One patient with a hypoplastic thyroid gland had a *de novo* Arg108Stop mutation. Another had a dysgenetic eutopic thyroid gland and an Arg31His mutation. A Leu63Arg mutation was found in one allele of this gene in a mother and two of her children with dysgenetic eutopic thyroid glands, hypothyroidism, and low serum thyroglobulin concentrations; the father was normal. *In vitro* expression experiments revealed that the differently mutated PAX8 molecules were unable to bind DNA and activate gene expression (72). The dominant expression of the PAX8 inactivating mutations is noteworthy. One explanation for the severe changes is that transcription of one wild-type allele yields insufficient amounts of the gene product, perturbing the binding equilibrium with competitors or cofactors, a phenomenon called haploinsufficiency (73). Mutations in the genes for these competitors or cofactors would have a similar effect. One of these factors is Ref-1, a nuclear protein that augments the DNA binding of PAX8 (74).

Williams' syndrome is a complex multisystemic syndrome that includes a characteristic elfin facies, cardiovascular malformations, and mental and growth retardation. The prevalence is between 1:10,000 and 1:20,000; almost all cases are sporadic. The syndrome arises because of a deletion that includes the elastin gene (*ELN*). Mild hypothyroidism has been recognized as a component of this syndrome; some patients have had thyroid dysgenesis (sublingual rudiment, hemiagenesis) (75).

The Young-Simpson syndrome is a rare syndrome characterized by thyroidal congenital hypothyroidism, mental retardation, peculiar facies, growth retardation, cryptorchidism, congenital heart defects, and many other milder malformations (76). The reported cases have all been sporadic. The congenital hypothyroidism is detectable by neonatal screening. Its severity varies considerably, depending on the extent of thyroid dysgenesis, which varies from agenesis to mild hypoplasia (77).

Finally, congenital hypothyroidism due to thyroid agenesis has been described in association with the CHARGE association (coloboma, heart defects, choanal atresia, retarded growth and development or central nervous system anomalies, genital hypoplasia, and ear anomalies or deafness) (78). The CHARGE association also has been associated with congenital hypopituitarism (79).

Hyporesponsiveness to Thyrotropin

Thyrotropin exerts its biologic activity by binding to the TSH receptor, a glycoprotein containing an extracellular amino-terminal region, seven transmembrane domains with three extra- and three intracellular loops, and an intracellular carboxyl-terminal domain. Activation of the receptor leads to activation of a stimulatory guanine nucleotide-binding (G) protein, resulting in stimulation of adenylyl cyclase and therefore increased production of cyclic adenosine monophosphate, and, at high TSH concentrations, stimulation of the phospholipase C and inositol pathway as well (see the section Thyrotropin Receptor in Chapter 10). Hyporesponsiveness (or resistance) to TSH may occur as a result of mutations in the TSH receptor, G protein, or specific proteins or factors further downstream in the signal transduction pathways.

Defects in the Thyrotropin Receptor

Mutations in the TSH receptor gene causing loss of function result in thyroidal congenital hypothyroidism. Patients with mutant receptors that can bind TSH, albeit with less affinity than normal receptors, may have, with

TSH stimulation, near-normal serum T_4 and T_3 concentrations and no thyroid enlargement (80). Patients whose mutant receptors have little or no affinity for TSH have severe hypothyroidism, despite high serum TSH concentrations (81–83). These patients have a normal-sized thyroid gland and low serum thyroglobulin concentrations. A list of the known mutations is available online (84). The inheritance is usually autosomal recessive; most patients have been found to be compound heterozygotes.

Abnormalities in the G Protein α Subunit

Another type of TSH hyporesponsiveness is found in patients with pseudohypoparathyroidism type 1a (Albright's hereditary osteodystrophy), a variably expressed disorder with autosomal-dominant inheritance (85,86). These patients have an approximately 50% reduction in the activity of the α-subunit of the stimulatory G protein. Multiple mutations have been found in the *GNAS1* gene coding for this protein. The patients often have low-normal serum T_4 concentrations, and little clinical evidence of hypothyroidism. Although early detection by neonatal screening has been described (4,87), the blood-spot TSH and T_4 concentrations usually do not reach the cut-off values for recall.

Several families have been reported in which some family members had congenital hypothyroidism with no goiter and in whom no TSH receptor or G protein mutations were detected (88). In two families the hyporesponsiveness was inherited as an autosomal-dominant trait. These findings suggest the presence of mutations in other steps in the TSH signaling pathway.

Defects in Thyroidal Iodide Transport

Iodide has to be transported from the extracellular fluid via thyroid follicular cells into the follicular lumen before it can be used to form T_4 and T_3. Therefore, iodide has to cross both the basolateral and apical membranes of the cells, after which it is oxidized and bound to tyrosine residues in thyroglobulin (see sections Thyroid Iodine Transport and Thyroid Hormone Synthesis in Chapter 4).

Iodide transport across the basolateral membrane, the crucial first step in thyroid hormone synthesis, is mediated by the sodium-iodide symporter (89). Iodide transport across the apical membrane is mediated by pendrin (90), and perhaps also another apical iodide transporter (AIT, SLC5A8) (91,92). Pendrin is encoded by the *PDS* gene (SLC26A4) (93–95).

The transport of iodide from the circulation into the thyroid can be traced by administration of radioiodide. Inhibition of radioiodide uptake by anions of similar molecular size and charge, such as perchlorate or thiocyanate, allows detection of the efflux of any accumulated iodide back into the circulation, and thus provides indirect information about the activity of the oxidation and organification processes.

Defects in Basolateral Iodide Transport

The postulated existence of genetic defects in thyroidal iodide transport in 1956 (96) has been confirmed by studies in patients with congenital hypothyroidism who had a low thyroid radioiodide uptake and a well-developed, often enlarged thyroid gland (97–99). In the first months of life, when the thyroid gland may not yet be visible or palpable, it can be difficult to distinguish iodide transport defects from thyroid agenesis. Measurement of serum thyroglobulin and ultrasonography of the thyroid can help to discriminate between the two disorders (99) (Table 48.1). The iodide transport defect is characterized by hypothyroidism, gradual goiter formation, low or very low serum T_4 concentrations, high serum TSH and thyroglobulin concentrations, undetectable or very low radioiodide uptake by the thyroid, and a saliva/serum ratio of radioiodide of about 1. The inheritance pattern is autosomal recessive (Table 48.1). The severity of the hypothyroidism, and as a consequence the neurodevelopmental impairment of affected patients, varies considerably, in part because of variation in dietary iodine intake. The patients can be treated with large doses of iodine, but treatment with T_4 is preferable, especially at young ages.

The sodium-iodide symporter gene was cloned in 1996, and since then some patients with this defect have been found to have mutations in this gene (89). The structural change has been defined for a few mutations. For instance, in the Thr235Pro mutation (100), the substituted threonine lies in the middle of a well-conserved putative transmembrane segment of the symporter that is essential for transport function, most likely for Na^+ binding and translocation (101). Another amino acid important for symporter activity is the glycine residue at position 395. Substitutions of large amino acid residues at this position diminished the maximal transport rate without affecting the Michaelis-Menten constant (K_m) values for I^- or Na^+ (102). One patient with an iodide transport defect was heterozygous for two different mutations. The paternally derived allele had a Gln267Glu mutation, resulting in an inactive cotransporter, and the maternally derived allele had a C1940G transversion, which created a downstream cryptic splice acceptor site in exon 13, resulting in a 67-bp deletion and a frame shift resulting in an unstable messenger RNA (mRNA). The predicted transcript would code for a truncated protein lacking 129 amino acids (103).

Defects in Apical Iodide Transport

Over 100 years ago Pendred described a syndrome characterized by overt, or more often subclinical, hypothyroidism, goiter, and moderate to severe sensorineural hearing loss (104). This syndrome has an autosomal-recessive inheritance. The prevalence varies between 1:15,000 and 1:100,000; it may be the most common genetic defect causing congenital hypothyroidism. Usually thyroid hormone synthesis is only mildly impaired, and therefore few patients with Pendred's syndrome are detected by neonatal screening (4).

One of the characteristic features of Pendred's syndrome is partial discharge of thyroidal radioiodide after administration of perchlorate, indicating that defective pendrin molecules result in intracellular iodide accumulation (105) (Table 48.1). This explains why, before the molecular defect was elucidated, Pendred's syndrome was classified as a partial iodide organification defect. Even in patients in whom the PDS gene mutation results in complete loss of function of pendrin, the radioiodide discharge after perchlorate is partial (90), an (indirect) indication that pendrin is not the exclusive apical cell membrane transporter.

PDS mutation analysis has been performed in many families. Frame shift mutations, mutations leading to aberrant splicing, and nonsense and missense mutations have been found. Two of them, Leu236Pro and Thr416Pro, are recurrent mutations (106). Recently a Val138Phe mutation was described as a founder mutation in German families (107). Usually, mutations in the PDS gene cause subclinical hypothyroidism and gradual thyroid enlargement combined with hearing loss, but mutations in the PDS gene have also been found in patients with large vestibular aqueduct defects who have normal thyroid function (108).

No mutations in the apical iodide transporter gene have been reported.

Defects in Iodide Organification

Iodine oxidation and organification are catalyzed by thyroid peroxidase. This enzyme is located primarily in the apical cell membrane, but its active center protrudes into the follicular lumen. It catalyzes not only iodide oxidation and organification, but also the coupling of iodotyrosine residues in thyroglobulin to form iodothyronines, mainly T_4 (109,110). The oxidizing agent used for iodination and coupling of iodotyrosine residues is hydrogen peroxide, synthesized by the thyroid oxidases THOX1 and THOX2 (111–113) (see section Thyroid Hormone Synthesis in Chapter 4).

In patients with defects in iodide oxidation and organification, little or no iodide is oxidized and organified, and T_4 and T_3 production is decreased or even absent, whereas iodide transport and thyroglobulin synthesis are strongly stimulated by TSH. Therefore, radioiodide uptake and serum thyroglobulin concentrations are high. The block in iodide oxidation and organification results in increased intracellular iodide concentrations, which can be quantified by measuring the amount of radioiodide lost from the gland after the administration of sodium or potassium perchlorate (Table 48.1).

Iodide oxidation and organification defects can be the result of abnormalities of thyroid peroxidase (114) or the H_2O_2 generating system (115,116).

Defects in Thyroid Peroxidase

Iodide oxidation and organification defects, transmitted as autosomal-recessive traits, are caused by abnormalities in thyroid peroxidase. The abnormalities include the inability to produce the enzyme, defects in its heme- or substrate-binding site, and abnormalities in the distribution of the enzyme in the thyroid (114,117–120). Most of the patients have a total inability to oxidize and organify iodide and consequently cannot produce T_4 or T_3 (Fig. 48.2). In a study of 29 Dutch families with this disorder, 16 different mutations in the thyroid peroxidase gene were found; 13 families were homozygous, and 16 were compound heterozygous (121). In four families only one mutated allele could be detected; in one family with a total iodide organification defect no mutation in the gene could be found (116). The most frequent mutation (14 of 36 alleles) was duplication of a GGCC sequence in exon 8. In one patient with severe hypothyroidism due to a total organification defect, partial maternal isodisomy of chromosome 2p was demonstrated. The mother was heterozygous for the same mutation (T2512del in exon 14) as her son had in both alleles, whereas the father had normal alleles (122). Apparently partial maternal isodisomy (2pter-2p12) is compatible with normal physical and mental development (122). Another total iodide organification defect was found in three siblings with a single mutated allele (Arg693Trp) inherited from the unaffected father; mutations in the maternal allele, maternal imprinting, and major deletions of the maternal chromosome at 2p25 were excluded (123). Several other inactivating mutations have been described in patients with total or partial iodide organification defects, including monoallelic and biallelic mutations, indicative of substantial allelic heterogeneity (124,125).

Mutations in thyroid peroxidase have also been reported in three siblings with onset of mild hypothyroidism in childhood and a partial iodide organification defect. The patients were compound heterozygous for a missense mutation (G1687T, exon 9) and a deletion (1808–13del, exon 10) (126). In expression studies, the protein with the missense mutation was retained in the cytoplasm of the cell, and the deleted protein had diminished enzyme activity.

Defects in Thyroid Oxidase

One patient with a total iodide organification defect has been described who was homozygous for a premature stop codon in the *THOX2* gene. The resulting truncated pro-

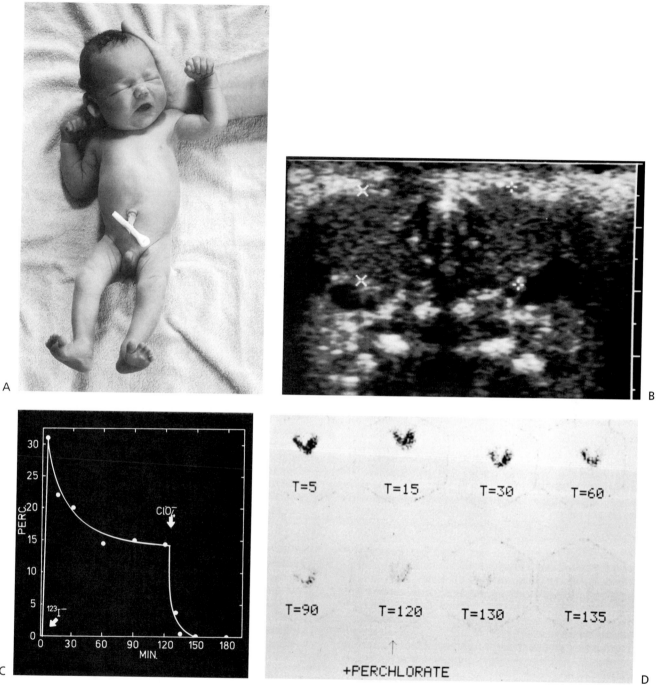

FIGURE 48.2. Newborn infant with congenital hypothyroidism due to a total iodide organification defect caused by mutations in both alleles of the thyroid peroxidase (TPO) gene (maternal allele, 20-bp duplication in exon 2, most likely resulting in a stop codon in exon 3; paternal allele, G2485A mutation translated into a Glu799Lys substitution, rendering TPO inactive, as proven by *in vitro* expression) (114). Because it was already known that the infant's brother had this disease, diagnosis could be made immediately after birth. **A:** Photograph of the infant showing periorbital edema and depressed nasal bridge, indicative of delayed bone maturation. **B:** Ultrasound image showing a symmetric, enlarged thyroid gland, not detected by physical examination. **C:** Plot of serial measurements of thyroidal ^{123}I uptake after intravenous administration of ^{123}I$^-$ [25 μCi (0.9 MBq)] and then, at 120 minutes, administration of NaClO$_4$ (100 mg intravenously). The ^{123}I was taken up more rapidly than normal, and then some was released. Blocking the uptake with NaClO$_4$ resulted in immediate release of the remaining ^{123}I, indicating that it was nonoxidized and nonorganified iodide. The release of all ^{123}I within 30 minutes after NaClO$_4$ administration indicates the complete inability of the patient's thyroid to oxidize and organify iodide. **D:** Images of the patient's thyroid during the ^{123}I$^-$ uptake and release study showing rapid uptake, and then rapid release after administration of NaClO$_4$ at 120 minutes. (From De Vijlder JJM, Vulsma T. Congenitale hypothyreoïdie. In: Wiersinga WM, Krenning EP, eds. *Schildklierziekten*. Houten, The Netherlands: Bohn, Stafleu & Van Loghum, 1998, with permission.)

tein had no functional domain. Monoallelic inactivating THOX2 mutations were found in three other patients who had a partial iodide organification defect. These patients had mild hypothyroidism at birth but were euthyroid later in childhood (116).

Questions remain about the role of THOX1 in thyroid physiology; no patients with mutations in the THOX1 gene have been reported.

Defects in Thyroglobulin Synthesis

Thyroglobulin is exclusively synthesized in the thyroid gland, and its production is essential for thyroid hormone synthesis. The thyroglobulin gene is greater than 300,000 bp in size, and the coding sequence has 8307 nucleotides, divided over 48 exons, of which 66 are triplets coding for tyrosine (127,128). Thyroglobulin is a homodimer with subunits of 330,000 daltons (330 kd) that contains several repeated amino acid sequences, about 60 disulfide bridges, and 10% carbohydrate (129) (see Chapter 5). Its structural conformation, which is dependent on the extent of glycosylation, is important for T_4 and T_3 synthesis. Defects in transcription, translation, or posttranslational processing cannot be distinguished by clinicopathologic classification; therefore, all these defects are classified as being defects in thyroglobulin synthesis (130).

Patients with defects in thyroglobulin synthesis have moderate to severe hypothyroidism. Most have low serum thyroglobulin concentrations, especially in relation to the degree of TSH stimulation (4); iodoproteins (mainly iodoalbumin) may be found in the circulation and iodopeptides in the urine (131,132). The processes of iodide uptake, oxidation, and organification are intact.

The exceptional size of the thyroglobulin gene has made it difficult to identify mutations in the regulatory or coding regions of the gene. Several mutations have been described in animals (see reference 133 for review); five mutations have been described in humans. A homozygous Arg227Stop mutation resulted in a short 30-kd fragment of thyroglobulin; the patients had mild hypothyroidism (134). Another patient had a homozygous mutation at the acceptor site of intron 3, resulting in an in-frame deletion of exon 4. The aberrant thyroglobulin lacked the donor tyrosine 130, resulting in less efficient T_4 and T_3 production, and a Cys-TrpCys repeat that could lead to misfolding and accumulation of the protein in the endoplasmic reticulum and subsequent proteolysis; this patient had severe hypothyroidism (135). In a third patient, a homozygous Arg1510Stop mutation gave rise to a truncated thyroglobulin molecule missing 57 amino-acid residues due to alternative splicing of exon 22; the patients had hypothyroidism and large goiters (136). A Cys1263Arg mutation in thyroglobulin caused a defect in intracellular transport due to an arrest in the endoplasmic reticulum; the patients had mild hypothyroidism, indicating that some thyroglobulin reached the follicular lumen (137). In a family with severe hypothy-

roidism, the thyroglobulin mRNA lacked 138 nucleotides between positions 5590 and 5727, resulting in retention of the protein in the endoplasmic reticulum (138,139). Based on the location of the mutations, it seems that shorter thyroglobulin molecules are associated with less severe hypothyroidism. It may be that shorter molecules are more easily secreted into the follicular lumen, where T_4 and T_3 are formed (133).

In six patients with the clinicopathologic features of a thyroglobulin synthesis defect, no mutations in the thyroglobulin gene other than polymorphisms were detected (130). These patients may have defects in posttranslational processing of thyroglobulin, for example, in glycosylation or intracellular chaperoning, or deficiencies of transcription factors such as NKX2.1 (140).

PERIPHERAL CONGENITAL HYPOTHYROIDISM

Defects in Recycling of Iodide

Thyroglobulin, after internalization by pinocytosis from the follicular lumen into thyroid follicular cells, is incorporated into early and late endosomes. These organelles, containing proteolytic enzymes, hydrolyze thyroglobulin to its constituent amino acids, including monoiodotyrosine (MIT) and diiodotyrosine (DIT), as well as T_4 and T_3. Subsequently, the iodotyrosines are deiodinated by specific dehalogenases present not only in the thyroid but also in peripheral tissues. Genetic defects in dehalogenases lead to loss of the iodotyrosines from the thyroid and their rapid excretion by the kidneys. The result is excessive loss of iodine, mimicking hypothyroidism due to iodine deficiency (141–144) (Table 48.1).

The inheritance is autosomal recessive, but some features of the disorder are expressed in heterozygotes, for example, goitrogenesis, a relatively high thyroid radioiodide uptake, and increased urinary excretion of DIT (144). The clinical expression depends strongly on the dietary iodine intake, which may explain why autosomal-dominant inheritance has been suggested (145). The disorder is not detected by neonatal screening, probably because maternal dehalogenase activity prevents loss of the iodotyrosines prenatally.

A single case report described a remarkable young woman with goitrous hypothyroidism due to a dehalogenase defect who also had hypogonadotropic hypogonadism, hyperprolactinemia, and hyperaldosteronism. She had very high serum MIT and DIT concentrations, which apparently inhibited tyrosine hydroxylase activity, decreasing dopamine synthesis, which in turn caused the hyperprolactinemia and hyperaldosteronism. The latter resolved with T_4 therapy (146).

Mutations in the *DEHAL1* gene, isolated from a thyroid library, are the likely cause of thyroid dehalogenase defects (147). This gene encodes a protein with a conserved nitroreductase domain that is capable of dehalogenating iodotyrosines (147,148); however, no mutations have as yet been detected.

Defects in Transmembrane Transport of Thyroxine and Triiodothyronine

T_4 and T_3 are carried into cells by several cell membrane transport systems. They include monocarboxylate transporter 8 (MCT8), located on the X chromosome (149,150). Males with MCT8 mutations have severe neurologic defects, psychomotor retardation, and mild hypothyroidism, with high serum T_3 concentrations (151, 152). The MCT8 genes of these patients contained deletions, frame shifts, and missense and nonsense mutations. Whether all the abnormalities are a result of decreased T_4 transport into the brain or other substances important in neurodevelopment are not transported normally, is not clear. What is clear is that these males are not protected against neurologic defects and hypothyroidism *in utero* by maternal-fetal transfer of T_4.

MISCELLANEOUS DEFECTS

Newborn and older infants with Down syndrome may have slightly high serum TSH concentrations and slightly low serum total and free T_4 concentrations, which tend to disappear as the infants age (153). The etiology is unclear. The infants do not have thyroid enlargement, and TSH bioactivity is normal (154). Although the relationship with trisomy 21 is obscure, the changes seem to be specific for Down's syndrome.

The Wolcott-Rallison syndrome is a rare autosomal-recessive disorder characterized by infancy-onset type 1 diabetes mellitus, spondyloepiphyseal dysplasia with short-trunk dwarfism, recurrent hepatitis, renal insufficiency, and developmental delay. The presence of collagen fibers of varying thickness and intracellular collagen-like fibers suggest an abnormality in collagen synthesis or processing. The syndrome is associated with mutations in the EIF2AK3 gene, which encodes translation initiation factor 2α kinase-3 (155). Some patients also have central hypothyroidism, with no MRI abnormalities (156).

The Pallister-Hall syndrome has as its common features hypothalamic hamartoma, mental retardation, seizures, polydactyly, bifid epiglottis, imperforate anus, and cardiac, renal, and pulmonary anomalies. The syndrome is often sporadic, but is sometimes inherited in an autosomal-dominant pattern. Mutations in the GLI3 gene are thought to be responsible for the syndrome. Some patients have pituitary dysgenesis, and as a consequence multiple pituitary hormone deficiencies, and others have thyroid dysgenesis (157).

The Johanson-Blizzard syndrome is a rare syndrome characterized by multiple anomalies, with autosomal-recessive inheritance (158–160). Approximately 25% of patients have thyroidal hypothyroidism, of unknown cause. Other features include intrauterine and postnatal growth retardation, developmental brain defects, midline ectodermal scalp defects, aplasia or hypoplasia of the nasal alae, congenital sensorineural hearing loss, absent permanent teeth, pancreatic exocrine insufficiency with malabsorption, and rectourogenital abnormalities. A few autopsy reports mention grossly and microscopically normal thyroid glands with abundant scalloping of colloid (161–163). In some of these infants thyroid function is sufficiently abnormal at birth that the hypothyroidism can be detected by neonatal screening.

Patients with several other syndromes (e.g., the Beckwith-Wiedemann syndrome, Ascher syndrome, and hypohydrotic ectodermal dysplasia syndrome) sometimes have hypothyroidism as one of many abnormalities (164). No doubt other syndromes that include congenital hypothyroidism will be recognized (165).

Finally, infants with congenital hypothyroidism detected by neonatal screening have a high frequency of additional congenital anomalies. In a large group of infants with congenital hypothyroidism in Italy, the prevalence of congenital malformations was more than four times higher than in the normal population (166). They included cardiac anomalies, anomalies of the nervous system and eyes, and multiple congenital malformations.

TREATMENT

In general, treatment of a patient with a genetic defect in thyroid hormone secretion is similar to the treatment of any other patient of the same age with hypothyroidism. In the neonatal period, the primary goal of treatment is prevention of brain damage, with irreversible motor and cognitive impairment. That these problems occur in infants with severe hypothyroidism is clear. Although the risk for lesser degrees of hypothyroidism is less clear, prudence dictates that treatment be initiated immediately in any infant with hypothyroidism, irrespective of severity and etiology (167). As noted above, treatment can be stopped at age 3 to 4 years, and the child evaluated in detail to confirm, or refute, the diagnosis of hypothyroidism, and if it is present to determine its cause.

The goal of treatment in infants with thyroidal hypothyroidism should be to normalize serum TSH concentrations; for infants with central hypothyroidism the goal should be a serum free T_4 concentration near the upper limit of the normal range for age (168). The details of treatment and follow-up are discussed in detail in the section on congenital hypothyroidism in Chapter 75.

In most of the genetic disorders that impair thyroid hormone synthesis, the thyroid gland will eventually become hyperplastic and nodular if serum TSH concentrations are even slightly elevated for a prolonged period. However, if

T_4 treatment is started at a very young age, and serum TSH concentrations are maintained within the normal range, goitrogenesis should not occur.

The treatment of infants with peripheral congenital hypothyroidism depends on the underlying defect. In case of an iodide recycling defect, euthyroidism can be restored by administration of high doses of iodine, but it is easier to give T_4. Treatment of thyroid hormone resistance depends on its severity and the relative responsiveness of peripheral tissues and the pituitary; judicious administration of T_4 may be indicated in infants with marked resistance (see Chapter 81).

Whether infants with defects in the thyroid hormone transmembrane transport might benefit from T_4 (or T_3) therapy is not known.

REFERENCES

1. Vulsma T, Gons MH, De Vijlder JJM. Maternal-fetal transfer of thyroxine in congenital hypothyroidism due to a total organification defect or thyroid agenesis. *N Engl J Med* 1989;321:13.
2. Morreale de Escobar G, Obregón MJ, et al. Maternal thyroid hormones early in pregnancy and fetal brain development. *Baillieres Best Pract Res Clin Endocrinol Metab* 2004;18:225.
3. Kooistra L, Laane C, Schellekens JMH, et al. Motor and cognitive development in congenital hypothyroidism: a long-term evaluation of the effects of neonatal treatment. *J Pediatr* 1994;124:903.
4. Rovet JF, Ehrlich RM. Long-term effects of L-thyroxine therapy for congenital hypothyroidism. *J Pediatr* 1995;126:380.
5. Vulsma T. Etiology and pathogenesis of congenital hypothyroidism. Evaluation and examination of patients detected by neonatal screening in The Netherlands [Ph.D. thesis]. Amsterdam: University of Amsterdam, 1991.
6. Lanting CI, van Tijn DA, Loeber JG, et al. Screening for CH in the Netherlands: use of thyroxine/TBG ratio [Abstract P24]. Presented at the Proceedings of the 5th Meeting of the International Society for Neonatal Screening, Genova, Italy, June 2002, p. 93.
7. De Vijlder JJM. Primary congenital hypothyroidism, defects in iodine pathways. *Eur J Endocrinol* 2003;149:247.
8. Grüters A. Diagnostic tests of thyroid function in children and adolescents. In: Ranke MB, ed. *Diagnostics of endocrine function in children and adolescents*. Basel, Switzerland: Karger, 2003:93.
9. Moreno JC, de Vijlder JJM, Vulsma T, et al. Genetic basis of hypothyroidism: recent advances, gaps and strategies for future research. *Trends Endocrinol Metab* 2003;14:318.
10. Fisher DA, Klein AH. Thyroid development and disorders of thyroid function in the newborn. *N Engl J Med* 1981;304:702.
11. Hanna CE, Krainz PL, Skeels MR, et al. Detection of congenital hypopituitary hypothyroidism: ten-year experience in the Northwest Regional Screening Program. *J Pediatr* 1986;109:959.
12. Vulsma T, Delemarre HA, de Muinck Keizer SMPF, et al. Detection and classification of congenital thyrotropin deficiency in The Netherlands. In: *The thyroid gland, environment and autoimmunity*. Amsterdam: Excerpta Medica, International Congress Series, 1989;896:343.
13. Mitchell LA, Thomas PQ, Zacharin MR, et al. Ectopic posterior pituitary lobe and periventricular heterotopia: cerebral malformations with the same underlying mechanism? *AJNR* 2002;23:1475.
14. Chen S, Leger J, Garel C, et al. Growth hormone deficiency with ectopic neurohypophysis: anatomical variations and relationship between the visibility of the pituitary stalk asserted by magnetic resonance imaging and anterior pituitary function. *J Clin Endocrinol Metab* 1999;84:2408.
15. Machinis K, Pantel J, Netchine I, et al. Syndromic short stature in patients with a germline mutation in the LIM homeobox LHX4. *Am J Hum Genet* 2001;69:961.
16. Dattani MT, Martinez-Barbera JP, Thomas PQ, et al. Mutations in the homeobox gene HESX1/hesx1 associated with septo-optic dysplasia in human and mouse. *Nat Genet* 1998;19:125.
17. Dattani MT, Robinson IC. HESX1 and septo-optic dysplasia. *Rev Endocrinol Metab Disorders* 2002;3:289.
18. Tajima T, Hattorri T, Nakajima T, et al. Sporadic heterozygous frameshift mutation of HESX1 causing pituitary and optic nerve hypoplasia and combined pituitary hormone deficiency in a Japanese patient. *J Clin Endocrinol Metab* 2003;88:45.
19. Netchine I, Sobrier M-L, Krude H, et al. Mutations in LHX3 result in a new syndrome revealed by combined pituitary hormone deficiency. *Nat Genet* 2000;25:182.
20. Turner G, Gedeon A, Mulley J, et al. I. Börjeson-Forssman-Lehmann syndrome: clinical manifestations and gene localization to Xq26–27. *Am J Med Genet* 1989;34:463.
21. Lower KM, Turner G, Kerr BA, et al. Mutations in PHF6 are associated with Börjeson-Forssman-Lehmann syndrome. *Nat Genet* 2002;32:661.
22. Birrell G, Lampe A, Richmond S, et al. Börjeson-Forssman-Lehmann syndrome and multiple pituitary hormone deficiency. *J Pediatr Endocrinol Metab* 2003;16:1295.
23. Baumstark A, Lower KM, Sinkus A, et al. Novel PHF6 mutation p.D333del causes Börjeson-Forssman-Lehmann syndrome. *J Med Genet* 2003;40:e50.
24. Gecz J, Baker E, Donnelly A, et al. Fibroblast growth factor homologous factor 2 (FHF2): gene structure, expression and mapping to the Borjeson-Forssman-Lehmann syndrome region in Xq26 delineated by a duplication breakpoint in a BFLS-like patient. *J Hum Genet* 1999;104:56.
25. Lagerstrom-Fermer M, Sundvall M, Johnsen E, et al. X-linked recessive panhypopituitarism associated with a regional duplication in Xq25-q26. *Am J Hum Genet* 1997;60:910.
26. Solomon NM, Nouri S, Warne GL, et al. Increased gene dosage at Xq26-q27 is associated with X-linked hypopituitarism. *Genomics* 2002;79:553.
27. Collu R. Genetic aspects of central hypothyroidism. *J Endocrinol Invest* 2000;23:125.
28. D'Elia AV, Tell G, Paron I, et al. Missense mutations of human homeoboxes: a review. *Hum Mutat* 2001;18:361.
29. Hendriks-Stegeman BI, Augustijn KD, Bakker B, et al. Combined pituitary hormone deficiency caused by compound heterozygosity for two novel mutations in the POU domain of the Pit1/POU1F1 gene. *J Clin Endocrinol Metab* 2001;86:1545.
30. Blankenstein O, Muhlenberg R, Kim C, et al. A new C-terminal located mutation (V272ter) in the PIT-1 gene manifesting with severe congenital hypothyroidism. Possible functionality of the PIT-1 C-terminus. *Horm Res* 2001;56:81.
31. Gat-Yablonski G, Lazar L, Pertzelan A, et al. A novel mutation in PIT-1: phenotypic variability in familial combined pituitary hormone deficiencies. *J Pediatr Endocrinol Metab* 2002;15:325.
32. McLennan K, Jeske Y, Cotterill A, et al. Combined pituitary hormone deficiency in Australian children: clinical and genetic correlates. *Clin Endocrinol (Oxf)* 2003;56:785.
33. Radovick S, Nations M, Du Y, et al. A mutation in the POU-homeodomain of Pit-1 responsible for combined pituitary hormone deficiency. *Science* 1992;292:1115.

34. Mody S, Brown MR, Parks JS. The spectrum of hypopituitarism caused by PROP1 mutations. *Best Pract Res Clin Endocrinol Metab* 2002;16:421.

35. Arroyo A, Pernasetti F, Vasilyev VV, et al. A unique case of combined pituitary hormone deficiency caused by a PROP1 gene mutation (R120C) associated with normal height and absent puberty. *Clin Endocrinol (Oxf)* 2002;57:283.

36. Voutetakis A, Maniati-Christidi M, Kanaka-Gantenbein C, et al. Prolonged jaundice and hypothyroidism as the presenting symptoms in a neonate with a novel Prop1 gene mutation (Q83X). *Eur J Endocrinol* 2004;150:257.

37. Voutetakis A, Argyropoulou M, Sertedaki A, et al. Pituitary magnetic resonance imaging in 15 patients with Prop1 gene mutations: pituitary enlargement may originate from the intermediate lobe. *J Clin Endocrinol Metab* 2004;89:2200.

38. Lo FS, Lee YJ, Lin SP, et al. Solitary maxillary central incisor and congenital nasal pyriform aperture stenosis. *Eur J Pediatr* 1998;157:39.

39. Nanni L, Ming JE, Du Y, et al. SHH mutation is associated with solitary median maxillary central incisor: a study of 13 patients and review of the literature. *Am J Med Genet* 2001;102:1.

40. Yamada M, Satoh T, Mori M. Mice lacking the thyrotropin-releasing hormone gene: what do they tell us? *Thyroid* 2003;13:1111.

41. Collu R, Tang J, Castagne J, et al. A novel mechanism for isolated central hypothyroidism: inactivating mutations in the thyrotropin-releasing hormone receptor gene. *J Clin Endocrinol Metab* 1997;82:1561.

42. Spitz IM, Le Roith D, Hirsch H, et al. Increased high-molecular weight thyrotropin with impaired biologic activity in a euthyroid man. *N Engl J Med* 1981;304:278.

43. Miyai K, Azukizawa M, Kumahara Y. Familial isolated thyrotropin deficiency with cretinism. *N Engl J Med* 1971;285:1043.

44. Dacou-Voutetakis C, Feltquate DM, Drakopoulou M, et al. Familial hypothyroidism caused by a nonsense mutation in the thyroid-stimulating hormone beta-subunit gene. *Am J Hum Genet* 1990;46:988.

45. Hayashizaki Y, Hiraoka Y, Tatsumi K, et al. Deoxyribonucleic acid analyses of five families with familial inherited thyroid stimulating hormone deficiency. *J Clin Endocrinol Metab* 1990;71:792.

46. Bonomi M, Proverbio MC, Weber G, et al. Hyperplastic pituitary gland, high serum glycoprotein hormone alpha-subunit, and variable circulating thyrotropin (TSH) levels as a hallmark of central hypothyroidism due to mutations of the TSH beta gene. *J Clin Endocrinol Metab* 2001;86:1600.

47. Vuissoz JM, Deladouy J, Buyukgebiz A, et al. New autosomal recessive mutation of the TSH-beta subunit gene causing central isolated hypothyroidism. *J Clin Endocrinol Metab* 2001;86:4468.

48. Sertedaki A, Papadimitriou A, Voutetakis A, et al. Low TSH congenital hypothyroidism: identification of a novel mutation of the TSH beta-subunit gene in one sporadic case (C85R) and of mutation Q49stop in two siblings with congenital hypothyroidism. *Pediatr Res* 2002;52:935.

49. Pohlenz J, Dumitrescu A, Aumann U, et al. Congenital secondary hypothyroidism caused by exon skipping due to a homozygous donor splice mutation in the TSH-beta-subunit gene. *J Clin Endocrinol Metab* 2002;87:336.

50. Medeiros-Neto G, Herodotou DT, Rajan S, et al. A circulating biologically inactive thyrotropin caused by a mutation in the beta subunit gene. *J Clin Invest* 1996;97:1250.

51. Doeker BM, Pfäffle RW, Pohlenz J, et al. Congenital central hypothyroidism due to a homozygous mutation in the thyrotropin beta-subunit gene follows an autosomal recessive inheritance. *J Clin Endocrinol Metab* 1998;83:1762.

52. Biebermann H, Liesenkotter KP, Emeis M, et al. Severe congenital hypothyroidism due to a homozygous mutation of the betaTSH gene. *Pediatr Res* 1999;46:170.

53. Heinrichs C, Parma J, Scherberg NH, et al. Congenital isolated hypothyroidism caused by a homozygous mutation in the TSH-beta subunit gene. *Thyroid* 2000;10:387.

54. McDemott MT, Haugen BR, Black JN, et al. Congenital isolated central hypothyroidism caused by a "hot spot" mutation in the thyrotropin-beta gene. *Thyroid* 2002;12:1141.

55. Deladoey J, Vuissoz JM, Domene HM, et al. Congenital secondary hypothyroidism due to a mutation C105Vfs114X thyrotropin-beta mutation: genetic study of five unrelated families from Switzerland and Argentina. *Thyroid* 2003;13:553.

56. Morales AE, Shi JD, Wang CY, et al. Novel TSH beta subunit gene mutation causing congenital central hypothyroidism in a newborn male. *J Pediatr Endocrinol Metab* 2004;17:355.

57. Brumm H, Pfeufer A, Biebermann H, et al. Congenital central hypothyroidism due to homozygous thyrotropin beta 313 delta T mutation is caused by a founder effect. *J Clin Endocrinol Metab* 2002;87:4811.

58. Devos H, Rodd C, Gagne N, et al. A search for the possible molecular mechanism of thyroid dysgenesis: sex ratios and associated malformations. *J Clin Endocrinol Metab* 1999;84:2502.

59. Perry R, Heinrichs C, Bourdoux P, et al. Discordance of monozygotic twins for thyroid dysgenesis: implications for screening and for molecular pathophysiology. *J Clin Endocrinol Metab* 2002;87:4072.

60. McLean R, Howard N, Murray IP. Thyroid dysgenesis in monozygotic twins: variants identified by scintigraphy. *Eur J Nucl Med* 1985;10:346.

61. Pan Q, Li C, Xiao J, et al. *In vivo* characterization of the Nkx2.1 promoter/enhancer elements in transgenic mice. *Gene* 2004;331:73.

62. De Felice M, Ovitt C, Biffali E, et al. A mouse model for hereditary thyroid dysgenesis and cleft palate. *Nat Genet* 1998;19:395.

63. Mansouri A, Chowdhury K, Gruss P. Follicular cells of the thyroid gland require Pax8 gene function. *Nat Genet* 1998;19:87.

64. Fagman H, Grande M, Gritli-Linde A, et al. Genetic deletion of sonic hedgehog causes hemiagenesis and ectopic development of the thyroid in mouse. *Am J Pathol* 2004;164:1865.

65. Postiglione MP, Parlato R, Rodriguez-Mallon A, et al. Role of the thyroid-stimulating hormone receptor signaling in development and differentiation of the thyroid gland. *Proc Natl Acad Sci U S A* 2002;99:15462.

66. Devriendt K, Vanhole C, Matthijs G, et al. Deletion of thyroid transcription factor-1 gene in an infant with neonatal thyroid dysfunction and respiratory failure. *N Engl J Med* 1998;338:1317.

67. Iwatani N, Mabe H, Devriendt K, et al. Deletion of NKX2.1 gene encoding thyroid transcription factor-1 in two siblings with hypothyroidism and respiratory failure. *J Pediatr* 2000;137:272.

68. Krude H, Schütz B, Biebermann H, et al. Choreoathetosis, hypothyroidism and pulmonary alterations due to human NKX2–1 haploinsufficiency. *J Clin Invest* 2002;109:475.

69. Pohlenz J, Dumitrescu A, Zundel D, et al. Partial deficiency of thyroid transcription factor 1 produces predominantly neurological defects in humans and mice. *J Clin Invest* 2002;109:469.

70. Clifton-Bligh RJ, Wentworth JM, Heinz P, et al. Mutation of the gene encoding human TTF-2 associated with thyroid agenesis, cleft palate and choanal atresia. *Nat Genet* 1998;19:399.

71. Castanet M, Park S-M, Smith A, et al. A novel loss-of-function mutation in TTF-2 is associated with congenital hypothyroidism, thyroid agenesis and cleft palate. *Hum Mol Genet* 2002;11:2051.

72. Macchia PE, Lapi P, Krude H, et al. PAX8 mutations associated with congenital hypothyroidism caused by thyroid dysgenesis. *Nat Genet* 1998;19:83.

73. Damante G. Thyroid defects due to Pax8 gene mutations. *Eur J Endocrinol* 1998;139:563.

74. Tell G, Pellizarri L, Cimarosti D, et al. Ref-1 controls Pax-8 DNA-binding activity. *Biochem Biophys Res Commun* 1998; 252:178.

75. Bini R, Pela I. New case of thyroid dysgenesis and clinical signs of hypothyroidism in Williams syndrome. *Am J Med Genet* 2004;127A:183.

76. Masuno M, Imaizumi K, Okada T, et al. Young-Simpson syndrome: further delineation of a distinct syndrome with congenital hypothyroidism, congenital heart defects, facial dysmorphism and mental retardation. *Am J Med Genet* 1999;84:8.

77. Kondoh T, Kinoshita E, Moriuchi H, et al. Young-Simpson syndrome comprising transient hypothyroidism, normal growth, macular degeneration and torticollis. *Am J Med Genet* 2000;90:85.

78. Marin JF, Garcia B, Quintana A, et al. The CHARGE association and athyreosis. *J Med Genet* 1991;28:207.

79. August GP, Rosenbaum KN, Friendly D, et al. Hypopituitarism and the CHARGE association. *J Pediatr* 1983;103:424.

80. Sunthornthepvarakul T, Gottschalk ME, Hayashi Y, et al. Resistance to thyrotropin caused by mutations in the thyrotropin receptor gene. *N Engl J Med* 1995;332:155.

81. Biebermann H, Schöneberg T, Krude H, et al. Mutations of the human thyrotropin receptor gene causing thyroid hypoplasia and persistent congenital hypothyroidism. *J Clin Endocrinol Metab* 1997;82:3471.

82. Gagné N, Parma J, Deal G, et al. Apparent congenital athyreosis contrasting with normal plasma thyroglobulin levels and associated with inactivating mutations in the thyrotropin receptor gene: are athyreosis and ectopic thyroid distinct entities? *J Clin Endocrinol Metab* 1998;83:1771.

83. Park SM, Clifton-Bligh RJ, Betts P, et al. Congenital hypothyroidism and apparent athyreosis with compound heterozygosity or compensated hypothyroidism with probable hemizygosity for inactivating mutations of the TSH receptor. *Clin Endocrinol (Oxf)* 2004;60:220.

84. *www.uni-leipzig.de/ninnere/tsh/frame.html;* accessed September 27, 2004.

85. Albright F, Burnett CH, Smith PH, et al. Pseudohypoparathyroidism an example of "Seabright-Bantam syndrome." Report of three cases. *Endocrinology* 1942;30:922.

86. Davies SJ, Hughes HE. Imprinting in Albright's hereditary osteodystrophy. *J Med Genet* 1993;30:101.

87. Levine MA, Jap TS, Hung W. Infantile hypothyroidism in two sibs: an unusual presentation of pseudohypoparathyroidism type Ia. *J Pediatr* 1985;107:919.

88. Xie J, Pannain S, Pohlenz J, et al. Resistance to thyrotropin (TSH) in three families is not associated with mutations in the TSH receptor or TSH. *J Clin Endocrinol Metab* 1997;82:3933.

89. Dohan O, De la Vieja A, Paroder V, et al. The sodium/iodide symporter (NIS): characterization, regulation, and medical significance. *Endocr Rev* 2003;24:48.

90. Gillam MP, Sidhaye AR, Lee EJ, et al. Functional characterization of pendrin in a polarized cell system. Evidence for pendrin-mediated apical iodide efflux. *J Biol Chem* 2004;279:13004.

91. Rodriquez A, Perron B, Lacroix L, et al. Identification and characterization of a putative human iodide transporter located at the apical membrane of thyrocytes. *J Clin Endocrinol Metab* 2002;87:3500.

92. Lacroix L, Pourcher T, Magnon C, et al. Expression of the apical iodide transporter in human thyroid tissues: a comparison study with other iodide transporters. *J Clin Endocrinol Metab* 2004;89:1423.

93. Everett LA, Glaser B, Beck JC, et al. Pendred syndrome is caused by mutations in a putative sulphate transporter gene (PDS). *Nat Genet* 1997;17:411.

94. Lacroix L, Mian C, Caillou B, et al. Na(+)/I(-) symporter and Pendred syndrome gene and protein expressions in human extra-thyroidal tissues. *Eur J Endocrinol* 2001;144:297.

95. Scott DA, Wang R, Kreman TM, et al. The Pendred syndrome gene encodes a chloride-iodide transport protein. *Nat Genet* 1999;21:440.

96. Stanbury JB, Querido A. Genetic and environmental factors in cretinism: a classification. *J Clin Endocrinol Metab* 1956;16: 1522.

97. Federman D, Robbins J, Rall JE. Some observations on cretinism and its treatment. *N Engl J Med* 1958;259:610.

98. Stanbury JB, Chapman EM. Congenital hypothyroidism with goitre. Absence of an iodide-concentrating mechanism. *Lancet* 1960;1:1162.

99. Vulsma T, Rammeloo JA, Gons MH, et al. The role of serum thyroglobulin concentration and thyroid ultrasound imaging in the detection of iodide transport defects in infants. *Acta Endocrinol (Copenh)* 1991;124:405.

100. Fujiwara H, Tatsumi K, Miki K, et al. Congenital hypothyroidism caused by a missense mutation in the Na+/I- symporter. *Nat Genet* 1997;16:124 [erratum in *Nat Genet* 1997;17: 122].

101. Levy O, Ginter CS, De la Vieja A, et al. Identification of a structural requirement for thyroid Na+/I- symporter (NIS) function from analysis of a mutation that causes human congenital hypothyroidism. *FEBS Lett* 1998;429:36.

102. Dohán O, Gavrielides MV, Ginter C, et al. Na+/I- symporter activity requires a small and uncharged amino acid residue at position 395. *Mol Endocrinol* 2002;16:1893.

103. Pohlenz J, Rosenthal IM, Weiss RE, et al. Congenital hypothyroidism due to mutations in the sodium/iodide symporter. Identification of a nonsense mutation producing a downstream cryptic 3' splice site. *J Clin Invest* 1998;101:1028.

104. Pendred V. Deaf mutism and goitre. *Lancet* 1896;2:532.

105. Reardon W, Trembath RC. Pendred syndrome. *J Med Genet* 1996;33:1037.

106. Van Hauwe P, Everett LA, Coucke P, et al. Two frequent missense mutations in Pendred syndrome. *Hum Mol Genet* 1998;7: 1099.

107. Borck G, Roth C, Martine U, et al. Mutations in the PDS gene in German families with Pendred's syndrome: V138F is a founder mutation. *J Clin Endocrinol Metab* 2003;88:2916.

108. Spitzweg C, Heufelder AE, Morris JC. Thyroid iodine transport. *Thyroid* 2000;10:321.

109. De Vijlder JJM, den Hartog MT. Anionic iodotyrosine residues are required for iodothyronine synthesis. *Eur J Endocrinol* 1998;138:227.

110. Kimura S, Hong YS, Kotani T, et al. Structure of the human thyroid peroxidase gene: comparison and relationship to the human myeloperoxidase gene. *Biochemistry* 1989;28:4481.

111. Dupuy C, Ohayon R, Valent A, et al. Purification of a novel flavoprotein involved in the thyroid NADPH oxidase. Cloning of the porcine and human cDNAs. *J Biol Chem* 1999;274: 37265.

112. DeDeken X, Wang D, Costagliola S, et al. Cloning of two hyman thyroid cDNAs encoding new members of the NADPH oxidase family. *J Biol Chem* 2000;275:23227.

113. Moreno JC, Pauws E, van Kampen AHC, et al. Cloning of tissue-specific genes using serial analysis of gene expression and a novel computational subtraction approach. *Genomics* 2001; 75:70.

114. Bikker H, Baas F, de Vijlder JJM. Molecular analysis of mutated thyroid peroxidase detected in patients with total iodide organification defects. *J Clin Endocrinol Metab* 1997;82:649.

115. Niepomniszcze H, Targovnik HM, Gluzman BE, et al. Abnormal H_2O_2 supply in the thyroid of a patient with goiter and iodine organification defect. *J Clin Endocrinol Metab* 1987;65:344.

116. Moreno JC, Bikker H, Kempers MJ, et al. Inactivating mutations in the gene for thyroid oxidase 2 (THOX2) and congenital hypothyroidism. *N Engl J Med* 2002;347:95.

117. Kimura S, Hong YS, Kotani T, et al. Structure of the human thyroid peroxidase gene: comparison and relationship to the human myeloperoxidase gene. *Biochemistry* 1989;28:4481.

118. Ambrugger P, Stoeva1 I, Biebermann H, et al. Novel mutations of the thyroid peroxidase gene in patients with permanent congenital hypothyroidism. *Eur J Endocrinol* 2001;145:19.

119. Umeki K, Kotani T, Kawano J, et al. Two novel missense mutations in the thyroid peroxidase gene, R665W and G771R, result in a localization defect and cause congenital hypothyroidism. *Eur J Endocrinol* 2002;146:491.

120. Niu DM, Hwang B, Chu YK, et al. High prevalence of a novel mutation (2268insT) of the thyroid peroxidase gene in Taiwanese patients with total iodide organification defect and evidence for a founder effect. *J Clin Endocrinol Metab* 2002;87:4208.

121. Bakker B, Bikker H, Vulsma T, et al. Two decades of screening for congenital hypothyroidism in The Netherlands: TPO gene mutations in total iodide organification defects (an update). *J Clin Endocrinol Metab* 2000;85:3708.

122. Bakker B, Bikker H, Hennekam RC, et al. Maternal isodisomy for chromosome 2p causing severe congenital hypothyroidism. *J Clin Endocrinol Metab* 2001;86:1164.

123. Fugazzola L, Cerutti N, Mannavola D, et al. Monoallelic expression of mutant thyroid peroxidase allele causing total iodide organification defect. *J Clin Endocrinol Metab* 2003;88:3264.

124. Rivolta CM, Esperante SA, Gruñeiro-Papendieck L, et al. Five novel inactivating mutations in the thyroid peroxidase gene responsible for congenital goiter and iodide organification defect. *Hum Mutat* 2003;22:259.

125. Nascimento AC, Guedes DR, Santos CS, et al. Thyroperoxidase gene mutations in congenital goitrous hypothyroidism with total and partial iodide organification defect. *Thyroid* 2003;13:1145.

126. Kotani T, Umeki K, Kawano J, et al. Partial iodide organification defect caused by a novel mutation of the thyroid peroxidase gene in three siblings. *Clin Endocrinol (Oxf)* 2003;59:198.

127. Van de Graaf SAR, Pauws E, de Vijlder JJM, et al. The revised 8307 base pair coding sequence of human thyroglobulin, transiently expressed in eukaryotic cells. *Eur J Endocrinol* 1997;136:508.

128. Mendive FM, Rivolta CM, Vassart G, et al. Genomic organization of the 3′ region of the human thyroglobulin gene. *Thyroid* 1999;9:903.

129. Malthièry Y, Lissitzky S. The primary structure of human thyroglobulin deduced from the sequence of its 8448 base complementary DNA. *Eur J Biochem* 1987;165:491.

130. Van de Graaf SAR, Cammenga M, Ponne NJ, et al. The screening for mutations in the thyroglobulin cDNA from six patients with congenital hypothyroidism. *Biochimie* 1999;81:425.

131. De Vijlder JJM, Veenboer GJM, van Dijk JE. Thyroid albumin originates from blood. *Endocrinology* 1992;131:578.

132. Gons MH, Kok JH, Tegelaers WHH, et al. Concentration of plasma thyroglobulin and urinary excretion of iodinated material in the diagnosis of thyroid disorders in congenital hypothyroidism. *Acta Endocrinol (Copenh)* 1983;104:27.

133. De Vijlder JJM. Primary congenital hypothyroidism: defects in iodine pathways. *Eur J Endocrinol* 2003;149:247.

134. Van de Graaf SAR, Ris-Stalpers C, Veenboer GJM, et al. A premature stopcodon in thyroglobulin mRNA results in familial goiter and moderate hypothyroidism. *J Clin Endocrinol Metab* 1999;84:2537.

135. Ieiri T, Cochaux R, Targovnik HM, et al. A 38 splice site mutation in the thyroglobulin gene responsible for congenital goiter with hypothyroidism. *J Clin Invest* 1991;88:1901.

136. Targovnik HM, Medeiros-Neto G, Varela V, et al. A nonsense mutation causes human hereditary congenital goiter with preferential production of a 171-nucleotide-deleted thyroglobulin ribonucleic acid messenger. *J Clin Endocrinol Metab* 1993;77:210.

137. Hishinuma A, Takamatsu J, Ohyama Y, et al. Two novel cysteine substitutions (C1263R and C1995S) of thyroglobulin cause a defect in intracellular transport of thyroglobulin in patients with congenital goiter and the variant type of adenomatous goiter. *J Clin Endocrinol Metab* 1999;84:1438.

138. Targovnik HM, Vono J, Billerbeck AEC, et al. A 138-nucleotide-deletion in the thyroglobulin ribonucleic acid messenger in a congenital goiter with defective thyroglobulin synthesis. *J Clin Endocrinol Metab* 1995;80:3356.

139. Medeiros-Neto G, Kim PS, Yoo SE, et al. Congenital hypothyroid goiter with deficient thyroglobulin. Identification of an endoplasmic reticulum storage disease with induction of molecular chaperones. *J Clin Invest* 1996;15:2838.

140. Acebron A, Aza-Blanc P, Rossi DL, et al. Congenital human thyroglobulin defect due to low expression of thyroid-specific transcription factor TTF-1. *J Clin Invest* 1995;96:781.

141. Stanbury JB, Kassenaar AAH, Meijer JWA, et al. The occurrence of mono- and di-iodotyrosine in the blood of a patient with congenital goiter. *J Clin Endocrinol Metab* 1955;15:1216.

142. Choufour JC, Kassenaar AAH, Querido A. The syndrome of congenital hypothyroidism with defective dehalogenation of iodotyrosines: further observations and a discussion of the pathophysiology. *J Clin Endocrinol Metab* 1960;20:983.

143. Hutchison JH, McGirr EM. Hypothyroidism as an inborn error of metabolism. *J Clin Endocrinol Metab* 1954;14:869.

144. McGirr EM, Hutchison JH, Clement WE. Sporadic goitrous cretinism. Dehalogenase deficiency in the thyroid gland of a goitrous cretin and in heterozygous carriers. *Lancet* 1959;2:823.

145. Ismail-Beigi F, Rahimifar M. A variant of iodotyrosine-dehalogenase deficiency. *J Clin Endocrinol Metab* 1977;44:499.

146. Tan SA, Tan LG. Hyperiodotyrosinemia-induced hyperprolactinemia and hyperaldosteronism. *Horm Res* 1990;34:83.

147. Moreno JC. Novel thyroid specific transcripts identified by SAGE: implications for congenital hypothyroidism [Thesis]. University of Amsterdam. 2003, p. 93.

148. Moreno JC, Keijser R, Aarraas S, et al. Cloning an characterization of a novel thyroidal gene encoding proteins with a conserved nitroreductase domain [Abstract]. *J Endocrinol Invest* 2002;25:23.

149. Friesema ECH, Gruters A, Halestrap A, et al. Mutations in a thyroid hormone transporter in patients with severe psychomotor retardation and high serum T_3 levels [Abstract]. *Thyroid* 2003;13:672.

150. Friesema ECH, Gruters A, Biebermann H, et al. Severe X-linked psychomotor retardation caused by mutations in a thyroid hormone transporter. *Lancet* 2004 (in press).

151. Dumitrescu AM, Liao XH, Best TB, et al. A novel syndrome combining thyroid and neurological abnormalities is associated with mutations in a monocarboxylate transporter gene. *Am J Hum Genet* 2004;74:168.

152. Friesema ECH, Ganguly S, Abdalla A, et al. Identification of nonocarboxylate transporter 8 as a specific thyroid hormone transporter. *J Biol Chem* 2003;278:40128.

153. Van Trotsenburg ASP, Vulsma T, Van Santen HM, et al. Lower neonatal screening thyroxine concentrations in Down syndrome newborns. *J Clin Endocrinol Metab* 2003;88:1512.

154. Konings CH, Van Trotsenburg ASP, Ris-Stalpers C, et al. Plasma thyrotropin bioactivity in Down's syndrome children with subclinical hypothyroidism. *Eur J Endocrinol* 2001;144:1.

155. Delepine M, Nicolino M, Barrett T, et al. EIF2AK3, encoding translation initiation factor 2-alpha kinase 3, is mutated in patients with Wolcott-Rallison syndrome. *Nat Genet* 2000;25:406.

156. Bin-Abbas B, Al-Mulhim A, Al-Ashwal A. Wolcott-Rallison syndrome in two siblings with isolated central hypothyroidism. *Am J Med Genet* 2002;111:187.

157. Ng D, Johnston JJ, Turner JT, et al. Gonadal mosaicism in severe Pallister-Hall syndrome. *Am J Med Genet* 2004;124A:296.

158. Johanson AJ, Blizzard RM. A syndrome of congenital aplasia of the alae nasi, deafness, hypothyroidism, dwarfism, absent permanent teeth, and malabsorption. *J Pediatr* 1971;79:982.

159. Park IJ, Johanson AJ, Jones HW Jr, et al. Special female hermaphroditism associated with multiple disorders. *Obstet Gynecol* 1972;39:100.

160. Vieira MW, Lopes VLGS, Teruya H, et al. Johanson-Blizzard syndrome: the importance of differential diagnostic in pediatrics. *J Pediatr (Rio J)* 2002;78:433.

161. Daentl DL, Frias JL, Gilbert EF, et al. The Johanson-Blizzard syndrome: case report and autopsy findings. *Am J Med Genet* 1979;3:129.

162. Hurst JA, Baraitser M. Johanson-Blizzard syndrome. *J Med Genet* 1989;26:45.

163. Alpay F, Gul D, Lenk MK, et al. Severe intrauterine growth retardation, aged facial appearance, and congenital heart disease in a newborn with Johanson-Blizzard syndrome. *Pediatr Cardiol* 2000;21:389.

164. Gorlin RJ, Cohen MM Jr, Hennekam RCM, eds. *Syndromes of the head and neck,* 4th ed. Oxford University Press, 2001.

165. Taha D, Barbar M, Kanaan H, et al. Neonatal diabetes mellitus, congenital hypothyroidism, hepatic fibrosis, polycystic kidneys, and congenital glaucoma: a new autosomal recessive syndrome? *Am J Med Genet* 2003;122A:269.

166. Olivieri A, Stazi MA, Mastroiacovo P, et al. Study group for congenital hypothyroidism: a population-based study on the frequency of additional congenital malformations in infants with congenital hypothyroidism: data from the Italian registry for congenital hypothyroidism (1991–1998). *J Clin Endocrinol Metab* 2002;87:557.

167. Working Group on Neonatal Screening of the ESPE. Revised guidelines for neonatal screening programmes for primary congenital hypothyroidism. *Horm Res* 1999;52:49.

168. Alexopoulou O, Beguin C, De Nayer P, et al. Clinical and hormonal characteristics of central hypothyroidism at diagnosis and during follow-up in adult patients. *Eur J Endocrinol* 2004;150:1.

49

ENDEMIC CRETINISM

FRANÇOIS M. DELANGE

Many people with severe endemic goiter have irreversible impairment of intellectual and physical development. These abnormalities are extremely polymorphous and have been grouped under the general heading of endemic cretinism. The prevalence of the disorders may reach 5% to 15% of the population. It is by far the most serious complication of endemic goiter and represents a veritable scourge, both medically and socially (1–3).

Despite recent experimental data, the etiopathogenesis of endemic cretinism remains only partly understood (see later sections Etiology and Pathogenesis), and information on its pathology is scanty (4–6). For these reasons, the diagnosis of the condition is still mostly descriptive.

This chapter summarizes the present knowledge on the epidemiology and clinical manifestations, laboratory data, etiology, pathogenesis, therapy, and prevention of endemic cretinism. A comprehensive bibliography, including the historical aspects, is available in more extensive reviews on the topic (1–11).

EPIDEMIOLOGY, CLINICAL MANIFESTATIONS, AND LABORATORY DATA

In 1986, a study group of the Pan American Health Organization (PAHO) formulated the following definition of endemic cretinism (12) :

> The condition of endemic cretinism is defined by three major features:
>   A. Epidemiology. It is associated with endemic goiter and severe iodine deficiency.
>   B. Clinical manifestations. These comprise mental deficiency, together with either:
>   1) A predominant neurological syndrome including defects of hearing and speech and characteristic disorders of stance and gait of varying degree; or
>   2) Predominant hypothyroidism and stunted growth.
>   Although in some regions, one of the two types may predominate, in other areas a mixture of the two syndromes will occur.
>   C. Prevention. In areas where adequate correction of iodine deficiency has been achieved, endemic cretinism has been prevented.

The clinical manifestations of endemic cretinism summarized in the PAHO definition correspond to the two extreme types of endemic cretinism initially defined in the pioneering work of McCarrison in 1908 (13) in the Himalayas and subsequently reported in the studies of endemic goiter and cretinism conducted in other parts of the world, for example, New Guinea (14,15) and the Democratic Republic of Congo (DRC, formerly Zaire) (16–23). The first type is marked by neurologic disorders (neurologic cretinism) and the second by symptoms of severe thyroid insufficiency (myxedematous cretinism).

Figure 49.1 shows the typical picture of neurologic cretinism as seen in New Guinea (14,15): the cretins in this endemia are extremely mentally retarded, and most of them are reduced to a vegetative existence. Almost all are deaf-mutes and have the following neurologic defects: (a) impaired voluntary motor activity, usually involving the pyramidal track, chiefly affecting the lower limbs, with hypertonia, clonus, and plantar cutaneous reflexes in extension—extrapyramidal signs are occasional; (b) spastic or ataxic gait—in the severest cases, walking or even standing is impossible; and (c) strabismus.

The prevalence of goiter in these cretins is as high as in the noncretin population of the area, and they are clinically euthyroid. Thyroid function is usually normal (14,15), but subclinical hypothyroidism with high basal serum thyrotropin (TSH) or exaggerated TSH response to thyrotropin-releasing hormone (TRH) may occur (24,25).

Figure 49.2 shows the typical picture of myxedematous endemic cretinism as most typically seen in the DRC (3,7, 16–23). These cretins have less mental retardation than the neurologic cretins; they are often capable of performing simple manual tasks. All have major symptoms of longstanding hypothyroidism: dwarfism, myxedema, dry skin, sparseness of hair and nails, retarded sexual development, and retarded maturation of body proportions and of nasoorbital configuration. The initial reports from the DRC indicated that myxedematous cretins occasionally had neurologic signs, including spasticity of the lower limbs, jerky movements, Babinski's sign, and shifting gait (18,23).

The prevalence of goiter in the myxedematous cretins is much lower than in the noncretin population. Many have palpable thyroid tissue, although thyroid scintigrams show

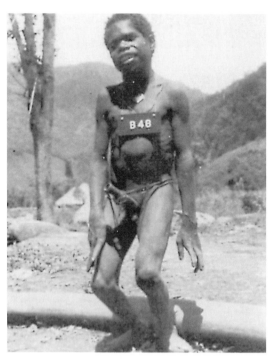

FIGURE 49.1. A 14-year-old boy with neurologic endemic cretinism, Mulia Valley, Western New Guinea. The boy has severe mental retardation, deaf-mutism, spastic diplegia, and strabismus. There are no clinical signs of hypothyroidism. Serum protein bound iodine (*PBI*) 1.7 μg/dL. (Photograph courtesy of Professor A. Querido, Leiden, The Netherlands.)

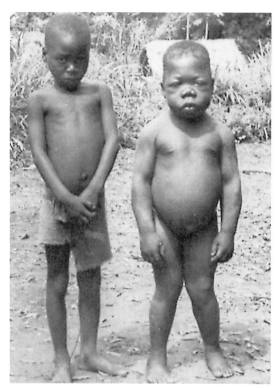

FIGURE 49.2. Myxedematous endemic cretinism in children in Ubangi, northwestern DRC. On the left, a clinically euthyroid 6-year-old girl with a height of 105 cm (50th percentile for age for the local population). On the right, a 17-year-old girl with a height of 100 cm, severe mental retardation, myxedema, markedly delayed puberty, flat and broad nose, hypoplastic mandibule, dry and scaly skin, dry and brittle hair, and prominent abdomen. Pseudomuscular hypertrophy, muscular weakness, flat feet, and genu valgum are present; no deaf-mutism. The thyroid gland was not palpable. Har serum concentration of thyrotropin was 288 μU/mL, thyroxine 0.1 μldl (1.29), and triiodothyronine 10 ngldl (0.154 n*M*).

small amounts of thyroid tissue located in normal position (18,23), precluding thyroid dysgenesis (agenesis, ectopic thyroid) as the cause of hypothyroidism.

The clinical diagnosis of hypothyroidism in myxedematous cretins is confirmed by a biochemical picture of thyroid failure with almost undetectable serum concentrations of thyroxine (T_4) and triiodothyronine (T_3) and extremely elevated serum levels of TSH (Table 49.1). The iodine pool of the thyroid is drastically reduced with a particularly fast turnover rate of iodine, as indicated by elevated serum radiolabeled protein bound iodine ($PB^{131}I$). The diagnosis of severe and long-standing hypothyroidism is further confirmed by a very important retardation in bone maturation and epiphyseal dysgenesis, indicating hypothyroidism of perinatal onset, and by characteristic changes in the electrocardiogram (23).

The review of the world literature on endemic cretinism up to the late 1970s indicated that the frequency distribution of the two extreme types of endemic cretinism varied markedly from one endemic area to another. In most of them, the neurologic type predominated, while in others, especially in DRC, myxedematous endemic cretinism was most frequently encountered. The reasons for these geographical variations in the epidemiologic pattern of endemic cretinism were unknown. It was also agreed that, between the two extreme types of cretinism, there were mixed forms characterized by dominant neurologic disorders or dominant hypothyroidism in the same individual (8,14–23,26–36).

It was then thought that neurologic and myxedematous endemic cretinism, in fact, constituted the extreme aspects of a continuous spectrum of developmental abnormalities, between which there were numerous intermediate forms (7,8,37). A similar variability in the geographic pattern of endemic cretinism has been reported from China: neurologic cretinism has been found in almost all the cretin endemias of China; the myxedematous type was less frequent and was found principally in the northwestern part of the country (38–40).

The results of subsequent detailed studies of cretinism in Ecuador (41–43), China (44–47), Indonesia (48), and Thailand (49,50) vigorously challenged the concept of a continuous spectrum of developmental abnormalities in

TABLE 49.1. THYROID FUNCTION TESTS AND CLINICAL AND RADIOLOGIC DATA IN HYPOTHYROID ENDEMIC CRETINS IN DRC, CHINA, AND INDONESIA

Variables	Belgian Controls (*n* = 12–255)	Noncretin Iodine-Deficient Adults (DRC) (*n* = 30–358)	Hypothyroid Endemic Cretins		
			DRC Idjwi-Ubangi (*n* = 6–120)	China Qinghai (*n* = 25)	Indonesia Bandung (*n* = 3)
Thyroid function tests					
Serum concentration of					
T_4 (n*M*)	104.2 ± 1.3	63.1 ± 2.6	6.4 ± 0.1	53.9 ± 7.1	
FT_4 (p*M*)	8.4 ± 1.3				
T_3 (n*M*)	2.21 ± 0.05	2.55 ± 0.04	0.70 ± 0.05	2.1 ± 0.2	11.2
TSH (μU/mL)	1.7 ± 0.1	18.6 ± 2.1	303 ± 20	123.8 ± 23.0	40.1
Protein bound [131]I (% dose/liter)	0.06 ± 0.01	0.17 ± 0.02	1.09 ± 0.18		
24-hour ^{131}I thyroid uptake (% dose)	46.4 ± 1.1	65.2 ± 0.9	28.3 ± 2.6		
Thyroid organic iodine pool (mg)	15.8 ± 3.5	1.60 ± 0.3	0.01–0.1		
Clinical and radiologic data					
Age (yr)			16.8	31.6	33.3
Clinical myxedema (%)			100	54	
Height (cm)			103	131	144
Bone maturation (yr)			2.8	26.2	
Epiphyseal dysgenesis			+++	±	±
Mental development vs. euthyroid cretins			Higher	Equal	Equal

DRC, Democratic Republic of Congo
Values recorded as mean ± SEM.
Data from references 18, 20, 44, 48, 114, 116, and 125.

endemic cretinism between two extreme types, myxedematous and neurologic. The main reason is that in their studies in China and Indonesia, the Australian researchers reported an identical pattern of intensity of neurologic, intellectual, and audiometric deficits in all cretins examined, regardless of type (myxedematous or neurologic) and current thyroid function (44,48). The neurologic aspects of both euthyroid and hypothyroid cretins are polymorphous and vary widely from one subject to another: in the 139 subjects they investigated in China and Indonesia, Halpern and colleagues (48) reported significant pyramidal dysfunction in a proximal distribution and exaggeration of the tendon reflexes, more commonly encountered in the lower limbs than in the upper. The posture is typical, with hips and knees flexed and the trunk tilted forward. The gait is broad based and knock-kneed. The arms are held with the shoulders abducted and the elbows flexed. These signs indicate extrapyramidal features. All the cretins have severe intellectual impairment, with a mean IQ of about 29. About half the patients have impaired hearing, and nearly one third have a squint. Musculoskeletal abnormalities are common and predominantly involve the weight-bearing joints, with excessive laxity of the hips, feet, and ankles. There are no signs of cerebellar dysfunction.

Subsequently, Rajatanavin and colleagues (49) reported a similar frequency of low intelligence, defects in visual perceptive neuromanual ability, sensorineural hearing loss, and neurologic defects in 57 neurologic, 19 myxedematous, and 36 mixed cretins in northern Thailand.

In another study conducted in China, in an attempt to better define the underlying pathology in the nervous system causing the functional deficits and to determine the developmental timing of the critical neurologic events, DeLong and colleagues (47) identified five patterns of neurologic involvement in these cretins:

1. "Typical" pattern, with hearing and speech deficit, proximal spastic rigid motor disorder, and mental retardation
2. "Thalamic" posturing, with undermost limbs extended and uppermost limbs flexed, together with severe mental retardation, marked microcephaly, inability to sit, stand, or walk, and primitive facial reflexes including a marked sucking or rooting reflex elicited by bringing an object into the visual field near the face
3. An autistic pattern, with severe mental deficiency aggravated by deaf-mutism and an almost total disregard of their surroundings and absence of purposeful activity
4. A cerebellar pattern, with marked abnormalities in standing, walking, and sitting, hypotonic truncal tone,

tremor, and dysmetria that are typical of cerebellar dysfunction

5. A hypotonic pattern, with marked truncal hypotonia and delayed sitting, standing, and walking

The hypothesis was proposed that the typical pattern may represent an insult occurring principally during the second trimester of pregnancy; that the severe thalamic form may represent a longer period of insult; that deafness results from a cochlear lesion occurring during the first and second trimesters; that the cerebellar form may result from a postnatal insult; and that the autistic form may depend on a severe insult to the cerebral cortex as well as the hippocampus, both pre- and postnatally (47,51).

In contrast to the exhaustive clinical descriptions of the nervous system defects in cretins and the diversity and severity of these deficits, information on brain pathology is scanty and does not elucidate entirely the anatomic locations of the injury: computed tomographic (CT) scans of cretins from Ecuador showed widespread atrophy that included the cerebral cortex and subcortical structures of the brainstem, with corresponding enlargement of the basal cisternae, the lateral ventricles, and the sulci over the surface of the cerebral cortex (52). Basal ganglia calcifications and cerebral atrophy were occasionally observed by Halpern et al (48), but there was no correlation between the CT scan abnormalities and the clinical signs. Magnetic resonance imaging in three cretins from China appeared remarkably normal (47).

On the basis of the observations in China, Indonesia, and Thailand, the concept was proposed that all cretins, including the so-called myxedematous form, belong to the neurologic type (44,48,50). The reason for the discrepancy between this concept and the concept of a spectrum with two extreme types is unclear. One possible explanation could be an underevaluation or misinterpretation of the neurologic signs in myxedematous cretins in DRC by the different Belgian and African teams (43) which investigated the Uele, Idjwi Island, and Ubangi areas during the past 40 years (16–23). If so, the same mistakes were also made by the team from Washington, which again investigated the Uele area and obtained exactly the same epidemiologic findings (53). It has to be recognized that at least some of the neurologic signs found in the myxedematous cretins of the DRC, including flat feet, knock knees, hyperreflexia, ataxia, strabismus, nystagmus, and hearing defects, have been occasionally reported in the past in unrecognized and consequently untreated children with sporadic congenital hypothyroidism (54,55).

Another possible explanation of the difference between the two concepts could be that the term "myxedematous cretinism" has been applied in China and Indonesia to patients with predominantly neurologic cretinism and post-

natally acquired hypothyroidism with moderate biochemical impairment of thyroid function, similar to that found in neurologic cretinism in other parts of the world and in noncretin, severely iodine-deficient adults (Table 49.1). In fact, the degree of hypothyroidism reported in the hypothyroid cretins in China and Indonesia is much milder than the hypothyroidism observed in Africa. The difference in severity is reflected by the results obtained for the biochemical tests and could explain why the retardation in height and especially in bone maturation is much less marked in hypothyroid cretins in China than in the DRC, where hypothyroidism is of perinatal onset. Only half of the myxedematous cretins in China are clinically myxedematous, while, by definition, all of them are in DRC.

The most probable explanation for the discrepancy between the two concepts, however, is that, although severe iodine deficiency is the main cause of all types of cretinism, additional causes, varying from place to place, may modulate the clinical expression of the disorder (see later sections Etiology and Pathogenesis).

ENDEMIC MENTAL RETARDATION IN SEVERE ENDEMIC GOITER

The statement that "feeble mindedness, a part of cretinism, arises distinctly in areas of endemic goiter" (56) has been rather difficult to confirm on an objective basis, particularly because of major technical limitations in the assessment of intelligence in preindustrialized societies (6,57).

Table 49.2 summarizes data available in the literature on the neuromotor and intellectual development in noncretinous people in areas with severe endemic goiter and cretinism. The same tests (optimally with no "cultural bias" or as little as possible) were administered to two groups of noncretinous subjects living in the same environmental conditions except for the goitrogenic factors: a test group was exposed to these factors, while in a control group, exposure was prevented by iodine prophylaxis, or these factors had never been present. In the test groups, neuromotor and intellectual deficits were frequently observed in subjects who did not have any of the other signs of endemic cretinism.

Thus, endemic cretinism only constitutes the extreme expression of a spectrum of abnormalities in physical and intellectual development and in the functional capacities of the thyroid gland in the inhabitants of severe endemic goiter areas.

ETIOLOGY

Iodine Deficiency

Iodine deficiency is fundamental in the etiology of endemic cretinism. This conclusion rests on (a) the correla-

TABLE 49.2. INTELLECTUAL, COGNITIVE, AND NEUROLOGIC DEFICITS IN NONCRETINS IN SEVERE ENDEMIC GOITER REGIONS

Regions	Tests	Findings	References
Ecuador	Goodenough Draw-a-man Stanford-Binet Gesell Leiter Bender-Gestalt	Low DQ, IQ, and visual-motor performances	57,123 126–128
Bolivia	Stanford-Binet Bender-Gestalt	Low IQ and visual-motor performances	129
Chile	Wechsler Bender Kopitz	Low IQ	130
Papua-New Guinea	Motor performances	Low motor skill	96,131,132
DRC (Zaire)	Brunet-Lezine	Low DQ	133
Java-Spain	Locally adapted "culture-free" intelligence tests Wechsler Catell Raven Ozeretsky	Low IQ Low perceptual and neuromotor abilities	134
China	Griffith Hiskey-Nebraska	Low IQ—Relationship between IQ and nerve deafness and abnormal neurologic signs	48,135,136
India	Bhatia Malin Bender-Gestalt Verbal, pictorial learning tasks Test of motivation	Low IQ Low rates of hearing Low motivation	137,138
Iran	Bender-Gestalt Raven	Low IQ	139

tion between the degree of iodine deficiency and the frequency of cretinism (3,8,11); (b) the prophylactic action of iodine on the incidence of cretinism (see later section Prevention); and (c) the emergence of cretinism in previously unaffected populations as a consequence of iodine deficiency of recent onset, as observed in the Jimi valley in New Guinea after replacement of natural rock salt rich in iodine with low-iodine industrial salt (58) (see section Iodine Deficiency in Chapter 11).

In addition, iodine deficiency during gestation in animals results in thyroid deficiency in the offspring. All the models used mimic the myxedematous type of cretinism; none was able to reproduce the neurologic type (59–61).

Naturally Occurring Goitrogens

The additional role played by naturally occurring goitrogens in the etiology of endemic cretinism has been established for a cyanogenic glucoside (linamarin) present in cassava, a staple food in many tropical areas (19,20). Linamarin yields cyanide on hydrolysis. This is metabolized to thiocyanate (SCN), which is well known for its goitrogenic effects. The role of SCN in the etiology of endemic cretinism in Africa has been proposed from the observation that people in areas with severe but uniform iodine defi-

ciency had cretinism only when a certain critical threshold in the dietary intake of SCN is reached (62). It has been shown experimentally in the rat that SCN affects the development of the central nervous system during fetal life (20). The action of SCN is entirely due to an aggravation of iodine deficiency resulting in fetal hypothyroidism.

Thyroid Autoimmunity

Boyages and colleagues (63) reported that purified immunoglobulin G (IgG) fractions of serum from patients with myxedematous endemic cretinism inhibited TSH-induced DNA synthesis and, consequently, growth of guinea pig thyroid segments in a sensitive cytochemical assay. By contrast, no growth-blocking effect was observed with IgGs from euthyroid subjects or neurologic cretins from the same area. These IgGs, often called thyroid growth-blocking immunoglobulins (TGBIs), are similar to those found by the same researchers in sporadic congenital hypothyroidism (64). The antigenic stimulus is unknown, as is the timing of appearance of these IgG fractions during pregnancy and fetal or postnatal life. Serum TGBIs were also detected using rat thyroid FRTL-5 cells in cretins in Brazil with atrophic thyroids (65). However, TGBI could not be found in sporadic congenital hypothyroidism or myxedematous endemic cretinism in Peru and Italy by other researchers (66–68); consequently, the possible role of thyroid autoimmunity in the etiology of endemic cretinism remains controversial.

Trace Elements

One question about the etiology of both myxedematous and neurologic endemic cretinism concerns the role of combined iodine and selenium deficiencies (69–73). In the DRC, myxedematous cretinism is found only in severe iodine-deficient areas that are also deficient in selenium (69,73) (Table 49.3). Selenium is present in high concentrations (0.72 µg/g) in the normal thyroid (74). It is present in glutathione peroxidase (GPX) and superoxide dismutase, the enzymes of the thyroid responsible for the detoxification of toxic derivates of oxygen (H_2O_2 and perhaps O_2^-) (75). It is also present in both iodothyronine 5'-deiodinases responsible for the conversion of T_4 to T_3 (76).

The following scheme has been proposed to explain the frequency of myxedematous cretinism and the relative rarity of neurologic cretinism in areas such as the DRC where both iodine and selenium are deficient (69–72) (Fig. 49.3): iodine deficiency results in hyperstimulation of the thyroid by TSH and consequently in increased production of H_2O_2 within the cells. Selenium deficiency results in GPX deficiency and consequently in accumulation of H_2O_2. Excess H_2O_2 could induce thyroid cell destruction and thyroid fibrosis, resulting in myxedematous cretinism. The re-

cent observation that the necrotizing effect of a high dose of iodide on the thyroid cells is much greater in selenium-deficient than in selenium-supplemented rats is consistent with this hypothesis, suggesting that the selenium-deficient thyroid gland is more sensitive to oxidative stress (77). The necrotizing effect is aggravated in the presence of SCN overload (78).

On the other hand, in pregnant women deficiency of the selenoenzyme iodothyronine 5'-deiodinase induced by selenium deficiency causes decreased catabolism of T_4 to T_3 and thus increased availability of maternal T_4 for the fetus and its brain. Indeed, despite a similar degree of iodine deficiency, serum T_4 levels are higher in selenium-deficient pregnant women in the DRC than in pregnant women in New Guinea (51). This mechanism could prevent the development of neurologic cretinism. Combined iodine and selenium deficiencies together with SCN overload due to the chronic consumption of cassava could thus explain the large predominance of the myxedematous type of endemic cretinism, rather than the neurologic type, in the DRC.

PATHOGENESIS

Endemic cretinism results from an insufficient supply of thyroid hormone to the developing brain. The physiologic role of thyroid hormones is to ensure the timed coordination of different developmental events through specific ef-

TABLE 49.3. COMPARISON BETWEEN AN AREA WITH SEVERE DEFICIENCIES IN IODINE AND SELENIUM AND OVERLOAD IN THIOCYANATE (UBANGI, NORTHERN DRC) AND CONTROL OF AREAS (BRUSSELS OR KIKWIT, DRC)

	Controls	
Variables	(Brussels, Kikwit) (*n* = 38–204)	Ubangi (*n* = 140–243)
Prevalence of goiter (%)	3	76.8
Prevalence of cretinism (%)	0	4.7
Urinary concentration of		
Iodine (µg/dL)	5.3 ± 0.7	2.3 ± 0.1
SCN (mg/dL)	0.60 ± 0.07	1.82 ± 0.10
Serum concentration of		
Selenium (ng/mL)	201.9 ± 5.23	27.1 ± 1.9
RBC-GPX (U/g Hb)	15.0 ± 0.8	3.3 ± 0.3
Cord serum concentration of		
TSH (µU/mL)	8.2 ± 0.4	70.7 ± 13.1
T_4 (n*M*/L)	146.7 ± 2.6	95.2 ± 5.1
T_3 (n*M*/L)	0.57 ± 0.01	1.47 ± 0.10

Epidemiologic data, variables exploring the nutritional status in iodine, SCN, and selenium (including RBC-GPX) and variables exploring thyroid function in cord blood. Values recorded as mean ± SEM. All the differences between the two groups are highly significant ($p < .01$ to $p < .001$).
RBC-GPX, red blood cell–glutathione peroxidase ; SCN, thiocyanate; T_3, triiodothyronine; T_4, thyroxine; TSH, thyrotropin.
Data from references 69, 71, and 99.

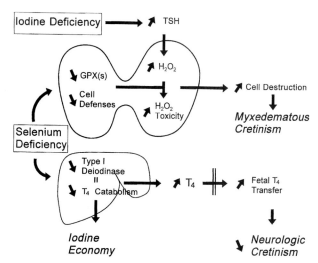

FIGURE 49.3. Effects of selenium deficiency on thyroid function and thyroxine metabolism in the presence of severe iodine deficiency. *GPX*, glutathione peroxidase. (From Contempré B, Many MC, Vanderpas J et al. Interaction between two trace elements: selenium and iodine. Implications of both deficiencies. In: Stanbury JB, ed. *The damaged brain and iodine deficiency.* New York: Cognizant Communication, 1994:133, with permission.)

fects on the rate of cell differentiation and gene expression (79). Thyroid hormone action is exerted through the binding of T_3 to nuclear receptors, which regulate the expression of specific genes in different brain regions following a precise development schedule (79). During the fetal and early postnatal life, T_3 bound to nuclear receptors is entirely dependent on its local production from T_4 via type 2 deiodinase (D2) (80) (see Chapter 74).

Maternal and Fetal Hypothyroxinemia before Onset of Fetal Thyroid Function

Despite the independence of maternal and fetal hypothalamus–pituitary–thyroid feedback mechanisms (81), maternal thyroid hormone is involved in the development and thyroid hormone economy of the fetus.

In rats, thyroid hormones are found in embryonic and fetal tissues before the onset of fetal thyroid function, which occurs at day 18 (82). The hormones are thus of maternal origin. Their concentrations remain fairly constant until day 18, when the fetal thyroid secretion begins (83). After day 18, the fetal thyroidal T_4 and T_3 pools as well as the circulating T_4 level increase steadily (84). At term, 17.5% of the fetal extrathyroidal T_4 is still of maternal origin (85).

In iodine deficiency, the rat embryo is T_4 deficient, and its brain is exposed to variable T_3 deficiency not only because of its own impairment of T_4 synthesis but also, and perhaps predominantly, because of maternal hypothyroxinemia and

insufficient transfer of T_4 from mother to fetus in early pregnancy, before the onset of fetal thyroid activity (86).

The key role of maternal T_4 during early gestation on the brain development of the fetus is demonstrated by the observation that in the 40-day-old progeny of hypothyroxinemic iodine-deficient pregnant rats, there is a significant proportion of neurons that are aberrant or inappropriate locators with respect to their birthdate (87). This is the first direct evidence of an alteration in fetal brain histogenesis and cytoarchitecture that can be only related to early maternal hypothyroxinemia.

An additional cause of fetal hypothyroxinemia in iodine deficiency is that the fetal thyroid, contrasting with the maternal thyroid, is unable to increase its avidity for iodide, that is, its iodide clearance rate in case of decreased serum concentration of iodide (88), despite up-regulation of Na^+/I^- symporter expression in fetal thyroid and placenta during iodine deficiency (89). This will further decrease the iodine stores of the fetal thyroid and, consequently, T_4 synthesis.

A partial mechanism of adaptation to fetal hypothyroxinemia in rats is that, in these circumstances, there is an increase in fetal brain deiodinase type 2 activity that protects the fetal brain from T_3 deficiency, even when euthyroidism is not maintained in other fetal tissues (90). In contrast, the transfer of maternal T_3 does not protect the hypothyroid fetal brain from T_3 deficiency.

In humans, T_4 is present in coelomic fluid 6 weeks of gestational age (91). Nuclear T_3 receptors are present in the brain of 10-week-old fetuses, and increase more than sixfold by 12 weeks and tenfold by 16 weeks (92), largely before the onset of fetal thyroid function, which occurs by 14 weeks of gestation. However, evaluation of fetal tissue exposure to maternal thyroid hormones up to midgestation indicated that first-trimester human fetal tissues are exposed to concentrations of T_4 of at least one third of those in their euthyroid mothers (93). These findings further underline the critical role of maternal thyroxinemia on the timely sequence of brain development in the human fetus. Fetal plasma T_4 is low although detectable up to the 14th week of gestation. After the onset of fetal thyroid function, T_4 increases steadily, reaching adult values by 36 weeks (94). However, transfer of maternal T_4 continues until birth, when it still represents 20% to 50% of cord serum T_4 (95).

Maternal hypothyroxinemia is rare in nonendemic areas, but it can result in impaired neurointellectual development in the offspring (5,96–98). In contrast, maternal hypothyroxinemia is extremely frequent in endemic areas (99,100). It is associated with increased mortality and morbidity in offspring (101,102), and increased incidence of hypothyroidism in neonates (99,103).

A unifying concept has been proposed that the neurologic defects, present in all cretins, are due to maternal and fetal hypothyroxinemia (48,50). This would account for

the picture of cretinism as found in China and Indonesia. In Africa, as indicated earlier, brain damage during early fetal life could be mitigated by concomitant selenium deficiency, which impairs peripheral conversion of T_4 to T_3 and consequently increases the availability of the prohormone T_4 to the fetal brain.

Fetal and Neonatal Hypothyroidism after Onset of Fetal Thyroid Function

Even a moderate degree of iodine deficiency during pregnancy, as occurs in Western Europe, can be accompanied by indexes of hyperstimulation of the thyroid in the neonates, as indicated by high serum levels of TSH and thyroglobulin (Tg) and by a slight enlargement of the thyroid. These abnormalities are prevented by the daily administration of a physiologic dose of iodide to pregnant women throughout pregnancy (104).

As noted above, the myxedematous endemic cretinism results from severe thyroid failure occurring during late fetal or early postnatal life: data from China have shown hypothyroxinemia and retardation in brain growth in human fetuses from the sixth month of gestation in re-

gions of severe iodine deficiency and myxedematous endemic cretinism (105). Thyroid failure at birth due to iodine deficiency occurs in several endemic areas with myxedematous endemic cretinism, such as the DRC (99, 103), India (106), Algeria (107), and even some parts of Europe such as Sicily (108). The most dramatic picture of neonatal hypothyroidism has been reported from DRC, where the frequency of myxedematous endemic cretinism is the highest: in this area, about 10% of unselected newborns and infants 1 to 24 months of age have both serum TSH above 100 μU/mL and T_4 levels below 3.1 μg/dL (40 nM) (99,103), a biochemical picture characteristic of congenital hypothyroidism in Western countries (109,110). About 10% of infants under 12 months of age are clinically hypothyroid, and nearly half have a marked delay in bone maturation, which is directly correlated with serum TSH and inversely correlated with serum T_4 (99,103). Finally, correction of iodine deficiency in pregnant women by injections of iodized oil results in a complete normalization of the biochemical and radiologic indexes of hypothyroidism in newborns and infants (103,111).

The presence of epiphyseal dysgenesis in x-ray studies of the knees (Fig. 49.4B) of some adult myxedematous en-

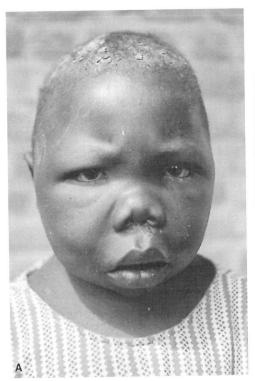 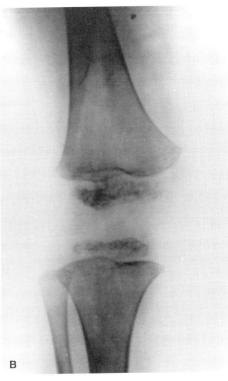

FIGURE 49.4. Clinical appearance **(A)** and knee x-ray **(B)** of a 17-year-old myxedematous cretin of Idjwi Island, DRC, with a height of 87.5 cm (56% of normal for the local population) and a serum protein bound iodine (*PBI*) of 1.0 μg/dL. Bone maturation is estimated at 2 to 5 years. The x-ray film shows failure of modeling, and tibial and femoral epiphyseal dysgenesis. The immaturity of the naso-orbital configuration, the mandibular hypoplasia, and the epiphyseal dysgenesis indicate hypothyroidism of pre- or perinatal onset.

demic cretins with clinical, biochemical, and radiologic signs of long-standing hypothyroidism suggests that hypothyroidism was present before or around birth (112). Also, the direct correlations observed in these cretins between mental retardation and both height retardation and retardation in bone maturation indicate that hypothyroidism present in early life would account for their mental deficiency (17).

In some infants in the Ubangi area in DRC, the biochemical signs of thyroid failure disappeared spontaneously within 6 to 10 weeks of life (113). The hypothesis has been proposed that permanent thyroid failure from birth results in myxedematous endemic cretinism, whereas transient hypothyroxinemia occurring during the critical period of brain development explains the endemic mental retardation in this population (114).

The cause of fetal hypothyroidism in the DRC is most likely the combined action of iodine deficiency and SCN overload. The latter results from the chronic consumption of cassava, which aggravates the effects of iodine deficiency (19,20). SCN freely crosses the placenta (115), and its concentration in cord blood is three times higher in Ubangi than in Brussels (99). The importance of this SCN overload in the impairment of thyroid function of the newborn is strongly suggested by the observation that, in severely iodine-deficient pregnant women, high urinary SCN values are associated with very high serum TSH and very low cord serum T4 levels (99). The hypersensitivity of the newborn to the antithyroid action of SCN probably results from the fact that this ion interferes with the trapping of iodide by both the placenta and the thyroid gland of the newborn. These two factors probably critically reduce the buildup of iodine stores within the thyroid gland during fetal and early postnatal life. This mechanism is consistent with the low iodine content of the thyroid gland reported in myxedematous cretins (116) (Table 49.1).

As discussed earlier, selenium deficiency could further aggravate thyroid failure during the late fetal and neonatal periods by damaging the hyperstimulated gland through the accumulation of H_2O_2 derivatives. This process, called exhaustion atrophy, would explain the usual absence of goiter in the myxedematous cretins in the DRC.

In addition, iodine deficiency can induce thyroid failure at any time, including after brain development, resulting in infantile hypothyroidism without the irreversible brain damage characteristic of cretinism (28,117,118).

This unifying view of the pathogenesis of endemic cretinism would account for the differences in the epidemiologic and clinical aspects of cretinism seen around the world. Iodine deficiency is a prerequisite. When present during early gestation before onset of fetal thyroid function, it would account for the neurologic aspects of cretinism via maternal and fetal hypothyroxinemia. Selenium deficiency could mitigate the neurologic picture by increasing the availability of the prohormone T_4 to the developing brain. It also could induce irreversible damage of the thyroid. Severe iodine and selenium deficiencies aggravated by SCN overload present during late pregnancy, after the onset of active fetal thyroid function, would account for the myxedematous component of cretinism.

It thus appears that the particular situation reported in the DRC with less neurologic damage and severe thyroid failure could be explained by a combination of severe iodine and selenium deficiencies complicated by SCN overload. The consequences of these three conditions are prevented by the correction of iodine deficiency in the pregnant mother.

THERAPY

There is no specific therapy for neurologic endemic cretinism. These patients need rehabilitation as do patients with cerebral palsy in Western countries. Thyroid function may improve after iodine supplementation in myxedematous cretins under 4 years of age but not in older patients, suggesting that in this type of cretinism the atrophic thyroid progressively loses its functional capacity (119,120). Some researchers, however, have reported significant improvement in neuromotor and physical appearance even in 30- to 40-year-old myxedematous endemic cretins treated with injections of iodized oil (53).

PREVENTION

Endemic cretinism is prevented when iodine deficiency has been corrected (3,5,8,11,111,121). Iodization of salt introduced independently in various Swiss cantons between 1922 and 1925 resulted in a decline in endemic deaf-mutism in these cantons that could be correlated with the extent of salt iodination (122). However, it must be pointed out that in Switzerland endemic cretinism started to diminish about 10 years before the introduction of iodine prophylaxis (5), probably because of improved socioeconomic conditions, resulting in a "silent iodine prophylaxis."

Table 49.4 summarizes the results of the controlled trials conducted during the past 20 years on the effect of iodine prophylaxis on the incidence of endemic cretinism. In Ecuador, in an attempt to study the effectiveness of iodine supplementation in early fetal life, pregnant women in the test village (Tocachi) were given iodine supplementation. Mothers who were in the sixth, seventh, eighth, and ninth months of pregnancy at the time of iodization were excluded. There have been no new cases of endemic cretinism among the infants investigated in the treated village, whereas six instances of severe and persistent mental and neuromotor deficiencies have appeared in the control village (123). The

TABLE 49.4. PREVENTION OF ENDEMIC CRETINISM BY INJECTIONS OF IODIZED OIL

Regions	Methods	Findings	References
Neurologic cretinism			
Ecuador	One village injected (Tocachi). One village not injected (La Esperanza). Follow-up of the children born in the two villages up to 60 mo of age.	No cretin among the 205 children born in the treated village. Six neurologic cretins among the 447 children born in the untreated village.	123
Papua-New Guinea	Families injected or not injected at random. Follow-up of the children up to 60 mo of age.	Six neurologic cretins among the 687 children in the treated group; in five of the six, the mother was pregnant at the time of injection. Thirty-one cretins among the 688 children in the untreated group.	124
Myxedematous cretinism			
DRC			
Idjwi Island	Two villages injected. One village not injected. Surveys after 1, 3.5, and 5 yr in the treated villages and after 5 yr in the untreated village.	No cretin born in the treated villages. Three myxedematous cretins were born in the untreated village during the fifth year of the investigation.	140
Ubangi	Pregnant women injected at random between the 20th and 36th wk of gestation (mean 28th wk).		103,111
	Follow-up of 99 infants age 1.5–15 mo (mean 6.5 mo).	One myxedematous cretin among 44 infants in the treated group (mother injected during the last month of gestation). Four myxedematous cretins among 45 infants in the untreated group.	
	Follow-up of 671 infants and children age 0–7 yr.	In infants 0–2 yr, myxedematous cretinism in 1/192 in the treated group and 10/109 in the untreated group ($p < .01$). The difference disappeared in children 3–7 yr.	

data of Pharoah and colleagues (124) indicate that iodized oil injections prevent neurologic endemic cretinism in offspring only if administered before pregnancy, indicating that the damage occurs during early fetal life.

The data from DRC show that correction of iodine deficiency prevents myxedematous endemic cretinism in the offspring even if administered during pregnancy (103). Subsequent studies showed that correction of iodine deficiency in pregnant mothers does not protect the infants against hypothyroidism for more than 2 to 3 years (111). The possibility that in some children, hypothyroidism could start after the age of 3 years is consistent with the observation of Goslings and colleagues (28) that hypothyroid patients in severe endemic goiter are not necessarily affected by severe and irreversible mental retardation and of Boyages and colleagues (44) that cretins with thyroid failure may have only moderate retardation in height and bone maturation (Table 49.1).

CONCLUSION

The epidemiology, clinical manifestation, laboratory data, therapy, and prevention of endemic cretinism are presently well established. Its etiopathogenesis is much better understood. Iodine deficiency appears to be an essential factor and, if severe enough, may be the sole factor in its causation. Selenium deficiency, if present, is an additional factor that results, on the one hand, in a risk of thyroid damage during the perinatal period and, on the other hand, in an increased availability of the prohormone T_4 of maternal origin to the fetal brain. Thiocyanate, if present, aggravates the effects of both iodine and selenium deficiencies, both in the mother and the fetus, as it freely crosses the placenta.

Distinction between the neurologic and myxedematous types of endemic cretinism is not required any longer for two reasons: (a) it is difficult to justify from an epidemiologic and clinical point of view, and (b) the various manifestations of cretinism are critically related to the degree, timing, and duration of the action of the different dietary goitrogenic factors, including iodine deficiency. The level of serum T_4 of the mother during gestation and the transfer of maternal T_4 to the fetus and neonate, especially during early gestation even before the onset of fetal thyroid function, are the determining factors in the occurrence of irreversible brain damage. The second trimester appears as the period of maximum vulnerability of the brain. Maternal hypothyroxinemia appears as the determining factor in the pathogenesis of the neurologic picture and selenium deficiency in the thyroid damage and failure in endemic cretinism, respectively. The respective importance of these two factors depends on the local goitrogenic factors in the diet.

Because of the gravity of the condition and the well-established preventive action of iodine, an efficient iodine prophylaxis is urgently needed in areas affected by endemic goiter and cretinism.

REFERENCES

1. Stanbury JB, Ermans AM, Hetzel BS, et al. Endemic goitre and cretinism: public health significance and prevention. *WHO Chron* 1974;28:220.
2. Hetzel BS, Dunn JT, Stanbury JB. *The prevention and control of iodine deficiency disorders.* Amsterdam: Elsevier, 1987.
3. Delange F. Endemic cretinism. An overview. In: Delong GR, Robbins J, Condliffe, eds. *Iodine and the brain.* New York: Plenum, 1989:219.
4. De Quervain F, Wegelin C. *Der Endemische Kretinismus.* Berlin: Springer Verlag, 1936.
5. König MP. *Die Kongenitale Hypothyreose und der Endemische Kretinismus.* Berlin: Springer Verlag, 1968.
6. Stanbury JB. *The damaged brain of iodine deficiency.* New York: Cognizant Communication, 1994:1–335.
7. Dumont JE, Delange F, Ermans AM. Endemic cretinism. In: Stanbury JB, ed. *Endemic goiter.* Washington, DC: Pan American Health Organization (publication no. 193), 1969:91.
8. Pharoah P, Delange F, Fierro-Benitez R, et al. Endemic cretinism. In: Stanbury JB, Hetzel BS, eds. *Endemic goiter and endemic cretinism: iodine nutrition in health and disease.* New York: John Wiley, 1980:395.
9. Hetzel BS, Querido A. Iodine deficiency, thyroid function, and brain development. In: Stanbury JB, Hetzel BS, eds. *Endemic goiter and endemic cretinism.* New York: John Wiley & Sons, 1980:461.
10. Hetzel BS. *The story of iodine deficiency.* Oxford, UK: Oxford University Press, 1989.
11. Querido A. History of iodine prophylaxis with regard to cretinism and deaf-mutism. In: Stanbury JB, Kroc RL, eds. *Human development and the thyroid gland: relation to endemic cretinism.* New York: Plenum, 1972:191.
12. Delange F, Bastani S, Benmiloud M, et al. Definitions of endemic goiter and cretinism, classification of goiter size and severity of endemias, and survey techniques. In: Dunn JT, Pretell E, Daza CH, et al., eds. *Towards the eradication of endemic goiter, cretinism and iodine deficiency.* Washington, DC: Pan American Health Organization (publication no. 502), 1986:373.
13. McCarrison R. Observations on endemic cretinism in the Chitral and Gilgit valleys. *Lancet* 1908;2:1275.
14. Choufoer JC, Van Rhijn M, Querido A. Endemic goiter in Western New Guinea. II. Clinical picture, incidence and pathogenesis of endemic cretinism. *J Clin Endocrinol Metab* 1965;25:385.
15. Buttfield IH, Hetzel BS. Endemic cretinism in Eastern New Guinea. *Aust Ann Med* 1969;18:217.
16. Bastenie PA, Ermans AM, Thys O, et al. Endemic goiter in the Uele region. III. Endemic cretinism. *J Clin Endocrinol Metab* 1962;22:187.
17. Dumont JE, Ermans AM, Bastenie PA. Thyroidal function in a goiter endemic. IV. Hypothyroidism and endemic cretinism. *J Clin Endocrinol Metab* 1963;23:325.
18. Delange F, Ermans AM, Vis HL, et al. Endemic cretinism in Idjwi Island (Kivu Lake, Republic of the Congo). *J Clin Endocrinol Metab* 1972;34:1059.
19. Ermans AM, Mbulamoko NM, Delange F, et al. *Role of cassava in the etiology of endemic goitre and cretinism.* Ottawa, Ontario, Canada: International Development Research Centre, 1980.
20. Delange F, Iteke FB, Ermans AM. *Nutritional factors involved in the goitrogenic action of cassava.* Ottawa, Ontario, Canada: International Development Research Centre, 1982.
21. Vanderpas JB, Rivera-Vanderpas MT, Bourdoux P, et al. Reversibility of severe hypothyroidism with supplementary iodine in patients with endemic cretinism. *N Engl J Med* 1986;315:791.
22. Vanderpas JB, Contempré B, Duale NL et al. Iodine and selenium deficiency associated with cretinism in Northern Zaire. *Am J Clin Nutr* 1990;52:1087.
23. Delange F. Endemic goitre and thyroid function in Central Africa. In: *Monographs in paediatrics.* Vol. 2. Basel, Switzerland: Karger, 1974.
24. Shenkman L, Medeiros-Neto GA, Mitsuma T, et al. Evidence for hypothyroidism in endemic cretinism in Brazil. *Lancet* 1973;2:67.
25. Zhu XY. Endemic goiter and cretinism in China with special reference to changes of iodine metabolism and pituitary-thyroid function two years after iodine prophylaxis in Gui-Zhou. In: Ui N, Torizuka K, Nagataki S, Miyai K, eds. *Current problems in thyroid research.* Amsterdam: Excerpta Medical, 1983:13.
26. Fierro-Benitez R, Ramirez I, Garces J, et al. The clinical pattern of cretinism as seen in Highland Ecuador. *Am J Clin Nutr* 1974;27:531.
27. Lobo LCG, Pompeu F, Rosenthal D. Endemic cretinism in Goiaz, Brazil. *J Clin Endocrinol Metab* 1963;23:407.
28. Goslings BM, Djokomoeljanto R, Doctor R, et al. Hypothyroidism in an area of endemic goiter and cretinism in Central Java, Indonesia. *J Clin Endocrinol Metab* 1977;44:481.
29. Costa A, Cottino F, Mortara M et al. Endemic cretinism in Piedmont. *Panminerva Med* 1964;6:250.
30. Squatrito S, Delange F, Trimarchi F, et al. Endemic cretinism in Sicily. *J Endocrinol Invest* 1981;4:295.
31. Delange F, Valeix P, Bourdoux P, et al. Comparison of the epidemiological and clinical aspects of endemic cretinism in Central Africa and in the Himalayas. In: Hetzel BS, Smith RM, eds. *Fetal brain disorders: recent approaches to the problem of mental deficiency.* Amsterdam: Elsevier North Holland, 1981:243.
32. Ibbertson HK, Tait JM, Pearl M, et al. Himalayan cretinism. In: Stanbury JB, Kroc RL, eds. *Human development and the thyroid gland: relation to endemic cretinism.* New York: Plenum, 1972:51.
33. Stanbury JB, Fierro-Benitez R, Estrella E, et al. Endemic goiter with hypothyroidism in three generations. *J Clin Endocrinol Metab* 1969;29:1596.
34. Lagasse R, Roger G, Delange F, et al. Continuous spectrum of physical and intellectual disorders in severe endemic goitre. In: Ermans AM, Mbulamoko NM, Delange F, et al, eds. *Role of cassava in the etiology of endemic goitre and cretinism.* Ottawa, Ontario, Canada: International Development Research Centre, 1980:135.
35. Trimarchi F, Vermiglio F, Finocchrio MD, et al. Epidemiology and clinical characteristics of endemic cretinism in Sicily. *J Endocrinol Invest* 1990;13:543.
36. Donati L, Antonelli A, Bertoni F, et al. Clinical picture of endemic cretinism in Central Apennines (Montefeltro). *Thyroid* 1992;2:283.
37. Delange F, Costa A, Ermans AM, et al. Clinical and metabolic patterns of endemic cretinism. In: Stanbury JB, Kroc RL, eds. *Human development and the thyroid gland: relation to endemic cretinism.* New York: Plenum, 1972:175.

38. Wang HM, Ma T, Li XT, et al. A comparative study of endemic myxedematous and neurological cretinism in Hetian and Luopu, China. In: Ui N, Torizuka K, Nagataki S, et al., eds. *Current problems in thyroid research.* Amsterdam: Excerpta Medica, 1983:349.

39. Shi ZF, Zeng GH, Zhang JX, et al. Endemic goiter and cretinism in Guizhou: clinical analysis of 247 cretins. *Chin Med J* 1984;97:689.

40. Ma T, Lu TZ, Tan YB, et al. Neurological cretinism in China. In: Kochupillai N, Karmakar MG, Ramalingaswami V, eds. *Iodine nutrition, thyroxine and brain development.* New Delhi: Tata McGraw-Hill, 1986:28.

41. DeLong GR, Stanbury JB, Fierro-Benitez R. Neurological signs in congenital iodine-deficiency disorder (endemic cretinism). *Dev Med Child Neurol* 1985;27:317.

42. DeLong GR. Observations on the neurology of endemic cretinism. In: DeLong GR, Robbins J, Condliffe PG, eds. *Iodine and the brain.* New York: Plenum, 1989:231.

43. DeLong GR. Neurological involvement in iodine deficiency disorders. In: Hetzel BS, Dunn JT, Stanbury JB, eds. *The prevention and control of iodine deficiency disorders.* Amsterdam: Elsevier, 1987:49.

44. Boyages SC, Halpern JP, Maberly GF, et al. A comparative study of neurological and myxedematous endemic cretinism in Western China. *J Clin Endocrinol Metab* 1988;67:1262.

45. Halpern JP, Morris JGL, Boyages S, et al. Neurological aspects of cretinism in Qinghai Province. In: DeLong GR, Robbins J, Condliffe PG, eds. *Iodine and the brain.* New York: Plenum, 1989:239.

46. Boyages SC. Iodine deficiency disorders. *J Clin Endocrinol Metab* 1993;77:587.

47. De Long GR, Ma T, Cao Xy, et al. The neuromotor deficit in endemic cretinism. In: Stanbury JB, ed. *The damaged brain of iodine deficiency.* New York: Cognizant Communication, 1994:9.

48. Halpern JP, Boyages SC, Maberly GF, et al. The neurology of endemic cretinism. *Brain* 1991;114:825.

49. Rajatanavin R, Chailurkit L, Winichakoon P, et al. Endemic cretinism in Thailand: a multidisciplinary survey. *Eur J Endocrinol* 1997;137:349.

50. Boyages S. Iodine and the brain: evidence from the mountains of Thailand. *Eur J Endocrinol* 1997;137:336.

51. Morreale de Escobar G, Obregon MJ, Escobar del Rey F. Is neuropsychological development related to maternal hypothyroidism or to maternal hypothyroxinemia? *J Clin Endocrinol Metab* 2000;85:3975.

52. Ramirez I, Cruz M, Varea J. Endemic cretinism in the Andean region: new methodological approaches. In: Delange F, Ahluwalia R, eds. *Cassava toxicity and thyroid: research and public health issues.* Ottawa, Ontario, Canada: International Development Research Centre, 1983:73.

53. Downing D, Geel Hoed GW. Goiter and cretinism in the Uele Zaire endemia: studies of an iodine deficient population with changes following intervention. II. Functional and behavioral aspects. In: Stanbury JB, ed. *The damaged brain of iodine deficiency.* New York: Cognizant Communication, 1994:233.

54. Smith DW, Blizzard RM, Wilkins L. The mental prognosis in hypothyroidism of infancy and childhood: a review of 128 cases. *Pediatrics* 1957;19:1011.

55. Vanderschueren-Lodeweyckx M, Debruyne F, Dooms L, et al. Sensorineural hearing loss in sporadic congenital hypothyroidism. *Arch Dis Child* 1983;58:419.

56. Raman G, Beierwaltes WH. Correlation of goiter, deafmutism and mental retardation with serum thyroid hormone levels in non-cretinous inhabitants of a severe endemic goiter area in India. *J Clin Endocrinol Metab* 1959;19:228.

57. Trowbridge FL. Intellectual assessment in primitive societies, with a preliminary report of a study of the effects of early iodine supplementation on intelligence. In: Stanbury JB, Kroc RL, eds. *Human development and the thyroid gland: relation to endemic cretinism.* New York: Plenum Press, 1972:137.

58. Pharoah POD, Hornabrook RW. Endemic cretinism of recent onset in New Guinea. *Lancet* 1973;2:1038.

59. Hetzel BS, Hay ID. Thyroid function, iodine nutrition and fetal brain development. *Clin Endocrinol (Oxf)* 1979;11:445.

60. Smith RM. Thyroid hormones and brain development. In: Hetzel BS, Smith RM, eds. *Fetal brain disorders: recent approaches to the problem of mental deficiency.* Amsterdam: Elsevier/North Holland Biomedical Press, 1981:149.

61. Potter BJ, McIntosh, Hetzel BS. The effect of iodine deficiency on fetal brain development in the sheep. In: Hetzel BS, Smith RM, eds. *Fetal brain disorders: recent approaches to the problem of mental deficiency.* Amsterdam: Elsevier/North Holland Biomedical Press, 1981:119.

62. Courtois P, Bourdoux P, Lagasse R, et al. Role of the balance between the dietary supplies of iodine and thiocyanate in the etiology of endemic goitre in the Ubangi area. In: Delange F, Iteke FB, Ermans AM, eds. *Nutritional factors involved in the goitrogenic action of cassava.* Ottawa, Ontario, Canada: International Development Research Centre, 1982:65.

63. Boyages SC, Maberly GF, Chen J, et al. Endemic cretinism: possible role for thyroid autoimmunity. *Lancet* 1989;2:529.

64. Boyages SC, Lens JW, Van Der Gaag RD, et al. Sporadic and endemic congenital hypothyroidism: evidence for autosensitization. In: Delange F, Fisher DA, Glinoer D, eds. *Research in congenital hypothyroidism.* New York: Plenum, 1989:123.

65. Medeiros-Neto G, Tsuboi K, Lima N. Thyroid autoimmunity and endemic cretinism. *Lancet* 1989;1:111.

66. Brown RS, Keating P, Mitchell E. Maternal thyroid-blocking immunoglobulins in congenital hypothyroidism. *J Clin Endocrinol Metab* 1990;70:1341.

67. Chiovato L, Vitti P, Marcocci C, et al. TSH-blocking antibodies and congenital hypothyroidism. In: Delange F, Fisher DA, Glinoer D, eds. *Research in congenital hypothyroidism.* New York: Plenum, 1989:141.

68. Chiovato L, Vitti P, Bendinelli G, et al. Humoral thyroid autoimmunity is not involved in the pathogenesis of myxedematous endemic cretinism. *J Clin Endocrinol Metab* 1995;80:1509.

69. Vanderpas JB, Contempré B, Duale NL, et al. Iodine and selenium deficiency associated with cretinism in Northern Zaire. *Am J Clin Nutr* 1990;52:1087.

70. Corvilain B, Contempré B, Longombe AO, et al. Selenium and the thyroid: how the relationship was established. *Am J Clin Nutr Suppl* 1993;57:244S.

71. Contempré B, Many MC, Vanderpas J et al. Interaction between two trace elements: selenium and iodine: implications of both deficiencies. In: Stanbury JB, ed. *The damaged brain and iodine deficiency.* New York: Cognizant Communication, 1994:133.

72. Dumont JE, Corvilain B, Contempré B. Endemic cretinism: the myxedematous and neurologic forms of a disease caused by severe iodine deficiency. In: Stanbury JB, ed. *The damaged brain and iodine deficiency.* New York: Cognizant Communication, 1994:133.

73. Goyens P, Golstein J, Nsombola B, et al. Selenium deficiency as possible factor in the pathogenesis of myxedematous endemic cretinism. *Acta Endocrinol (Copenh)* 1987;114:497.

74. Aaseth J, Frey H, Glattre E, et al. Selenium concentrations in the human thyroid. *Biol Trace Elem Res* 1990;24:147.

75. Dumont JE. The action of thyrotropin on thyroid metabolism. *Vitam Horm* 1971;29:287.

76. Arthur JR, Nicol F, Beckett GJ. Hepatic iodothyronine 5′-deiodinase: the role of selenium. *Biochem J* 1990;272:537.

77. Contempré B, Denef JF, Dumont JE, et al. Selenium deficiency aggravates the necrotizing effects of a high iodide dose in iodine deficient rats. *Endocrinology* 1993;132:1866.

78. Contempré B, Morreale de Escobar G, Denef JF, et al. Thiocyanate induces cell necrosis and fibrosis in selenium- and iodine-deficient rat thyroids: a potential experimental model for myxedematous endemic cretinism in Central Africa. *Endocrinology* 2004; 145:994.

79. Bernal J, Nunez J. Thyroid hormones and brain development. *Eur J Endocrinol* 1995;133:390.

80. Calvo R, Obregon MJ, Ruiz de Ona C, et al. Congenital hypothyroidism, as studied in rats: crucial role of maternal thyroxine but not of 3,5,3'-triiodothyronine in the protection of the fetal brain. *J Clin Invest* 1990;86:889.

81. Fisher DA, Klein AH. Thyroid development and disorders of thyroid function in the newborn. *N Engl J Med* 1981;304:702.

82. Obregon MJ, Mallol J, Pastor R, et al. L-thyroxine and 3,5,3' triiodo-L-thyroxine in rats embryos before onset of fetal thyroid function. *Endocrinology* 1984;114:305.

83. Morreale de Escobar G, Pastor R, Obregon MJ, et al. Effects of maternal hypothyroidism on the weight and thyroid hormone content of rat embryonic tissues, before and after onset of fetal thyroid function. *Endocrinology* 1985;117:1890.

84. Ruiz de Ona C, Morreale de Escobar G, Galvo RM, et al. Thyroid hormones and 5'-deiodinase in the rat fetus late in gestation: effects of maternal hypothyroidism. *Endocrinology* 1991; 128:422.

85. Morreale de Escobar G, Calvo RM, Obregon MJ, et al. Contribution of maternal thyroxine to fetal thyroxine pools in normal rats near term. *Endocrinology* 1990;126:2765.

86. Escobar del Rey F, Pastor R, Mallol J, et al. Effects of maternal iodine deficiency on the L-thyroxine and 3,5,3'-triiodo-L-thyroxine contents of rat embryonic tissues before and after onset of fetal thyroid function. *Endocrinology* 1986;118:1259.

87. Lavado-Autric R, Auso E, Garcia-Velasco JV, et al. Early maternal hypothyroxinemia alters histogenesis and cerebral cortex cytoarchitecture of the progeny. *J Clin Invest* 2003;111:1073.

88. Versloot PM, Schröder-Van Der Elst JP, Van Der Heide D, et al. Effects of marginal iodine deficiency during pregnancy: iodide uptake by the maternal and fetal thyroid. *Am J Physiol* 1997;273:E1121.

89. Schröder-Van Der Elst JP, Vanderheiden D, Kastelijn J, et al. The expression of the sodium/iodide symporter is up-regulated in the thyroid of the fetuses of iodine-deficient rats. *Endocrinology* 2001;142:3736.

90. Morreale de Escobar G, Obregon MJ, Escobar del Rey F. Hormone nurturing of the developing brain: the rat model. In: Stanbury JB, ed. *The damaged brain of iodine deficiency.* New York: Cognizant Communication, 1994:103.

91. Contempré B, Jauniaux E, Calvo R, et al. Detection of thyroid hormones in human embryonic cavities during the first trimester of gestation. *J Clin Endocrinol Metab* 1993;77:1719.

92. Bernal J, Pekonen F. Ontogenesis of the nuclear 3,5,3'-triiodothyronine receptor in the human fetal brain. *Endocrinology* 1984;114:677.

93. Calvo RM, Jauniaux E, Gulbis B, et al. Fetal tissues are exposed to biologically relevant free thyroxine concentrations during early phases of development. *J Clin Endocrinol Metab* 2002;87:1768.

94. Thorpe-Beeston JG, Nicolaides KH, Felton CV, et al. Maturation of the secretion of thyroid hormone and thyroid-stimulating hormone in the fetus. *N Engl J Med* 1991;324:532.

95. Vulsma T, Gons MH, De Vijlder JJM. Maternal-fetal transfer of thyroxine in congenital hypothyroidism due to a total organification defect or thyroid agenesis. *N Engl J Med* 1989;321:13.

96. Man EB, Jones WS, Holden RH, et al. Thyroid function in human pregnancy. VIII. Retardation of progeny aged 7 years: relationship to maternal age and maternal thyroid function. *Am J Obstet Gynecol* 1971;111:905.

97. Matsuura N, Konishi J. Transient hypothyroidism in infants born to mothers with chronic thyroiditis: a nationwide study of twenty-three cases. *Endocrinol Japon* 1990;37:369.

98. Glinoer D, Delange F. The potential repercussions of maternal, fetal and neonatal hypothyroxinemia on the progeny. *Thyroid* 2000;10:871.

99. Delange F, Thilly C, Bourdoux P, et al. Influence of dietary goitrogens during pregnancy in humans on thyroid function of the newborn. In: Delange F, Iteke FB, Ermans AM, eds. *Nutritional factors involved in the goitrogenic action of cassava.* Ottawa, Ontario, Canada: International Development Research, 1982:40.

100. Pharoah POD, Connolly KJ, Ekins RP, et al. Maternal thyroid hormone levels in pregnancy and the subsequent cognitive and motor performance of the children. *Clin Endocrinol* 1984;21:265.

101. Pharoah POD, Ellis SM, Ekins RP, et al. Maternal thyroid function, iodine deficiency and fetal development. *Clin Endocrinol (Oxf)* 1976;5:159.

102. Thilly CH, Swennen B, Moreno-Reyes R, et al. Maternal, fetal and juvenile hypothyroidism: birth weight, and infant mortality in the etiopathogenesis of the IDD spectrum in Zaire and Malawi. In: Stanbury JB, ed. *The damaged brain of iodine deficiency.* New York: Cognizant Communication, 1994:241.

103. Thilly CH, Delange F, Lagasse R, et al. Fetal hypothyroidism and maternal thyroid status in severe endemic goiter. *J Clin Endocrinol Metab* 1978;47:354.

104. Glinoer D, De Nayer P, Delange F, et al. A randomized trial for the treatment of mild iodine deficiency during pregnancy: maternal and neonatal effects. *J Clin Endocrinol Metab* 1995;80:258.

105. Liu JL, Tan YB, Zuang ZL, et al. Morphologic study of development of cerebral cortex of therapeutically aborted fetuses in endemic region, Gui-Zhou Province, China. In: Ui N, Torizuka K, Nagataki S, Miyai K, eds. *Current problems in thyroid research.* Amsterdam: Excerpta Medica, 1983:390.

106. Kochupillai N, Pandav CS. Neonatal chemical hypothyroidism in iodine-deficient environments. In: Hetzel BS, Dunn JT, Stanbury JB, eds. *The prevention and control of iodine deficiency disorders.* Amsterdam: Elsevier, 1987:85.

107. Chaouki ML, Delange F, Maoui R, et al. Endemic cretinism and congenital hypothyroidism in endemic goiter in Algeria. In: Meideiros-Neto GA, Gaitan E, eds. *Frontiers of thyroidology.* New York: Plenum Press, 1986:1055.

108. Sava L, Delange F, Belfiore, et al. Transient impairment of thyroid function in newborn from an area of endemic goiter. *J Clin Endocrinol Metab* 1984;59:90.

109. Delange F, Beckers C, Höfer R, et al. Progress report on neonatal screening for congenital hypothyroidism in Europe. In: Burrow GN, Dussault JH, eds. *Neonatal thyroid screening.* New York: Raven, 1980:107.

110. Dussault JH, Mitchell ML, La Franchi S, et al. Regional screening for congenital hypothyroidism: results of screening one million North American infants with filter paper spot T_4-TSH. In: Burrow GN, Dussault JH, eds. *Neonatal thyroid screening.* New York: Raven, 1980:155.

111. Thilly C, Vanderpas J, Bourdoux P, et al. Prevention of myxedematous cretinism with iodized oil during pregnancy. In: Ui N, Torizuka K, Nagataki S, Miyai K, eds. *Current problems in thyroid research.* Amsterdam: Excerpta Medica, 1983:386.

112. Wilkins L. Epiphyseal dysgenesis associated with hypothyroidism. *Am J Dis Child* 1941;61:13.

113. Courtois P, Delange F, Bourdoux P, et al. Significance of neonatal thyroid screening tests in severe endemic goiter [Abstract 81]. *Ann Endocrinol* 1982;43:51.

114. Delange F. Adaptation to iodine deficiency during growth: etiopathogenesis of endemic goiter and cretinism. In: Delange F, Fisher D, Malvaux P, eds. *Pediatric thyroidology.* Basel, Switzerland: Karger, 1985:295.

115. Braverman LE. Placental transfer for substances from mother to fetus affecting fetal pituitary-thyroid function. In: Delange F, Fisher DA, Glinoer D, eds. *Research in congenital hypothyroidism.* New York: Plenum, 1989:3.

116. Dumont JE, Ermans AM, Bastenie PA. Thyroid function in a goiter endemic. V. Mechanism of thyroid failure in the Uele endemic cretins. *J Clin Endocrinol Metab* 1963;23:847.

117. Vanderpas J, Bourdoux P, Lagasse R, et al. Endemic infantile hypothyroidism in a severe endemic goitre area of Central Africa. *Clin Endocrinol (Oxf)* 1984;20:327.

118. Moreno-Reyes R, Boelaert M, El Badawi S, et al. Endemic juvenile hypothyroidism in a severe endemic goitre area in Sudan. *Clin Endocrinol (Oxf)* 1993;38:19.

119. Vanderpas JB, Rivera-Vanderpas MT, Bourdoux P et al. Reversibility of severe hypothyroidism with supplementary iodine in patients with endemic cretinism. *N Engl J Med* 1986; 315:791.

120. Boyages SC, Halpern JP, Maberly GF, et al. Supplementary iodine fails to reverse hypothyroidism in adolescents and adults with endemic cretinism. *J Clin Endocrinol Metab* 1990;70:336.

121. Hetzel BS, Thilly CH, Fierro-Benitez R, et al. Iodized oil in the prevention of endemic goiter and cretinism. In: Stanbury JB, Hetzel BS, eds. *Endemic goiter and endemic cretinism.* New York: John Wiley & Sons, 1980:513.

122. Wespi HJ. Abnahme der Taubstumnheit in der Schweiz als Folge der Kropfprophylaxe mit iodertem Kochsalz. *Schweiz Med Wochenschr* 1945;75:625.

123. Ramirez I, Fierro-Benitez R, Estrella E, et al. The results of prophylaxis of endemic cretinism with iodized oil in rural Andean Ecuador. In: Stanbury JB, Kroc RL, eds. *Human development and the thyroid gland: relation to endemic cretinism.* New York: Plenum, 1972:223.

124. Pharoah POB, Buttfield IH, Hetzel BS. Neurological damage to the fetus resulting from severe iodine deficiency during pregnancy. *Lancet* 1971;1:308.

125. Ermans AM, Kinthaert J, Delcroix C, et al. Metabolism of intrathyroidal iodine in normal men. *J Clin Endocrinol Metab* 1968;28:169.

126. Fierro-Benitez R, Ramirez I, Estrella E, et al. The role of iodine deficiency in intellectual development in an area of endemic goiter. In: Dunn JT, Medeiros-Neto GA, eds. *Endemic goiter and cretinism: continuing threats to world health.* Washington, DC: Pan American Health Organization (publication no. 292), 1974:135.

127. Dodge PR, Palkes H, Fierro-Benitez R, et al. Effect on intelligence of iodine in oil administered to young Andean children: a preliminary report. In: Stanbury JB, ed. *Endemic goiter.* Washington, DC: Pan American Health Organization (publication no. 193), 1969:378.

128. Greene LS. Physical growth and development, neurological maturation and behavioral functioning in two Andean communities in which goiter is endemic. *Am J Phys Anthropol* 1973;38:119.

129. Bautista A, Barker PA, Dunn JT, et al. The effects of oral iodized oil on intelligence, thyroid status, and somatic growth in school-age children from an area of endemic goiter. *Am J Clin Nutr* 1982;35:127.

130. Muzzo S, Leiva L, Carrasco D. Possible etiological factors and consequences of a moderate iodine deficiency on intellectual coefficient of school-age children. In: Meideiros-Neto GA, Gaitan E, eds. *Frontiers of thyroidology.* New York: Plenum, 1985:1001.

131. Connolly KJ, Pharoah POD, Hetzel BS. Fetal iodine deficiency and motor performance during childhood. *Lancet* 1979;2: 1149.

132. Pharoah POD, Connolly K, Hetzel B, et al. Maternal thyroid function and motor competence in the child. *Dev Med Child Neurol* 1981;23:76.

133. Thilly CH, Roger G, Lagasse R, et al. Fetomaternal relationship, fetal hypothyroidism, and psychomotor retardation. In: Ermans AM, Mbulamoko NM, Delange F, et al, eds. *Role of cassava in the etiology of endemic goitre and cretinism.* Ottawa, Ontario, Canada: International Development Research, 1980:111.

134. Bleichrodt N, Garcia I, Rubio C, et al. Developmental disorders associated with severe iodine deficiency. In: Hetzel BS, Dunn JT, Stanbury JB, eds. *The prevention and control of iodine deficiency disorders.* Amsterdam: Elsevier, 1987:65.

135. Boyages SC, Collins JK, Maberly GF, et al. Iodine deficiency impairs intellectual and neuromotor development in apparently normal persons. *Med J Aust* 1989;150:676.

136. Ma T, Wang YY, Wang D, et al. Neuropsychological studies in iodine deficiency areas in China. In: DeLong GR, Robbins J, Condliffe G, eds. *Iodine and the brain.* New York: Plenum, 1989:259.

137. Kochupillai N, Pandav CS, Godbole MM, et al. Iodine deficiency and neonatal hypothyroidism. *Bull WHO* 1986;64: 547.

138. Tiwari BD, Godbole MM, Chattopadhyay N, et al. Learning disabilities and poor motivation to achieve due to prolonged iodine deficiency. *Am J Clin Nutr* 1996;63:782.

139. Azizi F, Sarshar A, Nafarabadi M, et al. Impairment of neuromotor and cognitive development in iodine-deficient schoolchildren with normal physical growth. *Acta Endocrinol (Copenh)* 1993;125:501.

140. Thilly CH, Delange F, Golstein-Golaire J, et al. Endemic goiter prophylaxis by iodized oil: a reassessment. *J Clin Endocrinol Metab* 1973;36:1196.

PRIMARY HYPOTHYROIDISM DUE TO OTHER CAUSES

PETER A. SINGER

Spontaneous primary hypothyroidism, which is nearly always due to chronic autoimmune (Hashimoto's) thyroiditis, is the most common cause of hypothyroidism in many countries. In the United States alone, cross-sectional studies of the elderly have demonstrated high serum thyrotropin (TSH) levels in from 6.7% to 19% of people, with a greater prevalence in women (1–3). Iodine deficiency is the principal cause of hypothyroidism in underdeveloped areas in the world, and may be present in as many as 1 billion people worldwide, although the actual prevalence of hypothyroidism in affected individuals is not known. (These disorders are discussed in detail in the section Iodine Deficiency in Chapter 11 and Chapter 49.)

This chapter will discuss other types of primary hypothyroidism, ranging from those encountered commonly, such as following radioactive iodine therapy (RAI) or thyroidectomy, and uncommon and even rare forms of hypothyroidism, including some due to infiltrative and inherited disorders (Table 50.1). Some types of hypothyroidism are so rare that they are unlikely to be encountered by a practicing physician, and are of academic interest only.

For the purpose of this discussion, hypothyroidism is defined as a sustained elevation of serum TSH. Thus, subclinical hypothyroidism, which is characterized by normal serum levels of free thyroxine and high serum levels of TSH (see Chapter 78) will be included, along with overt hypothyroidism.

HYPOTHYROIDISM DUE TO THYROID ABLATION

Treatment of Graves' Disease

Radioactive Iodine Therapy

Iodine 131 (^{131}I) therapy for thyrotoxic Graves' disease is the most common cause of nonspontaneous hypothyroidism in the United States, probably because of physician preference for ^{131}I, due to the relatively high relapse rate (~60%) of thyrotoxicosis following withdrawal of antithyroid drug therapy (4). An international survey of thyroid specialists over a decade ago revealed that ^{131}I was chosen by 69% of physicians in the United States as the primary

form of treatment for a typical 43-year-old woman with Graves' thyrotoxicosis (5). In contrast, only 22% of physicians from Europe, 17% from Latin America, and 11% from Asia, selected ^{131}I as the primary form of therapy (6,7). This therapy almost always results in hypothyroidism, necessitating othyroxine (T$_4$) treatment. Indeed, most physicians in North America recommend a dose of ^{131}I sufficient to ensure hypothyroidism, so that the need for T$_4$ replacement will be predictable (8). Efforts to restore long-term euthyroidism with smaller doses of ^{131}I have generally been unsuccessful, resulting in either persistent or recurrent thyrotoxicosis, or later onset of hypothyroidism. In one study of 187 patients in the United States treated with low doses of ^{131}I, 12% become hypothyroid after 1 year, and 76% were hypothyroid at the end of 11 years of follow-up (9). A similar study in England yielded similar results, with 11% of patients becoming hypothyroid after 1 year, and 55% developing hypothyroidism after 15 years (10). Recently, high-dose ^{131}I (128–155 µCi/g) was shown to result in cure of Graves' thyrotoxicosis in 90% of patients, and the development of hypothyroidism in approximately 80% (1–3). Because hypothyroidism develops so frequently, regardless of the dose used, the goal of long-term euthyroidism with ^{131}I is not only difficult but is probably unwise, because patients treated with lower ^{131}I doses require more careful long-term surveillance.

Surgery

Surgery was the choice of treatment for the above-mentioned 43-year-old woman with Graves' thyrotoxicosis by only approximately 1% of physicians in the United States, whereas it was the preferred method of treatment by physicians in Latin America, Europe, and Asia (11). Although euthyroidism after surgery is desirable, hypothyroidism usually develops; 59% of 81 patients who underwent subtotal thyroidectomy in the United States, and 51% of 216 patients who underwent similar surgery in Japan, developed hypothyroidism within several years (11,12). In both studies, a thyroid remnant of less than 6 g was left in order to avoid recurrent thyrotoxicosis. Other studies have yielded similar findings, including two studies from Europe, in

TABLE 50.1. OTHER CAUSES OF PRIMARY HYPOTHYROIDISM

Thyroid ablation
  Radioactive iodine therapy or surgery for
    Graves' thyrotoxicosis
    Toxic nodular goiter
    Nontoxic nodular goiter
  External radiotherapy for
    Hodgkin's and non-Hodgkin's lymphoma
    Solid cancers of the head and neck
    Aplastic anemia
    Leukemia
Pharmacologic agents
  Lithium carbonate
  Cytokines (interferon-α, interleukin-2)
  Other drugs (aminogluthamide, ethionamide, sulfonamides)
Infiltrative disorders
  Riedel's (invasive fibrous) thyroiditis
  Amyloidosis
  Sarcoidosis
  Hemochromatosis
  Cystinosis
  AIDS (including *Pneumocystis infection*)
  Primary thyroid lymphoma
Toxic substances
  Cigarettes
  Industrial and environmental agents
Embryologic variants
  Lingual thyroid

which nearly 50% of patients who underwent subtotal thyroidectomy eventually became hypothyroid (13,14). It is my practice to recommend near-total thyroidectomy for Graves' disease, so that the need for T_4 therapy will be more predictable. Thus, both ^{131}I and surgical treatment for thyrotoxic Graves' disease usually result in the need for T_4 replacement.

Treatment of Toxic Nodular Goiter

Both ^{131}I and surgery are commonly used for the treatment of patients with thyrotoxicosis due to either single or multiple autonomously functioning thyroid nodules. Because ^{131}I is mainly concentrated in autonomously functioning tissue, extranodular thyroid tissue should theoretically be spared the effects of ^{131}I. Between 6% and 36% of patients have been reported to become hypothyroid following ^{131}I treatment, however, regardless of the dose of ^{131}I administered (15,16). Patients who become hypothyroid are likely those in whom ^{131}I uptake in nonnodular thyroid tissue was not completely suppressed (16). Radioactive iodine accumulation in the contralateral lobe assumes additional importance in younger patients, who may be subject to nodule formation many years following ^{131}I therapy; hence the common recommendation that younger patients (perhaps <30 years of age) be treated surgically (17,18). It has

been suggested that administration of low doses of ^{131}I (5–15 mCi) to patients with autonomous nodules minimizes the likelihood of posttreatment hypothyroidism (19).

Treatment of Nontoxic Nodular Goiter

Patients undergoing near-total thyroidectomy for nontoxic nodular goiter usually develop hypothyroidism, whereas partial thyroidectomy results in a lower incidence (20,21). Incomplete surgery, however, increases the possibility of recurrence, with regrowth reported to be as high as 10% to 20% of patients approximately 10 years after surgery, and 40% to 45% 30 years after surgery (22). Radioiodine treatment of nontoxic nodular goiter also appears to result in an appreciable incidence of hypothyroidism, with approximately 20% to 30% developing high serum TSH levels within 5 years after therapy (23). This form of treatment has been used in the United States less often than in Europe (24–27). Since the recent availability of recombinant TSH there has been more interest in the use of ^{131}I for treatment of nontoxic goiter, because uptake of ^{131}I can be increased with recombinant TSH administration, including previously nonfunctioning tissue, and lower doses of ^{131}I may be required (28).

Euthyroid patients undergoing lobectomy for single nodules may develop hypothyroidism when exposed to pharmacologic doses of iodides, suggesting that patients with apparent uninodular disease may have a more diffuse underlying thyroid abnormality (29).

Radiation Exposure

Hypothyroidism is common after external radiotherapy with doses of 25 Gy (2,500 rad) or more to the head and neck area for malignant tumors, including Hodgkin's and non-Hodgkin's lymphoma, and solid cancers of the head and neck. Hypothyroidism may develop within the first year after radiotherapy, especially in patients under 20 years of age (30) but it typically develops within 3 to 5 years, and it may continue to develop many years later. In a review of 1,677 Hodgkin's lymphoma patients treated with external radiotherapy, the risk of hypothyroidism was 52% after 20 years, and 67% 26 years after therapy (31). This risk appears to be dose dependent (32).

When laryngectomy or partial thyroidectomy is done in addition to external radiotherapy, the likelihood of hypothyroidism increases to 65% to 70% (33,34). Hypothyroidism occurs in 30% to 40% of children and adolescents who receive whole-body irradiation for either aplastic anemia or leukemia, and in approximately 6% of children who receive craniospinal radiation for brain tumors (35,36). Hypothyroidism also occurs in 9% to 16% of adults who undergo total body irradiation following bone marrow transplantation (37).

Internal radiation to the thyroid from ^{131}I may also induce the formation of thyroid antibodies. Children exposed to radioactive fallout following the 1986 Chernobyl disaster had an increased prevalence of both thyroglobulin and thyroid peroxidase antibodies 6 to 8 years later (19.5% in exposed children vs. 3.8% in unexposed controls) (33). Their thyroid function was normal at the time of study, but they are probably at greater risk for the development of hypothyroidism.

Chemotherapy also appears to be associated with the development of hypothyroidism in patients with lymphoma (30,38), and the combination of chemotherapy and external radiotherapy results in a greater incidence of hypothyroidism than occurs with either chemotherapy or external radiotherapy alone (31,39,40).

Because hypothyroidism may be either an early or late sequela of external radiotherapy, long-term surveillance of irradiated patients with serum TSH testing is indicated.

HYPOTHYROIDISM DUE TO THERAPEUTIC PHARMACOLOGIC AGENTS

Iodides, thionamide drugs, and other agents used in the treatment of thyroid disorders are discussed in Chapter 45. This section will focus on agents not used primarily for the treatment of thyroid disease.

Lithium Carbonate

Lithium carbonate is usually prescribed for the treatment of manic-depressive disorders, and may be associated with the development of both goiter and hypothyroidism. Goiter has been reported in 4% to 60% of patients receiving lithium, and is due primarily to its inhibitory effect on thyroid hormone secretion, resulting in TSH stimulation of the thyroid (41–44). The goiter is typically diffuse. A review of 4,681 lithium-treated patients revealed the overall prevalence of hypothyroidism to be 3.4%, with a range of 0% to 23.3% (45). Risk factors for the development of hypothyroidism include female sex and the presence of thyroid antibodies; patients who develop hypothyroidism during lithium therapy likely have underlying chronic autoimmune (Hashimoto's) thyroiditis (46,47). Lithium-treated patients with no thyroid antibodies may have transient increases in serum TSH (48). Most lithium-treated patients who develop hypothyroidism have subclinical hypothyroidism, with only mild to moderate increases in serum TSH and normal serum thyroid hormone concentrations, although overt hypothyroidism may occur (49,50). Exogenous iodides act synergistically with lithium, resulting in greater serum TSH increases than with lithium alone (51). Because of lithium's effects on the thyroid, patients for whom the drug is prescribed should have a serum TSH

determination at the time of initiation of therapy, and every 6 to 12 months thereafter, or more frequently, as the clinical situation dictates. Lithium therapy is also associated with a greater prevalence of painless thyroiditis than in the general population (52). Although the mechanism for this in unclear, it might be due to induction of an autoimmune process, or to a direct toxic effect on thyroid cells (52,53) (see Chapter 27).

Cytokines

Interferon-α

Interferon-α (IFN-α) is used for the treatment of hepatitis B and C, as well as for various tumors, including malignant carcinoid, Kaposi's sarcoma, chronic myelogenous leukemia, and hairy cell leukemia (54). It is also used in combination with interleukin-2 (IL-2), a cytokine sometimes used in the treatment of tumors (55).

Hypothyroidism was initially described as a side effect of IFN-α therapy in patients receiving long-term IFN-α treatment for breast cancer (56). Thyroid dysfunction due to IFN-α is now more commonly associated with its use in the treatment of chronic hepatitis C virus (HCV) infection (57). IFN-α-associated abnormalities include both thyrotoxicosis and hypothyroidism, with the latter being much more common (57). A biphasic pattern of thyroid dysfunction, with thyrotoxicosis followed by hypothyroidism, is often seen, similar to that observed with silent thyroiditis (58). The observed incidence of IFN-α-associated hypothyroidism in patients with HCV has been reported to vary from 7% to 39% (54,57–60). The addition of ribavirin to IFN-α therapy may increase the risk of hypothyroidism (61).

Risk factors associated with the development of hypothyroidism include female sex, longer duration of IFN-α treatment, presence of HCV, older age, and the preexisting presence of thyroid antibodies, especially antithyroid peroxidase (anti-TPO) antibodies (57). A recent study suggested that Asian origin is an independent risk factor for IFN-α-induced hypothyroidism (62). The presence of anti-TPO antibodies may be the most important risk factor; in one study, thyroid dysfunction occurred in 60% of patients receiving IFN-α who had anti-TPO antibodies before therapy, compared with only 3.3% of patients who did not have anti-TPO antibodies at that time (63).

Transient hypothyroidism occurs more commonly with IFN-α therapy than does persistent hypothyroidism, although pooled data from several series indicate that 30% to 44% of patients who develop hypothyroidism during IFN-α treatment have persistent thyroid failure (54,57). The presence of thyroid antibodies at the end of IFN-α treatment is a positive predictive factor for persistent hypothyroidism (64).

The precise mechanism of IFN-α-induced thyroid dysfunction is not known, although it is probably related to activation or enhancement of the autoimmune process, As mentioned, patients with HCV are more susceptible than patients with other types of hepatitis (e.g., HBV) to develop thyroid dysfunction during IFN-α treatment. They also have a higher baseline prevalence of anti-TPO antibodies, suggesting an association between HCV and underlying thyroid autoimmunity (60). In addition, IFN-α therapy induces the production of thyroid antibodies in patients with HCV who had no prior thyroid abnormalities (57).

In addition to affecting the autoimmune process, IFN-α may exert a direct effect on the thyroid gland. In one study, perchlorate discharge test results were positive in 7 of 32 patients who were being treated with IFN-α, all of whom had negative test results prior to IFN-α, suggesting an IFN-α-induced organification defect of iodine (58).

Interleukin-2

Patients treated with IL-2 for various tumors have an increased risk of hypothyroidism. In one series, 32% of 111 patients with cancer developed hypothyroidism during IL-2 treatment, and 14% had hypothyroidism posttherapy, persisting from 44 to more than 149 days (median 54 days) (65). As with IFN-α-treated patients, positive thyroid antibodies and female sex are risk factors for thyroid dysfunction, whereas the type of tumor is not a predisposing factor (66,67). Patients who developed persistent hypothyroidism had more severe biochemical hypothyroidism during IL-2 treatment than those who had transient hypothyroidism (68).

As with IFN-α, IL-2 treatment likely activates the autoimmune process. Administration of IL-2 is associated with both the development of thyroid antibodies and increased titers of thyroid antibodies in patients who had antibodies or baseline (55,66). Combination therapy with IFN-α and IL-2 leads to an even greater prevalence of thyroid dysfunction than with either alone (69,70).

Because thyroid dysfunction is so common in patients treated with IFN-α or IL-2, measurements of serum TSH and anti-TPO antibodies before initiation of therapy may be indicated, especially in patients with HCV. One group recommends thyroid antibody and TSH testing before and during IFN-α, and 6 months after its withdrawal (60). Several months after treatment with IFN-α or IL-2 has been completed, T_4 should be withdrawn to determine whether or not hypothyroidism is persistent.

Other Drugs

Several other drugs have been occasionally associated with hypothyroidism, including aminoglutethimide (71), ethionamide (72), and sulfonamides and sulfonylureas (73), by interfering with thyroid hormone biosynthesis. Generally, these drugs result in only mild increases in serum TSH, and overt hypothyroidism is very rare (71). One study reported that 31% of 29 men with prostate cancer treated with aminoglutethamide developed clinical or biochemical findings of hypothyroidism (71). Recently, therapy with thalidomide associated with hypothyroidism, although the mechanism is not known (74).

HYPOTHYROIDISM DUE TO INFILTRATIVE DISORDERS

Riedel's Thyroiditis (Invasive Fibrous Thyroiditis)

This rare disorder has a reported prevalence of 0.06% to 0.3% in surgical series (75–77). It is characterized pathologically by replacement of the thyroid gland with dense fibrous tissue, which often invades adjacent soft tissue and muscle, hence the term *invasive fibrous thyroiditis.* Significant thyroid destruction with resultant hypothyroidism occurs in approximately 30% to 40% of cases (75,78). Hypoparathyroidism has been reported in a few patients in whom the destructive process involved the parathyroid glands (79).

The signs and symptoms of Riedel's thyroiditis include the development of an enlarging, hard neck mass associated with tracheoesophageal compression, findings suggestive of the possibility of poorly differentiated thyroid cancer and thyroid lymphoma (78). Riedel's thyroiditis is often associated with extracervical fibrosis, and within 10 years of the diagnosis approximately 30% of patients develop retroperitoneal or mediastinal fibrosis (77).

The etiology of Riedel's thyroiditis is not known; debate continues as to whether or not it is an autoimmune or a fibrotic disorder (80,81). An autoimmune etiology has been suggested because of the presence of thyroid antibodies, as well as histologic findings of lymphocytes and plasma cells (79).

Riedel's thyroiditis is usually slowly progressive, but it may also regress spontaneously. Treatment is focused on relief of obstruction; surgery may be necessary to relieve tracheal or esophageal compression, but the results may be unsatisfactory (82). Treatment with glucocorticoids has been used successfully (83), and the antiestrogen tamoxifen also has been used with some success (82,84). Although the mechanism for tamoxifen's beneficial effect is not known, it may be related to its stimulatory effect on production of transforming growth factor-β, a potent growth inhibitor (85,86).

Amyloidosis

Amyloid deposition in the thyroid is relatively common, reported to occur in 1.9% of 376 thyroidectomy specimens in one surgical series (87). Thyroid amyloid may occur in the context of either primary or secondary amyloidosis, with the latter being much more common, usually in patients with rheumatoid arthritis, although it occurs in patients with other chronic diseases as well, including tuberculosis, multiple myeloma, and inflammatory bowel disease (88–91). Clinically, asymptomatic diffuse or nodular thyroid enlargement is frequent, having been reported in 63% of 30 patients in one retrospective series (88). Thyroid function was abnormal in 10 of 30 patients with biopsy-proven amyloid deposits, including hypothyroidism in 5, thyrotoxicosis in 1, and painless thyroiditis in 1 patient (88). However, other reports suggest that thyroid dysfunction is rare in patients with amyloidosis (89,92).

Sarcoidosis

Approximately 4% of patients with sarcoidosis have histologic changes of sarcoid in the thyroid (93). Hypothyroidism is the fact that thyroid autoantibodies are relatively common. In one report, 17 of 62 patients with pulmonary sarcoidosis had positive thyroid autoantibodies (94), with a higher prevalence of antibodies in men (54.5%) than in women (32.4%) over 40 years of age, in contrast to the usually greater prevalence of antibodies in women. Only one of the 17 patients had hypothyroidism, however (94).

Hemochromatosis

Hemochromatosis may be associated with either secondary or primary hypothyroidism. Primary hypothyroidism in patients with hereditary hemochromatosis is associated with iron deposition in the thyroid gland, as well as in other tissues. The thyroid gland shows histologic evidence of fibrosis and lymphocytic infiltration (95,96). In one report, primary hypothyroidism was present in 3 of 17 adolescents who required multiple blood transfusions because of thalassemia major (97). These patients also are susceptible to hypothyroidism when given excess quantities of iodide (98). A study of 34 men with hemochromatosis revealed hypothyroidism in 3 patients, all of whom had high serum titers of anti-TPO antibodies, and histologic examination of one patient's thyroid revealed lymphocytic infiltration as well as iron deposition. The risk for hypothyroidism in men with hereditary hemochromatosis is about 80 times that of men in the general population (95).

Cystinosis

Nephropathic cystinosis is a rare autosomal-dominant cystine storage disease resulting from deficiency of the normal carrier-mediated system that transports cystine out of lysosomes (99,100). As a result, there is an accumulation of cystine in various tissues, especially the kidneys, resulting in severe renal damage (99). The thyroid glands in these patients also commonly contain cystine deposits, and in one review of eight children with cystinosis, six had elevations in serum TSH (100). Among 36 adult patients who had undergone renal transplantation due to cystinosis revealed that 31 had hypothyroidism (96). The availability of renal transplantation fortunately allows for survival into adulthood of patients with cystinosis, and most of them develop hypothyroidism.

Other Infiltrative or Infectious Disorders

Hypothyroidism may occur as a result of opportunistic infections. Hypothyroidism due to *Pneumocystis carinii* involvement of the thyroid has been reported in several patients with acquired immunodeficiency syndrome (AIDS) (101–103). We reported three patients with *Pneumocystis carinii* thyroiditis, two of whom developed persistent hypothyroidism (103). Destruction of the thyroid gland by Kaposi's sarcoma, with resultant hypothyroidism, also has been reported in a patient with AIDS (104).

Primary thyroid lymphoma is associated with hypothyroidism. In one study 119 patients with primary thyroid lymphoma, overt hypothyroidism was present in 27% and subclinical hypothyroidism in 14% (105). Thyroid lymphoma occurs almost exclusively in patients with underlying chronic autoimmune (Hashimoto's) thyroiditis, which probably explains the high prevalence of hypothyroidism; thyroid antibodies are present in the serum in the majority of patients who have thyroid lymphoma (105–107).

HYPOTHYROIDISM DUE TO TOXINS

Cigarette Smoking

Cigarette smoking increases the risk of hypothyroidism in patients who have underlying Hashimoto's thyroiditis. In a study from Japan of 380 women with Hashimoto's thyroiditis, 76% of 110 women who were smokers had hypothyroidism, in contrast to 35% of 256 nonsmokers (108). Also, 62% of 21 ex-smokers with Hashimoto's had hypothyroidism, suggesting that cessation of smoking does not result in restoration of normal thyroid function. In a study from Switzerland, 23% of 135 women with hypothyroidism were smokers. Those with subclinical hypothyroidism who smoked had higher serum TSH concentrations than nonsmokers, higher ratios of serum T_3 to serum T_4, and higher total and low-density lipoprotein cholesterol levels. Smoking had no effect on serum TSH, T_4, or T_3 levels in patients with overt hypothyroidism (109). A recent Danish study, on the other hand, found that mean serum TSH levels were lower among smokers than nonsmokers, although there was no association between smoking and either thyrotoxicosis or hypothyroidism (110). Another study from Denmark, however, did show a relationship between smoking and autoimmune thyrotoxicosis (111). A recent meta-analysis described an association between cigarette smoking and Graves' thyrotoxicosis and ophthalmopathy, Hashimoto's disease, and postpartum thyroiditis, but not hypothyroidism (112).

The mechanism for the effects of smoking on the thyroid is not entirely clear, but it may be related to higher concentrations of thiocyanate (113,114), which decreases iodide transport into the thyroid (115,116). In addition, other elements of tobacco smoke, including hydroxypyridine metabolites and benzopyrenes, may interfere with thyroid function (117,118). High concentrations of nicotine in rats do not affect thyroid function, the metabolism of thyroid hormones, or thyroid hormone action (119).

Industrial and Environmental Agents

Numerous synthetic and natural chemicals have been reported to cause goiter or hypothyroidism, including various pesticides, herbicides, industrial chemicals, and naturally occurring environmental chemicals. This topic has been discussed in comprehensive reviews (120,121).

The clinical importance of industrial agents on thyroid function is not clear, although there appears to be an increased incidence of autoimmune hypothyroidism in people exposed to polybrominated biphenyls (122). Resorcinol, which occurs in relatively high concentrations in watershed areas of coal-rich regions, has been associated with a higher prevalence of goiter (123).

Among naturally occurring substances, cassava has an antithyroid affect, probably by releasing thiocyanate, and is associated with a higher prevalence of goiter in areas of iodine deficiency (124). Pearlmilate, a fruit staple in iodine-deficient areas of sub-Saharan Africa, is rich in flavonites, which have an antithyroid effect (125). It is not clear whether hypothyroidism results from ingesting cassava and pearlmilate, although such substances enhance goitrogenesis in iodine-deficient areas (124).

EMBRYOLOGIC VARIANTS

Lingual Thyroid

Thyroid tissue restricted to the lingual region is rare, occurring in 1 in 100,000 persons, with a female predominance of 3:1 to 7:1 (126–129). Approximately one third of the patients have hypothyroidism at the time of the diagnosis, and in more than two thirds there is no other thyroid tissue (129).

Lingual thyroid is characterized by the presence of thyroid tissue at the base of the tongue in the midline and results from failure of the normal migration of thyroid tissue from its origin at the base of the tongue to the normal pretracheal location.

Symptoms of lingual thyroid, in addition to those associated with hypothyroidism, include the sensation of a foreign body in the posterior pharynx. If the mass is sufficiently large, signs and symptoms of obstruction of the throat especially when recumbent, may occur (130).

The diagnosis of lingual thyroid is usually made clinically, and radionuclide scanning may be used to confirm the diagnosis. Small asymptomatic lingual thyroid masses may be treated with T_4 to decrease their size or prevent further growth. In patients with symptomatic lesions, surgery is preferred, although radioactive iodine also has been used (131–133).

REFERENCES

1. Bagchi N, Brown TR, Parish RF. Thyroid dysfunction in adults over age 55 years: a study in an urban U.S. community. *Arch Intern Med* 1990:150:785.
2. Bacharach P. The aging thyroid. Thyroid deficiency in the Framingham Study. *Arch Intern Med* 1985;145:1386.
3. Canaris GJ, Manowitz NR, Mayor G, et al. The Colorado thyroid disease prevalence study. *Arch Intern Med* 2000;160:526.
4. Franklyn JA: The management of hyperthyroidism. *N Engl J Med* 1994;330:1731.
5. Wartofsky L, Glinoer D, Solomon B, et al. Differences and similarities in the diagnosis and treatment of Graves' disease in Europe, Japan, and the United States. *Thyroid* 1991;1:129.
6. Tominaga T, Yokoyama N, Nagataki S, et al. International difference in approaches to ^{131}I therapy for Graves' disease: case selection and restrictions recommended in patients in Japan, Korea, and China. *Thyroid* 1997;7:217.
7. Romaldini JH. Case selection and restrictions recommended to patients with hyperthyroidism in South America. *Thyroid* 1997;7:225.
8. Singer PA, Cooper DS, Levy EG, et al. Treatment guidelines for patients with hyperthyroidism and hypothyroidism. *JAMA* 1995;273:808.
9. Sridama V, McCormick M, Kaplan EL, et al. Long term follow up study of compensated low dose ^{131}I therapy for Graves' disease. *N Engl J Med* 1984;311:426.
10. Goolden AW, Stewart JS. Long term results from graded low dose radioactive iodine therapy for thyrotoxicosis. *Clin Endocrinol (Oxf)* 1986;24:217.
11. Patwardhan NA, Moront M, Rao S, et al. Surgery still has a role in Grave's hyperthyroidism. *Surgery* 1993;114:1108.
12. Sugino K, Mimura T, Toshima K, et al. Follow up evaluation of patients with Graves' disease treated by subtotal thyroidectomy and risk factor for post operative thyroid dysfunction. *J Endocrinol Invest* 1993;16:1995.
13. Menegaux F, Ruprecht T, Chigot JP. The surgical treatment of Graves' disease. *Surg Gynecol Obstet* 1993;176:277.
14. Miccoli P, Vitti P, Rago T, et al. Surgical treatment of Graves' disease: subtotal or total thyroidectomy? *Surgery* 1996;120:1020.
15. Huysmans DA, Corstens FH, Kloppenborg PW. Long term follow up in toxic solitary autonomous thyroid nodules treated with radioactive iodine. *J Nucl Med* 1991;32:27.
16. Goldstein R, Hart JR. Follow up of solitary autonomous thyroid nodules treated with [131]I. *N Engl J Med* 1983;309:1473.
17. Miller JM. Radioiodine therapy of the autoimmune functioning thyroid. *Semin Nucl Med* 1971;1:432.
18. Ziliotto D, Scandellari C, Conte N. Radioiodine therapy of toxic adenoma of the thyroid. *Acta Isotop (Padova)* 1964;4:223.

19. Ross DS, Ridgway EC, Daniels GH. Successful treatment of solitary toxic thyroid nodules with relatively low dose iodine 131 with low prevalence of hypothyroidism. *Ann Intern Med* 1984;101:488.

20. Berghout A, Wiersinga WM, Drexhage HA. The long-term outcome of thyroidectomy for sporadic non-toxic goitre. *Clin Endocrinol* 1989;31:193.

21. Berglund J, Bondesson L, Christensen SB, et al. Indication for thyroxine therapy after surgery for nontoxic benign goitre. *Acta Chir Scand* 1990;156:433.

22. Röjdmark J, Jarhult J. High long term recurrence rate after subtotal thyroidectomy for nodular goitre. *Eur J Surg* 1995;161;725.

23. Huysmans D, Hermus A, Edelbrock M, et al. Radioiodine for nontoxic multinodular goiter. *Thyroid* 1997;7:235.

24. Huysmans DA, Hermus AR, Corstens FH, et al. Large, compressive goiters treated with radioiodine. *Ann Intern Med* 1994;121:757.

25. Wesche MF, Tiel-V-Buul MM, Smits NJ, et al. Reduction in goiter size by ^{131}I therapy in patients with non-toxic multinodular goiter. *Eur J Endocrinol* 1995;132.

26. Nygaard B, Faber J, Hegedus L, et al. [131]I treatment of nodular non-toxic goiter. *Eur J Endocrinol* 1996;134:15.

27. Wesche MF, Tiel-V-Buul MM, Lips P, et al. A randomized trial comparing levothyroxine with radioactive iodine in the treatment of sporadic nontoxic goiter. *J Clin Endocrinol Metab* 2001;86:998.

28. Nieuwlaat WA, Huysmans DA, van den Bosch HC, et al. Pretreatment with a single low dose of recombinant human thyrotropin allows dose reduction of radioiodine therapy in patients with nodular goiter. *J Clin Endocrinol Metab* 2003;88: 3121–3129.

29. Clark OH, Cavalieri RR, Moser C, et al. Iodide-induced hypothyroidism in patients after thyroid resection. *Eur J Clin Invest* 1990;20:573.

30. Glatstein E, McHardy-Young S, Brast N, et al. Alterations in serum thyrotropin (TSH) and thyroid function following radiotherapy in patients with malignant lymphoma. *J Clin Endocrinol Metab* 1971;32:833.

31. Hancock SL, Cox RS, McDougall IR. Thyroid disease after treatment of Hodgkin's disease. *N Engl J Med* 1991;325:559.

32. Constine LS, Donaldson SS, McDougall IR. Thyroid dysfunction after radiotherapy in children with Hodgkin's disease. *Cancer* 1984;53:878.

33. Pacini F, Verontsova T, Molinaro E, et al. Prevalence of thyroid autoantibodies in children and adolescents from Belarus exposed in the Chernobyl radioactive fallout. *Lancet* 1998;352:763.

34. Liening DA, Duncan NO, Blakeslee DB, et al. Hypothyroidism following radiotherapy for head and neck cancer. *Otolaryngol Head Neck Surg* 1990;103:10.

35. Locatelli F, Giorgiani G, Pession A, et al. Late effects in children after bone marrow transplantation: a review. *Haematologica* 1993;78:319.

36. Chin D, Sklar C, Donahue B, et al. Thyroid dysfunction as a late effect in survivors of pediatric medulloblastoma primitive neuroectodermal tumors: a comparison of hyperfractionated versus conventional radiotherapy. *Cancer* 1997;80:798.

37. Al-Fiar FZ, Colwill R, Lipton JH, et al. Abnormal thyroid stimulating hormone (TSH) levels in adults following allogeneic bone marrow transplants. *Bone Marrow Transplant* 1997;19:1019.

38. Maarcial-Vega VA, Order SE, Lasmer G, et al. Prevention of hypothyroidism related to mantle irradiation for Hodgkin's disease: preparative phantom study. *Int J Radiat Oncol Biol Phys* 1990;18:613.

39. Pasqualini T, Ioncansky S, Gruneiro L, et al. Thyroid dysfunction in Hodgkin's disease. *Cancer* 1989;63:335.

40. Devney RB, Sklar CA, Nesbit ME, et al. Serial thyroid function measurements in children with Hodgkin's disease. *J Pediatr* 1984;105:223.

41. Lazarus JH. The effects of lithium therapy on thyroid and thyrotropin releasing hormone. *Thyroid* 1998;8:909:913.

42. Perrild H, Hegedus L, Baastrup PC, et al. Thyroid function and ultrasonically determined thyroid size in patients receiving long-term lithium treatment. *Am J Psychiatry* 1990;147:1518.

43. Bocchetta A, Bernardi F, Burrai C, et al. Thyroid abnormalities during lithium treatment. *Acta Psychiatr Scand* 1991;83: 193.

44. Lee S, Chow CC, Wing YK, et al. Thyroid abnormalities during chronic lithium treatment in Hong Kong Chinese: a controlled study. *J Affect Disord* 1992;26:173.

45. Lazarus JH. The effect of lithium on the thyroid gland. In: Weetman AP, Grossman A, eds. *Pharmacotherapy of the thyroid gland: handbook of experimental pharmacology.* Vol. 128. Berlin: Springer-Verlag, 1998:207.

46. Bagchi N, Brown JR, Mack RE. Studies on the mechanism of inhibition of thyroid function by lithium. *Biochim Biophys Acta* 1978;542:163.

47. Berens SC, Berstein RS, Robbins J, et al. Antithyroid effects of lithium. *J Clin Invest* 1970;49:1357.

48. Bocchetta A, Bernardi F, Burrai C, et al. The course of thyroid abnormalities during lithium treatment: a two year follow up study. *Acta Psychiatr Scand* 1992;86:38.

49. Schou M. Lithium prophylaxis: myths and realities. *Am J Psychiatry* 1989;146:573.

50. Lindstedt G, Nilsson LA, Walinder J, et al. On the prevalence, diagnosis and management of lithium induced hypothyroidism in psychiatric patients. *Br J Psychiatry* 1977;130:452.

51. Shopsin B, Shenkman I, Blum M, et al. Iodine and lithium induced hypothyroidism. *Am J Med* 1973;55:697.

52. Miller KK, Daniels GH. Association between lithium use and thyrotoxicosis caused by silent thyroiditis. *Clin Endocrinol (Oxf)* 2001;55:501–508.

53. Mizukami Y, Michigishi T, Nonomura A, et al. Histological features of the thyroid gland in a patient with lithium-induced thyrotoxicosis. *J Clin Pathol* 1995;48:582–584.

54. Koh LKH, Greenspan FS, Yoo PP. Interferon-α induced thyroid dysfunction: three clinical presentations and a review of the literature. *Thyroid* 1997;7:891.

55. Sauter NP, Atkins MB, Mier JW, et al. Transient thyrotoxicosis and persistent hypothyroidism due to acute autoimmune thyroiditis after interleukin-2 and interferon-α therapy for metastatic carcinoma: a case report. *Am J Med* 1992;92:441.

56. Fentiman IS, Thomas BS, Bulkwill FR, et al. Primary hypothyroidism associated with interferon therapy of breast cancer. *Lancet* 1985;1:1166.

57. Preziati D, La Rosa L, Covini G, et al. Autoimmunity and thyroid function in patients with chronic active hepatitis treated with recombinant interferon alpha 2a. *Eur J Endocrinol* 1995; 132:587.

58. Roti E, Minelli R, Giubert T, et al. Multiple changes in thyroid function in patients with chronic active HCV hepatitis treated with recombinant interferon-alpha. *Am J Med* 1996;101:482.

59. Deutsch M, Dourakis S, Manesis EK, et al. Thyroid abnormalities in chronic viral hepatitis and their relationship to interferon-alpha therapy. *Hepatology* 1997;26:206.

60. Fernandez-Soto L, Gonzalez A, Escobar-Jimenes F, et al. Increased risk of autoimmune thyroid disease in hepatitis C vs hepatitis B before, during, and after discontinuing interferon therapy. *Arch Intern Med* 1998;158:1445.

61. Carell C, Mazziotti G, Morisco F, et al. The addition of rib-avirin to interferon-alpha therapy in patients with hepatitis C virus related chronic hepatitis does not modify the thyroid autoantibody pattern but increases the risk of developing hypothyroidism. *Eur J Endocrinol* 2002;146:743–749.

62. Dalgard O, Bjoro K, Hellum K, et al. Thyroid dysfunction during treatment of chronic hepatitis C with interferon alpha: no association with either interferon dosage or efficacy of therapy. *J Intern Med* 2002;251:400–406.

63. Marazuela M, Garcia-Buey L, Gonzalez-Fernandez B, et al. Thyroid autoimmune disorders in patients with chronic hepatitis C before and during interferon-α therapy. *Clin Endocrinol (Oxf)* 1996;44:635.

64. Carella C, Mazziotti G, Morisco F, et al. Long term outcome of interferon alpha induced thyroid autoimmunity and prognostic influence of thyroid autoantibody pattern at the end of treatment. *J Clin Endocrinol Metab* 2001;86:1925–1929.

65. Schwartzentruber DJ, White DE, Zweig MH, et al. Thyroid dysfunction associated with immunotherapy for patients with cancer. *Cancer* 1991;115:178.

66. Fentiman IS, Balkwill FR, Thomas BS, et al. An autoimmune etiology for hypothyroidism following interferon therapy for breast cancer. *Eur J Cancer Clin Oncol* 1988;24:1299.

67. Pichert G, Jost LM, Zobeli L, et al. Thyroiditis after treatment with interleukin-2 and interferon α-2. *Br J Cancer* 1991;62:100.

68. Vialettes B, Guillerand MA, Viens P, et al. Incidence rate and risk factors for thyroid dysfunction during recombinant interleukin-2 therapy in advanced malignancies. *Acta Endocrinol (Copenh)* 1993;129:31.

69. Rosenberg SA, Lotze MT, Yang JC, et al. Experience with the use of high dose interleukin-2 in the treatment of 653 cancer patients. *Ann Surg* 1989;210:474.

70. Reid I, Sharpe I, McDevitt J, et al. Thyroid dysfunction can predict response to immunotherapy with interleukin-2 and interferon-α-2. *Br J Cancer* 1991;64:915.

71. Figg WD, Thibault A, Sartor AO, et al. Hypothyroidism associated with aminoglutethimide in patients with prostate cancer. *Arch Intern Med* 1994;154:1023.

72. Drucker D, Eggo MC, Salit IE, et al. Ethionamide induced goitrous hypothyroidism. *Ann Intern Med* 1984;100:837.

73. Gupta A, Eggo MC, Uetrecht JP, et al. Drug induced hypothyroidism: the thyroid as a target organ in hypersensitivity reactions to anticonvulsants and sulfonamides. *Clin Pharmacol Ther* 1992;51:56.

74. Badros AZ, Siegal E, Bodenner D, et al. Hypothyroidism in patients with multiple myeloma following treatment with thalidomide. *Ann Intern Med* 2002;112:412.

75. Woolner LB, et al. Invasive fibrous thyroiditis (Riedel's struma). *J Clin Endocrinol Metab* 1957;17:201.

76. Joll CA. The pathology, diagnosis and treatment of Hashimoto's disease (struma lymphomatosa). *Br J Surg* 1939;27:351.

77. Hay ID. Thyroiditis: a clinical uptake. *Mayo Clin Proc* 1985;60:836.

78. DeLange WE, Freling NJ, Molenaar WM, et al. Invasive fibrous thyroiditis (Riedel's struma): a manifestation of multifocal fibrosclerosis? A case report with review of the literature. *QJM* 1989;72:709.

79. Best TB, Munro RE, Burwell S, et al. Riedel's thyroiditis associated with Hashimoto's thyroiditis, hypoparathyroidism, and retroperitoneal fibrosis. *J Endocrinol Invest* 1991;14:767.

80. Zimmermann-Belsing T, Feldt-Rasmussen U. Riedel's thyroiditis: an autoimmune or primary fibrous disease? *J Intern Med* 1994;235:271.

81. Heufelder AE, Hay ID. Further evidence for autoimmune mechanisms in the pathogenesis of Riedel's invasive fibrous thyroiditis. *J Intern Med* 1995;238:85.

82. Few J, Thompson NW, Angelos P, et al. Reidel's thyroiditis: treatment with tamoxifen. *Surgery* 1996;120:993.

83. Bagnasco M, Passalacqua G, Pronzato C, et al. Fibrous invasive (Riedel's) thyroiditis with critical response to steroid treatment. *J Endocrinol Invest* 1995;18:305.

84. Clark CP, Vanderpool D, Preskin JT. The response of retroperitoneal fibrosis to tamoxifen. *Surgery* 1991;109:502.

85. Arteaga CL, Tandon AK, Von Hoff DD, et al. Transforming growth factor beta: potential autocrine growth inhibitor of estrogen receptor-negative human breast cancer cells. *Cancer Res* 1988;48:3898.

86. Butta A, MacLennan K, Flanders KC, et al. Induction of transforming growth factor beta 1 in human breast cancer *in vivo* following tamoxifen treatment. *Cancer Res* 1992;52:4261.

87. Sinha SN, Sengupta SK. Surgical thyroid disease in Papua New Guinea. *Aust N Z J Surg* 1993;63:878.

88. Kimura H, Yamashita S, Ashizawa K, et al. Thyroid dysfunction in patients with amyloid goitre. *Clin Endocrinol (Oxf)* 1997;46:769.

89. James PD. Amyloid goiter. *J Clin Pathol* 1972;25:683.

90. Hirotu S, Miyamoto M, Kasugai T, et al. Crystalline light-chain deposition and amyloidosis in the thyroid gland and kidneys of a patient with myeloma. *Arch Pathol Lab Med* 1990;14:429.

91. Greenstein AJ, Sachar DB, Panday AK, et al. Amyloidosis and inflammatory bowel disease: a 50 year experience with 25 patients. *Medicine* 1992;75:261.

92. Kneebone RL, Greeff H, Mannell A. Amyloid goiter: a case report. *S Afr Med J* 1984;65:931.

93. Harach HR, Williams ED. The pathology of granulomatous diseases of the thyroid gland. *Sarcoidosis* 1990;7:19.

94. Nakamura H, Genma R, Mikami T, et al. High incidence of positive autoantibodies against thyroid peroxidase and thyroglobulin in patients with sarcoidosis. *Clin Endocrinol (Oxf)* 1997;48:467.

95. Edwards CQ, Kelly TM, Ellwein G, et al. Thyroid disease in hemochromatosis. *Arch Intern Med* 1983;143:1890.

96. Moerman P, Pauwels P, Vandenberghe K, et al. Neonatal haemochromatosis. *Histopathology* 1990;17:345.

97. Oerter KE, Kamp GA, Munson PJ, et al. Multiple hormone deficiencies in children with hemochromatosis. *J Clin Endocrinol Metab* 1993;75:357.

98. Alexandrides T, Georgopoulos N, Yermenitis S, et al. Increased sensitivity to the inhibitory effect of excess iodide on thyroid function in patients with beta-thalassemia major and iron overload and the subsequent development of hypothyroidism. *Eur J Endocrinol* 2000;143:319.

99. Theodoropoulos DS, Krasnewich D, Kaiser-Kupfer MI, et al. Classic nephropathic cystinosis as an adult disease. *JAMA* 1993;270:2200.

100. Burke JR, El-Bishti MM, Maisey MN, et al. Hypothyroidism in children with cystinosis. *Arch Dis Child* 1978;53:947.

101. Guttler R, Singer PA, Axline SG, et al. *Pneumocystis carinii* thyroiditis. *Arch Intern Med* 1993;153:393.

102. Ragni MV, Dekker A, DeRubertis FR, et al. *Pneumocystis carinii* infection presenting as necrotizing thyroiditis and hypothyroidism. *Am J Clin Pathol* 1991;95:489.

103. Spitzer RD, Chan JC, Marks JB, et al. Case report: hypothyroidism due to *Pneumocystis carinii* thyroiditis in a patient with acquired immunodeficiency syndrome. *Am J Med Sci* 1991;302:98.

104. Mollison LC, Mijch A, McBride G, et al. Hypothyroidism due to destruction of the thyroid by Kaposi's sarcoma. *Rev Infect Dis* 1991;13:826.

105. Matsuzuka F, Miyauchi A, Katayama S, et al. Clinical aspects of primary thyroid lymphoma: diagnosis and treatment based on our experience of 119 patients. *Thyroid* 1993;3:93.

106. Limanova Z, Neuwirtova R, Smejkal V. Malignant lymphoma of the thyroid. *Exp Clin Endocrinol* 1987;90:113.

107. Ansocombe AM, Wright DH. Primary, malignant lymphoma of the thyroid—a tumor of mucosa associated lymphoid tissue: review of seventy six cases. *Histopathology* 1985;9:81.

108. Fukata S, Kuma K, Sugawara M. Relationship between cigarette smoking and hypothyroidism in patients with Hashimoto's thyroiditis. *J Endocrinol Invest* 1996;19:607.

109. Muller B, Zulewski H, Huber P, et al. Impaired action of thyroid hormones associated with smoking in women with hypothyroidism. *N Engl J Med* 1995;333:964.

110. Knudsen N, Bulow I, Laurberg P, et al. High occurrence of thyroid multinodularity and low occurrence of subclinical hypothyroidism among tobacco smokers in a large population study. *J Endocrinol* 2002;175:571–6.

111. Vestergaard P, Rejnmark L, Weeke J, et al. Smoking as a risk factor for Graves' disease, toxic nodular goiter, and autoimmune thyroiditis. *Thyroid* 2002;12:69–75.

112. Vestergaard P. Smoking and thyroid disorders—a meta-analysis. *Eur J Endocrinol* 2002;146:153–161.

113. Bertelsen JB, Hegedus H. Cigarette smoking and the thyroid. *Thyroid* 1994;4:327.

114. Cooper DS. Tobacco and Graves' disease: smoking gun or smoke and mirrors? *JAMA* 1993;269:518.

115. Fukuyama H, Nasu M, Murakami S, et al. Examination of antithyroid effects of smoking products in cultured thyroid follicles only thiocyanate is a potent antithyroid agent. *Acta Endocrinol (Copenh)* 1992;127:520.

116. Sepkovic DW, Haley NJ, Wynder El. Thyroid activity and cigarette smokers. *Arch Intern Med* 1984;144:501.

117. Ericsson UB, Lindgarde F. Effects of cigarette smoking on thyroid function and the prevalence of goitre, thyrotoxicosis and autoimmune thyroiditis. *J Intern Med* 1991;229:67.

118. Sugawara M, Park DL, Hersman JM. Antithyroid effect of 2,3-dihydroxypyridine *in vivo* and *in vitro*. *Proc Soc Exp Biol Med* 1982;170:431.

119. Colzani R, Fang SL, Alex S, et al. The effect of nicotine on thyroid function in rats. *Metabolism* 1998;47:154.

120. Engel A, Lamm SH, Gaitan E. Goitrogens in the environment. In: Braverman LE, ed. *Contemporary endocrinology: diseases of the thyroid.* Totowa, NJ: Humana, 2003.

121. Brucker-Davis F. Effects of environmental synthetic chemicals on thyroid function. *Thyroid* 1998;8:827.

122. Bahn AK, Mills JL, Snyder PJ, et al. Hypothyroidism in workers exposed to polybrominated biphenyls. *N Engl J Med* 1980; 302:31.

123. Jolley RL, et al. Identification of organic pollutants in drinking waters from areas with endemic thyroid disorders and potential pollutants of drinking water sources associated with coal processing areas. *Am Chem Soc Environ Chem* 1986; 26:59.

124. Delange F. Cassava and the thyroid. In: Gaitan E, ed. *Environmental goitrogenesis.* Boca Raton, FL: CRC Press, 1989:173.

125. Gaitan E, Lindsay RH, Reichert RD, et al. Antithyroid and goitrogenic effects of millet: role of C-glycosylflavones. *J Clin Endocrinol Metab* 1989;68:707.

126. Noyek AM, Friedberg J. Thyroglossal duct and ectopic thyroid disorders. *Otolaryngol Clin North Am* 1981;14:187.

127. Pollice L, Caruso G. Struma cordis: ectopic thyroid goitre in the right ventricle. *Arch Pathol Lab Med* 1986;110:452.

128. Kamat M, Kulkarni JN, Desai PB, et al. Lingual thyroid: a review of 12 cases. *Br J Surg* 1979;66:537.

129. Neinas FW, Gorman CA, Devine KD, et al. Lingual thyroid: clinical characteristics of 15 cases. *Ann Intern Med* 1973;79: 205.

130. Arancibia P, Veliz J, Barria M, et al. Lingual thyroid: report of three cases. *Thyroid* 1998;8:1055.

131. Farrell ML, Forer M. Lingual thyroid. *Aust N Z J Surg* 1994; 64:135.

132. Kansal P, Sakati N, Rifai A, et al. Lingual thyroid: diagnosis and treatment. *Arch Intern Med* 1987;147:2046.

133. Williams JD, Sclafani AP, Slupchinski O, et al. Evaluation and management of the lingual thyroid gland. *Ann Otol Rhinol Laryngol* 1996;105:312.

CENTRAL HYPOTHYROIDISM

ENIO MARTINO
ALDO PINCHERA

Central hypothyroidism is defined as reduced thyroid hormone secretion resulting from deficient stimulation of an intrinsically normal thyroid gland by thyroid-stimulating hormone (thyrotropin, TSH). This condition can be the consequence of an anatomic or functional disorder of the pituitary gland, the hypothalamus, or both. Because the final result in both cases is deficient TSH secretion, the formerly used terms, "secondary hypothyroidism of pituitary origin, and tertiary hypothyroidism of hypothalamic origin," resulting from absent or insufficient TSH stimulation by thyrotropin-releasing hormone (TRH), are no longer recommended. In addition, the pituitary and hypothalamic forms of central hypothyroidism cannot be distinguished easily on the basis of the serum TSH response to exogenous TRH administration, as suggested in the past. It had been thought that an increase in serum TSH after TRH administration indicated hypothalamic hypothyroidism, and the lack of a serum TSH response indicated pituitary hypothyroidism. It is now established that considerable overlap exists between the profile of serum TSH responses to TRH in the two conditions. Finally, TSH secretion can be impaired not only quantitatively but also qualitatively as a result of secretion of TSH that is biologically inactive (1,2). For these reasons, the term "central hypothyroidism" is now preferred because it includes both quantitative and qualitative abnormalities of TSH secretion, irrespective of the hypothalamic or pituitary origin of the disorder.

Central hypothyroidism is rarely an isolated defect, most often being part of a more complex deficit in pituitary hormone secretion, hypopituitarism, which can also affect gonadotropin, corticotropic hormone (ACTH), and growth hormone (GH) secretion. The hypothyroidism may be mild and overshadowed by the clinical features of other pituitary hormone defects, or it may be so severe as to dominate the clinical picture. Isolated TSH deficiency can occur as an autosomal-recessive trait resulting from a TSH-β subunit gene abnormality (3–7).

The prevalence of central hypothyroidism is unknown, but it is much rarer than primary hypothyroidism. The latter is found in about 1% to 2% of the general population. Based on the prevalence of pituitary tumors, central hypothyroidism has been estimated to occur in 0.0002% of the general population, but the true prevalence is probably higher considering that pituitary tumors are not the only cause of this disorder. In our experience, the frequency of central hypothyroidism in the general population is about 0.005%. Central hypothyroidism is distributed equally between the sexes, with an age peak in childhood for the idiopathic and genetic forms and a peak between 30 and 60 years of age for cases caused by lesions of the pituitary and hypothalamus.

Although central hypothyroidism is rare, from a clinical standpoint it is important to recognize it because it is often associated with defects of other pituitary hormones, and correction of hypothyroidism by thyroxine (T_4) alone can precipitate acute adrenocortical insufficiency.

ETIOLOGY

Table 51.1 shows the different causes of central hypothyroidism, subdivided according to the main location of the lesion. Because several of these conditions can affect both the hypothalamus and the pituitary either simultaneously or sequentially, it is often impossible to locate the precise anatomic site of the deficiency. For example, in the presence of a large pituitary tumor, hypothyroidism may be caused by an intrinsic deficiency of the pituitary thyrotrophs or interruption of hypothalamic TRH input.

Pituitary adenoma is the most frequent cause of central hypothyroidism, accounting for more than half the cases (8). The tumor may be nonfunctioning or it may secrete GH, prolactin (PRL), or both, or, less frequently, ACTH or gonadotropins. Varying degrees of hypopituitarism may result from compression of the nontumorous portion of the pituitary. The pituitary stalk and the hypothalamus also may be involved by suprasellar extension of the tumor. Interference with the adenohypophyseal blood flow is an additional factor. Rarely, hypopituitarism may result from hemorrhage within a pituitary adenoma (pituitary apoplexy) (8).

Primary extrasellar brain tumors can cause central hypothyroidism (8–10). Metastases to the hypothalamic–pituitary region arising from carcinomas of the breast, lung, and

TABLE 51.1. CAUSES OF CENTRAL HYPOTHYROIDISM

Pituitary disorders
  Tumors
    Pituitary adenoma (functioning and nonfunctioning)
    Craniopharyngioma
    Meningioma
    Dysgerminoma
    Metastatic tumor
  Ischemic necrosis
    Postpartum (Sheehan's syndrome)
    Severe shock
    Diabetes mellitus
  Trauma
  Aneurysm of internal carotid artery
  Iatrogenic
    Radiation therapy
    Surgery
  Infectious diseases
    Abscesses
    Tuberculosis
    Syphilis
    Toxoplasmosis
    Trypanosomiasis
  Sarcoidosis
  Histiocytosis (Hand-Schüller-Christian disease)
  Hemosiderosis
  Chronic lymphocytic hypophysitis
  Pituitary aplasia or hypoplasia
  Idiopathic
Hypothalamic disorders
  Tumors
  Suprasellar extension of pituitary adenoma
  Craniopharyngioma
  Meningioma
  Glioma and other brain tumors
  Metastatic tumor
  Trauma
  Ischemic necrosis
  Iatrogenic
    Radiation therapy
    Surgery
  Infections
    Abscesses
    Tuberculosis
    Syphilis
    Toxoplasmosis
  Sarcoidosis
  Histiocytosis
  Congenital malformations
    Basal encephalocele
    Septo-optic dysplasia
  Idiopathic

occasionally other sites are infrequent and usually reflect the presence of advanced disease. Hypopituitarism is rare because of the limited survival of these patients and, when present, usually is preceded or accompanied by diabetes insipidus. Craniopharyngioma is a relatively frequent cause of central hypothyroidism, especially in younger patients.

Meningiomas, gliomas, and nontumorous mass lesions are rare causes of central hypothyroidism.

Postpartum pituitary necrosis (Sheehan's syndrome) is now rare in developed countries as a result of improved health care, but it remains a relatively common cause of adult panhypopituitarism (8,11,12). Pituitary insufficiency does not occur unless most of the anterior pituitary is affected. In Sheehan's syndrome, increased serum TSH levels in the afternoon and a loss of the nocturnal TSH surge have been described (13).

Although less frequent, pituitary necrosis also may occur in patients with severe shock resulting from nonobstetric conditions, such as diabetes mellitus, traumatic head injury, and in association with cerebrovascular accidents, increased intracranial pressure, or epidemic hemorrhagic fever (8), and in patients who are being maintained on mechanical respirators (14). Other rare disorders that lead to central hypothyroidism include vasculitis, aneurysms of the internal carotid artery, and rupture of an aneurysm of the circle of Willis. Hypothalamic rather than pituitary lesions can also be the cause of central hypothyroidism in patients who have had severe head injury. Indeed, the first case of documented hypothalamic hypothyroidism was ascribed to a lesion in the hypothalamus resulting from head trauma (15). In addition, central hypothyroidism, often associated with various defects of pituitary function, may be due to closed head injury (16).

External radiotherapy for tumors of the head and neck can affect the hypothalamus, the pituitary, and the thyroid, and hypothyroidism often results from damage of one or more of these structures. Hypothyroidism resulting from pituitary or hypothalamic dysfunction was observed in 20% to 53% of patients irradiated for nasopharyngeal or paranasal sinus tumors (17) and in 65% of patients, both children and adults, irradiated for brain tumors (18). On the contrary, other researchers (19,20) reported a 6% incidence of central hypothyroidism in two series of patients irradiated for childhood brain tumor, after a mean follow-up of 12 years. TSH deficiency also can result from direct irradiation of the pituitary, either by conventional external radiotherapy or by computed tomography (CT)–particle radiotherapy for GH-secreting adenomas or other pituitary tumors (8). Overall, the risk of the development of central hypothyroidism is related to the total radiation dose, being higher for intracranial solid tumors, which are treated with higher radiation doses (21–23).

If not present initially, central hypothyroidism may result from surgical therapy of pituitary tumors. Radical excision of large pituitary tumors induces hypothyroidism in about 10% of patients, but selective removal of microadenomas rarely is followed by impaired TSH secretion.

Purulent hypophysitis may occur in patients with septicemia or by direct extension of infection from neighboring areas (24). Abscesses also may develop in pituitary tumors or craniopharyngiomas (8). Granulomatous lesions of diverse etiology, including tuberculosis, syphilis, and giant cell granuloma, are rare causes of pituitary insufficiency (8). Pituitary sarcoidosis often is associated with granulomatous lesions in the neurohypophysis and the hypothalamus (25). Histiocytosis (Hand-Schüller-Christian disease) may involve the pituitary and result in varying degrees of hypopituitarism (8). The neurohypophysis also is affected in most patients, leading to diabetes insipidus. In hemochromatosis, iron pigment accumulates in the cytoplasm of anterior pituitary cells and can lead to fibrosis of the anterior pituitary and hypopituitarism. Central hypothyroidism may occur in thalassemia patients treated with frequent blood transfusions (26,27) and in patients with African trypanosomiasis (28). Chronic lymphocytic hypophysitis has been described with or without pituitary insufficiency in association with autoimmune thyroiditis or adrenalitis (8).

Pituitary aplasia or hypoplasia is a rare congenital defect, usually associated with other severe malformations (8,29). These infants usually die shortly after birth, and evidence of multiple endocrine failure is found at autopsy.

Rare cases of hereditary panhypopituitarism have been reported in association with a small but normally shaped sella turcica (30).

Idiopathic hypopituitarism indicates a deficiency of one or more of the anterior pituitary hormones in the absence of any demonstrable pathology. Idiopathic TSH deficiency usually occurs in association with GH deficiency (31), but secretion of other pituitary hormones also may be deficient. An autosomal-recessive deficiency of pituitary hormones (except ACTH) was reported in a consanguineous Brazilian kindred (32). The finding of a normal, exaggerated, or delayed serum TSH response to TRH in most of these patients suggests the presence of a hypothalamic lesion (33). Birth trauma has been implicated as the etiologic factor secondary to the use of vacuum extraction or breech delivery in the histories of many of these patients.

Isolated TSH deficiency has been reported in patients with a pituitary tumor, empty sella (34), or diabetes mellitus (35), but in most instances no apparent cause has been identified, and the anatomic site of the lesion was not identified (36). A few of these patients had an increased serum TSH response to TRH, but most had no change in serum TSH, suggesting that the defect was at the level of the pituitary (8). The defect may be partial rather than complete, and therapy with thyroid hormone may facilitate the release of small amounts of TSH after TRH administration (36). Although more common in adults, isolated TSH deficiency also occurs in children and may result in a secondary impairment of GH secretion, simulating primary deficiency of TSH and GH (8). In these patients, GH secretion is restored after initiation of T_4 therapy.

Inherited isolated TSH deficiency resulting in congenital central hypothyroidism has been described in a few families (3–5). It is due to single-base substitutions, nonsense mutations, or deletions in the TSH-β subunit (3–5). These abnormalies are inherited or autosomal-recessive traits (37). Mutations in the *TSH*-β gene have been reported with increasing frequency, suggesting that they might be more common than previously thought (6,7,38, 39). Recently, defects in pituitary-specific transcription factors (Pit-1 and PROP-1) have been described (40–47). Pit-1 is a pituitary-specific transcription factor belonging to the POU family, which regulates mammalian development. It binds to the promoter region of the GH and PRL genes and plays an important role in regulation of the expression of the *TSH*-β gene. PROP-1 leads to ontogenesis of pituitary cells, and inactivating mutations result in several degree of hypopituitarism. A rare cause of isolated central hypothyroidism recently is an inactivating mutation of the TRH receptor gene (48). Otherwise genetic causes of central hypothyroidism include mutations of the *LHX3* gene (associated with rigid cervical spine) (49), of the *HESX1* gene (associated with septoptic dysplasia) (50,51) and of the leptin receptor gene (associated with obesity) (52). A summary of the reported genetic abnormalities are shown in Table 51.2 (see Chapter 2).

PATHOGENESIS

Hyposecretion of TSH in pituitary hypothyroidism may be ascribed to a reduced mass of functioning thyrotrophs as a consequence of various lesions, including mechanical compression by tumor, destruction by vascular, inflammatory, or physical injuries, aplasia, or hypoplasia. In these patients, low serum TSH levels and no response to TRH are the expected findings.

Several explanations are possible for idiopathic isolated TSH deficiency. Provided that the thyrotrophs are present and morphologically intact, the abnormality could reside in the TRH receptor or at some subsequent step in the transmission of the hypothalamic message, in the process of TSH synthesis, or in the mechanism of TSH release. Iso-

TABLE 51.2. GENETIC ABNORMALITIES IN THYROTROPIN SYNTHESIS

Mutations in the thyrotropin-releasing hormone receptor
Mutations in the *PROP*-1 gene
Mutations in the *Pit-1* gene
Mutations in the *TSH*-β gene
Mutations in the *HESX1* gene
Mutations in the *LHX3* gene
Mutations in the leptin receptor

TABL
OF T

Use o
L-th
Glu
Dop
Gro
Retin
Suppr
Anti
Radi
Suba
Nonth
Majo
Majo
Bone
Burn
AIDS
Depr
Anor
Fasti
Agin

AIDS, a
rotropir

clinical
Cushin
surge i
with bc
tumors
tern is
sol sec
surge o
major s
surge ar
reporte
subclini
hormon
that the
early sta
Patie
chemica
TSH res
serum T
idiopath
peutic d
occasion
pothyroi
firm this
sive effe
somatost
(98), and
increase
tions (63

lated TSH deficiency in children has been found in association with pseudohypoparathyroidism (53); other patients with this disorder have had primary hypothyroidism (54).

In inherited TSH deficiency resulting from an abnormal TSH-β subunit, a few families had a single-base mutation in nucleotide 145 of exon 2 of the gene, with substitution of glycine for arginine in the 29th amino acid. This substitution causes a conformational change in TSH-β that hampers its dimerization with the α subunit to form a complete TSH molecule. In two families, the molecular abnormality was a nonsense mutation in nucleotide 94 of exon 2, leading to premature termination of TSH-β synthesis at amino acid 11 (4,5,55). With the increasing reports of TSH-β mutations, it appears that many of the mutations are clustered in a "hot spot" involving codon 105 in exon 3. This results in a truncated TSH-β subunit that is unable to dimerize with the α subunit. Central hypothyroidism has been related to a mutation in the pituitary specific transcription factor POU1F1, in the context of multiple pituitary hormone deficiencies (40–43). This clinical picture also may result from mutations of the *PROP1* gene (45–47), which encodes a homeodomain protein expressed briefly in the embryonic pituitary and necessary for *POU1F1* expression (56). The hormonal phenotype consists of gonadotropin, PRL, GH, and TSH deficiency. The pituitary usually is normal in size, albeit a family with *PROP-1* gene mutations and an enlarged anterior pituitary has been reported (57). Recently, Riepe et al. (58) reported variations in pituitary size in two brothers with inactivating *PROP-1* deletions, the gland being enlarged at an early age and hypoplastic after 12 years. Vallette-Kasic et al. (59) reported that nine patients from eight unrelated families who had homozygous *PROP-1* gene defects located in exon 2. The clinical manifestations of GH and TSH deficiency are variable, as is hypogonadism. Late-onset hypocortisolism has been reported as a part of combined pituitary hormone deficiency in two patients with a homozygous deletion of the *PROP-1* gene (60).

Hypothalamic hypothyroidism is commonly attributed to TRH deficiency, whether from acquired or congenital abnormalities of the hypothalamus. These patients have low or normal serum TSH levels that increase after the administration of TRH. No evidence directly supports the concept of TRH deficiency as the cause of hypothalamic hypothyroidism, because of the interference of various serum components in the available TRH radioimmunoassays, the rapid degradation of TRH by serum, and the uncertain origin of TRH in the peripheral blood. Indeed, most TRH is derived from extrahypothalamic sources (61). Indirect evidence favoring TRH deficiency as the cause of hypothyroidism in these patients has come from the demonstration that their hypothyroidism can be corrected by the repetitive administration of TRH (62, 63). The causes of TRH deficiency are unknown but might be re-

lated to reduced TRH synthesis resulting from some destructive lesions of the hypophysiotropic areas of the hypothalamus. In addition, a single patient with TRH receptor gene mutation has been reported (48). The patient was a 9-year-old boy with a compound heterozygous inactivating mutation of the TRH receptor gene.

Reduced stimulation of the pituitary by TRH also may result from suprasellar lesions preventing TRH from reaching the anterior pituitary, as in tumorous or vascular lesions involving the pituitary stalk. The delayed serum TSH response to TRH in these patients could be explained by the fact that TRH reaches the pituitary through the systemic circulation and not through the hypothalamic–pituitary portal system.

A possible explanation for idiopathic hypothalamic hypothyroidism is the excessive production of substances, such as dopamine or somatostatin, that inhibit TSH secretion (64,65). Some indirect support for this concept was provided by the demonstration that naloxone pretreatment resulted in the normalization of a subnormal serum TSH response to TRH in a patient with hypothyroidism (66). The effect of naloxone might be related to the experimental evidence indicating that opiates inhibit TSH secretion by increasing production of a hypothalamic TSH inhibitory factor, such as dopamine (67).

In central hypothyroidism, irrespective of the underlying lesion, the nocturnal surge of serum TSH that occurs in normal subjects (68,69) is reduced or abolished (69–72), although this finding may be equivocal in some patients (72). This loss is due to diminished TSH pulse amplitude with relatively preserved pulse frequency. The loss of the nocturnal surge in TSH secretion may contribute to thyroid hypofunction because it appears that the thyroid is most stimulated at night after the nocturnal surge. Evaluation of the nocturnal serum TSH surge appears to be a sensitive diagnostic test in children with central hypothyroidism (73).

Administration of GH to children with idiopathic GH deficiency may result in central hypothyroidism (74). It has been postulated that GH administration leads to increased secretion of somatostatin, thereby blocking TSH release (74). Other studies documented a subnormal nocturnal TSH surge in GH-deficient children prior to GH therapy, with no further changes in the pituitary–thyroid axis function after GH administration (75). GH therapy also increases peripheral conversion of T_4 to triiodothyronine (T_3), which may result in biochemical changes that mimic central hypothyroidism, such as low serum T_4 concentrations and impaired TSH secretion (76,77). GH therapy of GH-deficient children does not require thyroid hormone therapy (78). Recently, Porretti et al (79) reported the effects of recombinant human GH replacement therapy on thyroid function in a series of 66 adult GH-deficient patients, 49 of whom had central hypothyroidism adequately

ciated with an increased TSH responsiveness to TRH and a normal nocturnal TSH surge (115).

Aging is associated with a variety of hypothalamic–pituitary–thyroid axis changes, but in many instances these are related to concomitant NTI, drug administration, or the increased prevalence of primary hypothyroidism in elderly patients. In male Fisher rats, aging has been associated with decreased synthesis of hypothalamic TRH and consequently with decreased pituitary TSH-β mRNA levels and TSH content, suggesting a defect at the hypothalamic level (116). Evaluation of the pituitary–thyroid axis in healthy elderly subjects, including centenarians, showed a complex derangement of thyroid function, probably resulting from a combination of defective peripheral metabolism of thyroid hormones and of decreased thyroid hormone secretion of central origin. As a consequence, a slight but progressive decrease in serum TSH concentration was observed with age in these healthy subjects; this finding might be related to a resetting of the pituitary threshold of TSH suppression (117). Alcoholism has been associated with varying hypothalamic–pituitary–thyroid axis abnormalities (118). About 60% of subjects with chronic alcoholism have a blunted serum TSH response to TRH, which was more frequent after a short period of abstinence (118).

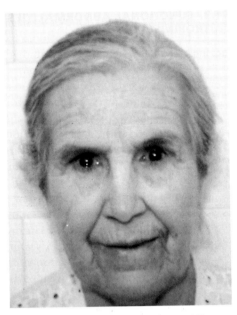

FIGURE 51.1. Patient with central hypothyroidism caused by a nonfunctioning pituitary tumor. The patient had low serum thyroid hormone and thyrotropin (TSH) concentrations; no serum TSH response to thyrotropin-releasing hormone; and corticotropin, growth hormone, and gonadotropin deficiency.

CLINICAL FEATURES

The clinical picture of central hypothyroidism varies widely, depending on the severity of the thyroid failure, the extent of the associated hormone deficiencies, the age of the patient at the time of onset, and the nature of the underlying lesion (101). The clinical features of thyroid insufficiency resulting from TSH deficiency are similar to those of primary hypothyroidism, although generally less pronounced. Patients may complain of cold intolerance, constipation, fatigue, lethargy, and mental dullness. Physical findings include bradycardia, hypothermia, slow speech, and a prolonged relaxation phase of the deep tendon reflexes. Children may present with stunted growth and delay in sexual maturation and bone development. Dwarfism and cretinism occur in the rare patient with familial inherited TSH deficiency. Several differentiating features, largely related to hyposecretion of other pituitary hormones, help to distinguish central hypothyroidism from primary hypothyroidism. The skin is pale and cool but not as coarse and dry as in primary hypothyroidism. The face is characteristically covered with fine wrinkles, but periorbital and peripheral edema are uncommon in patients with central hypothyroidism (Fig. 51.1). Loss of axillary, pubic, and facial hair and thinning of the lateral eyebrows are usually more pronounced, and the texture of the remaining hair is thinner than in primary hypothyroidism. The tongue is not enlarged, and hoarseness of the voice is not prominent in patients with central hypothyroidism. The

heart tends to be small, and blood pressure is low. Pericardial, pleural, and peritoneal effusions are rare in these patients (119). Atrophic breasts and amenorrhea, rather than metrorrhagia, are found in premenopausal women. Body weight is more likely to be reduced than increased. The severity of the hypothyroid state ranges from mild to severe, but, in general, is mild. Although residual hormone secretion from the unstimulated thyroid gland may account for the mild degree of hypothyroidism in most patients, early recognition is also an important factor. In fact, most patients have other endocrine and nonendocrine manifestations of the hypothalamic or pituitary disease that lead them to seek medical attention before their hypothyroidism becomes severe.

Defects in GH and gonadotropin secretion usually precede TSH deficiency as hypopituitarism develops, and ACTH secretion is usually the last to be affected. Growth failure with delayed skeletal maturation is the result of GH deficiency in children, but it has few manifestations in adults. Hypoglycemia may occur, especially if hypocortisolism is also present. In diabetic patients, GH deficiency decreases insulin requirements. Gonadotropin insufficiency results in impotence, loss of libido, diminished beard growth, and testicular atrophy in men; amenorrhea, infertility, and atrophy of the breasts in women; and loss of pubic and axillary hair in both sexes. Delayed sexual maturation is the result of gonadotropin insufficiency in children. ACTH deficiency leads to weakness, postural hypotension, and depigmentation of the areolae and other normally pigmented areas of the skin. Dangerous and potentially lethal adrenal crisis may be precipitated by trauma, intercurrent infection, or surgery.

Symptoms and signs that arise directly from the hypothalamic or pituitary lesion may precede, accompany, and even obscure the manifestations of pituitary failure. Headache and visual field defects are often the presenting symptoms in patients with nonfunctioning pituitary adenomas that extend beyond the sella turcica. As a rule, hormone-secreting adenomas manifest themselves through the consequences of pituitary hormone hypersecretion before symptoms of pituitary insufficiency become apparent. This may not be the case, however, in men with PRL-secreting adenomas. In addition to headache and visual loss, diabetes insipidus occurs frequently in patients with craniopharyngioma, in association with growth failure in children and hypogonadism in adults. Diabetes insipidus is also a prominent feature of histiocytosis and of sarcoidosis involving the hypothalamus. In patients with tumors arising in the hypothalamus or in the region of the third ventricle, meningeal signs may occur early in the course of the disease. Rarely, hypothalamic lesions may cause obesity and abnormal temperature regulation. Patients with postpartum pituitary necrosis have a history of hemorrhage and shock after delivery, followed by deficient lactation, persistent amenorrhea, and other signs of hypogonadism. Severe headache is usually the predominant symptom of pituitary apoplexy, whereas a sudden decrease in insulin requirement may be the first indication of pituitary infarction in a diabetic patient. In other cases, a history of head injury, pituitary surgery, or radiation to the head or neck suggests the underlying lesion. Patients with idiopathic hypopituitarism may have a history of breech delivery or birth by vacuum extraction.

The rate of progression and the degree of central hypothyroidism are influenced markedly by the nature of the underlying disease. Clinical features of thyroid failure are usually detectable within 1 month after hypophysectomy. The development of hypothyroidism is less abrupt in Sheehan's syndrome, but in most instances it is relatively rapid compared with the slow, insidious onset of primary hypothyroidism resulting from atrophic autoimmune thyroiditis. It is not infrequent, however, that several years elapse after a postpartum hemorrhage before hypothyroidism, adrenal insufficiency, and hypogonadism become clinically apparent. A long latency period also may occur in patients who develop central hypothyroidism after a head injury or radiation. In patients with pituitary or hypothalamic tumors, the course and severity of hypopituitarism depend on the rate of tumor growth and the degree of compression of adjacent structures. Overt manifestations of central hypothyroidism are rare in patients with metastatic pituitary tumors or in infants with pituitary aplasia or hypoplasia because of the short life span.

Central hypothyroidism that results from prolonged thyroid hormone therapy is characteristically transient and is usually more evident at the biochemical than the clinical level. Similarly, clinical evidence of central hypothyroidism is rare in patients with other functional abnormalities of TSH secretion, such as endogenous depression and endogenous or exogenous hypercortisolism.

DIAGNOSIS AND LABORATORY TESTS

Central hypothyroidism must be suspected when symptoms and signs of hypothyroidism are associated with manifestations of other hormonal deficiencies or pituitary mass lesions. Because the clinical expression of thyroid insufficiency may be obscured by the features of other hormonal deficiencies or features arising directly from the underlying disease, thyroid function should be evaluated in any patient suspected of having a hypothalamic or pituitary disorder. The possibility of central hypothyroidism also should be considered in hypothyroid patients with no evidence of pituitary failure because it may be difficult, if not impossible, to clinically distinguish central from primary hypothyroidism.

The diagnosis of central hypothyroidism is based on the demonstration of low serum thyroid hormone concentrations in the presence of inappropriately low serum TSH values. Laboratory evaluation of this condition should include assessment of (a) serum thyroid hormone concentrations and TSH secretion, (b) the secretion of the other pituitary hormones, and (c) the anatomy of the hypothalamic and pituitary region.

Serum Thyroid Hormone Concentrations and Thyrotropin Secretion

The prerequisite for the diagnosis of central hypothyroidism is the finding of low serum total and free T_4 concentrations. Measurements of serum total and free T_3 concentrations are much less useful because they are frequently within the normal range. The reduction of serum thyroid hormone concentrations in central hypothyroidism usually is less pronounced than in primary hypothyroidism, although extremely low concentrations are found occasionally in patients with severe, long-standing central hypothyroidism. In newborns, a low serum reverse T_3 concentration may help to distinguish infants with central hypothyroidism from sick and well infants (120).

Basal serum TSH values are inappropriately low with respect to the low serum thyroid hormone concentrations and are either undetectable or within the normal range in most patients (8,121,122). Serum TSH values may be slightly high in some patients (100,123), but not to the levels commonly found in patients with primary hypothyroidism who have a comparable reduction of serum T_4. This finding may be explained by the secretion of immunoreactive but biologically inactive TSH, as discussed previously. Considerable overlap exists in basal serum TSH values between the two types of central hypothyroidism. Thus, determination of basal serum TSH is essential for the differentiation between primary and central hypothyroidism but does not allow the distinction between hypothalamic and pituitary hypothyroidism.

Measurements of the serum TSH response to TRH (200–500 μg or 5 μg/kg administered intravenously) have been used in an attempt to identify the site of the primary lesion. On the basis of the classic concept of the control mechanism of TSH secretion, it was anticipated that the serum TSH response to TRH would be impaired in pituitary hypothyroidism but preserved in hypothalamic hypothyroidism. However, as noted previously, serum TSH responses to TRH differ little in patients with hypothalamic or pituitary disorders. As shown in Figure 51.2, serum TSH responses to TRH may be subdivided into several categories according to the magnitude of the increase in serum TSH after TRH administration and the pattern of the response curve (64). Although absent and impaired responses have been encountered more frequently in hypothyroid patients who have pituitary lesions (64), they also have been found in some patients with hypothalamic disorders who have no apparent pituitary involvement. Conversely, normal or even exaggerated serum TSH responses are found in some hypothyroid patients with hypothalamic disorders (64,124) and in occasional patients with documented primary pituitary disease with no apparent hypothalamic involvement (64). Thus, it appears that the pattern of the serum TSH response to TRH does not reliably distinguish between hypothalamic and pituitary lesions. For this reason, analysis of the entire clinical picture and the results of other tests of pituitary function are required. Some euthyroid patients with hypothalamic–pituitary disorders (e.g., empty sella) also have abnormal serum TSH responses to TRH, for which

there is no satisfactory explanation. Whether these abnormalities predict the subsequent development of central hypothyroidism remains to be clarified (64). The usefulness of the TRH test was further questioned in a recent report (125). A normal TRH test was found in 23% of patients with central hypothyroidism; brisk, absent-blunted, and delayed responses were present in the remaining 77%. In addition, the response to the TRH test did not differentiate between hypothalamic and pituitary disease (125).

In normal subjects, TSH secretion is characterized by a nocturnal surge that begins in the evening and reaches a peak at the time of onset of sleep (68–70,126). This surge does not occur in central hypothyroidism. A reasonable assessment of the nocturnal surge of TSH may be obtained by measuring serum TSH in samples taken every 30 minutes from 11:00 p.m. to 2:00 a.m. (68,69). Evaluation of the nocturnal TSH peak is a more reliable test for confirming the diagnosis of central hypothyroidism than is the TRH test (68, 69). Finally, TRH is no longer available in the United States for clinical use.

Biologic Assay of Serum Thyrotropin

The paradoxic finding of measurable and even slightly high serum immunoreactive TSH concentrations in patients with central hypothyroidism (see previous discussion) stimulated study of the biologic activity of circulating TSH in this condition. Bioassayable serum TSH may be determined by cytochemical assay, based on the ability of TSH to increase lysosomal membrane permeability in thyroid follicular cells (78,81). Less sensitive but more feasible assays are based on the stimulation of adenylyl cyclase activity in human thyroid membranes or cells (82,83) and in continuously cultured rat thyroid cells (FRTL-5) (82,83) or CHO-R cells (83) (Fig. 51.3). These assays require preliminary concentration and purification of serum TSH by immunoaffinity chromatography. Using these techniques, reduced biologic activity of immunoreactive serum TSH was documented in several patients with central hypothyroidism (1,80). These tests, although important for the assessment of TSH biologic activity, are not widely available.

Serum Triiodothyronine Response to Thyrotropin-Releasing Hormone

The release of T$_3$ from the thyroid in response to the increase in serum TSH that follows TRH administration may provide an indirect assessment of the bioactivity of endogenous TSH. In normal subjects, serum T$_3$ concentrations increase from 30% to 100% above the baseline values 120 to 180 minutes after intravenous injection of 200 μg of TRH. An impaired or absent serum T$_3$ response is indicative of central hypothyroidism, provided that a primary thyroid lesion has been excluded (2). The coexistence

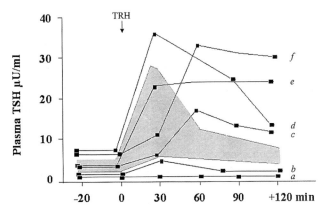

FIGURE 51.2. Patterns of serum thyrotropin (TSH) response to thyrotropin-releasing hormone (TRH) (200 μg administered intravenously) in patients with central hypothyroidism. Type of TSH response: *a,* absent; *b,* impaired; *c,* delayed; *d,* exaggerated; *e,* prolonged; *f,* delayed and prolonged (and exaggerated). The shaded area represents the normal response.

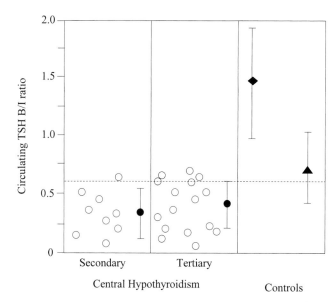

FIGURE 51.3. The ratio between biologic (*B*) and immunologic (*I*) activities of serum thyrotropin (TSH) in patients with central hypothyroidism and in control subjects. The open circles refer to single cases, and the filled circle, triangle, and diamond refer to mean ± SD in central hypothyroidism, primary hypothyroidism, and normal subjects, respectively. The dotted line indicates the lower limit of the normal range. Patients with central hypothyroidism have B/I ratios lower than those in normal or primary hypothyroid subjects (Adapted from Persani L, Ferretti E, Borgato S, et al. Circulating thyrotropin in sporadic central hypothyroidism. *J Clin Endocrinol Metab* 2000;85:3631, with permission.)

of a normal or exaggerated serum immunoreactive TSH response with an abnormally low serum T_3 response suggests the secretion of bioactive TSH (2,80).

Measurement of Thyrotropin-Releasing Hormone

Attempts to measure serum or urine TRH by radioimmunoassay have been made by several investigators (127). TRH is widely distributed throughout the brain and several other tissues, which suggests that most of the TRH in peripheral blood is derived from nonhypothalamic sources (50,127). Thus, measurement of serum or urinary TRH cannot be used as a reliable test for the evaluation of the hypothalamic–pituitary–thyroid axis.

Other Tests

Serum antibodies against to thyroglobulin and thyroid peroxidase are present in a high proportion of patients with primary hypothyroidism (128), but they are usually undetectable in patients with central hypothyroidism (80).

Routine laboratory tests are of little value in the differentiation between primary and central hypothyroidism.

Hypercholesterolemia is commonly regarded as characteristic of primary hypothyroidism, but mild to moderate elevations of serum cholesterol occur in some patients with central hypothyroidism (129).

In the rare forms of inherited TSH deficiency, recently developed molecular biology methodology allows identification of the affected subjects, identification of the mutated gene carriers, and prenatal diagnosis in at-risk pregnancies, which is of the greatest value for the early institution of T_4 replacement therapy.

Tests of Other Pituitary Hormones

In hypothyroid patients with impaired TSH secretion, deficiency of other pituitary hormones should be sought by specific tests for each hormone. Evaluation of GH and PRL secretion under basal conditions and after appropriate stimulation, as well as tests of the pituitary–adrenal and pituitary–gonadal axes, should be performed. Abnormalities of various degrees in these tests are common in patients with central hypothyroidism. Caution should be used, however, in the interpretation of the results because some of these abnormalities may be due to hypothyroidism itself. A low serum GH concentration and a blunted GH response to hypoglycemia are frequent findings in central hypothyroidism, but may also occur in patients with primary hypothyroidism. In the latter condition, as in patients with isolated TSH deficiency, GH secretion is restored to normal by T_4 therapy. High basal serum PRL concentrations with an increased response to TRH frequently are associated with hypothalamic–pituitary disorders, but they too may occur in primary hypothyroidism. Serum follicle-stimulating hormone and luteinizing hormone concentrations are low in most patients with central hypothyroidism, but some reduction and an impaired response to gonadotropin-releasing hormone are found in patients with primary hypothyroidism. In postmenopausal women with primary hypothyroidism, however, serum gonadotropin concentrations remain high.

Serum cortisol concentrations are characteristically reduced in hypopituitarism and are usually normal in primary hypothyroidism. Measurements of serum cortisol may help to differentiate the hypothyroxinemia of central hypothyroidism (low to normal serum cortisol) from the low T_4 state due to nonthyroidal illness, which generally is associated with high serum cortisol values. The response to metyrapone is frequently subnormal in hypopituitarism, reflecting diminished ACTH reserve. The response is usually normal in primary hypothyroidism, although delayed or subnormal responses occur in some patients. Similarly, the serum cortisol response to insulin-induced hypoglycemia may be impaired in hypopituitarism as well as in some patients with primary hypothyroidism (130).

Location of the Hypothalamic–Pituitary Lesion

Various imaging techniques may be used to identify lesions in the hypothalamic and pituitary region. Skull radiography and tomography have been largely replaced by more sensitive procedures, such as computed tomography (CT) and magnetic resonance imaging (MRI). Indirect signs of pituitary tumors detectable by the older techniques include enlargement of the sella, erosion of its floor, and erosion or elevation of the clinoid processes. The presence of soft tissue densities within the sphenoid sinus suggests the presence of extrasellar extension of a pituitary tumor. Suprasellar calcification is a common finding in craniopharyngioma. Long-standing primary hypothyroidism also may be associated with enlargement of the pituitary gland that can be reversed by T_4 therapy (131). A normal or small sella turcica is found in patients with central hypothyroidism attributable to nontumorous lesions (132). CT and MRI have the advantage of visualizing the pituitary gland directly and therefore may provide direct evidence of pituitary tumors or other abnormalities, such as an empty sella turcica. CT and MRI are especially useful in the evaluation of extrasellar extension of pituitary tumors.

THERAPY

Therapy of central hypothyroidism should be directed toward restoring and maintaining euthyroidism. In addition, hypofunction of other endocrine glands resulting from pituitary hormone deficiencies should be corrected and the pituitary or hypothalamic cause of the central hypothyroidism treated appropriately.

Patients with central hypothyroidism should be treated with T_4 in the same way as are patients with primary hypothyroidism, except when there is coexisting ACTH deficiency. Before T_4 therapy is initiated, pituitary-adrenal function should be evaluated by measurement of serum cortisol and assessment of ACTH reserve. If ACTH deficiency is present, cortisol replacement should be initiated before any T_4 is given because of the risk of precipitating an adrenal crisis. In addition, if gonadotropin, GH (especially in children), and antidiuretic hormone deficiencies are present, appropriate replacement therapy should be instituted after the adrenal steroid and T_4 are given. Patients with isolated TSH deficiency require only T_4 therapy, but should be evaluated carefully at least twice a year to detect further loss of pituitary function. Transient functional TSH deficiency usually does not require any treatment.

Although other thyroid preparations can be used, T_4 is the preparation of choice (see Chapter 67). The initial dose of T_4 should be based on the age and cardiovascular status of the patient. In young adults who do not have ACTH deficiency, therapy may be initiated at a daily dose of 1.4 to 1.6 mg/kg T_4 for 4 to 6 weeks; the dose then may be adjusted on the basis of its peripheral effects. In patients with cardiovascular disease or ACTH deficiency and in elderly patients, therapy should be begun with 0.3 to 0.7 mg/kg of T_4; after 3 to 4 weeks, the dose can be increased progressively until an optimal effect is achieved. In infants and children, the dose of T_4 should be relatively higher because T_4 clearance is more rapid and underreplacement may result in mental retardation and impaired physical growth.

Serum TSH measurements cannot be used as in primary hypothyroidism to determine the adequacy of T_4 therapy. Instead, the correct dosage should be determined by clinical response and by measurements of serum free T_4, and together with some biochemical indexes of thyroid hormone action (133).

REFERENCES

1. Beck-Peccoz P, Amr S, Menezes-Ferreira NM, et al. Decreased receptor binding of biologically inactive thyrotropin in central hypothyroidism: effect of treatment with thyrotropin-releasing hormone. *N Engl J Med* 1985;312:1085.
2. Collu R. Genetic aspects of central hypothyroidism. *J Endocrinol Invest* 2000;23:125.
3. Dacou-Votetakis C, Felquate DM, Drakopoulos M, et al. Familial hypothyroidism caused by a nonsense mutation in thyroid-stimulating hormone beta subunit gene. *Am J Human Genet* 1990;46:988.
4. Hayashizaky J, Hiraoka Y, Fndo Y, et al. Thyroid-stimulating hormone (TSH) deficiency caused by a single base substitution in the Cagyc region of the B-subunit. *EMBO J* 1989;8:2291.
5. Hayashizaky J, Hiraoka Y, Tatsumi K, et al. DNA analysis of five families with familial inherited thyroid stimulating hormone (TSH) deficiency. *J Clin Endocrinol Metab* 1990;71:792.
6. Vuissoz JM, Deladoey J, Buyukbebiz A, et al. New autosomal recessive mutation of the TSHbeta subunit gene causing central isolated hypothyroidism. *J Clin Endocrinol Metab* 2001;86:4468.
7. McDermott MT, Haugen BR, Black JN, et al. Congenital isolated central hypothyroidism caused by a "hot spot" mutation in the thyrotropin-beta gene. *Thyroid* 2002;12:1141.
8. Samuels MH, Ridgway EC. Central hypothyroidism. *Endocrinol Metabol Clin North Am* 1992;21:903.
9. Rivarola MA, Mendilaharzou H, Warman M, et al. Endocrine disorders in 66 suprasellar and pineal tumors of patients with prepubertal and pubertal ages. *Horm Res* 1992;37:1.
10. Mathiasen RA, Jarrahy R, Tae Cha S, et al. Pituitary lymphoma: a case report and literature review. *Pituitary* 2000;4:283.
11. Leiba S, Schindel B, Weinstein R, et al. Spontaneous post-partum regression of pituitary mass with return of function. *JAMA* 1986;255:230.
12. Sheehan HL, Davis JC. Pituitary necrosis. *Br Med Bull* 1968;24:59.
13. Abuchan J, Catro V, Maccagnan P, et al. Increased thyrotrophin levels and loss of the nocturnal thyrotrophin surge in Sheehan's syndrome. *Clin Endocrinol (Oxf)* 1997;47:515.
14. Daniel PM, Spicer EJF, Treip CS. Pituitary necrosis in patients maintained on mechanical respirators. *J Pathol* 1973;111:135.

15. Pittman JA Jr, Haigler ED, Hershman JM, et al. Hypothalamic hypothyroidism. *N Engl J Med* 1971;285:844.

16. Segal-Lieberman G, Karasik A, Shimon I. Hypopituitarism following closed head injury. *Pituitary* 2000;3:181.

17. Samaan NA, Cangir A, Maor MH, et al. Effect of irradiation on the hypothalamic, pituitary and thyroid function in patients with tumors of the head and neck. In: Linfoot JA, ed. *Recent advances in the diagnosis and treatment of pituitary tumors.* New York: Raven, 1979:148.

18. Constine LS, Woolf PD, Cann D, et al. Hypothalamic-pituitary dysfunction after radiation for brain tumors. *N Engl J Med* 1993;328:87.

19. Schmiegelow M, Feldt-Rasmussen U, Rasmussen AK, et al. A population-based study of thyroid function after radiotherapy and chemotherapy for a childhood brain tumor. *J Clin Endocrinol Metab* 2003;88:136.

20. Spoudeas HA, Charmandari E, Brook CGD. Hypothalamo-pituitary-adrenal axis integrity after cranial irradiation for childhood posterior fossa tumours. *Med Pediatr Oncol* 2003; 40:224.

21. Rose SR. Cranial irradiation and central hypothyroidism. *Trends Endocrinol Metab* 2001;12:97.

22. Rose SR, Lustig RH, Pitukcheewanont P, et al. Diagnosis of hidden central hypothyroidism in survivors of childhood cancer. *J Clin Endocrinol Metab* 1999;84:4472.

23. Kanumakata S, Warme GL, Zacharin MR. Evolving hypopituitarism following cranial irradiation. *J Paediatr Child Health* 2003;39:232.

24. Dominique JN, Wilson CB. Pituitary abscesses: report of seven cases and review of the literature. *J Neurosurg* 1977;46:601.

25. Bell NH. Endocrine complications of sarcoidosis. *Endocrinol Metabol Clin North Am* 1991;20:645.

26. Lai ME, Balzano S, Murtas ML, et al. High incidence of primary not autoimmune hypothyroidism in adult thalassemia major patients. In: Nagataki S, Torizuka K, eds. *The thyroid.* Amsterdam: Excerpta Medica, 1988:487.

27. Zervas A, Katopodi A, Protonotariou A, et al. Assessment of thyroid function in two hundred patients with beta-thalassemia major. *Thyroid* 2002;12:151.

28. Reincke M, Arit W, Heppner C, et al. Neuroendocrine dysfunction in African trypanosomiasis: the role of cytokines. *Ann NY Acad Sci* 1998;840:809.

29. Salazar H, MacAulay MA, Charles D, et al. The human hypophysis in anencephaly. *Arch Pathol* 1969;87:201.

30. Schimke RN, Spaulding JJ, Hollowell JB. X-linked congenital panhypopituitarism. *Birth Defects* 1971;7:21.

31. Gharib H, Abboud CF. Primary idiopathic hypothalamic hypothyroidism. *Am J Med* 1987;83:171.

32. Nogueira CR, Leite CC, Chedid EPT, et al. Autosomal recessive deficiency of combined pituitary hormones (except ACTH) in a consanguineous Brazilian kindred. *J Endocrinol Invest* 1998;21:386.

33. Proulx F, Weber ML, Collu R, et al. Hypothalamic dysfunction in a child: a distinct syndrome. *Eur J Pediatr* 1993;152: 526.

34. Cannavò S, Curtò L, Venturino M, et al. Abnormalities of hypothalamic-pituitary-thyroid axis in patients with primary empty sella. *J Endocrinol Invest* 2002;25:236.

35. Chandra M, Lifshitz F, Fort P, et al. Isolated thyrotropin deficiency in diabetes mellitus. *Acta Endocrinol (Copenh)* 1977; 84:80.

36. Boehm TM, Dimond RC, Wartofsky L. Isolated thyrotropin deficiency with thyrotropin releasing hormone induced TSH secretion and thyroidal reserve. *J Clin Endocrinol Metab* 1976; 43:1041.

37. Heinrichs C, Parma J, Scherberg NH, et al. Congenital central isolated hypothyroidism caused by a homozygous mutation in the TSH-beta subunit gene. *Thyroid* 2000;10:387.

38. Bonomi M, Proverbio MC, Weber G, et al. Hyperplastic pituitary gland, high serum glycoprotein hormone alpha-subunit, and variable circulating thyrotropin (TSH) levels as hallmark of central hypothyroidism due to mutations of the TSHbeta gene. *J Clin Endocrinol Metab* 2001;86:1600.

39. Doeker RM, Pfaffle RW, Pohlenz J, et al. Congenital central hypothyroidism due to a homozygous mutation in the thyrotropin β-subunit gene follows an autosomal recessive inheritance. *J Clin Endocrinol Metab* 1998;83:1762.

40. Pfaffle RW, Di Mattia GE, Parks JS, et al. Mutation of the POU-specific domain of Pit 1 and hypopituitarism without pituitary hypoplasia. *Science* 1992;257:1118.

41. Pfaffle RW, Parks JS, Brown MR, et al. Pit 1 and pituitary function. *J Pediatr Endocrinol* 1993;6:229.

42. Tatsumi K, Miyai K, Notomi T, et al. Cretinism with combined hormone deficiency caused by a mutation in the *Pit1* gene. *Nat Genet* 1992;1:56.

43. Pellegrini-Bouiller I, Bélicar P, Barrier A, et al. A new mutation of the gene encoding the transcription factor *Pit-1* is responsible for combined pituitary hormone deficiency. *J Clin Endocrinol Metab* 1996;81:2790.

44. Brown MR, Parks JS, Addesses ME, et al. Central hypothyroidism reveals compound heterozygous mutations in the *Pit-1* gene. *Horm Res* 1998;49:98.

45. Wu W, Cogan JD, Pfaffle RW, et al. Mutations in *PROP1* cause familial combined pituitary hormone deficiency. *Nat Genet* 1998;18:147.

46. Fofanova O, Takamura N, Kinoshita E, et al. Compound heterozygous deletion of the *PROP1* gene in children with combined pituitary hormone deficiency. *J Clin Endocrinol Metab* 1998;83:2601.

47. Rosenbloom AL, Selman Almonte A, Brown MR, et al. Clinical and biochemical phenotype of familial anterior hypopituitarism from mutation of the *PROP1* gene. *J Clin Endocrinol Metab* 1999;84:50.

48. Collu R, Tang J, Castagné J, et al. A novel mechanism for isolated central hypothyroidism: inactivating mutations in the thyrotropin-releasing hormone receptor gene. *J Clin Endocrinol Metab* 1997;82:1361.

49. Netchine I, Sobrier M-L, Krude H, et al. Mutations in LHX3 results in a new syndrome revealed by combined pituitary hormone deficiency. *Nat Genet* 2000;25:182.

50. Carvalho LR, Woods KS, Mendonca BB, et al. A homozygous mutation in HESX1 is associated with evolving hypopituitarism due to impaired represor-corepressor interaction. *J Clin Invest* 2003;112:1192.

51. Tajima T, Hattorri T, Nakajima T, et al. Sporadic heterozygous frameshift mutation of HESX1 causing pituitary and optic nerve hypoplasia and combined pituitary hormone deficiency in a Japanese patient. *J Clin Endocrinol Metab* 2003; 88:45.

52. Clement K, Vaisse C, Lahlou N, et al. A mutation in the human leptin receptor gene causes obesity and pituitary dysfunction. *Nature* 1998;392:398.

53. Zisman E, Lotz M, Jenkins ME, et al. Studies in pseudohypoparathyroidism: two new cases with a probable selective deficiency of thyrotropin. *Am J Med* 1969;46:464.

54. Mallet E, Carayon P, Amr S, et al. Coupling defects of thyrotropin receptor and adenylate cyclase in pseudohypoparathyroid patients. *J Clin Endocrinol Metab* 1982;54:1028.

55. Tatsumi K, Hayashizaki Y, Hiraoka Y, et al. The structure of the thyrotropin β-subunit gene. *Gene* 1988;73:489.

56. Sornson MW, Wu W, Dasen JS, et al. Pituitary lineage determination by the Prophet of *Pit-1* homeodomain factor defective in Ames dwarfism. *Nature* 1996;384:327.

57. Mendoca BB, Osorio MGF, Latronico AC et al. Longitudinal hormonal and pituitary imaging changes in two females with combined pituitary hormone deficiency due to a deletion of A301G302 in PROP1 gene. *J Clin Endocrinol Metab* 1999;84:942.

58. Riepe FG, Partsch C-J, Blankenstein O, et al. Longitudinal imaging reveals pituitary enlargement preceding hypoplasia in two brothers with combined pituitary hormone deficiency attributable to PROP1 mutation. *J Clin Endocrinol Metab* 2001;86:4353.

59. Vallette-Kasic S, Barlier A, Teinturier C, et al. PROP1 gene screening in patients with multiple pituitary hormone deficiency reveals two sites of hypermutability and a high incidence of corticotroph deficiency. *J Clin Endocrinol Metab* 2001;86:4529.

60. Asteria C, Persani L, Beck-Peccoz P. Central hypothyroidism: consequences in adult life. *J Pediatr Endocrinol Metab* 2001;14:1263.

61. Martino E, Bartalena L, Gasperi M. Extrapituitary effects of thyrotropin-releasing hormone. In: Monaco F, Satta MA, Shapiro BS, Troncone L, eds. *Thyroid diseases: clinical fundamentals and therapy.* Boca Raton: CRC Press, 1993:595.

62. Faglia G, Beck-Peccoz P, Ballabin M, et al. Excess of beta-subunit of thyrotropin in patients with idiopathic central hypothyroidism due to the secretion of TSH with reduced biological activity. *J Clin Endocrinol Metab* 1983;56:908.

63. Van den Berghe G, De Zegher F, Baxter RC, et al. Neuroendocrinology of prolonged critical illness: effects of exogenous thyrotropin-releasing hormone and its combination with growth hormone secretagogues. *J Clin Endocrinol Metab* 1998;83:309.

64. Faglia G, Beck-Peccoz P, Ferrari C, et al. Plasma thyrotropin response to thyrotropin releasing hormone in patients with pituitary and hypothalamic disorders. *J Clin Endocrinol Metab* 1973;37:595.

65. Van den Berghe G, De Zegher F, Lauwers P. Dopamine and the sick euthyroid syndrome in critical illness. *Clin Endocrinol (Oxf)* 1994;41:731.

66. Dunger DB, Leonard JW, Wolff OH, et al. Effect of naloxone in a previously undescribed hypothalamic syndrome. *Lancet* 1980;1:1277.

67. Morley JE. Neuroendocrine control of thyrotropin secretion. *Endocr Rev* 1981;2:396.

68. Bartalena L, Martino E, Falcone M, et al. Evaluation of the nocturnal serum thyrotropin (TSH) surge, as assessed by TSH ultrasensitive assay, in patients receiving long term L-thyroxine suppression therapy and in patients with various thyroid disorders. *J Clin Endocrinol Metab* 1987;65:1265.

69. Caron PJ, Lynette KN, Rose SR, et al. Deficient nocturnal surge of thyrotropin in central hypothyroidism. *J Clin Endocrinol Metab* 1986;62:969.

70. Rose SR, Manasco PK, Pearce S, et al. Hypothyroidism and deficiency of the nocturnal thyrotropin surge in children with hypothalamic pituitary disorders. *J Clin Endocrinol Metab* 1990;70:1750.

71. Samuels MH, Lillehei K, Kleinschmidt-Demasters BK, et al. Patterns of pulsatile pituitary glycoprotein secretion in central hypothyroidism and hypogonadism. *J Clin Endocrinol Metab* 1990;70:391.

72. Adriaanse R, Romijn JA, Endert E, et al. The nocturnal thyroid-stimulating hormone surge is absent in overt, present in mild primary and equivocal in central hypothyroidism. *Acta Endocrinol (Copenh)* 1992;126:206.

73. Pitukcheewanont P, Rose SR. Nocturnal TSH surge: a sensitive diagnostic test for central hypothyroidism in children. *Endocrinologist* 1997;7:226.

74. Lippe BM, Van Herle AJ, La Franchi SH, et al. Reversible hypothyroidism in growth hormone-deficient children treated with human growth hormone. *J Clin Endocrinol Metab* 1975;40:612.

75. Maghnie M, Triulzi F, Larizza D, et al. Hypothalamic-pituitary dysfunction in growth hormone-deficient patients with pituitary abnormalities. *J Clin Endocrinol Metab* 1991;73:79.

76. Jorgensen JO, Pedersen SA, Lauerberg P, et al. Effects of growth hormone therapy on thyroid function of growth hormone deficient adults with and without concomitant thyroxine substituted central hypothyroidism. *J Clin Endocrinol Metab* 1989;69:1127.

77. Sato T, Suzuki Y, Taketani T, et al. Enhanced peripheral conversion of thyroxine to triiodothyronine during hCG therapy in GH deficient children. *J Clin Endocrinol Metab* 1977;45:324.

78. Wyatt DT, Gesundheit N, Sherman B. Changes in thyroid hormone levels during growth hormone therapy in initially euthyroid patients: lack of need for thyroxine supplementation. *J Clin Endocrinol Metab* 1998;83:3493.

79. Porretti S, Giavoli C, Ronchi C, et al. Recombinant human GH replacement therapy and thyroid function in a large group of adult GH-deficient patients: when does L-T$_4$ therapy become mandatory? *J Clin Endocrinol Metab* 2002;87:2042.

80. Faglia G, Bitensky L, Pinchera A, et al. Thyrotropin secretion in patients with central hypothyroidism: evidence for reduced biological activity of immunoreactive thyrotropin. *J Clin Endocrinol Metab* 1979;48:989.

81. Illig R, Krawczynka M, Torresani T, et al. Elevated plasma TSH and hypothyroidism in children with hypothalamic hypothyroidism. *J Clin Endocrinol Metab* 1975;41:722.

82. Vitti P, Valente WA, Ambesi-Impiombato FS, et al. Graves' IgG stimulation of continuously cultured rat thyroid cells: a sensitive and potentially useful clinical assay. *J Endocrinol Invest* 1982;5:179.

83. Persani L, Ferretti E, Borgato S, et al. Circulating thyrotropin in sporadic central hypothyroidism. *J Clin Endocrinol Metab* 2000;85:3631.

84. Persani L, Tonacchera M, Beck-Peccoz P, et al. Measurement of cAMP accumulation in Chinese hamster ovary cells transfected with the recombinant human TSH receptor (CHO-R): a new bioassay for human thyrotropin. *J Endocrinol Invest* 1993;16:511.

85. Taylor T, Weintraub BD. Altered thyrotropin (TSH) carbohydrate structures in hypothalamic hypothyroidism created by paraventricular nuclear lesions are corrected by *in vivo* TSH-releasing hormone administration. *Endocrinology* 1989;125:2189.

86. Magner J, Klibanski A, Fein H, et al. Ricin and lentil lectin affinity chromatography reveals oligosaccharide heterogeneity of thyrotropin secreted by 12 human pituitary tumors. *Metabolism* 1992;41:1109.

87. Miura Y, Perkel VS, Papenberg KA, et al. Concanavalin-A, lentil, and ricin lectin affinity binding characteristic of human thyrotropin: differences in the sialylation of thyrotropin in sera of euthyroid, primary, and central hypothyroid patients. *J Clin Endocrinol Metab* 1989;69:985.

88. Papandreou MJ, Persani L, Asteria C, et al. Variable carbohydrate structures of circulating thyrotropin as studied by lectin affinity chromatography in different clinical conditions. *J Clin Endocrinol Metab* 1993;77:393.

89. Faglia G, Beck-Peccoz R. Thyrotropin, thyrotropin beta and alpha-subunit secretion in central hypothyroidism. In: Motta M, Zanisi M, Piva F, eds. *Pituitary hormones and related peptides*. London: Academic, 1982:353.

90. Medeiros-Neto G, Herodotou DT, Ryan S, et al. A circulating biologically inactive thyrotropin caused by a mutation in the β-subunit gene. *J Clin Invest* 1996;97:1250.

91. Vagenakis AG, Braverman LE, Azizi F, et al. Recovery of pituitary thyrotropic function after withdrawal of prolonged thyroid-suppression therapy. *N Engl J Med* 1975;293:681.

92. Bartalena L, Martino E, Petrini L, et al. The nocturnal serum thyrotropin surge is abolished in patients with ACTH-dependent or ACTH-independent Cushing's syndrome. *J Clin Endocrinol Metab* 1991;72:1203.

93. Benker G, Raida M, Olliright T, et al. TSH secretion in Cushing's syndrome: relation to glucocorticoid excess, diabetes, goiter, and the "sick euthyroid syndrome." *Clin Endocrinol (Oxf)* 1990;33:777.

94. Bartalena L, Martino E, Brandi LS, et al. Lack of nocturnal serum thyrotropin surge after surgery. *J Clin Endocrinol Metab* 1990;70:293.

95. Coiro V, Volpi R, Capretti L, et al. The nocturnal serum thyrotropin surge is inhibited in patients with adrenal incidentaloma. *J Investig Med* 2002;50:350.

96. Porter BA, Refetoff S, Rosenfield RL, et al. Abnormal thyroxine metabolism in hyposomatrophic dwarfism and inhibition of responsiveness to TRH during GH therapy. *Pediatrics* 1973; 51:668.

97. Municchi G, Malozowski S, Nisula BC, et al. Nocturnal thyrotropin surge in growth hormone-deficient children. *J Pediatr* 1992;121:214.

98. Pasqualini T, Zantleifer D, Balzaretti M, et al. Evidence of hypothalamic-pituitary thyroid abnormalities in children with end-stage renal disease. *J Pediatr* 1991;118:873.

99. Kaptein EM, Spencer CA, Kamiel MB, et al. Prolonged dopamine administration and thyroid economy in normal and critically ill subjects. *J Clin Endocrinol Metab* 1980;51:387.

100. Docter R, Krenning EP, De Jong M, et al. The sick euthyroid syndrome: changes in thyroid hormone serum parameters and hormone metabolism. *Clin Endocrinol (Oxf)* 1993;39:499.

101. DeGroot LJ. Dangerous dogmas in medicine: the nonthyroidal illness syndrome. *J Clin Endocrinol Metab* 1999;84: 151.

102. Bartalena L, Cossu E, Grasso L, et al. Relationship between nocturnal serum thyrotropin peak and metabolic control in diabetic patients. *J Clin Endocrinol Metab* 1993;76:983.

103. Bartalena L, Pacchiarotti A, Palla R, et al. Lack of nocturnal serum thyrotropin (TSH) surge in patients with chronic renal failure undergoing regular maintenance hemofiltration: a case of central hypothyroidism. *Clin Nephrol* 1990;34:30.

104. Custro N, Scafidi V, Gallo S, et al. Deficient pulsatile thyrotropin secretion in the low thyroid hormone state of severe nonthyroidal illness. *Eur J Endocrinol* 1994;130:132.

105. Adriaanse R, Romijn JA, Brabant G, et al. Pulsatile thyrotropin secretion in nonthyroidal illness. *J Clin Endocrinol Metab* 1993; 77:1313.

106. Vaughan GM, Pruitt BA. Thyroid function in critical illness and burn injury. *Semin Nephrol* 1993;13:359.

107. Coiro V, Volpi R, Marchesi C, et al. Influence of residual C-peptide secretion on nocturnal serum TSH peak in well-controlled diabetic patients. *Clin Endocrinol (Oxf)* 1997;47: 305.

108. Bartalena L, Martino E, Placidi GF, et al. Nocturnal serum thyrotropin (TSH) and the TSH response to TSH-releasing hormone: dissociated behavior in untreated depressives. *J Clin Endocrinol Metab* 1990;71:650.

109. Bartalena L, Brogioni S, Grasso L, et al. Interleukin-6 and the thyroid. *Eur J Endocrinol* 1995;132:386.

110. Bartalena L, Brogioni S, Grasso L, et al. Relationship of the increased serum interleukin-6 to changes of thyroid function in nonthyroidal illness. *J Endocrinol Invest* 1994;17:269.

111. Boelen A, Platvoet-ter Schiphorst MC, Wiersinga WM. Association between serum interleukin-6 and serum 3,5,3'-triiodothyronine in nonthyroidal illness. *J Clin Endocrinol Metab* 1993;77:1695.

112. Sherman SI, Gopal J, Haugen BR, et al. Central hypothyroidism associated with retinoid X receptor-selective ligands. *N Engl J Med* 1999;340:1075.

113. Macchia PE, Jiang P, Yuan Y-D, et al. RXR receptor agonist suppression of thyroid function: central effects in the absence of thyroid hormone receptor. *Am J Physiol Endocrinol Metab* 2001;283:E326.

114. Merenich JA. Hypothalamic and pituitary function in AIDS. *Baillieres Clin Endocrinol Metab* 1994;8:757.

115. Lambert M. Thyroid dysfunction in HIV infection. *Baillieres Clin Endocrinol Metab* 1994;8:825.

116. Cizza G, Brady LS, Calogero AE, et al. Central hypothyroidism is associated with advanced age in male Fisher 344/N rats: *in vivo* and *in vitro* studies. *Endocrinology* 1992;131:2672.

117. Mariotti S, Barbesino G, Caturegli P, et al. Complex alteration of thyroid function in healthy centenarians. *J Clin Endocrinol Metab* 1993;77:1130.

118. Hermann D, Heinz A, Mann K. Dysregulation of the hypothalamic-pituitary-thyroid axis in alcoholism. *Addiction* 2002; 97:1369.

119. Parker DR, Shabourry AH. Central hypothyroidism presenting with pericardial and pleural effusions. *J Intern Med* 1993;234: 429.

120. Faase EM, Meacham LR, Novack CM, et al. Decreased reverse T_3 levels in neonates with central hypothyroidism. *J Perinatol* 1997;17:15.

121. Ehrman DA, Weinberg N, Sarne DH. Limitations to the use of a sensitive assay for serum thyrotropin in the assessment of thyroid status. *Arch Intern Med* 1989;149:369.

122. Demers LM, Spencer CA. Laboratory medicine practice guidelines—laboratory support for the diagnosis and monitoring of thyroid disease. *Thyroid* 2003;13:33.

123. Spencer CA, Schwarzbein D, Guttler RB, et al. Thyrotropin (TSH)-releasing hormone stimulation test responses employing third and fourth generation TSH assays. *J Clin Endocrinol Metab* 1993;76:494.

124. Mills GH, Ellis RD, Beck PR. Exaggerated and prolonged thyrotrophin-releasing hormone (TRH) test responses in tertiary hypothyroidism. *J Clin Pathol* 1991;44:522.

125. Mehta A, Hindmarsh PC, Stanhope RG, et al. Is the thyrotropin-releasing hormone test necessary in the diagnosis of central hypothyroidism in children. *J Clin Endocrinol Metab* 2003;88:5696.

126. Brabant G, Prank K, Hoang-vu C, et al. Hypothalamic regulation of pulsatile thyrotropin secretion. *J Clin Endocrinol Metab* 1991;72:145.

127. Engler D, Scanlon MF, Jackson IMD. Thyrotropin-releasing hormone in the systemic circulation of the neonatal rat is derived from the pancreas and other extraneural tissues. *J Clin Invest* 1981;67:800.

128. Mariotti S, Caturegli P, Piccolo P, et al. Antithyroid peroxidase autoantibodies in thyroid disease. *J Clin Endocrinol Metab* 1990;71:661.

129. O'Brien T, Dinneem SF, O'Brien PC, et al. Hyperlipidemia in patients with primary and secondary hypothyroidism. *Mayo Clin Proc* 1993;68:860.

130. Rosen HN, Greenspan SL, Landsberg L, et al. Distinguishing hypothyroxinemia due to euthyroid sick syndrome from pituitary insufficiency. *Isr J Med Sci* 1994;30:746.

131. Vagenakis AG, Dole K, Braverman LE. Pituitary enlargement, pituitary failure and primary hypothyroidism. *Ann Intern Med* 1976;85:195.

132. Meador CK, Worrel JL. The sella turcica in postpartum pituitary necrosis (Sheehan's syndrome). *Ann Intern Med* 1966;65.

133. Ferretti E, Persani L, Jaffrain-Rea M-L, et al. Evaluation of the adequacy of levothyroxine replacement therapy in patients with central hypothyroidism. *J Clin Endocrinol Metab* 1999; 84:924.

ORGAN SYSTEM MANIFESTATIONS OF HYPOTHYROIDISM

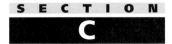

52

THE SKIN AND CONNECTIVE TISSUE IN HYPOTHYROIDISM

JOSHUA D. SAFER

The skin characteristics associated with thyroid dysfunction are classic. The term "myxedema," the original name for hypothyroidism, refers to the edema-like associated skin condition caused by increased glycosaminoglycan deposition in the skin. In 1878, Ord published the first comprehensive description of myxedematous skin (1). Horsley connected myxedema to the thyroid in 1885 (2). Still the classic cutaneous sign of hypothyroidism, generalized myxedema is caused by deposition of dermal acid mucopolysaccharides, especially hyaluronic acid. The entire skin is firm to the touch, appearing swollen, dry, pale, and waxy. Despite its edematous appearance, the skin does not pit with pressure. There is also a typical facial appearance manifested by a broad nose, swollen lips, macroglossia, and puffy eyelids (3).

More generally, skin manifestations of hypothyroidism may be divided into three categories (Table 52.1): (a) direct action of thyroid hormone on skin tissues, (b) skin manifestations of direct thyroid hormone action on nonskin tissues, and (c) autoimmune skin disease associated with hypothyroidism of autoimmune etiology.

DIRECT THYROID HORMONE ACTION ON SKIN TISSUES

Thyroid hormone acts directly on skin, mediating its effect through the thyroid hormone receptor (TR). The TR has been identified in both epidermis and dermis. Hair, which has important relationships with both epidermis and dermis, is a site where TR has also been identified. Immunohistochemical localization and quantitative polymerase chain reaction (PCR) have demonstrated all three thyroid hormone–binding TR isoforms in skin tissues (4–7). TRs have been detected in epidermal keratinocytes, skin fibroblasts, hair arrector pili muscle cells, other smooth muscle cells, sebaceous gland cells, vascular endothelial cells, Schwann's cells, and cell types composing the hair follicle (see Fig. 30.1). Several thyroid hormone responsive genes have been identified in skin (see Chapter 30).

Epidermal Changes

Thyroid hormone is an important regulator of epidermal growth, differentiation, and homeostasis. Epidermal manifestations of thyroid hormone deficiency are evident in that the skin in hypothyroidism is rough and covered with fine superficial scales, especially on the extensor extremities (8). Xerosis may be severe enough to resemble an acquired ichthyosis. The dryness of the palms and soles may be extensive (9). Histologic examination reveals epidermal thinning and hyperkeratosis (10).

In the 1970s, investigators reported conversion of thyroxine (T_4) to either triiodothyronine (T_3) or rT_3 in skin

TABLE 52.1. SKIN MANIFESTATIONS OF HYPOTHYROIDISM

Direct thyroid hormone action on skin tissues
  Epidermal changes
    Coarsened, thin, scaly skin
  Dermal changes
    Nonpitting edema (myxedema)
    Edema (hands, face, eyelids)
    Carotenemia
    Pallor
  Hair and nail changes
    Dry, brittle, coarse hair
    Alopecia
    Loss of lateral third of eyebrows
    Coarse, dull, thin, brittle nails
  Sweat gland changes
    Dry skin (xerosis)
    Decreased sweating
Skin manifestation of thyroid hormone action on other tissues
  Cold intolerance
  Pallor
  Purpura
  Drooping of upper eyelids
  Nerve entrapment syndromes
Associated autoimmune phenomena
  Urticaria, pruritis
  Vitiligo
  Pernicious anemia
  Bullous disorders
  Eczema
  Connective tissue diseases

cultures, thus demonstrating indirectly the presence of thyroid hormone deiodinases in skin (11–13). RNA expression of both deiodinase types II and III has been found in human skin (14). In one study in goats, investigators found that deiodinase type III was most active in skin (15) followed by deiodinase type II. An *in vivo* study in humans (16) provided further evidence that deiodinase type III is functionally dominant in skin. Women receiving supraphysiologic doses of T_4 in a topical cream did not have detectable changes in circulating TSH, T_4, or T_3 concentrations. Only serum rT_3 levels increased significantly, strongly suggesting the dominance in skin of type III (inner ring) deiodinase activity.

In tissue culture studies, thyroid hormone stimulates growth of both epidermal keratinocytes and dermal fibroblasts (4,17,18). However, thyroid hormone–mediated inhibition of keratinocyte growth has been observed when keratinocytes were cocultured with dermal fibroblasts (18).

Up to 90% of hypothyroid patients may have scaly skin (19). In addition to the thyroid hormone–mediated growth characteristics noted above, *in vitro* keratinocyte studies have shown that depletion of T_3 results in elevated levels of transglutaminase, an enzyme involved in the formation of the cornified envelope. Further *in vitro* analysis has suggested that T_3-depleted keratinocytes have diminished lev-

els of plasminogen activator, a putative enzyme implicated in the corneocyte shedding process (20).

Other contributory factors in the development of xerosis involve epidermal lipids. Studies of thyroidectomized rats have suggested that sterol synthesis is altered in epidermal keratinocytes deprived of thyroid hormone (21). Thyroid hormone accelerates barrier formation by increasing the activity of enzymes in the cholesterol sulfate cycle. Thus, a deficiency of thyroid hormone may hinder the epidermal barrier function (22). Hypothyroidism also may affect the development of the lamellar granules (Odland bodies), which are vital in the establishment of a normal stratum corneum (23).

Dermal Changes

In hypothyroidism, the skin tends to be pale both because of the dermal mucopolysaccharides and increased dermal water content. In addition, increased dermal carotene content may be evident, appearing as a prominent yellow hue on the palms, soles, and nasolabial folds (19).

The seminal histologic evaluation of the skin of a patient with hypothyroidism was done by Reuter in 1931 (10). Reuter was able to demonstrate increased hyaluronic acid in hypothyroid dermis. Gabrilove and Ludwig (24) examined via biopsy the skin of individuals with hypothyroidism before and after treatment. Histologic changes were observed within 3 to 4 weeks of thyroid hormone changes (24).

Hyaluronic acid is the predominant glycosaminoglycan that accumulates in myxedema (25). Its hygroscopic nature allows it to swell to 1,000 times its dry weight when hydrated. Mucin deposition is extensive and involves not only the skin but also the tongue, myocardium, kidney, and most other organs of the body. Although the hygroscopic nature of hyaluronic acid may partly explain the presence of cutaneous edema, increased transcapillary escape of albumin, resulting in extravascular accumulation, may also contribute to the edema. In addition, inadequate lymphatic drainage may further explain the formation of exudates in the serous cavities that are apparent in the myxedematous state (26).

Since the early histologic studies, there have been a number of systematic evaluations of the glycosaminoglycans (GAGs) present in the skin of hypothyroid patients (25). Most researchers record increased hyaluronic acid in the absence of thyroid hormone (27–29). *In vitro* studies suggest that thyroid hormone decreases synthesis of hyaluronic acid by inhibiting action of hyaluronan synthetase. Thyroid hormone also increases hyaluronic acid degradation. Chondroitin sulfate and dermatan sulfate are reported to be unchanged in hypothyroidism. Heparan sulfate is reported to be either stable or decreased. Data are contradictory for thyroid hormone action on collagen synthesis in skin fibroblasts (30,31).

Hypothyroid dermis is further characterized by a scarcity of dermal fibroblasts. Indeed, *in vitro* studies confirm that thyroid hormone deficiency retards dermal fibroblast proliferation (4,17,18). Among the fibroblasts present, there can be both decreased activity and absence of new collagen deposition. Abnormal fibroblast function may be the cause of decreased and irregularly shaped elastic microfibrils demonstrated in patients with myxedema (32).

Although the data favor a role for thyroid hormone in normal healing (33), the importance of thyroid hormone to wound healing is debated. Diminished wound healing rates have been reported in both hypothyroid mice (33) and rats (34). There are also reports that several hypothyroid patients required thyroid hormone to achieve healing of radiation-induced neck fistulae (35,36). Conversely, Cannon (37) reported that hypothyroidism did not diminish wound strength in pigs, and Ladenson et al (38) reported an absence of wound healing deficits in hypothyroid humans.

Hair and Nail Changes

In hypothyroidism, hair can be dry, coarse, dull, and brittle. The rate of hair growth is slowed (39,40). Similarly, nails may be thickened, brittle, and slow growing (41). Diffuse or partial alopecia may be observed, and loss of the lateral third of the eyebrow (madarosis) is reported. The alopecia associated with hypothyroidism may be mediated by hormone effects on the initiation as well as the duration of hair growth.

In the 1950s and 1960s, Hale and Ebling documented the impact of thyroid hormone on rat hair growth cycles (39). With the addition of thyroid hormone, they demonstrated decreased resting phase of the hair growth cycle (telogen) and decreased growth phase of the hair growth cycle (anagen). Although there was enhanced turnover, the net hair length at any given time was unchanged from that of untreated animals. Importantly, the time to regrowth of hair following epilation was shortened. The induction of hypothyroidism with the antithyroid drug propylthiouracil significantly increased the time to the restoration of hair.

In vitro studies on human tissue suggest slowed hair growth rates in hypothyroidism. DNA flow cytometry studies on dissected anagen hair follicles from hypothyroid patients (compared with follicles taken from euthyroid controls) demonstrated a 15% decrease in the S and G2 + M phases of the cell cycle (40).

There is a report of long, terminal hairs on the backs and extremities of hypothyroid children (42). The hair disappeared following thyroid hormone replacement, but no mechanism was determined.

Hypothyroid patients may sometimes manifest *Candida* folliculitis. It has been theorized that because the sebaceous glands of hypothyroid patients secrete less sebum than those of euthyroid persons, the hair follicles may develop a flora depleted of lipophilic organisms, which are replaced by *Candida albicans* (43).

Sweat Gland Changes

The dryness of hypothyroid skin results from decreased eccrine gland secretion. The mechanism for decreased sweating is not clear, although the hypothyroid glands are atrophic on histologic examination. A role may also be played by a periodic acid–Schiff-positive material that can accumulate in the eccrine apparatus of hypothyroid patients (44). Hypothyroidism has been reported to be a cause of increased sweat electrolytes, requiring differentiation from cystic fibrosis (45).

SKIN MANIFESTATION OF THYROID HORMONE ACTION ON OTHER TISSUES

Several dermatologic manifestations of hypothyroidism derive from hypothyroidism in nonskin tissues. Thyroid hormone–mediated changes to the basal metabolic, vascular, and sympathetic nervous systems are evident when the skin is examined (see Chapters 53, 60, and 63).

Cool, pale skin may result from decreased skin perfusion in hypothyroidism. The decreased skin perfusion has been documented with both nailfold capillaroscopy (46) and laser Doppler techniques (47). It has been suggested that the diminished skin perfusion is a reflex vasoconstriction compensatory to diminished core temperature. The diminished core temperature itself may be secondary to the reduced thermogenesis of the hypometabolic state (48). Occasionally, purpura may be noted in hypothyroid patients as a result of diminished levels of clotting factors or the loss of vascular support secondary to the dermal mucin (49,50).

Drooping of the upper lids has been attributed to decreased sympathetic stimulation of the superior palpebral muscle (19). Entrapment syndromes, such as carpal tunnel syndrome and facial nerve palsy, have been reported (51).

ASSOCIATED AUTOIMMUNE PHENOMENA

When hypothyroidism is of autoimmune etiology, additional skin findings may be evident that reflect associated autoimmune diseases (52). Although patients with autoimmune thyroid disease are at increased risk for other tissue-specific autoimmune diseases and are even at a slightly increased risk for more generalized autoimmune diseases, screening hypothyroid patients for other autoimmune disease is not cost effective. Conversely, autoimmune thyroid disease is sufficiently common that patients with other autoimmune disease deserve screening for thyroid dysfunction.

A list of autoimmune conditions apparent when examining the skin includes alopecia areata, pernicious anemia, bullous disorders (pemphigus, bullous pemphigoid, dermatitis herpetiformis), connective tissue diseases (lupus erythematosus, scleroderma), lichen sclerosus et atrophicus, palmoplantar pustulosis, and urticaria. Some patients with autoimmune dermatologic diseases may present with pitting nails (53) independent of the dry, brittle nails associated with direct thyroid hormone action. It has been reported that a subset of patients with chronic urticaria and angioedema associated with thyroid autoimmunity may have their urticaria abate with the administration of thyroid hormone (54). The mechanism by which thyroid hormone may alleviate this process remains speculative.

REFERENCES

1. Ord WM. On myxoedema, term proposed to be applied to an essential condition in the "cretinoid" affection occasionally observed in middle-aged women. *Med Chir Trans Lond* 1878;61:57–78.

2. Horsley V. The thyroid gland: its relation to the pathology of myxoedema and cretinism, to the question of surgical treatment of goitre, and to the general nutrition of the body. *BMJ* 1885;1:111–115.

3. Maize J, Metcalf J. Metabolic diseases of the skin. In: Elder D, ed. *Lever's histopathology of the skin,* 8th ed. Philadelphia: Lippincott-Raven, 1997:369.

4. Ahsan MK, Urano Y, Kato S, et al. Immunohistochemical localization of thyroid hormone nuclear receptors in human hair follicles and *in vitro* effect of L-triiodothyronine on cultured cells of hair follicles and skin. *J Med Invest* 1998;44:179–184.

5. Torma H, Rollman O, Vahlquist A. Detection of mRNA transcripts for retinoic acid, vitamin D$_3$, and thyroid hormone (c-erb-A) nuclear receptors in human skin using reverse transcription and polymerase chain reaction. *Acta Derm Venereol* 1993;73:102–107.

6. Billoni N, Buan B, Gautier B, et al. Thyroid hormone receptor beta-1 is expressed in the human hair follicle. *Br J Dermatol* 2000;142:645–652.

7. Torma H, Karlsson T, Michaelsson G, et al. Decreased mRNA levels of retinoic acid receptor-alpha, retinoid X receptor-alpha and thyroid hormone receptor-alpha in lesional psoriatic skin. *Acta Derm Venereol* 2000;80:4–9.

8. Heymann WR. Cutaneous manifestations of thyroid disease. *J Am Acad Dermatol* 1992;26:885.

9. Hodak E, David M, Feuerman EJ. Palmoplantar keratoderma in association with myxedema. *Acta Derm Venereol (Stockh)* 1986;66:354.

10. Reuter MJ. Histopathology of the skin in myxedema. *Arch Dermatol Syphilol* 1931;24:55–71.

11. Refetoff S, Matalon R, Bigazzi M. Metabolism of L-thyroxine (T$_4$) and L-triiodothyronine (T$_3$) by human fibroblasts in tissue culture: evidence for cellular binding proteins and conversion of T$_4$ to T$_3$. *Endocrinology* 1972;91:934–947.

12. Huang TS, Chopra IJ, Beredo A, et al. Skin is an active site for the inner ring monodeiodination of thyroxine to 3,3′,5′-triiodothyronine. *Endocrinology* 1985;117:2106–2113.

13. Kaplan MM, Pan C, Gordon PR, et al. Human epidermal keratinocytes in culture convert thyroxine to 3,5,3′-triiodothyronine by type II iodothyronine deiodination: a novel endocrine function of skin. *J Clin Endocrinol Metab* 1988;66:815–822.

14. Slominski A, Wortsman J, Kohn L, et al. Expression of hypothalamic-pituitary-thyroid axis related genes in human skin. *J Invest Dermatol* 2002;119:1449–1455.

15. Villar D, Nichols F, Arthur JR, et al. Type II and type III monodeiodinase activities in the skin of untreated and propylthiouracil-treated cashmere goats. *Res Vet Sci* 2000;68:119–123.

16. Santini F, Vitti P, Chiovato L, et al. Role for inner ring deiodination preventing transcutaneous passage of thyroxine. *J Clin Endocrinol Metab* 2003;88:2825–2830.

17. Holt PJA. *In vitro* responses of the epidermis to triiodothyronine. *J Invest Dermatol* 1978;71:202–204.

18. Safer JD, Crawford TM, Fraser LM, et al. Thyroid hormone action on skin: diverging effects of topical versus intraperitoneal administration. *Thyroid* 2003;13:159–165.

19. Freinkel RK. Cutaneous manifestations of endocrine disease. In: Freedberg IM, Jisen AZ, Wolff K, et al, eds., *Dermatology in general medicine,* 4th ed. New York: McGraw-Hill, 1993:2113.

20. Isseroff RR, Chun KT, Rosenberg RM. Triiodothyronine alters the cornification of cultured human keratinocytes. *Br J Dermatol* 1989;120:503–510.

21. Rosenberg RM, Isseroff RR, Ziboh VA, et al. Abnormal lipogenesis in thyroid hormone-deficient epidermis. *J Invest Dermatol* 1986;86:244.

22. Hanley K, Jiang Y, Katagiri C, et al. Epidermal steroid sulfatase and cholesterol sulfotransferase are regulated during late gestation in the fetal rat. *J Invest Dermatol* 1997;108:871.

23. Hanley K, Devaskar UP, Hicks SJ, et al. Hypothyroidism delays fetal stratum corneum development in mice. *Pediatr Res* 1997;42:610.

24. Gabrilove JL, Ludwig AW. The histogenesis of myxedema. *J Clin Endocrinol Metab* 1957;17:925–932.

25. Smith TJ, Bahn RS, Gorman CA. Connective tissue, glycosaminoglycans and diseases of the thyroid. *Endocr Rev* 1989;10:366–391.

26. Parving H-H, Hansen JM, Nielsen SL, et al. Mechanisms of edema formation in myxedema: increased protein extravasation and relatively slow lymphatic drainage. *N Engl J Med* 1979;301:460.

27. Kofoed JA. The acidic glycosaminoglycans in the skin of athyroid rats: the effects of l-tri-iodothyronine. *Experientia* 1971;27:702–703.

28. Smith TJ, Murata Y, Horwitz AL, et al. Regulation of glycosaminoglycan synthesis by thyroid hormone *in vitro*. *J Clin Invest* 1982;70:1066–1073.

29. Smith TJ. Dexamethasone regulation of glycosaminoglycan synthesis in cultured human skin fibroblasts: similar effects of glucocorticoid and thyroid hormones. *J Clin Invest* 1984;74:2157–2163.

30. De Rycker C, Vandelem J-L, Hennen G. Effect of 3,5,3′-triiodothyronine on collagen synthesis by cultured human skin fibroblasts. *FEBS Lett* 1984;174:34.

31. Yazdanparest P, Carlsson B, Oikarinen A, et al. The thyroid hormone analogues triiodothyroacetic acid, corrects corticosteroid-downregulated collagen synthesis. *Thyroid* 2004;14:345–353.

32. Matsuoka LY, Wortsman J, Uitto J, et al. Altered skin elastic fibers in hypothyroid myxedema and pretibial myxedema. *Arch Intern Med* 1985;145:117.

33. Safer JD, Crawford TM, Holick MF. A role for thyroid hormone in wound healing through keratin gene expression. *Endocrinology* 2004;145:2359–2360.

34. Lennox J, Johnston ID. The effect of thyroid status on nitrogen balance and the rate of wound healing after injury in rats. *Br J Surg* 1973;60:309.

35. Alexander MV, Zajtchuk JT, Henderson RL. Hypothyroidism and wound healing: occurrence after head and neck radiation and surgery. *Arch Otolaryngol* 1982;108:289–291.

36. Talmi YP, Finkelstein Y, Zohar Y. Pharyngeal fistulas in postoperative hypothyroid patients. *Ann Otol Rhinol Laryngol* 1989;98:267–268.

37. Cannon CR. Hypothyroidism in head and neck cancer patients: experimental and clinical observations. *Laryngoscope* 1994;104:1–22.

38. Ladenson, PW, Levin AA, Ridgeway EC, et al. Complications of surgery in hypothyroid patients. *Am J Med* 1984;77:261–266.

39. Hale PA, Ebling FJ. The effect of a single epilation on successive hair eruptions in normal and hormone-treated rats. *J Exp Zool* 1979;207:49–72.

40. Schell H, Kiesewetter F, Seidel C, et al. Cell cycle kinetics of human anagen scalp hair bulbs in thyroid disorders determined by DNA flow cytometry. *Dermatologica* 1991;182:23.

41. Mullin GE, Eastern JS. Cutaneous signs of thyroid disease. *Am Fam Physician* 1986;34:93.

42. Perloff WH. Hirsutism: a manifestation of juvenile hypothyroidism. *JAMA* 1955;157:651.

43. Dekio S, Imaoka C, Jidoi J. Candida folliculitis associated with hypothyroidism. *Br J Dermatol* 1987;117:663.

44. Means MA, Dobson RL. Cytological changes in the sweat gland in hypothyroidism. *JAMA* 1963;186:113.

45. Squires L, Dolan TF. Abnormal sweat chloride in auto-immune hypothyroidism. *Clin Pediatr* 1989;28:535.

46. Pazos-Moura CC, Moura EG, Breitenbach MMD, et al. Nailfold capillaroscopy in hypothyroidism: blood flow velocity during rest and postocclusive reactive hyperemia. *Angiology* 1998;49:471.

47. Weiss M, Milman B, Rosen B, et al. Quantitation of thyroid hormone effect on skin perfusion by laser Doppler flowmetry. *J Clin Endocrinol Metab* 1993;76:680.

48. Silva JE. The thermogenic effect of thyroid hormone and its clinical implications. *Ann Intern Med* 2003;139:205–213.

49. Christianson HB. Cutaneous manifestations of hypothyroidism including purpura and ecchymoses. *Cutis* 1976;17:45.

50. Feingold KR, Elias PM. Endocrine-skin interactions. *J Am Acad Dermatol* 1987;17:921.

51. Diven DG, Gwinup G, Newton RC. The thyroid. *Dermatol Clin* 1989;7:547–557.

52. Ai J, Leonhardt JM, Heymann WR. Autoimmune thyroid diseases: etiology, pathogenesis, and dermatologic manifestations. *J Am Acad Dermatol* 2003;48:641–659.

53. Barth JH, Telfer NR, Dawber RP. Nail abnormalities and autoimmunity. *J Am Acad Dermatol* 1988;18:1062

54. Heymann WR. Chronic idiopathic urticaria and angioedema associated with thyroid autoimmunity: review and therapeutic implications. *J Am Acad Dermatol* 1999;40:229.

THE CARDIOVASCULAR SYSTEM
IN HYPOTHYROIDISM

IRWIN L. KLEIN

The changes in cardiovascular function that occur in patients with hypothyroidism are opposite those of thyrotoxicosis (see Chapter 31) (1). Symptoms and signs related to cardiovascular dysfunction are much less prominent in patients with hypothyroidism than in those with thyrotoxicosis. This chapter reviews the pathophysiologic basis for the cardiac findings of hypothyroidism and the potential of hypothyroidism as a risk factor for accelerated atherosclerosis.

CARDIOVASCULAR HEMODYNAMICS

The hemodynamic changes associated with hypothyroidism are listed in Table 53.1. Compared with normal subjects, patients with hypothyroidism have an increase of 50% to 60% in peripheral vascular resistance; this increase is accompanied by a 30% to 50% decrease in resting cardiac output (2,3). The net effect of the decrease in blood flow and the decrease in tissue oxygen consumption that occurs in hypothyroidism is that arteriovenous oxygen extraction across major organs is similar in patients with hypothyroidism and normal subjects (2). Studies of the molecular mechanism underlying the increase in systemic vascular resistance suggest that thyroid hormone, specifically triiodothyronine (T_3), may have a direct vasodilator action on vascular smooth muscle cells (4,5). In addition endothelium-derived vascular relaxation, which involves nitric oxide release and action, is impaired in both mild and overt hypothyroidism (6,7). Thus, in the absence of T_3, vascular smooth muscle tone and systemic vascular resistance may increase. This increase can in part be reversed by acute T_3 administration (8).

All measurements of left ventricular contractility and performance are lower in patients with both acute and chronic hypothyroidism (9–12). Cardiac output (index) is decreased as a result of decreases in both stroke volume and, to a lesser extent, heart rate (1,12). The duration of both the preejection period and the isovolumic contraction time is prolonged compared with normal subjects, and these times decrease in response to thyroid hormone therapy (9,12). In addition, and perhaps more important, the rate of ventricular relaxation during diastole is slower, and diastolic filling and compliance are impaired (3,6). The

rate of diastolic filling may decrease from normal values of 400 mL per second to less than 300 mL per second. The mechanisms underlying the impaired ventricular performance in patients with hypothyroidism are multifactorial and appear to result from changes in the expression of important myocyte-specific regulatory proteins and in pre- and afterload (1,12–14). As noted in Chapter 31, the expression of many cardiac genes is modulated by thyroid hormone, and in experimental animals, lowering serum concentrations of thyroxine (T_4) and T_3 alters the expression of the distribution of the heavy chain isoforms of myosin and of the calcium regulatory proteins (15–17). Myocyte nuclei contain T_3 receptors that bind to specific DNA sequences of several genes, and thus many of the cardiac actions of T_3 occur at the level of gene transcription. Decreases in the expression of the genes for the sarcoplasmic reticulum calcium adenosine triphosphatase (ATPase), Na^+,K^+-ATPase, β-adrenergic receptors, and voltage-gated potassium channels (Kv) all may play a role in the altered cardiac physiology in patients with hypothyroidism (see Chapter 8 and Chapter 31) (1,13,17).

The rate of tension development during cardiac systole is determined in part by the rate at which myosin catalyzes the hydrolysis of ATP. There are two isoforms of myosin ATPase, α and β, in cardiac myocytes. The predominant form in human ventricular tissue is β-myosin (18,19). In one hypothyroid patient with severe left ventricular dysfunction, the content of α-myosin in ventricular muscle increased slightly during treatment with T_4, but β-myosin predominated at both times (17). The patient's left ventricular contractile function improved during treatment, most probably a result of improved calcium handling (cycling) in cardiac muscle cells (20). The activities of several enzymes involved in regulating calcium fluxes in the heart are controlled by thyroid hormone. These include the calcium-activated ATPase of the sarcoplasmic reticulum and phospholamban (21,22). In addition, in hypothyroidism, the increase in systemic vascular resistance (afterload) and decrease in blood volume and venous return (preload) impair cardiovascular hemodynamics (1,11,12).

As a result of the increase in systemic vascular resistance and decrease in cardiac output, mean blood pressure is largely unaltered in hypothyroidism (1,2). There may be

TABLE 53.1. CARDIOVASCULAR HEMODYNAMICS IN HYPOTHYROIDISM

	Finding	Comments
Systemic vascular resistance	↑	50%–60% above normal
Cardiac output	↓	30%–50% below normal
Blood pressure		
Systolic	↓ or normal	Narrowed pulse pressure
Diastolic	↑ or normal	20% prevalence of diastolic hypertension
Heart rate	↓ or normal	
Cardiac contractility	↓ or normal	Systolic and diastolic function both impaired
Cardiac mass	↓	Pericardial effusion may suggest cardiomegaly
Blood volume	↓	Decreased preload

an increase in diastolic pressure and a decrease in systolic pressure, so the pulse pressure is low. Hypothyroid patients may have diastolic hypertension that declines, sometimes to normal, during treatment with thyroid hormone as systemic vascular resistance decreases (23,24).

Plasma volume is decreased in patients with hypothyroidism (11), an unexpected finding because some patients have pitting edema suggestive of fluid overload. Capillary permeability is increased, and therefore the albumin and water content in the interstitial space is increased. Fluid may accumulate not only in gravity-dependent regions, but also in the pericardial pleural and other spaces (25). Patients with hypothyroidism also have nonpitting edema (myxedema), caused by the accumulation of hydrophilic glycosaminoglycans in the interstitial space (see Chapter 52).

The response of hypothyroid patients to exercise supports the hypothesis that peripheral circulatory changes mediate many of the changes in cardiac performance. Exercise lowers systemic vascular resistance in patients with hypothyroidism, causing an increase in cardiac index, heart rate, and stroke volume to 85% to 90% of the responses in normal subjects (26). These observations indicate that the reduced left ventricular function in hypothyroid patients at rest is at least partially the result of a decrease in hemodynamic loading.

CLINICAL MANIFESTATIONS

Most patients with hypothyroidism have few symptoms directly referable to the cardiovascular system (27). Although fatigue, lack of energy, exertional dyspnea, and exercise intolerance have been attributed to impaired cardiac performance, they are more likely to be related to psychological or skeletal muscle dysfunction (28). Whether or not congestive heart failure with orthopnea and paroxysmal nocturnal dyspnea occurs solely as a result of hypothyroidism is discussed later.

Patients with hypothyroidism can have angina-like pain (26), and many have hypercholesterolemia (see Chapter 60). Various metabolic changes and cardiac risk factors predisposing to atherosclerosis are present in patients even with mild hypothyroidism (Table 53.2) (29). An occa-

sional patient with normal coronary arteries has angina that resolves with thyroid hormone therapy (26).

Physical Examination

The abnormalities that may be found on physical examination of the cardiovascular system in patients with hypothyroidism include bradycardia, narrow pulse pressure, low-amplitude pulse, diminished apical impulse, and distant heart sounds (1,2,3,10) (Table 53.1). The bradycardia may result from a loss of the chronotropic action of thyroid hormone directly on the sinoatrial pacemaker cells (1); heart rate analysis reveals changes in both sympathetic and parasympathetic tone (30). The abnormal heart sounds may be caused by decreased left ventricular contractility or a pericardial effusion (9,10,25,31). From 20% to 40% of patients with hypothyroidism have a diastolic blood pressure greater than 90 mm Hg (11,23,32,33). Patients not only complain of cold intolerance but also may have cold feet and hands because of decreased skin blood flow.

Patients with hypothyroidism may have edema of the extremities or presacral region, mostly caused by increased extravasation of albumin and water. Myxedema, the characteristic nonpitting edema of the face, hands, and feet, occurs only in patients with severe, long-standing untreated hypothyroidism, and is rarely seen now (see Chapter 52).

TABLE 53.2. CARDIOVASCULAR RISK ASSOCIATED WITH HYPOTHYROIDISM AND EFFECT OF THYROID HORMONE THERAPY

Risk Factor	Response to Thyroid Hormone Therapy
Diastolic hypertension	+
Left ventricular diastolic dysfunction	++
Impaired endothelium-mediated vasodilatation	++
Hypercoagulable state	++
Hypercholesterolemia	++
High serum homocysteine concentration	+

+, modest improvement; ++, marked improvement.

Pericardial effusions occur in a variable frequency in patients with hypothyroidism (3,25). The effusions are usually small and escape detection, but occasional patients with severe, long-standing hypothyroidism have large effusions (25,34). However, even large effusions rarely affect cardiac function (35,36). The protein content of the fluid tends to be high, most likely because of an increase in albumin transudation. The fluid usually has a high cholesterol concentration and may be viscous. The pericardial effusions disappear gradually during treatment with T_4 (25). Rare patients with severe, long-standing hypothyroidism have effusions in other spaces, including the peritoneal cavity, pleural cavities, and joints (36).

Laboratory Tests

Hemoglobin and hematocrit values may be slightly low (see Chapter 57) (36). The partial thromboplastin time and other measures of coagulation may be prolonged in overt hypothyroidism (37). Serum total and low-density lipoprotein cholesterol, lipoprotein(a), and apolipoprotein B concentrations are often high, and some patients have high serum triglyceride concentrations (see Chapter 60). There is a progressive increase in serum total cholesterol concentrations across the entire spectrum of hypothyroidism (38).

Serum creatine kinase concentrations are high in as many as 30% of patients (28,36). Most of the increase is in the MM fraction, indicating that its source is skeletal rather than cardiac muscle (39). Serum myoglobin concentrations and urinary myoglobin excretion also may be high. These findings indicate that the permeability of muscle cell membranes is increased. The half-life of creatine kinase in serum is prolonged, which contributes to the high serum concentration (28). The serum concentrations of other muscle-related enzymes, such as aldolase, may also be high (see Chapter 63).

Electrocardiography

Hypothyroidism classically has been associated with bradycardia, but the degree of slowing of the heart rate is often modest (30,40). The function of the atrial pacemaker is normal and atrial ectopy is rare, but premature ventricular beats and occasionally ventricular tachycardia can occur (3). This is in contrast to thyrotoxicosis, in which atrial tachyarrhythmias are common and ventricular arrhythmias are rare. The syndrome of torsade de pointes with a long QT interval and ventricular tachycardia can occur with hypothyroidism and resolve with T_4 treatment alone (41). The duration of the action potential may be prolonged, perhaps reflecting a decrease in voltage-gated potassium channels.

Low-voltage and nonspecific ST wave changes are other electrocardiographic abnormalities found in some patients with hypothyroidism (3,34,36). Although occasionally suggestive of myocardial ischemia (29), these changes are more likely to disappear during T_4 treatment than with antiangina drug treatment (26). The low voltage may be a result of pericardial effusion, altered myocyte ion conduction, or cardiac atrophy (25,34).

Noninvasive Evaluation

All measures of left ventricular contractility and cardiac workload, as determined by echocardiography, are decreased in patients with hypothyroidism (10,12,14,42–44). These include systolic time intervals and measures of diastolic performance, such as isovolumic filling and compliance. Whereas cardiac contractility and work are impaired at rest, they increase during exercise (26), confirming the importance of loading conditions and heart rate as determinants of cardiac output (12). Even mild degrees of hypothyroidism of short duration are associated with predictable prolongation in the isovolumic relaxation time (14,44); thus, diastolic relaxation appears to be a sensitive and specific measurement of the cardiovascular response to thyroid hormone (3). The latter in turn most likely reflects the decrease in cardiac myocyte calcium cycling (45). Positron emission tomography and magnetic resonance imaging of the heart in patients with hypothyroidism demonstrate the expected decreases in oxidative metabolism and cardiac contractility and work. With the accompanying increase in systemic vascular resistance and afterload, the net effect is to render the heart energy inefficient (46).

Asymmetric hypertrophy of the intraventricular septum has been reported in patients with hypothyroidism, but evidence that it is caused by thyroid hormone deficiency is lacking (47). It is not likely to be responsible for the abnormalities in left ventricular function that occur in hypothyroidism, because these abnormalities often occur in the absence of any changes in cardiac morphology.

Hypertension

From 20% to 40% of patients with hypothyroidism have hypertension; diastolic pressure is increased more than systolic pressure (11). The increase in diastolic pressure is due primarily to the increase in systemic vascular resistance. As noted above, T_3 may act as a direct vasodilator, and therefore vascular tone may increase in its absence (4,5,11,24). The blood pressure in these patients is less sensitive to variations in salt intake, as reflected by changes in blood pressure in response to sodium restriction, as compared with other hypertensive patients (3,11,33).

In large series of hypertensive patients, varying degrees of hypothyroidism were a contributing factor in about 3% to 5% (see Chapter 55) (23). This is a low-renin form of hypertension that may occur early in the course of the hypothyroidism (32,33). Among hypothyroid patients with hypertension, some have normal or near-normal blood pressure after treatment with T_4 alone (11,23,32).

Heart Failure

The presence of impaired left ventricular contractility, diastolic hypertension, increased systemic vascular resistance, and peripheral edema suggests that hypothyroidism can cause heart failure (2,17,48). However, documentation of hypothyroidism as the sole cause of congestive heart failure is rare (1,3,49,50). Arteriovenous oxygen extraction is normal in hypothyroid patients, whereas it is increased in patients with organic heart disease and heart failure (2). Patients with hypothyroidism have an increase in cardiac output and a decrease in systemic vascular resistance in response to exercise, unlike patients with heart failure (2,10). Also, in contrast to patients with heart failure, patients with hypothyroidism are able to excrete a sodium load (51) and do not develop signs of pulmonary fluid overload characteristic of intrinsic heart disease. As noted above, limitations of exercise capacity are more likely the result of skeletal muscle fatigue and weakness and from pulmonary-related causes than from cardiac insufficiency (See Chapters 54 and 63). Although histologic changes in the heart of patients dying of profound hypothyroidism include myocyte swelling and mucinous edema (52), the most characteristic findings are the functional abnormalities related to impaired diastolic relaxation (1,3,14).

TREATMENT

All the changes in cardiovascular function in patients with hypothyroidism improve in response to treatment with T_4 or T_3 (see Chapter 67) (31,49). In most patients the symptoms are chronic, and hemodynamic performance is not impaired sufficiently to require urgent therapy (3,8,9,53). Young patients can be given full replacement doses of T_4, for example, 100 to 150 µg daily. Older patients initially should be given lower doses, for example, 50 µg daily, and older patients with coronary artery disease even lower doses, for example, 25 µg daily. In patients with severe hypothyroidism treated with high doses of T_3, cardiovascular performance improves within 48 to 96 hours (49). T_4 treatment reverses not only the abnormalities in cardiac contractility and systemic vascular resistance, often including blood pressure, but also the high serum lipid concentrations and other biochemical abnormalities in weeks or months (11,23,25,28).

SPECIAL CLINICAL SITUATIONS

Hypothyroidism, Thyroid Hormone Therapy, and Coronary Artery Disease

Patients with hypothyroidism might be expected to have an increased risk for coronary artery disease, since they may have hypertension and they often have hypercholesterol-emia (11,34,38,40). In a case control autopsy study, coro-nary artery disease was more prevalent in hypothyroid patients with coexistent hypertension, but not in normotensive hypothyroid patients, compared with euthyroid patients (54). In a cross-sectional study of 280 nursing home patients there was an increase in the frequency of hypercholesterolemia and coronary artery disease in patients with hypothyroidism, as compared with patients with normal thyroid function (53,54a). Similarly, an increase in abdominal aortic calcification and incident myocardial infarction was noted in a study of women 55 years of age or older with subclinical hypothyroidism in Amsterdam (see Chapters 77 and 78) (55).

Hypothyroidism may predispose to the development of atherosclerosis and coronary artery disease by several mechanisms (11,29,56) (Table 53.2). Hypercholesterolemia [and high serum lipoprotein(a) concentrations] and increased systemic vascular resistance with diastolic hypertension are well-recognized cardiovascular risk factors. In addition, hypothyroidism is associated with slightly high serum homocysteine concentrations (perhaps secondary to decreased folic acid absorption) and impaired endothelium-mediated vasodilatation (6,7). Although patients with overt hypothyroidism have abnormal platelet function and impaired hemostasis, subclinical hypothyroidism is associated with increased platelet aggregation and impaired fibrinolysis, changes that could be proatherogenic (57). In one study, the serum concentrations of C-reactive protein, an acute inflammatory marker associated with risk for cardiovascular disease, were slightly higher in patients with both overt and subclinical hypothyroidism than normal subjects; the concentrations did not decrease during T_4 therapy in the patients with subclinical hypothyroidism (the only group studied) (58).

In patients with coronary artery disease who develop hypothyroidism, the decreases in cardiac work and oxygen demand were previously thought to promote better tolerance of decreases in myocardial blood flow. These considerations led some clinicians either to not treat or to give only a low dose of T_4 to patients with known or suspected coronary artery disease (26). [Hypothyroid dogs tolerate myocardial ischemia less well than do euthyroid dogs, and myocardial damage is more extensive and ventricular arrhythmias are more common after experimentally induced myocardial infarction than in euthyroid animals (59)]. However, given the deleterious effects of hypothyroidism on cardiac function and the debilitating effects of hypothyroidism per se, it is not reasonable to withhold or limit T_4 replacement for a theoretic benefit on myocardial ischemia (1,3).

With regard to angina pectoris, the effects of thyroid hormone treatment are mostly beneficial. In the largest study of this issue, 1,503 hypothyroid patients received thyroid hormone therapy and subsequently were evaluated for angina pectoris and myocardial infarction (60). Of the 55 patients with known symptomatic coronary artery disease, 38% improved with treatment, 46% had no change, and only 16% had more symptoms. Thirty-five patients had chest pain after thyroid hormone therapy was begun, but in two thirds of them the pain began more than 1 year after initiation of treatment. Considering the demographics of the overall study group, several hundred patients were probably at risk for coronary artery disease; thus, the overall incidence of symptoms attributable to coronary artery disease after initiation of thyroid hormone therapy was low. Thyroid hormone therapy should not be withheld on the grounds that angina pectoris might occur.

Occasional hypothyroid patients have sufficiently extensive coronary artery disease to justify coronary artery bypass surgery before or soon after T_4 therapy is begun (3,61). The operation can be performed safely and without excessive morbidity in these patients (61,62), as can coronary angioplasty or stenting (63). Postoperatively, full-dose T_4 therapy is most likely to prevent progression of coronary artery disease (64).

Thyroid Hormone Therapy in Heart Disease and After Cardiac Surgery

Thyroid hormone metabolism, specifically the extrathyroidal conversion of T_4 to T_3, is altered in patients with both chronic and acute cardiac disease, as in many other illnesses (see section on Nonthyroidal Illness in Chapter 11). A study of 573 patients with all types of cardiac disease identified a low serum free T_3 concentration as a predictor of death; during a mean follow-up period of 11 months, 14% of the patients with a low serum free T_3 concentration at base line died, as compared with 3% of the patients with normal serum free T_3 concentrations (65). In a study of patients with congestive heart failure, serum total and free T_3 concentrations were inversely related to the degree of heart failure, as assessed by New York Heart Association scoring criteria (66). Short-term treatment of heart failure patients with intravenous T_3 increases cardiac output and reduces systemic vascular resistance, and has no adverse effects (67,68). Whether the illness- or surgery-related decrease in serum T_3 concentrations results in thyroid deficiency in the heart or other organs is debated. In one study in animals, induction of nonthyroidal illness resulted in changes in gene expression in cardiac muscle and changes in cardiac function similar to those that occur in hypothyroidism, and administration of low doses of T_3 reversed the changes (69). All these findings, and the reports that T_3 administration after experimental myocardial infarction in animals improved cardiovascular hemodynamics, suggest that low serum T_3 concentrations may have deleterious effects on cardiac function (70).

Serum T_3 concentrations decrease acutely after cardiopulmonary surgery in both children and adults; the decrease is greater and more prolonged in children, especially those with complicated congenital heart defects (8,24, 71–73). This decline, and the marked effect of thyroid hor-

mone on cardiac contractility, provided the rationale for administering T_3 as a potential positive inotropic agent and a novel vasodilator in these patients. Children with serum T_3 concentrations less than 40 ng/dL (0.6 nM) who were given T_3 intravenously for 48 to 96 hours after surgery had improved cardiovascular hemodynamics and renal perfusion, with a reduced need for inotropic support (71,72). Among patients with coronary artery disease undergoing elective coronary artery bypass grafting, intravenous administration of high doses of T_3 immediately after surgery was associated with an increase in cardiac output and a decrease in systemic vascular resistance during the first 24 hours after surgery, as compared with placebo (24). In addition, the frequency of postoperative atrial fibrillation was reduced by 50%; postoperative mortality in the two groups was similar (74).

Subclinical Hypothyroidism

Patients with subclinical hypothyroidism have changes in cardiovascular function and risk factors for cardiovascular disease that are similar to but smaller in magnitude to those of patients with overt hypothyroidism described above (see Chapter 78) (12,14). In a study of these patients, the rate of isovolumic relaxation, diastolic flow, and systemic vascular resistance improved during thyroid hormone therapy (14). Long-term benefits of T_4 therapy in these patients have not been documented (75). Nonetheless, the improvement in cardiac dynamics and the at least partial reversal of some of the risk factors (e.g., serum cholesterol) that occur during T_4 therapy suggest that these patients should have long-term cardiovascular benefits from therapy.

REFERENCES

1. Klein I, Ojamaa K. Thyroid hormone and the cardiovascular system. *N Engl J Med* 2001;344:501.
2. Graettinger JS, Muenster JJ, Checchia CS, et al. A correlation of clinical and hemodynamic studies in patients with hypothyroidism. *J Clin Invest* 1957;37:502.
3. Klein I. Endocrine disorders and cardiovascular disease. In: Braunwald E, Zipes DP, Libby P, eds *Heart disease,* 7th ed. New York: WB Saunders, 2004 (in press).
4. Ojamaa K, Balkman C, Klein I. Acute effects of triiodothyronine on arterial smooth muscle cells. *Ann Thorac Surg* 1993; 56(suppl):61.
5. Park KW, Dai HB, Ojamaa K, et al. The direct vasomotor effect of thyroid hormones on rat skeletal muscle resistance arteries. *Anesth Analg* 1997;85:734.
6. Lekakis J, Papamichael C, Alevizaki M, et al. Flow mediated endothelium dependent vasodilatation is impaired in subjects with hypothyroidism. *Thyroid* 1997;7:411.
7. Taddei S, Caraccio N, Virdis A, et al. Impaired endothelial-dependent vasodilatation in subclinical hypothyroidism. *J Clin Endocrinol Metab* 2003;88:3731.
8. Klemperer JD, Ojamaa K, Klein I. Thyroid hormone therapy in cardiovascular disease. *Prog Cardiovasc Dis* 1996;38:329.

9. Crowley WF Jr, Ridgway EC, Bough EW, et al. Non-invasive evaluation of cardiac function in hypothyroidism. *N Engl J Med* 1977;296:1.

10. Wieshammer S, Keck F, Waitzinger J, et al. Acute hypothyroidism slows the rate of left ventricular diastolic relaxation. *Can J Physiol Pharmacol* 1988;67:1007.

11. Danzi S, Klein I. Thyroid hormone and blood pressure regulation. In: *Curr Hypertension Rep* 2003;5:513.

12. Biondi B, Palmieri EA, Lombardi L, et al. Effects of thyroid hormone on cardiac function. *J Clin Endocrinol Metab* 2002;87:968.

13. Bluhm WF, Meyer M, Sayen MR, et al. Over-expression of SERCA improves cardiac contractile function in hypothyroid mice. *Cardiovasc Res* 1999;43:382.

14. Biondi B, Palmieri EA, Lombardi L, et al. Effects of subclinical thyroid dysfunction on the heart. *Ann Intern Med* 2002;137:904.

15. Ojamaa K, Klein I. *In vivo* regulation of recombinant cardiac myosin heavy chain gene expression by thyroid hormone. *Endocrinology* 1993;132:1002.

16. Danzi S, Klein I. Thyroid hormone-regulated cardiac gene expression and cardiovascular disease. *Thyroid* 2002;12:467.

17. Ladenson PW, Sherman SI, Baughman KL, et al. Reversible alterations in myocardial gene expression in a young man with dilated cardiomyopathy and hypothyroidism. *Proc Natl Acad Sci U S A* 1992;89:5251.

18. Reiser PJ, Portman MA, Ning X, et al. Human cardiac myosin heavy chain isoforms in fetal and failing adult atria and ventricles. *Am J Physiol* 2001;280:H1814.

19. Magner JA, Clark W, Allenby P. Congestive heart failure and sudden death in a young woman with thyrotoxicosis. *West J Med* 1990;8:553.

20. Khoury SF, Hoit BD, Dave V, et al. Effect of thyroid hormone on left ventricular performance and regulation of contractile and calcium cycling proteins in the baboon. *Circ Res* 1996;79:727.

21. Carr AN, Kranias EG. Thyroid hormone regulation of calcium cycling proteins. *Thyroid* 2002;12:453.

22. Ojamaa K, Klein I. Thyroid hormone regulation of phospholamban phosphorylation in the rat heart. *Endocrinology* 2000;141:2139.

23. Streeten DHP, Anderson GH Jr, Howland T, et al. Effects of thyroid function on blood pressure: recognition of hypothyroid hypertension. *Hypertension* 1988;11:78.

24. Klemperer JD, Klein I, Gomez M, et al. Thyroid hormone treatment after coronary-artery bypass surgery. *N Engl J Med* 1995;333:1522.

25. Kabadi UM, Kumar SP. Pericardial effusion in primary hypothyroidism. *Am Heart J* 1990;120:159.

26. Myerowitz P, Kamienski R, Swanson D, et al. Diagnosis and management of the hypothyroid patient with chest pain. *J Thorac Cardiovasc Surg* 1983;86:57.

27. Zulewski H, Muller B, Eter P. Estimation of tissue hypothyroidism by a new clinical score: Evaluation of patients with various grades of hypothyroidism and controls. *J Clin Endocrinol Metab* 1997;82:771.

28. Klein I, Mantell P, Parker M, et al. Resolution of abnormal muscle enzymes in hypothyroidism. *Am J Med Sci* 1980;279:159.

29. Biondi B, Klein I. Hypothyroidism as a risk factor for cardiovascular disease. *Endocrine* 2004;24:1.

30. Inukai T, Takanashi K, Kobayashi H, et al. Power spectral analysis of heart rate in hyperthyroidism and hypothyroidism. *Horm Metab Res* 1998;30:531.

31. Bough EW, Crowley WF, Ridgway E, et al. Myocardial function in hypothyroidism. *Arch Intern Med* 1978;138:1476.

32. Dernellis J, Panaretou M. Effects of thyroid replacement therapy on arterial blood pressure in patients with hypertension and hypothyroidism. *Am Heart J* 2002;143:718.

33. Marcisz C, Jonderko G, Kucharz EJ. Influence of short-time application of a low sodium diet on blood pressure in patients with hyperthyroidism or hypothyroidism during therapy. *Am J Hypertens* 2001;14:995.

34. Zimmerman J, Yahalom J, Bron H. Clinical spectrum of pericardial effusion as the presenting feature of hypothyroidism. *Am Heart J* 1984;106:770.

35. Oliver C, Martin F. Low QRS voltage in cardiac tamponade: a study of 70 cases. *Int J Cardiol* 2002;83:93.

36. Klein I, Levey GS. Unusual manifestations of hypothyroidism. *Arch Intern Med* 1984;144:123.

37. Attivissimo LA, Lichtman SM, Klein I. Acquired von Willebrand's syndrome causing a hemorrhagic diathesis in a patient with hypothyroidism. *Thyroid* 1995;5:399.

38. Canaris GJ, Manowitz NR, Ridgway EC. The Colorado thyroid disease prevalence study. *Arch Intern Med* 2000;160:526.

39. Madariaga MG. Polymyositis-like syndrome in hypothyroidism. *Thyroid* 2002;12:381.

40. Staub JJ, Althaus BU, Engler H, et al. Spectrum of subclinical and overt hypothyroidism: effect on thyrotropin, prolactin and thyroid reserve and metabolic impact on peripheral target tissues. *Am J Med* 1992;92:631.

41. Fredlund B, Olsson SB. Long QT interval and ventricular tachycardia of "torsade de pointe" type in hypothyroidism. *Acta Med Scand* 1983;213:231.

42. Virtanen VK, Saha HH, Groundstroem KW, et al. Thyroid hormone substitution therapy rapidly enhances left ventricular diastolic function in hypothyroid patients. *Cardiology* 2001;96:59.

43. Tielens E, Pillay M, Storm C, et al. Changes in cardiac function at rest before and after treatment of hypothyroidism. *Am J Cardiol* 2000, 85:376.

44. Brenta G, Mutti LA, Schnitman M, et al. Assessment of left ventricular diastolic function by radionuclide ventriculography at rest and exercise in subclinical hypothyroidism and its response to l-thyroxine therapy. *Am J Cardiol* 2003;91:1327.

45. Dillmann WH. Cellular action in primary thyroid hormone on the heart. *Thyroid* 2002;12:447.

46. Bengel FM, Nekolla SG, Ibrahim T, et al. Effect of thyroid hormones on cardiac function, geometry, and oxidative metabolism assessed non-invasively by positron emission tomography and magnetic resonance imaging. *J Clin Endocrinol Metab* 2000;85:1822.

47. Bernstein R, Muller C, Midtbo K, et al. Coronary dysfunction in severe hypothyroidism. In: Braverman LE, Eber O, Langsteger W, eds. *Heart and thyroid*. Vienna: Blackwell, 1994:154.

48. Lowes BD, Minobe W, Abraham WT, et al. Changes in gene expression in the intact human heart: downregulation of α-myosin heavy chain in hypertrophied, failing ventricular myocardium. *J Clin Invest* 1997;100:2315.

49. Ladenson PW, Goldenheim PD, Ridgway EC. Rapid pituitary and peripheral tissue responses to intravenous l-triiodothyronine in hypothyroidism. *J Clin Endocrinol Metab* 1983;56:1252.

50. Tielens ET, Pillay M, Storm C, et al. Cardiac function at rest in hypothyroidism evaluated by equilibrium radionuclide angiography. *Clin Endocrinol (Oxf)* 1999;50:497.

51. DeRubertis FR Jr, Michelis MF, Bloom ME, et al. Impaired water excretion in myxedema. *Am J Med* 1971;51:41.

52. LaDue JS. Myxedema heart: a pathological and therapeutic study. *Ann Intern Med* 1943;18:332.

53. Klein I, Danzi S. Evaluation of the therapeutic efficacy of different levothyroxine preparations in the treatment of human thyroid disease. *Thyroid* 2003;13:1127.

54. Steinberg AD. Myxedema and coronary artery disease: a comparative autopsy study. *Ann Intern Med* 1968;68:338.

54a. Mya MM, Aronow WS. Subclinical hyperthyroidism is associated with coronary artery disease in older persons. *J Gerontol A Biol Sci Med Sci* 2002;57:M658.

55. Hak AE, Pols HA, Visser TJ, et al. Subclinical hypothyroidism is an independent risk factor for atherosclerosis and myocardial infarction in elderly women: the Rotterdam Study. *Ann Intern Med* 2000;132:270.

56. Cappola AR, Ladenson PW. Hypothyroidism and atherosclerosis. *J Clin Endocrinol Metab* 2003;88:2438.

57. Chadarevian R, Bruckert E, Leenhardt L, et al. Components of the fibrinolytic system are differently altered in moderate and severe hypothyroidism. *J Clin Endocrinol Metab* 2001;86:732.

58. Christ-Crain M, Meier C, Guglielmetti M, et al. Elevated C-reactive protein and homocysteine values: cardiovascular risk factors in hypothyroidism? A cross-sectional and a double-blind, placebo-controlled trial. *Atherosclerosis* 2003;166:379.

59. Karlsberg RA, Friscia DA, Aronow WS, et al. Deleterious influence of hypothyroidism on evolving myocardial infarction in conscious dogs. *J Clin Invest* 1981;67:1024.

60. Keating FR Jr, Parkin TW, Selby JB, et al. Treatment of heart disease associated with myxedema. *Prog Cardiovasc Dis* 1961;3:364.

61. Drucker DJ, Burrow GD. Cardiovascular surgery in the hypothyroid patient. *Arch Intern Med* 1985;145:1585.

62. Ladenson PW, Levin AA, Ridgway EC, et al. Complications of surgery in hypothyroid patients. *Am J Med* 1984;77:261.

63. Sherman SI, Ladenson PW. Percutaneous transluminal coronary angioplasty in hypothyroidism. *Am J Med* 1991;90:367.

64. Pek M, O'Neill BJ. Effect of thyroid hormone therapy on angiographic coronary artery disease progression. *Can J Cardiol* 1997;13:273.

65. Iervasi G, Pingitore A, Landi P, et al. Low T_3 syndrome: a strong prognostic predictor of death in patients with heart disease. *Circulation* 2003;107:708.

66. Asheim DD, Hyrniewicz K. Thyroid hormone metabolism in patients with congestive heart failure: the low triiodothyronine state. *Thyroid* 2002 12(6):511.

67. Hamilton MA, Stevenson LW. Thyroid hormone abnormalities in heart failure: possibilities for therapy. *Thyroid* 1996;6:527.

68. Hamilton MA, Stevenson LW, Fonarow GC, et al. Safety and hemodynamic effects of intravenous triiodothyronine in advanced congestive heart failure. *Am J Cardiol* 1998;81:443.

69. Katzeff HL, Powell SR, Ojamaa K. Alterations in cardiac contractility and gene expression during low-T_3 syndrome: prevention with T_3. *Am J Physiol* 1997;273:E951.

70. Ojamaa K, Kenessey A, Shenoy R, et al. Thyroid hormone metabolism and cardiac gene expression after acute myocardial infarction in the rat. *Am J Physiol* 2000;279:E1319.

71. Chowdhury D, Parnell V, Ojamaa K, et al. Usefulness of triiodothyronine (T_3) treatment after surgery for complex congenital heart disease in infants and children. *Am J Cardiol* 1999;84:1107.

72. Portman MA, Fearneyhough C, Ning X-H, et al. Triiodothyronine repletion in infants during cardiopulmonary bypass for congenital heart disease. *J Thorac Cardiovasc Surg* 2000;120:604.

73. Mainwaring RD, Lamberti JJ, Carter TL Jr, et al. Reduction in triiodothyronine levels following modified Fontan procedure. *J Card Surg* 1994;9:322.

74. Klemperer JD, Klein IL, Ojamaa K, et al. Triiodothyronine therapy lowers the incidence of atrial fibrillation after cardiac operations. *Ann Thorac Surg* 1996;61:1323.

75. Surks MI, Ortiz E, Daniels GH, et al. Subclinical thyroid disease: scientific review and guidelines for diagnosis and management. *JAMA* 2004;291:228.

THE PULMONARY SYSTEM
IN HYPOTHYROIDISM

DAVID H. INGBAR

Respiratory manifestations are seldom the major complaint of patients with hypothyroidism; nonetheless, the pulmonary system may be affected in many ways. Fatigue and dyspnea on exertion are frequent symptoms (1). Occasionally, pulmonary involvement is major and life threatening, as in the patient with myxedema coma and CO_2 retention.

The roles of thyroid hormone in lung development, respiratory muscle function, and regulation of ventilation during sleep and wakefulness are of interest to multiple specialties. All these subjects are brought together in the patient with hypothyroidism. This chapter examines the ways that the respiratory system can be affected in hypothyroid patients. The pulmonary consequences of hypothyroidism can be categorized as those that directly affect the lung and those that result from changes in the function of other organ systems. Table 54.1 classifies these consequences.

ALTERATIONS IN PULMONARY FUNCTION IN ADULTS

Pulmonary Function Tests and Gas Exchange

Analysis of changes in pulmonary function is complicated by an increased frequency of obesity in hypothyroid patients. Abnormalities attributed in the literature to hypothyroidism actually may have been due to obesity. Obesity alone frequently may decrease one of more of the following: diffusing capacity of the lung for carbon monoxide (DLCO), vital capacity (VC), total lung capacity (TLC), functional residual capacity (FRC), and especially expiratory reserve volume. All these abnormalities do not necessarily occur together in the individual patient.

In an old study contrasting patients with either hypothyroidism alone or hypothyroidism accompanied by obesity, the 16 patients with hypothyroidism alone had normal lung volumes and arterial blood gases (ABG), but decreased DLCO (2). After replacement with thyroid hormone, the patients lost a mean of 6 kg from their initial mean weight of 71 kg, and the DLCO returned to normal. Pretherapy, patients with hypothyroidism and obesity had hypercapnia (arterial P_{CO_2} 55 mm Hg), hypoxemia (83%

oxygen saturation), and diminished lung volumes, DLCO, peak expiratory flow rate, and maximal voluntary ventilation. After hormone replacement and weight loss, the DLCO, Pa_{CO_2}, and lung volumes returned to normal.

The few studies of resting pulmonary function in nonobese patients with hypothyroidism have found minor abnormalities; they included a decrease in VC, slightly decreased Pa_{O_2}, a decreased DLCO corrected for hemoglobin, and a widened alveolar-arterial (A-a) DO_2 (oxygen partial pressure) gradient. Some researchers propose that microatelectasis that is not radiographically visualized exists and that this results from either respiratory muscle weakness or a deficiency of surfactant; altered muscle function, abnormal surfactant production, or an opening of anatomic shunts in the lung has not been documented.

Exercise Capacity

Many patients with hypothyroidism complain of fatigue and exercise intolerance. These subjective sensations could arise from limited pulmonary reserve, limited cardiac reserve, decreased muscle strength, or increased muscle fatigue. Although there are few clinical studies of exercise in hypothyroid patients, the most detailed study suggested that the primary problem is cardiac limitation resulting from an inability to increase stroke volume (3). Maximal oxygen consumption and workload were diminished significantly, and arterial lactate levels rose more than normal. Abnormalities of blood flow distribution, especially to muscles, also may be present. On return to euthyroid status, some, but not all, exercise parameters returned to normal. For example, the A-a O_2 gradient worsened, and the lactate levels remained high (3).

Hypothyroid rats have decreased endurance. Biochemical changes observed have included decreases in muscle oxidation of pyruvate and palmitate, with more rapid use of glycogen stores and diminished fatty acid mobilization (4), and increased activity of enzymes of glycolysis, the tricarboxylic acid cycle, and fatty acid oxidation in resting diaphragm muscle (5).

Hypothyroidism may reduce the severity of dyspnea in patients with severe chronic obstructive pulmonary disease

TABLE 54.1. PULMONARY CONSEQUENCES OF HYPOTHYROIDISM

Direct effects
  Altered pulmonary function tests
    Increased (A-a) O_2 gradient
    Decreased DLCO (?)
    Decreased maximal exercise capacity
  Depressed ventilatory drives
  Pleural effusions
  Decreased surfactant production in the neonate
  Upper airway obstruction (goiter, enlarged tongue, or
     pharyngeal muscle dysfunction)
  Sleep apnea syndrome, obstructive > central type
Indirect effects
  Phrenic nerve paralysis
  Neuromuscular weakness or dyscoordination (?)
  Obesity causing atelectasis
  Congestive heart failure causing pulmonary edema
  Difficulty in weaning from mechanical ventilation
  Tendency toward theophylline intoxication

A-a, alveolar-arterial; DLCO, diffusing capacity of the lung for carbon monoxide.

(COPD) (6,7). However, these reports provide little information on changes in pulmonary functions, ABG, responses to exercise, or ventilatory drives. One study of 10 euthyroid COPD patients treated with carbimazole in a double-blind crossover trial found no effect on ABG, dyspnea, 12-minute walking distance, or resting minute ventilation (8). It is unknown whether the increased dyspnea with an increase in thyroid hormone results either from greater work of breathing with higher minute ventilation or from a mismatch of increased ventilatory drive to breath more than the augmented ventilatory capacity.

In summary, limited data suggest that decreased stroke volume and cardiac output play greater roles than pulmonary dysfunction in limiting the exercise capacity of hypothyroid patients. The roles of abnormal muscle function, blood flow distribution, and energy metabolism are not yet well defined. Some patients with severe lung disease may have increased dyspnea upon correction of hypothyroidism as a result of increases in either oxygen consumption or ventilatory drive.

VENTILATORY CONTROL

Patients with myxedema coma first were noted to retain CO_2 in the late 1950s (9), and in the mid-1960s diminished ventilatory responses to hypercapnia in hypothyroidism were reported, which improved after thyroid hormone replacement therapy (10,11). This finding led to interest in ventilatory control in hypothyroid patients without myxedema coma.

Ventilatory drive is the net output of the respiratory centers in response to a given physiologic stimulus, as mea-

sured indirectly by examining the change in function of the pulmonary system when the respiratory center input is changed. Ventilatory drive output measured as ventilatory response to either progressive hypercapnia (HCVR) or isocapneic hypoxia (HVR) includes minute ventilation (liters per minute), transdiaphragmatic pressure (Pdi), percentage of inspiratory time per respiratory cycle, diaphragmatic electromyogram (EMG), and inspiratory mouth occlusion pressure in the first 0.1 second (Po.1).

Patients with hypothyroidism have depressed HVR and HCVR (12). In one study, the HVR was more severely depressed in the patients with idiopathic primary hypothyroidism, but both the HVR and HCVR rapidly returned to normal with therapy. In patients with iatrogenic hypothyroidism, the HVR, but not the HCVR, increased significantly after 3 to 9 months of therapy but did not return to normal. Lung volumes and ABGs did not improve with therapy in either group, and muscle weakness was not assessed.

In the largest study, ventilatory drive was decreased in 34% of 38 hypothyroid patients (13). Depressed responses to hypercapnia or hypoxia often did not occur in the same patients. In almost all these patients, ventilatory drive normalized after 1 week of replacement therapy, and HVR often returned more rapidly than HCVR.

A detailed study (14) of 13 patients with severe hypothyroidism identified two abnormal patient subsets with slight overlap: muscle weakness and depressed ventilatory drive. Seven patients had a normal ventilatory drive, but four of them had decreased maximal inspiratory pressures (Pi_{max}). The other six patients had decreased HCVR, as assessed by minute ventilation and diaphragmatic EMG, but only two Pi_{max}. The HCVR increased after thyroid hormone replacement, but Pi_{max} did not increase in patients with low pretreatment values. These results suggest that the low HCVR in some patients is not due to impaired respiratory muscle function, but is more likely a central nervous system effect. The lack of correlation between respiratory muscle strength and ventilatory drive indicates that these abnormalities occur independently and are not directly related.

In summary, patients with hypothyroidism often have depressed HVR or HCVR. Usually, there is rapid reversibility of at least the hypercapneic component with hormone replacement. The mechanism by which thyroid hormone influences ventilatory drive is unknown. It also is unclear why these changes occur only in some patients.

PULMONARY FUNCTION IN MYXEDEMA COMA

The role of pulmonary dysfunction resulting from hypothyroidism in causing myxedema coma is not clearly defined and remains controversial. Not only is coma a rare complication of hypothyroidism, but the analysis of cause and effect is difficult. Depressed ventilatory drive also may result from the central nervous system damage causing coma, obesity–hypoventilation syndrome, chronic CO_2 retention, or sleep apnea. The many other potential precipitants of coma in hypothyroidism include decreased cerebral oxygen delivery, sedative and respiratory depressant drug treatment, hyponatremia, adrenal insufficiency, infection, heart failure, hypoglycemia, and hypothermia (15–17). Because many of these factors occur together in the seriously ill patient, it is difficult to ascribe causality to a single factor. Hypercapnic patients with myxedema coma almost always have at least one other factor causing hypoventilation, such as lung disease, central nervous system disease, neuromuscular weakness, obesity, kyphoscoliosis, or pleural restrictive disease (11, 18).

In summary, all reported cases of myxedema coma with severe CO_2 retention have had at least one additional potential cause for hypoventilation. Although some causes of hypoventilation, such as respiratory depressant drug treatment, are avoidable, most are not. It seems likely that hypothyroidism contributes to coma in some patients by decreasing the HVR and HCVR. Alone, however, it probably is not sufficient to cause CO_2 retention and thereby precipitate myxedema coma. Thus, a careful review of all potential contributing causes of an elevated $PaCO_2$ is worthwhile in the patient with respiratory failure and myxedema coma.

PLEURAL EFFUSIONS

Effusions may occur at many sites in patients with hypothyroidism. Most common among them is the pericardial space, but peritoneal, pleural, middle ear, and uveal effusions also occur (19–21). Whereas pericardial exudative effusions are typical, in the few well-characterized cases with hypothyroidism as the sole cause of pleural effusion, both transudates and exudative pleural effusions are well reported (22). In most patients, congestive heart failure, pericardial effusion, or transdiaphragmatic passage of ascitic fluid contributes to the pleural effusions (22). The pleural effusion in patients with hypothyroidism may be either bilateral or unilateral, it is usually small, and it usually does not cause symptoms (22,23). Chylous effusions occur rarely in hypothyroidism.

The reason effusions occur in patients with hypothyroidism is not well established, but changes in the capillaries may be involved. Extrapulmonary capillary structure is altered in patients with hypothyroidism, with a probable decrease in number, a narrowed diameter (24), and an increase in permeability (25). No histopathologic studies of the pulmonary capillary bed in patients with hypothyroidism have been done.

SLEEP APNEA AND OBESITY–HYPOVENTILATION SYNDROMES

Sleep apnea syndrome (SAS) is prevalent in the population, and obesity is a major predisposition. The three forms of SAS are obstructive, central, and mixed sleep apnea. In obstructive apnea, decreased ventilatory drive is a secondary consequence of the effect of recurrent hypoxia on brain neurochemistry.

Obesity–hypoventilation syndrome (or pickwickian syndrome) is defined as daytime resting hypercapnia while awake and upright in obese individuals with normal pulmonary function and no underlying lung disease. Their diminished ventilatory drive may be a primary pathogenic factor or acquired from a chronic increase in $PaCO_2$, neurologic dysfunction, hypoxemia, or increased work of breathing with an increased ventilatory load.

How are these two disorders related to hypothyroidism? Many patients with myxedema coma described in the 1960s were obese and probably had the obesity–hypoventilation syndrome. It is not surprising that the increased work of breathing and increased CO_2 production rate found in obese patients combine with the diminished HCVR in patients with myxedema to cause CO_2 retention.

Hypothyroidism is a well-recognized cause of obstructive sleep apnea (OSA) (26–28). In all reported cases, the patient's sleep apnea responded to thyroid therapy or weight loss. Sleep apnea may improve with treatment of hypothyroidism without weight change (29). The moderate degree of weight loss with thyroid replacement probably is not sufficient to account for significant improvement in sleep apnea (26). The prevalence of sleep apnea in hypothyroidism is not well defined. Recent studies of 1,000 and 290 sleep clinic found that 1.2% to 2.4% of patients diagnosed with OSA had undiagnosed hypothyroidism (30–32). Conversely, 9 of 11 consecutive patients newly diagnosed with hypothyroidism had sleep apnea, with much worse severity of apnea in the six patients who also were obese (28). All patients improved significantly, with a sixfold reduction in sleep apnea after thyroxine (T_4) replacement, even without weight loss. Ventilatory drive also increased after therapy. Of 26 consecutive Finnish patients with hypothyroidism screened with polysomnography, nocturnal breathing abnormalities were seen in 50% and severe obstructive apnea in 7.7% (29). However, male sex and obesity were stronger independent predictors of nocturnal breathing abnormalities than hypothyroidism.

Hypothyroidism may predispose to upper airway obstruction by several mechanisms: increased size of the tongue and other pharyngeal skeletal muscles, a slow and sustained pharyngeal muscle contraction pattern, or diminished neural output of the respiratory center. Most patients have had an enlarged tongue. Decreased neural output likely plays a role in some patients, because there may be a favorable response to the respiratory stimulant medroxyprogesterone alone (26). One hypothyroid patient with purely central sleep apnea has been reported (33).

UPPER AIRWAY EFFECTS

Minor complaints referable to the upper airway, ear, nose, and throat are common in hypothyroidism. Patients frequently have nasal stuffiness, recurrent colds, voice change, foreign body sensation, and discomfort or dryness of the throat (34). However, it is not proven that these complaints truly are more prevalent in hypothyroidism, and their cause is uncertain. Secretion of nasal mucus may be increased, and 20% of patients have tonsillar enlargement. Although myxedematous thickening of the vocal cords or larynx or stretching of the recurrent laryngeal nerves by an enlarging thyroid gland have been proposed, little evidence supports either theory.

NEUROMUSCULAR DYSFUNCTION

Hypothyroid myopathy may involve the respiratory muscles and the diaphragm, slowing contraction and relaxation and decreasing maximal power. It can occur in either children or adults. In adults, it may be accompanied by an increased muscle volume, in which case it is known as Hoffman's syndrome.

Respiratory muscle dysfunction clinically manifests as hypoventilation, atelectasis, or easy fatigability. Values for many classic pulmonary function tests usually decrease: peak expiratory flow, compliance, DLCO, Pi_{max}, and all lung volumes except residual volume (RV). The RV/TLC ratio increases, and the $PaCO_2$ may be elevated. The most sensitive readily available test of diaphragmatic function is measurement of Pi_{max} and maximal expiratory pressure (Pe_{max}). The Pdi and diaphragmatic EMG are noninvasive methods for early detection of myopathy.

Diaphragm dysfunction resulting from hypothyroidism was reported in the 1980s (35,36). The abnormalities returned toward or to normal with thyroid replacement therapy, although there also was an average 7 kg weight loss. In 43 hypothyroid patients, the mean pretreatment values for VC, forced vital capacity, and forced expiratory volume in 1 second were within the normal range, but each variable increased significantly after thyroid therapy (37). Before treatment, both the Pi_{max} and Pe_{max} were reduced. After 3 months of treatment, there was almost a 50% increase in both pressures, even though only half the patients had normal serum thyrotropin (TSH) concentrations and there was almost no mean weight change. It is difficult to estimate the prevalence of respiratory muscle dysfunction in

hypothyroidism, but this study suggests it may be common. Other respiratory system abnormalities (e.g., obesity, ventilatory drive) need to be looked for carefully in these patients, because they also generate a restrictive physiologic pattern and predispose to hypoventilation and a shallow, rapid respiratory pattern.

The mechanism of thyroid myopathy remains undefined. The activity of muscle 1,4-glucosidase (acid maltase) may be decreased. This enzyme also is deficient in Pompe's disease, the rare, recessive disease of generalized glycogenolysis; these patients may present with acute hypercapneic respiratory failure without glycogen accumulation in the heart, liver, or brain (38). Hamsters have a recessive genetic dystrophy accompanied by abnormal thyroid metabolism, decreased ventilatory drive, and abnormal diaphragm morphology and function (39). Hypothyroidism also may alter the balance of fast and slow muscle fibers in the diaphragm, favoring slow fibers; type I heavy-chain myosin (40,41) shifting the myosin heavy chain isoforms (42), or the expression of peroxisome proliferator–activated receptor gamma coactivator 1-alpha (43). Hypothyroid rats also have significantly reduced maximal shortening velocity, tension, and specific force of the diaphragm.

Two patients with orthopnea and dyspnea on exertion had bilateral phrenic nerve paralysis resulting from hypothyroidism (44). One patient had return of normal phrenic nerve function after 4 months of thyroid hormone therapy. The other patient died in an accident; autopsy revealed demyelination and fibrosis of the phrenic nerves.

In summary, weakness of the diaphragm is likely one of the most common respiratory system abnormalities of hypothyroidism.

MISCELLANEOUS PULMONARY CONSEQUENCES OF HYPOTHYROIDISM

Hypothyroidism slows theophylline metabolism and therefore predisposes patients to theophylline intoxication if they are given usual daily doses (45). Hypothyroidism may limit weaning patients from mechanical ventilation by a combination of the mechanisms discussed previously: decreased VC, respiratory muscle weakness, decreased ventilatory drive, and pleural effusions. Screening of 121 ventilator-dependent patients in a long-term ventilator care unit found four hypothyroid patients (46). The weaning of three of these patients was facilitated by treatment of their hypothyroidism. Finally, the response to sepsis may be altered by hypothyroidism. Rats with hypothyroidism and sepsis had decreased survival, as compared with euthyroid septic rats (30% vs. 65% survival), possibly related to decreases in oxygen consumption (47) or more severe pulmonary edema (48).

LUNG MATURATION AND SURFACTANT PRODUCTION

After the pioneering discovery that glucocorticoids accelerated surfactant production by type II pneumocytes, studies in the early 1970s demonstrated that thyroid hormone accelerates surfactant production and fetal lung maturation (49,50). The role of the thyroid hormones in lung development and their effects of thyroid hormones on type II alveolar epithelial cells are discussed in Chapter 32, but studies important for understanding the consequences of hypothyroidism on developmental lung problems are summarized herein.

Injection of T_4 into rabbit fetuses *in utero* led to earlier appearance of both surface-active material in lung washes and lamellar bodies in type II alveolar epithelial cells (50). Exogenous T_4 given subcutaneously to adult rats for 14 days increased type II cell size, lamellar body size and number, and surfactant per unit wet weight of lung; hypothyroidism led to the converse changes (49). Acceleration of fetal lung maturation and surfactant production occurs in many *in vitro* model systems, including fetal rat lung explants and cultures of mixed fetal rabbit lung cells or fetal type II cells (51,52). The ability of triiodothyronine (T_3) or T_4 to cross the placenta in different species remains controversial, although small quantities of T_4 do so (53). It is not clear whether it is fetal or maternal hormone that may be physiologically important in normal development or whether T_3 or T_4 is involved. A T_4 analogue that readily crosses the placenta, 3,5-dimethyl-3'-isopropyl-l-thyronine, increases fetal rabbit phosphatidylcholine synthesis (54). Exogenous thyrotropin-releasing hormone (TRH) also crosses the placenta. Lung lavage from the fetuses of mothers given TRH displayed increases in phosphatidylcholine, total phospholipids, and the phosphatidylcholine:sphingomyelin ratio (55). The lung tissue itself did not reveal a change in any of these variables, suggesting an effect on surfactant release but not synthesis. Whether or not thyroid hormones affect the production of any of the surfactant apoproteins is uncertain.

Beyond promoting early alveolar development before birth, thyroid hormones modulate postnatal alveolar development. Rat pups given exogenous T_3 postnatally have a greater than normal increase in their alveolar gas exchange surface area and the surface:volume ratio, whereas postnatal propylthiouracil (PTU) has the opposite effect (56).

Other hormones interact with thyroid hormones to influence lung development. Thyroid hormones may potentiate glucocorticoid promotion of surfactant and lung maturation (57–60). In fetal sheep, the β-adrenergic-induced increase in lung liquid resorption that normally occurs before birth is inhibited by fetal thyroidectomy (61). *In vitro*, dexamethasone, T_3, and theophylline synergistically promote phospholipid release in organ cultures of fetal rat lung explants (60,62), human lung explants (62,63), and

fetal rat cells *in vitro* (57). This combined effect is faster and greater than the impact of glucocorticoids alone (59).

Although thyroid hormones can affect lung lipid biosynthesis, their physiologic roles in normal lung maturation and surfactant synthesis are not clear and may differ at different ages. The responsible form of the hormone also is uncertain. In the adult, this is likely to be T_3 rather than T_4, because high-affinity nuclear receptors for T_3 exist in lung cells (55,64). T_3 stimulates transcription and activity of the key surfactant phospholipid synthesis enzyme cholinephosphotransferase (65) and may act at other biochemical loci. Finally, the effects of thyroid hormones could be exerted indirectly, such as serving as a permissive factor in the regulation of lung β-adrenergic receptors (66), or potentiating the action of glucocorticoids or fibroblast-pneumocyte factor. Multiple steps in type II pneumocyte development and surfactant synthesis likely are regulated in a complex and interactive fashion by different hormones, including thyroid hormones.

In summary, there is good *in vitro* evidence for thyroid hormone stimulation of type II pneumocyte differentiation and function in the fetus and adult. The *in vivo* physiologic significance of thyroid hormones in this role, however, apart from interactions with glucocorticoids, is not yet clear for any age group. Their significance may depend on the stage of lung development.

RESPIRATORY DISTRESS SYNDROME OF THE NEWBORN

The stimulation of surfactant production by type II pneumocytes by thyroid hormones raises the question of whether hypothyroidism *in utero* or in the early postnatal period contributes to the pathogenesis of respiratory distress syndrome (RDS) in preterm infants. Preterm infants at less than 30 weeks have lower initial and postnatal surge thyroid hormone levels than full-term infants (67). Early studies supported an association of hypothyroidism with an increased frequency of RDS. Cord serum values for total T_4 and free T_4 index were lower in premature infants with RDS than in premature infants without RDS (68). In premature infants born at 33 to 37 weeks with and without RDS, those with RDS had lower values for serum T_3, and free T_3 index; serum TSH levels and the T_4:T_3 ratio were increased, but the free T_4 index was unchanged (69). The same investigators later reconfirmed these results, except that the postnatal TSH surge in infants with RDS was less than that in control infants of the same gestational age (70).

Other data raised uncertainty about the physiologic significance of these associations. Klein and colleagues found that the initial cord serum TSH levels and the increases after birth were the same in RDS and normal premature infants, although the increase was less than that seen in mature-term infants (71,72). The reverse T$_3$ level gradually increased after birth only in the infants with RDS. A later case control study (73) showed a lower cord serum T$_3$ level at birth in the infants with RDS but no difference in serum total, reverse T$_3$, or TSH levels. Lower fetal and neonatal T$_3$ levels may have been due to altered peripheral thyroid hormone metabolism associated with nonthyroidal illness, rather than hypothyroidism, given the lack of an elevated serum TSH level. The incidence of RDS has not been explained as a function of maternal thyroid status. Thus, the role of fetal hypothyroidism predisposing to RDS is uncertain.

Treatment with thyroid hormone for prevention of RDS in high-risk premature infants has been studied. In a small number of infants, intra-amniotic injection of 200 μg of T$_4$ was performed in eight mothers with nine fetuses at high-risk for RDS who required early delivery (73). In seven of eight cases, repeat amniocentesis yielded fluid with improved parameters of fetal lung maturity. None of the nine fetuses developed RDS, but no control group was included in this study. Eighteen mothers with severe toxemia of pregnancy received intra-amniotic injections of T$_4$ for immature amniotic lipid profiles (74). Within 24 hours, the lecithin:sphingomyelin ratios of the amniotic fluid increased at least twofold in all cases. Only one child died, and none of the others had RDS. In a recent randomized trial of postnatal oral or intravenous T$_4$ treatment of 49 newborns less than 32 weeks' gestation, there was no benefit of T$_4$ on chronic lung disease or other complications of prematurity (75).

Another important question is whether there is an additive or synergistic effect on lung maturation when thyroid hormone and glucocorticoids are given in combination. *In vitro* studies suggest that there may be little additive benefit in midgestation. Thyroid hormone also may have adverse effects, slowing increases in lung glycogen stores (76) and antioxidant enzymes (77). Inhibition of thyroid hormone synthesis with PTU in premature rats increased their antioxidant enzymes and promoted survival in hyperoxia (78). In contrast, considerable experimental data suggest that combined use of thyroid hormone and glucocorticoids accelerates lung epithelial maturation, surfactant production, and surfactant release (79). Two early randomized clinical trials used maternal antenatal treatment with TRH combined with glucocorticoids. Combined therapy reduced adverse outcomes, including ventilator days and bronchopulmonary dysplasia (80,81). However, despite these encouraging results, large trials of combining either TRH or T$_3$ with glucocorticoids have not shown large clinical benefits thus far. The North American TRH Study Group found that antenatal maternal administration of TRH and glucocorticoids was not more beneficial in reducing infant RDS, death, or chronic lung disease than treatment with glucocorticoids alone (82). Infants of TRH-treated mothers had reduced postnatal surge in

serum TSH and T$_3$ concentrations, but recovered within 28 days. The THORN trial of T$_3$ and hydrocortisone treatment of preterm infants of less than 30 weeks' gestation did not demonstrate outcome benefits of T$_3$ treatment, but higher serum free T$_3$ or T$_4$ levels were statistically associated with better outcome (83). Despite these discouraging results, intra-amniotic combined therapy enhances lung maturation in the preterm rhesus fetal monkey compared with maternal injection (84). Thus, studies of combined treatment should not yet be abandoned.

The complex interactions of thyroid hormones with multiple other hormone systems during fetal lung development are not yet well defined. Clearly, thyroid hormones can influence development of the lung and the response to prematurity, but to affect development favorably, the degree of benefit, optimal timing, and best agent for exogenous stimulation of the fetal thyroid axis need to be determined. Clinical studies thus far do not support an additive or synergistic effect of combined thyroid axis and glucocorticoid treatment. Because complications of perinatal glucocorticoid therapy are being appreciated, there still is a potential role for thyroid hormone prevention or treatment of the lung disease of prematurity.

REFERENCES

1. Hall R, Scanlon MF. Hypothyroidism: clinical features and complications. *Clin Endocrinol Metab* 1979;8:29.
2. Wilson WR, Bedell GN. The pulmonary abnormalities in myxedema. *J Clin Invest* 960;39:42.
3. Burack R, Edwards RHT, Green M, et al. The response to exercise before and after treatment of myxedema with thyroxine. *J Pharmacol Exp Ther* 1971;176:212.
4. Baldwin KM, Hooker AM, Herrick RE, et al. Respiratory capacity and glycogen depletion in thyroid deficient muscle. *J Appl Physiol* 1980;49:102.
5. Ianuzzo CD, Chen V, O'Brien P, et al. Effect of experimental dysthyroidism on the enzymatic character of the diaphragm. *J Appl Physiol* 1984;56:117.
6. Bercu BA, Mandell HN. Radioactive iodine for chronic lung disease [Abstract]. *J Clin Invest* 1954;33:917.
7. Hurst A, Levine MH, Rich DR. Radioactive iodine in the management of patients with severe emphysema. *Ann Allergy* 1955;13:393.
8. Butland RJA, Pang JA, Geddes DM. Carbimazole and exercise tolerance in chronic airflow obstruction. *Thorax* 1982;37:64.
9. Nordqvist P, Dhuner KG, Stenberg K, et al. Myxedema coma and CO2 retention. *Acta Med Scand* 1960;166:189.
10. Massumi RA, Winnacker JL. Severe depression of the respiratory center in myxedema. *Am J Med* 1964;36:876.
11. Weg JG, Calverly JR, Johnson C. Hypothyroidism and alveolar hypoventilation. *Arch Intern Med* 1965;115:302.
12. Zwillich CW, Pierson DJ, Hofeldt FD, et al. Ventilatory control in myxedema and hypothyroidism. *N Engl J Med* 1975;292:662.
13. Ladenson PW, Goldenheim PD, Ridgway EC. Prediction and reversal of blunted ventilatory responsiveness in patients with hypothyroidism. *Am J Med* 1988;84:877.
14. Duranti R, Gheri RG, Gorini M, et al. Control of breathing in patients with severe hypothyroidism. *Am J Med* 1993;95:29.

15. Blum M. Myxedema coma. *Am J Med Sci* 1972;264:432.
16. Forester CF. Coma in myxedema. *Arch Intern Med* 1963;111:100.
17. Royce PC. Severely impaired consciousness in myxedema: a review. *Am J Med Sci* 1971;261:46.
18. Domm BM, Vassallo CL. Myxedema coma with respiratory failure. *Am Rev Respir Dis* 1973;107:842.
19. Marzullo ER, Franco S. Myxedema with multiple serous effusions and cardiac involvement (myxedema heart). *Am Heart J* 1939;17:360.
20. Schneierson SJ, Katz M. Solitary pleural effusion due to myxedema. *JAMA* 1958;168:1003.
21. Sachdev Y, Hall R. Effusions into body cavities in hypothyroidism. *Lancet* 1975;1:564.
22. Gottehrer A, Roa J, Stanford G, et al. Hypothyroidism and pleural effusions. *Chest* 1990;98:1130.
23. Brown SD, Brashear RE, Schnute RB. Pleural effusion in a young woman with myxedema. *Arch Intern Med* 1983;143:1458.
24. Zondek H, Michael M, Kaatz A. The capillaries in myxedema. *Am J Med Sci* 1941;202:435.
25. Lange K. Capillary permeability in myxedema. *Am J Med Sci* 1944;208:5.
26. Orr WC, Males JL, Imes NK. Myxedema and obstructive sleep apnea. *Am J Med* 1981;70:1061.
27. Skatrud J, Iber C, Ewart R, et al. Disordered breathing during sleep in hypothyroidism. *Am Rev Respir Dis* 1981;124:325.
28. Rajagopal KR, Albrecht PH, Derderian SS, et al. Obstructive sleep apnea in hypothyroidism. *Ann Intern Med* 1984;101:491.
29. Pelttari L, Rauhala E, Polo O, et al. Upper airway obstruction in hypothyroidism. *J Intern Med* 1994;236:177.
30. Kapur VK, Koepsell TD, deMaine J, et al. Association of hypothyroidism and obstructive sleep apnea. *Am J Respir Crit Care Med* 1998;158:1379–1383.
31. Mickelson SA, Lian T, Rosenthal L. Thyroid testing and thyroid hormone replacement in patients with sleep disordered breathing. *ENTechnology* 1999;78(10):768–771, 774–775.
32. Skjodt NM, Atkar R, Easton PA. Screening for hypothyroidism in sleep apnea. *Am J Respir Crit Care Med* 1999;160:732–735.
33. Millman RP, Bevilacqua J, Peterson DD, et al. Central sleep apnea in hypothyroidism. *Am Rev Respir Dis* 1983;127:504.
34. Gupta OP, Bhatia PL, Agarwal MK, et al. Nasal, pharyngeal, and laryngeal manifestations of hypothyroidism. *Ear Nose Throat J* 1977;56:349.
35. Laroche CM, Cairns T, Moxham J, et al. Hypothyroidism presenting with respiratory muscle weakness. *Am Rev Respir Dis* 1988;138:472.
36. Martinez FJ, Bermudez-Gomez M, Celli BR. Hypothyroidism: a reversible cause of diaphragmatic dysfunction. *Chest* 1989;96:1059.
37. Siafakas NM, Salesiotou V, Filaditaki V. Respiratory muscle strength in hypothyroidism. *Chest* 1992;102:189.
38. Rosenow EC, Engel AG. Acid maltase deficiency in adults presenting as respiratory failure. *Am J Med* 1978;64:485.
39. Schlenker EH, Burbach, JA. Thyroxine affects ventilation, lung morphometry and necrosis of diaphragm in dystrophic hamsters. *Am J Physiol* 1995;268:R779.
40. Gosselin LE, Zhan W-Z, Sieck GC. Hypothyroid-mediated changes in adult rat diaphragm muscle contractile properties and MHC isoform expression. *J Appl Physiol* 1996;80:1934.
41. Herb RA, Powers SK, Criswell DS, et al. Alterations in phenotypic and contractile properties of the rat diaphragm: influence of hypothyroidism. *J Appl Physiol* 1996;80:2163.
42. Caiozzo VJ, Haddad F, Baker M, et al. MHC polymorphism in rodent plantaris muscle: effects of mechanical overload and hypothyroidism. *Am J Physiol (Cell)* 2000;278:C709–C717.
43. Irrcher I, Adhihetty PJ, Sheehan DA, et al. PPARgamma coactivator-1 alpha expression during thyroid hormone– and contractile activity–induced mitochondrial adaptations. *Am J Physiol (Cell)* 2003;284:C1669.
44. Hamly FH, Timms RM, Mihn VD, et al. Bilateral phrenic paralysis in myxedema [Abstract]. *Am Rev Respir Dis* 1975;111:911.
45. Aderka D, Shavit G, Garfinkel D, et al. Life-threatening theophylline intoxication in a hypothyroid patient. *Respiration* 1985;44:77.
46. Pandya K, Lal C, Scheinhorn D, et al. Hypothyroidism and ventilator dependency. *Arch Intern Med* 1989;149:2115.
47. Moley JR, Ohkawa M, Chaudry IH, et al. Hypothyroidism abolishes the hyperdymanic phase and increases susceptibility to sepsis. *J Surg Res* 1984;36:265.
48. Dulchavsky SA, Hendrick SR, Dutta S. Pulmonary biophysical effects of triiodothyronine augmentation during sepsis-induced hypothyroidism. *J Trauma* 1993;35:104.
49. Redding RA, Douglas WHJ, Stein M. Thyroid hormone influence on lung surfactant metabolism. *Science* 1972;175:994.
50. Wu B, Kikkawa Y, Drzaleski MM, et al. The effect of thyroxine on the maturation of fetal rabbit lungs. *Biol Neonate* 1973;22:161.
51. Ballard PL, Hovey ML, Gonzales LK. Thyroid hormone stimulation of phosphatidylcholine synthesis in cultured fetal rabbit lung. *J Clin Invest* 1984;74:898.
52. Rooney SA, Marino PA, Bogran LI, et al. Thyrotropin-releasing hormone increases the amount of surfactant in lung lavage from fetal rabbits. *Pediatr Res* 1979;13:623.
53. Burrow GN, Fisher DA, Larsen PR. Maternal and fetal thyroid function. *N Engl J Med* 1994;331:1072.
54. Ballard PL, Benson BJ, Bichjen A, et al. Transplacental stimulation of lung development in the fetal rabbits by 3,5-dimethyl, 3'-isopropyl-l-thyronine. *J Clin Invest* 1980;65:1407.
55. Hitchcock KR. Hormones and the lung. I. Thyroid hormones and glucocorticoids in lung development. *Anat Rec* 1979;194:15.
56. Massaro D, Teich N, Massaro GD. Postnatal development of pulmonary alveoli: modulation in rats by thyroid hormones. *Am J Physiol* 1986;250:R51.
57. Gross I, Dynia DW, Wilson CM, et al. Glucocorticoid–thyroid hormone interactions in fetal rat lung. *Pediatr Res* 1984;18:191.
58. Smith BT, Sabry K. Glucocorticoid-thyroid synergism in lung maturation: a mechanism involving epithelial-mesenchymal interaction. *Proc Natl Acad Sci USA* 1983;80:1951.
59. Ballard PL. Combined hormonal treatment and lung maturation. *Semin Perinatol* 1984;8:283.
60. Gonzales LW, et al. Glucocorticoids and thyroid hormone stimulate biochemical and morphological differentiation of human fetal lung in organ culture. *J Clin Endocrinol Metab* 1986;62:687.
61. Barker PM, Brown MJ, Ramsden CA, et al. The effect of thyroidectomy in the fetal sheep on lung liquid reabsorption induced by adrenaline or cyclic AMP. *J Physiol* 1988;407:373.
62. Gross I, Wilson CM. Fetal lung in organ culture. IV. Supra-additive hormone interactions. *J Appl Physiol* 1982;52:1421.
63. Gross I, Wilson CM, Ingleson LD, et al. Fetal lung in organ culture. III. Comparison of dexamethasone, thyroxine, and methylxanthines. *J Appl Physiol* 1980;48:872.
64. Gonzales VW, Ballard PL. Identification and characterizations of nuclear T$_3$-binding sites in fetal human lung. *J Clin Endocrinol Metab* 1981;53:21.
65. Chatterjee D, Mukherjee S, Das SK. Regulation of cholinephosphotransferase by thyroid hormone. *Biochem Biophys Res Commun* 2001;282:861.
66. Whitsett J, Darovec-Beckerman C, Manton M, et al. Thyroid dependent maturation of adrenergic receptors in the rat lung. *Biochem Biophys Res Commun* 1980;97:913.
67. Biswas S, Buffery J, Enoch H. et al. A longitudinal assessment of thyroid hormone concentrations in preterm infants younger than 30 weeks' gestation during the first 2 weeks of life and their relationship to outcome. *Pediatrics* 2002;109(2):222.

68. Redding RA, Pereira C. Thyroid function in respiratory distress syndrome of the newborn. *Pediatrics* 1974;54:423.

69. Cuestas RA, Lindall A, Engel RR. Low thyroid hormones and respiratory distress syndrome of the newborn: studies on cord blood. *N Engl J Med* 1976;295:297.

70. Cuestas RA, Engel RR. Thyroid function in preterm infants with respiratory distress syndrome. *J Pediatr* 1979;94:643.

71. Klein AH, Stinson D, Foley B, et al. Thyroid function studies in pre-term infants recovering from the respiratory distress syndrome. *J Pediatr* 1977;91:261.

72. Klein AH, Foley B, Foley TP, et al. Thyroid function studies in cord blood from premature infants with and without respiratory distress syndrome. *J Pediatr* 1981;98:818.

73. Mashiach S, Barkai G, Sack J, et al. Enhancement of fetal lung maturity by intraamniotic administration of thyroid hormone. *Am J Obstet Gynecol* 1979;130:289.

74. Veszelovszky I, Nagy ZB, Bodis L. Effects of intraamniotically administered thyroxine on acceleration of fetal pulmonary maturity in preeclamptic toxemia. *J Perinatol Med* 1986;14:227.

75. Smith LM, Leake RD, Berman N, et al. Postnatal thyroxine supplementation in infants less than 32 weeks' gestation: effects on pulmonary morbidity. *J Perinatol* 2000;20:427.

76. Rooney SA, Gobran LI, Chu AJ. Thyroid hormone opposes some glucocorticoid effects on glycogen content and lipid synthesis in developing fetal rat lung. *Pediatr Res* 1986;20:545.

77. Sosenko IRS, Frank L. Thyroid inhibition and developmental increases in fetal rat lung antioxidant enzymes. *Am J Physiol* 1989;257:L94.

78. Chen Y, Sosenko IRS, Frank L. Premature rats treated with propylthiouracil show enhanced pulmonary antioxidant enzyme gene expression and improved survival during prolonged exposure to hyperoxia. *Pediatr Res* 1995;38:292.

79. Liggins, GC. Thyrotrophin-releasing hormone and lung maturation. *Reprod Fertil Dev* 1995;7:443.

80. NIH Consensus Panel. Effect of corticosteroids for fetal maturation on perinatal outcomes. *JAMA* 1995;273:413.

81. Moya FR, Gross I. Combined hormonal therapy for the prevention of respiratory distress syndrome and its consequences. *Semin Perinatol* 1993;17:267.

82. Ballard RA, Ballard PL, Cnaan A, et al. Antenatal thyrotropin-releasing hormone to prevent lung disease in preterm infants. *N Engl J Med* 1998; 338:493.

83. Biswas S, Buffery J, Enoch H, et al. Pulmonary effects of T_3 and hydrocortisone supplementation in preterm infants less than 30 weeks gestation: results of the THORN trial—thyroid hormone replacement in neonates. *Pediatr Res* 2003;53:48.

84. Gilbert WM, Eby-Wilkens E, Plopper C, et al. Fetal monkey surfactants after intra-amniotic or maternal administration of betamethasone and thyroid hormone. *Obstet Gynecol* 2001;98:466.

55

THE KIDNEYS AND ELECTROLYTE METABOLISM IN HYPOTHYROIDISM

ELAINE M. KAPTEIN

Hypothyroidism, particularly severe primary hypothyroidism, is associated with multiple alterations in cardiovascular function, renal hemodynamics, and renal tubular reabsorption, as well as endocrine and metabolic alterations. Renal function is altered due to a combination of direct and indirect effects of hypothyroidism on the kidney (Fig. 55.1). The direct effects relate to alterations in glomerular and tubular function, and the indirect effects to changes in cardiovascular hemodynamics. Reversible alterations in sodium and water, calcium, phosphate, vitamin D, and uric acid homeostasis also occur.

HEMODYNAMIC CHANGES

Patients with hypothyroidism have decreases in myocardial contractility and cardiac output, and in peripheral oxygen consumption, with an increase in peripheral vascular resistance (see Chapter 53). These changes result in hypertension, decreased renal blood flow, and decreased glomerular filtration (1–3). The increase in peripheral vascular resistance is caused by a combination of decreased relaxation of vascular smooth muscle cells, increased catecholamine activity, and decreased effective blood volume (3). Plasma renin activity is decreased, and serum concentrations of endothelin-1 (vasoconstricting) and adrenomedullin (vasodilating) are normal (3). Hypothyroidism attenuates the responsiveness of resistance vessels to the endothelium-dependent vasodilator acetylcholine (4).

Nitric oxide is an important regulator of vascular tone, renal sodium excretion, and the pressure diuresis-natriuresis response (4) and, therefore, arterial blood pressure. In rats with hypothyroidism, nitric oxide synthase activity is decreased in large vessels, which may contribute to the increase in peripheral vascular resistance and decrease in responsiveness to acetylcholine in hypothyroidism (4).

RENAL TUBULAR FUNCTION

Hypothyroidism is associated with decreased renal tubular reabsorption of several solutes. In rats, fractional excretion of sodium is increased, despite renal vasoconstriction and a decrease in glomerular filtration rate, due to decreased Na^+, K^+-ATPase activity, and reduced activity of transporter proteins (5) (Fig. 55.1). In humans with hypothyroidism, the fractional excretion of sodium also is increased, whereas fractional excretion of potassium is decreased; in one study there was a 22% decrease that was reversed during thyroxine (T_4) therapy (6). The increase in sodium excretion is due to decreased proximal tubular sodium reabsorption and decreased Na^+,K^+ pump activity in the collecting tubules (6,7). Na^+,H^+ exchange activity (amiloride-sensitive Na^+ and H^+ flux) in brush border membrane vesicles of proximal tubular cells also is decreased in hypothyroid rats (8,9). The Na^+,H^+ exchanger is responsible for the largest portion of sodium transport in this segment of the nephron. The function of other sodium-dependent transporters also is decreased; for example, the Na^+-dependent transport of adenosine is decreased in brush border membrane vesicles (10).

Hypothyroid rats have other defects of renal tubular function. For example, renal responsiveness to arginine vasopressin is decreased, primarily in the medullary portion of the thick ascending limb of the loop of Henle (11,12). As a result, generation of a hypertonic medullary interstitium is impaired (12), which impairs generation of free water and reduces maximal urine concentrating ability. These defects are corrected by thyroid hormone (11–14). Patients with hypothyroidism also have decreased free water and osmolar clearance (6) and decreased renal responsiveness to parathyroid hormone (15), which are reversed by T_4 therapy.

Threats to sodium balance include a decrease in glomerular filtration, and hence in the filtered load of sodium, and changes in sodium intake. Normally, these changes are counterbalanced by appropriate alterations in glomerulotubular balance, autoregulation of the glomerular filtration rate, the activity of the renin–angiotensin–aldosterone system, and redistribution of blood flow to individual nephrons. In hypothyroid rats, plasma renin activity, plasma angiotensin concentrations, and serum aldosterone concentrations are low (16). Similarly, patients with hypothyroidism often have low plasma renin activity and serum aldosterone concentrations, which normalize with T_4 ther-

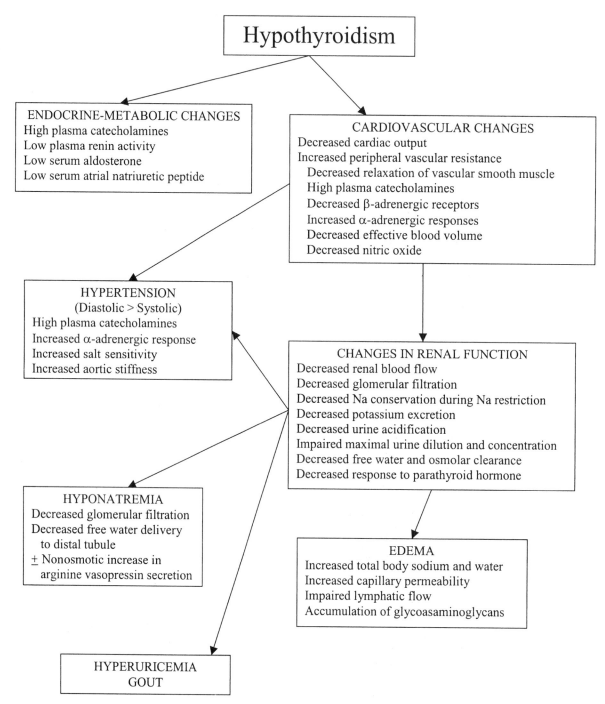

FIGURE 55.1. Diagram of the cardiovascular and other changes affecting renal function in patients with hypothyroidism.

apy (6,17,18). Perhaps as a result of the hormonal changes, or because of decreased sodium reabsorption caused by defects in sodium transport, hypothyroid animals and patients have an impaired ability to conserve sodium during sodium restriction (13,19–21). Serum atrial natriuretic peptide concentrations are low (6,22–24). The natriuretic response to a saline load is exaggerated (23).

GLOMERULAR FUNCTION

The hemodynamic changes of hypothyroidism, notably decreased cardiac output and increased peripheral resistance, lead to decreases in glomerular filtration rate (by 20% to 30%) and effective renal plasma flow (by 25%) (1,2,6). Other factors contributing to the decrease in glomerular filtration rate are low serum atrial natriuretic peptide concentrations, afferent renal arteriolar constriction, and thickening of the glomerular basement membrane (2). Micropuncture studies have revealed a marked reduction in single-nephron glomerular filtration rate in thyroidectomized rats, due to decreased renal plasma flow, increased vascular resistance of both afferent and efferent arterioles, and reduced glomerular ultrafiltration coefficient, which were reversed with inhibition of generation of angiotensin II (19). Activation of adenosine-A1 receptors also may contribute to the changes (25).

In a group of elderly patients with long-standing hypothyroidism (mean age, 63 years), the mean creatinine clearance was 62 mL/min, and 54% had serum creatinine concentrations above 1.2 mg/dL (106 μ*M*) (1). After treatment with T_4 for 2 months, their mean creatinine clearance increased to 90 mL/min, and their mean serum creatinine concentration was 0.9 mg/dL (80 μ*M*). In a group of young women with hypothyroidism (mean age, 31 years), the mean creatinine clearance was 97 mL/min, and it increased to 118 mL/min after treatment with T_4 for 4 months; their mean serum creatinine concentrations decreased from 0.8 to 0.7 mg/dL (71–62 μ*M*) during the same interval (6).

Similar changes occur in patients with hypothyroidism of short duration. Among 128 athyreotic patients with thyroid carcinoma in whom T_4 therapy was stopped for 4 weeks, 19% had high serum creatinine concentrations (26). Similarly, the mean serum creatinine concentration was 1.2 mg/dL (106 μM) in 24 athyreotic patients 2 weeks after withdrawal of T_4, and it decreased to 0.9 mg/dL (80 μ*M*) after resumption of therapy (27). These small but significant increases in serum creatinine concentrations induced by acute hypothyroidism are associated with significant decreases in glomerular filtration rate, which in turn may result in a decrease in radioiodine clearance (28). Thus, unless formal dosimetry studies are performed, larger than intended doses of radioactivity may be delivered to the gastrointestinal tract, salivary glands, and bone marrow when radioiodine is given to patients with thyroid carcinoma after T_4 withdrawal (see section Radioiodine and Other Treatments and Outcomes in Chapter 70) (28).

In patients with chronic renal failure, hypothyroidism may result in deterioration of renal function, which improves during T_4 therapy (29,30). Thus, serum thyrotropin (TSH) should be measured in patients with unexplained deterioration in renal function to rule out hypothyroidism.

Many patients with hypothyroidism have high serum myoglobin and creatine kinase concentrations, thought to be due to increased release from muscle and slowed clearance from the circulation (see Chapter 63). Rare patients with hypothyroidism who had the sudden, seemingly spontaneous, onset of rhabdomyolysis and acute renal failure have been described (31–34).

HYPERTENSION

In a study of 688 patients with hypertension, 3.6% had previously unrecognized hypothyroidism (35). Among different groups of patients with hypothyroidism, 10% to 40% had hypertension, predominantly diastolic hypertension (36–38). In one study of patients with hypothyroidism and hypertension, T_4 treatment lowered diastolic blood pressure to below 90 mm Hg in all patients who were under 45 years of age, but in only 23% of the older patients (39). Others have found no significant change in blood pressure during hypothyroidism, as compared with T_4 therapy for 4 months (6).

Mechanisms that might contribute to hypertension in patients with hypothyroidism include activation of the autonomic nervous system, increased activity of the renin–angiotensin–aldosterone system, increased sensitivity to salt, increased vascular reactivity and compliance, and decreased renal function. In a study of patients with thyroid carcinoma in whom T_4 therapy was stopped for 6 weeks, one third had hypertension. In the group as a whole, mean daytime systolic blood pressure increased by 5 to 126 mm Hg, and daytime diastolic blood pressure increased by 8 to 85 mm Hg, whereas nighttime values did not change (38). Plasma norepinephrine concentrations increased 1.9-fold, and plasma epinephrine concentrations increased 2.0-fold. Plasma renin activity did not change, but serum aldosterone and cortisol concentrations decreased during hypothyroidism.

Patients with hypothyroidism have a decreased response to β-adrenergic stimulation, despite high plasma catecholamine concentrations, due to a decreased number of β-adrenergic receptors; they have increased responses to α-adrenergic stimulation, which may contribute to the increased peripheral vascular resistance and hypertension of hypothyroidism (36).

Intravascular volume, plasma volume, and red cell mass are decreased in patients with hypothyroidism (2). Furthermore, in one study 52% of hypothyroid patients had salt-sensitive hypertension, as compared with 24% of normal subjects, and salt restriction lowered diastolic pressure in the patients (37). This suggests that hypothyroidism increases the blood pressure response to salt restriction. Hypothyroid patients with salt-resistant hypertension had slightly higher plasma renin activity during sodium restriction, whereas their serum aldosterone and atrial natriuretic peptide and plasma arginine vasopressin concentrations were similar before and after salt restriction (37). The response of blood pressure to sodium restriction may relate to activity of the sympathetic nervous system.

In addition to the factors cited above, the predominance of diastolic hypertension in patients with hypothyroidism may be caused by increased aortic stiffness, as measured by echocardiography in one study (36). During T_4 therapy, the patients in this study had a decrease in aortic stiffness as well as systemic vascular resistance, and 50% of them became normotensive.

HYPONATREMIA

Hyponatremia is an occasional finding in patients with hypothyroidism, mostly in patients with severe primary hypothyroidism or myxedema coma (Fig. 55.1) (see Chapter 65) (40). In one study it was twice as common in patients who also had high serum creatinine concentrations, as compared with those in whom serum creatinine concentrations were normal (1). Among athyreotic patients in whom T_4 therapy was stopped for 5 weeks, 4% had hyponatremia (serum sodium concentration, <135 mEq/L) (26). However, in a survey of hyponatremia in a large hospital, the frequency of hyponatremia was similar in patients with hypothyroidism and in all other patients (41). In patients with hypopituitarism who have hyponatremia, it is nearly always associated with corticotropin deficiency and is corrected by glucocorticoid, not thyroid, replacement therapy (42).

When present, hyponatremia in hypothyroidism has been attributed to water retention. Patients with hypothyroidism, whether or not they have hyponatremia, have diminished ability to excrete free water, impaired maximum urinary dilution, and delayed excretion of a water load (43,44). In one study of water loading in patients with hypothyroidism, maximum urinary flow was 51%, free water clearance was 39%, and minimum urinary osmolality was 186% of the values in normal subjects (44).

The major postulated causes for these changes are decreased renal blood flow and glomerular filtration rate. Some patients have had inappropriately high plasma vasopressin concentrations (43), but most have not (1,45). Indeed, in several studies of patients with mild to moderately severe hypothyroidism, plasma arginine vasopressin concentrations were low both before and after oral water loading, during which the patients had a low rate of free water clearance and low serum osmolality; these abnormalities were reversed by T_4 therapy (44,46). These changes in water metabolism may be caused by increased renal sensitivity to arginine vasopressin, decreased free water delivery to the distal tubules, or functional abnormalities of the distal tubules. Infusion of 5% hypertonic saline over 120 minutes in hypothyroid patients raised plasma arginine vasopressin concentrations, but to a lesser extent than in normal subjects, despite similar increases in serum osmolality; this abnormality normalized during T_4 therapy (46). There were no differences in basal or stimulated serum atrial natriuretic peptide concentrations, plasma renin activity, or serum aldosterone concentrations in the patients with hypothyroidism and the normal subjects, and the serum os-

molality values associated with perception of thirst and an increase in arginine vasopressin secretion were similar in the two groups (46).

Among hypothyroid patients and euthyroid patients with chronic renal disease who had comparable decreases in glomerular filtration rate, both had decreased proximal tubular sodium reabsorption and increased distal tubular sodium reabsorption (beyond the loop of Henle) (47). Maximal urinary flow rate and free water clearance were similarly reduced in both groups of patients. Proximal sodium reabsorption and maximal urinary volume were directly correlated with the glomerular filtration rates, and distal sodium reabsorption was proportionate to delivery of sodium from the proximal tubule. Thus, abnormalities in sodium and water handling in hypothyroidism may be a direct consequence of decreased glomerular filtration. In both normal rats and rats with congenital hypothalamic diabetes insipidus, hypothyroidism impairs free water excretion and reduces inulin, free water, and sodium clearance (48). When distal delivery of sodium is increased by an intravenous infusion of a carbonic anhydrase inhibitor or by removal of one kidney, free water clearance increases greatly. Thus, the major cause of diminished water excretion is a reduction in glomerular filtration rate, which limits delivery of glomerular filtrate to distal diluting segments and thus impairs the ability to create and excrete free water.

High plasma arginine vasopressin concentrations in hypothyroid patients, when present (43), are most likely due to nonosmotic stimuli, such as low cardiac output or decreased blood volume (6,46,49,50). In a group of hypothyroid patients studied before and during T_4 therapy, the mean serum sodium concentration increased from 136 to 142 mEq/L, whereas mean serum osmolality increased from 286 to 291 mosmol/kg H_2O; the mean plasma arginine vasopressin concentration was slightly increased [8.3 pg/mL (7.6 pM)], and it decreased to 3.2 pg/ml (2.9 pM) during T_4 therapy (6). Free water clearance was impaired during hypothyroidism, and it increased from −1.03 to +0.89 mL/min during therapy (6). There was no correlation between plasma arginine vasopressin concentrations and serum osmolality, supporting the suggestion that nonosmotic factors are responsible for any excess arginine vasopressin secretion in patients with hypothyroidism.

EDEMA

Edema is a common manifestation of hypothyroidism (Fig. 55.1). A few patients have myxedema, nonpitting edema of the hands, feet, and face, especially the eyelids. Many more note mild swelling of their hands and feet, which may or may not be pitting. These changes resolve in response to T_4 therapy. Patients with hypothyroidism have an increase in total body sodium and water content (44). Protein-rich fluid accumulates most commonly in subcutaneous tissues, but at times as a pericardial or pleural effusion or ascites (51).

The edema in patients with myxedema has multiple causes, including increased capillary permeability, impaired lymphatic flow, and sodium retention, as well as accumulation of hydrophilic glycosaminoglycans in the interstitial space (myxedema). Increased transcapillary escape of albumin during hypothyroidism was suggested by the finding that plasma volumes in hypothyroid patients, as determined by dilution of radiolabeled albumin over 30 minutes, were 13% higher than when measured using labeled red blood cells, whereas values were similar using these two methods after euthyroidism was achieved during T_4 therapy (2). These results confirmed previous studies using radiolabeled albumin that indicated that patients with hypothyroidism have large extravascular accumulations of albumin and presumably other proteins (50).

The interstitial fluid of the skin and muscle is the major site of albumin accumulation, possibly as a result of decreased barrier function of endothelial cells, leading to an increase in the transcapillary escape of albumin (50,52). This extravascular escape of albumin during hypothyroidism is reversed by T_4 (2). Furthermore, the transcapillary escape rate of albumin and extravascular albumin mass are higher in hypothyroid patients than in those with other causes of edema, and the albumin transit time through the extravascular space is lower, suggesting absence of a compensatory increase in lymphatic drainage in hypothyroidism (50). Thus, decreased renal function, increased transcapillary escape rates for plasma proteins such as albumin, plus inadequate lymphatic drainage may result in sodium and water retention by the kidneys and contribute to interstitial edema and accumulation of fluid in body cavities in hypothyroidism (1,2).

POTASSIUM

Urinary potassium excretion is low in hypothyroidism and increases during T_4 therapy (6). The low excretion correlates with low serum aldosterone concentrations. The increase during T_4 therapy may relate to an increase in serum aldosterone concentrations, increased delivery of sodium to the collecting duct, increased fluid flow to the distal tubule, and increased osmolar excretion (6). Hypothyroidism does not cause abnormal serum potassium concentrations (6). When hyperkalemia is associated with hypothyroidism, adrenal insufficiency should be suspected.

MINERAL METABOLISM

Serum calcium and phosphate concentrations are nearly always normal in patients with hypothyroidism. Hypothy-

roidism is associated with decreased bone turnover, which tends to lower serum calcium concentrations; however, normocalcemia is maintained by a small increase in parathyroid secretion (see Chapter 62) (53,54). Urinary calcium excretion is often low in patients with hypothyroidism, due to a decreased filtered load of calcium and increased parathyroid hormone secretion.

Even though hypothyroidism does not cause hypocalcemia, the two conditions occasionally are found together. For example, hypoparathyroidism may be a complication of thyroidectomy, or may be due to pseudohypoparathyroidism type 1a (McCune-Albright syndrome), which is caused by deficient activity of guanine nucleotide–binding stimulatory protein (Gs) (55,56). In pseudohypoparathyroidism, peptide hormone receptors become uncoupled from adenylyl cyclase, resulting in impaired production of cyclic adenosine monophosphate in response to parathyroid hormone in the kidney and similarly impaired responses to tropic hormone stimulation in other tissues, including an impaired thyroidal response to TSH. Few of these patients have overt hypothyroidism, but subclinical hypothyroidism, or at least an excessive serum TSH response to thyrotropin-releasing hormone (TRH), indicative of very mild hypothyroidism, is common (55).

Although hypercalcemia is rare in patients with hypothyroidism, it can occur if calcium intake is high or if hypocalciuria is marked and parathyroid hormone secretion is not normally suppressible (57,58). Infants with congenital hypothyroidism also may have mild hypercalcemia (59). Other situations in which hypercalcemia may occur in a patient with hypothyroidism are primary hyperparathyroidism, which rarely occurs after radioactive iodine therapy (so rarely that it is likely to be a coincidence) (60); sarcoidosis, with increased 1,25-dihydroxyvitamin D (calcitriol) production and concomitant TSH or TRH deficiency (61); and therapy with lithium, a well-known cause of hypothyroidism (see Chapter 50).

Serum and erythrocyte magnesium concentrations may be slightly high in patients with hypothyroidism, perhaps because of decreased renal clearance of magnesium (62). In a series of 84 patients with a variety of thyroid diseases, both serum and erythrocyte magnesium concentrations were negatively correlated with serum thyroid hormone concentrations. Serum zinc concentrations and urinary zinc excretion are low in hypothyroidism (63). The clinical importance of these alterations in magnesium and zinc metabolism is not known.

URIC ACID METABOLISM

Among patients with gout, 20% to 30% have hypothyroidism (64). In a group of 28 patients with hypothyroidism, 32% had hyperuricemia, as compared with 2% to

10% in the general population, and 7% had gout (64). The patients with hypothyroidism and hyperuricemia had a higher mean serum creatinine concentration [1.9 mg/dL (168 μ*M*)], lower creatinine clearance (59 mL/min), and lower urinary uric acid excretion, as compared with hypothyroid patients with normal serum uric acid concentrations. The hyperuricemia was attributed to decreased renal plasma flow and impaired glomerular filtration (64). T_4 therapy resulted in normalization of serum uric acid and creatinine concentrations, urinary uric acid excretion, and creatinine clearance.

IMMUNE COMPLEX GLOMERULONEPHRITIS

Proteinuria and immune complex glomerulonephritis have been reported in patients with both thyrotoxicosis and hypothyroidism. The renal abnormalities, therefore, more likely reflect the presence of autoimmune thyroid disease than thyroid dysfunction per se. In one study, 11 of 25 patients with chronic autoimmune thyroiditis had proteinuria, most of whom were receiving thyroid hormone therapy (65). Membranous glomerulonephritis was described in a hypothyroid patient who earlier had Graves' thyrotoxicosis; the mesangial immune complex deposits in this patient stained positively for thyroglobulin and thyroid peroxidase (66).

REFERENCES

 1. Montenegro J, Gonzalez O, Saracho R, et al. Changes in renal function in primary hypothyroidism. *Am J Kidney Dis* 1996;27:195.
 2. Villabona C, Sahun M, Roca M, et al. Blood volumes and renal function in overt and subclinical primary hypothyroidism. *Am J Med Sci* 1999;318:277.
 3. Diekman MJ, Harms MP, Endert E, et al. Endocrine factors related to changes in total peripheral vascular resistance after treatment of thyrotoxic and hypothyroid patients. *Eur J Endocrinol* 2001;144:339.
 4. Quesada A, Sainz J, Wangensteen R, et al. Nitric oxide synthase activity in hyperthyroid and hypothyroid rats. *Eur J Endocrinol* 2002;147:117.
 5. McDonough AA, Brown TA, Horowitz B, et al. Thyroid hormone coordinately regulates Na⁺-K⁺-ATPase alpha- and beta-subunit mRNA levels in kidney. *Am J Physiol* 1988;254:C323.
 6. Park CW, Shin YS, Ahn SJ, et al. Thyroxine treatment induces upregulation of renin-angiotensin-aldosterone system due to decreasing effective plasma volume in patients with primary myxoedema. *Nephrol Dial Transplant* 2001;16:1799.
 7. Garg LC, Tisher CC. Effects of thyroid hormone on Na-K-adenosine triphosphatase activity along the rat nephron. *J Lab Clin Med* 1985;106:568.
 8. Kinsella J, Sacktor B. Thyroid hormones increase Na⁺H⁺ exchange activity in renal brush border membranes. *Proc Natl Acad Sci USA* 1985;82:3606.
 9. Marcos Morales M, Purchio Brucoli HC, Malnic G, et al. Role of thyroid hormones in renal tubule acidification. *Mol Cell Biochem* 1996;154:17.
10. Martinez F, Franco M, Quintana A, et al. Sodium-dependent adenosine transport is diminished in brush border membrane vesicles from hypothyroid rat kidney. *Pflugers Arch* 1997;433:269.
11. Harkcom TM, Kim JK, Palumbo PJ, et al. Modulatory effect of thyroid function on enzymes of the vasopressin-sensitive adenosine 3′,5′-monophosphate system in renal medulla. *Endocrinology* 1978;102:1475.
12. Kim JK, Summer SN, Schrier RW. Cellular action of arginine vasopressin in the isolated renal tubules of hypothyroid rats. *Am J Physiol* 1987;253:F104.
13. Vaamonde CA, Michael UF, Oster JR, et al. Impaired renal concentrating ability in hypothyroid man. *Nephron* 1976;17:382.
14. Bradley SE, Stephan F, Coelho JB, et al. The thyroid and the kidney. *Kidney Int* 1974;6:346.
15. Fraser WD, Logue FC, MacRitchie K, et al. Intact parathyroid hormone concentration and cyclic AMP metabolism in thyroid disease. *Acta Endocrinol* (Copenh) 1991;124:652.
16. Marchant C, Brown L, Sernia C. Renin-angiotensin system in thyroid dysfunction in rats. *J Cardiovasc Pharmacol* 1993;22:449.
17. Hauger-Klevene JH, Brown H, Zavaleta J. Plasma renin activity in hyper- and hypothyroidism: effect of adrenergic blocking agents. *J Clin Endocrinol Metab* 1972;34:625.
18. Resnick LM, Laragh JH. Plasma renin activity in syndromes of thyroid hormone excess and deficiency. *Life Sci* 1982;30:585.
19. Gillum DM, Falk SA, Hammond WS, et al. Glomerular dynamics in the hypothyroid rat and the role of the renin-angiotensin system. *Am J Physiol* 1987;253:F170.
20. Katz AI, Lindheimer MD. Renal sodium- and potassium-activated adenosine triphosphate and sodium reabsorption in the hypothyroid rat. *J Clin Invest* 1973;52:796.
21. Katz AI, Emmanouel DS, Lindheimer MD. Thyroid hormone and the kidney. *Nephron* 1975;15:223.
22. Rolandi E, Santaniello B, Bagnasco M, et al. Thyroid hormones and atrial natriuretic hormone secretion: study in hyper- and hypothyroid patients. *Acta Endocrinol* (Copenh) 1992;127:23.
23. Barna I, Foldes J, Toth M, et al. Atrial natriuretic peptide (ANP) responsiveness in patients with hypothyroidism. *Acta Med Hung* 1994;50:23.
24. Ota K, Kimura T, Sakurada T, et al. Effects of an acute water load on plasma ANP and AVP, and renal water handling in hypothyroidism: comparison of before and after L-thyroxine treatment. *Endocr J* 1994;41:99.
25. Franco M, Bobadilla NA, Suarez J, et al. Participation of adenosine in the renal hemodynamic abnormalities of hypothyroidism. *Am J Physiol* 1996;270:F254.
26. Baajafer FS, Hammami MM, Mohamed GE. Prevalence and severity of hyponatremia and hypercreatininemia in short-term uncomplicated hypothyroidism. *J Endocrinol Invest* 1999;22:35.
27. Kreisman SH, Hennessey JV. Consistent reversible elevations of serum creatinine levels in severe hypothyroidism. *Arch Intern Med* 1999;159:79.
28. Kaptein EM. Thyroid hormone metabolism and thyroid diseases in chronic renal failure. *Endocr Rev* 1996;17:45.
29. Makino Y, Fujii T, Kuroda S, et al. Exacerbation of renal failure due to hypothyroidism in a patient with ischemic nephropathy. *Nephron* 2000;84:267.
30. Nakahama H, Sakaguchi K, Horita Y, et al. Treatment of severe hypothyroidism reduced serum creatinine levels in two chronic renal failure patients. *Nephron* 2001;88:264.
31. Kung AW, Ma JT, Yu YL, et al. Myopathy in acute hypothyroidism. *Postgrad Med J* 1987;63:661.

32. Jain S, Bhargava K, Sawlani KK, et al. Myoglobinuria and transient acute renal failure in a patient revealing hypothyroidism. *J Assoc Physicians India* 1999;47:444.

33. Barahona MJ, Mauri A, Sucunza N, et al. Hypothyroidism as a cause of rhabdomyolysis. *Endocr J* 2002;49:621.

34. Kisakol G, Tunc R, Kaya A. Rhabdomyolysis in a patient with hypothyroidism. *Endocr J* 2003;50:221.

35. Streeten DHP, Anderson GH Jr, Howland T, et al. Recognition of hypothyroid hypertension. *Hypertension* 1988;11:78.

36. Dernellis J, Panaretou M. Effects of thyroid replacement therapy on arterial blood pressure in patients with hypertension and hypothyroidism. *Am Heart J* 2002;143:718.

37. Marcisz C, Jonderko G, Kucharz EJ. Influence of short-time application of a low sodium diet on blood pressure in patients with hyperthyroidism or hypothyroidism during therapy. *Am J Hypertens* 2001;14:995.

38. Fommei E, Iervasi G. The role of thyroid hormone in blood pressure homeostasis: evidence from short-term hypothyroidism in humans. *J Clin Endocrinol Metab* 2002;87:1996.

39. Streeten DHP, Anderson GH Jr, Elias MF. Prevalence of secondary hypertension and unusual aspects of the treatment of hypertension in elderly individuals. *Geriatr Nephrol Urol* 1992;2:91.

40. Macaron C, Famuyiwa O. Hyponatremia of hypothyroidism: appropriate suppression of antidiuretic hormone levels. *Arch Intern Med* 1978;138:820.

41. Croal BL, Blake AM, Johnston J, et al. Absence of relation between hyponatraemia and hypothyroidism. *Lancet* 1997;350:1402.

42. Moses AM, Gabrilove JL, Soffer LJ. Simplified water loading test in hypoadrenocorticism and hypothyroidism. *J Clin Endocrinol Metab* 1958;18:1413.

43. Skowsky WR, Kikuchi TA. The role of vasopressin in the impaired water excretion of myxedema. *Am J Med* 1978;64:613.

44. Hierholzer K, Finke R. Myxedema. *Kidney Int Suppl* 1997;59:82.

45. Iwasaki Y, Oiso Y, Yamauchi K, et al. Osmoregulation of plasma vasopressin in myxedema. *J Clin Endocrinol Metab* 1990;70:534.

46. Sahun M, Villabona C, Rosel P, et al. Water metabolism disturbances at different stages of primary thyroid failure. *J Endocrinol* 2001;168:435.

47. Allon M, Harrow A, Pasque CB, et al. Renal sodium and water handling in hypothyroid patients: the role of renal insufficiency. *J Am Soc Nephrol* 1990;1:205.

48. Emmanouel DS, Lindheimer MD, Katz AI. Mechanism of impaired water excretion in the hypothyroid rat. *J Clin Invest* 1974;54:926.

49. Schrier RW, Goldberg JP. The physiology of vasopressin release and the pathogenesis of impaired water excretion in adrenal, thyroid, and edematous disorders. *Yale J Biol Med* 1980;53:525.

50. Parving HH, Hansen JM, Nielsen SL, et al. Mechanisms of edema formation in myxedema-increased protein extravasation and relatively slow lymphatic drainage. *N Engl J Med* 1979;301:460.

51. Sachdev Y, Hall R. Effusions into body cavities in hypothyroidism. *Lancet* 1975;1:564.

52. Wheatley T, Edwards OM. Mild hypothyroidism and oedema: evidence for increased capillary permeability to protein. *Clin Endocrinol* (Oxf) 1983;18:627.

53. Castro JH, Genuth SM, Klein L. Comparative response to parathyroid hormone in hyperthyroidism and hypothyroidism. *Metabolism* 1975;24:839.

54. Bouillon R, De Moor P. Influence of thyroid function on the serum concentration of 1,25-dihydroxyvitamin D_3. *J Clin Endocrinol Metab* 1980;51:793.

55. Levine MA, Downs RW Jr, Moses AM, et al. Association with deficient activity of guanine nucleotide regulatory protein. *Am J Med* 1983;74:545.

56. Levine MA, Schwindinger WF, Downs RW Jr, et al. Pseudohypoparathyroidism: clinical, biochemical, and molecular features. In: Bilezikian JP, Marcus R, Levine MA, eds. *The parathyroids: basic and clinical concepts.* New York: Raven, 1994:781.

57. Lowe CE, Bird ED, Thomas WC. Hypercalcemia in myxedema. *J Clin Endocrinol Metab* 1962;22:261.

58. Zaloga GP, Eil C, O'Brian JT. Reversible hypocalciuric hypercalcemia associated with hypothyroidism. *Am J Med* 1984;77:1101.

59. Tau C, Garabedian M, Farriaux JP, et al. Hypercalcemia in infants with congenital hypothyroidism and its relation to vitamin D and thyroid hormones. *J Pediatr* 1986;109:808.

60. Bondeson AG, Bondeson L, Thompson NW. Hyperparathyroidism after treatment with radioactive iodine: not only a coincidence? *Surgery* 1989;106:1025.

61. Porter N, Beymon HL, Randeva HS. Endocrine and reproductive manifestations of sarcoidosis. *Q J Med* 2003;96:553.

62. Shibutani Y, Yokota T, Iijima S, et al. Plasma and erythrocyte magnesium concentrations in thyroid disease: relation to thyroid function and the duration of illness. *Jpn J Med* 1989;28:496.

63. Dolev E, Deuster PA, Solomon B, et al. Alterations in magnesium and zinc metabolism in thyroid disease. *Metabolism* 1988;37:61.

64. Giordano N, Santacroce C, Mattii G, et al. Hyperuricemia and gout in thyroid endocrine disorders. *Clin Exp Rheumatol* 2001;19:661.

65. Weetman AP, Tomlinson K, Amos N, et al. Proteinuria in autoimmune thyroid disease. *Acta Endocrinol* (Copenh) 1985;109:341.

66. Jordan SC, Johnston WH, Bergstein JM. Immune complex glomerulonephritis mediated by thyroid antigens. *Arch Pathol Lab Med* 1978;102:530.

THE GASTROINTESTINAL TRACT AND LIVER IN HYPOTHYROIDISM

SANJEEV M. WASAN
JOSEPH H. SELLIN
RENA VASSILOPOULOU-SELLIN

The sluggish and slow response characteristic of the patient with hypothyroidism in general marks the major gastrointestinal (GI) manifestations of hypothyroidism: sluggish intestinal motility ranging from mild obstipation to paralytic ileus and intestinal pseudo-obstruction. Hypothyroidism most often afflicts elderly persons, who frequently discount the significance of an insidious decrease in bowel movements. Severe constipation unresponsive to laxatives, therefore, may be a prominent finding at diagnosis. Younger patients with hypothyroidism secondary to treatment for thyrotoxicosis or thyroid cancer frequently gain weight because of decreased physical activity coupled with unchanged food intake. In infants, the observation of infrequent hard stools should serve as a clue to the diagnosis.

Hypothyroidism affects the GI tract in several additional ways. As with thyrotoxicosis, atrophic gastritis and pernicious anemia may be associated findings. Therefore, prompt investigation of gastric histology and vitamin B_{12} metabolism should follow the discovery of megaloblastic anemia in the hypothyroid patient. Although there may be a specific hepatic lesion of hypothyroidism, associated autoimmune liver disease is probably more common. In the hypothyroid patient with liver function abnormalities, particular diagnostic efforts should be directed toward the possibility of primary biliary cirrhosis or autoimmune hepatitis.

INTESTINAL MOTILITY IN HYPOTHYROIDISM

Although most patients with hypothyroidism average one bowel movement daily, about one eighth have fewer than three movements weekly; also, laxative use increases significantly (1). Insidious symptoms of vague abdominal pain and distention may be present and often are diagnosed as functional bowel disease. Unusual GI manifestations, such as a gastric phytobezoar (2) or a lesion mimicking carci-

noma of the sigmoid colon (3), have been reported. Rectal prolapse, sigmoid volvulus, and intestinal pseudo-obstruction (4) occasionally are seen. Severe cases may present with intestinal atony and ileus (5), often misinterpreted as intestinal obstruction. In recent years, earlier diagnosis of hypothyroidism resulted in fewer cases progressing to pseudo-obstruction. Radiologic studies reveal generalized dilatation of the GI tract, especially the colon. Pathologic examination of the intestine demonstrated a thickened, pale, leathery colon that is generally lengthened; microscopically, myxedema and round cell infiltration of the submucosal and muscle layers is evident. A decrease in colonic crypts suggests mucosal atrophy.

The motility of the GI tract may be assessed using several different methods (see Chapter 34). Studies of hypothyroid humans and dogs demonstrated a decrease in the electric and motor activity of the esophagus, stomach, small intestine, and colon (6–8). Dysphagia is not uncommon in hypothyroidism and may be related to esophageal motility abnormalities, including decreases in the amplitude and velocity of peristalsis and a decrease in lower esophageal sphincter pressure. These abnormalities correct with thyroid replacement (6). Gastric emptying as measured with a liquid meal of glucose is prolonged in hypothyroidism and returns to normal with therapy (9). The neuropeptide thyrotropin-releasing hormone (TRH) has a central effect on gastric emptying; injected into the cerebrospinal fluid (CSF), TRH increases phasic motor activity of the stomach, mediated by TRH receptors on postsynaptic vagal neurons (10). Orocecal (intestinal) transit time, as measured by a lactulose-hydrogen breath test, decreased significantly in one study when hypothyroid patients were given thyroid hormone replacement (11), but was normal in another study in the hypothyroid state and was not altered significantly by thyroid hormone replacement (12). In the sigmoid colon and rectum, the number and amplitude of muscular contractions are decreased. The relative importance of the small bowel and colon in the "sluggish gut" of hypothyroidism remains to be determined. Several theories have been proposed to explain the changes of the intestine in hypothyroidism, including autonomic neuropathy, altered impulse transmission at the myoneural junction, intestinal ischemia, and intestinal myopathy.

ABSORPTION IN HYPOTHYROIDISM

In most patients, intestinal absorption is normal. The malabsorption occasionally reported in severely hypothyroid patients remains poorly understood but has been attributed to myxedematous infiltration of the mucosa, decreased intestinal motility, or associated autoimmune phenomena. Intestinal handling of D-xylose is normal, although renal clearance after both intravenous and oral administration is lower as a result of a decrease in glomerular filtration rate. In addition, glucose absorption is normal overall, whereas net transmural transport is enhanced, in part because of decreased glucose utilization (13). Hypercalcemia may occur as a result of increased absorption of dietary calcium in conjunction with a decrease in calcium incorporation into bone (14). Pancreatic function is generally normal in hypothyroidism; hypothermia associated with severe hypothyroidism occasionally may result in hyperamylasemia, probably secondary to pancreatitis (15). The intestinal epithelium may be less responsive to secretory stimuli, such as vasoactive intestinal peptide, suggesting a possible pathophysiologic mechanism for some of the intestinal alterations of hypothyroidism (16). Although rare in hypothyroidism, diarrhea can occur and may be due to bacterial overgrowth from small bowel hypomotility, corrected with antibiotic therapy (17). In hypothyroid patients who receive thyroid hormone replacement, the addition of other pharmacologic agents (e.g., bile acid sequestrants, sucralfate, ferrous sulfate, or aluminum hydroxide) may impair thyroxine T_4 absorption and complicate management (18,19). Thyroid function may be altered in inflammatory and immune-mediated diseases of the intestine (see Chapter 34).

THYROID FUNCTION IN MALABSORPTION AND INTESTINAL DISEASE

An enterohepatic circulation of thyroid hormone has been described (20) in which thyroid hormone secreted into bile is delivered into the intestinal lumen, reabsorbed, and delivered back to the liver (see Chapter 34). This system is similar to that described for other hormones, such as vitamin D and estrogens. Interactions of the gut with thyroid hormone, the potential role of the intestine both as a reservoir for thyroid hormones and as a regulator of hormone activity (21), and the presence of the enterohepatic circulation raise several interesting questions: Does intraluminal thyroid hormone affect intestinal function? Does thyroid hormone delivered to the liver through the enterohepatic circulation and portal vein in relatively high concentration have an effect on hepatic function? Given the ability of intestinal bacteria to bind and degrade thyroid hormones (22), is there a clinically important, although indirect, effect of intestinal hypomotility on thyroid hormone economy?

Significant adaptation in fecal losses of thyroid takes place in hypothyroidism (23) both through decreased excretion and increased absorption. Nevertheless, intestinal diseases and malabsorption may affect the metabolism of thyroid hormone. Increased fecal T_4 losses may occur in pancreatic steatorrhea, celiac sprue (24), and inflammatory bowel disease (25). In addition, autoimmune thyroid disease (hypothyroidism more frequently than thyrotoxicosis) may be more prevalent in patients with celiac disease (26). Given the association between celiac sprue and thyroid disease, this may be a confounding variable to consider when oral thyroid replacement is difficult. Malabsorption of oral thyroid medication is seen after jejunoileal bypass (27,28). In balance, the euthyroid patient is generally capable of compensating for intestinal losses with increased endogenous thyroid secretion, whereas the hypothyroid patient may require an increase in thyroid hormone replacement dosage.

EPITHELIAL TRANSPORT AND GUT FUNCTION

Because Na^+,K^+-adenosine triphosphatase (ATPase) is pivotal to both thyroid hormone–regulated thermogenesis and epithelial ion transport, the linkage between thyroid hormone and ion transport has been investigated (29). Thyroid hormone stimulates both Na^+,K^+-ATPase activity and electrogenic Na absorption in the intestine (30,31). The effect may be due to enhanced message of the β subunit of Na^+,K^+-ATPase (31). Thyroid hormone also induces Na pump activity, enhances bile flow, and increases the messenger RNA (mRNA) for α and β subunits of Na^+,K^+-ATPase in the liver (32,33).

Thyroid hormone also may stimulate the activity of apical, amiloride-sensitive Na^+ channels in the colon (34). These effects may be indirect; thyroid hormone may function by increasing the sensitivity of these transporters to aldosterone, one of the principal regulators of Na^+ absorption in the gut (35,36). Aldosterone has effects on both the amiloride-sensitive Na channel and the Na^+ pump. T_4 also may have a role in regulating anion transport in the intestine by inhibiting an apical $Cl:HCO_3$ exchanger (37). The effects on nutrient transport are complex. Animal studies have demonstrated complex and conflicting effects on active, electrogenic transfer of amino acids and sugars (38, 39).

Triiodothyronine (T_3) down-regulates lactase, stimulates alkaline phosphatase, and does not affect sucrase gene expression (40). T_3 causes epithelial hypertrophy and villus hyperplasia with minimal change in the morphometry of the crypts (40). Thyroid-associated changes in colonic epithelial membrane lipid composition and fluidity may exert generalized functional changes on epithelial function (41). In sum, the effects of thyroid hormone on intestinal function are significant and complex; their clinical implications are not so clear.

GUT AND LIVER DEVELOPMENT

Intestinal development is physiologically regulated by thyroid hormone at multiple levels (42–47). In developing animals, hypothyroidism results in decreased mucosal thickness and villous height, weight, and protein content of the small intestine (48) and in abnormal peptide content and binding properties (16,49,50). As for the converse, experimental hyperthyroidism in developing animals leads to mucosal hypertrophy and epithelial hyperplasia. In humans, however, fetal hypothyroidism does not appear to affect the gut seriously.

Overall, thyroid hormone alone has only modest effects on intestinal maturation but, when combined with glucocorticoids, may have a synergistic effect on multiple enzymes, including lactose, sucrase, maltase, and alkaline phosphatase. Thyroid hormone has a role in both gene expression and protein abundance (40,45–47,51). In the presence of glucocorticoids, thyroid hormone appears to accelerate the maturation process, changing the programmed alterations in specific enzyme levels during the weaning period.

Although diet may have a role in this modulation, thyroid hormone appears to have a direct effect on the intestine (44,52). Changes in hormonal responsiveness of the intestine during development may reflect changes in the forms of T_3 receptors found in the intestine, with fairly constant levels of TR-β_1 but decreases in *c-erbA* levels (44).

Most studies have focused on the effect of thyroid hormone on intestinal brush-border enzymes. Recent observations suggest that thyroid hormone may have a similar permissive effect in the developmental changes of electrogenic Na transport in the weanling colon (53). Thus, thyroid hormone is an important developmental modifier of the biologic effects of other hormones, primarily glucocorticoids and mineralocorticoids.

GASTRIC FUNCTION IN HYPOTHYROIDISM

Immune gastritis coexists with hypothyroidism in about 11% of patients. This association is probably due to the propensity of such patients for autoimmune disease (54). As with thyrotoxicosis, abnormalities of vitamin B_{12} metabolism without overt anemia, antiparietal cell antibodies, and hypochlorhydria or achlorhydria have been reported much more commonly. Similarly, there is a high incidence of thyroid antibodies in patients with pernicious anemia (55). The mechanism of gastric acid secretory dysfunction is also not clear. The observation that thyrotoxicosis is associated with hypergastrinemia (56,57), whereas patients with hypothyroidism have subnormal serum gastrin levels (58), implies that the pathophysiology of achlorhydria differs in the two conditions. The embryologic similarity between thyroid and gastric tissue, their mutual iodine-concentrating ability, and their similar histologic abnormalities led many investigators to consider that thyrogastric autoimmune disorders are linked pathophysiologically; to date, no human lymphocyte antigen (HLA) association has been found. An association between atrophic autoimmune thyroiditis and *Helicobacter pylori* infection has been observed (59). In fact, recent studies suggest infection by *H. pylori* strains expressing CagA is prevalent in patients with autoimmune thyroid disease. *H. pylori* organisms possessing pathogenicity carry a gene encoding for an endogenous peroxidase, which tends to increase the organism's inflammatory potential (60).

LIVER IN HYPOTHYROIDISM

An association exists between Hashimoto's thyroiditis and hypothyroidism with autoimmune liver diseases such as chronic active hepatitis (61,62) and primary biliary cirrhosis (63,64). Hypothyroidism is seen in approximately 5% to 20% of patients with primary biliary cirrhosis (65,66). Primary biliary cirrhosis may be associated with other organ-specific autoimmune diseases and thus with autoimmune polyglandular syndrome (67). In addition, 8% to 12% of patients with autoimmune hepatitis have been found to have hypothyroidism, especially chronic thyroiditis (66,68). Liver, gastric, and thyroid dysfunction in autoimmune disease may constitute a constellation of coexisting abnormalities (see Chapter 34 for a discussion of thyroid and liver interactions). Thyroid hormones have a significant impact in the regulation of hepatic mitochondrial metabolism (69,70). Hypothyroid animals have decreased resting metabolic rate with decreased hepatocyte oxygen consumption (71). A specific hypothyroid hepatic lesion of central congestive fibrosis without myxedematous infiltration has been reported (72). Persistent hyperbilirubinemia in the newborn may suggest the diagnosis of congenital hypothyroidism.

Ascites is a rare and poorly understood complication of severe hypothyroidism (73); it consists of a yellow, gelatinous peritoneal exudate. There is a high protein content of the fluid (>2.5 g/dL), a high serum-ascites albumin gradient, a long duration of the ascites, and resolution with thyroid replacement (72). It has been suggested that the ascites is related to congestive heart failure, enhanced capillary permeability, or the inappropriate secretion of antidiuretic hormone associated with hypothyroidism.

Reversible abnormalities of liver function tests are common, although usually mild, in hypothyroidism. In addition, there is abnormal fuel use with significant decrease in gluconeogenesis (74). Hypothyroid patients have specific defects in hepatic handling of amino acids resulting in decreased urea nitrogen generation (75).

Thyroid status clearly affects bile flow and composition. In experimental models of hypothyroidism, a decrease in bile flow is due primarily to a decrease in the bile salt–independent component (32). Additionally, the biliary excretion of bilirubin is diminished in association with some subtle alterations of hepatic bilirubin metabolism (76). Hypothyroidism may alter several critical steps in cholesterol and bile acid synthesis (77). In addition, thyroid hormone modifies lipoprotein metabolism in the liver (78–84). It is unclear whether this is a direct thyroid effect on liver enzymes or secondary to altered intestinal handling of cholesterol and bile acids (85,86). The changes in enzyme activities, the hypercholesterolemia of myxedema, and the hypotonia of the gallbladder in hypothyroidism suggest the possibility of increased cholesterol saturation of bile (85,86) and a higher incidence of gallstones. Direct measurements of the lithogenicity of hypothyroid bile are not available, however.

HEPATITIS C, INTERFERON, AND THE THYROID

Although autoimmune liver disease has long been associated with thyroid disease, the increasingly frequent diagnosis of hepatitis C and its treatment with interferon-α has suggested novel and different linkages between the thyroid and viral hepatitis. A relationship exists between the low thyroid hormone levels (free T_4, T_4, T_3) and the degree of hepatic dysfunction based on the Child-Pugh classification in chronic viral hepatitis (87). There is an increased incidence of both thyroid antibodies and clinically significant thyroid disease in patients with hepatitis C prior to treatment. The incidence of anti-TPO (thyroid peroxidase) antibodies is about 10% to 15% (88–92), whereas overt thyroid dysfunction occurs in 0% to 4% of patients. Antithyroid antibodies are found more frequently in hepatitis C virus–positive women when compared with men (92).

Thyroid dysfunction and antithyroid antibodies, especially anti-TPO antibodies, both increase with interferon treatment, which generally lasts up to 12 months in treatment of hepatitis C. Anti-TPO antibodies occur in 20% to 30% of patients, although titers may vary considerably during treatment (91). Clinical manifestations of thyroid dysfunction occur in 10% to 15% of patients and may

present as either hyperthyroidism or hypothyroidism (90–93). Thyrotoxicosis usually occurs due to silent thyroiditis, but Graves' disease during interferon therapy has been reported. Hypothyroidism occurs from 2 months to 2 years after initiating interferon-α therapy and thyrotoxicosis from 6 weeks to 6 months. Thyroid dysfunction is transient in greater than two thirds of cases; however, thyroid function tests may not return to normal until up to as many as 17 months after discontinuation of therapy (94). From studies in a Japanese population, HLA-A2 is highly linked to autoimmune thyroid disease induced by interferon-α therapy in patients with chronic hepatitis C (95).

Whereas some investigators have found a higher incidence of anti-TPO and anti-thyroglobulin antibodies in hepatitis C compared with hepatitis B (88), others have not (89). Interferon therapy in a variety of other diseases also has been associated with thyroid abnormalities; however, the problem appears to be more common with hepatitis C, suggesting that some specific (but as yet undefined) factors that may be involved. The mechanisms for interferon-induced thyroid disease are unknown but may involve increased expression of major histocompatability (MHC) class I antigens, induction of autoantibodies, or a direct effect of interferon on the thyroid. There are some suggestions that interferon may interfere with iodide organification (95,95).

The major risk factor implicated in the development of thyroid disease during interferon treatment has been the presence of a high titer anti-TPO antibodies (88,90); however, it is clear that patients with preexisting thyroid disease do not necessarily worsen on interferon, and most patients who develop thyroid disease do not have preexisting antibodies. Cessation of interferon treatment usually leads to resolution of thyroid dysfunction.

SUMMARY

Hypothyroidism appears to affect the GI tract more profoundly than thyrotoxicosis. Hypomotility with constipation is a fairly frequent, although usually mild, manifestation of hypothyroidism. Associated gastric, liver, and thyroid dysfunctions are often due to systemic autoimmune diseases. Although the clinical picture of hypothyroidism has been well characterized, the mechanisms of thyroid action on the gut and liver remain poorly understood.

REFERENCES

1. Baker JT, Harvey RF. Bowel habits in thyrotoxicosis and hypothyroidism. *BMJ* 1971;1:322.
2. Kaplan LR. Hypothyroidism presenting as a gastric phytobezoar. *Am J Gastroenterol* 1980;74:168.

3. Duks S, Pitlik S, Rosenfeld JB. Hypothyroidism mimicking a tumor of the sigmoid colon. *Mayo Clin Proc* 1979;54:623.

4. Bassotti G, et al. Intestinal pseudoobstruction secondary to hypothyroidism. Importance of small bowel manometry. *J Clin Gastroenterol* 1992;14(1):56.

5. Abbasi AA, Douglass RC, Bissel GW, et al. Myxedema ileus. *JAMA* 1975;234:181.

6. Eastwood GL, Braverman LG, White EM, et al. Reversal of lower esophageal sphincter hypotension and esophageal aperistalsis after treatment for hypothyroidism. *J Clin Gastroenterol* 1982;4:307.

7. Karaus M, Wienbeck M, Grussendorf M, et al. Intestinal motor activity in experimental hyperthyroidism in conscious dogs. *Gastroenterology* 1989;97:911.

8. Kowalewski K, Kolodej A. Myoelectrical and mechanical activity of stomach and intestine in hypothyroid dogs. *Am J Dig Dis* 1977;22:235.

9. Kahraman H, Kaya N, Demircali A, et al. Gastric emptying time in patients with primary hypothyroidism. *Eur J Gastroenterol Hepatol* 1997;9:901.

10. Raybould HE, Jacobsen LJ, Tache J. TRH stimulation and L-glutamic acid inhibition of proximal gastric motor activity in the rat dorsal vagal complex. *Brain Res* 1989;49:319.

11. Shafer RB, Prentiss RA, Bond JH. Gastrointestinal transit in thyroid disease. *Gastroenterology* 1994;86:852.

12. Tobin MV, Fisken RA, Diggory RT, et al. Orocecal transit time in health and disease. *Gut* 1989;30:26.

13. Khoja SM, Kellett GL. Effects of hypothyroidism on glucose transport and metabolism in rat small intestine. *Bioch Biophys Acta* 1993;1179:76.

14. Lekkerkerker JF, Van Woudenberg F, Beekhuis H, et al. Enhancement of calcium absorption in hypothyroidism. *Isr J Med Sci* 1971;7:399.

15. Maclean D, Murison J, Griffiths PD. Acute pancreatitis and diabetic ketoacidosis in accidental hypothermia and hypothermic myxedema. *BMJ* 1973;4:757.

16. Molinero P, Calvo JR, Jimenez J, et al. Decreased binding of vasoactive intestinal peptide to intestinal epithelial cells from hypothyroid rats. *Biochem Biophys Res Commun* 1989;162:701.

17. Goldin E, et al. Diarrhea in hypothyroidism: Bacterial overgrowth as a possible etiology. *J Clin Gastroenterol* 1990;12:98.

18. Shakir KM, Michaels RD, Hays JH, et al. The use of bile acid sequestrants to lower serum thyroid hormones in introgenic hyperthyroidism. *Ann Intern Med* 1993;118:112.

19. Sherman SI, Tielens ET, Ladenson RW. Sucralfate causes malabsorption of L-thyroxine. *Am J Med* 1994;96:531.

20. Miller JL, Gorman CA, Go VLM. Thyroid-gut interrelationships. *Gastroenterology* 1978;75:901.

21. Hays MT. Thyroid hormone and the gut. *Endocr Res* 1988;14:203.

22. Distefano JJ III, De Luze A, Nguyen TT. Binding and degradation of 3,5,38-triiodothyronine and thyroxine by rat intestinal bacteria. *Am J Physiol* 1993;264:E966.

23. Distefano JJ III, Morris WL, Nguyen TT, et al. Enterophepatic regulation and metabolism of 3,5,38-triiodothyronine in hypothyroid rats. *Endocrinology* 1993;132:1665.

24. Vanderschuren-Lodeweyckx M, Eggermont E, Cornette C, et al. Decreased serum thyroid hormone levels and increased TSH response to TRH in infants with coeliac disease. *Clin Endocrinol* 1977;6:361.

25. Janerot G, Kagedal B, Von Schenk H, et al. The thyroid in ulcerative colitis and Crohn's disease. *Acta Med Scand* 1976;199:229.

26. Counsell CE, Taha A, Rudell WJJ. Coeliac disease and autoimmune thyroid disease. *Gut* 1994;35:844.

27. Azisi F, Belur R, Albano J. Malabsorption of thyroid hormones after jejunoileal bypass for obesity. *Ann Intern Med* 1979;90:941.

28. Topliss DJ, Wright JA, Volpe R. Increased requirements for thyroid hormone after a jejuno-ileal bypass operation. *Can Med Assoc J* 1978;123:765.

29. Edelman IS, Ismail-Beigi F. Thyroid thermogenesis and active sodium transport. *Rec Prog Horm Res* 1974;30:235.

30. Giannella RA, Orlowski J, Jump ML, et al. Na⁺-K⁺-ATPase gene expression in rat intestine Caco-2 cells: response to thyroid hormone. *Am J Physiol* 1993;265:G775.

31. Wiener H, Nielsen JM, Klaerke DA, et al. Aldosterone and thyroid hormone modulation of alpha 1, beta 1-mRNA and Na, K pump sits in rabbit distal colon epithelium: evidence for a novel mechanism of escape from the effects of hyperaldosteronemia. *J Membr Biol* 1993;133:203.

32. Layden TJ, Boyer JL. Effect of thyroid hormone on bile-salt-independent bile flow and Na⁺-K⁺-ATPase activity in liver plasma membrane enriched bile canaliculi. *J Clin Invest* 1976;57:1009.

33. Gick GG, Ismail-Beigi F. Thyroid hormone induction of Na(+)-K(+)-ATPase and its mRNAs in a rat liver cell line. *Am J Physiol* 1990;258:C544.

34. Pacha J, Pohlova I, Zemanova Z. Hypothyroidism affects the expression of electrogenic amiloride-sensitive sodium transport in rat colon. *Gastroenterology* 1996;111:1551.

35. Edmonds CJ, Willis CJ. Aldosterone and thyroid hormone interaction on the sodium and potassium transport pathways of rat colonic epithelium. *J Endocrinol* 1990;124:47.

36. Barlet C, Doucet A. Triiodothyronine enhances renal response to aldosterone in the rabbit collecting tubule. *J Clin Invest* 1987;79:629.

37. Tenore A, Fasano A, Gasparini N, et al. Thyroxine effects on intestinal Cl-HCO3-exchange in hypo- and hyperthyroid rats. *J Endocrinol* 1996:151:431.

38. Levin RJ, Syme G. Differential changes in the "apparent Km" and maximum potential differences of the hexose and amino acid electrogenic transfer mechanisms of the small intestine, induced by fasting and hypothyroidism. *J Physiol* 1971;213:46.

39. Syme G, Levin RJ. The effects of hypothyroidism and fasting on electrogenic amino acid transfer. *Biochim Biophys Acta* 1977;464:620.

40. Hodin RA, Chamberlain SM, Uptan MP. Thyroid hormone differentially regulates rat intestinal brush border enzyme gene expression. *Gastroenterology* 1992;103:1529.

41. Brasitus TA, Dudeja PH. Effect of hypothyroidism on the lipid composition and fluidity of rat colonic apical membranes. *Biochim Biophys Acta* 1988;939:189.

42. Galton VA, McCarthy PT, St. Germain DL. The ontogeny of iodothyronine deiodinase systems in liver and intestine of the rat. *Endocrinology* 1991;128:1717.

43. Henning JJ. Permissive role of thyroxine in the ontogeny of jejunal sucrase. *Endocrinology* 1978:102:9.

44. Hodin RA, Meng S, Chamberlain SM. Thyroid hormone responsiveness is developmentally regulated in the rat small intestine: a possible role for the α-2 receptor variant. *Endocrinology* 1994;135:564.

45. Yeh KY, Yeh M, Holt PR. Differential effects of thyroxine and cortisone on jejunal sucrase expression in suckling rats. *Am J Physiol* 1989;256:G604.

46. Yeh KY, Yeh M, Holt PR. Thyroxine and cortisone cooperate to modulate postnatal intestinal enzyme differential in the rat. *Am J Physiol* 1991;260:371.

47. Leeper LL, McDonald MC, Heath JP, et al. Sucrase-isomaltase ontogeny: synergism between glucocorticoids and thyroxine re-

flects increased mRNA and no change in migration. *Biochem Biophys Res Commun* 1998;246:765.

48. Blanes A, Martinez A, Bujan J, et al. Intestinal mucosal changes following induced hypothryroidism in the developing rat. *Virchows Arch A* 1977;375:233.

49. Shi YN, Hayes WP. Thyroid hormone-dependent regulation of the intestinal fatty acid-binding protein gene during amphibian metamorphosis. *Dev Biol* 1994;161:48.

50. Zheng B, Eng J, Yalow RS. Cholecystokinin and vasoactive intestinal peptide in brain and gut of the hypothyroid neonatal rat. *Horm Metab Res* 1989;21:127.

51. Brewer LM, Betz TW. Thyroxine and duodenal development in chicken embryos. *Can J Zool* 1979;57:416.

52. Hodin RA, Shei A, Morin M, et al. Thyroid hormone and the gut: selective transcriptional activation of a villus-enterocyte marker. *Surgery* 1996;120:138.

53. Pacha J. Ontogeny of Na$^+$ transport in rat colon. *Comp Biochem Physiol A Physiol* 1997;118:209.

54. Irvine WJ. The association of atrophic gastritis with autoimmune thyroid disease. *J Clin Endocrinol Metab* 1975;4:351.

55. Markson JL, Moore JM. Thyroid auto-antibodies in pernicious anemia. *BMJ* 1962;2:1352.

56. Muller MK, Pederson R, Olbricht T, et al. Increased release of gastrin in hyperthyroid rats *in vitro*. *Horm Metab Res* 1986;18:675.

57. Noll B, Goke B, Printz H, et al. Influence of experimental hyperthyroidism on the adult rat pancreas, small intestine, and blood gastrin levels. *J Gastroenterol* 1988;26:331.

58. Seino Y, Matsukura S, Inoue Y, et al. Hypogastrinemia in hypothyroidism. *Dig Dis* 1978;23:189.

59. deLuis DA, Varela C, de La Calle H, et al. *Helicobacter pylori* infection is markedly increased in patients with autoimmune atrophic thyroiditis. *J Clin Gastroenterol* 1998;26:249.

60. Figura N, et al. The infection by *Helicobacter pylori* strains expressing CagA is highly prevalent in women with autoimmune thyroid disorders. *J Physiol Pharm* 1999;50(5):817.

61. Doniach D, Roitt IM, Walkers JG, et al. Tissue antibodies in primary biliary cirrhosis, active chronic hepatitis, cryptogenic cirrhosis. *Clin Exp Immunol* 1966;237:262.

62. Tran A, Quaranta HF, Benzaken S, et al. High prevalence of thyroid autoantibodies in a prospective series of patients with chronic hepatitis C before interferon therapy. *Hepatology* 1993;18:253.

63. Crowe JP, Christensen E, Butler J, et al. Primary biliary cirrhosis: prevalence of hypothyroidism and its relationship to thyroid antibodies. *Gastroenterology* 1980:78:1437.

64. Culp KS, Fleming CR, Duffy J, et al. Autoimmune association in primary biliary cirrhosis. *Mayo Clin Proc* 1982;57:365.

65. Elta GH, et al. Increased incidence of hypothyroidism in primary biliary cirrhosis. *Dig Dis Sci* 1983;28:971.

66. Zeniya M. Thyroid disease in autoimmune liver diseases. *Nippon Rinsho* 1999;57(8):1882.

67. Borgaonkar MR, Morgan DG. Primary biliary cirrhosis and type II autoimmune polyglandular syndrome. *Can J Gastroenterol* 1999;13(9):767.

68. Cindoruk M, et al. The prevalence of autoimmune hepatitis in Hashimoto's thyroiditis in a Turkish population. *Acta Gastroenterol Belg* 2002;65(3):143.

69. Paradies G, Ruggiero FM, Dinoi P. The influence of hypothyroidism on the transport of phosphate and on the lipid composition in rat-liver mitochondria. *Biochem Biophys Acta* 1991;1070:180.

70. Sobol S. Long-term and short-term changes in mitochondrial parameters by thyroid hormones. *Biochem Soc Trans* 1993;21:799.

71. Liverini G, Iossa S, Barletta A. Relationship between resting metabolism and hepatic metabolism: effect of hypothyroidism and 24 hours fasting. *Horm Res* 1992;38:154.

72. De Castro F, et al. Myxedema ascites. Report of two cases and review of the literature. *J Clin Gastroenterol* 1991;13(4):411.

73. Clancy RL, MacKay IR. Myxoedematous ascites. *Med J Aust* 1979;2:415.

74. Comte B, Vidal H, Laville M, et al. Influence of thyroid hormones on gluconeogenesis from glycerol in rat hepatocytes: a dose-response study. *Metabolism* 1990;39:259.

75. Marchesini G, Fabbri A, Bianchi GP, et al. Hepatic conversion of amino nitrogen to urea nitrogen in hypothyroid patients and upon L-thyroxine therapy. *Metabolism* 1993:42:1263.

76. Van Steenbergen W, Fevery J, DeVos R, et al. Thyroid hormones and the hepatic handling of bilirubin. *Hepatology* 1989;9:314.

77. Balasubramaniam S, Mitropoulous KA, Myant NB. Hormonal control of the activities of cholesterol-7 α-hydroxylase and hydroxy methylglutaryl-CoA reductase in rats. In: Matern S, Hachenschmidt J, Back P, et al., eds. *Advances in bile acid research*. Stuttgart: Schattauer Verlag, 1975:61.

78. Caro JF, Cecchin F, Folli F, et al. Effect of T$_3$ on insulin action, insulin binding, and insulin receptor kinase activity in primary cultures of rat hepatocytes. *Horm Metab Res* 1988;20:327.

79. Dang AQ, Fass FH, Carter WJ. Effects of experimental hypo- and hyperthyroidism on hepatic long-chain fatty Acyl-CoA synthetase and hydrolase. *Metabol Res* 1989;21:359.

80. Davidson NO, Carlos RC, Drewek MJ, et al. Apolipoprotein gene expression in the rat is regulated in a tissue-specific manner by thyroid hormone. *J Lipid Res* 1988;29:1511.

81. Hoogenbrugge van der Linden H, Jansen H, Hulsmann WC, et al. Relationship between insulin-like growth factor-I and low density lipoprotein cholesterol levels in primary hypothyroidism in women. *J Endocrinol* 1989;123:341.

82. Lin-Lee YC, Strobl W, Soyal S, et al. Role of thyroid hormone in the expression of apolipoprotein A-IV and C-III Genes in rat liver. *J Lipid Res* 1993;34:249.

83. Staels B, Tol AV, Chan L, et al. Alterations in thyroid status modulate apolipoprotein, hepatic tryglyceride lipase, and low density lipoprotein receptor in rats. *Endocrinology* 1990:127:1144.

84. Strobl W, Gorder NL, Lin-Lee YC, et al. Role of thyroid hormones in apolipoprotein A-I gene expression in rat liver. *J Clin Invest* 1990;85:659.

85. Gebhart RL, Stone BG, Andreini JP, et al. Thyroid hormone differentially augments biliary sterol secretion in the rat. I: The isolated-perfused liver model. *J Lipid Res* 1992;33:1459.

86. Goldfarb S. Regulation of hepatic cholesterogenesis. In: Javitt NB, ed. *Liver and biliary tract: physiology I.* Baltimore: University Park Press, 1980:317.

87. Novis M, et al. Thyroid function tests in viral chronic hepatitis. *Arq Gastroenterol* 2001;38(4):254.

88. Fernandez-Soto L, Gonzalez A, Escobar-Jimenez F, et al. Increased risk of autoimmune thyroid disease in hepatitis C vs. hepatitis B before, during, and after discontinuing interferon therapy. *Arch Intern Med* 1998;158:1445.

89. Deutsch M, Dourakis S, Manesis EK, et al. Thyroid abnormalities in chronic viral hepatitis and their relationship to interferon alpha therapy. *Hepatology* 1997;26:206.

90. Watanabe U, Hashimoto E, Hisamitsu T, et al. The risk factor for development of thyroid disease during interferon-alpha therapy for chronic hepatitis C. *Am J Gastroenterol* 1994;89:399.

91. Kiehne I, Kloehn S, Hinrichesen H, et al. Thyroid autoantibodies and thyroid dysfunction during treatment with interferon-alpha for chronic hepatitis C. *Endocrine* 1997;6:231.

92. Ploix C, et al. Hepatitis C virus infection is frequently associated with high titers of anti-thyroid antibodies. *Int J Immunopharmacol* 1999;12(3):121.

93. Roti E, Minelli R, Giuberti T, et al. Multiple changes in thyroid function in patients with chronic active HCV hepatitis treated with recombinant interferon-alpha. *Am J Med* 1996; 101:482.

94. Braga-Basaria M, Basaria S. Interferon-alpha-induced transient severe hypothyroidism in a patient with Graves' disease. *J Endocrinol Invest* 2003;26(3):261.

95. Kakizaki S, et al. HLA antigens in patients with interferon-alpha-induced autoimmune thyroid disorders in chronic hepatitis C. *J Hepatol* 1999;30(5):794.

THE BLOOD IN HYPOTHYROIDISM

ELLEN MARQUSEE
SUSAN J. MANDEL

Hypothyroidism has several effects on hematopoiesis, the peripheral blood elements, and the coagulation system.

ERYTHROCYTES

Some patients with hypothyroidism have an anemia. In older studies, it was found in 25% to 50% of patients (1,2), but the percentage is lower now because relatively few patients have either severe or long-standing hypothyroidism. In a 1981 study of children and adolescents with severe hypothyroidism, based on the presence of height below the third percentile, 65% had anemia (3), but there was no correlation between the severity of anemia and serum thyroxine (T_4) concentrations. Anemia was present in 13% to 36% of infants with congenital hypothyroidism; in this group, serum T_4 concentrations were correlated with hemoglobin concentrations (4).

Anemia in patients with hypothyroidism to some extent may be physiologic, that is, a result of reduced need for delivery of oxygen to peripheral tissues. On the other hand, a reduction in plasma volume may mask a reduction in red cell mass (1). Thus, few patients have hematocrit values below 35%.

The anemia of hypothyroidism is caused by a decrease in erythropoiesis. Serum erythropoietin concentrations are low (1). The bone marrow is hypocellular, with normal red blood cell differentiation and a normal myeloid:erythroid ratio (5). Erythroblast proliferation, as measured by ^{3}H-thymidine incorporation into erythroblast DNA, is decreased, as is the incorporation of iron into red cell precursors (1). These patients usually have normal iron stores, and normal serum iron, vitamin B_{12}, and folate concentrations, and red cell survival is normal (1,6). Their anemia is normochromic and normocytic or slightly macrocytic, and it improves in several weeks or months in response to treatment with T_4.

In an early study, patients with hypothyroidism had low red cell concentrations of 2,3-diphosphoglycerate (2,3-DPG), which alter red cell oxygen transport to shift the oxyhemoglobin dissociation curve to the left, thereby reducing the release of oxygen from hemoglobin (7). Such a change would be consistent with the reduced tissue need for oxygen in hypothyroidism; however, in a more recent study, red cell 2,3-DPG concentrations were normal (8).

In addition to the nonspecific anemia described above, some patients with hypothyroidism have iron deficiency anemia and others have megaloblastic anemia. Iron deficiency anemia may be either microcytic or normocytic. The cause may be blood loss, notably menorrhagia, but more often is poor iron absorption (2), caused at least in part by achlorhydria. In thyroidectomized rats, gastrointestinal iron absorption is decreased, and it increases in response to thyroid hormone (9). Similarly, in a group of hypothyroid patients with low serum iron concentrations, the hemoglobin concentrations increased in response to T_4, but the increase was greater in response to T_4 and iron (2).

Most patients with hypothyroidism have normal serum vitamin B_{12} and folate concentrations, but the dietary intake or absorption of either substance may be reduced, resulting in macrocytic, and sometimes megaloblastic, anemia (10,11). In these patients, T_4 treatment alone may reverse the anemia, but supplementation with vitamin B_{12} or folate is advisable as well. About 10% of patients with hypothyroidism caused by chronic autoimmune thyroiditis have true pernicious anemia (12). Conversely, about 12% of patients with pernicious anemia have overt hypothyroidism, and an additional 15% have subclinical hypothyroidism (11); thus, screening patients with pernicious anemia for hypothyroidism is recommended (11,13). In patients with pernicious anemia and hypothyroidism, both vitamin B_{12} and T_4 therapy are needed for complete resolution of the anemia (12). In rats, T_4 increases absorption of vitamin B_{12} from the gastrointestinal tract and facilitates mobilization of vitamin B_{12} from stores in the liver (14).

LEUKOCYTES

Granulocyte and lymphocyte counts are normal in patients with hypothyroidism. Examination of the bone marrow may reveal an increase in the proportion of differentiated myeloid cells. Hypothyroidism has been considered to cause basophilia (15), but a 1993 study revealed no difference in basophil counts in normal subjects and patients with hypothyroidism (16). Similarly, T- and B-lymphocyte counts and the ratio of T cells to B cells are normal in patients with hypothyroidism (17).

HEMOSTASIS

Bleeding problems such as easy bruising, prolonged bleeding after dental or other procedures or minor injuries, and menorrhagia occur occasionally in hypothyroid patients.

CLOTTING FACTORS AND WARFARIN THERAPY

The biological half-lives of several coagulation factors, including factors II, VII, and X, are prolonged in patients with hypothyroidism (18). The plasma concentrations of these and other factors have been reported as normal or slightly reduced (19–23). These disparities may be due to differences in assay methods or in the duration and degree of hypothyroidism. The most consistent abnormalities in patients with hypothyroidism are a decrease in plasma factor VIII concentrations (19,24) and a prolonged partial thromboplastin time (19–21). Slight decreases in plasma factor VIII activity can occur in a few weeks in severely hypothyroid patients with thyroid carcinoma in whom T_4 is discontinued to administer radioiodine therapy (24).

Acquired von Willebrand's disease, with decreases in plasma factor VIII coagulant activity and von Willebrand antigen activity, can occur in patients with hypothyroidism (21,25). Proposed mechanisms include a decreased response to adrenergic stimulation (which stimulates release of factor VIII coagulant activity from endothelial cells) or decreased protein synthesis (22). As in patients with other coagulation disorders, a surgical procedure may unmask the clinical manifestations. Most hypothyroid patients with acquired von Willebrand's disease presented with prolonged bleeding after a dental procedure (21,26). The abnormalities are reversed by T_4 therapy (21,25,26).

Desmopressin has been used to treat patients with acquired von Willebrand's disease caused by disorders other than hypothyroidism because it stimulates release of factor VIII from endothelial cells and platelets (27). Its efficacy in hypothyroid patients with this disorder is not known, but it could be of value if treatment other than T_4 was considered necessary.

A recent study described biphasic alterations in the fibrinolytic system depending on the degree of hypothyroidism (28). Compared with patients with severe hypothyroidism [serum thyrotropin (TSH) concentrations greater than 50 mU/L], those with milder hypothyroidism (mean serum TSH, 21 mU/L) had lower plasma concentrations of D-dimers, higher plasma α_2-antiplasmin activity, and higher plasma concentrations of plasminogen acti-

vator inhibitor type 1 (PAI-1) and tissue plasminogen activator antigen. This profile in patients with mild hypothyroidism may indicate a relative hypofibrinolytic state, and provide insight into the association between mild hypothyroidism and cardiovascular disease (29). Whether the seeming activation of the fibrinolytic system in patients with severe hypothyroidism confers any protection against myocardial infarction is not known (28).

Patients with hypothyroidism are relatively refractory to the hypoprothrombinemic effects of warfarin, because the clearance of coagulation factors is slowed. Therefore, it may take longer to prolong the prothrombin time with warfarin in these patients than in euthyroid patients (18). In a warfarin-treated woman who became hypothyroid, a dose of warfarin three times higher than the original dose was required to maintain adequate anticoagulation until one was treated with T_4, after which the original warfarin dose was again adequate (30). Hypothyroidism should be considered in patients who seem to become "resistant" to warfarin. In patients beginning heparin and warfarin therapy, it may be necessary to administer heparin longer than the usual 4 to 5 days (18).

BLEEDING TIME

A few patients with hypothyroidism note increased bruising or bleeding, and more have prolonged bleeding times, with a rough correlation between the bleeding time and the severity and duration of hypothyroidism (21,31,32). Prolonged bleeding times may be present in patients with normal plasma factor VIII activity (31). In addition, severely hypothyroid patients may be more sensitive to aspirin and therefore have a prolonged bleeding time after aspirin ingestion (33). There are reports of untreated or partially treated hypothyroid patients who bled profusely after taking aspirin (33). Therefore, aspirin should be given cautiously to patients with hypothyroidism.

PLATELETS

Platelet counts are usually normal in hypothyroid patients, although the bone marrow megakaryocyte count may be low (5). Mean platelet volume is also normal (22). Hypothyroidism, however, may alter platelet function, with increased adenosine diphosphate– and collagen-induced aggregation of platelets (34). This increase may be due to an increase in platelet myosin light-chain kinase, which increases the activity of the contractile proteins of platelets (35). On the other hand, ristocetin-induced platelet aggregation is impaired in hypothyroid patients; however, ristocetin induces aggregation by facilitating platelet interaction with factor VIII (32), and the low plasma factor VIII activity found in hypothyroid patients probably accounts for the diminished ristocetin response. All these abnormalities improve during T_4 treatment.

AUTOIMMUNE ASSOCIATIONS

In a group of 12 patients with chronic autoimmune thyroiditis, of whom two were hypothyroid and ten euthyroid, serum levels of platelet-bound immunoglobulin G were high in six, of whom two had thrombocytopenia (36). Autoimmune thrombocytopenic purpura only rarely is associated with chronic autoimmune thyroiditis (37). In addition, low serum concentrations of anticardiolipin antibodies were found in two of five patients with chronic autoimmune thyroiditis (38), but there are no reports of the antiphospholipid syndrome in hypothyroid or euthyroid patients with autoimmune thyroiditis.

REFERENCES

1. Das KC, Mukherjee, Sarkar TK, et al. Erythropoiesis and erythropoietin in hypo- and hyperthyroidism. *J Clin Endocrinol Metab* 1975;40:211.
2. Horton l, Coburn RJ, England JM, et al. The hematology of hypothyroidism. *Q J Med* 1976;45:101.
3. Chu JY, Monteleone JA, Peden VH, et al. Anemia in children and adolescents with hypothyroidism. *Clin Pediatr* 1981;20:696.
4. Franzese A, Salerno A, Angenziano A, et al. Anemia in infants with congenital hypothyroidism diagnosed by neonatal screening. *J Endocrinol Invest* 1996;19:613.
5. Axelrod AR, Berman L. The bone marrow in hyperthyroidism and hypothyroidism. *Blood* 1951;6:436–453.
6. Kiley JM, Purnell DC, Owen CA. Erythrokinetics in myxedema. *Ann Intern Med* 1967;67:533.
7. Grosz HJ. Reduction-oxidation potential of blood determined by oxygen releasing factor in thyroid disorders. *Nature* 1969; 222:875.
8. Zaroulis CG, Kourides IA, Valeri CR. Red cell 2,3-diphosphoglycerate and oxygen affinity of hemaglobin in patients with thyroid disorders. *Blood* 1978;53:181.
9. Donati RM, Fletcher JW, Warnecke MA, et al. Erythropoiesis in hypothyroidism. *Proc Soc Exp Biol Med* 1973;144:78.
10. Hines JD, Halsted Ch, Griggs RC, et al. Megaloblastic anemia secondary to folate deficiency associate with hypothyroidism. *Ann Intern Med* 1968;68:792.
11. Carmel R, Spencer CA. Clinical and subclinical thyroid disorders associated with pernicious anemia. *Arch Intern Med* 1982; 142:1465.
12. Tudhope GR, Wilson GM. Deficiency of vitamin B_{12} in hypothyroidism. *Lancet* 1962;1;703.
13. Ottesen M, Feldt-Rasmussen U, Andersen J, et al. Thyroid function and autoimmunity in pernicious anemia before and during cyanocobalamin treatment. *J Endocrinol Invest* 1995;18:91.
14. Okuda K, Chow BF. The thyroid and absorption of vitamin B_{12} in rats. *Endocrinology* 1961;68:607.
15. Athens JW. Variation of leukocytes in disease. In: Lee GR, Bithell TC, Foerster J, et al., eds. *Wintrobe's Clinical Hematology.* Philadelphia/London: Lea & Febiger, 1993:1564.
16. Petrasch SG, Mlynek-Kersjes ML, Haase R, et al. Basophilic leukocytes in hypothyroidism. *Clin Invest* 1993;71:27.
17. Urbaniak SJ, Penhale WJ, Irvine WJ. Peripheral blood T and B lymphocytes in patients with thyrotoxicosis and Hashimoto's thyroiditis and in normal subjects. *Clin Exp Immunol* 1974;18:449.
18. Loeliger EA, vanderEsch B, Mattern MJ, et al. The biological disappearance rate of prothrombin, factors VII, IX, and X from plasma in hypothyroidism, hyperthyroidism and during fever. *Thrombosis Diath Hemorrh* 1964;10:267.
19. Simone JV, Abildgaard CF, Schulman I. Blood coagulation in thyroid dysfunction. *N Eng J Med* 1965;237:1057.
20. Edson JR, Fecher DR, Doe RP. Low platelet adhesiveness and other hemostatic abnormalities in hypothyroidism. *Ann Intern Med* 1975;82:342.
21. Dalton RG, Dewar MS, Savidge GF, et al. Hypothyroidism as a cause of acquired von Willebrand's disease. *Lancet* 1987;1:1007.
22. Ford HC, Carter JM. Haemostasis in hypothyroidism. *Postgrad Med J* 1990;66:280.
23. Farid NR, Griffiths BL, Collins JR, et al. Blood coagulation and fibrinolysis in thyroid disease. *Thromb Haemost* 1976;35:415.
24. Palareti G, Biagi G, Legnani C, et al. Association of reduced factor VIII with impaired platelet reactivity to adrenaline and collagen after total thyroidectomy. *Thromb Heamost* 1989;62:1053.
25. Michiels JJ, Schroyens W, Berneman Z, et al. Acquired von Willebrand syndrome type 1 in hypothyroidism: reversal after treatment with thyroxine. *Clin Appl Thromb Hemost* 2001; 7:113.
26. Attivissimo LA, Lichtman SM, Klein I. Acquired von Willebrand's syndrome causing a hemorrhagic diathesis in a patient with hypothyroidism. *Thyroid* 1995;5:399.
27. Erfurth EM, Ericsson UC, Egervall K, et al. Effect of acute desmopressin and of long term thyroxine replacement on haemostasis in hypothyroidism. *Clin Endocrinol (Oxf)* 1995;42:373.
28. Chadarevian R, Bruckert E, Leenhardt L, et al. Components of the fibrinolytic system are differently altered in moderate and severe hypothyroidism. *J Clin Endocrinol Metab* 2001;86:732.
29. Hak AE, Pols HAP, Visser TJ, et al. Subclinical hypothyroidism is an independent risk factor for atherosclerosis and myocardial infarction in elderly women: the Rotterdam Study. *Ann Intern Med* 2000;132:270.
30. Stephens MA, Self TH, Lancaster D, et al. Hypothyroidism: effect on warfarin anticoagulation. *South Med J* 1989;82:1585.
31. Zeigler Z, Hasiba U, Lewis J, et al. Exaggeration of defective platelet function by methyldopa in hypothyroidism. *Am J Hematol* 1984;17:209.
32. Myrup B, Bregengard C, Faber J. Primary haemostasis in thyroid disease. *J Intern Med* 1995;238:59.
33. Zeigler ZR, Hasiba U, Lewis JH, et al. Hemostatic defects in response to aspirin challenge in hypothyroidism. *Am J Hematol* 1986;23:391.
34. Masunaga R, Nagasaka A, Nakai A, et al. Alteration of platelet aggregation in patients with thyroid disorders. *Metabolism* 1997; 46:1128.
35. Mamiya S, Hagiwara M, Inoue S, et al. Thyroid hormones inhibit platelet function and myosin light chain kinase. *J Biol Chem* 1989; 264:8575.
36. Hymes K, Blum M, Lackner H, et al. Easy bruising, thrombocytopenia, and elevated platelet immunoglobulin G in Graves' disease and Hashimoto's thyroiditis. *Ann Intern Med* 1981;94:27.
37. Robbins JB. Autoimmune thrombocytopenia purpura and Hashimoto's thyroiditis. *Ann Intern Med* 1975;83:371.
38. Paggi A, Caccavo D, Ferri GM, et al. Anti-cardiolipin antibodies in autoimmune thyroid diseases. *Clin Endocrinol (Oxf)* 1994;40:329.

58

THE PITUITARY IN HYPOTHYROIDISM

PETER J. SNYDER

Hypothyroidism affects the secretion of all pituitary hormones. This chapter discusses the effects of hypothyroidism on the secretion of growth hormone (GH) and prolactin as well as the clinical consequences of these effects. The effects of hypothyroidism on the secretion of vasopressin, corticotropin, and follicle-stimulating hormone and luteinizing hormone are discussed elsewhere (see Chapters 55, 59, and 61, respectively).

GROWTH HORMONE

Clinical Features

Suspicion that hypothyroidism decreases GH secretion is based on the dramatic retardation of growth that occurs in children with hypothyroidism (see Chapter 75), followed by the equally dramatic increase in growth when they are treated with thyroid hormone. The degree of growth retardation, which may be severe, is accompanied by a corresponding decrease in bone age.

The growth curve of a child who has hypothyroidism (Fig. 58.1) is characterized by normal growth until onset of the hypothyroidism, then abrupt cessation of growth, and rapid catch-up growth after initiation of thyroid hormone replacement therapy. The final height may be normal, especially if treatment is begun before the anticipated age of puberty. Final height may be less than normal, however, if treatment is not begun until after the anticipated age of puberty because secretion of gonadal steroids, which increases after correction of the hypothyroidism, may cause epiphyseal closure before catch-up growth can occur.

Hormonal Abnormalities

The growth retardation caused by hypothyroidism appears to result from deficient secretion of GH as well as from impaired action of GH. Many but not all children with hypothyroidism have subnormal serum GH responses to insulin-induced hypoglycemia and arginine (1–3), and not all of those who have impaired responses have an increase in GH secretion after treatment with thyroid hormone.

Spontaneous GH secretion is usually greatest at night, especially during stages 3 and 4 of sleep, in normal children and young adults; therefore, it seems especially important that in a study of nocturnal serum GH concentrations in

seven children with primary hypothyroidism, all had higher values after they were treated with thyroxine (T_4) and were euthyroid; the mean serum GH concentration in the group increased more than twofold (4). The nocturnal pattern of GH secretion in one of the patients before and during thyroid hormone treatment is shown in Figure 58.2. The serum GH response to growth hormone–releasing hormone (GHRH) in two groups of hypothyroid adults increased twofold to threefold after treatment with thyroid hormone (5,6).

The mechanism by which impaired GH secretion impairs growth in hypothyroidism is likely decreased production of insulin-like growth factor-1 (IGF-1). Normally, GH stimulates skeletal growth because it increases the production of IGF-1 by the liver and other tissues. Thyroid hormone treatment of three groups of patients, including both adults and children, with hypothyroidism increased the serum IGF-1 concentrations in each group twofold to fourfold (4,5,7). When six of the untreated hypothyroid patients in one group were given a single injection of GH, their serum IGF-1 concentrations increased fourfold (7). This increase suggests that hypothyroidism does not impair IGF-1 responsiveness to GH. By exclusion, these results suggest that decreased IGF-1 secretion results from decreased GH secretion, a conclusion corroborated by the decreased nocturnal serum GH concentrations in hypothyroid patients described previously (4).

Decreased GH secretion in hypothyroidism probably results from a direct effect of thyroid hormone deficiency on the pituitary somatotrophs and perhaps also from an effect on hypothalamic GHRH secretion. The marked improvement in GH responsiveness to GHRH administration when hypothyroid adults were treated with thyroid hormone (6) suggests that thyroid hormone directly affects GH secretion by the pituitary. The molecular mechanism by which thyroid hormone permits normal GH secretion is not clear, especially in humans. Although triiodothyronine (T_3) increases the expression of the promoter region of the rat GH gene after transfection of rat pituitary tumor cells, it does not increase expression of the promoter region of the human GH gene when it is similarly transfected (8). This effect of T_3 requires the presence of the transcription factor *Pit1*, which is expressed in somatotroph cells; without it, T_3 inhibits the promoter (9).

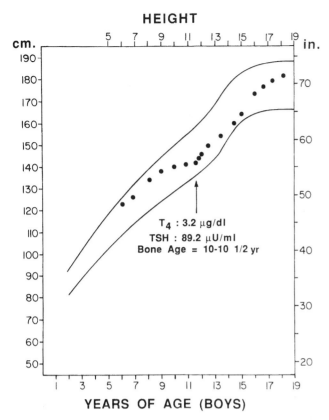

HEIGHT

YEARS OF AGE (BOYS)

T₄ : 3.2 µg/dl
TSH : 89.2 µU/ml
Bone Age = 10-10 1/2 yr

FIGURE 58.1. The growth curve of a boy found to have primary hypothyroidism at age 11.5 years. Growth virtually ceased after age 9 years until the diagnosis was made. After treatment was initiated (*arrow*), growth resumed at an accelerated rate. To convert the serum thyroxine (T₄) value to n*M*, multiply by 12.9. (Courtesy of Dr. Thomas Moshang, Children's Hospital of Philadelphia.)

The effect of thyroid hormone on GHRH secretion has not been studied in humans, but it has been studied in rats. Hypothyroidism in rats decreases the hypothalamic content of GHRH, but it increases GHRH messenger RNA content and GHRH release *in vitro* (10,11). These abnormalities are restored to normal by thyroid hormone and also by GH treatment, suggesting that the abnormal GHRH secretion in hypothyroidism is the result, not the cause, of decreased GH secretion. The effect of hypothyroidism on hypothalamic somatostatin has not been studied.

Hypothyroidism also impairs growth by impairing the response of cartilage to IGF-1. Administration of GH to children with hypothyroidism does not stimulate growth, even though serum IGF-1 concentrations increase. When cartilage is incubated *in vitro,* the addition of T₃ to the incubation medium is necessary for the full effect of IGF-1. The diminished response of cartilage to GH also could be related to diminished GH receptors on cartilage cells, because the serum concentrations of GH-binding protein, which is the extracellular domain of the GH receptor, are less than normal in hypothyroidism and increase during

treatment with thyroid hormone (12,13). Hypothyroidism, in summary, impairs growth by impairing the secretion of GH, which results in decreased IGF-1 secretion by the liver, as well as by impairing the response of cartilage to IGF-1 and possibly GH.

PROLACTIN

Clinical Features

Galactorrhea is the only clinical manifestation of the effect of hypothyroidism on prolactin secretion, although even this does not occur often. Galactorrhea occurred in about 5% of cases in three series of patients with hypothyroidism comprising 56 to 235 patients, but it did not occur in any of 1,005 patients in a fourth series (14). One factor that appears to influence which hypothyroid patients develop galactorrhea is the duration of their hypothyroidism. In one study, galactorrhea occurred in 7 of 27 women who had spontaneous hypothyroidism for an estimated mean duration of 72 months, but in none of 16 women who had iatrogenic hypothyroidism for an estimated mean duration of 7 months (15).

When galactorrhea occurs in patients with long-standing primary hypothyroidism who also have sellar enlargement attributable to thyrotroph hyperplasia, a prolactin-secreting adenoma may be diagnosed erroneously. This misdiagnosis has been reported in women who presented with amenorrhea and galactorrhea and had serum prolactin concentrations of 35 to 85 ng/mL. These values are compatible with small prolactin-secreting adenomas, which are what the women were thought to have when modest enlargement of their pituitary gland was seen by imaging (16,17). The true diagnosis, severe primary hypothyroidism causing pituitary enlargement as a result of thyrotroph hyperplasia and simultaneously causing hyperprolactinemia, was made in each of these women only when their serum T₄ concentrations were found to be extremely low and their serum thyrotropin (TSH) concentrations quite high. The diagnosis was confirmed when treatment with T₄ alone decreased the serum concentrations of TSH and prolactin and decreased the size of the pituitary gland to normal (Fig. 58.3).

Hormonal Abnormalities

The mechanism by which galactorrhea occurs in patients with hypothyroidism most likely is hyperprolactinemia, which is also the mechanism by which other causes of galactorrhea occur. When serum prolactin concentrations were measured in unselected patients with primary hypothyroidism, the values were normal in most patients but mildly supranormal in a few (18–20). In patients, nearly all of whom were women, with galactorrhea thought to be caused by hypothyroidism, values were normal to mildly supranormal (21–23). Even when the serum prolactin concentrations in hypothyroidism are supranormal, however,

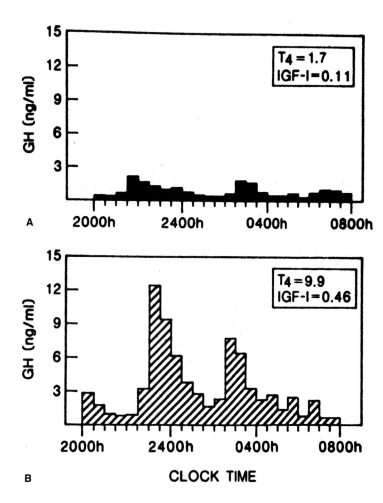

A

B

CLOCK TIME

FIGURE 58.2. The nocturnal pattern of growth hormone secretion in a patient with primary hypothyroidism before **(A)** and during **(B)** treatment with thyroid hormone. The serum thyroxine (T_4) and insulin-like growth factor-1 (IGF-1) concentrations at these times were 1.7 µg/dL and 0.11 U/mL and 9.9 µg/dL and 0.46 U/mL, respectively. To convert the serum T_4 values to n*M*, multiply by 12.9. (From Chernausek SD, Turner R. Attenuation of spontaneous, noctural growth hormone secretion in children with hypothyroidism and its correlation with plasma insulin-like growth factor-1 concentrations. *J Pediatr* 1989; 114:968, with permission.)

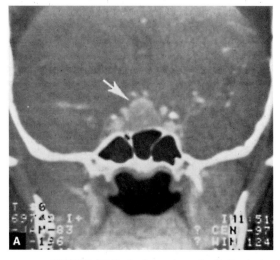

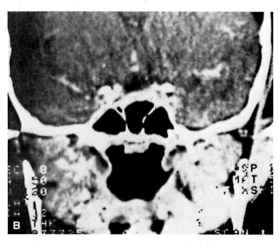

FIGURE 58.3. A: An enlarged pituitary gland in a 24-year-old woman who presented with amenorrhea and galactorrhea and was found to have primary hypothyroidism and hyperprolactinemia. **B:** After treatment with thyroxine (T_4) for 2 months, the patient's pituitary gland was no longer enlarged, and her serum thyrotropin concentration was normal. (From Groff TR, Shulkin BL, Utiger RD, et al. Amenorrhea-galactorrhea, hyperprolactinemia, and suprasellar pituitary enlargment as presenting features of primary hypothyroidism. *Obstet Gynecol* 1984;63 (suppl):86, with permission.)

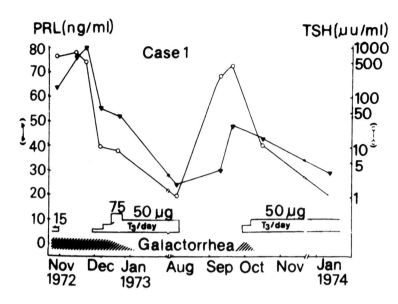

FIGURE 58.4. Serum prolactin (*PRL*) and thyrotropin (*TSH*) concentrations in a woman who presented with galactorrhea and primary hypothyroidism. When she was treated with triiodothyronine (T$_3$), her serum prolactin and TSH concentrations decreased, and the galactorrhea disappeared. When treatment was discontinued, serum PRL and TSH concentrations both increased again. When treatment was resumed, both declined again. (From Onishi T, Miyai K, Aono T, et al. Primary hypothyroidism and galactorrhea. *Am J Med* 1977;63:373, with permission.)

they are usually less than 100 ng/mL, and so a higher value should raise the suspicion of a prolactin-secreting adenoma. In one study of serum prolactin concentrations in hypothyroid men, the values were normal in magnitude, pulsatility, and circadian pattern (24), suggesting that hypothyroidism alone is not sufficient to cause hyperprolactinemia; rather, another stimulus, such as estrogen, is required. The strongest evidence for concluding that hypothyroidism is the cause of the hyperprolactinemia in patients who have both hypothyroidism and hyperprolactinemia is that their serum prolactin concentrations decline to normal when they are treated with thyroid hormone (14,16,17,25, 26) (Fig. 58.4).

The mechanism by which hypothyroidism causes hyperprolactinemia is not known, but it is probably due to a direct effect on the pituitary gland. Patients who are hypothyroid have greater than normal serum prolactin responses to thyrotropin-releasing hormone (TRH), and the responses decrease to normal during thyroid hormone therapy (18,19). The molecular mechanism by which thyroid hormone inhibits prolactin secretion may involve interaction with both activating and inhibitory elements in the proximal promoter region of the prolactin gene (27). Thyroid hormone may also influence prolactin secretion through an effect on TRH secretion, because T$_3$ decreases the expression of the messenger RNA for the TRH precursor in the hypothalamus (28).

REFERENCES

1. Katz HP, Youltan R, Kaplan SL, et al. Growth and growth hormone. III. Growth hormone release in children with primary hypothyroidism and thyrotoxicosis. *J Clin Endocrinol Metab* 1969; 29:346.

2. MacGillivray MH, Aceto T, Frohman LA. Plasma growth hormone responses and growth retardation in hypothyroidism. *Am J Dis Child* 1968;115:273.

3. Root AW, Rosenfeld RL, Bongiovanni AM, et al. The plasma growth hormone response to insulin-induced hypoglycemia in children with retardation of growth. *Pediatrics* 1967;39:844.

4. Chernausek SD, Turner R. Attenuation of spontaneous, nocturnal growth hormone secretion in children with hypothyroidism and its correlation with plasma insulin-like growth factor I concentrations. *Pediatrics* 1989;114:968.

5. Valcavi R, Dieguez C, Preece M, et al. Effect of thyroxine replacement therapy on plasma insulin-like growth factor I levels and growth hormone responses to growth hormone releasing factor in hypothyroid patients. *Clin Endocrinol (Oxf)* 1987;27: 85.

6. Williams T, Maxon H, Thorner MO, et al. Blunted growth hormone (GH) response to GH-releasing hormone in hypothyroidism resolves in the euthyroid state. *J Clin Endocrinol Metab* 1985;61:454.

7. Chernausek SD, Underwood LE, Utiger RD, et al. Growth hormone secretion and plasma somatomedin-C in primary hypothyroidism. *Clin Endocrinol (Oxf)* 1983;19:337.

8. Brent GA, Harney JW, Moore DD, et al. Multihormonal regulation of the human, rat, and bovine growth hormone promoters: differential effects of 3',5' cyclic adenosine monophosphate, thyroid hormone, and glucocorticoids. *Mol Endocrinol* 1988;2:792.

9. Palamino T, Barettino D, Aranda A. Role of GHF-1 in the regulation of the rat growth hormone gene promoter by thyroid hormone and retinoic acid receptors. *J Biol Chem* 1998;273: 27541.

10. Katakami H, Downs TR, Frohman LA. Decreased hypothalamic growth hormone-releasing hormone content and pituitary responsiveness in hypothyroidism. *J Clin Invest* 1987;77:1704.

11. Downs TR, Chomczynski P, Frohman LA. Effects of thyroid hormone deficiency and replacement on rat hypothalamic growth hormone (GH)–releasing hormone gene expression *in vivo* are mediated by GH. *Mol Endocrinol* 1990;4:402.

12. Amit T, Hertz P, Ish-Shalom S, et al. Effects of hypo- or hyperthyroidism on growth hormone-binding protein. *Clin Endocrinol (Oxf)* 1991;35:159.

13. Miell JP, Taylor AM, Zini M, et al. Effects of hypothyroidism and hyperthyroidism on insulin-like growth factors (IGFs) and

complex regulation by glucagon, norepinephrine, glucocorticoids, and TH, all of which concur to stimulate activity, as well as by insulin, which represses the activity of the enzyme (16). The PEPCK gene has a complex promoter/enhancer region with regulatory elements for the hormones mentioned above or their intracellular messengers. Triiodothyronine (T_3) stimulates the gene directly via its corresponding response element (17) and amplifies the responses of the gene to other stimuli, most notably to cyclic adenosine monophosphate (cAMP) generated in response to glucagon or epinephrine (18), but also enhances the response to glucocorticoids (19). As it occurs with UCP1, and discussed in Chapter 38, the effect of each stimulus is relatively modest, but together their effects are synergistic (T_3 and cAMP) or additive (glucocorticoids). This multiplicity of influences allows a more flexible response tuned to the physiologic needs, so that TH will not increase glucose production exaggeratedly in a postprandial status, when signals stimulating gluconeogenesis are low and signals inhibiting glucose production, such as glucose itself and insulin, are high. On the other hand, when this balance fails, such as in diabetes, the stimulatory effect of TH on PEPCK and glucose production resulting from elevated TH levels becomes clinically relevant. In hypopituitarism, the risk for fasting hypoglycemia is enhanced by the concomitant lack of glucocorticoids and TH. In severe primary hypothyroidism, hypoglycemia results from the blunted response of the PEPCK to fasting-induced signals such as glucagon, epinephrine, and glucocorticoids, as well as from the limited supply of gluconeogenic precursors, namely amino acids and glycerol, in turn resulting from reduced protein turnover and limited lipolysis.

Effects of Thyroid Hormone on Lipid Metabolism

As occurs with protein and carbohydrate metabolism, TH stimulates both the *de novo* synthesis of fatty acids (lipogenesis) and the degradation of lipids (lipolysis and fatty acid oxidation). Lipogenesis is stimulated by T_3 mainly in liver, with rather limited effect in white adipose tissue, kidney, and heart, and this is the result of the stimulation of synthesis of key lipogenic enzymes at the transcriptional level (20–22). Such enzymes include among others malic enzyme, glucose-6-phosphate dehydrogenase, acetyl CoA carboxylase, and the protein Spot 14, whose stimulation by T_3 bears a close relationship with the stimulation of lipogenesis (23). As measured by the incorporation of ^3H_2O into fatty acids, TH stimulates liver lipogenesis 16-fold between the hypothyroid state and a short-term thyrotoxicosis (20). In this transition, liver contribution to total lipogenesis increases by 5% to 50% (20), whereas the relative contribution of white adipose tissue and other organs decreases. Brown adipose tissue global lipogenesis is increased in hypothyroidism, but this is probably due to a complex interaction with the sympathetic nervous system, the activity of which is markedly enhanced in the hypothyroid state (24). If the adrenergic stimulation is prevented, for example by denervation, the stimulatory effect of TH on brown adipose tissue lipogenesis is readily demonstrable (24). Overall lipogenesis increases promptly after T_3 injection in rats, which protects the stores of fat before food intake is increased (25). The induction of the hyperthyroid state is immediately associated with increased use of fat as fuel (25), which comes both from increased synthesis in the liver and from hydrolysis of triglycerides (lipolysis) in white adipose tissue. TH stimulates lipolysis indirectly, by enhancing the catecholamine-induced stimulation of the hormone-sensitive lipase in adipose tissue. This results from amplification of the effect of catecholamines at the adrenergic receptor level and, most importantly, at postreceptor levels (see Chapter 38). In rats fasted for 15 hours, white adipose tissue lipolysis is increased. Under such conditions about 55% of the fatty acids are reesterified. TH increases lipolysis and reduces the fraction of fatty acids that is reesterified *in situ* (26). Interestingly, neither fasting nor TH stimulates reesterification of fatty acids in the liver and its incorporation into very-low-density lipoprotein particles, consistent with the concept that fatty acids are being used as fuel in various tissues. TH actually decreases fatty acid reesterification in liver and increases its oxidation (26).

Although much of the information on the effect of TH on lipid metabolism has been obtained in animal models with short-term experimental thyrotoxicosis, the dose-related manner in which TH stimulates these processes and observations on hypothyroid animals make it reasonable to assume those effects are physiologic. *De novo* lipogenesis is reduced in hypothyroidism, particularly in the liver, and this is corrected by thyroid hormone (20,27). TH action on lipid metabolism and adipose tissue has also been demonstrated in humans, wherein stimulation of the same relevant genes and lipolysis have been documented (28,29).

There seems to be a distinct difference between rodent models and humans in the response of lipoprotein lipase (LPL) to hypothyroidism. In humans, hypothyroidism is associated with reduced LPL and hepatic lipase activities, both of which respond to TH replacement (30–32) and continue to increase, in a T_3 concentration-dependent manner in the transition to thyrotoxicosis (33). Such observation may explain the elevation in serum triglyceride levels frequently seen in hypothyroid patients (31,32). In contrast, rat white adipose tissue LPL is inhibited by TH and is, hence, increased in the hypothyroid state (34). TH is believed to induce a messenger RNA (mRNA)–binding protein that inhibits the translation of LPL mRNA upon binding to a specific sequence in the 3′-untranslated region of the LPL mRNA. The low concentration of this protein in hypothyroidism is the cause of the higher LPL abundance and activity (35). LPL mass and activity are much higher in the heart and in oxidative muscle (e.g., soleus) than in the fast twitch muscle extensor digitorum longus (EDL) in euthyroid rats, and hypothyroidism further stimulates activity in heart and soleus but not in EDL (36). It was interesting in these studies that heart, but not EDL or soleus LPL, increased by fasting (36). It has been suggested that the increase in LPL activity in hypothyroid rats results in part from the marked reduction in food intake observed in such rats, because the differences with euthyroid controls are attenuated when these are pair fed with hypothyroid rats (37). Such interspecies difference has no apparent explanation.

Serum cholesterol levels have long been known to be sensitive to thyroid status. Total serum cholesterol is reduced in thyrotoxicosis and increased in hypothyroidism. TH indeed increases cholesterol synthesis, stimulating the rate-limiting enzyme 3-OH-methyl glutaryl CoA reductase (HMG CoA reductase) (38,39). However, the net effect of TH is to reduce cholesterol serum concentrations in a dose-dependent manner (40), which is largely the result of a more vigorous stimulation by TH of the removal of cholesterol by the liver via LDL receptors. TH increases the concentration of these via the stimulation of the expression of sterol regulatory element binding protein-2 (SREBP-2), a transcription factor that enhances LDL gene transcription and expression (see reference 41 and references therein). The stimulation by TH of HMG CoA reductase has a double meaning. All cells produce cholesterol, which is an essential element on plasma membrane. Plasma membrane is a very dynamic cell structure, in constant renovation at rates that are proportional to the metabolic activity of the cells. By stimulating the synthesis of cholesterol (and the other basic components of plasma membrane), TH facilitates its effects and those of other hormones in cell function, remodeling, and differentiation. In addition, cholesterol constitutes the foundation for the synthesis of steroid hormones. From a clinical point of view, higher levels of HMG CoA reductase expand the range where intracellular cholesterol concentration can negatively feed back into its synthesis and cell import of cholesterol. Statins, the collective name of widely used drugs to reduce serum cholesterol levels, work by inhibiting this enzyme. Its effect will depend, therefore, on how much cholesterol synthesis is contributing to its turnover and plasma levels (42).

THE SYMPATHOADRENAL SYSTEM IN HYPOTHYROIDISM

As noted above and in Chapter 38, TH interacts with catecholamines and the sympathoadrenal system (as defined in Chapter 38) at different levels, most notably in the control of metabolism and cardiovascular function. At a central level, TH in general has an inhibitory role over the sympathetic output to the periphery by mechanisms that remain largely undefined. Peripherally and in general terms, TH enhances the responses to catecholamines mediated by β-adrenergic receptors while inhibiting those mediated by α-adrenergic receptors. This dual control allows a synergistic interaction in a controlled manner. Such homeostatic interaction is impaired in hypothyroidism or thyrotoxicosis, as discussed at length in Chapter 38. This chapter briefly summarizes those aspects that relate specifically to catecholamines and hypothyroidism.

Hypothyroidism influences the sympathetic nervous system basically in a direction opposite that of thyrotoxicosis. At the cell and tissue levels, the responses to catecholamines are reduced, whereas the central sympathetic output reaching the tissues is, in general, enhanced. The mechanisms leading to decreased responsiveness or sensitivity to catecholamines vary according to tissue and species. These mechanisms include a reduced number of β-adrenergic receptors and an increased number of α-adrenergic receptors (43); enhanced inhibitory responses to adenosine (44–46), probably related to increases in Giα or Gβ protein subunits (47–50); enhanced phosphodiesterase activity (51); and lack of T_3 potentiation of cAMP effects at the gene level (17,52,53). A novel β-adrenergic receptor, the β_3-receptor, is receiving much attention (reviewed in reference 54). This receptor is coupled to adenylyl cyclase by G_s-proteins as the β_1 and β_2 counterparts and is abundantly expressed in brown fat and less so in white adipose tissue. This receptor and its mRNA are increased in rat hypothyroid brown fat and are rapidly reduced by T_3, whereas the opposite occurs in white adipose tissue (55), adding another bit of complexity to the intricate thyroid–adrenergic interactions. The α_2-adrenergic receptor, which causes inhibition of the cAMP production through coupling to Gi-proteins, is affected little by thyroid dysfunction (56,57).

In contrast to the overall depression of the adrenergic responses at the peripheral level, there is an increase in efferent sympathetic activity reaching virtually every tissue that has been investigated (48,58–61). Kinetic studies in hypothyroid patients show that the clearance of norepinephrine is not reduced and that the overall production rate of norepinephrine is faster than normal (61,62). Accordingly, plasma levels of norepinephrine are elevated in these patients (63–65). Furthermore, the increase in the production rate is selective for norepinephrine because epinephrine turnover is not affected (66). The increase in sympathetic activity appears to be compensatory in nature and may come about in response to the deficient peripheral responses to catecholamines, the thermal stress derived from the lack of the thermogenic effect of thyroid hormone, the reduction in cardiac output, or the lack of T_3 in critical regulatory centers of the central nervous system. Some of the abnormalities in the norepinephrine signaling pathway in hypothyroidism may not be caused directly by the lack of thyroid hormone in the tissues but by the increased sympathetic tone; that is, they may represent desensitization. Thus, brown fat–reduced β_1- and β_2-adrenergic receptors are normalized in athyreotic rats when sympathetic activity is reduced by placing them at 30°C, whereas the number of these receptors decreases in euthyroid rats placed at 4°C (67). Desensitization at a postreceptor level also has been described in brown fat of cold-exposed hamsters (68).

Severely hypothyroid patients may develop hypothermia and myxedema coma after exposure to low environmental temperatures or to medications that compromise heat conservation. Thermogenesis is markedly reduced in these patients: obligatory thermogenesis because of the slow rate of metabolism and facultative thermogenesis because of the diminished response to catecholamines and limited substrate availability due to the lack of thyroid hormone (see Chapter 38 and reference 69 for review). In hypothyroid rats, brown adipose tissue, the main site of facultative thermogenesis, does not respond to cold exposure, exogenous norepinephrine, or nerve stimulation (70–75). In humans with hypothyroidism, direct or indirect evidence has been found that metabolic responses to adrenergic stimulation involved in facultative thermogenesis, such as glycogenolysis, lipolysis, gluconeogenesis, and intracellular calcium mobilization, are reduced in hypothyroidism (76–81). Reduced heat loss through the skin becomes an essential mechanism for hypothyroid patients to maintain their body temperature. These patients have intense skin and subcutaneous tissue vasoconstriction (82), probably caused by an elevated sympathetic tone (83), increased α_1-adrenergic receptors (43), and reduced responses to vasodilating stimuli (84). These findings suggest that peripheral vasculature is under maximal stimulation, although postreceptor defects in the α_1-adrenergic pathway may limit the responses to the enhanced sympathetic input (80,85). In the clinical situation of severe, profound hypothyroidism, therefore, it would seem more prudent to treat the thyroid insufficiency as aggressively as possible, to provide glucose and other supportive treatment, and not to rely on catecholamines to improve the hemodynamic condition or thermogenesis.

In addition to the depressed peripheral vascular response to α_1-adrenergic agonists, the responsiveness of the heart to catecholamines is reduced markedly in hypothyroidism. Although the common belief is that this is caused by a reduced number of β-adrenergic receptors in the myocardium (43), there is evidence to indicate important postreceptor defects (45,47,86–88). Even though sympathetic stimulation of the heart is increased in hypothyroidism (59,89), the contractility (90) and functional reserve of the heart are severely compromised (91) because of both the direct biochemical consequences of the lack of thyroid hormone and the reduced sympathetic responsiveness. This condition easily can become clinically relevant in cases of bleeding or contraction of the extracellular volume or in cases of rapid reduction of peripheral vascular resistance, as may occur when patients with severe hypothyroidism are rapidly rewarmed. Likewise, volume or pressure overloads may precipitate congestive heart failure. The solutions to such problems are to avoid situations that require important hemodynamic adjustments and to provide thyroid hormone as rapidly as possible. Even though type II 5'-deiodinase mRNA has been identified in the human

heart (92), the contribution of this enzyme to nuclear T_3 in this organ has not yet been documented, and because thyroxine (T_4) to T_3 conversion by type I 5'-deiodinase is reduced in hypothyroidism (see Chapter 7), in situations of severely depressed myocardial function, it may be necessary to add small doses of T_3 to the initial treatment to accelerate the recovery of the heart (see Chapters 53 and 67).

A number of metabolic abnormalities are also caused in part by the negative effect of hypothyroidism in several signal transduction pathways. Lipolytic responses to catecholamines and glucagon are decreased largely because of postreceptor defects in the cAMP production in animals as well as in humans (51,81,93,94). Glocyogenolysis of muscle and liver also are reduced in part because of defects in the β-adrenergic cAMP pathway and Ca^{2+} mobilization (80,95). Insulin secretory responses are diminished in part because of defects in the cAMP signaling pathway (96,97). Gluconeogenic responses to glucagon and epinephrine are limited in hypothyroidism in part because of defects in the cAMP cascade and partly because of the lack of thyroid hormone at the level of the PEPCK gene, as discussed above (17,18). As mentioned previously, brown adipose tissue is indeed under maximal adrenergic stimulation in the hypothyroid rat, and yet its responses are depressed dramatically (52,75,98,99). Brown fat lipolytic, respiratory (100), and uncoupling protein responses (101) are also curtailed in brown adipocytes isolated from hypothyroid rats. Despite a clear reduction in β_1- and β_2-adrenergic receptors (102) and in cAMP accumulation (67,103), these defects do not seem to account for much of the reduced uncoupling protein responses because by the time thyroid hormone administration has completely restored the response of this protein to norepinephrine, neither the receptor number nor cAMP production has been normalized (52,55,67,75). Rather, the dominant defect in hypothyroid brown fat thermogenic responses to adrenergic stimulation seems to reside distal to the generation of cAMP (52,53, 100), pointing again to the physiologic relevance of interactions between cAMP and T_3 at levels further beyond, probably the genes themselves. Even though brown adipose tissue may not be as important in human facultative thermogenesis as it is in rodents, these observations underscore the importance of postreceptor defects in the poor responsiveness to catecholamines seen in hypothyroidism.

Thyroid hormone is also important for the development of the sympathetic nervous system. Abundant evidence has been found to show that congenital hypothyroidism results in numerous and ubiquitous abnormalities of the sympathoadrenal system, including the receptors and signaling pathways as well as enzymes involved in the synthesis of catecholamines (104–106). Neonatal rat hypothyroidism is associated with reduced β-adrenergic receptor and Gsα proteins, whereas Giα2 and Giα3 proteins are increased and the inotropic responses to isoproterenol are reduced (107). Except for a reduction in β-adrenergic receptor that persists into adulthood, these abnormalities are corrected with treatment and the responses to isoproterenol of the heart of these rats when adults is normal.

REFERENCES

1. Morrison WL, Gibson JN, Jung RT, et al. Skeletal muscle and whole body protein turnover in thyroid disease. *Eur J Clin Invest* 1988;18:62–68.
2. Brown JG, Millward DJ. Dose response of protein turnover in rat skeletal muscle to triiodothyronine treatment. *Biochim Biophys Acta* 1983;757:182–190.
3. Tauveron I, Charrier S, Champredon C, et al. Response of leucine metabolism to hyperinsulinemia under amino acid replacement in experimental hyperthyroidism. *Am J Physiol* 1995;269:E499–E507.
4. Lovejoy JC, Smith SR, Bray GA, et al. A paradigm of experimentally induced mild hyperthyroidism: effects on nitrogen balance, body composition, and energy expenditure in healthy young men. *J Clin Endocrinol Metab* 1997;82:765–770.
5. Grofte T, Wolthers T, Moller N, et al. Moderate hyperthyroidism reduces liver amino nitrogen conversion, muscle nitrogen contents and overall nitrogen balance in rats. *Eur J Clin Invest* 1997;27:85–92.
6. Wolman SI, Sheppard H, Fern M, et al. The effect of triiodothyronine (T_3) on protein turnover and metabolic rate. *Int J Obes* 1985;9:459–463.
7. Wood DF, Franklyn JA, Docherty K, et al. The effect of thyroid hormones on growth hormone gene expression *in vivo* in rats. *J Endocrinol* 1987;112:459–463.
8. Burstein PJ, Draznin B, Johnson CJ, et al. The effect of hypothyroidism on growth, serum growth hormone, the growth hormone–dependent somatomedin, insulin-like growth factor, and its carrier protein in rats. *Endocrinology* 1979;104:1107–1111.
9. Katz HP, Youlton R, Kaplan SL, et al. Growth and growth hormone. 3. Growth hormone release in children with primary hypothyroidism and thyrotoxicosis. *J Clin Endocrinol Metab* 1969; 29:346–351.
10. Cattini PA, Anderson TR, Baxter JD, et al. The human growth hormone gene is negatively regulated by triiodothyronine when transfected into rat pituitary cells. *J Biol Chem* 1986;261: 13367–13372.
11. Morin A, Louette J, Voz ML, et al. Triiodothyronine inhibits transcription from the human growth hormone promoter. *Mol Cell Endocrinol* 1990;71:261–267.
12. Belkhou R, Bechet D, Cherel Y, et al. Effect of fasting and thyroidectomy on cysteine proteinase activities in liver and muscle. *Biochim Biophys Acta* 1994;1199:195–201.
13. Rochon C, Tauveron I, Dejax C, et al. Response of leucine metabolism to hyperinsulinemia in hypothyroid patients before and after thyroxine replacement. *J Clin Endocrinol Metab* 2000; 85:697–706.
14. Rochon C, Tauveron I, Dejax C, et al. Response of glucose disposal to hyperinsulinaemia in human hypothyroidism and hyperthyroidism. *Clin Sci (Lond)* 2003;104:7–15.
15. Shulman GI, Ladenson PW, Wolfe MH, et al. Substrate cycling between gluconeogenesis and glycolysis in euthyroid, hypothyroid, and hyperthyroid man. *J Clin Invest* 1985;76:757–764.
16. Hanson RW, Reshef L. Regulation of phosphoenolpyruvate carboxykinase (GTP) gene expression. *Annu Rev Biochem* 1997; 66:581–611.
17. Giralt M, Park EA, Gurney AL, et al. Identification of a thyroid hormone response element in the phospho*enol*pyruvate car-

18. boxykinase (GTP) gene. Evidence for synergistic interaction between thyroid hormone and cAMP *cis*-regulatory elements. *J Biol Chem* 1991;266:21991–21996.
18. Hoppner W, Sussmuth W, Seitz HJ. Effect of thyroid state on cyclic AMP-mediated induction of hepatic phosphoenolpyruvate carboxykinase. *Biochem J* 1985;226:67–73.
19. Hoppner W, Sussmuth W, O'Brien C, et al. Cooperative effect of thyroid and glucocorticoid hormones on the induction of hepatic phosphoenolpyruvate carboxykinase *in vivo* and in cultured hepatocytes. *Eur J Biochem* 1986;159:399–405.
20. Blennemann B, Moon YK, Freake HC. Tissue-specific regulation of fatty acid synthesis by thyroid hormone. *Endocrinology* 1992;130:637–643.
21. Blennemann B, Leahy P, Kim TS, et al. Tissue-specific regulation of lipogenic mRNAs by thyroid hormone. *Mol Cell Endocrinol* 1995;110:1–8.
22. Feng X, Jiang Y, Meltzer P, et al. Thyroid hormone regulation of hepatic genes *in vivo* detected by complementary DNA microarray. *Mol Endocrinol* 2000;14:947–955.
23. Freake HC, Oppenheimer JH. Stimulation of S14 mRNA and lipogenesis in brown fat by hypothyroidism, cold exposure, and cafeteria feeding: evidence supporting a general role for S14 in lipogenesis and lipogenesis in the maintenance of thermogenesis. *Proc Natl Acad Sci USA* 1987;84:3070–3074.
24. Yeh W-J, Leahy P, Freake HC. Regulation of brown adipose tissue lipogenesis by thyroid hormone and the sympathetic nervous system. *Am J Physiol Endocrinol Metab* 1993;265:E252–E258.
25. Oppenheimer JH, Schwartz HL, Lane JT, et al. Functional relationship of thyroid hormone-induced lipogenesis, lipolysis and thermogenesis in the rat. *J Clin Invest* 1991;87:125–132.
26. Kalderon B, Mayorek N, Berry E, et al. Fatty acid cycling in the fasting rat. *Am J Physiol Endocrinol Metab* 2000;279:E221–E227.
27. Freake HC, Schwartz HL, Oppenheimer JH. The regulation of lipogenesis by thyroid hormone and its contribution to thermogenesis. *Endocrinology* 1989;125:2868–2874.
28. Viguerie N, Millet L, Avizou S, et al. Regulation of human adipocyte gene expression by thyroid hormone. *J Clin Endocrinol Metab* 2002;87:630–634.
29. Hellstrom L, Wahrenberg H, Reynisdottir S, et al. Catecholamine-induced adipocyte lipolysis in human hyperthyroidism. *J Clin Endocrinol Metab* 1997;82:159–166.
30. Pykalisto O, Goldberg AP, Brunzell JD. Reversal of decreased human adipose tissue lipoprotein lipase and hypertriglyceridemia after treatment of hypothyroidism. *J Clin Endocrinol Metab* 1976;43:591–600.
31. Valdemarsson S, Hedner P, Nilsson-Ehle P. Reversal of decreased hepatic lipase and lipoprotein lipase activities after treatment of hypothyroidism. *Eur J Clin Invest* 1982;12:423–428.
32. Valdemarsson S, Hansson P, Hedner P, et al. Relations between thyroid function, hepatic and lipoprotein lipase activities, and plasma lipoprotein concentrations. *Acta Endocrinol (Copenh)* 1983;104:50–56.
33. Lam KS, Chan MK, Yeung RT. High-density lipoprotein cholesterol, hepatic lipase and lipoprotein lipase activities in thyroid dysfunction—effects of treatment. *Q J Med* 1986;59:513–521.
34. Redgrave TG, Elsegood CL, Mamo JC, et al. Effects of hypothyroidism on the metabolism of lipid emulsion models of triacylglycerol-rich lipoproteins in rats. *Biochem J* 1991;273: 375–381.
35. Kern PA, Ranganathan G, Yukht A, et al. Translational regulation of lipoprotein lipase by thyroid hormone is via a cytoplasmic repressor that interacts with the 3′ untranslated region. *J Lipid Res* 1996;37:2332–2340.
36. Ong JM, Simsolo RB, Saghizadeh M, et al. Expression of lipoprotein lipase in rat muscle: regulation by feeding and hypothyroidism. *J Lipid Res* 1994;35:1542–1551.

37. Hansson P, Nordin G, Nilsson-Ehle P. Influence of nutritional state on lipoprotein lipase activities in the hypothyroid rat. *Biochim Biophys Acta* 1983;753:364–371.

38. Choi JW, Choi HS. The regulatory effects of thyroid hormone on the activity of 3-hydroxy-3-methylglutaryl coenzyme A reductase. *Endocr Res* 2000;26:1–21.

39. Ness GC, Lopez D, Chambers CM, et al. Effects of L-triiodothyronine and the thyromimetic L-94901 on serum lipoprotein levels and hepatic low-density lipoprotein receptor, 3-hydroxy-3-methylglutaryl coenzyme A reductase, and apo A-I gene expression. *Biochem Pharmacol* 1998;56:121–129.

40. Bantle JP, Dillmann WH, Oppenheimer JH, et al. Common clinical indices of thyroid hormone action: relationships to serum free 3,5,3′-triiodothyronine concentration and estimated nuclear occupancy. *J Clin Endocrinol Metab* 1980;50:286–293.

41. Shin DJ, Osborne TF. Thyroid hormone regulation and cholesterol metabolism are connected through sterol regulatory element-binding protein-2 (SREBP-2). *J Biol Chem* 2003;278:34114–34118.

42. Ness GC, Chambers CM. Feedback and hormonal regulation of hepatic 3-hydroxy-3-methylglutaryl coenzyme A reductase: the concept of cholesterol buffering capacity. *Proc Soc Exp Biol Med* 2000;224:8–19.

43. Bilezikian JP, Loeb JN. The influence of hyperthyroidism and hyperthyroidism on α- and β-adrenergic receptor systems and adrenergic responsiveness. *Endocr Rev* 1983;4:378–388.

44. Bumgarner JR, Ramkumar V, Stiles GL. Altered thyroid status regulates the adipocyte A1 adenosine receptor-adenylate cyclase system. *Life Sci* 1989;44:1705–1712.

45. Kaasik A, Seppet EK, Ohisalo JJ. Enhanced negative inotropic effect of an adenosine A1-receptor agonist in rat left atria in hypothyroidism. *J Mol Cell Cardiol* 1994;26:509–517.

46. Woodward JA, Saggerson ED. Effect of adenosine deaminase, N6-phenylisopropyladenosine and hypothyroidism on the responsiveness of rat brown adipocytes to noradrenaline. *Biochem J* 1986;238:395–403.

47. Levine MA, Feldman AM, Robishaw JD, et al. Influence of thyroid hormone status on expression of genes encoding G proteins subunits in rat heart. *J Biol Chem* 1990;265:3553–3560.

48. Michel-Reher MB, Gross G, Jasper JR, et al. Tissue- and subunit-specific regulation of G-protein expression by hypo- and hyperthyroidism. *Biochem Pharmacol* 1993;45:1417–1423.

49. Orford M, Mazurkiewicz D, Milligan G, et al. Abundance of the alpha-subunits of Gi1, Gi2 and Go in synaptosomal membranes from several regions of the rat brain is increased in hypothyroidism. *Biochem J* 1991;275:183–186.

50. Rapiejko PJ, Watkins DC, Ros M, et al. Thyroid hormones regulate G-protein β-subunit mRNA expression *in vivo*. *J Biol Chem* 1989;264:16183–16189.

51. Goswami A, Rosenberg IN. Effects of thyroid status on membrane-bound low Km cyclic nucleotide phosphodiesterase activities in rat adipocytes. *J Biol Chem* 1985;260:82–85.

52. Bianco AC, Sheng X, Silva JE. Triiodothyronine amplifies norepinephrine stimulation of uncoupling protein gene transcription by a mechanism not requiring protein synthesis. *J Biol Chem* 1988;263:18168–18175.

53. Silva JE, Rabelo R. Regulation of the uncoupling protein gene expression. *Eur J Endocrinol* 1997;136:251–264.

54. Lowell BB, Flier JS. Brown adipose tissue, beta 3-adrenergic receptors, and obesity [Review]. *Annu Rev Med* 1997;48:307–316.

55. Rubio A, Raasmaja A, Silva JE. Effects of thyroid hormone on norepinephrine signalling in brown adipose tissue. II. Differential effects of thyroid hormone on β3-adrenergic receptors in brown and white adipose tissue. *Endocrinology* 1995;136:3277–3284.

56. Del Rio G, Zizzo G, Marrama P, et al. Alpha 2-adrenergic activity is normal in patients with thyroid disease. *Clin Endocrinol (Oxf)* 1994;40:235–239.

57. Richelsen B, Sorensen NS. Alpha 2- and beta-adrenergic receptor binding and action in gluteal adipocytes from patients with hypothyroidism and hyperthyroidism. *Metabolism* 1987;36:1031–1039.

58. Gripois D, Valens M. Uptake and turnover rate of norepinephrine in interscapular brown adipose tissue of the young rat: influence of hypothyroidism. *Biol Neonate* 1982;42:113–119.

59. Landsberg L, Axelrod J. Influence of pituitary, thyroid and adrenal hormones on norepinephrine turnover and metabolism in the rat heart. *Circ Res* 1968;22:559–571.

60. Matsukawa T, Mano T, Gotoh E, et al. Altered muscle sympathetic nerve activity in hyperthyroidism and hypothyroidism. *J Auton Nerv Syst* 1993;42:171–175.

61. Polikar R, Kennedy B, Ziegler M, et al. Plasma norepinephrine kinetics, dopamine-beta-hydroxylase, and chromogranin-A, in hypothyroid patients before and following replacement therapy. *J Clin Endocrinol Metab* 1990;70:277–281.

62. Coulombe P, Dussault JH. Catecholamine metabolism in thyroid disease. II. Norepinephrine secretion rate in hyperthyroidism and hypothyroidism. *J Clin Endocrinol Metab* 1977;44:1185–1189.

63. Brown RT, Lakshmanan MC, Baucom CE, et al. Changes in blood pressure and plasma noradrenaline in short-term hypothyroidism. *Clin Endocrinol (Oxf)* 1989;30:635–638.

64. Coulombe P, Dussault JH, Walker P. Plasma catecholamine concentrations in hyperthyroidism and hypothyroidism. *Metabolism* 1976;25:973–979.

65. Manhem P, Bramnert M, Hallengren B, et al. Increased arterial and venous plasma noradrenaline levels in patients with primary hypothyroidism during hypothyroid as compared to euthyroid state. *J Endocrinol Invest* 1992;15:763–765.

66. Coulombe P, Dussault JH, Letarte J, et al. Catecholamine metabolism in thyroid diseases. I. Epinephrine secretion rate in hyperthyroidism and hypothyroidism. *J Clin Endocrinol Metab* 1976;42:125–131.

67. Rubio A, Raasmaja A, Maia AL, et al. Effects of thyroid hormone on norepinephrine signalling in brown adipose tissue. I. β1- and β2-adrenergic receptors and cyclic adenosine monophosphate generation. *Endocrinology* 1995;136:3267–3276.

68. Svoboda P, Unelius L, Cannon B, et al. Attenuation of Gsa coupling efficiency in brown-adipose-tissue plasma membranes from cold-acclimated hamsters. *Biochem J* 1993;295:655–661.

69. Silva JE. The thermogenic effect of thyroid hormone and its clinical implications. *Ann Intern Med* 2003;139:205–213.

70. Bianco AC, Silva JE. Intracellular conversion of thyroxine to triiodothyronine is required for the optimal thermogenic function of brown adipose tissue. *J Clin Invest* 1987;79:295–300.

71. Carvalho SD, Kimura ET, Bianco AC, et al. Central role of brown adipose tissue thyroxine 5′deiodinase on thyroid hormone-dependent thermogenic response to cold. *Endocrinology* 1991;128:2149–2159.

72. Mory G, Ricquier D, Pesquies P, et al. Effects of hypothyroidism on the brown adipose tissue of adult rats: comparison with the effects of adaptation to the cold. *J Endocrinol* 1981;91:515–524.

73. Seydoux J, Giacobino J-P, Girardier L. Impaired metabolic response to nerve stimulation in brown adipose tissue of hypothyroid rats. *Mol Cell Endocrinol* 1982;25:213–226.

74. Triandafillou J, Gwilliam C, Himms-Hagen J. Role of thyroid hormone in cold-induced changes in rat brown adipose tissue mitochondria. *Can J Biochem* 1982;60:530–537.

75. Silva JE. Full expression of uncoupling protein gene requires the concurrence of norepinephrine and triiodothyronine. *Mol Endocrinol* 1988;2:706–713.

76. Clausen T, van Hardeveld C, Everts ME. Significance of cation transport in control of energy metabolism and thermogenesis. *Physiol Rev* 1991;71:733–774.

77. Leijendekker WJ, van Hardeveld C, Elzinga G. Heat production during contraction in skeletal muscle of hypothyroid mice. *Am J Physiol* 1987;253(part 1):E214–E220.

78. McCulloch AJ, Johnston DG, Baylis PH, et al. Evidence that thyroid hormones regulate gluconeogenesis from glycerol in man. *Clin Endocrinol (Oxf)* 1983;19:67–76.

79. Sestoft L. Metabolic aspects of the calorigenic effect of thyroid hormone in mammals. *Clin Endocrinol (Oxf)* 1980;13:489–506.

80. Storm H, van Hardeveld C. Effect of thyroid hormone on intracellular Ca^{2+} mobilization by noradrenaline and vasopressin in relation to glycogenolysis in rat liver. *Biochim Biophys Acta* 1985;846:275–285.

81. Wahrenberg H, Wennlund A, Arner P. Adrenergic regulation of lipolysis in fat cells from hyperthyroid and hypothyroid patients. *J Clin Endocrinol Metab* 1994;78:898–903.

82. Vagn NH, Hasselstrom K, Feldt-Rasmussen U, et al. Increased sympathetic tone in forearm subcutaneous tissue in primary hypothyroidism. *Clin Physiol* 1987;7:297–302.

83. Fagius J, Westermark K, Karlsson A. Baroreflex-governed sympathetic outflow to muscle vasculature is increased in hypothyroidism. *Clin Endocrinol (Oxf)* 1990;33:177–185.

84. McAllister RM, Grossenburg VD, Delp MD, et al. Effects of hyperthyroidism on vascular contractile and relaxation responses. *Am J Physiol* 1998;274:E946–E953.

85. Daza FJ, Parrilla R, Martin-Requero A. Influence of thyroid status on hepatic alpha 1-adrenoreceptor responsiveness. *Am J Physiol* 1997;273:E1065–E1072.

86. Beekman RE, van Hardeveld C, Simonides WS. On the mechanism of the reduction by thyroid hormone of beta-adrenergic relaxation rate stimulation in rat heart. *Biochem J* 1989;259:229–236.

87. Daly MJ, Dhalla NS. Alterations in the cardiac adenylate cyclase activity in hypothyroid rat. *Can J Cardiol* 1985;1:288–293.

88. Zhang Y, Xu K, Han C. Alterations of cardiac α1-adrenoceptor subtypes in hypothyroid rats. *Clin Exp Pharmacol Physiol* 1997;24:481–486.

89. Tu T, Nash CW. The influence of prolonged hyper- and hypothyroid states on the noradrenaline content of rat tissues and on the accumulation and efflux rates of tritiated noradrenaline. *Can J Physiol Pharmacol* 1975;53:74–80.

90. Buccino RA, Spann JF Jr, Pool PE, et al. Influence of the thyroid state on the intrinsic contractile properties and energy stores of the myocardium. *J Clin Invest* 1967;46:1669–1682.

91. Bramnert M, Hallengren B, Lecerof H, et al. Decreased blood pressure response to infused noradrenaline in normotensive as compared to hypertensive patients with primary hypothyroidism. *Clin Endocrinol (Oxf)* 1994;40:317–321.

92. Salvatore D, Bartha T, Harney JW, et al. Molecular biological and biochemical characterization of the human type 2 selenodeiodinase. *Endocrinology* 1996;137:3308–3315.

93. Milligan G, Saggerson ED. Concurrent up-regulation of guanine-nucleotide-binding proteins Gi1 alpha, Gi2 alpha and Gi3 alpha in adipocytes of hypothyroid rats. *Biochem J* 1990;270:765–769.

94. Saggerson ED. Sensitivity of adipocyte lipolysis to stimulatory and inhibitory agonists in hypothyroidism and starvation. *Biochem J* 1986;238:387–394.

95. Chu DT, Shikama H, Khatra BS, et al. Effects of altered thyroid status on beta-adrenergic actions on skeletal muscle glycogen metabolism. *J Biol Chem* 1985;260:9994–10000.

96. Diaz GB, Paladini AA, Garcia ME, et al. Changes induced by hypothyroidism in insulin secretion and in the properties of islet plasma membranes. *Arch Int Physiol Biochim Biophys* 1993;101:263–269.

97. Young JB, Landsberg L. Catecholamines and the regulation of hormone secretion [Review]. *Clin Endocrinol Metab* 1977;6:657–695.

98. Arieli A, Chinet A. Brown adipose tissue heat production in heat acclimated and perchlorate treated rats. *Horm Metab Res* 1985;17:12–15.

99. Ilyes I, Yahata T, Stock M. Brown adipose tissue cell respiration in hypo- and hyperthyroidism after stimulation with selective and non selective beta-adrenergic agonists. *Acta Biol Hungar* 1991;42:345–355.

100. Sundin U, Mills I, Fain JN. Thyroid-catecholamine interactions in isolated brown adipocytes. *Metabolism* 1984;33:1028–1033.

101. Bianco AC, Kieffer JD, Silva JE. Adenosine 3′,5′-monophosphate and thyroid hormone control of uncoupling protein messenger ribonucleic acid in freshly dispersed brown adipocytes. *Endocrinology* 1992;130:2625–2633.

102. Revelli JP, Pescini R, Muzzin P, et al. Changes in β1- and β2-adrenergic receptor mRNA levels in brown adipose tissue and heart of hypothyroid rats. *Biochem J* 1991;277:625–629.

103. Raasmaja A, Larsen PR. α1- and β-adrenergic agents cause synergistic stimulation of the iodothyronine deiodinase in rat brown adipocytes. *Endocrinology* 1989;125:2502–2509.

104. Blouquit MF, Gripois D. Norepinephrine and dopamine content in the brown adipose tissue of developing eu- and hypothyroid rats. *Horm Metab Res* 1991;23:326–328.

105. Blouquit MF, Gripois D. Activity of enzymes involved in norepinephrine biosynthesis in the brown adipose tissue of the developing rat. Influence of hypothyroidism. *Horm Metab Res* 1990;22:423–425.

106. Diarra A, Lefauconnier JM, Valens M, et al. Tyrosine content, influx and accumulation rate, and catecholamine biosynthesis measured *in vivo*, in the central nervous system and in peripheral organs of the young rat: influence of neonatal hypo- and hyperthyroidism. *Arch Int Physiol Biochim* 1989;97:317–332.

107. Novotny J, Bourova L, Malkova O, et al. G proteins, β-adrenoreceptors and β-adrenergic responsiveness in immature and adult rat ventricular myocardium: influence of neonatal hypo- and hyperthyroidism. *J Mol Cell Cardiol* 1999;31:761–772.

THE MALE AND FEMALE REPRODUCTIVE SYSTEM IN HYPOTHYROIDISM

GERASIMOS E. KRASSAS

Hypothyroidism affects the reproductive system in women more than in men. Clinicians have long recognized that thyroid diseases in general and hypothyroidism in particular in premenopausal women are often associated with menstrual abnormalities. A review of the physiology of the female reproductive system from fetal to adult life is given in Chapter 39.

REPRODUCTIVE EFFECTS OF HYPOTHYROIDISM IN FEMALES

Animal Studies

In the rat, fetal hypothyroidism results in small ovaries deficient in lipid and cholesterol (1). Propylthiouracil (PTU)-induced hypothyroidism or thyroidectomy of sexually immature rats results in delayed vaginal opening and sexual maturation, smaller ovaries and follicles than in controls (2), and poorly developed uteri and vaginas. When adult female rats are made hypothyroid, their estrous cycles become irregular and their ovaries become atrophic (3,4). Also, an enhanced response to human chorionic gonadotropin (hCG) with the development of large cystic ovaries but few corpora lutea have also been described in hypothyroid rats (5). In the mature female rat, hypothyroidism does not result in sterility, but it does interfere with gestation, especially in the first half of pregnancy (6), with resorption of the embryo and subsequent reduction in litter size and an increase in stillbirths (7). Ruh et al (8) reported increased estradiol (E_2) binding in the uteri of hypothyroid rats, which has not been confirmed by others (9).

In sheep, fetal hypothyroidism does not interfere with reproductive tract development. The uterus in hypothyroid sheep shows endometrial hyperplasia and smooth muscle hypertrophy, perhaps related to the prolonged estrous noted in hypothyroid ewes (10).

Human Studies

Hormonal Changes

Women with hypothyroidism have decreased rates of metabolic clearance of androstenedione and estrone and an increase in peripheral aromatization (11). The $5\alpha/5\beta$ ratio of the metabolites of androgens is decreased in hypothyroid women, and there is an increase in the excretion of 2-oxygenated estrogens (12). The binding activity of sex hormone–binding globulin (SHBG) in plasma is decreased, which results in decreased plasma concentrations of both testosterone and E_2, but their unbound fractions are increased. The alterations in steroid metabolism disappear when the euthyroid state is restored (13).

Gonadotropin levels are usually normal (14). However, blunted or delayed luteinizing hormone (LH) response to gonadotropin-releasing hormone (GnRH) has been reported in some female patients with hypothyroidism (15,16). When there is a delayed LH response, the serum prolactin (PRL) concentration may be increased (17). This may be due to the fact that hypothalamic thyrotropin-releasing hormone (TRH) increases the secretion of both thyrotropin (TSH) and PRL. Galactorrhea may occur. These disturbances usually disappear after thyroxine (T_4) administration (17).

Effects of Hypothyroidism in Early Life

The reproductive tract appears to develop normally in cretins; thus, hypothyroidism during fetal life does not appear to interfere with the normal development of the reproductive tract. Hypothyroidism in prepubertal years generally leads to short stature and may result in a delay in sexual maturation (18). An interesting syndrome, described by Kendle (19) and Van Wyk and Grumbach (20), may be seen occasionally; it is characterized by precocious menstruation, galactorrhea, and sella enlargement in girls with juvenile hypothyroidism. This is probably due to a "spillover" effect, because TSH, PRL, follicle-stimulating hormone (FSH), and LH are all glycoproteins and may have interlapping actions. However, axillary and public hair are usually not affected because there is no pubertal increase in the adrenal production of androgen precursors (18). Therapy with T_4 in proper dosage results in prompt alleviation of the symptomatology.

Menstrual Function and Fertility

In women of fertile age, hypothyrodism results in changes in cycle length and amount of bleeding (i.e., oligomenorrhea and amenorrhea, polymenorrhea, and menorrhagia). The latter is probably due to estrogen breakthrough bleeding secondary to anovulation (21). Defects in hemostasis, such as the decreased levels of factors VII, VIII, IX, and XI that may occur in hypothyroidism, may also contribute to polymenorrhea and menorrhagia (22).

More precisely, Goldsmith et al (23) found that 8 (80%) of 10 patients with primary myxedema had menstrual disturbances. Specifically, one patient had amenorrhea, five had clinical metropathia hemorrhagica, and two had menorrhagia. Benson and Dailey (24) studied the menstrual pattern in hyperthyroidism and subsequent posttherapy hypothyroidism. Menorrhagia, polymenorrhea, or both were noted in 18 (58.6%) of 31 women during the period of decreased thyroid function subsequent to specific therapy for hyperthyroidism.

Scott and Mussey (25) found that 28 (56%) of 50 hypothyroid patients had menstrual irregularities, mainly metrorrhagia or menorrhagia, alone or combined. Joshi et al (26) found that 15 (68.2%) of 22 patients with hypothyroidism had menstrual irregularities in comparison with 6 (12.2%) of 49 controls. Of those, 8 had oligohypomenorrhea, 2 amenorrhea, and 5 polymenorrhea and menorrhagia.

In a recent study (21), we found that 40 (23.4%) of 171 hypothyroid women had irregular cycles. Of those, 17 had oligomenorrhea, 6 hypomenorrhea, 5 amenorrhea, and 12 hypermenorrhea/menorrhagia. None had polymenorrhea or hypermenorrhea. For the purpose of the study, 214 normal controls with similar age and body mass index were investigated concerning their menstrual history. We found that only 18 (8.4%) had irregular periods. Although this finding indicates that the frequency of menstrual disturbances in hypothyroidism is approximately three times greater than in the normal population, this is still much lower than the findings in previous similar studies. Furthermore, we found that the main menstrual irregularity in these patients was oligomenorrhea (42.5%), which is also inconsistent with what is generally believed. Moreover, as expected, patients with more severe hypothyroidism had higher TSH levels. Although there was a tendency for patients with higher serum TSH levels to have more menstrual disturbances, these differences were not statistically significant. Finally, we found that thyroid antibodies are unimportant in the development of menstrual abnormalities in hypothyroidism. The fewer menstrual abnormalities in these more recent studies may be attributed to genetic and other factors among the populations studied or to the more delayed diagnosis of hypothyroidism in the earlier studies, which would result in a more severe clinical picture in the newly diagnosed patient.

In women, severe hypothyroidism is commonly associated with diminished libido and failure of ovulation (23).

Hypothyroid women who become pregnant have more fetal wastage (27). Ovulation and conception can occur in mild hypothyroidism, but in the past those pregnancies that did occur were often associated with abortions in the first trimester, stillbirths, or prematurity (28,29). Recent studies indicate that these events may be less common but that gestational hypertension often occurs in pregnant women with untreated hypothyroidism (30). Data from two studies indicate that large medical centers are likely to care for one or two women each year who are hypothyroid at the time that they become pregnant (31,32), and a report of a screening study described an incidence rate of 0.4% in pregnant women (33). Hyperprolactinemia resulting from long-standing primary hypothyroidism has been implicated in ovulatory dysfunction ranging from inadequate corpus luteal progesterone secretion when mildly elevated (34) to oligomenorrhea or amenorrhea when circulating PRL levels are high. Adequate thyroid supplementation restores PRL levels and normalizes ovulatory function. In some cases the latter may be delayed (35).

Goldsmith et al (23) reported that 7 of 10 patients with myxedema had no evidence of ovulation and one demonstrated inadequate corpus luteum effect. The anovulation was reflected in the frequent finding of a proliferative endometrium on endometrial biopsy. All 7 patients had menstrual irregularities. Joshi et al (26) found that only 1 of 16 patients with hypothyroidism was infertile.

Bohnet et al (36) investigated 150 unselected women 25 to 34 years of age with long-standing (>2 years) primary or secondary infertility due to anovulation or luteal insufficiency. A 400-μg TRH test was performed in all. In patients with subclinical hypothyroidism, a PRL stimulation test (metoclopramide) was done. They found that subclinical hypothyroidism may be of greater clinical importance in infertile women with menstrual disorders—especially when the luteal phase is inadequate—than is usually thought. They concluded that a TRH stimulation test in such patients should be mandatory. This was also confirmed in a recent study (37) reporting that mean serum TSH levels and antithyroid peroxidase antibodies were higher among women with infertility compared with controls. It must be emphasized, however, that the use of T_4 is not helpful in treating euthyroid patients for infertility or menstrual irregularity.

Earlier work indicated that T_4 enhanced the action of gonadotropins on luteinization and progestin secretion by cultured granulosa cells (38). It has recently been reported that in a group of infertile women, those with elevated TSH levels had a higher incidence of out-of-phase biopsies than women with normal serum TSH concentrations (39). These data support the suggestion that women presenting with menstrual irregularities or conception difficulties should be examined in depth for thyroid dysfunction before specific T_4 treatment is considered. Hypothyroidism during and after pregnancy is discussed in detail in Chapters 27 and 80.

In summary, contemporary studies have shown that the frequency of menstrual irregularities in hypothyroidism is far less than reported earlier. Moreover, the most common manifestation is oligomenorrhea. Also, hypothyroidism is commonly associated with failure of ovulation. Ovulation and conception can occur in mild hypothyroidism. However, these pregnancies are often associated with abortions, stillbirths, or prematurity. Subclinical hypothyroidism may be of significant clinical importance in infertile women with "unexplained" infertility, and such patients should be investigated in depth for thyroid dysfunction.

REPRODUCTIVE EFFECTS OF HYPOTHYROIDISM IN MALES

Although less common in men than in women, hypothyroidism, whether induced or spontaneous, affects the male reproductive tract in a number of ways, depending in part on the age at onset. A review of the physiology of the male reproductive system from fetal to adult life is given in Chapter 39.

Animal Studies

Hypothyroidism, induced or occurring soon after birth, is associated with a marked delay in sexual maturation and development (40). When rats are made hypothyroid with PTU administered from birth to 24 to 26 days of age, testicular size is decreased, Sertoli cell differentiation is retarded, and the time of Sertoli cell proliferation is prolonged (41,42). Transient hypothyroidism also alters the expression of a number of mRNAs in the Sertoli cell (43). Testis size, Sertoli cell number, and sperm production are increased as these rats become older and euthyroid (43). Hardy et al (44) found that Leydig cell numbers are increased, testosterone secretion per cell is decreased, although total testosterone secretion remains the same as controls. FSH and LH levels tend to remain low throughout treatment and recovery periods, whereas inhibin levels are increased (41).

If hypothyroidism persists untreated, there is an arrest of sexual maturity, and libido and ejaculate are absent (45). The interstitial cells of the testis are reduced in number, and the arrested growth of the accessory male sex organs indicates a decrease in the production of testosterone (45). The longer the hypothyroidism persists, the greater the degree of damage to the testes (45), although genetically induced hypothyroidism in male mice is associated with normal fertility (46). In the mature male rat, the induction of hypothyroidism has little effect on the pathology of the testes, spermatogenesis, or serum testosterone concentrations (47), although the LH response to GnRH may be blunted (48). In the adult ram, hypothyroidism is associated with a decrease in testosterone concentration but normal spermatogenesis (49). Thus, it would appear that

hypothyroidism can affect the immature, but not the mature, testis.

Human Studies

Hormonal Changes

Hypothyroidism is associated with a decrease in serum total testosterone (50,51). SHBG is usually low (50,52, 53). Dehydroepiandrosterone (DHEA), DHEA sulphate, estrogenic metabolites of DHEA (androstenediol and its sulphate), and pregnenolone sulphate are decreased in the serum of men with hypothyroidism compared with normal controls (54). In a prospective study of 10 men with primary hypothyroidism, plasma free testosterone levels were low, and they increased after beginning T_4 therapy (55). Gonadotropin levels were not elevated, consistent with a state of hypogonadotropic hypogonadism (55). In addition, a marked decrease in the $5\alpha:5\beta$ ratio of the metabolites of androstenedione and testosterone has been reported in hypothyroidism, which is the reverse of that seen in hyperthyroidism (56). A small study of hypothyroid men showed an attenuated LH response to GnRH, which improved after thyroid hormone therapy (52). These findings suggest an effect of hypothyroidism on gonadotropin secretion at the level of the hypothalamus–pituitary. In rare cases of severe prolonged primary hypothyroidism, pituitary hyperplasia may occur, causing multiple pituitary hormone deficiencies, including gonadotropin and corticotropin deficiencies (57,58). Circulating androgenic steroids may also be reduced by hyperprolactinemia caused by hypothyroidism (17,59).

Effects of Hypothyroidism in Early Life

Congenital hypothyroidism is not associated with abnormal development of the male reproductive tract (40). This is not surprising because small but adequate amounts of maternal thyroid hormones cross the placenta to satisfy fetal demands (60). Maternal hypothyroidism during pregnancy and cretinism are also not associated with abnormal male reproductive tract development (61). When adequately treated with thyroid hormone, boys with congenital hypothyroidism progress through puberty normally and at the appropriate time (62,63). Untreated hypothyroidism in early childhood can result in delay in sexual maturation, which can be reversed by thyroid hormone therapy (64). It has been known for many years that severe juvenile hypothyroidism is associated with precocious pseudopuberty (19,40). External genitalia develop early, but without axillary or pubic hair, and there is often macro-orchidism (65). The serum gonadotropins are usually normal, and serum testosterone is in the prepubertal range. It is proposed that cross-reactivity of TSH with the FSH receptor may be responsible for this rare phenomenon (66).

Spermatogenesis and Fertility

Hypothyroidism is associated with decreased libido (50, 52,67) or impotence (50,67). However, little is known about the effects of hypothyroidism on human spermatogenesis and fertility. Griboff (68) investigated five men with primary hypothyroidism who were 30 to 64 years of age. All demonstrated normal sperm counts. However, exposure of semen to room air revealed a rapid drying of the material and loss of sperm motility in two of the five specimens. A study by De la Balze et al (69) investigated six adult male hypothyroid patients 17 to 59 years of age. Thyroid insufficiency had occurred before puberty in five subjects and in childhood in one. All patients demonstrated features of hypogonadotropic hypogonadism. Testicular biopsies revealed histologic abnormalities in all patients. It was concluded that severe and prolonged thyroid insufficiency occurring early in life resulted in moderate failure of pituitary gonadotropins secretion and abnormal testicular biopsy results. Wortsman et al (50) studied eight hypothyroid men 37 to 77 years of age. All patients had evidence of hypogonadism, five were hypergonadotropic, and the remaining three hypogonadotropic. Seven of eight patients had varying degrees of testicular atrophy. Serum testosterone and SHBG concentrations were low in four of the patients. Sperm analyses were not performed. They concluded that abnormalities of gonadal function are common in men with primary hypothyroidism. Corrales Hernandez et al (51) studied spermatogesis in 10 patients with a history of hypothyroidism treated with T_4. Hypothyroidism was induced by discontinuation or a decrease of the dose of T_4 over at least one spermatogenic cycle. A decrease in seminal volume, progressive forward motility, and cumulative percentage of mobile forms was observed compared with controls. There were no abnormalities in sperm density or percentage of spermatozoa with normal morphology. Induction of hypothyroidism did not lead to seminal changes compared with the same patients when euthyroid. Serum concentrations of testosterone and gonadotropin were normal during the hypothyroid phase. It appears, therefore, that short-term postpubertal hypothyroidism does not cause seminal alterations sufficiently intense to impair male fertility. Jaya Kumar et al (52) studied the reproductive and endocrine function of eight men with primary hypothyroidism during the hypothyroid phase and after achieving euthyroid status with T_4 substitution therapy. They found high mean levels of gonadotropins, low serum testosterone, low SHBG, and subnormal testosterone response to hCG. Semen analysis was performed in five of eight patients, but these data were not presented, although the authors claimed that "some improvement in sperm count and motility was observed."

In summary, the data so far suggest that short-term hypothyroidism in adults has no significant effect on reproductive function. Severe, prolonged hypothyroidism, particularly when the onset occurs in childhood, may impair reproductive function. However, more studies are needed with a larger number of patients to define the effects of hypothyroidism on male reproductive function.

REFERENCES

1. Leathem JH. Extragonadal factors in reproduction. In: Lloyd CW, ed. *Recent progress in the endocrinology of reproduction.* New York: Academic, 1959:179.
2. Dijkstra G, De Rooij DG, de Jong FH, et al. Effect of hypothyroidism on ovarian follicular development, granulosa cell proliferation, and peripheral hormone levels in the prepubertal rat. *Eur J Endocrinol* 1996;134:649.
3. Mattheij JA, Swarts JJ, Lokerse P, et al. Effect of hypothyroidism on the pituitary-gonadal axis in the adult female rat. *J Endocrinol* 1995;146:87.
4. Tohei A, Imai A, Watanabe G, et al. Influence of thiouracil-induced hypothyroidism on adrenal and gonadal functions in adult female rats. *J Vet Med Sci* 1998;60:439.
5. Bagavandoss P, England B, Asirvatham A, et al. Transient induction of polycystic ovary-like syndrome in immature hypothyroid rats. *Proc Soc Exp Biol Med* 1998;219:77.
6. Bonet B, Herrera E. Maternal hypothyroidism during the first half of gestation compromises normal catabolic adaptations of late gestation in the rat. *Endocrinology* 1991;129:210.
7. Rao PM, Panda JN. Uterine enzyme changes in thyroidectomized rats at parturition. *J Reprod Fertil* 1981;61:109.
8. Ruh MF, Ruh TS, Klitgaard HM. Uptake and retention of estrogens by uteri from rats in various thyroid states. *Proc Soc Exp Biol Med* 1970;134:558.
9. Kirkland JL, Gardner RM, Mukku VR, et al. Hormonal control of uterine growth: the effect of hypothyroidism on estrogen-stimulated cell division. *Endocrinology* 1981;108:2346.
10. Nesbitt REL, Abdul-Karim RW, Prior JT, et al. Study of the effect of experimentally induced endocrine insults upon pregnant and nonpregnant ewes. III. ACTH and propylthiouracil administration and the production of polycystic ovaries. *Fertil Steril* 1967;18:739.
11. Longcope C, Abend S, Braverman LE, et al. Androstenedione and estrone dynamics in hypothyroid women. *J Clin Endocrinol Metab* 1990;70:903.
12. Gallagher TF, Fukushima DK, Noguchi S, et al. Recent studies in steroid hormone metabolism in man. *Rec Prog Horm Res* 1966;22:283.
13. Gordon GG, Southern AL. Thyroid-hormone effects on steroid hormone metabolism. *Bull NY Acad Med* 1977;53:241.
14. Larsen PR, Davies TF, Hay ID. The thyroid gland. In: Wilson JD, Foster DW, Kronenberg HM, et al, eds. *Williams textbook of endocrinology,* 9th ed. Philadelphia: WB Saunders, 1998:389.
15. Distiller LA, Sagel J, Morley JE. Assessment of pituitary gonadotropin reserve using luteinizing hormone–releasing hormone (LRH) in states of altered thyroid function. *J Clin Endocrinol Metab* 1975;40:512.
16. Valenti G, Ceda GP, Denti L, et al. Gonadotropin secretion in hyperthyroidism and hypothyroidism. *La Ric Clin Lab* 1984;14:53.
17. Honbo KS, van Herle AJ, Kellett KA. Serum prolactin levels in untreated primary hypothyroidism. *Am J Med* 1978;64:782.
18. Krassas GE. Thyroid disease and female reproduction. *Fertil Steril* 2000;74:1063.
19. Kendle F. Case of precocious puberty in a female cretin. *BMJ* 1905;1:246.
20. Van Wyk J, Grumbach MM. Syndrome of precocious menstruation and galactorrhea in juvenile hypothyroidism: an example of hormonal overlap pituitary feedback. *J Pediatr* 1960;57:416.

21. Krassas GE, Pontikides N, Kaltsas Th, et al. Disturbances of menstruation in hypothyroidism. *Clin Endocrinol* 1999;50:655.

22. Ansell JE. The blood in the hypothyroidism. In: Braverman L, Utiger R, eds. *Werner and Ingbar's The thyroid, a fundamental and clinical text,* 7th ed. Philadelphia: Lippincott-Raven, 1996: 821.

23. Goldsmith RE, Sturgis SH, Lerman J, et al. The menstrual pattern in thyroid disease. *J Clin Endocrinol Metab* 1952;12:846.

24. Benson RC, Dailey ME. Menstrual pattern in hyperthyroidism and subsequent post-therapy hypothyroidism. *Surg Gynaecol Obstet* 1955;100:19.

25. Scott JC, Mussey E. Menstrual patterns in myxedema. *Am J Obstet Gynecol* 1964;90:161.

26. Joshi JV, Bhandakar SD, Chadha M, et al. Menstrual irregularities and lactation failure may precede thyroid dysfunction or goitre. *J Postgrad Med* 1993;39:137.

27. Niswander KR. Metabolic and endocrine conditions In: Niswander KR, Gordon M, eds. *The women and their pregnancies.* Philadelphia: WB Saunders, 1972:246.

28. Thomas R, Reid RL. Thyroid disease and reproductive dysfunction: a review. *Obstet Gynecol* 1987;70:789.

29. Davis LE, Leveno KJ, Cunningham FG. Hypothyroidism complicating pregnancy. *Obstet Gynecol* 1988;72:108.

30. Leung AS, Millar LK, Koonings PP, et al. Perinatal outcome in hypothyroid pregnancies. *Obstet Gynecol* 1993;81:349.

31. Montoro M, Collea JV, Frasier SD, et al. Successful outcome of pregnancy in women with hypothyroidism. *Ann Intern Med* 1981;94:31.

32. Pekonen F, Teramo K, Ikonen E, et al. Women on thyroid hormone therapy: pregnancy course, fetal outcome, and amniotic fluid thyroid hormone level. *Obstet Gynecol* 1984;63:635.

33. Klein RZ, Haddow JE, Faix JD, et al. Incidence of thyroid deficiency in pregnancy. *Pediatr Res* 1990;27:79A.

34. del Pozo E, Wyss H, Tollis G, et al. Prolactin and deficient luteal function. *Obstet Gynecol* 1979;53:282.

35. Stoffer SS, McKeel DW Jr, Randall RV, et al. Pituitary prolactin cell hyperplasia with autonomous prolactin secretion and primary hypothyroidism. *Fertil Steril* 1981;36:682.

36. Bohnet HG, Fielder K, Leidenberger FA. Subclinical hypothyroidism and infertility [Letter]. *Lancet* 1981;2:1278.

37. Poppe K, Velkeniers B. Thyroid disorders in infertile women. *Ann Endocrinol* 2003;64:45.

38. Channing CP, Tsai V, Sachs D. Role of insulin, thyroxine and cortisol in luteinization of porcine granulosa cells grown in chemically defined media. *Biol Reprod* 1976;15:247.

39. Gerhard I, Becker T, Eggert-Kruse W, et al. Thyroid and ovarian function in infertile women. *Hum Reprod* 1991;6:338.

40. Jannini EA, Ulisse S, D'Armiento M. Thyroid hormone and male gonadal function. *Endocr Rev* 1995;16:443.

41. Kirby JD, Jetton AE, Cooke PS, et al. Developmental hormonal profiles accompanying the neonatal hypothyroidism-induced increase in adult testicular size and sperm production in the rat. *Endocrinology* 1992;131:559.

42. Van Haaster LH, de Jong FH, Docter R, et al. The effect of hypothyroidism on Sertoli cell proliferation and differentiation and hormone levels during testicular development in the rat. *Endocrinology* 1992;131:1574.

43. Bunick D, Kirby J, Hess RA, et al. Developmental expression of testis messenger ribonucleic acids in the rat following propylthiouracil-induced neonatal hypothyroidism. *Biol Reprod* 1994; 51:706.

44. Hardy MP, Kirby JD, Hess RA, et al. Leydig cells increase their numbers but decline in steroidogenic function in the adult rat after neonatal hypothyroidism. *Endocrinology* 1993;132:2417.

45. Gomes WR. Metabolic and regulatory hormones influencing testis function. In: Johnson AD, Gomes WR, Vandemark NL,

eds. *The testis.* Vol. III. *Influencing factors.* New York: Academic, 1970:67.

46. Chubb C, Henry L. The fertility of hypothyroid male mice. *J Reprod Fertil* 1988;83:819.

47. Weiss SR, Burns JM. The effect of acute treatment with two goitrogens on plasma thyroid hormones, testosterone and testicular morphology in adult male rats. *Comp Biochem Physiol* 1988; 90A:449.

48. Tohei A, Akai M, Tomabechi T, et al. Adrenal and gonadal function in hypothyroid adult male rats. *J Endocrinol* 1997;152: 147.

49. Chandrasekhar Y, Holland MK, D'Occhio MJ, et al. Spermatogenesis, seminal characteristics and reproductive hormone levels in mature rams with induced hypothyroidism and hyperthyroidism. *J Endocrinol* 1985;105:39.

50. Wortsman J, Rosner W, Dufau ML. Abnormal testicular function in men with primary hypothyroidism. *Am J Med* 1987;82: 207–212.

51. Corrales Hernandez JJ, Miralles Garcia JM, Garcia Diez LC. Primary hypothyroidism and human spermatogenesis. *Arch Androl* 1990;25:21.

52. Jaya Kumar B, Khurana ML, Ammini AC, et al. Reproductive endocrine functions in men with primary hypothyroidism: effect of thyroxine replacement. *Horm Res* 1990;34:215.

53. Cavaliere H, Abelin N, Medeiros-Neto G. Serum levels of total testosterone and sex hormone binding globulin in hypothyroid patients and normal subjects treated with incremental doses of L-T$_4$ or L-T$_3$. *J Androl* 1988;9:215.

54. Tagawa N, Takano T, Fukata S, et al. Serum concentration of androstenediol and androstenediol sulfate in patients with hyperthyroidism and hypothyroidism. *Endocr J* 2001;48:345.

55. Donnelly P, White C. Testicular dysfunction in men with primary hypothyroidism: reversal of hypogonadotrophic hypogonadism with replacement thyroxine. *Clin Endocrinol (Oxf)* 2000; 52:197.

56. Gallagher TF, Fukushima DK, Noguchi S, et al. Recent studies in steroid hormone metabolism in man. *Rec Prog Horm Res* 1966;22:283.

57. Horvath E, Kovacs K, Scheithauer BW. Pituitary hyperplasia. *Pituitary* 1999;1:169.

58. Kocova M, Netkov S, Sukarova-Angelovska E. Pituitary pseudotumor with unusual presentation reversed shortly after the introduction of thyroxine replacement therapy. *J Pediatr Endocrinol Metab* 2001;14:1665.

59. Notsu K, Ito Y, Furuya H, et al. Incidence of hyperprolactinemia in patients with Hashimoto's thyroiditis. *Endocr J* 1997;44:89–94.

60. Vulsma T, Gons MH, de Vijlder JJM. Maternal-fetal transfer of thyroxine in congenital hypothyroidism due to a total organification defect or thyroid agenesis. *N Engl J Med* 1989;321:13.

61. Longcope C. The male and female reproductive systems in hypothyroidism. In: Braverman LE, Utiger RD, eds. *Werner & Ingbar's The thyroid: a fundamental and clinical text,* 8th ed. Philadelphia: Lippincott Williams & Wilkins, 2000:824.

62. Salerno M, Micillo M, Di Maio S, et al. Longitudinal growth, sexual maturation and final height in patients with congenital hypothyroidism detected by neonatal screening. *Eur J Endocrinol* 2001;145:377.

63. Dickerman Z, De Vries L. Prepubertal and pubertal growth, timing and duration of puberty and attained adult height in patients with congenital hypothyroidism (CH) detected by the neonatal screening programme for CH-a longitudinal study. *Clin Endocrinol (Oxf)* 1997;47:649.

64. Hanna CE, LaFranchi SH. Adolescent thyroid disorders. *Adolesc Med* 2002;13:13.

65. Panidis DK, Rousso DH. Macro-orchidism in juvenile hypothyroidism. *Arch Androl* 1999;42:85.

66. Grossman M, Weintraub BD, Szkudlinski MW. Novel insights into the molecular mechanisms of human thyrotropin action: structural, physiological, and therapeutic implications for the glycoprotein hormone family. *Endocr Rev* 1997;18:476.
67. Krassas GE, Perros P. Thyroid disease and male reproductive function. *J Endocrinol Invest* 2003;26:372.
68. Griboff SI. Semen analysis in myxedema. *Fertil Steril* 1962;13:436.
69. De la Balze EA, Arrilaga F, Mancini RE, et al. Male hypogonadism in hypothyroidism: a study of six cases. *J Clin Endocrinol Metab* 1962;22:212.

THE SKELETAL SYSTEM IN HYPOTHYROIDISM

NEIL J.L. GITTOES
MICHAEL C. SHEPPARD

Skeletal growth is the result of a complex interplay of nutritional, genetic, and hormonal factors. Linear growth occurs throughout development and the childhood years until epiphyseal fusion occurs as the result of endochondral ossification in the growth plates of long bones. Thyroid hormones are essential for normal skeletal development, as is evidenced by poor bone growth and mineralization, delayed bone age, epiphyseal dysgenesis, and immature body proportions in children with hypothyroidism (1). Thyroxine (T_4) replacement therapy in these children induces a rapid phase of catch-up growth that is often incomplete because bone age advances more rapidly than height, leading to early fusion of the epiphyseal growth plates. Catch-up growth may be particularly compromised when treatment is initiated at the onset of puberty; it may be appropriate to treat pubertal children with hypothyroidism with lower doses of T_4 and add therapy to slow pubertal development and hence delay epiphyseal fusion. The deficit in final height correlates with the duration of untreated hypothyroidism (2). Other important endocrine regulators of skeletal development and growth are growth hormone, insulin-like growth factor 1 (IGF-1), glucocorticoids, and sex steroids, and their production may be decreased by hypothyroidism (see the section Acquired Hypothyroidism in Children in Chapter 75).

BONE REMODELING IN HYPOTHYROIDISM

Hypothyroidism decreases recruitment, maturation, and activity of bone cells, leading to decreased bone resorption and bone formation (3). Despite the decrease in bone resorption, trabecular bone volume (3) and bone mineral density (4) are comparable with those of age-matched normal subjects, presumably because there is a corresponding decrease in osteoblastic activity. Biochemical markers of bone metabolism also suggest that skeletal turnover is decreased in hypothyroidism. Serum alkaline phosphatase concentrations are often low (5–8), as are serum osteocalcin concentrations (6,8,9). Urinary excretion of hydroxyproline also is decreased in both adults and children with hypothyroidism (8,10–12).

The decrease in bone resorption in hypothyroidism results in a tendency for serum calcium concentrations to decline, but in fact serum calcium concentrations are usually normal (13). Serum parathyroid hormone concentrations tend to be increased (14,15), presumably as a result of the decrease in bone resorption (16). Induction of hypocalcemia acutely in patients with hypothyroidism results in a greater decline in serum calcium concentrations, and the concentrations return to normal more slowly, as compared with normal subjects (14). Urinary and fecal calcium excretion tends to be low, presumably due to increased parathyroid hormone secretion (13).

THYROID HORMONE AND INTERACTIONS WITH OTHER HORMONES IN BONE

The skeletal abnormalities of hypothyroidism may be mediated, at least in part, by decreased growth hormone and IGF-1 production and signaling (see Chapter 58). Thyroid hormone has little effect on growth in hypophysectomized rats (17,18). In contrast, growth hormone stimulates growth in thyroid hormone–deficient rats (18), and the effect of growth hormone is augmented when thyroid hormone is given with growth hormone (19–21). In thyroparathyroidectomized rats treated with growth hormone, T_4, or both, T_4 reversed the decrease in growth plate width, articular cartilage thickness, and trabecular bone volume (22). Growth hormone had no effect on the growth plate but partially restored trabecular bone volume, and growth hormone and T_4 in combination increased growth plate width and trabecular bone volume more than did T_4 alone. Thyroid hormone thus appears to have some direct effects on the growth plate and trabecular bone formation, independent of growth hormone (22). However, the two hormones also appear to potentiate each other's effects not only in rats (17,18,20), but also in humans (19,21).

The effects of thyroid hormone on cartilage and bone may be mediated in part through stimulation of IGF-1 production. Serum IGF-1 concentrations tend to be low in patients with hypothyroidism (23–31), although whether this is directly related to thyroid deficiency per se or is secondary to growth hormone deficiency remains unclear. The serum growth hormone response to stimulation in patients with hypothyroidism is diminished, suggesting that the low serum IGF-1 concentrations in hypothyroidism may be caused by decreased growth hormone secretion (32–34). However, thyroid hormone directly increases the expression of several components of IGF-1 signaling in bone. It increases IGF-1 mRNA expression and IGF-1 production in osteoblastic cells (35), IGF-1 receptor mRNA in chondrocytes (36), and IGF binding protein 4 in osteoblastic cells (37). This binding protein is an inhibitor of cell proliferation, and it may contribute to the antiproliferative effect of thyroid hormone in osteoblasts. Thyroid hormone also stimulates IGF-1 production in rat calvarial osteoblasts, whereas growth hormone has no effect (38). *In vivo*, T_4 increases the production of IGF-1 and IGF binding protein 3 in patients with congenital hypothyroidism (39,40).

LESSONS FROM GENE KNOCKOUT/ KNOCK-IN STUDIES IN ANIMALS

Impaired skeletal development and growth is a key feature of untreated hypothyroidism (see sections Congenital Hypothyroidism and Acquired Hypothyroidism in Children in Chapter 75). Studies of mice in which the different iso-forms of the thyroid receptor (TR) have been knocked out have provided information about the effects of thyroid hormone deficiency on bone, and at the same time have highlighted some of the complexities of thyroid hormone action (Table 62.1) (see Chapter 8). Selective inactivation of the α_1 isoform of TR [with preservation of the α_2 isoform, which does not bind triiodothyronine (T_3)] results in normal skeletal development (41), suggesting that the β isoforms of the receptor are functional in bone in the absence of $TR\alpha_1$. Mice with no $TR\alpha$ isoforms ($TR\alpha^{0/0}$) do, however, have growth delay, defective bone mineralization, and disorganized growth plate architecture (42). $TR\beta^{0/0}$ mice have no developmental abnormalities in bone and cartilage (43). Combined $TR\alpha^{0/0}/\beta^{0/0}$ mice have more severe growth retardation than their $TR\alpha^{0/0}$ counterparts (44). Taken together, these results suggest that $TR\alpha$ is functionally predominant in bone, and that its deficiency can be partly compensated for by $TR\beta$. However, skeletal development in $TR\alpha^{0/0}/\beta^{0/0}$ mice is not as poor as it is in $Pax8^{-/-}$ mice, which have severe congenital hypothyroidism as a result of agenesis of thyroid follicular cells (see Chapter 2). Possible explanations for this difference are signaling through an as yet unidentified TR, nongenomic actions of thyroid hormone (45), and an action of unliganded TRs (46). The latter possibility is supported by the observation that $Pax8^{-/-}/TR\alpha^{0/0}$ mice have fairly normal skeletal development (47).

TABLE 62.1. EFFECTS OF MUTATIONS IN THE GENES FOR THYROID HORMONE RECEPTORS AND THYROID DEVELOPMENT ON THE SKELETON IN MICE

Mouse Model	Endocrine Status	Skeletal Consequences	References
$TR\alpha^{-/-}$	Hypothyroidism	Growth retardation, delayed endochondral bone formation, ossification, and mineralization; reduced bone mass and disorganized growth plate	42, 63
$TR\alpha_1^{-/-}$	Mild hypothyroidism	Normal	41
$TR\alpha_2^{-/-}$	Mild hypothyroidism	Abnormal mineralization	64
$TR\alpha^{0/0}$	Euthyroid	Growth retardation. Growth plate disorganized; reduced mineralization and reduced bone mineral density	65
$TR\beta^{-/-}$	RTH + goiter	Normal	43,44
$TR\beta_2^{-/-}$	Mild RTH	Normal	66,67
$TR\alpha^{-/-}/TR\beta^{-/-}$	RTH + goiter	Similar to $TR\alpha^{-/-}$; no abnormalities at birth; delayed ossification and mineralization, and growth arrest and death at weaning; phenotype not rescued by T_4 treatment	44
$TR\alpha_1^{-/-}/TR\beta^{-/-}$	RTH + goiter	Growth retardation, delayed ossification, and disorganized growth plate; delayed bone age	68,69
$TR\alpha^{0/0}/TR\beta^{-/-}$	RTH + goiter	More severe phenotype than $TR\alpha^{0/0}$; impaired ossification and delayed bone maturation	65
$Pax8^{-/-}$	No thyroid	Severe growth retardation; mice die at weaning; rescued by T_4 treatment	47,70
$Pax8^{-/-}/TR\alpha^{0/0}$	No thyroid	Growth retardation less than $Pax8^{-/-}$ mice; mice survived to adulthood	47
$Pax8^{-/-}/TR\beta^{-/-}$	No thyroid	Similar phenotype to $Pax8^{-/-}$ mice; mice die before weaning	47
$TR\beta^{PV/PV}$	Severe RTH + goiter	Growth retarded, advanced bone age and craniosynostosis	71
$TR\beta^{PV/+}$	Mild RTH + goiter	Similar but less severe phenotype than homozygous mice	71
$TR\alpha^{PV/+}$	Mild hypothyroidism	Severe growth retardation from shortly after birth, suggesting a hypothyroid bone phenotype	50

PV, a dominant-negative mutation of $TR\beta$ that results in severe thyroid hormone resistance in humans; RTH, resistance to thyroid hormone; T_4, thyroxine; TR, thyroid hormone receptor; $TR\alpha^{0/0}$ mice, mice that express no $TR\alpha$ gene products; $TR^{-/-}$ mice, mice that express $TR\Delta\alpha1$ and $TR\Delta\alpha2$. Modified from Duncan Bassett J, Williams G. The molecular actions of thyroid hormone in bone. *Trends Endocrinol Metab* 2003;14:356, with permission.

Gene knock-in studies, using mutant TRβ genes derived from patients with resistance to thyroid hormone, have afforded further insight into the molecular mechanisms of thyroid hormone action in bone. Many patients with resistance to thyroid hormone have short stature and epiphyseal dysgenesis, indicating that TRβ is important in mediating thyroid hormone effects on skeletal development (see Chapter 81) (48). However, knock-in mice with a TRβ mutation associated with severe resistance to thyroid hormone in humans have advanced bone age, craniosynostosis, and growth retardation (features more suggestive of thyrotoxicosis than hypothyroidism) (49). When this TRβ mutation is introduced into the TRα$_1$ gene in mice, the result is severe growth retardation, a phenotype suggestive of hypothyroidism (50). These results further support the importance of TRα$_1$ in mediating the effects of thyroid hormone in bone.

HYPOTHYROIDISM AND SKELETAL MATURATION

Skeletal maturation, defined as the appearance of secondary centers of ossification, depends largely on the presence of thyroid hormone (51–55), and the retardation of skeletal maturation in children with hypothyroidism manifests itself as a delay in ossification at epiphyseal centers (see sections Congenital Hypothyroidism and Acquired Hypothyroidism in Children in Chapter 75). When ossification does occur, the pattern is irregular and mottled, with multiple foci that coalesce to give a porous or fragmented appearance known as epiphyseal dysgenesis (56, 57) (Fig. 62.1). These changes are most often noted in large cartilaginous centers, such as the head of the femur and the tarsal navicular bone. Changes in the upper lumbar vertebrae result in wedge-shaped anterior margins, which appear between the ages of 6 months and 2 years, and may lead to spondylolisthesis (58).

The onset of thyroid deficiency can be determined by the presence of dysgenesis at an epiphyseal ossification site. Absence of osseous retardation excludes the diagnosis of hypothyroidism unless thyroid deficiency is of recent onset (57). Because the various epiphyseal centers begin to ossify at different times during childhood, the presence of epiphyseal dysgenesis at a particular site will date the onset of thyroid deficiency. For example, the presence of stippled epiphyses in the femoral head of a 4-year-old child indicates that thyroid deficiency began before the 9th to 12th month, the age when these centers usually ossify. Likewise, the presence of dysgenesis in centers that ossify before birth suggests prenatal hypothyroidism. The observation that epiphyseal dysgenesis occurs in infants with thyroid agenesis whose mothers had normal thyroid function during pregnancy indicates that the maternal thyroid is not able to protect the fetal skeleton fully against hypothyroidism. Normal infants born of hypothyroid mothers do not have retardation of epiphyseal ossification.

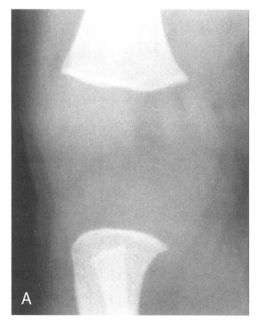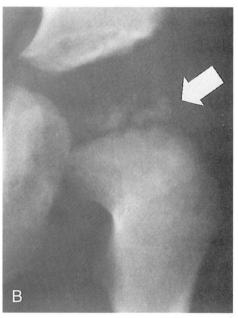

FIGURE 62.1. Skeletal abnormalities in children with hypothyroidism. **A:** Radiograph of the knee in a 2-year-old boy with delayed bone maturation due to hypothyroidism. There is no ossification of the epiphysis of the distal femur and that of the proximal tibia. Both epiphyses should be ossified by 1 month of age. **B:** Anteroposterior radiograph of the left hip in another child with hypothyroidism showing a fragmented, irregular (*arrow*) proximal femoral epiphysis.

CLINICAL CONSEQUENCES OF HYPOTHYROIDISM

In patients with hypothyroidism, trabecular bone turnover is decreased and cortical thickness is increased, as determined by histomorphometry (59,60). T_4 therapy results in rapid increases in resorption of trabecular bone and in cortical porosity, and after therapy for 6 months in trabecular and cortical bone loss, as compared with pretreatment measurements (60).

Fracture risk and risk factors for fractures were studied in 412 patients with primary hypothyroidism seen in five Danish hospitals between 1990 and 1998 (61). Overall fracture risk was increased in the patients as compared with normal subjects (relative risk 1.6). However, the increase was limited to the 2-year period after the diagnosis of hypothyroidism; the risk before diagnosis and more than 2 years after diagnosis was similar to that in normal subjects. The increase was significant only in patients over 50 years of age and was limited to the forearm. Although serum thyrotropin (TSH) was not measured in these patients, only 8% had to have their dose of T_4 reduced, suggesting that overtreatment was not a major determinant of fracture (see Chapter 40).

A further extensive study from Denmark (62) illustrated some of the risks associated with hypothyroidism, but also accentuated the difficulty in separating the effects of hypothyroidism from those of T_4 therapy. All patients with autoimmune hypothyroidism diagnosed for the first time between 1983 and 1996 in Denmark were identified through the National Patient Discharge Register. Each patient was matched with three age- and sex-matched normal subjects. Among the 4,473 patients with hypothyroidism (mean age 66 years), the frequency of fracture was significantly increased both before and after diagnosis, with a peak at about the time of diagnosis (incidence rate ratio 2.2–2.4). Fractures were increased at most skeletal sites, including the spine and hip. In the small number of patients who underwent bone densitometry several years after diagnosis and treatment, the mean Z score did not deviate from that of the general population. These results indicate that fracture risk is increased in both untreated and treated hypothyroid patients. The more marked increase in fracture risk and the increased distribution of sites affected compared with the earlier study were probably due to a more reliable population-based estimate and more complete follow-up.

In patients with hypothyroidism, bone turnover is reduced and bone mass is normal or slightly increased (16). The most plausible explanation for the increase in fracture risk in untreated hypothyroid patients is reduced renewal of bone, leading to accumulation of stress fractures. An additional factor may be an increased risk for falling because of poor muscular function, poor coordination, increased sensitivity to sedating drugs, and other illnesses. After initiation of T_4 therapy, an increase in bone turnover, a decrease in bone mass, and an increased risk for falls may contribute to the increased fracture risk.

REFERENCES

1. Reiter EO, Rosenfeld RG. Normal and aberrant growth. In: Wilson JD, Foster DW, Kronenberg HM, et al., eds. *Williams textbook of endocrinology*. Philadelphia: WB Saunders,1998:1427.
2. Rivkees SA, Bode HH, Crawford JD. Long-term growth in juvenile acquired hypothyroidism: the failure to achieve normal adult stature. *N Engl J Med* 1988;318:599.
3. Eriksen EF, Mosekilde L, Melsen F. Kinetics of trabecular bone resorption and formation in hypothyroidism: evidence for a positive balance per remodeling cycle. *Bone* 1986;7:101.
4. Krolner B, Jorgensen JV, Nielsen SP. Spinal bone mineral content in myxoedema and thyrotoxicosis: effects of thyroid hormone(s) and antithyroid treatment. *Clin Endocrinol (Oxf)* 1983;18:439.
5. Krane SM, Brownell GL, Stanbury JB, et al The effect of thyroid disease on calcium metabolism in man. *J Clin Invest* 1956;35:874.
6. Brixen K, Nielsen HK, Eriksen EF, et al. Efficacy of wheat germ lectin-precipitated alkaline phosphatase in serum as an estimator of bone mineralization rate: comparison to serum total alkaline phosphatase and serum bone Gla-protein. *Calcif Tissue Int* 1989;44:93.
7. Cassar J, Joseph S. Alkaline phosphatase levels in thyroid disease. *Clin Chim Acta* 1969;23:33.
8. Charles P, Poser JW, Mosekilde L, et al. Estimation of bone turnover evaluated by ^{47}Ca-kinetics: efficiency of serum bone gamma-carboxyglutamic acid-containing protein, serum alkaline phosphatase, and urinary hydroxyproline excretion. *J Clin Invest* 1985;76:2254.
9. Verrotti A, Greco R, Altobelli E, et al. Bone metabolism in children with congenital hypothyroidism—a longitudinal study. *J Pediatr Endocrinol Metab* 1998;11:699.
10. Kivirikko KI. Urinary excretion of hydroxyproline in health and disease. *Int Rev Connect Tissue Res* 1970;5:93.
11. Kivirikko KI, Laitinen O, Lamberg BA. Value of urine and serum hydroxyproline in the diagnosis of thyroid disease. *J Clin Endocrinol Metab* 1965;25:1347.
12. Siersbaek-Nielsen K, Skovsted L, Hansen JM, et al. Hydroxyproline excretion in the urine and calcium metabolism during long-term treatment of thyrotoxicosis with propylthiouracil. *Acta Med Scand* 1971;189:485.
13. Aub JC, Bauer W, Heath C, et al. Studies of calcium and phosphorous metabolism. III. The effects of thyroid hormone and thyroid disease. *J Clin Invest* 1929;7:97.
14. Bouillon R, De Moor P. Parathyroid function in patients with hyper- or hypothyroidism. *J Clin Endocrinol Metab* 1974;38:999.
15. Castro JH, Genuth SM, Klein L. Comparative response to parathyroid hormone in hyperthyroidism and hypothyroidism. *Metabolism* 1975;24:839.
16. Mosekilde L, Eriksen EF, Charles P. Effects of thyroid hormones on bone and mineral metabolism. *Endocrinol Metab Clin North Am* 1990;19:35.
17. Scow RO. Effect of growth hormone and thyroxine on growth and chemical composition of muscle, bone and other tissues in thyroidectomized-hypophysectomized rats. *Am J Physiol* 1959;196:859.
18. Thorngren KG, Hansson LI. Effect of thyroxine and growth hormone on longitudinal bone growth in the hypophysectomized rat. *Acta Endocrinol (Copenh)* 1973;74:24.
19. Harada Y, Okada Y, Hikita T, et al. Comparison of growth acceleration of pituitary dwarfs treated with anabolic steroid and thy-

roid hormone with normal growth spurt. *Acta Endocrinol (Copenh)* 1973;74:237.

20. Lewinson D, Bialik GM, Hochberg Z. Differential effects of hypothyroidism on the cartilage and the osteogenic process in the mandibular condyle: recovery by growth hormone and thyroxine. *Endocrinology* 1994;135:1504.

21. Van den Brande JL, Van Wyk JJ, French FS, et al. Advancement of skeletal age of hypopituitary children treated with thyroid hormone plus cortisone. *J Pediatr* 1973;82:22.

22. Lewinson D, Harel Z, Shenzer P, et al. Effect of thyroid hormone and growth hormone on recovery from hypothyroidism of epiphyseal growth plate cartilage and its adjacent bone. *Endocrinology* 1989;124:937.

23. Westermark K, Alm J, Skottner A, et al. Growth factors and the thyroid: effects of treatment for hyper- and hypothyroidism on serum IGF-I and urinary epidermal growth factor concentrations. *Acta Endocrinol (Copenh)* 1988;118:415.

24. Burstein PJ, Draznin B, Johnson CJ, et al. The effect of hypothyroidism on growth, serum growth hormone, the growth hormone-dependent somatomedin, insulin-like growth factor, and its carrier protein in rats. *Endocrinology* 1979;104:1107.

25. Cavaliere H, Knobel M, Medeiros-Neto G. Effect of thyroid hormone therapy on plasma insulin-like growth factor I levels in normal subjects, hypothyroid patients and endemic cretins. *Horm Res* 1987;25:132.

26. Chernausek SD, Turner R. Attenuation of spontaneous, nocturnal growth hormone secretion in children with hypothyroidism and its correlation with plasma insulin-like growth factor I concentrations. *J Pediatr* 1989;114:968.

27. Draznin B, Burstein PJ, Heinrich UE, et al. Insulin-like growth factor and its carrier protein in hypopituitary and hypothyroid children and adults. *Clin Endocrinol (Oxf)* 1980;12:137.

28. Hoogerbrugge-vd Linden N, Jansen H, Hulsmann WC, et al. Relationship between insulin-like growth factor-I and low-density lipoprotein cholesterol levels in primary hypothyroidism in women. *J Endocrinol* 1989;123:341.

29. Ren SG, Malozowski S, Simoni C, et al. Dose-response relationship between thyroid hormone and growth velocity in cynomolgus monkeys. *J Clin Endocrinol Metab* 1988;66:1010.

30. Valcavi R, Dieguez C, Preece M, et al. Effect of thyroxine replacement therapy on plasma insulin-like growth factor 1 levels and growth hormone responses to growth hormone releasing factor in hypothyroid patients. *Clin Endocrinol (Oxf)* 1987;27:85.

31. Valimaki M, Liewendahl, Karonen SL, et al. Concentrations of somatomedin-C and triiodothyronine in patients with thyroid dysfunction and nonthyroidal illnesses. *J Endocrinol Invest* 1990; 13:155.

32. Chernausek SD, Underwood LE, Utiger RD, et al. Growth hormone secretion and plasma somatomedin-C in primary hypothyroidism. *Clin Endocrinol (Oxf)* 1983;19:337.

33. Clemmons DR, Van Wyk JJ. Factors controlling blood concentration of somatomedin C. *Clin Endocrinol Metab* 1984;13:113.

34. Williams T, Maxon H, Thorner MO, et al. Blunted growth hormone (GH) response to GH-releasing hormone in hypothyroidism resolves in the euthyroid state. *J Clin Endocrinol Metab* 1985;61:454.

35. Varga F, Rumpler M, Klaushofer K. Thyroid hormones increase insulin-like growth factor mRNA levels in the clonal osteoblastic cell line MC3T3-E1. *FEBS Lett* 1994;345:67.

36. Ohlsson C, Nilsson A, Isaksson O, et al. Effects of tri-iodothyronine and insulin-like growth factor-I (IGF-I) on alkaline phosphatase activity, [3H]thymidine incorporation and IGF-I receptor mRNA in cultured rat epiphyseal chondrocytes. *J Endocrinol* 1992;135:115.

37. Glantschnig H, Varga F, Klaushofer K. Thyroid hormone and retinoic acid induce the synthesis of insulin-like growth factor-

binding protein-4 in mouse osteoblastic cells. *Endocrinology* 1996;137:281.

38. Schmid C, Schlapfer I, Futo E, et al. Triiodothyronine (T_3) stimulates insulin-like growth factor (IGF)-1 and IGF binding protein (IGFBP)-2 production by rat osteoblasts *in vitro*. *Acta Endocrinol (Copenh)* 1992;126:467.

39. Kandemir N, Yordam N, Oguz H. Age-related differences in serum insulin-like growth factor-I (IGF-I) and IGF-binding protein-3 levels in congenital hypothyroidism. *J Pediatr Endocrinol Metab* 1997;10:379.

40. Bona G, Rapa A, Boccardo G, et al. IGF-1 and IGFBP-3 in congenital and acquired hypothyroidism after long-term replacement treatment. *Panminerva Med* 1998;40:103.

41. Wikstrom L, Johansson C, Salto C, et al. Abnormal heart rate and body temperature in mice lacking thyroid hormone receptor alpha 1. *EMBO J* 1998;17:455.

42. Fraichard A, Chassande O, Plateroti M, et al. The T_3R alpha gene encoding a thyroid hormone receptor is essential for postnatal development and thyroid hormone production. *EMBO J* 1997;16:4412.

43. Forrest D, Hanebuth E, Smeyne RJ, et al. Recessive resistance to thyroid hormone in mice lacking thyroid hormone receptor beta: evidence for tissue-specific modulation of receptor function. *EMBO J* 1996;15:3006.

44. Gauthier K, Chassande O, Plateroti M, et al. Different functions for the thyroid hormone receptors TRalpha and TRbeta in the control of thyroid hormone production and post-natal development. *EMBO J* 1999;18:623.

45. Davis PJ, Davis FB. Nongenomic actions of thyroid hormone. *Thyroid* 1996;6:497.

46. Brent GA, Dunn MK, Harney JW, et al. Thyroid hormone aporeceptor represses T_3-inducible promoters and blocks activity of the retinoic acid receptor. *New Biol* 1989;1:329.

47. Flamant F, Poguet AL, Plateroti M, et al. Congenital hypothyroid Pax8(−/−) mutant mice can be rescued by inactivating the TRalpha gene. *Mol Endocrinol* 2002;16:24.

48. Weiss RE, Refetoff S. Effect of thyroid hormone on growth. Lessons from the syndrome of resistance to thyroid hormone. *Endocrinol Metab Clin North Am* 1996;25:719.

49. O'Shea PJ, Harvey CB, Suzuki H, et al. A thyrotoxic skeletal phenotype of advanced bone formation in mice with resistance to thyroid hormone. *Mol Endocrinol* 2003;17:1410.

50. Kaneshige M, Suzuki H, Kaneshige K, et al. A targeted dominant negative mutation of the thyroid hormone alpha 1 receptor causes increased mortality, infertility, and dwarfism in mice. *Proc Natl Acad Sci USA* 2001;98:15095.

51. Hamburgh M. An analysis of the action of thyroid hormone on development based on *in vivo* and *in vitro* studies. *Gen Comp Endocrinol* 1968;10:198.

52. Walker DG. An assay of the skeletogenic effect of L-triiodothyronine and its acetic acid analogue in immature rats. *Bull Johns Hopkins Hosp* 1957;101:101.

53. Fell HB, Mellanby E. The effect of L-triiodothyronine on the growth and development of embryonic chick limb-bones in tissue culture. *J Physiol* 1956;133:89.

54. Burch WM, Lebovitz HE. Triiodothyronine stimulates maturation of porcine growth-plate cartilage *in vitro*. *J Clin Invest* 1982; 70:496.

55. Burch WM, Lebovitz HE. Triiodothyronine stimulation of *in vitro* growth and maturation of embryonic chick cartilage. *Endocrinology* 1982;111:462.

56. Edeiken J, Hodes PJ. Skeletal maturation. In: Robbins LL, ed. *Roentgen diagnosis of diseases of bone*. Baltimore: Williams & Wilkins,1973:8.

57. Wilkins LW. Hormonal influences on skeletal growth. *Ann New York Acad Sci* 1955;60:763.

58. Fourman P, Royer P, Levell MJ, et al. *Calcium metabolism and the bone.* Oxford: Blackwell Scientific Publications, 1968.

59. Mosekilde L, Melsen F. Morphometric and dynamic studies of bone changes in hypothyroidism. *Acta Pathol Microbiol Scand [A]* 1978;86:56.

60. Coindre JM, David JP, Riviere L, et al. Bone loss in hypothyroidism with hormone replacement: a histomorphometric study. *Arch Intern Med* 1986;146:48.

61. Vestergaard P, Weeke J, Hoeck HC, et al. Fractures in patients with primary idiopathic hypothyroidism. *Thyroid* 2000;10:335.

62. Vestergaard P, Mosekilde L. Fractures in patients with hyperthyroidism and hypothyroidism: a nationwide follow-up study in 16,249 patients. *Thyroid* 2002;12:411.

63. Chassande O, Fraichard A, Gauthier K, et al. Identification of transcripts initiated from an internal promoter in the c-erbA alpha locus that encode inhibitors of retinoic acid receptor-alpha and triiodothyronine receptor activities. *Mol Endocrinol* 1997; 11:1278.

64. Salto C, Kindblom JM, Johansson C, et al. Ablation of TR alpha2 and a concomitant overexpression of alpha1 yields a mixed hypo- and hyperthyroid phenotype in mice. *Mol Endocrinol* 2001;15:2115.

65. Gauthier K, Plateroti M, Harvey CB, et al. Genetic analysis reveals different functions for the products of the thyroid hormone receptor alpha locus. *Mol Cell Biol* 2001;21:4748.

66. Abel ED, Boers ME, Pazos-Moura C, et al. Divergent roles for thyroid hormone receptor beta isoforms in the endocrine axis and auditory system. *J Clin Invest* 1999;104:291.

67. Ng L, Hurley JB, Dierks B, et al. A thyroid hormone receptor that is required for the development of green cone photoreceptors. *Nat Genet* 2001;27:94.

68. Gothe S, Wang Z, Ng L, et al. Mice devoid of all known thyroid hormone receptors are viable but exhibit disorders of the pituitary-thyroid axis, growth, and bone maturation. *Genes Dev* 1999;13:1329.

69. Kindblom JM, Gothe S, Forrest D, et al. GH substitution reverses the growth phenotype but not the defective ossification in thyroid hormone receptor alpha 1−/− beta−/− mice. *J Endocrinol* 2001;171:15.

70. Mansouri A, Chowdhury K, Gruss P. Follicular cells of the thyroid gland require Pax8 gene function. *Nat Genet* 1998;19:87.

71. Kaneshige M, Kaneshige K, Zhu X, et al. Mice with a targeted mutation in the thyroid hormone beta receptor gene exhibit impaired growth and resistance to thyroid hormone. *Proc Natl Acad Sci USA* 2000;97:13209.

63

THE NEUROMUSCULAR SYSTEM AND BRAIN IN HYPOTHYROIDISM

DAVID F. GARDNER

Hypothyroidism may result in a wide spectrum of reversible abnormalities in neuromuscular function in adults. In infants and young children, however, hypothyroidism has devastating effects on the developing nervous system that are irreversible. The focus of this chapter will be a review of the muscular and neurologic sequelae of hypothyroidism in adult patients. The frequency and severity of the abnormalities that have been described have varied considerably, undoubtedly due to variations in the severity of hypothyroidism and the ways it was identified. The effects of thyroid hormone deficiency on children and newborns are discussed in detail in Chapter 49 and the section on congenital hypothyroidism in Chapter 75.

MUSCLE DISORDERS

Hypothyroid Myopathy

Muscle-related symptoms are common in patients with hypothyroidism. Typical symptoms include weakness, which is usually proximal, stiffness, cramps, myalgia, and muscle fatigue. The prevalence of these symptoms has varied in different series, but they appear to be common, ranging from 79% to 100% in studies published over the past 50 years (1–6). Most patients with myopathic symptoms also report the more typical symptoms of hypothyroidism such as lethargy, constipation, weight gain, and cold intolerance. However, myopathy may be the sole clinical manifestation of hypothyroidism (7), suggesting that all patients with unexplained muscular symptoms should be screened for thyroid dysfunction.

Although muscle weakness may be severe, objective findings on physical examination are often unimpressive. In a recent series in which 79% of patients reported symptoms suggestive of myopathy, only 37% had decreased strength on manual muscle testing (6). This may be because many patients perceive fatigue and lack of energy as muscle weakness. Physical examination may reveal evidence of proximal muscle weakness, hypokinesis, and delayed relaxation of the deep tendon reflexes. The pathophysiology of the delayed deep tendon reflex appears to be related to underlying muscle disease rather than slowing of nerve conduction, because there is no difference in the latency from the tapping of the tendon to the onset of muscle contraction in hyperthyroid, euthyroid, and hypothyroid patients (8,9). Slow relaxation of tendon reflexes is not unique to hypothyroidism; it also occurs in normal older people, pregnant women, patients with diabetes mellitus, and patients receiving a β-adrenergic antagonist drug (10,11). Rare patients have muscle atrophy (4), and other, rarer patients have frank muscle enlargement; this is actually pseudohypertrophy (see later discussion on Hoffman's and Kocher-Debré-Sémélaigne syndromes). Patients with severe hypothyroidism may have myoedema, a focal contraction and mounding of muscle tissue occurring after the muscle is tapped with a reflex hammer. The mounding is typically followed by slow relaxation, which may last from seconds to minutes (12,13). This phenomenon also occurs in occasional normal subjects and patients with muscle wasting associated with malnutrition or cancer (14,15).

In the late 1800s, Hoffman and Kocher described hypothyroid patients with enlarged, apparently hypertrophied muscles, weakness, muscle stiffness, and slow movements (16,17). Debré and Sémélaigne described similar findings in infants with cretinism in 1935 (18). Today, the term "Hoffman's syndrome" is applied to adults with hypothyroidism who have increased muscle mass, severe muscle stiffness, varying degrees of weakness, and often painful muscle cramps (19,20). The increased muscle mass is not associated with increased muscle strength, and therefore is referred to as pseudohypertrophy. The gastrocnemius, deltoid, and trapezius muscles are typically involved. On examination, involved muscles are firm to palpation, usually weak, and contract slowly. The Kocher-Debré-Sémélaigne or Hercules syndrome is a similar syndrome described in children with cretinism, although it differs clinically in that painful muscle cramps are typically absent (21). Transition from the Kocher-Debré-Sémélaigne syndrome to Hoffman's syndrome has been described, and the only difference between these syndromes may be the age of the patient (13,20). In both children and adults the findings of pseudohypertrophy resolve with correction of hypothyroidism, although resolution may take many months (19). The pathophysiology of pseudohypertrophy remains unexplained; most studies have not revealed any increase in the size or number of muscle fibers, or an increase in mucinous deposits or the amount of connective tissue present in muscle.

The most common laboratory abnormality indicative of muscle dysfunction in patients with hypothyroidism is a high serum creatine kinase concentration. However, the concentrations also are high in as many as 70% to 90% of patients with hypothyroidism who have no clinical evidence of muscle involvement (22–25). The increase is almost invariably in the MM isoenzyme of skeletal muscle origin (22,26). Occasional patients have strikingly high serum creatine kinase concentrations, occasionally more than 100 times the upper limit of normal (27–29); the severity of symptoms associated with these markedly high values varies tremendously, from virtually no symptoms to substantial muscle weakness, muscle cramps, and myalgia (29). In most, but not all (30), studies there was little correlation between the magnitude of the elevation in serum creatine kinase concentration and the severity of hypothyroidism, as determined by measurements of either serum thyroxine (T_4) or thyrotropin (TSH). The mechanism underlying the high serum creatine kinase concentrations is not clear; possibilities include muscle fiber degeneration (29), altered muscle energy metabolism (31), and decreased clearance of creatine kinase from the circulation (32). High serum myoglobin concentrations have also been reported in hypothyroid patients, but the degree of elevation is considerably less than that of creatine kinase (33).

The histopathologic changes in muscle in patients with hypothyroidism are variable and nonspecific. The most consistent findings are atrophy or loss of type 2 muscle fibers, resulting in predominance of type 1 muscle fibers, and increased numbers of central nuclei (3,13,15,21,34–36). Additional findings have included sporadic areas of muscle fiber necrosis and regeneration, glycogen accumulation, and mitochondrial disruption. A clinical and pathologic study of 13 patients with hypothyroid myopathy revealed inflammatory changes, consistent with an underlying myositis, in 5 patients (35). The researchers emphasized the importance of considering other causes of myopathy in hypothyroid patients, particularly those who do not improve in response to thyroid hormone replacement therapy. Reported ultrastructural changes have included myofibrillar disorganization and fragmentation evidenced by the presence of "corelike" structures, increased numbers of mitochondria in the sarcolemmic region, glycogen accumulation, vacuolization, lipid accumulation, and proliferation of sarcoplasmic reticulum and T tubules (5,13,21,34–36).

The prevalence of electromyographic abnormalities in hypothyroid myopathy has varied substantially in different studies, ranging from 7% to 88%, undoubtedly due to varying methods of recruitment (e.g., all patients encountered, or only those with definite muscle weakness) (13, 21). The most common abnormalities are low-amplitude, short-duration polyphasic motor unit action potentials, consistent with a nonspecific myopathy. In a recent study of 19 hypothyroid patients, one third had these "myopathic" abnormalities (6). Other changes have included increased insertional activity and repetitive positive waves (37). Muscle fasciculations or fibrillations are extremely rare, and probably related to coincident neuropathy rather than intrinsic muscle disease (21). Perhaps the most unique electromyographic abnormality is the "electrical silence" associated with myoedema (14,38). Overall, electromyography is not very revealing in patients with hypothyroidism, and should be done only in patients in whom the clinical findings are atypical and who may have a treatable myopathy unrelated to hypothyroidism.

Acute rhabdomyolysis has been described in a few patients with hypothyroidism, including one patient who developed acute renal failure (39–43). Most of the patients have had severe hypothyroidism of recent onset; possible precipitating factors have included exercise (40,44), hypolipidemic drug therapy (41), and preexisting renal failure (45). In virtually all patients, the muscle injury resolved with correction of hypothyroidism.

Although most of the preceding discussion relates to patients with overt hypothyroidism, patients with subclinical hypothyroidism may have similar, although usually less severe, findings (see Chapter 78) (30,31,46–48). The prevalence of muscle symptoms in these patients has ranged from 26% to 75%, and in one study muscle weakness was more prevalent in patients with subclinical hypothyroidism than in those with overt hypothyroidism (48). As in overt hypothyroidism, symptoms resolve in most patients with correction of the thyroid dysfunction.

The mechanisms underlying abnormal muscle function in hypothyroidism are not known. Possibilities include impaired glycogenolysis (49,50), alterations in myosin heavy chain gene expression (51), and reduced mitochondrial activity, with a decrease in production of adenosine triphosphate (52,53). A recent study in patients with subclinical hypothyroidism documented increased lactate production during exercise, as compared with normal subjects, findings consistent with impaired mitochondrial oxidative function (31).

NEUROLOGIC DISORDERS

Neuropathy

Neuropathic symptoms including paresthesias and painful dysesthesias have been reported in patients with hypothyroidism. The patients may have symptoms and signs of a mononeuropathy, polyneuropathy, or cranial nerve neuropathy. Older series suggest a prevalence of neuropathic complaints in 40% to 60% of patients (1,54,55), but these patients undoubtedly had more severe hypothyroidism than do patients today (56). In a recent study of 19 patients with overt hypothyroidism, only 29% had symptoms of sensory nerve dysfunction (6).

The most common mononeuropathy encountered in hypothyroid patients is the carpal tunnel syndrome associated with median nerve compression as it traverses the volar aspect of the wrist. Typical symptoms include tingling, numbness, and pain in the sensory distribution of the distal median nerve, affecting the first, second, and third digits; other findings are wrist pain, nocturnal worsening of symptoms, and occasionally clumsiness of the hand and fingers (56). On examination there may be loss of sensation over the first three digits, weakness and atrophy of thenar muscles, and positive Tinel's and Phalen's signs. The symptoms and signs are identical to those in any patient with the carpal tunnel syndrome, and typically resolve with correction of the hypothyroidism (8). The pathophysiology of this disorder appears to be mechanical compression of the median nerve caused by edema and myxedema of perineural, endoneural, and synovial tissue within the carpal tunnel (2,57). Electrophysiologic studies document delayed distal median sensory nerve conduction, and less often delayed distal motor nerve conduction. The prevalence of the carpal tunnel syndrome in patients with hypothyroidism varies considerably; in three older series of unselected patients it varied from 27% to 45% (55,58,59), and in two more recent series it was 25% and 26% (6,60).

Other mononeuropathies that have been reported in association with hypothyroidism include the tarsal tunnel syndrome (61) and meralgia paresthetica (62), secondary to compression of the posterior tibial nerve and lateral femoral cutaneous nerves, respectively.

Generalized peripheral neuropathy is far less common than entrapment mononeuropathies in hypothyroid patients, although many patients have symptoms suggestive of a polyneuropathy. Distal paresthesias and pain were present in 48% to 100% of patients in three older series (2,54,55), but in a recent study distal sensory symptoms were present in only 29% of patients, nearly all of whom had the carpal tunnel syndrome rather than a more generalized sensorimotor polyneuropathy (6). Findings on examination that suggest peripheral neuropathy vary considerably; most often there is distal sensory loss and diminished deep tendon reflexes (6,8,56). A recent study of 19 hypothyroid patients documented distal sensory disturbances in the limbs or depressed deep tendon reflexes in 42%, although there was no significant symptomatology associated with these findings (6). Nerve conduction study results may be abnormal; they typically reveal decreased nerve conduction velocity, as well as diminished amplitude or complete absence of sensory nerve action potentials (6, 54,58,63–66). Pathologic findings have varied, with some showing segmental demyelination (64,65) and others suggesting axonal degeneration as the primary process (63,67).

Although polyneuropathy has clearly been described in case reports and small groups of patients with hypothyroidism, it is rarely an important clinical problem. In a recent study of 16 patients, 44% had the carpal tunnel syndrome, but none had polyneuropathy (68). The absence of any recent case series suggests that polyneuropathy may occur only in patients with much more severe hypothyroidism than is less usually encountered in clinical practice now.

Although most studies have focused on the peripheral nervous system, there are several studies that document abnormalities in nerve conduction in the central nervous system. The findings were usually prolongation of the latencies of visual evoked potentials and brainstem auditory evoked potentials (60,69). The clinical consequences of these findings are not known, and not all studies have confirmed the findings (70).

Isolated mononeuropathies involving cranial nerves II, V, VII, and VIII have been reported, but with the exception of hearing loss, these syndromes are extremely rare (1,2,13). Hearing loss has been reported in 31% to 85% of patients with hypothyroidism (1,71,72) and tinnitus in 7% to 29% (1,72); on the other hand one group found no evidence of hearing loss when hypothyroid patients were compared with age and sex-matched normal subjects (73). However, an etiologic role for hypothyroidism in causing deafness, at least in some patients, is strongly suggested by studies documenting improvement in hearing during thyroid hormone therapy (71). Hearing loss appears to be sensorineural rather than conductive, but its anatomic basis is not known.

Ataxia

In a report published by the Committee of the Clinical Society of London in 1888, more than one third of hypothyroid patients were found to have gait unsteadiness (74). Since that initial description there have been numerous descriptions of gait ataxia and poor coordination of the extremities, suggesting cerebellar dysfunction, in patients with hypothyroidism (1,75–78). Typical findings on examination have included gait unsteadiness with impaired tandem walking, generalized incoordination of the extremities, dysmetria, and rarely, dysarthric speech. In a single study of 24 patients with hypothyroidism and ataxia, prompt and almost complete clearing of symptoms occurred in the majority of patients after the initiation of thyroid hormone therapy (76). Proposed mechanisms for this syndrome include degenerative changes in the cerebellum, impaired cerebellar blood flow, deposition of glycogen within the cerebellum, and primary muscle dysfunction. A recent report described six euthyroid patients with chronic autoimmune thyroiditis who developed progressive nonfamilial adult-onset cerebellar degeneration (79). Posterior fossa magnetic resonance imaging (MRI) revealed cerebellar degeneration in all six patients, and all had a strong family history of autoimmune disease, suggesting an immune-mediated process for the cerebellar changes.

Mental Status Changes

Neurocognitive impairment may be a prominent feature of hypothyroidism, particularly in elderly patients. Slowness in comprehension, diminished attention span, poor recent memory, difficulty with word fluency, and impaired abstract thinking may all be present (80–82), and indeed may be among the patients' more prominent symptoms. Most patients improve substantially when treated with thyroid hormone, but resolution may be slow or incomplete (82). Hypothyroidism is often considered a cause of reversible dementia in the elderly, and thyroid function is often routinely assessed in the evaluation of patients with cognitive impairment. The incidence of hypothyroidism in demented patients is actually low, ranging from 1.5% to 4.2%, even when patients with subclinical hypothyroidism are included (83–85). Consistent improvement in cognitive function in patients with dementia after correction of hypothyroidism has not been demonstrated, suggesting that other factors are contributing to mental impairment in these patients (82–84).

Alterations in cognition have been reported in patients with subclinical hypothyroidism as well as those with overt hypothyroidism (see Chapter 78). In a study of 19 women with subclinical hypothyroidism (mean serum TSH concentration 12.0 mU/L), there was evidence of memory impairment that improved significantly during thyroid hormone therapy (86).

The behavioral and psychiatric abnormalities associated with hypothyroidism are reviewed in detail in Chapter 64.

Hashimoto's Encephalopathy

Since an initial case report in 1966 (87), about 100 patients have been described with an encephalopathy associated with high serum antithyroid antibody concentrations, responsiveness to glucocorticoid therapy, and no other definable neurologic disorder. The term "Hashimoto's encephalopathy" has been applied to these patients. A recent review of the literature identified 85 patients who met strict criteria for this diagnosis (encephalopathy, high serum concentrations of either antithyroid peroxidase or antithyroglobulin antibodies, and no other neurologic disorder); they had the following clinical findings: stroke-like signs (27%), psychosis (38%), seizures (66%), high cerebrospinal fluid protein concentrations (78%), and abnormal electroencephalograms (98%) (88). The clinical course of the disorder is characterized by remissions and relapses, generalized and focal seizures, focal and often transient neurologic deficits, and a variety of psychiatric manifestations, including hallucinations, dementia, and acute psychosis (89,90).

The diagnosis is based on the characteristic neurologic findings reviewed above, high serum antithyroid antibody concentrations, and exclusion of other causes of encephalopathy. Thyroid function varies; among the 85 patients referred to above, 30% had normal serum free T_4 and TSH concentrations, 55% had either overt or subclinical hypothyroidism, and the remainder had biochemical evidence of hyperthyroidism (88). The neurologic presentation does not appear to be influenced by the patient's thyroid status. Cerebrospinal fluid protein levels are typically high, but most patients do not have pleocytosis. Brain imaging studies (MRI and computed tomography) are normal or show nonspecific findings. Electroencephalography typically reveals diffuse abnormalities with excess slow wave activity (89).

A high percentage of patients appear to respond to glucocorticoid therapy (88), and some researchers have suggested that an underlying vasculitis is responsible for this encephalopathy. However, there is no compelling clinical or pathologic evidence to support a diagnosis of vasculitis, and the pathophysiology of this disorder is not known. The high serum antithyroid antibody concentrations, part of the definition of the disorder, suggest the possibility of an immune-mediated central nervous system process, but there is no evidence that any antithyroid antibody reacts with neural or meningeal tissue, and antineuronal antibodies have not been detected.

Miscellaneous Neurologic Abnormalities

Seizures are a rare neurologic complication of hypothyroidism, and when they do occur it is almost always in patients who have myxedema coma or Hashimoto's encephalopathy. The few isolated case reports of seizures in hypothyroidism suggest that this may be a coincidental rather than an etiologic association, although in three reported patients seizures did not recur after thyroid hormone therapy had been initiated (91–93). In a study of 23 hypothyroid patients without seizures, 35% had electroencephalographic abnormalities; the most common abnormality was diffuse slowing of background activity, and epileptiform foci were not recorded (60).

A high cerebrospinal fluid protein concentration has been a consistent finding in studies of hypothyroid patients (1,2,8). In a study of nine patients with overt hypothyroidism, all had high cerebrospinal fluid albumin and immunoglobulin G concentrations that returned to normal during thyroid hormone therapy (94). The high protein concentrations are not related to thyroid autoimmunity per se; patients with subclinical hypothyroidism and high serum antithyroid antibody concentrations do not have high cerebrospinal albumin or immunoglobulin G concentrations. Presumably, hypothyroidism results in increased permeability of the blood–brain barrier.

The clinical features of myxedema coma are reviewed in detail in Chapter 65.

REFERENCES

1. Nickel SN, Frame B. Neurologic manifestations of myxedema. *Neurology* 1958;8:511.
2. Nickel SN, Frame B, Bebin J, et al. Myxedema neuropathy and myopathy: a clinical and pathologic study. *Neurology* 1961;11:125.
3. McKeran RO, Slavin G, Ward P, et al. Hypothyroid myopathy: a clinical and pathological study. *J Pathol* 1980;132:35.
4. Khaleeli AA, Griffith DF, Edwards RHT. The clinical presentation of hypothyroid myopathy and its relationship to abnormalities in structure and function of skeletal muscle. *Clin Endocrinol (Oxf)* 1983;19:365.
5. Modi G. Cores in hypothyroid myopathy: a clinical, histological, and immunofluorescence study. *J Neurol Sci* 2000;175:28.
6. Duyff RF, Van den Bosch J, Laman DM. Neuromuscular findings in thyroid dysfunction: a prospective clinical and electrodiagnostic study. *J Neurol Neurosurg Psychiatry* 2000;68:750.
7. Rodolico C, Toscano A, Benvenga S, et al. Myopathy as the persistently isolated symptomatology of primary autoimmune hypothyroidism. *Thyroid* 1998;8:1033.
8. Laureno R. Neurologic manifestations of thyroid disease. *Endocrinologist* 1996;6:467.
9. Lambert EH, Underdahl LO, Beckett S, et al. A study of the ankle jerk in myxedema. *J Clin Endocrinol* 1951;11:1186.
10. Wise MP, Blunt S, Lane RJ. Neurologic presentations of hypothyroidism: the importance of slow relaxing reflexes. *J R Soc Med* 1995;88:272.
11. Reinfrank RF, Kaufman RP, Wetstone HJ, et al. Observations of the Achilles reflex test. *JAMA* 1967;199:59.
12. Swanson JW, Kelly JJ, McConahey WM. Neurologic aspects of thyroid dysfunction. *Mayo Clin Proc* 1981;56:504.
13. Laycock MA, Pascuzzi RM. The neuromuscular effects of hypothyroidism. *Semin Neurol* 1991;11:288.
14. Salick AI, Pearson CM. Electrical silence of myoedema. *Neurology* 1967;17:899.
15. Salick AI, Colachis SC, Pearson CM. Myxedema myopathy: clinical, electrodiagnostic, and pathologic findings in an advanced case. *Arch Phys Med Rehabil* 1968;49:230.
16. Hoffman J. Weitere Beitrag zur Lehre von der Tetanie. *Deutsche Z Nervenheilk* 1897;9:278.
17. Kocher T. Zur Verhutung der Cretinismus und cretinoider Zustande nach neuen Forschungen. *Deutsch Z Chir* 1892;26:556.
18. Debre F, Semelaigne G. Syndrome of diffuse muscular hypertrophy in infants causing athletic appearance: its connection with congenital myxedema. *Am J Dis Child* 1935;50:1351.
19. Klein I, Parker M, Shebert R, et al. Hypothyroidism presenting as muscle stiffness and pseuohypertrophy: Hoffman's syndrome. *Am J Med* 1981;70:891.
20. Norris FH, Panner BJ. Hypothyroid myopathy: clinical, electromyographical, and ultrastructural observations. *Arch Neurol* 1966;14:574.
21. Kaminski HJ, Ruff RL. Endocrine myopathies (hyper- and hypofunction of adrenal, thyroid, pituitary, and parathyroid glands and iatrogenic corticosteroid myopathy). In: Engel AG, Franzini-Armstrong C, eds. *Myology: basic and clinical,* 2nd ed., Vol. 2. New York: McGraw-Hill, 1994:1726.
22. Burnett JR, Crooke MJ, Delahunt JW, et al. Serum enzymes in hypothyroidism. *N Z Med J* 1994;107:355.
23. Graig FA, Smith JC. Serum creatine phosphokinase activity in altered thyroid states. *J Clin Endocrinol Metab* 1965;25:723.
24. Fleisher GA, McConahey WM, Pankow M. Serum creatine kinase, lactic dehydrogenase, and glutamic-oxaloacetic transaminase in thyroid diseases and pregnancy. *Mayo Clin Proc* 1965;40:300.
25. Giampietro O, Clerico A, Buzzigoli G, et al. Detection of hypothyroid myopathy by measurements of various serum muscle markers—myoglobin, creatine kinase, lactic dehydrogenase, and their isoenzymes. *Horm Res* 1984;19:232.
26. Goti I. Serum creatine phosphokinase isoenzymes in hypothyroidism, convulsions, myocardial infarction, and other diseases. *Clin Chim Acta* 1974;52:27.
27. Goldman J, Matz R, Mortimer R, et al. High elevations of creatine phosphokinase in hypothyroidism: an isoenzyme analysis. *JAMA* 1977; 238:325.
28. Finsterer J, Stollberger C, Grossegger C, et al. Hypothyroid myopathy with unusually high serum creatine kinase values. *Horm Res* 1999;52:205.
29. Scott KR, Simmons Z, Boyer PJ. Hypothyroid myopathy with a strikingly elevated creatine kinase level. *Muscle Nerve* 2002; 26:141.
30. Beyer IW, Karmali R, Demeester-Mirkine N, et al. Serum creatine kinase levels in overt and subclinical hypothyroidism. *Thyroid* 1998;8:1029.
31. Monzani F, Caraccio N, Siciliano G, et al. Clinical and biochemical features of muscle dysfunction in subclinical hypothyroidism. *J Clin Endocrinol Metab* 1997;82:3315.
32. Karlsberg RP, Roberts R. Effect of altered thyroid function on plasma creatine kinase clearance in the dog. *Am J Physiol* 1978; 235:E614.
33. Karlsson FA, Dahlberg PA, Venge P, et al. Serum myoglobin in thyroid disease. *Acta Endocrinol* (Copenh) 1980;94:184.
34. Khaleeli AA, Gohil K, McPhail G, et al. Muscle morphology and metabolism in hypothyroid myopathy. *J Clin Pathol* 1983;36:519.
35. Mastaglia FL, Ojeda VJ, Sarnat HB, et al. Myopathies associated with hypothyroidism: a review based upon 13 cases. *Aust N Z J Med* 1988;18:799.
36. Ono S, Inouye K, Mannen T. Myopathology of hypothyroid myopathy. *J Neurol Sci* 1987;77:237.
37. Klein I, Levey GS. Unusual manifestations of hypothyroidism. *Arch Intern Med* 1984;144:123.
38. Mizusawa H, Takagi A, Sugita H, et al. Mounding phenomenon: an experimental study *in vitro. Neurology* 1983;33:90.
39. Halverson PB, Kozin F, Ryan LM, et al. Rhabdomyolysis and renal failure in hypothyroidism. *Ann Intern Med* 1979;91:57.
40. Riggs JE. Acute exertional rhabdomyolysis in hypothyroidism: the result of a reversible defect in glycogenolysis? *Milit Med* 1990;155:171.
41. Clouatre Y, Lebland M, Quimet D, et al. Fenofibrate-induced rhabdomyolysis in two dialysis patients with hypothyroidism. *Nephrol Dial Transplant* 1999;14:1047.
42. Barahona MJ, Mauri A, Sucunza N, et al. Hypothyroidism as a cause of rhabdomyolysis. *Endocr J* 2002;49:621.
43. Kisakol G, Tunc R, Kaya A. Rhabdomyolysis in a patient with hypothyroidism. *Endocr J* 2003;50:221.
44. Nelso SR, Phillips AO, Hendry BM. Hypothyroidism and rhabdomyolysis in a marathon runner. *Nephrol Dial Transplant* 1993; 8:375.
45. Leonetti F, Dussol B, Berland Y. Rhabdomyolyse et insuffisance renale au cours d'une hypothyroidie. *Presse Med* 1992;21:31.
46. Rodolico C, Toscano A, Benvenga S, et al. Skeletal muscle disturbances may precede clinical and laboratory evidence of autoimmune hypothyroidism. *J Neurol* 1998;245:555.
47. Monzani F, Caraccio N, Del Guerra P, et al. Neuromuscular symptoms and dysfunction in subclinical hypothyroid patients: beneficial effect of L-T$_4$ replacement therapy. *Clin Endocrinol (Oxf)* 1999;51:237.

48. Hartl E, Finsterer J, Grossegger C, et al. Relationship between thyroid function and skeletal muscle involvement in subclinical and overt hypothyroidism. *Endocrinologist* 2001;11:217.

49. McDaniel HG, Pittman CS, Oh SJ, et al. Carbohydrate metabolism in hypothyroid myopathy. *Metabolism* 1977;26:867.

50. Taylor DJ, Rajagopalan B, Radda GK. Cellular energetics in hypothyroid muscle. *Eur J Clin Invest* 1992;22:358.

51. Caiozzo VJ, Baker MJ, Baldwin KM. Novel transformation in MHC isoforms: separate and combined effects of thyroid hormone and mechanical unloading. *J Appl Physiol* 1998;85:2237.

52. Kaminsky P, Robin-Lherbier B, Brunotte F, et al. Energetic metabolism in hypothyroid skeletal muscle, as studied by phosphorus magnetic resonance spectroscopy. *J Clin Endocrinol Metab* 1992;74:124.

53. Argov Z, Renshaw PF, Boden B, et al. Effects of thyroid hormones on skeletal muscle bioenergetics: *in vivo* phosphorus-31 magnetic resonance spectroscopy study of humans and rats. *J Clin Invest* 1988;81:1695.

54. Crevasse LE, Logue RB. Peripheral neuropathy in myxedema. *Ann Intern Med* 1959;50:1433.

55. Rao SN, Katiyar BC, Nair KRP, et al. Neuromuscular studies in hypothyroidism. *Acta Neurol Scand* 1980;61:167.

56. Crum BA, Bolton CF. Peripheral neuropathy in systemic disease. In: Brown WF, Bolton CF, Aminoff MJ, eds. *Neuromuscular function and disease: basic, clinical and electrodiagnostic aspects.* Vol. 2. Philadelphia: WB Saunders, 2002:1081.

57. Purnell DC, Daly D, Lipscomb PR. Carpal tunnel syndrome associated with myxedema. *Arch Intern Med* 1961;108:751.

58. Fincham RW, Cape CA. Neuropathy in myxedema: a study of sensory nerve conduction in the upper extremities. *Arch Neurol* 1968;19:464.

59. Murray IPC, Simpson JA. Acroparesthesias in myxoedema: a clinical and electromyographic study. *Lancet* 1958;1:1360.

60. Khedr EM, El Toony LF, Tarkhan MN, et al. Peripheral and central nervous system alterations in hypothyroidism: electrophysiological findings. *Neuropsychobiology* 2000;41:88.

61. Schwartz MS, Mackworth-Young CG, McKeran R. The tarsal tunnel syndrome in hypothyroidism. *J Neurol Neurosurg Psychiatry* 1983;46:440.

62. Suarez G, Sabin TD. Meralgia paresthetica and hypothyroidism [Letter]. *Ann Intern Med* 1990;112:149.

63. Pollard JD, McLeod JG, Honnibal TGA, et al. Hypothyroid polyneuropathy: clinical, electrophysiological, and nerve biopsy findings in two cases. *J Neurol Sci* 1982;53:461.

64. Dyck PJ, Lambert ED. Polyneuropathy associated with hypothyroidism. *J Neuropathol Exp Neurol* 1970;29:631.

65. Shirabe T, Tawara S, Terao A, et al. Myedematous polyneuropathy: a light and electron microscopic study of the peripheral nerve and muscle. *J Neurol Neurosurg Psychiatry* 1975;38:241.

66. Nemni R, Bottacchi E, Fazio R, et al. Polyneuropathy in hypothyroidism: clinical, electrophysiological, and morphological findings in four cases. *J Neurol Neurosurg Psychiatry* 1987;50:1454.

67. Meier C, Bischoff A. Polyneuropathy in hypothyroidism: clinical and nerve biopsy study of four cases. *J Neurol* 1977;215:103.

68. Cruz MW, Tendrich M, Vaisman M, et al. Electroneuromyography and neuromuscular findings in 16 primary hypothyroidism patients. *Arq Neuropsiquiatr* 1996;54:12.

69. Huang TS, Chang YC, Lee SH, et al. Visual, brainstem auditory and somatosensory evoked potential abnormalities in thyroid disease. *Thyroidology* 1989;1:137.

70. Vanesse M, Fischer C, Berthezene F, et al. Normal brainstem evoked potential in adult hypothyroidism. *Laryngoscope* 1989;99:302.

71. Van't Hoff W, Stuart DW. Deafness in myxoedema. *Q J M* 1979;48:361.

72. Bhatia PL, Gupta DP, Agrawal MK, et al. Audiological and vestibular function tests in hypothyroidism. *Laryngoscope* 1977;87:2082.

73. Parving A, Ostri B, Hansen JM, et al. Audiological and temporal bone findings in myxedema. *Ann Otol Rhinol Laryngol* 1986;95:278.

74. Clinical Society of London. Report on myxedema. *Trans Clin Soc Lond* 1888;21(suppl):1–215.

75. Jellinek EH, Kelly RE. Cerebellar syndrome in myxedema. *Lancet* 1960;2:225.

76. Cremer GM, Goldstein NP, Paris J. Myxedema and ataxia. *Neurology* 1969;19:37.

77. Blume WT, Grabow JD. The "cerebellar" signs of myxedema. *Dis Nerv Syst* 1969;30:55.

78. Westphal SA. Unusual presentations of hypothyroidism. *Am J Med Sci* 1997;314:333.

79. Selim M, Drachman DA. Ataxia associated with Hashimoto's disease: progressive non-familial adult onset cerebellar degeneration with autoimmune thyroiditis. *J Neurol Neurosurg Psychiatry* 2001;71:81.

80. Kornstein SG, Sholar EF, Gardner DF. Endocrine disorders. In: Stoudemire A, Fogel BS, Greenberg DB, eds. *Psychiatric care of the medical patient,* 2nd ed. New York: Oxford University Press, 2000:801.

81. Osterweil D, Syndulko K, Cohen SN, et al. Cognitive function in non-demented older adults with hypothyroidism. *J Am Geriatr Soc* 1992;40:325.

82. Dugbartey AT. Neurocognitive aspects of hypothyroidism. *Arch Intern Med* 1998;158:1413.

83. Larson EB, Reifler BV, Featherstone HJ, et al. Dementia in elderly outpatients: a prospective study. *Ann Intern Med* 1984;100:417.

84. Larson EB, Reifler, Sumi SM, et al. Diagnostic evaluation of 200 elderly outpatients with suspected dementia. *J Gerontol* 1985;40:536.

85. D'Angelo R, Fogato E, Balzaretti M, et al. Screening for hypothyroidism in institutionalized elderly people with cognitive and functional impairment. *J Endocrinol Invest* 1999;22(suppl 10):42.

86. Baldini IM, Vita A, Mauri MC, et al. Psychopathological and cognitive features in subclinical hypothyroidism. *Prog Neuropsychopharmacol Biol Psychiatry* 1997;21:925.

87. Brain L, Jellinek EH, Ball K. Hashimoto's disease and encephalopathy. *Lancet* 1966;2:512.

88. Chong JY, Rowland LP, Utiger RD. Hashimoto encephalopathy: syndrome or myth? *Arch Neurol* 2003;60:164.

89. Shaw PJ, Walls TJ, Newman PK, et al. Hashimoto's encephalopathy: a steroid responsive disorder associated with high antithyroid antibody titers—report of five cases. *Neurology* 1991;41:228.

90. Kothbauer-Margreiter I, Sturzenegger M, Komor J, et al. Encephalopathy associated with Hashimoto thyroiditis: diagnosis and treatment. *J Neurol* 1996;243:585.

91. Evans EC. Neurologic complications of myxedema: convulsions. *Ann Intern Med* 1960;52:434.

92. Rowell NP, Clarke SW. Myxoedema presenting as epilepsy. *Postgrad Med J* 1984;60:605.

93. Bryce GM, Poyner F. Myxoedema presenting with seizures. *Postgrad Med J* 1992;68:35.

94. Nystrom E, Hamberger A, Linstedt G, et al. Cerebrospinal fluid proteins in subclinical and overt hypothyroidism. *Acta Neurol Scand* 1997;95:311.

BEHAVIORAL AND PSYCHIATRIC ASPECTS OF HYPOTHYROIDISM

PETER C. WHYBROW
MICHAEL BAUER

The prevalence, nature, and clinical course of the behavioral and psychological changes that occur in adults with primary hypothyroidism were first described in the latter half of the nineteenth century (1–4). In 1888, the Clinical Society of London described myxedematous (hypothyroid) patients, most of whom had some mental disturbance, ranging from irritability and agoraphobia to dementia and melancholia (3). Subsequently, it became generally accepted that hypothyroidism had severe effects on brain function and could irreversibly damage the developing brain. In adults with hypothyroidism, the subtle behavioral and psychological changes, especially during the early stages of the illness, confounded the clinical diagnosis, and people with "myxedematous madness" were commonly found on careful evaluation of patients in mental hospitals (5). Objective laboratory tests have improved this situation enormously, but isolated case reports of patients with hypothyroidism who present with severe mental disturbance continue to appear, and it remains important that the clinician be aware of the wide range of behavioral disturbances that can occur in patients with hypothyroidism (6–8).

NEUROPSYCHIATRIC FEATURES

The initial behavioral and neuropsychological changes in adults with primary hypothyroidism are nonspecific and ill-defined complaints (e.g., weakness, fatigue) and disturbances in cognition. The latter include inattentiveness, inability to concentrate, slowing of thought processes, and inability to calculate and to understand complex questions. Memory for recent events is frequently poor, and eventually memory for remote events also may become impaired. Ability to perform everyday, routine tasks is decreased. The patient becomes less responsive to others, less interested in his or her surroundings, and less capable of learning and performing new tasks. There is a paucity of speech, frequently with perseveration. Motor functions are slowed. Alterations in the accuracy of perception with an increased tendency toward illusion formation may appear; still later, visual and other hallucinatory distortions may occur that result in bizarre behavior and paranoid ideas. We know

from historical descriptions that as hypothyroidism becomes more severe, progressive drowsiness, with lethargy and difficulty in arousal, occurs. The patient may sleep for long periods during the day and, finally, may lapse into stupor and even coma (see Chapter 65) (9). Convulsions also can occur (10).

Because of slowing of thought and speech, decreased attentiveness, poor concentration, and diminished interest in and responsiveness to others, the diagnosis initially may be confused with that of a depressive mood state (Fig. 64.1). Indeed, hypothyroidism may induce a specific melancholic disorder in some patients (11), with crying, loss of appetite, constipation, insomnia, delusions of self-reproach, and suicidal ideation (7,12–14). The picture is not consistently one of depression; a disorganized agitated state also has been described. In case vignettes of hypothyroid patients with psychosis (5,15–17), insomnia, hyperactivity, irritability, anger, and both auditory and visual hallucinations are described. Other patients become fearful, suspicious, and delusional. Hence, although depressed mood seems to predominate, the specific mental state and thought content varies with the individual patient. Cognitive changes, however, with alterations in attention, concentration, perception, and speed of thought, appear to be the most common of the clinical manifestations.

OBJECTIVE BEHAVIORAL ASSESSMENT

These clinical observations are confirmed by the few objective studies of behavior that have been conducted in patients with hypothyroidism. Taken together, the symptoms and signs are diverse, and the mental state of hypothyroid patients thus has much in common with other organic syndromes of brain dysfunction. The results of electroencephalographic studies reflect this, with low-voltage θ and δ waves predominating (18,19). Stages 3 and 4 of sleep may be reduced (13), and evoked responses also are slowed (20–22). The electroencephalographic changes can be correlated with the mental status examination and particularly with tests of cognitive function, such as mental arithmetic or short-term memory and attention (23). More recently,

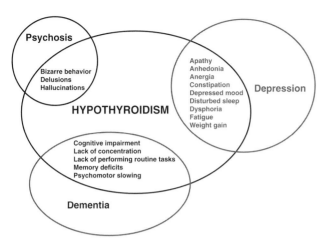

FIGURE 64.1. The symptoms of hypothyroidism overlap with those of dementia, psychosis, and depression.

studies using positron emission tomography have revealed a reduction of brain activity in association with the behavioral symptoms in severe hypothyroidism, but with varying results in different regions of the brain (24–26).

Objective psychological testing has revealed impairment in cognitive function with deficits in memory and learning, attention, visuoperceptual and construction skills, and psychomotor slowing (27,28). In most patients the deficits in cognitive function improve markedly with treatment (14, 27,29–33). Some investigators have suggested that treatment with a combination of thyroxine (T_4) and triiodothyronine (T_3) improves performance in cognitive tasks more than does treatment with T_4 alone (34). Subsequent analysis suggested that the combination had a greater effect in those patients with thyroid carcinoma than in those with autoimmune thyroiditis (35). Subsequent studies, however, have not confirmed the benefit of combined T_4 and T_3 therapy (36,37). Not all cognitive dysfunction, however, is reversed by therapy, suggesting that chronic deficiency of thyroid hormone may induce irreversible deficits in central nervous system (CNS) function (14,27,28,38).

Few behavioral studies have been conducted in hypothyroid patients unselected for psychiatric disorder, and hence the incidence of psychosis in hypothyroidism is difficult to estimate. Among the hypothyroid patients studied in 1888, it was about 15% (3). A study in the 1920s described hallucinations in 26% of patients (39). Improvements in laboratory tests that aid in the early diagnosis of hypothyroidism have reduced the incidence substantially, probably to less than 5%.

ASSOCIATED PSYCHIATRIC SYNDROMES

Schizophrenic and Affective Psychoses

The psychoses that occur in patients with hypothyroidism are nonspecific, representing a final common path of neu-

robiologic disorganization. Thus, they may mimic schizophrenic, paranoid, and affective psychoses. Although a careful history and physical examination usually reveal at least a few stigmata of hypothyroidism, the florid and acute nature of the psychotic disturbance may distract the physician or preclude such detailed clinical examination. Of special importance in clarifying the differential diagnosis is the impairment of cognitive function that is found in hypothyroidism. Even though confusion occurs in acute schizophrenia, together with distractibility that may masquerade as poor memory, visual hallucinations with profound and persistent cognitive disturbance (including memory and orientation) are rare. Thus, formal neuropsychological testing can be helpful. The very low amplitude waves present on electroencephalography in patients with severe hypothyroidism suggest an underlying delirium (18), but this test cannot be considered a reliable differential diagnostic procedure.

In patients with affective psychoses, cognitive impairment or pseudodementia is more common, especially in elderly persons, in whom it may be dismissed as the dementia of old age. Indeed, the symptoms of hypothyroid psychosis may mimic so closely those of the severely psychotic affective states that routine thyroid screening should be performed in all patients over 60 years of age who present with the clinical syndrome of affective psychosis and intellectual impairment.

The Depressive Syndrome and Manic Depression

Several metabolic and behavioral disturbances are common to hypothyroidism and affective illness, even in the absence of psychosis, suggesting that changes in pituitary–thyroid secretion may play an important role in the modulation of mood (40,41).

Patients with depression have a spectrum of abnormalities in thyroid test results, the most common of which is a slightly high serum T_4 concentration (40–42), with a decline during treatment that correlates with the clinical response to antidepressant drug therapy (42,43). The serum thyrotropin (TSH) response to thyrotropin-releasing hormone (TRH) is blunted in approximately 25% of patients with depression, even though their serum T_4 concentrations are within normal limits (44,45). Finally, as part of the disturbed circadian endocrine profile, the nocturnal surge in serum TSH concentrations is lost in depression, but returns with recovery (46).

Hypothyroidism is a graded phenomenon, and changes in serum T_4 and especially TSH concentrations can be detected before the appearance of any clinical evidence of hypothyroidism. About 10% of 250 consecutive patients referred to a psychiatric hospital for treatment of depression or anergia had evidence of subclinical hypothyroidism (high serum TSH concentrations alone) or overt hypothyroidism (high serum TSH and low T_4 concentrations) (47).

Furthermore, T_3 given as an adjunct to tricyclic antidepressant drug treatment speeds recovery in some patients with depression (48), especially women (43,49). Some depressed patients resistant to therapeutic doses of antidepressant drugs may respond when T_3 or high doses of T_4 are added to the therapeutic regimen (50–53). Other patients with subclinical hypothyroidism complain of anergia and depressive-like symptoms that fall short of the classic depressive syndromes (see Chapter 78). However, the effect of T_4 therapy on these symptoms in patients with subclinical hypothyroidism has been mixed (54–58).

Among women with postpartum depression, some also have postpartum thyroiditis, which occurs in about 5% of postpartum women (see Chapter 27). Each of these disorders can occur separately, but postpartum women with high serum antithyroid antibody concentrations are more likely to be depressed. In a study of 145 women who had high serum antithyroid antibody concentrations 6 weeks postpartum, 47% later had significant depressive symptoms, as compared with 32% of women with normal serum antibody concentrations (59). In a randomized double-blind placebo-controlled trial of 446 thyroid antibody–positive women, however, administration of 100 µg of T_4 per day failed to diminish the incidence of depressive symptomatology (60).

Thyroid dysfunction is particularly important in the clinical course of manic-depressive (bipolar) illness, especially in rapid cycling, a severe form of the illness. Patients with the rapid cycling pattern, 70% to 90% of whom are women, by definition have more than four episodes of bipolar illness per year (61). They have a much higher incidence (~25%) of hypothyroidism than depressed patients in general (2%–5%) or those taking lithium carbonate (9%) (62,63). Administration of therapeutic doses of lithium carbonate, an established drug for the prophylaxis of bipolar disorder that also has antithyroid properties (64), resulted in significantly higher serum TSH responses to TRH stimulation in otherwise untreated patients with rapid cycling bipolar disease, as compared with normal subjects (65). This difference suggests that small degrees of hypothyroidism play a key role in the development of a rapid cycling pattern in patients with bipolar disorder. High doses of T_4 added to the established treatment with lithium and other psychotropic drugs can reverse the rapid cycling pattern (66,67) and reduce the number of episodes in otherwise refractory bipolar disorder (68,69).

In addition to its antithyroid activity (70), lithium may inhibit type 2 deiodinase activity, the predominant deiodinase in the brain and pituitary (see Chapter 7) (71,72). Hence, the treatment of bipolar illness with lithium may impair brain thyroid economy and thus complicate the clinical course of the mood disturbance itself (73). Conversely, in some hypothyroid patients with a family history of bipolar affective illness, rapid replacement with T_4 can induce mania (74). Tricyclic antidepressant drugs, which can precipitate rapid cycling disease (62,74), may also inhibit T_4 conversion to T_3 in the brain (75).

Taken together, these studies suggest that thyroid abnormalities, including overt and subclinical hypothyroidism, may contribute to psychiatric disability. Therefore, thyroid screening by measurement of serum TSH is warranted in all patients with syndromes of affective illness, especially women, who are resistant to antidepressant drugs and in those with atypical psychoses with a substantial cognitive disorder.

PATHOPHYSIOLOGY OF BEHAVIORAL DYSFUNCTION IN HYPOTHYROIDISM

The specific pathophysiology responsible for the behavioral disturbances of patients with hypothyroidism is unknown. It is probable that the general decline in cognitive and behavioral function is an integral part of the hypometabolic state characteristic of the disorder.

It has long been recognized that thyroid hormone is essential for the normal development of the central nervous system (see Chapter 74) (76,77). T_4 is taken up avidly by the developing rat brain, and brain T_3 content in these animals is higher than in mature animals (10). During development, T_4 and T_3 determine the rate and completeness of neuronal cell division and stimulate the activity of many enzyme systems in the brain, by exerting major effects on both nucleic acid and protein synthesis (78).

In an early study in adults with hypothyroidism, cerebral blood flow was reduced 38% below normal, as were oxygen and glucose consumption (27% below normal), and cerebrovascular resistance was increased twofold (79). All of the patients in this study had evidence of cognitive impairment. The three patients studied after treatment had normal values for those measurements. These changes, coupled with the electroencephalographic disturbances noted earlier (13,18,20–22), suggest delirium as the nonspecific final common path to mental dysfunction in patients with hypothyroidism.

Currently, there is no way to measure the effects of thyroid hormone on brain metabolism, but novel brain imaging techniques for evaluating the relationship between cerebral metabolism and thyroid status are being developed. In a study of hypothyroid patients using phosphorus 31 magnetic resonance spectroscopy, frontal lobe phosphate metabolism increased during T_4 (80). Data from studies using positron emission spectroscopy also indicate a close relationship between thyroid status and cerebral blood flow and cerebral glucose metabolism in depression. Serum TSH concentrations were inversely related to both global and regional cerebral blood flow and cerebral glucose metabolism, a relationship that was most pronounced in the prefrontal cortex and independent of the severity of depression (81). More recently, positron imaging of blood flow using [18F]-fluorodeoxyglucose in patients with hypothyroidism has confirmed frontal lobe dysfunction, which improved when the patients were treated with T_4 (25,82) (Fig. 64.2).

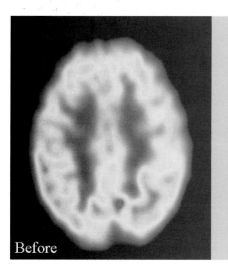
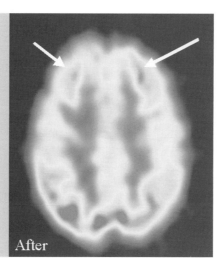

FIGURE 64.2. Positron emission tomography scans after administration of [^{18}F]-fluorodeoxyglucose in a 35-year-old woman with hypothyroidism before and after thyroxine treatment. Note increase in frontal lobe uptake of the fluorodeoxyglucose (*arrows*), indicative of increased metabolic activity, during treatment.

Both T_4 and T_3 regulate cellular function in most organs, including the brain (83). T_3 nuclear receptors are prominent in brain tissue, particularly in neurons, but they are not evenly distributed; high concentrations are found in the amygdala and hippocampus—regions of importance in the modulation of mood—and low concentrations in the brainstem and cerebellum (84). T_3 receptor complexes regulate expression of various proteins (83) and, in the brain, T_3 receptor binding is sensitive to the local thyroid hormone economy (see Chapter 8) (85).

About half of the T_3 in brain nuclei is produced within the neurons by deiodination of T_4, a reaction catalyzed by type 2 deiodinase (see Chapter 7) (85). The activity of this enzyme is increased in hypothyroidism and decreased in thyrotoxicosis. This precise autoregulatory mechanism not only underscores the importance of T_4 and its deiodination to optimal brain function, but also suggests that minor changes in local T_3 production can lead to major changes in behavior (86). Thus, in hypothyroidism, intracerebral generation of T_3 from T_4 increases as serum T_4 declines, but intracellular T_3 concentrations decline little until serum T_4 is virtually exhausted (87).

Are changes in thyroid economy in the brain important to the aberrant behavior of patients with hypothyroidism and psychiatric disease? Until brain T_4 and T_3 metabolism can be quantified *in vivo,* this question cannot be answered; however, strong clinical evidence in support of such speculation exists. This evidence includes the role of mild hypothyroidism in depressive illness and in postpartum depressive states associated with thyroiditis, the association of the rapid cycling variant of bipolar illness with hypothyroidism, the adjunctive therapeutic role of thyroid hormones in both depression and rapid cycling bipolar illness, and the profound disturbances that are found in hypothyroidism.

The depressive mood disturbances that occur in patients with hypothyroidism are of great interest to psychiatrists because they suggest the possibility of a common pathophysiology of the affective disorders and thyroid disease.

The biogenic amines, putatively disturbed in both disorders, may form a linkage (41). The interaction of thyroid state and sympathetic nervous system activity has been recognized for many years (88,89). The biochemical activity of noradrenergic neurons and thyroid function are inversely related. For example, in hypothyroid rats, norepinephrine synthesis from tyrosine in increased in the heart, spleen, and adrenal tissue, as compared with normal rats (90). Conversely, in rats given T_4 for 10 days, norepinephrine synthesis in the heart and brain is decreased by 30% and 15%, respectively (91). The activity of the enzyme dopamine β-hydroxylase also decreases in response to thyroid hormone in animals and humans (92).

This paradox, in which the biochemical activity of the adrenergic nervous system is apparently inversely related to thyroid state, whereas physiologic activity is directly related, is possibly explained by changes in adrenergic receptor function. In the heart and adipose tissue, increasing thyroid activity increases the number of β-adrenergic receptors, whereas the number of α-adrenergic receptors declines; decreasing thyroid hormone activity leads to the reverse (93). In rat brain, both the serotonergic and noradrenergic systems are responsive to changes in hypothalamic–pituitary–thyroid function (94–96). Thyroidectomy decreases ligand binding to β- and α_2-adrenergic receptors in the limbic regions of the brain, and increases ligand binding to 5-hydroxytryptamine (5-HT)$_{1A}$ receptors in the cortex and hippocampus, changes that can be reversed by the administration of T_4. In *in vivo* microdialysis studies in rats, coadministration of the tricyclic antidepressant drug clomipramine and T_3 raised 5-hydroxytryptamine concentrations in the frontal cortex more than either alone (97). Furthermore, the decrease in 5-hydroxytryptamine concentrations in the frontal cortex induced by an injection of a receptor agonist was significantly less in rats given T_3 compared with control animals (97). In challenge experiments with *d*-fenfluramine, a centrally acting 5-hydroxytryptamine agonist, T_4 increased central serotonergic activ-

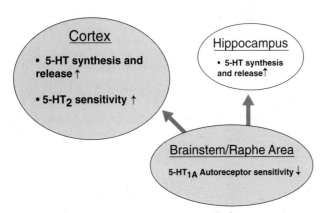

FIGURE 64.3. Increased availability of thyroid hormone decreases 5-hydroxytryptamine (5-HT)$_{1A}$ receptor sensitivity in the brainstem, thus stimulating the synthesis and release of serotonin (5-HT) in the cortex and hippocampus.

ity in hypothyroid patients (98). Thus, a careful review of the available animal and human studies suggests that T$_3$ may act presynaptically in the brainstem through the inhibition of 5-HT$_{1A}$ receptors to increase serotonergic activity in the cerebral cortex and hippocampus (95) (Fig. 64.3).

These results from animal and human studies suggest that there are neuromodulatory links among the serotonergic and adrenergic systems and thyroid state. Furthermore, thyroid hormones may also influence affective state through postreceptor mechanisms, for example, changes in guanine-nucleotide-binding (G) protein synthesis and adenylyl cyclase activity, that facilitate signal transduction (99,100). The sensitivity of Purkinje neurons in the cerebellum of hypothyroid rats to iontophoretically applied norepinephrine is decreased in association with decreased adenylyl cyclase activity and returns to normal after the administration of T$_3$ (101). Whether these changes in serotonergic and adrenergic brain mechanisms are the principal pathway mediating the melancholic symptoms that commonly occur in patients with hypothyroidism remains to be determined.

TREATMENT AND OUTCOME

The behavioral disturbances of hypothyroidism in adults respond to adequate T$_4$ replacement therapy unless there is underlying depression unrelated to the hypothyroidism, in which case cognition may improve, but the depressed mood persists (17,37). Exacerbation of the psychosis may occur soon after T$_4$ treatment is initiated (18), and thus, ideally, severely disturbed patients should be hospitalized. Therapy with a major tranquilizing drug may be necessary in a few patients, but the drug should be given with great caution and in conjunction with T$_4$ to avoid precipitating myxedema coma. Haloperidol or other dopamine-blocking agents are the preferred drugs to be used in the treatment

of the psychosis. The patients should be monitored carefully for cardiac arrhythmias, especially in those patients given a phenothiazine; there is a case report of cardiac arrest in such a situation (102).

When a patient with hypothyroidism has a strong family history of affective disorder, especially bipolar in character, the initiation of T$_4$ treatment may precipitate manic excitement (73). In such a patient, it may be necessary to add lithium or an anticonvulsant drug to the treatment regimen. Parenthetically, when a patient who is receiving lithium develops a severe depressive state, cognitive confusion, and anergy, the clinician should think of the possibility of lithium-induced hypothyroidism (see Chapter 50).

When hypothyroidism is mild and complicating a predominantly depressive syndrome, the therapeutic goal is to provide sufficient T$_4$ to reduce the serum TSH concentration to normal. However, when the melancholia persists, an antidepressant drug or even electroconvulsive therapy may be necessary.

REFERENCES

1. Gull WW. On a cretinoid state supervening in adult life in women. *Trans Clin Soc (Lond)* 1873;7:180.
2. Inglis T. Two cases of myxoedema. *Lancet* 1880;2:496.
3. Report of a committee of the Clinical Society of London. Report on myxedema. *Trans Clin Soc (Suppl) (Lond)* 1888;21:18.
4. Savage GH. Myxoedema and its nervous symptoms. *J Ment Sci* 1880;25:417
5. Asher R. Myxoedematous madness. *BMJ* 1949;2:555.
6. Granet RB, Kalman JP. Hypothyroidism and psychosis: a case illustration of the diagnostic dilemma in psychiatry. *J Clin Psychiatry* 1978;39:260.
7. McNamara ME, Southwick SM, Fogel BS. Sleep apnea and hypothyroidism presenting as depression in 2 patients. *J Clin Psychiatry* 1987;48:164.
8. Vieweg WV, Yank GR, Steckler TL, et al. Grades 1 and 2 hypothyroidism in a state mental hospital: risk factors and clinical findings. *Psych Q* 1987;58:135.
9. Levin ME, Daughaday WH. Fatal coma due to myxedema. *Am J Med* 1955;18:1017.
10. Jellinek EH. Fits, faints, coma and dementia in myxoedema. *Lancet* 1962;2:1010.
11. Shaw C. Case of myxedema with restless melancholia treated by injections of thyroid juice. *BMJ* 1892;2:451.
12. Jain V. A psychiatric study of hypothyroidism. *Psychiatr Clin* 1972;5:121.
13. Kales A, Henze G, Jacobson A, et al. All night sleep studies in hypothyroid patients before and after treatment. *J Clin Endocrinol Metab* 1967;27:1593.
14. Whybrow PC, Prange AJ, Treadway CR. Mental changes accompanying thyroid gland dysfunction. *Arch Gen Psychiatry* 1969;20:48.
15. Easson WM. Myxedema with psychosis. *Arch Gen Psychiatry* 1966;14:277.
16. Karnosh LJ, Stout RE. Psychoses of myxoedema. *Am J Psychiatry* 1934;91:1263.
17. Treadway CR, Prange AJ, Duehne EF, et al. Myxedema psychosis: clinical and biochemical changes during recovery. *J Psychiatr Res* 1967;5:289.

18. Browning TB, Atkins RW, Weiner H. Cerebral metabolic disturbances in hypothyroidism: clinical and electroencephalographic studies in the psychosis of myxoedema and hypothyroidism. *Arch Intern Med* 1954;93:938.

19. Neiman EA. The electroencephalogram in myxoedema coma: clinical and electroencephalographic study of three cases. *BMJ* 1959;1:1204.

20. Himelfarb MZ, Lakretz T, Gold S, et al. Auditory brain stem responses in thyroid dysfunction. *J Laryngol Otol* 1981; 95: 679.

21. Huang TS, Chang YC, Lee SH, et al. Evoked potential abnormalities in thyroid disorders. In: Nagataki S, Torizuka K, eds. *The thyroid*. Amsterdam: Elsevier, 1988:411.

22. Ladenson PW, Stakes JW, Ridgway EC. Reversible alteration of the visual evoked potential in hypothyroidism. *Am J Med* 1984; 77:1010.

23. Logothetis J. Psychotic behavior as the initial indicator of adult myxoedema. *J Nerv Ment Dis* 1963;36: 561.

24. Constant EL, de Volder AG, Ivanoiu A, et al. Cerebral blood flow and glucose metabolism in hypothyroidism: a positron emission tomography study. *J Clin Endocrinol Metab* 2001;86: 3864.

25. Bauer M, Whybrow PC. Thyroid hormone and mood modulation: new insights from functional brain imaging techniques. *Curr Psych Rep* 2003:5:163.

26. Bauer M, London ED, Rasgon N, et al. Supraphysiological doses of levothyroxine alter regional cerebral metabolism and improve mood in women with bipolar depression (*Mol Psychiatry* 2004; in press).

27. Osterweil D, Syndulko K, Cohen SN, et al. Cognitive function in non-demented older adults with hypothyroidism. *J Am Geriatr Soc* 1992;40:325.

28. Dugbartey AT. Neurocognitive aspects of hypothyroidism. *Arch Intern Med* 1998;158:1413.

29. Crown S. Notes on an experimental study of intellectual deterioration. *BMJ* 1949;2:684.

30. Reitan RM. Intellectual functions in myxoedema. *Arch Neurol Psychiatry* 1953;69:436.

31. Schon M, Sutherland AM, Rawson RW. Hormones and neuroses—the psychological effects of thyroid deficiency. In: *Proceedings of the Third World Congress of Psychiatry*. Vol. 2. Montreal, Canada: McGill University Press/University of Toronto Press, 1961:835.

32. Haggerty JJ Jr., Garbutt JC, Evans DL, et al. Subclinical hypothyroidism: a review of neuropsychiatric aspects. *Int J Psychiatry Med* 1990;20:193.

33. Burmeister LA, Ganguli M, Dodge HH, et al. Hypothyroidism and cognition: preliminary evidence for a specific defect in memory. *Thyroid* 2001;11:1177.

34. Bunevicius R, Kazanavicius G, Zalinkevicius R, et al. Effects of thyroxine as compared with thyroxine plus triiodothyronine in patients with hypothyroidism. *N Engl J Med* 1999; 340:424.

35. Bunevicius R, Prange AJ. Mental improvement after replacement therapy with thyroxine plus triiodothyronine: relationship to cause of hypothyroidism. *Int J Neuropsychopharmacol* 2000;3:167.

36. Walsh JP, Shiels L, Lim EM, et al. Combined thyroxine/liothyronine treatment does not improve well-being, quality of life, or cognitive function compared to thyroxine alone: a randomized controlled trial in patients with primary hypothyroidism. *J Clin Endocrinol Metab* 2003;88:4543.

37. Sawka AM, Gerstein HC, Marriott MJ, et al. Does a combination regimen of thyroxine (T$_4$) and 3,5,3'-triiodothyronine improve depressive symptoms better than T$_4$ alone in patients with hypothyroidism? Results of a double-blind, randomized, controlled trial. *J Clin Endocrinol Metab* 2003; 88:4551.

38. Mennemeier M, Garner RD, Heilman KM. Memory, mood and measurement in hypothyroidism. *J Clin Exp Neuropsychol* 1993;15:822.

39. Beck HG. The hallucinations of myxedema. *Med Times* 1926; 54:201.

40. Bauer MS, Whybrow PC. Thyroid hormones and the central nervous system in affective illness: interactions that may have clinical significance. *Integr Psychiatry* 1988;6:75.

41. Whybrow PC, Prange AJ. A hypothesis of thyroid-catecholamine-receptor interaction: its relevance to affective illness. *Arch Gen Psychiatry* 1981;38:106.

42. Whybrow PC, Coppen A, Prange AJ Jr, et al. Thyroid function and the response of L-liothyronine in depression. *Arch Gen Psychiatry* 1972;26:242.

43. Coppen A, Whybrow PC, Noguera R, et al. The comparative antidepressant value of L-tryptophan and imipramine with and without attempted potentiation by liothyronine. *Arch Gen Psychiatry* 1972;26:234.

44. Jackson IMD. The thyroid axis and depression. *Thyroid* 1998; 8:951.

45. Kirkegaard C, Faber J. The role of thyroid hormones in depression. *Eur J Endocrinol* 1998;138:1.

46. Bartalena L, Placidi GF, Martino E, et al. Nocturnal serum thyrotropin (TSH) surge and the TSH response to TSH-releasing hormone: dissociated behavior in untreated depressives. *J Clin Endocrinol Metab* 1990;71:650.

47. Gold MS, Pottash ALC, Extein I. Hypothyroidism and depression: evidence from complete thyroid function evaluation. *JAMA* 1981;245:1919.

48. Prange AJ Jr, Wilson IC, Rabon AMN, et al. Enhancement of imipramine antidepressant activity by thyroid hormone. *Am J Psychiatry* 1969;126:457.

49. Altshuler LL, Bauer M, Frye MA, et al. Does thyroid supplementation accelerate tricyclic antidepressant response? A review and meta-analysis of the literature. *Am J Psychiatry* 2001;158:1617.

50. Goodwin FK, Prange AJ Jr, Post RM, et al. Potentiation of antidepressant effects by triiodothyronine in tricyclic nonresponders. *Am J Psychiatry* 1982;139:34.

51. Joffe RT, Singer W, Levitt A, et al. A placebo-controlled comparison of lithium and triiodothyronine augmentation of tricyclic antidepressants in unipolar refractory depression. *Arch Gen Psychiatry* 1993;50:387.

52. Aronson R, Offman HJ, Joffe RT, et al. Triiodothyronine augmentation in the treatment of refractory depression. *Arch Gen Psychiatry* 1996;53:842.

53. Bauer M, Hellweg R, Gräf KJ, et al. Treatment of refractory depression with high-dose thyroxine. *Neuropsychopharmacology* 1998;18:444.

54. Jaeschke R, Guyatt G, Gerstein H, et al. Does treatment with L-thyroxine influence health status in middle-aged and older adults with subclinical hypothyroidism? *J Gen Intern Med* 1996;11:744.

55. Prinz PN, Scanlan JM, Vitaliano PP, et al. Thyroid hormones: positive relationships with cognition in healthy, euthyroid older men. *J Gerontol A Biol Sci Med Sci* 1999;54:M111.

56. Pollock MA, Sturrock A, Marshall K, et al. Thyroxine treatment in patients with symptoms of hypothyroidism but thyroid function tests within the reference range: randomised double blind placebo controlled crossover trial. BMJ 2001;323:891.

57. Kong WM, Sheikh MH, Lumb PJ, et al. A 6-month randomized trial of thyroxine treatment in women with mild subclinical hypothyroidism. *Am J Med* 2002;112:348.

58. Saravanan P, Chau WF, Roberts N, et al. Psychological well-being in patients on 'adequate' doses of L-thyroxine: results of a

large, controlled community-based questionnaire study. *Clin Endocrinol (Oxf)* 2002;57:577.

59. Harris B, Othman S, Davies JA, et al. Association between postpartum thyroid dysfunction and thyroid antibodies and depression. *BMJ* 1992;305:152.

60. Harris B, Oretti R, Lazarus J, et al. Randomised trial of thyroxine to prevent postnatal depression in thyroid-antibody-positive women. *Br J Psychiatry* 2002;180:327.

61. Bauer MS, Whybrow P. Rapid cycling bipolar disorder: clinical features, treatment and etiology. In: Amsterdam J, ed. *Refractory depression: frontiers in research and treatment.* New York: Raven, 1991:191.

62. Bauer MS, Whybrow PC, Winokur A. Rapid cycling bipolar affective disorder. I. Association with grade I hypothyroidism. *Arch Gen Psychiatry* 1990;47:427.

63. Cowdry RW, Wehr TA, Zis AP, et al. Thyroid abnormalities associated with rapid cycling bipolar illness. *Arch Gen Psychiatry* 1983;40:414.

64. Rogers M, Whybrow PC. Clinical hypothyroidism occurring during lithium treatment: two case histories and a review of thyroid function in 19 patients. *Am J Psychiatry* 1971;128:158.

65. Gyulai L, Bauer M, Bauer MS, et al. Thyroid hypofunction in patients with rapid-cycling bipolar disorder after lithium challenge. *Biol Psychiatry* 2003;53:899.

66. Bauer MS, Whybrow PC. Rapid cycling bipolar affective disorder. II. Treatment of refractory rapid cycling with high dose levothyroxine: a preliminary study. *Arch Gen Psychiatry* 1990;4:435.

67. Whybrow PC. The therapeutic use of triiodothyronine and high-dose thyroxine in psychiatric disorder. *Acta Med Aust* 1994;21:47.

68. Baumgartner A, Bauer M, Hellweg R. Treatment of intractable non-rapid cycling bipolar affective disorder with high-dose thyroxine: an open clinical trial. *Neuropsychopharmacology* 1994;10:183.

69. Bauer M, Berghöfer A, Bschor T, et al. Supraphysiological doses of L-thyroxine in the maintenance treatment of prophylaxis-resistant affective disorders. *Neuropsychopharmacology* 2002;27:620.

70. Lazarus JH. The effects of lithium therapy on thyroid and thyrotropin-releasing hormone. *Thyroid* 1998;8:909.

71. St Germain D. Regulatory effect of lithium on thyroxine metabolism in murine neural and anterior pituitary tissue. *Endocrinology* 1987;120:1430.

72. Baumgartner A, Pinna G, Hiedra L, et al. Effects of lithium and carbamazepine on thyroid hormone metabolism in rat brain. *Neuropsychopharmacology* 1997;16:25.

73. Josephson AM, McKenzie TB. Thyroid induced manias in hypothyroid patients. *Br J Psychiatry* 1980;137:222.

74. Wehr TA, Goodwin FK. Rapid cycling in manic-depressives induced by tricyclic antidepressants. *Arch Gen Psychiatry* 1979;36:555.

75. Dratman M, Crutchfield F. Thyroid hormones and adrenergic neurotransmittors. In: Usdin E, Kopin I, eds. *Catecholamines basic and clinical. Fourth International Catecholamine Symposium.* Elmsford, NY: Pergamon, 1978:1155.

76. Timiras PS. Thyroid hormones and nervous system development. *Biol Neonate* 1989;55:376.

77. Porterfield SP, Hendrich CE. The role of thyroid hormones in prenatal and neonatal neurological development—current perspectives. *Endocr Rev* 1993;14:94.

78. Berti CN, Sato C, Gomez CL, et al. Thyroid hormone effects on RNA synthesis in brain and liver of neonatal hypothyroid rats. *Horm Metab Res* 1981;13:691.

79. Scheinberg P, Stead EA Jr, Brannon ES, et al. Correlative observations on cerebral metabolism and cardiac output in myxedema. *J Clin Invest* 1950;29:1139.

80. Smith CD, Ain KB. Brain metabolism in hypothyroidism studied with ^{31}P magnetic-resonance spectroscopy. *Lancet* 1995;345:619.

81. Marangell LB, Ketter TA, George MS, et al. Inverse relationship of peripheral thyrotropin-stimulating hormone levels to brain activity in mood disorders. *Am J Psychiatry* 1997;154:224.

82. Bauer M, London ED, Silverman DH, et al. Thyroid, brain and mood modulation in affective disorder: insights from molecular research and functional brain imaging. *Pharmacopsychiatry* 2003;36(suppl 3);5215.

83. Oppenheimer JH, Schwartz HL, Mariash CN, et al. Advances in our understanding of thyroid hormone action at the cellular level. *Endocr Rev* 1987;8:288.

84. Ruel J, Faure R, Dussault JH. Regional distribution of nuclear T_3 receptors in rat brain and evidence for preferential localization in neurons. *J Endocrinol Invest* 1985;8:343.

85. Larsen PR. Thyroid hormone metabolism in the central nervous system. Proceedings of the 2nd Thyroid Symposium: Peripheral thyroid hormone metabolism, Graz, Austria. *Acta Med Aust* 1988;15:5.

86. Dratman MB, Crutchfield FL, Gordon JT, et al. Iodothyronine homeostasis in rat brain during hypo- and hyperthyroidism. *Am J Physiol* 1983;245:R185.

87. Dratman MB, Crutchfield FL. Interactions of adrenergic and thyroergic systems in the development of the low T_3 syndrome. In: Hesch R, ed. *The low T_3 syndrome.* London: Academic, 1981:115.

88. Goetsch E. New methods in the diagnosis of thyroid disorders: pathological and clinical. *NY State Med J* 1918;18:257.

89. Harrison TS. Adrenal medullary and thyroid relationships. *Physiol Rev* 1964;44:161.

90. Lipton MA, Prange AJ, Dairman W. Increased rate of norepinephrine biosynthesis in hypothyroid rats. *Fed Proc* 1968;27:399.

91. Prange AJ Jr, Meek JL, Lipton MA. Catecholamines: diminished rate of norepinephrine biosynthesis in rat brain and heart after thyroxine pretreatment. *Life Sci* 1970;9:901.

92. Stolk JM, Whybrow PC. Clinical and experimental interrelationships between sympathetic nervous activity and pituitary thyroid function. In: *Proceedings of the Academiai Kiado Symposium of the International Society of Psychoneuroendocrinology.* Budapest: Hungarian Academy of Sciences, 1976:273.

93. Scarpace P, Abrass I. Thyroid hormone regulations of rat heart, lymphocyte and lung beta-adrenergic receptors. *Endocrinology* 1981;108:1007.

94. Tejani-Butt SM, Yang J, Kaviani A. Time course of altered thyroid states on 5-HT$_{1A}$ receptors and 5-HT uptake sites in rat brain: an autoradiographic analysis. *Neuroendocrinology* 1993;57:1011.

95. Tejani-Butt SM, Yang J. A time course of altered thyroid states on the noradrenergic system in rat brain by quantitative autoradiography. *Neuroendocrinology* 1994;59:235.

96. Bauer M, Heinz A, Whybrow PC. Thyroid hormones, serotonin and mood: of synergy and significance in the adult brain. *Mol Psychiatry* 2002;7:140.

97. Gur E, Lerer B, Newman ME. Chronic clomipramine and triiodothyronine increase serotonin levels in rat frontal cortex *in vivo*: relationship to serotonin autoreceptor activity. *J Pharmacol Exp Ther* 1999;288:81.

98. Cleare AJ, McGregor A, Chambers SM, et al. Thyroxine replacement increases central 5-hydroxytryptamine activity and

reduces depressive symptoms in hypothyroidism. *Neuroendocrinology* 1996;64:65.

99. Orford M, Mazurkiewicz D, Milligan G, et al. Abundance of the α-subunits of G$_i$1, G$_i$2 and G$_0$ in synaptosomal membranes from several regions of the rat brain is increased in hypothyroidism. *Biochem J* 1991;275:183.

100. Henley WN, Koehnle TJ. Thyroid hormones and the treatment of depression: an examination of basic hormonal actions in the mature mammalian brain. *Synapse* 1997;27:36.

101. Marwaha J, Prasad KN. Hypothyroidism elicits electrophysiological noradrenergic subsensitivity in rat cerebellum. *Science* 1981;214:675.

102. Gomez ST. Hypothyroidism, psychotropic drugs and cardiotoxicity. *Br J Psychiatry* 1980;136.

65

MYXEDEMA COMA

LEONARD WARTOFSKY

Myxedema coma is severe, life-threatening hypothyroidism. It was probably first reported in 1879 by Ord from the St. Thomas Hospital, London. Two of 12 patients with fatal hypothyroidism described in a report of the Clinical Society of London in 1888 appeared to have died in coma (1). Remarkably, the next cases did not appear in the literature until 1953 (2,3), and about 200 cases have been reported subsequently. Additional references may be obtained from earlier reviews (4,5).

Most patients with myxedema coma are elderly women with long-standing hypothyroidism and who therefore usually have myxedema and other characteristic clinical manifestations of hypothyroidism. Once considered, the diagnosis should be easy to establish on the basis of both clinical and laboratory findings; despite vigorous therapy, the mortality rate may be high.

CLINICAL FEATURES: PRECIPITATING EVENTS

Myxedema coma is more likely to occur in the winter than in the summer, suggesting that low environmental temperature may somehow precipitate the syndrome, and hypothermia is a cardinal clinical finding. Other events that may trigger the onset of myxedema coma include pulmonary and other infections, cerebrovascular accidents, and congestive heart failure (Table 65.1). Pulmonary infection may occur as a secondary event because of hypoventilation due to somnolence, as can aspiration pneumonia. Similarly, it may be difficult to determine whether other abnormalities, such as hypoglycemia, hyponatremia, hypoxemia, and hypercapnia, which often are present in patients with myxedema coma, contributed to the onset of the coma or are consequences of it. In other patients, sedative, analgesic, antidepressant, hypnotic, and anesthetic drugs have been incriminated as precipitating or exacerbating myxedema coma because of their ability to depress respiration. Drug-induced myxedema coma is particularly likely to occur in hospitalized patients because these types of drugs are more likely to be dispensed there than outside of the hospital, and the patients are typically not known to have hypothyroidism.

GENERAL DESCRIPTION

Most patients with myxedema coma have had symptoms of hypothyroidism for many months, and the onset of stupor or coma is precipitated by cold exposure, infection, or other systemic disease or by drugs, as noted above. There may be a past history of antecedent thyroid disease, thyroid hormone therapy that was discontinued for no apparent reason, or radioiodine therapy. Examination of the neck may reveal a surgical scar and no palpable thyroid tissue or a goiter. Approximately 5% to 10% of patients have hypothalamic or pituitary disease as the cause of their hypothyroidism.

A survey of hospitals in Germany (1993–1995) identified 24 patients with myxedema coma, probably the largest number ever analyzed together, although the authors reclassified 12 patients as having severe hypothyroidism but not coma (6). The mean age of the 24 patients (20 women, 4 men) was 73 years. Twenty-three had primary hypothyroidism and one central hypothyroidism; nine were known to have hypothyroidism before the episode of coma. With respect to clinical findings, 80% had hypoxemia, 54% had hypercapnia, and 21 had a temperature less than 94°F. All received some thyroid hormone therapy, and six (25%) died.

The course often is one of lethargy progressing to stupor and then coma, with respiratory failure and hypothermia, all of which may be hastened by the administration of drugs that depress respiration and other central nervous system (CNS) functions. Most patients have the characteristic features of severe hypothyroidism, such as dry, coarse, and scaly skin; sparse or coarse hair; nonpitting edema (myxedema) of the periorbital regions, hands, and feet; macroglossia; hoarseness; and delayed deep-tendon reflexes. Moderate to profound hypothermia is common.

Respiratory System

Respiratory depression, common in patients with myxedema coma, is caused by decreased hypoxic respiratory drive and a decreased ventilatory response to hypercapnia (7) (see Chapter 54). The resulting alveolar hypoventilation leads to progressive hypoxemia, and ultimately to CO_2

TABLE 65.1. MYXEDEMA COMA: PRECIPITATING AND EXACERBATING FACTORS

Hypothermia
Infections
Cerebrovascular accidents
Congestive heart failure
Drugs
   Anesthetics
   Sedatives
   Tranquilizers
   Narcotics
   Amiodarone
Trauma
Gastrointestinal bleeding
Metabolic disturbances exacerbating myxedema coma
   Hypoglycemia
   Hyponatremia
   Hypoxemia
   Hypercapnia
   Acidosis
   Hypercalcemia

narcosis and coma. Impaired respiratory muscle function may exacerbate the hypoventilation (8,9). Obesity also can exacerbate hypoventilation, although its importance has been questioned (10). With respect to coma, the principal factor seems to be a depressed respiratory center response to CO_2 (11,12). Whether attributable to central respiratory depression or to respiratory muscle dysfunction, hypoventilation is sufficiently severe in most patients with myxedema coma to require mechanically assisted ventilation. Other factors that may impair respiration in severely hypothyroid patients include pleural effusions or ascites, by reducing lung volume, and macroglossia and myxedema of the nasopharynx and larynx by reducing the lumen of the airway. Recovery from respiratory failure may be slow (13) despite apparently adequate therapy.

Cardiovascular Manifestations

The findings considered typical of hypothyroid heart disease also are found in myxedema coma and include cardiac enlargement, bradycardia, decreased cardiac contractility, and nonspecific electrocardiographic abnormalities (see Chapter 53). The cardiac enlargement may be due to either ventricular dilatation or pericardial effusion. The decrease in cardiac contractility results in a low stroke volume and low cardiac output, but frank congestive heart failure is rare.

Patients with myxedema coma may have hypotension because of decreased intravascular volume, and cardiovascular collapse and shock may occur late in the course. If at all, the latter characteristically responds only when both a vasopressor drug such as dopamine and thyroid hormone are given.

Gastrointestinal Manifestations

A neurogenic oropharyngeal dysphagia has been described that is associated with delayed swallowing, aspiration, and risk of aspiration pneumonia (14). Decreased intestinal motility is common in hypothyroidism, and its most severe manifestations, paralytic ileus and megacolon, can occur in patients with myxedema coma. Thus, many patients have anorexia, nausea, abdominal pain, constipation, and a distended, quiet abdomen. Gastric atony also occurs and can be a particularly troublesome problem because it may serve to reduce absorption of oral medications.

Renal and Electrolyte Manifestations

Hyponatremia and a decreased glomerular filtration rate are rather consistent findings among patients with myxedema coma. The hyponatremia is due to the inability to excrete a water load, caused both by decreased delivery of water to the distal nephron (15) and excess vasopressin secretion (16) (see Chapter 55). Urinary sodium excretion is normal or increased, urinary osmolality is high relative to plasma osmolality, and there may be bladder atony, with urinary retention. Hyponatremia alone may cause lethargy and confusion, and it undoubtedly contributes further to these problems in patients who have them as a result of hypothyroidism.

Neuropsychiatric Manifestations

Just as is seen in other patients with hypothyroidism (see Chapter 64). Patients with myxedema coma may have a history of lethargy, slowed mentation, poor memory, cognitive dysfunction, depression, or even psychosis. They do not complain of these symptoms, however, because of their impaired state of consciousness. Up to 25% of patients with myxedema coma have focal or generalized seizures caused by CNS dysfunction per se, hyponatremia, or hypoxemia resulting from decreased cerebral blood flow (17).

Infections

The high mortality rate of myxedema coma may be due, at least in part, to infection. Complicating our ability to detect infection is the hypothermia commonly present in hypothyroidism, and even if the patient is normothermic, the temperature may not be increased much by an infection. Thus, infection may be difficult to recognize or even overlooked entirely and antibiotic treatment consequently delayed or not given at all. Similarly, the patients often perspire little, and their pulse rate tends to be slow, both of which may result in the likelihood that the physician will overlook the possibility of an acute infection. Pulmonary infections may aggravate or even cause hypoventilation, and susceptibility to these infections may be increased because of aspiration caused by neurogenic dysphagia, semicoma, or seizures (14,17).

These considerations led to the suggestion that all patients with myxedema coma be given antibiotic therapy (18). A more prudent approach is to search vigorously for infection but to initiate antibiotic therapy only when some evidence of infection is present.

Hypothermia

Hypothermia is present in about three fourths of patients. It may be dramatic (<80°F), and it may be the first clinical clue to the diagnosis of myxedema coma. Conversely, the diagnosis should be considered seriously in any unconscious patient with an infection who does not have fever. There is a correlation of survival with presenting body temperature, with patients having core temperatures below 90°F having the poorest prognosis. Hypoglycemia may decrease body temperature further. It is fortunate that old-style mercury thermometers are rarely used today because the degree of hypothermia may be underestimated if the mercury column has not been lowered to well below normal before the patient's temperature is measured. Moreover, these thermometers do not record below 94°F, and therefore the degree of hypothermia may be underestimated. Electronic thermometers record temperature over a much wider range.

DIAGNOSIS

The presence of marked stupor, confusion, or coma in a patient with a history and physical findings of hypothyroidism, especially if the patient has hypothermia, should suggest the diagnosis of myxedema coma. Treatment should be initiated immediately, without awaiting the results of measurements of serum thyrotropin (TSH) and thyroxine (T_4). Marked fatigue and somnolence often occur in patients with severe hypothyroidism, and a clear distinction between them and coma may be neither practical nor sensible. Because of the risks for high-dose thyroid hormone therapy in elderly patients, therapy should not be undertaken lightly. Therefore, in a lethargic or somnolent but not comatose patient, the presence of abnormalities often present in myxedema coma, such as hypothermia, hypoventilation, and hyponatremia, should be used to determine whether or not to initiate high-dose thyroid hormone therapy.

As mentioned, the typical patient is an older woman who is brought to the hospital during the winter in a severely obtunded state, if not comatose. If a history can be elicited, there often is a history of thyroid disease. Physical examination may reveal bradycardia and the skin and other abnormalities described earlier, in addition to hypoventilation and hypothermia. Routine laboratory evaluation may reveal ane-

mia, hyponatremia, hypercholesterolemia, and high serum lactate dehydrogenase and creatine kinase concentrations.

In many patients, the clinical features may be sufficiently clear to make measurements of serum TSH and T_4 necessary only for confirmation of the diagnosis. Nonetheless, in many hospitals, both can be measured in several hours on an emergency basis. Although a high serum TSH concentration is the most important laboratory evidence of the diagnosis, severe systemic illness can lower TSH secretion in hypothyroid patients, and therefore the values may not be notably high (19,20). Also, as noted, a few patients with myxedema coma have central hypothyroidism, with normal or low serum TSH concentrations (see Chapter 51). Nearly all patients with myxedema coma have very low serum total and free T_4 and triiodothyronine (T_3) concentrations, and associated nonthyroidal illness will contribute to the observed reduction in serum T_3 concentration.

TREATMENT

In view of the high mortality rate among patients with myxedema coma, treatment should be instituted promptly as soon as the diagnosis is strongly suspected. Treatment with thyroid hormone alone without addressing all of the physiologic and metabolic derangements described herein is inadequate therapy, and will likely contribute to a poor prognosis. All patients should be admitted to an intensive care unit so that their pulmonary and cardiac status can be monitored continuously. A central venous pressure line should be used to monitor volume repletion therapy, and placement of a Swan-Ganz catheter is justifiable in patients with cardiac disease.

Ventilatory Support

Hypoventilation is an important component of myxedema coma and is a common cause of death in these patients. Evaluation of respiratory function should include assessment of not only pulmonary function (blood gas measurements), but also the possibility of pulmonary infection and airway obstruction by macroglossia or myxedema of the larynx. Thus, in addition to ventilatory support to relieve or prevent hypoxemia and hypercapnia, antibiotic therapy and steps to maintain an open upper airway may be indicated. Most patients require mechanical ventilatory support for 24 to 48 hours, especially those in whom the hypoventilation was caused by drug-related respiratory depression, and some may require it for several weeks (13).

During the period of ventilatory support, arterial blood gases should be measured frequently, and it may be necessary to insert an endotracheal tube or even perform tracheostomy to ensure adequate oxygenation. The tube should not be removed until the patient is fully conscious and there is evidence that the removal will be successful. Very rarely, a patient with myxedema coma may require emergency surgery and management of these patients should adhere to the same general principles (21).

Hyponatremia

Hyponatremia undoubtedly contributes to the mental status changes in patients with myxedema coma, especially in patients with serum sodium concentrations of less than 120 mEq/L. Therefore, although comatose patients must be given some saline (and glucose) intravenously to replace daily losses, the volume should be limited in those with mild to moderate hyponatremia (serum sodium concentrations of 120–130 mEq/L) such that all water lost is not replaced. In patients with serum sodium concentrations of less than 120 mEq/L, it may be appropriate to administer a small amount of hypertonic saline (50–100 mL of 3% sodium chloride), followed by an intravenous bolus dose of 40 to 120 mg of furosemide to promote a water diuresis (22).

Hypothermia

Thyroid hormone must be given to restore body temperature to normal, but its action is slow. Therefore, warming of patients with hypothermia and maintaining normal temperature in the others with an electric blanket is advisable, but should be done cautiously so as not to cause vasodilatation with a decrease in peripheral vascular resistance and hypotension.

Hypotension

Hypotension should be corrected by judicious administration of intravenous fluid, initially 5% to 10% glucose in half-normal sodium chloride or as isotonic sodium chloride if hyponatremia is present. Administration of hydrocortisone (100 mg intravenously every 8 hours) is indicated if there is any suspicion of adrenal insufficiency. Rare patients may require vasopressor drug therapy to maintain a blood pressure sufficient to sustain adequate perfusion until thyroid hormone action begins. Although an adverse interaction between administered vasopressor drug and thyroid hormone is possible, this risk is counterbalanced by the high mortality rate among patients with myxedema coma who have hypotension unresponsive to initial fluid therapy.

Glucocorticoid Therapy

The few patients with myxedema coma who have central hypothyroidism are likely to have corticotropin (ACTH) deficiency as well as TSH deficiency. Some patients with primary hypothyroidism also have primary adrenal insufficiency (Schmidt's syndrome) (see Chapter 59). The coexis-

tence of adrenal insufficiency in patients with myxedema coma may be suggested by the presence of hypotension, hypoglycemia, hyponatremia, hyperkalemia, and azotemia; however, most patients with myxedema coma have normal serum cortisol concentrations, although their ACTH and cortisol responses to stress may be slightly impaired.

It is prudent to administer hydrocortisone or another glucocorticoid to patients with myxedema coma based on the occasional presence of definite adrenal insufficiency, the possibility of impaired ACTH and cortisol responses to stress, and the possibility that thyroid hormone therapy may increase cortisol clearance. Moreover, short-term glucocorticoid therapy is safe and can be discontinued when the patient has improved and pituitary–adrenal function has been assessed to be adequate. Hydrocortisone usually is given intravenously in a dosage of 50 to 100 mg every 6 to 8 hours for several days, after which it is tapered and discontinued on the basis of clinical response and plans for further diagnostic evaluation.

Thyroid Hormone Therapy

The most controversial aspect of the treatment of patients with myxedema coma concerns what may be the most appropriate method for restoring to normal the low serum and tissue thyroid hormone concentrations. The main controversy concerns whether to administer T_4 alone, with conversion to T_3 being dependent on the deiodinase activity in the patient, or to directly administer T_3 itself. Secondary concerns include dose, frequency, and route of administration (of either hormone). Different approaches to treatment are based on balancing concerns for the high mortality of untreated myxedema coma and the obvious need for attaining effective thyroid hormone concentrations in different tissues fairly rapidly, against the risks of high-dose thyroid hormone therapy, which may include atrial tachyarrhythmias or myocardial infarction. Because of the rarity of myxedema coma and the paucity of studies of the effects of treatment, the optimal therapy remains uncertain and several different approaches have been used.

Advocates of administering T_4 alone point out that it provides a steady and smooth, but rather slow, onset of action with low risk for adverse effects. Conversely, the onset of action of T_3 is quicker, and its serum (and probably tissue) concentrations fluctuate more between doses. Another argument for using T_4 is because it is somewhat easier to measure than is serum T_3, and the results are easier to interpret because the values vary less between doses. In either case, serum TSH values should provide information about the impact of treatment at the tissue level, with the caveat that the sick patient may exhibit TSH suppression as part of the nonthyroidal illness syndrome.

Although T_4 (or T_3) tablets can be given by nasogastric tube, administration by this route has the risks for aspiration and uncertain absorption, particularly in patients with gastric atony. Preparations of T_4 for parenteral administration are available in vials containing 100 and 500 µg. A high dose, given as a single intravenous bolus dose, was popularized by a report suggesting that replacement of the entire extrathyroidal pool of T_4 (usually 300–600 µg) was desirable to restore near-normal hormonal status as rapidly as possible, with the pool then maintained by administration of 50 to 100 µg daily given either intravenously or orally (23). With this regimen, serum T_4 concentrations increase abruptly to supranormal values and decrease to within normal range in 24 hours as the administered T_4 is distributed throughout the extracellular and then intracellular spaces, serum T_3 concentrations increase slightly, and serum TSH concentrations decrease substantially (24). Although the importance of extrathyroidal T_4 conversion to T_3 was not known when this regimen was proposed, the approach proved effective. The 24 patients with myxedema coma or severe hypothyroidism reported from Germany (described earlier) were treated initially with T_4, in doses ranging from 25 to 500 µg, with six deaths (6).

The important potential drawback to total reliance on generation of T_3 from T_4 is that the rate of extrathyroidal conversion of T_4 to T_3 is reduced in patients with virtually all illnesses, including hypothyroidism (20) (see section on nonthyroidal illness in Chapter 11D). Furthermore, the onset of action of T_3 is considerably more rapid than is that of T_4, which some argue may be crucial to increasing survival (22), and in baboons it crosses the blood–brain barrier more readily than does T_4 (25).

For intravenous administration, T_3 is available in vials containing 10 µg. When given alone, the usual dose is 10 to 20 µg followed by 10 µg every 4 hours for the first 24 hours, then 10 µg every 6 hours for a day or two, after which oral administration should be feasible. Increases in body temperature and oxygen consumption may occur 2 to 3 hours after intravenous administration of T_3, compared with 8 to 14 hours after intravenous administration of T_4. Significant clinical improvement may be seen within 24 hours with T_3 (26), but the more rapid action of T_3 may be associated with a higher risk of adverse cardiovascular actions, and in one report high serum T_3 concentrations during treatment with T_4 alone were associated with fatal outcome in several patients (27). In another series of eight patients, two of three patients treated with high-dose T_4 died, whereas the other five who were treated with smaller doses of T_4 or T_4 survived (28). These researchers reviewed 82 cases from the literature and found that advanced age, high-dose T_4 therapy, and cardiac complications were associated with mortality. They concluded that a 500 µg dose of T_4 should be safe in younger patients, but lower doses are safer in the elderly.

Consequently, our approach to therapy is to administer both T_4 and T_3. The T_4 is given intravenously in a dose of 4 µg/kg lean body weight (or about 200–250 µg), followed by 100 µg 24 hours later and then 50 µg daily, either intra-

venously or orally, as appropriate. The dose subsequently is adjusted on the basis of clinical and laboratory results, as in any other hypothyroid patient. With respect to T_3, the initial intravenous dose is 10 µg, and the same dose is given every 8 to 12 hours until the patient can take maintenance oral doses of T_4.

No general guide to treatment can take into account all the factors that might affect sensitivity to thyroid hormone, such as age, intrinsic cardiovascular function, and neuropsychiatric status. Hence, patients should be monitored closely before each dose of thyroid hormone is administered. In addition to the specific treatments considered above, attention should be given to any comorbid conditions, recognizing that drug dosages may need to be modified because hypothyroidism can result in altered drug distribution and metabolism.

With aggressive comprehensive treatment, most patients with myxedema coma should recover. Better, however, that it be prevented, by recognition of hypothyroidism earlier and by ensuring that patients with hypothyroidism do not discontinue therapy because they feel well.

REFERENCES

1. Report of a committee of the Clinical Society of London to investigate the subject of myxedema. *Trans Clin Soc (Lond) (Suppl)* 1888:21.
2. LeMarquand HS, Hausmann W, Hemstead EH. Myxedema as a cause of death. *BMJ* 1953;1:704.
3. Summers VK. Myxedema coma. *BMJ* 1953;2:336.
4. Ringel MD. Management of hypothyroidism and hyperthyroidism in the intensive care unit. *Crit Care Clin* 2001;17:59–74.
5. Nicoloff JT, LoPresti JS. Myxedema coma: a form of decompensated hypothyroidism. *Endocrinol Metab Clin North Am* 1993; 22:279.
6. Reinhardt W, Mann K. Incidence, clinical picture, and treatment of hypothyroid coma: results of a survey. *Med Klin* 1997; 92:521.
7. Zwillich CW, Pierson DJ, Hofeldt FD, et al. Ventilatory control in myxedema and hypothyroidism. *N Engl J Med* 1975;292:662.
8. Martinez FJ, Bermudez-Gomez M, Celli BR. Hypothyroidism: a reversible cause of diaphragmatic dysfunction. *Chest* 1989;96:1059.
9. Wilson WR, Bedell GM. The pulmonary abnormalities in myxedema. *J Clin Invest* 1960;39:42.
10. Massumi RA, Winnacker JL. Severe depression of the respiratory center in myxedema. *Am J Med* 1964;36:876.
11. Ladenson PW, Goldenheim PD, Ridgway EC. Prediction of reversal of blunted respiratory responsiveness in patients with hypothyroidism. *Am J Med* 1988;84:877.
12. Domm BB, Vassallo CL. Myxedema coma with respiratory failure. *Am Rev Respir Dis* 1973;107:842.
13. Yamamoto T. Delayed respiratory failure during the treatment of myxedema coma. *Endocrinol Jpn* 1984;31:769.
14. Urquhart AD, Rea IM, Lawson LT, Skipper M. A new complication of hypothyroid coma: neurogenic dysphagia: presentation, diagnosis, and treatment. *Thyroid* 2001;11:595–598.

15. DeRubertis FR Jr, Michelis MF, Bloom MG, et al. Impaired water excretion in myxedema. *Am J Med* 1971;51:41.

16. Skowsky RW, Kikuchi TA. The role of vasopressin in the impaired water excretion of myxedema. *Am J Med* 1978;64:613.

17. Sanders V. Neurologic manifestations of myxedema. *N Engl J Med* 1962;266:547.

18. Lindberger K. Myxoedema coma. *Acta Med Scand* 1975;198:87.

19. Hooper MJ. Diminished TSH secretion during acute non-thyroidal illness in untreated primary hypothyroidism. *Lancet* 1976;1:48.

20. Wartofsky L, Burman KD. Alterations in thyroid function in patients with systemic illness: the euthyroid sick syndrome. *Endocr Rev* 1982;3:164.

21. Mathes DD Treatment of myxedema coma for emergency surgery. *Anesth Analg* 1997;85:30–36, and 1998;86:450–451.

22. Pereira VG, Haron ES, Lima-Neto N, et al. Management of myxedema coma: report on three successfully treated cases with nasogastric or intravenous administration of triiodothyronine. *J Endocrinol Invest* 1982;5:331.

23. Holvey DN, Goodner CJ, Nicoloff JT, et al. Treatment of myxedema coma with intravenous thyroxine. *Arch Intern Med* 1964; 113:89.

24. Ridgway EC, McCammon JA, Benotti J, et al. Metabolic responses of patients with myxedema to large doses of intravenous L-thyroxine. *Ann Intern Med* 1972;77:549.

25. Chernow B, Burman KD, Johnson DL, et al. T_3 may be a better agent than T_4 in the critically ill hypothyroid patient: evaluation of transport across the blood–brain barrier in a primate model. *Crit Care Med* 1983;11:99.

26. MacKerrow SD, Osborn LA, Levy H, Eaton RP, Economou P. Myxedema-associated cardiogenic shock treated with intravenous triiodothyronine. *Ann Int Med* 1992;117:1014–1015.

27. Hylander B, Rosenqvist U. Treatment of myxoedema coma: factors associated with fatal outcome. *Acta Endocrinol* 1985; 108: 65.

28. Yamamoto T, Fukuyama J, Fujiyoshi A. Factors associated with mortality of myxedema coma: report of eight cases and literature survey. *Thyroid* 1999;9:1167–1174.

MANAGEMENT OF HYPOTHYROIDISM

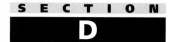

66

DIAGNOSIS OF HYPOTHYROIDISM

PAUL W. LADENSON

Since the syndrome of myxedema was described more than a century ago, criteria for the diagnosis of hypothyroidism have evolved from clinical observation to bioassays, increasingly specific measurements of thyroid hormones in serum, and quantitation of endogenous thyrotropin (thyroid-stimulating hormone, TSH) production. Accurate diagnosis of hypothyroidism requires awareness of the clinical features that define a patient's risk for thyroid hormone deficiency and proper use of the two tests usually required to confirm the disorder: serum TSH and free thyroxine (T_4) assays. These sensitive and specific measures of thyroid function have largely resolved the inaccuracy associated with the clinical diagnosis of hypothyroidism. However, they also have introduced new diagnostic challenges. First, we now appreciate that there are many patients with few clinical manifestations of hypothyroidism and mild thyroid hormone deficiency that is revealed only by serum TSH measurements—a disorder defined as mild or subclinical hypothyroidism (1). Second, thyroid test abnormalities are common in patients with nonthyroidal illness (2). Consequently, clinicians must still integrate clinical observations with laboratory test results to properly diagnose and manage patients with hypothyroidism.

CLINICAL DIAGNOSIS

Three types of clinical evidence suggest hypothyroidism: symptoms and signs consistent with thyroid hormone defi-

ciency; evidence of disease, previous treatment, or exposure known to cause thyroid or pituitary failure; and the presence of disorders associated with increased risk of chronic autoimmune thyroiditis.

CLINICAL MANIFESTATIONS

Thyroid hormone deficiency may present as an obvious clinical syndrome (e.g., cretinism or myxedema). Clinical manifestations are also often present in patients with mild to moderate hypothyroidism. In one large population survey, individuals with a greater number of typical symptoms, particularly if they were new complaints, were more likely to have thyroid function test results that confirm the diagnosis (3). However, symptoms were present in only 30% of biochemically hypothyroid patients, whereas 17% of euthyroid people had the same complaints. As a result, the positive predictive value of individual symptoms was only 8% to 12%. Consequently, although symptom scoring scales with significant predictive power have been described (4), they remain too insensitive and nonspecific for definitive diagnosis (5).

Even in patients with overt biochemical hypothyroidism, symptoms and signs may be minimal or absent (5a). Several factors account for the subtlety with which hypothyroidism can present: its insidious onset, the presence of mild thyroid hormone deficiency, and the passivity that accompanies hypothyroidism in many patients. Furthermore, many of the symptoms of hypothyroidism are nonspecific (e.g., fatigue and constipation), as are several of the physical findings (e.g., dry skin and weight gain). Among patients with symptoms potentially attributable to hypothyroidism in a primary care setting, the diagnosis is established in only 1% to 4% (6,7). Moreover, hypothyroidism can have age- and sex-specific presentations (e.g., impaired growth in children, menorrhagia in menstruating women, and dementia in the elderly).

Predisposition to Hypothyroidism

Hypothyroidism should be suspected when there is evidence of an underlying thyroid, pituitary, or hypothalamic disorder known to cause thyroid failure, or when some previous treatment has destroyed thyroid, pituitary, or hypothalamic tissue. For example, the presence of a diffuse goiter, a common manifestation of chronic autoimmune thyroiditis, should prompt laboratory evaluation for hypothyroidism (see Chapter 47). A history of previous thyroid surgery or radioactive iodine therapy likewise suggests possible primary hypothyroidism, which can occur both soon or many years after either treatment. This is particularly true in patients with Graves' disease, which may eventually cause hypothyroidism even without destructive therapy (8). Neck surgery and external radiation therapy for lymphoma (9) and head and neck cancer (10) also frequently cause hypothyroidism (see Chapter 50).

Clinical evidence of hypothalamic or pituitary disease should raise suspicion of central hypothyroidism, also known as secondary or hypothyrotropic hypothyroidism (see Chapter 51) (7). Hypothalamic disorders that can cause thyrotropin-releasing hormone (TRH) deficiency include tumors and granulomatous diseases. The pituitary's thyrotropic cells can be affected by endocrine and other tumors, treatment for them, inflammation, or hemorrhage. Therefore, other evidence of hypopituitarism, such as growth failure, hypogonadism, adrenal insufficiency, or diabetes insipidus; an expanding sellar mass lesion (e.g., headache, bitemporal hemianopsia); or a pituitary tumor secreting hormones other than TSH should prompt evaluation for hypothyroidism.

Risk factors for hypothyroidism include a variety of drugs, of which lithium carbonate and amiodarone are the most commonly used (11) (see Chapter 11C). Iodine in pharmacologic quantities, such as occurs with amiodarone therapy (12), can cause hypothyroidism in patients with underlying thyroid disease by interfering with thyroid hormone synthesis and release (see Chapter 11F). Phenytoin, carbamazepine, and rifampin, which increase the clearance of T_4, can cause hypothyroidism in patients with limited thyroid reserve (13) (see Chapter 11C). Patients with mycosis fungoides who are treated with the selective retinoid-X receptor ligand bexarotene can develop central hypothyroidism due to the drug's suppression of TSH production (13a).

Chronic Autoimmune Thyroiditis and Hypothyroidism

The patient's personal and family histories and presence of a goiter on physical examination may provide clues to the presence of chronic autoimmune thyroiditis and therefore the presence of hypothyroidism. Treatment with interferon-α has been associated with a high incidence of autoimmune thyroiditis and hypothyroidism that can be reversible after use of the agent is discontinued (14). Because of the genetic predisposition to chronic autoimmune thyroiditis, patients with affected family members are at increased risk for having hypothyroidism. Certain other endocrine deficiencies believed to have an autoimmune pathogenesis also are associated with chronic autoimmune thyroiditis, including idiopathic adrenal insufficiency, autoimmune diabetes mellitus, hypoparathyroidism, and primary ovarian failure. Patients with several other autoimmune disorders, including vitiligo, atrophic gastritis, pernicious anemia, systemic sclerosis, and Sjögren's syndrome, are also at increased risk of autoimmune thyroiditis.

LABORATORY TESTING

Several laboratory test abnormalities may suggest hypothyroidism but are not specific tests for it. They include hypercholesterolemia, hyperprolactinemia, anemia, hyponatremia, hyperhomocysteinemia, and elevated levels of the skeletal muscle–associated isoenzymes creatine phosphokinase and lactic dehydrogenase. Other abnormalities that may indicate the presence of hypothyroidism are x-ray or echocardiographic evidence of pericardial effusion or impaired myocardial contractility. Diffuse flat T waves and low voltage are also present in patients with more overt hypothyroidism.

Failure of thyroid hormone production causes a decline in serum (and plasma) T_4 concentrations. Serum triiodothyronine (T_3) concentrations also decline, but not until hypothyroidism is severe. Most patients with overt hypothyroidism have primary thyroid disease, which results in low serum T_4 and high serum TSH concentrations. In contrast, the infrequent patients with central hypothyroidism most often have low serum T_4 concentrations and low or normal serum TSH concentrations. It is important to remember, however, that even these serum thyroid function test findings are not entirely specific for hypothyroidism. Abnormal serum thyroid hormone–binding protein concentrations may mask or falsely suggest hypothyroidism (see next section). Serum TSH concentrations may be elevated despite normal serum T_4 concentrations when hypothyroidism is mild (subclinical hypothyroidism). Furthermore, some patients with central hypothyroidism actually have slightly elevated serum TSH concentrations due to secretion of TSH that is immunoreactive but bioinactive (15).

Serum Thyroxine Determinations

The serum total T_4 concentration can be measured accurately by competitive protein-binding assays that use either anti-T_4 antibodies or serum thyroid hormone–binding proteins (see Chapter 13). Because most (99.97%) of the T_4 in serum is bound to thyroxine-binding globulin (TBG), transthyretin (TTR, or thyroxine-binding prealbumin), and albumin, low concentrations of one or more of these serum proteins and drug-induced inhibition of T_4 binding to them result in low serum total T_4 concentrations (hypothyroxinemia) that can be misconstrued as indicating hypothyroidism (Table 66.1). Conversely, increased serum protein binding of T_4 may mask hypothyroidism.

Measurement of serum free T_4 resolves most of these problems. Although equilibrium dialysis and ultrafiltration are the most accurate methods for determining serum free T_4, serum free T_4 radioimmunoassays and the serum free T_4 index are adequate for this purpose in most circumstances, and they are simpler, quicker, and less costly. Almost all serum free T_4 assays have excellent sensitivity for detection of hypothyroidism in symptomatic patients. The serum free T_4 index is the product of the serum total T_4 and the thyroid hormone–binding ratio (THBR, also known as the T_3 uptake or T_4 uptake) (16) (see Chapter 13). Serum free T_4 assay techniques usually yield comparable values. The THBR value, however, can sometimes provide additional useful information in patients with nonthyroidal illness, in whom the values are often normal or high despite low calculated serum free T_4 index values and free

T_4 concentrations; in contrast, THBR values are low in most patients with hypothyroidism (17).

The principal shortcoming of serum T_4 determinations is the prevalence of low values in hospitalized patients with nonthyroidal illness. For example, in one study about 20% of patients admitted to an inpatient medical service had low serum total T_4 concentrations, and 12% of these patients had low free T_4 index values (18).

Serum TSH Determinations

Assay of serum TSH is an exquisitely sensitive test for identifying patients with any degree of primary hypothyroidism. As thyroid hormone production decreases in patients with any form of thyroid injury, serum TSH increases. The decrease in thyroid secretion may be small and not sufficient to reduce the serum total or free T_4 concentration to below the reference range. Because an elevated serum TSH concentration identifies primary hypothyroidism, the analytic sensitivity of the TSH assay (i.e., the least detectable TSH concentration) is not critical in using this test to study patients suspected of having hypothyroidism.

The combination of an elevated serum TSH with a normal free T_4 value defines the syndrome of mild or subclinical hypothyroidism. Several small studies have shown that some of these patients have symptoms (19,20) or hypercholesterolemia (1,21) that respond specifically to T_4 therapy. Furthermore, patients with an isolated elevation of the serum TSH concentration are at increased risk for progression to hypothyroidism (22), particularly if they also have circulating antithyroid antibodies indicative of autoimmune thyroiditis (see Chapter 47) (23,24).

Serum TSH measurements alone do not identify all patients with hypothyroidism. Some patients with central hypothyroidism have normal serum TSH concentrations, although in others they are low or even modestly elevated. Furthermore, serum TSH concentrations may be high in conjunction with high total and free serum T_4 concentrations in patients with two unusual conditions: generalized thyroid hormone resistance and TSH-induced thyrotoxicosis, which can, in turn, be caused by TSH-secreting pituitary adenomas or by isolated pituitary resistance to thyroid hormone (25,26). However, in T_4-treated hypothyroid patients, this combination of results is most often due to erratic ingestion of T_4 medication (27). Serum TSH concentrations may also be transiently elevated during recovery from nonthyroidal illness (28) and painful subacute and postpartum lymphocytic thyroiditis (see Chapter 11D).

Serum TSH concentrations are often low in patients with nonthyroidal illness (29), but suppression of TSH secretion is seldom, if ever, great enough to mask primary hypothyroidism. The exception to this rule may be the hypothyroid patient who has a severe nonthyroidal illness and

TABLE 66.1. ABNORMALITIES IN SERUM THYROID HORMONE BINDING THAT CAN MIMIC OR MASK HYPOTHYROIDISM

Mimicking conditions—hypothyroxinemia
  Decreased serum TBG concentration
    Inherited
    Drugs: androgens, glucocorticoids
    Nephrotic syndrome
    Severe liver dysfunction
  Competitive inhibition of T_4 binding
    Drugs: salicylate, furosemide
    Nonthyroidal illnesses
Masking conditions
  Increased serum TBG concentration
    Inherited
    Estrogen: pregnancy, exogenous, tumoral production
    Hepatitis, hepatoma
    HIV infection
    Drugs: methadone, heroin, clofibrate, 5-fluorouracil
  Familial dysalbuminemic hyperthyroxinemia
  Increased transthyretin binding
    Inherited
    Pancreatic and hepatic tumors

HIV, human immunodeficiency virus; TBG, thyroxine-binding globulin; T_4, thyroxine.

who is receiving dopamine or glucocorticoid therapy, each of which inhibit TSH secretion. Differentiating the hypothyroxinemia of nonthyroidal illness from central hypothyroidism can often be accomplished by serial testing of thyroid function. It also requires careful consideration of clinical and laboratory clues suggesting hypothalamic or pituitary disease (e.g., atrophic testes in men, a low serum cortisol concentration or lack of an elevated serum follicle-stimulating hormone concentration in postmenopausal women). In some patients, cranial imaging is required to exclude disorders causing central hypothyroidism.

Other Measures of Thyroid Hormone Action

A variety of physiologic measures and serum constituents have been used to quantify thyroid hormone action in peripheral tissues, among them determinations of serum cholesterol, ankle reflex relaxation time, and myocardial contractility. The accuracy of these tests has been evaluated in management of central hypothyroidism (30), for which they would theoretically be particularly useful in the absence of reliable TSH guidance. However, none of these peripheral tissue response parameters is sufficiently sensitive or specific for hypothyroidism to be useful clinically. Similarly, measurement of basal body temperature is a very poor diagnostic test for hypothyroidism.

SCREENING, CASE FINDING, AND DIAGNOSIS

It is important to distinguish between case finding and screening for hypothyroidism. Case finding refers to laboratory testing of individual patients or well-defined populations (e.g., those previously treated with radioiodine), whereas screening implies wide-scale testing of large populations, either indiscriminately or based on broad demographic criteria (e.g., older women). Two strategies may be used in case finding or screening: measurement of serum TSH or free T_4. The choice should be based on the pretest probability of hypothyroidism, the potential for confounding influences in assay interpretation, and cost. With respect to case finding, patients can be categorized as having low, moderate, or high risk for hypothyroidism based on published studies of patients with different conditions (Table 66.2). In patients with a low risk for hypothyroidism, a single test should be used. The serum TSH is preferable when detection of subclinical hypothyroidism is important, when coexisting nonthyroidal illness may cause hypothyroxinemia, or when both hypothyroidism and thyrotoxicosis must be excluded. The serum free T_4 index or free T_4 should be used when central hypothyroidism is a

TABLE 66.2. SCREENING AND CASE FINDING FOR HYPOTHYROIDISM IN VARIOUS PATIENTS AND CONDITIONS

Patients or conditions with low risk (prevalence < 2%)
　Adults and children at routine visits
　Dementia
　Psychiatric patients
　Elderly patients
　Hypercholesterolemia
　Sleep apnea
Patients or conditions with moderate risk (prevalence 3%–10%)
　Goiter or thyroid nodular disease
　Lithium carbonate therapy
　Associated autoimmune diseases, such as pernicious anemia
　Graves' ophthalmopathy
　Postpartum women
Patients or conditions with high risk (prevalence > 10%)
　Chronic autoimmune thyroiditis
　Previous treatment for thyrotoxicosis
　Previous high-dose neck radiation therapy
　Suspected hypopituitarism
　Amiodarone therapy

possibility. If either test result is abnormal, the other measurement should be done before any intervention is undertaken. In patients at moderate or high risk for hypothyroidism or those who have symptoms or signs of hypothyroidism in the absence of any of the risk factors listed in Table 66.2, serum TSH and free T_4 or free T_4 index should both be measured (Fig. 66.1). A high serum TSH value and a low serum free T_4 value nearly always confirm the diagnosis of primary hypothyroidism; the rare exception is a patient who has central hypothyroidism and is producing bioinactive TSH. A high serum TSH value—albeit usually less than 25 mU/L—and a normal serum free T_4 value are diagnostic of mild or subclinical hypothyroidism. If the serum TSH is low or normal and the serum free T_4 is low, the diagnosis is central hypothyroidism, nonthyroidal illness, or the thyroxine-lowering effect of certain drugs, such as phenytoin. The distinction between these two possibili-

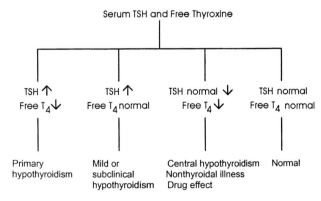

FIGURE 66.1. Laboratory assessment of hypothyroidism.

ties must be based on the context in which the patient is encountered, the presence of other manifestations of hypothalamic or pituitary disease, and the results of follow-up determinations.

With regard to population screening for hypothyroidism, or thyroid dysfunction in general, the recommendations of professional societies and expert consensus panels differ widely (Table 66.3). One society recommends TSH screening of all adults over 35 years (31), whereas another supports screening only for women over 50 years of age (32). Some panels restrict their recommendations for thyroid function screening to women before or during early pregnancy (33,34). Others advise against laboratory screening for adults under 60 years of age (35), or find insufficient evidence to support population screening for thyroid dysfunction at all (36,37). A decision and cost-effectiveness model of every-5-year TSH screening for women and men beginning at age 35 estimated the cost of this intervention to be $9,200 and $22,300 per quality-adjusted life-year in women and men, respectively (38). These amounts are considerably less than those widely considered reasonable for detection of other conditions, such as hypertension, hypercholesterolemia, and breast cancer, in asymptomatic adult populations.

It is important for health professionals and payers responsible for developing policies related to thyroid screening procedures to appreciate two things. First, their protocols should not interfere with the ability of practitioners to pursue appropriate case finding for hypothyroidism in individual patients or populations at high risk. Second, the recommendations of professional societies differ widely, and those guidelines that do not currently support screening do

so because of a lack of evidence, not because studies have shown that the practice is futile or harmful. Decision makers should pay attention to new data addressing this issue, particularly concerns regarding undiagnosed hypothyroidism in women who are or plan to become pregnant.

DIAGNOSIS OF DIFFERENT CAUSES OF HYPOTHYROIDISM

Although clinical findings suggest the cause of hypothyroidism in most patients, it is crucial that these be supported by the serum TSH to exclude those with central hypothyroidism. These latter patients may be endangered by the failure to recognize and treat other consequences of hypopituitarism, particularly adrenal insufficiency and pituitary mass lesions.

Antithyroid thyroid peroxidase (anti-TPO or antimicrosomal) or antithyroglobulin antibodies are present in more than 90% of patients with chronic autoimmune thyroiditis. Although detection of these antibodies indicates that this disorder is the probable cause of primary hypothyroidism, the practical value of these assays is greater in other settings, for example, in predicting the likelihood of progression of mild thyroid failure (22–24), increasing suspicion of underlying thyroid disease in hypothyroxinemic patients with nonthyroidal illness, and predicting postpartum thyroiditis (39).

Several tests have little or no value in diagnosing or defining the cause of hypothyroidism, or are outmoded. Serum T_3 measurements are insensitive because the values

TABLE 66.3. RECOMMENDATIONS REGARDING LABORATORY SCREENING FOR HYPOTHYROIDISM

Authority	Summary of Recommendation
American College of Physicians, 1998 (32)	Only office-based screening for women 50 years and older is recommended.
American Thyroid Association, 2000 (31)	Adults, particularly women, should be screened for thyroid dysfunction by measurement of the serum thyroid-stimulating hormone (TSH) concentration beginning at age 35 years and every 5 years thereafter in the context of the periodic health examination. Individuals with clinical manifestations potentially attributable to thyroid dysfunction and those with risk factors for its development may require more frequent TSH testing.
American Association of Clinical Endocrinologists, 2002 (33)	Screening for thyroid dysfunction by TSH measurement should be routine in women before or during the first trimester of pregnancy.
American Academy of Family Physicians, 2002 (35)	Screening for thyroid dysfunction at the periodic health examination for individuals under 60 years of age (except neonates) is not recommended.
National Academy of Clinical Biochemistry, 2003 (34)	Women should be screened for screening for thyroid dysfunction using serum TSH and thyroperoxidase autoantibodies (TPOAb) either prepregnancy or during first trimester to detect mild thyroid insufficiency and assess their risk for postpartum thyroiditis.
Consensus Development Conference, 2004[a] (36)	There is insufficient evidence to support population-based screening. Aggressive case finding is appropriate in pregnant women, women over 60 years of age, and others at high risk for thyroid dysfunction.
U.S. Preventive Services Task Force (USPSTF), 2004 (37)	There is insufficient evidence to recommend for or against routine screening for thyroid disease in adults.

[a]Expert panel nominated by a planning committee composed of representatives of the American Thyroid Association, the American Association of Clinical Endocrinologists, and the Endocrine Society.

are normal in about one third of overtly hypothyroid patients. Furthermore, they are nonspecific because the values are subnormal in many patients with nonthyroidal illness (Chapter 11D). TRH stimulation testing can be helpful in identifying patients with mild central hypothyroidism, but it is no more useful than basal serum TSH measurements in identifying subclinical primary hypothyroidism. TRH tests also fail to distinguish reliably between hypothalamic and pituitary hypothyroidism, and between these two disorders and nonthyroidal illness (2).

FUTURE ADVANCES IN LABORATORY ASSESSMENT

Despite the several sensitive and usually specific tests for accurate evaluation of patients with potential hypothyroidism, certain clinical problems occasionally remain unresolved. The evaluation of hypothyroxinemic patients with nonthyroidal illness would be aided by more practical techniques to quantify the biologically active free thyroid hormone fractions in serum and tissues. Simple methods of quantifying tissue thyroid hormone responsiveness—in addition to serum TSH assay—would be very useful, but all foreseeable approaches are nonspecific and, like serum TSH, may not be generalizable beyond the organ system assessed.

REFERENCES

1. Staub JJ, Althaus BU, Engler H, et al. Spectrum of subclinical and overt hypothyroidism: effect on thyrotropin, prolactin, and thyroid reserve, and metabolic impact in target tissues. *Am J Med* 1992;92:631.
2. Docter R, Krenning EP, deJong M, et al. The sick euthyroid syndrome: changes in serum thyroid hormone parameters and hormone metabolism. *Clin Endocrinol* 1993;39:499.
3. Canaris GJ, Steiner JF, Ridgway EC. Do traditional symptoms of hypothyroidism correlate with biochemical disease? *J Gen Intern Med* 1997;12:544.
4. Zulewski H, Muller B, Exer P, et al. Estimation of tissue hypothyroidism by a new clinical score: evaluation of patients with various grades of hypothyroidism and controls. *J Clin Endocrinol Metab* 1997;82:771.
5. Seshadri MS, Samuel BU, Kanagasabapathy AS, et al. Clinical scoring system for hypothyroidism: is it useful? *J Gen Intern Med* 1989;4:490.
5a. Zargar AH, Laway BA, Bashir MI, et al. Clinical spectrum of adult onset spontaneous hypothyroidism. *Saud Med J* 1999;20:870.
6. Goldstein BJ, Mushlin AL. Use of a single thyroxine test to evaluate ambulatory patients for suspected hypothyroidism. *J Gen Intern Med* 1987;2:20.
7. Schectman JM, Kallenberg GA, Shumacher RJ, et al. Yield of hypothyroidism in symptomatic primary care patients. *Arch Intern Med* 1989;149:861.
8. Murakami M, Koizumi Y, Aizawa T, et al. Studies of thyroid function and immune parameters in patients with hyperthyroid Graves' disease in remission. *J Clin Endocrinol Metab* 1988;66: 103.
9. Sears JD, Greven KM, Ferree CR, et al. Definitive irradiation in the treatment of Hodgkin's disease: analysis of outcome, prognostic factors, and long-term complications. *Cancer* 1997;79:145.
10. Tell R, Sjodin H, Lundell G, et al. Hypothyroidism after external radiotherapy for head and neck cancer. *Int J Radiat Oncol Biol Phys* 1997;39:303.
11. Myers DH, Carter RA, Burns BH, et al. A prospective study of the effect of lithium on thyroid function and on the prevalence of antithyroid antibodies. *Psychol Med* 1985;15:55.
12. Martino E, Safran M, Aghini-Lombardi F, et al. Environmental iodine intake and thyroid dysfunction during chronic amiodarone therapy. *Ann Intern Med* 1984;101:28.
13. Curran PG, De Groot LJ. The effect of hepatic enzyme-inducing drugs on thyroid hormones and the thyroid gland. *Endocr Rev* 1991;12:135.
13a. Sherman SI, Gopal J, Haugen BR, Chiu AC, Whaley K, Nowlakha P, Duvic M. Central hypothyroidism associated with retinoid X receptor-selective ligands. *N Engl J Med* 1999;340:1075–1079.
14. Custro N, Montalto G, Scafidi V, et al. Prospective study on thyroid autoimmunity and dysfunction related to chronic hepatitis C and interferon therapy. *J Endocrinol Invest* 1997;20:374.
15. Horimoto M, Nishikawa M, Ishihara T, et al. Bioactivity of thyrotropin (TSH) in patients with central hypothyroidism: comparison between the *in vivo* 3,5,38-triiodothyronine response to TSH and *in vitro* bioactivity of TSH. *J Clin Endocrinol Metab* 1995;80:1124.
16. Larsen PR, Alexander NM, Chopra IJ, et al. Revised nomenclature for tests of thyroid hormones and thyroid related proteins in serum. *J Clin Endocrinol Metab* 1987;64:1089.
17. Kaptein EM, MacIntyre SS, Weiner JM, et al. Free thyroxine estimates in nonthyroidal illness: comparison of eight methods. *J Clin Endocrinol Metab* 1981;52:1073.
18. Gooch BR, Isley WL, Utiger RD. Abnormalities in thyroid function tests in patients admitted to a medical service. *Arch Intern Med* 1982;142:1801.
19. Cooper DS, Halpern R, Wood LC, et al. L-thyroxine therapy in subclinical hypothyroidism: a double-blind, placebo controlled trial. *Ann Intern Med* 1984;101:18.
20. Nystrom E, Caidahl K, Fager G, et al. A double-blind cross over 12-month study of L-thyroxine treatment of women with "subclinical" hypothyroidism. *Clin Endocrinol* 1988;29:63.
21. Tanis BC, Westendorp GJ, Smelt AHM. Effect of thyroid substitution on hypercholesterolemia in patients with subclinical hypothyroidism: a reanalysis of intervention studies. *Clin Endocrinol* 1996;44:643.
22. Tunbridge WMG, Evered DC, Hall R, et al. The spectrum of thyroid disease in a community: the Whickham survey. *Clin Endocrinol* 1977;7:481.
23. Rosenthal MJ, Hunt WC, Garry PJ, et al. Thyroid failure in the elderly: microsomal antibodies as discriminant for therapy. *JAMA* 1987;258:209.
24. Vanderpump MPJ, Tunbridge WMG, French JM, et al. The incidence of thyroid disorders in the community: a twenty-year follow-up of the Whickham Survey. *Clin Endocrinol* 1995;43:55.
25. Refetoff S, Usala SJ. The syndromes of resistance to thyroid hormones. *Endocr Rev* 1993;14:348.
26. Gesundheit N, Petrick PA, Nissim M, et al. Thyrotropin-secreting pituitary adenomas: clinical and biochemical heterogeneity. Case reports and follow-up of nine patients. *Ann Intern Med* 1989;111:827.
27. England ML, Hershman JM. Serum TSH concentration as an aid to monitoring compliance with thyroid hormone therapy in hypothyroidism. *Am J Med Sci* 1986;292:264.
28. Hamblin PS, Dyer SA, Mohr VS, et al. Relation between serum thyrotropin and thyroxine changes during recovery from severe

hypothyroxinemia of critical illness. *J Clin Endocrinol Metab* 1986;62:717.

29. Spencer CA, Eigen A, Shen D, et al. Specificity of sensitive assays of thyrotropin (TSH) used to screen for thyroid disease in hospitalized patients. *Clin Chem* 1987;33:1391.

30. Ferretti E, Persani L, Jaffrain-Rea ML, et al. Evaluation of the adequacy of levothyroxine replacement therapy in patients with central hypothyroidism. *J Clin Endocrinol Metab* 1999;84:924.

31. Ladenson PW, Singer PA, Ain KB, Bagchi N, Bigos ST, Levy EG, Smith SA, Daniels GH, Cohen HD. American Thyroid Association guidelines for detection of thyroid dysfunction. *Arch Intern Med* 2000;160:1573–5.

32. Helfand M, Redfern C. Clinical Guideline. II. Screening for thyroid disease: an update. *Ann Intern Med* 1998;129:144.

33. AACE Thyroid Task Force. American Association of Clinical Endocrinologists medical guidelines for clinical practice for the evaluation and treatment of hyperthyroidism and hypothyroidism. *Endocr Pract* 2002;8:457–469.

34. Baloch Z, Carayon P, Conte-Devolx B, et al.; Guidelines Committee, National Academy of Clinical Biochemistry. Laboratory medicine practice guidelines: laboratory support for the diagnosis and monitoring of thyroid disease. *Thyroid* 2003;13:3–126.

35. American Academy of Family Physicians (AAFP). Summary of policy recommendations for periodic health examinations. Leawood, KS: Author, 2002:15.

36. Surks MI, Ortiz E, Daniels GH, et al. Subclinical thyroid disease: scientific review and guidelines for diagnosis and management. *JAMA* 2004;291:228–238.

37. U.S. Preventive Services Task Force. Screening for thyroid disease: recommendation statement. *Ann Intern Med* 2004;140:125–127. *www.ahrq.gov/clinic/uspstf/uspsthyr.htm.*

38. Danese MD, Powe NR, Sawin CT, et al. Screening for mild thyroid failure at the periodic health examination: a decision and cost-effectiveness analysis. *JAMA* 1996;276:285.

39. Hayslip CC, Fein HG, O'Donnell VM, et al. The value of serum antimicrosomal antibody testing in screening for symptomatic postpartum thyroid dysfunction. *Am J Obstet Gynecol* 1988;159:203.

TREATMENT OF HYPOTHYROIDISM

KENNETH A. WOEBER

Hypothyroidism was the first endocrine disorder to be treated with replacement of the deficient hormone. More than 100 years have elapsed since extracts of animal thyroid glandular tissue were found to be effective in treating hypothyroidism. Subsequently, chemically synthesized thyroid hormone preparations were developed, and these have largely replaced the use of thyroid extracts. In addition, the elucidation of thyroid hormone economy in humans and the ability to accurately measure serum thyrotropin (TSH) have made it possible to virtually mimic normal thyroid physiology (1,2). Accordingly, the treatment of hypothyroidism has become straightforward. Nevertheless, various clinical circumstances and drugs can affect the absorption, metabolism, and action of administered thyroid hormone and may necessitate adjustment of dosage. This chapter will review the treatment of hypothyroidism in the adult. The treatment of hypothyroidism in the infant and child is presented in Chapter 75, and the treatment of myxedema coma in Chapter 65.

PHARMACOLOGIC CONSIDERATIONS

We now know that in the normal adult about 100 μg of L-thyroxine (T_4) is secreted by the thyroid daily and that about 30 μg of L-triiodothyronine (T_3) is produced daily, 80% arising from the 5′-deiodination of T_3 in the peripheral tissues and 20%, or about 6 μg daily, from thyroid secretion (1). Thus, T_4 is the principal product of thyroid glandular secretion and serves as the prohormone for T_3, which is the principal arbiter of thyroid hormone action (3).

Various thyroid hormone preparations are available for the treatment of hypothyroidism. They include levothyroxine sodium (L-thyroxine, T_4), liothyronine sodium (L-triiodothyronine, T_3), liotrix (a 1:4 combination of T_3 and T_4), and thyroid USP (a porcine thyroid glandular extract containing T_3 and T_4 in a ratio of ~1:4).

T_4 is the preferred drug because its administration mostly closely mimics glandular secretion and because its conversion to T_3 will be appropriately regulated in the tissues. Approximately 70% of an administered dose is absorbed, principally in the jejunum (4). The advantages of T_4 include its long half-life in blood (~7 days), small (~13%) fluctuations in serum concentration between single daily doses, and ease of titration of dosage because of

the availability of multiple tablet strengths. An additional important advantage of T_4 is the stable serum T_3 concentration between T_4 doses (Fig. 67.1).

T_3 and the T_3-containing preparations have several drawbacks to their use. T_3 is rapidly and virtually completely absorbed and has a half-life in blood of approximately 1 day. Accordingly, serum levels attain a peak in 2 to 4 hours, and a dose of 25 μg will produce supranormal serum concentrations for 6 to 8 hours, often accompanied by precordial palpitations. Moreover, currently available T_3-containing preparations (liotrix and thyroid USP) contain T_3 and T_4 in a ratio of approximately 1:4, whereas the ratio of T_3 to T_4 in thyroid glandular secretion is much less, approximately 1:15.

The T_4 content of tablets is standardized by high-performance liquid chromatography and, as stipulated by the USP, must conform to between 90% and 110% of the stated amount. Because reformulation of T_4 tablets by various manufacturers had previously resulted in changes in stability and potency, the U.S. Food and Drug Administration recently enacted legislation to ensure that the amount of available drug is consistent with a given tablet strength and that the tablets from various manufacturers be bioequivalent (5). Numerous brand-name and some generic preparations are available in 12 strengths ranging from 25 to 300 μg, which allows precise replacement in most patients. The 12 strengths of the more common brand-name preparations in the United States are similarly color coded. T_4 tablets are stable with a finite shelf-life at 15° to 30°C, but may lose potency if exposed to light or moisture. T_4 is also available as a lyophilized preparation for injection.

T_3 tablets are available in three strengths—5, 25, and 50 μg—and are not color coded. T_3 is also available in an injectable preparation. Liotrix tablets are available in five color-coded strengths, ranging from tablets containing 3.1 μg of T_3 and 12.5 μg of T_4 to tablets containing 50 μg of T_3 and 200 μg of T_4. Thyroid USP is available in eight strengths, ranging from 0.25 gr to 5 gr and containing 9 μg of T_3 and 38 μg of T_4 per grain. The approximate bioequivalence of the various thyroid hormone preparations is 100 μg T_4, approximately 37.5 μg T_3, liotrix-1, and 1.5 gr (90 mg) thyroid USP.

Combination T_4 and T_3 treatment in the form of thyroid USP was used before chemically synthesized T_4 became available. Although T_4 has become the recommended

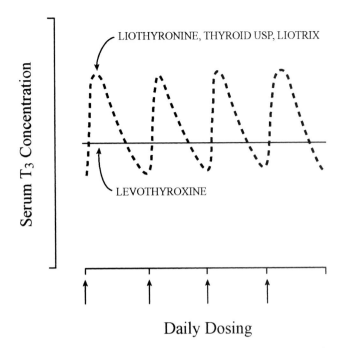

FIGURE 67.1. Schema depicting the effects of daily dosing with various thyroid hormone preparations on serum triiodothyronine concentration.

form of replacement therapy, interest in the use of a combination of T_4 and T_3 has resurfaced. This interest has its basis in the observation that in thyroidectomized rats normal serum and tissue T_3 concentrations can only be achieved with either supraphysiologic doses of T_4 or a combination of T_4 and T_3 (6). One short-term study in hypothyroid patients has suggested that partial substitution of T_3 for T_4 resulting in a T_3 to T_4 ratio of approximately 1:10 in the total replacement dosage improves mood and cognitive performance (7). This observation, however, was not corroborated in more recent studies (8,9,9a).

APPROACH TO TREATMENT

The goal of treatment is to restore a normal (euthyroid) state of the tissues with resolution of the symptoms and signs of hypothyroidism. This goal is accomplished by administering sufficient T_4 so that the serum TSH in patients with primary hypothyroidism is reduced to within the normal range. The dosage of T_4 that results in a normal serum TSH will increase the serum free T_4 concentration to well within the normal range and the serum free T_3 concentration into the low normal range, this discordance reflecting the lack of the thyroidal contribution to serum T_3 concentration (10). Serum TSH bears a negative logarithmic-linear relationship to serum free T_4 and is therefore a more sensitive index of the thyroid state than serum free T_4 (2). At present, no sufficiently sensitive measurements exist for assessing the metabolic effects of T_4 on the tissues. Thus,

measurement of serum TSH is the best way to identify patients who are taking too much T_4 (low serum TSH) or too little T_4 (high TSH).

Serum TSH concentration does not reflect the thyroid state in patients with central hypothyroidism, and measurement of serum free T_4 must be used to monitor treatment in this circumstance. Similarly, in patients recently treated for hyperthyroidism, delayed recovery of pituitary TSH secretion may result in a low serum TSH concentration for several months, necessitating measurement of serum free T_4 to assess the thyroid state.

Patients who have taken thyroid USP or combined T_4 and T_3 preparations for many years may be reluctant to switch to T_4 despite its advantages. However, such preparations can be continued provided that measurement of serum TSH, but not serum free T_4 or free T_3, is used to monitor therapy

INITIATION OF TREATMENT

The initial dosage of T_4 should be based on the age of the patient, the severity and duration of hypothyroidism, and the presence of concurrent disorders. In healthy young patients with mild disease, treatment can be initiated with a dosage that approaches a full replacement dosage of approximately 1.6 µg/kg/day (11). In patients over 60 years of age without clinically overt cardiac disease and in patients with disease of long duration, treatment should be initiated with 50 µg of T_4 per day. Treatment of patients with cardiac disease is discussed in a subsequent section.

T_4 is taken in a single daily dose. Ideally, it should be taken alone on arising and at least 30 minutes before breakfast because some fiber and bran products as well as certain medications and dietary supplements can impede its absorption.

Because it takes about 2 months for serum TSH to attain a new steady state, the initial dosage of T_4 should not be increased earlier. Thereafter, the dosage of T_4 is gradually increased at about 2-month intervals until the patient is clinically euthyroid with serum TSH in the normal range.

MAINTENANCE AND
MONITORING OF TREATMENT

With the exception of certain disorders that lead to self-limited hypothyroidism, such as recovery from thyroiditis or resolution of iodine-induced hypothyroidism, treatment will be lifelong. Because of the negative logarithmic-linear relationship between serum TSH and serum free T_4, measurement of serum TSH is used to monitor replacement. Because serum TSH and free T_4 levels are influenced by T_4 administration, blood should be collected before the T_4 is taken (12). Dosage adjustments should be limited to 25 µg/day or less and should not occur more frequently than at 2-month intervals to permit serum TSH to stabilize. Similarly, if the brand of T_4 is changed, measurement of serum TSH is advisable about 2 months later. Because normal values for serum TSH display a logarithmic normal distribution between approximately 0.5 and 5.0 mU/L with a tail at the upper end, a target range of 0.5 to 2.0 mU/L is the desired goal of treatment in otherwise healthy patients and is associated with optimal general well-being (13). Thereafter, the patient should be followed up at 6- to 12-month intervals with measurement of serum TSH and free T_4 levels.

The replacement dosage of T_4 may be affected by several factors. Patients with hyperthyroidism rendered hypothyroid with iodine 131 or subtotal thyroidectomy may initially require a lower dosage of T_4 than patients with hypothyroidism due to chronic thyroiditis or following total thyroidectomy because of persistence of an autonomously functioning thyroid remnant. Progressive failure of a functioning thyroid remnant will necessitate an increase in dosage. Patients over 60 years of age may require a lower dosage of T_4 because of its reduced metabolic disposition (14). Substantial changes in body weight may require an adjustment in T_4 dosage.

Patients who forget or are unable to take T_4 for several days should not be concerned because of the approximately 7-day half-life of T_4. However, in patients who are unable to take T_4 orally for prolonged periods, T_4 can be given intravenously in a dosage of approximately 70% of the oral dose, reflecting the fractional absorption of an oral dose.

The response to treatment should be assessed both clinically and biochemically. Resolution of the symptoms and signs of hypothyroidism lags behind the return to normal of serum TSH concentration, and complete resolution requires at least 3 months. Many patients with hypothyroidism complain of weight gain and expect to lose substantial weight after treatment is initiated. Because most of the weight gain is due to fluid retention, the diuresis following treatment results in weight loss that seldom exceeds 10% of body weight.

FACTORS AFFECTING BIOAVAILABILITY OF THYROXINE

Various clinical circumstances and drugs can affect the bioavailability of T_4 and may necessitate an adjustment of dosage (Table 67.1). Pregnancy results in an increased dosage requirement for T_4 in women being treated for hypothyroidism. The increased requirement is due to an increase in serum thyroxine-binding globulin (TBG) concentration and to placental transfer of T_4 to the fetus as well as placental 5'-deiodination of T_4 to inactive reverse T_3 (see Chapter 80). Oral, but not transdermal, estrogen, tamoxifen, and raloxifene also induce an increase in TBG and may result in an increased dosage requirement for T_4 (15–17).

TABLE 67.1. FACTORS THAT INCREASE THYROXINE REQUIREMENT

Pregnancy, estrogen, tamoxifen, raloxifene
Small bowel disease
Drugs or dietary supplements that reduce absorption
  Fiber, bran, soy protein
  Calcium carbonate
  Ferrous sulfate
  Aluminum hydroxide
  Cholestyramine
  Sucralfate
  Sodium polystyrene sulfonate
Drugs that increase metabolic disposition
  Rifampin
  Carbamazepine
  Phenytoin
  Phenobarbital
Mechanism not known
  Sertraline
  Lovastatin

Conversely, oral androgens, which induce a decrease in TBG, may result in a decreased requirement for T_4.

Patients who have extensive small bowel disease or who consume large quantities of fiber, bran, or soy protein may absorb T_4 less effectively and require more T_4 (18–20). Many drugs and dietary supplements can reduce the bioavailability of T_4 through various mechanisms. Ferrous sulfate and calcium carbonate reduce T_4 absorption and are especially noteworthy because many older women consume these supplements and are the group in which hypothyroidism is most prevalent (21,22). Moreover, these compounds are present in prenatal vitamins and may contribute to the increased requirement for T_4 in pregnancy if concurrently taken with T_4 (23). Accordingly, T_4 should be taken at least 4 hours apart from the ingestion of drugs or dietary supplements that impede its absorption.

Drugs that induce hepatic microsomal enzymes, such as rifampin and anticonvulsants, increase the metabolic disposition of T_4 and may increase its dosage requirement (24–26). Other drugs have been reported to increase T_4 requirements, but these reports have been limited to a single patient or very few patients.

TREATMENT IN SPECIAL CIRCUMSTANCES
Central Hypothyroidism

In patients with central hypothyroidism, measurement of serum TSH is not useful for monitoring treatment with T_4. Instead, measurement of both serum free T_4 and free T_3 before the daily dose of T_4 is taken should be used to assess the adequacy of replacement, the target being normal serum values for both hormones (27). Because patients with central hypothyroidism have limited or no adrenal reserve, treatment with T_4 alone may precipitate adrenal insufficiency by accelerating the metabolic disposition of cortisol as a euthyroid state is approached. Accordingly, hydrocortisone should be given until pituitary–adrenal function can be properly evaluated.

Pregnancy

As noted earlier, pregnancy results in an increased dosage requirement for T_4, which becomes evident early in the first trimester. During the first trimester, serum TSH normally decreases because of the presence of high concentrations of chorionic gonadotropin, which has thyroid-stimulating activity. Accordingly, measurement of serum free T_4 before the daily dose of T_4 is taken should be used in conjunction with serum TSH to monitor treatment. Patients should be monitored at 6-week intervals until they are well into the second trimester, the target being the maintenance of a high normal serum free T_4 and a low normal serum TSH. After parturition, the dosage of T_4 can be reduced to the dosage before pregnancy.

Cardiac Disease

Hypothyroidism is a risk factor for accelerated atherosclerosis and coronary artery disease. These adverse consequences result from the dyslipidemia, increased total homocysteine, increased C-reactive protein, and increased prevalence of diastolic hypertension (28–30). Accordingly, in patients over 60 years of age with long-standing hypothyroidism, treatment should be initiated with 50 µg or less of T_4 daily. In patients with known coronary heart disease, the initial dosage of T_4 should not exceed 25 µg daily. Treatment will aggravate angina in about one fifth of patients with preexisting angina and result in no change or improvement in the remainder. In some patients without preexisting angina, treatment will provoke angina. Angina should be managed with aspirin and lower than normal dosages of nitrate and a β-adrenergic blocker and the dosage of T_4 gradually increased at about 2-month intervals. If angina cannot be controlled, percutaneous transluminal coronary angioplasty or coronary artery bypass grafting should be considered. A recent study has shown that the mortality rate in men on T_4 replacement undergoing bypass grafting was not increased, but that the mortality rate in women was increased, and this increase appeared to be due to insufficient replacement (31).

The dosage requirement for warfarin is increased in hypothyroidism because of the reduced metabolic disposition of the vitamin K–dependent clotting factors (32). Accordingly, in hypothyroid patients who are taking warfarin, the international normalized ratio should be closely monitored because warfarin dosage will need to be lowered as the euthyroid state is approached.

ADVERSE EFFECTS OF THYROXINE

Although hypersensitivity reactions to the inactive ingredients of a specific brand of T_4 tablet or to the dye have been reported, these are exceedingly rare. On the other hand, adverse effects resulting from an excessive dosage of T_4 are very common. It has been estimated that more than one fifth of patients taking thyroid medication for hypothyroidism have a subnormal serum TSH and therefore are either clinically or subclinically thyrotoxic (33). The adverse consequences of a low serum TSH are principally manifested on the skeleton and heart. In women over 65 years of age, a low serum TSH (<0.1 mU/L) has been shown to result in a threefold increased risk for hip fracture and a fourfold increased risk for vertebral fracture (34). In persons over 60 years of age, a low serum TSH (<0.1 mU/L) has been shown to be associated with a threefold increased risk for atrial fibrillation during the ensuing 10 years of follow-up (35). Moreover, subclinical thyrotoxicosis due to an excessive dosage of T_4 has been reported to lead to an increase in resting heart rate, to a decrease in exercise capacity, and to an increase in left ventricular mass index with the potential for reduced diastolic function (36). Whether lesser degrees of TSH suppression are associated with fewer adverse consequences is uncertain. Nevertheless, the foregoing observations indicate the importance of avoiding a suppressed TSH value, the only exception being the patient who has undergone ablative treatment for thyroid cancer.

APPARENT FAILURE OF THYROXINE TREATMENT

Persistent Elevation of Serum Thyroid-Stimulating Hormone

Some patients display a persistently elevated serum TSH despite being prescribed a dosage of T_4 that should be adequate. The most common reason for this phenomenon is partial compliance, and is suggested by a discordance between the serum TSH and free T_4 values. As the TSH response to treatment is delayed, serum TSH will remain elevated in the presence of a normal serum free T_4 if the daily dosage of T_4 is taken on an irregular basis.

Persistent elevation of serum TSH despite patient compliance may be due to one or more of the factors affecting bioavailability of the T_4 preparation described earlier. In their absence, changing the brand of T_4 should be considered as the dissolution time, which is a function of the inactive ingredients, varies among different preparations, and this phenomenon could be a factor in the patient with rapid intestinal transit.

Persistence of Symptoms Despite Normal Serum TSH

Some patients continue to display symptoms suggesting a persistent hypothyroid state after serum TSH has been restored to within the normal reference range with treatment. Several reasons may account for this phenomenon. First, it is important to recognize that each patient has a unique set point for free T_4 in relation to TSH within the reference ranges for the laboratory (37). Accordingly, adjustment of T_4 dosage to maintain the serum TSH between 0.5 and 2.0 mU/L, which is the reference range for a rigorously screened normal population (38), may serve to attenuate the patient's symptoms. Second, there is evidence to suggest that some patients on an optimal replacement dosage of T_4 fail to attain a sense of normal general wellbeing (39). This observation might be due to preexisting comorbidity, such as depression. Indeed, the presence of antithyroid peroxidase antibodies has been shown to be an independent risk factor for depression (40).

Finally, the possibility exists that in some patients an optimal dosage of T_4 does not provide through peripheral conversion a quantity of T_3 that is sufficient to sustain a euthyroid state. In fact, in most patients on T_4 replacement, serum free T_3 is at the lower end of the normal reference range and in a small number of patients subnormal (10). One short-term study had suggested that partial substitution of T_3 for T_4 in the total replacement dosage of T_4 improved mood and cognitive performance (7). This observation, however, has been refuted in 3 recent studies (8,9,9a). Thus, in most patients with hypothyroidism, combined treatment with T_4 and T_3 cannot be currently recommended over treatment with T_4 alone.

REFERENCES

1. Pilo A, Iervasi G, Vitek F, et al. Thyroidal and peripheral production of 3,5,3'-triiodothyronine in humans by multicompartmental analysis. *Am J Physiol* 1990;258:E715–E726.
2. Spencer CA, Lopresti JS, Patel A, et al. Applications of a new chemiluminometric thyrotropin assay to subnormal measurement. *J Clin Endocrinol Metab* 1990;70:453–460.
3. Koenig RJ. Ubiquinated deiodinase: not dead yet. *J Clin Invest* 2003;112:145–147.
4. Hays MT, Nielsen KRK. Human thyroxine absorption: age effects and methodological analyses. *Thyroid* 1994;4:55–64.
5. Hennessey JV. In my view . . . Levothyroxine a new drug? Since when? How could that be? *Thyroid* 2000;13:279–282.
6. Escobar-Morreale HF, Escobar del Rey F, Obregon MJ, et al. Only the combined treatment with thyroxine and triiodothyronine ensures euthyroidism in all tissues of the thyroidectomized rat. *Endocrinology* 1996;137:2490–2502.
7. Bunevicius R, Kazanavicius G, Zalinkevicius R, et al. Effects of thyroxine as compared with thyroxine plus triiodothyronine in patients with hypothyroidism. *N Engl J Med* 1999;340:424–429.
8. Walsh JP, Shiels L, Mun Lim E, et al. Combined thyroxine/liothyronine treatment does not improve well-being, quality of life,

or cognitive function compared to thyroxine alone: a randomized controlled trial in patients with primary hypothyroidism. *J Clin Endocrinol Metab* 2003;88:4543–4550.
9. Sawka AM, Gerstein HC, Marriott MJ, et al. Does a combination regimen of thyroxine (T4) and 3,5,3'-triiodothyronine improve depressive symptoms better than T4 alone in patients with hypothyroidism? Results of a double-blind, randomized, controlled trial. *J Clin Endocrinol Metab* 2003;88:4551–4555.
9a. Clyde PW, Harari AE, Getka EJ, et al. Combined levothyroxine plus liothyronine compared with levothyroxine alone in primary hypothyroidism. A randomized controlled trial. *JAMA* 2003; 290:2952–2958.
10. Woeber KA. Levothyroxine therapy and serum free thyroxine and free triiodothyronine concentrations. *J Endocrinol Invest* 2002;25:106–109.
11. Fish LH, Schwartz HL, Cavanaugh J, et al. Replacement dose, metabolism, and bioavailability of levothyroxine in the treatment of hypothyroidism. *N Engl J Med* 1987;316:764–770.
12. Ain KB, Pucino F, Shiver, T, et al. Thyroid hormone levels affected by time of blood sampling in thyroxine-treated patients. *Thyroid* 1993;3:81–85.
13. Hollowell JG, Staehling NW, Hannon WH, et al. Serum thyrotropin, thyroxine and thyroid antibodies in the United States population (1988–1994): NHANES III. *J Clin Endocrin Metab* 2002;87:489–499.
14. Sawin CT, Herman T, Molitch ME, et al. Aging and the thyroid. Decreased requirement for thyroid hormone in older hypothyroid patients. *Am J Med* 1983;75:206–209.
15. Arafah BM. Increased need for thyroxine in women with hypothyroidism during estrogen therapy. *N Engl J Med* 2001;344: 1743–1749.
16. Kostoglou-Athanassiou I, Ntalles K, Markopoulos C, et al. Thyroid function in postmenopausal women with breast cancer on tamoxifen. *Eur J Gynaecol Oncol* 1998;19:150–154.
17. Duntas LH, Mantzou E, Koutras DA. Lack of substantial effects of raloxifene on thyroxine-binding globulin in postmenopausal women: dependency on thyroid status. *Thyroid* 2001;11:779–782.
18. d'Esteve-Bonetti L, Bennet AP, Malet D, et al. Gluten-induced enteropathy (coeliac disease) revealed by resistance to treatment with levothyroxine and alfacalcidol in a sixty-eight-year-old patient: a case report. *Thyroid* 2002;12:633–636.
19. Liel Y, Harman-Boehm I, Shany S. Evidence for a clinically important adverse effect of fiber-enriched diet on the bioavailability of levothyroxine in adult hypothroid patients. *J Clin Endocrinol Metab* 1996;80:857–859.
20. Bell DSH, Ovalle F. Use of soy protein supplement and resultant need for increased dose of levothyroxine. *Endocr Pract* 2001;7: 193–194.
21. Campbell NRC, Hasinoff BB, Stalts H, et al. Ferrous sulfate reduces thyroxine efficacy in patients with hypothyroidism. *Ann Intern Med* 1992;117:1010–1013.
22. Singh N, Singh PN, Hershman JM. Effect of calcium carbonate on the absorption of levothyroxine. *JAMA* 2000;283:2822–2825.
23. Chopra IJ, Baber K. Treatment of primary hypothyroidism during pregnancy: is there an increase in thyroxine dose requirement in pregnancy? *Metabolism* 2003;52:122–128.
24. Nolan SR, Self TH, Norwood JM. Interaction between rifampin and levothyroxine. *South Med J* 1999;92:529–531.
25. Curran PG, DeGroot LJ. The effect of hepatic enzyme-inducing drugs on thyroid hormones and the thyroid gland. *Endocr Rev* 1991;12:135–150.
26. Isojarvi JI, Turrka J, Pakarinen AJ, et al. Thyroid function in men taking carbamazepine, oxcarbazepine, or valproate for epilepsy. *Epilepsia* 2001;42:930–934.

27. Ferretti E, Persani L, Jaffrain-Rea M-L, et al. Evaluation of the adequacy of levothyroxine replacement therapy in patients with central hypothyroidism. *J Clin Endocrinol Metab* 1999;84:924–929.
28. Duntas LH. Thyroid disease and lipids. *Thyroid* 2002;12:287–293.
29. Christ-Crain M, Meier C, Guglielmetti M, et al. Elevated C-reactive protein and homocysteine values: cardiovascular risk factors in hypothyroidism? A cross-sectional and a double-blind, placebo-controlled trial. *Atheroscloerosis* 2003;166:379–386.
30. Dernellis J, Panaretou M. Effects of thyroid replacement therapy on arterial blood pressure in patients with hypertension and hypothyroidism. *Am Heart J* 2002;143:718–724.
31. Zindrou D, Taylor KM, Peder Bagger J. Excess coronary artery bypass graft mortality among women with hypothyroidism. *Ann Thorac Surg* 2002;74:2121–2125.
32. Stephens MA, Self TH, Lancaster D, et al. Hypothyroidism: effect on warfarin anticoagulation. *South Med J* 1989;82:1585–1586.
33. Canaris GJ, Manowitz NR, Mayor G, et al. The Colorado thyroid disease prevalence study. *Arch Intern Med* 2000;160:526–534.
34. Bauer DC, Ettinger B, Nevitt MC, et al. Risk for fracture in women with low serum levels of thyroid-stimulating hormone. *Ann Intern Med* 2001;134:561–568.
35. Sawin CT, Geller A, Wolf PA, et al. Low serum thyrotropin concentrations as a risk factor for atrial fibrillation in older patients. *N Engl J Med* 1994;331:1249–1252.
36. Biondi B, Palmieri EA, Lombardi G, et al. Effects of subclinical thyroid dysfunction on the heart. *Ann Intern Med* 2002;137:903–914.
37. Andersen S, Pedersen KM, Bruun NH, et al. Narrow individual variations in serum T_4 and T_3 in normal subjects: a clue to the understanding of subclinical thyroid disease. *J Clin Endocrinol Metab* 2002;87:1068–1072,
38. Spencer C, Hollowell J, Nicoloff J, et al. NHANES III: Impact of TSH: TPOAb relationships on redefining the serum TSH normal reference range. Presented at the American Thyroid Association 74th Annual Meeting, 2002. Program No. 2, p. 111.
39. Saravanan P, Chau W-F, Roberts N, et al. Psychological well-being in patients on "adequate" doses of L-thyroxine: results of a large, controlled community-based questionnaire study. *Clin Endocrinol* 2002;57:577–585.
40. Pop VJ, Maartens LH, Leusink G, et al. Are autoimmune thyroid dysfunction and depression related. *J Clin Endocrinol Metab* 1998;83:3194–3197.

THYROID DISEASES: NONTOXIC DIFFUSE AND MULTINODULAR GOITER

Nontox
largeme
thyroto
mune c
is used
age witl
"sporad
　Both
the patl
wide, tl
ing to
ciency
some io
contain
growth
the abs
tors for
cigarett
ium anc
and Otl
Metabo
tional fa
nontoxi
commo
disorder
(see Ch
goiter ir
have prc
the etiol
in none
interest,
chromos
but it is
role in tl

NATUF

In the e
diffuse
prevalen

the trachea or esophagus and venous outflow obstruction. Therapy should also be considered when there is progressive growth of the entire goiter or of individual nodules, especially when there is substantial intrathoracic extension of the goiter. The intrathoracic parts of these goiters cannot be examined by palpation and fine-needle aspiration biopsy, and they may cause acute and life-threatening tracheal compression due to hemorrhage into a nodule or a cyst. Sometimes treatment is indicated because of neck discomfort or cosmetic concerns.

The main therapeutic options are thyroidectomy, administration of radioiodine, or administration of T_4. In patients with a small, diffuse, nontoxic goiter due to iodine deficiency, an additional option is low-dose iodine treatment (14). However, when the goiter is multinodular, iodine supplementation is not advisable because it is rarely effective and it may induce thyrotoxicosis.

Thyroidectomy

Surgical treatment leads to rapid decompression of vital structures and provides tissue for pathologic examination (15,16). Usually bilateral subtotal thyroidectomy is performed, with removal of all grossly abnormal tissue. Some surgeons advise more extensive resection (near-total or even total thyroidectomy) in order to minimize the risk for recurrent goiter (17–19). Nearly all nontoxic goiters can be removed through a collar incision, even those with substantial intrathoracic extension. However, thoracotomy must be performed in the rare patients who have goiters that arise from aberrant thyroid tissue within the thorax or who have recurrent intrathoracic goiter after earlier thyroidectomy (3,4,15,20).

The mortality rate after thyroid surgery in patients with nontoxic goiter is low (<1%) (15,16). The most important complications of thyroid surgery for nontoxic goiter are tracheal obstruction due to hemorrhage, tracheomalacia, recurrent laryngeal nerve injury, hypoparathyroidism, and hypothyroidism (15,16). Permanent lesions of the recurrent laryngeal nerve and the parathyroid glands occur in less than 1% of patients treated in specialized units (21). Persistent voice changes (dysphonia, hoarseness, fatigue, or reduction of voice range) are not uncommon. The rate of postoperative hypothyroidism is determined mainly by the extent of surgery. Surgical morbidity is highest in patients with large goiters and in those who undergo reoperation (21–24).

The rate of goiter recurrence depends on the duration of follow-up after surgery. With adequate surgery, the recurrence rate should not be higher than approximately 10% after 10 years (25). Postoperatively, T_4 is often prescribed to prevent goiter recurrence, but at best it seems only modestly effective for this purpose (26,27). Therefore, there is no indication for routine T_4 therapy after surgery for nontoxic goiter (27,28). An exception should be made for patients who had previous head and neck radiation for be-

nign conditions; in one large, randomized study of these patients, T_4 therapy prevented goiter recurrence after subtotal thyroidectomy for benign nodular disease (29).

Radioiodine

During the 1990s, measurements of thyroid volume (see Chapter 16) convincingly demonstrated that radioiodine treatment is effective in reducing thyroid volume in over 90% of patients with nontoxic goiter (30–39). Usually single doses of approximately 100 to 120 mCi (3.7–4.4 MBq) of radioiodine (^{131}I) per gram of thyroid tissue (corrected for the percentage uptake of radioiodine in the thyroid at 24 hours) are given, but multiple fractionated doses also may be effective (40).

In patients with nontoxic diffuse goiters treated in this way, thyroid volume decreases on average by 50% to 60% in 12 to 18 months (35,36). In patients with nontoxic multinodular goiters, radioiodine treatment results in a reduction in goiter volume of approximately 40% after 1 year (30–34,37,38) and 50% to 60% after 3 to 5 years (31,41) (Fig. 69.3). Half of the effect appears within the first 3 months (31). The decrease in goiter size is positively correlated with the dose of radioiodine per gram of thyroid tissue (34,39) and negatively correlated with pretreatment goiter volume (37–39).

In the majority of patients, radioiodine treatment decreases not only thyroid volume, but also compressive symptoms (32,39). The decreases in compressive symptoms are accompanied by substantial tracheal widening, as measured by MRI (32) and improvement in respiratory function (32,42).

Early side effects (radiation thyroiditis and esophagitis) are usually mild and transient (32,41,43). Exacerbation of compressive symptoms after radioiodine administration is

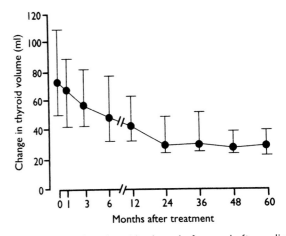

FIGURE 69.3. Median thyroid volume before and after radioiodine treatment in 39 patients with nontoxic multinodular goiter who remained euthyroid after a single dose. Bars are quartiles. (From Nygaard B, Hegedüs L, Gervil M, et al. Radioiodine treatment of multinodular non-toxic goitre. *BMJ* 1993;307:828, with permission.)

rare; therefore, glucocorticoids should not be given routinely. The development of autoimmune (Graves') hyperthyroidism, with thyrotoxicosis presumably triggered by radiation-induced release of thyroid antigens, is the most important late complication, occurring several or more months after radioiodine therapy in approximately 5% of patients (44, 45). The thyrotoxicosis may be severe. Therefore, informing patients to be alert to symptoms and signs of thyrotoxicosis is important to recognize this complication promptly. Patients with high serum antithyroid peroxidase antibody concentrations before treatment are at greater risk for this complication (44). The incidence of posttreatment hypothyroidism is 20% to 50% at 5 years (31,39); it is more common in patients with small goiters and those with high pretreatment serum antithyroid peroxidase antibody concentrations (39,44). In approximately 10% of patients the nodular goiters enlarge again after 3 to 5 years (39), and in them a second dose of radioiodine may be effective (33).

There are no follow-up data on the risk of thyroid or other cancers after radioiodine treatment of patients with nontoxic goiter. The lifetime risk for radiation-induced cancer depends not only on the administered dose of radioiodine but also on the age of the patient. It has been estimated that the lifetime risk for radiation-induced cancer in extrathyroidal tissues in people 65 years of age or older who are treated with high doses of radioiodine is similar to the surgical mortality of subtotal thyroidectomy (46).

Until now, most clinicians have restricted radioiodine therapy for nontoxic goiter to elderly patients, especially those who have a high operative risk or refuse surgery. In these patients, the benefit of noninvasive radioiodine treatment outweighs the lifetime risk for this mode of therapy. However, radioiodine may prove to be an attractive alternative to surgery in younger patients, provided that the dose of radioiodine administered is relatively low (e.g., in patients with small goiters and sufficient radioiodine uptake). In this respect, the observations that pretreatment with a single, low dose (0.01 or 0.03 mg) of recombinant human TSH doubles thyroid radioiodide uptake (47) and results in a more homogeneous uptake of radioiodide (48) in nontoxic goiter is of interest. Indeed, pretreatment with these doses allowed a 50% to 60% reduction of the therapeutic dose of radioiodine without compromising the efficacy of thyroid volume reduction in patients with nontoxic nodular goiters (49). Such a strategy decreases the radiation dose to extrathyroidal organs (50). Alternatively, one may hypothesize that the efficacy of thyroid volume reduction can be increased when pretreatment with recombinant human TSH is given without reducing the therapeutic dose of radioiodine (50,51).

Thyroxine

Thyrotropin is the main stimulator of growth of normal thyroid tissue. The hypothesis underlying T_4 treatment in patients with nontoxic goiter is that growth of goitrous tissue is also dependent on TSH and therefore that suppression of TSH secretion will result in a decrease in goiter size or at least prevent further enlargement of the goiter.

Thyroxine therapy may be effective in reducing the thyroid volume in patients with diffuse nontoxic goiters, as measured by ultrasonography (52,53). Nonrandomized studies suggest that it is also effective in some patients with multinodular goiters (26). However, most of the studies did not exclude patients with iodine deficiency or subclinical hypothyroidism (i.e., those with TSH-dependent thyroid enlargement), and none had adequate control groups or objective measurements of thyroid volume. Only two randomized trials on the effect of T_4 therapy in patients with nontoxic goiter using objective thyroid volume measurements have been reported. In a placebo-controlled double-blind randomized trial in patients with relatively small nontoxic multinodular goiters, thyroid volume, as measured by ultrasonography, decreased substantially in 58% of the T_4-treated patients, as compared with 5% of those given placebo (54); the mean decrease in thyroid volume in the patients who responded was 25% after 9 months of T_4 treatment. Goiter size returned to baseline within 9 months after discontinuation of therapy, demonstrating that maintenance of volume reduction requires long-term T_4 treatment. In a more recent study (37), a significant decrease in goiter size was observed in 43% of patients after 2 years of T_4 therapy (mean decrease 22% in the responders). In the nonresponders, a mean increase in thyroid volume of 16% was found.

Long-term T_4 therapy in doses sufficient to reduce serum TSH concentrations to below normal may have adverse skeletal and cardiac effects. It may decrease bone mineral density, particularly in postmenopausal women (55). Furthermore, it increases left ventricular mass, causes cardiac dysfunction or arrhythmias, especially atrial fibrillation (56–58) (see Chapter 79).

Before T_4 therapy is begun in patients with nontoxic goiter, serum TSH should be measured. Many patients with multinodular goiters have autonomous thyroid hormone production and subclinical thyrotoxicosis. In them, T_4 therapy is inadvisable because it is likely to cause overt thyrotoxicosis, and no shrinkage of the goiter can be expected when TSH secretion is already suppressed (59). For patients who have normal serum TSH concentrations, the optimal level of TSH suppression has not been defined. Suppression of serum TSH concentrations to less than 0.1 mU/L is probably unnecessary; lowering the concentrations to between 0.1 and 0.5 mU/L may be adequate and is safer (28).

Choice of Treatment

The advantages and disadvantages of the three treatments—thyroidectomy, radioiodine, and T_4—should be carefully weighed when advising an individual patient with

TABLE 69.1. TREATMENT OPTIONS FOR PATIENTS WITH NONTOXIC GOITER

Treatment	Advantage	Disadvantages	Comments
Surgery	Rapid decompression of vital structures; allows pathologic examination	Surgical mortality (<1%); postoperative tracheal obstruction; recurrent laryngeal nerve injury (1%–2%); hypoparathyroidism (0.5%–5%); hypothyroidism[a]; goiter recurrence[a]	Standard therapy, especially when rapid decompression of vital structures is required
Radioiodine	Substantial decrease in thyroid volume and improvement of compressive symptoms in most patients	Only gradual decrease in thyroid volume; radiation thyroiditis (usually mild); radiation-induced thyroid dysfunction (thyrotoxicosis in 5%, hypothyroidism in 20%–50%); theoretic risk for radiation-induced cancer (<1% in elderly people)	Alternative to surgery in older patients and those with cardiac or pulmonary disease
Thyroxine	Easiest treatment option	Only small decrease in thyroid volume; probably only effective if goiter is small; long-term efficacy unknown; decrease in bone mineral density in postmenopausal women; possible cardiac side effects	Alternative to surgery in young patients with a small, diffuse goiter

[a]The percentage of patients affected depends on the extent of surgery.
Modified from Hermus AR, Huysmans DA. Treatment of benign nodular thyroid disease. *N Engl J Med* 1998;338:1438, with permission.

a nontoxic goiter (60) (Table 69.1). Thyroidectomy is standard therapy for young and otherwise healthy patients, especially when prompt decompression of vital structures is required. Radioiodine therapy is an attractive alternative to surgery in older patients, in those with cardiopulmonary disease, and in those with recurrent goiter. The indication for T$_4$ therapy in patients with nontoxic goiter is limited. It may be tried in young patients with small, diffuse goiters who have normal serum TSH concentrations. In patients with nodular goiters, it is less effective and associated with significantly more adverse effects than radioiodine treatment (37). Therefore, T$_4$ therapy should no longer be recommended for patients with nodular goiters.

REFERENCES

1. Vander JB, Gaston EA, Dawber TR. Significance of solitary nontoxic thyroid nodules: preliminary report. *N Engl J Med* 1954;251:970.
2. Vanderpump MPJ, Tunbridge WMG, French JM, et al. The incidence of thyroid disorders in the community: a twenty-year follow-up of the Whickham Survey. *Clin Endocrinol (Oxf)* 1995; 43:55.
3. Katlic MR, Wang C, Grillo HC. Substernal goiter. *Ann Thorac Surg* 1985;39:391.
4. Katlic MR, Grillo HC, Wang C. Substernal goiter: analysis of 80 patients from Massachusetts General Hospital. *Am J Surg* 1985; 149:283.
5. Humphrey ML, Burman KD. Retrosternal and intrathoracic goiter. *Endocrinologist* 1992;2:195.
6. Blum M, Biller BJ, Bergman DA. The thyroid cork: obstruction of the thoracic inlet due to retroclavicular goiter. *JAMA* 1974; 227:189.
7. Pemberton HS. Sign of submerged goitre. *Lancet* 1946;251:509.
8. Hegedüs L, Bonnema SJ, Bennedbaek FN. Management of simple nodular goiter: current status and future perspectives. *Endocr Rev* 2003;24:102.
9. Miller MR, Pincock AC, Oates GD, et al. Upper airway obstruction due to goitre: detection, prevalence and results of surgical management. *Q J Med* 1990;74:177
10. Rojeski MT, Gharib H. Nodular thyroid disease: evaluation and management. *N Engl J Med* 1985;313:428.
11. Belfiore A, La Rosa GL, La Porta GA, et al. Cancer risk in patients with cold thyroid nodules: relevance of iodine intake, sex, age, and multinodularity. *Am J Med* 1992;93:363.
12. Franklyn JA, Daykin J, Young J, et al. Fine needle aspiration cytology in diffuse or multinodular goitre compared with solitary thyroid nodules. *BMJ* 1993;307:240.
13. Singer PA, Cooper DS, Daniels GH, et al. Treatment guidelines for patients with thyroid nodules and well-differentiated thyroid cancer. *Arch Intern Med* 1996;156:2165.
14. Kahaly G, Dienes HP, Beyer J, et al. Randomized, double blind, placebo-controlled trial of low dose iodide in endemic goiter. *J Clin Endocrinol Metab* 1997;82:4049.
15. Studley J, Lynn J. Surgical anatomy of the thyroid gland and the technique of thyroidectomy. In: Lynn J, Bloom SR, eds. *Surgical endocrinology.* Oxford, UK: Butterworth-Heinemann, 1993:231.
16. Kaplan EL, Shukla M, Hara H, et al. Surgery of the thyroid. In: DeGroot LJ, ed. *Endocrinology,* 3rd ed. Vol. 1. Philadelphia: WB Saunders, 1995:900.
17. Delbridge L, Guinea AI, Reeve TS. Total thyroidectomy for bilateral benign multinodular goiter: effect of changing practice. *Arch Surg* 1999;134:1389.
18. Mishra A, Agarwal A, Agarwal G, et al. Total thyroidectomy for benign thyroid disorders in an endemic region. *World J Surg* 2001;25:307.
19. Hisham AN, Azlina AF, Aina EN, et al. Total thyroidectomy: the procedure of choice for multinodular goitre. *Eur J Surg* 2001; 167:403.
20. Mack E. Management of patients with substernal goiters. *Surg Clin North Am* 1995;75:377.
21. Al Suliman NN, Ryttov NF, Qvist N, et al. Experience in a specialist thyroid surgery unit: a demographic study, surgical complications, and outcome. *Eur J Surg* 1997;163:13.
22. Thomusch O, Machens A, Sekulla C, et al. Multivariate analysis of risk factors for postoperative complications in benign goiter surgery: prospective multicenter study in Germany. *World J Surg* 2000;24:1335.

23. Beahrs OH, Vandertoll DJ. Complications of secondary thyroidectomy. *Surg Gynecol Obstet* 1963;117:535.

24. Wilson DB, Staren ED, Prinz RA. Thyroid reoperations: indications and risks. *Am Surgeon* 1998;64:674.

25. Röjdmark J, Järhult J. High long term recurrence rate after subtotal thyroidectomy for nodular goitre. *Eur J Surg* 1995;161:725.

26. Ross DS. Thyroid hormone suppressive therapy of sporadic nontoxic goiter. *Thyroid* 1992;2:263.

27. Hegedüs L, Nygaard B, Hansen JM. Is routine thyroxine treatment to hinder postoperative recurrence of nontoxic goiter justified? *J Clin Endocrinol Metab* 1999;84:756.

28. Gharib H, Mazzaferri EL. Thyroxine suppressive therapy in patients with nodular thyroid disease. *Ann Intern Med* 1998;128:386.

29. Fogelfeld L, Wiviott MB, Shore-Freedman E, et al. Recurrence of thyroid nodules after surgical removal in patients irradiated in childhood for benign conditions. *N Engl J Med* 1989;320:835.

30. Hegedüs L, Hansen BM, Knudsen N, et al. Reduction of size of thyroid with radioactive iodine in multinodular non-toxic goitre. *BMJ* 1988;297:661.

31. Nygaard B, Hegedüs L, Gervil M, et al. Radioiodine treatment of multinodular non-toxic goitre. *BMJ* 1993;307:828.

32. Huysmans DAKC, Hermus ARMM, Corstens FHM, et al. Large, compressive goiters treated with radioiodine. *Ann Intern Med* 1994;121:757.

33. Wesche MF, Tiel-van Buul MM, Smits NJ, et al. Reduction in goiter size by ^{131}I therapy in patients with non-toxic multinodular goiter. *Eur J Endocrinol* 1995;132:86.

34. de Klerk JMH, van Isselt JW, van Dijk A, et al. Iodine-131 therapy in sporadic nontoxic goiter. *J Nucl Med* 1997;38:372.

35. Nygaard B, Faber J, Veje A, et al. Thyroid volume and function after ^{131}I treatment of diffuse non-toxic goitre. *Clin Endocrinol (Oxf)* 1997;46:493.

36. Hegedüs L, Bennedbaek FN. Radioiodine for non-toxic diffuse goitre. *Lancet* 1997;350:409.

37. Wesche MFT, Tiel-van Buul MMC, Lips P, et al. A randomized trial comparing levothyroxine with radioactive iodine in the treatment of sporadic nontoxic goiter. *J Clin Endocrinol Metab* 2001;86:998.

38. Bonnema SJ, Bertelsen H, Mortensen J, et al. The feasibility of high dose iodine 131 treatment as an alternative to surgery in patients with a very large goiter: effect on thyroid function and size and pulmonary function. *J Clin Endocrinol Metab* 1999;84:3636.

39. Le Moli R, Wesche MF, Tiel-van Buul MM, et al. Determinants of longterm outcome of radioiodine therapy of sporadic nontoxic goiter. *Clin Endocrinol (Oxf)* 1999;50:783.

40. Howarth DM, Epstein MT, Thomas PA, et al. Outpatient management of patients with large multinodular goitres treated with fractionated radioiodine. *Eur J Nucl Med* 1997;24:1465.

41. Huysmans D, Hermus A, Edelbroek M, et al. Radioiodine for nontoxic multinodular goiter. *Thyroid* 1997;7:235.

42. Nygaard B, Søes-Petersen U, Høilund-Carlsen PF, et al. Improvement of upper airway obstruction after ^{131}I-treatment of multinodular nontoxic goiter evaluated by flow volume loop curves. *J Endocrinol Invest* 1996;19:71.

43. Nygaard B, Faber J, Hegedüs L. Acute changes in thyroid volume and function following ^{131}I therapy of multinodular goitre. *Clin Endocrinol (Oxf)* 1994;41:715.

44. Nygaard B, Knudsen JH, Hegedüs L, et al. Thyrotropin receptor antibodies and Graves' disease, a side-effect of ^{131}I treatment in patients with nontoxic goiter. *J Clin Endocrinol Metab* 1997;82:2926.

45. Huysmans DAKC, Hermus ARMM, Edelbroek MAL, et al. Autoimmune hyperthyroidism occurring late after radioiodine treatment for volume reduction of large multinodular goiters. *Thyroid* 1997;7:535.

46. Huysmans DAKC, Buijs WCAM, van de Ven MTJ, et al. Dosimetry and risk estimates of radioiodine therapy for large, multinodular goiters. *J Nucl Med* 1996;37:2072.

47. Huysmans DA, Nieuwlaat W-A, Erdtsieck RJ, et al. Administration of a single low dose of recombinant human thyrotropin significantly enhances thyroid radioiodide uptake in nontoxic nodular goiter. *J Clin Endocrinol Metab* 2000;85:3592.

48. Nieuwlaat W-A, Hermus AR, Sivro-Prndelj F, et al. Pretreatment with recombinant human thyrotropin changes the regional distribution of radioiodine on thyroid scintigrams of nodular goiters. *J Clin Endocrinol Metab* 2001; 86:5330.

49. Nieuwlaat W-A, Huysmans DA, van den Bosch HC, et al. Pretreatment with a single, low dose of recombinant human thyrotropin allows dose reduction of radioiodine therapy in patients with nodular goiter. *J Clin Endocrinol Metab* 2003;88:3121.

50. Huysmans DA, Nieuwlaat WA, Hermus AR. Towards larger volume reduction of nodular goitres by radioiodine therapy; a role for pretreatment with recombinant human thyrotropin? *Clin Endocrinol (Oxf)* 2004;60:297.

51. Silva MNC, Rubió IGS, RomMão R, et al. Administration of a single dose of recombinant human thyrotropin enhances the efficacy of the radioiodine treatment of large compressive multinodular goitres. *Clin Endocrinol (Oxf)* 2004;60:300.

52. Hansen JM, Kampmann J, Madsen SN, et al. L-thyroxine treatment of diffuse non-toxic goitre evaluated by ultrasonic determination of thyroid volume. *Clin Endocrinol (Oxf)* 1979; 10:1.

53. Perrild H, Hansen JM, Hegedüs L, et al. Triiodothyronine and thyroxine treatment of diffuse non-toxic goitre evaluated by ultrasonic scanning. *Acta Endocrinol (Copenh)* 1982;100:382.

54. Berghout A, Wiersinga WM, Drexhage HA, et al. Comparison of placebo with L-thyroxine alone or with carbimazole for treatment of sporadic non-toxic goitre. *Lancet* 1990;336:193.

55. Uzzan B, Campos J, Cucherat M, et al. Effects on bone mass of long term treatment with thyroid hormones: a meta-analysis. *J Clin Endocrinol Metab* 1996;81:4278.

56. Biondi B, Fazio S, Carella C, et al. Cardiac effects of long term thyrotropin-suppressive therapy with levothyroxine. *J Clin Endocrinol Metab* 1993;77:334.

57. Ching GW, Franklyn JA, Stallard TJ, et al. Cardiac hypertrophy as a result of long-term thyroxine therapy and thyrotoxicosis. *Heart* 1996;75:363.

58. Shapiro LE, Sievert R, Ong L, et al. Minimal cardiac effects in asymptomatic athyreotic patients chronically treated with thyrotropin-suppressive doses of L-thyroxine. *J Clin Endocrinol Metab* 1997;82:2592.

59. Toft AD. Thyroxine therapy. *N Engl J Med* 1994;331:174.

60. Hermus AR, Huysmans DA. Treatment of benign nodular thyroid disease. *N Engl J Med* 1998;338:1438.

THYROID DISEASES: TUMORS

CARCINOMA OF FOLLICULAR EPITHELIUM

70A EPIDEMIOLOGY AND PATHOGENESIS

ARTHUR B. SCHNEIDER
ELAINE RON

The thyroid gland is an uncommon site of cancer, accounting for only 0.85% and 2.5% new cases of cancers among men and women, respectively, in the United States. Because of its favorable prognosis, thyroid carcinoma causes an even lower percentage of cancer deaths, 0.21% and 0.30% for men and women, respectively (1). Since 1980, the incidence of thyroid carcinoma in the United States has been increasing rapidly (2) (Fig. 70A.1). As shown in Figure 70A.1, among women the increase has been particularly steep since 1993 (4.3% per year, $p < .05$), whereas among men the rate has been increasing 1.9% per year ($p < .05$) since 1980. Thyroid carcinoma was the most rapidly increasing malignancy in women and the second most rapidly increasing in the general population (2) (Fig. 70A.2).

In contrast to incidence, the changes in mortality rates were much smaller. From the 1980s to 2000, the mortality rate for thyroid carcinoma increased by 1.0% per year ($p < .05\%$) among men, whereas there was no change (0.0% per year) in women. The increasing incidence is due in part to more sensitive diagnostic methods that find thyroid carcinomas with little or no propensity to progress. Improved treatment, a decline in anaplastic thyroid carcinoma (3), and the fact that the increase is primarily in early stage papillary carcinomas explain why, despite the increasing incidence, there has been little or no change in mortality.

The increasing incidence of thyroid carcinoma is not confined to the United States, as seen in Table 70A.1. To understand this apparently uniform increase in thyroid carcinoma incidence, birth cohort analyses have been performed. In Connecticut, where the incidence of papillary thyroid carcinoma in both women and men has been increasing since 1935, while the rates for other histologic types generally have been stable for the past two to three decades, the results of a birth cohort analysis fit the hypothesis that the increase was due to radiation treatment to the head and neck area of children, which is the only proven carcinogen (8). Similar results were observed in Canada and Norway (4,9). However, other factors, such as improved diagnosis, may be important as well. In some countries the incidence of thyroid carcinoma is no longer increasing (10,11).

Papillary thyroid carcinoma is the predominant histologic form in most parts of the world (12–14). The distribution has changed over time due to an increase in papillary carcinoma and a decrease in anaplastic carcinoma. From 1993 to 1997 the U.S. Surveillance, Epidemiology, and End Results (SEER) cancer registries reported 85.3% papillary (compared with 73.0% during 1973–1987), 10.9% follicular, 1.7% medullary, 0.78% anaplastic, and 1.3% other thyroid carcinomas in whites and 72.3% papillary, 20.5% follicular, 3.0% medullary, 0.5% anaplastic, and 4.2% other thyroid carcinomas in blacks (12,14). The worldwide distribution is similar, although in some areas the papillary/follicular ratio is smaller. In Sweden, from 1958 to 1987 there were 7,906 thyroid carcinomas reported to the national cancer registry. After excluding 947 (12%) that were actually follicular adenomas, 52% were classified as papillary thyroid carcinoma, 28% as follicular thyroid carcinoma, and 20% as anaplastic or medullary thyroid carcinoma (15). During this interval, the overall incidence of thyroid carcinoma increased, the incidence of papillary carcinoma increased, and the incidence of anaplastic carcinoma decreased (3). Similarly, in Canada and Switzerland, the increases over similar periods of time were confined to papillary carcinomas (Table 70A.1). A limitation in interpreting these trends is that a new histologic classification was published in 1988 (16). This caused some follicular carcinomas to be reclassified as a follicular variant of papillary carcinoma.

In the United States, thyroid carcinoma occurs about three times more frequently in women than in men, and this ratio is relatively constant over differ racial and ethnic groups. However, thyroid carcinoma incidence varies

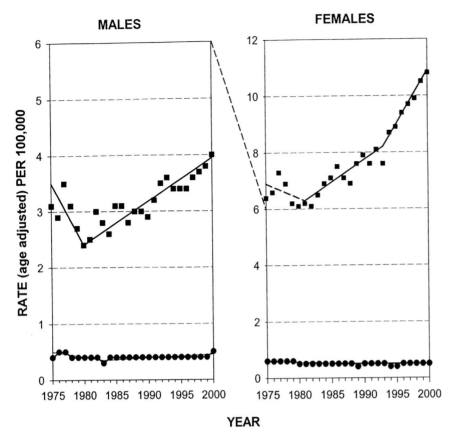

FIGURE 70A.1. Time trend in the United States for thyroid carcinoma incidence and mortality for men **(left)** and women **(right)** by year. The vertical scale for women is reduced by twofold compared with men. The data are fit with a program set to allow up to three connected lines. (Data from Ries LAG, Eisner MP, Kosary CL, et al. *SEER Cancer Statistics Review, 1975–2000.* Bethesda, MD: National Cancer Institute, 2003.)

among racial and ethnic groups (2). Age-adjusted rates are about twofold higher in white men and women compared with black men and women, whereas white Hispanics have nearly the same rates as non-Hispanic whites. The highest rates among U.S. residents are found in Filipino men and women, about twice those of whites.

External radiation is the clearest pathogenetic factor associated with thyroid carcinoma. Because thyroid carci-

noma is two to three times more common in women than in men, especially during the reproductive ages (17), hormonal factors probably are involved (Fig. 70A.3). However, after years of study, epidemiologic data are still inconclusive. Other environmental factors (e.g., diet) have been implicated in the etiology of thyroid carcinoma. Many of these factors are thought to operate through the action of thyrotropin (TSH). There is considerable evidence from

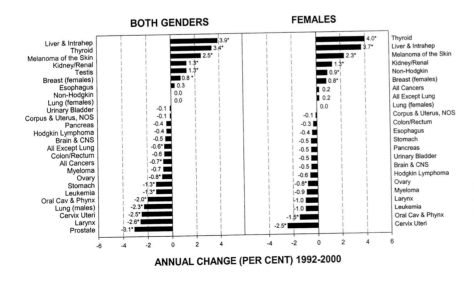

FIGURE 70A.2. Change in the incidence of various malignancies in the United States over the time interval 1975 to 2000. (Data from Ries LAG, Eisner MP, Kosary CL, et al. *SEER Cancer Statistics Review, 1975–2000.* Bethesda, MD: National Cancer Institute, 2003.)

TABLE 70A.1. TIME TRENDS FOR THYROID CARCINOMA IN VARIOUS PARTS OF THE WORLD

Geographical Area	Time Interval	Rate of Increase (%/yr)	
		Women	Men
United States (2)	1993–2000; 1980–2000	4.3	1.9
Canada (4)	1970–1996	2.7	2.9
Australia (5)	1982–1997	10.7	8.3
France (6)[a]	1978–1997	8.1	6.2
Sweden (3)	1958–1981	2.0	1.7
Vaud, Switzerland (7)[a]	1974–1998	2.8	2.9

[a]Papillary only.

animal experiments that prolonged TSH stimulation can cause thyroid carcinoma, but in humans the evidence is not as clear (18). Inherited genetic factors are related to thyroid carcinoma in familial adenomatous polyposis syndrome, Cowden's disease, and probably in other familial occurrences of thyroid carcinoma.

RADIATION

Although radiation can damage cells in several ways, it is generally accepted that it primarily causes carcinoma by its effects on DNA. The site of this initial DNA damage and the path leading to the eventual carcinoma involve multiple, as yet incompletely understood, steps (19). While radiation can initiate and possibly promote thyroid carcinogenesis, additional factors probably are required before clinically evident carcinoma occurs. Factors that increase TSH secretion may not be sufficient to cause thyroid carcinoma, but may stimulate tumorigenic growth. Thus, even after radiation damage has occurred, giving thyroid hormone treatment may prevent the progression to clinically important thyroid tumors.

External Radiation and Thyroid Carcinoma

The relationship between radiation and thyroid carcinoma was first recognized by Duffy and Fitzgerald in 1950 (20). They found that an unusually large fraction of their childhood thyroid carcinoma patients had a history of radiation therapy for benign conditions of the head and neck. This relationship was subsequently confirmed by many epidemiologic studies (21,22).

Several difficulties arise in studying the relationship between radiation exposure and thyroid carcinoma. Because thyroid carcinoma is a rare disease, few studies have sufficient statistical power to adequately quantify risk; the very good survival rate of thyroid carcinoma patients requires that incidence rather than mortality be assessed; because radiation exposure frequently occurs at a young age, people often are unaware of, or uncertain about, their exposure; and finally, the diagnosis of thyroid tumors is highly dependent on the extent of the procedures used to look for them (diagnostic bias). In the case control studies, cases of thyroid carcinoma were identified by their entry into a tumor registry or by their admission to a hospital. The control subjects were comparable subjects without thyroid carcinoma. Information on risk factors, such as radiation exposure, was obtained retrospectively and the distribution in the two groups compared. In case control studies, cases may report exposure to risk factors more completely than controls (recall bias). In the cohort studies, exposure to radiation generally was documented, and the characteristics and amount of exposure was known. The frequency of thyroid carcinoma in the radiation-exposed group was compared with a group of similar subjects who had little or no exposure. Therefore, in cohort studies, recall bias was minimized, but diagnostic bias could have been important. The evidence in Table 70A.2 is especially strong because multiple studies conducted in various locations using different methodologies report similar findings.

Ron et al (23) conducted a comprehensive analysis of radiation exposure and thyroid carcinoma, combining the data from seven studies that had individual thyroid dose estimates. Their analysis of childhood exposure, which included nearly 500 patients with thyroid carcinomas, demonstrated a strong positive association between radiation dose and thyroid carcinoma. Based on an excess relative risk model (i.e., risk increases multiplicatively with dose), a linear dose-response relationship fit the data well. A consistent and strong relationship between radiation exposure, possibly at doses as low as 0.1 Gy (10 rad) and thyroid carcinoma was found (21–23). At doses below 0.1 Gy, results have been equivocal, but a linear nonthreshold dose-response relationship fits the data well.

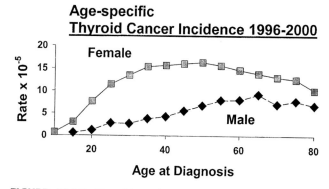

FIGURE 70A.3. Thyroid carcinoma incidence in the United States by age and sex. (Data from Ries LAG, Eisner MP, Kosary CL, et al. *SEER Cancer Statistics Review, 1975–2000.* Bethesda, MD: National Cancer Institute, 2003.)

TABLE 70A.2. SELECTED EPIDEMIOLOGIC STUDIES OF THE RELATIONSHIP BETWEEN EXTERNAL RADIATION AND THYROID CARCINOMA

Location (reference)	Study Population			Comments
	Age at Exposure	Exposed (*n*)	Nonexposed (*n*)	
Cohort studies[a]				
Boston, tonsils (24)	Children	1,192	1,063	Elevated risk for nodules
Chicago, tonsils (25)	Children	2,643	0	ERR/Gy = 2.5
China, background radiation (26)	All ages	1,001	1,005	No effect
China, radiology workers (27)	Adults	27,000	26,000	Doses unknown, relative risk = 2.1
Israel, tinea capitis (28)	Children	10,834	16,226	ERR/Gy = 32.5
Japan, atomic bomb (29)	All ages	41,234	38,738	ERR/Gy = 4.7 (children), 0.4 (adults)
Marshall Islands, fallout (30)	All ages	250	600	ERR/Gy = 0.3 (children), 0.5 (adults)
New York City, tinea capitis (21)	Children	2,200	1,400	ERR/Gy = 7.7 (not significant)
Rochester NY, thymus (31)	Children	2,475	4,991	ERR/Gy = 9.1
Utah-Nevada-Arizona, fallout (32)	Children	1,055	1,418	ERR/Gy = 7 for benign and malignant neoplasms combined, carcinoma not significant
		Cases (*n*)	Controls (*n*)	
Nested case control studies[a]				
International, cervical cancer (33)	Adults	43	81	ERR/Gy = 34.9
International, childhood cancer (34)	Children	22	82	ERR/Gy = 1.1

[a]In the cohort studies, individual doses were estimated, and dose-response relationships were evaluated. In the nested case control studies, cases had thyroid carcinoma, and controls did not. In the two case control studies, the cases were derived from 150,000 patients treated for carcinoma of the uterine cervix and 9,170 children treated for carcinoma, respectively. Controls in the Japan atomic bomb study were exposed to <0.01 Sv and in the Utah-Nevada-Arizona fallout study to <0.05 Gy. ERR, excess relative risk. All of the estimates of ERR are taken from reference 15, except for the Marshall Island study taken from reference 30 and the Utah-Nevada-Arizona study taken from reference 32.

Several additional observations, with important clinical implications, follow from the analysis of the pooled data. First, there is a strong inverse relationship between age at exposure and risk. In fact, there was little evidence for a radiation effect among persons exposed after age 15 years (Fig. 70A.4). Second, women tended to be more sensitive to the effects of radiation overall, although the difference between men and women is not statistically significant and is not consistent across studies. Third, the risk remains elevated several decades after the initial exposure. Between 5 and 30 years after exposure the risk is essentially constant. After 30 years, it appears to decline, but still remains elevated. However, depending on the model used to describe the data, the magnitude and duration of the risk can vary considerably, and more work is needed to determine which model is most appropriate (35).

Internal Radiation and Thyroid Carcinoma

It is now clear from the Chernobyl accident experience that exposure to radioactive iodine (RAI) during childhood is associated with an increased risk for thyroid carcinoma (36,37). Nevertheless, in the past few years, additional evidence has been obtained that adds support to the safety of using iodine 131 in the clinical setting. The following two sections summarize the evidence for both of these observations and discuss the likely explanations for this apparent paradox.

Iodine 131 Releases into the Environment

Even prior to the Chernobyl accident, there was concern about the carcinogenic potential of ^{131}I. In part, this came from experiments in animals, but it was unclear if these findings could be extrapolated to humans (38). Some people living on certain atolls of the Marshall Islands who were exposed to fallout from a nuclear test explosion in 1954 subsequently developed thyroid tumors, including carcinomas (30,39,40). However, their radiation exposure came from a combination of ^{131}I, other more rapidly decaying isotopes of iodine, and external gamma radiation.

Shortly after the accident at the Chernobyl power plant, which released an estimated 23 to 46 MCi of ^{131}I, reports began to appear of thyroid carcinoma occurring in exposed children. Because of the unusually short latency and the intense thyroid screening performed in the area, it was not immediately clear whether these carcinomas were attributable to exposure to ^{131}I from the accident. The data collected during the years since the accident now indicate that the sharp increase in childhood thyroid carcinoma is asso-

Dose-response by age at exposure

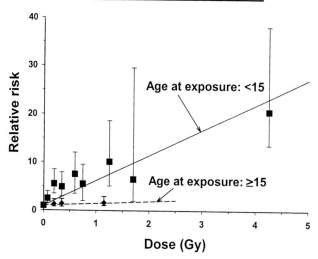

FIGURE 70A.4. Relative risk for thyroid carcinoma by age at radiation exposure. The dose-response relationship for age at exposure <15 years is compared with the dose-response for age at exposure ≥15 years. (Data from Ron E, Lubin JH, Shore RE, et al. Thyroid cancer after exposure to external radiation: a pooled analysis of seven studies. *Radiat Res* 1995;141:259.)

ciated with exposure to ^{131}I from Chernobyl (41–45). This conclusion is drawn from several lines of evidence. An international panel of pathologists has reviewed the thyroid carcinoma diagnoses and has confirmed about 95% them. The incidence of childhood thyroid neoplasms is far higher than the incidence prior to the accident, and the cases have been confined almost exclusively to children who were alive, or in utero, at the time of the accident. As has been demonstrated in studies of external radiation, the risk for developing thyroid carcinoma in the Chernobyl area has been found to increase with decreasing age at exposure. Furthermore, studies have linked thyroid dose with thyroid carcinoma incidence (44,46,47). For example, a case control study conducted in Belarus has demonstrated a statistically significant relationship between childhood thyroid carcinoma and individually estimated radiation doses (46). In addition, based on detailed dose reconstruction data from Ukraine, Belarus, and Russia, Jacob et al (47) correlated mean regional thyroid doses with thyroid carcinoma incidence and found a linear dose-response relationship. The risk estimates were similar to those reported for external radiation (23,48). However, only carefully conducted long-term studies will provide an accurate and complete account of the dose-response relationships.

There are several distinctive features of the Chernobyl-related cases of childhood thyroid carcinoma. The latency was shorter than previously reported for external radiation–related cases. This may be a result of intense thyroid screening, the promotion of thyroid tumorigenesis by iodine deficiency (43,49–55), or the extremely large number

of exposed individuals, which increases the chance to observe an uncommon disease. Furthermore, many of the cases had a unique histologic pattern of papillary carcinoma with a large solid component (56–60), and cases appeared to be rapidly growing and aggressive, with infiltration and lymph node involvement. Some of these findings are similar to those of thyroid carcinoma in children in general (61). Finally, the pattern of somatic mutations in the carcinomas, particularly in the *ret* proto-oncogene, appeared to be distinctive (see Chapter 70B).

In addition to the Marshall Islands and Chernobyl, ^{131}I was widely dispersed into the environment in the United States and elsewhere by above-ground nuclear tests (62) and as a by-product of plants preparing isotopes for use in nuclear weapons (63). An epidemiologic study of children exposed to nuclear fallout from weapons testing at the Nevada Test Site found a significant association between all thyroid nodules and dose, but not for thyroid carcinoma separately (32). In a detailed evaluation of thyroid doses received by Americans during the testing period, the estimated average collective dose was 2.0 cGy. For people under age 20 at the time of exposure, the mean dose was about 10 cGy (62). An ecologic study of U.S. thyroid carcinoma incidence and mortality rates and ^{131}I doses from the bomb tests was recently conducted (64). No association with cumulative dose was found, but associations were observed for children exposed under 1 year of age and those in the 1950 to 1959 birth cohort. Although it is impossible to determine the number of potential excess thyroid carcinomas caused by exposure to the tests, a National Academy of Sciences (USA) committee calculated that, if there is an excess, it is probably no more than 11,000 cases and that about 45% of them have already been diagnosed (65).

The Hanford nuclear site released ^{131}I into the atmosphere, particularly in its early years, as part of the process of preparing fissionable materials for the U.S. atomic program. Prior to studying the potential consequences of the resulting exposure, methods were devised to estimate ("reconstruct") individual thyroid doses. Subsequently, study individuals were selected to represent the spectrum of doses, to determine if there were any dose-response relationships for several thyroid diseases, particularly thyroid carcinoma. In the Hanford Thyroid Disease Study, the thyroid glands of 3,441 people who were born in the vicinity of the Hanford nuclear plant between 1940 and 1946 were thoroughly examined, including by ultrasound imaging. Among the 3,193 participants who lived in the Hanford site region during the years of atmospheric emissions, the mean and median thyroid doses were 18.6 and 10.0 cGy, respectively. No evidence of an increased risk for developing benign or malignant thyroid neoplasms associated with childhood exposure to the atmospheric releases of RAI from the Hanford Nuclear site was found (66).

The reasons for the apparent differences in the findings at Chernobyl and at Hanford are not clear. The roles of short-lived isotopes, iodine deficiency (43,49–55), and genetic predisposition need to be elucidated before the Chernobyl or the Hanford findings can confidently be extrapolated to other settings.

Medical Uses of Iodine 131

A great deal of effort has gone into assessing the relationship between ^{131}I used for therapeutic or diagnostic medical purposes and the development of thyroid carcinoma (67–78). These studies generally have been reassuring about the use of ^{131}I, but small increased risks for anaplastic thyroid carcinoma have been reported following ^{131}I therapy for hyperthyroidism (75,76). The U.S. Thyrotoxicosis Therapy Follow-up Study Group reported that among 35,593 hyperthyroid patients treated during 1946 to 1964 and followed through 1990, 63% of whom were treated with ^{131}I, total carcinoma mortality was not associated with ^{131}I use (76). However, the standardized mortality rate for thyroid carcinoma was slightly, but significantly, elevated, resulting in a very small number of excess thyroid carcinomas (76). Most of the deaths occurred soon after ^{131}I treatment, suggesting that the underlying thyroid disease may have been involved in the development of thyroid carcinoma or may have influenced the surveillance or reporting on death certificates (74). In a study conducted in Birmingham, England, 634 cancers were diagnosed among 7,417 hyperthyroid patients treated with [131]I (75,79). Although the overall cancer incidence and mortality rates were lower than expected compared with age, sex, and period-specific national rates, both the thyroid cancer incidence and mortality rate were significantly higher than expected.

In a study of 10,552 hyperthyroid patients treated with ^{131}I in Sweden, there was a nonsignificant 30% increased risk for thyroid carcinoma that was more pronounced among the toxic nodular goiter patients (69). No dose-response relationship was demonstrated. Although the number of excess cases of thyroid cancer was small in these investigations, the increased relative risk suggests that these patients need continued follow-up.

The health effects following diagnostic ^{131}I have been studied most thoroughly in Sweden (72,73,78). Among 36,792 predominantly adult patients administered diagnostic ^{131}I and followed through 1998, 24,010 had scans for reasons other than suspicion of a thyroid tumor and did not have a history of exposure to external radiation. The average absorbed thyroid dose was estimated to be 0.94 Gy. The number of observed thyroid carcinomas was very close to the number expected [respectively, 36 vs. 39.5 SIR (standardized incidence ratio) = 0.91; confidence interval (CI) 0.64–1.26]. In contrast, there was an increased risk among patients whose scan was performed due to suspicion of a tumor. Among patients with a his-

tory of external radiation exposure, the risk was about 10-fold. However, there was no evidence that the ^{131}I exposure contributed to the risk, because there was no effect of age or dose of ^{131}I exposure (78). When a sample of approximately 1,005 female patients examined with ^{131}I and 248 nonexposed female patient controls were examined for palpable thyroid nodularity, no excess was found among exposed women compared with nonexposed women. However, among the exposed women there was a significant relationship between ^{131}I dose and the prevalence of nodules (72).

It is of special interest to know if diagnostic ^{131}I exposure in children is associated with thyroid carcinoma; however, the available data are too sparse for any conclusions. After a mean of 20 years, examinations were performed on 789 people who had a history of diagnostic ^{131}I procedures (mean thyroid dose of 100 cGy) before age 18 and 1,118 controls who had other thyroid-related tests. Although no radiation effect was observed based on two exposed and three nonexposed cases (relative risk 0.86; CI 0.14–5.13), this study provides little relevant information (77). In this study, only 147 people were no more than 10 years of age at the time of ^{131}I administration, and the study was severely limited by the low and differential participation rates for exposed and nonexposed subjects (35% and 41%, respectively), which could result in substantial selection bias.

In general, studies of adult ^{131}I exposure for therapeutic and diagnostic purposes continue to be reassuring, but some aspects of the studies suggest a small effect, apparently related to ^{131}I exposure, on thyroid nodularity, thyroid carcinoma incidence, and thyroid carcinoma mortality. Although a causal relationship is possible, it may be that the observations represent the nature of the underlying thyroid condition or an increase in surveillance and diagnostic misclassification.

Comparison of External and Internal Radiation

The reasons for the apparent difference between external and internal radiation are not known with certainty. One factor is undoubtedly age at exposure, which has a very strong modifying effect for external radiation (Fig. 70A.4). Because most of the patients included in studies of the medical uses of ^{131}I have been adults, the results cannot be extrapolated to children. Another factor is that compared with the instantaneous dose received from external radiation, the lower dose rate of ^{131}I may allow repair of radiation damage. Finally, when ^{131}I is administered, it results in a wide range of doses to different areas of the thyroid, whereas external radiation exposes the entire thyroid to the same dose, making it difficult to compare the two types of radiation. Exposures to ^{131}I, as occurs in the medical setting, may not be applicable to the more prolonged exposures people generally receive from fallout or living near nuclear production facilities.

Preventing Radiation-Related Thyroid Carcinoma

Functioning nuclear plants continue to generate iodine isotopes in large quantities that could, in the case of an accident or terrorist attack, pose a threat to the surrounding population. Potassium iodide (KI), if taken promptly, effectively reduces the dose to the thyroid (80). Following the Chernobyl accident, KI was widely administered to residents of Poland (81). The success of the program and the rarity of observed side effects support the distribution of KI as an effective means of reducing ^{131}I exposure in the event of a nuclear accident (82). The World Health Organization and the U.S. Food and Drug Administration have both adopted age-based guidelines for the use of KI in case of an emergency, taking into account the varying sensitivity of the thyroid shown in Figure 70A.4 (83). In some countries the distribution of KI has been achieved, whereas in the United States evaluation is continuing, and implementation varies from state to state (84).

Evaluation of Irradiated Patients

An essential part of evaluating a person with a history of irradiation is determining the type of radiation, the site or sites treated, the age at treatment, and the dose (21,23, 85,86). Among these factors, the dose received by the thyroid is the most important, because risk increases linearly with increasing dose. The dose timing may modify risk, with fractionation possibly reducing it. Age at the time of radiation exposure is an independent risk factor, with younger age at exposure associated with greater risk. There is a greater spontaneous thyroid carcinoma risk for women than men, but it is unclear whether radiation increases the risk for thyroid carcinoma equally for women and men.

External irradiation formerly was used to treat a wide range of benign conditions during childhood. These included enlargement of the thymus, tonsils, adenoids, and cervical lymph nodes, as well as pertussis, asthma, bronchitis, tinea capitis, and acne. In most cases the radiation treatment resulted in an increased risk for thyroid carcinoma. Other commonly used forms of radiotherapy involved local application of radioactive plaques to treat hemangiomas, other localized lesions, and enlarged tonsils, as well as radium rods inserted through the nose into the nasopharynx as treatment for impaired eustachian tube function and hearing loss. Following treatment for hemangioma, the mean dose to the thyroid was about 0.2 Gy, and the excess relative risks were significantly increased (87,88) and consistent with those from the pooled analysis of exter-

nal radiation (23). In contrast, treatment with nasopharyngeal radium rods resulted in very low doses to the thyroid (mean dose < 0.02 Gy) and no excess of thyroid carcinomas (89–92).

Currently, external radiation of the neck for malignant conditions such as childhood cancer, Hodgkin's disease, and carcinoma of the larynx is used widely. Such treatment often results in subclinical or overt hypothyroidism (93–95), and sometimes in nodular thyroid disease and thyroid carcinoma (96,97). Although the dose to the thyroid following radiation therapy for breast carcinoma frequently is high, no dose-related excess of thyroid carcinoma was found in two recent studies (98,99). Although diagnostic radiologic examinations may confer some risk for thyroid carcinoma, a large case control study in Sweden (484 cases of thyroid carcinoma and 484 controls) found no association with prior diagnostic radiography (100). A smaller case control study from Sweden, using medical records and dentist cards to estimate radiation exposure, reached the same conclusion (101). Thus, it is important to obtain the best radiation history possible, because it is needed to decide whether further evaluation, particularly thyroid imaging, should be performed.

How to examine a patient with a history of radiation exposure is a deceptively simple question (102). Thyroid palpation has limited sensitivity, but whether imaging should be used remains controversial. The limitations of palpation are shown by the following illustrative studies involving radiation-exposed individuals. In one small series, about half of the nodules found by ultrasonography that were larger than 1.5 cm were not palpable (103). In a larger series, about two thirds of the palpable nodules were not confirmed by ultrasonography (104). The use of imaging is supported by the observation that many people with nodular thyroid disease, including carcinoma, were discovered solely by imaging (103,105). On the other hand, ultrasonography is associated with considerable observer variation and may be too sensitive because approximately one third of adult women have ultrasound-detectable thyroid nodules (106,107). Some clinicians believe that even if imaging identifies otherwise undetectable nodules, they are too small to be of clinical consequence and can be safely ignored until they become palpable.

To determine the clinical importance of a nonpalpable nodule larger than 10 mm in diameter, ultrasound-guided fine-needle aspiration (FNA) is the method of choice (108). However, it is important to know if FNA is as reliable in radiation-exposed patients. Two reports provide some reassurance, although they also point out the limitations of FNA (109,110). The sensitivity and specificity rates of FNA were similar for a given size of nodule to those reported for nodules not associated with radiation, but because radiation-exposed thyroids frequently have multiple nodules, small carcinomas are more likely to be missed.

However, these small carcinomas may not be clinically important. A reasonable approach is to reserve ultrasound imaging for irradiated patients who are at especially high risk (102,111).

There is no evidence that subclinical or overt hypothyroidism or thyrotoxicosis result from the level of radiation dose used to treat benign childhood conditions (112). However, there is some, as yet unconfirmed, data suggesting a relationship between autoimmune thyroid disease and radiation (113,114). The evaluation and treatment of patients with nodular disease is discussed further in Chapters 68 and 69 and in the next section of this chapter.

Patients with a currently normal thyroid and a history of irradiation should be examined periodically. Radiation-related nodular disease continues to occur for as long as it has been possible to study patients irradiated between 1939 and 1962 (25,115,116). Patients at especially high risk should have thyroid ultrasound imaging as part of their follow-up examination. Ultrasound results should be interpreted with caution, given the high prevalence of abnormalities found in the general adult population. Examples of high-risk patients are those with one or more of the factors listed in Table 70A.3. An examination interval of 1 to 2 years and an imaging interval of 3 to 5 years, continued indefinitely, seem prudent.

Prophylactic therapy to prevent the occurrence of nodular thyroid disease should be considered in patients who received radiation treatment (117,118). One report demonstrated the effectiveness of thyroid hormone therapy in preventing the appearance of nodules in irradiated patients, but this was not confirmed by another (119,120). In patients at high risk, thyroxine (T_4) therapy has potential benefits that probably outweigh its risks. In this instance a reasonable definition of high risk is more than one of the factors listed in Table 70A.3. Also, an abnormal or equivocal thyroid imaging finding, such as a nodule seen by ultrasonography that is too small to aspirate, would contribute to a classification of high risk. Even if only benign nodules occur less frequently in T_4-treated patients, the reduction of both anxiety and the likelihood of surgery is important.

Other head and neck tumors may arise in patients with a history of childhood radiation exposure, some of which can have equal or greater clinical consequence for the patient than thyroid tumors. Parathyroid adenomas and hyperparathyroidism have been reported in people who received radiation therapy (121–124). Whether the parathyroid glands show the marked age-related sensitivity characteristic of the thyroid gland is not clear. After radiation exposure, salivary gland tumors most commonly occur in the parotid glands and are usually readily evident to the patient. About two thirds are benign, and most of these are of the mixed cell variety. Mucoepidermoid carcinomas were the most common malignant form. A dose-response relationship was observed among atomic bomb survivors and the Michael Reese patients (125,126). Salivary gland neoplasms can occur many years after radiation exposure (125–128). Benign and malignant neural tumors also can be radiation related (129–131). Benign neural tumors, particularly neurilemomas and acoustic neuromas, occasionally occur as multiple tumors in an individual following childhood radiation therapy (130,131). Finally, an elevated risk of nonmelanoma skin carcinoma has been observed on the face and scalp among several of the irradiated groups studied (29,132–134).

Clinical Features of Radiation-Related Thyroid Neoplasms

A history of radiation exposure has two major clinical implications: the increased risk for developing thyroid nodules and the increased risk for a thyroid nodule being malignant. In the Michael Reese tonsil group (mean dose to the thyroid ~60 cGy), more than one third of radiation-exposed patients who had thyroidectomies had a thyroid carcinoma (116).

Follow-up studies so far indicate that external radiation-related thyroid carcinomas behave the same as other thyroid carcinomas in both children and adults (135–138). A nested case control study of 364 thyroid carcinomas (91 in radiation-exposed patients vs. 273 matched unexposed controls) was performed in France. Cases had a higher frequency of multifocal carcinomas and more frequent local residual carcinoma. However, the rates of recurrence and thyroid carcinoma-related mortality did not differ. Therefore, therapy and follow-up should be similar to that provided to other patients with thyroid carcinoma. As mentioned above, the behavior of the Chernobyl-related carcinomas may be especially aggressive. Whether this behavior is due to the young age at diagnosis and iodine deficiency at the time of exposure remains to be determined.

The thyroid carcinomas that arise in relation to radiation treatment are almost all well-differentiated papillary or papillary-follicular carcinomas. Case reports of anaplastic thyroid carcinoma occurring after radiation treatment are rare (139). There is no evidence that the well-differentiated radiation-related thyroid carcinomas are more likely to undergo transition to more aggressive or less differentiated malignancies. It is possible, however, that as the population ages, more aggressive carcinomas will be seen, as occurs in the general population (140).

All irradiated patients who have had nodular thyroid disease treated by thyroidectomy should receive thyroid hormone treatment, even if enough of the gland remains to maintain normal thyroid hormone secretion. This recom-

TABLE 70A.3. RISK FACTORS ASSOCIATED WITH RADIATION-INDUCED THYROID TUMORS

Amount of radiation exposure
Young age at exposure to radiation
High serum thyroglobulin concentration
Other radiation-related tumor(s)

mendation is based on the observation that nodules continue to occur in these patients with equal or greater frequency compared with patients who did not have surgery. When thyroid hormone therapy is given after thyroidectomy, the frequency of recurrence is reduced (141).

The carcinomas in the children from the Chernobyl region have presented with a high frequency of advanced features. Of the approximately 1,500 cases from Belarus, Ukraine, and Russia, 45% were classified as pT4 (142). Treatment of more advanced cases has included RAI. In 249 patients treated with one or more courses of RAI, only 129 (51.8%) were completely ablated, suggesting increased resistance to RAI therapy (143). In another group of 209 Belarus children treated in Germany with 755 RAI treatment courses, 84% of the carcinomas were ablated and none progressed following the treatment (142).

FAMILIAL THYROID CARCINOMA

The existence of two familial syndromes that include carcinoma of the thyroid of follicular cell origin supports the existence of genetic factors in the pathogenesis of thyroid carcinoma. Thyroid carcinomas occur in association with familial adenomatous polyposis (FAP) and its subtype, Gardner's syndrome, which is FAP associated with osteomas, epidermoid cysts, and desmoid tumors. Both are dominantly inherited conditions with mutations in the *APC* gene. In fact, thyroid carcinoma is considered to be the most common noncolonic malignancy in these syndromes. As reviewed by Hizawa et al (144), the risk for thyroid carcinoma is increased by more than 100-fold over the general population. In the Leeds Castle Polyposis database, 45 patients (1.2%) had thyroid carcinoma (145). Because there was only one death from thyroid carcinoma and the frequency was relatively low, Bulow et al concluded that screening for thyroid carcinoma is not indicated. However, it seems prudent to perform careful palpation of the thyroid in any patient with these syndromes. The thyroid carcinomas in these syndromes have two distinguishing features. They tend to occur at an early age, often before 35 years (146), and they have a distinct histologic pattern (147,148). The carcinomas are papillary carcinomas with a cribriform pattern and solid, spindle cell–containing areas. One clue to the pathogenesis of these carcinomas comes from the observation that the germline mutations in *APC* of cases with thyroid carcinoma tend to cluster in a region of the gene associated with extracolonic features of the disease (149). Another clue is that there is no loss of heterozygosity or biallelic mutations in the *APC* gene (in six cases) and that ret/ptc1 activation is often (in four of the six cases) found (150). Whether reduced *APC* activity facilitates *ret* translocaction remains to be determined.

The second familial syndrome associated with thyroid carcinoma is Cowden's disease, a rare autosomal-dominant disorder involving the development of multiple hamartomatous polyps, mucocutaneous pigmentation, and extraintestinal manifestations. Thyroid abnormalities, including thyroid carcinomas, are common in these cases (151, 152). Mutations in the *PTEN* gene, a tumor suppressor gene that functions as a protein phosphatase, cause the syndrome.

Studies of family patterns of nonmedullary thyroid carcinoma have provided increasing evidence supporting the existence of additional hereditary factors. In a systematic study of 576 people with thyroid carcinoma in Utah, using extensive family history records and the state tumor registry, 28 first-degree relatives were found to have thyroid carcinoma (153). The expected number of cases was only 3.3, and compared with 27 other sites of malignancy, this was the largest increase found. In Norway, the number of thyroid carcinomas in 5,457 first-degree relatives of patients with thyroid carcinoma was about fivefold greater than expected (154). Using the Swedish Family Cancer Registry covering 9.6 million people, Hemminki and colleagues have examined the familial risk for thyroid carcinoma (155). When a parent had papillary or follicular thyroid carcinoma, the risk for an offspring developing thyroid carcinoma was 7.8 (95% CI 3.9–13.2) for a son and 2.8 (95% CI 1.4–4.5) for a daughter. These familial risks were higher than for any other cancer site.

There have been multiple reports of family aggregates of papillary thyroid carcinoma. For example, in a clinical study, 6% of 226 patients with papillary carcinoma reported having at least one relative who also had a papillary thyroid carcinoma (156). In two case control studies, relative risks of 5 and 10 were found in close relatives of patients with nonmedullary thyroid carcinoma (157,158).

There is some debate about the behavior of the thyroid carcinomas found in family clusters. In one series, the high frequency of lymph node and local invasion was cited as reason for aggressive treatment (159). In a review of 15 case series, containing 87 families with 178 cases, evidence for aggressive presentation was present in only 6 (160). Although the investigator did not advocate therapy more aggressive than usual, it should be noted that the overall frequency, where it was reported, of distant metastases (10%) and recurrences (29%) was high. Two other studies showed high rates of recurrence (16% and 44%) and advocated aggressive therapy (161,162). So far, other than *APC* and *PTEN*, mentioned above, no gene, including the two potential candidate genes, *FAP* and *ret*, has been identified as a cause of familial thyroid carcinoma (163–165).

It has been hypothesized that there are genetic factors related to the probability of developing radiation-induced thyroid tumors. If so, then patients who have one radiation-associated tumor (thyroid, salivary, or benign neural) might be more likely to develop a second tumor than other patients without a tumor but with comparable radiation exposure and other risk factors. Although earlier observations supported this possibility (130,166), more recent data do not (167). Another way to evaluate a genetic sensitivity to radiation tumorigenesis is to see whether siblings who were both irradiated had a higher rate of concordance than expected. Earlier analysis of thyroid nodules, but not thyroid carcinoma, showed that concordance occurred more often than would be expected by chance (168). However, when all radiation-related neoplasms are considered together and other known risk factors are taken into account, more recent analyses show that there is no excess concordance.

PREEXISTING THYROID DISEASE

Thyroid carcinoma is often preceded by other thyroid abnormalities, including endemic and sporadic goiter, benign thyroid nodules, lymphocytic thyroiditis, and Graves' disease, all of which are common. Whether patients with these abnormalities should be considered at increased risk for developing thyroid carcinoma is uncertain. Despite considerable efforts to resolve this question, results remain inconclusive. Many case control studies of thyroid carcinoma have revealed more preexisting benign thyroid nodules and goiter in the carcinoma patients than in the control subjects (157,169–176). The risks have been high, especially for nodules. A pooled analysis of 14 case control studies (177–180) with 2,725 cases and 4,776 controls was conducted to allow a systematic approach to analyzing and interpreting major hypotheses for thyroid carcinoma etiology. Large risks were associated with a self-reported history of goiter (odds ratio 5.9) or benign nodules (odds ratio 30) among women (177). Case control studies, however, are especially subject to recall bias, in which cases may remember all previous thyroid diseases while controls may forget them. This is less of a problem in prospective studies. In one prospective study of women with benign thyroid conditions in Boston, there was a significant excess of thyroid carcinoma mortality among patients with thyroid adenomas (181). In a cohort study of 204,964 members of a large health plan, 196 thyroid carcinomas occurred, and a history of goiter (as well as Asian race, educational attainment, family history, and radiation exposure) was a risk factor (relative risk 3.36; CI 1.82–6.20) (182). In a multi-ethnic case control study designed to explain the higher incidence of thyroid carcinoma among Asian women living in the San Francisco area, prior goiter and nodules were significant explanatory factors (183). Perhaps the most convincing study is one from Denmark (184,185). In the period 1977 to 1991 there were 57,326 patients discharged from Danish hospitals with a diagnosis of myxedema, thyrotoxicosis, or goiter. The subsequent incidence of thyroid carcinoma was ascertained through the Danish Cancer Registry and compared with thyroid carcinoma incidence in the general population. The incidence of thyroid carci-

noma was increased among all three patient groups but was substantially higher among goiter patients. However, prospective studies remain subject to potential ascertainment bias (i.e., one thyroid disorder could draw attention to another). In the Danish study, the thyroid carcinoma risk decreased with time following hospital discharge, but the risk remained elevated even 10 years later. The cumulated data now suggest that a history of goiter or benign thyroid nodules is a strong thyroid carcinoma risk factor.

Recent genetic data suggest that thyroid neoplasms may progress from benign tumors to well-differentiated carcinomas to anaplastic carcinomas, as somatic mutations accumulate (see next section). The epidemiologic data relating previous nodular thyroid disease to thyroid carcinoma are consistent with this model.

HORMONAL AND REPRODUCTIVE FACTORS

Thyroid carcinoma, like most other thyroid diseases, occurs more frequently in women than men, suggesting that hormonal factors are involved in its pathogenesis. In England and Wales, the female to male ratio was highest at the time of puberty. From puberty to menopause, the difference between females and males declined consistently (17). In Switzerland, the female to male ratio at puberty for papillary carcinoma was high, but for follicular carcinoma the ratio was highest between the ages of 25 and 44 years (186). These findings suggest that hormonal events occurring at puberty or during the early reproductive years might be important in influencing the development of papillary thyroid carcinoma, but few significant relationships between hormonal and reproductive factors and thyroid carcinoma have been found, and often the findings have not been consistent across studies (157,170,171, 173,174,187–190). In a pooled analysis of thyroid carcinoma etiology, there was a small but significantly positive trend for risk to increase with increasing age at menarche (179).

Results from some, but not all, epidemiologic studies indicate that parity may increase the risk for thyroid carcinoma (157,170,171,173,191–193). The pooled analysis found a slightly elevated risk associated with having had at least one child but no relationship with number of children (179). The most convincing data come from a prospective study of 1.1 million Norwegian women of reproductive age. Based on almost 1,000 thyroid carcinomas, a significant trend for increasing risk with increasing parity was demonstrated (191). In an attempt to distinguish the role of the biologic effects of pregnancy from lifestyle or environmental exposures, the number of children of male thyroid carcinoma patients was studied (194). No trend was found, which led the researchers to conclude that the parity effect was due to biologic changes during pregnancy.

Results from the pooled analysis also suggest that thyroid carcinoma occurs more often among women who are older when they first give birth (179). Data from some studies suggest that women with a history of spontaneous or induced abortion, particularly during the first pregnancy, have an enhanced risk for thyroid carcinoma (31,157,170, 189,190), that the risk of thyroid carcinoma may be elevated among women seeking medical care for fertility problems (195,196), and that women undergoing hysterectomy may be at increased risk for developing thyroid carcinoma (192,197), but these findings were not confirmed in the pooled analysis (179).

Three studies, from Washington State, the San Francisco area, and Kuwait, each suggest that recent pregnancy, within about 5 years, is a thyroid carcinoma risk factor and that the risk is even higher with more than one recent pregnancy (198–200). Whether these observations are confirmed and, if so, whether they are related to hormonal effects or are incidental to increased pregnancy-related medical attention, remains to be seen.

Other suggested risk factors for thyroid carcinoma in women are exogenous estrogens, including oral contraceptives (170,173,201), lactation suppressant drugs (201), postmenopausal estrogen therapy (201), and fertility drugs (189). These associations, however, were usually weak and not dose dependent. In the recent pooled analysis, current oral contraceptive users had a moderately increased risk, which disappeared 10 or more years after discontinuing use (178). No significant risks were reported for use of hormone replacement therapy or fertility drugs, but the odds ratio for drugs used to suppress lactation was elevated. Although positive associations between hormonal and reproductive factors and the incidence of thyroid carcinoma have been found in some studies, they are generally weak and not always consistent across studies.

Two studies, both conducted among irradiated individuals, have looked at reproductive factors and benign thyroid tumors (202,203). One study showed a protective effect of pregnancy, whereas, in apparent contradiction, both showed a nonsignificant increase in risk with number of pregnancies.

DIETARY FACTORS

Iodine

A relationship between iodine-deficient endemic goiter and thyroid carcinoma has been suspected since Wegelin (204) reported more thyroid carcinoma at autopsy in Bern, an endemic goiter area, compared with Berlin, a nonendemic goiter area. Since then, several studies of the effects of iodine supplementation on the incidence of thyroid carcinoma have, with at least one exception, failed to show a decline. In Switzerland, thyroid carcinoma mortality de-

creased after the introduction of iodized salt (205), but it did not decrease in Italy or the United States (206,207). In Austria, the incidence continued to increase after the introduction of iodine prophylaxis (208). In Sweden, the incidence of thyroid carcinoma has continued to increase in both iodine-deficient and iodine-sufficient areas (3).

The effects of iodine intake on specific histologic types of thyroid carcinomas are clearer. In endemic goiter areas, follicular and, perhaps, anaplastic thyroid carcinoma predominate. When iodine supplementation is introduced, the proportion of papillary carcinomas increases and that of follicular carcinomas decreases (18,209,210). In Hawaii, where iodine intake is extremely high, the proportion of papillary carcinoma is also high (189). In Sweden, the risk for follicular carcinoma was higher in iodine-deficient areas than in iodine-sufficient areas, whereas the pattern was opposite for papillary carcinoma (211). Similar findings were reported in Sicily (212). These data suggest that follicular carcinomas are related to iodine deficiency and prolonged TSH stimulation.

There are several studies in which iodine intake was evaluated, and a pooled analysis of case control studies of fish and shellfish intake has recently appeared (213). In a case control study in Hawaii in which iodine intake from food sources and supplements was quantitated, iodine intake was higher in the patients with thyroid carcinoma than in the control subjects (189). There have been seven case control studies in which fish and shellfish consumption was examined as a surrogate measure of iodine intake. In all but the Hawaiian study the dietary data were extremely limited and, therefore, the findings should be interpreted with caution. Because shellfish generally have a higher iodine content than fish, they are a better indication of high iodine intake. Although the results were not always statistically significant, fish or shellfish consumption was reported more frequently among cases than controls in four studies (157,173,189,214). In a Norwegian population-based study a similar conclusion was reached based on the observation that among women, being married to a fisherman was a risk factor for thyroid carcinoma (215). In contrast, results from northern Italy and Vaud, Switzerland, indicated a protective effect of fish (216). In a study conducted in northern Sweden, the results were equivocal: adult consumption of fish appeared to be associated with a slightly decreased risk for thyroid carcinoma, and shellfish intake with a higher risk (188). The pooled analysis of these studies suggests that high fish consumption is not associated with thyroid carcinoma, except in areas of iodine deficiency, where it may have a beneficial effect (213).

Other Dietary Factors

Some dietary factors have been related to thyroid carcinoma, but many findings have been reported in single studies or have been inconsistent. In most studies, vegetables, particularly cruciferous ones, appear to be associated with a reduced risk for thyroid carcinoma (157,189,216). This would be a somewhat surprising finding, since these vegetables contain natural goitrogens. However, in a pooled analysis of 10 case control studies, the risk reduction associated with cruciferous vegetables is of borderline significance for moderate consumption (odds ratio 0.87; CI 0.75–1.01) and not significant for high consumption (odds ratio 0.94; CI 0.80–1.10) (217). In another pooled analysis, of Italian and Swiss studies, pasta, bread, pastry, and potatoes were associated with an increased risk (216), and in studies from Norway and Sweden, consumption of butter and cheese was associated with an increased risk (218). In a study from Hawaii, the cases reported eating more fat, protein, and carbohydrates than the control subjects. The higher total calorie intake among cases is consistent with an association of thyroid carcinoma with obesity seen in the Hawaiian study (189), as well as two other epidemiologic studies (157,201). Finally, in studies conducted in Greece and Japan, coffee consumption appeared to protect against thyroid carcinoma, but not in Los Angeles County (219–221).

SMOKING, PHARMACEUTICAL AGENTS, AND TOXINS

Cigarette smoking has been associated with a decreased risk for thyroid carcinoma in three recently reported case control studies (192,222,223). In Washington state 410 women with papillary carcinoma were compared with 574 controls. Ever having smoked 100 cigarettes was associated with a decreased odds ratio of 0.7 (CI 0.5–0.9) (223). In Northern Norway and Central Sweden 191 papillary and follicular cases were compared with 341 controls (192). Smoking was associated with an odds ratio of 0.69 (CI 0.47–1.01), and in premenopausal women it was 0.60 (CI 0.38–0.96). In Canada, 1,224 cases were compared with 2,659 controls (222). The risk ratios were reduced in male (0.77; CI 0.58–1.02) and female (0.71; CI 0.60–0.84) smokers. Notably, there were dose-response relationships for the duration and amount smoked. The relative uniformity of the estimates of risk reduction and the dose-response relationships support the physiologic relevance of the observation. However, two other recent reports, from the San Francisco area and Los Angeles County, did not find an effect of smoking (182,221). It is not clear why cigarette smoking should reduce the risk for thyroid carcinoma, but current smoking has been shown to reduce TSH levels in some studies (224).

Although no pharmaceutical agent or toxin has been implicated in the etiology of thyroid carcinoma in humans, there is reason to remain open to this possibility. Drugs such as lithium and phenobarbital are known to cause goiter and increased serum TSH concentrations, making it reasonable to suspect that certain drugs could cause or promote the growth of thyroid carcinoma. In rodents, a variety of drugs and other chemicals cause thyroid growth and thyroid neoplasms (225). None of them have been shown to be thyroid mutagens. Rather, they appear to act by interfering with the synthesis of thyroid hormones or by altering the peripheral metabolism of thyroid hormones (226). In either case, the increased TSH secretion, possibly combined with subsequent random events or events promoted by the TSH stimulation, may lead to thyroid neoplasms (227,228). Patients with congenital goiter have thyroid glands that are subjected to intense TSH stimulation until appropriate treatment is given. Rarely, such patients develop thyroid carcinoma, supporting the possibility that intense TSH stimulation contributes to thyroid carcinogenesis in humans (229,230).

SUMMARY

Radiation is the clearest risk factor for thyroid carcinoma in humans, but a history of goiter or benign nodules also appears to significantly increase the risk for developing thyroid carcinoma. One of the major problems in understanding the pathogenesis of thyroid carcinoma is the need to take histology into account. The four major histologic types of thyroid carcinoma (papillary, follicular, anaplastic, and medullary) may have different risk factors, and the rarity of the disease makes it extremely difficult to study the histologic types separately. Although pooling data from several studies of radiation-induced thyroid carcinoma has helped resolve questions regarding the shape of the dose-response curve and effect modification, similar pooling of data from etiologic studies of thyroid carcinoma so far has been less informative. The roles of iodine, diet, reproductive and hormonal factors, and genetics still remain unclear.

REFERENCES

1. Jemal A, Murray T, Samuels A, et al. Cancer statistics, 2003. *CA Cancer J Clin* 2003;53:5–26.
2. Ries LAG, Eisner MP, Kosary CL, et al. SEER Cancer Statistics Review, 1975–2000. Bethesda, MD: National Cancer Institute, 2003. *seer.cancer.gov/csr/1975_2000*.
3. Pettersson B, Coleman MP, Ron E, et al. Iodine supplementation in Sweden and regional trends in thyroid cancer incidence by histopathologic type. *Int J Cancer* 1996;65:13–19.
4. Liu S, Semenciw R, Ugnat AM, et al. Increasing thyroid cancer incidence in Canada, 1970–1996: time trends and age-period-cohort effects. *Br J Cancer* 2001;85:1335–1339.
5. Burgess JR. Temporal trends for thyroid carcinoma in Australia: an increasing incidence of papillary thyroid carcinoma (1982–1997). *Thyroid* 2002;12:141–149.
6. Colonna M, Grosclaude P, Remontet L, et al. Incidence of thyroid cancer in adults recorded by French cancer registries (1978–1997). *Eur J Cancer* 2002;38:1762–1768.
7. Levi F, Randimbison L, Te VC, et al. Thyroid cancer in Vaud, Switzerland: an update. *Thyroid* 2002;12:163–168.

8. Zheng TZ, Holford TR, Chen YT, et al. Time trend and age-period-cohort effect on incidence of thyroid cancer in Connecticut, 1935–1992. *Int J Cancer* 1996;67:504–509.

9. Akslen LA, Haldorsen T, Thoresen SØ, et al. Incidence pattern of thyroid cancer in Norway—influence of birth cohort and time period. *Int J Cancer* 1993;53:183–187.

10. Hrafnkelsson J, Jonasson JG, Sigurdsson G, et al. Thyroid cancer in Iceland 1955–1984. *Acta Endocrinol (Copenh)* 1988;118:566–572.

11. Akslen LA, Haldorsen T, Thoresen SO, et al. Incidence of thyroid cancer in Norway 1970–1985: population review on time trend, sex, age, histological type and tumour stage in 2625 cases. *APMIS* 1990;98:549–558.

12. Correa P, Chen VW. Endocrine gland cancer. *Cancer* 1995;75:338–352.

13. Ron E. Thyroid cancer. In: Schottenfeld D, Fraumeni Jr JF, eds. *Cancer epidemiology and prevention,* 2nd ed. New York: Oxford University Press, 1996:1000–1021.

14. Parkin DM, Whelan SL, Ferlay J, et al. *Cancer incidence in five continents.* Vol. VIII. Lyon: IARC Scientific, 2002.

15. Lundgren CI, Hall P, Ekbom A, et al. Incidence and survival of Swedish patients with differentiated thyroid cancer. *Int J Cancer* 2003;106:569–573.

16. Hedinger C, Williams ED, Sobin LH. *International histological typing of thyroid tumours,* 2nd ed. Berlin: Springer-Verlag, 1988.

17. dos Santos Silva I, Swerdlow AJ. Sex differences in the risks of hormone-dependent cancers. *Am J Epidemiol* 1993;138:10–28.

18. Williams ED. TSH and thyroid cancer. *Horm Metab Res Suppl* 1990;23:72–75.

19. Schneider AB, Robbins J. Ionizing radiation and thyroid cancer. In: Fagin J, ed. *Thyroid cancer.* Boston: Kluwer Academic, 1998:27–57.

20. Duffy BJ, Fitzgerald P. Thyroid cancer in childhood and adolescence: a report on twenty-eight cases. *Cancer* 1950;10:1018–1032.

21. Shore RE. Issues and epidemiological evidence regarding radiation-induced thyroid cancer. *Radiat Res* 1992;131:98–111.

22. UNSCEAR (United Nations Scientific Committee on the Effects of Radiation). *Sources and effects of ionizing radiation.* New York: United Nations, 2000.

23. Ron E, Lubin JH, Shore RE, et al. Thyroid cancer after exposure to external radiation: a pooled analysis of seven studies. *Radiat Res* 1995;141:259–277.

24. Pottern LM, Kaplan MM, Larsen PR, et al. Thyroid nodularity after childhood irradiation for lymphoid hyperplasia—a comparison of questionnaire and clinical findings. *J Clin Epidemiol.* 1990;43:449–460.

25. Schneider AB, Ron E, Lubin J, et al. Dose-response relationships for radiation-induced thyroid cancer and thyroid nodules: evidence for the prolonged effects of radiation on the thyroid. *J Clin Endocrinol Metab* 1993;77:362–369.

26. Wang Z, Boice JD Jr, Wei L, et al. Thyroid nodularity and chromosome aberrations among women in areas of high background radiation in China. *J Natl Cancer Inst* 1990;82:4784–185.

27. Wang JX, Boice JD Jr, Li BX, et al. Cancer among medical diagnostic X-ray workers in China. *J Natl Cancer Inst* 1988;80:344–350.

28. Ron E, Modan B, Preston D, et al. Thyroid neoplasia following low-dose radiation in childhood. *Radiat Res* 1989;120:516–531.

29. Thompson DE, Mabuchi K, Ron E, et al. Cancer incidence in atomic bomb survivors. II. Solid tumors, 1958–1987. *Radiat Res* 1994;137(2 suppl):17–67

30. Robbins J, Adams WH. Radiation effects in the Marshall Islands. In: Nagataki S, ed. *Radiation and the thyroid.* Amsterdam: Excerpta Medica, 1989:11–24.

31. Shore RE, Hildreth N, Dvoretsky PM, et al. Thyroid cancer among persons given x-ray treatment in infancy for an enlarged thymus gland. *Am J Epidemiol* 1993;137:1068–1080.

32. Kerber RA, Till JE, Simon SL, et al. A cohort study of thyroid disease in relation to fallout from nuclear weapons testing. *JAMA* 1993;270:2076–2082.

33. Boice JD, Jr., Engholm G, Kleinerman RA, et al. Radiation dose and second cancer risk in patients treated for cancer of the cervix. *Radiat Res* 1988;116:3–55.

34. Tucker MA, Jones PH, Boice JD Jr, et al. Therapeutic radiation at a young age is linked to secondary thyroid cancer: the Late Effects Study Group. *Cancer Res* 1991;51:2885–2888.

35. Shore RE, Xue X. Comparative thyroid cancer risk of childhood and adult radiation exposure and estimation of lifetime risk. In: Thomas G, Karaoglou A, Williams ED, eds. *Radiation and thyroid cancer.* Singapore: World Scientific, 1999:491–498.

36. Robbins J, Schneider AB. Thyroid cancer following exposure to radioactive iodine. *Rev Endocrin Metab Dis* 2000;1:197–203.

37. Williams ED. Chernobyl, 15 years later, correlation of clinical, epidemiological and molecular outcomes. *Ann Endocrinol* 2003;64:72

38. National Council on Radiation Protection and Measurement. *Induction of thyroid cancer by ionizing radiation.* NCRP Report No. 80. Bethesda, MD: National Council on Radiation Protection and Measurement, 1985.

39. Conard RA. Late radiation effects in Marshall Islanders exposed to fallout 28 years ago. In: Boice JD Jr, Fraumeni JR, eds. *Radiation carcinogenesis: epidemiology and biological significance.* New York: Raven, 1984:57–71.

40. Takahashi T, Schoemaker MJ, Trott KR, et al. The relationship of thyroid cancer with radiation exposure from nuclear weapon testing in the Marshall Islands. *J Epidemiol* 2003;13:99–107.

41. Becker DV, Robbins J, Beebe GW, et al. Childhood thyroid cancer following the Chernobyl accident: a status report. *Endocrinol Metab Clin North Am* 1996;25:197–211.

42. Robbins J. Lessons from Chernobyl: the event, the aftermath fallout: radioactive, political, social. *Thyroid* 1997;7:189–192.

43. Robbins J, Schneider AB. Radioiodine-induced thyroid cancer: studies in the aftermath of the accident at Chernobyl. *Trends Endocrinol Metab* 1998;9:87–94.

44. Sobolev B, Heidenreich WF, Kairo I, et al. Thyroid cancer incidence in the Ukraine after the Chernobyl accident: comparison with spontaneous incidences. *Radiat Environ Biophys* 1997;36:195–199.

45. Buglova EE, Kenigsberg JE, Sergeeva NV. Cancer risk estimation in Belarussian children due to thyroid irradiation as a consequence of the Chernobyl nuclear accident. *Health Phys* 1996;71:45–49.

46. Astakhova LN, Anspaugh LR, Beebe GW, et al. Chernobyl-related thyroid cancer in children of Belarus: a case-control study. *Radiat Res* 1998;150:349–356.

47. Jacob P, Goulko G, Heidenreich WF, et al. Thyroid cancer risk to children calculated. *Nature* 1998;392:31–32.

48. Jacob P, Kenigsberg Y, Goulko G, et al. Thyroid cancer risk in Belarus after the Chernobyl accident: comparison with external exposures. *Radiat Environ Biophys.* 2000;39:25–31.

49. Ashizawa K, Shibata Y, Yamashita S, et al. Prevalence of goiter and urinary iodine excretion levels in children around Chernobyl. *J Clin Endocrinol Metab* 1997;82:3430–3433.

50. Kasatkina EP, Shilin DE, Rosenbloom AL, et al. Effects of low level radiation from the Chernobyl accident in a population with iodine deficiency. *Eur J Pediatr* 1997;156:916–920.

51. Bleuer JP, Averkin YI, Abelin T. Chernobyl-related thyroid cancer: What evidence for role of short-lived iodines? *Environ Health Perspect* 1997;105:1483–1486.

52. Gembicki M, Stozharov AN, Arinchin AN, et al. Iodine deficiency in Belarussian children as a possible factor stimulating

the irradiation of the thyroid gland during the Chernobyl catastrophe. *Environ Health Perspect* 1997;105:1487–1490.

53. Karaoglou A, Chadwick KH. Health consequences of Chernobyl and other radiation accidents—Report on the European Union Cluster Contractors' workshop (San Miniato, Italy, 17–22 June 1997). *Radiat Environ Biophys* 1998;37: 1–9.

54. Ishigaki K, Namba H, Takamura N, et al. Urinary iodine levels and thyroid diseases in children; comparison between Nagasaki and Chernobyl. *Endocr J* 2001;48:591–595.

55. Robbins J, Dunn JT, Bouville A, et al. Iodine nutrition and the risk from radioactive iodine: a workshop report in the Chernobyl long-term follow-up study. *Thyroid* 2001;11:487–491.

56. Nikiforov YE, Rowland JM, Bove KE, et al. Distinct pattern of ret oncogene rearrangements in morphological variants of radiation-induced and sporadic thyroid papillary carcinomas in children. *Cancer Res* 1997;57:1690–1694.

57. Williams ED, Tronko ND. *Molecular, cellular, biological characterization of childhood thyroid cancer. International Scientific Collaboration on Consequences of Chernobyl Accident.* Luxembourg: European Commission, 1996.

58. Nikiforov Y, Gnepp DR. Pediatric thyroid cancer after the Chernobyl disaster—pathomorphologic study of 84 cases (1991–1992) from the Republic of Belarus. *Cancer* 1994;74: 748–766.

59. Lushnikov EF, Abrossimov AY. Histological characterization of papillary thyroid carcinoma in children, adolescents and young adults in Russia after the Chernobyl accident. In: Yamushita S. *Chernobyl: message for the 21st century.* New York: Elsevier Amsterdam, 2002:239–244.

60. Williams D. Cancer after nuclear fallout: lessons from the Chernobyl accident. *Nat Rev Cancer* 2002;2:543–549.

61. Harach HR, Williams ED. Childhood thyroid cancer in England and Wales. *Br J Cancer* 1995;72:777–783.

62. National Cancer Institute. *Estimated exposures and thyroid doses received by the American people from I-131 in fallout following Nevada atmospheric nuclear bomb tests.* Bethesda, MD: National Institutes of Health, 1997.

63. Shipler DB, Napier BA, Farris WT, et al. Hanford environmental dose reconstruction project: an overview. *Health Phys* 1996; 71:532–544.

64. Gilbert ES, Tarone R, Bouville A, et al. Thyroid cancer rates and I-131 doses from Nevada atmospheric nuclear bomb tests. *J Natl Cancer Inst* 1998;90:1654–1660.

65. National Research Council and Institute of Medicine. *Exposure of the American people to iodine-131 from Nevada nuclear-bomb tests: review of the National Cancer Institute report and public health implications.* Washington, DC: National Academy Press, 1999.

66. Davis S, Kopecky KJ, Hamilton TE. *Hanford Thyroid Disease Study Final Report.* Seattle: Fred Hutchinson Cancer Research Center, 2002.

67. Dobyns BM, Sheline GE, Workman JB, et al. Malignant and benign neoplasms of the thyroid in patients treated for hyperthyroidism: a report of the Cooperative Thyrotoxicosis Therapy Study. *J Clin Endocrinol Metab* 1974;38:976–998.

68. Holm L-E, Wilkund KE, Lundell GE, et al. Thyroid cancer after diagnostic doses of iodine-131: a retrospective cohort study. *J Natl Cancer Inst* 1988;80:1132–1138.

69. Holm L-E, Hall P, Wiklund K, et al. Cancer risk after iodine-131 therapy for hyperthyroidism. *J Natl Cancer Inst* 1991;83: 1072–1077.

70. Hall P, Berg G, Bjelkengren G, et al. Cancer mortality after iodine-131 therapy for hyperthyroidism. *Int J Cancer* 1992;50: 886–890.

71. Hall P, Lundell G, Holm L-E. Mortality in patients treated for hyperthyroidism with iodine-131. *Acta Endocrinol* 1993;128: 230–234.

72. Hall P, Furst CJ, Mattsson A, et al. Thyroid nodularity after diagnostic administration of iodine-131. *Radiat Res* 1996;146: 673–682.

73. Hall P, Mattsson A, Boice JD Jr. Thyroid cancer after diagnostic administration of iodine-131. *Radiat Res* 1996;145:86–92.

74. Cooper DS. Radioiodine for hyperthyroidism—where do we stand after 50 years? *JAMA* 1998;280:375–376.

75. Franklyn JA, Maisonneuve P, Sheppard MC, et al. Mortality after the treatment of hyperthyroidism with radioactive iodine. *N Engl J Med* 1998;338:712–718.

76. Ron E, Doody MM, Becker DV, et al. Cancer mortality following treatment for adult hyperthyroidism. *JAMA* 1998;280:347–355.

77. Hahn K, Schnell-Inderst P, Grosche B, et al. Thyroid cancer after diagnostic administration of iodine-131 in childhood. *Radiat Res* 2001;156:61–70.

78. Dickman PW, Holm LE, Lundell G, et al. Thyroid cancer risk after thyroid examination with I-131: a population-based cohort study in Sweden. *Int J Cancer* 2003;106:580–587.

79. Franklyn JA, Maisonneuve P, Sheppard M, et al. Cancer incidence and mortality after radioiodine treatment for hyperthyroidism: a population-based cohort study. *Lancet* 1999;353: 2111–2115.

80. Becker DV, Braverman LE, Dunn JT, et al. The use of iodine as a thyroid blocking agent in the event of a reactor accident. Report of the Environmental Hazards Committee of the American Thyroid Association. *JAMA* 1984:659–661.

81. Nauman J, Wolff J. Iodide prophylaxis in Poland after the Chernobyl reactor accident: benefits and risks. *Am J Med* 1993; 94:524–532.

82. Becker DV, Zanzonico P. Potassium iodide for thyroid blockade in a reactor accident: administrative policies that govern its use. *Thyroid* 1997;7:193–197.

83. US Food and Drug Administration Center for Drug Evaluation Branch. *Guidance: potassium iodide as a thyroid blocking agent in radiation emergencies.* Rockville, MD: 2001.

84. Schneider AB, Becker DV, Robbins J. Protecting the thyroid from accidental or terrorist-instigated ^{131}I releases. *Thyroid* 2002; 12:271–272.

85. UNSCEAR (United Nations Scientific Committee on the Effects of Radiation). *Sources and effects of ionizing radiation.* New York: United Nations, 1994.

86. Hall P, Holm L-E. Radiation-associated thyroid cancer—facts and fiction. *Acta Oncol* 1998;37:325–330.

87. Lundell M, Hakulinen T, Holm L-E. Thyroid cancer after radiotherapy for skin hemangioma in infancy. *Radiat Res* 1994; 140:334–339.

88. Lindberg S, Karlsson P, Arvidsson B, et al. Cancer incidence after radiotherapy for skin haemangioma during infancy. *Acta Oncol* 1995;34:735–740.

89. Ronckers CM, van Leeuwen FE, Hayes RB, et al. Cancer incidence after nasopharyngeal radium irradiation. *Epidemiology* 2002;13:552–560.

90. Ronckers CM, Land CE, Hayes RB, et al. Late health effects of childhood nasopharyngeal radium irradiation: nonmelanoma skin cancers, benign tumors, and hormonal disorders. *Pediatr Res* 2002;52:850–858.

91. Sandler DP, Comstock GW, Matanoski GM. Neoplasms following childhood radium irradiation of the nasopharynx. *J Natl Cancer Inst* 1982;68:3.

92. Yeh H, Matanoski GM, Wang N, et al. Cancer incidence after childhood nasopharyngeal radium irradiation: a follow-up study in Washington County, Maryland. *Am J Epidemiol* 2001; 153:749–756.

93. Kaplan MM, Garnick MB, Gelber R, et al. Risk factors for thyroid abnormalities after neck irradiation for childhood cancer. *Am J Med* 1983;74:272–280.

94. Fleming ID, Black TL, Thompson EI, et al. Thyroid dysfunction and neoplasia in children receiving neck irradiation for cancer. *Cancer* 1985;55:1190–1194.

95. Pasqualini T, Iorcansky S, Gruneiro L, et al. Thyroid dysfunction in Hodgkin's disease. *Cancer* 1989;63:335–339.

96. Schneider AB. Cancer therapy and endocrine disease: radiation-induced thyroid tumours. In: Sheaves R, Jenkins PJ, Wass JA, eds. *Clinical endocrine oncology.* Oxford: Blackwell Science, 1997:514–517.

97. Hancock SL, Cox RS, Mcdougall IR. Thyroid diseases after treatment of Hodgkin's disease. *N Engl J Med* 1991;325:599–605.

98. Huang J, Walker R, Groome PG, et al. Risk of thyroid carcinoma in a female population after radiotherapy for breast carcinoma. *Cancer* 2001;92:1411–1418.

99. Adjadj E, Rubino C, Shamsaldim A, et al. The risk of multiple primary breast and thyroid carcinomas—role of the radiation dose. *Cancer* 2003;98:1309–1317.

100. Inskip PD, Ekbom A, Galanti MR, et al. Medical diagnostic x rays and thyroid cancer. *J Natl Cancer Inst* 1995;87:1613–1621.

101. Hallquist A, Nasman A. Medical diagnostic x-ray radiation—an evaluation from medical records and dentist cards in a case-control study of thyroid cancer in the northern medical region of Sweden. *Eur J Cancer Prev* 2001;10:147–152.

102. Sarne DH, Schneider AB. External radiation and thyroid neoplasia. *Endocrinol Metab Clin North Am* 1996;25:181–195.

103. Schneider AB, Bekerman C, Leland J, et al. Thyroid nodules in the follow-up of irradiated individuals: comparison of thyroid ultrasound with scanning and palpation. *J Clin Endocrinol Metab* 1997;82:4020–4027.

104. Inskip PD, Hartshorne MF, Tekkel M, et al. Thyroid nodularity and cancer among Chernobyl cleanup workers from Estonia. *Radiat Res* 1997;147:225–235.

105. Favus M, Schneider A, Stachura M, et al. Thyroid cancer occurring as a late consequence of head-and-neck irradiation. *N Engl J Med* 1976;294:1019–1025.

106. Brander A, Viikinkoski P, Nickels J, et al. Thyroid gland—US screening in middle-aged women with no previous thyroid disease. *Radiology* 1989;173:507–510.

107. Jarløv AE, Nygård B, Hegedus L, et al. Observer variation in ultrasound assessment of the thyroid gland. *Br J Radiol* 1993;66:625–627.

108. Fischer AH, Bond JA, Taysavang P, et al. Papillary thyroid carcinoma oncogene (RET/PTC) alters the nuclear envelope and chromatin structure. *Am J Pathol* 1998;153:1443–1450.

109. Hatipoglu BA, Gierlowski T, Shore-Freedman E, et al. Fine-needle aspiration of thyroid nodules in radiation-exposed patients. *Thyroid* 2000;10:63–69.

110. Kikuchi S, Perrier ND, Ituarte PHG, et al. Accuracy of fine-needle aspiration cytology in patients with radiation-induced thyroid neoplasms. *Br J Surg* 2003;90:755–758.

111. Sarne DH, Schneider AB. Evaluation and management of patients exposed to childhood head and neck irradiation. *Endocrinologist* 1995;5:304–307.

112. Schneider AB, Favus MJ, Stachura ME, et al. Plasma thyroglobulin in detecting thyroid carcinoma after childhood head and neck irradiation. *Ann Intern Med* 1977;86:29–34.

113. Nagataki S, Shibata Y, Inoue S, et al. Thyroid diseases among atomic bomb survivors in Nagasaki. *JAMA* 1994;272:364–370.

114. Pacini F, Vorontsova T, Molinaro E, et al. Prevalence of thyroid autoantibodies in children and adolescents from Belarus exposed to the Chernobyl radioactive fallout. *Lancet* 1998;352:763–766.

115. Schneider A, Bekerman C, Favus M, et al. Continuing occurrence of thyroid-nodules after head and neck irradiation: relationship to plasma thyroglobulin concentration. *Ann Intern Med* 1981;94:176–180.

116. Schneider AB, Shore-Freedman E, Ryo UY, et al. Radiation-induced tumors of the head and neck following childhood irradiation: prospective studies. *Medicine* 1985;64:1–15.

117. Kaplan MM. Thyroid hormone prophylaxis after radiation exposure. In: Robbins J, ed. *Treatment of thyroid cancer in childhood.* Springfield, VA: National Technical Information Service, 1994:143.

118. Robbins J. Thyroid suppression therapy for prevention of thyroid tumors after radiation exposure. In: Degroot LJ, Frohman LA, Kaplan EL, et al, eds. *Radiation-associated thyroid carcinoma.* New York: Grune & Stratton, 1976:419.

119. Murphy ED, Scanlon EF, Garces RM, et al. Thyroid hormone administration in irradiated patients. *J Surg Oncol* 1986;31:214–217.

120. Degroot LJ. Diagnostic approach and management of patients exposed to irradiation to the thyroid. *J Clin Endocrinol Metab* 1989;69:925–928.

121. Tisell LE, Carlsson S, Fjalling M, et al. Hyperparathyroidism subsequent to neck irradiation: risk factors. *Cancer* 1985;56:1529–1533.

122. Fujiwara S, Sposto REH, Akiba S, et al. Hyperparathyroidism among atomic bomb survivors in Hiroshima. *Radiat Res* 1992;130:372–378.

123. Schneider AB, Gierlowski TC, Shore-Freedman E, et al. Dose-response relationships for radiation-induced hyperparathyroidism. *J Clin Endocrinol Metab* 1995;80:254–257.

124. Rasmuson T, Damber L, Johansson L, et al. Increased incidence of parathyroid adenomas following x-ray treatment of benign diseases in the cervical spine in adult patients. *Clin Endocrinol (Oxf)* 2002;57:731–734.

125. Land CE, Saku T, Hayashi Y, et al. Incidence of salivary gland tumors among atomic bomb survivors, 1950–87: evaluation of radiation-related risk. Radiat Res 1996;146:28–36.

126. Schneider AB, Lubin J, Ron E, et al. Salivary gland tumors after childhood radiation treatment for benign conditions of the head and neck: dose-response relationships. *Radiat Res* 1998;149:625–630.

127. Saku T, Hayashi Y, Takahara O, et al. Salivary gland tumors among atomic bomb survivors, 1950–1987. *Cancer* 1997;79:1465–1475.

128. Modan B, Chetrit A, Alfandary E, et al. Increased risk of salivary gland tumors after low-dose irradiation. *Laryngoscope* 1998;108:1095–1097.

129. Ron E, Modan B, Boice JD Jr, et al. Tumors of the brain and nervous system after radiotherapy in childhood. *N Engl J Med* 1988;319:1033–1039.

130. Schneider AB, Shore-Freedman E, Weinstein R. Radiation-induced thyroid and other head and neck tumors: occurrence of multiple tumors and analysis of risk factors. *J Clin Endocrinol Metab* 1986;63:107–112.

131. Sznajder L, Abrahams C, Parry DM, et al. Multiple schwannomas and meningiomas associated with irradiation in childhood. *Arch Intern Med* 1996;156:1873–1878.

132. Shore RE, Albert RE, Reed M, et al. Skin cancer incidence among children irradiated for ringworm of the scalp. *Radiat Res* 1984;100:192–204.

133. Ron E, Modan B, Preston D, et al. Radiation-induced skin carcinomas of the head and neck. *Radiat Res* 1991;125:318–325.

134. Ron E, Preston DL, Kishikawa M, et al. Skin tumor risk among atomic-bomb survivors in Japan. *Cancer Causes Control* 1998;9:393–401.

135. Schneider AB, Recant W, Pinsky S, et al. Radiation-induced thyroid carcinoma: clinical course and results of therapy in 296 patients. *Ann Intern Med* 1986;105:405–412.

136. Rubino C, Cailleux AF, Abbas M, et al. Characteristics of follicular cell–derived thyroid carcinomas occurring after external radiation exposure: results of a case control study nested in a cohort. *Thyroid* 2002;12:299–304.

137. Samaan N, Schultz P, Ordonez N, et al. A comparison of thyroid carcinoma in those who have and have not had head and neck irradiation in childhood. *J Clin Endocrinol Metab* 1987; 64:219–223.

138. Viswanathan K, Gierlowski TC, Schneider AB. Childhood thyroid cancer—characteristics and long-term outcome in children irradiated for benign conditions of the head and neck. *Arch Pediatr Adolesc Med* 1994;148:260–265.

139. Shimaoka K, Getaz EP, Rao U. Anaplastic carcinoma of thyroid: radiation-associated. *NY State J Med* 1979;79:874–877.

140. Mazzaferri EL, Young RL. Papillary thyroid carcinoma: a 10 year follow-up report of the impact of therapy in 576 patients. *Am J Med* 1981;70:511–518.

141. Fogelfeld L, Wiviott MBT, Shore-Freedman E, et al. Recurrence of thyroid nodules after surgical removal in patients irradiated in childhood for benign conditions. *N Engl J Med* 1989; 320:835–840.

142. Reiners C, Biko J, Demidchik EP, et al. Results of radioactive iodine treatment in children from Belarus with advanced stages of thyroid cancer after the Chernobyl accident. In: Yamushita S. *Chernobyl: message for the 21st century*. New York: Elsevier Amsterdam, 2002:205–214.

143. Oliynyk V, Epshtein O, Sovenko T, et al. Post-surgical ablation of thyroid residues with radioiodine in Ukrainian children and adolescents affected by post-Chernobyl differentiated thyroid cancer. *J Endocrinol Invest* 2001;24:445–447.

144. Hizawa K, Iida M, Aoyagi K, et al. Thyroid neoplasia and familial adenomatous polyposis/Gardner's syndrome. *J Gastroenterol* 1997;32:196–199.

145. Bulow C, Bulow S, Berk T, et al. Is screening for thyroid carcinoma indicated in familial adenomatous polyposis? *Int J Colorectal Dis* 1997;12:240–242.

146. Perrier ND, van Heerden JA, Goellner JR, et al. Thyroid cancer in patients with familial adenomatous polyposis. *World J Surg* 1998;22:738–743.

147. Harach HR, Williams GT, Williams ED. Familial adenomatous polyposis associated thyroid carcinoma: a distinct type of follicular cell neoplasm. *Histopathology* 1994;25:549–561.

148. Fenton PA, Clarke SEM, Owen W, et al. Cribriform variant papillary thyroid cancer: a characteristic of familial adenomatous polyposis. *Thyroid* 2001;11:193–197.

149. Cetta F, Montalto G, Gori M, et al. Germline mutations of the APC gene in patients with familial adenomatous polyposis-associated thyroid carcinoma: results from a European cooperative study. *J Clin Endocrinol Metab* 2000;85:286–292.

150. Cetta F, Curia MC, Montalto G, et al. Thyroid carcinoma usually occurs in patients with familial adenomatous polyposis in the absence of biallelic inactivation of the adenomatous polyposis coli gene. *J Clin Endocrinol Metab* 2001;86:427–432.

151. Thyresson HN, Doyle JA. Cowden's disease (multiple hamartoma syndrome). *Mayo Clin Proc* 1981;56:179–184.

152. McIver B, Eberhardt NL. Cowden disease and the PTEN/MMAC1 gene. In: Akamizu T, Kasuga M, Davies TF (eds), *Genetics of Complex Thyroid Diseases*. New York, Tokyo: Springer. 2002: 151–175.

153. Goldgar DE, Easton DF, Cannon-Albright LA, et al. Systematic population-based assessment of cancer risk in first-degree relatives of cancer probands. *J Natl Cancer Inst* 1994;86: 1600–1608.

154. Frich L, Glattre E, Akslen LA. Familial occurrence of nonmedullary thyroid cancer: a population-based study of 5673 first-degree relatives of thyroid cancer patients from Norway. *Cancer Epidemiol Biomarkers Prev* 2001;10:113–117.

155. Hemminki K, Dong CH. Familial relationships in thyroid cancer by histo-pathological type. *Int J Cancer* 2000;85:201–205.

156. Stoffer SS, Van Dyke DL, Bach JV, et al. Familial papillary carcinoma of the thyroid. *Am J Med Genet* 1986;25:775–782.

157. Ron E, Kleinerman R, Boice JD Jr, et al. A population-based case-control study of thyroid cancer. *J Natl Cancer Inst* 1987;79:1–12.

158. Pal T, Vogl FD, Chappuis PO, et al. Increased risk for non-medullary thyroid cancer in the first degree relatives of prevalent cases of nonmedullary thyroid cancer: a hospital-based study. *J Clin Endocrinol Metab* 2001;86:5307–5312.

159. Grossman RF, Tu SH, Duh QY, et al. Familial nonmedullary thyroid cancer: an emerging entity that warrants aggressive treatment. *Arch Surg* 1995;130:892–899.

160. Loh KC. Familial nonmedullary thyroid carcinoma: a meta-review of case series. *Thyroid* 1997;7:107–113.

161. Alsanea O. Familial nonmedullary thyroid cancer. *Curr Treat Options Oncol* 2000;1:345–351.

162. Uchino S, Noguchi S, Kawamoto H, et al. Familial nonmedullary thyroid carcinoma characterized by multifocality and a high recurrence rate in a large study population. *World J Surg* 2002;26:897–902.

163. Brunaud L, Zarnegar R, Wada N, et al. Chromosomal aberrations by comparative genomic hybridization in thyroid tumors in patients with familial nonmedullary thyroid cancer. *Thyroid* 2003;13:621–629.

164. Kraimps JL, Bouin-Pineau MH, Amati P, et al. Familial papillary carcinoma of the thyroid. *Surgery* 1997;121:715–718.

165. Malchoff CD, Sarfarazi M, Tendler B, et al. Familial papillary thyroid carcinoma is genetically distinct from familial adenomatous polyposis coli. *Thyroid* 1999;9:247–252.

166. Cohen J, Gierlowski TC, Schneider AB. A prospective study of hyperparathyroidism in individuals exposed to radiation in childhood. *JAMA* 1990;264:581–584.

167. Mihailescu D, Shore-Freedman E, Mukani S, et al. Multiple neoplasms in an irradiated cohort: pattern of occurrence and relationship to thyroid cancer outcome. *J Clin Endocrinol Metab* 2002;87:3236–3241.

168. Perkel V, Gail MH, Lubin J, et al. Radiation-induced thyroid neoplasm: evidence for familial susceptibility factors. *J Clin Endocrinol Metab* 1988;66:1316–1322.

169. McTiernan AM, Weiss NS, Daling JR. Incidence of thyroid cancer in women in relation to previous exposure to radiation therapy and history of thyroid disease. *J Natl Cancer Inst* 1984; 73:575–581.

170. Preston-Martin S, Bernstein L, Pike MC, et al. Thyroid cancer among young women related to prior thyroid disease and pregnancy history. *Br J Cancer* 1987;55:191–195.

171. Franceschi S, Fassina A, Talamini R, et al. Risk factors for thyroid cancer in Northern-Italy. *Int J Epidemiol* 1989;18:578–584.

172. Levi F, Franceschi S, Lavecchia C, et al. Previous thyroid disease and risk of thyroid cancer in Switzerland. *Eur J Cancer* 1991; 27:85–88.

173. Preston-Martin S, Jin F, Duda MJ, et al. A case-control study of thyroid cancer in women under age 55 in Shanghai (People's Republic of China). *Cancer Causes Control* 1993;4:431–440.

174. Wingren G, Hatschek T, Axelson O. Determinants of papillary cancer of the thyroid. *Am J Epidemiol* 1993;138:482–491.

175. Akslen LA, Sothern RB. Seasonal variations in the presentation and growth of thyroid cancer. *Br J Cancer* 1998;77:1174–1179.

176. Memon A, Varghese A, Suresh A. Benign thyroid disease and dietary factors in thyroid cancer: a case-control study in Kuwait. *Br J Cancer* 2002;86:1745–1750.

177. Franceschi S, Preston-Martin S, Dal Maso L, et al. A pooled analysis of case-control studies of thyroid cancer. IV. Benign thyroid diseases. *Cancer Causes Control* 1999;10:583–595.

178. La Vecchia C, Ron E, Franceschi S, et al. A pooled analysis of case-control studies of thyroid cancer. III. Oral contraceptives,

menopausal replacement therapy and other female hormones. *Cancer Causes Control* 1999;10:157–166.

179. Negri E, Dal Maso L, Ron E, et al. A pooled analysis of case-control studies of thyroid cancer. II. Menstrual and reproductive factors. *Cancer Causes Control* 1999;10:143–155.

180. Negri E, Ron E, Franceschi S, et al. A pooled analysis of case-control studies of thyroid cancer. I. Methods. *Cancer Causes Control* 1999;10:131–142.

181. Goldman MB, Monson RR, Maloof F. Cancer mortality in women with thyroid disease. *Cancer Res* 1990;50:2283–2289.

182. Iribarren C, Haselkorn T, Tekawa IS, et al. Cohort study of thyroid cancer in a San Francisco Bay area population. *Int J Cancer* 2001;93:745–750.

183. Haselkorn T, Stewart SL, Horn-Ross PL. Why are thyroid cancer rates so high in Southeast Asian women living in the United States? The bay area thyroid cancer study. *Cancer Epidemiol Biomarkers Prev* 2003;12:144–150.

184. Mellemgaard A, From G, Jorgensen T, et al. Cancer risk in individuals with benign thyroid disorders. *Thyroid* 1998;8:751–754.

185. From G, Mellemgaard A, Knudsen N, et al. Review of thyroid cancer cases among patients with previous benign thyroid disorders. *Thyroid* 2000;10:697–700.

186. Levi F, Franceschi S, Te VC, et al. Descriptive epidemiology of thyroid cancer in the Swiss canton of Vaud. *J Cancer Res Clin Oncol* 1990;116:639–647.

187. Akslen LA, Nilssen S, Kvåle G. Reproductive factors and risk of thyroid cancer: a prospective study of 63,090 women from Norway. *Br J Cancer* 1992;65:772–774.

188. Hallquist A, Hardell L, Degerman A, et al. Thyroid cancer: reproductive factors, previous diseases, drug intake, family history and diet: a case-control study. *Eur J Cancer Prev* 1994;3:481–488.

189. Kolonel LN, Hankin JH, Wilkens LR, et al. An epidemiologic study of thyroid cancer in Hawaii. *Cancer Causes Control* 1990;1:223–234.

190. Levi F, Franceschi S, Gulie C, et al. Female thyroid cancer: the role of reproductive and hormonal factors in Switzerland. *Oncology* 1993;50:309–315.

191. Kravdal Ø, Glattre E, Haldorsen T. Positive correlation between parity and incidence of thyroid cancer: new evidence based on complete Norwegian birth cohorts. *Int J Cancer* 1991;49:831–836.

192. Galanti MR, Hansson L, Lund E, et al. Reproductive history and cigarette smoking as risk factors for thyroid cancer in women: a population-based case-control study. *Cancer Epidemiol Biomarkers Prev* 1996;5:425–431.

193. Modan B, Ron E, Lerner-Geva L, et al. Cancer incidence in a cohort of infertile women. *Am J Epidemiol* 1998;147:1038–1042.

194. Glattre E, Kravdal Ø. Male and female parity and risk of thyroid cancer. *Int J Cancer* 1994;58:616–617.

195. Brinton LA, Melton LJ III, Malkasian GD Jr, et al. Cancer risk after evaluation for infertility. *Am J Epidemiol* 1989;129:712–722.

196. Ron E, Lunenfeld B, Menczer J, et al. Cancer incidence in a cohort of infertile women. *Am J Epidemiol* 1987;125:780–790.

197. Luoto R, Grenman S, Salonen S, et al. Increased risk of thyroid cancer among women with hysterectomies. *Amer J Obstet Gynecol* 2003;188:45–48.

198. Memon A, Darif M, Al Saleh K, et al. Epidemiology of reproductive and hormonal factors in thyroid cancer: evidence from a case-control study in the Middle East. *Int J Cancer* 2002;97:82–89.

199. Rossing MA, Voigt LF, Wicklund KG, et al. Reproductive factors and risk of papillary thyroid cancer in women. *Am J Epidemiol* 2000;151:765–772.

200. Sakoda LC, Horn-Ross PL. Reproductive and menstrual history and papillary thyroid cancer risk: the San Francisco Bay Area thyroid cancer study. *Cancer Epidemiol Biomarker Prev* 2002;11:51–57.

201. McTiernan AM, Weiss NS, Daling JR. Incidence of thyroid cancer in women in relation to reproductive and hormonal factors. *Am J Epidemiol* 1984;120:423–435.

202. Shore RE, Hildreth N, Dvoretsky P, et al. Benign thyroid adenomas among persons X-irradiated in infancy for enlarged thymus glands. *Radiat Res* 1993;134:217–223.

203. Wong FL, Ron E, Gierlowski T, et al. Benign thyroid tumors: general risk factors and their effects on radiation risk estimation. *Am J Epidemiol* 1996;144:728–733.

204. Wegelin C. Malignant disease of the thyroid and its relation to goiter in men and animals. *Cancer Rev* 1928;3:297.

205. Wynder EL. Some practical aspects of cancer prevention. *N Engl J Med.* 1952;246:573

206. Franceschi S, Talamini R, Fassina A, et al. Diet and epithelial cancer of the thyroid gland. *Tumori* 1990;76:331–338.

207. Pendergrast WJ, Milmore BK, Marcus SC. Thyroid cancer and thyrotoxicosis in the United States: their relation to endemic goiter. *J Chronic Dis* 1961;13:22

208. Bacher-Stier C, Riccabona G, Totsch M, et al. Incidence and clinical characteristics of thyroid carcinoma after iodine prophylaxis in an endemic goiter country. *Thyroid* 1997;7:733– 741.

209. Bakiri F, Djemli FK, Mokrane LA, et al. The relative roles of endemic goiter and socioeconomic development status in the prognosis of thyroid carcinoma. *Cancer* 1998;82:1146–1153.

210. Feldt-Rasmussen U. Iodine and Cancer. *Thyroid* 2001;11:483–486.

211. Pettersson B, Adami HO, Wilander E, et al. Trends in thyroid cancer incidence in Sweden, 1958–1981, by histopathologic type. *Int J Cancer* 1991;48:28–33.

212. Belfiore A, La Rosa GL, Padova G, et al. The frequency of cold thyroid nodules and thyroid malignancies in patients from an iodine-deficient area. *Cancer* 1987;60:3096–3102.

213. Bosetti C, Kolonel L, Negri E, et al. A pooled analysis of case-control studies of thyroid cancer. VI. Fish and shellfish consumption. *Cancer Cause Control* 2001;12:375–382.

214. Glattre E, Haldorsen T, Berg JP, et al. Norwegian case-control study testing the hypothesis that seafood increases the risk of thyroid cancer. *Cancer Causes Control* 1993;4:11–16.

215. Frich L, Akslen LA, Glattre E. Increased risk of thyroid cancer among Norwegian women married to fishery workers—a retrospective cohort study. *Br J Cancer* 1997;76:385–389.

216. Franceschi S, Levi F, Negri E, et al. Diet and thyroid cancer: a pooled analysis of four European case-control studies. *Int J Cancer* 1991;48:395–398.

217. Bosetti C, Negri E, Kolonel L, et al. A pooled analysis of case-control studies of thyroid cancer. VII. Cruciferous and other vegetables (International). *Cancer Cause Control* 2002;13:765–775.

218. Galanti MR, Hansson L, Bergstrom R, et al. Diet and the risk of papillary and follicular thyroid carcinoma: a population-based case-control study in Sweden and Norway. *Cancer Cause Control* 1997;8:205–214.

219. Linos A, Linos DA, Vgotza N, et al. Does coffee consumption protect against thyroid disease? *Acta Chir Scand* 1989;155:317–320.

220. Takezaki T, Hirose K, Inoue M, et al. Risk factors of thyroid cancer among women in Tokai, Japan. *J Epidemiol* 1996;6:140–147.

221. Mack WJ, Preston-Martin S, Bernstein L, et al. Lifestyle and other risk factors for thyroid cancer in Los Angeles county females. *Ann Epidemiol* 2002;12:395–401.

222. Kreiger N, Parkes R. Cigarette smoking and the risk of thyroid cancer. *Eur J Cancer* 2000;36:1969–1973.

223. Rossing MA, Cushing KL, Voigt LF, et al. Risk of papillary thyroid cancer in women in relation to smoking and alcohol consumption. *Epidemiology* 2000;11:49–54.

224. Fisher CL, Mannino DM, Herman WH, et al. Cigarette smoking and thyroid hormone levels in males. *Int J Epidemiol* 1997; 26:972–977.

225. Capen CC. Mechanisms of chemical injury of thyroid gland. *Prog Clin Biol Res* 1994;387:173–191.

226. Hurley PM. Mode of carcinogenic action of pesticides inducing thyroid follicular cell tumors in rodents. *Environ Health Perspect* 1998;106:437–445.

227. Capen CC. Mechanistic data and risk assessment of selected toxic end points of the thyroid gland. *Toxicol Pathol* 1997;25:39–48.

228. Williams ED. Mechanisms and pathogenesis of thyroid cancer in animals and man. *Mutat Res* 1995;333:123–129.

229. Cooper DS, Axelrod L, Degroot LJ, et al. Congenital goiter and the development of metastatic follicular carcinoma with evidence for a leak of nonhormonal iodide: clinical, pathological, kinetic, and biochemical studies and a review of the literature. *J Clin Endocrinol Metab* 1981;52:294–306.

230. Medeiros-Neto G, Gil-Da-Costa MJ, Santos CLS, et al. Metastatic thyroid carcinoma arising from congenital goiter due to mutation in the thyroperoxidase gene. *J Clin Endocrinol Metab* 1998;83:4162–4166.

70B   MOLECULAR GENETICS OF TUMORS OF THYROID FOLLICULAR CELLS

JAMES A. FAGIN

Thyroid follicular cells can give rise to tumors with distinct pathologic and clinical features, as discussed in Chapter 21. Benign and malignant thyroid neoplasms consist of clonal cell populations (1–3). This points to their derivation from single precursor cells, with the initial step in tumor development involving the acquisition of a somatic mutation that alters the structure of a gene that confers cells with a growth advantage. Many of the genes involved in the pathogenesis of thyroid tumors have been identified, and found to be preferentially associated with certain tumor types. Cell proliferation is stimulated by extracellular growth factors that activate specific signaling cascades that dictate the orderly sequence of events needed for DNA synthesis and cell division. Molecules acting at multiple steps along growth signaling pathways can function as oncogenes when their structure is disrupted. In addition, loss-of-function mutations of genes coding for growth-inhibitory proteins involved in cell cycle checkpoints or cell survival contribute significantly to tumorigenesis. In the first section of this chapter, the contribution of growth and survival molecules to thyroid cancer pathogenesis based on their cellular function will be discussed.

GROWTH FACTORS AND EICOSANOIDS AS THYROID TUMOR PROGRESSION FACTORS AND PROMOTERS OF ANGIOGENESIS

The abundance of thyroid-stimulating hormone (TSH, or thyrotropin) in plasma is an important determinant of the mitotic rate of thyroid cells (4). High TSH levels promote progression of certain thyroid neoplasms, including many thyroid cancers. By contrast, the role of growth factors present in the tumor environment is not as well defined. Whereas growth of normal cells is highly dependent on external mitogenic stimulation by growth factors, a classical feature of cancer cells is that they are to a large extent released from this constraint. Nevertheless, tumor cells retain variable degrees of responsiveness to polypeptide growth factors, and these may contribute to tumor progression or development. Fibroblast growth factors (FGF) 1 and 2 are mitogens for thyroid follicular cells (5), and are overexpressed in multinodular goiters as well as benign and malignant thyroid neoplasms (6–8). TSH requires the presence of insulin-like growth factor-I (IGF-I) to exert its full mitogenic effect in human thyroid cells. Moreover, overexpression of IGF-I and the IGF-I receptor in thyroid cells of transgenic mice induces goiter formation (9). Both IGF-I and IGF-II are overexpressed in human thyroid cancers (10,11). Whereas IGF-I is primarily produced by cells in the tumor stroma (12), thyroid cancer cells are believed to be the source of local IGF-II production (10). Transforming growth factor-α (TGF-α, and its close relative epidermal growth factor, EGF) is also a mitogen for thyroid follicular cells *in vitro*, and is locally expressed within the thyroid (13,14). The mechanism by which tumor cells overexpress growth factors does not involve primary modifications of the growth factor genes themselves. Rather, growth factor overexpression is secondary to oncogenic activation of other signaling pathways. For example, mutations of *RAS* result in increased TGF-α gene expression in rat thyroid FRTL-5 cells (15), and of IGF-I in human thyroid cells (16).

For cancer clones to progress, tumor cells promote growth of capillaries and larger vessels from adjacent tissue in order to deliver nutrients and oxygen and eliminate metabolic waste. Some of the most prominent signals driving the process of angiogenesis have been identified in other cancer types (17,18), and are likely to play similar roles in the thyroid. Vascular endothelial cell growth factors (VEGFs) comprise a family of at least five structurally related polypeptides—VEGF-A, VEGF-B, VEGF-C, VEGF-D, and placental growth factor (PIGF)—that modulate blood and lymphatic vessel growth (19). VEGF-A is expressed at higher levels in thyroid cancers than in normal thyroid cells or benign thyroid tumors (20–22). VEGF-C, which primarily stimulates lymphangiogenesis, is also overexpressed in thyroid cancers, although this alone is unlikely to account for the predisposition to undergo lymphatic spread, since not all thyroid tumor types prone to lymph node metastasis overexpress this growth factor (23). Besides its mitogenic effects on thyroid cells, FGF-2 is also a potent angiogenic factor (24). TGF-β, which despite inhibiting thyroid cell growth and differentiated function (25) has been implicated in pathogenesis of multinodular goiters (26,27), could play a role in vascular remodeling. It is important to consider the role of stromal-derived growth factors in tumor evolution, as illustrated by recent evidence indicating that modulation of TGF-β signaling in stromal fibroblasts can impact the oncogenic potential of adjacent epithelial cells (28). In addition to polypeptide growth factors, other secreted products present in the tumor microenvironment can promote neovascularization. Thyroid cancers, like other epithelial malignancies, have higher expression of cyclooxygenase-2 (COX-2), the enzyme catalyzing the initial step in prostanoid biosynthesis from arachidonic acid (29–32). Tumor-derived prostanoid production is a significant contributor to colorectal tumorigenesis in animals and humans (33–36). Prostaglandin E_2 (PGE$_2$), the major product of COX-2 acting via microsomal prostaglandin E synthase (mPGES), has been implicated as a key mediator of these effects. Among other properties, PGE$_2$ is a powerful stimulus for angiogenesis. Recent evidence shows that expression of Ret or Ras mutants induces PGE$_2$ production via increased expression of COX-2 and mPGES1 in rat thyroid cells, thus providing a link between oncogenic tumor initiation, activation of prostaglandin biosynthesis, and tumor neovascularization (37).

DEFECTS IN SIGNAL RECEPTION FROM EXTRACELLULAR LIGANDS

Tyrosine Kinase Receptors

Polypeptide growth factor receptors are common targets of oncogenesis. This can occur through gene amplification of a tyrosine kinase receptor of normal structure, resulting in an increase in the total number of receptors in the plasma membrane. For example, the epidermal growth factor receptor (EGFR, or Erb1) is overexpressed in certain epithelial malignancies and in glioblastomas, and its close relative Erb-B2/neu is amplified and overexpressed in breast and ovarian cancer (38–40). Even though in most cases these receptors are structurally intact, their increased abundance favors a higher amplitude of signaling through effector pathways that can favor cell transformation (41). So far, gene amplification of growth factor receptors has not proven to be a common feature of thyroid neoplasms. However, all members of the EGFR family have been reported to be overexpressed in papillary thyroid cancers (42,43). Overexpression of Met, the receptor for hepatocyte growth factor (HGF), is also highly prevalent in these cancers (44,45). This is not due to amplification of the *MET* or *EGFR* genes, but may instead be secondary to induction of gene expression, possibly as a result of illegitimate signaling from mutant *RAS* or *RET/PTC* oncogenes (46,47). The predicted increase in responsiveness to the respective ligands for these tyrosine kinase receptors may thus participate in the tumorigenic process.

Growth factor receptors can also lead to cell transformation when their structure is modified through activating mutations. The most significant example relevant to the pathogenesis of papillary thyroid carcinomas are the *RET/PTC* oncogenes (48), mutant forms of the tyrosine kinase receptor *RET*. The *RET* gene encodes a transmembrane tyrosine kinase receptor whose expression is normally restricted to a subset of neuronal and neuroendocrine cells, and to the collecting duct of the kidney. Ret is a receptor for growth factors belonging to the glial cell–derived neurotropic growth factor (GDNF) family, which also includes neurturin, persephin, and artemin (49). The Ret protein is not normally present in thyroid follicular cells. Chromosomal rearrangements linking the promoter and N-terminal domains of unrelated genes to the C-terminal fragment of *RET* result in the aberrant production of a chimeric form of the receptor in thyroid cells. Rearrangements of *RET* resulting in its constitutive activation are believed to play a causative role in the pathogenesis of a significant proportion of papillary carcinomas of the thyroid (PTC) (50). Several forms have been identified that differ according to the 5′ partner gene involved in the rearrangement. *RET/PTC1* is formed by an intrachromosomal inversion of the long arm of chromosome 10, leading to fusion of *RET* with a gene named *H4/D10S170* (51). *RET/PTC2* is formed by a reciprocal translocation between chromosomes 10 and 17, resulting in the juxtaposition of the TK domain of *RET* with a portion of the regulatory subunit of *PKAR1A* (52). *RET/PTC3* is also a result of an intrachromosomal rearrangement and is formed by fusion with the *RFG/ELE1* gene (53,54) (Fig. 70B.1). Recently, several additional variants of *RET/PTC* have been observed in papillary carcinomas from individuals exposed to ionizing radiation as well as in sporadic cases (55–61). The fusion proteins generated

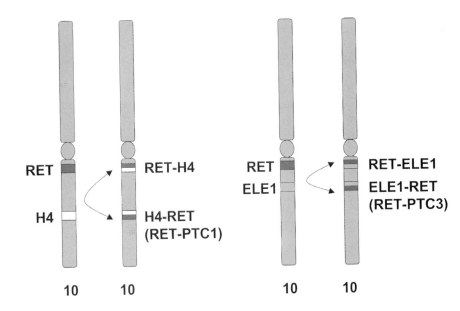

FIGURE 70B.1. The *RET* oncogene is activated by intrachromosomal inversions in papillary thyroid cancers. Reciprocal rearrangements of the tyrosine kinase receptor gene *RET* with partners in the same arm of chromosome 10 are the most common genetic defects in radiation-induced thyroid cancers, and they are also found in a smaller fraction of sporadic cases. Recombination with *H4* **(left)** gives rise to the *RET/PTC1* gene, which consists of a fusion between the promoter and N-terminal coding domains of *H4* with the tyrosine kinase domain of *RET*. Recombination with the promoter and N-terminal coding domains of *ELE1* with the same region of *RET* gives rise to *RET/PTC3* **(right)**.

by these recombinant genes homodimerize in a ligand-independent manner through the action of coiled-coil motifs in the N-termini donated by the respective upstream fusion partners (62), resulting in constitutive activation of the tyrosine kinase function of Ret.

RET/PTC rearrangements are found in 5% to 40% of PTC in the adult population (48). By contrast, *RET* rearrangements are more common in pediatric PTC, and in cancers from children exposed to ionizing radiation (63–67). There are several lines of evidence pointing to *RET/PTC* as one of the key first steps in thyroid cancer pathogenesis:

1. Thyroid-specific overexpression of either RET/PTC1 (68,69) or RET/PTC3 (70), in transgenic mice leads to development of tumors with histologic features consistent with PTC.
2. There is a high prevalence of RET/PTC expression in occult or microscopic PTC (71,72).
3. Exposure of cell lines (73) and fetal thyroid explants (74) to ionizing radiation results in expression of RET/PTC within hours, supporting a direct role for radiation in the illegitimate recombination of *RET*.
4. The breakpoints in the *RET* and *ELE1/RFG* genes resulting in the *RET/PTC3* rearrangements of radiation-induced pediatric thyroid cancers from Chernobyl are consistent with direct double-stranded DNA break, resulting in illegitimate reciprocal recombination (75).

Moreover, the *H4* and *RET* genes, although lying at a considerable linear distance from each other within chromosome 10, are spatially juxtaposed during interphase in thyroid cells and presumably present a target for simultaneous double strand breaks in each gene after ionizing radia-

tion, thus giving rise to the *RET/PTC1* rearrangement (76). Several groups have examined whether RET/PTC may serve as a prognostic marker for papillary thyroid cancers, and although the results are controversial, the preponderance of the evidence is that sporadic PTCs with this rearrangement have a more favorable natural history (77).

Somatic rearrangements of another member of the tyrosine kinase receptor gene family, the protooncogene *NTRK1*, which codes for the receptor for nerve growth factor (NGF), are also seen in papillary thyroid cancers, albeit with a far lower prevalence (78). *NTRK1* encodes for the receptor for NGF. Several thyroid-specific TRK oncogenes, named *TRK*, *TRK-T1*, *TRK-T2*, and *TRK-T3*, have been isolated (79–81). All contain a variable portion of NTRK1, including the tyrosine kinase domain, and differ in the 5′-upstream sequences, contributed by the tropomyosin (*TPM3*), translocated promoter region (*TPR*), and TRK-fused (*TFG*) genes, respectively. Targeted overexpression of *TRK-T1* induces lesions resembling PTC in transgenic mice, supporting a role for this oncogene as an alternative pathway in tumor initiation (82).

The *RET* gene also plays a prominent role in the pathogenesis of medullary thyroid cancer. Germline mutations of *RET* confer predisposition to all forms of familial medullary thyroid carcinoma (MTC), either as part of the multiple endocrine neoplasia type 2 (MEN-2) syndromes or when MTC is the sole manifestation of the disease (83–85). Acquired somatic mutations of *RET* are also found in a large fraction of sporadic medullary thyroid carcinomas. *RET* is activated by point mutations in MTC, resulting in a gain of function of the receptor. The genetic basis of MTC is of great clinical relevance, and genotyping is used as a basis for prophylactic thyroidectomy in *RET* mutation gene carriers. Readers are referred to Chapter 71 for a more comprehensive discussion of the molecular genetics of *RET* in MTC, genotype/phenotype correlations, and relevance to patient management.

G Protein–Coupled Receptors

Growth of pituitary, thyroid, and adrenal cells is controlled in part through polypeptide ligands that activate G protein–coupled receptors of the seven-transmembrane domain family, and that signal in part through stimulation of adenylyl cyclase activity. The TSH receptor (TSHR) can be activated by point mutations leading to amino acid substitutions that either abrogate the requirement for ligand or enhance responses to ligand-mediated activation (86). Germline mutations of this receptor are associated with syndromes of familial hyperthyroidism (87). More relevant to neoplasia, somatic mutations of the *TSHR* are observed in many autonomously functioning thyroid nodules (AFTNs). These benign tumors are characterized by progressive growth and the ability to synthesize hormones in the absence of TSH stimulation. Activating mutations of *TSHR* result in amino acid substitutions at multiple sites of the receptor protein, including the third, sixth, and seventh transmembrane domains, and the first, second, and third intracellular loops (88). Mutations of *TSHR* are believed to release the receptor protein from structural constraints present in its unliganded form, thus allowing it to activate Gsα in a constitutive manner (89). Although there is general agreement that *TSHR* mutations play an important role in pathogenesis of AFTNs, there is some debate about the actual prevalence of these abnormalities (90,91). About 50% to 80% of solitary AFTNs have *TSHR* mutations, whereas in autonomous nodules present in multinodular goiters the frequency appears to be less (92). The consensus from clinical studies is that AFTNs have a low probability of malignant transformation (93). Accordingly, activating point mutations of *TSHR* are rare in differentiated thyroid carcinomas (94–100).

Nuclear Receptors

Peroxisome proliferator-activated receptors (PPARs) are nuclear receptors that bind to DNA as heterodimers with the retinoid X receptors. The activity of PPARγ is regulated by binding to small lipophilic ligands, mainly fatty acids derived from nutritional intake or metabolism (101). PPARγ has been shown to play an important role in regulating genes involved in adipocyte differentiation and lipid metabolism. An involvement of this nuclear receptor in thyroid cancer was recently discovered by the characterization of a translocation in a subset of human thyroid follicular carcinomas, t(2;3)(q13;p25), which results in fusion of the DNA binding domains of the thyroid transcription factor PAX8 to domains A to F of PPARγ1 (102). PAX8-PPARγ1 messenger RNA (mRNA) and protein are present

specifically in follicular neoplasms, particularly in follicular carcinomas. Based on the studies published so far, prevalence of the *PAX8-PPARγ1* rearrangement is 10% (11/112) in follicular adenomas, and 41% (34/82) in follicular carcinomas (102–106), suggesting a role for this fusion protein in malignant transformation. The mechanism of transformation induced by PAX8-PPARγ1 is unclear, although it has been shown to have a dominant negative effect on thiazolidinedione-induced transactivation by PPARγ1 (102). Overexpression of wild-type PPARγ1 in thyroid cancer cell lines inhibits cell growth, an effect that is further enhanced by PPARγ1 agonists (107). Taken together, these data suggest that the PAX8-PPARγ1 fusion protein may derepress growth inhibitory controls requiring PPARγ1.

Recently, a remarkably high prevalence (>90%) of mutant of thyroid hormone receptor (TR) α1 and β1 transcripts was reported in human papillary thyroid carcinomas (108). Many of these mutant TRs had impaired transactivation properties, and were predicted to act in a dominant negative fashion. However, these findings were not confirmed in a separate independent study, in which no such mutations were found despite full-length sequencing of TRβ1 complementary DNAs from a similar number of thyroid cancers (109). Homozygous gene–targeted mice with a mutant *TR*β (*TR*β*PV* mice) develop invasive thyroid cancers late in life (110). Although this is consistent with a role for TRβ in thyroid cancer progression, it should be noted that these mice have extreme thyroid hormone resistance and high TSH levels throughout life. In summary, a role for TR loss-of-function mutations in thyroid cancer is intriguing but remains controversial.

DEFECTS IN THE INTRACELLULAR TRANSMISSION OF THE SIGNAL

RAS Oncogenes

After ligand binding, tyrosine kinase receptors dimerize and become autophosphorylated on selected tyrosine residues within their cytoplasmic region. The phosphorylated tyrosines create high-affinity binding sites for proteins containing Src homology 2 (SH2) domains. Recruitment of SH2-containing proteins represents the initial link in a chain of phosphorylation reactions that relay and amplify the growth factor receptor signal. Coupling to Ras takes place through the SH2/SH3 adaptor protein Grb2, which is in turn linked to Sos proteins that activate Ras by exchange of guanosine diphosphate (GDP) for guanosine triphosphate (GTP). GTP-bound Ras is inactivated by hydrolysis of its associated GTP to GDP, which is dependent on its intrinsic GTPase activity, and on interaction with proteins (GTPase-activating proteins, or GAPs) that markedly increase the hydrolysis of Ras-bound GTP. Three

RAS genes are prominent in cancer pathogenesis: *H-RAS*, *K-RAS* and *N-RAS*. From a biochemical standpoint their properties are quite similar, and all can be converted to an oncogenic form. Point mutations in discrete domains within *RAS* that increase protein affinity for GTP, or inactivate its GTPase function, permanently switch the protein to the "on" position. Activation of Ras leads to the activation of mitogen-activated protein (MAP) kinases, thus linking the activity of cell surface receptors to critical intracellular targets. MAP kinase activity is regulated through the sequential activation of three kinases, which in the case of extracellular signal–related kinases (ERKs) includes successive activation of Raf and MEK kinases. As discussed in greater detail below, this pathway is believed to be central to Ras-mediated dedifferentiation and transformation (111,112). Remarkably, 30% of all human tumors contain a mutation in a *RAS* allele, making *RAS* the most widely mutated human protooncogene (113). Mutations of all three *RAS* oncogenes have been reported in thyroid neoplasms (prevalence is *N-RAS* > *H-RAS* > *K-RAS*) (114, 115). *RAS* mutations are fairly common in both follicular adenomas and carcinomas, but are more prevalent in the latter (116–118). In addition, they are present in a small subset of papillary carcinomas (114,119), particularly in follicular variant PTCs (120). The fact that *RAS* mutations are present in both benign and malignant thyroid neoplasms suggests that *RAS* activation may be an early step in thyroid tumor development (119,121). In support of this, transgenic mice with thyroid-specific expression of mutant K-Ras develop benign thyroid lesions (122), which tend to become more prevalent and undergo malignant transformation after prolonged goitrogen stimulation. Despite early onset of Ras activation in human thyroid tumor development and progression, *RAS* mutations may confer cancers with more aggressive properties, because undifferentiated and anaplastic cancers have a higher prevalence of these genetic defects (116,123).

The functional consequences of mutagenic Ras activation in thyrocytes are only partially understood. Activation of Ras induces cell proliferation in primary cultures of human thyrocytes (124,125) and in rat thyroid cell lines (126,127). In human thyroid cells Ras-induced proliferation is self-limited through a mechanism that may require reactivation of expression of the cyclin-dependent kinase inhibitor p16(INK4a) (124,128). By contrast, in immortalized rat thyroid cell lines, Ras-induced cell proliferation is followed by genomic instability (129) and apoptosis (126,127). Mutant Ras is not by itself sufficient to induce thyroid cell transformation, as determined by the ability to form tumors in athymic mice or colonies in soft agar (130). In primary cultures of human thyroid cells, Ras activation does not impair thyroid-differentiated function, whereas in immortalized rat thyroid cell lines, Ras inhibits TSH-induced iodine uptake, and expression of thyroglobulin (Tg) and thyroid peroxidase (TPO) (131). The differ-ences between human thyroid cells and immortalized rat thyroid cell lines suggest that Ras requires an as yet un-identified cooperating event to induce thyroid dedifferentiation. Ras-mediated dedifferentiation in PCCL3 cells requires Raf-MEK-ERK (111,112), and may occur in part by interference with cyclic adenosine monophosphate (cAMP)–dependent signaling, through exclusion of the catalytic domain of protein kinase A from the nucleus (132, 133). Ras activation interferes with phosphorylation and activation of TTF-1, a transcription factor necessary for expression of thyroid-specific genes such as the TSH receptor, thyroglobulin, and thyroid peroxidase (111).

BRAF

There are three isoforms of the serine-threonine kinase Raf in mammalian cells: ARaf, BRaf, and CRaf or Raf1, with different tissue distribution of expression (134). Although all Raf isoforms activate MEK phosphorylation, they are differentially activated by oncogenic Ras. In addition, BRaf has higher affinity for MEK1 and MEK2 and is more efficient in phosphorylating MEKs than other RAF isoforms (135). *BRAF* somatic mutations were recently reported in a high proportion of benign nevi (136) and malignant melanomas (137), and in a smaller subset of colorectal and ovarian cancers (137). A total of 98% of the mutations in melanomas resulted from thymine-to-adenine transversions at nucleotide position 1796, resulting in a valine-to-glutamate substitution at residue 599 (V599E). This mutation is believed to mimic the phosphorylation in the activation segment by insertion of an acidic residue close to a site of regulated phosphorylation at serine 598. BRaf ^{V599E} exhibits elevated basal kinase activity, and has diminished responsiveness to stimulation by oncogenic H-Ras. BRaf ^{V599E} also transformed NIH3T3 cells with higher efficiency than the wild-type form of the kinase, consistent with it functioning as an oncogene. This same somatic mutation of *BRAF* is the most common genetic change in PTC, and present in about 40% of cases (138–145). *BRAF* ^{T1796A} mutations are unique to PTC, and not found in any other form of well-differentiated follicular neoplasm arising from the same cell type. There is practically no overlap between PTC with *RET/PTC, BRAF,* or *RAS* mutations, which altogether are found in about 70% of cases (138,144). The lack of concordance for these mutations provides compelling genetic evidence for the requirement of this signaling system for transformation to PTC. Because these signaling proteins function along the same pathway in thyroid cells, this represents a unique paradigm of human tumorigenesis through mutation of three signaling effectors lying in tandem (Fig. 70B.2). *BRAF* mutations can occur early in development of PTC, based on evidence that they are present in microscopic PTC (140). Moreover, PTC with BRAF mutations have more aggressive properties and can transform to undifferentiated or

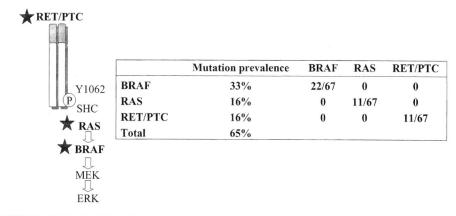

FIGURE 70B.2. Papillary thyroid cancers have non-overlapping mutations of *RET/PTC*, *RAS*, or *BRAF*. Signaling via RAS-RAF-MAP kinase may be required for some of the transforming properties of the RET/PTC oncoproteins *in vitro* **(left)**. Three of the effectors in this pathway—*RET/PTC*, *RAS*, and *B-RAF* (*stars*)—can be activated by mutations in papillary carcinomas. Surveys of papillary carcinoma tissue samples showed no overlap in mutation of these genes **(right)**, providing strong genetic evidence for the requirement of this pathway in thyroid tumorigenesis. (Right panel reproduced from Kimura ET, Nikiforova MN, Zhu Z, et al. High prevalence of BRAF mutations in thyroid cancer: genetic evidence for constitutive activation of the RET/PTC-RAS-BRAF signaling pathway in papillary thyroid carcinoma. *Cancer Res* 2003;63:1454–1457, with permission.)

anaplastic carcinomas (140,142), whereas PTC with RET/PTC rearrangements do not.

The *GSP* Oncogene

As discussed, *TSHR* is subject to somatic activating mutations in autonomously functioning thyroid adenomas, indicating that intermediates along the cAMP-dependent signal transduction cascade can function as oncogenes when their structure is modified in a manner that renders them constitutively active. After ligand activation, the TSHR associates with the heterotrimeric G-protein complex, which in turn transmits the signal by stimulating the catalytic activity of adenylyl cyclase. The Gsα subunit of this complex is also a target of activating point mutations in autonomously functioning thyroid adenomas (146,147), as well as in growth hormone–secreting pituitary tumors (148). The resulting *GSP* oncogene has mutations that are confined to one of two possible hot spots, which either inactivate the intrinsic GTPase activity of the protein (Arg201), or alter the affinity of Gsα for guanine nucleotides (Gln227). Mutations of Gsα are uncommon in thyroid carcinomas (97,98,147), again attesting to the fact that constitutive activation of intermediates along the adenylyl cyclase signaling cascade may not be a frequent harbinger of malignant transformation.

β-catenin

β-catenin is a ubiquitously expressed cytoplasmic protein involved in cell-cell adhesion and regulation of gene transcription as a downstream signaling molecule in the wingless pathway. Inappropriate stabilization of β-catenin fol-

lowed by nuclear translocation has been proposed as an important step in oncogenesis. Stabilization may occur through activating mutations in exon 3 at the phosphorylation sites for ubiquitination and degradation of β-catenin. Somatic mutations in exon 3 of β-catenin associated with nuclear localization were reported in about 25% of poorly differentiated and 60% of anaplastic carcinomas (149,150), but not in well-differentiated cancers (151), strongly implicating the Wnt-β catenin pathway in late-stage progression of thyroid cancer (152).

Other Candidate Oncogenes

The oncogenes discussed so far have been shown to play a role in the pathogenesis of thyroid neoplasms based on the fact that they are subject to genetic modifications that are selected during tumor microevolution. In some cases, there is controversy as to whether a particular oncogene is subject to mutations in thyroid cancer. Other signaling effectors may play critically important roles, and be required for oncogenesis, but not be subject to illegitimate activation through mutations. Because of space limitations these will not be described here, and the reader is referred to other papers and reviews for a more expanded discussion (153–157).

TUMOR SUPPRESSOR GENES

Tumor suppressor genes code for proteins that normally inhibit or restrict cell division. Cells must overcome a series of barriers that normally restrain growth in order to progress toward malignancy. Whereas oncogenes act in a dominant fashion, that is, a disruption in one allele is sufficient to promote the neoplastic phenotype, tumor suppressor genes have a recessive mode of action. In familial syndromes, such as in congenital retinoblastoma or MEN-1, one of the alleles of the tumor suppressor gene (i.e., *RB, MENIN*) is already mutated in the germline, but cells remain normal unless the second allele is also damaged, which often takes place postnatally. Structural inactivation of both alleles of a tumor suppressor gene can also arise as an acquired event during the course of sporadic tumor evolution.

Retinoblastoma

The normal counterparts of several tumor suppressor genes play important roles in control of cell cycle progression. The retinoblastoma (*RB*) gene product, the first tumor suppressor to be identified (158), serves as a gatekeeper between the G1 and S phases of the cell cycle. During G1, Rb is underphosphorylated, and prevents entry into S by binding and sequestering transcription factors needed to activate DNA synthesis. Rb is inactivated by phosphorylation when the cell has completed the preparation to replicate its DNA (159). Inactivating mutations of both copies of *RB* illegitimately release this cell cycle block. *RB* mutations are seen not only in retinoblastomas, but in common cancers as well. Viral oncoproteins such as the SV40 large T antigen, adenoviral E1A, and the human papilloma virus E7 can also functionally inactivate Rb, in part by their ability to bind to the underphosphorylated domains of the protein (160–162). Cancer cell lines lacking functional Rb can be growth arrested by reintroduction of a normal copy of the gene (163). Although mice with homozygous germline inactivation of *RB* are not viable, heterozygous *RB*-null mice develop intermediate lobe pituitary tumors (164), and when crossed with *P53*-null heterozygotes, they also develop medullary thyroid cancers (165). A role for *RB* mutations in development of human medullary thyroid cancers has not been established firmly, although clonal loss of *RB* alleles has been reported in early stages of development of familial forms of the disease. In tumors derived from thyroid follicular cells, the role of Rb is controversial. Targeted expression of the E7 oncoprotein of human papilloma virus to thyroid cells of transgenic mice is associated with development of a colloid goiter, and progressive occurrence of differentiated malignant lesions, indirectly implicating Rb inactivation in this process (166). However, in human thyroid cancers *RB* gene allelic losses are either absent (167) or relatively infrequent (168,169). One study reported *RB* gene mutations, but it remains unclear whether both alleles were inactivated (170). In addition, a subset of thyroid cancers have decreased immunohistochemical staining for Rb (171), but this again is controversial (172).

p16^INK4A

The D-type cyclins, in association with the cyclin-dependent kinases cdk4 and cdk6, promote progression through the G1 phase of the cell cycle. p15^INK4b and p16^INK4a are cyclin-dependent kinase inhibitors that prevent Rb phosphorylation by specifically antagonizing the activity of the cyclin D/cdk4 or cdk6 holoenzymes. Loss of function of p15^INK4b or p16^INK4a impairs the G1/S cell cycle checkpoint and contributes to the transformation of several cell types. Mutations of *P16* have been found in many thyroid cancer cell lines, but only rarely in primary tumors (173–176). Interestingly, the *P16* gene is frequently hypermethylated in thyroid cancers, suggesting that loss of expression of this critical cell cycle checkpoint gene may occur more commonly as an epigenetic event during tumor evolution (176–178).

The *p53* Tumor Suppressor Gene

P53 is the most commonly mutated gene in human cancer (179). The fact that many cancers have lost p53 function points to the cardinal role it plays in the maintenance of cell homeostasis. The p53 protein is a transcriptional activator, and this property is needed for preservation of its tumor suppressing properties. Most inactivating mutations of the gene nullify one of the sequence-specific DNA binding domains of the protein. In some cell types, a single mutant *P53* allele can generate a product that complexes with the wild-type form of the protein to functionally inactivate it. In this circumstance, p53 has a dominant negative effect, and violates the paradigm that tumor suppressor genes are invariably recessive (i.e., both copies must be mutated for the phenotype to manifest). The p53 protein is involved in control of cell cycle progression, largely by its ability to transactivate expression of genes coding for proteins such as p21/WAF1, that induce G1 arrest by inhibiting cyclin-dependent kinase complexes (180,181). In addition, p53 can help trigger a program of apoptosis. The ability to arrest the cell cycle, and under certain conditions to activate a program of cell death, place p53 at a major crossroads in the determination of cell survival. A fuller picture emerges by understanding the conditions that lead to p53 expression. Levels of p53 increase after exposure to agents that induce DNA damage, such as ionizing radiation and certain drugs used in cancer chemotherapy. Presumably, p53 acts to allow DNA repair to proceed under more favorable conditions (182). However, if the damage is overwhelming, p53 can initiate apoptosis to prevent perpetuation of the flawed cell. Interestingly, mice with homozygous disruption of both *P53* alleles develop normally, but get cancers at many sites after birth (183). Affected members of families with Li-Fraumeni syndrome inherit a single mutant *P53* allele, and have a high predisposition to cancers of several organs (these tumors exhibit somatic mutations in the other *P53* allele). Thus, it appears that p53 is required in cellular emergencies. In its absence, cells that would normally be removed survive, and occasionally give rise to cancers.

Inactivating point mutations of the *P53* tumor suppressor gene are highly prevalent in anaplastic and poorly differentiated thyroid tumors, but not in well-differentiated papillary or follicular carcinomas (184–187). These data implicate p53 inactivation as an important step in late-stage progression of thyroid cancer. Besides impairing apoptosis and removing an important cell cycle checkpoint, loss of function of p53 predisposes cells to additional genetic damage, and is therefore commonly associated with cancers displaying aggressive behavior (188). In addition, loss of function of p53 may impair thyroid cell–differentiated gene expression. Introduction of mutant p53 expression vectors into the well-differentiated thyroid cell line PCCL3 results in loss of expression of thyroglobulin, thyroid peroxidase, and the TSH receptor, and preferential impairment of expression of the thyroid-specific transcription factor Pax-8 (189). Conversely, reexpression of wild-type p53 in undifferentiated thyroid carcinoma cell lines is associated with restoration of Pax-8 production, and of expression of thyroid peroxidase (190,191). The precise mechanism by which loss of function of p53 interferes with thyroid-specific gene expression is not known. However, because p53 does not appear to be required for thyroid development, it is likely that loss of function of p53 does not directly impact thyroid-differentiated gene expression.

PTEN

Germline mutations of the *PTEN* gene confer predisposition to Cowden's disease, a condition characterized by development of hamartomas in multiple organs, and increased risk of breast, thyroid, and other cancers (192, 193). *PTEN* codes for a dual specificity lipid and tyrosine phosphatase, which dephosphorylates phosphatidylinositol 3,4,5 trisphosphate and antagonizes the phosphatidylinositol-3 kinase (PI3K)-protein kinase B (Akt) signaling pathway. Hamartomas and cancers developing in these patients acquire loss-of-function mutations or deletions affecting the remaining *PTEN* allele (194,195). A role for *PTEN* on development of sporadic thyroid neoplasms has not yet been firmly established. Allelic loss of the *PTEN* locus in 10q23.3 is seen in about a quarter of sporadic non-medullary thyroid cancers, yet this is not coupled with mutations in the hemizygous *PTEN* allele. Loss or reduction of PTEN protein expression as well as inappropriate subcellular compartmentalization has been reported in non-medullary thyroid cancers (196–198), and may occur in part through epigenetic silencing. The absence of somatic *PTEN* mutations in thyroid cancer has prompted a screen

for other candidate tumor suppressor genes close to the *PTEN* locus on 10q23.3. *MINPP1* has also been localized to this region, and codes for a phosphatase that has the ability to remove the 3-phosphate from inositol phosphate substrates, a function that overlaps that of PTEN. One follicular carcinoma with loss of heterozygosity at this locus had a somatic point mutation in the other *MINPP1* allele, but the functional consequences of this are not known (199). Despite these issues, the potential relevance of the PI3K-Akt pathway in thyroid tumorigenesis is supported by the observation that Akt expression and activation is increased in thyroid cancers, particularly in follicular carcinomas (200).

Other Candidate Tumor Suppressor Genes

As mentioned above, loss of function of tumor suppressor genes usually requires structural inactivation of both alleles. One of these is usually lost as part of a large deletion of chromosomal material. Based on this paradigm, the hunt for tumor suppressor genes has been conducted using approaches to identify regions of chromosomal loss that are common in particular forms of tumors. Papillary carcinomas have a low prevalence of chromosomal or allelic losses (201,202). By contrast, follicular neoplasms, particularly follicular carcinomas, exhibit more frequent allelic deletions (202,203). Using polymorphic molecular probes to scan the genome, some of the regions preferentially affected lie within chromosomes 2p, 2q, 3p, 7q, 10q, 11q, and 17p (202–208). There has been considerable effort to identify potential tumor suppressor genes lying within those regions. No mutations of either the von Hippel-Lindau (*VHL*) or the *FHIT* genes were found in follicular neoplasms with 3p deletions, possibly excluding these candidate tumor suppressors as significant in the pathogenesis of differentiated thyroid cancer (204).

Epigenetic Changes: Abnormalities in DNA Methylation

The majority of human gene promoters lie within chromosome areas rich in CG dinucleotides, referred to as CG islands. Most of these CG sites are demethylated, with the exception of genes located on the X chromosome, and certain imprinted loci (209). CG island methylation results in heritable inhibition of gene transcription and has been proposed as an alternative mechanism of gene inactivation in neoplasia (210,211). Increased DNA methylation has been reported to inhibit expression of tumor suppressor genes (212) and to predispose to transitional point mutations at methylated cytosines (213). Abnormal CpG methylation is a common event in neoplasia, usually occurring as an early event (211,214). The mechanism for these methylation changes is unknown. Thyroid tumors are no exception to this paradigm, because they exhibit a high prevalence of methylation abnormalities, occurring early in tumor progression and affecting loci of potential pathogenetic significance (176–178,215–218).

DISRUPTION OF PROGRAMMED CELL DEATH

Tissue homeostasis is maintained in part by factors that control the appropriate balance between cell proliferation and cell death. Apoptosis is a physiologic process that requires sequential expression of gene products that induce chromatin condensation, DNA cleavage, and cytosolic shrinkage. Within endocrine tissues, for instance, apoptosis is required for breast and prostatic involution after lactation, and androgen withdrawal, respectively. As mentioned previously, apoptosis is triggered to prevent proliferation of damaged cells, such as occurs after exposure to ionizing radiation. If tumors are to arise they must successfully bypass the cell-killing program that is activated in response to particular cues. In certain cancers, mutations of genes involved in the regulation of cell death appear to be primary mediators of tumorigenesis. Perhaps the most significant example is the overexpression of *bcl-2* in follicular lymphomas that occurs as a result of a translocation between the immunoglobulin heavy chain gene promoter and the *bcl-2* gene (219,220). The normal function of *bcl-2* in B-lymphocytes is to promote cell survival, presumably as a mechanism to perpetuate immune memory. Illegitimate overexpression of *bcl-2* is not in itself sufficient to induce tumorigenesis, but favors the perpetuation of a neoplastic clone by impairing apoptosis, and allowing the survival of cells that accumulate mutations affecting genes involved in growth control. There is presently only sketchy information on the possible role of apoptosis in thyroid tumor evolution. However, initiation of programmed cell death is a key protective mechanism evoked after oncogene activation in thyroid cells (125,126,221,222). For tumor clones to develop and expand, it is likely that the apoptotic program must be disabled through secondary genetic or epigenetic events that are yet to be identified.

FACTORS THAT MAINTAIN THE INTEGRITY OF THE GENOME

Mismatch Repair Deficiency Causing Microsatellite Instability

Hereditary nonpolyposis colorectal cancer (HNPCC) is an autosomal-dominant disease associated with early onset of colorectal cancer. The genes responsible for conferring this predisposition, *hMSH2, hMLH1, hPMS1,* and *hPMS2,* code for enzymes that correct nucleotide mismatches that occur during DNA synthesis (223,224). A homozygous disruption of one of these genes (one allele mutated in the germline, the other as an acquired somatic event) results in microsatellite instability (RER), a tendency to acquire alterations at mononucleotide, dinucleotide, or trinucleotide repeat sequences (microsatellites), which are widespread throughout the genome. These regions are more prone to error during DNA replication, and the mismatches cannot be efficiently corrected when the appropriate enzymatic complex is defective. It is thought that the RER genome results in mutations of genes important in growth control, as demonstrated for the *TGFβII* receptor in colorectal cancers (225). Microsatellite instability is uncommon in sporadic papillary thyroid carcinomas (226–231), and probably not a major mechanism of transformation in follicular neoplasms, although the latter findings are not conclusive (227). Whether radiation-induced papillary thyroid cancers exhibit microsatellite instability is somewhat controversial, with some studies failing to find evidence of RER (226), and others finding a low prevalence (231). Perhaps tellingly, patients with HNPCC do not appear to have a higher incidence of thyroid cancer, and none of the studies of sporadic or radiation-induced thyroid cancers has identified mutations of any of the genes coding for mismatch repair enzymes.

Chromosomal Instability

Genetic instability in cancer more commonly manifests as alterations in chromosome number (aneuploidy) (232, 233). Follicular carcinomas are more frequently aneuploid than papillary carcinomas, a phenomenon that has been proposed to be due to chromosome nondisjunction (201, 234,235). There is reason to believe that aneuploidy may have a genetic etiology, based primarily on studies in yeast in which mutations of over 100 genes can cause chromosomal instability. These include genes involved in chromosome metabolism, spindle assembly, chromosome segregation, and checkpoint control (236). In human cancers, this notion has gained experimental support (232). A predisposition to gain or lose whole chromosomes in colorectal cell lines has been linked to abnormalities in the mitotic checkpoint (237), which is activated by the presence of unattached kinetochores (238). In *Saccharomyces cerevisiae,* the "budding uninhibited by benzimidazole" (BUB1, 2, and 3), and the mitotic-arrest defective (MAD1, 2, and 3) proteins are intermediates in signal transduction cascades that are activated by mitotic spindle damage and delay onset of anaphase (239,240). This pathway also responds to defects in the structure of centromeres and kinetochores, and is thought to be responsible for the mitotic checkpoint activated by unattached or misaligned chromosomes. In *Drosophila,* animals with near-null mutations of *BUB1* die during late larval stages due to mitotic abnormalities, indicative of bypass of the mitotic checkpoint function (241). Mutations of a human homologue of *BUB1* have been identified in a subset of colorectal cancer cell lines with chromosomal instability (237), and in one sporadic rectal cancer (242). Somatic mutations of *hBUB1* have also been reported in primary lung cancers and lung cancer cell lines (243). However, subsequent studies have not found this to be a common abnormality in these and other tumor types (244,245). This is also the case in aneuploid thyroid neoplasms and thyroid cancer cell lines with mitotic checkpoint dysfunction, in which mutations of *BUB1* or its homologue *BUBR1* are largely absent (246). It remains to be seen whether or not somatic mutations of other genes coding for components of the mitotic checkpoint pathway may play a role in aneuploidy. An alternative explanation for the chromosomal instability of colorectal cancers has recently been advanced based on the discovery of a new property of the adenomatous polyposis coli tumor suppressor gene product (APC). A complex of proteins that includes APC may function as adaptors that allow the kinetochore to attach to microtubules. Mutations in APC domains involved in these associations may disrupt normal chromosome alignment and segregation in metaphase, thus predisposing to polyploidy (247).

Overexpression of the pituitary tumor transforming gene product (PTTG), the mammalian homologue of the yeast protein securin, has been reported in different tumor types, including pituitary adenomas (248,249) and thyroid neoplasms (250). Separation of sister chromatids in anaphase is mediated by separase, an endopeptidase that cleaves the chromosomal cohesin complexes that bridge the aligned sister chromatids. Separase is in turn inhibited by securin, which is degraded at the metaphase–anaphase transition. Overexpression of PTTG/securin induces aneuploidy in certain cell types (251). Curiously, mice lacking PTTG/securin are viable, and embryonic *PTGG* (−/−) fibroblasts have numerous chromosomal abnormalities (252). Thus, disruption of factors involved in sister chromatid separation can result in aneuploidy. So far there are no reports of tumor-promoting mutations of PTTG/securin, and most cancers exhibit primarily higher levels of expression. Interestingly, PTTG/securin overexpression in cell lines induces FGF2 production, and increased abundance of these gene products is a negative prognostic indicator in differentiated thyroid cancers (253).

Some of the early genetic events involved in tumor initiation could confer cells with a "mutator" phenotype, characterized by loss of genomic stability and a higher rate of mutations than normal cells (254). The standard interpretation of this hypothesis is that genes conferring cells with a "mutator" phenotype are likely to be directly involved in DNA repair (e.g., mismatch repair enzymes) or in cell cycle checkpoints. However, there is evidence that constitutive activation of oncogenes such as Ras may also disrupt genomic stability. A key role for Ras in mitotic spindle assembly has been reported in fission yeast (255,256). In mammalian cells, MAP kinases may also play a direct role in mitosis and chromosome segregation. Activated MAP kinase localizes to kinetochores in early and midmitosis, in

asters during all stages of mitosis, and in the chromosome midbody in late anaphase (257). Evidence for a temporal sequence of localization of activated MAP kinase in different nuclear compartments during mitosis (257,258) suggests that phosphorylation-dephosphorylation steps are needed for orderly progression, a step that may be disrupted when MAPK activation is constitutive. Induction of expression of the human H-Ras oncogene in p53-null cells leads to premature entry of cells into S phase, increased permissivity for gene amplification, and generation of aberrant chromosomes within a single cell cycle (259, 260). Overexpression of oncogenic Ras has also been shown to produce chromosome aberrations in rat mammary carcinoma cells (261), rat prostatic tumor cells (262), and in a human colon carcinoma cell line (263). In thyroid PCCL3 cells, acute H-Ras^{v12} activation induces chromosome missegregation, centrosome amplification, and chromosome misalignment within two cell cycles after activation (129). A putative role of *RAS* as a mutator gene has not been studied in animal models or in human studies.

EVENTS PREDISPOSING TO THYROID NEOPLASIA

Genetic Predisposition to Nonmedullary Thyroid Cancer

There are several familial syndromes of neoplasia that exhibit increased incidence of tumors of thyroid follicular cells (Table 70B.1). An increased predisposition to papillary carcinoma is well established in certain families with adenomatous polyposis (FAP), an autosomal condition characterized by the presence of multiple adenomatous polyps of the intestine (264–266). The association with thyroid cancer extends to Gardner's syndrome, a variant of FAP characterized by numerous intestinal adenomas, osteomas, soft tissue lesions, and other extracolonic neoplasms (267,268). Thyroid cancers in FAP exhibit a marked female preponderance (female:male ratio 8:1) and are more common under the age of 30. Women under 35 years of age with FAP have been estimated to have a 160-fold higher risk for thyroid carcinoma than normal individuals (265). Papillary carcinomas from patients with FAP are commonly multifocal, well encapsulated, and often display unusual histopathologic features, such as areas of cribriform, solid, and spindle cells within the tumors (269). Predisposition to FAP is conferred by germline-inactivating mutations of *APC*, which maps to chromosome 5q21 (270,271). Colorectal neoplasms from patients with FAP frequently exhibit loss of heterozygosity at this locus, consistent with a role for APC as a tumor suppressor gene, requiring loss of function of both alleles in order for the recessive phenotype to emerge. However, no biallelic inactivation of the APC gene was found in thyroid cancers from four patients in two FAP kindreds (272). Most patients with FAP developing papillary thyroid carcinomas

TABLE 70B.1. FAMILIAL SYNDROMES ASSOCIATED WITH TUMORS OF THYROID FOLLICULAR CELLS

Disease Entity	Manifestations	Chromosomal Location	Gene	Function
Familial polyposis coli	Polyps in large intestine, papillary thyroid cancer	5q21	APC	Cell adhesion, mitotic checkpoint
Gardner's syndrome	Polyps in small and large intestine, osteomas, fibromas, lipomas, ampullary cancers, papillary thyroid cancer	5q21, others(?)	APC	Cell adhesion, mitotic checkpoint
Turcot's syndrome	Polyps in large intestine, brain tumors, papillary thyroid cancer	5q21, others(?)	APC	Cell adhesion, mitotic checkpoint
Multiple endocrine neoplasia type I	Parathyroid adenomas, pituitary adenomas, pancreatic endocrine tumors, follicular adenomas (?)	11q13	Menin	Transcriptional regulation, telomerase activity
Cowden's disease	Multiple hamartomas, follicular adenomas, goiter, follicular carcinomas	10q22-23	PTEN	Dual-specificity phosphatase
Carney complex	Spotty skin pigmentation, myxomas, schwannomas, pigmented adrenocortical nodules, hypercortisolism, follicular adenomas, follicular carcinomas	2p16, 17q23	PKARIA	cAMP signaling
Familial non-medullary thyroid cancer syndromes	Papillary thyroid carcinoma, non-toxic multinodular goiter	14q	MNGI (unknown)	
	Papillary thyroid cancer and papillary renal neoplasms	1q21	PTC (unknown)	
	Benign and malignant tumors with oxyphilia	19p13.2	TCO (unknown)	

have *APC* defects lying outside of the mutation cluster region (codons 1286–1513), considered the hot spot mutation area for extracolonic manifestations of FAP (273). The existence of "modifier" genes that act in concert with *APC* to alter the predisposition to tumor formation at extracolonic sites, such as the thyroid gland, has been proposed. This is supported by analysis of FAP kindreds with family members inheriting the same *APC* mutation but differing dramatically in tumor burden (i.e., number of polyps). It is noteworthy that mutations of *APC* are not common in sporadic thyroid cancers, suggesting that inactivation of this gene is not likely to be a major pathogenetic event in thyroid tumorigenesis (274,275).

Thyroid tumors have also been reported in other familial syndromes. They are a frequent extracutaneous manifestation of Cowden's disease (multiple hamartoma syndrome), being observed in two thirds of patients; they include benign thyroid lesions (adenomas, goiter, thyroglossal duct cyst), and follicular thyroid carcinoma (276). As mentioned above, the gene for Cowden's disease has recently been identified (*PTEN*), and found to function as a dual-specificity phosphatase. There are case reports describing the association of thyroid carcinoma in patients with Peutz-Jeghers syndrome (277) and ataxia-telangiectasia (278).

It is controversial whether there is a significant increase in prevalence of thyroid tumors in patients with multiple endocrine neoplasia type 1 (MEN-1). When present, thyroid disease is observed mostly as benign lesions (nodular

hyperplasia, goiter, adenoma), and far more rarely as a malignancy (279). The gene conferring predisposition to MEN-1 (*MENIN*) is located on chromosome 11q13 (280,281), and believed to function as a tumor suppressor through mechanisms that may involve interference with control of gene transcription (282,283), DNA replication/repair (284,285), and telomerase activity (286, 287). Pancreatic, pituitary, and parathyroid tumors from patients with MEN-1 frequently exhibit loss of heterozygosity at this locus, leading to loss of function of the normal allele. Loss of heterozygosity at chromosome 11q13 is also found in sporadic follicular thyroid neoplasms, but to our knowledge no intragenic *MENIN* mutations have been reported in these tumors (206,208). However, a role for *MENIN* in thyroid tumor development is supported by data from heterozygous *MENIN* knockout mice, which develop thyroid neoplasms (288).

Carney complex is an autosomal-dominant disorder associated with cardiac myxomas and endocrine tumors caused in part by inactivating mutations of the gene encoding the regulatory subunit 1A of the cAMP-dependent protein kinase (*PKAR1A*), resulting in its inappropriate activation (289,290). Although the Carney complex is primarily associated with benign endocrine neoplasms, thyroid follicular carcinomas may also be observed (291).

There have been multiple reports of familial clustering of papillary carcinomas (292–296). Most of the literature consists of descriptions of individual family pedigrees. This has resulted in uncertainty as to whether the familial association represents evidence of genetic predisposition to the disease, exposure to a common environmental triggering event, increased susceptibility to environmental effects, or a chance occurrence. A comprehensive analysis of families of all cases of papillary carcinoma diagnosed in Iceland between 1955 and 1984 revealed that 3.8% of the propositi had a first-degree relative with thyroid carcinoma, a higher than expected frequency that was not, however, statistically significant (although there was a significantly increased risk in male relatives) (297). Stoffer et al studied families from 226 consecutive papillary thyroid carcinoma patients from a private practice, and concluded that 3.5% to 6.2% had at least one affected relative (298). Ron et al reported a population-based case control study of the Connecticut Tumor Registry, in which a fivefold excess risk for nonmedullary thyroid cancer was found in close relatives (299,300). On balance, the evidence for a genetic basis for familial non-medullary thyroid carcinoma is quite supportive. The transmission of susceptibility to familial nonmedullary thyroid cancer is compatible with autosomal-dominant inheritance with reduced penetrance, or with complex inheritance (301). Linkage studies have identified the putative locations of three genes for familial NMTC: *MNG1* (302), *TCO* (303, 304), and *PTC* (305). A large Canadian family of German origin showed linkage of *MNG1* to chromosome 14q (302). This family included 18 cases of nontoxic multinodular goiter, with 2 individuals having papillary lesions suggestive of papillary thyroid cancer. A gene conferring predisposition to benign and malignant tumors with oxyphilia in a French family was mapped to chromosome 19p13.2 by linkage analysis (303). In a three-generation family with five cases of papillary thyroid cancer, three cases of thyroid nodules, and two cases of papillary renal neoplasia, linkage was found to 1q21 (putative *PTC* gene) (305).

Radiation-Induced Thyroid Cancer

The major known risk factor for papillary thyroid carcinoma is prior exposure to radiation. The most significant sources of exposure have been after therapeutic irradiation and through environmental disasters (306–308). The effects of radiation on thyroid cancer risk are dose dependent (307,308). A lower age at the time of exposure has been consistently associated with a higher relative risk for thyroid cancer, a phenomenon that was clearly apparent in the pediatric thyroid carcinomas arising after the Chernobyl nuclear disaster (309–311). As a result of the accident at the Chernobyl nuclear power plant, 8×10^{18} Bq of radioactivity were released, most in the form of radioiodine isotopes. The absorption of radioiodines from ingestion of contaminated food and water and through inhalation led to internal exposure to the thyroid gland, which was 3 to 10 times higher in children than in adults. An increased incidence of thyroid cancer in children from Belarus and Ukraine was noted as early as 4 to 5 years after the accident (312), and the risk

was higher in the most contaminated regions. Between 1990 and 1998, the incidence of childhood thyroid cancer in Belarus was at least 60-fold greater than prior to the disaster (309), and this increase extends to contaminated regions of Ukraine and Southwest Russia. More than 95% of post-Chernobyl thyroid cancers are papillary carcinomas. Radiation is known to induce DNA strand breaks, and it was therefore fitting that *RET/PTC* rearrangements were highly prevalent in cancers from children exposed to radiation after the Chernobyl nuclear accident (64,65,313), or to external irradiation for treatment of benign diseases of the head and neck (64,314,315). It should be noted that *RET* rearrangements are also found with high prevalence in pediatric papillary thyroid carcinomas with no documented history of radiation exposure, so it cannot be assumed that this genetic recombination is specific to radiation-induced DNA damage (63). There are several lines of evidence indicating that *RET/PTC* rearrangements are likely caused directly by ionizing irradiation:

1. Irradiation of human fetal thyroid explants, undifferentiated thyroid carcinoma, or fibrosarcoma cells *in vitro* induces *RET/PTC1* rearrangements in a dose-dependent fashion within a short time frame (73,74).
2. The pattern of breakpoints in *ELE1* and *RET* intronic DNA, the target genes involved in the *RET/PTC3* recombination, revealed that in each tumor the position of the break in one gene corresponded to the position of the break in the other gene. This tendency suggests that the two genes may lie next to each other in the nucleus. Such a structure would facilitate formation of *RET/PTC3* rearrangements because a single radiation track could produce concerted breaks in both genes, leading to intrachromosomal inversion due to reciprocal exchange via end-joining.
3. Juxtaposition of chromosomal loci participating in the *RET/PTC1* rearrangement (i.e., *RET* and *H4*) during interphase in normal human thyroid cells was later demonstrated, further suggesting that chromosomal architecture during interphase may be an important prerequisite for *RET* recombination after radiation in thyroid cells (76) (Fig. 70B.3).

A distinguishing feature of these pediatric radiation-induced tumors is the high prevalence of solid pattern growth manifesting as sheets of malignant epithelial cells surrounded by varying amounts of fibrotic stroma. A solid growth pattern was seen in almost half of all Chernobyl cancers (64). By contrast, this type of histologic appearance is rare in sporadic adult and pediatric papillary carcinomas. Solid variant papillary carcinomas are primarily associated with *RET/PTC3*, whereas tumors with typical papillary morphology more commonly have *RET/PTC1* rearrangements (64,316,317). These data suggest that these two fusion genes may have distinct functional properties. This is supported by the observation that transgenic mice with

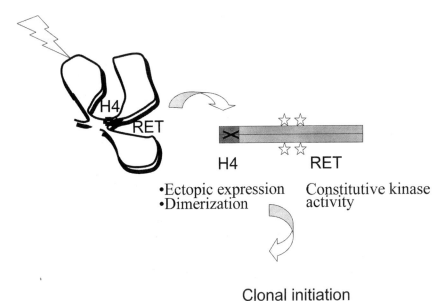

FIGURE 70B.3. Chromosomal architecture during interphase may predispose thyroid cells to *RET* activation by recombination after radiation exposure. The *RET* and *H4* genes, despite being at a considerable distance from each other on chromosome 10, are spatially juxtaposed during interphase in normal human thyroid cells. This could presumably generate a target for a single radiation track to produce concerted breaks in both genes, leading to intrachromosomal inversion and activation of expression of the H4-RET fusion protein (RET/PTC1). The N-terminal domain of H4 donates a coiled-coil motif, thus allowing constitutive dimerization, and activation of tyrosine kinase activity in an unregulated fashion.

thyroid-specific expression of *RET/PTC1* develop typical papillary carcinomas (68,69), whereas those expressing *RET/PTC3* develop solid-variant tumors (318). There are preliminary indications that solid-variant tumors may carry a worse prognosis (319).

Mutations of *RAS* or *P53* were not involved in the generation of radiation-induced PTC (320,321).

CONCLUSIONS: AN INTEGRATED PERSPECTIVE OF THYROID TUMOR PATHOGENESIS

It may be enlightening to attempt to recreate the natural history of thyroid cancers based on available epidemiologic and genetic information. However, it is important to emphasize that there is much we do not know. Progression of thyroid tumors is mostly interrupted when they are removed at surgery, making data on prognostic implications of particular genotypes difficult to evaluate. Although in part speculative, this remains a worthwhile exercise, because it may point to some unresolved questions and areas of opportunity for the future.

Papillary Thyroid Carcinomas

A general assumption in tumor genetics is that a single oncogenic mutation is not sufficient to induce malignant transformation. It follows that sequential abnormalities must take place. The evidence that activating rearrangements of tyrosine kinase receptors (i.e., *RET/PTCs* and *NTRK*) are likely early events in papillary thyroid cancer has been reviewed, and is now quite compelling. Similarly, recent studies indicating that papillary cancers harbor mutually exclusive mu-

tations of *RET/PTC* or *RAS* or *B-RAF* point to a requirement for constitutive activation of this signaling pathway (presumably acting via MEK-ERK) in tumor initiation. PTCs harboring different *RET/PTC* variants, *RAS,* or *BRAF* mutations often exhibit distinct pathologic features, and may also differ in their biologic behavior, indicating that the nature of the tumor-initiating event is important. Thus, most solid-variant PTCs harbor the *RET/PTC3* rearrangement, follicular variant PTCs commonly have *RAS* mutations, and tall cell variant PTCs have *BRAF* mutations. Clearly, other cooperating genetic events must take place, but these are yet to be discovered. There is now an abundance of information on global gene expression changes and epigenetic modifications of putative tumor suppressor genes in PTC, but their significance to tumor progression has not been studied. Papillary carcinomas have a low rate of aneuploidy, loss of heterozygosity, and microsatellite instability. This predicts that the tumor clone will remain fairly homogeneous, and explains in part the excellent prognosis and response to therapy of this type of thyroid cancer.

Follicular Thyroid Carcinomas

Follicular carcinomas are believed to arise from benign adenomas. Absolute proof of the adenoma–carcinoma transition is lacking, but the existence of intermediate phenotypes (i.e., minimally invasive follicular carcinomas) is consistent with this microevolution. Follicular carcinomas are more common in iodine deficiency regions, suggesting that the proliferative drive may be a factor in their development. Mutations of all three mammalian *RAS* genes (*H-RAS, N-RAS,* and to a lesser extent *K-RAS*) are seen in follicular adenomas and carcinomas, although they appear to be more prevalent in the latter. It is unclear why *RAS* mutations are associated with both PTC and FTC. One can speculate that the impact of *RAS* mutations on tumor phenotype may differ according to whether they occur early or later in tumor progression, and with which other cooperating genetic event they are associated. PAX8-PPARγ1 rearrangements are present specifically in follicular neoplasms, particularly follicular carcinomas. Based on the observation that FTC either have *RAS* mutations or *PAX8-PPARγ1* rearrangements, but rarely both, the existence of two distinct and virtually nonoverlapping molecular pathways initiated by these oncoproteins has been proposed (322). FTC have higher rates of allelic loss and aneuploidy, consistent with chromosomal instability.

Undifferentiated or Anaplastic Thyroid Carcinomas

The end-stage forms of thyroid cancer are characterized by loss of differentiated properties, greater tumor invasiveness, and metastatic spread. Both FTC and PTC can progress to undifferentiated or anaplastic carcinomas. Mutations of the *P53* tumor suppressor gene are a common feature of undifferentiated thyroid cancers, and this tumor suppressor is a strong candidate for the transition from well-differentiated to anaplastic carcinoma.

REFERENCES

1. Namba H, Matsuo K, Fagin JA. Clonal composition of benign and malignant human thyroid tumors. *J Clin Invest* 1990; 86:120–125.
2. Fey MF, Peter HJ, Hinds HL, et al. Clonal analysis of human tumors with M27 beta, a highly informative polymorphic X chromosomal probe. *J Clin Invest* 1992;89:1438–1444.
3. Aeschimann S, Kopp PA, Kimura ET, et al. Morphological and functional polymorphism within clonal thyroid nodules. *J Clin Endocrinol Metab* 1993;77:846–851.
4. Wynford-Thomas D, Stringer BM, Williams ED. Dissociation of growth and function in the rat thyroid during prolonged goitrogen administration. *Acta Endocrinol (Copenh)* 1982;101:210–216.
5. Black EG, Logan A, Davis JR, et al. Basic fibroblast growth factor affects DNA synthesis and cell function and activates multiple signalling pathways in rat thyroid FRTL-5 and pituitary GH3 cells. *J Endocrinol* 1990;127:39–46.
6. Eggo MC, Hopkins JM, Franklyn JA, et al. Expression of fibroblast growth factors in thyroid cancer. *J Clin Endocrinol Metab* 1995;80:1006–1011.
7. Shingu K, Sugenoya A, Itoh N, et al. Expression of basic fibroblast growth factor in thyroid disorders. *World J Surg* 1994; 18:500–505.
8. Boelaert K, McCabe CJ, Tannahill LA, et al. Pituitary tumor transforming gene and fibroblast growth factor-2 expression: potential prognostic indicators in differentiated thyroid cancer. *J Clin Endocrinol Metab* 2003;88:2341–2347.
9. Clement S, Refetoff S, Robaye B, et al. Low TSH requirement and goiter in transgenic mice overexpressing IGF-I and IGF-Ir receptor in the thyroid gland. *Endocrinology* 2001;142:5131–5139.
10. Vella V, Sciacca L, Pandini G, et al. The IGF system in thyroid cancer: new concepts. *Mol Pathol* 2001;54:121–124.
11. van der Laan BF, Freeman JL, Asa SL. Expression of growth factors and growth factor receptors in normal and tumorous human thyroid tissues. *Thyroid* 1995;5:67–73.
12. Belfiore A, Pandini G, Vella V, et al. Insulin/IGF-I hybrid receptors play a major role in IGF-I signaling in thyroid cancer. *Biochimie* 1999;81:403–407.
13. Lemoine NR, Hughes CM, Gullick WJ, et al. Abnormalities of the EGF receptor system in human thyroid neoplasia. *Int J Cancer* 1991;49:558–561.
14. Aasland R, Akslen LA, Varhaug JE, et al. Co-expression of the genes encoding transforming growth factor-alpha and its receptor in papillary carcinomas of the thyroid. *Int J Cancer* 1990; 46:382–387.
15. Colletta G, Cirafici AM, Di Carlo A, et al. Constitutive expression of transforming growth factor alpha does not transform rat thyroid epithelial cells. *Oncogene* 1991;6:583–587.
16. Dawson TP, Radulescu A, Wynford-Thomas D. Expression of mutant p21ras induces insulin-like growth factor 1 secretion in thyroid epithelial cells. *Cancer Res* 1995;55:915–920.
17. Ferrara N. VEGF and the quest for tumour angiogenesis factors. *Nat Rev Cancer* 2002;2:795–803.
18. Kerbel R, Folkman J. Clinical translation of angiogenesis inhibitors. *Nat Rev Cancer* 2002;2:727–739.
19. Jussila L, Alitalo K. Vascular growth factors and lymphangiogenesis. *Physiol Rev* 2002;82:673–700.
20. Viglietto G, Maglione D, Rambaldi M, et al. Upregulation of vascular endothelial growth factor (VEGF) and downregulation of placenta growth factor (PlGF) associated with malignancy in human thyroid tumors and cell lines. *Oncogene* 1995; 11:1569–1579.
21. Soh EY, Duh QY, Sobhi SA, et al. Vascular endothelial growth factor expression is higher in differentiated thyroid cancer than in normal or benign thyroid. *J Clin Endocrinol Metab* 1997;82: 3741–3747.
22. Shushanov S, Bronstein M, Adelaide J, et al. VEGFc and VEGFR3 expression in human thyroid pathologies. *Int J Cancer* 2000;86:47–52.
23. Hung CJ, Ginzinger DG, Zarnegar R, et al. Expression of vascular endothelial growth factor-C in benign and malignant thyroid tumors. *J Clin Endocrinol Metab* 2003;88:3694–3699.
24. Friesel RE, Maciag T. Molecular mechanisms of angiogenesis: fibroblast growth factor signal transduction. *FASEB J* 1995; 9:919–925.
25. Franzen A, Piek E, Westermark B, et al. Expression of transforming growth factor-beta1, activin A, and their receptors in thyroid follicle cells: negative regulation of thyrocyte growth and function. *Endocrinology* 1999;140:4300–4310.
26. Grubeck-Loebenstein B, Buchan G, Sadeghi R, et al. Transforming growth factor beta regulates thyroid growth. Role in the pathogenesis of nontoxic goiter. *J Clin Invest* 1989;83:764–770.
27. Kimura ET, Kopp P, Zbaeren J, et al. Expression of transforming growth factor beta1, beta2, and beta3 in multinodular goiters and differentiated thyroid carcinomas: a comparative study. *Thyroid* 1999;9:119–125.
28. Bhowmick NA, Chytil A, Plieth D, et al. TGF-beta signaling in fibroblasts modulates the oncogenic potential of adjacent epithelia. *Science* 2004;303:848–851.
29. Nose F, Ichikawa T, Fujiwara M, et al. Up-regulation of cyclooxygenase-2 expression in lymphocytic thyroiditis and thyroid tumors: significant correlation with inducible nitric oxide synthase. *Am J Clin Pathol* 2002;117:546–551.
30. Cornetta AJ, Russell JP, Cunnane M, et al. Cyclooxygenase-2 expression in human thyroid carcinoma and Hashimoto's thyroiditis. *Laryngoscope* 2002;112:238–242.

31. Specht MC, Tucker ON, Hocever M, et al. Cyclooxygenase-2 expression in thyroid nodules. *J Clin Endocrinol Metab* 2002; 87:358–363.

32. Bauer AJ, Patel A, Terrell R, et al. Systemic administration of vascular endothelial growth factor monoclonal antibody reduces the growth of papillary thyroid carcinoma in a nude mouse model. *Ann Clin Lab Sci* 2003;33:192–199.

33. Seno H, Oshima M, Ishikawa TO, et al. Cyclooxygenase 2- and prostaglandin E(2) receptor EP(2)-dependent angiogenesis in Apc(Delta716) mouse intestinal polyps. *Cancer Res* 2002;62: 506–511.

34. Oshima M, Murai N, Kargman S, et al. Chemoprevention of intestinal polyposis in the Apcdelta716 mouse by rofecoxib, a specific cyclooxygenase-2 inhibitor. *Cancer Res* 2001;61:1733–1740.

35. Baron JA, Cole BF, Sandler RS, et al. A randomized trial of aspirin to prevent colorectal adenomas. *N Engl J Med* 2003;348: 891–899.

36. Sandler RS, Halabi S, Baron JA, et al. A randomized trial of aspirin to prevent colorectal adenomas in patients with previous colorectal cancer. *N Engl J Med* 2003;348:883–890.

37. Puxeddu E, Mitsutake N, Knauf JA, et al. Microsomal prostaglandin E$_2$ synthase-1 is induced by conditional expression of RET/PTC in thyroid PCCL3 cells through the activation of the MEK-ERK pathway. *J Biol Chem* 2003;278:52131–52138.

38. Collins VP. Epidermal growth factor receptor gene and its transcripts in glioblastomas. *Rec Results Cancer Res* 1994;135:17–24.

39. Di Fiore PP, Kraus MH. Mechanisms involving an expanding erbB/EGF receptor family of tyrosine kinases in human neoplasia. *Cancer Treat Res* 1992;61:139–160.

40. Pegram MD, Konecny G, Slamon DJ. The molecular and cellular biology of HER2/neu gene amplification/overexpression and the clinical development of herceptin (trastuzumab) therapy for breast cancer. *Cancer Treat Res* 2000;103:57–75.

41. Habib AA, Chun SJ, Neel BG, et al. Increased expression of epidermal growth factor receptor induces sequestration of extracellular signal-related kinases and selective attenuation of specific epidermal growth factor-mediated signal transduction pathways. *Mol Cancer Res* 2003;1:219–233.

42. Chen BK, Ohtsuki Y, Furihata M, et al. Co-overexpression of p53 protein and epidermal growth factor receptor in human papillary thyroid carcinomas correlated with lymph node metastasis, tumor size and clinicopathologic stage. *Int J Oncol* 1999;15:893–898.

43. Haugen DR, Akslen LA, Varhaug JE, et al. Expression of c-erbB-3 and c-erbB-4 proteins in papillary thyroid carcinomas. *Cancer Res* 1996;56:1184–1188.

44. Di Renzo MF, Olivero M, Ferro S, et al. Overexpression of the c-MET/HGF receptor gene in human thyroid carcinomas. *Oncogene* 1992;7:2549–2553.

45. Belfiore A, Gangemi P, Costantino A, et al. Negative/low expression of the Met/hepatocyte growth factor receptor identifies papillary thyroid carcinomas with high risk of distant metastases. *J Clin Endocrinol Metab* 1997;82:2322–2328.

46. Ivan M, Bond JA, Prat M, et al. Activated ras and ret oncogenes induce over-expression of c-met (hepatocyte growth factor receptor) in human thyroid epithelial cells. *Oncogene* 1997;14: 2417–2423.

47. Croyle ML, Knauf JA, Fagin JA. RET/PTC induces EGF receptor expression and formation of RET/PTC-EGFR heterodimers in thyroid PCCL3 cells. Presented at the 75th Annual Meeting of the American Thyroid Association, 2003.

48. Santoro M, Melillo RM, Carlomagno F, et al. Molecular mechanisms of RET activation in human cancer. *Ann NY Acad Sci* 2002;963:116–121.

49. Airaksinen MS, Saarma M. The GDNF family: signalling, biological functions and therapeutic value. *Nat Rev Neurosci* 2002; 3:383–394.

50. Santoro M, Melillo RM, Carlomagno F, et al. Molecular mechanisms of RET activation in human cancer. *Ann NY Acad Sci* 2002;963:116–121.

51. Grieco M, Santoro M, Berlingieri MT, et al. PTC is a novel rearranged form of the ret proto-oncogene and is frequently detected *in vivo* in human thyroid papillary carcinomas. *Cell* 1990;60:557–563.

52. Bongarzone I, Monzini N, Borello MG, et al. Molecular characterization of a thyroid tumor-specific transforming sequence formed by the fusion of ret tyrosine kinase and the regulatory subunit RI alpha of cyclic AMP-dependent protein kinase A. *Mol Cell Biol* 1993;13:358–366.

53. Minoletti F, Butti MG, Coronelli S, et al. The two genes generating RET/PTC3 are localized in chromosomal band 10q11.2. *Genes Chromosomes Cancer* 1994;11:51–57.

54. Santoro M, Dathan NA, Berlingieri MT, et al. Molecular characterization of RET/PTC3; a novel rearranged version of the RETproto-oncogene in a human thyroid papillary carcinoma. *Oncogene* 1994;9:509–516.

55. Klugbauer S, Lengfelder E, Demidchik EP, et al. A new form of RET rearrangement in thyroid carcinomas of children after the Chernobyl reactor accident. *Oncogene* 1996;13:1099–1102.

56. Klugbauer S, Demidchik EP, Lengfelder E, et al. Detection of a novel type of RET rearrangement (PTC5) in thyroid carcinomas after Chernobyl and analysis of the involved RET-fused gene RFG5. *Cancer Res* 1998;58:198–203.

57. Klugbauer S, Rabes HM. The transcription coactivator HTIF1 and a related protein are fused to the RET receptor tyrosine kinase in childhood papillary thyroid carcinomas. *Oncogene* 1999;18:4388–4393.

58. Saenko V, Rogounovitch T, Shimizu-Yoshida Y, et al. Novel tumorigenic rearrangement, Delta rfp/ret, in a papillary thyroid carcinoma from externally irradiated patient. *Mutat Res* 2003;527:81–90.

59. Corvi R, Berger N, Balczon R, et al. RET/PCM-1: a novel fusion gene in papillary thyroid carcinoma. *Oncogene* 2000;19: 4236–4242.

60. Salassidis K, Bruch J, Zitzelsberger H, et al. Translocation t(10;14)(q11.2:q22.1) fusing the kinetin to the RET gene creates a novel rearranged form (PTC8) of the RET proto-oncogene in radiation-induced childhood papillary thyroid carcinoma. *Cancer Res* 2000;60:2786–2789.

61. Klugbauer S, Jauch A, Lengfelder E, et al. A novel type of RET rearrangement (PTC8) in childhood papillary thyroid carcinomas and characterization of the involved gene (RFG8). *Cancer Res* 2000;60:7028–7032.

62. Tong Q, Xing S, Jhiang SM. Leucine zipper-mediated dimerization is essential for the PTC1 oncogenic activity. *J Biol Chem* 1997;272:9043–9047.

63. Bongarzone I, Fugazzola L, Vigneri P, et al. Age-related activation of the tyrosine kinase receptor protooncogenes RET and NTRK1 in papillary thyroid carcinoma. *J Clin Endocrinol Metab* 1996;81:2006–2009.

64. Nikiforov YE, Rowland JM, Bove KE, et al. Distinct pattern of ret oncogene rearrangements in morphological variants of radiation-induced and sporadic thyroid papillary carcinomas in children. *Cancer Res* 1997;57:1690–1694.

65. Fugazzola L, Pilotti S, Pinchera A, et al. Oncogenic rearrangement of the RET proto-oncogene in papillary thyroid carcinomas from children exposed to the Chernobyl nuclear accident. *Cancer Res* 1995;55:5617–5620.

66. Elisei R, Romei C, Vorontsova T, et al. RET/PTC rearrangements in thyroid nodules: studies in irradiated and not irradi-

ated, malignant and benign thyroid lesions in children and adults. *J Clin Endocrinol Metab* 2001;86:3211–3216.

67. Bounacer A, Wicker R, Caillou B, et al. High prevalence of activating ret proto-oncogene rearrangements, in thyroid tumors from patients who had received external radiation. *Oncogene* 1997;15:1263–1273.

68. Jhiang SM, Sagartz JE, Tong Q, et al. Targeted expression of the ret/PTC1 oncogene induces papillary thyroid carcinomas. *Endocrinology* 1996;137:375–378.

69. Santoro M, Chiappetta G, et al. Development of thyroid papillary carcinomas secondary to tissue-specific expression of the RET/PTC1 oncogene in transgenic mice. *Oncogene* 1996;12:1821–1826.

70. Powell DJJ, Russell J, Nibu K, et al. The RET/PTC3 oncogene: metastatic solid-type papillary carcinomas in murine thyroids. *Cancer Res* 1998;58:5523–5528.

71. Viglietto G, Chiappetta G, Martinez-Tello FJ, et al. RET/PTC oncogene activation is an early event in thyroid carcinogenesis. *Oncogene* 1995;11:1207–1210.

72. Sugg SL, Ezzat S, Rosen IB, et al. Distinct multiple RET/PTC gene rearrangements in multifocal papillary thyroid neoplasia. *J Clin Endocrinol Metab* 1998;83:4116–4122.

73. Ito T, Seyama T, Iwamoto KS, et al. *In vitro* irradiation is able to cause RET oncogene rearrangement. *Cancer Res* 1993;53:2940–2943.

74. Mizuno T, Kyoizumi S, Suzuki T, et al. Continued expression of a tissue specific activated oncogene in the early steps of radiation-induced human thyroid carcinogenesis. *Oncogene* 1997;15:1455–1460.

75. Nikiforov YE, Koshoffer A, Nikiforova M, et al. Chromosomal breakpoint positions suggest a direct role for radiation in inducing illegitimate recombination between the ELE1 and RET genes in radiation-induced thyroid carcinomas. *Oncogene* 1999;18:6330–6334.

76. Nikiforova MN, Stringer JR, Blough R, et al. Proximity of chromosomal loci that participate in radiation-induced rearrangements in human cells. *Science* 2000;290:138–141.

77. Tallini G, Santoro M, Helie M, et al. RET/PTC oncogene activation defines a subset of papillary thyroid carcinomas lacking evidence of progression to poorly differentiated or undifferentiated tumor phenotypes. *Clin Cancer Res* 1998;4:287–294.

78. Bongarzone I, Pierotti MA, Monzini N, et al. High frequency of activation of tyrosine kinase oncogenes in human papillary thyroid carcinoma. *Oncogene* 1989;4:1457–1462.

79. Greco A, Pierotti MA, Bongarzone I, et al. TRK-T1 is a novel oncogene formed by the fusion of TPR and TRK genes in human papillary thyroid carcinomas. *Oncogene* 1992;7:237–242.

80. Pierotti MA, Bongarzone I, Borello MG, et al. Cytogenetics and molecular genetics of carcinomas arising from thyroid epithelial follicular cells. *Genes Chromosomes Cancer* 1996;16:1–14.

81. Greco A, Mariani C, Miranda C, et al. The DNA rearrangement that generates the TRK-T3 oncogene involves a novel gene on chromosome 3 whose product has a potential coiled-coil domain. *Mol Cell Biol* 1995;15:6118–6127.

82. Russell JP, Powell DJ, Cunnane M, et al. The TRK-T1 fusion protein induces neoplastic transformation of thyroid epithelium. *Oncogene* 2000;19:5729–5735.

83. Brandi ML, Gagel RF, Angeli A, et al. Guidelines for diagnosis and therapy of MEN type 1 and type 2. *J Clin Endocrinol Metab* 2001;86:5658–5671.

84. Eng C. RET proto-oncogene in the development of human cancer. *J Clin Oncol* 1999;17:380–393.

85. Hoff AO, Cote GJ, Gagel RF. Multiple endocrine neoplasias. *Annu Rev Physiol* 2000;62:377–411.

86. Parma J, Duprez L, Van Sande J, et al. Somatic mutations in the thyrotropin receptor gene cause hyperfunctioning thyroid adenomas. *Nature* 1993;365:649–651.

87. Duprez L, Parma J, Van Sande J, et al. Germline mutations in the thyrotropin receptor gene cause non-autoimmune autosomal dominant hyperthyroidism. *Nat Genet* 1994;7:396–401.

88. Parma J, Duprez L, Van Sande J, et al. Diversity and prevalence of somatic mutations in the thyrotropin receptor and Gs alpha genes as a cause of toxic thyroid adenomas. *J Clin Endocrinol Metab* 1997;82:2695–2701.

89. Rodien P, Ho SC, Vlaeminck V, et al. Activating mutations of TSH receptor. *Ann Endocrinol (Paris)* 2003;64:12–16.

90. Arturi F, Scarpelli D, Coco A, et al. Thyrotropin receptor mutations and thyroid hyperfunctioning adenomas ten years after their first discovery: unresolved questions. *Thyroid* 2003;13:341–343.

91. Krohn K, Paschke R. Clinical review 133: progress in understanding the etiology of thyroid autonomy. *J Clin Endocrinol Metab* 2001;86:3336–3345.

92. Vanvooren V, Uchino S, Duprez L, et al. Oncogenic mutations in the thyrotropin receptor of autonomously functioning thyroid nodules in the Japanese population. *Eur J Endocrinol* 2002;147:287–291.

93. Mazzaferri EL. Management of a solitary thyroid nodule [see comments] [Review]. *N Engl J Med* 1993;328:553–559.

94. Bourasseau I, Savagner F, Rodien P, et al. No evidence of thyrotropin receptor and G(s alpha) gene mutation in high iodine uptake thyroid carcinoma. *Thyroid* 2000;10:761–765.

95. Cetani F, Tonacchera M, Pinchera A, et al. Genetic analysis of the TSH receptor gene in differentiated human thyroid carcinomas. *J Endocrinol Invest* 1999;22:273–278.

96. Russo D, Arturi F, Schlumberger M, et al. Activating mutations of the TSH receptor in differentiated thyroid carcinomas. *Oncogene* 1996;11:1907–1911.

97. Spambalg D, Sharifi N, Elisei R, et al. Structural studies of the thyrotropin receptor and Gs alpha in human thyroid cancers: low prevalence of mutations predicts infrequent involvement in malignant transformation. *J Clin Endocrinol Metab* 1996;81:3898–3901.

98. Esapa C, Foster S, Johnson S, et al. G protein and thyrotropin receptor mutations in thyroid neoplasia. *J Clin Endocrinol Metab* 1997;82:493–496.

99. Russo D, Wong MG, Costante G, et al. A Val 677 activating mutation of the thyrotropin receptor in a Hurthle cell thyroid carcinoma associated with thyrotoxicosis. *Thyroid* 1999;9:13–17.

100. Baloch Z, LiVolsi VA. Detection of an activating mutation of the thyrotropin receptor in a case of an autonomously hyperfunctioning thyroid insular carcinoma. *J Clin Endocrinol Metab* 1997;82:3906–3908.

101. Cock TA, Houten SM, Auwerx J. Peroxisome proliferator-activated receptor-gamma: too much of a good thing causes harm. *EMBO Rep* 2004;5:142–147.

102. Kroll TG, Sarraf P, Pecciarini L, et al. PAX8-PPARgamma1 fusion oncogene in human thyroid carcinoma [corrected]. *Science* 2000;289:1357–1360.

103. Nikiforova MN, Biddinger PW, Caudill CM, et al. PAX8-PPARgamma rearrangement in thyroid tumors: RT-PCR and immunohistochemical analyses. *Am J Surg Pathol* 2002;26:1016–1023.

104. Marques AR, Espadinha C, Catarino AL, et al. Expression of PAX8-PPAR gamma 1 rearrangements in both follicular thyroid carcinomas and adenomas. *J Clin Endocrinol Metab* 2002;87:3947–3952.

105. Dwight T, Thoppe SR, Foukakis T, et al. Involvement of the PAX8/peroxisome proliferator-activated receptor gamma rearrangement in follicular thyroid tumors. *J Clin Endocrinol Metab* 2003;88:4440–4445.

106. Cheung L, Messina M, Gill A, et al. Detection of the PAX8-PPAR gamma fusion oncogene in both follicular thyroid carcinomas and adenomas. *J Clin Endocrinol Metab* 2003;88:354–357.

107. Martelli ML, Iuliano R, Le PI, et al. Inhibitory effects of peroxisome poliferator-activated receptor gamma on thyroid carcinoma cell growth. *J Clin Endocrinol Metab* 2002;87:4728–4735.

108. Puzianowska-Kuznicka M, Krystyniak A, Madej A, Cheng SY, Nauman J. Functionally impaired TR mutants are present in thyroid papillary cancer. *J Clin Endocrinol Metab* 2002;87:1120–1128.

109. Takano T, Miyauchi A, Yoshida H, et al. Expression of TRbeta1 mRNAs with functionally impaired mutations is rare in thyroid papillary carcinoma. *J Clin Endocrinol Metab* 2003;88:3447–3449.

110. Suzuki H, Willingham MC, Cheng SY. Mice with a mutation in the thyroid hormone receptor beta gene spontaneously develop thyroid carcinoma: a mouse model of thyroid carcinogenesis. *Thyroid* 2002;12:963–969.

111. Missero C, Pirro MT, Di Lauro R. Multiple ras downstream pathways mediate functional repression of the homeobox gene product TTF-1. *Mol Cell Biol* 2000;20:2783–2793.

112. Knauf JA, Kuroda H, Basu S, et al. RET/PTC-induced dedifferentiation of thyroid cells is mediated through Y1062 signaling through SHC-RAS-MAP kinase. *Oncogene* 2003;22:4406–4412.

113. Medema RH, Bos JL. The role of p21ras in receptor tyrosine kinase signaling [Review]. *Crit Rev Oncogenesis* 1993;4:615–661.

114. Lemoine NR, Mayall ES, Wyllie FS, et al. Activated ras oncogenes in human thyroid cancers. *Cancer Res* 1988;48:4459–4463.

115. *www.sanger.ac.uk/genetics/CGP/cosmic/*, 2004.

116. Esapa CT, Johnson SJ, Kendall-Taylor P, et al. Prevalence of Ras mutations in thyroid neoplasia. *Clin Endocrinol (Oxf)* 1999;50:529–535.

117. Karga H, Lee J-K, Vickery AL, et al. Ras oncogene mutations in benign and malignant thyroid neoplasms. *J Clin Endocrinol Metab* 1991;73:832–836.

118. Suarez HG, du Villard JA, Severino M, et al. Presence of mutations in all three ras genes in human thyroid tumors. *Oncogene* 1990;5:565–570.

119. Namba H, Rubin SA, Fagin JA. Point mutations of ras oncogenes are an early event in thyroid tumorigenesis. *Mol Endocrinol* 1990;4:1474–1479.

120. Zhu Z, Gandhi M, Nikiforova MN, et al. Molecular profile and clinical-pathologic features of the follicular variant of papillary thyroid carcinoma: in unusually high prevalence of ras mutations. *Am J Clin Pathol* 2003;120:71–77.

121. Lemoine NR, Mayall ES, Wyllie FS, et al. High frequency of ras oncogene activation in all stages of human thyroid tumorigenesis. *Oncogene* 1989;4:159–164.

122. Santelli G, Franciscis V, Portella G, et al. Production of transgenic mice expressing the Ki-ras oncogene under the control of a thyroglobulin promoter. *Cancer Res* 1993;53:5523–5527.

123. Garcia-Rostan G, Zhao H, Camp RL, et al. ras mutations are associated with aggressive tumor phenotypes and poor prognosis in thyroid cancer. *J Clin Oncol* 2003;21:3226–3235.

124. Jones CJ, Kipling D, Morris M, et al. Evidence for a telomere-independent "clock" limiting RAS oncogene-driven proliferation of human thyroid epithelial cells. *Mol Cell Biol* 2000;20:5690–5699.

125. Gire V, Marshall CJ, Wynford-Thomas D. Activation of mitogen-activated protein kinase is necessary but not sufficient for proliferation of human thyroid epithelial cells induced by mutant Ras. *Oncogene* 1999;18:4819–4832.

126. Shirokawa JM, Elisei R, Knauf JA, et al. Conditional apoptosis induced by oncogenic ras in thyroid cells. *Mol Endocrinol* 2000;14:1725–1738.

127. Cheng G, Meinkoth JL. Enhanced sensitivity to apoptosis in Ras-transformed thyroid cells. *Oncogene* 2001;20:7334–7341.

128. Bond J, Jones C, Haughton M, et al. Direct evidence from siRNA-directed "knock down" that p16(INK4a) is required for human fibroblast senescence and for limiting ras-induced epithelial cell proliferation. *Exp Cell Res* 2004;292:151–156.

129. Saavedra HI, Knauf JA, Shirokawa JM, et al. The RAS oncogene induces genomic instability in thyroid PCCL3 cells via the MAPK pathway. *Oncogene* 2000;19:3948–3954.

130. Fusco A, Berlingieri MT, Di Fiore PP, et al. One- and two-step transformations of rat thyroid epithelial cells by retroviral oncogenes. *Mol Cell Biol* 1987;7:3365–3370.

131. Francis-Lang H, Zannini M, De Felice M, et al. Multiple mechanisms of interference between transformation and differentiation in thyroid cells. *Mol Cell Biol* 1992;12:5793–5800.

132. Avvedimento VE, Musti AM, Ueffing M, et al. Reversible inhibition of a thyroid-specific trans-acting factor by Ras. *Genes Dev* 1991;5:22–28.

133. Gallo A, Benusiglio E, Bonapace IM, et al. v-Ras and protein kinase C dedifferentiate thyroid cells by down-regulating nuclear cAMP-dependent protein kinase A. *Genes Dev* 1992;6:1621–1630.

134. Daum G, Eisenmann-Tappe I, Fries HW, et al. The ins and outs of Raf kinases. *Trends Biochem Sci* 1994;19:474–480.

135. Peyssonnaux C, Eychene A. The Raf/MEK/ERK pathway: new concepts of activation. *Biol Cell* 2001;93:53–62.

136. Pollock PM, Harper UL, Hansen KS, et al. High frequency of BRAF mutations in nevi. *Nat Genet* 2003;33:19–20.

137. Davies H, Bignell GR, Cox C, et al. Mutations of the BRAF gene in human cancer. *Nature* 2002;417:949–954.

138. Kimura ET, Nikiforova MN, Zhu Z, et al. High prevalence of BRAF mutations in thyroid cancer: genetic evidence for constitutive activation of the RET/PTC-RAS-BRAF signaling pathway in papillary thyroid carcinoma. *Cancer Res* 2003;63:1454–1457.

139. Trovisco V, Vieira DCI, Soares P, et al. BRAF mutations are associated with some histological types of papillary thyroid carcinoma. *J Pathol* 2004;202:247–251.

140. Nikiforova MN, Kimura ET, Gandhi M, et al. BRAF mutations in thyroid tumors are restricted to papillary carcinomas and anaplastic or poorly differentiated carcinomas arising from papillary carcinomas. *J Clin Endocrinol Metab* 2003;88:5399–5404.

141. Fukushima T, Suzuki S, Mashiko M, et al. BRAF mutations in papillary carcinomas of the thyroid. *Oncogene* 2003;22:6455–6457.

142. Namba H, Nakashima M, Hayashi T, et al. Clinical implication of hot spot BRAF mutation, V599E, in papillary thyroid cancers. *J Clin Endocrinol Metab* 2003;88:4393–4397.

143. Xu X, Quiros RM, Gattuso P, et al. High prevalence of BRAF gene mutation in papillary thyroid carcinomas and thyroid tumor cell lines. *Cancer Res* 2003;63:4561–4567.

144. Soares P, Trovisco V, Rocha AS, et al. BRAF mutations and RET/PTC rearrangements are alternative events in the etiopathogenesis of PTC. *Oncogene* 2003;22:4578–4580.

145. Cohen Y, Xing M, Mambo E, et al. BRAF mutation in papillary thyroid carcinoma. *J Natl Cancer Inst* 2003;95:625–627.

146. Lyons J, Landis CA, Harsh G, et al. Two G protein oncogenes in human endocrine tumors. *Science* 1990;249:655–659.

147. O'Sullivan CO, Barton CM, Staddon SL, et al. Activating point mutations of the gsp oncogene in human thyroid adenomas. *Mol Carcinogenesis* 1991;4:345–349.

148. Landis CA, Masters SB, Spada A, et al. GTPase inhibiting mutations activate the α chain of Gs and stimulate adenylyl cyclase in human pituitary tumours. *Nature* 1989;340:692–696.

149. Garcia-Rostan G, Camp RL, Herrero A, et al. Beta-catenin dysregulation in thyroid neoplasms: down-regulation, aberrant nuclear expression, and CTNNB1 exon 3 mutations are markers for aggressive tumor phenotypes and poor prognosis. *Am J Pathol* 2001;158:987–996.

150. Garcia-Rostan G, Tallini G, Herrero A, et al. Frequent mutation and nuclear localization of beta-catenin in anaplastic thyroid carcinoma. *Cancer Res* 1999;59:1811–1815.

151. Miyake N, Maeta H, Horie S, et al. Absence of mutations in the beta-catenin and adenomatous polyposis coli genes in papillary and follicular thyroid carcinomas. *Pathol Int* 2001;51:680–685.

152. Ishigaki K, Namba H, Nakashima M, et al. Aberrant localization of beta-catenin correlates with overexpression of its target gene in human papillary thyroid cancer. *J Clin Endocrinol Metab* 2002;87:3433–3440.

153. Dumont JE, Lamy F, Roger P, et al. Physiological and pathological regulation of thyroid cell proliferation and differentiation by thyrotropin and other factors. *Physiol Rev* 1992;72:667–697.

154. Stergiopoulos SG, Stratakis CA. Human tumors associated with Carney complex and germline PRKAR1A mutations: a protein kinase A disease! *FEBS Lett* 2003;546:59–64.

155. Fagin JA. Minireview: branded from the start-distinct oncogenic initiating events may determine tumor fate in the thyroid. *Mol Endocrinol* 2002;16:903–911.

156. Kimura T, Van Keymeulen A, Golstein J, et al. Regulation of thyroid cell proliferation by TSH and other factors: a critical evaluation of *in vitro* models. *Endocr Rev* 2001;22:631–656.

157. Takahashi M. The GDNF/RET signaling pathway and human diseases. *Cytokine Growth Factor Rev* 2001;12:361–373.

158. Friend SH, Bernards R, Rogelj S, et al. A human DNA segment with properties of the gene that predisposes to retinoblastoma and osteosarcoma. *Nature* 1986;323:643–646.

159. Chen PL, Scully P, Shew JY, et al. Phosphorylation of the retinoblastoma gene product is modulated during the cell cycle and cellular differentiation. *Cell* 1989;58:1193–1198.

160. Dyson N, Bernards R, Friend SH, et al. Large T antigens of many polyomaviruses are able to form complexes with the retinoblastoma protein. *J Virol* 1990;64:1353–1356.

161. Whyte P, Buchkovich KJ, Horowitz JM, et al. Association between an oncogene and an anti-oncogene: the adenovirus E1A proteins bind to the retinoblastoma gene product. *Nature* 1988;334:124–129.

162. Chellappan S, Kraus VB, Kroger B, et al. Adenovirus E1A, simian virus 40 tumor antigen, and human papillomavirus E7 protein share the capacity to disrupt the interaction between transcription factor E2F and the retinoblastoma gene product. *Proc Natl Acad Sci U S A* 1992;89:4549–4553.

163. Huang HJ, Yee JK, Shew JY, et al. Suppression of the neoplastic phenotype by replacement of the RB gene in human cancer cells. *Science* 1988;242:1563–1566.

164. Hu N, Gutsmann A, Herbert DC, et al. Heterozygous Rb-1 delta 20/+ mice are predisposed to tumors of the pituitary gland with a nearly complete penetrance. *Oncogene* 1994;9:1021–1027.

165. Harvey M, Vogel H, Lee EY, et al. Mice deficient in both p53 and Rb develop tumors primarily of endocrine origin. *Cancer Res* 1995;55:1146–1151.

166. Ledent C, Franc B, Parmentier M. [Transgenic mouse models: their interest in thyroid tumors]. *Arch Anat Cytol Pathol* 1998;46:31–37.

167. Bartolone L, Vermiglio F, Finocchiaro MD, et al. Thyroid follicular oncogenesis in iodine-deficient and iodine-sufficient areas: search for alterations of the ras, met and bFGF oncogenes and of the Rb anti-oncogene. *J Endocrinol Invest* 1998;21:680–687.

168. Zedenius J, Wallin G, Svensson A, et al. Deletions of the long arm of chromosome 10 in progression of follicular thyroid tumors. *Hum Genet* 1996;97:299–303.

169. Omura K, Nagasato A, Kanehira E, et al. Retinoblastoma protein and proliferating-cell nuclear antigen expression as predictors of recurrence in well-differentiated papillary thyroid carcinoma. *J Clin Oncol* 1997;15:3458–3463.

170. Zou M, Shi Y, Farid NR, et al. Inverse association between cyclin D1 overexpression and retinoblastoma gene mutation in thyroid carcinomas. *Endocrine* 1998;8:61–64.

171. Anwar F, Emond MJ, Schmidt RA, et al. Retinoblastoma expression in thyroid neoplasms. *Mod Pathol* 2000;13:562–569.

172. Holm R, Nesland JM. Retinoblastoma and p53 tumour suppressor gene protein expression in carcinomas of the thyroid gland. *J Pathol* 1994;172:267–272.

173. Jones CJ, Shaw JJ, Wyllie FS, et al. High frequency deletion of the tumour suppressor gene P16INK4a (MTS1) in human thyroid cancer cell lines. *Mol Cell Endocrinol* 1996;116:115–119.

174. Tung WS, Shevlin DW, Bartsch D, et al. Infrequent CDKN2 mutation in human differentiated thyroid cancers. *Mol Carcinogenesis* 1996;15:5–10.

175. Calabro V, Strazzullo M, La Mantia G, et al. Status and expression of the p16INK4 gene in human thyroid tumors and thyroid-tumor cell lines. *Int J Cancer* 1996;67:29–34.

176. Elisei R, Shiohara M, Koeffler HP, et al. Genetic and epigenetic alterations of the cyclin-dependent kinase inhibitors p15INK4b and p16INK4a in human thyroid carcinoma cell lines, and in primary thyroid cancers. *Cancer* 1998;83:2185–2193.

177. Schagdarsurengin U, Gimm O, Hoang-Vu C, et al. Frequent epigenetic silencing of the CpG island promoter of RASSF1A in thyroid carcinoma. *Cancer Res* 2002;62:3698–3701.

178. Boltze C, Zack S, Quednow C, et al. Hypermethylation of the CDKN2/p16INK4A promotor in thyroid carcinogenesis. *Pathol Res Pract* 2003;199:399–404.

179. Greenblatt MS, Bennett WP, Hollstein M, et al. Mutations in the p53 tumor suppressor gene: clues to cancer etiology and molecular pathogenesis [Review]. *Cancer Res* 1994;54:4855–4878.

180. el-Deiry WS, Harper JW, O'Connor PM, et al. WAF1/CIP1 is induced in p53-mediated G1 arrest and apoptosis. *Cancer Res* 1994;54:1169–1174.

181. el-Deiry WS, Tokino T, Velculescu VE, et al. WAF1, a potential mediator of p53 tumor suppression. *Cell* 1993;75:817–825.

182. Lane DP. Cancer. p53, guardian of the genome [News; Comment]. Nature 1992;358:15–16.

183. Donehower L, Donehower LA, Harvey M, et al. Mice deficient for p53 are developmentally normal but susceptible to spontaneous tumours. *Nature* 1992;356:215–220.

184. Ito T, Seyama T, Mizuno T, et al. Genetic alterations in thyroid tumor progression: association with p53 gene mutations. *Jpn J Cancer Res* 1993;84:526–531.

185. Ito T, Seyama T, Mizuno T, et al. Unique association of p53 mutations with undifferentiated but not with differentiated carcinomas of the thyroid gland. *Cancer Res* 1992;52:1369–1371.

186. Fagin JA, Matsuo K, Karmakar A, et al. High prevalence of mutations of the p53 gene in poorly differentiated human thyroid carcinomas. *J Clin Invest* 1993;91:179–184.

187. Donghi R, Longoni A, Pilotti S, et al. Gene p53 et al. *J Clin Invest* 1993;91:1753–1760.

188. Livingstone LR, White A, Sprouse J, et al. Altered cell cycle arrest and gene amplification potential accompany loss of wild-type p53. *Cell* 1992;70:923–935.

189. Battista S, Martelli ML, Fedele M, et al. A mutated p53 gene alters thyroid cell differentiation. *Oncogene* 1995;11:2029–2037.

190. Fagin JA, Tang SH, Zeki K, et al. Reexpression of thyroid peroxidase in a derivative of an undifferentiated thyroid carcinoma cell line by introduction of wild-type p53. *Cancer Res* 1996; 56:765–771.

191. Moretti F, Farsetti A, Soddu S, et al. p53 re-expression inhibits proliferation and restores differentiation of human thyroid anaplastic carcinoma cells. *Oncogene* 1997;14:729–740.

192. Eng C. Genetics of Cowden syndrome: through the looking glass of oncology [Review]. *Int J Oncol* 1998;12:701–710.

193. Liaw D, Marsh DJ, Li J, et al. Germline mutations of the PTEN gene in Cowden disease, an inherited breast and thyroid cancer syndrome. *Nat Genet* 1997;16:64–67.

194. Marsh DJ, Dahia PL, Coulon V, et al. Allelic imbalance, including deletion of PTEN/MMACI, at the Cowden disease locus on 10q22–23, in hamartomas from patients with Cowden syndrome and germline PTEN mutation. *Genes Chromosomes Cancer* 1998;21:61–69.

195. Lynch ED, Ostermeyer EA, Lee MK, et al. Inherited mutations in PTEN that are associated with breast cancer, Cowden disease, and juvenile polyposis. *Am J Hum Genet* 1997;61:1254–1260.

196. Bruni P, Boccia A, Baldassarre G, et al. PTEN expression is reduced in a subset of sporadic thyroid carcinomas: evidence that PTEN-growth suppressing activity in thyroid cancer cells mediated by p27kip1. *Oncogene* 2000;19:3146–3155.

197. Gimm O, Perren A, Weng LP, et al. Differential nuclear and cytoplasmic expression of PTEN in normal thyroid tissue, and benign and malignant epithelial thyroid tumors. *Am J Pathol* 2000;156:1693–1700.

198. Frisk T, Foukakis T, Dwight T, et al. Silencing of the PTEN tumor-suppressor gene in anaplastic thyroid cancer. *Genes Chromosomes Cancer* 2002;35:74–80.

199. Gimm O, Chi H, Dahia PL, et al. Somatic mutation and germline variants of MINPP1, a phosphatase gene located in proximity to PTEN on 10q23.3, in follicular thyroid carcinomas. *J Clin Endocrinol Metab* 2001;86:1801–1805.

200. Ringel MD, Hayre N, Saito J, et al. Overexpression and overactivation of Akt in thyroid carcinoma. *Cancer Res* 2001;61:6105–6111.

201. Califano JA, Johns MM III, Westra WH, et al. An allelotype of papillary thyroid cancer. *Int J Cancer* 1996;69:442–444.

202. Ward LS, Brenta G, Medvedovic M, et al. Studies of allelic loss in thyroid tumors reveal major differences in chromosomal instability between papillary and follicular carcinomas. *J Clin Endocrinol Metab* 1998;83:525–530.

203. Tung WS, Shevlin DW, Kaleem Z, et al. Allelotype of follicular thyroid carcinomas reveals genetic instability consistent with frequent nondisjunctional chromosomal loss. *Genes Chromosomes Cancer* 1997;19:43–51.

204. Grebe SK, McIver B, Hay ID, et al. Frequent loss of heterozygosity on chromosomes 3p and 17p without VHL or p53 mutations suggests involvement of unidentified tumor suppressor genes in follicular thyroid carcinoma. *J Clin Endocrinol Metab* 1997;82:3684–3691.

205. Chen XN, Knauf JA, Gonsky R, et al. From amplification to gene in thyroid cancer: a high resolution mapped BAC resource for cancer chromosome aberrations guides gene discovery after comparative genome hybridization (CGH). *Am J Hum Genet* 1998.

206. Matsuo K, Tang SH, Fagin JA. Allelotype of human thyroid tumors: loss of chromosome 11q13 sequences in follicular neoplasms. *Mol Endocrinol* 1991;5:1873–1879.

207. Herrmann MA, Hay ID, Bartelt DH Jr, et al. Cytogenetic and molecular genetic studies of follicular and papillary thyroid cancers. *J Clin Invest* 1991;88:1596–1604.

208. Zedenius J, Wallin G, Svensson A, et al. Allelotyping of follicular thyroid tumors. *Hum Genet* 1995;96:27–32.

209. Eden S, Cedar H. Genomic imprinting. Action at a distance [News; Comment]. *Nature* 1995;375:16–17.

210. Issa JP, Vertino PM, Wu J, et al. Increased cytosine DNA-methyltransferase activity during colon cancer progression. *J Natl Cancer Inst* 1993;85:1235–1240.

211. Baylin SB, Herman JG, Graff JR, et al. Alterations in DNA methylation: a fundamental aspect of neoplasia [Review]. *Adv Cancer Res* 1998;72:141–196.

212. Herman JG, Merlo A, Mao L, et al. Inactivation of the CDKN2/p16/MTS1 gene is frequently associated with aberrant DNA methylation in all common human cancers. *Cancer Res* 1995;55:4525–4530.

213. Rideout WM3, Coetzee GA, Olumi AF, et al. 5-Methylcytosine as an endogenous mutagen in the human LDL receptor and p53 genes. *Science* 1990;249:1288–1290.

214. Counts JL, Goodman JI. Alterations in DNA methylation may play a variety of roles in carcinogenesis [Review]. *Cell* 1995; 83:13–15.

215. Matsuo K, Tang SH, Zeki K, et al. Aberrant deoxyribonucleic acid methylation in human thyroid tumors. *J Clin Endocrinol Metab* 1993;77:991–995.

216. Graff JR, Greenberg VE, Herman JG, et al. Distinct patterns of E-cadherin CpG island methylation in papillary, follicular, Hurthle's cell, and poorly differentiated human thyroid carcinoma. *Cancer Res* 1998;58:2063–2066.

217. Xing M, Usadel H, Cohen Y, et al. Methylation of the thyroid-stimulating hormone receptor gene in epithelial thyroid tumors: a marker of malignancy and a cause of gene silencing. *Cancer Res* 2003;63:2316–2321.

218. Xing M, Tokumaru Y, Wu G, et al. Hypermethylation of the Pendred syndrome gene SLC26A4 is an early event in thyroid tumorigenesis. *Cancer Res* 2003;63:2312–2315.

219. McDonnell TJ, Korsmeyer SJ. Progression from lymphoid hyperplasia to high-grade malignant lymphoma in mice transgenic for the t(14; 18). *Nature* 1991;349:254–256.

220. Hockenbery D, Nunez G, Milliman C, et al. Bcl-2 is an inner mitochondrial membrane protein that blocks programmed cell death. *Nature* 1990;348:334–336.

221. Castellone MD, Cirafici AM, De Vita G, et al. Ras-mediated apoptosis of PC CL 3 rat thyroid cells induced by RET/PTC oncogenes. *Oncogene* 2003;22:246–255.

222. Wang J, Knauf JA, Basu S, et al. Conditional expression of RET/PTC induces a weak oncogenic drive in thyroid PCCL3 cells and inhibits thyrotropin action at multiple levels. *Mol Endocrinol* 2003;17:1425–1436.

223. Nicolaides NC, Papadppoulos N, et al. Mutations of two PMS homologues in hereditary nonpolyposis colon cancer. *Nature* 1994;371:75–80.

224. Parsons R, Li GM, Longley M, et al. Mismatch et al. *Science* 1995;268:738–740.

225. Markowitz S, Wang J, Myeroff L, et al. Inactivation of the type II TGF-beta receptor in colon cancer cells with microsatellite instability [Comments]. *Science* 1995;268:1336–1338.

226. Nikiforov YE, Nikiforova M, Fagin JA. Prevalence of minisatellite and microsatellite instability in radiation-induced post-Chernobyl pediatric thyroid carcinomas. *Oncogene* 1998;17: 1983–1988.

227. Lazzereschi D, Palmirotta R, Ranieri A, et al. Microsatellite instability in thyroid tumours and tumour-like lesions. *Br J Cancer* 1999;79:340–345.

228. Rodrigues-Serpa A, Catarino A, Soares J. Loss of heterozygosity in follicular and papillary thyroid carcinomas. *Cancer Genet Cytogenet* 2003;141:26–31.

229. Bauer AJ, Cavalli LR, Rone JD, et al. Evaluation of adult papillary thyroid carcinomas by comparative genomic hybridization and microsatellite instability analysis. *Cancer Genet Cytogenet* 2002;135:182–186.

230. Stoler DL, Datta RV, Charles MA, et al. Genomic instability measurement in the diagnosis of thyroid neoplasms. *Head Neck* 2002;24:290–295.

231. Richter HE, Lohrer HD, Hieber L, et al. Microsatellite instability and loss of heterozygosity in radiation-associated thyroid carcinomas of Belarussian children and adults. *Carcinogenesis* 1999;20:2247–2252.

232. Lengauer C, Kinzler KW, Vogelstein B. Genetic instability in colorectal cancers. *Nature* 1997;386:623–627.

233. Jallepalli PV, Lengauer C. Chromosome segregation and cancer: cutting through the mystery. *Nat Rev Cancer* 2001;1:109–117.

234. Tung WS, Shevlin DW, Kaleem Z, et al. Allelotype of follicular thyroid carcinomas reveals genetic instability consistent with frequent nondisjunctional chromosomal loss. *Genes Chromosomes Cancer* 1997;19:43–51.

235. Ward LS, Brenta G, Medvedovic M, et al. Studies of allelic loss in thyroid tumors reveal major differences in chromosomal instability between papillary and follicular carcinomas. *J Clin Endocrinol Metab* 1998;83:525–530.

236. Spencer F, Gerring SL, Connelly C, et al. Mitotic chromosome transmission fidelity mutants in *Saccharomyces cerevisiae*. *Genetics* 1990;124:237–249.

237. Cahill DP, Lengauer C, Yu J, et al. Mutations of mitotic checkpoint genes in human cancers [Comments]. *Nature* 1998;392:300–303.

238. Taylor SS, McKeon F. Kinetochore localization of murine Bub1 is required for normal mitotic timing and checkpoint response to spindle damage. *Cell* 1997;89:727–735.

239. Hoyt MA, Totis L, Roberts BT. *S. cerevisiae* genes required for cell cycle arrest in response to loss of microtubule function. *Cell* 1991;66:507–517.

240. Roberts BT, Farr KA, Hoyt MA. The *Saccharomyces cerevisiae* checkpoint gene BUB1 encodes a novel protein kinase. *Mol Cell Biol* 1994;14:8282–8291.

241. Basu J, Bousbaa H, Logarinho E, et al. Mutations in the essential spindle checkpoint gene bub1 cause chromosome missegregation and fail to block apoptosis in *Drosophila*. *J Cell Biol* 1999;146:13–28.

242. Imai Y, Shiratori Y, Kato N, et al. Mutational inactivation of mitotic checkpoint genes, hsMAD2 and hBUB1, is rare in sporadic digestive tract cancers. *Jpn J Cancer Res* 1999;90:837–840.

243. Gemma A, Seike M, Seike Y, et al. Somatic mutation of the hBUB1 mitotic checkpoint gene in primary lung cancer [in process citation]. *Genes Chromosomes Cancer* 2000;29:213–218.

244. Yamaguchi K, Okami K, Hibi K, et al. Mutation analysis of hBUB1 in aneuploid HNSCC and lung cancer cell lines. *Cancer Lett* 1999;139:183–187.

245. Ohshima K, Haraoka S, Yoshioka S, et al. Mutation analysis of mitotic checkpoint genes (hBUB1 and hBUBR1) and microsatellite instability in adult T-cell leukemia/lymphoma [in process citation]. *Cancer Lett* 2000;158:141–150.

246. Ouyang B, Knauf JA, Ain K, et al. Mechanisms of aneuploidy in thyroid cancer cell lines and tissues: evidence for mitotic checkpoint dysfunction without mutations in BUB1 and BUBR1. *Clin Endocrinol (Oxf)* 2002;56:341–350.

247. Pellman D. Cancer. A CINtillating new job for the APC tumor suppressor. *Science* 2001;291:2555–2556.

248. Pei L, Melmed S. Isolation and characterization of a pituitary tumor-transforming gene (PTTG). *Mol Endocrinol* 1997;11:433–441.

249. Zhang X, Horwitz GA, Heaney AP, et al. Pituitary tumor transforming gene (PTTG) expression in pituitary adenomas. *J Clin Endocrinol Metab* 1999;84:761–767.

250. Heaney AP, Nelson V, Fernando M, et al. Transforming events in thyroid tumorigenesis and their association with follicular lesions. *J Clin Endocrinol Metab* 2001;86:5025–5032.

251. Yu R, Heaney AP, Lu W, et al. Pituitary tumor transforming gene causes aneuploidy and p53-dependent and p53-independent apoptosis. *J Biol Chem* 2000;275:36502–36505.

252. Wang Z, Yu R, Melmed S. Mice lacking pituitary tumor transforming gene show testicular and splenic hypoplasia, thymic hyperplasia, thrombocytopenia, aberrant cell cycle progression, and premature centromere division. *Mol Endocrinol* 2001;15:1870–1879.

253. Boelaert K, McCabe CJ, Tannahill LA, et al. Pituitary tumor transforming gene and fibroblast growth factor-2 expression: potential prognostic indicators in differentiated thyroid cancer. *J Clin Endocrinol Metab* 2003;88:2341–2347.

254. Loeb LA. Cancer cells exhibit a mutator phenotype. *Adv Cancer Res* 1998;72:25–56.

255. Segal M, Clarke DJ. The Ras pathway and spindle assembly collide? *Bioessays* 2001;23:307–310.

256. Li YC, Chen CR, Chang EC. Fission yeast Ras1 effector Scd1 interacts with the spindle and affects its proper formation. *Genetics* 2000;156:995–1004.

257. Zecevic M, Catling AD, Eblen ST, et al. Active MAP kinase in mitosis: localization at kinetochores and association with the motor protein CENP-E. *J Cell Biol* 1998;142:1547–1558.

258. Shapiro PS, Vaisberg E, Hunt AJ, et al. Activation of the MKK/ERK pathway during somatic cell mitosis: direct interactions of active ERK with kinetochores and regulation of the mitotic 3F3/2 phosphoantigen. *J Cell Biol* 1998;142:1533–1545.

259. Denko N, Stringer J, Wani M, et al. Mitotic and post mitotic consequences of genomic instability induced by oncogenic Ha-ras. *Somat Cell Mol Genet* 1995;21:241–253.

260. Wani MA, Xu X, Stambrook PJ. Increased methotrexate resistance and dhfr gene amplification as a consequence of induced Ha-ras expression in NIH 3T3 cells. *Cancer Res* 1994;54:2504–2508.

261. Ichikawa T, Kyprianou N, Isaacs JT. Genetic instability and the acquisition of metastatic ability by rat mammary cancer cells following v-H-ras oncogene transfection. *Cancer Res* 1990;50:6349–6357.

262. Ichikawa T, Schalken JA, Ichikawa Y, et al. H-ras expression, genetic instability, and acquisition of metastatic ability by rat prostatic cancer cells following v-H-ras oncogene transfection. *Prostate* 1991;18:163–172.

263. de Vries JE, Kornips FH, Marx P, et al. Transfected c-Ha-ras oncogene enhances karyotypic instability and integrates predominantly in aberrant chromosomes. *Cancer Genet Cytogenet* 1993;67:35–43.

264. Bell B, Mazzaferri EL. Familial adenomatous polyposis (Gardner's syndrome) and thyroid carcinoma. *Dig Dis Sci* 1993;38:185–190.

265. Plail RO, Bussey HJR, Glazer G, et al. Adenomatous polyposis: an association with carcinoma of the thyroid. *Br J Surg* 1987;74:377–380.

266. Iwama T, Mishima Y, Utsunomiya J. The Impact of familial adenomatous polyposis on the tumorigenesis and mortality at the several organs. its rational treatment. *Ann Surg* 1993;217:101–108.

267. Camiel MR, Mule JE, Alexander LL, et al. Association of thyroid carcinoma with Gardner's syndrome in siblings. *N Engl J Med* 1968;278:1056–1059.

268. Bell B, Mazzaferri EL. Familiar adenomatous polyposis (Gardner's syndrome) and thyroid carcinoma. A case report and review of the literature. *Dig Dis Sci* 1993;38:185–190.

269. Harach HR, Williams GT, Williams ED. Familial adenomatous polyposis associated thyroid carcinoma: a distinct type of follicular cell neoplasm [Review]. *Histopathology* 1994;25:549–561.

270. Kinzler KW, Nilbert MC, Su NKL. Identification of FAP locus genes from chromosome 5q21. *Science* 1991;253:661–664.

271. Groden J, Thliveris A, Samowitz W, et al. Identification and characterization of the familial adenomatous polyposis coli gene. *Cell* 1991;66:589–600.

272. Cetta F, Olschwang S, Petracci M, et al. Genetic alterations in thyroid carcinoma associated with familial adenomatous polyposis: clinical implications and suggestions for early detection. *World J Surg* 1998;22:1231–1236.

273. Cetta F, Montalto G, Gori M, et al. Germline mutations of the APC gene in patients with familial adenomatous polyposis–associated thyroid carcinoma: results from a European cooperative study. *J Clin Endocrinol Metab* 2000;85:286–292.

274. Zeki K, Spambalg D, Sharifi N, et al. Mutations of the adenomatous polyposis coli gene in sporadic thyroid neoplasms. *J Clin Endocrinol Metab* 1994;79:1317–1321.

275. Colletta G, Sciacchitano S, Palmirotta R, et al. Analysis of adenomatous polyposis coli gene in thyroid tumours. *Br J Cancer* 1994;70:1085–1088.

276. Mallory SB. Cowden syndrome (multiple hamartoma syndrome). *Dermatol Clin* 1995;13:27–31.

277. Reed MWR, Harris SC, Quayle AR, et al. The association between thyroid neoplasia and intestinal polyps. *Ann R Coll Surg Engl* 1990;72:357–359.

278. Ohta S, Katsura T, Shimada M, et al. Ataxia-telangiectasia with papillary carcinoma of the thyroid. *Am J Pediatr Hematol Oncol* 1986;8:255–268.

279. DeLellis RA. Biology of disease. Multiple endocrine neoplasia syndromes revisited. *Lab Invest* 1995;72:494–505.

280. Larsson C, Skogseid B, Oberg K, et al. Multiple endocrine neoplasia type 1 gene maps to chromosome 11 and is lost in insulinoma. *Nature* 1988;332:85–87.

281. Chandrasekharappa SC, Guru SC, Manickam P, et al. Positional cloning of the gene for multiple endocrine neoplasia type 1. *Science* 1997;276:404–407.

282. Agarwal SK, Guru SC, Heppner C, et al. Menin interacts with the AP1 transcription factor JunD and represses JunD-activated transcription. *Cell* 1999;96:143–152.

283. Heppner C, Bilimoria KY, Agarwal SK, et al. The tumor suppressor protein menin interacts with NF-kappaB proteins and inhibits NF-kappaB-mediated transactivation. *Oncogene* 2001;20:4917–4925.

284. Jin S, Mao H, Schnepp RW, et al. Menin associates with FANCD2, a protein involved in repair of DNA damage. *Cancer Res* 2003;63:4204–4210.

285. Sukhodolets KE, Hickman AB, Agarwal SK, et al. The 32-kilodalton subunit of replication protein A interacts with menin, the product of the MEN1 tumor suppressor gene. *Mol Cell Biol* 2003;23:493–509.

286. Suphapeetiporn K, Greally JM, Walpita D, et al. MEN1 tumor-suppressor protein localizes to telomeres during meiosis. *Genes Chromosomes Cancer* 2002;35:81–85.

287. Lin SY, Elledge SJ. Multiple tumor suppressor pathways negatively regulate telomerase. *Cell* 2003;113:881–889.

288. Bertolino P, Tong WM, Galendo D, et al. Heterozygous Men1 mutant mice develop a range of endocrine tumors mimicking multiple endocrine neoplasia type 1. *Mol Endocrinol* 2003;17:1880–1892.

289. Kirschner LS, Sandrini F, Monbo J, et al. Genetic heterogeneity and spectrum of mutations of the PRKAR1A gene in patients with the carney complex. *Hum Mol Genet* 2000;9:3037–3046.

290. Kirschner LS, Carney JA, Pack SD, et al. Mutations of the gene encoding the protein kinase A type I-alpha regulatory subunit in patients with the Carney complex. *Nat Genet* 2000;26:89–92.

291. Nwokoro NA, Korytkowski MT, Rose S, et al. Spectrum of malignancy and premalignancy in Carney syndrome. *Am J Med Genet* 1997;73:369–377.

292. Ozaki O, Ito K, Kobayashi K, et al. Familial occurrence of differentiated, nonmedullary thyroid carcinoma. *World J Surg* 1988;12:565–571.

293. Nemec J, Soumar J, Zamrazil V, et al. Familial occurrence of differentiated (non-medullary) thyroid cancer. *Oncology* 1975;32:151–157.

294. Samaan NA. Papillary carcinoma of the thyroid: hereditary or radiation-induced? *Cancer Invest* 1996;7:399–400.

295. Lote K, Andersen K, Nordal E, et al. Familial occurrence of papillary thyroid carcinoma. *Cancer* 1980;46:1291–1297.

296. Kwok CG, McDougall IR. Familial differentiated carcinoma of the thyroid: report of five pairs of siblings. *Thyroid* 1995;5:395–397.

297. Hrafnkelsson J, Tulinius H, Jonasson JG, et al. Papillary thyroid carcinoma in Iceland. *Acta Oncol* 1989;28:785–788.

298. Stoffer SS, Van Dyke DL, Vaden Bach J, et al. Familial papillary carcinoma of the thyroid. *Am J Med Genet* 1986;25:775–782.

299. Ron E, Kleinerman RA, Boice JD Jr, et al. A population-based case-control study of thyroid cancer. *J Natl Cancer Inst* 1987;79:1–12.

300. Ron E, Kleinerman RA, LiVolsi VA, et al. Familial nonmedullary thyroid cancer. *Oncology* 1991;48:309–311.

301. Fagin JA. Familial nonmedullary thyroid carcinoma—the case for genetic susceptibility [Editorial] [Review]. *J Clin Endocrinol Metab* 1997;82:342–344.

302. Bignell GR, Canzian F, Shayeghi M, et al. Familial nontoxic multinodular thyroid goiter locus maps to chromosome 14q but does not account for familial nonmedullary thyroid cancer. *Am J Hum Genet* 1997;61:1123–1130.

303. Canzian F, Amati P, Harach HR, et al. A gene predisposing to familial thyroid tumors with cell oxyphilia maps to chromosome 19p13.2. *Am J Hum Genet* 1998;63:1743–1748.

304. Bevan S, Pal T, Greenberg CR, et al. A comprehensive analysis of MNG1, TCO1, fPTC, PTEN, TSHR, and TRKA in familial nonmedullary thyroid cancer: confirmation of linkage to TCO1. *J Clin Endocrinol Metab* 2001;86:3701–3704.

305. Malchoff CD, Sarfarazi M, Tendler B, et al. Papillary thyroid carcinoma associated with papillary renal neoplasia: genetic linkage analysis of a distinct heritable tumor syndrome. *J Clin Endocrinol Metab* 2000;85:1758–1764.

306. Schneider AB, Fogelfeld L. Radiation-induced endocrine tumors. *Cancer Treat Res* 1997;89:141–161.

307. Ron E, Lubin JH, Shore RE, et al. Thyroid cancer after exposure to external radiation: a pooled analysis of seven studies. *Radiat Res* 1995;141:259–277.

308. Schneider AB, Ron E, Lubin J, et al. Dose-response relationships for radiation-induced thyroid cancer and thyroid nodules: evidence for the prolonged effects of radiation on the thyroid. *J Clin Endocrinol Metab* 1993;77:362–369.

309. Williams D. Cancer after nuclear fallout: lessons from the Chernobyl accident. *Nat Rev Cancer* 2002;2:543–549.

310. Nikiforov Y, Gnepp DR, Fagin JA. Thyroid lesions in children and adolescents after the Chernobyl disaster: implications for the study of radiation carcinogenesis. *J Clin Endocrinol Metab* 1996;81:9.

311. Farahati J, Demidchik EP, Biko J, et al. Inverse association between age at the time of radiation exposure and extent of disease in cases of radiation-induced childhood thyroid carcinoma in Belarus. *Cancer* 2000;88:1470–1476.

312. Kazakov VS, Demidchik EP, Astakhova LN. Thyroid cancer after Chernobyl. *Nature* 1992;359:21.

313. Klugbauer S, Lengfelder E, Demidchik EP, et al. High prevalence of RET rearrangement in thyroid tumors of children

from Belarus after the Chernobyl reactor accident. *Oncogene* 1995;11:2459–2467.

314. Bounacer A, Wicker R, Caillou B, et al. High prevalence of activating ret proto-oncogene rearrangements, in thyroid tumors from patients who had received external radiation. *Oncogene* 1997;15:1263–1273.

315. Fugazzola L, Pilotti S, Pinchera A, et al. Oncogenic rearrangements of the RET proto-oncogene in papillary thyroid carcinomas from children exposed to the Chernobyl nuclear accident. *Cancer Res* 1995;55:5617–5620.

316. Rabes HM, Demidchik EP, Sidorow JD, et al. Pattern of radiation-induced RET and NTRK1 rearrangements in 191 post-Chernobyl papillary thyroid carcinomas: biological, phenotypic, and clinical implications. *Clin Cancer Res* 2000;6:1093–1103.

317. Thomas GA, Bunnell H, Cook HA, et al. High prevalence of RET/PTC rearrangements in Ukrainian and Belarussian post-Chernobyl thyroid papillary carcinomas: a strong correlation between RET/PTC3 and the solid-follicular variant. *J Clin Endocrinol Metab* 1999;84:4232–4238.

318. Powell DJ Jr, Russell J, Nibu K, et al. The RET/PTC3 oncogene: metastatic solid-type papillary carcinomas in murine thyroids. *Cancer Res* 1998;58:5523–5528.

319. Nikiforov YE, Erickson LA, Nikiforova MN, et al. Solid variant of papillary thyroid carcinoma: incidence, clinical-pathologic characteristics, molecular analysis, and biologic behavior. *Am J Surg Pathol* 2001;25:1478–1484.

320. Nikiforov YE, Nikiforova MN, Gnepp DR, et al. Prevalence of mutations of ras and p53 in benign and malignant thyroid tumors from children exposed to radiation after the Chernobyl nuclear accident. *Oncogene* 1996;13:687–693.

321. Suchy B, Waldmann V, Klugbauer S, et al. Absence of RAS and p53 mutations in thyroid carcinomas of children after Chernobyl in contrast to adult thyroid tumours. *Br J Cancer* 1998;77:952–955.

322. Nikiforova MN, Lynch RA, Biddinger PW, et al. RAS point mutations and PAX8-PPARgamma rearrangement in thyroid tumors: evidence for distinct molecular pathways in thyroid follicular carcinoma. *J Clin Endocrinol Metab* 2003;88:2318–2326.

70C CARCINOMA OF FOLLICULAR EPITHELIUM: SURGICAL THERAPY

ROBERT M. BEAZLEY

A thyroid nodule of uncertain nature is a frequent indication for thyroidectomy. Clinically detectable thyroid nodules are relatively common, with an estimated prevalence in U.S. adults of 2.1% to 4.2% (1,2). Based on 2000 U.S. Bureau of the Census Data, one might predict that 5.8 to 11.7 million Americans harbor clinical thyroid nodules. The American Cancer Society estimates 22,000 new thyroid cancers will be diagnosed in 2003 (3). The clinical challenge, because of the relative rarity of thyroid malignancy, is detecting malignant nodules or those that have a high likelihood of malignancy. Overall, 5% to 10% of thyroid nodules presenting for surgical consultation will ultimately be determined to be cancerous.

EVALUATION OF PATIENTS WITH THYROID NODULES

Initial evaluation of a patient with a thyroid nodule consists of a thorough history and physical. A number of aspects of the patient's history are important in the workup of a suspected malignant nodule. Age is significant in that nodules in the young (under 14 years of age) and old (over 65 years) are more likely to be malignant than those in intervening age groups. Sex is of interest in that although thyroid nodules are more common in females, nodules in males are more likely to be malignant. A family history of multinodular goiter might tend to predict a benign lesion, whereas documented thyroid cancer in a first-degree relative increases the likelihood of a malignant nodule. A history of pain suggests inflammation and may be indicative of thyroiditis. Sudden rapid appearance of a nodule is commonly associated with hemorrhage into a preexisting colloid nodule. A diffuse goiter with signs of metabolic hyperactivity suggests Graves' disease. If hyperactivity is associated with multinodular goiter, one must consider Plummer's syndrome. Goiter patients presenting with atrial fibrillation or heart failure should also be evaluated for a hyperfunctioning thyroid nodule. Rapid enlargement of a long-standing goiter, particularly in an elderly patient, may predict thyroid malignancy. Past history of external radiation exposure in childhood significantly increases the likelihood that a thyroid nodule is cancerous or that subclinical cancer may be located elsewhere in the thyroid gland. Although in the distant past external beam radiation therapy was used in the head and neck region for a variety of dermatologic and lymphatic conditions, it is seldom used today. The most recent internal radiation experience occurred following exposure of a large population after the Chernobyl accident, resulting in an epidemic of pediatric thyroid cancer. Cowden's disease, characterized by multiple cutaneous facial papules and oral papillomatosis, may be associated with toxic and nontoxic goiters, thyroid adenomas, and a high incidence of follicular carcinomas. Pendred's syndrome is an autosomal-recessive disorder presenting with deafness, hypothyroidism, and goiter. Patients with a family history of multiple endocrine neoplasia type 1 or familial hyperparathyroidism may be at risk for developing carcinoma of follicular cell origin. Papillary thyroid cancer is recognized as the third most common malignancy associated with Gardner's syndrome after colon and ampullary carcinoma. It is multifocal, more aggressive, and appears one third of the time before the diagnosis of Gardner's is established. Papillary thyroid cancer is reported to occur at more than 100 times the expected incidence in females under 35 years of age with Gardner's syndrome (4). Patients who have had thyroid cancer in the past treated by lobectomy are at increased risk for having recurrence in the thyroid remnant.

Physical Examination

Patients presenting with a multinodular goiter have a lower incidence of malignancy than individuals presenting with a solitary nodule. Those presenting with a solitary nodule and cervical lymphadenopathy, particularly involving the lower jugular chain, should be considered as having thyroid malignancy until proven otherwise. Clinical presentation with bilateral cervical adenopathy and rapid thyroid enlargement is suspect for lymphoma, especially if there is a history of Hashimoto's disease. Hard nodules, which are adherent or fixed to surrounding tissues are highly suggestive of malignancy. Patients presenting with a solitary thyroid nodule and fracture or bone pain should also be suspected of harboring a thyroid malignancy. Patients with thyroid nodules may present with signs of cervicothoracic venous obstruction, particularly if the lesion is in the mediastinum, so-called Pemberton's sign. Dysphagia and dyspnea may accompany large goiters occurring in the neck or those with a significant mediastinal component. Likewise, recurrent nerve palsy with hoarseness and Horner's syndrome from cervical sympathetic involvement may occasionally accompany large benign multinodular goiters, although these signs are more likely to be predictors of malignancy.

Evaluation

Fine-needle aspiration biopsy (FNAB) is the key to characterizing the nature of thyroid nodules. However, the inability to distinguish between benign follicular lesions and follicular carcinoma remains the major shortcoming of this technique. As a result, most patients with the diagnosis of follicular lesion are advised to have surgery. Ultimately, only 15% to 20% of follicular lesions will be found to be malignant. Intraoperative frozen section determination of malignancy may be difficult and can be impossible with follicular carcinomas. Several studies have concluded that both the increased operative time and pathology charges do not support routine frozen section analysis, especially if FNAB is malignant or benign (5,6). Frozen section may be helpful in FNAB classified as suspicious (7). Frequently the surgeon must wait for permanent section to obtain the diagnosis. The false-positive rate for FNAB is in the 1% range, whereas the false-negative rate is about 5%, probably resulting from sampling error or misinterpretation.

Ultrasonography (US) is especially useful in the management of thyroid nodules because it is noninvasive and may be quickly performed in the outpatient setting. Thyroid US allows discrimination between cystic, mixed, and solid nodules, as well as evaluation of regional nodal beds. A recent study from M.D. Anderson Cancer Center documented lymph node metastases by preoperative US in 34% of thyroid cancer patients felt to be node negative by physical examination (8). US is extremely helpful in accurately directing FNAB. Additionally, US may be repeated so that existing nodules (FNAB negative) may be monitored for future size change. Simple cysts smaller than 4 cm, which are nearly always benign, may be managed by aspiration or tetracycline sclerosis, thus avoiding surgery. US allows lesions located on the edge of a cystic nodule to be accurately sampled by FNAB.

Owing to the widespread acceptance and utilization of FNAB, traditional nuclear thyroid scans are performed much less frequently. They are useful for evaluating hot nodules, in the workup of Plummer's disease, and with goiters suspected of having mediastinal extension. In the past few years, positron emission tomography (PET) has become available in many centers. A recent paper by Kresnik et al reported a group of 24 patients with follicular cytology in whom preoperative PET accurately predicted cancer in 9. All remaining 15 patients had benign lesions (9). Other reports have similarly suggested potential usefulness for PET in evaluating thyroid nodules. This new modality may aid in discriminating benign follicular lesions from malignant lesions, allowing more selective surgical management of the "follicular lesion."

Preoperative computed tomography (CT) can be helpful in determining the extent of disease and involvement of adjacent tissue and lymph nodes. Preoperative awareness of tracheal deviation or compression is especially important from an anesthesia standpoint. One must ensure that intravenous contrast media is not used during CT studies because the high iodine load of the contrast will interfere with pre- and postoperative isotopic scanning.

Routine chest x-rays that include the neck can show tracheal deviation, intrathoracic extension, and pulmonary metastases. Occasionally, fine calcifications are seen within the thyroid gland, which may be associated with papillary or medullary thyroid carcinomas.

PREOPERATIVE PREPARATION

Preoperative preparation for thyroidectomy is not especially involved and does not differ from that for any other major surgical procedure. Cardiopulmonary function needs to be assessed, and problems like chronic lung disease, asthma, and cardiac instability addressed prospectively. Any hyperthyroid state should be treated as necessary us beta-blockers, antithyroid drugs, and iodine depending on time constraints. Anticoagulants and aspirin should be stopped approximately 1 week prior to the planned procedure. Laryngoscopy should be considered in those patients manifesting or complaining of voice changes as well as patients undergoing reoperative surgery.

Preoperative patient counseling should include a discussion of the conduct of surgery, essentially what patients will experience from the time they enter the hospital until the time they leave. Additionally, patients should be told what they may expect at home in the way of recovery and when to return to work. Patients with "follicular lesions or suspicious" FNAB diagnosis should be reassured that they may not necessarily have cancer, although many are quite anxious because they are convinced they already have it. A 1 in 5 or less risk for cancer may be quoted for these anxious patients. Additionally, one must alert them to the fact that frozen section may not be helpful and that a reoperation might be necessary when the permanent section report is obtained. At this juncture many patients will request that if there is a question or ambiguity at the time of frozen section that a total thyroidectomy be performed rather than chancing the necessity of a second procedure.

Clearly the major operative risks of bleeding, infection, nerve injury, and hypoparathyroidism must be discussed in detail, including treatments for these various complications. This discussion should take place with the patient and a family member or friend because the accompanying person will hear and retain more of the explanation than the patient. It is useful to use diagrams and illustrative materials during this portion of the interview. Written material, which the patient may take home, can also be of great help.

THYROIDECTOMY

Thyroid surgical procedures generally follow a series of technical steps, which are invariably the same with every procedure. First is that of anatomic exposure; second, identification of structures to be preserved (i.e., nerves, parathyroid glands); and lastly, excision of pathologic tissues. As patients undergoing thyroid surgery are frequently young women, cosmetic considerations related to the incision are a major concern. A symmetric "collar" incision utilizing a visible skin crease or in the plane of Langer's skin lines offers the best option for a pleasing cosmetic result.

The incision should be located on the anterior neck approximately one finger breadth above the clavicular heads. The majority of thyroidectomies can be performed through a skin incision of 6 to 8 cm. Skin flaps are raised under the plane of the platysma muscle, cephalad, caudally, and laterally. The sternohyoid and sternothyroid muscles are liberally divided vertically along the median raphe from the sternal notch to the superior portion of the thyroid cartilage. In most cases transection of these muscles is not required for exposure, but doing so will enhance exposure, particularly of the upper thyroid pole region. If surgical division is elected, the muscles should be divided cephalad because the ansa cervicalis innervation takes place toward the caudal portion of the muscles. The functional morbidity of dividing, denervating, or even excising the sternohyoid or sternothyroid muscles is relatively minimal. Muscle found to be adherent to underlying tumor nodules should be divided and allowed to remain on the resection specimen. Exposure continues by dissecting the overlying strap muscles off the anterior capsular surface of the thyroid gland.

The thyroid gland is invested by the deep layer of cervical fascia, which forms a "filmy" capsule over the gland projecting into the thyroid substance, dividing the gland into irregularly shaped and sized lobules. The capsule provides a plane of surgical dissection between the gland and the strap muscles, which are retracted laterally as the capsular dissection progresses over the surface of the gland. The superficial surface of the gland is covered with multiple veins of varying size and numerous small lymphatic vessels. Early in this lateral dissection, a middle thyroid vein or veins are encountered, which upon ligation and division allows more lateral and dorsal capsular dissection with additional mobilization and exposure of the gland. At this juncture, the carotid artery will be visualized laterally and the tracheoesophageal groove medially (Fig. 70C.1).

Exposure is enhanced at this point by dissection of the upper pole of the thyroid lobe and ligation of the superior thyroid artery (first branch of the external carotid) and the superior thyroid veins, which may be multiple. Lateral and caudal retraction of the thyroid lobe permits visualization of the superior pole vessels and helps to identify the relative avascular "medial cricothyroid space" (between upper pole and cricothyroid muscle), facilitating individual ligation of the vascular structures on the surface of the thyroid capsule. In this region the surgeon must be aware of the external branch of superior laryngeal nerve, which innervates the cricothyroid muscle and is a tensor of the vocal cord responsible for the timbre or pitch of the voice. This nerve is especially important in individuals who are singers or public speakers. Identification of the nerve may be difficult with large goiters or fibrosis associated with radiation or Hashimoto's disease. Approximately 50% of the time the nerve courses more than a centimeter superior to the site of vessel ligation and hugs the larynx medially, and is thus not

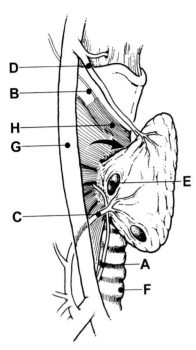

FIGURE 70C.1. Anatomy on medial rotation of the thyroid gland. **A:** Recurrent laryngeal nerve. **B:** Superior laryngeal nerve. **C:** Inferior thyroid artery. **D:** Superior thyroid artery. **E:** Superior parathyroid gland. **F:** Trachea. **G:** Carotid artery. **H:** Cricothyroid muscle.

likely to be injured. Fifty percent of the time the course of the nerve is such that injury may occur if ligation of the superior pole vessels is not immediately performed on the thyroid capsule (10). It is not possible to estimate the frequency of inadvertent injury to the superior laryngeal nerve, because the ensuing morbidity may be subtle and laryngoscopic findings minimal. However, one might speculate that such injury could account for the occasional ill-defined dysphonia and dysphagia complaints manifested following thyroidectomy. The surgeon must be diligent in ensuring that the nerve does not traverse close to the gland prior to ligating the superior pole vessels.

Mobilization of the upper pole permits the thyroid lobe to be retracted medially, exposing the tracheoesophageal groove and providing visualization of the posterior thyroid capsule. At this point parathyroid tissue lying on the posterior surface of the thyroid near the inferior thyroid artery may become visible. The inferior thyroid artery may be localized laterally, coursing medially toward the thyroid lobe. As the recurrent nerve crosses the inferior thyroid artery at an acute angle in its course to the cricothyroid membrane, careful dissection of the vessel can be helpful in localizing the nerve with minimal undue trauma. The recent availability of intraoperative neuromonitoring of vocal cord muscle responsiveness has provided an aid in early nerve identification, especially in conditions of fibrosis and scarring, thus preserving nerves and saving time (11). Another successful anatomic approach to nerve iden-

tification is the tubercle of Zuckerkandl. The tubercle is a thickening on the posterior thyroid surface, which is a remnant of the fusion of the lateral thyroid anlage and ultimobranchial body to the median thyroid analage. The recurrent nerve lies in a "fissure" in the tubercle between the lateral and posterior surfaces of the thyroid or trachea. Gentle "unroofing" of the overlying tubercle from the nerve is a safe and effective technique of nerve identification and exposure (12).

Terminally the nerve may vary in size from a few millimeters to 3 to 4 mm in some cases. It usually is a bright white color with distinguishing "racing stripes"—vaso nervorum—running on the surface. Frequently the nerve branches prior to entering the cricothyroid membrane, occasionally caudal to the junction with the inferior thyroid artery, which if unrecognized may put one or both nerve branches at risk. With large goiters, nodules, or fibrosis the nerve may be adherent or incorporated into the thyroid capsule in the lower pole region and mistaken for a vascular structure, with disastrous outcome. The current standard of care is to identify and dissect the nerve before thyroid resection while leaving the surrounding connective tissue and attachments to the trachea intact, basically atraumatically unroofing the nerve in order to preserve its blood supply. Some difficulty may be encountered in the area of the posterior suspensory ligament (ligament of Berry), which attaches the thyroid lobe to the side of the cricoid cartilage as well as the first and second tracheal rings and the esophagus. This firm fibrous attachment to the laryngoskeleton is responsible for the movement of the thyroid gland experienced during swallowing. The recurrent nerve can pass deep to the ligament of Berry or between the ligament and its lateral fascial leaf. This is a sticky area where identification and dissection may be difficult, especially with cancer and fibrosis from radiation or Hashimoto's disease.

It is nearly impossible to perform thyroid surgery without encountering and having to deal with the parathyroid glands. Eighty percent of the time the upper parathyroids will be found within a 1 cm radius of the junction of the inferior thyroid artery and the recurrent laryngeal nerve. Embryologically, the lower parathyroid develops and descends with the thymus, separating to remain near the lower pole of the thyroid as the thymus continues descending into the mediastinum. However, the lower parathyroid gland may be found within the thyroid gland, the thymus, or anywhere from the angle of the mandible to the deep mediastinum, including the pericardium and even the heart. Once the parathyroid glands are identified, they may need to be dissected from the thyroid capsule, using great care to preserve their delicate blood supply, generally end arterial branches of the inferior thyroid artery. Inadvertent devascularization dictates parathyroid autotransplantation into the adjacent sternocleidomastoid muscle. A postoperative serum (parathyroid hormone) PTH level may be useful in clinical management and patient counseling if postoperative hypocalcemia is experienced.

Veins accompanying the inferior thyroid artery are ligated on the capsule of the thyroid, carefully avoiding branches of the recurrent laryngeal nerve. Careful attention should be practiced in controlling the small branch of the inferior thyroid artery and accompanying vein within Berry's ligament. This branch is usually quite close to the nerve and if torn nearly always appears to retract under the nerve, necessitating control by local pressure and hemostatics. Point suture ligation under loup magnification may be required to control bleeding and avoid nerve injury.

Having identified and exposed the recurrent nerve and controlled the vascular supply, one is ready to resect the lobe. The status of the parathyroid glands should be reevaluated to ensure that the glands have a satisfactory blood supply. If in doubt, a devascularized gland should be removed, minced into 1 to 2 mm pieces, and transplanted into the ipsilateral sternocleidomastoid muscle. At this point, resection of the lobe is performed by retracting the thyroid lobe medially and elevating it from the underlying trachea. This fibrous pretracheal plane is easily dissected with electrocautery or the scalpel. The pyramidal lobe, a cephalad extension from the isthmus or medial aspect of the thyroid lobe, lying on the anterior surface of the cricoid cartilage and the larynx is dissected and included with the specimen. Failure to excise the pyramidal lobe is a recognized cause of "incomplete" total thyroidectomy. Any nodal tissues associated with the isthmus and the pyramidal lobe should also be resected. At times, particularly with papillary thyroid cancer, an enlarged pretracheal node in this area will contain metastatic disease. This node has been dubbed the delphian node after the Oracle of Delphi, who was able to predict what the future held.

EXTENT OF THYROIDECTOMY

If a total thyroidectomy is planned, the contralateral lobe is removed using the same extracapsular technique and maneuvers as described above. If the planned operation is a lobectomy, the isthmus is divided at the junction with the contralateral lobe, the cut edge being suture ligated. The other surgical option at this point is a near-total thyroidectomy, in which varying amounts of contralateral thyroid tissue are left in place, usually requiring intraglandular resection as opposed to the extracapsular approach described above.

No clear consensus exists of the definition of the extent of thyroidectomy. Bliss et al have proposed a classification of extent of thyroidectomy as follows (12). Partial thyroidectomy is defined as removal of neoplasm with a margin of normal thyroid tissue. Subtotal thyroidectomy is described as bilateral excision of more than 50% of each lobe, including the isthmus, whereas a lobectomy or hemithyroidectomy is a total extracapsular excision, including the isthmus. Total thyroidectomy is the extracapsular removal of both lobes and the isthmus (Fig. 70C.2). Bliss et al define near-total thyroidectomy as the extracapsular removal

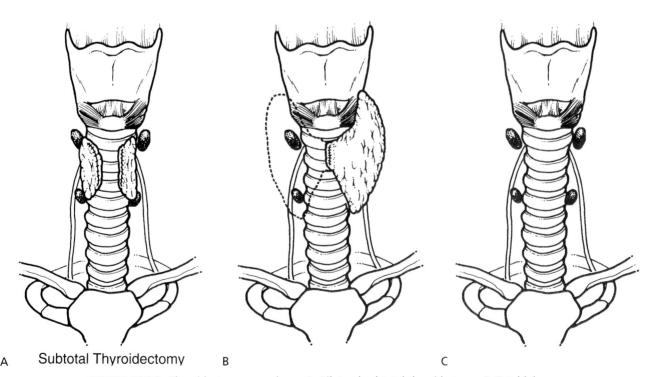

A   Subtotal Thyroidectomy   B   C

FIGURE 70C.2. Thyroidectomy procedures. **A:** Bilateral subtotal thyroidectomy. **B:** Total lobectomy and isthmusectomy. **C:** Total thyroidectomy.

of one lobe and up to 90% of the contralateral lobe, leaving behind approximately 1 g of thyroid tissue (12).

Considerable debate continues in the literature concerning the appropriate surgical procedure for thyroid carcinoma of follicular epithelium. The controversy is between two ideologies, that of management by lobectomy or by total thyroidectomy. Arguments for lobectomy include the fact that overall survival appears uninfluenced by the extent of surgical resection in low-risk patients. A number of prognostic systems have been proposed for defining risk level in thyroid malignancy (13–15). Although there are some individual differences between the prognostic systems, all use patient age, size of tumor, extent of disease, and metastases. Low-risk female patients, of age less than 50, with well-differentiated tumors without tumor extension outside the thyroid gland, and without metastases, are predicted to have an excellent prognosis with either lobectomy or total thyroidectomy. The majority of patients with thyroid carcinomas of follicular epithelium fall into this favorable category. On the other hand, patients deemed to be high risk have been found to do equally poorly with either limited or total thyroidectomy. Additional recognized advantages of lobectomy are decreased morbidity from nerve injury, negligible hypoparathyroidism, no absolute need for thyroid replacement therapy, and the lack of potential risks from adjuvant ^{131}I treatment.

The advantages of total thyroidectomy include the ability to remove occult multicentric disease, present in over 30% of cases, thus reducing remnant recurrences; the ability to postoperatively scan patients for residual thyroid-bred tissue and distant disease, and to treat if necessary with radioactive iodine; and the ability to monitor for tumor recurrence with serum thyroglobulin levels following removal of all thyroid tissue.

At Boston University School of Medicine we have favored the more aggressive regimen of total thyroidectomy for all but minimal lesions (i.e., <1 cm well-differentiated without capsular invasion) in patients under 40 years of age, thereby accepting the studies of Mazzaferri and others that document both decreased local recurrence and improved survival with combined total thyroidectomy and ^{131}I therapy (16–18).

Occasionally, patients with thyroid cancer require reoperation, either a completion procedure to remove a thyroid remnant or a procedure to excise recurrent local disease. Reoperative thyroid surgery presents a number of technical challenges, which in some instances are best managed by an experienced endocrine surgeon. In the hands of such an individual, surgery can be performed successfully with minimal morbidity (19).

LYMPH NODE DISSECTION

Patients with known thyroid malignancy or who have suspicious appearing tracheoesophageal (TE) nodes should have a lymph node dissection. At a minimum, dissection should include all the nodes on the epsilateral TE groove and a bilateral dissection if the contralateral nodes are grossly suspicious or the opposite thyroid lobe appears to contain multicentric disease. Nodes anterior to the trachea, above the isthmus and under the sternal notch, also should be removed. Nodal resection carried out between both carotid vessels and from the sternal notch to the thyroid cartilage constitute what is known as a central compartment resection and are indicated in patients with high-grade lesions or larger tumors, as well as in men over 40 and women over 50. The use of sentinel lymph node techniques have been proposed to identify drainage nodes and aid in sampling, particularly if lymph nodes are clinically not involved (20).

Patients with suspicious or enlarged nodes in the lateral neck or with biopsy-proven metastatic disease are candidates for a modified neck dissection, which would include lymph nodes in levels III, IV, and V, preserving the jugular vein, sternocleidomastoid muscle, and accessory nerve.

Individuals with clinically negative lateral lymph nodes who have positive central nodes may be treated with ^{131}I in observation. In most instances, subclinical disease will be adequately successfully controlled by ^{131}I and TSH suppression. Postoperative monitoring with clinical examination, cervical ultrasound evaluation of the neck, and serum thyroid-binding globulins should be used.

COMPLICATIONS OF THYROIDECTOMY

In general, complications of thyroidectomy may be related to disease type, size of the gland, degree of technical difficulty (i.e., reoperative surgery), surgical training, and volume of surgical work (21). Three major complications need to be highlighted in any preoperative discussion with the patient: postoperative recurrent nerve dysfunction, hypoparathyroidism, and bleeding complications, which may occur during or following thyroidectomy. Permanent unilateral recurrent nerve palsy is perhaps the most disabling. Bilateral nerve palsy, although rare, even of a transient nature, on the other hand, may be life threatening. Such an injury may become immediately apparent with the patient developing significant stridor within minutes or hours following extubation. Reintubation or possibly immediate tracheotomy may be required to save the patient's life.

Identification and dissection of the recurrent laryngeal nerve does not increase the risk for either transient or permanent nerve palsy; indeed, it has been found to decrease the incidence of these complications. Ideally, the nerve should be exposed over its entire course from the jugular angle to insertion into the cricothyroid membrane while leaving surrounding supporting connective tissues intact to minimize the risk for devascularization. When the nerve is visualized to be intact, any ensuing palsy will be almost uniformly transient. The nerve is most commonly injured at the junction with the inferior thyroid artery and the ligament of Berry or near the inferior pole of the thyroid. About 60% of the time, extralaryngeal branching occurs near the inferior thyroid artery or the ligament of Berry, significantly increasing the risk for nerve damage. In the majority of cases, the most ventral nerve branch innervates the intrinsic laryngeal muscles. Obviously, the anterior location of the ventral branch makes it vulnerable to suture injuries when less than a lobectomy is performed. Failure to recognize adherence of the nerve to an enlarged lower pole nodule or the occurrence of an aberrant nonrecurring laryngeal nerve (1%) are other causes of nerve injury. Permanent nerve palsy is cited in the literature to occur from 0% to 2.1%, with the average of approximately 0.5% to 1%. Temporary palsy varies from 2.9% to over 10% (12).

The second feared adverse result of thyroidectomy is temporary or permanent hypoparathyroidism. Obviously this is only a consideration in bilateral procedures or patients having central neck dissection for cancer. Careful identification and ligation of the terminal branches of the inferior thyroid artery with preservation of vascular pedicles, especially to the inferior parathyroid gland, and liberal employment of autotransplantation of damaged or devascularized glands will minimize this difficult complication. Transient hypocalcaemia, frequently asymptomatic, may be related to intraoperative manipulation, vitamin D deficiency, or hypomagnesemia and may be observed in up to 7.3% of patients. If a patient is symptomatic, treatment with calcium and 1,25-dihydroxy vitamin D is indicated. On the other hand, in the asymptomatic individual one might argue for expectant observation. However, in this day of outpatient or short-stay surgery, the clinician does not have the luxury of additional observation days. Therefore, many patients, asymptomatic or otherwise, will get outpatient calcium supplementation. A postoperative serum PTH determination may reassure the physician enough to follow an outpatient observation course.

Bleeding or hematoma is an infrequent but potentially serious complication of thyroidectomy. The signs of postoperative bleeding can be respiratory distress, pain, pressure, and dysphagia, with symptoms sometimes appearing 4 to 18 hours after wound closure. Meticulous hemostasis is the best technique to avoid hematoma, and wound drainage should not to be used routinely. Although drainage will not prevent hemorrhage, it can alert the staff to the occurrence of postoperative bleeding. If a hematoma is not visible, but the patient complains of pain out of proportion to the operation, US of the neck may reveal a developing hematoma and lessen treatment delay. Some surgeons have used fibrin glue application to the thyroid resection bed as an adjunct to hemostasis, particularly in patients with large glands or a bleeding disorder such as low platelets. Other rare complications include pneumothorax, pneumomedi-

astinum, and wound infection. With large glands, Hashimoto's disease, or cancer, injury to the sympathetic nerves, esophagus, and trachea are possibilities that must be avoided.

THYROID SURGERY IN THE ELDERLY

When thyroid problems occur in the elderly, the risk for malignancy is higher and the end results are generally poorer. Questions often are raised as to the patient's ability to tolerate thyroid surgery based on age and concomitant diseases. A recent study evaluated morbidity following thyroidectomy in patients 75 years of age and over and concluded that it was no greater than in patients under the age of 75 years (22). These results were obtained in the face of comorbidity rates of 80%, including essential hypertension (52.7%), coronary arteriosclerosis (30.9%), cardiac arrhythmias (21.8%), diabetes (5.5%), Parkinson's disease (9.1%), and chronic obstructive pulmonary disease (12.7%). Forty-two percent of individuals had two or more comorbidity's in the elderly group. When the two groups were compared, no statistical differences were documented in postoperative course or morbidity. As expected, in the elderly population there were more reinterventions and an increased occurrence of large goiters with associated mechanical symptoms, substernal thyroid tumors, and cancer, particularly of the undifferentiated variety. Fortunately, even the frail elderly tolerate modern anesthesia and expert thyroid surgery quite well if the procedure is an elective one. The aim should be to manage these patients electively rather than on an emergency basis.

NEW DIMENSIONS

The future holds a number of technological changes that will impact thyroid surgery. The first is the increased use of the harmonic scalpel, which employs US to simultaneously cut and coagulate tissue. Recently it was documented in a large series to reduce operative time by at least 30 minutes for the standard thyroidectomy (23).

Increased use of intraoperative neuromonitoring has decreased operative time while lowering the morbidity of both transient and permanent nerve palsy. High-risk groups for postoperative palsy are the reoperative patient and those undergoing extended surgeries for nodular disease, Hashimoto's disease, and cancer. Nerve monitoring facilitates earlier, easier, and less traumatic identification of the recurrent laryngeal nerve and allows the surgeon to reassure those patients who may be hoarse following surgery that electrical continuity exists with an excellent possibility of full voice recovery (24).

Finally, video-assisted surgery has found a role in nearly every surgical specialty. With evolution of advanced video operative skills, reports have appeared showing that video-assisted thyroid lobectomy leads to better cosmetic outcome and is associated with less postoperative pain and reduces postoperative hospital stays when compared with standard open lobectomy. Bellantone et al concluded thatt could be "a valid alternative to conventional surgery in patients with small solitary nodular thyroid lesions" (25). At this time the operation appears best suited to those patients with solitary nodules smaller than 3 cm, cysts, and small toxic nodules. This area is currently developing and may expand when surgical robotics become more widely available.

REFERENCES

1. Vander JB, Gaston EA, Dawber TR. The significance of nontoxic thyroid nodules. Final report of a 15-year study of the incidence of thyroid malignancy. *Ann Intern Med* 1968;69: 537–540.
2. Rallison ML, Dobyns BM, Meikle AW, et al. Natural history of thyroid abnormalities: prevalence, incidence, and regression of thyroid diseases in adolescents and young adults. *Am J Med* 1991;91:363–370.
3. Jemal A, Murray T, Samuels A, et al. Cancer statistics, 2003. *CA Cancer J Clin* 2003;53:5–26
4. Perrier ND, vanHeerden JA, Goellner JR, et al. Thyroid cancer in patients with familial adenomatous polyposis. *World J Surg* 1998;22:738–743.
5. Udelsman R, Westra WH, Donovan PI, et al. Randomized prospective evaluation of frozen-section analysis for follicular neoplasms of the thyroid. *Ann Surg* 2001;233:716–722.
6. Richards ML, Chisolm R, Bruder JM, et al. Is thyroid frozen section too much for too little? *Am J Surg* 2002;184:510–514.
7. Chen H, Zeiger MA, Clark DP, et al. Papillary thyroid cancer: can operative management be solely based on fine needle aspiration? *J Am Coll Surg* 1997;184:605–610.
8. Kouvaraki MA, Shapiro SE, Fornage BD, et al. Role of preoperative ultrasonography in the surgical management of patients with thyroid cancer. *Surgery* 2003;134:946–953.
9. Kresnik E, Gallowitsch HJ, Mikosch P, et al. Fluorine-18-fluorodeoxyglucose positron emission tomography in the preoperative assessment of thyroid nodules in an endemic goiter area. *Surgery* 2003;133:294–299.
10. Kierner AC, Aigner M, Burian M. The external branch of the superior laryngeal nerve. Its topographical anatomy as related to surgery of the neck. *Arch Otolaryngol Head Neck Surg* 1998; 124:301–303.
11. Jonas J, Bahr R, Intraoperative electromyographic identification of the recurrent laryngeal nerves. *Chirurgie* 2000;71:534–538.
12. Bliss RD, Gauger PG, Delbridge LW. Surgeon's approach to the thyroid gland: surgical anatomy and the importance of technique. *World J Surg* 2000;24:891–897.
13. Hay ID, Grant CS, Taylor WF, et al. Ipsilateral lobectomy versus bilateral lobar resection in papillary thyroid carcinoma: a retrospective analysis of surgical outcome using a novel prognostic scoring system. *Surgery* 1987;102:1088–1095.
14. Cady B, Rossi R. An expanded view of risk-group definition in differentiated thyroid carcinoma. *Surgery* 1988;104:947–953.
15. Shaha AR, Loree TR, Shah JP. Intermediate risk group for differentiated carcinoma of the thyroid. *Surgery* 1994;116:1036–1041.
16. Mazzaferri EL, Young RL. Papillary thyroid carcinoma: a 10-year follow-up report of the impact of therapy in 576 patients. *Am J Med* 1981;70:511–518.
17. Degroot LJ, Kaplan EL, McCormick M, et al. Natural history, treatment and course of papillary thyroid carcinoma. *Clin Endocrinol Metab* 1990;71:414–424.
18. Kebebew E, Clark OH. Differentiated thyroid cancer: "Complete" rational approach. *World J Surg* 2000;24:942–951.
19. Levin KE, Clark AH, Duh Q-Y, et al. Reoperative thyroid surgery. *Surgery* 1992;111:604–609.
20. Arch-Ferrer J, Velaquez D, Fajardo R, et al. Accuracy of sentinel lymph node in papillary thyroid carcinoma. *Surgery* 2001;130: 907–913.
21. Henry CR, Patient volumes and complications in thyroid surgery. *Br J Surg* 2002;89:821–823.
22. Passler C, Avanessian R, Kaczirek K, et al. Thyroid surgery in the geriatric patent. *Arch Surg* 2002;137:1243–1248.
23. Siperstein AE, Berber E, Morkoyun E. The use of the Harmonic scalpel vs conventional knot tying for vessel ligation in thyroid surgery. *Arch Surg* 2002;137:137–142.
24. Thomusch O, Sehulla C, Walls G, et al. Intraoperative neuromonitoring of surgery for benign goiter. *Am J Surg* 2002;183: 673–678.
25. Bellantone R, Lombardi CP, Bossola M, et al. Video-assisted conventional thyroid lobectomy: a randomized trial. *Arch Surg* 2002;137:301–305.

70D CARCINOMA OF FOLLICULAR EPITHELIUM: RADIOIODINE AND OTHER TREATMENTS AND OUTCOMES

ERNEST L. MAZZAFERRI
RICHARD T. KLOOS

Papillary and follicular thyroid carcinomas, termed differentiated thyroid carcinoma (DTC), typically have a prolonged course and are asymptomatic for long periods. The tumor usually presents as a thyroid nodule and is identified by fine-needle aspiration (FNA) cytology, often when it is confined to the thyroid or has metastasized only to regional lymph nodes, giving an ample opportunity to cure the disease. Distant metastases or tumor that aggressively invades the neck is the presenting manifestation in about 5% of patients with papillary carcinoma and up to 10% with follicular carcinoma, which drastically lowers the likelihood of cure. Choice of therapy rests on an understanding of the natural history of these tumors and on the premise that prognosis can be altered by early intervention. The treatment of choice is surgery, whenever possible, usually followed by radioactive iodine (^{131}I) and thyroxine (T_4) therapy, but external radiation and chemotherapy have a role in management of some patients.

Papillary carcinoma comprises about 80% of all thyroid carcinomas, follicular carcinoma about 10%, and Hürthle cell carcinoma about 3% (1). Although these are distinct pathologic entities, their clinical features and outcomes are similar when the tumor is confined to the thyroid. Much of the following discussion refers to DTC, because the approach to treatment of these tumors is similar (2). Where there are substantial differences among the three tumors in treatment, prognosis, or behavior, the differences have been highlighted.

CHANGING INCIDENCE AND MORTALITY RATES

During the years from 1973 to 2003, the incidence of thyroid cancer increased steadily in North America (3) and Europe (4). It is the fastest rising cancer in women in the United States (5). Why this has happened is unknown, but it may be partially the result of exposure of the population to radiation fallout (6). During this same time, the mortality rates of thyroid cancer have declined significantly (~20%) in women (3). This is likely due to early diagnosis and effective treatment in women but not in men. The peak age at the time of diagnosis of thyroid carcinoma is around 45 years in women and 75 years in men (3). At the time of diagnosis, men have 25% more locoregional metastases and more than a 200% greater rate of distant metastases than do women, resulting in thyroid cancer mortality rates that are twice as high in men as in women (3). In the United States, this is the fastest rising cause of cancer death in men (7). These statistics are driven by papillary, follicular, and Hürthle cell carcinomas, which comprised about 95% of thyroid cancers and accounted for about 76% of all thyroid cancer deaths between 1985 and 1995 (1). Yet these thyroid tumors are the most amenable to treatment when identified at an early stage.

CONTEMPORARY VIEWS CONCERNING THERAPY

Prognosis of DTC is typically so favorable that it is difficult to demonstrate a beneficial effect of therapy unless very

large cohorts are studied for several decades. No prospective randomized clinical trials have been done, so that all contemporary views of the efficacy of different treatments are based on retrospective studies.

Several studies shed light on the current practice. A study of 5,583 cases of thyroid carcinoma treated in over 1,500 hospitals in the United States during 1996 found that total or near-total thyroidectomy was performed in the vast majority (~75%) of patients with DTC (8). After surgery at least half were treated with ^{131}I and were given T_4 to suppress thyrotropin (TSH), but this was underreported in the study. A report from Germany (9) of 2,376 patients with DTC treated in 1996 indicated that total thyroidectomy was performed in about 90% of the patients and that ^{131}I was almost always administered postoperatively (74% papillary, over 90% follicular). Lymph node dissection was performed in 22% of those with papillary carcinoma.

Current guidelines on the treatment of DTC from the United States (10) and Europe (11) advise total or near-total thyroidectomy followed by ^{131}I ablation of the thyroid remnant for most patients. Although the treatment of children has been more controversial, many clinicians now recommend that they be treated the same as adults (12).

PROGNOSTIC FEATURES

The distinction between aggressive and slow-growing tumors becomes less clear when multiple and opposing prognostic features intermingle to shape the final outcome. The three main features determining prognosis, however, are tumor stage, age at the time of diagnosis, and treatment. The most disagreement stems from the weight clinicians allocate to these variables when planning initial therapy.

Mortality Rates

A study of 53,856 cases of thyroid carcinoma treated in the United States during 1985 to 1995 found 10-year cancer mortality rates of about 7% for papillary carcinoma, 15% for follicular carcinoma, and 24% for Hürthle cell carcinoma (1). Prognosis is less favorable in older patients and among those with certain histologic variants. In our 1,355 patients with DTC whose mean age at diagnosis was only 36 years, the 30-year cancer-specific mortality rates were 6% for papillary and 15% for follicular carcinoma (13). Cancer mortality rates are even lower for children (12), except for those under age 10, in whom the prognosis may be less favorable (14).

Recurrence Rates

Depending on the initial therapy and tumor stage, about 20% to 30% of patients have recurrences over several decades, two thirds of which occur within the first decade

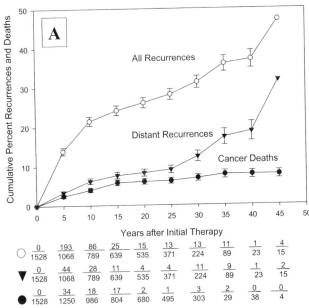

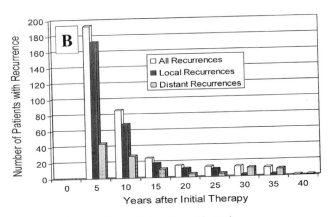

FIGURE 70D.1. Tumor recurrence and cancer death rates from differentiated thyroid carcinoma. **A:** The vertical bars represent standard errors. Numerators are the number of events during the previous interval, and denominators the number of patients at the beginning of the next time interval. **B:** Recurrences at 5-year intervals. All recurrences, local recurrences, and distant recurrences are shown for each time interval. [Modified from Mazzaferri EL, Kloos RT. Current approaches to primary therapy for papillary and follicular thyroid cancer. *J Clin Endocrinol Metab* 2001;86(4):1447–1463. 2001, with permission.]

after initial therapy (13) (Fig. 70D.1). Although not usually fatal, a neck recurrence is not a trivial event and may be the first sign of a lethal outcome. In our patients who had local recurrences, 74% were in cervical lymph nodes, 20% were in thyroid remnants, and 6% were in trachea or muscle; 7% of this group died of cancer (13). The tumors recurred at distant locations in 21%, most often in the lungs alone (63%); half died of carcinoma. Recurrent tumor caused over half the cancer deaths in our patients. The other deaths were due to recognized persistent disease.

TUMOR FEATURES THAT INFLUENCE OUTCOME

Features of the tumor often play a major role in decisions regarding therapy. What follows are summaries considered more or less independently of variations in therapy.

Typical Papillary Tumors

This tumor has distinctive cellular features that can be recognized by fine-needle aspiration biopsy or frozen section in 95% of cases (see Chapter 28) (15). Most are mixed papillary-follicular tumors, while a few have a purely papillary pattern, features that have no bearing on prognosis. Most are unencapsulated tumors that are 2 to 3 cm in diameter and tend to infiltrate the thyroid, but are confined by its capsule. This tumor invades lymphatics and blood

vessels and is commonly found in multiple sites within the thyroid and in regional lymph nodes. Those that metastasize to the lung typically appear as diffuse bilateral pulmonary nodules on chest x-ray or are visible only by ^{131}I scans. Hematogenous spread to bone, central nervous system, and other sites can also occur. These features have important prognostic implications, as noted below.

Papillary Carcinoma Variants

Survival rates vary considerably among certain subsets of patients with papillary carcinoma (16). About 10% of papillary carcinomas have a well-defined capsule, which is a particularly favorable prognostic sign, even in tumors with cellular features suggesting otherwise (17). Other variants have a more serious prognosis. Anaplastic tumor transformation, a rare event occurring in fewer than 1% of papillary carcinomas, is associated with p53 oncogene expression and causes death within a year (18). Tall cell papillary carcinomas, which are large tumors in older patients that can be identified by FNA, have up to a 25% 10-year mortality rate (16). The outcome is even worse with columnar-variant papillary carcinoma, which has a 90% mortality rate unless the tumor is encapsulated (17). About 2% of papillary carcinomas are diffuse sclerosing variants that infiltrate the entire gland and may cause a diffuse goiter without a palpable nodule, which may be mistaken for goitrous autoimmune thyroiditis (15). Most metastasize to lymph nodes, and about 25% have distant metastases (15).

Mainly affecting younger persons, about 10% of the tumors found in children following the Chernobyl accident were of this type (19). They are aggressive tumors that may have a poor prognosis; however, with aggressive treatment the prognosis is as good as that of classical papillary carcinoma (20). Follicular-variant papillary carcinomas have typical papillary nuclear features and follicular architecture that may suggest a follicular neoplasm on FNA, although the cellular features may identify this as follicular-variant papillary carcinoma (21); their clinical behavior resembles that of typical papillary more than follicular carcinoma (22).

Follicular Carcinoma Histology

This is usually a solitary encapsulated tumor with a microfollicular histologic pattern that is slightly more aggressive than papillary carcinoma. Widely invasive tumors have a poor prognosis and are easily recognized by their aggressive extension into surrounding tissues. Up to 80% of patients with such tumors develop metastases, and more than 15% die of their disease within 10 years (1,2). However, most follicular carcinomas are minimally invasive encapsulated tumors that closely resemble follicular adenomas, and the distinction can be made only by review of the permanent histologic sections and not by FNA or frozen-section study, which poses a serious management predicament at the time of surgery. The main diagnostic criteria for follicular carcinoma are cells penetrating the tumor capsule or invading blood vessels within or beyond its capsule. The latter has a worse prognosis than capsular penetration alone (23). Still, a few patients with minimally invasive follicular carcinomas, the main type diagnosed in recent years, have distant metastases or die of their disease (24).

The poorer prognosis of follicular carcinoma is more closely related to the patient's older age at the time of diagnosis and advanced tumor stage than its histology alone (13). The survival rates of patients with papillary or follicular carcinomas are similar in patients of comparable age and disease stage (2,13). Both have an excellent prognosis if they are confined to the thyroid, are small tumors (≥1.0 cm), or are minimally invasive (13). Both have poor outcomes if they are widely invasive (papillary carcinoma invading the thyroid capsule and adjacent structures, and follicular carcinoma invading blood vessels and the tumor capsule) or metastatic to distant sites (2,13).

The 30-year survival rate in our series was 76%, and the cancer-specific death rate was 8% in 1,355 patients, of whom 79% had papillary and 21% follicular carcinoma (13). The mortality rate in patients with follicular carcinoma was over twofold that of the patients with papillary carcinoma; however, those with follicular carcinoma were older than patients with papillary carcinoma and had larger tumors and more advanced disease at presentation. Patients with tumors of similar stage had 30-year recurrence and cancer-specific mortality rates that were the same, regardless of the tumor's papillary or follicular histology (13).

Hürthle (Oncocytic) Cell Follicular Variant

These cells may constitute most (>75%) or all of a tumor; such tumors are sometimes classified as Hürthle cell carcinoma or as variants of follicular carcinoma. Although there has been some controversy about their diagnosis, management, and outcome, more recent large series clarify some of these issues. A study of 1,585 cases of Hürthle cell carcinoma found the 10-year cancer mortality rate was 25%, compared with a 15% rate in 5,271 patients with follicular carcinoma (1). Pulmonary metastases occur in 20% to 35% of patients with Hürthle cell carcinoma, about twice that of follicular carcinoma (25). Hürthle cell–variant papillary carcinoma is even less common, but may have higher than usual recurrence and mortality rates (2).

Tumor Size

Papillary carcinomas smaller than or equal to 1 cm, termed microcarcinomas, are often found unexpectedly during surgery for benign thyroid conditions. Although they usually pose no threat to survival and ordinarily require no further surgery (26), about 20% are multifocal and as many as 60% have cervical lymph node metastases that may be the presenting feature (27). Lung metastases occur rarely, except for multifocal tumors with cervical metastases, which are the only microcarcinomas with significant morbidity and mortality (27,28). Otherwise, the recurrence and cancer-specific mortality rates are near zero (26,27). In our series, 30-year recurrence rates with DTC smaller than 1.5 cm were one-third those associated with larger tumors (13). The small tumors rarely metastasized to distant sites and had low cancer-specific mortality rates (0.4% vs. 7% for tumors ≥ 1.5 cm, $p < .001$) (13). There is a linear relationship between tumor size and cancer recurrence and mortality for both papillary and follicular carcinomas (13) (Fig. 70D.2).

Multiple Intrathyroidal Tumors

Multicentric tumors are found in about 20% of patients with papillary carcinoma when the thyroid is examined routinely and in up to 80% if the thyroid is examined with great care (2). Although regarded as intrathyroidal metastases in the past, multiple distinct *RET/PTC* gene rearrangements found in the majority of multifocal papillary carcinomas proves that they are individual tumors that arise independently in a background of genetic or environmental susceptibility (29). Their presence cannot be predicted on the basis of clinical risk stratification (30), and is thus not apparent until the final histologic sections of the entire thyroid gland have been studied, which has a bearing on the need to surgically excise the contralateral lobe and to ablate the thyroid remnant with [131]I. Among patients un-

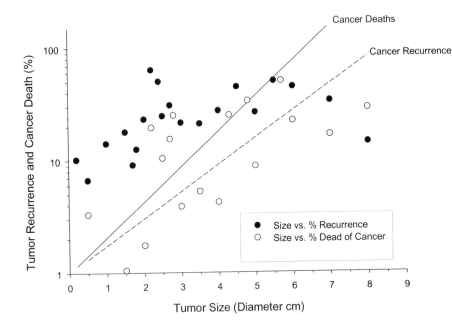

FIGURE 70D.2. Primary tumor size as it affects cancer recurrence (●) and cancer death rates (○) from DTC. Regression lines are for cancer death (*solid line*) and tumor recurrence (*dashed line*). Each point represents the percentage of events for tumor size in more than one patient. (Drawn from data in Mazzaferri EL, Kloos RT. Current approaches to primary therapy for papillary and follicular thyroid cancer. *J Clin Endocrinol Metab* 2001;86 (4):1447–1463.)

dergoing routine completion thyroidectomy for presumed unilateral DTC, about half have a tumor in the contralateral lobe (2,30,31); however, when multifocal disease is present in the thyroid lobe first excised, or when the tumor has recurred in any site, bilateral multifocal tumors are almost always found (32). Thus, the prognosis may be more serious than usual with this feature, even when there are multicentric microcarcinomas. There is a higher incidence of recurrent regional lymph node metastases in multicentric microcarcinomas than in single 1 cm tumors, and the presence of lymph node metastases increases the likelihood of distant metastases from microscopic multicentric tumors (28,33,34). Multicentric microcarcinomas are often found in patients with familial nonmedullary thyroid carcinoma, which tends to be more aggressive than usual (34).

Those who find few recurrences in the contralateral thyroid lobe after hemithyroidectomy argue that multiple microscopic tumors are of little clinical consequence (35). Others find recurrence rates ranging from 5% to 20% in large thyroid remnants and that pulmonary metastases occur more frequently after subtotal than total thyroidectomy (36–38). In one study, patients with multiple intrathyroidal tumors had almost twice the incidence of nodal metastases and three times the rate of pulmonary and other distant metastases than those with single tumors, and the likelihood of persistent disease was three times more likely in those with multiple tumors (38). Another study found a 1.7-fold higher risk for recurrence in multifocal compared with unifocal tumors (39). Another study found that the only two parameters significantly influencing tumor recurrence of papillary microcarcinomas were the number of histologic foci (*p* < .002) and the extent of initial thyroid surgery (27). The 30-year cancer mortality rates among our

patients with multiple tumors were two times those in the patients with a single tumor (13). At 30 years, the recurrence rate among 436 patients who had undergone subtotal thyroidectomy was significantly higher than that among 698 patients who had undergone total or near-total thyroidectomy (40% vs. 26%, *p* < .002); cancer-specific mortality rates were also higher in the subtotal thyroidectomy group (9% and 6%, *p* = .02) (13).

Lymphocytic Infiltration of Tumor

Lymphocytic infiltration ranging from focal areas of lymphocytes and plasma cells to classic Hashimoto's disease, which is often seen in papillary carcinoma, is associated with a lower than usual tumor stage and may be an independent predictor of a favorable prognosis (40).

Local Tumor Invasion

About 5% to 10% of tumors grow directly into surrounding tissues, increasing both morbidity and mortality. Local invasion, which can occur with both papillary and follicular carcinoma, ranges from microscopic to gross tumor invasion (13). The most commonly invaded structures are the neck muscles and vessels, recurrent laryngeal nerves, larynx, pharynx, and esophagus, but tumor can extend into the spinal cord and brachial plexus. The symptoms are usually hoarseness, cough, dysphagia, hemoptysis, airway insufficiency, or neurologic dysfunction. Extrathyroidal tumor extension is a key risk factor leading to lymph node and distant metastasis (41). The tumor was locally invasive in 115 of our patients (8% of those with papillary and 12% of those with follicular carcinoma); 10-year recurrence rates were 1.5 times and cancer-specific death rates were 5 times those of patients without local tumor invasion, and nearly all with tumor invasion died within the first decade (13).

Lymph Node Metastases

The first sign of thyroid carcinoma may be an enlarged cervical lymph node; in such a patient, multiple nodal metastases are usually found at surgery. About 33% of metastatic lymph nodes from papillary carcinoma are partly cystic (42). The incidence and location of lymph node metastases varies with the tumor type, patient age, and the extent of lymph node surgery. For example, gross lymph node metastases are found in about 36% of adults and in up to 80% of children with papillary carcinoma, and in about 17% with follicular carcinoma (12,43) (Table 70D.1). Micrometastases are found even more often. In one series of 119 patients in which 21% were known preoperatively to have lymph nodes metastases, almost 61% were found to have micrometastases after undergoing bilateral lateral neck compartment dissection; 41% were bilateral (44). Another study (45) of 2,551 cervical lymph nodes obtained from 80 patients with papillary thyroid carcinoma also found micrometastases in 60% of the lymph nodes. Tumors located in the upper third of the thyroid were found to metastasize in the direction of upward lymphatic flow, whereas tumors located in the lower third or isthmus metastasized inferiorly (45).

The prognostic importance of regional lymph node metastases is controversial. Some find their presence has no impact on recurrence or survival (46). On the other hand an increasingly larger number of studies find nodal metastases are a risk factor for local or distant tumor recurrence and cancer-specific mortality, especially if there are bilateral cervical or mediastinal lymph node metastases or if tumor invades through the lymph node capsule (13,28, 47–50). In one study, 15% of patients with and none without cervical node metastases died of disease ($p < .02$) (51). Another study of patients with distantly metastatic papillary carcinoma reported that 80% had mediastinal node metastases at the time the carcinoma was diagnosed (52). Our patients with papillary or follicular carcinoma who had cervical or mediastinal lymph node metastases had significantly higher 30-year cancer mortality rates than those without them (10% vs. 6%, $p < .01$).

Distant Metastases

About 10% of patients with papillary carcinoma and up to 25% of those with follicular carcinoma develop distant metastases; half are present at the time of diagnosis (43) (Table 70D.1). They occur more often (35%) with Hürthle cell carcinoma and after the age of 40 years (25). Among 1,231 patients reported in 13 studies, 49% of the metastases were to lung, 25% to bone, 15% to both lung and bone, and 10% to the central nervous system or other soft tissues (43). The outcome is influenced mainly by the patient's age, the tumor's metastatic site(s), ability to concentrate ^{131}I, and tumor bulk (53,54). Although some patients survive for decades, especially younger patients, about half die within 5 years regardless of tumor histology (43). In a study from France, survival rates with distant metastases were 53% at 5 years, 38% at 10 years and 30% at 15 years (55). Survival is longest with diffuse microscopic lung metastases seen only on posttreatment ^{131}I imaging and not by x-ray (55–57). The prognosis is much worse when the metastases do not concentrate ^{131}I or appear as large lung nodules and is intermediate when the tumors are small nodules on x-ray that concentrate ^{131}I (53,57).

The 3-year survival rate for patients with ^{18}FDG-PET avid tumor metastasis volumes of 125 mL or less is 96% compared with 18% in patients with ^{18}FDG-PET volumes greater than 125 mL (58). Patients with multiple bone or central nervous system metastases have a poor prognosis (57). About half die within 3 years of discovery of the bone metastases (54) and survive about 1 year after the diagnosis of brain metastases (59). A study of 161 patients who died of thyroid carcinoma found that the main causes of death were respiratory insufficiency due to pulmonary metastasis (43%), circulatory failure due to vena cava obstruction by

TABLE 70D.1. REGIONAL AND DISTANT METASTASES AT DIAGNOSIS AND AFTER TUMOR RECURRENCE

	Papillary Carcinoma Metastases			Follicular Carcinoma Metastases		
	n^a	Nodal (%)^b	Distant (%)	n^a	Nodal (%)	Distant (%)
Presentation	7,845	36	5	1,437	17	13
Recurrence	4,165	9 (17)^c	4	1,185	7 (15)	12
Total	7,845	45 (53)	9	1,437	24 (32)	25

^{a}All patients in 13 series (43).
^{b}Rounded to nearest integer.
^{c}In parentheses are all local recurrences, including those in the contralateral thyroid lobe and other neck structures.

extensive mediastinal or sternal metastases (15%), and airway obstruction (13%) and massive hemorrhage (15%) due to uncontrolled local tumor (60).

Thyroglossal Duct Tumors

Small papillary carcinomas that arise in a thyroglossal duct remnant are typically encapsulated by the cyst and usually are not recognized until the permanent histologic sections are reviewed. Dissection of the tract and removal of the hyoid bone (Sistrunk operation) is adequate for most patients because these tumors rarely metastasize (61). However, one study found a high incidence of intrathyroidal carcinomas in such cases, some with aggressive behavior, suggesting that total thyroidectomy may be justified (62).

PATIENT FEATURES INFLUENCING PROGNOSIS

Age

Practically every study shows that the age of the patient at the time of diagnosis is an important prognostic variable. Thyroid carcinoma is more lethal after age 40 years. The risk for cancer death increases with each subsequent decade of life, dramatically rising after age 60 years (Fig. 70D.3). However, there is a remarkably different pattern of tumor recurrence: rates are highest (40%) at the extremes of life, before age 20 years and after age 60 years (12,13,43) (Fig. 70D.3). Despite the clear effect of age on survival, there is disagreement about how age should be factored into the treatment plan, especially in children and young adults. Children commonly present with more advanced disease than adults and have more tumor recurrences after therapy, yet their prognosis for survival is good (12). Some believe that young age has such a favorable influence on survival

that it overshadows the prognosis predicted by the tumor characteristics (46). The majority, however, believe that the tumor stage and histologic differentiation are as important as the patient's age in determining prognosis and management (10,12,13,63).

Gender

Men have a less favorable prognosis than women (13,46). The death rates from all types of thyroid cancer reported in the National Cancer Institute (NCI) Surveillance, Epidemiology, and End Results (SEER) database are twice as high in men as in women (3). In our study, the risk for thyroid cancer death was about twice as great in men as in women (13). Because of this, men with thyroid carcinoma should be regarded with special concern, especially those over age 50.

Graves' Disease

Thyrotropin receptor antibodies may promote tumor growth in patients with Graves' disease. Some find thyroid carcinoma in almost half of the palpable nodules in patients with Graves' disease (64). The tumors are larger and display more aggressive behavior than usual (64). Some, but not all, find that thyroid carcinoma occurring in patients with Graves' disease is more often invasive and metastatic to regional lymph nodes, even when the primary tumor is small (64,65).

CLINICAL STAGING SYSTEMS AND PROGNOSTIC INDEXES

Although the patient's age and tumor stage at the time of diagnosis are the most important variables predicting out-

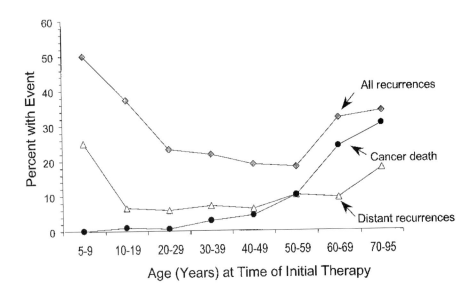

FIGURE 70D.3. Age stratified by decade at the time of initial treatment as it affects the percentage of patients with tumor recurrence, distant recurrence, and cancer deaths. (Modified from Mazzaferri EL, Kloos RT. Current approaches to primary therapy for papillary and follicular thyroid cancer. *J Clin Endocrinol Metab* 2001;86(4):1447–1463, with permission.)

come, their relative importance is debated. Several clinical staging and prognostic scoring systems have been proposed that use age over 40 years as a major feature to identify risk. When more weight is assigned to the patient's age, the relative importance of tumor stage tends to be decreased. This concept, however, does not appear to be widely accepted among practicing physicians because young patients with low prognostic scores often have tumor recurrence. At an international consensus conference in 1987, only 5 of 160 participants treated younger patients more conservatively (66). Similarly, in an international survey of thyroid specialists performed in 1988 (67) and in a survey of clinical members of the American Thyroid Association performed in 1996 (68), age was not used by the majority of respondents in their therapeutic decisions. Current recommendations for the treatment of children now suggest the same therapy as is given to adults with similarly stage tumors (12).

Eight schemes for clinically staging DTC are summarized in Table 70D.2 (69–76). When applied to the papillary carcinoma data from the Mayo Clinic, four of the schemes that use age (EORTC, TNM, AMES, AGES) were effective in separating low-risk patients in whom cancer-specific mortality was 1% at 20 years from high-risk patients in whom it was 30% to 40% at 20 years (73). Twenty-year survival rates for patients with MACIS of less than 6, 6 to 6.99, 7 to 7.99, and 8+ were 99%, 89%, 56%, and 24%, respectively (74). A study that categorized 269 patients with papillary carcinoma according to five differ-

ent prognostic scoring schemes found that some patients in the lowest risk group for each scheme died of cancer (70). This is particularly true of the schemes that simply categorize risk dichotomously as low or high (69,77). Moreover, these schemes do not consider tumor recurrence and are inaccurate in predicting disease-free survival. The latest American Joint Committee on Cancer (AJCC) TNM staging system (76) for thyroid cancer (Table 70D.2), classifies even more patients as being at low risk than did the former version. Staging systems derived from multivariate analyses that do not take into account the effects of therapy assume that treatment does not alter outcome. This is likely incorrect and suggests that none of the prognostic schemes permit clear decisions to be made for individual patients at the time of surgery based on risk group.

Ohio State University Staging System

This classification scheme is shown in Tables 70D.2 and 70D.3 (13). Stage 4 patients were significantly older than the others. After a median follow-up of almost 17 years, tumor recurrence and cancer-specific mortality rates were progressively and significantly greater with each tumor stage (Table 70D.3). Based on regression modeling on 1,501 patients, excluding those who presented with distant metastases and including therapy, the likelihood of death from thyroid carcinoma was increased if age is at least 40 years, the tumor is a folllicular thyroid cancer, tumor size is at least 1.5 cm, local tumor invasion or regional lymph

TABLE 70D.2. A. COMPONENTS OF STAGING SYSTEMS AND RATING SCHEMES FOR DEFINING RISK CATEGORY IN PATIENTS WITH DIFFERENTIATED THYROID CARCINOMA

Variable at Time of Diagnosis	Staging System and Rating Schemes							
	TNM[a,b]	EORTC[b]	AMES[b]	AGES[c]	MACIS[c]	NTCTCS[b]	University of Chicago[c]	Ohio State University[b]
Patient characteristics								
Age	X	X	X	X	X	X		
Sex	X	X	X					
Tumor characteristics								
Cell type	X	X						
Size	X		X	X	X		X	X
Grade (histologic)				X				
Extrathyroidal extension	X	X	X	X	X	X	X	X
Lymph node metastases						X	X	X
Distant metastases	X	X	X	X	X	X	X	X
Therapy characteristics								
Incomplete resection					X			

[a]T, primary tumor, T1, ≤2 cm; T2, >2–4 cm; T3, >4 cm; T4a, any size tumor to invade subcutaneous soft tissues, larynx, trachea, esophagus, or recurrent laryngeal nerve; T4b tumor invades prevertebral fascia or encases carotid artery or mediastinal vessels; all anaplastic tumors are considered T4. T4a intrathyroidal anaplastic carcinoma surgically resectable; T4b extrathyroidal anaplastic carcinoma surgically unresectable; regional lymph nodes are the central compartment, lateral cervical and upper mediastinal lymph nodes. N1a, metastases to level IV (pretracheal, paratracheal, and prelaryngeal/Delphian lymph nodes); N1b, metastases to unilateral, bilateral, or contralateral cervical or superior mediastinal lymph nodes; M0, distant metastases absent; M1, distant metastases present.
[b]Both papillary and follicular carcinoma.
[c]Only papillary carcinoma.

TABLE 70D.2. B. SCORING METHODS

TNM Stage	Papillary or Follicular		Medullary
	<45 years	≥45 years	
I	M0	T1+N0+M0	T1+N0+M0
II	M1	T2+N0+M0	T2+N0+M0
		T3+N0+M0	T3+N0+M0
		T1–3+N1a	T1+N1a+M0
III	None		T2+N1a+M0
			T3+N1a+M0
		T4a+N0+M0	T4a+N0+M0
		T4a+N1a+M0	T4a+N1a+M0
IVA		T1+N1b+M0	T1+N1b+M0
	None	T2+N1b+M0	T2+N1b+M0
		T3+N1b+M0	T3+N1b+M0
		T4a+N1b+M0	T4a+N1b+M0
IVB	None	T4b+Any N+M0	T4b+Any N+M0
IVC	None	Any T+Any N+M1	Any T+Any N+M1

TNM staging varies with cell type and age. Undifferentiated (anaplastic) carcinomas are stage IV.
EORTC (72). Age in years +12 if male, +10 if medullary, +10 if poorly differentiated follicular, +45 if anaplastic, +10 if extending beyond thyroid, +15 if one distant metastasis, +30 if multiple distant metastases.
AMES (Age-Metastasis-Extent-Size) (69). High risk is female >50 years of age, male > 40 years, tumor > 5 cm (if older age), distant metastases, substantial extension beyond tumor capsule (follicular) or gland capsule (papillary).
AGES (Age-Grade-Extent-Size) (73). Calculated from 0.5 × age in years (if > 40), +1 (if grade 2), +3 (if grade 3 or 4), +1 (if extra thyroidal), +3 (if distant spread), +0.2× maximum tumor diameter.
MACIS (Metastasis-Age-Completeness of resection, Invasion-Size) (74). MACIS = 3.1 (if ≤ 39 years of age) or 0.08 × age (if ≥ 40 years of age), +0.3 × tumor size (in centimeters), +1 (if incompletely resected), +1 (if locally invasive), +3 (if distant metastases present).
NTCTCS (National Thyroid Cancer Treatment Cooperative Study) (71). Staging variables (part A) not scored quantitatively.
University of Chicago system for papillary carcinoma (47). Staging variables (part A) not scored quantitatively.
The Ohio State system for papillary or follicular carcinoma (13).
Data from American Joint Committee on Cancer. *Manual for staging of carcinoma*, 6th ed. Chicago: Springer-Verlag, 2003.

TABLE 70D.3. OHIO STATE STAGING OF DIFFERENTIATED THYROID CARCINOMA (13)

Variables	Stage 1	Stage 2	Stage 3	Stage 4
Tumor size (cm)	<1.5	1.5–4.4[a] (or)	≥4.5 (or)	Any
Cervical metastases	No	Yes[a]	Any	Any
Multiple thyroidal tumors (>3) any size	No	Yes[a]	Any	Any
Local tumor invasion	No	No	Yes	Any
Distant metastases	No	No	No	Yes
No. of patients (%)	170 (13)	948 (83)	204 (15)	33 (2)
Age (mean yr)	38	34	38	48
p[b]	—	.001	<.05	.01
No. of recurrence n (%)[c]	10 (8)	210 (31)	59 (36)	10 (62)
p[b]	—	.001	.001	NS
No. of deaths from carcinoma (%)[c]	0	34 (6)	19 (14)	17 (65)
p[b]	—	.01	.001	.001

[a]Includes tumors < 1.5 cm with cervical metastases and palpable tumors of uncertain size confined to the thyroid; any tumor that fulfills one of the three criteria for size, cervical metastases, or multiple intrathyroidal tumors is considered stage 2.
[b]Wilcoxon rank-sum test comparing stage with preceding lower stage (left).
[c]30-year recurrence or carcinoma death rate, log rank test comparing stage with preceding lower stage (left).
NS, not significant

TABLE 70D.4. COX REGRESSION MODEL ON CANCER RECURRENCE, DISTANT METASTASIS RECURRENCE, AND DEATH DUE TO THYROID CANCER IN 1,501 PATIENTS WITHOUT DISTANT METASTASES AT THE TIME OF INITIAL THERAPY

Variable	Hazard Ratio	p	95% Confidence Interval
All cancer recurrence			
Age[a]	1.0	.2	0.9–1.3
Local tumor invasion	1.4	.01	1.1–2.2
Lymph node metastases[b]	1.3	.01	1.1–1.6
Follicular histology	0.8	.012	0.7–0.96
Tumor size[c]	1.2	.0001	1.1–1.3
Thyroid remnant ^{131}I ablation[d]	0.8	.016	0.7–0.97
Therapy with [131]I[d]	0.5	.0001	0.4–0.6
Surgery more than lobectomy[e]	0.7	.0001	0.6–0.9
Distant metastasis recurrence			
Age[a]	1.	.0001	1.2–1.5
Follicular histology	1.0	.864	0.8–1.2
Lymph node metastases[c]	1.6	.002	1.2–2.2
Local tumor invasion	1.6	.927	0.9–2.7
Tumor size[d]	1.2	.001	1.1–1.3
Thyroid remnant ^{131}I ablation[e]	0.6	.002	0.5–0.8
Therapy with [131]I[e]	0.4	.0001	0.2–0.6
Surgery more than lobectomy[f]	0.8	.379	0.6–1.2
Cancer mortality			
Age[a]	9.5	.0001	5.3–17.1
Time to treatment[b]	2.4	.0001	1.5–4.0
Follicular histology	1.4	.003	1.1–1.8
Lymph node metastases[c]	2.0	.006	1.2–3.4
Tumor size[d]	1.2	.025	1.02–1.3
Local tumor invasion	1.1	.002	1.0–1.2
Female (vs. male)	0.6	.046	0.4–0.99
Thyroid remnant ^{131}I ablation[e]	0.5	.0001	0.4–0.7
Surgery more than lobectomy[f]	0.5	.0001	0.4–0.7
Therapy with [131]I[e]	0.4	.010	0.2–0.8

[a]Age stratified as less than 40 years versus 40 years and older for cancer mortality, and by decade for recurrences and distant recurrences.
[b]Time to treatment ≤12 months versus >12 months.
[c]Lymph node metastases present versus absent.
[d]Tumor diameter stratified into 1-cm increments from tumors smaller than 1 cm to >5 cm.
[e]Remnant ablation is the use of ^{131}I in patients with uptake only in the thyroid bed and no evidence of residual tumor; therapy with ^{131}I is postoperative treatment of patients with known residual disease.
[f]Bilateral thyroid surgery versus lobectomy with or without isthmusectomy
From Mazzaferri EL, Kloos RT. Current approaches to primary therapy for papillary and follicular thyroid cancer. *J Clin Endocrinol Metab* 2001;86(4):1447–1463, with permission.

node metastases were present, or therapy had been delayed for at least 12 months. It was reduced in women, by surgery more extensive than lobectomy, by ^{131}I remnant ablation, and by ^{131}I and T$_4$ therapy for metastases (Table 70D.4).

The rigid application of staging systems in support of conservative treatment for low-risk patients may lead to inadequate initial therapy. Aggressive disease may occur in patients who appear to be at low risk at the time of diagnosis (13,27). Hundahl et al (1) reported 96% and 68% relative 10-year survival rates for patients categorized as low and high risk, respectively, according to the AMES classification; however, almost two thirds of the cancer deaths in this series occurred in the low-risk group because they outnumbered high-risk patients almost 15:1.

THERAPY

Delay in Therapy

The median time from the first detection of the tumor—nearly always a neck mass—to initial therapy in our patients was 4 months, but ranged from less than 1 month to 20 years (13). Delay in diagnosis correlated with cancer mortality (Fig. 70D.4). The median delay was 18 months in those patients who died of carcinoma compared with 4 months in those still living (*p* < .001). The cancer mortality rate was 4% in patients who underwent initial therapy within a year, as compared with 10% in the others; the 30-year cancer mortality rates in these two groups, respectively, were 6% and 13% (*p* < .001).

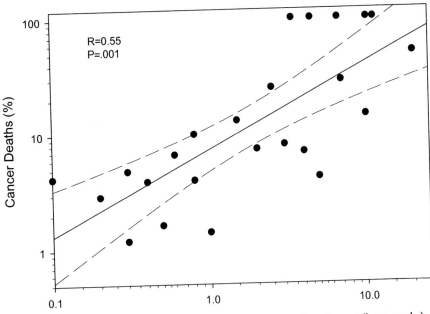

FIGURE 70D.4. Percentage of cancer deaths according to time (on a logarithmic scale) from the first manifestation of the tumor to initial therapy. Each data point represents one to three patients. (Drawn from data in Mazzaferri EL, Kloos RT. Current approaches to primary therapy for papillary and follicular thyroid cancer. *J Clin Endocrinol Metab* 2001;86 (4):1447–1463.)

Extent of Surgery

Clark discusses surgery for thyroid carcinoma in detail in Chapter 80, but it will be briefly summarized here because the extent of surgery has an impact on the subsequent medical therapy. Recurrence rates are high with large thyroid gland remnants. For example, in one study (78) of patients with papillary carcinoma, tumor recurrence rates during the first 2 years after surgery were about fourfold greater after unilateral lobectomy than after total or near-total thyroidectomy (26% vs. 6%, p = .01). In a subsequent report from the same institution, patients with papillary carcinoma whose AGES score was 4 or more had a 25-year cancer mortality rate almost twice as high after lobectomy than after bilateral thyroid resection (65% vs. 35%, p = .06) (79). In a study of AMES low-risk patients from the same institution, 20-year rates for local recurrence and nodal metastases were, respectively, 14% and 19% after unilateral lobectomy, which were significantly higher (p = .001) than the 2% and 6% rates after bilateral lobar resection (80). The researchers concluded that bilateral lobar resection probably represents the preferable initial surgical approach to patients with low-risk papillary thyroid carcinoma (80). In another study of patients with papillary carcinoma (47), near-total thyroidectomy decreased the risk for death from tumors larger than 1 cm and decreased the risk for recurrence as compared with lobectomy or bilateral subtotal thyroidectomy. We found that recurrence and cancer death rates were both about 50% lower after near-total or total thyroidectomy as compared with less surgery in patients with stage 2 and 3 tumors (13) and that surgery more extensive than lobectomy was an independent vari-

able that reduced the likelihood of carcinoma mortality rate by 50% (Table 70D.4). Thus, there is abundant evidence that microscopic residual disease remaining after initial surgery leads to high recurrence and carcinoma mortality rates.

Thyroxine Therapy

Effects of Thyrotropin Suppression on Tumor Growth

The idea that TSH stimulates both the iodine transport and growth of thyroid carcinoma forms the basis for the wide use of T_4 in treating this disease. Like normal thyroid tissue, most papillary and follicular carcinomas contain functional TSH receptors, but whether postoperative T_4 alone improves survival is less certain. There have been no prospective randomized trials of this question, but there is evidence that TSH stimulates tumor growth. Tumors in patients with Graves' disease may be more aggressive, presumably as a result of stimulatory effects of circulating TSH receptor antibodies (64). Rapid tumor growth sometimes follows T_4 withdrawal in preparation for ^{131}I therapy. Moreover, T_4 given as an adjuvant to surgical and ^{131}I therapy is effective. Tumor recurrence rates are higher if T_4 is not given after surgery. After 30 years' follow-up, we found that there were significantly fewer recurrences in patients treated with T_4 as compared with no adjunctive therapy (Fig. 70D.5, p < .01) and there were fewer cancer deaths in the T_4 group (6% vs. 12%, p < .001) (13).

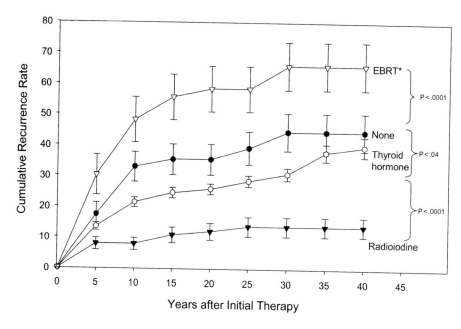

FIGURE 70D.5. Recurrence rates of differentiated thyroid carcinoma in 1,439 patients without distant metastases treated with surgery and no medical therapy (n = 101), or surgery and T$_4$ alone (n = 783), surgery and T$_4$ with ^{131}I (n = 503) for remnant ablation or treatment of metastases, or surgery and external radiation (n = 52). The vertical bars represent standard errors. [Drawn from data in Mazzaferri EL, Kloos RT. Current approaches to primary therapy for papillary and follicular thyroid cancer. *J Clin Endocrinol Metab* 2001;86 (4):1447–1463.)

Potential Adverse Effects of Thyroxine Therapy

Patients with thyroid carcinoma are usually treated with T$_4$ to lower TSH secretion below normal, thereby deliberately causing subclinical if not overt thyrotoxicosis (see Chapter 88). One potential consequence of this is bone mineral loss, even in children (12). It especially contributes to osteoporosis in postmenopausal women with thyroid carcinoma (81–83), which may be prevented by estrogen or antiresorptive therapy. However, using the smallest T$_4$ dose necessary to suppress TSH has no significant effects on bone metabolism and bone mass in men or women with thyroid carcinoma (84).

Cardiovascular abnormalities, well recognized in endogenous subclinical thyrotoxicosis, also occur in patients taking suppressive doses of T$_4$ and may be ameliorated by beta-adrenergic blockade. Subclinical thyrotoxicosis causes an increased risk for atrial fibrillation (85), a higher 24-hour heart rate, more atrial premature contractions, increased cardiac contractility and ventricular hypertrophy, systolic and diastolic dysfunction, and increased cardiovascular mortality (86–89).

Thyroxine Dose

Patients with thyroid carcinoma who have undergone total thyroid ablation require more T$_4$ than those with spontaneously occurring primary hypothyroidism. In one study, the average dosage of T$_4$ that resulted in an undetectable basal serum TSH concentration and no increase in serum TSH after thyrotropin-releasing hormone (TRH) was 2.7 ± 0.4 (SD) µg/kg/day (90). Younger patients needed larger doses than older patients did, and TSH suppression was more likely when the therapy had been prolonged. In a

comparative study of patients with thyroid carcinoma and patients with non-carcinoma-related hypothyroidism, the dose of T$_4$ needed to reduce serum TSH concentrations to normal was 2.11 and 1.62 µg/kg/day, respectively (91). These results suggest that some T$_4$ is secreted from residual thyroid tissue in patients who have spontaneously occurring hypothyroidism.

One study found that a constantly suppressed TSH (≤0.05 µU/mL) was associated with a longer relapse-free survival than when serum TSH levels were always 1 µU/mL or greater, and that the degree of TSH suppression was an independent predictor of recurrence (92). Another large study found that disease stage, patient age, and ^{131}I therapy independently predicted disease progression, but that the degree of TSH suppression did not (93).

As a practical matter, the most appropriate dose of T$_4$ for most patients with thyroid carcinoma reduces the serum TSH concentration to just below the lower limit of the normal range. Some prefer greater suppression, for example, serum TSH concentrations between 0.05 to 0.1 µU/mL in low-risk patients and less than 0.01 µU/mL in high-risk patients (81), and a few advocate the latter target for all patients. However, there is no published evidence that maintaining serum TSH concentrations less than 0.01 µU/mL has benefits, and it does have some risks.

Iodine 131 Therapy
Sodium Iodide Symporter

Therapy with ^{131}I requires optimal uptake of iodine by tumor cells, which is difficult because iodide is concentrated much less avidly by DTC than by normal thyroid tissue. Yet some studies of papillary thyroid carcinoma reported increased sodium iodide symporter (NIS) activity (94), whereas others reported reduced NIS activity and heterogeneous immunohistochemical NIS staining (95). There is a clinical correlation between immunohistochemical NIS staining and the ability of a tumor to concentrate [131]I (96). A more recent study (97) suggests that NIS is absent in about 30% and clearly expressed or even overexpressed in the rest of the thyroid cancer cells, but that malignant transformation often interferes with the proper targeting or retention of NIS to the plasma membrane. An improved response to ^{131}I therapy might result from enhanced NIS expression, function, and targeting to the plasma membrane.

Therapeutic ^{131}I has been used for over 50 years for patients with papillary and follicular thyroid carcinoma, both to ablate any remaining normal thyroid tissue and to treat residual thyroid carcinoma. It has gained wide use in part because it is the most effective systemic therapy, and because recurrence rates are high in patients treated with surgery and T_4 alone. Although eliminating residual normal thyroid tissue greatly simplifies follow-up and facilitates tumor detection, the explicit indications for its use continue to provoke debate (73).

Ablation of Residual Normal Thyroid Tissue

Routine thyroid remnant ablation with ^{131}I, although questioned by some (73), is widely used and has appeal for several reasons. First, it may destroy occult microscopic carcinoma within the thyroid remnant or elsewhere (2,30). Second, it enables later detection of recurrent or persistent disease, particularly in the neck and lung, by imaging studies (63). Third, it greatly facilitates the value of serum thyroglobulin (Tg) measurements during follow-up. Few metastases can be visualized by ^{131}I scanning when appreciable amounts of normal thyroid tissue remain after surgery. Moreover, serum Tg concentration—the most sensitive marker of recurrent or persistent disease—is less reliable with large thyroid remnants (98). Accordingly, ^{131}I is commonly used postoperatively to ablate thyroid gland remnants even in patients without known residual disease who have a very good prognosis (25,99,100). We found tumor recurrences in 7% of patients treated with 29 to 50 mCi (1,073–3,750 MBq) and in 9% after 51 to 200 mCi (1,887–7,400 MBq) [131]I given to ablate thyroid remnants. Both rates were significantly lower than that in patients receiving no ^{131}I ablation (Fig. 70D.6).

Iodine 131 Therapy for Thyroid Remnant Ablation

For many years, remnant ablation was performed with 75 to 150 mCi (2,775–5,550 MBq). However, clinicians began using 25 to 30 mCi (925–1,110 MBq) to avoid hospitalization, which is no longer necessary because of a change in federal regulations that permits the use of much larger ^{131}I doses (in this chapter, the term "dose" is used to describe ^{131}I activity and not the radiation dose expressed in rad) in ambulatory patients. Smaller doses of [131]I (<30 mCi, 1,110 MBq) can ablate thyroid remnants if the amount of thyroid tissue remaining after surgery is small. It has appeal because of the lower cost and the lower whole-body radiation dose. In a randomized prospective study of this question, the first dose ablated thyroid bed uptake in

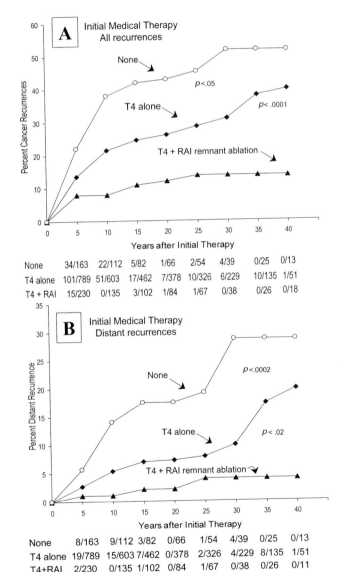

None	34/163	22/112	5/82	1/66	2/54	4/39	0/25	0/13
T4 alone	101/789	51/603	17/462	7/378	10/326	6/229	10/135	1/51
T4 + RAI	15/230	0/135	3/102	1/84	1/67	0/38	0/26	0/18

None	8/163	9/112	3/82	0/66	1/54	4/39	0/25	0/13
T4 alone	19/789	15/603	7/462	0/378	2/326	4/229	8/135	1/51
T4+RAI	2/230	0/135	1/102	0/84	1/67	0/38	0/26	0/11

FIGURE 70D.6. Tumor recurrence (±SEM) 16.7 years (median) after thyroid surgery and ^{131}I ablation of uptake in the thyroid bed compared with those treated with thyroid hormone alone. The numerator is the number of patients with recurrence, and the denominator is the number of patients in each time interval. **A:** All recurrences. **B:** Distant metastasis recurrences. Probability values are from log rank statistical analysis of 40-year life-table data. (From Mazzaferri EL, Kloos RT. Current approaches to primary therapy for papillary and follicular thyroid cancer. *J Clin Endocrinol Metab* 2001;86(4):1447–1463, with permission.)

81% of patients given 30 mCi (225 MBq) and in 84% treated with 100 mCi (3,700 MBq) (101).

Others have found that larger ^{131}I doses are necessary to ablate normal thyroid tissue and to treat residual microscopic carcinoma. Using a dosimetry approach, the ^{131}I must deliver about 30,000 rad (300 Gy) to ablate normal thyroid tissue (102).Using this approach, less than half the patients could be successfully treated with 30 mCi (102). A meta-analysis found a statistically significant advantage for a single high ^{131}I dose (75–100 mCi) over a single low (30–50 mCi) dose such that for every seven patients treated, one more would have successful thyroid ablation given a high rather than a low dose (103). The meta-analysis also found that the size of the thyroid remnant is important. Another study found that an average of 86.8 mCi (3,212 MBq) was more successful in ablating the thyroid remnant after near-total thyroidectomy than less extensive surgery (90% vs. 22%) (102). Stated in different terms, 94% of patients had successful ablation when the surgeon left less than 2 g of thyroid tissue as compared with a 68% success rate when the remnant was larger (102).

Some researchers did not find lower recurrence rates after ^{131}I ablation of the thyroid remnant. At the Mayo Clinic, the recurrence rates were about the same in 220 patients treated with surgery and ^{131}I ablation and 726 patients treated with surgery alone (13.3% vs. 9.6%); 10-year cancer-specific mortality rates were 3% and 2% in the two groups, respectively. These results contrast with those reported by others who found a more favorable effect of ^{131}I ablation. Indeed, ^{131}I remnant ablation conferred a survival benefit even in patients with Hürthle cell carcinoma (25).

Most researchers reported that tumor recurrence rates are lowered with ^{131}I remnant ablation. In one study, postoperative ^{131}I ablation of residual thyroid tissue decreased recurrence rates for tumors larger than 1 cm and reduced the risk for death in patients with stage I or II disease who had tumors larger than 1 cm (47). Among 831 patients with DTC in another series, pulmonary metastases developed in 58; they occurred in 11% after partial thyroidectomy, whereas the rate was reduced by more than half (5%) when subtotal thyroidectomy was supplemented with ^{131}I and was only 1.3% after total thyroidectomy and ^{131}I (38). Among 321 patients treated in 13 Canadian hospitals with ^{131}I mainly to ablate residual normal thyroid tissue in those with microscopic residual papillary or follicular carcinoma, local disease was controlled significantly more often with either postoperative external radiotherapy or ^{131}I therapy, or both together, than with T_4 alone ($p < .001$) (104). Survival at 20 years with microscopic residual disease treated by surgery alone was less favorable (~40%) than after treatment with either ^{131}I or external radiation (~90%, $p < .01$), but ^{131}I treatment of patients without obvious residual disease did not increase survival significantly (104). In a later study from Canada of 382 patients with DTC, initial thyroid ^{131}I ablation after total thyroidectomy was associated

with a significantly lower rate of local relapse that was independent of tumor stage (105). A study from Italy of 48 children who underwent near-total (44 patients) or partial (4 patients) thyroidectomy followed by ^{131}I ablation found only one tumor recurrence during an average follow-up of 5 years (106). Thyroid ^{131}I bed ablation has been shown to confer a survival benefit in patients with Hürthle cell carcinoma (25) and to reduce the tumor recurrence rates in patients with either papillary microcarcinomas or macrocarcinomas (20,107).

We studied 230 patients with no obvious residual disease who were given ^{131}I postoperatively to ablate presumably normal thyroid remnants (2). The 40-year rates of all recurrences and distant recurrences in patients treated with remnant ablation were each less than one-fourth that of patients treated with T_4 alone ($p < 0.0001$) (2) (Fig. 70D.6). The cancer death rate of those treated with T_4 alone was fourfold that of patients treated with ^{131}I ablation. In turn, the distant metastasis rates and cancer death rates were about 150% higher in patients not given T_4 postoperatively than it was in those treated with T_4 (Fig. 70D.6). Thyroid remnant ablation had an independent and favorable prognostic impact on tumor recurrence, distant metastases, and carcinoma deaths (Fig. 70D.6, Table 70D.4).

Patient Preparation

One must closely adhere to a protocol that ensures optimal preparation for ^{131}I scanning and therapy (Fig. 70D.7). To maximize ^{131}I uptake, total body ^{131}I scans are performed 4 to 6 weeks after surgery. At the time of the scan, the serum TSH concentrations should be above 30 µU/mL, and the total body iodine pool should be as low as possible. Urine iodine levels should be obtained if there is any question about iodine contamination from medications or iodinated contrast materials in the previous months leading up to therapy.

Triiodothyronine (T_3) may be given immediately after surgery. In a young adult the dosage is 100 µg/day in divided doses; older patients are given 50 to 75 µg/day. The T_3 is given for 4 weeks, then discontinued for 2 weeks. Other options include withdrawal of T_4 for 4 weeks, or to give no thyroid hormone postoperatively and just measure serum TSH after about 3 to 4 weeks. Serum TSH should increase above 30 µU/mL. Although the protocol that uses T_3 ensures the fewest symptoms, most patients develop overt hypothyroidism during the last week or two if they have undergone complete thyroidectomy. Furthermore, concern over stimulation of tumor growth during these weeks of TSH elevation remains a possibility.

Recombinant Human Thyrotropin

Intramuscular administration of recombinant human thyrotropin (rhTSH) stimulates thyroidal ^{131}I uptake and Tg

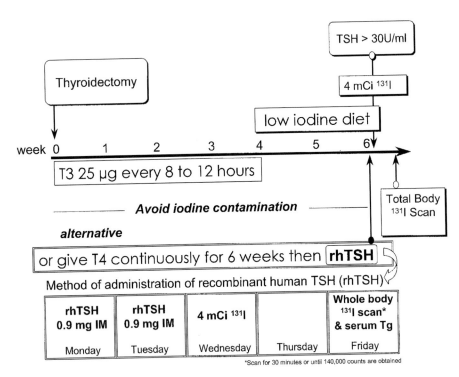

FIGURE 70D.7. Protocol for patient preparation for ^{131}I scan after initial thyroidectomy or at yearly follow-up intervals. Liothyronine (T_3) is given to alleviate symptoms of hypothyroidism. Recombinant human thyrotropin (*rhTSH*) used in preparation for ^{131}I ablation of normal thyroid bed tissue is an off-label use of the drug, but it is as effective as thyroxine (T_4) withdrawal if 100 mCi ^{131}I is used or T_4 is withdrawn for several days before and after treatment with 30 mCi ^{131}I. Another option is to give no thyroid hormone and just measure serum TSH about 3 weeks postoperatively. Serum TSH should increase above 30 μU/mL before the scan is done.

release while the patient continues T_4 therapy, thus avoiding symptomatic hypothyroidism (108). Now approved for diagnostic use, rhTSH has been tested in two large international multicenter studies. The first showed that rhTSH stimulates ^{131}I uptake for diagnostic whole-body scanning (DxWBS), but the sensitivity of scanning after its administration was less than after the T_4 withdrawal (108). A second multicenter international study tested the results of two dosing schedules of rhTSH on the DxWBS images and serum Tg levels compared with those obtained after T_4 withdrawal. The ^{131}I DxWBS method was more carefully standardized in this study than the first one (109). The DxWBS images in the second study were slightly better after T_4 withdrawal than rhTSH stimulation, but the differences were not statistically significant. The combination of DxWBS and serum Tg measurements detected 93% of the patients with tumor or tissue limited to the thyroid bed and detected 100% of those with metastases (109). There were no important differences between the two- and three-dose regimens. For diagnostic studies, 0.9 mg rhTSH is given intramuscularly every day for 2 days followed by a minimum of 4 mCi of ^{131}I on the third day and a DxWBS and Tg measurement on day 5 (Fig. 70D.7). DxWBS ^{131}I images must be acquired after a minimum scan time of 30 minutes or 140,000 counts. A serum Tg of 2 ng/mL or higher 72 hours after the last rhTSH injection indicates that thyroid remnant tissue or carcinoma is present, which may be identified on the rhTSH-stimulated DxWBS (109), especially in high-risk patients (110). The drug is well tolerated. Mild headache and nausea are its main ad-

verse effects, but rhTSH is associated with significantly fewer symptoms and dysphoric mood states than occur with T_4 withdrawal.

Although not yet approved for therapeutic purposes, rhTSH given according to the same protocol used for diagnostic studies has been shown to successfully prepare patients for ^{131}I remnant ablation. Complete ablation, defined as an absence of uptake on a 5 mCi ^{131}I DxWBS image 10 to 14 months after treatment, was achieved in 84.2% of patients prepared with T_4 withdrawal and 86.5% of those given rhTSH, who were treated, respectively, with an average of 126 and 119 mCi of ^{131}I (100). Another study found that 30 mCi ^{131}I given 48 hours instead of 24 hours after the last rhTSH injection failed to ablate the thyroid remnant when rhTSH was given (111). Still another study showed that 30 mCi of ^{131}I was successful when T_4 was stopped the day before the first injection of rhTSH and started again the day after the ^{131}I was administered, which was associated with a decline in urine iodine levels attributed to the approximate 50 μg iodine content in a daily dose of T_4 compared with the 5 μg content of ^{131}I (112).

Low-Iodine Diet

A daily diet of about 50 μg of iodine can increase ^{131}I uptake in normal subjects and can double the rad (Gy) per 100 mCi (3,700 MBq) of ^{131}I administered (113). However, total body radiation after therapeutic ^{131}I may be increased up to 70% as the result of delayed iodine clearance. Although this diet can be tedious for the patient, a daily io-

TABLE 70D.5. LOW-IODINE DIET

Avoid the following foods for 2 weeks prior to your radioactive iodine test and until your thyroid scan and treatment, if needed, are completed:

1. Iodized salt, sea salt
2. Milk or other dairy products, including ice cream, cheese, yogurt, etc.
3. Eggs
4. Seafood, including fish, shellfish, kelp, or seaweed
5. Foods that contain the additives carrageenan, agar-agar, algin, alginate
6. Cured and corned foods (ham, lox, corned beef, sauerkraut)
7. Breads made with iodate dough conditioners
8. Foods and medications containing red food dyes
9. Chocolate
10. Molasses
11. Soy products (soy sauce, soy milk)

Additional guidelines:

Avoid restaurant foods since there is no reasonable way to determine which restaurants use iodized salt.
Foods that contain small amounts of milk or eggs may be used.
Noniodized salt may be used as desired.
Consult your doctor before discontinuing any red-colored medication.

Sample meal patterns:

Breakfast	Lunch	Dinner
Orange juice	Turkey sandwich	London broil
Cream of wheat	Lettuce and tomato	Mushroom sauce
Whole wheat toast	Italian dressing	
Margarine	Fresh apple	Green beans
Coffee	Graham crackers	Cucumber vinaigrette
	Iced tea	Small roll with margarine
		Lemon sherbet
		Iced tea

From Pineda JD, Lee T. Robbins J. Treating metastatic thyroid cancer *Endocrinologist* 1992;6:433–442, with permission.

dine intake of 50 µg can be achieved by restricting the use of iodized salt, dairy products, eggs, and seafood (Table 70D.5). Patients should check the labels of prepared foods for algae derivatives, all breads for iodates, and avoid all red-colored foods and medicines, and should avoid eating in restaurants if possible. The diet is typically started 2 weeks before ^{131}I scanning and continued for several days thereafter. More complex regimens that include diuretics can be used, but are usually unnecessary unless tumor ^{131}I uptake is very low.

Lithium

This drug enhances tumor ^{131}I retention. At pharmacologic levels, it decreases the release of iodine from both the thyroid and tumors (114). Given at a dosage of 400 to 800 mg daily (10 mg/kg) for 7 days, lithium increases uptake in metastatic lesions while only slightly increasing ^{131}I uptake in normal tissue. Serum lithium concentrations should be measured daily and maintained between 0.8 and 1.2 nM. Radiation of tumors with a biologic half-life of iodine of less than 6 days is enhanced without increasing that to other organs. It should be considered when treating patients with metastases, particularly those that concentrate ^{131}I poorly.

Whole-Body Iodine 131 Scans

A DxWBS is only useful when there is little or no remaining normal thyroid tissue. Large amounts of normal thyroid tissue often prevent the TSH from rising above 30 µU/mL, and scanning should be postponed until the remnant is eliminated. DxWBS images are usually obtained 48 hours after the oral administration of 2 to 5 mCi (74 MBq) of [131]I. However, 2 mCi (74 MBq) doses of ^{131}I may fail to show thyroid bed or tumor uptake on the DxWBS, whereas larger doses have a sufficiently harmful effect to interfere with subsequent uptake of therapeutic doses of ^{131}I on the posttreatment whole-body scan (RxWBS), particularly in thyroid remnants and cervical lymph nodes (115). This effect, referred to as "thyroid stunning," occurs with 3 mCi doses and becomes progressively greater with larger ^{131}I doses, but is not produced by [123]I. An increase in serum Tg is observed for about 2 weeks after a scanning dose of ^{131}I, which in one study was associated with more frequent incomplete ablation than that in patients without an increase in serum Tg levels (116). More recent studies, however, suggest that stunning may not impair ^{131}I ablation (115). Moreover, tumors not visualized on the DxWBS, regardless of the scanning ^{131}I dose, not infrequently are visualized on the RxWBS images obtained after large therapeutic ^{131}I doses (2,117). Of perhaps greater importance are more recent studies suggesting that DxWBS is usually not necessary, even before the first postoperative ^{131}I treatment, in low-risk patients who are clinically free of residual tumor (117,118).

False-Positive Iodine 131 Scans

False-positive scans may be due to body secretions, pathologic transudates and inflammation, nonspecific mediastinal uptake, and uptake by thymus or tumors of nonthyroidal origin (118). Misleading scans can be caused by physiologic secretion of ^{131}I from the nasopharynx, salivary and sweat glands, stomach, genitourinary tract, and from skin or hair contamination with urine, sputum, or tears. Pulmonary transudates and inflammation due to cysts, as well as lung lesions caused by fungal and other inflammatory disease, may produce false-positive scans. Diffuse physiologic hepatic ^{131}I uptake is often seen on the RxWBS. The result of ^{131}I-labeled Tg, hepatic uptake in the RxWBS images is related to the ^{131}I dose, ranging from

40% with 30 mCi to 70% with 150 to 200 mCi of [131]I (119). Diffuse hepatic ^{131}I uptake without visible uptake in the thyroid bed usually represents extrahepatic metastases, not occult liver metastases (119).

Tumor Uptake of Iodine 131

The effect of ^{131}I therapy is related to the tumor's capacity to concentrate iodine. Even after meticulous preparation and large ^{131}I doses, many thyroid carcinomas do not concentrate ^{131}I in amounts sufficient for therapy. This is more common after the age of 40 years and in those with Hürthle cell tumors. For example, among 101 patients with distant metastases, 60% of papillary, 64% of follicular, and only 36% of Hürthle cell carcinomas concentrated [131]I (120). More recent series report similarly low ^{131}I uptake in Hürthle cell carcinoma (25). However, DTC lung or bone metastases in younger patients are more likely to trap [131]I (25,55).

Efficacy of Iodine 131 Therapy for Macroscopic Residual or Recurrent Disease

Although some studies find that total thyroidectomy and ^{131}I therapy does not have a favorable effect on outcome (121), long-term studies generally report a beneficial effect of ^{131}I therapy. For example, a long-term study of 1,599 patients with DTC treated between 1948 and 1989, ^{131}I therapy was the single most powerful prognostic indicator for increased disease-free survival (122). Low-risk patients had significantly fewer recurrences and lower death rates after ^{131}I and T_4 therapy than with T_4 alone, whereas ^{131}I therapy conferred only a slight advantage to high-risk patients.

Multivariate analyses show ^{131}I to have an independent prognostic effect when administered either to ablate the thyroid remnant or to treat metastases (2,25,107). In our study, ^{131}I given either to ablate the thyroid bed or to treat metastases each independently lowered the rates of all recurrences, distant recurrence, and cancer deaths (Table 70D.4). In studies with somewhat shorter follow-up than ours, multivariate analyses have shows that ^{131}I therapy lowers death rates in patients with bone (49,54) and lung (123) metastases providing they concentrate ^{131}I, and reduces locoregional recurrences, whether given to treat metastases or to ablate the thyroid remnant (36,105,107).

Therapeutic Iodine 131 Dosimetry

Of the three dosimetry methods available, the most widely used and simplest is to administer an empiric fixed dose. Most clinics use this method regardless of the percentage of

[131]I uptake in the thyroid remnant or metastatic lesion. Hospitalization was required in the past to administer therapeutic doses of ^{131}I larger than 30 mCi (1,110 MBq) in the United States, but is no longer necessary as long as the exposure to the public is calculated to be less than 5.0 mSv (124). From 30 to 100 mCi [131]I (1,110–3,700 MBq) is given to ablate a thyroid remnant (125). Lymph node metastases that are not excised are treated with 100 to 175 mCi (3,700–6,475 MBq). Tumor extending through the thyroid capsule and invading the neck is treated with 150 to 200 mCi (5,550–7,400 MBq), which typically will not induce radiation sickness or produce serious damage to other structures, although sialadenitis and xerostomia are common (126). Diffuse pulmonary metastases that concentrate 50% or more of the test dose of ^{131}I, which is very uncommon (127), are treated with 150 mCi [131]I (5,550 MBq) or less to avoid lung injury that may occur when more than 80 mCi (2,960 MBq) are retained in the whole body 48 hours after the dose. Distant metastases are usually treated with 200 mCi (7,400 MBq) [131]I.

A second approach is to use quantitative dosimetry methods to predict radiation doses to target tissues (e.g., thyroid remnant or metastases) and dose-limiting nontarget tissues (e.g., bone marrow, the lungs in those with diffuse pulmonary metastases, and the whole body). Lesional dosimetry is favored by some because radiation exposure from arbitrarily fixed doses of ^{131}I can vary considerably. If the calculated lesional dose is less than 3,500 rad (35 Gy) when reaching radiation limits in nontarget tissues, it is unlikely that the tumor will respond to ^{131}I therapy (102,124). Conversely, doses that will deliver 30,000 rad (300 Gy) to the thyroid remnant or 8,000 to 12,000 rad (80–120 Gy) to metastatic foci are likely to be effective. To make these calculations it is necessary to estimate tumor size.

In a third approach, which is based on dose-limiting toxicities to nontarget tissues, an upper ^{131}I dose is calculated to deliver a maximum of 200 rad (2 Gy) to the whole blood while keeping the whole body retention less than 120 mCi (4,440 MBq) at 48 hours, or less than 80 mCi (2,960 MBq) when there is diffuse pulmonary uptake. Some limit the maximum administered dose to 300 mCi (1,100 MBq) (128). In a more recent study (129) in which up to 300 rad (3 Gy) was delivered to the bone marrow, all patients developed transient bone marrow suppression that was severe enough in four to require hospitalization. Five patients with lung micrometastases had a Tg level of less than 1 ng/mL after treatment, but whether this could have been achieved with lower ^{131}I doses is uncertain.

Dosimetry is complicated and is performed in a limited number of large medical centers that have a dedicated team of physicists, nuclear medicine technologists, and physicians with thyroid cancer expertise. It is often reserved for patients with distant metastases or unusual circumstances such as concurrent renal failure. Comparison of outcomes between empiric fixed dose methods and dosimetric approaches is difficult and unreliable. Moreover, prospective randomized trials to address the optimal therapeutic approach have not been done (130). Those in favor of high-dose therapy cite the positive relationship between the total ^{131}I uptake per tumor mass and outcome (131), but this has not been confirmed (132,133).

After a therapeutic dose of ^{131}I is administered, oral fluid intake should be large enough to increase urine output and avoid bladder radiation injury. Also, the patient should suck on lemon drops to stimulate salivary flow to minimize the risk for radiation-induced sialadenitis. Constipation should be treated with cathartics to reduce colon and gonadal radiation. Radiation safety procedures must be followed carefully to minimize the risk for exposure to family members and personnel handling these patients. T_4 therapy is resumed 24 hours after ^{131}I therapy. It may take up to 2 months for serum TSH levels to decline to normal or below when T_4 doses of 100 to 200 µg are given, but this may be expedited by giving 300 to 400 µg of T_4 daily or 50 to 100 µg of T_3 daily in divided doses for several days. The use of rhTSH stimulation for imaging or therapy alleviates these untoward effects of iatrogenic hypothyroidism.

Choice of Therapy

An approach used in our clinic and consistent with the guidelines of the National Comprehensive Cancer Network (NCCN) (10), the American Thyroid Association (ATA) (134), the American Association of Clinical Endocrinologists (AACE) (135), and the British Thyroid Association (BTA) (11) is summarized in Table 70.D6. In our practice, patients with tumors of different stages are treated differently after having been fully informed of the potential risks and benefits. Dosimetry is often used in patients with distant metastases.

Stage 1 Tumors

Patients with small tumors [≤1.5 cm (many use a 1.0-cm cutoff)] that are single papillary carcinomas clearly confined to one lobe or follicular tumors with minimal capsular invasion may be adequately treated with lobectomy and T_4 alone (Table 70.D6). When discovered postoperatively after lobectomy, we do not advise ^{131}I therapy for stage 1 tumors because a large thyroid remnant often requires multiple or large doses for ablation and may cause severe radiation thyroiditis (136). Although one study reported minimal morbidity after 30 mCi ^{131}I ablation of lobar remnants in patients with minimally invasive follicular carcinoma (137), this strategy is not widely used. Instead, we

advise completion thyroidectomy and ^{131}I ablation for anyone with a small tumor that is metastatic or that invades the thyroid capsule, or for patients with a history of head and neck radiation or a family history of differentiated thyroid cancer or whose tumor is multifocal or has histology that suggests a more aggressive tumor, such as tall cell papillary carcinoma, tumor necrosis, marked nuclear atypia, or vascular invasion. If none of these features are present, the patient is advised that the only merit for performing completion thyroidectomy and ^{131}I ablation is to facilitate follow-up with sensitive tests, which is not ordinarily possible after subtotal thyroidectomy (138).

However, when the diagnosis of carcinoma is known preoperatively, we advise near-total thyroidectomy because tumor stage is not completely apparent until after the specimen has been studied by the pathologist and ^{131}I scanning has been done. If a small amount (<2 g) of thyroid is detected by thyroid ultrasonography (US) after near-total or completion thyroidectomy, we advise ^{131}I ablation. In this group, we maintain serum TSH in the low-normal range if the Tg level is undetectable during T_4 therapy. If the TSH-stimulated serum Tg is less than 2 ng/mL 1 year later, a second ablation is unlikely to be of further benefit (139,140).

Stage 2 Tumors

For tumors that are 1.5 to 4.4 cm in diameter that are not locally invasive, with or without regional lymph node metastases, we advise total or near-total thyroidectomy with compartmental lymph node dissections for metastases recognized at surgery followed by ^{131}I therapy (Table 70.D6). Small ablative doses of about 30 mCi (1,110 MBq) are used for tumors confined to the thyroid, whereas higher doses are given for the more aggressive tumors. Repeat ^{131}I therapy may be necessary 1 year later if the serum Tg concentration during T_4 withdrawal is greater than 10 ng/mL or Tg is over 2 ng/mL after rhTSH stimulation and resectable disease cannot be identified by neck US. T_4 is given at dosages sufficient to maintain the serum TSH concentrations just below normal for several years. Over the long-term, if rhTSH-stimulated Tg remains undetectable (<1 ng/mL), sufficient T_4 is given to keep serum TSH concentrations in the low-normal range.

Stage 3 Tumors

For tumors that are large (>4.5 cm) or invading local structures, we advise total thyroidectomy and compartmental neck dissection for lymph node metastases recognized at surgery followed by ^{131}I therapy (Table 70.D6). If there is any question that residual tumor remains after surgery, as with microscopic locally invasive tumors, at least 150 mCi

TABLE 70D.6. SUGGESTED TREATMENT OF PAPILLARY AND FOLLICULAR THYROID CARCINOMA

Clinical Stage	Thyroid Surgery	[131]I Dosage (mCi)	T₄ Therapy (Target Serum TSH and Tg Values)
1	Near-total thyroidectomy[a] (preferred if carcinoma identified at or before surgery, follicular thyroid carcinoma, age over 45, men, prior head and neck ERT, family history of thyroid carcinoma)	<30[b] to 100 (preferred)	TSH < 0.5 µU/mL Tg < 1 ng/mL[c]
	Lobectomy or subtotal thyroidectomy[a] (if a single nonmetastatic tumor < 1.5 cm without aggressive histology detected in a resected specimen from a young person; it is not necessary to complete thyroidectomy other than to facilitate follow-up at patient request)	None	TSH < 0.5 µU/mL Tg < 10 ng/mL[d] (after T₄ withdrawal) Tg < 5 ng/mL[d] (after rhTSH)
2	Near-total or total thyroidectomy, compartmental lymph node dissections as needed[e]	100–150	TSH < 0.5 µU/mL Tg < 1 ng/mL[c]
3	Near-total or total thyroidectomy, compartmental lymph node dissections as needed[e]	150–200	TSH < 0.5 µU/mL Tg < 1 ng/mL[c]
4	Near-total or total thyroidectomy, compartmental lymph node dissections as needed[e]	200 or more	TSH < 0.1 µU/mL Tg < 1 ng/mL[c]

Near-total thyroidectomy defined as an attempt to remove all thyroid tissue without damage to recurrent laryngeal nerves or parathyroid tissue, usually leaving portions of the posterior thyroid behind on the contralateral side.
[a]Subtotal thyroidectomy defined as lobectomy plus contralateral subtotal lobectomy.
[b]<30 mCi (1110 MBq) for patients without postoperative residual tumor; consider larger doses for patients with cervical or mediastinal nodes, or incompletely resected tumor. Serum TSH is maintained at low normal values over the long-term if serum Tg is < 1 ng/mL during T₄ suppression of TSH and after TSH stimulation by T₄ withdrawal or rhTSH.
[c]Serum Tg measured during T₄ therapy and after TSH-stimulation (T₄ withdrawal or rhTSH stimulation)
[d]Serum Tg after T₄ withdrawal or rhTSH stimulation. This is an arbitrary estimate not supported by studies.
[e]Central neck dissection (level VI, sparing the parathyroid glands and laryngeal nerves), lateral neck dissection (levels II–V, sparing spinal accessory nerve, internal jugular vein, and sternocleidomastoid muscle).
ERT, external radiation therapy; rhTSH, recombinant human thyrotropin; T₄, thyroxine; Tg, thyroglobulin; TSH, thyrotropin.

(5,550 MBq) [131]I should be given (assuming normal renal function) followed by doses of T₄ sufficient to maintain the serum TSH just below normal. If there is gross local tumor invasion, external beam radiotherapy (EBRT) is recommended in patients over age 45 following ^{131}I therapy. Long-term, serum TSH concentrations are maintained in the low normal range if serum Tg remains below 1 ng/mL on T₄ therapy and after TSH stimulation.

Stage 4 Tumors (Distant Metastases)

Treatment includes total thyroidectomy and compartmental neck dissections as required, followed by [131]I (Table 70D.6). T₄ is given in doses sufficient to maintain the serum TSH below normal, often less than 0.1 µU/mL. Over the long term, however, if serum Tg measured by a sensitive assay is maintained below the detection limit (≤1 ng/mL), and there is no clinical evidence of tumor, serum TSH is kept in the low normal range.

When tumor deposits are unresectable, treatment with ^{131}I is repeated at 6- to 12-month intervals until the tumor no longer concentrates it or there is no benefit from the previous therapy, large cumulative doses are reached, or there are serious adverse effects. We try to wait a full year between treatments and try to keep the cumulative dose under 500 mCi (18,500 MBq) in children and under 700 mCi

(25,900 MBq) in adults. However, there is no specific limit to the cumulative dose that can be administered safely, although the frequency of complications does increase.

Treatment of Patients with Negative Diagnostic Iodine 131 Scans (DxWBS) and High Serum Thyroglobulin Levels

After total thyroidectomy and thyroid remnant ^{131}I ablation, a detectable serum Tg during T₄ suppression of TSH or a Tg level greater than 2 ng/mL after rhTSH stimulation is sometimes associated with negative DxWBS ^{131}I scans. This may be caused by at least five different situations (141): (a) TSH is too low to stimulate tumor ^{131}I uptake; (b) iodine contamination, usually from radiographic contrast material; (c) tumor dedifferentiation with a reduction in or an absence of sodium iodine symporter function; (d) metastases too small to see on the body scans; or (e) heterophile antibody interference with Tg assays (142).

Patients with both negative [131]I DxWBS and neck US often are treated with ^{131}I to locate and treat persistent tumor (143). However, whether this benefits patients has sparked controversy (144–146) because of a lack of randomized prospective studies and the considerable differences in patient cohorts and end points among studies. Nonetheless, there is one consistent observation: serum Tg levels almost invariably decline when ^{131}I uptake is seen on the RxWBS, particularly in patients with lung metastases (144,146). Follow-up is so short in most studies that only a few find enhanced survival after empirically treating a high serum Tg level when the DxWBS is negative. Schlumberger (57) reported complete remission and 10-year survival rates, respectively, of 96% and 100% in 19 patients with tumor found only on a positive RxWBS, compared with 83% and 91% in 55 patients with metastases seen on DxWBS and RxWBS, and 53% and 63% in 64 patients with micronodules seen on chest x-ray, and with 14% and 11% in 77 patients with macronodules seen on chest x-ray.

A more recent study (147) of 56 patients with DTC who were treated with 150 mCi ^{131}I because of an elevated serum Tg level after T_4 withdrawal, despite having a negative 10 mCi [131]I DxWBS, found that half had ^{131}I uptake on the RxWBS and half did not. After a median of 4.2 years (range 0.5–13.5 years) and treatment with a median cumulative ^{131}I dose of 150 mCi (range 50–650 mCi), 64% of the 28 patients with positive RxWBS achieved complete remission (negative RxWBS and undetectable Tg), compared with only 36% of the 28 patients with a negative RxWBS. None of those with a positive RxWBS died of thyroid cancer, whereas 9 without uptake did so, producing 5-year survival rate of 100% in the former and 76% in the latter ($p < .001$).

The best responses to ^{131}I therapy occur in children and younger adults with diffuse pulmonary metastases not seen on any imaging studies except on the RxWBS (117,148). This is not uncommon. One study (149) reported that 15% of 45 children had lung metastases identified by a serum Tg greater than 10 ng/mL. We found that 13% of 89 consecutive paired DxWBS and RxWBS studies in 79 patients (15%) with high serum Tg levels (usually > 15 ng/mL after T_4 withdrawal) and a negative DxWBS had ^{131}I uptake in the lung on the RxWBS (2). Among 23 patients treated with ^{131}I for diffuse pulmonary metastases detected only by ^{131}I imaging, 87% had no lung uptake on subsequent scans (150). After ^{131}I therapy, serum Tg became undetectable and lung computed tomography (CT) scans showed disappearance of the micronodules in almost half the patients, whereas lung biopsy showed no evidence of disease in two. Others also report a substantial decrease in serum Tg levels after ^{131}I treatment of such patients (144). Others report a reduction of metastatic disease in most patients whose lung metastases concentrate ^{131}I, but find that a complete remission is uncommon (56,133). Still, a partial response with reduction of metastatic disease is usually possible, and patients generally have a good quality of life with no further disease progression.

Benefit from ^{131}I therapy is inversely related to tumor mass. When a large tumor is not visualized on a DxWBS, the implication is that its ^{131}I-concentrating ability is low and a poor response to ^{131}I therapy is anticipated. Patients with a high serum Tg and negative DxWBS should not be treated with ^{131}I when (a) there is no ^{131}I uptake on a previous RxWBS, (b) the Tg did not decrease despite optimal conditions of a high serum TSH level without iodine contamination, (c) [18]FDG-PET scanning shows intense uptake in metastases, or (d) anatomic imaging, such as US, shows tumor deposits amenable to surgery.

Treatment of Children and Adolescents

Treatment of children and adolescents is even more controversial than it is in adults because experience is more limited and there are no randomized studies. However, cohort studies provide some guidance about management. Hung and Sarlis (12) conceptually separated young patients with DTC into two groups: children under 10 years of age and teenagers and adolescents between 10 and 18 years of age, because DTC developing in the two groups have different clinical behaviors with regard to recurrence and mortality rates. They made treatment recommendations that were especially pertinent for younger children, because after mid-puberty patients have generally fully matured and their optimal treatment is addressed in the literature on adults with this malignancy (2).

Although younger children commonly present with more advanced clinical disease stage, perhaps due to late diagnosis (2), their prognosis for survival over several decades is usually excellent, even when distant metastases are present (151,152). Overall survival rates at 20 to 30 years in most series published since 1997 are over 95% (12). However, this gives an incomplete picture of the long-term prognosis of children. For example, in a study of 72 children under age 16 years, 42% developed distant metastases, mostly to lung, but 70% had a complete remission; nonetheless, their long-term mortality rate was eightfold that of healthy children (153).

Children under 10 years of age may have an even less favorable outcome. In a long-term study from London, the risk for recurrence in children 10 years of age or younger was almost 3.5-fold that of older children (154). In another study from England and Wales, 5 of 122 children died of DTC within 17 years of diagnosis: 25% of children ages 9 or younger died, compared with three deaths among 28 older children (14). Moreover, persistent disease is common in children, affecting 20% or more of all children with DTC and 50% or more with tumors of advanced stage at the time of diagnosis (133,155). Although lung metastases in children usually concentrate ^{131}I, almost one third (63,133) are not seen on x-ray or DxWBS and may be overlooked unless they are treated with near-total thyroidectomy and ^{131}I remnant ablation followed by Tg measurements and RxWBS scanning.

Surgery is the treatment of choice, but there is no clear consensus concerning the optimal procedure (152,156). Surgical complications occur more frequently in children than in adults, even at large centers (157). Because the risk for cancer death is low in children, the risk for complications thus constitutes the major reservation about performing more extensive surgery.

Strong arguments for an aggressive approach to the treatment of children include the high incidence of primary tumor multicentricity and metastases in children, the high recurrence rate, and the fact that life expectancy exceeds 60 years (12). For the majority of children, total or near-total thyroidectomy is recommended as the standard initial therapy, followed by ^{131}I to destroy the thyroid remnant (12). Because in adults with DTC completion thyroidectomy may result in lower mortality rates (31) and the same may be true for children and adolescents with radiation-induced DTC (63), completion thyroidectomy when less than near-total thyroidectomy has been performed is advised (12). Others propose a similarly aggressive approach to initial therapy (155,158,159). This is especially important for children with multifocal or invasive tumors, cervical lymph node metastases, or very high serum Tg levels after hemithyroidectomy. Although the indications for postoperative ^{131}I are controversial, ^{131}I ablation of the thyroid remnant with 30 mCi (1,110 MBq) (63,160) is safe. TSH should be maintained in the low normal range with T$_4$ therapy.

Persistent tumor not amenable to surgical resection should be treated with ^{131}I in doses adjusted for body surface area or total body weight (12,161). Some routinely treat distant metastases in children with 1 mCi/kg body weight (132), whereas others recommend dosimetry (162). About half the children become free of disease after ^{131}I treatment, usually after one or two additional therapies, although some may require more (12). The use of rhTSH has not been approved in children; if it is administered, however, the dose may be adjusted in proportion to the child's total body weight or body surface area (12).

Posttreatment Iodine 131 Scans

When ^{131}I therapy is given, RxWBS should always be performed to document ^{131}I uptake by the tumor. Up to 25% of RxWBS studies show lesions not detected by the DxWBS (117). Posttreatment ^{131}I scans are likely to yield the most important information when pretreatment scans are negative and serum Tg concentrations are very high.

Acute Complications of Iodine 131 Therapy

Radiation thyroiditis occurs in about 20% of patients, most often in those with large thyroid remnants given doses of ^{131}I that deliver about 50,000 rad (500 Gy) (136),

although this may occur less often when 30 mCi doses of ^{131}I are given (137). It usually appears within the first week after ^{131}I administration and is recognized by neck and ear pain, painful swallowing, thyroid swelling and tenderness, and transient mild thyrotoxicosis. Rarely, the thyroid remnant may swell enough to cause airway obstruction. Mild pain can be treated with analgesics, but severe pain or swelling requires prednisone at a dose of 30 mg daily for several days and then tapered over a week to 10 days.

Painless neck edema within 48 hours after ^{131}I administration is a rare and much different problem than radiation thyroiditis (163). It occurs after high radiation doses, sometimes rather rapidly, and may be accompanied by stridor, regardless of remnant size, and usually responds to corticosteroids.

Radiation sialadenitis involving either the parotid or submandibular glands may occur after ^{131}I therapy in up to 33% of patients, and may be either acute or chronic (126). Acute symptoms may occur within 24 hours and are more likely when large amounts of ^{131}I have been given to a patient with a small thyroid remnant (126). Chewing gum, lemon candies, and hydration may prevent the sialadenitis and xerostomia; however, most patients with sialadenitis experience intermittent painless salivary gland swelling that starts after several months and lasts a few hours, reminiscent of a salivary duct stone. There is a salty taste when the salivary pressure is reduced spontaneously or by manual pressure. Often misdiagnosed as infectious parotitis, it requires no therapy and improves spontaneously within about a year, but it may be associated with a chronic dry mouth or xerostomia (126).

About two thirds of patients given 200 mCi or more develop mild radiation sickness characterized by headache, nausea, and occasional vomiting, which begins about 4 hours after ^{131}I administration and resolves in about 24 hours, but rarely occurs with smaller doses (124). Some patients have transient tongue pain, whereas most have reduced taste for several weeks (126). Ocular dryness, conjunctivitis, and nasolacrimal drainage system obstruction may occur 3 to 16 months after ^{131}I treatment (164).

The most important acute complication is tumor edema or hemorrhage, which may result from ^{131}I effects or TSH stimulation. Serious symptoms can occur rapidly from tumor in a critical location such as the central nervous system, spinal cord, or airway (165). Similarly, pain may occur in bone metastases. Pretreatment with corticosteroids may minimize these hazards, but surgery for spinal lesions and isolated brain metastases should be considered before TSH stimulation or ^{131}I therapy (59). Vocal cord paralysis is reported in patients with a large amount of functioning thyroid tissue in close proximity to the vocal cords (124). Transient peripheral facial nerve palsy also occurs rarely after high-dose ^{131}I therapy (166).

Acute hematologic changes, especially a slight reduction in platelets and white blood cell counts, may follow ^{131}I therapy but are typically transient and asymptomatic (167). Severe pancytopenia can follow very large doses of ^{131}I, which may require transfusions, but this is typically reversible (129,167).

Late Complications of Iodine 131 Therapy

The main long-term complications of ^{131}I are damage to the gonads, bone marrow, and lungs, and the induction of other carcinomas. During the first year after ^{131}I therapy, middle-aged women may developed transient amenorrhea and elevated serum gonadotropin concentrations (168) and women of all ages have a higher than expected rate of spontaneous miscarriage (169), yet there are no measurable effects of ^{131}I on fertility, birth defect, birth weight, and prematurity rates (170). Also, ^{131}I therapy is associated with early menopause (171).

In men, the problem may be more severe (172), with permanent testicular damage or transiently reduced sperm counts roughly proportional to the ^{131}I dose administered (173). In 37% of 103 patients treated with ^{131}I for residual disease, the serum follicle-stimulating hormone (FSH) concentration was almost threefold higher than normal (174). In a longitudinal analysis of 21 men, 6 had no change or only a slight increase in serum FSH after ^{131}I therapy, whereas 11 others had a transient increase above normal 6 to 12 months after treatment. Four men treated with several doses of ^{131}I had a progressive increase in serum FSH, which eventually became permanent. Semen analysis performed in a small subgroup of men showed a consistent reduction in sperm motility. The serum testosterone concentrations in the treated and normal men were similar. A survey of 59 men treated with ^{131}I found they had fathered 106 children, none of whom was reported to have had major malformations (175). In 33 children treated at an average age of 14.6 years with a mean dose of 196 mCi (7,252 MBq) of ^{131}I, the frequency of infertility (12%), miscarriage (1.4%), prematurity (8%), and major congenital anomalies (1.4%) after an average of almost 19 years of follow-up was not significantly different from that in the general population (176). In another study, fertility was normal in 30 patients who were no more than 30 years of age when treated; they had 44 live births (177). Two men who had received a total of 972 and 1,432 mCi (35,964 and 52,984 MBq) between ages 10 and 19 years had fathered two and three children, respectively, up to 13 and 24 years later. Another treated at age 24 with 680 mCi had oligospermia with an elevated serum FSH. Thus, ^{131}I therapy occasionally impairs testicular germinal cell function, posing a significant risk for infertility. Young men should consider banking sperm specimens before therapy, particularly if larger cumulative doses of ^{131}I are to be given (172).

Persistent bone marrow damage and induction of other tumors are the most serious late problems of ^{131}I therapy. Large doses of ^{131}I (usually > 1,000 mCi, 37,000 MBq) can cause a small but significant excess of deaths from bladder carcinoma and leukemia (177). Bladder carcinoma occurs more often in those with relatively little ^{131}I uptake in the neck or metastases. In one report, 80% of 35 patients treated with ^{131}I had bone marrow abnormalities, including three with acute myeloid leukemia (178). Those with pancytopenia had received very high ^{131}I doses, all greater than 1,000 mCi (37,000 MBq) (178). In 13 large series comprising a total of 2,753 patients with thyroid carcinoma, 14 cases of leukemia were detected (179). The resulting prevalence of about five leukemia cases per 1,000 patients (0.5%) is higher than expected in the general population. Acute myeloid leukemia, the type associated with ^{131}I therapy, usually has occurred within 10 years of treatment. Leukemia was less likely when ^{131}I was given annually rather than every few months, and when total blood doses per administration was less than 200 rad (2 Gy). Despite this report, the lifetime risk for leukemia is so small (0.33%) that it does not outweigh the benefit of ^{131}I therapy (180). The absolute risk for life lost because of recurrent thyroid carcinoma exceeds that from leukemia by 4-fold to 40-fold, depending on the age at which the patient is treated (180). When lower total cumulative ^{131}I doses (600–800 mCi, 22,000–29,600 MBq) are given at widely spaced intervals (12 months), long-term effects on the bone marrow are minimal (167), and few cases of leukemia occur. Furthermore, one large population study did not find an increased risk for leukemia in patients with thyroid carcinoma treated with ^{131}I (181).

Pulmonary fibrosis occurs rarely in patients with diffuse pulmonary metastases treated with ^{131}I (182). It can be avoided by using ^{131}I doses that result in a whole body retention of less than 80 mCi 48 hours after its administration when there is diffuse ^{131}I uptake in the lungs seen on the DxWBS, recognizing that retention of greater than 50% at 48 hours is uncommon (127).

Treatment of Persistent Disease Not Amenable to Iodine 131 Therapy

Whenever possible, surgery is the treatment of choice for recurrent or residual tumor. Before other therapies are given, surgical excision or external irradiation should be considered for focal lesions that do not concentrate ^{131}I adequately and isolated skeletal or brain metastases (10). A few patients with tumor that does not concentrate ^{131}I may benefit from 13-cis retinoic acid therapy, which partly redifferentiates follicular thyroid carcinoma *in vitro*. In an early study, when retinoic acid was given orally for at least 2 months to 12 patients with differentiated carcinoma that could not be treated with other modalities, significant ^{131}I uptake was induced in 2 patients, and a faint response was seen in 3 (183). However, subsequent studies have shown the effect is less than previously reported (184).

Octreotide inhibits the growth of DTC *in vitro* (185). Although there are a few examples of patients with DTC who have responded to this therapy (186), it has not been effective in most patients (187). Those with an impending fracture should receive prompt orthopedic stabilization. They also should receive antiresorptive therapy that may improve their quality of life and has induced clinical remission in some patients (188). Patients with pain or symptoms of compression from metastases should be considered for surgery, embolization, EBRT, and ^{131}I (189).

External Beam Radiation Therapy

Selected bone metastases and postoperative macroscopic residual disease that does not concentrate ^{131}I may respond to EBRT (104,105). It improves locoregional control and is particularly effective in the treatment of patients over age 45 years with incompletely resected gross residual cervical tumor (107,190), including tumors that invade the aerodigestive tract, or in the treatment of microscopic perithyroidal tumor that is invading muscle or fat tissues (105). Patients with microscopic residual papillary carcinoma after surgery are more commonly rendered disease free when EBRT is given (90%) than when it is not (26%) (104). This is also true for patients with microscopically invasive follicular carcinoma, more of whom are disease free when postoperative EBRT is given (53%) than when it is not (38%) (104). In another study of patients who had incomplete surgical resection of their tumors, although the irradiated tumors were larger and more extensive than those treated with surgery alone, the 15-year local recurrence rate after EBRT was about half that of patients treated with surgery alone (11% vs. 23%) (191). Two studies found that EBRT had an independent therapeutic effect on the control of locoregional tumor: in one (190) the 5-year control rates were 95% in those treated with EBRT and 68% in those not so treated, and in the other (107) EBRT reduced the risk for locoregional failure to 35% that of patients not so treated. Some have also observed improved survival rates in patients with residual disease treated with EBRT (191).

Although children and young adults may be treated with EBERT if they have macroscopically invasive neck tumor that is unresponsive to other therapy (12), its side effects are significant, and it is generally recommended mainly for those over age 45 years (10). A few children and young adults have been reported to develop neck sarcomas decades after EBRT therapy (192).

Chemotherapy

Experience with chemotherapy in patients with DTC is limited, because most tumors grow slowly and respond well to conventional therapy (e.g., surgery, ^{131}I therapy, or EBRT). Chemotherapy is mainly for tumors that are progressive and have failed conventional therapy. Among 49 patients with metastatic DTC treated with five chemotherapy protocols, only two (3%) patients had objective responses (193). In a review of published series, 38% of patients had a response to doxorubicin defined as a reduction in tumor mass (194). Low-dose doxorubicin has been used with EBRT as a radiation sensitizer, but usually is no better than radiotherapy alone. A recent study found that the combination of carboplatin and epirubicin with TSH stimulation to promote cell proliferation produced temporary complete or partial remission or tumor stabilization in 81% of the patients with advanced DTC, although no long-term cures were achieved and one third of the patients died after a short follow-up time (195). Interested and informed patients should be encouraged to participate in appropriate clinical trials.

FOLLOW-UP

Follow-up can be divided onto three stages: 4 to 6 weeks postoperatively, 6 to 12 months postoperatively, and thereafter annual long-term follow-up (Fig. 70D.8). Until recently, this was usually done with serum Tg determinations and ^{131}I DxWBS imaging. More recently, however, follow-up has become more complex, and substantially more accurate. Older antithyroglobulin antibody (TgAb) assays did not detect low levels of TgAb, which factitiously lower serum Tg results from immunometric assays (IMAs). Also, 3 to 5 mCi ^{131}I DxWBS, CT, and magnetic resonance imaging (MRI), the mainstays of imaging in the past, are far less capable of locating tumor than are newer more sensitive US and Doppler techniques, ^{131}I RxWBS, and ^{18}FDG PET imaging studies. Identifying persistent DTC late in its course was the inevitable consequence of using insensitive tests: long-term studies show that late tumor recurrences, some as long as 45 years after initial treatment, are common (Fig. 70D.1B) (196). Many were probably persistent tumors that had fallen below the detection limits of older tests. Newer follow-up paradigms identify persistent tumor 6 to 18 months after total thyroid ablation, permitting the application of earlier therapy with the hope of improving outcome.

Serum Thyroglobulin

The paradigm for the follow-up of patients who appear to be free of tumor after thyroid ablation has shifted to performing neck US and measuring Tg during TSH suppression and after rhTSH stimulation or T_4 withdrawal, although the latter produces symptomatic hypothyroidism that many patients choose to avoid (109). Accurate serum Tg measurement is the cornerstone of this follow-up paradigm (see Chapter 20). Done accurately, serum Tg and US

A

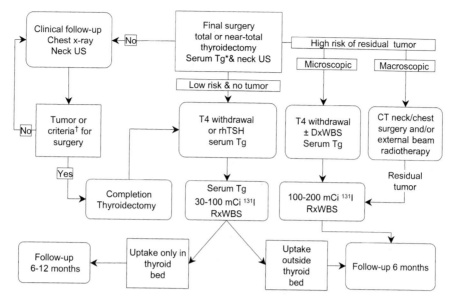

Phase 1
Follow-up 4 to 6 Weeks after Surgery Evaluation for Completeness of Tumor Resection

FIGURE 70D.8. The three phases of follow-up of patients after thyroidectomy for differentiated thyroid carcinoma. **A:** Phase 1: rhTSH is recombinant human thyrotropin (see Fig. 70D.7 and text for dosage schedules). DxWBS is diagnostic ^{131}I whole-body scan, which after withdrawal of thyroid hormone is performed with 2 to 3 mCi [131]I (74–185 MBq) or with 4 mCi of ^{131}I if rhTSH is given for preparation of the scan. Treatment with 30 mCi [131]I (1,110–3,700 MBq), 75 to 100 mCi (2,775–3,700 MBq), or 200 mCi (2,775 MBq) [131]I is given, depending on the clinical situation (see text and Figure 70D.8). *Serum TSH and antithyroglobulin antibody (*TgAb*) levels should be performed any time serum Tg is determined. US is neck ultrasonography. †See text for criteria for completion thyroidectomy. **B:** Phase 2 follow-up. **C:** Phase 3 follow-up. (Reproduced from Mazzaferri EL, et al. A consensus report of the role of serum thyroglobulin as a monitoring method for low-risk patients with papillary thyroid carcinoma. *J Clin Endocrinol Metab* 2003;88(4): 1433–1441, with permission.)

B

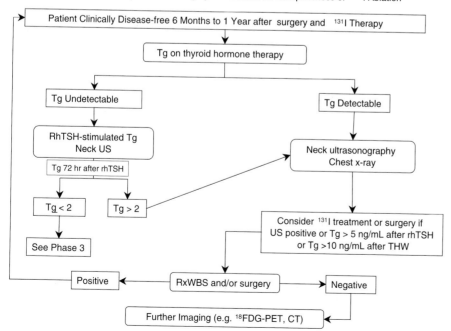

Phase 2
Follow-up 6 to 12 months After surgery - Evaluation for Completeness of [131]I Ablation

FIGURE 70D.8. *Continued*

C

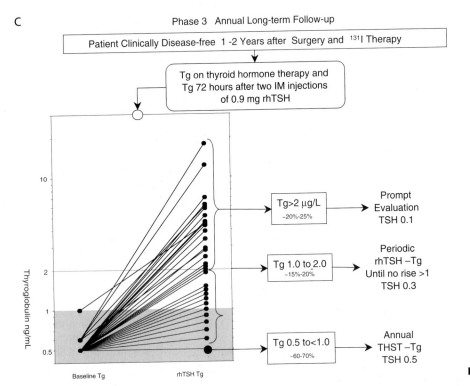

Phase 3   Annual Long-term Follow-up

Patient Clinically Disease-free 1 -2 Years after Surgery and [131]I Therapy

Tg on thyroid hormone therapy and
Tg 72 hours after two IM injections
of 0.9 mg rhTSH

Tg>2 µg/L
~20%-25%

Prompt
Evaluation
TSH 0.1

Tg 1.0 to 2.0
~15%-20%

Periodic
rhTSH –Tg
Until no rise >1
TSH 0.3

Tg 0.5 to<1.0
~60-70%

Annual
THST –Tg
TSH 0.5

Thyroglobulin ng/mL

Baseline Tg   rhTSH Tg

FIGURE 70D.8. *Continued*

identifies almost all patients with residual tumor, thus preventing unnecessary additional testing in those who are cured. However, Tg measurements may be misleading. Tg is now usually measured by IMA, which may be altered by failure to use the CRM-457 international standard, poor assay functional sensitivity, a "hook" effect, or the presence of serum TgAb that falsely lowers Tg results (98), or, conversely, serum heterophile human antianimal antibodies that factitiously increase Tg levels measured in some Tg IMA systems (142). Serial Tg measurements in a patient should be made in the same laboratory using the same assay method (98) because methodologies standardized to CRM-457 may still yield different results, and the trend in Tg levels is often more important than a single Tg measurement (139). Circulating Tg messenger RNA is a potentially more sensitive marker of thyroid tissue or carcinoma than Tg by IMA, particularly during T_4 treatment or with circulating TgAb, but it is not yet ready for clinical use and remains controversial (197).

Measuring serum Tg during T_4 suppression of TSH and performing DxWBS after T_4 withdrawal or rhTSH administration often fail to identify persistent DTC (140,143, 198,199), whereas a TSH-stimulated serum Tg level above 2 µg/L, achieved either after T_4 withdrawal or rhTSH injection, is highly accurate in identifying persistent tumor (139,140,200). For example, eight studies comprising 1,029 patients showed that 21% of 784 patients who had no clinical evidence of tumor with baseline serum Tg levels usually less than 1 ng/mL during T_4 suppression of TSH

had an rhTSH-stimulated serum Tg of greater than 2 ng/mL. When this happened, 36% of the patients were found to have metastases, including 36% to distant sites. A rhTSH-stimulated Tg level of greater than 2 ng/mL identified 91% of the patients with metastases, whereas DxWBS, after either rhTSH or T_4 withdrawal, identified only 19% (200). Ten studies comprising 1,599 patients found that using a TSH-stimulated Tg cutoff of 2 ng/L, either after T_4 withdrawal or 72 hours after rhTSH, is sufficiently sensitive to be used as the principal test in the follow-up of low-risk patients with DTC without routine use of DxWBS (200). Still, some patients with tumor, especially those with lymph node metastases (201,202), may have a false-negative TSH-stimulated serum Tg level, which in almost all reported cases was measured by recovery Tg assays performed on sera with TgAb (139,140, 202,203), a controversial practice (98).

Imaging Studies

Based on these observations, a follow-up guideline is proposed using Tg levels during T_4 suppression and after rhTSH stimulation (200) (Fig. 70D.8). Patients who have no clinical evidence of residual tumor, negative serum TgAb, and a serum Tg of less than 1 µg/L during T_4 suppression of TSH usually do not require DxWBS (139,140, 200). An injection of 0.9 mg rhTSH is given on 2 consecutive days and a serum Tg level is measured 72 hours after the last injection (Fig. 70D.7). If the Tg level increases above 2 ng/mL, then further testing is advised. This can also be done with T_4 withdrawal.

Neck Ultrasonography

Study of the central and lateral cervical compartments by US usually detects malignant lymph nodes and other neck tumors. The classic criterion for differentiating benign from malignant lymph nodes is a size cutoff of about 1 cm, but this misses the majority of tumors. Benign lymph nodes tend to be elongated (oval to fusiform) with a Solbiati index (SI = ratio of largest to smallest diameter) greater than 2 and show a stringlike hyperechoic central structure (hilar sign) with a central hilar-oriented pattern of blood flow on power Doppler (204). Malignant lymph nodes have a rounded or oval appearance with an SI less than or equal to 2 in over 80% of cases and do not have a hilar sign (204). The best indicators of malignancy, however, are a heterogenous echo pattern or irregular hyperechoic small intranodal structures and the presence of irregular diffuse intranodal blood flow on power Doppler (204).

Neck US combined with TSH-stimulated Tg has the highest diagnostic accuracy for detecting persistent cervical tumor. A study of 294 patients with DTC found that three patients with a serum Tg of less than 1 ng/mL had tiny lymph node metastases identified by US (110). The sensitivity and negative predictive values were, respectively, 85% and 98% for Tg alone, 96% and 99.5% for US and rhTSH-stimulated Tg together, and 21% and 99% for rhTSH-stimulated DxWBS alone, and 93% and 99% with rhTSH-stimulated Tg and DxWBS combined.

Another study (140) of 99 patients found that US identified small lymph node metastases missed by all other tests. Six to 12 months after total thyroidectomy and ^{131}I ablation, rhTSH-stimulated DxWBS was negative in all patients with persistent DTC (sensitivity = 0%); however, neck US identified lymph node metastases in 67% with rhTSH-Tg levels of greater than 5 ng/mL, in 13% with Tg levels greater than 1 but less than 5 ng/mL, and in 3% with undetectable Tg levels. The serum Tg was measured by a recovery Tg IMA method, which might account for some of the undetectable serum Tg levels.

A third study (203) of 494 patients with DTC found that 10% had recurrent neck tumor after total thyroidectomy and ^{131}I ablation. After T_4 withdrawal, the sensitivity for detecting neck metastases was 57% for Tg greater than 2 ng/mL (measured by recovery Tg assay), 45% for ^{131}I DxWBS, and 94% for neck US. A fourth study (149) of 45 children treated with total thyroidectomy for papillary carcinoma found that 22 had cervical lymph node metastases. After T_4 withdrawal, the sensitivity for detecting lymph node metastases was 68% for US, 82% for DxWBS and 77% for Tg, but the lower detection limit of the Tg assay was 3 ng/mL, and Tg was measured in sera that tested pos-

itive for TgAb. Still, either Tg or US detected 100% of the lymph node metastases.

Radioiodine (^{131}I and ^{123}I) Scans

Although we prefer ^{131}I DxWBS for patients at high risk for having persistent tumor, other imaging studies may be useful. DxWBS imaging with ^{131}I may pose the problems of stunning and undesirable beta radiation, but also requires a low-iodine diet and TSH stimulation. Although ^{123}I and ^{131}I DxWBS studies are comparable, even after rhTSH stimulation (205), ^{123}I for this use is expensive and has not gained wide use. The main problem with ^{131}I DxWBS is its low sensitivity in detecting residual tumor discussed above. Other scans may be done but also have limitations.

18-Fluorodeoxyglucose Positron Emission Tomography

The most consistent data concerning 18-fluorodeoxyglucose positron emission tomography (^{18}FDG-PET) scanning is that it localizes foci of persistent DTC in patients with elevated serum Tg levels and a negative DxWBS (206). It is thus widely used in follow-up, specifically when the serum Tg is greater than 10 ng/mL in patients with no other clinical evidence of tumor, including both a negative neck US and a 100-mCi RxWBS (206–208). Although ^{18}FDG-PET may not identify miliary lung metastases, it usually makes more sense than performing a CT at this point because ^{18}FDG-PET provides information about both the location (208–211) and prognosis of a tumor (58). Persistent tumor identified as a hot spot on the ^{18}FDG PET scan is typically resistant to ^{131}I therapy but may be amenable to surgery or EBRT (207,212). A large multicenter study (213) found the sensitivity of ^{18}FDG-PET for identifying DTC was 75% in 222 patients and 85% in a subset of 166 patients with a negative DxWBS. Although ^{111}In DTPA-octreotide scintigraphy or conventional radiographic imaging may locate metastatic DTC, both are less sensitive than ^{18}FDG-PET (214). The Centers for Medicare and Medicaid Services recently approved coverage for ^{18}FDG-PET by dedicated full or partial ring scanners in patients who have an elevated or increasing serum Tg of greater than 10 µg/L and negative RxWBS, but not for other indications such as initial staging. Because of their cost, however, dedicated PET systems are not available in all institutions. Coincidence ^{18}FDG imaging with a triple-head scintillation camera does not require a dedicated PET scanner and is much less costly than conventional ^{18}FDG-PET. Its sensitivity was 100% in a retrospective study (215) of 10 patients with serum Tg levels ranging from less than 0.5 to 54.2 µg/L. However, it is likely not as sensitive as a dedicated PET scanner, particularly for tumors smaller than 1.5 cm. TSH stimulates ^{18}FDG uptake by DTC (211), making ^{18}FDG-PET more accurate in DTC after rhTSH

(211) or T$_4$ withdrawal (216) than it is when the TSH is suppressed.

^{99m}Tc-Tetrofosmin, ^{99m}Tc-MIBI, and ^{201}Tl and ^{111}In DTPA-Octreotide Scintigraphy

These isotopes might be considered for localizing tumor in patients with an elevated serum Tg concentration and negative US, ^{131}I RxWBS, and chest CT results, but they are less sensitive than ^{18}FDG-PET or conventional radiographic studies(214).

Computed Tomography and Magnetic Resonance Imaging

Although chest x-rays can be useful for evaluating the response to treatment of macronodular pulmonary metastases, their sensitivity is low, and other imaging studies are generally used for follow-up. CT and MRI scans yield high-resolution cross-sectional images of the thyroid bed and neck and may be particularly helpful in evaluating the extent of local invasion of a tumor prior to surgery (217). CT scanning of the lungs does not require contrast and may reveal micronodular lesions better than MRI. Iodinated radiographic contrast agents are useful for CT of the neck, mediastinum, and abdomen but seriously interfere with ^{131}I uptake for at least 6 to 12 weeks. MRI offers certain advantages because it can be performed in transaxial, coronal, and sagittal planes, and vascular structures are well defined without contrast material. MRI can detect cervical, mediastinal, and hepatic metastases not revealed by CT. Bone metastases usually are detected with ^{131}I scanning or ^{18}FDG-PET, but may be found by ^{99m}Tc-pyrophosphate scan.

Follow-up Paradigm

In our clinic we depend heavily on neck US and a sensitive Tg IMA test with a detection limit of 0.9 ng/mL, which is highly reliable unless TgAb levels are detected in the serum sample.

Phase 1 begins about 4 to 6 weeks after surgery when the completeness of thyroidectomy is evaluated by reviewing the surgery and pathology reports and by performing a serum Tg and neck US examination, which provide guidance for subsequent decisions (Fig. 70.8A). A large (>2 g) thyroid remnant usually requires larger than usual amounts of ^{131}I for ablation. If an entire thyroid lobe is present, completion thyroidectomy should be considered.

Phase 2 begins about 9 to 12 months after surgery when patients are evaluated for completeness of ^{131}I ablation and for residual tumor (Fig. 70.8B). Patients who had no uptake outside the thyroid bed on the phase 1 RxWBS and are now clinically free of disease undergo neck US and serum Tg and TSH measurements. If the serum Tg is undetectable (<1 ng/mL) during thyroid hormone suppres-

sive therapy (THST) and neck US shows no tumor, serum Tg is remeasured under TSH stimulation, usually with rhTSH. If the serum Tg increases by more than 2 ng/mL after rhTSH or more than 10 ng/mL after T$_4$ withdrawal, normal or malignant thyroid tissue is often found (2, 109, 132,218). When malignant lymph nodes are found on US-guided FNA, ipsilateral modified neck dissection is usually performed. If the US result is negative but the Tg is high, we usually give therapeutic ^{131}I—usually 100 mCi (3,700 MBq)—and perform an RxWBS. Up to 15% of such patients have lung metastases (2). Others use different Tg cutoff values and different doses of ^{131}I, but the Tg levels that trigger treatment have been gradually coming down in recent years (117). We continue ^{131}I treatment until the RxWBS is negative. When the serum Tg is undetectable during THST and fails to increase above 2 ng/mL during rhTSH stimulation, patients undergo annual long-term follow-up.

Phase 3 occurs 18 to 24 months after initial therapy (Fig. 70D.8C). In this phase, neck US and serum Tg measurements are made during THST. If the rhTSH-stimulated serum Tg was undetectable in phase 2 and remains so during THST in phase 3, the dose of thyroid hormone is reduced to maintain the serum TSH level around 0.5 ng/mL and patients are seen thereafter at about 12-month intervals. In contrast, if during phase 2 the rhTSH-stimulated serum Tg increased after rhTSH but did not increase above 2 ng/mL and does the same during phase 2, then the TSH is maintained at around 0.3 µU/mL. If rhTSH-stimulated Tg increases above 2 ng/mL, then the phase 2 protocol is followed.

REFERENCES

1. Hundahl SA, Fleming ID, Fremgen AM, et al. A National Cancer Data Base report on 53,856 cases of thyroid carcinoma treated in the US, 1985–1995. *Cancer* 1998;83:2638–2648.
2. Mazzaferri EL, Kloos RT. Current approaches to primary therapy for papillary and follicular thyroid cancer. *J Clin Endocrinol Metab* 2001;86(4):1447–1463.
3. Ries LAG, Eisner MP, Kosary CL, et al. *SEER Cancer Statistics Review, 1973–1997*. Bethesda, MD: National Cancer Institute, 2000.
4. Colonna M, Grosclaude P, Remontet L, et al. Incidence of thyroid cancer in adults recorded by French cancer registries (1978–1997). *Eur J Cancer* 2002;38(13):1762–1768.
5. National Cancer Institute DSRPCSB. Surveillance, Epidemiology, and End Results (SEER) Program, November 2002 (1973–2000). April 1, 2003.
6. Institute of Medicine, Committee on Thyroid Screening Related to, National Research Council (U.S.), Committee on Exposure of the American People to Iodine-131 from Nevada Nuclear-Bomb Tests. *Review of the National Cancer Institute report and public health implications*. Washington, DC: National Academy Press, 1999.
7. National Cancer Institute DSRPCSB. Surveillance, Epidemiology, and End Results (SEER) Program, November 2002 (1973–2000). April 1, 2003.

8. Hundahl SA, Cady B, Cunningham MP, et al. Initial results from a prospective cohort study of 5583 cases of thyroid carcinoma treated in the United States during 1996. U.S. and German Thyroid Cancer Study Group. An American College of Surgeons Commission on Cancer Patient Care Evaluation study. *Cancer* 2000;89(1):202–217.

9. Holzer S, Reiners C, Mann K, et al. Patterns of care for patients with primary differentiated carcinoma of the thyroid gland treated in Germany during 1996. U.S. and German Thyroid Cancer Group. *Cancer* 2000;89(1):192–201.

10. Mazzaferri EL. NCCN thyroid carcinoma practice guidelines. NCCN Proceedings. *Oncology* 1999;13(suppl 11A):391–442. *www.nccn.org/physician_gls/f_guidelines.html.*

11. British Thyroid Association. Guidelines for the Management of Differentiated Thyroid Cancer in adults. *www.british-thyroid-association.org/guidelines.htm,* 2002.

12. Hung W, Sarlis NJ. Current controversies in the management of pediatric patients with well-differentiated non-medullary thyroid cancer: a review. *Thyroid* 2002;12:683–702.

13. Mazzaferri EL, Jhiang SM. Long-term impact of initial surgical and medical therapy on papillary and follicular thyroid cancer. *Am J Med* 1994;97:418–428.

14. Harach HR, Williams ED. Childhood thyroid cancer in England and Wales. *Br J Cancer* 1995;72:777–783.

15. LiVolsi VA. Unusual variants of papillary thyroid carcinoma. In: Mazzaferri EL, Kreisberg RA, Bar RS, eds. *Advances in endocrinology and metabolism.* St. Louis: Mosby-Year Book, 1995:39–54.

16. Burman KD, Ringel MD, Wartofsky L. Unusual types of thyroid neoplasms. *Endocrinol Metabol Clin North Am* 1996;25:49–68.

17. Evans HL. Encapsulated columnar-cell neoplasms of the thyroid—a report of four cases suggesting a favorable prognosis. *Am J Surg Pathol* 1996;20:1205–1211.

18. Rüter A, Dreifus J, Jones M, et al. Overexpression of p53 in tall cell variants of papillary thyroid carcinoma. *Surgery* 1996;120:1046–1050.

19. Nikiforov Y, Gnepp DR. Pediatric thyroid cancer after the Chernobyl disaster: pathomorphologic study of 84 cases (1991–1992) from the Republic of Belarus. *Cancer* 1994;74:748–766.

20. Chow SM, Chan JK, Law SC, et al. Diffuse sclerosing variant of papillary thyroid carcinoma—clinical features and outcome. *Eur J Surg Oncol* 2003;29(5):446–449.

21. Baloch ZW, Gupta PK, Yu GH, et al. Follicular variant of papillary carcinoma—cytologic and histologic correlation. *Am J Clin Pathol* 1999;111:216–222.

22. Zidan J, Karen D, Stein M, et al. Pure versus follicular variant of papillary thyroid carcinoma. *Cancer* 2003;97(5):1181–1185.

23. van Heerden JA, Hay ID, Goellner JR, et al. Follicular thyroid carcinoma with capsular invasion alone: a nonthreatening malignancy. *Surgery* 1992;112:1130–1138.

24. Thompson LD, Wieneke JA, Paal E, et al. A clinicopathologic study of minimally invasive follicular carcinoma of the thyroid gland with a review of the English literature 2. *Cancer* 2001;91(3):505–524.

25. Lopez-Penabad L, Chiu AC, Hoff AO, et al. Prognostic factors in patients with Hurthle cell neoplasms of the thyroid. *Cancer* 2003;97(5):1186–1194.

26. Moosa M, Mazzaferri EL. Occult thyroid carcinoma. *Cancer J* 1997;10:180–188.

27. Baudin E, Travagli JP, Ropers J, et al. Microcarcinoma of the thyroid gland—the Gustave-Roussy Institute experience. *Cancer* 1998;83:553–559.

28. Chow SM, Law SC, Chan JK, et al. Papillary microcarcinoma of the thyroid—prognostic significance of lymph node metastasis and multifocality. *Cancer* 2003;98(1):31–40.

29. Sugg SL, Ezzat S, Rosen IB, et al. Distinct multiple RET/PTC gene rearrangements in multifocal papillary thyroid neoplasia. *J Clin Endocrinol Metab* 1998;83:4116–4122.

30. Pacini F, Elisei R, Capezzone M, et alet al. Contralateral papillary thyroid cancer is frequent at completion thyroidectomy with no difference in low- and high-risk patients. *Thyroid* 2001;11(9):877–881.

31. Scheumann GFW, Seeliger H, Musholt TJ, et al. Completion thyroidectomy in 131 patients with differentiated thyroid carcinoma. *Eur J Surg* 1996;162:677–684.

32. Pasieka JL, Thompson NW, McLeod MK, et al. The incidence of bilateral well-differentiated thyroid cancer found at completion thyroidectomy. *World J Surg* 1992;16:711–716.

33. Furlan JC, Bedard Y, Rosen IB. Biologic basis for the treatment of microscopic, occult well-differentiated thyroid cancer. *Surgery* 2001;130(6):1050–1054.

34. Lupoli G, Vitale G, Caraglia M, et al. Familial papillary thyroid microcarcinoma: a new clinical entity. *Lancet* 1999;353:637–639.

35. Cady B, Hay ID, Shaha AR, et al. Unilateral total lobectomy: is it sufficient surgical treatment for patients with AMES low-risk papillary thyroid carcinoma? Discussion. *Surgery* 1998;124:964–966.

36. Taylor T, Specker B, Robbins J, et al. Outcome after treatment of high-risk papillary and non-Hurthle-cell follicular thyroid carcinoma. *Ann Intern Med* 1998;129:622–627.

37. Mazzaferri EL. Thyroid remnant ^{131}I ablation for papillary and follicular thyroid carcinoma. *Thyroid* 1997;7:265–271.

38. Massin JP, Savoie JC, Garnier H, et al. Pulmonary metastases in differentiated thyroid carcinoma. Study of 58 cases with implications for the primary tumor treatment. *Cancer* 1984;53:982–992.

39. Loh KC, Greenspan FS, Gee L, Miller TR, Yeo PPB. Pathological tumor-node-metastasis (pTNM) staging for papillary and follicular thyroid carcinomas: A retrospective analysis of 700 patients. *J Clin Endocrinol Metab* 1997;82:3553–3562.

40. Gupta S, Patel A, Folstad A, Fenton C, Dinauer CA, Tuttle RM et al. Infiltration of differentiated thyroid carcinoma by proliferating lymphocytes is associated with improved disease-free survival for children and young adults. *J Clin Endocrinol Metab* 2001;86(3):1346–1354.

41. Machens A, Holzhausen HJ, Lautenschlager C, et al. Enhancement of lymph node metastasis and distant metastasis of thyroid carcinoma. *Cancer* 2003;98(4):712–719.

42. Wunderbaldinger P, Harisinghani MG, Hahn PF, et al. Cystic lymph node metastases in papillary thyroid carcinoma. *AJR* 2002;178(3):693–697.

43. Mazzaferri EL. Thyroid carcinoma: papillary and follicular. In: Mazzaferri EL, Samaan N, eds. *Endocrine tumors.* Cambridge, MA: Blackwell Scientific, 1993:278–333.

44. Mirallie E, Visset J, Sagan C, et al. Localization of cervical node metastasis of papillary thyroid carcinoma. *World J Surg* 1999;23(9):970–973.

45. Qubain SW, Nakano S, Baba M, et al. Distribution of lymph node micrometastasis in pN0 well-differentiated thyroid carcinoma. *Surgery* 2002;131(3):249–256.

46. Cady B. Staging in thyroid carcinoma. *Cancer* 1998;83:844–847.

47. DeGroot LJ, Kaplan EL, McCormick M, et al. Natural history, treatment, and course of papillary thyroid carcinoma. *J Clin Endocrinol Metab* 1990;71:414–424.

48. Yamashita H, Noguchi S, Murakami N, et al. Extracapsular invasion of lymph node metastasis is an indicator of distant metastasis and poor prognosis in patients with thyroid papillary carcinoma. *Cancer* 1997;80:2268–2272.

49. Bernier MO, Leenhardt L, Hoang C, et al. Survival and therapeutic modalities in patients with bone metastases of differentiated thyroid carcinomas. *J Clin Endocrinol Metab* 2001;86 (4):1568–1573.

50. Voutilainen PE, Multanen MM, Leppaniemi AK, et al. Prognosis after lymph node recurrence in papillary thyroid carcinoma depends on age. *Thyroid* 2001;11(10):953–957.

51. Sellers M, Beenken S, Blankenship A, et al. Prognostic significance of cervical lymph node metastases in differentiated thyroid cancer. *Am J Surg* 1992;164:578–581.

52. Lindegaard MW, Paus E, Hie J, et al. Thyroglobulin radioimmunoassay and ^{131}I scintigraphy in patients with differentiated thyroid carcinoma. *Acta Chir Scand* 1988;154:141–115.

53. Schlumberger M, Challeton C, De Vathaire F, et al. Treatment of distant metastases of differentiated thyroid carcinoma. *J Endocrinol Invest* 1995;18:170–172.

54. Pittas AG, Adler M, Fazzari M, et al. Bone metastases from thyroid carcinoma: clinical characteristics and prognostic variables in one hundred forty-six patients. *Thyroid* 2000;10(3):261–268.

55. Schlumberger M, Tubiana M, De Vathaire F, et al. Long-term results of treatment of 283 patients with lung and bone metastases from differentiated thyroid carcinoma. *J Clin Endocrinol Metab* 1986;63:960–967.

56. Sisson JC, Giordano TJ, Jamadar DA, et al. 131-I treatment of micronodular pulmonary metastases from papillary thyroid carcinoma. *Cancer* 1996;78:2184–2192.

57. Schlumberger MJ. Diagnostic follow-up of well-differentiated thyroid carcinoma: historical perspective and current status. *J Endocrinol Invest* 1999;22(suppl):3–7.

58. Wang W, Larson SM, Fazzari M, et al. Prognostic value of [18F]fluorodeoxyglucose positron emission tomographic scanning in patients with thyroid cancer. *J Clin Endocrinol Metab* 2000;85(3):1107–1113.

59. Chiu AC, Delpassand ES, Sherman SI. Prognosis and treatment of brain metastases in thyroid carcinoma. *J Clin Endocrinol Metab* 1997;82:3637–3642.

60. Kitamura Y, Shimizu K, Nagahama M, et al. Immediate causes of death in thyroid carcinoma: clinicopathological analysis of 161 fatal cases. *J Clin Endocrinol Metab* 1999;84:4043–4049.

61. Patel SG, Escrig M, Shaha AR, et al. Management of well-differentiated thyroid carcinoma presenting within a thyroglossal duct cyst. *J Surg Oncol* 2002;79(3):134–139.

62. Miccoli P, Pacini F, Basolo S, et al. [Thyroid carcinoma in a thyroglossal duct cyst: tumor resection alone or a total thyroidectomy?]. *Ann Chir* 1998;52(5):452–454.

63. Miccoli P, Antonelli A, Spinelli C, et al. Completion total thyroidectomy in children with thyroid cancer secondary to the Chernobyl accident. *Arch Surg* 1998;133:89–93.

64. Belfiore A, Russo D, Vigneri R, et al. Graves' disease, thyroid nodules and thyroid cancer. *Clin Endocrinol (Oxf)* 2001;55(6):711–718.

65. Ohta K, Pang XP, Berg L, et al. Growth inhibition of new human thyroid carcinoma cell lines by activation of adenylate cyclase through the β-adrenergic receptor. *J Clin Endocrinol Metab* 1997;82:2633–2638.

66. Van De Velde CJH, Hamming JF, Goslings BM, et al. Report of the consensus development conference on the management of differentiated thyroid cancer in the Netherlands. *Eur J Cancer Clin Oncol* 1988;24:287–292.

67. Baldet L, Manderscheid JC, Glinoer D, et al. The management of differentiated thyroid cancer in Europe in 1988. Results of an international survey. *Acta Endocrinol (Copenh)* 1989;120:547–558.

68. Solomon BL, Wartofsky L, Burman KD. Current trends in the management of well differentiated papillary thyroid carcinoma. *J Clin Endocrinol Metab* 1996;81:333–339.

69. Cady B, Sedgwick CE, Meissner WA, et al. Risk factor analysis in differentiated thyroid cancer. *Cancer* 1979;43:810–820.

70. DeGroot LJ, Kaplan EL, Straus FH, et al. Does the method of management of papillary thyroid carcinoma make a difference in outcome? *World J Surg* 1994;18:123–130.

71. Sherman SI, Brierley JD, Sperling M, et al. Prospective multicenter study of thyroid carcinoma treatment—initial analysis of staging and outcome. *Cancer* 1998;83:1012–1021.

72. Byar DP, Green SB, Dor P, et al. A prognostic index for thyroid carcinoma. A study of the E.O.R.T.C. Thyroid Cancer Cooperative Group. *Eur J Cancer* 1979;15:1033–1041.

73. Hay ID. Papillary thyroid carcinoma. *Endocrinol Metab Clin North Am* 1990;19(3):545–576.

74. Hay ID, Bergstralh EJ, Goellner JR, et al. Predicting outcome in papillary thyroid carcinoma: development of a reliable prognostic scoring system in a cohort of 1779 patients surgically treated at one institution during 1940 through 1989. *Surgery* 1993;114:1050–1058.

75. Cady B, Rossi R. An expanded view of risk-group definition in differentiated thyroid carcinoma. *Surgery* 1988;104:947–953.

76. Greene FL, Page DL, Fleming ID, et al. *AJCC cancer staging manual*, 6th ed. Chigago: Springer-Verlag, 2003.

77. American Joint Committee on Cancer. Head and neck tumors. Thyroid gland. In: Beahrs OH, Henson DE, Hutter RVP, eds. *Manual for staging of cancer*. Philadelphia: JB Lippincott, 1992:53–54.

78. McConahey WM, Hay ID, Woolner LB, et al. Papillary thyroid cancer treated at the Mayo Clinic, 1946 through 1970: initial manifestations, pathologic findings, therapy and outcome. *Mayo Clin Proc* 1986;61:978–996.

79. Hay ID, Grant CS, Taylor WF, et al. Ipsilateral lobectomy versus bilateral lobar resection in papillary thyroid carcinoma: a retrospective analysis of surgical outcome using a novel prognostic scoring system. *Surgery* 1987;102:1088–1095.

80. Hay ID, Grant CS, Bergstralh EJ, et al. Unilateral total lobectomy: is it sufficient surgical treatment for patients with AMES low-risk papillary thyroid carcinoma? *Surgery* 1998;124:958–966.

81. Dulgeroff AJ, Hershman JM. Medical therapy for differentiated thyroid carcinoma. *Endocrinol Rev* 1994;15:500–515.

82. Faber J, Galloe AM. Changes in bone mass during prolonged subclinical hyperthyroidism due to L-thyroxine treatment: a meta-analysis. *Acta Endocrinol (Copenh)* 1994;130:350–356.

83. Uzzan B, Campos J, Cucherat M, et al. Effects on bone mass of long term treatment with thyroid hormones: a meta-analysis. *J Clin Endocrinol Metab* 1996;81:4278–4289.

84. Marcocci C, Golia F, Vignali E, et al. Skeletal integrity in men chronically treated with suppressive doses of L-thyroxine. *J Bone Miner Res* 1997;12:72–77.

85. Sawin CT, Geller A, Wolf PA, et al. Low serum thyrotropin concentrations as a risk factor for atrial fibrillation in older persons. *N Engl J Med* 1994;331:1249–1252.

86. Parle JV, Maisonneuve P, Sheppard MC, et al. Prediction of all-cause and cardiovascular mortality in elderly people from one low serum thyrotropin result: a 10-year cohort study. *Lancet* 2001;358(9285):861–865.

87. Biondi B, Fazio S, Carella C, et al. Cardiac effects of long term thyrotropin-suppressive therapy with levothyroxine. *J Clin Endocrinol Metab* 1993;77:334–338.

88. Fazio S, Biondi B, Carella C, et al. Diastolic dysfunction in patients on thyroid-stimulating hormone suppressive therapy with levothyroxine: beneficial effect of β-blockade. *J Clin Endocrinol Metab* 1995;80:2222–2226.

89. Shapiro LE, Sievert R, Ong L, et al. Minimal cardiac effects in asymptomatic athyreotic patients chronically treated with thyrotropin-suppressive doses of L-thyroxine. *J Clin Endocrinol Metab* 1997;82:2592–2595.

90. Bartalena L, Martino E, Pacchiarotti A, et al. Factors affecting suppression of endogenous thyrotropin secretion by thyroxine treatment: retrospective analysis in athyreotic and goitrous patients. *J Clin Endocrinol Metab* 1987;64:849–855.

91. Burmeister LA, Goumaz MO, Mariash CN, et al. Levothyroxine dose requirements for thyrotropin suppression in the treatment of differentiated thyroid cancer. *J Clin Endocrinol Metab* 1992;75:344–350.

92. Pujol P, Daures JP, Nsakala N, et al. Degree of thyrotropin suppression as a prognostic determinant in differentiated thyroid cancer. *J Clin Endocrinol Metab* 1996;81:4318–4323.

93. Cooper DS, Specker B, Ho M, et al. Thyrotropin suppression and disease progression in patients with differentiated thyroid cancer: results from the National Thyroid Cancer Treatment Cooperative Registry. *Thyroid* 1999;8:737–744.

94. Saito T, Endo T, Kawaguchi A, et al. Increased expression of the sodium/iodide symporter in papillary thyroid carcinomas. *J Clin Invest* 1998;101:1296–1300.

95. Jhiang SM, Cho JY, Ryu K-Y, et al. An immunohistochemical study of Na+/I− symporter in human thyroid tissues and salivary gland tissues. *Endocrinology* 1998;139:4416–4419.

96. Caillou B, Troalen F, Baudin E, et al. Na+/I− symporter distribution in human thyroid tissues: an immunohistochemical study. *J Clin Endocrinol Metab* 1998;83(11):4102–4106.

97. Dohan O, Baloch Z, Banrevi Z, et al. Rapid communication: predominant intracellular overexpression of the Na(+)/I(−) symporter (NIS) in a large sampling of thyroid cancer cases. *J Clin Endocrinol Metab* 2001;86(6):2697–2700.

98. Baloch Z, Carayon P, Conte-Devolx B, et al. Laboratory medicine practice guidelines. Laboratory support for the diagnosis and monitoring of thyroid disease. *Thyroid* 2003;13(1):3–126.

99. Koh JM, Kim ES, Ryu JS, et al. Effects of therapeutic doses of ^{131}I in thyroid papillary carcinoma patients with elevated thyroglobulin level and negative ^{131}I whole-body scan: comparative study. *Clin Endocrinol (Oxf)* 2003;58(4):421–427.

100. Robbins RJ, Larson SM, Sinha N, et al. A retrospective review of the effectiveness of recombinant human TSH as a preparation for radioiodine thyroid remnant ablation. *J Nucl Med* 2002;43(11):1482–1488.

101. Johansen K, Woodhouse NJ, Odugbesan O. Comparison of 1073 MBq and 3700 MBq iodine-131 in postoperative ablation of residual thyroid tissue in patients with differentiated thyroid cancer. *J Nucl Med* 1991;32:252–254.

102. Maxon HR, Englaro EE, Thomas SR, et al. Radioiodine-131 therapy for well-differentiated thyroid cancer—a quantitative radiation dosimetric approach: outcome and validation in 85 patients. *J Nucl Med* 1992;33:1132–1136.

103. Doi SA, Woodhouse NJ. Ablation of the thyroid remnant and ^{131}I dose in differentiated thyroid cancer. *Clin Endocrinol (Oxf)* 2000;52(6):765–773.

104. Simpson WJ, Panzarella T, Carruthers JS, et al. Papillary and follicular thyroid cancer: impact of treatment in 1578 patients. *Int J Radiat Oncol Biol Phys* 1988;14:1063–1075.

105. Tsang TW, Brierley JD, Simpson WJ, et al. The effects of surgery, radioiodine, and external radiation therapy on the clinical outcome of patients with differentiated thyroid carcinoma. *Cancer* 1998;82:375–388.

106. Danese D, Gardini A, Farsetti A, et al. Thyroid carcinoma in children and adolescents. *Eur J Pediatr* 1997;156:190–194.

107. Chow SM, Law SC, Mendenhall WM, et al. Papillary thyroid carcinoma: prognostic factors and the role of radioiodine and external radiotherapy. *Int J Radiat Oncol Biol Phys* 2002;52(3):784–795.

108. Ladenson PW, Braverman LE, Mazzaferri EL, et al. Comparison of administration of recombinant human thyrotropin with withdrawal of thyroid hormone for radioactive iodine scanning in patients with thyroid carcinoma. *N Engl J Med* 1997;337:888–896.

109. Haugen BR, Pacini F, Reiners C, et al. A comparison of recombinant human thyrotropin and thyroid hormone withdrawal for the detection of thyroid remnant or cancer. *J Clin Endocrinol Metab* 1999;84:3877–3885.

110. Pacini F, Molinaro E, Castagna MG, et al. Recombinant human thyrotropin-stimulated serum thyroglobulin combined with neck ultrasonography has the highest sensitivity in monitoring differentiated thyroid carcinoma. *J Clin Endocrinol Metab* 2003;88(8):3668–3673.

111. Pacini F, Molinaro E, Castagna MG, et al. Ablation of thyroid residues with 30 mCi (131)I: a comparison in thyroid cancer patients prepared with recombinant human TSH or thyroid hormone withdrawal. *J Clin Endocrinol Metab* 2002;87(9):4063–4068.

112. Barbaro D, Boni G, Meucci G, et al. Radioiodine treatment with 30 mCi after recombinant human thyrotropin stimulation in thyroid cancer: effectiveness for postsurgical remnants ablation and possible role of iodine content in L-thyroxine in the outcome of ablation. *J Clin Endocrinol Metab* 2003;88(9):4110–4115.

113. Maxon HR, Boehringer TA, Drilling J. Low iodine diet in I-131 ablation of thyroid remnants. *Clin Nucl Med* 1983;8:123–126.

114. Koong SS, Reynolds JC, Movius EG, et al. Lithium as a potential adjuvant to ^{131}I therapy of metastatic, well differentiated thyroid carcinoma. *J Clin Endocrinol Metab* 1999;84:912–916.

115. Morris LF, Waxman AD, Braunstein GD. Thyroid stunning. *Thyroid* 2003;13(4):333–340.

116. Muratet JP, Giraud P, Daver A, et al. Predicting the efficacy of first iodine-131 treatment in differentiated thyroid carcinoma. *J Nucl Med* 1997;38:1362–1368.

117. Schlumberger M, Mancusi F, Baudin E, et al. 131-I therapy for elevated thyroglobulin levels. *Thyroid* 1997;7:273–276.

118. Greenler DP, Klein HA. The scope of false-positive iodine-131 images for thyroid carcinoma. *Clin Nucl Med* 1989;14:111–117.

119. Chung JK, Lee YJ, Jeong JM, et al. Clinical significance of hepatic visualization on iodine-131 whole-body scan in patients with thyroid carcinoma. *J Nucl Med* 1997;38:1191–1195.

120. Samaan NA, Schultz PN, Haynie TP, et al. Pulmonary metastasis of differentiated thyroid carcinoma: treatment results in 101 patients. *J Clin Endocrinol Metab* 1985;60:376–380.

121. Hay ID, Thompson GB, Grant CS, et al. Papillary thyroid carcinoma managed at the Mayo Clinic during six decades (1940–1999): temporal trends in initial therapy and long-term outcome in 2444 consecutively treated patients. *World J Surg* 2002;26(8):879–885.

122. Samaan NA, Schultz PN, Hickey RC, et al. Well-differentiated thyroid carcinoma and the results of various modalities of treatment: a retrospective review of 1599 patients. *J Clin Endocrinol Metab* 1992;75:714–720.

123. Schlumberger M, Challeton C, De Vathaire F, et al. Radioactive iodine treatment and external radiotherapy for lung and bone metastases from thyroid carcinoma. *J Nucl Med* 1996;37:598–605.

124. Brierley J, Maxon HR. Radioiodine and external radiation therapy. In: Fagin JA, ed. *Thyroid cancer*. Boston: Kluwer Academic, 1998:285–317.

125. Hodgson DC, Brierley JD, Tsang RW, et al. Prescribing ^{131}iodine based on neck uptake produces effective thyroid ablation and reduced hospital stay. *Radiother Oncol* 1998;47:325–330.

126. Alexander C, Bader JB, Schaefer A, et al. Intermediate and long-term side effects of high-dose radioiodine therapy for thyroid carcinoma. *J Nucl Med* 1998;39:1551–1554.

127. Sisson JC. Practical dosimetry of ^{131}I in patients with thyroid carcinoma. *Cancer Biother Radiopharm* 2002;17(1):101–105.

128. Benua RS, Cicale NR, Sonenberg M, et al. The relation of radioiodine dosimetry to results and complications in the treatment of metastatic thyroid cancer. *AJR* 1962;87:171–178.

129. Dorn R, Kopp J, Vogt H, et al. Dosimetry-guided radioactive iodine treatment in patients with metastatic differentiated thyroid cancer: largest safe dose using a risk-adapted approach. *J Nucl Med* 2003;44(3):451–456.

130. Van Nostrand D, Atkins F, Yeganeh F, et al. Dosimetrically determined doses of radioiodine for the treatment of metastatic thyroid carcinoma. *Thyroid* 2002;12(2):121–134.

131. Maxon HR, Thomas SR, Hertzberg VS, et al. Relation between effective radiation dose and outcome of radioiodine therapy for thyroid cancer. *N Engl J Med* 1983;309:937–941.

132. Schlumberger MJ. Medical progress—papillary and follicular thyroid carcinoma. *N Engl J Med* 1998;338:297–306.

133. Samuel AM, Rajashekharrao B, Shah DH. Pulmonary metastases in children and adolescents with well-differentiated thyroid cancer. *J Nucl Med* 1998;39:1531–1536.

134. Singer PA, Cooper DS, Daniels GH, et al. Treatment guidelines for patients with thyroid nodules and well-differentiated thyroid cancer. *Arch Intern Med* 1996;156:2165–2172.

135. AACE/AAES medical/surgical guidelines for clinical practice: management of thyroid carcinoma. *Endo Pract* 2001;7(3): 202–220.

136. Burmeister LA, duCret RP, Mariash CN. Local reactions to radioiodine in the treatment of thyroid cancer. *Am J Med* 1991; 90:217–222.

137. Randolph GW, Daniels GH. Radioactive iodine lobe ablation as an alternative to completion thyroidectomy for follicular carcinoma of the thyroid. *Thyroid* 2002;12(11):989–996.

138. Van Wyngaarden K, McDougall IR. Is serum thyroglobulin a useful marker for thyroid cancer in patients who have not had ablation of residual thyroid tissue? *Thyroid* 1997;7(3):343–346.

139. Baudin E, Cao CD, Cailleux AF, et al. Positive predictive value of serum thyroglobulin levels, measured during the first year of follow-up after thyroid hormone withdrawal, in thyroid cancer patients. *J Clin Endocrinol Metab* 2003;88(3):1107–1111.

140. Torlontano M, Crocetti U, D'Aloiso L, et al. Serum thyroglobulin and 131I whole body scan after recombinant human TSH stimulation in the follow-up of low-risk patients with differentiated thyroid cancer. *Eur J Endocrinol* 2003;148(1):19–24.

141. Mazzaferri EL. Treating high thyroglobulins with radioiodine. A magic bullet or a shot in the dark? *J Clin Endocrinol Metab* 1995;80:1485–1487.

142. Preissner CM, O'Kane DJ, Singh RJ, et al. Phantoms in the assay tube: heterophile antibody interferences in serum thyroglobulin assays. *J Clin Endocrinol Metab* 2003;88(7):3069–3074.

143. Cailleux AF, Baudin E, Travagli JP, et al. Is diagnostic iodine-131 scanning useful after total thyroid ablation for differentiated thyroid cancer? *J Clin Endocrinol Metab* 2000;85(1):175–178.

144. Pineda JD, Lee T, Ain K, et al. Iodine-131 therapy for thyroid cancer patients with elevated thyroglobulin and negative diagnostic scan. *J Clin Endocrinol Metab* 1995;80:1488–1492.

145. Fatourechi V, Hay ID, Javedan H, et al. Lack of impact of radioiodine therapy in Tg-positive, diagnostic whole-body scan-negative patients with follicular cell-derived thyroid cancer. *J Clin Endocrinol Metab* 2002;87(4):1521–1526.

146. Pacini F, Agate L, Elisei R, et al. Outcome of differentiated thyroid cancer with detectable serum Tg and negative diagnostic 131-I whole body scan: comparison of patients treated with high 131-I activities versus untreated patients. *J Clin Endocrinol Metab* 2001;86(9):4092–4097.

147. Van Tol KM, Jager PL, De Vries EG, et al. Outcome in patients with differentiated thyroid cancer with negative diagnostic whole-body scanning and detectable stimulated thyroglobulin. *Eur J Endocrinol* 2003;148(6):589–596.

148. Casara D, Rubello D, Saladini G, et al. Different features of pulmonary metastases in differentiated thyroid cancer: natural history and multivariate statistical analysis of prognostic variables. *J Nucl Med* 1993;34:1626–1631.

149. Antonelli A, Miccoli P, Fallahi P, et al. Role of neck ultrasonography in the follow-up of children operated on for thyroid papillary cancer. *Thyroid* 2003;13(5):479–484.

150. Schlumberger M, Arcangioli O, Piekarski JD, et al. Detection and treatment of lung metastases of differentiated thyroid carcinoma in patients with normal chest x-rays. *J Nucl Med* 1988; 29:1790–1794.

151. Brink JS, van Heerden JA, McIver B, et al. Papillary thyroid cancer with pulmonary metastases in children: long-term prognosis. *Surgery* 2000;128(6):881–886.

152. Dottorini ME, Vignati A, Mazzucchelli L, et al. Differentiated thyroid carcinoma in children and adolescents: a 37-year experience in 85 patients. *J Nucl Med* 1997;38:669–675.

153. Schlumberger M, De Vathaire F, Travagli JP, et al. Differentiated thyroid carcinoma in childhood: long term follow-up of 72 patients. *J Clin Endocrinol Metab* 1987;65:1088–1094.

154. Landau D, Vini L, A'Hern R, et al. Thyroid cancer in children: the Royal Marsden Hospital experience. *Eur J Cancer [A]* 2000;36(2):214–220.

155. Jarzab B, Handkiewicz JD, Wloch J, et al. Multivariate analysis of prognostic factors for differentiated thyroid carcinoma in children. *Eur J Nucl Med* 2000;27(7):833–841.

156. Zimmerman D, Hay ID, Gough IR, et al. Papillary thyroid carcinoma in children and adults: long- term follow-up of 1039 patients conservatively treated at one institution during three decades. *Surgery* 1988;104:1157–1166.

157. Zimmerman D, Hay I, Bergstralh E. Papillary thyroid carcinoma in children. In: Robbins J, ed. *Treatment of thyroid cancer in childhood.* Proceedings of a workshop held September 10–11, 1992, at the NIH in Bethesda, MD. DOE/EH-0406, Springfield, VA: US Department of Commerce, 1992:3–10.

158. Haveman JW, Van Tol KM, Rouwe CW, et al. Surgical experience in children with differentiated thyroid carcinoma. *Ann Surg Oncol* 2003;10(1):15–20.

159. La Quaglia MP, Black T, Holcomb GW III, et al. Differentiated thyroid cancer: clinical characteristics, treatment, and outcome in patients under 21 years of age who present with distant metastases. A report from the Surgical Discipline Committee of the Children's Cancer Group [in process citation]. *J Pediatr Surg* 2000;35(6):955–959.

160. Stael APM, Plukker JTM, Piers DA, et al. Total thyroidectomy in the treatment of thyroid carcinoma in childhood. *Br J Surg* 1995;82:1083–1085.

161. Reynolds JC. Comparison of I-131 absorbed radiation doses in children and adults: a tool for estimating therapeutic I-131 doses in children. In: Robbins J, ed. *Treatment of thyroid cancer in childhood.* Springfield, VA: US Department of Commerce, Technology Administration, National Technical Information Service, 1994:127–135.

162. Maxon HR. Quantitative radioiodine therapy in the treatment of differentiated thyroid cancer. *Q J Nucl Med* 1999;43(4): 313–323.

163. Goolden AWG, Kam KC, Fitzpatrick ML, et al. Oedema of the neck after ablation of the thyroid with radioactive iodine. *Br J Radiol* 1986;59:583–586.

164. Kloos RT, Duvuuri V, Jhiang SM, et al. Nasolacrimal drainage system obstruction from radioactive iodine therapy for thyroid carcinoma. *J Clin Endocrinol Metab* 2002;87(12):5817–5820.

165. Datz FL. Cerebral edema following iodine-131 therapy for thyroid carcinoma metastatic to the brain. *J Nucl Med* 1986;27: 637–640.

166. Levenson D, Gulec S, Sonenberg M, et al. Peripheral facial nerve palsy after high-dose radioiodine therapy in patients with papillary thyroid carcinoma. *Ann Intern Med* 1994;120:576–578.

167. Van Nostrand D, Neutze J, Atkins F. Side effects of "rational dose" iodine-131 therapy for metastatic well-differentiated thyroid carcinoma. *J Nucl Med* 1986;27:1519–1527.

168. Raymond JP, Izembart M, Marliac V, et al. Temporary ovarian failure in thyroid cancer patients after thyroid remnant ablation with radioactive iodine. *J Clin Endocrinol Metab* 1989;69:186–190.

169. Schlumberger M, De Vathaire F, Ceccarelli C, et al. Exposure to radioactive iodine-131 for scintigraphy or therapy does not preclude pregnancy in thyroid cancer patients. *J Nucl Med* 1996;37:606–612.

170. Dottorini ME, Lomuscio G, Mazzucchelli L, et al. Assessment of female fertility and carcinogenesis after iodine-131 therapy for differentiated thyroid carcinoma. *J Nucl Med* 1995;36:21–27.

171. Ceccarelli C, Bencivelli W, Morciano D, et al. ^{131}I therapy for differentiated thyroid cancer leads to an earlier onset of menopause: results of a retrospective study. *J Clin Endocrinol Metab* 2001;86(8):3512–3515.

172. Mazzaferri EL. Gonadal damage from ^{131}I therapy for thyroid cancer. *Clin Endocrinol (Oxf)* 2002;57(3):313–314.

173. Handelsman DJ, Turtle JR. Testicular damage after radioactive iodine (I-131) therapy for thyroid cancer. *Clin Endocrinol* 1983;18:465–472.

174. Pacini F, Gasperi M, Fugazzola L, et al. Testicular function in patients with differentiated thyroid carcinoma treated with radioiodine. *J Nucl Med* 1994;35:1418–1422.

175. Hyer S, Vini L, O'Connell M, et al. Testicular dose and fertility in men following I(131) therapy for thyroid cancer. *Clin Endocrinol (Oxf)* 2002;56(6):755–758.

176. Sarkar SD, Beierwaltes WH, Gill SP, et al. Subsequent fertility and birth histories of children and adolescents treated with ^{131}I for thyroid cancer. *J Nucl Med* 1976;17:460–464.

177. Edmonds CJ, Smith T. The long-term hazards of the treatment of thyroid cancer with radioiodine. *Br J Radiol* 1986;59:45–51.

178. Gunter HH, Schober O, Schwarzrock R, et al. Hematologic long-term modifications after radio-iodine therapy in carcinoma of the thyroid gland. II. Modifications of the bone marrow including leukemia. *Strahlenther Onkol* 1986;163:475–485.

179. Maxon H III, Smith HS. Radioiodine-131 in the diagnosis and treatment of metastatic well differentiated thyroid cancer. *Endocrinol Metabol Clin North Am* 1990;19:685–718.

180. Wong JB, Kaplan MM, Meyer KB, et al. Ablative radioactive iodine therapy for apparently localized thyroid carcinoma: a decision analytic perspective. *Endocrinol Metabol Clin North Am* 1990;19:741–760.

181. Hall P, Holm L-E. Cancer in iodine-131 exposed patients. *J Endocrinol Invest* 1995;18:147–149.

182. Brown AP, Greening WP, McCready VR, et al. Radioiodine treatment of metastatic thyroid carcinoma: the Royal Marsden Hospital experience. *Br J Radiol* 1984;57:323–327.

183. Grünwald F, Menzel C, Bender H, et al. Redifferentiation therapy-induced radioiodine uptake in thyroid cancer. *J Nucl Med* 1998;39:1903–1906.

184. Gruning T, Tiepolt C, Zophel K, et al. Retinoic acid for redifferentiation of thyroid cancer—does it hold its promise? *Eur J Endocrinol* 2003;148(4):395–402.

185. Hoelting T, Duh QY, Clark OH, et al. Somatostatin analog octreotide inhibits the growth of differentiated thyroid cancer cells *in vitro,* but not *in vivo. J Clin Endocrinol Metab* 1996;81(7):2638–2641.

186. Robbins RJ, Hill RH, Wang W, et al. Inhibition of metabolic activity in papillary thyroid carcinoma by a somatostatin analogue. *Thyroid* 2000;10(2):177–183.

187. Sarlis NJ. Metastatic thyroid cancer unresponsive to conventional therapies: novel management approaches through translational clinical research. *Curr Drug Targets Immune Endocr Metabol Disord* 2001;1(2):103–115.

188. Vitale G, Fonderico F, Martignetti A, et al. Pamidronate improves the quality of life and induces clinical remission of bone metastases in patients with thyroid cancer. *Br J Cancer* 2001;84(12):1586–1590.

189. Eustatia-Rutten CF, Romijn JA, Guijt MJ, et al. Outcome of palliative embolization of bone metastases in differentiated thyroid carcinoma. *J Clin Endocrinol Metab* 2003;88(7):3184–3189.

190. Kim TH, Yang DS, Jung KY, et al. Value of external irradiation for locally advanced papillary thyroid cancer. *Int J Radiat Oncol Biol Phys* 2003;55(4):1006–1012.

191. Tubiana M, Haddad E, Schlumberger M, et al. External radiotherapy in thyroid cancers. *Cancer* 1985;55:2062–2071.

192. Vassilopoulou-Sellin R, Goepfert H, Raney B, et al. Differentiated thyroid cancer in children and adolescents: clinical outcome and mortality after long-term follow-up. *Head Neck* 1998;20(6):549–555.

193. Droz JP, Schlumberger M, Rougier P, et al. Chemotherapy in metastatic nonanaplastic thyroid cancer: experience at the Institut Gustave-Roussy. *Tumori* 1990;76:480–483.

194. Ahuja S, Ernst H. Chemotherapy of thyroid carcinoma. *J Endocrinol Invest* 1987;10:303–310.

195. Santini F, Bottici V, Elisei R, et al. Cytotoxic effects of carboplatinum and epirubicin in the setting of an elevated serum thyrotropin for advanced poorly differentiated thyroid cancer. *J Clin Endocrinol Metab* 2002;87(9):4160–4165.

196. Mazzaferri EL, Kloos RT. Using recombinant human TSH in the management of well-differentiated thyroid cancer: current strategies and future directions. *Thyroid* 2000;10(9):767–778.

197. Ringel M, Ladenson P, Levine MA. Molecular diagnosis of residual and recurrent thyroid cancer by amplification of thyroglobulin messenger ribonucleic acid in peripheral blood. *J Clin Endocrinol Metab* 1998;83:4435–4442.

198. Pacini F, Capezzone M, Elisei R, et al. Diagnostic 131-iodine whole-body scan may be avoided in thyroid cancer patients who have undetectable stimulated serum Tg levels after initial treatment. *J Clin Endocrinol Metab* 2002;87(4):1499–1501.

199. Mazzaferri EL, Kloos RT. Is diagnostic iodine-131 scanning with recombinant human TSH (rhTSH) useful in the follow-up of differentiated thyroid cancer after thyroid ablation? *J Clin Endocrinol Metab* 2002;87:1490–1498.

200. Mazzaferri EL, Robbins RJ, Spencer CA, et al. A consensus report of the role of serum thyroglobulin as a monitoring method for low-risk patients with papillary thyroid carcinoma. *J Clin Endocrinol Metab* 2003;88(4):1433–1441.

201. Bachelot A, Cailleux AF, Klain M, et al. Relationship between tumor burden and serum thyroglobulin level in patients with papillary and follicular thyroid cancer. *Thyroid* 2002;12(8):707–711.

202. Robbins RJ, Chon JT, Fleisher M, et al. Is the serum thyroglobulin response to recombinant human TSH sufficient, by itself, to monitor for residual thyroid carcinoma? *J Clin Endocrinol Metab* 2002;87:3242–3247.

203. Frasoldati A, Pesenti M, Gallo M, et al. Diagnosis of neck recurrences in patients with differentiated thyroid carcinoma. *Cancer* 2003;97(1):90–96.

204. Gorges R, Eising EG, Fotescu D, et al. Diagnostic value of high-resolution B-mode and power-mode sonography in the follow-up of thyroid cancer. *Eur J Ultrasound* 2003;16(3):191–206.

205. Anderson GS, Fish S, Nakhoda K, et al. Comparison of I-123 and I-131 for whole-body imaging after stimulation by recombinant human thyrotropin: a preliminary report. *Clin Nucl Med* 2003;28(2):93–96.

206. Hooft L, Hoekstra OS, Deville W, et al. Diagnostic accuracy of 18F-fluorodeoxyglucose positron emission tomography in the follow-up of papillary or follicular thyroid cancer. *J Clin Endocrinol Metab* 2001;86(8):3779–3786.

207. Alnafisi NS, Driedger AA, Coates G, et al. FDG PET of recurrent or metastatic ^{131}I-negative papillary thyroid carcinoma. *J Nucl Med* 2000;41(6):1010–1015.

208. Chung JK, So Y, Lee JS, et al. Value of FDG PET in papillary thyroid carcinoma with negative ^{131}I whole-body scan. *J Nucl Med* 1999;40:986–992.

209. Wang W, Macapinlac H, Larson SM, et al. [18F]-2-fluoro-2-deoxy-D-glucose positron emission tomography localizes residual thyroid cancer in patients with negative diagnostic (131)I whole body scans and elevated serum thyroglobulin levels. *J Clin Endocrinol Metab* 1999;84(7):2291–2302.

210. Van den Bruel A, Maes A, De Potter T, et al. Clinical relevance of thyroid fluorodeoxyglucose-whole body positron emission tomography incidentaloma. *J Clin Endocrinol Metab* 2002; 87(4):1517–1520.

211. Petrich T, Borner AR, Otto D, et al. Influence of rhTSH on [(18)F]fluorodeoxyglucose uptake by differentiated thyroid carcinoma. *Eur J Nucl Med* 2002;29(5):641–647.

212. Muros MA, Llamas-Elvira JM, Ramirez-Navarro A, et al. Utility of fluorine-18-fluorodeoxyglucose positron emission tomography in differentiated thyroid carcinoma with negative radioiodine scans and elevated serum thyroglobulin levels. *Am J Surg* 2000;179(6):457–461.

213. Grünwald F, Kaelicke T, Feine U, et al. Fluorine-18 fluorodeoxyglucose positron emission tomography in thyroid cancer: results of a multicentre study. *Eur J Nucl Med* 1999;26 (12):1547–1552.

214. Sarlis NJ, Gourgiotis L, Guthrie LC, et al. In-111 DTPA-octreotide scintigraphy for disease detection in metastatic thyroid cancer: comparison with F-18 FDG positron emission tomography and extensive conventional radiographic imaging. *Clin Nucl Med* 2003;28(3):208–217.

215. Gaw-Gonzalo IT, Litti E, Mikotic A, et al. [18F]Fluorodeoxyglucose triple-head coincidence imaging as an adjunct to ^{131}I scanning for follow-up of papillary thyroid carcinoma. *Endo Pract* 2003;9(4):273–279.

216. Moog F, Linke R, Manthey N, et al. Influence of thyroid-stimulating hormone levels on uptake of FDG in recurrent and metastatic differentiated thyroid carcinoma. *J Nucl Med* 2000; 41(12):1989–1995.

217. Burman KD, Anderson JH, Wartofsky L, et al. Management of patients with thyroid carcinoma: application of thallium-201 scintigraphy and magnetic resonance imaging. *J Nucl Med* 1990;31:1958–1964.

218. Spencer CA, Wang CC. Thyroglobulin measurement—techniques, clinical benefits, and pitfalls. *Endocrinol Metabol Clin North Am* 1995;24:841–863.

MEDULLARY THYROID CARCINOMA

ROBERT F. GAGEL
ANA O. HOFF
GILBERT J. COTE

Medullary thyroid carcinoma (MTC) is an uncommon malignant tumor derived from the calcitonin-producing cells (C cells) of the thyroid gland. It is notable for being one of the last forms of thyroid carcinoma to be identified. The first description by Hazard et al in 1959 separated this form of aggressive thyroid carcinoma from other poorly differentiated or anaplastic forms of thyroid carcinoma (1). This description of MTC presaged two periods of intense study over a period of almost a half century that has brought our understanding of the pathogenesis of this unusual thyroid carcinoma to a remarkable level.

The first period, during the 1960s and early 1970s, was initiated by a report from Sipple (2) describing the association of MTC and pheochromocytoma in a single patient and several other examples from the literature, an association we now know as multiple endocrine neoplasia type 2A (MEN2A). Although the thyroid carcinoma was not identified as MTC, others (3–5) quickly pieced together the association of MTC and pheochromocytoma and correctly hypothesized that MTC was derived from the parafollicular or C cells, a cell type that produced the newly discovered peptide, calcitonin (6–8). During the next 3 to 5 years this hypothesis was confirmed by the demonstration that the carcinomas produce calcitonin (9,10) and that measurement of serum calcitonin could be used to diagnose MTC (11).

The second intense period of discovery followed the mapping of the gene for MEN2 and the discovery that mutations of the *RET* protooncogene (12,13), a tyrosine kinase (TK) receptor (14), were present in the germ line of patients with MEN2 and also as somatic mutations in approximately 25% of sporadic MTCs (15). The recognition of *RET* mutations as the major cause of MTC led to the identification of all the major components of the RET receptor system, an understanding of the role of the receptor system in the development of the sympathetic nervous system, and the beginnings of an understanding of how mutations of *RET* cause cell transformation. More importantly, these discoveries created a new paradigm for management of patients with genetic tumor syndromes: identification of gene carriers and removal of the organ containing cells at risk for transformation early in life.

The remainder of this chapter chronicles these events and, more importantly, attempts to place the discoveries into a context of clinical usefulness.

THE THYROIDAL C CELL

C cells are neuroendocrine cells that constitute less than 1% of the cells in the thyroid gland. They are distinct and separable from the more ubiquitous thyroid follicular cells. The precursors of the C cells originate in the neural crest and migrate to the ultimobranchial body, a discrete and separable entity in the neck, where they differentiate into C cells. The ultimobranchial body is the repository of C cells in birds and fish (16,17), whereas in mammals these cells migrate into the thyroid gland during development. There they occupy a characteristic central location at the junction of the upper one third and lower two thirds of each lobe. This developmental pattern explains the characteristic location of hereditary MTC (Fig. 71.1).

C cells are neuroendocrine cells with quasineuronal properties (uptake of biogenic amines and neuronal features when placed in tissue culture) combined with endocrine secretory peptide production analogous to adrenal chromaffin, pancreatic or gastrointestinal neuroendocrine, and certain pituitary cells. C cells secrete calcitonin and other small peptides (somatostatin) directly into blood vessels. In the past, members of this class of neuroendocrine cells were called APUD cells (amine precursor uptake and decarboxylation) (18), but this term has fallen out of favor as the complexity and differences between members of this group of cells have been elucidated.

Unique Features of C Cells

C cells, be they located in the ultimobranchial body (birds and fish) or distributed throughout the thyroid gland (mammals), are characterized by the production of calcitonin. This small 32–amino acid peptide lowers serum calcium concentrations when injected into rodents (6,8). This effect is mediated through binding of calcitonin to a specific calcitonin receptor on osteoclasts (19), causing them to retract and cease bone resorption (20). Recent studies

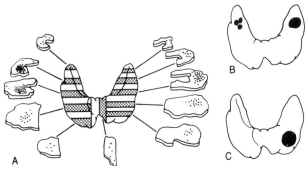

FIGURE 71.1. Distribution of C cells in the thyroid gland. **A:** In the normal human thyroid gland, the concentration of C cells is highest at the junction of the upper one third and lower two thirds of the gland, and this is where most medullary carcinomas of the thyroid (*MCT*) are located. **B:** Hereditary medullary carcinoma is almost always bilateral, although the extent of involvement may be asymmetric. **C:** Sporadic medullary carcinoma is usually unilateral, and may occur anywhere in the thyroid gland. (Adapted from Grauer A, Friedhelm R, Gagel RF. Changing concepts in the management of hereditary and sporadic medullary thyroid carcinoma. *Endocrinol Metab Clin North Am* 1990;19:3, with permission.)

suggest a more complicated role for calcitonin in bone remodeling. Deletion of the calcitonin/calcitonin gene–related peptide (CT/CGRP) gene in mice leads to a higher bone mass (21), as does deletion of the calcitonin receptor (22). Thus, disruption of the calcitonin signaling pathway leads to increased bone formation, suggesting that calcitonin may inhibit bone formation. The major physiologic effects of calcitonin appear to be short-term inhibition of bone resorption, perhaps to protect against hypercalcemia, and a more subtle and potentially more important long-term effect to regulate bone formation.

Although calcitonin is produced in multiple neuroendocrine cell types in mammals [neuroendocrine cells in the adrenal, pancreas, lung, prostate, and other tissues, and in any cell type during sepsis (23,24)], under normal physiologic conditions the C cells of the thyroid are the predominant source. Removal of the thyroid gland in mammals lowers serum calcitonin concentrations to nearly undetectable levels. Non–C cell production of calcitonin during infection or inflammation may explain the persistent elevations of serum calcitonin concentrations after thyroidectomy in some patients with MTC (25).

The CT/CGRP gene (*CALCA*) contains 6 exons (Fig. 71.2). Alternative RNA processing of the primary transcript by inclusion of exons 1 through 4 with polyadenylation following exon 4 produces a messenger RNA (mRNA) that encodes the precursor for calcitonin; processing the same transcript to exclude exon 4 produces an mRNA that encodes the precursor for CGRP. The splice signals surrounding exon 4 are weak, particularly an atypical pyrimidine branch point instead of the usual adenine, making inclusion of exon 4 in the final transcript an unfavored event. This suggests that exon 4 exclusion is the default pathway.

Therefore, the inclusion of this exon to produce calcitonin requires a mechanism that enhances recognition of the splicing and polyadenylation sequences and is ubiquitous. Selective interaction of transacting factors with repeating sequences within exon 4 by a *tra*-like protein and Srp55 (26) increases recognition of the splice site, whereas a large complex of factors bound to a novel intronic sequence downstream of the exon 4 polyadenylation signal increases polyadenylation and simultaneously inhibits splicing to the CGRP exon (27,28). This ultimately leads to selective inclusion of exon 4 in C cells and production of calcitonin. The mechanisms involved in the production of CGRP are less well studied, but are thought to involve the disruption of enhancer complexes (28,29). In MTC there is disordered splicing that causes production of a higher percentage of CGRP; at present there is no evidence that the disordered splicing plays a pathogenic role in transformation of the C cells.

Calcitonin gene expression is increased by activators of protein kinase A (30), protein kinase C (31), and mitogen-activated protein (MAP) kinases (32). It is inhibited by 1,25-dihydroxyvitamin D, retinoic acid analogues, nerve growth factor, and 5-hydroxytryptamine agonists (33–37). Glucocorticoids have complex effects on transcription (38–40). Tissue-specific expression of the calcitonin gene is regulated by two widely separated enhancer regions. The first (distal enhancer) is located 1000 nucleotides (41,42), and the second (proximal enhancer) approximately 250 nucleotides (30) upstream of the transcription start site. The distal enhancer is composed of three functional CANNTG or E-box motifs that bind helix-loop-helix (HLH) transcription factors (41). Members of the USF-1 and USF-2 HLH family of proteins, in combination with other undefined proteins, constitute the major transcription complex regulating the distal enhancer and likely confer tissue specificity (43). The proximal site contains cyclic adenosine monophosphate (cyclic AMP) response elements (CREs) and an overlapping octamer homeodomain-like binding site (CREL/O). These sequences mediate the cyclic AMP/protein kinase A responsiveness of cells (30). MAP kinase activation of CT/CGRP gene transcription is mediated through a Ras interacting site near the CRE that binds a novel and as yet unidentified zinc-fingered protein (32). The active metabolite of vitamin D, 1,25-dihydroxyvitamin D, inhibits transcription of the calcitonin gene by interfering with the interaction between the transcription complexes that occupy the upstream and downstream enhancers (34).

Calcitonin secretion is regulated primarily by the extracellular calcium concentration. An increase in serum calcium concentration above normal activates the calcium-sensing receptor (CaSR) (44,45), a G protein–coupled receptor that facilitates increased calcitonin secretion. Binding of calcitonin to its receptor on the osteoclast inhibits bone resorption (46). The resulting reduction in serum calcium concentration leads to lowered calcitonin secretion. Other stimuli that increase calcitonin secretion

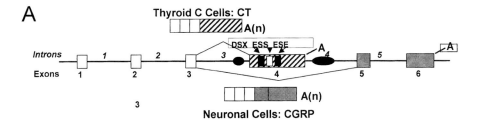

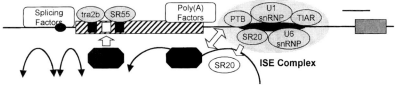

FIGURE 71.2. Alternative splicing of the calcitonin/CGRP (*CALCA*) gene. **A:** Transcripts derived from the six-exon *CALCA* gene are alternatively spliced to produce messenger RNAs (mRNAs) encoding either calcitonin (CT) or calcitonin gene-related peptide (CGRP). In thyroid C cells, CT is produced by RNA splicing that includes exon 4; in neuronal cells, CGRP is produced by skipping this exon. Studies of the rat and human genes have identified five key sequences that are involved in recognition of exon 4. These sequences include a pyrimidine branch point, which creates a "weak" 3' splice site, a double-sex repeat element (DSX), an exonic splicing silencer (ESS), an exonic splicing enhancer (ESE), and an intronic splicing enhancer (ISE). **B:** The production of calcitonin mRNA requires facilitated recognition of exon 4. The binding of tra2b to the DSX and SRp55 to the ESE is thought to facilitate recognition of the 3' splice site by splicing factors. The downstream ISE element forms a large complex that binds several factors. The binding of polypyrimidine-binding protein (PTB), SR20, and U1 snRNP is thought to stimulate polyadenylation, whereas binding of U6 snRNP and TIAR is thought to inhibit recognition of the exon 5 splice site. The production of CGRP requires the blocking or disruption of enhancer complexes. A brain-specific candidate splicing repressor (CSR) has been demonstrated to bind the ESS sequence and to prevent the binding of tra2b and SRp55, as discussed in the text. In addition, formation of the ISE complex is disrupted in neural cells due to the presence of a neural-specific PTB (nPTB) and reduced levels of SR20. In the absence of facilitated recognition, exon 4 skipping is thought to be the default pathway.

include supraphysiologic concentrations of glucagons, 5-hydroxytryptamine receptor agonists, gastrin (and pentagastrin), alcohol, and exercise (47–51). A detailed discussion of these stimuli has been published (52).

The recognition that more than 90% of calcitonin is derived from the thyroid (except during periods of inflammation or sepsis) and that serum calcitonin concentrations are high in patients with MTC has made it a useful tumor marker. The sensitivity of calcitonin measurements as an indicator of MTC was further increased by measurements after administration of calcium (11) or pentagastrin (49), and, at a time when serum calcitonin assays lacked sensitivity, these stimulation tests formed the basis for early identification of tumor in patients with hereditary MTC. Serum calcitonin measurements are used less frequently for early diagnosis of MTC today, largely replaced by genetic tests for diagnosis of hereditary MTC, although some have recommended that serum calcitonin be measured in all patients with thyroid nodules (see below and Chapter 73).

Serum calcitonin measurements are also used to follow patients with residual or metastatic MTC. Measurements over extended periods of time are useful for quantitation of tumor mass; there is an almost direct correlation between serum calcitonin concentrations and tumor volume (Fig. 71.3). There are several points to keep in mind regarding serum calcitonin measurements. The first is that in normal subjects (or patients with some normal thyroid tissue) calcitonin secretion may be episodic; it also may be affected by the ambient serum calcium concentration, exercise, eating (gastrin stimulation), or other poorly defined stimuli. Serum calcitonin concentrations may vary by two- or threefold, and therefore direct comparison of any two serum calcitonin measurements provides little useful information. A second consideration, although infrequent, is that more aggressive and dedifferentiated MTCs may lose the ability to transcribe the CT/CGRP gene, and therefore a decreasing serum calcitonin concentration value may be an indicator of a poor prognosis (53). Another pragmatic

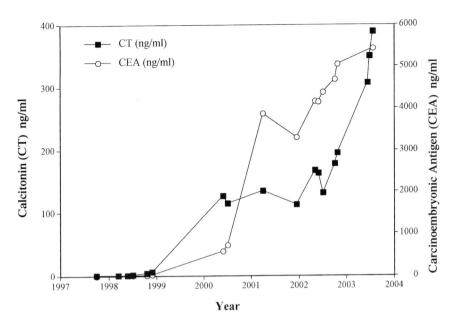

FIGURE 71.3. Measurements of serum calcitonin (CT) and carcinoembryonic antigen (CEA) in a patient with progressive medullary thyroid carcinoma (MTC) showing a progressive increase in serum calcitonin and carcinoembryonic antigen concentrations. Note the point-to-point variability in the values, although the trend over the 6 years of observation is clear. The patient died from hepatic failure caused by metastatic MTC shortly after the last measurements.

observation: patients with MTC who have serum calcitonin concentrations greater than 5,000 pg/mL (normal 2–30 pg/mL in most assays) after total thyroidectomy and lymph node dissection usually have metastatic disease outside the neck. In such patients, neck tumors can usually be detected by ultrasonography, and mediastinal, pulmonary, and abdominal disease by computed tomography. In patients in whom these radiographic studies are negative, the most likely site of metastasis is the liver, in which microscopic metastases are difficult to detect.

Carcinoembryonic antigen (CEA) is another useful tumor marker for monitoring the growth of MTC (54,55) (Fig. 71.3). There is less day-to-day variation in serum CEA concentrations than in serum calcitonin concentrations. However, CEA is made throughout the gastrointestinal tract and in the liver, and may be secreted in excess in cigarette smokers and in patients with other tumors, making it an insensitive and inaccurate marker for detection of early MTC.

Other substances produced by normal C cells that may be produced in excess by MTC include somatostatin, histaminase, and chromogranin A (56–58), but none are specific for MTC. Other substances produced by occasional MTCs are propopiomelanocortin (POMC), vasoactive intestinal peptide (VIP), neurotensin, and bombesin (59–61). Approximately 5% of patients with the ectopic corticotropin (ACTH) syndrome have MTC (62).

HISTOLOGIC FEATURES OF MEDULLARY THYROID CARCINOMA

Medullary thyroid carcinoma develops as a firm, white, almost chalky tumor within the thyroid gland. The transformed C cells are usually polyhedral or polygonal in shape and may be arranged in a variety of patterns (1,63) (see Chapter 21). Amyloid, dispersed between pockets of tumor cells, is commonly seen in slowly growing tumors (64), whereas cellular components predominate in more rapidly growing tumors. Tumor calcification is common and may be detected by x-ray.

The derivation of MTC from C cells provides its most characteristic feature, the presence of calcitonin, which can be detected by immunohistochemical staining (65). The combination of amyloid and immunohistochemical staining for calcitonin are the most characteristic features of MTC. Rare, poorly differentiated MTCs lose the ability to produce calcitonin, a finding that generally indicates a poor prognosis. Other tumors that produce calcitonin and should be considered in the differential diagnosis in a patient found to have a high serum calcitonin concentration include breast, prostate, and small cell lung carcinomas and other neuroendocrine tumors, including pheochromocytomas, islet cell carcinomas, and carcinoid tumors (65). The diagnosis of MTC can be made easily by fine-needle aspiration biopsy, based on immunohistochemical staining for calcitonin and the presence of amyloid (66).

CLINICAL PRESENTATION OF MEDULLARY THYROID CARCINOMA

The most common presentation of MTC is as a single or multiple thyroid nodules, with or without palpable lymph nodes. This tumor may also present in the context of a known kindred with hereditary MTC. In most such patients, early screening by genetic testing will result in a thyroidectomy before the presence of any detectable disease. Rare patients with hereditary MTC may present with clinical features of a pheochromocytoma (MEN2A or MEN2B), Hirschsprung's disease with intestinal obstruction or pseudoobstruction (MEN2A or MEN2B), or hyperparathyroidism (MEN2A). A few patients, generally with widespread disease and hepatic metastases, may present with diarrhea (67–69). Perhaps the most unusual example was a patient with breast cancer who had a high serum CEA concentration for years, and was presumed to have metastatic breast cancer, who then presented with diarrhea and was belatedly discovered to have MTC (70).

CLINICAL SYNDROMES ASSOCIATED WITH MEDULLARY THYROID CARCINOMA

Sporadic Medullary Carcinoma

Sporadic MTC is the most common form of this tumor. It arises, *de novo*, as a result of a somatic mutation of the *RET* protooncogene in a single C cell or by other undefined mechanisms. Sporadic MTC is most commonly unicentric, but a small percentage are multicentric. Six percent to 10% of patients with apparently sporadic MTC are subsequently found to have a germline *RET* mutation indicative of hereditary disease (discussed in detail below) (15).

Most patients with sporadic MTC present with a thyroid nodule. MTCs have no distinguishing ultrasound features, and they do not concentrate iodide, and therefore they are hypofunctioning on ^{131}I, ^{123}I, or $^{99m}TcO_4$ imaging. The diagnosis is most commonly made by fine-needle aspiration biopsy and confirmed by measurement of serum calcitonin. The cytologic diagnosis of MTC may be difficult. MTCs are rare and may be diagnosed as a parathyroid tumor, poorly differentiated carcinoma of unknown etiology, or rarely anaplastic carcinoma. Any biopsy that reveals cells that are not obviously of thyroid follicular origin should be immunostained for calcitonin, CEA, or chromogranin A.

At the time of diagnosis, 80% of patients with an MTC greater than 1 cm in diameter have lymph node metastases (71–73). Lymph node metastases are often not apparent to the surgeon, and may be missed by the pathologist unless each node removed is carefully examined. The most common pattern of metastasis is to ipsilateral lymph nodes in levels II through VI (see Chapter 17); metastases to contralateral nodes occur in approximately 40% of patients in whom the primary MTC is palpable (71,72). Another common pattern of metastasis is to mediastinal lymph nodes. Hepatic and pulmonary parenchymal metastases are commonly vascular. Clinicians should be aware that even experienced radiologists often report a small focus of hepatic metastasis, as defined by contrast-enhanced computed tomography, as a hemangioma. Another pattern of metastasis is miliary spread to the liver. This pattern is difficult to identify by any currently available imaging technique; it is usually identified by laparoscopic biopsy (74). Bone metastases are most commonly lytic; spinal metastases are uncommon, but of particular concern because of the potential for neurologic deficit.

Hereditary Medullary Carcinoma

Sipple's description in 1961 provided the first compilation of the association between thyroid carcinoma and pheochromocytoma (now known as MEN2A) (2,75). The subsequent separation of MEN1 from MEN2 (76) and the separation of MEN2A and MEN2B (77–81) provided further clarification of the distinctions between these clinical syndromes. The addition of several variants: familial MTC (without other manifestations of MEN2A) (82), MEN2A with Hirschsprung's disease (83), and MEN2A with cutaneous lichen amyloidosis (84,85) have added further complexity to the classification system. The discovery of *RET* mutations and insight gained from the correlation of clinical phenotype with specific molecular changes has led to the current classification system (86) (Table 71.1).

Multiple Endocrine Neoplasia Type 2A

The association of MTC, pheochromocytoma, and hyperparathyroidism is classified as MEN2A (Table 71.1). The complete syndrome develops most often in the third and fourth decades of life. It is characterized by bilateral and multicentric MTC in more than 90% of gene carriers, unilateral or bilateral multicentric pheochromocytomas in approximately 50%, and hyperparathyroidism in 5% to 10%. MTC is nearly always the first manifestation of the syndrome. Before this syndrome was recognized, death was as likely to be sudden, caused by a pheochromocytoma, as by metastatic thyroid carcinoma.

The recognition of the clinical syndrome and its genetic nature has led to its earlier recognition in affected families. It is transmitted as an autosomal-dominant trait. The fact that both MTC and pheochromocytoma may occur late in the second decade or later ensured transmittal of this gene to the next generation and the existence of multigenerational kindreds; death from either MTC or pheochromo-

TABLE 71.1. HEREDITARY MEDULLARY THYROID CARCINOMA

Multiple endocrine neoplasia type 2 (MEN2)
Multiple endocrine neoplasia type 2A (MEN2A or Sipple's
  syndrome)
  Medullary thyroid carcinoma
  Pheochromocytoma
  Parathyroid neoplasia
Variants of MEN2A
  Familial medullary thyroid carcinoma (FMTC)
  MEN2A with cutaneous lichen amyloidosis (MEN2A/CLA)
  MEN2A with Hirschsprung's disease
Multiple endocrine neoplasia type 2B
  Medullary thyroid carcinoma
  Pheochromocytoma
  Absence of parathyroid disease
  Marfanoid habitus and tall stature
  Intestinal ganglioneuromatosis

cytoma most commonly occurred in the mid-fifties. Because the average life expectancy at the beginning of the twentieth century was 50 to 55 years, it is not surprising that the hereditary nature of this syndrome escaped detection then.

After or concurrent with Sipple's description in 1961, there followed the discovery of calcitonin (6,8), followed by recognition that it is produced by the parafollicular cells of the thyroid, that MTC is composed of transformed C cells (87), and that calcium and peptides such as glucagon and gastrin (or pentagastrin) stimulate release of calcitonin from C cells (49,88–90). These observations led to the use of calcium or pentagastrin in conjunction with measurements of serum calcitonin to define the spectrum of C-cell abnormalities in MTC.

The Natural History of Medullary Carcinoma in Multiple Endocrine Neoplasia Type 2A

The earliest histologic abnormality in thyroid glands removed from children and young adults with MEN2A is one or more foci of C-cell hyperplasia (91) (Fig. 71.4). These foci become nodular, so named because the growing mass of C cells appears to displace a thyroid follicle, creating the appearance of a nodule (65), then appear as microscopic MTC, and finally as a visible focus of MTC. Although the progression time is unclear, foci of microscopic

MTC have been observed in children as young as 3 years of age, implying progression from normal to carcinoma in a period of less than 4 years. The variability of the latent period for development of MTC (4–50 years) suggests that the presence of a mutant *RET* TK receptor is necessary but not sufficient for transformation.

When metastasis occurs in the evolution of MEN2A is not known. The youngest reported patient with metastatic disease to local lymph nodes was a 6-year-old child (92, 93), and unpublished reports describe metastatic MTC in 3-year-old children. Also unknown is when metastases progress beyond local lymph nodes, but it is known that metastases may be confined to local lymph nodes. Reports from the early 1970s and more recently described MEN2A patients with MTC and local lymph node metastases who underwent extensive lymph node dissection and remained free of disease for up to 30 years thereafter (73,94–98). These results provide a compelling argument for a thorough lymph node dissection at the time of initial surgery.

Pheochromocytoma in Multiple Endocrine Neoplasia Type 2A

Approximately one half of patients with MEN2A develop clinical evidence of a pheochromocytoma. These tumors evolve from adrenal medullary hyperplasia and may be

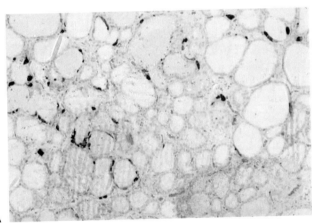

A

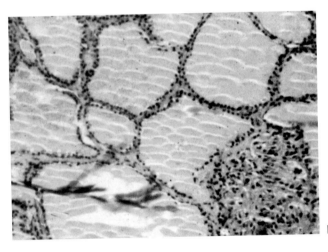

B

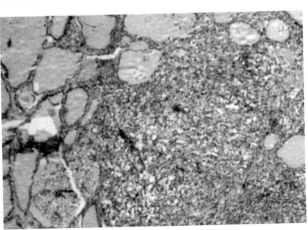

C

FIGURE 71.4. Progression of transformation in hereditary medullary thyroid carcinoma. **A:** A histologic section from a 3-year-old child with a germ line codon 634 mutation. The C cells were immunostained for calcitonin. The section shows a slight increase in number of C cells, which are clustered around the thyroid follicles. **B:** Nodular C-cell hyperplasia. In this section the C cells displace the thyroid follicle, creating the appearance of a nodule. **C:** A microscopic focus of medullary thyroid carcinoma, which obliterates the thyroid follicles.

multicentric. A detailed discussion of pheochromocytoma in MEN2 is beyond the scope of this chapter, and the reader is referred to other reviews (99–102). Several points are of relevance to the management of patients with MEN2A in this context. First, all patients should be screened for pheochromocytoma before undergoing thyroid surgery. Measurements of plasma or urinary metanephrines and catecholamines are sufficient for screening purposes. More often the question of pheochromocytoma is raised in the context of a planned thyroid surgical procedure, when the patient or surgeon opposes delay. In this situation, demonstration of normal adrenal glands by computed tomography will suffice, because in 99% of patients with MEN2A who have a pheochromocytoma the tumor is intraadrenal (the remainder are intraabdominal). If a pheochromocytoma is identified, the thyroid surgical procedure should be deferred until the pheochromocytoma is removed. The absence of hypertension does not exclude a MEN2-related pheochromocytoma. Unlike the clinical picture in sporadic pheochromocytoma or other hereditary pheochromocytoma syndromes (von Hippel-Lindau disease or hereditary paraganglioma), the disproportionate production of epinephrine associated with MEN2-related pheochromocytomas is more likely to cause palpitations than hypertension (Fig. 71.5).

Primary hyperparathyroidism is an uncommon manifestation of MEN2A, occurring in 5% to 10% of patients. Serum calcium should be measured preoperatively in patients with MTC, and the possibility of MEN2 should be considered in all patients with primary hyperparathyroidism.

Variants of Multiple Endocrine Neoplasia Type 2A

In addition to classic MEN2A, there are three distinct variants of MEN2A (Table 71.1). The first, familial MTC (82), is characterized by the presence of MTC without other manifestations of MEN2A. The reports describing this variant have usually encompassed three or four generations with 20 to 30 affected members with no evidence of pheochromocytoma or hyperparathyroidism. In these families, MTC tends to develop later and be less aggressive, as compared with MEN2A families. Before categorizing a particular kindred as having familial MTC, it is important to consider the fact that the penetrance of pheochromocytoma in MEN2A is only 50%. In a small kindred with predominantly young members, in whom pheochromocytomas may not have yet developed, miscategorization is possible. The important point is that screening for pheochromocytoma should continue in affected members unless there is multigenerational experience to exclude this possibility.

MEN2A with Hirschsprung's disease is also an uncommon variant in which affected family members develop Hirschsprung's disease (83,103). The penetrance varies considerably; in some large kindreds a high percentage have the disease, whereas in other equally large kindreds only one or two family members are affected (15,104).

The association of a cutaneous form of lichen amyloidosis with MEN2A is the most recently discovered variant (84,85). In a few kindreds, estimated to be fewer than 25 worldwide, affected people have pruritic papular lesions superimposed on a well-demarcated plaque, invariably over the upper back. The rash may be unilateral or bilateral, and may extend from C6 to approximately T5. Current evidence suggests that the rash results from continuous scratching and irritation of the skin, a condition analogous to "friction" amyloidosis, and is caused by deposition of amyloid in the skin (105,106). In some kindreds, the presence of localized pruritus is a phenotypic indicator of MEN2A (85).

Multiple Endocrine Neoplasia Type 2B

The association of MTC, pheochromocytoma, and ganglioneuromatosis has been classified as MEN2B. Williams and Pollock (107) were the first to piece together the components of this syndrome, although earlier reports exist. It is transmitted as an autosomal-dominant trait (78,108,109), although most identified cases represent *de novo* mutations (110). The presence of mucosal neuromas on the distal tongue, conjunctiva, and throughout the gastrointestinal tract give this clinical syndrome its most distinctive feature. Hyperparathyroidism is almost never found (111), but unilateral or bilateral pheochromocytomas occur in approximately half of affected patients.

This syndrome is most commonly identified in childhood as a result of gastrointestinal manifestations that may include colic, abdominal cramping, intestinal obstruction (pseudo or real), or diarrhea. These symptoms are most commonly related to intestinal dysfunction caused by neurologic dysfunction of the gastrointestinal tract (Hirschsprung-like) or intermittent physical obstruction caused by neuromas (80). Marfan-like features include long, thin arms and legs, a reduced upper/lower body ratio, pectus excavatum, and slipped femoral capital epiphyses (78). The lens and aortic manifestations of Marfan's syndrome are never seen. Approximately 5% of patients have a more subtle form of the disorder, with normal stature or barely detectable neuromas, making clinical diagnosis challenging.

MTC in patients with MEN2B is bilateral and multicentric, metastasizes early, and is usually more aggressive than in MEN2A (112,113). Metastasis to local lymph nodes during the first few years of life is common. Despite the high level of aggressiveness, there is considerable variability in outcome. Death from metastatic MTC most commonly occurs during the second or third decade, but some patients with metastatic disease have survived for long periods (109,114).

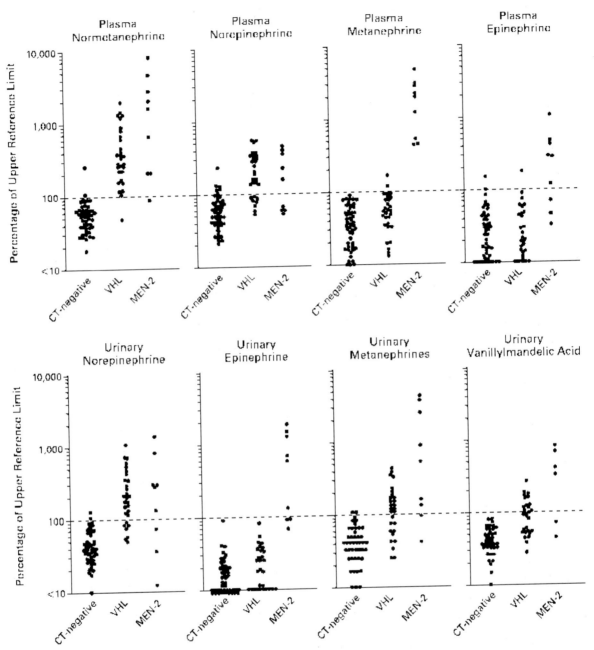

FIGURE 71.5. Plasma concentrations of normetanephrine, norepinephrine, metanephrine, and epinephrine **(top)** and urinary excretion of norepinephrine, epinephrine, metanephrines, and vanillylmandelic acid **(bottom)**. The values are expressed as percentages of the upper reference limit for each test. Data on individual patients are shown for three groups of patients with von Hippel-Lindau disease and multiple endocrine neoplasia type 2 (MEN2), as follows: patients with von Hippel-Lindau disease or MEN2 in whom a pheochromocytoma was ruled out on the basis of normal computed tomography (CT-negative), patients with von Hippel-Lindau disease who had histologically verified pheochromocytomas (VHL), and patients with MEN2 who had histologically verified pheochromocytomas (MEN2). The values for patients with pheochromocytoma were determined when the tumors were first identified by computed tomography. The dotted horizontal line represents the upper reference limit for each test. The y-axes are logarithmic. (Data from Eisenhofer G, Lenders JWM, Linehan WM, et al. Plasma normetanephrine and metanephrine for detecting pheochromocytoma in von Hippel-Lindau disease and multiple endocrine neoplasia type 2. *N Engl J Med* 1999;340:1872.)

THE GENETICS AND MOLECULAR CAUSATION OF MEDULLARY THYROID CARCINOMA

The availability of large and well-characterized kindreds with hereditary MTC made it an ideal candidate for genetic linkage analysis. The causative gene was mapped to chromosome 10q in 1987 (115,116), and mutations of the *RET* protooncogene were identified in 1993 (12,13). Since then, mutations of *RET* have been identified for each of the variants of MEN2. Current understanding of the genotype-phenotype relationships are shown in Fig. 71.6 and Table 71.1. Importantly, mutations of *RET* have been identified in greater than 98% of kindreds with hereditary MTC.

The *RET* (REarranged during Transfection) protooncogene is a transmembrane TK receptor (14). It has an extracellular domain with a cadherin-like portion and cysteine-rich region just external to the plasma membrane spanning region. The intracellular component is analogous to other TK receptors, particularly the epidermal growth factor receptor, and links to multiple signaling pathways (Fig. 71.7).

The *RET* gene occupies a unique place in thyroid oncogenesis. Not only are germ line mutations of this gene involved in the development of MTC, but rearrangements of *RET* that bring the TK domain under the control of one of several promoters expressed in thyroid follicular cells have been implicated in the causation of approximately one third of papillary thyroid carcinomas (PTCs)

(see section on oncogenes in Chapter 70). With the exception of a few reports of *RET* involvement in acute myeloid leukemia (117–119), papillary carcinoma and MTC are the only tumors caused by *RET* mutation/rearrangement.

What is unique about RET is that it is the backbone for a family of ligands and coreceptors that are involved in the development of specific components of the nervous system. RET partners with one of four proteins tethered to the extracellular membrane by a glycosyl-phosphatidylinositol (GPI) linkage (Fig. 71.7). These four coreceptors (GFRα-1, GFRα-2, GFRα-3, GFRα-4) together with the RET TK receptor form a receptor for one of four ligands (glial cell–derived neurotrophic factor (GDNF), neurturin (NTN), persephin (PSP), and artemin (ART) (120–121). GFRα-4 and *RET* may play a role in the normal development of C cells (22). These two proteins are expressed in C cells, adrenal chromaffin cells, and certain pituitary cells, and homologous inactivation of RET in mice causes a reduction in the numbers of C cells and adrenal chromaffin cells (122). This suggests that persephin, a ligand for the GFRα-4 and RET complex, is involved in normal differentiation of C cells and adrenal chromaffin cells (123).

There appear to be two fundamentally different mechanisms by which mutations of the RET protooncogene cause activation of this receptor system. Mutations of the extracellular domain, affecting predominantly cysteine residues at codons 533, 609, 611, 618, 620, 630, and 634, cause dimerization of the receptor in the absence of ligand. This leads to autophosphorylation of RET and activation of downstream signaling pathways (124–126) (Fig. 71.7). Mutations of the intracellular domain change the conformation of the TK domain, leading to activation of catalytic activity in the absence of receptor dimerization (124,125, 127).

Several different intracellular signaling pathways are activated by these mutations. There is general consensus that tyrosine 1062 (Fig. 71.7) is an important mediator of transformation and mediates activation of MAP kinase pathways through binding of shc (128–130). Tyrosine 1062 also mediates phosphatidyl inositol-3-kinase (PI-3-K) and activation of AKT (Fig. 71.7) (131). The nature of the complex that forms at tyrosine 1062 is still being investigated; there is some evidence that SNT/FRS2 is involved in MAP kinase but not PI-3-K activation (127,132). Most importantly, mutation of codon 1062 abrogates the transforming capability of RET (133). There is also evidence that *RET* mutations activate JNK through interaction with the p85 subunit; this effect also may be mediated through the tyrosine at codon 1062 (131,134).

The importance of tyrosine at codon 1062 for transformation is documented by the fact that *RET* protooncogenes in which this residue is deleted are incapable of causing transformation. However, this does not exclude a

Common Germline *RET* Tyrosine Kinase Receptor Mutations in Hereditary Medullary Thyroid Carcinoma

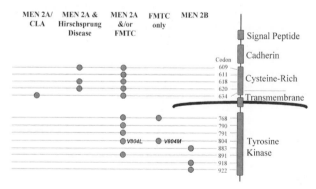

FIGURE 71.6. Common germ line *RET* protooncogene mutations in hereditary medullary thyroid carcinoma. The figure shows genotype-phenotype correlation for the most common mutations found in patients with multiple endocrine neoplasia type 2. Each of the specific mutations is described in Table 71.2. *MEN2A/CLA,* multiple endocrine neoplasia type 2A and cutaneous lichen amyloidosis; *MEN2A/Hirschsprung's disease,* the association of MEN2A with Hirschsprung's disease in affected kindreds; *FMTC,* familial medullary thyroid carcinoma with no other manifestations of MEN2A; *MEN2B,* multiple endocrine neoplasia type 2B.

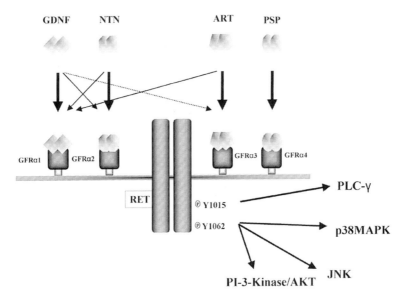

FIGURE 71.7. The *RET* tyrosine kinase receptor/glia cell–derived neurotrophic factor-α (GFRα) receptor system. The *RET* receptor forms the backbone for a complex signaling system. *RET* partners with one of four coreceptors (GFRα-1, GFRα-2, GFRα-3, or GFRα-4) to form a receptor for one of four ligands (GDNF, glial cell-derived neurotrophic factor; NTN, neurturin; ART, artemin; PSP, persephin). The GDNF family functions as neuronal survival factors and is intimately involved in the developmental embryology of the sympathetic nervous system. Activation of the *RET*/GFRα receptor system in the C cell leads to autophosphorylation and phosphorylation of downstream substrates from at least four different signaling pathways: phosphatidyl inositol-3-kinase (PI-3-K), jun activated kinases (JNK), mitogen-activated kinase (MAPK), and phospholipase Cγ, (PLCγ). Phosphorylation of tyrosine 1062 is required for transformation of C cells; mutation of this residue abrogates transformation. The activating mutations of *RET* lead to dimerization of the receptor in the absence of ligand (extracellular domain mutations) or modify the tyrosine kinase domain (intracellular domain mutations) to facilitate autophosphorylation and activation of downstream signaling pathways.

contribution by other tyrosine residues to the transformation process or some of the other manifestations found in the variant forms of MEN2.

Indirect evidence from studies of the *RET/PTC* rearrangements found in papillary carcinoma indicates that MAP kinase activation is important. Nearly all of these carcinomas have mutations of *RET* or one of the linker proteins (RAS or RAF) that activate MAP kinase (135–137). These observations have led to *in vitro* studies of small molecules that inhibit RET-TK activation (138,139), and several of these small molecules are now being investigated in phase I clinical trials.

Somatic *RET* Protooncogene Mutations in Sporadic Medullary Carcinoma

Approximately 25% of sporadic MTCs have a somatic *RET* protooncogene mutation, most commonly a Met918Thr *RET* mutation (140,141), identical to the germ line mutation that causes MEN2B. Furthermore, there is compelling evidence that codon 918 mutations are associated with a more aggressive form of MTC. Reports from several groups indicate that this mutation is associated with a greater extent of disease and a significant reduction in survival (142, 143). Indeed, the characteristic phenotype associated with

a somatic codon 918 mutation is the presence of extensive lymph node metastases in the neck, extension of disease into mediastinal and perihilar lymph nodes, and pulmonary, hepatic, and bony metastases. In one study, the 10-year survival in patients with a codon 918 mutation was 50%, as compared with 85% among patients without this mutation (143). Findings at the University of Texas M.D. Anderson Cancer Center are nearly identical (unpublished observations). Other *RET* codons mutated in sporadic MTC include 631, 634, 766, 768, 876, 804, 883, 884, 901, 922, and 930 (140,144–149).

There may be heterogeneity of somatic mutations. For example, there are reports that some metastatic foci had a codon 918 mutation, whereas the primary MTC or another metastatic focus did not. These results suggest that acquisition of *RET* mutations may be but one element in the progression of metastatic potential (150,151).

There are reports that polymorphism at codon 836 of *RET* is more frequent in patients with sporadic MTC (152,153). In addition, a codon 834 polymorphism has been associated with a codon 804 mutation, but does appear to affect the aggressiveness of an 804 mutation (154). A relationship between the 836 polymorphism and sporadic MTC is not proven, but is not unrealistic given the role of polymorphisms of *RET* in Hirschsprung's disease (155).

Other Molecular Abnormalities in the Progression of Medullary Thyroid Carcinoma

MTC is one of a small number of carcinomas in which an imbalance between the normal and mutant copy of the activated oncogene contributes to progression of the tumor. In MTC there are three identified mechanisms by which this occurs. The first is through a chromosomal duplicative event that results in a 2:1 ratio of mutant to normal RET receptors (156,157). A second variant is found in the TT cell line, derived from a human MTC with a codon 634 *RET* mutation. In this cell line there is a tandem duplication of the mutant *RET* locus, resulting in twice the level of expression of the mutant sequence (158). Finally, in some MTCs there is loss of part or all of the normal *RET* allele, creating a situation in which there is homogeneous expression of mutant allele (156,157,159). The implication of these findings is that the normal copy of *RET* functions as a tumor suppressor gene, and that its loss results in a greater mutant *RET* effect, analogous to earlier observations for the *MET* and *RAS* oncogenes (160,161).

Although no other specific causative loci have been identified in either hereditary or sporadic MTC, the finding of loss of heterozygosity at several chromosomal locations (chromosomes 1p, 3p, 9q, 17p, and 22q) suggests there are other tumor suppressor genes that are likely to be involved in the genesis of medullary thyroid carcinoma (162–165).

GENOTYPE-PHENOTYPE CORRELATION IN HEREDITARY MEDULLARY THYROID CARCINOMA

Since the discovery of *RET* mutations in MEN2, there has been a gradual refinement of the phenotypes associated with particular activating mutations of *RET* (Fig. 71.6 and Table 71.2).

The most commonly identified mutations in hereditary MTC are located in the extracellular cysteine-rich region of the receptor. Mutations of the cysteine at codon 634 account for approximately 80% of germ line *RET* mutations; substitution of arginine for cysteine accounts for more than one half of the mutations at this codon. The invariable clinical phenotype associated with any codon 634 *RET* mutation is the MEN2A syndrome (166). The next largest clustering of mutations, accounting for 10% to 15% of mutations, involves substitution of one of several amino acids for cysteine at codons 609, 611, 618, 620, and 630. Mutations at these codons may be associated with either MEN2A or familial MTC. There are clearly defined kindreds with either familial MTC or MEN2A with each of these substitutions. All patients with the MEN2A/CLA syndrome have been found to have one of several substitutions at codon 634 (166). Patients with the MEN2A/Hirschsprung variant have been found to have codon 609,

618, or 620 mutations; investigators studying Hirschsprung's disease have identified codon 609 or 620 *RET* mutations among kindreds with hereditary Hirschsprung's disease (167).

The remainder of mutations, mostly intracellular, account for no more than 5% to 10% of all mutations. Mutations at codons 883 and 918 are invariably associated with MEN2B (168–172). Mutations at codons 768 and V804M are invariably associated with familial MTC (166,173–175). Intracellular domain mutations that may be associated with either familial MTC or MEN2A include codons 790, 791, V804L, and 891 (176–178).

Although it is unlikely that there will be substantial change in the genotype-phenotype correlations described, there will be refinement. Two types of changes seem likely. The first is a gradual expansion of the phenotype associated with rare mutations. An example of this is the reclassification of the phenotype associated with a codon 891 mutation during the past year. Early reports of this mutation described five kindreds (175,179–182), and a single patient (181) in which the only manifestation was MTC. The identification of a kindred with this same mutation and a single member with a pheochromocytoma has necessitated reclassification of this mutation from familial MTC to MEN2A (178).

A second phenomenon has been the identification of rare germ line mutations or polymorphisms of the *RET* gene associated with hereditary MTC. Examples include germ line mutations at codon 666 associated with MTC in one kindred and an ACTH-secreting pheochromocytoma in a single person from another kindred (Table 71.2), a codon 912 mutation associated with MTC in a single kindred (183), a codon 778 mutation associated with MTC in a single patient (184), and an unusual variant of MEN2B in a kindred, namely codon 804 and 904 mutations on the same allele (185). The two largest compilations of genotype–phenotype information describing these rare mutations are at Online Mendelian Inheritance in Man (185a) and the Human Gene Mutation Database (185b), although neither is complete. Many of the rare mutations are listed in Table 71.2, and there are others scattered throughout the literature. It may take another decade or more before a complete understanding of the phenotypes associated with these rare mutations emerges.

UNUSUAL DIAGNOSTIC ISSUES IN THE EVALUATION OF MEDULLARY THYROID CARCINOMA

The Use of Serum Calcitonin Measurements in the Evaluation of Nodular Goiter

Several studies have described the results of measurements of serum calcitonin in patients with thyroid nodules, as

TABLE 71.2. MUTATIONS OF THE *RET* PROTOONCOGENE IN HEREDITARY MEDULLARY THYROID CARCINOMA

HGMD Accession No.	Affected Codon	Exon	Amino Acid Change Normal → Mutant	Nucleotide Change Normal → Mutant	Clinical Syndrome	Percentage of all MEN2 Mutations
CM961242	609	10	cys → arg	TGC → CGC	MEN2A/	0–1
CM961243			cys → gly	TGC → GGC	FMTC	
CM014088			cys → ser	TGC → TCC		
CM941226			cys → tyr	TGC → TAC[a]	MEN2A	2–3
CM961703	611	10	cys → arg	TGC → CGC		
CM961245			cys → gly	TGC → GGC		
CM961246			cys → phe	TGC → TTC		
CM930642			cys → ser	TGC → AGC[b]		
CM930642			cys → trp	TGC → TGG		
CM961244			cys → tyr	TGC → TAC	MEN2A/	3–5
CM941231	618	10	cys → arg	TGC → CGC[c]	FMTC	
CM941232			cys → gly	TGC → GGC[d]		
CM961248			cys → phe	TGC → TTC		
CM941230			cys → ser	TGC → AGC		
CM941229			cys → ser	TGC → TCC		
CM941228			cys → tyr	TGC → TAC	MEN2A/	6–8
CM941236	620	10	cys → arg	TGC → CGC	FMTC	
CM971302			cys → gly	TGC → GGC		
CM941234			cys → phe	TGC → TTC		
CM941233			cys → ser	TGC → TCC		
CM941235			cys → ser	TGC → AGC		
CM981704			cys → trp	TGC → TGG		
CM930643			cys → tyr	TGC → TAC	MEN2A/	<0.1
CM971305	630	11	cys → phe	TGC → TTC	FMTC	
CM971304			cys → ser	TGC → TCC		
CM971303			cys → tyr	TGC → TAC	MEN2A[5]	80–90
CM930644	634	10	cys → arg	TGC → CGC		
CM941242			cys → gly	TGC → GGC		
CM941239			cys → phe	TGC → TTC		
CM941241			cys → ser	TGC → AGC		
CM941238			cys → ser	TGC → TCC		
CM941240			cys → trp	TGC → TGG		
CM941237			cys → tyr	TGC → TAC	FMTC	0–1
CM020961	768	13	glu → asp	GAG → GAT		
CM951125			glu → asp	GAG → GAC	MEN2A/	<0.1
CM981706	790	13	leu → phe	TTG → TTT	FMTC	
CM981705			leu → phe	TTG → TTC	FMTC	<0.1
CM971306	791	13	tyr → phe	TAT → TTT	FMTC	
CM951126	804	14	val → leu	GTG → TTG		
CM981707			val → met	GTG → ATG	MEN2A/FMTC	0–1
CM971307	891	15	ser → val	TCG → GCG	MEN2B	10–20
CM941246	918	16	met → thr	ATG → ACG		

noted above. A consistent finding in these studies was the identification of MTC in a small number of patients, based on a high serum calcitonin concentration. In an early study, of 1385 patients, all 8 (0.5%) who had a high serum calcitonin value had MTC (186). Overall, there have been eight studies of over 6000 patients (186–193). All patients in these studies who had a serum calcitonin value of greater than 100 pg/mL, with the exception of a patient with pancreatic cancer, had MTC; in many of these patients the diagnosis of MTC was apparent by other clinical criteria or biopsy.

In these same studies there were 130 patients (2%) who had serum calcitonin values between 10 and 100 pg/mL; only 23 of these 130 patients (18%) were found to have MTC at surgery. The basal serum calcitonin concentrations plotted as a function of the size of the MTC in 21 of these patients are shown in Fig. 71.8. It is clear that in most of these patients the MTC was very small, and not likely to have been identified by any diagnostic technique. Furthermore, using a serum calcitonin cutoff value of 25 pg/mL, only 3 of the 21 MTCs would have been missed.

In one of these studies 1167 patients with one or more thyroid nodules underwent surgery, and the resected thyroid tissue was examined for the presence of MTC (191). Of the 1167 patients, 34 (3%) had a high basal serum calcitonin concentration. Fourteen of these 34 patients (41%)

TABLE 71.2. *CONTINUED*

			Rare RET Mutations (<0.1%)			
HGMD Accession No.	Affected Codon	Exon	Amino Acid Change Normal → Mutant	Nucleotide Change Normal → Mutant	Clinical Syndrome	Unique Manifestations
CI992071	533	8	gly → cys	GGC → TGC	FMTC	
	532/533	8	insertion	9 bp duplication GAGGAGTGT	FMTC	
CM014743	603	10	lys → gln	AAA → CAA	FMTC	
CX952207	631	11	Insertion/deletion	TGC ↑ GACGAgcgtgtGCC	FMTC	
CX942108	633	11	Insertion/deletion	GAG ↑ CTGTGccGCA	MEN2A	
	634/640	11	cys634arg/ala640gly	TGC634GGC/ GCC640GGC	MEN2A	Calcitonin-secreting pheochromocytoma
	634/648	11/11	cys634arg/val648ile		MEN2A	ACTH-secreting pheochromocytoma
CI972693	635	11	insertion	ACGAGCTGTGCC	MEN2A	
CI983210	637	11	insertion	TGCCGCACG	MEN2A	
	649	11	ser → leu	TCG → TTG	FMTC	Primary hyperparathyroidism (1 case)
	666	11	lys → glu	AAG → GAG	FMTC	ACTH-secreting pheochromocytoma
CM022982	778	13	val → ile	GTC → ATC	FMTC	
CM023442	781	13	gln → arg	CAG → CGG	FMTC	
CM001328	844	14	arg → leu	CGG → CTG	FMTC	
	804/844	14/14	val804met/arg844leu	GTG → ATG/	FMTC	
CX942108	882	15	Insertion/deletion	CTG ↑ GTAgcTGC	MEN2B	
	883	15	ala → phe	GCT → TTT	MEN2B	

[a,c] Mutations of these two codons have been reported in Hirschsprung's disease.
[a,b,d] Reported cases of MEN2A/Hirschsprung's disease variants have these mutations.
[e] A codon 634 cys ↑ arg (TGC ↑ CGC) mutation accounts for approximately 50% of all mutations associated with MEN 2A.
ACTH, corticotropin; MEN, multiple endocrine neoplasia; FMTC, familial medullary thyroid carcinoma.
Adapted from information available at the Human Gene Mutation Database (*www.HGMD.org*) and from Online Mendelian Inheritance in Man (*www.ncbi.nlm.nih.gov/entrez/query.fcgi?CMD=search&DB=omim*). In addition, the authors have added to this list from meeting abstracts and personal experience. This table describes *RET* mutations identified in 99.9% of germ line carriers of MEN2. In addition there are rare mutations that have been identified in individual patients or in sporadic tumors. In some cases the physical location of these rare coding changes adjacent to a sequence known to be mutated gives credibility to the role of the mutant sequence; in others the relevance is unclear. Further clarification of their relevance will await examination of their transforming abilities or additional genotype/phenotype correlation. It is likely there are other rare mutations.

had MTC. These findings indicate that a high serum calcitonin value has predictive value for the presence of MTC, but on the other hand high values are not specific for MTC. High values have been found in patients with all types of thyroid nodules, and perhaps most often in patients with autoimmune thyroiditis (193).

These collective results have led a German-based consensus group to recommend total thyroidectomy for patients with a pentagastrin-stimulated serum CT value greater than 100 pg/mL, and total thyroidectomy and lymph node dissection for patients with pentagastrin-stimulated serum CT values greater than 200 pg/mL (194). Pentagastrin is not available in the United States.

Despite the fact that approximately one in five patients with thyroid nodules who have a high basal serum calcitonin value will be found to have MTC, measurement of serum calcitonin in these patients has not been widely accepted in the United States. There are several reasons for this. First is the lack of specificity of measurements of basal

serum calcitonin (23,51,195,196). The finding that 1.7% of normal adults without evidence of thyroid disease had a serum calcitonin concentration of greater than 10 pg/mL (193) highlights the difficulty of differentiating between normal subjects and the 3.5% of patients with thyroid nodules who have similarly high values. Secondly, in none of the reported series was an attempt made to assess the risks (unnecessary surgery, hypoparathyroidism, recurrent laryngeal nerve injury, hypothyroidism) versus benefit (cure of MTC) of performing a thyroidectomy in a patient with a slightly high serum calcitonin concentration (197). Third, other than the axiom that "all carcinomas start small," there is little evidence that the small MTCs detected incidentally will in fact progress (198,199).

From a practical point of view, once the possibility of MTC has been raised, based on the finding of a high serum calcitonin value, however minimal the elevation may be, it is inevitable that the patient will eventually have a thyroidectomy. It is very difficult to reassure such a patient

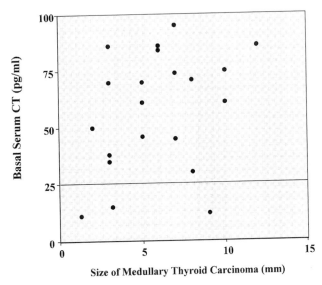

FIGURE 71.8. Basal serum calcitonin (CT) values plotted against size of the medullary thyroid carcinoma in 21 patients with a multinodular goiter who had basal serum calcitonin concentrations of 10 to 100 pg/mL. Note the limited correlation between serum calcitonin values and tumor size. Serum calcitonin concentrations ranged from less than 10 pg/mL to as high as 30 pg/mL in the normal subjects. All but three of the patients with goiter with MTC had values greater than 25 pg/mL (horizontal line).

that observation is a rational approach. The lack of availability of pentagastrin in the United States makes it necessary to base a decision on a basal serum calcitonin or a calcium-stimulated value. It is paradoxic that in an era when fine-needle aspiration biopsy is used routinely to reduce the need for thyroid surgery, use of a less specific test may increase the number of thyroid surgical procedures, without clear evidence of benefit. A reasonable course of action, based on the data in Fig. 71.8, is to follow patients with a serum calcitonin value of less than 25 pg/mL, particularly if the value is less than 100 pg/mL after calcium or pentagastrin stimulation. Those with basal values greater than 25 pg/mL or a stimulated value greater than 100 pg/mL could be followed or considered for surgery, dependent on other clinical factors. Finally, any patient with an unexplained elevation of serum calcitonin should have a *RET* protooncogene analysis.

Testing for Germline *RET* Protooncogene Mutations in Sporadic Medullary Carcinoma

A few patients with apparently sporadic MTC have a germ line *RET* mutation indicative of hereditary MTC (15,200–204). These findings have led to a consensus recommendation that all patients with apparently sporadic MTC have a DNA analysis for *RET* mutations (86). The rationale for this recommendation is based on the fact that patients with palpable MTC have a high rate of local or distant metasta-

tic disease. Identification of a germline mutation in these patients, thereby mandating mutation analysis in their offspring or relatives, should allow earlier identification of family members at risk, thereby improving their outcome. Hence, all patients with apparently sporadic MTC should have a germ line *RET* analysis. If a *RET* mutation is identified, first-degree relatives should also have a *RET* analysis, followed by appropriate evaluation and treatment for those with an identified mutation.

TREATMENT OF MEDULLARY THYROID CARCINOMA

Medullary Thyroid Carcinoma Presenting as a Thyroid Nodule

Patients with MTC can be classified into one of three groups: those with localized MTC in whom cure is possible, those with metastatic disease limited to the neck in whom cure may be possible, and those with evidence of metastases outside of the neck. Whenever possible, the diagnosis of MTC should be established preoperatively by biopsy, and the extent of disease evaluated by measurements of serum calcitonin and CEA and ultrasonography of the neck. In addition, a germ line analysis of the *RET* protooncogene should be performed, although it is unusual to have the result of this analysis before the primary surgical procedure. Consideration should also be given to the possibility of a pheochromocytoma, as discussed in an earlier section.

The appropriate surgical procedure for a patient with localized MTC without obvious metastatic disease (no abnormalities outside the neck on imaging studies and serum calcitonin values <500 pg/mL) is a total thyroidectomy with central (levels VI–VII) and bilateral lateral (levels II–V) node dissection (see Chapter 17). This is an extensive surgical procedure, but one that affords the highest probability of surgical cure, defined as an undetectable serum calcitonin concentration (<2 to 5 pg/mL). From 10% to 25% of patients can be cured by this approach (73,90,205–207).

The second group of patients, those with documented local metastatic disease, should be evaluated more carefully. Although surgical cure in these patients is possible, the probability is lower. Most patients in this group should be treated by total thyroidectomy and central (levels VI–VII) and bilateral lateral (levels II–V) node dissection. A question that arises in these patients is the extent of search for distant metastatic disease. If the patient's serum calcitonin value is greater than 500 pg/mL and there is no evidence of metastases in cervical lymph nodes, as assessed by ultrasonography, chest and abdominal computed tomography scans or positron-emission tomography (PET) should be performed (208,209). The high frequency of hepatic metastases has led to the recommendation that laparoscopic evaluation of the liver be performed as well (74,210).

The challenge is to differentiate between patients in whom there is a reasonable possibility of surgical cure and those with distant metastasis, in whom extensive neck surgery will not affect long-term outcome. The sensitivity of serum calcitonin measurements for detection of tumor is far greater than current imaging sensitivity, and as a result the number of patients with distant metastases is likely to be underestimated.

In those patients in whom cure by thyroidectomy and neck dissection is not possible, the goals change. In them, it is appropriate to perform a total thyroidectomy with surgical excision of identifiable disease, particularly if the disease is located so that it could impair the airway. There is little evidence that a mediastinal node dissection has curative value, and it is rarely performed as a part of a curative thyroidectomy.

The last group, those patients with clear evidence of distant metastases, is usually relatively easily identified. These are patients who have very high serum calcitonin concentrations (>5000 pg/mL), they may have diarrhea or flushing, and they have metastatic disease easily identified by imaging studies. In these patients, the goal of thyroid surgery is to remove all identifiable tumor in the neck and to protect the airway. Lymph nodes that obviously contain tumor should be resected, but extensive lymph node dissection probably has little value. Treatment of patients with mediastinal metastases should be individualized. In patients who have metastases in lymph nodes in the upper mediastinum or perihilar area that are likely to affect the airway, consideration should be given to a mediastinal lymph node dissection.

Surgical Treatment of Hereditary Medullary Thyroid Carcinoma

The identification of *RET* protooncogene mutations has provided a molecular basis not only for predicting a specific MEN2 phenotype, but also for providing insight into the clinical behavior of MTC. Some idea of the relative aggressiveness of MTC associated with specific *RET* mutations is provided by an examination of the earliest age at which MTC has been identified in patients with a specific mutation (211) (Fig. 71.9). Correlative studies indicate that the presence of a codon 918 mutation is indicative of an aggressive disease phenotype, whether the mutation is hereditary (MEN2B) or acquired as a somatic mutation. Children with MEN2B should have a total thyroidectomy and lymph node dissection performed in the first month of life or as soon as the germ line mutation is identified. Because most patients with MEN2B have *de novo* mutations, they are most commonly identified in the 3- to 10-year age period; in such children surgical cure is uncommon.

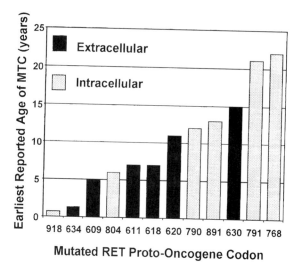

FIGURE 71.9. Plot showing the earliest age of identification of medullary thyroid carcinoma in patients with different germ line mutations in *RET*, derived from data presented in the EU-ROMEN study (referenced in text) and other reports. Note that the mutations are located in both the extra- and intracellular regions of the RET protein. (Modified from Cote GJ, Gagel RF. Lessons learned from the management of a rare genetic cancer. *N Engl J Med* 2003;349:1566, with permission.)

The next most aggressive phenotype is associated with a codon 634 *RET* mutation; this accounts for approximately 80% of hereditary MTC. Metastasis has been described in a 6-year-old child (92,93), and recent unpublished reports have described microscopic MTC with metastasis to at least one local lymph node in 3-year-old children. The EU-ROMEN consortium report described 196 children with codon 634 mutations; no one in this group under 14 years of age had metastasis (212). There is now consensus that thyroidectomy, with or without central lymph node dissection, should be performed by the age of 6 years (86), but some advocate earlier thyroidectomy, particularly in children with abnormal serum calcitonin responses to pentagastrin. Most clinicians would include children with mutations of codons 609, 611, 618, 620, 630, and 891 in this group, because of evidence of aggressive disease in a subset of these patients.

The final groups of children include those with mutations of codons 768, 790, 791, and 804. In some large kindreds with these mutations there has never been a death caused by MTC; in others metastases and death attributable to MTC occurred infrequently (213). If there has never been a death attributable to MTC in one of these kindreds (and the kindred is of sufficient size and the follow-up encompasses multiple generations), delaying thyroidectomy to a later age may be a reasonable course (213).

Twenty years ago, John Sipple, addressing the First International Workshop on Multiple Endocrine Neoplasia type 2, marveled at the progress toward understanding the syndrome he described some 22 years earlier (75). That morbidity and mortality would be eliminated for more than 90% of patients with disorder during his lifetime likely never entered his mind. Remarkably, it has happened for those kindreds with hereditary MTC who are prospectively screened and appropriately treated.

Medullary Thyroid Carcinoma and Persistent Elevations in Serum Calcitonin Concentrations

A common situation in MTC referral centers is a patient who had a total thyroidectomy with or without a neck dissection and is referred for evaluation of a persistently high serum calcitonin or CEA concentration. In evaluating such a patient, it is important to allow 3 to 4 months to elapse after thyroidectomy before concluding that the high serum value is related to the presence of MTC and not to a postoperative inflammatory stimulation of calcitonin production (23) or slow clearance of serum CEA due to its prolonged half-life (214,215).

The most common scenario is a patient who had a total thyroidectomy and a limited (or no) lymph node dissection. Among these patients, from 10% to 15% will in time have normal serum calcitonin concentrations (71–73, 96–98). Because the patient has received primary therapy (thyroidectomy) for MTC, the decision to perform a thorough lymph node dissection should be based on a realistic estimate of the probability of a surgical cure. Reasonable evaluation would consist of ultrasonography of the neck, chest and abdominal computed tomography, and nuclear imaging [PET, octreotide, or meta-iodobenzylguanidine (MIBG)]. Patients who have basal serum calcitonin concentrations of less than 100 pg/mL are unlikely to have any imaging abnormalities. Some clinicians would, in this situation, perform laparoscopy to examine the liver before proceeding to neck exploration (74). The major complication of reoperation in these patients is hypoparathyroidism (73); in addition, the operation is unlikely to result in normalization of serum calcitonin. In patients with obvious distant metastases, there is little if any reason to perform a detailed neck dissection; in such patients reoperation is appropriate to remove lymph nodes that may become problematic to patency of the airway if allowed to remain in place.

OTHER FORMS OF THERAPY FOR MEDULLARY THYROID CARCINOMA

Radiotherapy is routinely used as adjunctive palliative therapy for patients with extensive neck or mediastinal disease or a localized bony metastasis. It provides effective amelioration of MTC in both of these situations; but there is no evidence that it has any effect on survival (216,217). Targeted radiotherapy using radiolabeled somatostatin analogues (218,219), radiolabeled monoclonal antibodies directed against CEA (220), and radiolabeled MIBG (221) have been used with limited success.

Cytotoxic chemotherapy has a place in the treatment of patients with metastatic MTC. Approximately 30% of patients treated with dacarbazine (DTIC)-based chemotherapy have reductions in tumor size (222–224), and there are few reports of complete remission. Because MTC is most commonly a slowly progressive tumor, the challenge is to initiate therapy at an appropriate time. In patients with codon 918 *RET* mutations and rapidly progressive disease, early intervention with chemotherapy may delay tumor progression; in patients with more slowly progressive disease, intervention is advised at a point when there is substantial tumor mass, but before the patient's performance status has decreased appreciably.

Finally, the introduction of a variety of small molecules that inhibit signal transduction has opened a new era of investigation. Many of these drugs have limited side effects; patients with slowly growing MTC are being encouraged to participate in trials of selected drugs that target signal transduction pathways activated by the RET receptor.

REFERENCES

1. Hazard JB, Hawk WA, Crile G Jr. Medullary (solid) carcinoma of the thyroid: a clinicopathologic entity. *J Clin Endocrinol Metab* 1959;19:152.
2. Sipple JH. The association of pheochromocytoma with carcinoma of the thyroid gland. *Am J Med* 1961;31:163.
3. Williams ED. Histogenesis of medullary carcinoma of the thyroid. *J Clin Pathol* 1966;19:114.
4. Cushman P Jr. Familial endocrine tumors: report of two unrelated kindred affected with pheochromocytomas, one also with multiple thyroid carcinomas. *Am J Med* 1962;32:352.
5. Schimke RN, Hartmann WH. Familial amyloid-producing medullary thyroid carcinoma and pheochromocytoma: a distinct genetic entity. *Ann Intern Med* 1965;63:1027.
6. Copp DH, Davidson AGF, Cheney BA. Evidence for a new parathyroid hormone which lowers blood calcium. *Proc Can Fed Biol Soc* 1961;4:17.
7. Copp DH, Cameron EC, Cheney BA, et al. Evidence for calcitonin—a new hormone from the parathyroid that lowers blood calcium. *Endocrinology* 1962;70:638.
8. Hirsch PF, Voelkel EF, Munson PL. Thyrocalcitonin: hypocalcemic, hypophosphatemic principle of the thyroid gland. *Science* 1964;146:412.
9. Melvin KEW, Tashjian AH Jr. The syndrome of excessive thyrocalcitonin produced by medullary carcinoma of the thyroid. *Proc Natl Acad Sci U S A* 1968;59:1216.
10. Woodhouse NJ, Gudmundsson TV, Galante L, et al. Biochemical studies on four patients with medullary carcinoma of the thyroid. *J Endocrinol* 1969;45(suppl):xvi.
11. Melvin KEW, Miller HH, Tashjian AH Jr. Early diagnosis of medullary carcinoma of the thyroid gland by means of calcitonin assay. *N Engl J Med* 1971;285:1115.
12. Donis-Keller H, Dou S, Chi D, et al. Mutations in the RET proto-oncogene are associated with MEN 2A and FMTC. *Hum Mol Genet* 1993;2:851.

13. Mulligan LM, Kwok JB, Healey CS, et al. Germ-line mutations of the RET proto-oncogene in multiple endocrine neoplasia type 2A. *Nature* 1993;363:458.

14. Takahashi M, Ritz J, Cooper GM. Activation of a novel human transforming gene, *ret,* by DNA rearrangement. *Cell* 1985;42:581.

15. Wohllk N, Cote GJ, Bugalho MMJ, et al. Relevance of RET proto-oncogene mutations in sporadic medullary thyroid carcinoma. *J Clin Endocrinol Metab* 1996;81:3740.

16. Le Douarin N, Le Lievre C. Demonstration de l'origine neurales des cellules a calcitonine du corps ultimobranchial chez l'embryon de poulet. *Compt Rend* 1970;270:2857.

17. Le Douarin NM, Dupin E. Cell lineage analysis in neural crest ontogeny. *J Neurobiol* 1993;24:146.

18. Pearse AG, Takor TT. Neuroendocrine embryology and the APUD concept. *Clin Endocrinol (Oxf)* 1976;5(suppl):229.

19. Gorn AH, Lin HY, Yamin M, et al. Cloning, characterization, and expression of a human calcitonin receptor from an ovarian carcinoma cell line. *J Clin Invest* 1992;90:1726.

20. Wener JA, Gorton SJ, Raisz LG. Escape from inhibition or resorption in cultures of fetal bone treated with calcitonin and parathyroid hormone. *Endocrinology* 1972;90:752.

21. Hoff AO, Catala-Lehnen P, Thomas PM, et al. Increased bone mass is an unexpected phenotype associated with deletion of the calcitonin gene. *J Clin Invest* 2002;110:1849.

22. Dacquin R, Davey RA, Laplace C, et al. Amylin inhibits bone resorption while the calcitonin receptor controls bone formation *in vivo. J Cell Biol* 2004;164:509.

23. Muller B, White JC, Nylen ES, et al. Ubiquitous expression of the calcitonin-i gene in multiple tissues in response to sepsis. *J Clin Endocrinol Metab* 2001;86:396.

24. Nylen ES, Whang KT, Snider RH Jr, et al. Mortality is increased by procalcitonin and decreased by an antiserum reactive to procalcitonin in experimental sepsis. *Crit Care Med* 1998;26:1001.

25. Graze K, Spiler IJ, Tashjian AH Jr, et al. Natural history of familial medullary thyroid carcinoma: effect of a program for early diagnosis. *N Engl J Med* 1978;299:980.

26. Tran Q, Roesser JR. SRp55 is a regulator of calcitonin/CGRP alternative RNA splicing. *Biochemistry* 2003;42:951.

27. Lou H, Helfman DM, Gagel RF, et al. Polypyrimidine tract-binding protein positively regulates inclusion of an alternative 3′-terminal exon. *Mol Cell Biol* 1999;19:78.

28. Zhu H, Hasman RA, Young KM, et al. U1 snRNP-dependent function of TIAR in the regulation of alternative RNA processing of the human calcitonin/CGRP pre-mRNA. *Mol Cell Biol* 2003;23:5959.

29. Coleman TP, Tran Q, Roesser JR. Binding of a candidate splice regulator to a calcitonin-specific splice enhancer regulates calcitonin/CGRP pre-mRNA splicing. *Biochim Biophys Acta* 2003;1625:153.

30. Monla YT, Peleg S, Gagel RF. Cell type-specific regulation of transcription by cyclic adenosine 3′,5′-monophosphate-responsive elements within the calcitonin promoter. *Mol Endocrinol* 1995;9:784.

31. de Bustros A, Baylin SB, Berger CL, et al. Phorbol esters increase calcitonin gene transcription and decrease c-myc mRNA levels in cultured human medullary thyroid carcinoma. *J Biol Chem* 1985;260:98.

32. Thiagalingam A, De Bustros A, Borges M, et al. RREB-1, a novel zinc finger protein, is involved in the differentiation response to Ras in human medullary thyroid carcinomas. *Mol Cell Biol* 1996;16:5335.

33. Cote GJ, Rogers DG, Huang ES, et al. The effect of 1,25-dihydroxyvitamin D3 treatment on calcitonin and calcitonin gene-related peptide mRNA levels in cultured human thyroid C-cells. *Biochem Biophys Res Commun* 1987;149:239.

34. Peleg S, Abruzzese RV, Cooper CW, et al. Down-regulation of calcitonin gene transcription by vitamin D requires two widely separated enhancer sequences. *Mol Endocrinol* 1993;7:999.

35. Lanigan TM, Tverberg LA, Russo AF. Retinoic acid repression of cell-specific helix-loop-helix-octamer activation of the calcitonin/calcitonin gene-related peptide enhancer. *Mol Cell Biol* 1993;13:6079.

36. Watson A, Latchman D. The cyclic AMP response element in the calcitonin/calcitonin gene-related peptide gene promoter is necessary but not sufficient for its activation by nerve growth factor. *J Biol Chem* 1995;270:9655.

37. Durham PL, Russo AF. Serotonergic repression of mitogen-activated protein kinase control of the calcitonin gene-related peptide enhancer. *Mol Endocrinol* 1998;12:1002.

38. Cote GJ, Gagel RF. Dexamethasone differentially affects the levels of calcitonin and calcitonin gene-related peptide mRNAs expressed in a human medullary thyroid carcinoma cell line. *J Biol Chem* 1986;261:15524.

39. Muszynski M, Birnbaum RS, Roos BA. Glucocorticoids stimulate the production of preprocalcitonin-derived secretory peptides by a rat medullary thyroid carcinoma cell line. *J Biol Chem* 1983;258:11678.

40. Tverberg LA, Russo AF. Cell-specific glucocorticoid repression of calcitonin/calcitonin gene-related peptide transcription. Localization to an 18-base pair basal enhancer element. *J Biol Chem* 1992;267:17567.

41. Peleg S, Abruzzese RV, Cote GJ, et al. Transcription of the human calcitonin gene is mediated by a C cell-specific enhancer containing E-box-like elements. *Mol Endocrinol* 1990;4:1750.

42. de Bustros A, Lee RY, Compton D, et al. Differential utilization of calcitonin gene regulatory DNA sequences in cultured lines of medullary thyroid carcinoma and small-cell lung carcinoma. *Mol Cell Biol* 1990;10:1773.

43. Tverberg LA, Russo AF. Regulation of the calcitonin/calcitonin gene-related peptide gene by cell-specific synergy between helix-loop-helix and octamer-binding transcription factors. *J Biol Chem* 1993;268:15965.

44. Garrett JE, Tamir H, Kifor O, et al. Calcitonin-secreting cells of the thyroid express an extracellular calcium receptor gene. *Endocrinology* 1995;136:5202.

45. Freichel M, Zink-Lorenz A, Holloschi A, et al. Expression of a calcium-sensing receptor in a human medullary thyroid carcinoma cell line and its contribution to calcitonin secretion. *Endocrinology* 1996;137:3842.

46. Friedman J, Raisz LG. Thyrocalcitonin: inhibitor of bone resorption in tissue culture. *Science* 1965;150:1465.

47. Bell NH. Effects of glucagon, dibutyryl cyclic 3′,5′-adenosine monophosphate, and theophylline on calcitonin secretion *in vitro. J Clin Invest* 1970;49:1368.

48. Endo T, Saito T, Uchida T, et al. Effects of somatostatin and serotonin on calcitonin secretion from cultured rat parafollicular cells. *Acta Endocrinol (Copenh)* 1988;117:214.

49. Cooper CW, Schwesinger WH, Mahgoub AM, et al. Thyrocalcitonin: stimulation of secretion by pentagastrin. *Science* 1971;172:1238.

50. Dymling JF, Ljungberg O, Hillyard CJ, et al. Whisky: a new provocative test for calcitonin secretion. *Acta Endocrinol (Copenh)* 1976;82:500.

51. Aloia JF, Rasulo P, Deftos LJ, et al. Exercise-induced hypercalcemia and the calciotropic hormones. *J Lab Clin Med* 1985;106:229.

52. Russo AF, Gagel RF. Vitamin D control of the calcitonin gene in thyroid C cells. In: Feldman D, ed. *Vitamin D.* San Diego: Academic Press, 2004.

53. Mendelsohn G. Markers as prognostic indicators in medullary thyroid carcinoma. *Am J Clin Pathol* 1991;95:297.

54. DeLellis RA, Rule AH, Spiler I, et al. Calcitonin and carcinoembryonic antigen as tumor markers in medullary thyroid carcinoma. *Am J Clin Pathol* 1978;70:587.

55. Cox CE, VanVickle J, Froome LC, et al. Carcinoembryonic antigen and calcitonin as markers of malignancy in medullary thyroid carcinoma. *Surg Forum* 1979;30:120.

56. Gagel RF, Palmer WN, Leonhart K, et al. Somatostatin production by a human medullary thyroid carcinoma cell line. *Endocrinology* 1986;118:1643.

57. Mendelsohn G, Eggleston JC, Weisburger WR, et al. Calcitonin and histaminase in C-cell hyperplasia and medullary thyroid carcinoma: a light microscopic and immunohistochemical study. *Am J Pathol* 1978;92:35.

58. Deftos LJ, Woloszczuk W, Krisch I, et al. Medullary thyroid carcinomas express chromogranin A and a novel neuroendocrine protein recognized by monoclonal antibody HISL-19. *Am J Med* 1988;85:780.

59. Keusch G, Binswanger U, Dambacher MA, et al. Ectopic ACTH syndrome and medullary thyroid carcinoma. *Acta Endocrinol (Copenh)* 1977;86:306.

60. Zeytinoglu FN, Gagel RF, Tashjian AH Jr, et al. Characterization of neurotensin production by a line of rat medullary thyroid carcinoma cells. *Proc Natl Acad Sci U S A* 1980;77:3741.

61. Yamaguchi K, Abe K, Adachi I, et al. Concomitant production of immunoreactive gastrin-releasing peptide and calcitonin in medullary carcinoma of the thyroid. *Metabolism* 1984;33:724.

62. Rosenberg EM, Hahn TJ, Orth DN, et al. ACTH-secreting medullary carcinoma of the thyroid presenting a severe idiopathic osteoporosis and senile purpura: report of a case and review of the literature. *J Clin Endocrinol Metab* 1978;47:255.

63. Hazard JB. The C-cells (parafollicular cells) of the thyroid gland and medullary thyroid carcinoma: a review. *Am J Pathol* 1977;88:214.

64. Sletten K, Westermark P, Natvig JB. Characterization of amyloid fibril proteins from medullary carcinoma of the thyroid. *J Exp Med* 1976;143:993.

65. Wolfe HJ, DeLellis RA. Familial medullary thyroid carcinoma and C-cell hyperplasia. *Clin Endocrinol Metab* 1981;10:351.

66. Fadda G, LiVolsi VA. Histology and fine-needle aspiration cytology of malignant thyroid neoplasms. *Rays* 2000;25:139.

67. Cohen MS, Phay JE, Albinson C, et al. Gastrointestinal manifestations of multiple endocrine neoplasia type 2. *Ann Surg* 2002;235:648.

68. Cox TM, et al. Role of calcitonin in diarrhoea associated with medullary carcinoma of the thyroid. *Gut* 1979;20:629.

69. Aldrich LB, Moattari AR, Vinik AI. Distinguishing features of idiopathic flushing and carcinoid syndrome. *Arch Intern Med* 1988;148:2614.

70. Andry G, Wildschutz T, Chantrain G, et al. Elevated CEA in breast cancer patients with overlooked medullary thyroid carcinoma. *Eur J Surg Oncol* 1993;19:305.

71. Moley JF, DeBenedetti MK. Patterns of nodal metastases in palpable medullary thyroid carcinoma: recommendations for extent of node dissection. *Ann Surg* 1999;229:880.

72. Moley JF, Wells SA. Compartment-mediated dissection for papillary thyroid cancer. *Langenbecks Arch Surg* 1999;384:9.

73. Fleming JB, Lee JE, Bouvet M, et al. Surgical strategy for the treatment of medullary thyroid carcinoma. *Ann Surg* 1999;230:697.

74. Tung WS, Vesely TM, Moley JF. Laparoscopic detection of hepatic metastases in patients with residual or recurrent medullary thyroid cancer. *Surgery* 1995;118:1024.

75. Sipple JH. Multiple endocrine neoplasia type 2 syndromes: historical perspectives. *Henry Ford Hosp Med J* 1984;32:219.

76. Steiner AL, Goodman AD, Powers SR. Study of a kindred with pheochromocytoma, medullary carcinoma, hyperparathyroidism and Cushing's disease: multiple endocrine neoplasia, type 2. *Medicine (Baltimore)* 1968;47:371.

77. Williams ED, Brown CL, Doniach I. Pathological and clinical findings in a series of 67 cases of medullary carcinoma of the thyroid. *J Clin Pathol* 1966;19:103.

78. Rashid M, Khairi MR, Dexter RN, et al. Mucosal neuroma, pheochromocytoma and medullary thyroid carcinoma: multiple endocrine neoplasia type 3. *Medicine (Baltimore)* 1975;54:89.

79. Carney JA, Hayles AB. Alimentary tract manifestations of multiple endocrine neoplasia, type 2b. *Mayo Clin Proc* 1977;52:543.

80. Carney JA, Go VL, Sizemore GW, et al. Alimentary-tract ganglioneuromatosis. A major component of the syndrome of multiple endocrine neoplasia, type 2b. *N Engl J Med* 1976;295:1287.

81. Dyck PJ, Carney JA, Sizemore GW, et al. Multiple endocrine neoplasia, type 2b: phenotype recognition: neurological features and their pathological basis. *Ann Neurol* 1979;6:302.

82. Farndon JR, Leight GS, Dilley WG, et al. Familial medullary thyroid carcinoma without associated endocrinopathies: a distinct clinical entity. *Br J Surg* 1986;73:278.

83. Verdy M, Weber AM, Roy CC, et al. Hirschsprung's disease in a family with multiple endocrine neoplasia type 2. *J Pediatr Gastroenterol Nutr* 1982;1:603.

84. Gagel RF, Levy ML, Donovan DT, et al. Multiple endocrine neoplasia type 2a associated with cutaneous lichen amyloidosis. *Ann Intern Med* 1989;111:802.

85. Nunziata V, Giannattasio R, di Giovanni G, et al. Hereditary localized pruritus in affected members of a kindred with multiple endocrine neoplasia type 2A (Sipple's syndrome). *Clin Endocrinol (Oxf)* 1989;30:57.

86. Brandi ML, Gagel RF, Angeli A, et al. Guidelines for diagnosis and therapy of MEN type 1 and type 2. *J Clin Endocrinol Metab* 2001;86:5658.

87. Williams ED. A review of 17 cases of carcinoma of the thyroid and phaeochromocytoma. *J Clin Pathol* 1965;18:288.

88. Cooper CW, Deftos LJ, Potts JT Jr. Direct measurement of *in vivo* secretion of pig thyrocalcitonin by radioimmunoassay. *Endocrinology* 1971;88:747.

89. Hennessey JF, Gray TK, Cooper CW, et al. Stimulation of thyrocalcitonin secretion by pentagastrin and calcium in 2 patients with medullary thyroid carcinoma of the thyroid. *J Clin Endocrinol Metab* 1973;36:200.

90. Melvin KEW, Tashjian AH Jr, Miller HH. Studies in familial (medullary) thyroid carcinoma. *Rec Prog Horm Res* 1972;28:399.

91. Wolfe HJ, Melvin KEW, Cervi-Skinner SJ, et al. C-cell hyperplasia preceding medullary thyroid carcinoma. *N Engl J Med* 1973;289:437.

92. Graham SM, Genel M, Touloukian RJ, et al. Provocative testing for occult medullary carcinoma of the thyroid: findings in seven children with multiple endocrine neoplasia type IIa. *J Pediatr Surg* 1987;22:501.

93. Gill JR, Reyes-Mugica M, Iyengar S, et al. Early presentation of metastatic medullary carcinoma in multiple endocrine neoplasia, type IIA: implications for therapy. *J Pediatr* 1996;129:459.

94. Miller HH, Melvin KEW, Gibson JM, et al. Surgical approach to early familial medullary carcinoma of the thyroid gland. *Am J Surg* 1972;123:438.

95. Gagel RF, Tashjian AH Jr, Cummings T, et al. The clinical outcome of prospective screening for multiple endocrine neoplasia type 2a: an 18-year experience. *N Engl J Med* 1988;318:478.

96. Tisell L, Hansson G, Jansson S, et al. Reoperation in the treatment of asymptomatic metastasizing medullary thyroid carcinoma. *Surgery* 1986;99:60.

97. Moley JF, Debenedetti MK, Dilley WG, et al. Surgical management of patients with persistent or recurrent medullary thyroid cancer. *J Intern Med* 1998;243:521.

98. Moley JF, Wells SA, Dilley WG, et al. Reoperation for recurrent or persistent medullary thyroid carcinoma. *Surgery* 1993; 114:1090.

99. Lee JE, Curley SA, Gagel RF, et al. Cortical-sparing adrenalectomy for patients with bilateral pheochromocytoma. *Surgery* 1996;120:1064.

100. Brunt LM, Lairmore TC, Doherty GM, et al. Adrenalectomy for familial pheochromocytoma in the laparoscopic era. *Ann Surg* 2002;235:713.

101. Lairmore TC, Ball DW, Baylin SB, et al. Management of pheochromocytomas in patients with multiple endocrine neoplasia type 2 syndromes. *Ann Surg* 1993;217:595.

102. Gagel RF, Marx S. Multiple endocrine neoplasia. In: Larsen PR, Kronenberg H, Melmed S, et al., eds. *Williams textbook of endocrinology,* 10th ed. Philadelphia: WB Saunders, 2003:1717.

103. Borst M, Peacock BA, Minth C, et al. Mutational analysis of Hirschsprung's disease associated with multiple endocrine neoplasia type 2A [Abstract]. Presented at the Vth International Workshop on Multiple Endocrine Neoplasia, Stockholm, Sweden, 1994.

104. Borst MJ, Van Camp JM, Peacock ML, et al. Mutational analysis of multiple endocrine neoplasia type 2A associated with Hirschsprung's disease. *Surgery* 1995;117:386.

105. Wong C-K, Lin C-S. Friction amyloidosis. *Int J Dermatol* 1988;27:302.

106. Chabre O, Labat F, Pinel N, et al. Cutaneous lesion associated with multiple endocrine neoplasia type 2A: lichen amyloidosis or notalgia paresthetica. *Henry Ford Hosp J* 1992;40:245.

107. Williams ED, Pollock DJ. Multiple mucosal neuromata with endocrine tumours: a syndrome allied to Von Recklinghausen's disease. *J Pathol Bacteriol* 1966;91:71.

108. Aine E, Aine L, Huupponen T, et al. Visible corneal nerve fibers and neuromas of the conjunctiva-a syndrome of type-3 multiple endocrine adenomatosis in two generations. *Graefes Arch Clin Exp Ophthalmol* 1987;225:213.

109. Sizemore GW, Carney JA, Gharib H, et al. Multiple endocrine neoplasia type 2B: eighteen-year follow-up of a four-generation family. *Henry Ford Hosp J* 1992;40:236.

110. Carlson KM, Bracamontes J, Jackson CE, et al. Parent-of-origin effects in multiple endocrine neoplasia type 2B. *Am J Hum Genet* 1994;55:1076.

111. Carney JA, Sizemore GW, Hayles AB. Multiple endocrine neoplasia, type 2b. *Pathobiol Annu* 1978;8:105.

112. Stjernholm MR, Freudenbourg JC, Mooney HS, et al. Medullary carcinoma of the thyroid before age 2 years. *J Clin Endocrinol Metab* 1980;51:252.

113. Telander RL, Zimmerman D, van Heerden JA, et al. Results of early thyroidectomy for medullary thyroid carcinoma in children with multiple endocrine neoplasia type 2. *J Pediatr Surg* 1986;21:1190.

114. Vasen HFA, van der Feltz M, Raue F, et al. The natural course of multiple endocrine neoplasia type IIb: a study of 18 cases. *Arch Intern Med* 1992;152:1250.

115. Mathew CG, Chin KS, Easton DF, et al. A linked genetic marker for multiple endocrine neoplasia type 2A on chromosome 10. *Nature* 1987;328:527.

116. Simpson NE, Kidd KK, Goodfellow PJ, et al. Assignment of multiple endocrine neoplasia type 2A to chromosome 10 by linkage. *Nature* 1987;328:528.

117. Gattei V, Degan M, Aldinucci D, et al. Differential expression of the RET gene in human acute myeloid leukemia. *Ann Hematol* 1998;77:207.

118. Gattei V, Celetti A, Cerrato A, et al. Expression of the RET receptor tyrosine kinase and GDNFR-alpha in normal and leukemic human hematopoietic cells and stromal cells of the bone marrow microenvironment. *Blood* 1997;89:2925.

119. Nakayama S, Iida K, Tsuzuki T, et al. Implication of expression of GDNF/Ret signalling components in differentiation of bone marrow haemopoietic cells. *Br J Haematol* 1999;105:50.

120. Airaksinen MS, Saarma M. The GDNF family: signalling, biological functions and therapeutic value. *Nat Rev Neurosci* 2002; 3:383.

121. GFRa Nomenclature Committee. Nomenclature of GPI-linked receptors for the GDNF ligand family. *Neuron* 1997;19: 485.

122. Lindahl M, Timmusk T, Rossi J, et al. Expression and alternative splicing of mouse Gfra4 suggest roles in endocrine cell development. *Mol Cell Neurosci* 2000;15:522.

123. Enokido Y, de Sauvage F, Hongo JA, et al. GFR alpha-4 and the tyrosine kinase Ret form a functional receptor complex for persephin. *Curr Biol* 1998;8:1019.

124. Asai N, Iwashita T, Matsuyama M, et al. Mechansims of activation of the ret proto-oncogene by multiple endocrine neoplasia 2A mutations. *Mol Cell Biol* 1995;15:1613.

125. Santoro M, Carlomagno F, Romano A, et al. Activation of RET as a dominant transforming gene by germline mutations of MEN 2A and MEN 2B. *Science* 1995;267:381.

126. Asai N, Iwashita T, Murakami H, et al. Mechanism of Ret activation by a mutation at aspartic acid 631 identified in sporadic pheochromocytoma. *Biochem Biophys Res Commun* 1999;255: 587.

127. Ohiwa M, Murakami H, Iwashita T, et al. Characterization of Ret-Shc-Grb2 complex induced by GDNF, MEN 2A, and MEN 2B mutations. *Biochem Biophys Res Comm* 1997;237: 747.

128. Asai N, Murakami H, Iwashita T, et al. A mutation at tyrosine 1062 in MEN2A-Ret and MEN2B-Ret impairs their transforming activity and association with shc adaptor proteins. *J Biol Chem* 1996;271:17644.

129. Ishiguro Y, Iwashita T, Murakami H, et al. The role of amino acids surrounding tyrosine 1062 in *ret* in specific binding of the shc phosphotyrosine-binding domain. *Endocrinology* 1999; 140:3992.

130. Rossel M, Pasini A, Chappuis S, et al. Distinct biological properties of two RET isoforms activated by MEN 2A and MEN 2B mutations. *Oncogene* 1997;14:265.

131. De Vita G, Melillo RM, Carlomagno F, et al. Tyrosine 1062 of RET-MEN2A mediates activation of AKT (protein kinase B) and mitogen-activated protein kinase pathways leading to PC12 cell survival. *Cancer Res* 2000;60:3727.

132. Kurokawa K, Iwashita T, Murakami H, et al. Identification of SNT/FRS2 docking site on RET receptor tyrosine kinase and its role for signal transduction. *Oncogene* 2001;20:1929.

133. Hayashi Y, Iwashita T, Murakamai H, et al. Activation of BMK1 via tyrosine 1062 in RET by GDNF and MEN2A mutation. *Biochem Biophys Res Commun* 2001;281:682.

134. Chiariello M, Visconti R, Carlomagno F, et al. Signalling of RET receptor tyrosine kinase through the C-Jun NH2-terminal protein kinases (JNKS)—evidence for a divergence of the erks and jnks pathways induced by RET. *Oncogene* 1998;16: 2435.

135. Saavedra HI, Knauf JA, Shirokawa JM, et al. The RAS oncogene induces genomic instability in thyroid PCCL3 cells via the MAPK pathway. *Oncogene* 2000;19:3948.

136. Kimura ET, Nikiforova MN, Zhu Z, et al. High prevalence of BRAF mutations in thyroid cancer: genetic evidence for constitutive activation of the RET/PTC-RAS-BRAF signaling pathway in papillary thyroid carcinoma. *Cancer Res* 2003;63:1454.

137. Knauf JA, Kuroda H, Basu S, et al. RET/PTC-induced dedifferentiation of thyroid cells is mediated through Y1062 signaling through SHC-RAS-MAP kinase. *Oncogene* 2003;22:4406.

138. Strock CJ, Park JI, Rosen M, et al. CEP-701 and CEP-751 inhibit constitutively activated RET tyrosine kinase activity and block medullary thyroid carcinoma cell growth. *Cancer Res* 2003;63:5559.

139. Carlomagno F, Vitagliano D, Guida T, et al. ZD6474, an orally available inhibitor of KDR tyrosine kinase activity, efficiently blocks oncogenic RET kinases. *Cancer Res* 2002;62:7284.

140. Uchino S, Noguchi S, Adachi M, et al. Novel point mutations and allele loss at the RET locus in sporadic medullary thyroid carcinomas. *Jpn J Cancer Res* 1998;89:411.

141. Komminoth P, Roth J, Muletta-Feurer S, et al. RET protooncogene point mutations in sporadic neuroendocrine tumors. *J Clin Endocrinol Metab* 1996;81:2041.

142. Zedenius J, Larsson C, Bergholm U, et al. Mutations of codon 918 in the RET proto-oncogene correlate to poor prognosis in sporadic medullary thyroid carcinomas. *J Clin Endocrinol Metab* 1995;80:3088.

143. Schilling T, Burck J, Sinn HP, et al. Prognostic value of codon 918 (ATG→ACG) RET proto-oncogene mutations in sporadic medullary thyroid carcinoma. *Int J Cancer* 2001;95:62.

144. Scurini C, Quadro L, Fattoruso O, et al. Germline mutations and somatic mutations of the RET proto-oncogene in apparently sporadic medullary thyroid carcinoma. *Mol Cell Endocrinol* 1998;137:51.

145. Shirahama S, Ogura K, Takami H, et al. Mutational analysis of the RET proto-oncogene in 71 Japanese patients with medullary thyroid carcinoma. *J Hum Genet* 1998;43:101.

146. Marsh DJ, Learoyd DL, Andrew SD, et al. Somatic mutations in the RET proto-oncogene in sporadic medullary thyroid carcinoma. *Clin Endocrinol (Oxf)* 1996;44:249.

147. Uchino S, Noguchi S, Yamashita H, et al. Somatic mutations in RET exons 12 and 15 in sporadic medullary thyroid carcinomas: different spectrum of mutations in sporadic type from hereditary type. *Jpn J Cancer Res* 1999;90:1231.

148. Shan L, Nakamura M, Nakamura Y, et al. Somatic mutations in the RET protooncogene in Japanese and Chinese sporadic medullary thyroid carcinomas. *Jpn J Cancer Res* 1998;89:883.

149. Jindrichova S, Kodet R, Krskova L, et al. The newly detected mutations in the RET proto-oncogene in exon 16 as a cause of sporadic medullary thyroid carcinoma. *J Mol Med* 2003;81:819.

150. Eng C, Thomas GA, Neuberg DS, et al. Mutation of the RET proto-oncogene is correlated with RET immunostaining in subpopulations of cells in sporadic medullary thyroid carcinoma. *J Clin Endocrinol Metab* 1998;83:4310.

151. Eng C, Mulligan LM, Healey CS, et al. Heterogeneous mutation of the RET proto-oncogene in subpopulations of medullary thyroid carcinoma. *Cancer Res* 1996;56:2167.

152. Gimm O, Neuberg DS, Marsh DJ, et al. Over-representation of a germline RET sequence variant in patients with sporadic medullary thyroid carcinoma and somatic RET codon 918 mutation. *Oncogene* 1999;18:1369.

153. Elisei R, Cosci B, Romei C, et al. RET exon 11 (G691S) polymorphism is significantly more frequent in sporadic medullary thyroid carcinoma than in the general population. *J Clin Endocrinol Metab* 2004;89:3579.

154. Patocs A, Valkusz Z, Igaz P, et al. Segregation of the V804L mutation and S836S polymorphism of exon 14 of the RET gene in an extended kindred with familial medullary thyroid cancer. *Clin Genet* 2003;63:219.

155. Griseri P, Pesce B, Patrone G, et al. A rare haplotype of the RET proto-oncogene is a risk-modifying allele in Hirschsprung disease. *Am J Hum Genet* 2002;71:969.

156. Koch CA, Huang SC, Moley JF, et al. Allelic imbalance of the mutant and wild-type RET allele in MEN 2A-associated medullary thyroid carcinoma. *Oncogene* 2001;20:7809.

157. Huang SC, Koch CA, Vortmeyer AO, et al. Duplication of the mutant RET allele in trisomy 10 or loss of the wild-type allele in multiple endocrine neoplasia type 2-associated pheochromocytomas. *Cancer Res* 2000;60:6223.

158. Huang SC, Torres-Cruz J, Pack SD, et al. Amplification and overexpression of mutant RET in multiple endocrine neoplasia type 2-associated medullary thyroid carcinoma. *J Clin Endocrinol Metab* 2003;88:459.

159. Quadro L, Fattoruso O, Cosma MP, et al. Loss of heterozygosity at the RET protooncogene locus in a case of multiple endocrine neoplasia type 2A. *J Clin Endocrinol Metab* 2001;86:239.

160. Zhang Z, Wang Y, Vikis HG, et al. Wildtype Kras2 can inhibit lung carcinogenesis in mice. *Nat Genet* 2001;29:25.

161. Zhuang Z, Park WS, Pack S, et al. Trisomy 7-harbouring non-random duplication of the mutant MET allele in hereditary papillary renal carcinomas. *Nat Genet* 1998;20:66.

162. Khosla S, Patel VM, Hay ID, et al. Loss of heterozygosity suggests multiple genetic alterations in pheochromocytmoas and medullary thyroid carcinomas. *J Clin Invest* 1991;87:1691.

163. Cooley LD, Elder FF, Knuth A, et al. Cytogenetic characterization of three human and three rat medullary thyroid carcinoma cell lines. *Cancer Genet Cytogenet* 1995;80:138.

164. Moley JF, Brother MB, Fong CT, et al. Consistent association of 1p loss of heterozygosity with pheochromocytomas from patients with multiple endocrine neoplasia type 2 syndromes. *Cancer Res* 1992;52:770.

165. Takai S, Tateishi H, Nishisho I, et al. Loss of genes on chromosome 22 in medullary thyroid carcinoma and pheochromocytoma. *Jpn J Cancer Res* 1987;78:894.

166. Eng C, Clayton D, Schuffenecker I, et al. The relationship between specific RET proto-oncogene mutations and disease phenotype in multiple endocrine neoplasia type 2. International RET Mutation Consortium analysis. *JAMA* 1996;276:1575.

167. Angrist M, Bolk S, Thiel B, et al. Mutation analysis of the RET receptor tyrosine kinase in Hirschsprung disease. *Hum Mol Genet* 1995;4:821.

168. Eng C, Smith DP, Mulligan LM, et al. Point mutation within the tyrosine kinase domain of the RET proto-oncogene in multiple endocrine neoplasia type 2B and related sporadic tumours. *Human Mol Genet* 1994;3:237.

169. Maruyama S, Iwashita T, Imai T, et al. Germ line mutations of the ret proto-oncogene in Japanese patients with multiple endocrine neoplasia type 2A and type 2B. *Jpn J Cancer Res* 1994;85:879.

170. Hofstra RM, Landsvater RM, Ceccherini I, et al. A mutation in the RET proto-oncogene associated with multiple endocrine neoplasia type 2B and sporadic medullary thyroid carcinoma. *Nature* 1994;367:375.

171. Gimm O, Marsh DJ, Andrew SD, et al. Germline dinucleotide mutation in codon 883 of the RET proto-oncogene in multiple endocrine neoplasia type 2B without codon 918 mutation. *J Clin Endocrinol Metab* 1997;82:3902.

172. Smith DP, Houghton C, Ponder BA. Germline mutation of RET codon 883 in two cases of de novo MEN 2B. *Oncogene* 1997;15:1213.

173. Bolino A, Schuffenecker I, Luo Y, et al. RET mutations in exons 13 and 14 of FMTC patients. *Oncogene* 1995;10:2415.

174. Eng C, Smith DP, Mulligan LM, et al. A novel point mutation in the tyrosine kinase domain of the RET proto-oncogene in sporadic medullary thyroid carcinoma and in a family with FMTC. *Oncogene* 1995;10:509.

175. Hofstra RM, Fattoruso O, Quadro L, et al. A novel point mutation in the intracellular domain of the ret protooncogene in a family with medullary thyroid carcinoma. *J Clin Endocrinol Metab* 1997;82:4176.

176. Berndt I, Reuter M, Saller B, et al. A new hot spot for mutations in the ret protooncogene causing familial medullary thyroid carcinoma and multiple endocrine neoplasia type 2A. *J Clin Endocrinol Metab* 1998;83:770.

177. Nilsson O, Tisell LE, Jansson S, et al. Adrenal and extra-adrenal pheochromocytomas in a family with germline RET V804L mutation. *JAMA* 1999;281:1587.

178. Jimenez C, Habra MA, Huang SC, et al. Pheochromocytoma and medullary thyroid carcinoma: a new genotype-phenotype correlation of the RET protooncogene 891 germline mutation. *J Clin Endocrinol Metab* 2004;89:4142.

179. Kalinin VN, Amosenko FA, Puskas C, et al. [A new inherited RET proto-oncogene mutation associated with familial medullary thyroid carcinoma and polymorphisms in adjacent regions.] *Genetika* 1998;34:1157.

180. Fugazzola L, Cerutti N, Mannavola D, et al. Multigenerational familial medullary thyroid cancer (FMTC): evidence for FMTC phenocopies and association with papillary thyroid cancer. *Clin Endocrinol (Oxf)* 2002;56:53.

181. Dang GT, Cote GJ, Schultz PN, et al. A codon 891 exon 15 RET proto-oncogene mutation in familial medullary thyroid carcinoma: a detection strategy. *Mol Cell Probes* 1999;13:77.

182. Frank-Raue K, Heimbach A, Rondot S, et al. [Hereditary medullary thyroid carcinoma—genotype-phenotype characterization]. *Dtsch Med Wochenschr* 2003;128:1998.

183. Jimenez C, Dang GT, Schultz PN, et al. A novel point mutation of the RET protooncogene involving the second intracellular tyrosine kinase domain in a family with medullary thyroid carcinoma. *J Clin Endocrinol Metab* 2004;89:3521.

184. Miyauchi A, Matsuzuka F, Hirai K, et al. Prospective trial of unilateral surgery for nonhereditary medullary thyroid carcinoma in patients without germline RET mutations. *World J Surg* 2002;26:1023.

185. Menko FH, van der Luijt RB, de Valk IA, et al. Atypical MEN type 2B associated with two germline RET mutations on the same allele not involving codon 918. *J Clin Endocrinol Metab* 2002;87:393.

185a. *www.ncbi.nlm.nih.gov/entrez/query.fcgi?–OMIM,* accessed September 26, 2004.

185b. *www.archive.uwcm.ac.uk/wucm/mg/hgmd0.html,* accessed September 26, 2004.

186. Pacini F, Fontanelli M, Fugazzola L, et al. Routine measurement of serum calcitonin in nodular thyroid diseases allows the preoperative diagnosis of unsuspected sporadic medullary thyroid carcinoma. *J Clin Endocrinol Metab* 1994;78:826.

187. Rieu M, et al. Routine measurement of serum calcitonin in patients with thyroid nodules for the detection of medullary thyroid carcinoma. *Clin Endocrinol (Oxf)* 1995;42:453.

188. Vierhapper H, Raber W, Bieglmayer C, et al. Routine measurement of plasma calcitonin in nodular thyroid diseases. *J Clin Endocrinol Metab* 1997;82:1589.

189. Ozgen AG, Hamulu F, Bayraktar F, et al. Evaluation of routine basal serum calcitonin measurement for early diagnosis of medullary thyroid carcinoma in seven hundred seventy-three patients with nodular goiter. *Thyroid* 1999;9:579.

190. Hahm JR, Lee MS, Min YK, et al. Routine measurement of serum calcitonin is useful for early detection of medullary thyroid carcinoma in patients with nodular thyroid diseases. *Thyroid* 2001;11:73.

191. Niccoli P, Wion-Barbot N, Caron P, et al. Interest in routine measurement of serum calcitonin: study of a large series of thyroidectomized patients. The French Medullary Study Group. *J Clin Endocrinol Metab* 1997;82:338.

192. Kaserer K, Scheuba C, Neuhold N, et al. C-cell hyperplasia and medullary thyroid carcinoma in patients routinely screened for serum calcitonin. *Am J Surg Pathol* 1998;22:722.

193. Karanikas G, Moameni A, Poetzi C, et al. Frequency and relevance of elevated calcitonin levels in patients with neoplastic and nonneoplastic thyroid disease and in healthy subjects. *J Clin Endocrinol Metab* 2004;89:515.

194. Karges W, Dralle H, Raue F, et al. Calcitonin measurement to detect medullary thyroid carcinoma in nodular goiter: German evidence-based consensus recommendation. *Exp Clin Endocrinol Diabetes* 2004;112:52.

195. Nylen ES, Snider RH Jr, Thompson KA, et al. Pneumonitis-associated hyperprocalcitoninemia. *Am J Med Sci* 1996;312:12.

196. Nylen ES, al Arifi A, Becker KL, et al. Effect of classic heat-stroke on serum procalcitonin. *Crit Care Med* 1997;25:1362.

197. Sosa JA, Bowman HM, Tielsch JM, et al. The importance of surgeon experience for clinical and economic outcomes from thyroidectomy. *Ann Surg* 1998;228:320.

198. Raffel A, Cupisti K, Krausch M, et al. Incidentally found medullary thyroid cancer: treatment rationale for small tumors. *World J Surg* 2004;28:397.

199. Cupisti K, Simon D, Wolf A, et al. Surgical treatment of postoperative, incidentally diagnosed small sporadic C-cell carcinomas of the thyroid. *Langenbecks Arch Surg* 2000;385:526.

200. Wiench M, Wygoda Z, Gubala E, et al. Estimation of risk of inherited medullary thyroid carcinoma in apparent sporadic patients. *J Clin Oncol* 2001;19:1374.

201. Eng C, Mulligan LM, Smith DP, et al. Low frequency of germline mutations in the RET proto-oncogene in patients with apparently sporadic medullary thyroid carcinoma. *Clin Endocrinol (Oxf)* 1995;43:123.

202. Zedenius J, Wallin G, Hamberger B, et al. Somatic and MEN 2A de novo mutations identified in the RET proto-oncogene by screening of sporadic MTCs. *Hum Mol Genet* 1994;3:1259.

203. Komminoth P, Kunz EK, Matias-Guiu X, et al. Analysis of RET proto-oncogene point mutations distinguishes heritable from nonheritable medullary thyroid carcinomas. *Cancer* 1995; 76:479.

204. Decker RA, Peacock ML, Borst MJ, et al. Progress in genetic screening of multiple endocrine neoplasia type 2A: Is calcitonin testing obsolete? *Surgery* 1995;118:257.

205. Saad MF, Ordonez NG, Rashid RK, et al. Medullary carcinoma of the thyroid: a study of the clinical features and prognostic factors in 161 patients. *Medicine (Baltimore)* 1984;63: 319.

206. Cohen MS, Moley JF. Surgical treatment of medullary thyroid carcinoma. *J Intern Med* 2003;253:616.

207. Machens A, Hinze R, Thomusch O, et al. Pattern of nodal metastasis for primary and reoperative thyroid cancer. *World J Surg* 2002;26:22.

208. Szakall S Jr, Esik O, Bajzik G, et al. 18F-FDG PET detection of lymph node metastases in medullary thyroid carcinoma. *J Nucl Med* 2002;43:66.

209. Boer A, Szakall S Jr, Klein I, et al. FDG PET imaging in hereditary thyroid cancer. *Eur J Surg Oncol* 2003;29:922.

210. Evans DB, Fleming JB, Lee JE, et al. The surgical treatment of medullary thyroid carcinoma. *Semin Surg Oncol* 1999;16:50.

211. Cote GJ, Gagel RF. Lessons learned from the management of a rare genetic cancer. *N Engl J Med* 2003;349:1566.

212. Machens A, Niccoli-Sire P, Hoegel J, et al. Early malignant progression of hereditary medullary thyroid cancer. *N Engl J Med* 2003;349:1517.

213. Lombardo F, Baudin E, Chiefari E, et al. Familial medullary thyroid carcinoma: clinical variability and low aggressiveness associated with RET mutation at codon 804. *J Clin Endocrinol Metab* 2002;87:1674.

214. Choi JS, Min JS. Significance of postoperative serum level of carcinoembryonic antigen (CEA) and actual half life of CEA in colorectal cancer patients. *Yonsei Med J* 1997;38:1.

215. Saad MF, Fritsche HAJ, Samaan NA. Diagnostic and prognostic values of carcinoembryonic antigen in medullary carcinoma of the thyroid. *J Clin Endocrinol Metab* 1984;58:889.

216. Schlumberger M, Gardet P, de Vathaire F, et al. External radiotherapy and chemotherapy in MTC patients. In: Calmettes C, Guliana JM, eds. *Medullary thyroid carcinoma.* Vol. 211. Montrouge, France: Colloques INSERM/John Libbey Eurotext, 1991:213.

217. Brierley J, Tsang R, Simpson WJ, et al. Medullary thyroid cancer: analyses of survival and prognostic factors and the role of radiation therapy in local control. *Thyroid* 1996;6:305.

218. Diez JJ, Iglesias P. Somatostatin analogs in the treatment of medullary thyroid carcinoma. *J Endocrinol Invest* 2002;25:773.

219. Castellani MR, Alessi A, Savelli G, et al. The role of radionuclide therapy in medullary thyroid cancer. *Tumori* 2003;89:560.

220. Juweid ME, Hajjar G, Swayne LC, et al. Phase I/II trial of (131)I-MN-14F(ab)2 anti-carcinoembryonic antigen monoclonal antibody in the treatment of patients with metastatic medullary thyroid carcinoma. *Cancer* 1999;85:1828.

221. Monsieurs M, Brans B, Bacher K, et al. Patient dosimetry for 131I-MIBG therapy for neuroendocrine tumours based on 123I-MIBG scans. *Eur J Nucl Med Mol Imaging* 2002;29:1581.

222. Di Bartolomeo M, Bajetta E, Bochicchio AM, et al. A phase II trial of dacarbazine, fluorouracil and epirubicin in patients with neuroendocrine tumours: a study by the Italian Trials in Medical Oncology (I.T.M.O.) Group. *Ann Oncol* 1995;6:77.

223. Schlumberger M, Abdelmoumene N, Delisle MJ, et al. Treatment of advanced medullary thyroid cancer with an alternating combination of 5 FU-streptozocin and 5 FU-dacarbazine: the Groupe d'Etude des Tumeurs a Calcitonine (GETC). *Br J Cancer* 1995;71:363.

224. Wu LT, Averbuch SD, Ball DW, et al. Treatment of advanced medullary thyroid carcinoma with a combination of cyclophosphamide, vincristine, and dacarbazine. *Cancer* 1994;73:432.

MISCELLANEOUS TUMORS OF THE THYROID

NICHOLAS J. SARLIS
LOUKAS GOURGIOTIS

The overwhelming majority of thyroid carcinomas are well-differentiated and belong to one of three distinct histopathologic types: papillary, follicular, and medullary thyroid carcinomas. In this chapter, we review less common types of thyroid tumors, each with unique biologic behavior and treatment correlates (Table 72.1). These tumors should also be taken into consideration in the differential diagnosis of thyroid nodules.

ANAPLASTIC THYROID CARCINOMA

Prevalence

Anaplastic thyroid carcinoma (ATC) represents only 1.6% of all thyroid cancers, with an annual incidence of 2 per million (1). Its peak incidence is during the sixth and seventh decades of life, and it has a female:male ratio of 1.5:1. The incidence of ATC has been declining steadily over the past 20 years, for reasons that are unclear (2). Whether this trend will continue in the future remains unknown, depending on the relative impact on ATC incidence of the opposite effects of an aging population versus earlier detection/therapy of PTC (from which many ATCs are thought to originate).

Clinical Presentation

ATC is one of the most aggressive cancers, with rapid growth and tendency for disseminated metastases. Hence, its initial presentation is typically explosive (rapidly enlarging neck mass, with or without tracheal, esophageal, or thoracic inlet compressive symptoms). The average size of the primary tumor at diagnosis is 8 cm (3). Direct invasion of adjacent structures is present in more than 90% of patients at presentation, and 50% of patients have distant metastases at that time. Another 40% will develop them during the course of the disease, with deposits mainly in the lungs, bones, and brain (2,3). All ATCs by convention are assigned as clinical "stage IV" in current staging systems. A few ATCs are found incidentally in thyroidectomy specimens, typically as microscopic foci within a resected PTC.

Initial Diagnosis

Fine-needle aspiration biopsy of the primary mass is the method of choice for diagnosis. ATCs can be subdivided into four types, depending on the prevalent morphology of the cells on surgical pathology: spindle (53%), giant-cell (40%), squamoid (2%), and mixed (5%) (3). There is no correlation of the above types with survival (4). At diagnosis, careful staging with appropriate diagnostic imaging studies is needed for definition of the sites of disease, both locoregional and distant. Serum markers used in the evaluation of other types of thyroid cancer [i.e., thyroglobulin (Tg), calcitonin, and carcinoembryonic antigen (CEA)] are typically not useful for diagnosis or follow-up of ATC, because this type of cancer usually does not express or secrete these proteins (3).

Pathogenesis

Ras oncogene mutations occur infrequently in ATCs, whereas mutations in the tumor suppression gene *p53* are commonly found (5). Overexpression of RCAS1 (an antigen that can reduce the vigor of immune responses against tumors) is also present in ATC (6). The molecular phenotype of ATCs is characterized in most cases by complete loss of expression of thyroid-specific molecules, such as Tg, the sodium-iodide symporter (NIS), the thyrotropin receptor (TSH-R), and thyroid transcription factor-1 (TTF-1), and up-regulation of proliferative markers, such as Ki-67 and proliferative cell nuclear antigen (PCNA) (5) (see section Oncogenes in Chapter 70).

Treatment

ATC is an almost universally fatal disease, with median survival from diagnosis ranging from 3 to 7 months (2,3).

TABLE 72.1. MISCELLANEOUS TUMORS OF THE THYROID GLAND

Anaplastic carcinoma
Lymphoma
Mucoepidermoid carcinoma (± sclerosing features & peritumoral eosinophilia)
Primary squamous-cell carcinoma
Teratoma (including malignant variant in adults)
Mesenchymal tumors
Langerhans cell histiocytosis
Plasmacytoma
Paraganglioma
Metastases from other cancers

Due to the loss of NIS expression, iodine 131 (radioiodine) therapy has no role in management. Similarly, due to the loss of the TSH-R (or downstream effectors), thyroid hormone suppression therapy is inconsequential to final outcome. Usually, a multimodality approach is used, involving tailored combinations of surgery, external beam radiation therapy and chemotherapy (7). ATC management has two goals: prevention of local complications by the primary tumor, such as asphyxiation or erosion of major vessels, and palliation from distant metastatic disease.

Surgery

The role of primary surgery in ATC remains controversial. At the time of diagnosis, almost all patients have extensive locoregional involvement. Thus, even if thyroidectomy and associated neck dissection are technically feasible, these procedures have a palliative rather than curative intent. In a series of patients who did not initially have distant metastases, those who underwent extensive surgical debulking had an improved 1-year survival versus those who did not (60% vs. 21%) (8). Similarly, patients who have undergone surgery with a curative intent (followed by radiotherapy and chemotherapy) had a median survival of 43 months, compared with 3 months in those who had only palliative resection (9). Both studies were small and they may have favored ATC patients with smaller or less aggressive tumors. In fact, a recent retrospective analysis found that neither the extent of the operation nor the achieved completeness of resection had any significant impact on survival; in this series, median survival was 2.3 months for patients with gross residual disease after operation, and 4 months for those with "complete" tumor resection (10), reflecting the impact of rapid development of metastases in both groups. In contradistinction to the above considerations for macroscopic ATCs, in the rare cases of microscopic ATC incidentally discovered in association with a PTC, total thyroidectomy followed by ^{131}I therapy, possibly in addition to external beam radiotherapy, is usually adequate for local disease control.

Radiotherapy

External electron beam radiotherapy at total doses of 55 to 60 Gy is used for local disease control. Minimally prolonged survival has been reported when the cumulative dose exceeded 45 Gy (11). Hyperfractionated radiotherapy (1–1.5 Gy twice daily up to a total of 30 to 40 Gy over 3 weeks) has also been given in combination with doxorubicin, bleomycin, cisplatin, or 5-fluorouracil (5-FU) (used as radiosensitizers), although toxicity was severe in up to 50% of patients treated with these combinations (12). In small, noncontrolled studies, chemo- and radiotherapy resulted in local control rates as high as 80% (13). Combinations of paclitaxel and external radiotherapy have not proven effective. Newer techniques, such as intensity-modulated radiotherapy (IMRT), may enhance precision of delivery of radiotherapy to the targeted area, while minimizing the side effects. A preliminary feasibility study of IMRT for ATC patients was reported recently (14).

Chemotherapy

None of the currently available chemotherapeutic regimens has been shown to alter the overall survival of patients with metastatic or residual ATC. Doxorubicin, when used as monotherapy, has disappointing response rates, with no patient having complete response (2). The combination of doxorubicin with cisplatin or bleomycin was not superior to doxorubicin alone in one study (15). More recently, paclitaxel (a microtubule formation inhibitor) has been used in ATC patients with persistent or metastatic disease. Ten of 19 patients had partial responses to paclitaxel. Although this agent resulted in significant slowing of the rate of progression of the disease in the subgroup of "responders," it did not prevent an eventual fatal outcome in any of the patients (16). Based on the above results with paclitaxel, a combination of paclitaxel (or docetaxel) and carboplatin has been used empirically in large cancer centers in the United States, again with no sustained antitumor responses. A long-lasting complete response was reported in a single patient with ATC during a phase I clinical trial using combretastatin A4-phosphate. This agent is believed to act through a combination of direct cytotoxicity and angiogenesis inhibition (17). Gemcitabine, a deoxycytidine analogue, with or without cis-platinum has been shown to induce apoptosis in cell lines derived from ATC (18), although there is no published clinical experience. Of note, many of the patients with ATC are elderly (>70 years) and typically tolerate chemotherapy or multimodality approaches poorly, due to age-associated comorbidities. The above notwithstanding, a few ATC patients do respond remarkably well to aggressive multimodality therapy; this was evident in the paclitaxel study where one "responder" survived for 15.3 months (16).

Novel Therapies

Because none of the current therapies substantially improve survival in ATC, novel treatment agents are being actively sought. Gene therapy with functional p53 (with or without chemotherapy) (19), or interleukin-2 (IL-2) combined with herpes simplex virus thymidine kinase (HSV-TK) (20) has shown promising results in preclinical ATC tumor models. Peroxisome proliferator-activated receptor-γ agonists (21) or farnesyl transferase inhibitors (22) are also promising in ATCs, affecting differentiation status and *ras* signaling, respectively. The histone deacetylase inhibitor depsipeptide led to a significant increase in the expression of Tg and NIS in cell lines derived from ATC (23). Clinical trials using the above compounds and other biologic modifiers are needed to assess their clinical utility in ATC patients.

Until these new agents become clinically available, for patients with ATC, we recommend the following approach: (a) for locoregional disease, surgery (if technically feasible) followed promptly by external beam radiotherapy (with or without chemosensitizers) and then chemotherapy; and (b) for disseminated disease, systemic chemotherapy. Both approaches should be applied in conjunction with frequent and complete restaging with the appropriate diagnostic imaging tests.

THYROID LYMPHOMA

Prevalence

Thyroid lymphoma is an uncommon disorder, constituting less than 2% to 3% of all non-Hodgkin's lymphomas (24). Women are most commonly affected, with a peak incidence in the sixth decade of life (24). An association with chronic lymphocytic (Hashimoto's) thyroiditis can be found in 40% to 80% of cases, with the lymphoma typically developing 20 to 30 years after the onset of thyroiditis (25).

Clinical Presentation

The usual presentation is a rapidly enlarging, painless neck mass with prominent obstructive symptoms. Cervical lymphadenopathy is present in 40% to 50% of patients (25). Type B symptoms (fever, night sweats, weight loss) can also occur. Most patients have high serum antithyroid antibody concentrations.

Initial Diagnosis

Lymphoma may be suspected on the basis of cytomorphologic criteria alone, but immunophenotype analysis of cytopathology specimens is needed to provide the definitive diagnosis, as well to determine both the lineage and clonality of the cell population with an accuracy rate between 85% and 100% (26). In patients with lymphoma first seen by an endocrinologist or a surgeon, prompt referral to a medical oncologist is needed for optimal management.

Upon diagnosis, clinical staging is important. Staging is performed according to the Ann Arbor classification and includes blood count, liver function tests, serum lactic dehydrogenase and β$_2$-microglobulin measurements, serum protein electrophoresis, chest and abdominopelvic CT scan, as well as biopsies of the bone marrow and other potential sites of lymphomatous spread (24). The main adverse clinical prognostic factors are the presence of mediastinal lymphadenopathy, a low patient performance status, and the presence of type B symptoms, whereas a previous diagnosis of Hashimoto's thyroiditis is a favorable factor (27).

Pathogenesis

The presence of long-standing Hashimoto's thyroiditis has been associated with a several-fold increase in the relative risk for lifetime development of thyroid lymphoma (24). On a molecular level, Fas and Fas ligand (FasL) mutations have been implicated in the pathogenesis of the thyroiditis, leading to accumulation of apoptosis-resistant lymphoid cells harboring these mutations (28). Clonal expansion/immortalization of such cell populations through cytokine-mediated stimulation is believed to give rise to the lymphoma (29,30).

Thyroid lymphoma is a heterogeneous disease. The lymphoid infiltrates in Hashimoto's thyroiditis bear great resemblance to mucosa-associated lymphoid tissue (MALT). Until the late 1980s, according to earlier classifications of non-Hodgkin's lymphomas (such as the "Working Formulation" system), almost all thyroid lymphomas were considered MALT lymphomas (MALT-L or MALTomas) (31). However, since the mid-1990s, they have been reclassified according to the Revised European-American Classification of Lymphoid Neoplasms (REAL) (32), as well as the World Health Organization (WHO) Classification for Neoplastic Diseases of the Lymphoid Tissues (33). In these classification systems, MALTomas are categorized as marginal zone B-cell lymphoma of MALT-type (MZBL) and are considered "low-grade" lymphomas. Transformation of MZBLs to a large-cell morphologic phenotype can give rise to diffuse large B-cell lymphoma (DLBCL). According to the REAL/WHO classification scheme, the most common thyroid lymphoma subtype is DLBCL, either transformed from MZBL or occurring as such *de novo* (24,34). DLBCLs are considered "high-grade" lymphomas. Other subtypes include mixed MZBL/ DLBCL, follicular lymphoma, Burkitt's lymphoma, small lymphocytic lymphoma, and Hodgkin's disease (34). Determination of the exact subtype is of paramount importance for prognosis, treatment, and follow-up.

Treatment

Treatment of thyroid lymphoma is controversial, since the rarity of this condition precludes the conduct of clinical trials comparing the various available therapies. In general, treatment depends on the stage of the lymphoma and its subtype.

Localized (stages I and II) MZBLs can be controlled with regional therapy alone (i.e., radiotherapy) or, more rarely, surgery (35). Although surgery can result in a 95% to 100% survival rate at 5 years (36), the currently preferred treatment is radiotherapy (total dose of 40 Gy to the neck and upper mediastinum), with a similar 5-year survival (27,37), mainly because of the lower risk for local complications with radiotherapy. Disseminated (stages III and IV) thyroid MZBLs can be treated with surgery, followed by chemotherapy with a single agent, usually oral chlorambucil (38). As mentioned above, most thyroid lymphomas belong to the DLBCL subtype. Localized DLBCLs have been treated in the past with an anthracycline-containing regimen, such as CHOP (doxorubicin/ cyclophosphamide/vincristine/prednisone) or CHOP-like combinations, administered along with radiotherapy, with a survival rate of more than 90% at 5 years (39). Disseminated DLBCLs are treated with CHOP or CHOP-like chemotherapy alone (39). New treatments for non-Hodgkin's lymphomas are currently available, including the combination of rituximab (an anti-CD20 monoclonal antibody) and CHOP (the "R-CHOP" scheme) (40), which shows a survival advantage over CHOP-based regimens.

MISCELLANEOUS UNUSUAL THYROID TUMORS

Thyroid Mucoepidermoid Carcinoma

Mucoepidermoid carcinomas are rare tumors, primarily involving the salivary glands, and histologically characterized by a combination of mucin-producing cells and cells with squamous features (41). Occasionally, a sclerosing reaction can be seen within such tumors, along with peritumoral eosophilic infiltrates (41). Mucoepidermoid tumors exhibit a biologic behavior similar to that of papillary carcinomas, with local tissue invasion and lymph node metastasis (41). Primary therapy consists of total thyroidectomy and neck dissection (if there is locoregional dissemination). Postoperative ^{131}I therapy is considered inefficacious. Some patients may benefit from external beam radiotherapy, either postoperatively or as a primary therapy in unresectable tumors (41).

Primary Thyroid Squamous-Cell Carcinoma

This is an extremely rare tumor (42). Its differential diagnosis includes thyroid metastasis from a squamous cell carcinoma in the upper aerodigestive tract. Immunohistochemical study of cytokeratin expression can help in the diagnosis (43). Primary squamous-cell thyroid cancer is considered a lethal tumor, with aggressiveness similar to that of ATC. Complete or partial excision of the tumor with postoperative radiotherapy and chemotherapy [with a *cis*-platinum/5-fluorouracil (5-FU) combination] may provide short-term palliation (44).

Thyroid Teratoma

Most teratomas of the thyroid are benign, and occur in neonates and children. Teratomas in adults are extremely rare and, in contrast to such tumors in children, highly malignant (45). Treatment with surgery, radiation, and chemotherapy (*cis*-platinum/vincristine/cyclophosphamide actinomycin-D) has been used in these tumors, although most patients survive less than 24 months after diagnosis (46).

Mesenchymal Thyroid Tumors

Thyroid Carcinosarcoma

Fewer than 20 cases of this tumor have been reported to date. This mixed lineage carcinoma arises from both epithelial and stromal elements (47). It occurs predominantly in elderly women and is almost uniformly fatal. Treatment is similar to that of ATC, with surgery (whenever feasible), radiotherapy, and *cis*-platinum- or ifosfamide-based chemotherapy (48).

Thyroid Angiosarcoma

Most of these rare sarcomas occur in the iodopenic Alpine region of Europe, where they may account for up to 16% of all thyroid cancers in this part of the world (49). In cases occurring outside the Alpine region, thyroid angiosarcoma has been associated with exposure to arsenic, thorium dioxide, polyvinylchloride, and radiation (50). The expression of endothelium-specific markers by the tumor, as well as specific electron microscopic criteria, has been helpful for distinguishing between thyroid angiosarcomas and ATCs with epithelioid differentiation (50), although without any significant impact on prognosis, which is poor. Indeed, most patients have extensive local invasion at the time of diagnosis. Surgery (whenever feasible), radiotherapy, and doxorubicin- or paclitaxel-based chemotherapy can provide palliation (51). Other rare primary thyroid mesenchymal tumors include osteosarcomas, hemangiopericytomas, and fibrosarcomas.

Langerhans Cell Histiocytosis

Langerhans cell histiocytosis is characterized by accumulation or proliferation of a clonal population of histiocytes with a specific immunophenotype, which includes expression of the CD1a antigen (52). Thyroidal histiocystosis is extremely rare, even when there is involvement of multiple other organs by the histiocytic process, with fewer than 40 published cases. It presents as a diffuse or nodular goiter; pain or compressive symptoms are unusual (53). Diagnosis by biopsy can be difficult, and the disorder can be easily confused with other conditions, such as HT, lymphoma, and ATC (53). Treatment of isolated thyroidal LCH involves surgery, with or without postoperative radiotherapy, usually with good response (53). In cases of widespread disease, a variety of chemotherapeutic and immunosuppressive agents have been tried, such as 2′-chlorodeoxyadenosine, cyclosporine, etoposide, azathioprine, and methotrexate (54).

Other Primary Thyroid Tumors

Thyroid Plasmacytoma

Primary (extramedullary) thyroid plasmacytomas are rare. Progression to multiple myeloma can be found in 17% to 32% of cases (55). Serum protein electrophoresis universally reveals a monoclonal gammopathy (56). Treatment consists of total thyroidectomy with postoperative radiotherapy, with good prognosis in patients in whom there is no progression to myeloma (56).

Thyroid Neuroendocrine Tumors

In addition to C-cell lesions (C-cell hyperplasia, medullary thyroid carcinoma, and mixed C-cell/follicular cell carcinoma), paragangliomas, chemodectomas, and metastases from extrathyroidal neuroendocrine tumors can also occur in the thyroid (57). Thyroid paragangliomas are uncommon and typically present as painless neck masses (57,58). Immunocytochemistry reveals neuroendocrine markers (e.g., chromogranin-A), with concomitant lack of expression of Tg, calcitonin, or CEA (58). The primary therapy is surgery. Most paragangliomas are benign, as evidenced by lack of local invasion or development of metastases, but there is a tendency for local recurrence. A few paragangliomas have a truly malignant phenotype. In locally invasive tumors, postoperative radiation therapy may be beneficial. In metastatic disease, combination chemotherapy (cisplatin/doxorubicin/cyclophosphamide/dacarbazine) has been tried with variable success (59). Of note, a few thyroid paragangliomas secrete catecholamines, and patients with these tumors should be screened with the appropriate biochemical tests (60).

Intrathyroidal Metastases

Although the presence of metastases of nonthyroid cancers in the thyroid gland is a common autopsy finding (0.5%–1.5%) in patients with a history of disseminated cancer, a thyroid metastasis is an uncommon clinical finding (61). The primary tumors are usually carcinomas of the lung, kidney, breast, and stomach, but metastases of primary carcinomas of the colon, uterus, oral cavity, esophagus, skin (melanoma), neuroendocrine tissue, and unknown origin, as well as sarcomas, are seen rarely (62). If technically feasible, thyroidectomy can be effective for local control. Systemic therapy should always be considered and should include the treatment of choice for the primary tumor. Regional measures, such as resection of additional (extrathyroidal) metastatic deposits and radiotherapy, may also be used for palliation. Survival time after diagnosis of the thyroid metastasis is determined by the biology of the primary disease, but is typically short (6–9 months) (63).

REFERENCES

1. Gilliland FD, Hunt WC, Morris DM, et al. Prognostic factors for thyroid carcinoma: a population-based study of 15,698 cases from the Surveillance, Epidemiology and End Results (SEER) program 1973–1991. *Cancer* 1997;79:564–573.
2. Ain KB. Anaplastic thyroid carcinoma: behavior, biology, and therapeutic approaches. *Thyroid* 1998;8:715–726.
3. Pasieka JL. Anaplastic thyroid cancer. *Curr Opin Oncol* 2003; 15:78–83.
4. Sugitani I, Kasai N, Fujimoto Y, et al. Prognostic factors and therapeutic strategy for anaplastic carcinoma of the thyroid. *World J Surg* 2001;25:617–622.
5. Sarlis NJ. Expression patterns of cellular growth-controlling genes in non-medullary thyroid cancer: basic aspects. *Rev Endocr Metab Disord* 2000;1:183–196.
6. Ito Y, Yoshida H, Nakano K, et al. Overexpression of human tumor-associated antigen, RCAS1, is significantly linked to dedifferentiation of thyroid carcinoma. *Oncology* 2000;64:83–89.
7. Busnardo B, Daniele O, Pelizzo MR, et al. A multimodality therapeutic approach in anaplastic thyroid carcinoma: study on 39 patients. *J Endocrinol Invest* 2000;23:755–761.
8. Sugino K, Ito K, Mimura T, et al. The important role of operations in the management of anaplastic thyroid carcinoma. *Surgery* 2002;131:245–248.
9. Haigh PI, Ituarte PH, Wu HS, et al. Completely resected anaplastic thyroid carcinoma combined with adjuvant chemotherapy and irradiation is associated with prolonged survival. *Cancer* 2001;91:2335–2342.
10. McIver B, Hay ID, Giuffrida DF, et al. Anaplastic thyroid carcinoma: a 50-year experience at a single institution. *Surgery* 2001;130:1028–1034.
11. Pierie JP, Muzikansky A, Gaz RD, et al. The effect of surgery and radiotherapy on outcome of anaplastic thyroid carcinoma. *Ann Surg Oncol* 2002;9:57–64.
12. Heron DE, Karimpour S, Grigsby PW. Anaplastic thyroid carcinoma: comparison of conventional radiotherapy and hyperfractionation chemoradiotherapy in two groups. *Am J Clin Oncol* 2002;25:442–446.
13. Tennvall J, Lundell G, Wahlberg P, et al. Anaplastic thyroid carcinoma: three protocols combining doxorubicin, hyperfractionated radiotherapy and surgery. *Br J Cancer* 2002;86:1848–1853.
14. Nutting CM, Convery DJ, Cosgrove VP, et al. Improvements in target coverage and reduced spinal cord irradiation using intensity-modulated radiotherapy (IMRT) in patients with carcinoma of the thyroid gland. *Radiother Oncol* 2001;60:173–180.

15. De Besi P, Busnardo B, Toso S, et al. Combined chemotherapy with bleomycin, adriamycin, and platinum in advanced thyroid cancer. *J Endocrinol Invest* 1991;14:475–480.

16. Ain KB, Egorin MJ, DeSimone PA. Treatment of anaplastic thyroid carcinoma with paclitaxel: phase 2 trial using ninety-six-hour infusion. Collaborative Anaplastic Thyroid Cancer Health Intervention Trials (CATCHIT) Group. *Thyroid* 2000;10:587–594.

17. Dowlati A, Robertson K, Cooney M, et al. A phase I pharmacokinetic and translational study of the novel vascular targeting agent combretastatin a-4 phosphate on a single-dose intravenous schedule in patients with advanced cancer. *Cancer Res* 2002; 62:3408–3416.

18. Ringel MD, Greenberg M, Chen X, et al. Cytotoxic activity of 2′,2′-difluorodeoxycytidine (gemcitabine) in poorly differentiated thyroid carcinoma cells. *Thyroid* 2000;10:865–869.

19. Nagayama Y, Yokoi H, Takeda K, et al. Adenovirus-mediated tumor suppressor p53 gene therapy for anaplastic thyroid carcinoma *in vitro* and *in vivo*. *J Clin Endocrinol Metab* 2000;85: 4081–4086.

20. Barzon L, Bonaguro R, Castagliuolo I, et al. Gene therapy of thyroid cancer via retrovirally-driven combined expression of human interleukin-2 and herpes simplex virus thymidine kinase. *Eur J Endocrinol* 2003;148:73–80.

21. Chung SH, Onoda N, Ishikawa T, et al. Peroxisome proliferator-activated receptor gamma activation induces cell cycle arrest via the p53-independent pathway in human anaplastic thyroid cancer cells. *Jpn J Cancer Res* 2002;93:1358–1365.

22. Xu G, Pan J, Martin C, et al. Angiogenesis inhibition in the *in vivo* antineoplastic effect of manumycin and paclitaxel against anaplastic thyroid carcinoma. *J Clin Endocrinol Metab* 2001;86: 1769–1777.

23. Kitazono M, Robey R, Zhan Z, et al. Low concentrations of the histone deacetylase inhibitor, depsipeptide (FR901228), increase expression of the Na(+)/I(-) symporter and iodine accumulation in poorly differentiated thyroid carcinoma cells. *J Clin Endocrinol Metab* 2001;86:3430–3435.

24. Ansell SM, Grant CS, Habermann TM. Primary thyroid lymphoma. *Semin Oncol* 1999;26:316–323.

25. Wirtzfeld DA, Winston JS, Hicks WL Jr, et al. Clinical presentation and treatment of non-Hodgkin's lymphoma of the thyroid gland. *Ann Surg Oncol* 2001;8:338–341.

26. Cha C, Chen H, Westra WH, et al. Primary thyroid lymphoma: can the diagnosis be made solely by fine-needle aspiration? *Ann Surg Oncol* 2002;9:298–302.

27. Belal AA, Allam A, Kandil A, et al. Primary thyroid lymphoma: a retrospective analysis of prognostic factors and treatment outcome for localized intermediate and high grade lymphoma. *Am J Clin Oncol* 2001;24:299–305.

28. Dong Z, Takakuwa T, Takayama H, et al. Fas and Fas ligand gene mutations in Hashimoto's thyroiditis. *Lab Invest* 2002;82: 1611–1616.

29. Takakuwa T, Dong Z, Takayama H, et al. Frequent mutations of Fas gene in thyroid lymphoma. *Cancer Res* 2001;61:1382–1385.

30. Takakuwa T, Nomura S, Matsuzuka F, et al. Expression of interleukin-7 and its receptor in thyroid lymphoma. *Lab Invest* 2000; 80:1483–1490.

31. Laing RW, Hoskin P, Hudson BV, et al. The significance of MALT histology in thyroid lymphoma: a review of patients from the BNLI and Royal Marsden Hospital. *Clin Oncol* 1994;6: 300–304.

32. Harris NL, Jaffe ES, Stein H, et al. A revised European-American classification of lymphoid neoplasms: a proposal from the International Lymphoma Study Group. *Blood* 1994;84:1361–1392.

33. Jaffe ES, Harris NL, Diebold J, et al. World Health Organization classification of neoplastic diseases of the hematopoietic and lymphoid tissues: a progress report. *Am J Clin Pathol* 1999;111 (suppl):8–12.

34. Kossev P, Livolsi V. Lymphoid lesions of the thyroid: review in light of the revised European-American lymphoma classification and upcoming World Health Organization classification. *Thyroid* 1999;9:1273–1280.

35. Cheson BD. Hematologic malignancies: new developments and future treatments. *Semin Oncol* 2002;29:33–45.

36. Sippel RS, Gauger PG, Angelos P, et al. Palliative thyroidectomy for malignant lymphoma of the thyroid. *Ann Surg Oncol* 2002; 9:907–911.

37. Tsang RW, Gospodarowicz MK, Pintilie M, et al. Localized mucosa-associated lymphoid tissue lymphoma treated with radiation therapy has excellent clinical outcome. *J Clin Oncol* 2003; 21:4157–4164.

38. Thieblemont C, Mayer A, Dumontet C, et al. Primary thyroid lymphoma is a heterogeneous disease. *J Clin Endocrinol Metab* 2002;87:105–111.

39. Martelli M, De Sanctis V, Avvisati G, et al. Current guidelines for the management of aggressive non-Hodgkin's lymphoma. *Drugs* 1997;53:957–972.

40. Avivi I, Robinson S, Goldstone A. Clinical use of rituximab in haematological malignancies. *Br J Cancer* 2003;89:1389–1394.

41. Rhatigan RM, Roque JL, Bucher RL. Mucoepidermoid carcinoma of the thyroid gland. *Cancer* 1997;39:210–214.

42. Simpson WJ, Carruthers J. Squamous cell carcinoma of the thyroid gland. *Am J Surg* 1988;156:44–46.

43. Lam KY, Lo CY, Liu MC. Primary squamous cell carcinoma of the thyroid gland: an entity with aggressive clinical behaviour and distinctive cytokeratin expression profiles. *Histopathology* 2001;39:279–286.

44. Zimmer PW, Wilson D, Bell N. Primary squamous cell carcinoma of the thyroid gland. *Milit Med* 2003;168:124–125.

45. Djalilian HR, Linzie B, Maisel RH. Malignant teratoma of the thyroid: review of literature and report of a case. *Am J Otolaryngol* 2000;21:112–115.

46. Chen JS, Lai GM, Hsueh S. Malignant thyroid teratoma of an adult: a long-term survival after chemotherapy. *Am J Clin Oncol* 1998;21:212–214.

47. Giuffrida D, Attard M, Marasa L, et al. Thyroid carcinosarcoma, a rare and aggressive histotype: a case report. *Ann Oncol* 2000; 11:1497–1499.

48. Al-Sobhi SS, Novosolov F, Sabanci U, et al. Management of thyroid carcinosarcoma. *Surgery* 1997;122:548–552.

49. Rhomberg W, Bohler FK, Eiter H, et al. Das maligne Hämangioendotheliom der Schilddrüse: Neue Resultate zur Pathogenese, Therapie und Prognose. [German] *Wien Klin Wochenschr* 1998; 110:479–484.

50. Goh SG, Chuah KL, Goh HK, et al. Two cases of epithelioid angiosarcoma involving the thyroid and a brief review of non-Alpine epithelioid angiosarcoma of the thyroid. *Arch Pathol Lab Med* 2003;127:E70–E73.

51. Yu J, Steiner FA, Muench JP, et al. Juxtathyroidal neck soft tissue angiosarcoma presenting as an undifferentiated thyroid carcinoma. *Thyroid* 2002;12:427–432.

52. Willman CL, Busque L, Griffith BB, et al. Langerhans' cell histiocytosis (histiocytosis X)—a clonal proliferative disease. *N Engl J Med* 1994;331:154–160.

53. Behrens RJ, Levi AW, Westra WH, et al. Langerhans cell histiocytosis of the thyroid: a report of two cases and review of the literature. *Thyroid* 2001;11:697–705.

54. Malpas JS. Langerhans cell histiocytosis in adults. *Hematol Oncol Clin North Am* 1998;12:259–268.

55. Kovacs CS, Mant MJ, Nguyen GK, et al. Plasma cell lesions of the thyroid: report of a case of solitary plasmacytoma and a review of the literature. *Thyroid* 1994;4:65–71.

56. Galieni P, Cavo M, Pulsoni A, et al. Clinical outcome of extra-medullary plasmacytoma. *Haematologica* 2000;85:47–51.

57. Baloch ZW, LiVolsi VA. Neuroendocrine tumors of the thyroid gland. *Am J Clin Pathol* 2001;115(suppl):56–67.

58. LaGuette J, Matias-Guiu X, Rosai J. Thyroid paraganglioma: a clinicopathologic and immunohistochemical study of three cases. *Am J Surg Pathol* 1997;21:748–753.

59. Patel SR, Winchester DJ, Benjamin RS. A 15-year experience with chemotherapy of patients with paraganglioma. *Cancer* 1995;76:1476–1480.

60. Erickson D, Kudva YC, Ebersold MJ, et al. Benign paragangliomas: clinical presentation and treatment outcomes in 236 patients. *J Clin Endocrinol Metab* 2001;86:5210–5216.

61. Nakhjavani MK, Gharib H, Goellner JR, et al. Metastasis to the thyroid gland: a report of 43 cases. *Cancer* 1997;79:574–578.

62. Lin JD, Weng HF, Ho YS. Clinical and pathological characteristics of secondary thyroid cancer. *Thyroid* 1998;8:149–153.

63. Rosen IB, Walfish PG, Bain J, et al. Secondary malignancy of the thyroid gland and its management. *Ann Surg Oncol* 1995;2:252–256.

73

CLINICAL EVALUATION AND MANAGEMENT OF SOLITARY THYROID NODULES

MICHAEL M. KAPLAN

Many people have thyroid nodules. Estimates of the prevalence depend on the method of detection. Combined data from several studies in which ultrasonography was used reveal a roughly linear increase in the prevalence of thyroid nodules from near zero at age 15 years, to 50% by about age 60 to 65 years, and to even higher in older people (1). Only about 10% of these nodules are palpable, even by experienced examiners (1,2). The dilemma for the physician is to identify the few patients who have thyroid nodules that need treatment from the vast majority in whom the nodules pose no harm. Optimally, the selection process will have high diagnostic accuracy, minimize medical costs and patient anxiety, and lead to treatment that will improve the patient's health.

The most important consideration in evaluating patients with thyroid nodules is whether the nodule is a thyroid carcinoma. In addition, some thyroid nodules, although benign, reflect processes that can cause thyrotoxicosis or, rarely, hypothyroidism, or require treatment because their size causes an unacceptable appearance or compression of nearby structures in the neck and upper chest. This chapter discusses solitary thyroid nodules, the most important types of which are listed in Table 73.1. However, the distinction between solitary thyroid nodules and multiple nodules is artificial, because about 50% of patients thought on the basis of physical examination to have a solitary nodule have multiple nodules when studied by ultrasonography (2,3). Moreover, the likelihood that an individual nodule is a carcinoma is not much less in patients with a multinodular goiter than it is in patients with a solitary nodule. With respect to thyroid carcinoma, the concern is primarily for differentiated tumors of follicular cell origin, because they are far more common than medullary or anaplastic carcinoma (see Chapters 71 and 72). Patients with the latter types of carcinoma (and thyroid lymphoma) may present in the same way, and fine-needle aspiration biopsy may provide the diagnosis in the same way as in patients with differentiated thyroid carcinoma.

CLINICAL EVALUATION

Most patients with thyroid carcinoma present with an asymptomatic thyroid nodule, as do most patients with be-

nign thyroid nodules. Some clinical findings (Table 73.2) have long been thought to increase the likelihood that a nodule is a carcinoma (1,4). However, the relationship between most of these findings and the presence of carcinoma is not strong. Also, most studies of these factors predate the widespread use of thyroid ultrasonography and biopsy. Some more recent studies are reviewed below. Lastly, there are few data relating clinical variables and cancer risk in patients with small thyroid nodules discovered incidentally.

A thyroid nodule is more likely to be a thyroid carcinoma in patients under age 20 years and those over 60 years of age than in those in between, but overall most patients with thyroid carcinoma are in the age group of 20 to 60 years. Benign thyroid nodules are four to five times more common in women than men, but thyroid carcinomas are only two to three times more common in women; thus, a nodule is more likely to be a carcinoma in a man. A history of a benign thyroid nodule or goiter may increase the risk that a new nodule is a carcinoma, but ascertainment bias probably explains this increase. Hashimoto's thyroiditis can cause nodules, as a result of scarring and localized areas of hyperplasia or lymphocytic infiltration, and in addition it strongly predisposes to the rare thyroid lymphomas (see Chapter 72). Cancer metastatic to the thyroid gland is rare; when present, the primary tumor is usually a renal cell, colon, or breast carcinoma.

Radiation therapy directed to the head, neck, and upper chest increases the risk of both benign thyroid nodules and thyroid carcinoma (see section on pathogenesis in Chapter 70). In the past, most patients with radiation-related thyroid carcinoma had received radiation therapy for benign conditions, such as thymic or tonsillar enlargement, acne, or birthmarks in infancy, childhood, or adolescence. Radiation therapy for these conditions largely ceased 30 to 40 years ago; now radiation-related thyroid carcinoma occurs mostly in patients who received radiation therapy for lymphoma or head and neck cancer, although a high incidence of thyroid carcinoma occurred in children exposed to fallout from the Chernobyl nuclear power plant explosion in 1986. Although some studies suggest that up to 30% of patients with thyroid nodules and a history of radiation exposure in early childhood who undergo surgery have thyroid carcinoma, some of

TABLE 73.1. TYPES OF THYROID NODULES

Benign
  Adenomatous nodule (also called colloid nodule and
    hyperplastic nodule)
  Follicular adenoma
  Hürthle-cell adenoma
  Lymphocytic thyroiditis
  Thyroglossal duct cyst
Malignant
  Carcinomas of thyroid follicular-cell origin
    Papillary carcinoma
    Follicular carcinoma
    Hürthle-cell carcinoma
    Anaplastic carcinoma
  Carcinoma of C-cell origin
    Medullary carcinoma
  Lymphoma
  Cancer metastatic to the thyroid
Non-thyroid lesions
  Parathyroid cyst and adenoma
  Lymph node
  Branchial cleft cyst and other epithelial cysts

the carcinomas were incidental microcarcinomas distant from the nodule that prompted the surgery.

Large thyroid nodules, benign or malignant, can distort surrounding structures in the neck or upper mediastinum, causing difficulty breathing, shortness of breath or cough from tracheal compression, or difficulty swallowing from esophageal compression. The presence of these symptoms may increase the likelihood that a nodule is a carcinoma, but most carcinomas are small and do not cause these symptoms. Similarly, hoarseness or a change in voice can

TABLE 73.2. CLINICAL FINDINGS RELATED TO RISK OF CARCINOMA IN A THYROID NODULE

Age <20 or >60 years
Men > women (in terms of proportion of nodules that are a
  carcinoma)
History of benign or malignant thyroid disease
History of other cancer, especially kidney, breast, and colon
History of head or neck irradiation
Symptoms of possible compression of structures adjacent to
  the thyroid gland:
  Hoarseness or other change in voice
  Difficulty breathing
  Cough
  Dysphagia
Family history of benign or malignant thyroid disease,
  pheochromocytoma, hyperparathyroidism, familial
  adenomatous polyposis coli, Gardner's syndrome,
  Cowden's disease
Large size of nodule
Fixed nodule
Firm or hard nodule
Pain or tenderness in or around the nodule
Lymphadenopathy
Rapid growth
Growth during thyroid hormone treatment

be caused by infiltration or compression of the recurrent laryngeal nerve by a thyroid carcinoma, but other causes of a change in voice are much more common.

The family history is sometimes relevant. From 4% to 8% of patients with papillary thyroid carcinoma have a family history of the same tumor, although the genetics are not understood. In familial adenomatous polyposis and its variant, Gardner's syndrome, and in Cowden's disease, also called the multiple hamartoma syndrome, the prevalence of benign thyroid nodules and thyroid carcinoma is increased (see section Pathogenesis in Chapter 70). Medullary thyroid carcinoma can be familial (see Chapter 71), as part of the multiple endocrine neoplasia type 2 and related syndromes, in which there is a very high penetrance of medullary carcinoma, and less often pheochromocytoma and primary hyperparathyroidism.

Large nodules, nodules fixed to the surrounding tissue, and very firm nodules tend to be carcinomas, but some benign nodules have a calcified shell that makes them very hard. Some thyroid carcinomas are tender or cause pain, but these findings are much more likely to be caused by hemorrhage into a benign nodule. Subacute granulomatous thyroiditis is another cause of thyroid pain, usually bilateral but occasionally starting in one lobe and then affecting the other lobe. Rapid growth of a nodule is of concern, but the sudden appearance or increase in size of a nodule in a day or less is almost always due to hemorrhage into a benign nodule. Growth of a nodule during follow-up or thyroid hormone treatment has traditionally been considered to suggest that the nodule is a carcinoma, but benign nodules also grow (5). Conversely, some carcinomas do not grow during follow-up. The presence of cervical lymphadenopathy suggests that a thyroid nodule is a carcinoma.

Some clinical risk factors for thyroid carcinoma have been analyzed in several studies of patients who had surgery, partly on the basis of suspicious needle biopsy results (6–11). Four of these studies were retrospective, and none evaluated the putative risk factors prospectively in a separate set of patients, either in patients with inconclusive or suspicious biopsy results or those in whom biopsy revealed only benign thyroid cells. Despite these limitations, the studies consistently indicate that nodules that are fixed to surrounding structures and nodules that are larger than 4 cm in diameter are likely to be carcinomas. In three studies, age less than 20 years was a risk factor for carcinoma. The results were inconsistent with respect to whether the risk for carcinoma was higher in men, patients over 60 years of age, patients with rapidly growing nodules, those with solitary or multiple nodules, and patients in whom the nodule was firm in consistency.

LABORATORY EVALUATION

Serum Hormone and Other Measurements

Serum thyrotropin (TSH) should be measured in all patients with thyroid nodules (Table 73.3), to determine if

TABLE 73.3. DIAGNOSTIC TESTS FOR THYROID NODULES

Serum tests
  TSH, for assessment of thyroid function
  Antithyroid antibodies, for identification of autoimmune
    thyroiditis
  Calcitonin, for identification of medullary carcinoma
Imaging
  Scintiscanning
  Ultrasonography
  Computed tomography
  Magnetic resonance imaging
  Positron emission tomography
Fine-needle biopsy

the patient has an autonomously functioning thyroid adenoma causing subclinical thyrotoxicosis, and to identify unsuspected hypothyroidism, which may or may not be related to the patient's nodules. Measurements of serum antithyroid peroxidase antibodies may be indicated to distinguish between Hashimoto's thyroiditis and Hürthle-cell tumors; biopsies of both may contain many Hürthle cells. Measurements of serum thyroglobulin have little value in patients with thyroid nodules; the values may be normal or high in patients with either benign nodules or carcinoma.

Measurement of serum calcitonin is indicated in patients with a nodule if there is a family history of medullary thyroid cancer or other components of the multiple endocrine neoplasia type 2 syndrome, or a family history of thyroid carcinoma in which the type is not known. Some have recommended that serum calcitonin be measured in all patients with thyroid nodules, to identify patients with sporadic medullary carcinoma. In a study of 10,864 patients with thyroid nodules, 0.4% had high serum calcitonin concentrations and proved to have medullary thyroid carcinoma (12). However, about two thirds of those patients had suspicious needle biopsy results, and only 15 medullary thyroid carcinomas were identified solely by measurement of serum calcitonin (1 in 724 patients). In other, similar studies, measurements of serum calcitonin have identified patients with medullary carcinoma, but other patients with high serum calcitonin concentrations did not have medullary carcinoma (13). Because of the possibility of false-positive results and the lack of standardization of the measurement, it has not been widely adopted in the United States.

Imaging Tests

Radionuclide Imaging

About 5% to 10% of thyroid nodules are autonomously functioning thyroid nodules, nearly all of which are adenomas (14). In some of these tumors, activating mutations of the TSH receptor (15) or the G (guanine nucleotide-bind-ing) protein that links the TSH receptor with adenylyl cyclase (16) cause the TSH-independent function. In patients with thyroid nodules who have low serum TSH concentrations, a thyroid scintiscan, preferably with iodine 123, should be done to determine if the nodule is hyperfunctioning, that is, if it concentrates the radionuclide more than the rest of the thyroid gland (a so-called "hot" nodule) (see Chapter 12). If so, biopsy is not necessary unless there are findings suspicious of carcinoma, such as rapid growth or hypofunctioning areas within the nodule. In the past, a scintiscan was usually the first imaging study done in patients with thyroid nodules. However, since hyperfunctioning nodules are uncommon and scintiscans do not distinguish between benign and malignant hypofunctioning nodules, a scintiscan should be performed before needle biopsy only in patients with low serum TSH concentrations. If the practice is to biopsy all nodules, a scintiscan may be indicated in patients in whom the biopsy reveals a follicular tumor, because some autonomously functioning adenomas have this cytology (17), do not secrete enough thyroid hormone to lower TSH secretion, especially if less than 2.5 cm in diameter (14), and yet are active enough to be revealed as hyperfunctioning by scintiscan. The risk for carcinoma is low in this subset of patients, just as it is in those patients with an adenoma who have low serum TSH concentrations.

Ultrasonography

Thyroid ultrasonography is now widely used for evaluation of patients with thyroid nodules (see Chapter 16), although the most appropriate role of this test in the evaluation of patients with an apparently solitary thyroid nodule is not yet certain. The use of ultrasound guidance to perform needle biopsies of thyroid nodules is discussed later. Those who advocate diagnostic ultrasonography in all patients with a solitary nodule on physical examination argue that about 50% of the patients have other, nonpalpable nodules (4), and that some or even many of them are large enough to warrant biopsy, the latter depending on the size threshold considered to warrant biopsy.

For the most part, the ultrasonographic features of benign nodules and carcinomas are similar, but certain features increase the likelihood that a nodule is a carcinoma (18). These features are diffuse microcalcifications, hypoechogenicity, an irregular margin indicative of invasive growth, an irregular sonolucent halo or no halo around the nodule, and regional lymphadenopathy. However, calcifications and invasiveness are uncommon, even in malignant nodules. A search for lymph nodes is often omitted, but should be done routinely. Findings that make it unlikely that a nodule is a carcinoma are the presence of a well-defined sonolucent halo and a regular margin, and coarse calcification within the nodule or a rim of calcification surrounding the nodule. However, there are no ultrasound characteristics that definitively exclude carcinoma and therefore render biopsy unnecessary. Nonetheless, the ultrasonographic characteristics of a nodule may be of use in estimating cancer risk in patients in whom needle biopsy was inadequate and those who are hesitant to undergo or prefer to delay biopsy.

Thyroid ultrasonography has important limitations (18,19). The procedure is very operator dependent, and ultrasound reports often lack crucial information, such as the dimensions of nodules in all three planes (length, width, and depth), the location of a nodule in the thyroid lobe, comments about density or calcification, the appearance of the border of the nodule, and the presence of lymph nodes. Ultrasonography is usually performed as a diagnostic test, with no intent on the part of the ordering physician to have a biopsy done or no capability for biopsy at the ultrasound facility. Patients are better served if ultrasonography is done under conditions in which biopsy can be performed immediately if indicated. The operator must be interested in and knowledgeable about thyroid nodules, know what to look for, and be able to use the results to perform needle biopsy at the same time.

Computed tomography (CT), magnetic resonance imaging (MRI), and positron emission tomography (PET) using 19-fluorodeoxyglucose have no established role in the evaluation of patients with thyroid nodules. These tests are listed in Table 73.3 only because in some patients thyroid nodules are discovered when the test was performed for other reasons. A single thyroid nodule identified on a PET scan may be a carcinoma, but some benign nodules and Hashimoto's thyroiditis take up substantial quantities of 19-fluorodeoxyglucose as well.

FINE-NEEDLE BIOPSY

Fine-needle biopsy, which yields single cells or clumps of cells, is the standard test to determine whether a thyroid nodule is benign or malignant, and the test also has other uses (Table 73.4). It is often called fine-needle aspiration biopsy, but the more general term will be used here because aspiration by negative pressure is not always used. The pri-

mary goal of fine-needle biopsy is to reduce the number of unnecessary thyroid operations, by identifying those nodules that are benign or at least unlikely to be malignant. For this purpose, fine-needle biopsy is far more accurate than any other available test or combination of tests. Before the procedure was introduced, about half of patients with palpable thyroid nodules were referred for operation, but only about one fourth of those who underwent surgery had thyroid carcinoma. Hence, many patients with benign nodules were subjected to the costs, morbidity, and, rarely, risk for mortality of surgery (20, 21).

The use of fine-needle biopsy can reduce the proportion of nodules for which surgery is advised to less than 20%; at the same time, the proportion of resected nodules that are malignant is 50% or even higher. When an adequate sample is obtained, the reliability of fine-needle biopsy for excluding carcinoma is 98% to 99%. The second main use of fine-needle biopsy is to help plan the extent of surgery. Large-needle biopsy, which provides cores or fragments of tissue for conventional histologic evaluation, is rarely used now. Details of the methods can be found elsewhere (22).

Selection of Patients

Fine-needle biopsy is the most appropriate test for almost all patients with thyroid nodules, the exception being patients suspected to have an autonomously functioning thyroid adenoma. Biopsy is usually advised if the maximal diameter of the nodule is 1 cm or higher (23,24), but some researchers suggest a threshold of 1.5 or 2.0 cm (25,26). This distinction depends in part on the method of ascertainment. Nodules smaller than 1.5 cm are often not palpable, whereas much smaller nodules can be detected by ultrasonography. Even if ultrasonography is performed, or the nodule is detected incidentally when an imaging study of the neck is done for another purpose, nodules smaller than 1 cm in diameter are often not biopsied. The rationales for this threshold are that smaller nodules are so common that it is impractical to refer all of them for biopsy, and the risk for missing a carcinoma that will have adverse health consequences is low. Many people have small thyroid carcinomas that never become evident during life and cause no health problems. The prevalence of thyroid carcinoma at autopsy is about 4% in the United States (25), where there are currently about 2.5 million deaths per year, fewer than 24,000 incident cases of thyroid carcinoma diagnosed per year, and fewer than 1,500 deaths from thyroid carcinoma per year (27). Furthermore, among patients with thyroid carcinoma, the outcome is strongly influenced by the size of the tumor at the time of diagnosis: the life expectancy of patients with a tumor that is smaller than 1 cm in diameter is the same as that of the general population (see section Radioiodine and Other Treatments and Outcomes in Chapter 70).

TABLE 73.4. USES OF THYROID NEEDLE BIOPSY

Common
  Selection of therapy for a thyroid nodule
    Surgery versus observation
    Extent of surgery
Less common
  Diagnosis of the cause of thyroid enlargement
  Removal of fluid or blood from a cystic nodule
  Injection of a sclerosing agent for a recurrent cyst
  Ablation of a nodule by ethanol injection or laser
    coagulation
  Postoperative evaluation of cervical lymph nodes
  Diagnosis of infective thyroiditis

As noted above, incidental thyroid nodules may be detected by ultrasonography or other imaging procedures performed to evaluate neck structures other than the thyroid gland, or by thyroid ultrasonography done to evaluate neck pain, difficulty swallowing, or a known thyroid abnormality. Most of these nodules are too small to be detected by palpation, Others are located in the middle of a thyroid lobe (and do not distort its shape), or behind or below the lobe (28); have a soft consistency; or are hidden by subcutaneous fat, prominent neck muscles, or kyphosis of the cervical spine. These factors are independent of the biology of the nodule, and therefore it is likely that a nonpalpable nodule is a carcinoma as often as is a palpable nodule of the same size. The available data support this conclusion. Among patients with nonpalpable, incidentally discovered thyroid nodules who have undergone fine-needle biopsy—by necessity ultrasound-guided—4% to 10% have had thyroid carcinoma (3,29–32), very similar to the results in patients with palpable nodules. Therefore, the evaluation, including the size cut-off for biopsy, should be the same no matter how the nodule was detected.

Fine-needle biopsy is advisable in patients with a multinodular goiter who have a discrete hypofunctioning nodule within the goiter or a nodule of uncertain functional status that is growing, and patients with a partially cystic nodule after fluid has been removed. The prevalence of carcinoma in these nodules is similar to that in solitary solid nodules (3,6,7). Fine-needle biopsy is also indicated when a hypofunctioning area is seen in an otherwise hyperfunctioning nodule, although the great majority of these areas represent central degeneration within the nodule, not carcinoma. A few patients with thyrotoxicosis caused by Graves' disease also have hypofunctioning nodules, whether detected by palpation or scintiscan; these nodules should be biopsied because some are carcinomas. Patients treated with head and neck radiation for nonthyroid conditions, or accidentally exposed to radiation, who have thyroid nodules should be evaluated by biopsy like any other patient; biopsy results are as accurate in these patients as in patients without such a history (33,34).

Pregnant women found to have a thyroid nodule should undergo biopsy, like any other patient, for two reasons. First, the detection of the nodule raises concern about carcinoma that can usually be alleviated simply and quickly. Second, biopsy facilitates decisions regarding surgery in women whose nodules should be excised, including the options of surgery in the second trimester, as soon as possible after delivery, or at a time most consistent with plans for breast-feeding (35,36).

Fine-needle biopsy may not be as accurate in children as in adults, as discussed later.

Technique of Fine-Needle Biopsy

About two thirds of thyroid specialists in the United States currently perform fine-needle biopsy guided by palpation, whereas about two thirds in Europe use ultrasound guidance (37). The routine use of ultrasonography increases the expense of the procedure, usually requires advance scheduling, and requires an assistant. In a study from a single institution comparing the diagnostic accuracy of palpation-guided fine-needle biopsy of nearly 5,000 thyroid nodules with ultrasound-guided fine-needle biopsy of a similar number of nodules (38), the diagnostic accuracy was better when ultrasonography was used, but the differences between the two groups were small, and patients were not randomly allocated to each group. The biggest difference was in the frequency of biopsies in which the sample was inadequate; it was 3.5% for the ultrasound-guided biopsies versus 8.7% for the palpation-guided biopsies. The results were falsely negative (missed carcinoma) in 1% of nodules examined via biopsy with ultrasound guidance and in 2.3% of the nodules examined via biopsy with palpation guidance, although there were more nodules smaller than 1 cm in the ultrasound-guided biopsy group.

Palpation-guided fine-needle biopsy is satisfactory for nodules that are easily palpable. For nodules difficult to palpate, and of course those that are not palpable, the biopsy must be guided by ultrasonography. If palpation-guided biopsy yields an inadequate sample, an ultrasound-guided biopsy should be performed, especially if the nodule is relatively small. The alternate approach of doing only ultrasound-guided biopsies is favored by some physicians.

The actual procedure is performed with the patient supine, with a pillow under the shoulders to facilitate neck extension. The patient should be asked not to talk or swallow while the needle is in the neck. The skin is cleaned with alcohol, and the skin where the biopsy needle is to be inserted is infiltrated with 1 to 2 mL of 1% lidocaine (this may be omitted). The nodule is fixed by the fingers of one hand, and the needle in the other hand is inserted perpendicular to the anterior surface of the neck. Twenty-five-gauge, 1½-inch needles provide excellent specimens and are less likely than larger needles to cause bleeding that dilutes the specimens. The ease with which bleeding is induced depends on whether the nodule is dense and relatively avascular, or loosely organized and more vascular. Occasionally, 22- or 23-gauge needles may be needed to obtain adequate specimens from hard, fibrotic nodules.

The biopsy sample may be obtained without or with suction. In the nonsuction technique, the needle is gripped like a pencil, which facilitates precise needle placement for small nodules, and allows the needle to be moved both in and out over a few millimeters and rotated (39). This combined motion uses the bevel of the needle for cutting, which frees cells that flow into the needle by capillary action while the needle is held steady for about 10 seconds. Material can usually be seen entering the hub of the needle. Samples obtained in this way are less likely to be diluted with blood than samples obtained using suction. If the nonsuction method does not yield a satisfactory sample, or if cyst fluid requires removal, suction is used.

For the suction technique, a 10-mL syringe is used. Some operators put the syringe in a pistol grip designed to facilitate a one-handed biopsy. After the nodule is punctured, the plunger is withdrawn about two thirds of the way, and the needle is moved repeatedly in and out over a distance of 2 to 4 mm. At the first appearance of fluid, negative pressure is released and the needle is withdrawn. No fluid should enter the syringe. If this happens, the specimen may be too dilute and partly lost in the syringe. Material may appear in the syringe if too large a needle is used, if negative pressure is too vigorous, if the nodule is extensively degenerated or unusually vascular, or if the nodule is cystic. For the first two situations, adjustments can be made on subsequent aspirations. For the latter two situations it may help to insert the needle at the periphery of the nodule. The initial aspiration may yield no specimen if the needle is not in the nodule, if the needle is too fine, if negative pressure is not vigorous enough, or if the nodule is fibrotic. If the nodule is purely cystic, it will collapse with aspiration. The fluid should be sent for cytologic examination, although clear fluid is usually acellular. If there is a solid component, any residual mass should be examined via biopsy.

After needle withdrawal, 3 to 4 mL of air is forced through it to expel the specimen onto a glass slide. A grossly satisfactory specimen consists of a small amount of red-orange fluid. Voluminous bloody specimens or specimens that consist of watery, greenish brown fluid, crystal clear jellylike fluid, thick oily fluid, or cheesy white material usually contain insufficient epithelial cells for diagnosis. In some clinics, specimens are stained and examined immediately, so that if the biopsy specimen is inadequate the procedure can be repeated immediately.

Once the specimen is on the slide, it is smeared and fixed immediately to prevent air drying. Some pathologists use air-dried smears stained with May-Giemsa-Grunwald stain, which enhances cytoplasmic detail; some prefer the crisp nuclear detail obtained with the Papanicolaou stain, which requires immediate fixation before air drying occurs; and some use both stains or others. Alternatively, the biopsy specimens can be expelled from the needle directly into a fixative/preservative solution, and slides are later prepared in the laboratory. This permits the use of procedures that concentrate the thyroid cells and eliminate red blood cells. The choice of slide preparation technique needs to be made cooperatively between the person doing the biopsy and the cytopathologist.

Complications of thyroid fine-needle biopsy are exceedingly rare. Biopsy with a 25-gauge needle is safe even in patients taking anticoagulant drugs. Nevertheless, patients should be advised that trauma to adjacent structures is possible. Occasionally, a small hematoma forms at the biopsy site. An ice pack and pressure are adequate treatment. Occasional patients have mild pain that may radiate to the jaw or ear for a day or two, or rarely longer. Infection is rare. Seeding of carcinoma cells in the needle track has been reported in only three patients; two of the patients had large-needle biopsies (34) and one patient had a fine-needle biopsy (40). The reported seedings were excised and had no unfavorable impact on prognosis. Serum thyroglobulin concentrations may increase for a few days after a biopsy (41).

For adequate cytologic evaluation, the biopsy should yield at least six clusters of 20 or more thyroid cells on each of at least two separate aspirates. The guidelines for thyroid fine-needle biopsy of the Papanicolaou Society of Cytopathology cite this as one criterion of an adequate biopsy; alternate criteria are five to six clusters of at least 10 thyroid cells, or 10 clusters of at least 20 thyroid cells (42). When biopsy specimens can be examined immediately, sampling can stop as soon as adequate cellular material is collected. If immediate examination is not possible, sufficient aspirations to provide six separate specimens that appear grossly satisfactory yield adequate results in a high percentage of patients (43), although in many centers only two to four aspirations are performed routinely. For successive samples, the needle is aimed at a different part of the nodule, if size permits. A single aspiration with just one cluster of obviously malignant cells may be sufficient to diagnose a carcinoma, but many more cells are needed to exclude carcinoma, because benign thyroid cells adjacent to a carcinoma may be obtained or the needle may be misplaced. Also, within a carcinoma, the cells in some areas may look more normal than the cells in other areas.

Despite multiple aspirations, specimen cellularity is still sometimes unsatisfactory, and the biopsy is considered inadequate. In such patients, the biopsy should be repeated. A second attempt guided by palpation of a readily palpable nodule is successful in about half the patients, and ultrasound-guided biopsy was successful in 63% of second biopsies in one series (44). If two attempts fail, a third is occasionally successful (44).

After the biopsy, the patient's skin is dressed with an adhesive bandage, and the patient may depart after a few minutes of observation to let lightheadedness pass and to check for bleeding or local swelling.

Results of Fine-Needle Biopsy

Examples of the most common cytologic findings from fine-needle biopsies of thyroid nodules are shown in Fig. 73.1. The results of fine-needle biopsies are reported in various ways, and it is important that the clinician understand the terminology used by the cytopathologist. Inadequate biopsies, as noted above, are those in which too few cells are obtained to allow any interpretation. Other terms used include *normal* or *benign, papillary carcinoma* or *suspicious for papillary carcinoma,* and *follicular neoplasm* or *follicular tumor* (see Chapter 21). Some cytopathologists use the terms *nondiagnostic* or *inconclusive* instead of *follicular neoplasm* or *tumor,* because follicular adenomas and well-differentiated follicular carcinomas cannot be distinguished reliably by any cytologic criteria. *Nondiagnostic* should not be confused with *inadequate.*

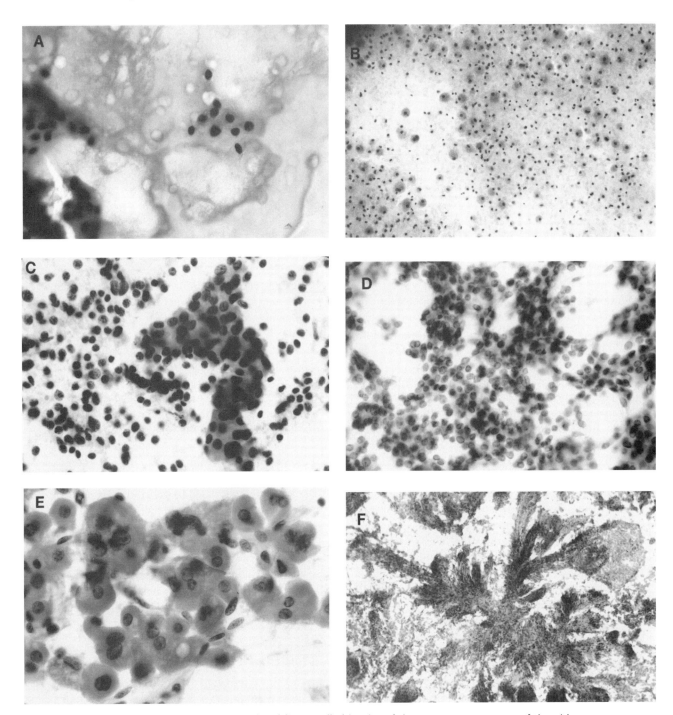

FIGURE 73.1. Photomicrographs of fine-needle biopsies of the most common types of thyroid nodules. A. Colloid nodule, colloid-rich type (magnification x400). B. Degenerating colloid nodule, colloid-poor type (x40). C. Hashimoto's thyroiditis (x400). D. Follicular tumor (x400). Most follicular tumors are adenomas, but the possibility of follicular thyroid carcinoma cannot be ruled out. E. Hürthle-cell nodule showing cells with abundant granular cytoplasm (x400). Some of these nodules are adenomas, others are carcinomas, and still others are aggregations of Hürthle cells in patients with Hashimoto's thyroiditis. F. Papillary carcinoma (x40). These photomicrographs were kindly provided by Edward Bernacki, M.D.

Table 73.5 shows the distribution of cytologic diagnoses in large studies of palpation-guided biopsies, studies of at least 100 patients with one or more palpable and nonpalpable nodules in whom all biopsies were ultrasound guided, and studies of nodules that could be examined via biopsied only with ultrasound guidance because they were difficult or impossible to palpate (3,30–32,37, 38,45–51). For each study, the average percentage of nodules in the four cytologic categories is similar; overall, 74% of the biopsies revealed benign cells, 4% revealed

TABLE 73.5. DISTRIBUTION OF CYTOLOGIC RESULTS IN REPRESENTATIVE THYROID FNB SERIES

Reference	Number of nodules	Benign %	Malignant %	Inconclusive or Suspicious %	Unsatisfactory (Inadequate) %
Guided by palpation					
37	4986	84	2	5	9
adapted from ref 45*	5605	74	3	17	6
46	7212	75	3	8	14
47	15210	64	4	11	21
Guided by ultrasound, palpable and non-palpable nodules					
3	205	63	3	17	16
38	4697	89	2	5	4
48	132	70	11	16	4
49	127	80	5	9	7
50	1135	82	4	13	0.1
Guided by ultrasound, difficult to palpate or non-palpable nodules					
30	450	65	2	14	19
31	110	80	5	2	13
32	48	85	4	2	8
51	32	69	3	9	19
Mean		75	4	10	11
SD		9	2	5	7

*Pooled data from several centers excluding the Mayo Clinic, from which more recent data (47) are listed separately. The values in some rows do not add to 100% because of rounding.

malignant cells, 10% were suspicious (follicular lesions), and 11% were inadequate. The variability of results between series is also reasonably similar within each of the three groups, notwithstanding differences in patient populations, criteria used for an adequate biopsy, and criteria used to differentiate between benign thyroid cells and follicular tumors. Even with repeated fine-needle biopsy and routine use of ultrasonography, there is probably an irreducible minimum of about 3% to 5% of nodules from which adequate fine-needle biopsy samples cannot be obtained.

Standard calculations of sensitivity, specificity, and false-positive and false-negative rates are complicated, and probably not of great utility. The reasons are that the great majority of patients with nodules with benign cytology do not undergo surgery; therefore, there is no reference standard for a benign final diagnosis, and on average about 10% to 12% of biopsies yield inadequate samples. In practical terms, about 2% to 3% of benign nodules, as determined by fine-needle biopsy, subsequently prove to be carcinomas. Conversely, about 2% to 5% of malignant nodules, as determined by fine-needle biopsy, prove to be benign on histologic study. Because a fine-needle biopsy diagnosis of follicular tumor does not exclude carcinoma, this biopsy result should only be considered as a guide to identify patients for whom surgery is probably advisable (52). There are as yet no cellular or molecular markers proven to distinguish reliably between follicular adenomas and follicular carcinomas.

There have been two studies of fine-needle biopsy in children with thyroid nodules. In the larger study, of 60 children, 50 of 51 nodules (98%) for which the biopsy revealed benign thyroid cells proved to be benign, and 8 of the 9 nodules (89%) that proved to be carcinomas were identified by biopsy (53). In the smaller study, benign needle biopsy diagnoses were correct in only 4 of 7 cases (57%), and only 2 of 5 thyroid carcinomas (40%) were identified by biopsy (54). Possible reasons that these results are not as good as those in adults include differences in patients, level of experience of the persons doing the biopsies, lack of cooperation of the children leading to fewer samples, and small numbers of patients.

Limitations of Fine-Needle Biopsy of Thyroid Nodules

There are some limitations of fine-needle biopsy of thyroid nodules (Table 73.6). The principal limitation is inexperience, both in obtaining adequate specimens and in interpreting the specimens. Instructional material is available, but there is no substitute for experience. Fine-needle biopsy is not applicable to all nodules. Some are too small and too inaccessible for accurate needle placement, or too far down in the chest to be aspirated safely. Others are so degenerated that useful material cannot be obtained. Finally, a fine-needle biopsy of one nodule provides no information about any other nodules that the patient may have.

TABLE 73.6. LIMITATIONS OF FINE-NEEDLE BIOPSY OF THE THYROID

Problem	Potential Solutions
Inaccurate, vague, or nonspecific reports	High level of interest and experience of clinician and pathologist and good communication between them
Adequate specimens with inconclusive cytology	Consider clinical features and other laboratory and imaging results
	Surgery may be appropriate
Inadequate specimens	Repeat the biopsy, with ultrasound guidance
Nonpalpable nodules	Observation or fine-needle biopsy with ultrasound guidance
Substernal nodules	Fine-needle biopsy with ultrasound guidance, if practical and safe
False negative and false positive results	Inform patient of possibility
	Use stringent criteria for adequacy
	Consider clinical features
	Perform follow-up evaluations, which may include repeat biopsy
Sampling limitations in large, heterogeneous nodules	Take multiple samples
	Perform biopsy with ultrasound guidance to sample non-cystic areas and areas of greatest concern according to appearance
Multiple nodules in one thyroid gland	Biopsy all that are accessible and of concern based on clinical and imaging criteria
Extreme patient anxiety about cancer despite biopsy finding of benign nodule	Consider surgery, using biopsy results to help decide on extent of resection

The legal consequences of false-positive or false-negative diagnoses, and therefore in advising patients to undergo, or to not undergo, surgery are of concern to some physicians. Fine-needle biopsy improves diagnostic precision and reduces the potential for error. However, patients should be informed that the procedure is not always successful or reliable.

COMBINED RESULTS OF SERUM, IMAGING, AND FINE-NEEDLE BIOPSY TESTING

For all adults with apparently solitary thyroid nodules, the combined results of serum measurements, imaging studies, and fine-needle biopsies lead to the following estimates:

Malignant nodules constitute approximately 3% to 6% of thyroid nodules at least 1 cm in maximum diameter. Most are differentiated thyroid carcinomas of follicular-cell origin.

Autonomously functioning adenomas account for approximately 5% to 10% of thyroid nodules in the United States. Their prevalence may differ in other geographic areas.

Cystic nodules, with more than 75% fluid content, account for 10% to 15% of thyroid nodules. Simple epithelial cysts are rare. The fluid in most cystic nodules is the result of hemorrhage or thyroid cell degeneration; either is as likely to occur in thyroid carcinomas as in benign nodules. Therefore, this category overlaps with the other types of thyroid nodules.

Benign thyroid nodules that are 75% cystic or less and are isofunctioning or hypofunctioning constitute the remaining 70% to 80%. This category includes adenomatous, colloid, and hyperplastic nodules and follicular adenomas (see Chapter 21).

APPLICATION OF FINE-NEEDLE BIOPSY TO THE MANAGEMENT OF PATIENTS WITH THYROID NODULES

Patients in whom an adequate biopsy reveals benign thyroid follicular cells do not need surgery based on risk for carcinoma. If surgery is chosen because of the appearance of the nodule, or the nodule compresses nearby structures, a lobectomy is usually the appropriate procedure. The chance of serious harm from a false-negative biopsy result in a patient who does not undergo surgery is less than the 2% to 3% frequency of false-negative biopsies, because thyroid carcinomas for which the biopsy was falsely negative are usually low-grade tumors that are still curable even if the diagnosis is delayed. If the patient returns for periodic reevaluation, a repeat biopsy can be performed if the nodule has enlarged. When repeat biopsies are performed, the biopsy diagnosis is more abnormal and suggests the need for surgery in 1% to 3% of patients (5,55–57).

A fine-needle biopsy diagnosis of papillary carcinoma is almost always confirmed at operation, and surgery is the initial treatment for patients with this tumor. A fine-needle biopsy diagnosis of medullary carcinoma or undifferentiated or anaplastic carcinoma is also nearly always confirmed at operation, and surgery is advised for patients with potentially resectable lesions. In the case of thyroid lymphoma, also reliably detected by fine-needle biopsy, open biopsy to obtain tissue for precise classification of the tumor using flow cytometry and immunohistochemical techniques is usually indicated.

In patients in whom the fine-needle biopsy diagnosis is suspicious for papillary carcinoma or follicular tumor (including Hürthle-cell tumor), the likelihood of carcinoma is high enough (25%–75%) that operation should be advised, unless there is a major contraindication to surgery. With respect to follicular tumors, the guidelines of the Papanicolaou Society of Cytopathology take note of two approaches to reporting cytologic findings: either making no further comment, or subdividing follicular tumors into two or three categories according to the degree of cellular atypia (42). If the cells show little or no atypia, about 5% to 15% of the nodules are follicular carcinomas. This risk is high enough to advise operation for most patients, but an 85% to 95% probability that the nodule is benign might make observation an acceptable choice for older patients or those with medical problems that increase the risk for complications of surgery. Higher degrees of atypia increase the likelihood that the nodule is a follicular carcinoma, and usually lead to a stronger recommendation for surgery. In patients with a fine-needle biopsy diagnosis of follicular tumor, repeating the biopsy rarely clarifies the nature of the nodule (58).

Among patients in whom the fine-needle biopsy was inadequate, thyroid carcinoma was found in an average of 14% of those selected for surgery, or 29 of 210 patients in data pooled from several studies (30,34,38,46,49,59,60). Patients whose biopsy results are inadequate may choose surgery because of fear of carcinoma, or may be advised to have surgery because of the presence of some clinical finding associated with a higher risk for carcinoma (Table 73.2).

In the past, many patients undergoing surgery for a thyroid nodule had a lobectomy (usually including the isthmus) with a frozen section, after which the operation was terminated or extended depending on the results of the histologic findings in the frozen sections of the nodule. This strategy has been largely abandoned; there is usually a firm biopsy diagnosis now, which is more reliable than frozen-section diagnosis (52). Although two recent studies report 78% and 88% accuracy of frozen-section diagnoses of thyroid nodules (61,62), most centers have less favorable results. Frozen-section diagnoses may be difficult to obtain, or the results may be erroneous, and reversed after review of the permanent sections (52). Frozen-section diagnosis is least reliable in distinguishing between follicular adenomas and follicular carcinomas, because this distinction is based primarily on the presence of vascular and capsular invasion by carcinomas.

These findings lead to the following conclusions:

If surgery is chosen despite a fine-needle biopsy diagnosis of a benign nodule, the operation can be a lobectomy; frozen-section analysis is not needed.

If surgery is chosen for a patient with a fine-needle biopsy diagnosis of follicular tumor, an initial lobectomy will be the correct procedure in about 85% of patients. Frozen-section is usually not helpful, as noted above. If the nodule is a small, low-grade follicular carcinoma, lobectomy may be an adequate operation.

For patients with a fine-needle biopsy diagnosis of Hürthle-cell tumor or suspected papillary carcinoma, the nodule is more likely to be a carcinoma, and the patient should be fully informed of the possible need for near-total thyroidectomy before the operation. Frozen-section diagnosis may or may not provide additional guidance. Many patients choose near-total thyroidectomy, accepting the additional risks to avoid the risks and unpleasantness of a second operation.

For patients with a fine-needle biopsy diagnosis of papillary or other carcinoma, the chance of a false-positive biopsy diagnosis is so small that near-total thyroidectomy or, for patients with medullary carcinoma, total thyroidectomy and extensive bilateral lymph node resection is indicated (see Chapter 71). The exact surgical procedure may be guided by frozen-section evaluation of lymph nodes, parathyroid glands, and tumor invasion into fat and muscle.

OTHER USES OF FINE-NEEDLE BIOPSY OF THE THYROID GLAND

Fine-needle biopsy can be used to evaluate diffuse enlargement of the thyroid gland or selective enlargement of one lobe, if serum tests and scintiscanning leave the etiology of the abnormality uncertain, or if the scintiscan shows a discrete area of hypofunction (Table 73.4). The area of concern is surveyed by aspirating six to eight sites, using the same technique as for nodules. Such survey biopsies can help distinguish patients with lymphoma from those with Hashimoto's thyroiditis, and patients with diffuse multifocal carcinoma from those with a colloid or adenomatous goiter.

Several types of thyroid nodules can be reduced in size and function, even destroyed, using fine-needle techniques. The most straightforward is aspiration of fluid or blood from a purely cystic or hemorrhagic nodule, which disappears and does not recur. However, about half of cystic thyroid nodules do recur each time that fluid is removed (63). Some patients in whom the cysts recur choose surgery, and some physicians recommend surgery for patients whose cysts reappear after two or three aspirations, but repeated aspirations may lead eventually to disappearance of the cyst (63). The solid portion of nodules that are largely cystic should be examined via biopsy, with ultrasound guidance, ideally when the cyst is first aspirated.

Sclerosing agents, such as tetracycline or ethanol, have been used to prevent recurrence of cystic thyroid nodules (63,64), although tetracycline may be no more effective than saline (65), and extravasation of the sclerosing agent may damage the recurrent laryngeal nerve. Several groups have been trying to destroy solid, autonomously functioning thyroid nodules, or hypofunctioning nodules with benign cytology, by repeated injections of ethanol into the nodules under ultrasound guidance, with some success (64,66–69). The procedure can be quite painful, and only a small amount of ethanol can be injected at a time, and therefore multiple injections are usually needed. The long-term efficacy and safety of this procedure remain to be established, and the cost may be considerable because of the need for repeated injections. A more recent innovation is the use of laser photocoagulation to destroy benign functioning or nonfunctioning nodules (70,71). The clinical effectiveness, safety, and cost of this technique have not yet been established.

The presence of crystal clear, colorless, watery fluid is diagnostic of a parathyroid cyst, and measurement of parathyroid hormone in the cystic fluid will confirm the diagnosis. Serum calcium concentrations are usually normal. The cyst can be drained, but may recur.

Fine-needle biopsy can be used in patients who have had surgery for thyroid carcinoma and who have cervical lymphadenopathy or possible recurrence of tumor in the bed of the thyroid gland. If the nodes are palpable, they can be examined via biopsy in the usual fashion. More often, the abnormal nodes are detected by ultrasonography, and biopsy must be ultrasound-guided. In clinics with extensive ultrasound experience, the yield of diagnostically useful material in these patients is high (72,73), and ethanol injection to destroy isolated foci of residual thyroid cancer has recently been reported (73).

If the rare entity of acute suppurative thyroiditis is suspected, fine-needle aspiration can provide material for Gram stain and culture, and special stains have identified *Pneumocystis carinii* as the cause of both painful and painless thyroid enlargement in patients with human immunodeficiency virus infection (74).

MANAGEMENT OF PATIENTS WITH BENIGN THYROID NODULES

Patients Who Do Not Undergo Surgery

Most patients who present with a thyroid nodule prove to have a benign nodule, receive a recommendation against surgery, and accept the recommendation. For this very large group, the management options are observation or thyroxine (T_4) therapy (ethanol injection or laser photocoagulation are other options currently available in a few cen-

ters). It is important to note that little is known about the natural history of benign thyroid nodules, although it is becoming clear that these nodules grow slowly in many, if not the majority of, patients (75–77).

For years, patients with benign thyroid nodules have been treated with T_4, in the hope that decreasing TSH secretion would result in a decrease in nodule size, or at least prevent further nodule growth. The results of some uncontrolled studies supported the benefit of T_4 therapy (78). Then, a series of controlled trials, most with a placebo group and all with repeated measurements of nodule volume by ultrasonography, found no effect or only modest benefit of T_4 therapy in reducing nodule volume, usually defined as a 50% or greater decrease in volume (79–83). Despite these results, in a survey published in 2000, a substantial minority of thyroidologists in the United States and Europe said that they still recommended T_4 therapy for selected patients with nodules (4). The main reasons for continued use of T_4 therapy are some patients' desire for treatment, even if the likelihood of benefit is small; the hope for decreasing the number of patients who ultimately have surgery for benign nodules, because nodule growth causes cosmetic or pressure symptoms or fear of cancer; the hope for decreasing the development of additional nodules; and a possibility of cost saving by avoiding repetitive imaging studies and biopsies for patients with stable or growing nodules whose physicians do not consider benign needle biopsy results sufficiently reassuring. T_4 treatment is ineffective in preventing the recurrence of cystic nodules (84). There is no reason to suppose that T_4 treatment would be effective in autonomously functioning nodules.

There have been four meta-analyses of controlled trials of T_4 therapy in patients with benign thyroid nodules, in which the number of nodules that decreased in volume by 50% or more was the measure of response (78,80–82). Each meta-analysis included at least one study that the others excluded for methodologic weaknesses or that was published afterward. In all these analyses the point estimate of relative likelihood of nodule shrinkage was in the 1.8 to 2.0 range in the T_4-treated patients, as compared with the control patients. Whether the higher response rate was statistically significant depended on the statistical model used. Thus, even meta-analysis has been inconclusive. In pooled data from six controlled studies of 11 to 18 months' duration (46,82,83,85–87), with ultrasound measurements of nodule volume, 52 of 210 nodules (25%) decreased in volume by more than 50% in the T_4 treatment groups, as compared with 22 of 205 (11%) in the control groups. Analysis of nodule growth in one meta-analysis revealed that T_4 therapy for 6 to 12 months was associated with a lower frequency of a 50% or more increase in nodule volume, as compared with no treatment (8% vs. 17%) (82).

Several individual trials of T_4 treatment that used other response measures, and, therefore, could not be combined with other studies, found statistically significant responses to

T_4 treatment. The only controlled long-term study (75) followed patients with 1- to 3-cm solitary nodules for 5 years and used a least-measurable size difference (12% change) end point. In this study, 20 of 42 nodules (48%) in the T_4-treated patients decreased in size, as compared with 9 of 41 nodules (22%) in the control patients; 12 nodules (29%) enlarged in the T_4-treated patients, as compared with 24 nodules (56%) in the control patients; and three new nodules greater than 1 cm developed in the T_4-treated patients, as compared with 12 new nodules in the control patients ($p < 0.05$, for all three comparisons). Two other uncontrolled observational studies using ultrasound measurements (76,77) similarly found that more than 50% of untreated nodules grew slowly. In the 5-year study (75) and two others, which were 12- and 18-month controlled trials of therapy (83,88), mean nodule volumes were significantly lower in the T_4 treated patients than in those given placebo or no treatment. In one 12-month study (85), which included some predominantly cystic nodules, there was no difference in mean nodule volume. One study with a crossover design found a significantly lower mean nodule volume in patients

treated with T_4 in doses that reduced serum TSH concentrations to low normal (0.4–0.6 mIU/L) for a year, as compared with a placebo period in the same patients (88). This approach is used by some American thyroidologists (37), and eliminates the potential for thyrotoxic symptoms and adverse skeletal and cardiac effects of suppressive doses of T_4.

Overall, the possibility that some patients might benefit from T_4 treatment has not been established, but has not yet been disproved either. Observation without treatment is currently the evidence-based choice.

More long-term studies of T_4 therapy in patients with benign thyroid nodules are needed. The studies should assess not only changes in nodule volume, but also the ultrasound characteristics of the nodules; the appearance of new nodules; clinical outcomes, such as the number of patients who come to surgery or have cosmetic or compressive symptoms; and patient satisfaction. The relationship of serum TSH concentrations to outcome should also be assessed.

For all patients with a thyroid nodule, whether treated with T_4 or not, nodule size should be reevaluated at regular intervals, at least annually. If T_4 is given, the patient should

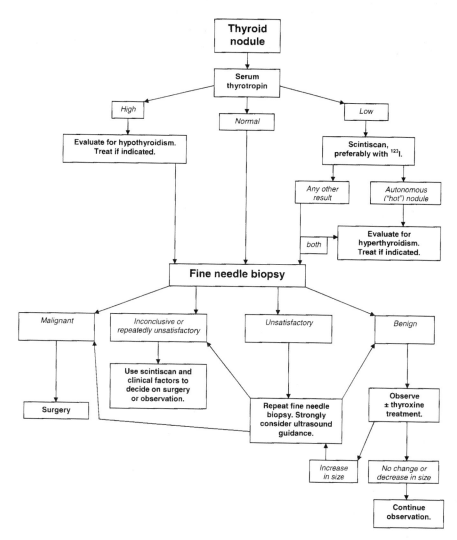

FIGURE 73.2. Scheme for evaluation and treatment of patients with solitary thyroid nodules.

have a measurement of serum TSH in 6 to 12 weeks, and periodically thereafter, to be sure that TSH secretion is not very low. Any patient in whom the nodule grows should have a repeat biopsy. If the biopsy again reveals benign thyroid cells in a patient who had not been treated, T_4 therapy can be considered then. If T_4 was given at the outset, yet the nodule enlarged, continuing T_4 is not a necessity, but is an option, since the nodule may have enlarged more had T_4 not been given. Whenever T_4 is given, the patient should be informed that the nodule may grow, and if the goal of therapy is a low serum TSH concentration, the risks of bone loss or cardiac arrhythmia should be discussed (see Chapter 40 and see Chapter 79).

Treatment after Thyroid Surgery

Patients who undergo thyroid lobectomy for what proves to be a benign thyroid nodule need no further therapy. These patients may have a small increase in serum TSH concentrations several months after surgery, but the increase is not sustained. Normal thyroid function should be verified by measurements of serum TSH 4 to 6 months after surgery. In the past, T_4 was given routinely to these patients, but a few controlled studies have provided no evidence that the therapy prevents the formation of new nodules. An exception is patients who had head or neck irradiation and a partial thyroidectomy for a benign nodule, in whom T_4 therapy does prevent new nodules (89). T_4 therapy should prevent compensatory enlargement of the contralateral thyroid lobe, and is safe so long as TSH secretion is not suppressed to below the normal range.

SUMMARY OF MANAGEMENT OF PATIENTS WITH THYROID NODULES

Figure 73.2 shows a flow diagram of management steps and options for patients who present with a solitary thyroid nodule. Although the many possibilities make it a complex scheme, the simplest pathway applies to the most common group of patients. They are patients who have a normal serum TSH concentration and a biopsy that revealed only benign thyroid follicular cells, and for whom observation is the most appropriate recommendation.

THYROGLOSSAL DUCT CYSTS

Thyroglossal duct cysts are collections of fluid in a persistent thyroglossal duct, the tract that forms as the thyroid gland descends from the base of the tongue to the lower neck during development (see Chapter 2). Most thyroglossal ducts disappear before birth, but they can persist and occasionally develop cysts, which are usually in the midline of the anterior neck, between the hyoid bone and the thyroid isthmus.

Most are asymptomatic and discovered during childhood or adolescence, but some are discovered later in life. If fluid is aspirated, it usually does not contain thyroid follicular cells. Because these cysts can become infected, they should usually be removed surgically. Rare cases of thyroid carcinoma have been reported in thyroglossal duct cysts (90).

REFERENCES

1. Mazzaferri EL. Management of a solitary thyroid nodule. *N Engl J Med* 1993;328:553.
2. Tan GH, Gharib H, Reading CC. Solitary thyroid nodule: comparison between palpation and ultrasonography. *Arch Intern Med* 1995;115:2418.
3. Marqusee E, Benson CB, Frates MC, et al. Usefulness of ultrasonography in the management of nodular thyroid disease. *Ann Intern Med* 2000;133:696.
4. Hegedüs L, Bonnema SJ, Bennedbaek FN. Management of simple nodular goiter: current status and future perspectives. *Endocr Rev* 2003;24:102.
5. Hamburger JI. Consistency of sequential needle biopsy findings for thyroid nodules. *Arch Intern Med* 1987;147:97.
6. Belfiore A, LaRosa GL, LaPorta GA, et al. Cancer risk in patients with cold thyroid nodules: relevance of iodine intake, sex, age, and multinodularity. *Am J Med* 1992;93:363.
7. Schlinkert RT, van Heerden JA, Goellner JR, et al. Factors that predict malignant thyroid lesions when fine-needle aspiration is "suspicious for follicular neoplasm." *Mayo Clin Proc* 1997;72:913.
8. Hamming JF, Goslings BM, van Steenis GJ, et al. The value of fine-needle aspiration biopsy in patients with nodular thyroid disease divided into groups of suspicion of malignant neoplasms on clinical grounds. *Arch Intern Med* 1990;150:113.
9. Tuttle RM, Lemar H, Burch HB. Clinical features associated with an increased risk of thyroid malignancy in patients with follicular neoplasia by fine-needle aspiration. *Thyroid* 1998;8:377.
10. Raber W, Kaserer K, Niederle B, et al. Risk factors for malignancy of thyroid nodules initially identified as follicular neoplasia by fine-needle aspiration: results of a prospective study of one hundred twenty patients. *Thyroid* 2000;10:709.
11. Chen H, Nicol TL, Zeiger MA, et al. Hürthle cell neoplams of the thyroid: are there factors predictive of malignancy? *Ann Surg* 1998;227:542.
12. Elisei R, Bottici V, Luchetti F, et al. Impact of routine measurement of serum calcitonin on the diagnosis and outcome of medullary thyroid cancer: experience in 10,684 patients with nodular thyroid disorders. *J Clin Endocrinol Metab* 2004;89:163.
13. Karanikas G, Moameni A, Poetai C, et al. Frequency and relevance of elevated calcitonin levels in patients with neoplastic and nonneoplastic thyroid disease and in healthy subjects. *J Clin Endocrinol Metab* 2004;89:515.
14. Hamburger JI. The autonomously functioning thyroid nodule: Goetsch's disease. *Endocr Rev* 1987;8:439.
15. Farfel Z, Bourne HR, Iiri T. The expanding spectrum of G protein diseases. *N Engl J Med* 1999;340:1012.
16. Porcellini A, Ciullo I, Laviola L, et al. Novel mutations of thyrotropin receptor gene in thyroid hyperfunctioning adenomas. *J Clin Endocrinol Metab* 1994;79:335.
17. Liel Y. The yield of adequate and conclusive fine-needle aspiration results in thyroid nodules is uniform across functional and goiter types. *Thyroid* 1999;9:25.
18. Hegedüs L. Thyroid ultrasound. *Endocrinol Metab Clin North Am* 2001;30:339.

19. Gallo M, Pesenti M, Valcavi R. Ultrasound thyroid nodule measurements: the "gold standard" and its limitations in clinical decision making. *Endocr Pract* 2003;9:194.

20. Zarnegar R, Brunaud L, Clark OH. Prevention, evaluation, and management of complications following thyroidectomy for thyroid carcinoma. *Endocrinol Metab Clin North Am* 2003;32:483.

21. Falk SA. Complications of thyroid surgery: an overview. In: Falk SA, ed. *Thyroid disease: endocrinology, surgery, nuclear medicine, and radiotherapy,* 2nd ed. Philadelphia: Lippincott-Raven, 1997:697.

22. LoGerfo P. Coarse needle biopsy of the thyroid. In: Hamburger JI, ed. *Diagnostic methods in clinical thyroidology.* New York: Springer-Verlag, 1989:205.

23. Singer PA, Cooper DS, Daniels GH, et al. Treatment guidelines for patients with thyroid nodules and well differentiated thyroid cancer. *Arch Intern Med* 1996;156:2165.

24. Feld S, Garcia M, Baskin HJ, et al. AACE clinical practice guidelines for the diagnosis and management of thyroid nodules. *Endocr Pract* 1996;2:78.

25. Tan GH, Gharib H. Thyroid incidentalomas: management approaches to nonpalpable nodules discovered incidentally on thyroid imaging. *Ann Intern Med* 1997;126:226.

26. Ezzat S, Sarti DA, Cain DR, et al. Thyroid incidentalomas: prevalence by palpation and ultrasonography. *Arch Intern Med* 1994;154:1838.

27. Jemal A, Tiwari RC, Ghafoor A, et al. Cancer statistics 2004. *CA Cancer J Clin* 2004;54:8.

28. Schneider AB, Bekerman C, Leland J, et al. Thyroid nodules in the follow-up of irradiated individuals: comparison of thyroid ultrasound with scanning and palpation. *J Clin Endocrinol Metab* 1997;82:4020.

29. Leinung MC, Gianoukakis A, Lee DW. Ultrasonography in management of nodular thyroid disease. *Ann Intern Med* 2001; 135:383.

30. Leenhardt L, Hejblum B, Franc B, et al. Indications and limits of ultrasound-guided cytology in the management of nonpalpable thyroid nodules. *J Clin Endocrinol Metab* 1999;84:24.

31. Hagag P, Strauss S, Weiss M. Role of ultrasound-guided fine-needle aspiration biopsy in evaluation of nonpalpable thyroid nodules. *Thyroid* 1998;8:989.

32. Khurana KK, Richards VI, Chopra PS, et al. The role of ultrasonography-guided fine-needle aspiration biopsy in the management of nonpalpable and palpable thyroid nodules. *Thyroid* 1998;8:511.

33. Hatipoglu BA, Gierlowski T, Shore-Freedman E, et al. Fine-needle aspiration of thyroid nodules in radiation-exposed patients. *Thyroid* 2000;10:63.

34. Hamburger JI, Kaplan MM, Husain M. Diagnosis of thyroid nodules by needle biopsy. In: Braverman LE, Utiger RD, eds. *Werner and Ingbar's the thyroid. A fundamental and clinical text,* 6th ed. Philadelphia: JB Lippincott, 1991:544.

35. Tan GT, Gharib H, Goellner JR, et al. Management of thyroid nodules in pregnancy. *Arch Intern Med* 1996;156:2317.

36. Rosen IB, Korman M, Walfish PG. Thyroid nodular disease in pregnancy: current diagnosis and management. *Clin Obstet Gynecol* 1997;40:81.

37. Bennedbaek FN, Hegedüs L. Management of the solitary thyroid nodule: results of a North American survey. *J Clin Endocrinol Metab* 2000;85:2493.

38. Danese D, Sciacchitano S, Farsetti A, et al. Diagnostic accuracy of conventional versus sonography-guided fine-needle aspiration biopsy of thyroid nodules. *Thyroid* 1998;8:15.

39. Santos JEC, Leiman G. Nonaspiration fine needle cytology. *Acta Cytol* 1988;32:353.

40. Hales MS, Hsu, FSF. Needle tract implantation of papillary carcinoma of the thyroid following aspiration biopsy. *Acta Cytol* 1990;34:801.

41. Lever EG, Refetoff S, Scherberg NH, et al. The influence of percutaneous fine needle aspiration on serum thyroglobulin. *J Clin Endocrinol Metab* 1983;56:26.

42. Guidelines of the Papanicolaou Society of Cytopathology for the examination of fine-needle aspiration specimens from thyroid nodules. The Papanicolaou Society of Cytopathology Task Force on Standards of Practice. *Diagn Cytopathol* 1996;15:84.

43. Hamburger JI, Husain M, Nishiyama R, et al. Increasing the accuracy of fine-needle biopsy for thyroid nodules. *Arch Pathol Lab Med* 1989;113:1035.

44. Alexander EK, Herring JP, Benson CB, et al. Assessment of nondiagnostic ultrasound-guided fine needle aspirations of thyroid nodules. *J Clin Endocrinol Metab* 2002;87:4924.

45. Gharib H, Goellner JR. Fine-needle aspiration biopsy of the thyroid: an appraisal. *Ann Intern Med* 1993;118:282.

46. La Rosa GL, Belfiore A, Giuffrida D, et al. Evaluation of the fine needle aspiration biopsy in the preoperative selection of cold thyroid nodules. *Cancer* 1991;67:2137.

47. Gharib H. Changing concepts in the diagnosis and management of thyroid nodules. *Endocrinol Metab Clin North Am* 1997;26: 777.

48. Cochand-Priollet B, Guillausseau P-J, Chagnon S, et al. The diagnostic value of fine-needle aspiration biopsy under ultrasonography in nonfunctional thyroid nodules: a prospective study comparing cytologic and histologic findings. *Am J Med* 1994;97:152.

49. Carmeci C, Jeffrey RB, McDougall IR, et al. Ultrasound-guided fine-needle aspiration biopsy of thyroid masses. *Thyroid* 1998; 8:283.

50. Yang GCH, Liebeskind D, Messina AV. Ultrasound-guided fine-needle aspiration of the thyroid assessed by ultrafast Papanicolaou stain: data from 1135 biopsies with a two- to six-year follow-up. *Thyroid* 2001;11:581.

51. Sanchez RB, vanSonnenberg E, D'Agostino HB, et al. Ultrasound guided biopsy of nonpalpable and difficult to palpate thyroid masses. *J Am Coll Surg* 1994;178:33.

52. LiVolsi VA. *Surgical pathology of the thyroid.* Philadelphia: WB Saunders, 1990.

53. Raab SS, Silverman JF, Elsheikh TM, et al. Pediatric thyroid nodules: disease demographics and clinical management as determined by fine needle aspiration biopsy. *Pediatrics* 1995; 95:46.

54. Degnan BM, McClellan DR, Francis GL. An analysis of fine-needle aspiration biopsy of the thyroid in children and adolescents. *J Pediatr Surg* 1996;31:903.

55. Chehade JM, Silverberg AB, Kim J, et al. Role of repeated fine-needle aspiration of thyroid nodules with benign cytologic features. *Endocr Pract* 2001;7:237.

56. Lucas A, Llatjos M, Salinas I, et al. Fine-needle aspiration cytology of benign nodular thyroid disease. Value of re-aspiration. *Eur J Endocrinol* 1995;132:677.

57. Erdogan MF, Kamel N, Aras D, et al. Value of re-aspirations in benign nodular thyroid disease. *Thyroid* 1998;8:1087.

58. Cersosimo E, Gharib H, Suman VJ, et al. "Suspicious" thyroid cytologic findings: outcome in patients without immediate surgical treatment. *Mayo Clin Proc* 1993;68:343.

59. McHenry CR, Walfish PG, Rosen IB. Non-diagnostic fine needle aspiration biopsy. A dilemma in management of thyroid disease. *Am Surgeon* 1993;59:415.

60. Baloch ZW, Sack MJ, Yu GH, et al. Fine-needle aspiration of thyroid: an institutional experience. *Thyroid* 1998;8:565.

61. Cheng H-Y, Lin J-D, Chen J-F, et al. Correlation of fine needle aspiration cytology and frozen section biopsies in the diagnosis of thyroid nodules. *J Clin Pathol* 1997;50:1005.

62. Paphavasit P, Thompson GB, Hay ID, et al. Follicular and Hürthle cell thyroid neoplasms. Is frozen section evaluation worthwhile? *Arch Surg* 1997;132:674.

63. Lee J-K, Tai F-T, Lin H-D, et al. Treatment of recurrent thyroid cysts by injection of tetracycline or minocycline. *Arch Intern Med* 1989;149:599.

64. Zingrillo M, Torlontano M, Ghiggi MR, et al. Percutaneous ethanol injection of large thyroid cystic nodules. *Thyroid* 1996;6:403.

65. Hegedüs L, Hansen JM, Karstrup S, et al. Tetracycline for sclerosis of thyroid cysts. A randomized study. *Arch Intern Med* 1988;148:1116.

66. Pacini F. Role of percutaneous ethanol injection in management of nodular lesions of the thyroid gland. *J Nucl Med* 2003;44:211.

67. Zingrillo M, Collura D, Ghiggi MR, et al. Treatment of large cold benign thyroid nodules not eligible for surgery with percutaneous ethanol injection. *J Clin Endocrinol Metab* 1998;83:3905.

68. Bennedbaek FN, Nielsen LK, Hegedüs L. Effect of percutaneous ethanol injection therapy versus suppressive doses of l-thyroxine on benign solitary solid cold thyroid nodules: a randomized trial. *J Clin Endocrinol Metab* 1998;83:830.

69. Caraccio N, Goletti O, Lippolis PV, et al. Is percutaneous ethanol injection a useful alternative for the treatment of the cold benign thyroid nodule? Five years' experience. *Thyroid* 1997;7:699.

70. Dossing H, Bennedbaek FN, Karstrup S, et al. Benign solitary solid cold thyroid nodules: US-guided interstitial laser photocoagulation—initial experience. *Radiology* 2002;225:53.

71. Dossing H, Bennedbaek FN, Hegedüs L. Ultrasound-guided interstitial photocoagulation of an autonomous thyroid nodule: the introduction of a novel alternative. *Thyroid* 2003;13:885.

72. Frasoldati A, Pesenti M, Gallo M, et al. Diagnosis of neck recurrences in patients with differentiated thyroid carcinoma. *Cancer* 2003;97:90.

73. Lewis BD, Hay ID, Charboneau JW, et al. Percutaneous ethanol injection for treatment of cervical lymph node metastases in patients with papillary thyroid carcinoma. *AJR* 2002;178:699.

74. Guttler R, Singer PA. *Pneumocystis carinii* thyroiditis: report of three cases and review of the literature. *Arch Intern Med* 1993;153:393.

75. Papini E, Petrucci L, Guglielmi R, et al. Long-term changes in nodular goiter: a 5-year prospective randomized trial of levothyroxine suppressive therapy for benign cold thyroid nodules. *J Clin Endocrinol Metab* 1998;83:780.

76. Alexander EK, Hurwitz S, Heering JP, et al. Natural history of benign solid and cystic thyroid nodules. *Ann Intern Med* 2003;138:315.

77. Quadbeck B, Pruellage J, Roggenbuck U, et al. Long-term follow-up of thyroid nodule growth. *Exp Clin Endocrinol Diabetes* 2002;110:348.

78. Richter B, Nesies G, Clar C. Pharmacotherapy for thyroid nodules: a systematic review and meta-analysis. *Endocrinol Metab Clin North Am* 2002;31:699.

79. Gharib H, Mazzaferri EL. Thyroxine suppressive therapy in patients with thyroid nodular disease. *Ann Intern Med* 1998;128:386.

80. Csako G, Byrd D, Wesley RA, et al. Assessing the effects of thyroid suppression on benign solitary thyroid nodules: a model for using quantitative research synthesis. *Medicine* 2000;79:9.

81. Castro MR, Caraballo PJ, Morris JC. Effectiveness of thyroid hormone suppressive therapy in benign solitary thyroid nodules: a meta-analysis. *J Clin Endocrinol Metab* 2002;87:4154.

82. Zelmanovitz F, Genro S, Gross JL. Suppressive therapy with levothyroxine for solitary thyroid nodules: a double-blind controlled clinical study and cumulative meta-analyses. *J Clin Endocrinol Metab* 1998;83:3881.

83. Wemeau J-L, Caron P, Schvartz C, et al. Effects of thyroid—stimulating hormone suppression with levothyroxine in reducing the volume of solitary thyroid nodules and improving extranodular nonpalpable changes: a randomized, double-blind, placebo-controlled trial by the French thyroid group. *J Clin Endocrinol Metab* 2002;87:4928.

84. McCowen K, Reed J, Fariss B. The role of thyroid therapy in patients with thyroid cysts. *Am J Med* 1980;68:853.

85. Larijani B, Pajouhi M, Bastanhagh MH, et al. Evaluation of suppressive therapy for cold thyroid nodules with levothyroxine: double-blind placebo-controlled clinical trial. *Endocr Pract* 1999;5:251.

86. Reverter J, Lucas A, Salinas I, et al. Suppressive therapy with levothyroxine for solitary thyroid nodules. *Clin Endocrinol (Oxf)* 1992;36:25.

87. Papini E, Bacci V, Panunzi C, et al. A prospective randomized trial of levothyroxine suppressive therapy for solitary thyroid nodules. *Clin Endocrinol (Oxf)* 1993;38:507.

88. Koc M, Ersoz HO, Akpinar I, et al. Effect of low- and high-dose levothyroxine on thyroid nodule volume: a crossover placebo-controlled trial. *Clin Endocrinol (Oxf)* 2002;57:621.

89. Fogelfeld L, Wiviott MBT, Shore-Freedman E, et al. Recurrence of thyroid nodules after surgical removal in patients irradiated in childhood for benign conditions. *N Engl J Med* 1989;320:835.

90. Doshi SV, Cruz RM, Hilsinger RL Jr. Thyroglossal duct carcinoma: a large case series. *Ann Otol Rhinol Laryngol* 2001;110:734.

THE THYROID IN INFANCY
AND CHILDHOOD

THE MATURATION OF THYROID FUNCTION IN THE PERINATAL PERIOD AND DURING CHILDHOOD

ROSALIND S. BROWN
STEPHEN A. HUANG
DELBERT A. FISHER

The maturation of thyroid function in the human fetus is a complex process that involves the growth and development not only of the thyroid gland itself but of the intricate network of regulatory systems required for mature activity as well. These include the development of the hypothalamus and pituitary gland, and, in addition, the coordinated maturation of mechanisms required for thyroid hormone transport, metabolism, and action. In general, fetal thyroid hormone levels are low in the first half of human pregnancy. During this period the fetus is entirely dependent on maternal thyroid hormone, the supply of which is controlled by the placenta and circulating maternal levels. Fetal thyroid hormone secretion increases in the second half of pregnancy, coincident with hypothalamic–pituitary–thyroid maturation. Despite the low serum concentrations of fetal thyroid hormones early in pregnancy, triiodothyronine (T_3) levels are well maintained in critical target tissues such as the fetal brain due to coordinate adjustments in the deiodinase system. Unique to the childhood years, thyroid hormone plays a critical role in the maturation of numerous target organs, including bone, brown adipose tissue, cochlea, retina, liver, lung, and heart, as well as brain. These maturational programs are precisely controlled and occur in developmental, regulated, tissue-specific windows of time. In this chapter, the intricate regulation of thyroid system development will be reviewed and recent important insights in our understanding discussed.

Much of our information about thyroid system development has derived from studies in two animal models, fetal-neonatal rodents and fetal sheep. Although the events of thyroid development are roughly comparable in rodents, sheep, and humans, important differences exist in both the structure of the placenta and the timing of development. In newborn rats, thyroid system development at birth (21 days) is relatively immature and is equivalent to the early third trimester human fetus. Therefore, it is possible to study much of the thyroid system development in the neonatal period in the absence of the placenta. Sheep fetuses on the other hand have more mature thyroid develop-

ment at birth and provides a model for intrauterine human thyroid development. The timing of thyroid hormone–dependent brain maturation relative to the intrauterine development also differs in the three species. In infant rats, from which much of our detailed information has been obtained, the major period of thyroid dependency of brain maturation extends from birth or slightly before to about 40 days of postnatal age. In sheep, thyroid-dependent brain maturation extends from 70 to 90 days of the 150-day gestation to several postnatal weeks. In human infants, the period of maximal thyroid-dependent brain development probably extends from midgestation to about 2 years of postnatal age. Recently, however, evidence has been provided in both rodents and humans to suggest that thyroid hormone may play an important role in fetal brain development much earlier than was appreciated previously and that this period might extend prior to the onset of fetal thyroid hormone production.

THYROID SYSTEM ONTOGENESIS

Hypothalamic–Pituitary Embryogenesis

The first trimester of human pregnancy is characterized by embryogenesis of the thyroid gland, hypothalamus, and pituitary. Glandular development is dependent on an orderly cascade of transcription factors and signaling molecules that determine organogenesis and cell determination and specification. Transcription factors involved in early human fetal forebrain and hypothalamic development include sonic hedgehog (SHH) and ZIC-2 (a homologue of the *Drosophila* odd-paired gene). These genes are first identified at about 3 weeks of gestation, when the hypothalamus starts to differentiate. Mutations of *SHH* and *ZIC-2* have been identified in familial and sporadic holoprosencephaly (1,2). Another important homeobox gene is *HESX-1,* mutations in which have been shown in siblings with septo-optic dysplasia involving midline brain defects and pituitary hypoplasia (3). SF-1, and the LIM class homeodomain factors LHX-3 and LHX-4 also play a role (4), but current understanding of the interaction of these factors is limited (see Chapter 2).

Considerable information has been developed in rodents regarding transcription factor programming of pituitary embryogenesis (5). The Rathke's pouch homeobox and the pituitary homeobox gene (*PTX-1*) are early factors in a cascade of determinants, including *TTF-1, LHX-3, LHX-4, Prop-1,* and *Pit-1,* and targeted disruption of these factors in mice leads to stillbirth or neonatal death (4). Thyroid transcription factor 1 (*TTF-1*) knockout leads to pituitary gland as well as thyroid gland aplasia. *LHX-3* and *LHX-4,* LIM-class homeodomain transcription factors, are also essential for normal pituitary embryogenesis. The terminal factors in the cascade are *Prop-1* and *Pit-1,* which program development and function of pituitary cells producing growth hormone (GH), prolactin, thyrotropin (TSH-β), and the growth hormone–releasing hormone (GHRH) receptor (4). Mutations in *Prop-1* and *Pit-1* have been described in patients with familial hypopituitarism (5).

Anatomically, the pituitary gland develops from two anlages: an evagination of the floor of the primitive forebrain and a ventral pouch from the ectoderm of the primitive oral cavity. The latter, Rathke's pouch, is visible by 5 weeks, evolving to a morphologically mature pituitary gland by 14 weeks. The pituitary–portal blood vessels have begun to develop by this time, and maturation continues through 30 to 35 weeks' gestation. The hypothalamic nuclei, median eminence, and supraoptic tract are identifiable by 15 to 18 weeks, and significant concentrations of thyrotropin-releasing hormone (TRH) and dopamine are detectable at this time. The anterior pituitary hormones, including TSH, can be identified by immunoassay at 10 to 17 weeks, and concentrations increase progressively thereafter (see Chapter 2).

Thyroid Gland Embryogenesis

The thyroid gland is derived from fusion of a medial outpouching from the floor of the primitive pharynx, the precursor of the thyroxine (T_4)-producing follicular cells, and bilateral evaginations of the fourth pharyngeal pouch, which give rise to the parafollicular, or calcitonin (C)-secreting cells (6). Analogous to pituitary gland development, commitment toward a thyroid-specific phenotype as well as the growth and descent of the thyroid anlage into the neck results from the coordinate action of multiple transcription factors, hormones, and growth factors. The approximate timing of molecular events controlling thyroid gland development in rats is summarized in Table 74.1. Three transcription factors, *TTF-1, TTF-2,* and *PAX-8,* are expressed before or just after the first appearance of the thyroid diverticulum on fetal day 9.5 to 10 and appear to be of major importance not only in early thyroid embryogenesis but in thyroid-specific gene expression as

well (7–11). *TTF-1,* a homeodomain-containing transcription factor, is expressed in both follicular cells and C cells. Targeted disruption of the *TTF-1* gene results in mice completely devoid of thyroid tissue (11). In contrast, *PAX-8,* a paired domain-containing transcription factor, is expressed only in thyroid follicular cell precursors and is involved in transcriptional regulation of the thyroglobulin and thyroid peroxidase genes but not the TSH receptor gene (10,12). The thyroid glands of mice lacking *PAX-8* are reduced in size, lack follicles, and are composed almost exclusively of C cells. A specific set of *HOX* genes (*HOX-A3* and the paralogous gene *HOX-B3*), members of a large family of genes that impart important patterning information in embryogenesis, appear to be important in the expression of *PAX-8* and *TTF-1,* respectively (13,14). Similarly, *NKX-2.5,* a member of the same family of genes as *TTF-1,* is expressed prior to *TTF-1* in the pharyngeal floor and thyroid primordium and may play a role in *TTF-1* regulation (15). It is of interest that both *TTF-1, TTF-2,* and *PAX-8* are also expressed in a limited number of other cell types, suggesting that it is the specific combination of transcription factors and possibly non-DNA binding cofactors acting coordinately that determine the specific genotype of a cell. For example, as noted, *TTF-1* is also expressed in the pituitary gland as well as the lungs, whereas *PAX-8* is expressed in the kidney (see Chapter 2).

Thyroid descent to the anterior neck is complete by fetal day 14.5 to 15 in rats; thyroglobulin, thyroid peroxidase, and TSH receptor gene expression can be demonstrated as early as fetal day 15 to 15.5 (7,16). In view of the 5- to 5.5-day delay between the first appearance of *TTF-1, TTF-2,* and *PAX-8* and thyroid-specific gene expression, additional factors must be involved. *TTF-2,* a forkhead domain–containing binding protein, is down-regulated between fetal day 13 and fetal day 15 in mice (equivalent to fetal day 14 and 16 in rats), and it has been proposed that, in addition to its role in the commitment to a thyroid-specific phenotype, *TTF-2* acts both to promote migration and repress thyroid-specific gene expression in thyroid follicular cell precursors (9). This interpretation is supported by findings in *TTF-2* null mice, which develop one of two phenotypes; either the thyroid gland fails to develop, or a sublingual thyroid gland is formed, demonstrating evidence of thyroid differentiation, at least as indicated by thyroglobulin expression (17).

At fetal day 15, despite early evidence of thyroid-specific gene expression, the rat thyroid gland is difficult to distinguish from the surrounding structures, and neither iodine organification, thyroid hormonogenesis, nor evidence of a follicular structure is present. Thus, *TTF-1* and *PAX-8* are necessary but not sufficient for expression of the fully differentiated thyroid phenotype. On day 17 to 18, TSH receptor gene expression is dramatically up-regulated, and this is accompanied by significant growth and rapid development of both structural and functional characteristics, suggesting that the TSH receptor plays a role at

TABLE 74.1   APPROXIMATE TIMING OF MOLECULAR EVENTS CONTROLLING THYROID GLAND DEVELOPMENT IN RATS

Fetal Age (Days)	Molecular Event	Development Concomitant
8.5–9.5	NKS-2.5, HOX-A3, and HOX-B3 genes expressed in primitive pharynx	
9.5–10	TTF-1, TTF-2, and PAX-8 genes expressed	
14–16[a]	TTF-2 expression decreases and disappears	Appearance of thyroid diverticulum
14.5–15	—	
15–15.5	Tg, TPO, TSH receptor expessed	Parathyroid glands join thyroid; migration completed
17–18	Tg, TPO, TSH receptor expression upregulated	Appearance of TSH in serum
		Appearance of thyroid follicles, iodine uptake, iodide uptake, and thyroid hormonogenesis
21	—	Delivery

[a]By analogy with data in mice.

Tt, thyroglobulin; TPO, thyroid peroxidase; TSH, thyrotropin; TTF,

this later stage of development (18). Expression of both thyroglobulin and thyroid peroxidase messenger RNA (mRNA) increase, thyroid follicles develop, thyroid peroxidase enzyme function can be demonstrated, and there is evidence of thyroid hormonogenesis (18–20). In contrast, hyt/hyt mice, which have a loss-of-function (Pro556-Leu) mutation in the transmembrane domain of the TSH receptor, have severe hypothyroidism and hypoplastic but normally located thyroid glands with a poorly developed follicular structure (21). Similar findings have been described in infants born to mothers with potent TSH receptor blocking antibodies and in infants with loss of function mutations of the TSH receptor (22,23). Up-regulation of TSH receptor gene expression on fetal days 17 to 18 in rats is coincident with the first appearance of pituitary TSH in the fetal circulation and implies that, unlike in adults, the TSH receptor in the fetus may be upregulated by TSH (18,24). Following fetal days 17 to 18, there is continuing maturation of thyroid gland morphology and function.

Information regarding the early phases of human fetal thyroid embryogenesis is limited, but thyroid gland embryogenesis and descent are largely complete by 10 to 12 weeks' gestation. At this stage, tiny follicle precursors can be seen, iodine uptake can be identified, and thyroglobulin is present in the follicular spaces (25–27). Thyroid hormonogenesis is detected by 11 to 12 weeks, coincident with the appearance of TSH in the fetal circulation.

Maturation of the Thyroid System Control

Hypothalamic–Pituitary Axis and Hormone Transport

The key events in thyroid development are summarized in Figure 74.1. The secretion of TSH and thyroid hormones is minimal until midgestation (28,29). At this time (18–20 weeks of gestation), fetal thyroid gland iodine uptake and serum T_4 concentrations begin to increase. The fetal serum TSH concentration progressively increases from a low value

at 16 to 18 weeks, associated with progressive increases in serum total and free T_4 concentrations between 20 weeks and term (28,29). Maturation of control of thyroid hormone secretion is superimposed on a progressive increase in fetal serum thyroxine-binding globulin (TBG) concentration caused by maturation of fetal hepatic TBG synthetic capacity. Pituitary TSH responsiveness to exogenous TRH is present early in the third trimester, and maturation of negative feedback control of pituitary TSH secretion develops progressively during the last half of gestation and the first 1 to 2 months of extrauterine life (28,30,31). Although immature, the fetal hypothalamic–pituitary system is capable of responding to hypothyroxinemia; congenital hypothyroidism in the 24-week fetus has been associated with a markedly increased serum TSH concentration (32).

During the neonatal period, the serum free T_4 concentration increases in response to an early neonatal TSH surge, and there is a marked increase in free T_4 concentration associated with a decline in TSH by 3 to 5 days (25,28,30) (Fig. 74.1). The free T_4:TSH and free T_3:TSH concentration ratios approximate adult values by 1 to 2 months of age (28). Thus, the human fetus matures from a state of combined primary and hypothalamic–pituitary hypothyroidism during the first trimester, through a period of hypothalamic hypothyroidism during the last half of gestation, to a state of mature function by 1 to 2 months of postnatal life.

Development of Thyroid Gland Responsiveness and Autonomy

The progressive increase in fetal serum free T_4 concentrations during the last half of gestation appears to be due to both increasing fetal serum TSH and progressive maturation of thyroid follicular cell responsiveness to TSH (29,33). There are no data regarding the thyroid response to TSH for the developing human fetus. Direct data are available, however, from fetal sheep, in which there is a progressive increase in the responses of serum T_4 and the serum T_4:TSH ratio to exogenous TRH during the last trimester of pregnancy (34).

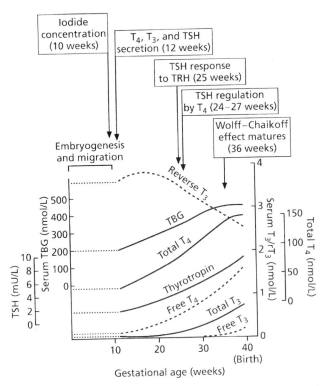

FIGURE 74.1. Maturation of thyroid gland development and function during gestation. During the first half of gestation the fetus is dependent on maternal thyroxine (T_4), the supply of which is regulated by placental deiodinase. Although first detected at 10 to 12 weeks, fetal T_4 and free T_4 concentrations do not begin to increase until 18 to 20 weeks, coincident with increasing hypothalamic-pituitary maturation. Serum levels of TRH and inactive T_4 metabolites, such as reverse triiodothyronine (T_3), are high in fetal life (not shown). (From Brown RS, Larsen R. Thyroid gland development and disease in infancy and childhood. In: DeGroot L, Hennemann G, eds. Thyroid *disease manager.* Accessed at http://*thyroidmanager.org,* accessed August 30, 2004.)

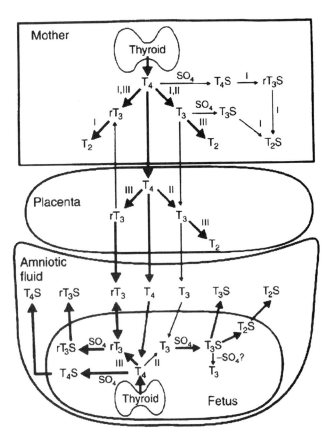

FIGURE 74.2. Differences in deiodinase activity in the maternal, placental, and fetal compartments. In the fetus, high levels of inactive thyroxine (T_4) metabolites and of sulfated analogues are present. This occurs because of increased activity of the inactivating deiodinase, D3, in fetal life, coupled with immaturity of D1, the major activating deiodinase in the adult. The placenta also contains high D3 activity that serves to inactivate most of the maternal T_4 presented to it. Nonetheless, significant maternal-fetal T_4 does occur, particularly when T_4 levels in the fetus are low. (From Burrow GN, Fisher DA, Larsen PR. Maternal and fetal thyroid function. *N Engl J Med* 1994;331:1072–1078, with permission.)

Thyroid gland maturation also includes maturation of thyroid autoregulation of iodine transport. The thyroid gland of adult mammals can modify iodine transport relative to dietary iodine intake and exclusive of variations in serum TSH. The developing mammalian thyroid gland lacks this autoregulatory mechanism and is thus susceptible to iodine-induced inhibition of thyroid hormone synthesis (35,36). The ability of the thyroid gland to defend against the thyroid-blocking effect of excessive iodide on thyroid hormone synthesis does not develop until after 36 to 40 weeks of gestation in the human fetus (35). Thus, premature infants under this age are at risk for the development of iodine-induced hypothyroidism.

Maturation of Thyroxine Metabolism

In adult humans, sequential monodeiodination, catalyzed by the iodothyronine deiodinase family of selenoenzymes,

is the main pathway of thyroid hormone metabolism. As detailed in Chapter 7, removal of an iodine atom from the outer ring of T_4 leads to substrate activation, a reaction catalyzed by types 1 (D1) and 2 (D2) deiodinase. Conversely, inner ring deiodination, catalyzed primarily by D3, leads to substrate inactivation. The three deiodinases share sequence homology around the active center, but different genes encode them and important differences exist with regard to their substrate affinity, tissue distribution, and sensitivity to inhibition by propylthiouracil. In the euthyroid state, approximately 80% of circulating T_3 is derived from the outer ring deiodination of T_4 in peripheral tissues (catalyzed by D1 and D2), and 80% of thyroid hormone is ultimately inactivated by inner ring deiodination (catalyzed by D3). In some tissues, such as the liver and kidney, most T_3 is derived from plasma and only 25% of the intracellular T_3 is generated from T_4. In contrast, in the pituitary gland and cerebral cortex, local conversion of T_4 to T_3 plays a significantly more important role.

Compared with adult serum, fetal serum has low concentrations of free T_4 and T_3 and high concentrations of several inactive iodothyronine metabolites (rT_3, T_2, T_3S, T_4S) (37) (Fig. 74.2). Although the physiologic significance of the low serum levels of T_3 is still unknown, it has been suggested that its function may be to avoid tissue thermogenesis and potentiate the anabolic state of the rapidly growing fetus. The low serum T_3 concentration is due both to increased activity of the inactivating deiodinase (D3) as well as to the low expression of D1, the major activating deiodinase in adults. Animal studies have documented D3 in the uteroplacental unit as well as in multiple embryonic structures, including the liver, brain, gonads, lung, heart, intestine, and skin (38–41). Of interest is the recent finding that D3 expression is localized in areas of the neonatal rat brain involved in sexual differentiation (42,43). In humans, studies have shown, similarly, high levels of D3 activity or protein in the fetal liver, the cerebral cortex, and the epithelial structures of the embryonic lung, intestine, skin, and urinary tract (44–47). The possibility that this increased D3 activity may protect the developing embryo from T_3 and T_4 is supported by findings in mice with a targeted disruption in D3 (48). These D3-deficient mice are exposed *in utero* to more maternal T_3 and T_4 levels and demonstrate significant growth retardation and perinatal mortality. Similarly, recent evidence suggests that the gene for D3 (*Dio3* in mice, *DIO3* in humans) is expressed preferentially from the paternal side. Disruption in the imprinting status of *Dio3* results in abnormal thyroid hormone levels and may explain, in part, the phenotypic abnormalities in mice with uniparental disomy 12 and its human equivalent uniparental disomy 14 (49).

In contrast to D3, D2 is the major activating deiodinase expressed in the fetus. D2 is present in brain, pituitary, cochlea, brown adipose tissue, keratinocytes, and placenta. In rats, D2 activity in fetal brain is relatively low early in gestation and increases markedly during neonatal life to reach maximal levels at 2 to 3 weeks of life (38). The increase in D2 activity is coincident with an 18-fold increase of brain T_3 content (50). In humans, both D2 and D3 activity are present in fetal brain as early as 7 to 8 weeks' gestation, indicating that the ability to convert T_4 to T_3 is present prior to the onset of fetal thyroid function (46). As in adults, the coordinated expression of these deiodinases throughout gestation determines the levels of the iodothyronines in fetal serum. Additionally, the tissue-specific expression of these enzymes allows the local concentration of T_3 to vary from one structure or compartment compared with another. For example, compared with adults, the human fetal cerebral cortex has a higher content of T_4 and T_3 with similar rT_3 content, despite the relatively low concentrations of T_4 and T_3 in fetal serum (45,51). This occurs because of the presence in fetal brain and pituitary of D2,

the activity of which increases when levels of T_4 are low. This represents an important level of prereceptor regulation of thyroid hormone action. In rodents, deiodinase activity in the fetal brain maintains local concentrations of in the normal range despite alternations in maternal thyroid status (52). A similar protective regulation in humans may explain the excellent neurologic outcome observed in infants with severe congenital hypothyroidism treated aggressively soon after birth.

Further evidence for the importance of the deiodinase system is the close temporal and spatial associations of the ontogeny of thyroid hormone metabolism and action. For example, in the mouse, D2 activity in the cochlea increases dramatically to reach a peak level at postnatal day 6, a few days prior to the onset of hearing (53). This is a critical period for the development of auditory function in rodents, and only thyroid hormone given to hypothyroid animals during the critical period prior to postnatal days 10 to 12 can rescue cochlear morphogenesis and auditory function (53). D2 expression is localized to connective tissue immediately adjacent to the sensory epithelium and spiral ganglion where thyroid hormone receptors (TRs) are found (53). Thus, it has been suggested that D2-containing cells in the connective tissue take up T_4 from the circulation, convert T_4 to T_3, and then release T_3 to the adjacent responsive cells. This provides an important degree of paracrine control of thyroid hormone action. A similar relationship is found in certain areas of the brain where D2 is expressed predominantly in glial cells, tanycytes (a specialized type of glial cells), and astrocytes, whereas TRs are found in the adjacent neurons and oligodendrocytes (42). Thus, T_4, which enters the developing brain more readily than T_3, is taken up from capillaries by glial cells, deiodinated to T_3, and then transferred to neurons for action (42). In other areas of the brain, such as the pituitary gland, hippocampus, and caudate nucleus, D2 and TRs are coexpressed (42). As described previously for the cochlea, the development of D2 activity in the cerebral cortex in rodents is temporally associated with the period of maximum sensitivity to thyroid hormone action (54). Unlike D2, D3 is coexpressed with TRs in neurons, perhaps underlying the importance of protecting them from the effects of excess thyroid hormone (42).

In addition to deiodination, sulfation is another important pathway of thyroid hormone metabolism in the fetus (31). In adults, the sulfation of T_4 and T_3 facilitates their degradation, because sulfated iodothyronines are excellent substrates for inner ring deiodination by D1. Sulfotransferase activity has been documented in human liver and kidney but, in adults, serum concentrations of sulfated iodothyronines are very low due to their rapid degradation by hepatic D1. The relatively high concentrations of these metabolites in fetal serum are presumably due to lower fetal hepatic D1 activity or decreased transport of T_4 and T_3 into fetal hepatocytes. Sulfation is reversible and, in settings where sulfated iodothyronines are not rapidly cleared, these conjugated thyroid hormones may serve as a local reserve of active hormone in tissues containing sulfatase enzymes (55).

Throughout pregnancy, the programmed expression of deiodinases permits the maternal and fetal thyroid axes to function relatively independently. Birth signals a rapid transition to adult thyroid hormone metabolism. In chickens, hatching is characterized by a rapid increase in serum T_3 that occurs in conjunction with a rapid decrease in hepatic D3 activity (56,57). Human birth is also associated with a rapid postnatal decline in hepatic and placental D3 activity and increase in brown-adipocyte D2 activity as part of adaptive thermogenesis. Both the decline in hepatic D3 and maturation of hepatic D1 activity contribute to a surge in serum levels of T_3 postnatally. Within a few weeks of life, serum T_3 concentrations in the newborn approximates these found in the adult, suggesting that maturation of deiodinase expression is complete (58).

Ontogenesis of Thyroid Receptors and Thyroid Hormone Actions

Receptor Maturation

As described in Chapter 8, the action of thyroid hormone is mediated primarily by specific nuclear receptors that function as ligand-mediated transcription factors to stimulate or inhibit expression of target genes (42). The binding of T_3 to thyroid hormone receptors (TRs) is at least 10 times higher than that of T_4. In addition to the four classical TRs—TRα1, TRα2, TRβ1, and TRβ2—multiple other transcripts that encode protein products have been identified. The gene encoding the TRα subtype is located on chromosome 17, whereas the gene encoding the TRβ subtype is on chromosome 3; the respective isoforms (1 and 2) result from alternative splicing of the initial mRNA transcripts. TRα2 and other splice variants, such as TRvα2 and TRvα3, do not bind T_3 and may inhibit the binding of the other TRs to DNA (dominant negative inhibition). The TRα gene also produces an orphan receptor, rev-erb αα, that plays a role in cerebellar development. TRs exist as monomers, homodimers, or heterodimers with other nuclear proteins such as retinoid X-receptors. The heterodimeric structure is the active form of the receptor. TR activity requires the interaction of numerous coactivators and corepressors. In the unliganded state, some TRs repress gene function (42).

Like the iodothyronine deiodinases discussed above, the various TRs are expressed developmentally and differentially in tissues. TRβ1 mRNA expression is particularly abundant in liver and kidney, but is also found in parts of the developing brain, hypothalamus, pituitary, ear, and heart. In contrast, TRβ2 mRNA expression is much more restricted, the highest concentration being found in the pituitary gland. TRα1 and TRα2 are widely distributed among tissues (42).

The temporal sequence of thyroid hormone-mediated effects on maturation is developmentally regulated and occurs during a critical window of time. Although thyroid hormone–dependent pituitary, brain, and bone development occur early, other effects, such as those on liver, brown adipose tissue, lung, and heart, are detected only later in gestation. In rats, receptors can be detected in brain by binding assay as early as 13.5 to 14 days postconception, prior to the onset of fetal thyroid function. The concentration is low initially but increases subsequently, to reach a maximum level on postnatal day 6, accompanied by increased hormone occupancy. The TRα1 isoform is the predominant variant in fetal rat brain, and TRα1 mRNA is detected as early as embryonic days 11.5 to 12.5. Expression of the TRβ1 isoform, first detected at the time of birth, increases dramatically; there is a 40-fold higher concentration in the early postnatal period, with maximal level at postnatal day 10. The increase in TRβ1 mRNA is coincident with the neonatal surge in serum T_3 and a postnatal increase in TR binding capacity. In contrast to the pituitary, hepatic nuclear T_3 receptors mature during the first 3 to 5 weeks of extrauterine life, a period equivalent to the last trimester and early postnatal period of human fetal development (59–61). Other thyroid hormone effects, such as those on thermogenesis, hepatic enzyme activities, growth hormone metabolism, and growth factor metabolism [insulin-like growth factors (IGFs), nerve growth factor, epidermal growth factor] appear during the first 4 weeks postnatally. In sheep, the pattern of thyroid ontogenesis is comparable with that in rats and humans; in this species, however, most of the events of thyroid maturation occur *in utero* (41).

Receptor ontogeny in the human fetus recapitulates the situation in rodents and sheep. Both the T_3 receptor, measured by binding assay, and the ligand T_3, presumably of maternal origin, have been detected in fetal brain as early as 10 weeks' gestation, with a 10-fold increase in receptor abundance at 16 to 18 weeks (42). Using more sensitive methods, TRα1, TRα2, and TRβ1 isoforms have been detected at both the mRNA and protein level even earlier, at 8 weeks' gestation (46). In humans, like in rodents, TRα1 is the preponderant isoform early in gestation. Liver, heart, and lung receptor binding, on the other hand, are only identified at 16 to 18 weeks (62).

Ontogenesis of Thyroid Hormone Action

Thyroid Hormone–Mediated Brain Maturation

Of the multiple actions of thyroid hormone, none is more critical than the effect on brain development, as demonstrated by the severe, irreversible mental retardation and deafness characteristic of patients with untreated congenital hypothyroidism. In the brain, thyroid hormone mediates the maturation of a diverse array of processes that follow a precise developmental program and lead to the es-

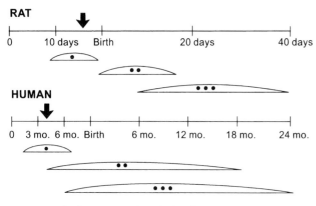

- • cerebral neurogenesis and migration
- •• neuronal differentiation, neurite outgrowth, synaptogenesis, cerebellar neurogenesis, gliogenesis
- ••• myelinogenesis
- ⬇ onset of fetal thyroid hormone secretion

FIGURE 74.3. Comparative central nervous system ontogenesis in rats and humans. In both species, cerebral neurogenesis and cell migration occur *in utero*. In rats, cerebellar maturation, neurite outgrowth, synaptogenesis, gliogenesis, and myelinogenesis are largely postnatal events. In humans, this period begins *in utero* at 6 months' gestation and extends to 1 to 2 years of postnatal life. During much of rat fetal development and the first half of human gestation, the fetus is dependent on maternal thyroid hormones. (Modified from Porterfield HP, Hendrick CE. The role of thyroid hormones in prenatal and neonatal neurological development—current perspectives. *Endocr Rev* 1993; 14:94, with permission.)

tablishment of neural circuits essential for normal central nervous system development. Several excellent recent reviews of this topic are available (42,43,63). Cerebral histogenesis and cell migration, beginning prior to the onset of fetal thyroid hormone production, are the first processes to occur (Fig. 74.3). Once these neurons have migrated to their final destination, multiple events take place, manifested in rodents during the first 2 to 3 weeks of postnatal life (equivalent to the last trimester of human pregnancy and the first few months postnatally). Neurons begin to differentiate, form dendritic processes, and develop synapses. Cerebellar and hippocampal granule cells proliferate, migrate, and differentiate, and Purkinje cells develop their characteristic dendritic tree. Myelin-forming oligodendroglia proliferate, migrate, and mature, and axonal myelination is initiated. Cochlear and retinal maturation and gliogenesis are additional processes that occur in this later phase of brain development (53,63–65).

Thyroid hormones provide the induction signal for the differentiation and maturation programs. In some cases, the absence of thyroid hormone appears to delay the timing rather than eliminate critical morphologic events or gene products, resulting in disorganization of intercellular communication. However, the molecular mechanisms by which this occurs are only now beginning to be understood. Consistent with a nuclear receptor mode of action,

thyroid hormone stimulates numerous developmentally regulated genes, including genes for myelin, neurotrophins and their receptors, cytoskeletal components, transcription factors, extracellular matrix proteins and adhesion molecules, intracellular signaling molecules, and mitochondrial and cerebellar genes. In some cases these genes appear to be direct targets of thyroid hormone action; thyroid hormone response elements can be detected in the DNA regulatory region, or the genes are stimulated in cell culture. In other cases, thyroid hormone control may occur secondarily as a consequence of effects on terminal differentiation. In addition, thyroid hormone regulates some genes at the level of mRNA stability or mRNA splicing.

One of the unexplained paradoxes has been the surprising lack of developmental abnormalities in mice lacking TRα1, TRβ, or both, in contrast to the severe abnormalities in hypothyroid animals (66). Emerging evidence suggests that the reason for the abnormal brain development observed after thyroid hormone deficiency but not TR deficiency is transcriptional repression or abnormal regulation by the unliganded TR (42,43). For example, when mice lacking the TRα1 receptor were made hypothyroid, no effects on cerebellar development were seen, contrary to findings in wild-type animals (67). Analogous results were obtained with euthyroid mice containing a knock-in TR mutation designed to inhibit T_3 binding but leave corepressor binding functions intact (68). As expected, these mice developed severe neurologic abnormalities. It is likely that the complexity of maturational control of thyroid hormone action involves developmental regulation of myriad factors that affect TR activity. These factors include corepressors and coactivators as well as transcription factors that compete with TRs for thyroid hormone response elements (TREs) on target genes, providing further levels of modulation (68).

There is also some evidence that the action of T_4 on the developing CNS involves, in part, a nonnuclear mechanism. The work of Farwell et al has shown that T_4-regulated actin polymerization plays an integral role in the regulation of deiodinase activity, and he and his colleagues have proposed that the action of T_4 on the actin cytoskeleton might be important in cellular migration, neurite outgrowth, and dendritic spine formation (69,70).

Thyroid Hormone–Mediated Growth

Thyroid hormones are critical for the normal growth and development of bone, as evidenced by the striking growth retardation, decreased growth velocity, and delayed ossification of the epiphyseal growth plate characteristic of long-standing, hypothyroidism in infancy and childhood. This growth-stimulatory actions of thyroid hormones occur in the context of a complex interplay of genetic, hormonal, and growth factor effects that are thyroid hormone independent (71,72). Thyroid hormone–mediated bone maturation involves both a direct and indirect action, the latter mediated by regulation of growth hormone gene expression and the IGF system (73). At a direct level, T_3 regulates endochondral ossification and controls chondrocyte differentiation in the growth plate both *in vitro* and *in vivo* (74,75). Both osteoblasts and growth plate chondrocytes express TRs, and several T_3-specific target genes have been identified in bone (66). T_3 also stimulates closure of the skull sutures *in vivo*, the basis for the enlarged anterior and posterior fontanelles characteristic of infants with congenital hypothyroidism (76). Complete deletion of TRβ does not cause growth or bone abnormalities, whereas mutant TRα mice exhibit growth retardation, poor bone mineralization, and an immature, disorganized growth plate, suggesting that the action of thyroid hormone on bone is mediated primarily by TRα gene products (66). However, the growth retardation in TRαβ double knockout mice is more severe than that seen in mice with a targeted disruption of TR alone, implying that some important growth-promoting actions are performed by TRβ (66). The growth retardation in hypothyroid mice is more severe than that in TRαβ double knockout mice, consistent with the effect of the unliganded receptor in mediating the deleterious effects of thyroid hormone deficiency (66).

Thyroid Hormone–Mediated Brown-Fat Thermogenesis

A third important action of thyroid hormone is on the development of nonshivering thermogenesis, a metabolic change of profound importance to the neonate as it transitions from fetal to neonatal life. The ability of human infants and selected other homeothermic newborn mammals to maintain body temperature in the immediate extrauterine environment depends on the presence and function of brown adipose tissue (BAT), the cells of which have high concentrations of mitochondria (77–79) (see Chapters 38 and 60). The oxidative degradation of substrate, predominantly lipid, in BAT mitochondria as in other mitochondria provides a nicotinamide dehydrogenase–linked supply of electrons to coenzyme Q (ubiquinone) and to the cytochrome system. This respiratory chain maintains a proton gradient across the mitochondrial membrane that provides for the phosphorylation of nucleotides and storage of energy as adenosine triphosphate (79). Mitochondria contain a unique 32,000 molecular weight protein (uncoupling protein, UCP1, or thermogenin) on the inner membrane. UCP1 catalyzes the uncoupling of oxidative phosphorylation by dissipating the proton gradient created by the respiratory chain, resulting in energy dissipation as heat (80,81).

Cold-induced, nonshivering adaptive thermogenesis depends on the synergistic stimulation of UCP1 gene transcription by catecholamines and thyroid hormones. There is one functional cyclic adenosine monophosphate (cyclic AMP) response element (CRE) and two thyroid hormone response elements (TREs) in the UCP1 gene promoter. In rodents, the normal response of UCP1 to cold is blunted in hypothyroidism and requires the complete saturation of BAT TRs for an effect. Normalizing the UCP1 response of hypothyroid rats with exogenous T_3 requires doses that cause systemic thyrotoxicosis, whereas the same results can be achieved with only physiologic replacement doses of T_4 (82–84). This thermogenic response in T_4-treated hypothyroid rats is due to the local conversion of T_4 to T_3 in BAT by D2, and can be blocked by the addition of the deiodinase inhibitor iopanoic acid (85,86). Experiments performed with D2 knockout mice have provided further direct evidence that D2 is required for the normal thermogenic response to cold stress. In the Dio2−/− knockout mice, cold exposure leads to hypothermia due to impaired BAT thermogenesis despite normal serum T_3 concentrations and normal basal mitochondrial concentrations of UCP1. The hypothyroid-like abnormalities of the Dio2−/− knockout mice are completely reversed by the administration of T_3 (87). The volume and functional activity of BAT, including D2 activity and UCP levels, increase progressively with fetal age so that BAT thermogenic activity is maximal in the perinatal period. As the human infant grows, shivering becomes the most important involuntary mechanism of cold-induced adaptive thermogenesis, and the anatomic distribution of BAT becomes restricted to the axillary, deep cervical, and perirenal adipose deposits (88).

Role of the Placenta

The placenta plays a vital role in fetal thyroid development and function by serving as an important site of thyroid hormone metabolism, by regulating the passage of substances from the maternal to the fetal circulation, and by synthesizing hormones that affect both maternal and fetal thyroid status (89). Much of our information has been derived from studies in rodents and sheep, but important differences exist in the structure of the placenta in humans and in these other species. Sheep have an epitheliochorial placenta in which the maternal and fetal circulations are separated by six tissue layers. Rats have a hemotrichorial placenta with four tissue layers separating the maternal and fetal circulation, whereas the human placenta is hemomonochorial with three tissue layers between the maternal and fetal circulations. Thus, differences in placental permeability to various substances, including drugs and hormones, might be expected among the three species.

Thyroid Hormone

Under normal circumstances, the placenta has only limited permeability to T_4 and T_3, and the fetal hypothalamic–pituitary–thyroid system develops relatively independent of maternal influence. Important species differences in the extent of maternal-fetal T_4 transfer exist, the order being rats > humans > sheep. The impermeability of the human placenta to thyroid hormone is due primarily to the high concentration of placental D3, which serves to inactivate most of the thyroid hormone presented from the maternal or fetal circulation, thereby protecting embryonic structures from the temporally inappropriate action of thyroid hormone (47). Immunostaining localizes D3 to the syncytiotrophoblast and cytotrophoblast layers of the placental membrane as well as to the fetal endothelium of the chorionic villi. Strong staining is also seen in the maternal decidua of human placentas and in the amniotic membranes. The iodide released serves to provide a continuing source of iodide for fetal thyroid hormone synthesis.

Human placental deiodination is a dynamic process, and activity varies throughout gestation. Specific activity is highest in the first trimester and then decreases as the pregnancy progresses. Although specific activity is decreased, total placental D3 activity is increased at term due to the concurrent increase in placental size. D2, which catalyzes the outer ring deiodination of T_4 to T_3, is also detectable in human placenta. However, placental D2 activity is approximately 200-fold lower than D3 activity throughout pregnancy, suggesting negligible contribution to the modulation of transplacental thyroid hormone transfer (90).

Recently, D2 and D3 activity has also been identified in the uterus (91–93). D3 activity is highest at the implantation site, but is also present in the endometrial glands of nonpregnant uteri. In rats, D3 activity at the implantation site is twice that in term placentas (94). In humans, the specific activity of endometrial homogenates from nonpregnant uteri exceeds that of term placenta (47). These data suggest that the uterus, like the placenta, also modulates the transfer of thyroid hormone to the fetus. Furthermore, the presence of high endometrial D3 activity in the nonpregnant state suggests that the local modulation of thyroid status is important at all stages of human reproduction, including implantation.

Importance of Maternal Thyroid Hormone

Despite the limited permeability of the placenta to T_4, significant maternal-to-fetal transfer does occur, and current evidence suggests that this is particularly important when serum T_4 concentrations in the fetus are low. For example, infants with the complete inability to synthesize T_4 due to an inborn error of thyroid hormonogenesis nonetheless have cord T_4 concentrations between 25% and 50% of normal (95). The results are similar in cord serum in infants with sporadic congenital athyreosis. This transplacental passage of maternal T_4 (coupled with the

coordinate adjustments in brain deiodinase activity discussed above) plays a critical role in minimizing the adverse effects of fetal hypothyroidism. Not only may it help to explain the normal or near-normal cognitive outcome of early-treated hypothyroid infants, but it also may provide a partial explanation for the relatively normal clinical appearance at birth of over 90% of infants with congenital hypothyroidism. In contrast, when both the mother and fetus are hypothyroid, such as in cases of iodine deficiency, potent TSH receptor blocking antibodies, or maternal-fetal PIT-1 deficiency, there is a significant impairment in neurointellectual development of the fetus despite the initiation of early and adequate postnatal thyroid replacement (96–98).

Recent evidence has suggested a role for maternal thyroid hormone on fetal brain maturation during the early stages of pregnancy as well. T_4, presumably of maternal origin, has been detected in embryonic coelomic fluid as early as 6 weeks' gestation and in fetal brain as early as 10 weeks' gestation, prior to the onset of fetal thyroid function (99). Furthermore, both D2 and D3 activity as well as TR isoforms are present in human fetal brain from the middle of the first trimester (46,70,99,100), indicating that the machinery to convert T_4 to T_3 and to respond to T_3 are present. In rodents, maternal hypothyroidism occurring prior to the onset of fetal thyroid function causes abnormal gene expression and aberrant cellular migration in the fetal cerebrum (101–103). Emerging evidence suggests that in humans, as well, both maternal hypothyroidism and even a low serum free T_4 unaccompanied by a high serum TSH early in pregnancy may cause significant cognitive or motor delay in the offspring, although the magnitude of the deficit is not as great as when both fetal and maternal hypothyroidism are present (104–106). However, mild overt maternal hypothyroidism is relatively common conditions, occurring in as many as 2.5% of pregnant women in the United States (107). In addition, maternal hypothyroidism has been associated with other adverse effects, including an increased risk for fetal loss. For these reasons universal screening for hypothyroidism during or prior to pregnancy has been suggested (108).

Other Hormones and Factors

In contrast to T_4 and T_3, the placenta is freely permeable to TRH and to iodide, the latter being essential for fetal thyroid hormone synthesis. The placenta is also permeable to certain drugs, and to immunoglobulins of the immunoglobulin G (IgG) class. Thus, administration to the mother of excess iodide, or drugs, or the transplacental passage of TSH receptor antibodies from mothers with Graves' disease or primary hypothyroidism may have significant effects on fetal and neonatal thyroid function. The placenta is not permeable to thyroglobulin.

Although the placenta is permeable to TRH, the maternal serum TRH concentration is low, and most of the peptide transferred to the placenta is degraded. Thus, maternal serum contributes little, if any, TRH to the fetus. The placenta, however, is capable of TRH synthesis, and combined placental and fetal extrahypothalamic TRH production, the latter from the fetal pancreas and gastrointestinal tissues, leads to high concentrations of TRH in fetal serum (89, 109). The high fetal TRH concentration is maintained in part because of absent or low concentrations of TRH-degrading activity in fetal serum (109,110).

The placenta also produces large amounts of chorionic gonadotropin (hCG), which has inherent albeit low level TSH bioactivity. The circulating maternal levels peak at the end of the first trimester, stimulating a transient increase in serum free T_4 and T_3 concentrations in maternal serum and transiently suppressing maternal TSH secretion. These changes are minimal, however, and there is little influence on fetal thyroid function (111).

NEONATAL PERIOD

Term Infants

The changes in thyroid function associated with extrauterine adaptation of the term infant are shown in Figure 74.4 (25). Delivery of the term fetus into the extrauterine environment is associated with a transient, marked increase in serum TSH (the neonatal TSH surge)

stimulated by neonatal cooling. This TSH surge, which peaks during the first 30 minutes at a secretory rate approximating 3 mU/L per minute, stimulates thyroidal release of T_4 and T_3 and a progressive increase in serum T_4 and T_3 concentrations during the first 24 to 36 hours of postnatal life (28,112). Umbilical cord occlusion triggers activation of BAT thermogenesis by removing placental inhibitors of BAT responsiveness to hormonal or neural stimuli (113). Both placental inhibitors and low fetal oxygen levels limit *in utero* catecholamine release and BAT thermogenesis. One of the placental factors appears to be adenosine, which inhibits BAT thermogenesis, and the levels of which rapidly decrease after umbilical cord occlusion (113). BAT thermogenesis also is augmented by vaginal versus cesarean section delivery, as a result of higher catecholamine concentrations in infants born vaginally (114).

In addition to the stimulation of BAT thermogenesis in newborn term infants, there is a dramatic and permanent increase in serum T_4 and T_3 concentrations (from 50 to 150 ng/dL) during the first 36 to 48 hours of postnatal life (28). This increase is due, at least in part, to increased secretion and to removal of the placenta from the fetal circulation, which reduces placental T_3 deiodination, further increasing serum T_3 concentrations (115). The progressive postnatal increase in serum T_3 concentrations to levels characteristic of the extrauterine state is due largely to increased activity of hepatic D1 activity. This increased activity is stimulated in part by the maturational increase in free T_4 concentrations.

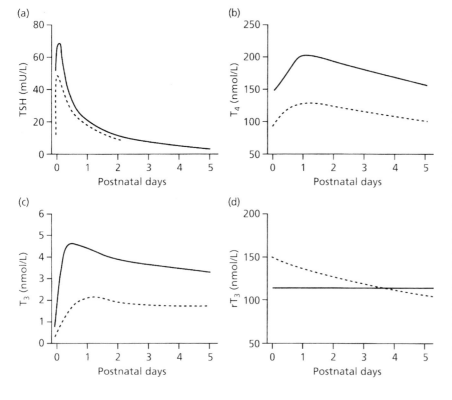

FIGURE 74.4. Postnatal changes in the serum concentration of TSH, thyroxine (T_4), triiodothyronine (T_3), and reverse T_3 (rT_3) in term infants (*continuous line*) versus premature infants (*broken line*) in the first week of life. Delivery is characterized by a postnatal surge in serum thyrotropin (TSH) that peaks at 30 minutes. This is followed by an increase in serum T_4 and T_3 concentrations in the first few days that subsequently decrease. The serum concentrations of T_4 and T_3 rise postnatally because of maturation of glandular secretion and coordinate adjustments in deiodinase activity. In contrast, levels of rT_3 decrease. Changes in premature infants are similar to those in term babies but are less marked. (From Fisher DA, Klein AH. Thyroid gland development and disorders of thyroid function in the newborn. *N Engl J Med* 1981; 304:702–712, as modified by Brown RS, Larsen PR. Thyroid gland development and disease in infancy and childhood. In: De-Groot L, Hennemann G, eds. *Thyroid disease manager.* Accessed at www.*thyroidmanager.org*, August 30, 2001, with permission.)

After the first 1 to 2 hours, serum TSH concentrations decrease progressively, falling to permanent values characteristic of the extrauterine environment and significantly below cord serum concentrations. The mechanisms for this reduction in serum TSH concentration are not clear. The increased serum free T_4 and free T_3 concentrations play a role, but newborn serum TSH concentrations remain at the new, lower level even after the transient neonatal hyperthyroxinemic state has resolved. A resetting of the hypothalamic–pituitary set point for free T_4 feedback control of TSH is involved, but maturative events are unclear. Umbilical cord cutting also removes the placental source of TRH (109). Whether this affects the TSH feedback control system is not known. Extrahypothalamic TRH could inhibit thyroid hormone suppression of TSH secretion, and reducing the prevailing intrauterine circulating extrahypothalamic TRH level tends to increase the FT_4: TSH ratio.

Finally, transition to the extrauterine environment and umbilical cord cutting are associated with a progressive decrease in production and concentrations of inactive thyroid hormone analogues. These include rT_3 and the sulfated metabolites T_4S, T_3S, rT_3S, and T_2S (115–117). This process occurs over several days to weeks and involves changes in activities of the deiodinase enzymes and perhaps tissue levels of sulfotransferase and sulfatase. The net effect is decreased production of bioactive thyroid hormone analogues and increased production of T_3.

Premature Infants

Preterm infants are delivered before full maturation of the hypothalamic–pituitary–thyroid system. They have qualitatively similar but quantitatively decreased changes in serum TSH and iodothyronine concentrations in the neonatal period (32,118,119). The serum TSH response to parturition is attenuated, and serum T_4 concentrations remain below those in full-term infants during the first few weeks of life. An abrupt early neonatal (2–4 hours) increase in serum T_3 concentrations also occurs in premature infants, but the increments are smaller and serum T_3 concentrations increase only slowly to the concentrations found in term infants. The timing of the decrease of the serum rT_3 is similar to that in term infants (25,115,116).

Relative to term infants at birth, serum TBG and total T_4 concentrations in premature infants are lower, tissue type I deiodinase activities and serum T_3 levels are lower, TRH and free T_4 concentrations are lower, bioactive thyroid hormone analogue levels are higher, BAT thermogenic mechanisms are immature, and tissue thyroid hormone response systems are variably immature (118). The extent of these immaturities is related inversely to gestational age. All but the largest premature infants are relatively hypothyroxinemic, with serum levels of TBG, T_4, and free T_4 directly related to gestational age at birth. Serum free T_4 concentrations in the most immature (24- to 27-week) infants are

twofold to threefold lower than values in term infants (120,121). This hypothyroxinemia, which is related to gestational age, is referred to as the hypothyroxinemia of prematurity. As indicated, it is characteristic of smaller low birth weight (LBW) infants (30–35 weeks' gestational age) and all very low birth weight (VLBW) infants (<30 weeks' gestational age) (118,120,121). The mechanisms are not entirely clear and differ to some degree in LBW and VLBW infants. Low TBG concentrations, decreased T_4 secretion largely resulting from inefficient thyroid gland synthesis, and decreased TSH secretion and action probably are involved (32,120–123).

Extrauterine hypothalamic–pituitary–thyroid adaptation in VLBW infants is more often compromised than in the more mature LBW infants. During the early neonatal period, the TSH surge and the early thyroidal response are limited and followed by a progressive decrease in serum T_4 and free T_4 concentrations, with a nadir at 1 to 2 weeks' postnatal age (120,124) (Fig. 74.5). The decrease in serum total T_4 concentrations is due to a transient decrease in TBG, which appears to reflect neonatal morbidity (32, 123). Serum TSH levels usually do not increase in response to the transient hypothyroxinemia, and serum free T_4 levels return to cord serum values by 3 to 4 weeks (121–123).

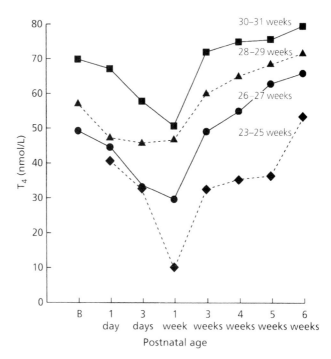

FIGURE 74.5. Postnatal changes in serum T_4 concentrations in very premature infants in the first 6 weeks of life. Unlike in older infants, no neonatal surge in thyroxine (T_4) is seen. Rather, the T_4 concentrations decrease in the first week of life to reach a nadir at 7 days. The extent of this decrease is related to the degree of prematurity. Values then normalize by 3 to 6 weeks of age. (From Mercado M, Yu VY, Francis I, et al. Thyroid function in very preterm infants. *Early Hum Dev* 1988;16:131–141, with permission.)

These very premature infants have a negative iodine balance during the early postnatal weeks, suggesting that they are unable to adapt to the extrauterine environment with augmentation of thyroidal iodine uptake and increased T_4 secretion as do the older LBW infants (122). Serum thyroglobulin concentrations also are high, implying increased production of poorly iodinated thyroid hormone precursors or inefficient metabolism of thyroglobulin by the thyroid follicular cells, in either case a hyperactive, inefficient thyroid hormone synthetic process (122,123). Serum T_3 concentrations also are low in VLBW infants as in older premature infants, but they fail to increase after T_4 administration (125). Thus, conversion of T_4 to T_3 by type I deiodinase is minimal and associated with relatively low levels of enzyme activity, particularly in liver. Most of the circulating T_3 in the very premature infant appears to be derived from thyroidal secretion (126).

Despite the reduced total T_4 in some preterm babies, the TSH concentration is not significantly elevated in most of these infants. In some babies, transient elevations in TSH are seen, the finding of a TSH concentration greater than 40 mU/L being more frequent the greater the degree of prematurity. In one study, for example, the prevalence of a TSH concentration greater than 40 mU/L in VLBW (<1.5 kg, i.e., very premature) infants was eightfold higher and in LBW (1.5–2.5 kg) infants twofold higher than in term infants (32). Whereas in some cases an elevated TSH concentration may reflect true primary hypothyroidism, in others this increase in TSH in preterm infants at several weeks of age may reflect the elevated TSH observed in adults who are recovering from severe illness. Such adults may have transient TSH elevations that are associated with still reduced serum T_4 and T_3 concentrations. These changes have been interpreted as reflecting a "reawakening" of the illness-induced suppression of the hypothalamic-pituitary axis. As the infant recovers from prematurity-associated illnesses such as respiratory distress syndrome (RDS), recovery of the illness-induced suppression of the hypothalamic-pituitary-thyroid axis also occur.

THYROID FUNCTION DURING INFANCY AND CHILDHOOD

During the prepubertal and pubertal periods of growth and development, there is progressive growth of the thyroid gland, a progressive increase in thyroglobulin and iodothyronine stores, and a progressive increase in production rate. The growth of the thyroid gland in residents of iodine-sufficient areas roughly parallels body growth. The gland volume, measured by ultrasonography, increases in size from about 1.0 g at birth to a mean of about 5 g at the age of 10 years (127). Average thyroid iodine content increases from 0.3 mg at birth to 16 mg in adolescents and adults. In areas of iodine deficiency, the average thyroid weight in newborn infants approximates 3 g, and iodine content may be as low as 0.04 mg. The iodide space increases progressively in volume. The relative size (liters per kilogram, expressed as percentage of body weight), however, decreases from about of 50% body weight at birth to 40% in 30 kg children (at about age 10 years). These values can be compared with the 33% body weight values in 65-kg adults.

Radioiodine uptake and clearance in children and adolescents vary with geographic location, diet, and iodine intake. Values have been reported both to decrease progressively with age during the first two decades and to remain relatively stable (128). This discrepancy is probably due largely to variations in iodine intake. The data showing a decrease with age were from areas of low iodine intake in Europe and Australia. A relatively high iodine intake could tend to mask differences in uptake with age.

Serum Thyroid Hormone Concentrations and Production Rates

During the first 20 years of life, serum total and free T_4 and T_3 concentrations decrease gradually (129–131). The decreases result largely from a decrease in serum TBG concentration that is progressive from early childhood through 15 to 16 years of age, when the mean serum TBG concentration is about the same as in adults. Reciprocal changes occur in serum transthyretin concentrations. These changes presumably reflect the effects of gonadal steroids, but other factors may be involved.

T_4 turnover and production rate on a body weight basis (μg/kg per day) also decrease with age during the first two decades (132). Estimated T_4 turnover or production rate values are 7 to 9 μg/kg per day in early infancy, 3 to 5 μg/kg per day at 1 to 3 years, 2 to 3 μg/kg per day at 3 to 9 years, and 1 μg/kg per day in adults.

The serum concentration of rT_3 remains unchanged or increases slightly during childhood and adolescence (129). The serum free rT_3 index (the product of the total rT_3 and fractional T_3 resin uptake) remains stable or increases slightly. Because circulating rT_3 is derived predominantly from peripheral deiodination of T_4, these observations and the fact that the mean calculated ratios of serum rT_3/T_4 and serum free rT_3 index/free T_4 index increase progressively with age suggest that the relative rate of T_4 conversion to rT_3 increases during childhood and adolescence (129). Direct measurements have not been made. The decreases with age in the ratios of serum T_3/rT_3 and free T_3 index/free rT_3 index suggest a progressive decrease in the relative conversion of T_4 to T_3 during the first 15 years of life.

The progressive decrease in serum free T_4, T_3 turnover, thyroglobulin, and thyroidal radioiodine uptake indicates a progressive relative decrease in thyroid function with age. The decreasing serum TSH concentration with age suggests that these decreases are mediated primarily by reduced TSH secretion. Whether this reflects decreased TRH secretion or non-TRH mechanisms is not clear. A progressive reduction in thyroid gland responsiveness to TSH also might be involved.

REFERENCES

1. Roessler E, Belloni E, Gaudenz K, et al. Mutations in the human Sonic Hedgehog gene cause holoprosencephaly. *Nat Genet* 1996;14:357–360.
2. Brown SA, Warburton D, Brown LY, et al. Holoprosencephaly due to mutations in ZIC2, a homologue of *Drosophila* odd-paired. *Nat Genet* 1998;20:180–183.
3. Dattani ML, Martinez-Barbera J, Thomas PQ, et al. Molecular genetics of septo-optic dysplasia. *Horm Res* 2000;53(Suppl 1): 26–33.
4. Lanctot C, Gauthier Y, Drouin J. Pituitary homeobox 1 (Ptx1) is differentially expressed during pituitary development. *Endocrinology* 1999;140:1416–1422.
5. Cohen LE, Radovick S. Molecular basis of combined pituitary hormone deficiencies. *Endocr Rev* 2002;23:431–442.
6. Missero C, Cobellis G, De Felice M, et al. Molecular events involved in differentiation of thyroid follicular cells. *Mol Cell Endocrinol* 1998;140:37–43.
7. Lazzaro D, Price M, de Felice M, et al. The transcription factor TTF-1 is expressed at the onset of thyroid and lung morphogenesis and in restricted regions of the foetal brain. *Development* 1991;113:1093–1104.
8. Plachov D, Chowdhury K, Walther C, et al. Pax8, a murine paired box gene expressed in the developing excretory system and thyroid gland. *Development* 1990;110:643–651.
9. Zannini M, Avantaggiato V, Biffali E, et al. TTF-2, a new forkhead protein, shows a temporal expression in the developing thyroid which is consistent with a role in controlling the onset of differentiation. *EMBO J* 1997;16:3185–3197.
10. Damante G, Di Lauro R. Thyroid-specific gene expression. *Biochim Biophys Acta* 1994;1218:255–266.
11. Kimura S, Hara Y, Pineau T, et al. The T/ebp null mouse: thyroid-specific enhancer-binding protein is essential for the organogenesis of the thyroid, lung, ventral forebrain, and pituitary. *Genes Dev* 1996;10:60–69.
12. Mansouri A, Chowdhury K, Gruss P. Follicular cells of the thyroid gland require Pax8 gene function. *Nat Genet* 1998;19: 87–90.
13. Manley NR, Capecchi MR. The role of Hoxa-3 in mouse thymus and thyroid development. *Development* 1995;121:1989–2003.
14. Guazzi S, Lonigro R, Pintonello L, et al. The thyroid transcription factor-1 gene is a candidate target for regulation by Hox proteins. *EMBO J* 1994;13:3339–3347.
15. Lints TJ, Parsons LM, Hartley L, et al. Nkx-2.5: a novel murine homeobox gene expressed in early heart progenitor cells and their myogenic descendants. *Development* 1993;119:969.
16. Rodriguez M, Santisteban P, Acebron A, et al. Expression of thyroglobulin gene in maternal and fetal thyroid in rats. *Endocrinology* 1992;131:415–422.
17. De Felice M, Ovitt C, Biffali E, et al. A mouse model for hereditary thyroid dysgenesis and cleft palate. *Nat Genet* 1998; 19:395–8.
18. Brown RS, Shalhoub V, Coulter S, et al. Developmental regulation of thyrotropin receptor gene expression in the fetal and neonatal rat thyroid: relation to thyroid morphology and to thyroid-specific gene expression. *Endocrinology* 2000;141:340–345.
19. Remy L, Michel-Bechet M, Athouel-Haon AM, et al. Critical study of endogenous peroxidase activity: its role in the morphofunctional setting of the thyroid follicle in the rat fetus. *Acta Histochem* 1980;67:159–172.
20. Kawaoi A, Tsuneda M. Functional development and maturation of the rat thyroid gland in the foetal and newborn periods: an immunohistochemical study. *Acta Endocrinol (Copenh)* 1985;108:518–524.
21. Stein SA, Shanklin DR, Krulich L, et al. Evaluation and characterization of the hyt/hyt hypothyroid mouse. II. Abnormalities of TSH and the thyroid gland. *Neuroendocrinology* 1989; 49:509–519.
22. Brown RS, Bellisario RL, Botero D, et al. Incidence of transient congenital hypothyroidism due to maternal thyrotropin receptor-blocking antibodies in over one million babies. *J Clin Endocrinol Metab* 1996;81:1147–1151.
23. Abramowicz MJ, Duprez L, Parma J, et al. Familial congenital hypothyroidism due to inactivating mutation of the thyrotropin receptor causing profound hypoplasia of the thyroid gland. *J Clin Invest* 1997;99:3018–3024.
24. Dussault JH, Labrie F. Development of the hypothalamic-pituitary-thyroid axis in the neonatal rat. *Endocrinology* 1975;97: 1321–1324.
25. Fisher DA, Klein AH. Thyroid development and disorders of thyroid function in the newborn. *N Engl J Med* 1981;304:702–712.
26. Costa A, Arisio R, Benedetto C, et al. Thyroid hormones in tissues from human embryos and fetuses. *J Endocrinol Invest* 1991;14:559–68.
27. Bocian-Sobkowska J, Malendowicz LK, Wozniak W. Morphometric studies on the development of human thyroid gland in early fetal life. *Histol Histopathol* 1992;7:415–420.
28. Fisher DA, Dussault JH, Sack J, et al. Ontogenesis of hypothalamic–pituitary–thyroid function and metabolism in man, sheep, and rat. *Rec Prog Horm Res* 1976;33:59–116.
29. Ballabio M, Nicolini U, Jowett T, et al. Maturation of thyroid function in normal human foetuses. *Clin Endocrinol (Oxf)* 1989;31:565–571.
30. Roti E. Regulation of thyroid-stimulating hormone (TSH) secretion in the fetus and neonate. *J Endocrinol Invest* 1988;11: 145–158.
31. Fisher DA, Nelson JC, Carlton EI, et al. Maturation of human hypothalamic-pituitary-thyroid function and control. *Thyroid* 2000;10:229–234.
32. Frank JE, Faix JE, Hermos RJ, et al. Thyroid function in very low birth weight infants: effects on neonatal hypothyroidism screening. *J Pediatr* 1996;128:548–54.
33. Thorpe-Beeston JG, Nicolaides KH, McGregor AM. Fetal thyroid function. *Thyroid* 1992;2:207–217.
34. Klein AH, Fisher DA. Thyrotropin-releasing hormone stimulated pituitary and thyroid gland responsiveness and 3,5,3′-triiodothyronine suppression in fetal and neonatal lambs. *Endocrinology* 1980;106:697–701.
35. Castaing H, Fournet JP, Leger FA, et al. [The thyroid gland of the newborn infant and postnatal iodine overload]. *Arch Fr Pediatr* 1979;36:356–368.
36. Theodoropoulos T, Braverman LE, Vagenakis AG. Iodide-induced hypothyroidism: a potential hazard during perinatal life. *Science* 1979;205:502–503.
37. Burrow GN, Fisher DA, Larsen PR. Maternal and fetal thyroid function. *N Engl J Med* 1994;331:1072–1078.
38. Bates JM, St Germain DL, Galton VA. Expression profiles of the three iodothyronine deiodinases, D1, D2, and D3, in the developing rat. *Endocrinology* 1999;140:844–851.

39. Van der Geyten S, Segers I, Gereben B, et al. Transcriptional regulation of iodothyronine deiodinases during embryonic development. *Mol Cell Endocrinol* 2001;183:1–9.

40. Van der Geyten S, Van den Eynde I, Segers IB, et al. Differential expression of iodothyronine deiodinases in chicken tissues during the last week of embryonic development. *Gen Comp Endocrinol* 2002;128:65–73.

41. Fisher DA, Polk DH, Wu SY. Fetal thyroid metabolism: a pluralistic system. *Thyroid* 1994;4:367–371.

42. Bernal J. Action of thyroid hormone in brain. *J Endocrinol Invest* 2002;25:268–288.

43. Bernal J, Guadano-Ferraz A, Morte B. Perspectives in the study of thyroid hormone action on brain development and function. *Thyroid* 2003;13:1005–1012.

44. Richard K, Hume R, Kaptein E, et al. Ontogeny of iodothyronine deiodinases in human liver. *J Clin Endocrinol Metab* 1998;83:2868–2874.

45. Karmarkar MG, Prabarkaran D, Godbole MM. 5′-Monodeiodinase activity in developing human cerebral cortex. *Am J Clin Nutr* 1993;57(suppl):291–294.

46. Chan S, Kachilele S, McCabe CJ, et al. Early expression of thyroid hormone deiodinases and receptors in human fetal cerebral cortex. *Brain Res Dev Brain Res* 2002;138:109–116.

47. Huang SA, Dorfman DM, Genest DR, et al. Type 3 iodothyronine deiodinase is highly expressed in the human uteroplacental unit and in fetal epithelium. *J Clin Endocrinol Metab* 2003;88:1384–1388.

48. Hernandez A, St Germain DL. Thyroid hormone deiodinases: physiology and clinical disorders. *Curr Opin Pediatr* 2003;15:416–420.

49. Tsai CE, Lin SP, Ito M, et al. Genomic imprinting contributes to thyroid hormone metabolism in the mouse embryo. *Curr Biol* 2002;12:1221–1226.

50. Ruiz de Ona C, Obregon MJ, Escobar del Rey F, et al. Developmental changes in rat brain 5′-deiodinase and thyroid hormones during the fetal period: the effects of fetal hypothyroidism and maternal thyroid hormones. *Pediatr Res* 1988;24:588–594.

51. Campos-Barros A, Hoell T, Musa A, et al. Phenolic and tyrosyl ring iodothyronine deiodination and thyroid hormone concentrations in the human central nervous system. *J Clin Endocrinol Metab* 1996;81:2179–2185.

52. Calvo R, Obregon MJ, Ruiz de Ona C, et al. Congenital hypothyroidism, as studied in rats: crucial role of maternal thyroxine but not of 3,5,3′-triiodothyronine in the protection of the fetal brain. *J Clin Invest* 1990;86:889–899.

53. Campos-Barros A, Amma LL, Faris JS, et al. Type 2 iodothyronine deiodinase expression in the cochlea before the onset of hearing. *Proc Natl Acad Sci USA* 2000;97:1287–92.

54. Obregon MJ, Ruiz de Ona C, Calvo R, et al. Outer ring iodothyronine deiodinases and thyroid hormone economy: responses to iodine deficiency in the rat fetus and neonate. *Endocrinology* 1991;129:2663–2673.

55. Kester MH, Kaptein E, Van Dijk CH, et al. Characterization of iodothyronine sulfatase activities in human and rat liver and placenta. *Endocrinology* 2002;143:814–819.

56. Darras VM, Visser TJ, Berghman LR, et al. Ontogeny of type I and type III deiodinase activities in embryonic and posthatch chicks: relationship with changes in plasma triiodothyronine and growth hormone levels. *Comp Biochem Physiol Comp Physiol* 1992;103:131–136.

57. Van der Geyten S, Sanders JP, Kaptein E, et al. Expression of chicken hepatic type I and type III iodothyronine deiodinases during embryonic development. *Endocrinology* 1997;138: 5144–5152.

58. Abuid J, Stinson DA, Larsen PR. Serum triiodothyronine and thyroxine in the neonate and the acute increases in these hormones following delivery. *J Clin Invest* 1973;52:1195–1199.

59. Coulombe P, Ruel J, Faure R, et al. Pituitary nuclear triiodothyronine receptors during development in the rat. *Am J Physiol* 1983;245:E81–E86.

60. Coulombe P, Ruel J, Dussault JH. Analysis of nuclear 5,5,3′-triiodothyronine-binding capacity and tissue response in the liver of the neonatal rat. *Endocrinology* 1979;105:952–959.

61. DeGroot LJ, Robertson M, Rue PA. Triiodothyronine receptors during maturation. *Endocrinology* 1977;100:1511–1515.

62. Gonzales LW, Ballard PL. Identification and characterization of nuclear 3,5,3′-triiodothyronine-binding sites in fetal human lung. *J Clin Endocrinol Metab* 1981;53:21–28.

63. Anderson GW, Schoonover CM, Jones SA. Control of thyroid hormone action in the developing rat brain. *Thyroid* 2003;13: 1039–1056.

64. Oppenheimer JH, Schwartz HL, Mariash CN, et al. Advances in our understanding of thyroid hormone action at the cellular level. *Endocr Rev* 1987;8:288–308.

65. Porterfield SP, Hendrich CE. The role of thyroid hormones in prenatal and neonatal neurological development—current perspectives. *Endocr Rev* 1993;14:94–106.

66. O'Shea PJ, Williams GR. Insight into the physiological actions of thyroid hormone receptors from genetically modified mice. *J Endocrinol* 2002;175:553–570.

67. Morte B, Manzano J, Scanlan T, et al. Deletion of the thyroid hormone receptor alpha 1 prevents the structural alterations of the cerebellum induced by hypothyroidism. *Proc Natl Acad Sci USA* 2002;99:3985–3989.

68. Hashimoto K, Curty FH, Borges PP, et al. An unliganded thyroid hormone receptor causes severe neurological dysfunction. *Proc Natl Acad Sci USA* 2001;98:3998–4003.

69. Farwell AP, Dubord-Tomasetti SA. Thyroid hormone regulates the expression of laminin in the developing rat cerebellum. *Endocrinology* 1999;140:4221–4227.

70. Farwell AP, Tranter MP, Leonard JL. Thyroxine-dependent regulation of integrin-laminin interactions in astrocytes. *Endocrinology* 1995;136:3909–3915.

71. Styne DM Fetal growth. *Clin Perinatol* 1998;25:917–938, vii.

72. Robson H, Siebler T, Shalet SM, et al. Interactions between GH, IGF-I, glucocorticoids, and thyroid hormones during skeletal growth. *Pediatr Res* 2002;52:137–147.

73. Ball SG, Ikeda M, Chin WW. Deletion of the thyroid hormone beta1 receptor increases basal and triiodothyronine-induced growth hormone messenger ribonucleic acid in GH3 cells. *Endocrinology* 1997;138:3125–3132.

74. Robson H, Siebler T, Stevens DA, et al. Thyroid hormone acts directly on growth plate chondrocytes to promote hypertrophic differentiation and inhibit clonal expansion and cell proliferation. *Endocrinology* 2000;141:3887–3897.

75. Stevens DA, Hasserjian RP, Robson H, et al. Thyroid hormones regulate hypertrophic chondrocyte differentiation and expression of parathyroid hormone-related peptide and its receptor during endochondral bone formation. *J Bone Miner Res* 2000;15:2431–2442.

76. Akita S, Nakamura T, Hirano A, et al. Thyroid hormone action on rat calvarial sutures. *Thyroid* 1994;4:99–106.

77. Klein AH, Reviczky A, Chou P, et al. Development of brown adipose tissue thermogenesis in the ovine fetus and newborn. *Endocrinology* 1983;112:1662–1666.

78. Himms-Hagen J. Brown adipose tissue metabolism and thermogenesis. *Annu Rev Nutr* 1985;5:69–94.

79. Klein AH, Reviczky A, Padbury JF. Thyroid hormones augment catecholamine-stimulated brown adipose tissue thermogenesis in the ovine fetus. *Endocrinology* 1984;114:1065–1069.

80. Casteilla L, Forest C, Robelin J, et al. Characterization of mitochondrial-uncoupling protein in bovine fetus and newborn calf. *Am J Physiol* 1987;252:E627–E636.

81. Silva JE. Full expression of uncoupling protein gene requires the concurrence of norepinephrine and triiodothyronine. *Mol Endocrinol* 1988;2:706–713.

82. Bianco AC, Silva JE. Optimal response of key enzymes and uncoupling protein to cold in BAT depends on local T_3 generation. *Am J Physiol* 1987;253:E255–E263.

83. Bianco AC, Sheng XY, Silva JE. Triiodothyronine amplifies norepinephrine stimulation of uncoupling protein gene transcription by a mechanism not requiring protein synthesis. *J Biol Chem* 1988;263:18168–18175.

84. Carvalho SD, Kimura ET, Bianco AC, et al. Central role of brown adipose tissue thyroxine 5′-deiodinase on thyroid hormone-dependent thermogenic response to cold. *Endocrinology* 1991;128:2149–2159.

85. Silva JE, Larsen PR. Adrenergic activation of triiodothyronine production in brown adipose tissue. *Nature* 1983;305:712–713.

86. Bianco AC, Silva JE. Intracellular conversion of thyroxine to triiodothyronine is required for the optimal thermogenic function of brown adipose tissue. *J Clin Invest* 1987;79:295–300.

87. de Jesus LA, Carvalho SD, Ribeiro MO, et al. The type 2 iodothyronine deiodinase is essential for adaptive thermogenesis in brown adipose tissue. *J Clin Invest* 2001;108:1379–1385.

88. Heaton JM. The distribution of brown adipose tissue in the human. *J Anat* 1972;112:35–39.

89. Roti E, Gnudi A, Braverman LE. The placental transport, synthesis and metabolism of hormones and drugs which affect thyroid function. *Endocr Rev* 1983;4:131–149.

90. Koopdonk-Kool JM, de Vijlder JJ, Veenboer GJ, et al. Type II and type III deiodinase activity in human placenta as a function of gestational age. *J Clin Endocrinol Metab* 1996;81:2154–2158.

91. Galton VA, Martinez E, Hernandez A, et al. The type 2 iodothyronine deiodinase is expressed in the rat uterus and induced during pregnancy. *Endocrinology* 2001;142:2123–2128.

92. Wasco EC, Martinez E, Grant KS, et al. Determinants of iodothyronine deiodinase activities in rodent uterus. *Endocrinology* 2003;144:4253–4261.

93. Carvalho DP. Modulation of uterine iodothyronine deiodinases—a critical event for fetal development? *Endocrinology* 2003;144:4250–4252.

94. Galton VA, Martinez E, Hernandez A, et al. Pregnant rat uterus expresses high levels of the type 3 iodothyronine deiodinase. *J Clin Invest* 1999;103:979–987.

95. Vulsma T, Gons MH, de Vijlder JJ. Maternal-fetal transfer of thyroxine in congenital hypothyroidism due to a total organification defect or thyroid agenesis. *N Engl J Med* 1989;321:13–16.

96. Cao XY, Jiang XM, Dou ZH, et al. Timing of vulnerability of the brain to iodine deficiency in endemic cretinism. *N Engl J Med* 1994;331:1739–1744.

97. de Zegher F, Pernasetti F, Vanhole C, et al. The prenatal role of thyroid hormone evidenced by fetomaternal Pit-1 deficiency. *J Clin Endocrinol Metab* 1995;80:3127–3130.

98. Matsuura N, Konishi J. Transient hypothyroidism in infants born to mothers with chronic thyroiditis—a nationwide study of twenty-three cases: the Transient Hypothyroidism Study Group. *Endocrinol Jpn* 1990;37:369–379.

99. Contempre B, Jauniaux E, Calvo R, et al. Detection of thyroid hormones in human embryonic cavities during the first trimester of pregnancy. *J Clin Endocrinol Metab* 1993;77:1719–1722.

100. Bernal J, Pekonen F. Ontogenesis of the nuclear 3,5,3′-triiodothyronine receptor in the human fetal brain. *Endocrinology* 1984;114:677–679.

101. Dowling AL, Martz GU, Leonard JL, et al. Acute changes in maternal thyroid hormone induce rapid and transient changes in gene expression in fetal rat brain. *J Neurosci* 2000;20:2255–2265.

102. Dowling AL, Zoeller RT. Thyroid hormone of maternal origin regulates the expression of RC3/neurogranin mRNA in the fetal rat brain. *Brain Res Mol Brain Res* 2000;82:126–132.

103. Lavado-Autric R, Auso E, Garcia-Velasco JV, et al. Early maternal hypothyroxinemia alters histogenesis and cerebral cortex cytoarchitecture of the progeny. *J Clin Invest* 2003;111:1073–1082.

104. Man EB, Brown JF, Serunian SA. Maternal hypothyroxinemia: psychoneurological deficits of progeny. *Ann Clin Lab Sci* 1991; 21:227–239.

105. Haddow JE, Palomaki GE, Allan WC, et al. Maternal thyroid deficiency during pregnancy and subsequent neuropsychological development of the child. *N Engl J Med* 1999;341:549–555.

106. Pop VJ, Kuijpens JL, van Baar AL, et al. Low maternal free thyroxine concentrations during early pregnancy are associated with impaired psychomotor development in infancy. *Clin Endocrinol (Oxf)* 1999;50:149–155.

107. Klein RZ, Haddow JE, Faix JD, et al. Prevalence of thyroid deficiency in pregnant women. *Clin Endocrinol (Oxf)* 1991;35: 41–46.

108. Smallridge RC, Ladenson PW. Hypothyroidism in pregnancy: consequences to neonatal health. *J Clin Endocrinol Metab* 2001;86:2349–2353.

109. Polk DH, Reviczky A, Lam RW, et al. Thyrotropin-releasing hormone in ovine fetus: ontogeny and effect of thyroid hormone. *Am J Physiol* 1991;260:E53–58.

110. Engler D, Scanlon MF, Jackson IM. Thyrotropin-releasing hormone in the systemic circulation of the neonatal rat is derived from the pancreas and other extraneural tissues. *J Clin Invest* 1981;67:800–808.

111. Ballabio M, Poshychinda M, Ekins RP. Pregnancy-induced changes in thyroid function: role of human chorionic gonadotropin as putative regulator of maternal thyroid. *J Clin Endocrinol Metab* 1991;73:824–831.

112. de Zegher F, Vanhole C, Van den Berghe G, et al. Properties of thyroid-stimulating hormone and cortisol secretion by the human newborn on the day of birth. *J Clin Endocrinol Metab* 1994;79:576–581.

113. Gunn TR, Gluckman PD. Perinatal thermogenesis. *Early Hum Dev* 1995;42:169–183.

114. Clarke L, Heasman L, Firth K, et al. Influence of route of delivery and ambient temperature on thermoregulation in newborn lambs. *Am J Physiol* 1997;272:R1931–R1939.

115. Santini F, Chiovato L, Ghirri P, et al. Serum iodothyronines in the human fetus and the newborn: evidence for an important role of placenta in fetal thyroid hormone homeostasis. *J Clin Endocrinol Metab* 1999;84:493–498.

116. Oddie TH, Bernard B, Klein AH, et al. Comparison of T_4, T_3, rT_3 and TSH concentrations in cord blood and serum of infants up to 3 months of age. *Early Hum Dev* 1979;3:239–244.

117. Chopra IJ, Wu SY, Teco GN, et al. A radioimmunoassay for measurement of 3,5,3′-triiodothyronine sulfate: studies in thyroidal and nonthyroidal diseases, pregnancy, and neonatal life. *J Clin Endocrinol Metab* 1992;75:189–194.

118. Fisher DA. Thyroid function in premature infants. The hypothyroxinemia of prematurity. *Clin Perinatol* 1998;25:999–1014, viii.

119. LaFranchi S Thyroid function in the preterm infant. *Thyroid* 1999;9:71–78.

120. Rooman RP, Du Caju MV, De Beeck LO, et al. Low thyroxinaemia occurs in the majority of very preterm newborns. *Eur J Pediatr* 1996;155:211–215.

121. van Wassenaer AG, Kok JH, de Vijlder JJ, et al. Effects of thyroxine supplementation on neurologic development in infants born at less than 30 weeks' gestation. *N Engl J Med* 1997;336: 21–26.

122. Ares S, Escobar-Morreale HF, Quero J, et al. Neonatal hypothyroxinemia: effects of iodine intake and premature birth. *J Clin Endocrinol Metab* 1997;82:1704–1712.

123. van Wassenaer AG, Kok JH, Dekker FW, et al. Thyroid function in very preterm infants: influences of gestational age and disease. *Pediatr Res* 1997;42:604–609.

124. Mercado M, Yu VY, Francis I, et al. Thyroid function in very preterm infants. *Early Hum Dev* 1988;16:131–141.

125. van Wassenaer AG, Kok JH, Endert E, et al. Thyroxine administration to infants of less than 30 weeks' gestational age does not increase plasma triiodothyronine concentrations. *Acta Endocrinol (Copenh)* 1993;129:139–146.

126. Pavelka S, Kopecky P, Bendlova B, et al. Tissue metabolism and plasma levels of thyroid hormones in critically ill very premature infants. *Pediatr Res* 1997;42:812–818.

127. Chanoine JP, Toppet V, Lagasse R, et al. Determination of thyroid volume by ultrasound from the neonatal period to late adolescence. *Eur J Pediatr* 1991;150:395–399.

128. Fields T, Kohlenbrener RM, Kunstadter RH, et al. Thyroid function studies in children: normal values for thyroidal I 131 uptake and PBI 131 levels up to the age of 18. *J Clin Endocrinol Metab* 1957;17:61–75.

129. Fisher DA, Sack J, Oddie TH, et al. Serum T_4, TBG, T_3 uptake, T_3, reverse T_3, and TSH concentrations in children 1 to 15 years of age. *J Clin Endocrinol Metab* 1977;45:191–198.

130. Nelson JC, Clark SJ, Borut DL, et al. Age-related changes in serum free thyroxine during childhood and adolescence. *J Pediatr* 1993;123:899–905.

131. Zurakowski D, Di Canzio J, Majzoub JA. Pediatric reference intervals for serum thyroxine, triiodothyronine, thyrotropin, and free thyroxine. *Clin Chem* 1999;45:1087–1091.

132. Oddie TH, Meade JH Jr, Fisher DA. An analysis of published data on thyroxine turnover in human subjects. *J Clin Endocrinol Metab* 1966;26:425–436.

HYPOTHYROIDISM IN INFANTS AND CHILDREN

75A HYPOTHYROIDISM IN INFANTS AND CHILDREN: NEONATAL SCREENING

GUY VAN VLIET

Mass biochemical screening of newborn infants for congenital hypothyroidism became possible after the development of methods for assaying thyrotropin (TSH) and thyroxine (T_4) in blood collected on filter paper in the 1970s [this type of blood sampling was originally introduced for the detection of phenylketonuria (1)]. The historical aspects of this important public health breakthrough have been recounted (2), and its results have been reviewed regularly (3,4). Screening for hypothyroidism among neonates has proven to be highly cost effective, because the societal burden of a person with mental deficiency caused by congenital hypothyroidism far exceeds the costs of the screening program (3).

RATIONALE FOR BIOCHEMICAL SCREENING FOR CONGENITAL HYPOTHYROIDISM

Most infants with congenital hypothyroidism appear normal at birth, and the diagnosis is rarely suspected clinically in the first few weeks of life. At my institution, only 2 of 200 cases of congenital hypothyroidism diagnosed by screening since 1987 were suspected clinically. Yet, it is during the first few months if not weeks of life that irreversible brain damage occurs in infants with hypothyroidism who are not treated. Before biochemical screening of newborn infants for hypothyroidism was introduced, the mean IQ of children with congenital hypothyroidism was less than 80 (5), mainly because less than 20% of affected infants were diagnosed within 3 months after birth; even those with an IQ above 80 had deficits in fine motor control and learning disabilities (6).

When biochemical screening was implemented, it became clear that the disorder was present at birth, no matter how normal the infant looked. It has subsequently also become clear that most infants with hypothyroidism treated soon after birth with high doses of T_4 can attain their full intellectual potential (7–9). However, some controversy remains as to whether the consequences of very severe congenital hypothyroidism can be entirely prevented (see section Congenital Hypothyroidism in this chapter).

BIOCHEMICAL AND CLINICAL ASPECTS OF SCREENING FOR CONGENITAL HYPOTHYROIDISM

Measurements of Thyroxine and Thyrotropin in Blood

Both T_4 and TSH can be measured accurately in blood spotted on filter paper, the standard method for sample collection from newborn infants for screening tests. T_4 refers to total T_4, because free T_4 cannot be measured reliably in blood spots (10). Initially, infants were screened by measurement of T_4, with measurement of TSH as a second step if the blood-spot T_4 value was below a certain cut-off point in the distribution of values measured that day (10), and this sequence is used now in many states in the United States and some European countries. In many places, however, TSH is measured first, with measurement of T_4 as a second step if the blood-spot TSH value is only slightly elevated (Fig. 75A.1).

The T_4-first approach misses some infants who have ectopic thyroid tissue that, when stimulated by TSH, produces enough T_4 so that the blood T_4 concentration is above the cut-off value (3). On the other hand, this approach detects infants who have low blood-spot T_4 values caused by prematurity, low serum thyroid hormone–binding proteins, central hypothyroidism, or severe nonthyroidal illness; these infants need second-step TSH measurements to exclude hypothyroidism (3). The TSH-first approach is designed to detect high blood-spot TSH values, and will miss infants with central hypothyroidism. Most programs using the latter approach consider a blood-

SCREENING FOR CONGENITAL HYPOTHYROIDISM

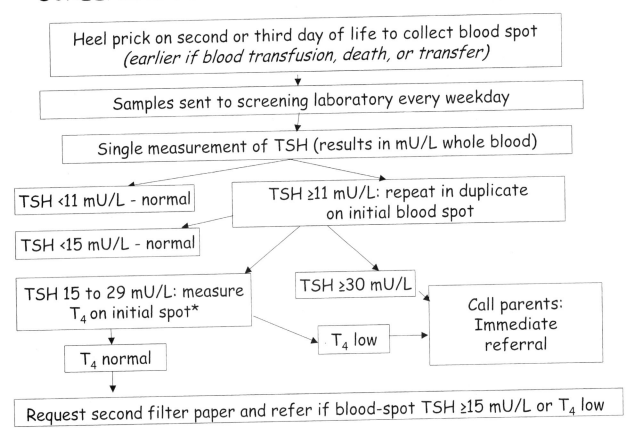

FIGURE 75A.1. Guidelines for biochemical screening for congenital hypothyroidism used in Quebec in 2003.

spot TSH value of greater than or equal to 30 mU/L as indicative of hypothyroidism, and values of 15 to 29 mU/L as highly suspicious of it; all these infants must be studied further (Fig. 75.1). The TSH-first approach also has the advantage that it can be used to monitor the iodine intake of a population, because even borderline iodine deficiency increases TSH secretion in neonates (11).

Although most screening programs measure T_4 or TSH in blood eluted from filter paper, a few use umbilical cord serum (12,13). One limitation of cord serum screening is that, in the case of twins discordant for congenital hypothyroidism, fetal blood mixing may result in a falsely normal serum TSH value in the hypothyroid twin (14).

Age at Screening for Congenital Hypothyroidism

As noted above, screening for congenital hypothyroidism started after screening for phenylketonuria, and this led to the use of the same filter paper blood spots, which were usually obtained several days after birth. As postnatal hos-

pital stays have shortened, blood sampling has been done sooner after birth. TSH secretion rises abruptly immediately after delivery (see Chapter 74), and, although the surge usually lasts only hours, it results in blood-spot TSH values of 15 mU/L or higher in 2% to 3% of normal infants sampled within 24 hours after birth (15). Therefore, in Quebec, infants who have blood-spot TSH values of greater than or equal to 15 mU/L in a first sample obtained within 24 hours after birth are recalled for a second filter paper sample before any further action is taken.

Sample collection for screening may be delayed or overlooked in newborn infants who are severely ill (16), but there is no reason for sample collection to be delayed in any infant, and it should not be overlooked just because an infant is ill. Sick infants who are to be transferred should be tested before transfer, even if the infant is not 24 hours old.

Very-Low-Birth-Weight Newborn Infants

The amplitude of the neonatal surge in TSH secretion is less in very-low-birth-weight infants who are born prematurely than in term newborn infants, but most TSH-screening programs use the same blood-spot TSH value as a cut-off in both groups. This policy has not resulted in permanent congenital hypothyroidism being missed (16), indicating that in these very-low-birth-weight infants TSH secretion increases appropriately when thyroid secretion is decreased. It has been suggested that the increase in TSH secretion might be delayed in these infants, so that congenital hypothyroidism could be missed if only a single sample were taken soon after birth (17), but this must be rare, and multiple sampling is not routinely indicated. These infants often have low serum T_4 concentrations, due primarily to decreased serum thyroid hormone binding; repeated measurements of serum T_4 are not indicated unless there is direct or indirect clinical evidence of hypothyroidism. Indeed, in a recent review of the large French database on congenital hypothyroidism, the disorder was associated with prolonged gestation and macrosomia, and not with low birth weight for gestational age (18). Furthermore, the lack of benefit of T_4 administration in very-low-birth-weight infants (19) suggests that those who have hypothyroxinemia, but no increase in TSH secretion, have physiologic delay in maturation of the hypothalamic–pituitary–thyroid system rather than true central hypothyroidism.

Newborn Infants with Trisomy 21

As a group, newborn infants with trisomy 21 have slightly higher blood-spot TSH concentrations and slightly lower T_4 concentrations than normal infants (20). At later ages, children with trisomy 21 have a propensity to develop autoimmune thyroid disease (see Chapter 75C), but congenital hypothyroidism is rare. There is not a single case of coexistence of permanent congenital hypothyroidism and of trisomy 21 in the Quebec database (21).

RESULTS OF BIOCHEMICAL SCREENING FOR CONGENITAL HYPOTHYROIDISM

Infants found to have screening values indicative of hypothyroidism should be recalled immediately for further study. This is often done through the family's physician, but time is saved if the staff of the screening laboratory contacts the family directly and advises referral to a pediatric endocrinology center. Many screening programs have been able to achieve recall in 8 to 14 days, ensuring prompt evaluation and initiation of therapy when appropriate. On recall, serum TSH and free T_4 should be measured. Other tests, for example, thyroid scintigraphy, are useful as well, but the two serum measurements are critical to confirm the screening results. Thyroid scintigraphy is important because the demonstration of ectopically located thyroid tissue immediately establishes that hypothyroidism will be permanent regardless of the degree of TSH elevation on

screening (see section Acquired Hypothyroidism in this chapter), and treatment should be started without waiting for the results of the serum studies. The same generally holds true when there is a goiter or when there is no detectable uptake on scintigraphy.

When scintigraphy shows a thyroid of normal shape, size, and position, the hypothyroidism may be transient. It is nevertheless prudent to begin T_4 treatment immediately if the results of screening were frankly abnormal (blood-spot TSH concentration ≥30 mU/L), whereas treatment may be withheld pending the results of measurements of serum TSH and free T_4 if the results of screening results were borderline (blood-spot TSH concentration 15 to 29 mU/L).

The prevalence and causes of transient primary congenital hypothyroidism vary according to the iodine intake of the population. In iodine-sufficient areas, the vast majority are infants born to mothers treated with an antithyroid drug or who have autoimmune thyroiditis. In areas of borderline or low iodine intake, they are most often infants exposed to acute iodine overload, whereas in areas of very low iodine intake they are a direct result of iodine deficiency compounded by thiocyanate overload (see section on iodine deficiency in Chapter 11 and Chapter 49).

False-negative results of blood-spot TSH screening are rare (3). Apart from the mixing of fetal blood between twins mentioned above, very few infants with blood-spot screening TSH values below the cut-off value have later proven to have severe hypothyroidism during infancy (at a time when it still has deleterious consequences for brain development). Most were infants with thyroid dyshormonogenesis in whom neonatal thyroid secretion was not severely impaired (16).

To minimize the risk for missing true congenital hypothyroidism while maintaining an acceptably low proportion of infants needing referral and retesting, most screening programs have adopted procedures for second-step screening, as described above and shown in Fig. 75.1. Nonetheless, clinical vigilance remains important, and serum TSH and free T_4 should be measured in any infant with symptoms and signs suggestive of hypothyroidism, even if neonatal screening was reported to be normal.

The most dramatic result of biochemical screening for congenital hypothyroidism is that, because it allows treatment to be started much earlier than in infants diagnosed on the basis of clinical findings, it effectively prevents severe mental deficiency. Fig. 75A.2 shows the distribution of IQ values of children with congenital hypothyroidism in the prescreening era and the results in children who, thanks to screening, were treated at a median age of 14 days after delivery. The impact of disease severity, age at diagnosis, and treatment factors on developmental outcome are discussed in detail in the next section of this chapter.

Another result of biochemical screening for congenital hypothyroidism is that it has revealed that the prevalence of permanent primary congenital hypothyroidism is re-

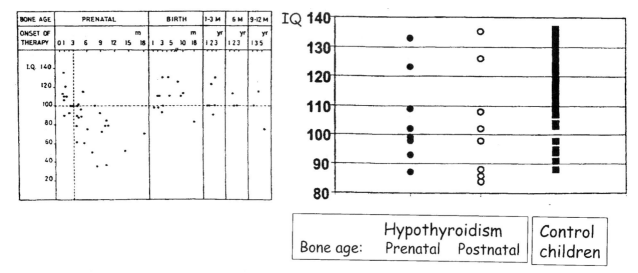

FIGURE 75A.2. IQ values in children with congenital hypothyroidism in the past (pre-screening era) and present (screening era). Left panel: individual IQ values of children aged 3 to 17 years with congenital hypothyroidism diagnosed clinically in the pre-screening era, as a function of bone age at diagnosis and age at onset of therapy. There was no control group in that study; the theoretical population mean of 100 is indicated by the dotted line. Note that IQ values below 80 were most common in the children with a prenatal bone age at diagnosis. Right panel: individual IQ values of children aged 5 years 9 months with congenital hypothyroidism identified by newborn biochemical screening, subdivided by bone age at diagnosis and compared with a control group matched for socioeducational level of the family. Note that, even in the subgroup with a prenatal bone age, the mean and the distribution of IQ values are indistinguishable from those of the control group. (Adapted from Wolter R, Noel P, De Cock P, et al. Neuropsychological study in treated thyroid dysgenesis. Acta Pediatr Scand, Suppl 1979;277:41. and Simoneau-Roy J, Marti S, Deal C, et al. Cognition and behavior at school entry in children with congenital hypothyroidism treated early with high-dose levothyroxine. *J Pediatr* 2004;144:747.)

markably similar around the world (1 in 3,500 newborn infants). The only exceptions are areas of severe iodine deficiency, in which the prevalence is higher (see section Iodine Deficiency in Chapter 11 and Chapter 49). Any differences in the proportions of infants in whom hypothyroidism was caused by thyroid ectopy and athyreosis likely reflect differences in the type and quality of the imaging tests done. The proportion of cases of dyshormonogenesis may vary slightly as a function of the background consanguinity of the population.

SUMMARY

By allowing treatment before the onset of any clinical manifestations of hypothyroidism, biochemical screening of neonates for congenital hypothyroidism has resulted in the disappearance of mental deficiency caused by this condition. However, this true public health triumph should not lead to complacency. Continuous auditing of all steps of the screening program is necessary to ensure that infants with congenital hypothyroidism are identified and treated with the least possible delay.

REFERENCES

1. McCabe LL, Therrell BL, McCabe ER. Newborn screening: rationale for a comprehensive, fully integrated public health system. *Mol Genet Metab* 2002;77:267.
2. Dussault JH. The anecdotal history of screening for congenital hypothyroidism. *J Clin Endocrinol Metab* 1999;84:4332.
3. Delange F. Neonatal screening for congenital hypothyroidism: results and perspectives. *Horm Res* 1997;48:51.
4. Van Vliet G, Czernichow P. Screening for neonatal endocrinopathies: rationale, methods and results. *Semin Neonatol* 2004;9:75.
5. Tillotson SL, Fuggle PW, Smith I, et al. Relation between biochemical severity and intelligence in early treated congenital hypothyroidism: a threshold effect. *BMJ* 1994;309:440.
6. Wolter R, Noel P, De Cock P, et al. Neuropsychological study in treated thyroid dysgenesis. *Acta Paediatr Scand Suppl* 1979; 277:41.
7. Dubuis JM, Glorieux J, Richer F, et al. Outcome of severe congenital hypothyroidism: closing the developmental gap with early high dose levothyroxine treatment. *J Clin Endocrinol Metab* 1996;81:222.
8. Bongers-Schokking JJ, Koot HM, Wiersma D, et al. Influence of timing and dose of thyroid hormone replacement on development in infants with congenital hypothyroidism. *J Pediatr* 2000; 136:292.
9. Simoneau-Roy J, Marti S, Deal C, et al. Cognition and behavior at school entry in children with congenital hypothyroidism

treated early with high-dose levothyroxine. *J Pediatr* 2004;144: 747.

10. Screening for congenital hypothyroidism. *Thyroid* 2003;13:87.
11. Delange F. Screening for congenital hypothyroidism used as an indicator of the degree of iodine deficiency and of its control. *Thyroid* 1998;8:1185.
12. Alvarez MA, Guell R, Gonzalez J, et al. Neuropsychological development during the first two years of life in children with congenital hypothyroidism screened at birth: the Cuban experience. *Screening* 1992;1:167.
13. Virtanen M, Maenpaa J, Pikkarainen J, et al. Aetiology of congenital hypothyroidism in Finland. *Acta Paediatr Scand* 1989; 78:67.
14. Perry R, Heinrichs C, Bourdoux P, et al. Discordance of monozygotic twins for thyroid dysgenesis: implications for screening and for molecular pathophysiology. *J Clin Endocrinol Metab* 2002;87:4072.
15. Dussault JH, Grenier A, Morissette J, et al. Preliminary report on filter paper TSH levels in the first 24h of life and the following days in a program screening for congenital hypothyroidism. In: Pass KA, Levy HL, eds. *Early hospital discharge: impact on newborn screening.* Atlanta: Council of Regional Networks for Genetics Services, Emory University School of Medicine, 1995:267.
16. Vincent MA, Rodd C, Dussault JH, et al. Very low birth weight newborns do not need repeat screening for congenital hypothyroidism. *J Pediatr* 2002;140:311.
17. Mandel SJ, Hermos RJ, Larson CA, et al. Atypical hypothyroidism and the very low birthweight infant. *Thyroid* 2000; 10:693.
18. Van Vliet G, Larroque B, Bubuteishvili L, et al. Sex-specific impact of congenital hypothyroidism due to thyroid dysgenesis on skeletal maturation in term newborns. *J Clin Endocrinol Metab* 2003;88:2009.
19. van Wassenaer AG, Kok JH, de Vijlder JJ, et al. Effects of thyroxine supplementation on neurologic development in infants born at less than 30 weeks' gestation. *N Engl J Med* 1997; 336:21.
20. van Trotsenburg AS, Vulsma T, Van Santen HM, et al. Lower neonatal screening thyroxine concentrations in Down syndrome newborns. *J Clin Endocrinol Metab* 2003;88:1512.
21. Devos H, Rodd C, Gagne N, et al. A search for the possible molecular mechanisms of thyroid dysgenesis: sex ratios and associated malformations. *J Clin Endocrinol Metab* 1999;84:2502.

75B HYPOTHYROIDISM IN INFANTS AND CHILDREN: CONGENITAL HYPOTHYROIDISM

GUY VAN VLIET

A relationship between an absent or defective thyroid gland and mental retardation was recognized long ago, but the most striking description of the clinical picture of "cretinism," as it was then called, was made by Sir William Osler in 1897, who then wrote, "No type of human transformation is more distressing to look at than an aggravated case of cretinism. The stunted stature, the semi-bestial aspect, the blubber lips, retroussé nose sunken at the root, the wide open mouth, the lolling tongue, the small eyes half-closed with swollen lids, the stolid, expressionless face, the squat figure, the muddy dry skin, combine to make the picture of what has been termed the 'pariah of nature'" (1).

A century ago, thyroid extract was found to normalize the physical appearance of patients with congenital hypothyroidism. However, the mental deficiency was irreversible, because treatment was started after the most critical period of sensitivity of the brain to thyroid hormone deficiency. Mental deficiency from congenital hypothyroidism was only eradicated when widespread mass biochemical screening of neonates was implemented in the 1980s (see section Neonatal Screening in this chapter).

During the same period, progress toward the elimination of iodine deficiency, the most important extrinsic factor causing congenital hypothyroidism, has been made in many countries (see section Iodine Deficiency in Chapter 11 and Chapter 49).

CLASSIFICATION OF CONGENITAL HYPOTHYROIDISM

Like acquired hypothyroidism, congenital hypothyroidism can be classified as primary (thyroidal), if the defect occurs at the level of the thyroid gland; peripheral, if the defect is in thyroid-hormone sensitive peripheral tissues; and central, if the defect involves the hypothalamus or pituitary gland (Table 75B.1). Central hypothyroidism may be further divided into secondary (pituitary causes) and tertiary (hypothalamic causes). Hypothyroidism can also be classified according to whether it is transient or permanent. Permanent primary congenital hypothyroidism is by far the most common form of congenital hypothyroidism, and is, in fact, the most common congeni-

TABLE 75B.1. CLASSIFICATION OF CONGENITAL HYPOTHYROIDISM

Permanent hypothyroidism
  Central (hypothalamic, pituitary) hypothyroidism
    Pituitary stalk interruption syndrome or other
      developmental defects
    Inactivating mutations:
      TRH receptor
      Transcription factors (HESX-1, LHX-3, LHX-4, PIT-1,
        PROP-1)
      β-subunit of TSH
  Primary (thyroidal) hypothyroidism
    Thyroid dysgenesis: ectopy, agenesis, hypoplasia,
      hemiagenesis
    Thyroid dyshormonogenesis
    Resistance to TSH from:
      Inactivating mutations of the TSH receptor
      Other mechanisms (e.g., pseudohypoparathyroidism)
Peripheral hypothyroidism
  Resistance to thyroid hormone
Transient hypothyroidism (all are of the primary type)
  Severe iodine deficiency
  Acute iodine load (usually on a background of borderline
    iodine deficiency)
  Maternal antithyroid drug therapy
  Transplacental transfer of TSH receptor-blocking antibodies
  Heterozygous mutations inactivating THOX2

TRH, thyrotropin-releasing hormone; TSH, thyrotropin.

tal endocrine disorder; it is found in approximately 1 in 3,500 newborn infants.

In 80% to 90% of infants, permanent primary congenital hypothyroidism is caused by thyroid dysgenesis, which includes multiple abnormalities in thyroid gland development. Among them, the most common is ectopic thyroid tissue (~60% of cases). The ectopic thyroid tissue is usually located above where the normal thyroid should be, as a result of an arrest in downward migration of the median thyroid anlagen during embryonic development; this ectopic tissue contains the only thyroid follicular cells in the affected infants (see Chapter 2). Approximately 20% of infants have complete absence of thyroid tissue (thyroid agenesis or athyreosis); this may result from a defect in the differentiation of thyroid follicular cells or from their disappearance during prenatal life. Less common are thyroid hypoplasia (<5% of cases), which is characterized by small thyroid lobes in the normal position, and thyroid hemiagenesis (<1% of cases), in which one lobe (usually the left), is missing. Ten percent to 20% of cases of permanent primary congenital hypothyroidism are due to defects in thyroid hormone biosynthesis (thyroid dyshormonogenesis), which, because of the trophic actions of thyrotropin (TSH), eventually lead to thyroid enlargement (see Chapter 48). However, thyroid enlargement is often not detected clinically at birth.

Permanent central hypothyroidism, resulting from defects at the level of the hypothalamus or pituitary, occurs in

less than 1 in 50,000 births. In addition to these permanent conditions, transient alterations in thyroid function are occasionally encountered.

ETIOLOGY AND PATHOGENESIS

Permanent Congenital Hypothyroidism

Thyroid dysgenesis was until recently considered a sporadic entity, although there had been some reports of familial occurrence. A systematic evaluation of the heritability of thyroid dysgenesis in France revealed that 48 of 2,472 infants with thyroid dysgenesis (2%) had an affected relative; this figure is 15-fold higher than predicted by chance alone (2). Pedigree analysis was most compatible with dominant inheritance with variable penetrance, although there was genetic heterogeneity and possible multigenic inheritance in some pedigrees (2,3). In another study by the same group, subclinical abnormalities of thyroid development (mostly persistence of thyroglossal duct remnants) were identified by ultrasonography in 8% of euthyroid first-degree relatives of children with thyroid dysgenesis, as compared with only 0.8% in a control population (4). On the other hand, a recent systematic survey of monozygotic twins revealed that discordance for thyroid dysgenesis was the rule, being observed in 12 of 13 reported twin pairs (92%) (5). Also incompatible with simple mendelian inheritance is the observation that thyroid dysgenesis (especially thyroid ectopy) has a marked female predominance (6).

Consistent with these epidemiologic findings, germ line mutations in genes known to be involved in thyroid development (*TTF-1, TTF-2, PAX-8,* and *TSH receptor*) have been identified in only about 50 patients with thyroid dysgenesis, among about 500 who were screened (see Chapter 2). Thus, alternative hypotheses have to be formulated to explain most cases of thyroid dysgenesis. These include epigenetic modifications, somatic mutations occurring early in embryogenesis in the parent thyroid follicular cell, or stochastic developmental events. The lines of evidence in favor of mendelian and nonmendelian mechanisms of thyroid dysgenesis are summarized in Table 75B.2 and are discussed in detail elsewhere (7,8).

Thyroid dyshormonogenesis results from a defect in any one of the steps involved in the biosynthesis of thyroid hormone, from the transport of iodine to the synthesis of thyroglobulin (see Chapter 48). These defects are inherited as autosomal-recessive traits, and they therefore occur at higher frequency in consanguineous families.

Given the different mechanisms underlying congenital hypothyroidism caused by thyroid dysgenesis and by dyshormonogenesis, it is essential that these two forms be distinguished when comparing prevalence figures between ethnic groups. Thus, evidence suggesting that congenital hypothyroidism is less prevalent among blacks should be viewed with caution because the etiology was not deter-

TABLE 75B.2. PROPOSED MECHANISMS OF THYROID DYSGENESIS AND SUPPORTING FINDINGS

	Mendelian Inheritance	Non-Mendelian Inheritance
Findings	2% of infants with thyroid dysgenesis have an affected relative (15-fold higher than chance)	Marked preponderance of females with ectopy (3 females for 1 male)
	Subclinical abnormalities of thyroid development in 8% of first- degree relatives of infants with thyroid dysgenesis (vs. 0.8 % in a control population)	92% discordance among monozygotic twin pairs
Mechanisms	Autosomal dominant with variable penetrance	Epigenetic
	Genetic heterogeneity	Early somatic mutations
	Multigenic	Stochastic events

mined (9). Although the prevalence of dyshormonogenesis is higher in inbred populations, the prevalence of thyroid ectopy does not seem to vary substantially around the world. The lack of consistent regional, and also seasonal, variation in the frequency of thyroid dysgenesis argues against an important role of environmental factors (10).

Congenital central hypothyroidism almost always occurs in conjunction with other pituitary hormone deficiencies, and it is usually caused by structural abnormalities of the pituitary or hypothalamus or functional abnormalities in hypothalamic or pituitary development (Table 75B.1). Isolated central hypothyroidism caused by mutations of the gene for the β-subunit of TSH is rare. These mutations result in the production of a TSH molecule with little biologic or immunologic activity, and affected infants usually have severe hypothyroidism (11,12). Other rare causes are inactivating mutations in the thyrotropin-releasing hormone receptor (13) and in pituitary transcription factors (14). TSH screening misses infants with these rare disorders.

Transient Congenital Hypothyroidism

Transient primary congenital hypothyroidism has been well described in areas where the iodine intake of the population is either severely or moderately deficient (see section Iodine Deficiency in Chapter 11 and Chapter 49). In the latter areas, it usually occurs in premature newborns and is associated with an acute iodine overload, most often from use of iodine-containing antiseptic agents in the infant or mother. Cessation of the use of these antiseptic agents in newborn nurseries has led to the almost complete disappearance of this form of transient primary hypothyroidism (15). It is rare in areas of iodine sufficiency such as North America.

In iodine-sufficient areas, the most common cause of transient primary hypothyroidism is maternal therapy with an antithyroid drug. These drugs are cleared rapidly from

the infant's circulation, and therefore the hypothyroidism is short-lived; most affected infants have normal serum TSH and free thyroxine (T_4) concentrations at recall. Transplacental transfer of maternal antibodies that block the action of TSH is a rare cause of transient primary hypothyroidism in newborn infants, causing only about 1% to 2% of cases (16); these infants may still have hypothyroidism at the time of recall because the antibodies are cleared relatively slowly. These antibodies do not interfere with the formation, migration, and growth of the thyroid gland, and therefore do not cause permanent primary congenital hypothyroidism. Transient primary congenital hypothyroidism from a heterozygous mutation in *THOX2*, the gene encoding one of the enzymes involved in the generation of H_2O_2 needed for iodine oxidation and organification in the thyroid (17), has recently been described. Its frequency remains to be determined.

CLINICAL PRESENTATION

Few infants with congenital hypothyroidism have an abnormal appearance or behavior at birth or even at recall when the diagnosis is confirmed and treatment started. On the other hand, the few newborn infants with clinical manifestations of hypothyroidism would probably benefit from diagnosis in the first days after birth and from treatment begun even earlier than can be achieved by screening programs (18). Thus, it is important to recognize the clinical manifestations of hypothyroidism in newborn infants. These include unexplained postmaturity, macrosomia, an open posterior fontanel, jaundice, and delayed skeletal maturation (19). A few infants have a goiter, but it is rarely of sufficient size to impede delivery or cause airway obstruction. Other symptoms and signs include poor feeding, hypothermia, lethargy, constipation, prolonged jaundice, abdominal distention, umbilical hernia, dry and mottled

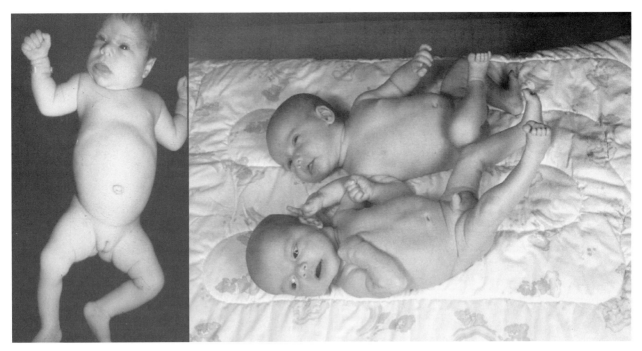

FIGURE 75B.1. Photographs of infants with congenital hypothyroidism. **Left:** 4-month-old infant with many signs of hypothyroidism, including puffy eyelids, macroglossia, and umbilical hernia. Treatment from this age onward results in disappearance of the physical stigmata of hypothyroidism, but irreversible brain damage has already occurred. **Right:** 14-day-old twin brothers, one of whom has severe congenital hypothyroidism due to thyroid agenesis. Note that they are clinically indistinguishable. Thanks to early treatment through biochemical screening, the intellectual development of the hypothyroid twin should be comparable with that of the euthyroid twin.

skin, macroglossia, a hoarse cry, and a myxedematous appearance (Fig. 75B.1).

A clinical suspicion of hypothyroidism in a newborn or very young infant should always lead to the immediate measurement of serum TSH and free T_4, even if the screening blood sample has already been collected. Also, the possibility of human or technical error in the screening process, of central hypothyroidism [in areas using a TSH-first screening approach (see section Neonatal Screening in this chapter)], or of falsely normal (false-negative) results should be kept in mind.

Among infants referred for an abnormal screening result, a family history should be obtained, with focus on consanguinity and on the existence of even distant relatives with congenital hypothyroidism (Table 75B.3). A family history of thyroid disorders with onset in later life is usually irrelevant, but a maternal history of thyroid disease, treatment for thyroid disease, or exposure to iodine-rich compounds such as radiographic contrast agents is relevant. An examination of the infant seeking the above-listed physical signs should be conducted. A goiter may be seen or palpated when the infant's neck is hyperextended. The only extrathyroid malformations consistently associated with thyroid dysgenesis are defects in heart septation (2,6,20); these are usually mild and not noted at the first visit.

Except when it is due to mutations of the β-subunit of TSH, congenital central hypothyroidism is clinically and biochemically mild and associated with other pituitary hormone deficiencies, the clinical expression of which leads to the diagnosis. Thus, the infant may have hypoglycemia caused by corticotropin (ACTH) or growth hormone deficiency, or micropenis and cryptorchidism caused by gonadotropin deficiency. The presence of midline malformations such as cleft lip or palate or optic nerve hypoplasia may also suggest the presence of these pituitary deficiencies.

DIAGNOSTIC EVALUATION

Serum TSH and free T_4 should be measured in all newborn infants recalled because of abnormal screening results, and also in any infant suspected clinically to have hypothyroidism immediately after birth (Table 75B.3). The biochemical severity of the hypothyroidism tends to be less in infants with thyroid ectopy or hypoplasia than in those with thyroid agenesis, and it is highly variable in infants with thyroid dyshormonogenesis. However, the overlap in values among infants with these different disorders is substantial; therefore, the cause of congenital hypothyroidism cannot be predicted reliably based on serum TSH and free T_4 concentrations.

TABLE 75B.3. DIAGNOSTIC EVALUATION OF A NEWBORN INFANT SUSPECTED TO HAVE CONGENITAL HYPOTHYROIDISM

Family history: especially sibling with congenital hypothyroidism or maternal thyroid disease
Infant history: length of gestation, birth weight, constipation, poor feeding
Physical examination: jaundice, open fontanels, goiter (neck hyperextended)
Obtain blood for measurements of serum TSH and free T_4
Anteroposterior x-ray of the knee
$^{99m}TcO_4$ (or ^{123}I) scintigraphy of cervical, lingual and mediastinal area (not required if goiter on clinical examination):
  If thyroid ectopy: permanent congenital hypothyroidism confirmed
  If $^{99m}TcO_4$ (or ^{123}I) uptake uindetectable, measure serum thyroglobulin:
    Serum thyroglobulin undetectable: thyroid agenesis confirmed
    Serum thyroglobulin detectable: thyroid tissue present
      Transplacental transfer of TSH receptor-blocking antibodies (transient hypothyroidism)
      Mutations in the TSH receptor or *PAX-8* (permanent hypothyroidism)
  If low uptake by a small or normal thyroid of normal shape:
    Iodine overload, TSH receptor–blocking antibodies (transient hypothyroidism)
    Mutations in the TSH receptor or *PAX-8* (permanent hypothyroidism)

T_4, thyroxine; TSH, thyrotropin.

The onset of hypothyroidism can be estimated from an anteroposterior x-ray of the knee. The absence of both the femoral and tibial epiphyseal centers in a term newborn infant suggests severe hypothyroidism, and these radiologic findings have consistently been found to be a reliable predictor of greater risk for developmental delay, even with early treatment (21,22). Unless a goiter is seen or palpated, scintigraphy should be performed to distinguish between the different types of thyroid dysgenesis. Detection of thyroid ectopy immediately establishes the permanent nature of the disorder (Table 75B.3) and allows estimation of the risk for recurrence in future pregnancies.

For scintigraphy, pertechnetate ($^{99m}TcO_4$) is preferred; it provides satisfactory images, is available daily in most nuclear medicine services, and the imaging can be completed in 15 to 30 minutes (Fig. 75B.2). $^{99m}TcO_4$ is also taken up by the salivary glands: it is therefore essential to feed the baby between the injection of the tracer and scanning, so that any uptake in the lingual area can be ascribed to thyroid tissue. Iodine 123 is satisfactory, but it usually must be specially ordered, and the test itself takes longer, because the imaging is done 4 to 6 or even 24 hours after ^{123}I administration. Difficulties in arranging for immediate imaging should never delay treatment, and it can be done during the first 3 to 4 days of treatment. Indeed, it is safer to start treatment in all infants referred for positive screening results immediately after the blood sample for measurement of serum TSH and free T_4 is obtained.

If scintigraphy cannot be done before or soon after treatment is started, it is done when the child is 3 years old. At that time, T_4 therapy can be safely discontinued for 1 month. If the diagnosis of hypothyroidism is confirmed by measurements of serum TSH and free T_4, its cause can be determined by scintigraphy. Infants with dyshormonogenesis are not studied routinely to determine the specific biosynthetic defect, for example, with a perchlorate dis-charge test, because a precise diagnosis of the defect has no impact on genetic counseling or treatment.

Thyroid ultrasonography is noninvasive, and no radioactivity is given, but it is less sensitive than scintigraphy in identifying small amounts of ectopic thyroid tissue (23), even when color Doppler ultrasonography is used (24). In infants in whom no thyroid tissue is detected by scintigraphy, serum thyroglobulin should be measured; only about 50% of these infants have complete thyroid agenesis as defined by an undetectable serum thyroglobulin concentration (25). The remainder have some thyroid tissue, however small in volume. Some of these infants have thyroid tissue that is not functioning (but should be detectable by ultrasonography) because of transplacentally transferred maternal TSH receptor-blocking antibodies (Table 75B.3).

Given the low yield of the searches for germline mutations discussed above, molecular genetic analyses are only performed on a research basis, and could probably be restricted to patients with positive family histories or suggestive phenotypes. Thus, unexplained respiratory distress, hypotonia, and choreoathetosis suggest a *TTF-1* mutation (26,27), and cleft palate and kinky hair a *TTF-2* mutation (28,29). In infants with isolated thyroid hypoplasia or apparent agenesis, a family history suggesting dominant inheritance points to a *PAX-8* mutation (30–33), whereas one suggesting recessive inheritance points to a *TSH receptor* mutation (34).

TREATMENT AND OUTCOME

As stated above, treatment should be started at recall regardless of whether imaging is done and without waiting for the results of the confirmatory serum tests. Every day of

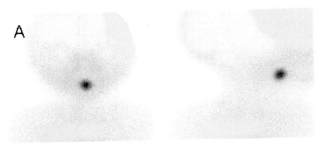

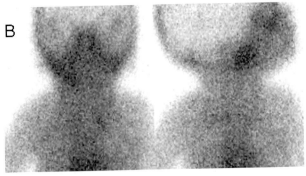

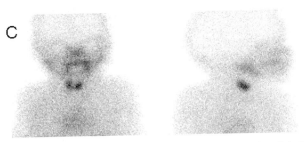

FIGURE 75B.2. Radionuclide images of the head and neck in infants with congenital hypothyroidism. **A:** Ectopic thyroid tissue in the lingual region. **B:** Athyreosis. Radioactivity is seen in the salivary glands, large vessels, and heart because the image was made at a high sensitivity in an effort to identify thyroid tissue. **C:** Normally located thyroid lobes. These images were made 30 minutes after intravenous administration of ^{99m}TcO$_4$-pertechnetate.

delay may result in loss of IQ; the loss is greater soon after birth than later (35). Therefore, it is safer to start treatment in all newborns, even those with marginal screening values; it can be stopped in the very few newborns who have normal serum TSH and T$_4$ concentrations at the time of the diagnostic evaluation.

The treatment of choice is T$_4$. The tablets should be crushed and given in water with a spoon or even given whole before feeding, but should never be added to a bottle of milk or formula that the infant may then not empty. Soy formulas tend to decrease the absorption of T$_4$, but are rarely used now. T$_4$ in solution for oral administration is available in some countries, but is not as stable as the tablet form. Compared with infants with thyroid ectopy, infants with thyroid agenesis usually need higher doses of T$_4$, whereas those with thyroid dyshormonogenesis need lower doses (36,37).

During chronic oral therapy, a missed dose can be given later that day, or two doses can be given the next day. However, mental retardation was attributed to more infrequent (i.e., weekly) dosing in one infant (38), and regular daily treatment is therefore recommended. The dose should be repeated if an infant or child vomits within an hour after taking T$_4$. If needed, which is rare, T$_4$ can be given as a daily intravenous injection; the dose should be about 75% of the oral dose. The addition of triiodothyronine (T$_3$) has no benefit (39).

In the first decade after screening was implemented, treatment was typically started at a mean age of 20 to 35 days and with doses of T$_4$ of 5 to 6 µg/kg/day. It was quickly noted that serum TSH concentrations remained high for weeks or even months with these doses. The persistent elevation was attributed to resistance to the negative feedback action of thyroid hormone on TSH secretion, rather than to inadequate treatment (40). Also, developmental problems and even premature fusion of the fontanels had been reported in infants with congenital thyrotoxicosis (41) and in infants treated with a total of 200 to 500 µg of T$_4$ for several months (42), so that iatrogenic thyrotoxicosis was considered to be as deleterious for the brain as hypothyroidism. It is now clear that only a minority of infants have resistance of TSH secretion to T$_4$ and that this resistance is transient (43).

More importantly, studies of outcome in infants and children treated with these doses of T$_4$ revealed that bone maturation remained delayed until 3 years of age (44), and that those with more severe congenital hypothyroidism (defined on the basis of retarded bone maturation or a very low serum T$_4$ concentration at diagnosis) had a clinically important loss of 6 to 22 IQ points (45–47). There seemed to be a threshold effect of severity of congenital hypothyroidism on IQ, superimposed on the well-known influence of socioeconomic status of the parents on the results of psychometric testing of their children (48). Some interpreted these findings as suggesting that irreparable brain damage would always occur before treatment could be started in infants with severe congenital hypothyroidism. However, before delivery, the brain of hypothyroid fetuses is protected to some extent by transplacental passage of maternal T$_4$ (49) and by local up-regulation of type 2 deiodinase (see Chapter 7). Indeed, newer studies suggest that normal intellectual potential can be reached in infants who are treated early and vigorously, as discussed below.

Since about 1990, most term newborn infants have been treated with T$_4$ in doses of 10 to 15 µg/kg/day (in practice, 50 µg/day for a term infant of normal weight) (50). The efficacy of these doses was confirmed in a study in which 47 infants weighing 3 to 4 kg were randomly assigned to treatment with 37.5 µg/day, 62.5 µg/day for 3 days then 37.5 µg/day, and 50 µg/day: only in the group treated with 50 µg/day was the mean serum TSH concentration normal within 2 weeks (51). There is no randomized study of different initial doses of T$_4$ on intellectual development, but observational studies strongly suggest that both initiation of treatment within 2 weeks after birth and a high initial dose are required for children with severe congenital hypothyroidism to develop normally (52–54).

Among infants in whom treatment is started, there is considerable variation in the frequency at which the infants are seen and the biochemical targets of treatment. Reference intervals for serum free T_4 and TSH are higher in infants than in older children and adults (55), but normative data for the first months of life are scarce, and the different commercially available serum free T_4 assays are variably influenced by changes in serum thyroid hormone–binding proteins (56). Based on the rule of thumb that four times the half-life of T_4 should elapse before steady state is achieved, it seems unnecessary to measure serum free T_4 before infants are treated for 2 or 3 weeks. In terms of what the target serum free T_4 value should be when the first follow-up sample is obtained, the study mentioned above (51) suggests that it should be about 5 ng/dL (65 pM) after treatment for 2 weeks if the serum TSH concentration is to be normal at that time.

With respect to chronic T_4 therapy, the required dose declines from 10 to 15 μg/kg/day in very young infants to about 4 to 5 μg/kg/day at age 5 years; this decrease is due to the progressive decrease in the turnover rate of T_4 with age (see Chapter 74). Conversely, the rate of weight gain decreases quickly in early infancy, so that a starting dose of 50 μg/day may not need to be changed for many months. Low serum TSH concentrations indicate subclinical thyrotoxicosis, but in rapidly growing infants the same dose of T_4 may soon be appropriate. Overt thyrotoxicosis is rare, perhaps because serum T_3 concentrations remain in the normal range even in infants with high serum free T_4 concentrations (50), but its presence should lead to a decrease in dose of T_4. The finding of a high serum TSH concentration should lead to inquiry about compliance, and if satisfactory the dose of T_4 should be increased to maintain serum TSH and free T_4 concentrations in the normal range for age, normal serum TSH values being more important than normal serum free T_4 values.

Although the frequency of follow-up visits varies considerably between clinics, there is no evidence that infants and children who are seen more often and have more dosage adjustments have a better developmental outcome. Based on the rapid growth rates of infants, it seems reasonable to reassess thyroid function at intervals of 3 months in the first year and of 6 months from age 1 to 3 years. After 3 years, because there is no irreversible effect of undertreatment on brain function, yearly assessments are probably sufficient. Poor compliance with treatment is associated with poorer developmental outcome (18,54). Therefore, a suspicion of poor compliance may justify more frequent visits.

If treatment is adequate, the mean height and weight are similar to those of normal children, but the mean head circumference of infants with congenital hypothyroidism is about 1 standard deviation above the mean of normal infants. This increase is likely related to differential maturation of the cranial base and of the skull and has no impact on the size of the brain or cerebral ventricles (52). However, it may sometimes be so marked in an individual infant as to lead to unnecessary imaging. Bone maturation at 3 years should be normal; in infants with delayed bone maturation at diagnosis, complete catch-up should occur. In the remainder, bone maturation is not advanced, confirming that the treatment regimen has not induced overt thyrotoxicosis (41,42).

Sensorineural hearing loss is a known consequence of congenital hypothyroidism, but does not seem to occur in children treated within 2 weeks after birth (57,58). As regards intellectual development, it appears that with the early high-dose regimen described above, the developmental gap between children with severe and those with moderate congenital hypothyroidism (or normal children) that was noted in children treated during the first decade of screening has now largely disappeared. In addition to cognitive performance, mean behavioral indexes up to school age are within normal limits, and there is no specific cognitive or behavioral trait that can be ascribed to congenital hypothyroidism or its treatment in any individual child (59). Thus, even among infants with severe congenital hypothyroidism, those who are treated vigorously and continuously from before 2 weeks of age should have growth, development, and behavior that proceed within normal limits.

Because of the recent studies on the genetic component of thyroid dysgenesis (2), the genetic counseling given to these families has changed. They should be told that the risk for congenital hypothyroidism is probably about 2% for subsequent siblings and for the offspring of the affected child. Because of the importance of euthyroidism in pregnant women from the beginning of gestation for the brain development of their offspring (60,61), girls with congenital hypothyroidism should be advised to have measurements of serum TSH and free T_4 when they contemplate pregnancy as well as throughout their pregnancies, because they may need a higher dose of T_4 during that time (see Chapter 80).

REFERENCES

1. Brown RS, Demmer LA. The etiology of thyroid dysgenesis—still an enigma after all these years. *J Clin Endocrinol Metab* 2002;87:4069.
2. Castanet M, Polak M, Bonaiti-Pellie C, et al. Nineteen years of national screening for congenital hypothyroidism: familial cases with thyroid dysgenesis suggest the involvement of genetic factors. *J Clin Endocrinol Metab* 2001;86:2009.
3. Castanet M. Mécanismes moléculaires impliqués dans les anomalies du développement de la glande thyroïde. Université René Descartes-Paris V, 2002.
4. Leger J, Marinovic D, Garel C, et al. Thyroid developmental anomalies in first degree relatives of children with congenital hypothyroidism. *J Clin Endocrinol Metab* 2002;87:575.

5. Perry R, Heinrichs C, Bourdoux P, et al. Discordance of monozygotic twins for thyroid dysgenesis: implications for screening and for molecular pathophysiology. *J Clin Endocrinol Metab* 2002;87:4072.

6. Devos H, Rodd C, Gagne N, et al. A search for the possible molecular mechanisms of thyroid dysgenesis: sex ratios and associated malformations. *J Clin Endocrinol Metab* 1999;84:2502.

7. Van Vliet G. Development of the thyroid gland: lessons from congenitally hypothyroid mice and men. *Clin Genet* 2003;63:445.

8. Van Vliet G. Molecular mechanisms of normal and abnormal thyroid gland development. In: Pescovitz OH, Eugster EE, eds. *Pediatric endocrinology: mechanisms, manifestations, and management.* Philadelphia: Lippincott Williams & Wilkins, 2004:479.

9. Brown AL, Fernhoff PM, Milner J, et al. Racial differences in the incidence of congenital hypothyroidism. *J Pediatr* 1981;99:934.

10. Toublanc JE. Comparison of epidemiological data on congenital hypothyroidism in Europe with those of other parts in the world. *Horm Res* 1992;38:230.

11. Brumm H, Pfeufer A, Biebermann H, et al. Congenital central hypothyroidism due to homozygous thyrotropin beta 313 delta T mutation is caused by a founder effect. *J Clin Endocrinol Metab* 2002;87:4811.

12. Deladoey J, Vuissoz JM, Domene HM, et al. Congenital secondary hypothyroidism due to a mutation C105Vfs114X thyrotropin-beta mutation: genetic study of five unrelated families from Switzerland and Argentina. *Thyroid* 2003;13:553.

13. Collu R, Tang J, Castagne J, et al. A novel mechanism for isolated central hypothyroidism: inactivating mutations in the thyrotropin-releasing hormone receptor gene. *J Clin Endocrinol Metab* 1997;82:1561.

14. Ward L, Chavez M, Huot C, et al. Severe congenital hypopituitarism with low prolactin levels and age-dependent anterior pituitary hypoplasia: a clue to a PIT-1 mutation. *J Pediatr* 1998;132:1036.

15. Chanoine JP, Pardou A, Bourdoux P, et al. Withdrawal of iodinated disinfectants at delivery decreases the recall rate at neonatal screening for congenital hypothyroidism. *Arch Dis Child* 1988;63:1297.

16. Brown RS, Bellisario RL, Botero D, et al. Incidence of transient congenital hypothyroidism due to maternal thyrotropin receptor-blocking antibodies in over one million babies. *J Clin Endocrinol Metab* 1996;81:1147.

17. Moreno JC, Bikker H, Kempers MJ, et al. Inactivating mutations in the gene for thyroid oxidase 2 (THOX2) and congenital hypothyroidism. *N Engl J Med* 2002;347:95.

18. New England Congenital Hypothyroidism Collaborative. Effects of neonatal screening for hypothyroidism: prevention of mental retardation by treatment before clinical manifestations. *Lancet* 1981;2:1095.

19. Van Vliet G, Larroque B, Bubuteishvili L, et al. Sex-specific impact of congenital hypothyroidism due to thyroid dysgenesis on skeletal maturation in term newborns. *J Clin Endocrinol Metab* 2003;88:2009.

20. Olivieri A, Stazi MA, Mastroiacovo P, et al. A population-based study on the frequency of additional congenital malformations in infants with congenital hypothyroidism: data from the Italian Registry for Congenital Hypothyroidism (1991–1998). *J Clin Endocrinol Metab* 2002;87:557.

21. Wolter R, Noel P, De Cock P, et al. Neuropsychological study in treated thyroid dysgenesis. *Acta Paediatr Scand Suppl* 1979;277:41.

22. Wasniewska M, De Luca F, Cassio A, et al. In congenital hypothyroidism bone maturation at birth may be a predictive factor of psychomotor development during the first year of life irrespective of other variables related to treatment. *Eur J Endocrinol* 2003;149:1.

23. Perry RJ, Maclennan A, Maroo S, et al. Ultrasound findings versus isotope scanning in neonates with TSH elevation. *Horm Res* 2002;58(suppl 2):64.

24. Ohnishi H, Sato H, Noda H, et al. Color Doppler ultrasonography: diagnosis of ectopic thyroid gland in patients with congenital hypothyroidism caused by thyroid dysgenesis. *J Clin Endocrinol Metab* 2003;88:5145.

25. Djemli A, Fillion M, Belgoudi J, et al. Twenty years later: a reevaluation of the contributon of plasma thyroglobulin to the diagnosis of thyroid dysgenesis in infants with congenital hypothyroidism. *Clin Biochem* 2004;37:818.

26. Pohlenz J, Dumitrescu A, Zundel D, et al. Partial deficiency of thyroid transcription factor 1 produces predominantly neurological defects in humans and mice. *J Clin Invest* 2002;109:469.

27. Krude H, Schutz B, Biebermann H, et al. Choreoathetosis, hypothyroidism, and pulmonary alterations due to human NKX2–1 haploinsufficiency. *J Clin Invest* 2002;109:475.

28. Clifton-Bligh RJ, Wentworth JM, Heinz P, et al. Mutation of the gene encoding human TTF-2 associated with thyroid agenesis, cleft palate and choanal atresia. *Nat Genet* 1998;19:399.

29. Castanet M, Park SM, Smith A, et al. A novel loss-of-function mutation in TTF-2 is associated with congenital hypothyroidism, thyroid agenesis and cleft palate. *Hum Mol Genet* 2002;11:2051.

30. Macchia PE, Lapi P, Krude H, et al. PAX8 mutations associated with congenital hypothyroidism caused by thyroid dysgenesis. *Nat Genet* 1998;19:83.

31. Vilain C, Rydlewski C, Duprez L, et al. Autosomal dominant transmission of congenital thyroid hypoplasia due to loss-of-function mutation of PAX8. *J Clin Endocrinol Metab* 2001;86:234.

32. Congdon T, Nguyen LQ, Nogueira CR, et al. A novel mutation (Q40P) in PAX8 associated with congenital hypothyroidism and thyroid hypoplasia: evidence for phenotypic variability in mother and child. *J Clin Endocrinol Metab* 2001;86:3962.

33. Komatsu M, Takahashi T, Takahashi I, et al. Thyroid dysgenesis caused by PAX8 mutation: the hypermutability with CpG dinucleotides at codon 31. *J Pediatr* 2001;139:597.

34. Abramowicz MJ, Duprez L, Parma J, et al. Familial congenital hypothyroidism due to inactivating mutation of the thyrotropin receptor causing profound hypoplasia of the thyroid gland. *J Clin Invest* 1997;99:3018.

35. Fisher DA. The importance of early management in optimizing IQ in infants with congenital hypothyroidism. *J Pediatr* 2000;136:273.

36. Germak JA, Foley TP Jr. Longitudinal assessment of L-thyroxine therapy for congenital hypothyroidism. *J Pediatr* 1990;117:211.

37. Hanukoglu A, Perlman K, Shamis I, et al. Relationship of etiology to treatment in congenital hypothyroidism. *J Clin Endocrinol Metab* 2001;86:186.

38. Rivkees SA, Hardin DS. Cretinism after weekly dosing with levothyroxine for treatment of congenital hypothyroidism. *J Pediatr* 1994;125:147.

39. Cassio A, Cacciari E, Cicognani A, et al. Treatment for congenital hypothyroidism: thyroxine alone or thyroxine plus triiodothyronine? *Pediatrics* 2003;111:1055.

40. Sack J, Shafrir Y, Urbach D, et al. Thyroid-stimulating hormone, prolactin, and growth hormone response to thyrotropin-releasing hormone in treated children with congenital hypothyroidism. *Pediatr Res* 1985;19:1037.

41. Daneman D, Howard NJ. Neonatal thyrotoxicosis: intellectual impairment and craniosynostosis in later years. *J Pediatr* 1980;97:257.

42. Penfold JL, Simpson DA. Premature craniosynostosis—a complication of thyroid replacement therapy. *J Pediatr* 1975;86:360.

43. Fisher DA, Schoen EJ, La Franchi S, et al. The hypothalamic-pituitary-thyroid negative feedback control axis in children with

treated congenital hypothyroidism. *J Clin Endocrinol Metab* 2000;85:2722.

44. Van Vliet G, Barboni Th, Klees M, et al. Treatment strategy and long term follow up of congenital hypothyroidism. In: Delange F, Fisher DA, Glinoer D, eds. *Research in congenital hypothyroidism*. New York: Plenum, 1989:245.

45. Glorieux J, Dussault J, Van Vliet G. Intellectual development at age 12 years of children with congenital hypothyroidism diagnosed by neonatal screening. *J Pediatr* 1992;121:581.

46. Derksen-Lubsen G, Verkerk PH. Neuropsychologic development in early treated congenital hypothyroidism: analysis of literature data. *Pediatr Res* 1996;39:561.

47. Oerbeck B, Sundet K, Kase BF, et al. Congenital hypothyroidism: influence of disease severity and L-thyroxine treatment on intellectual, motor, and school-associated outcomes in young adults. *Pediatrics* 2003;112:923.

48. Tillotson SL, Fuggle PW, Smith I, et al. Relation between biochemical severity and intelligence in early treated congenital hypothyroidism: a threshold effect. *BMJ* 1994;309:440.

49. Vulsma T, Gons MH, de Vijlder JJ. Maternal-fetal transfer of thyroxine in congenital hypothyroidism due to a total organification defect of thyroid agenesis. *N Engl J Med* 1989;321:13.

50. Fisher DA, Foley BL. Early treatment of congenital hypothyroidism. *Pediatrics* 1989;83:785.

51. Selva KA, Mandel SH, Rien L, et al. Initial treatment dose of L-thyroxine in congenital hypothyroidism. *J Pediatr* 2002;141:786.

52. Dubuis JM, Glorieux J, Richer F, et al. Outcome of severe congenital hypothyroidism: closing the developmental gap with early high dose levothyroxine treatment. *J Clin Endocrinol Metab* 1996;81:222.

53. Bongers-Schokking JJ, Koot HM, Wiersma D, et al. Influence of timing and dose of thyroid hormone replacement on development in infants with congenital hypothyroidism. *J Pediatr* 2000;136:292.

54. Leger J, Larroque B, Norton J. Influence of severity of congenital hypothyroidism and adequacy of treatment on school achievement in young adolescents: a population-based cohort study. *Acta Paediatr* 2001;90:1249.

55. Zurakowski D, Di Canzio J, Majzoub JA. Pediatric reference intervals for serum thyroxine, triiodothyronine, thyrotropin, and free thyroxine. *Clin Chem* 1999;45:1087.

56. Bongers-Schokking JJ, de Muinck Keizer-Schrama SM, Docter R. Pitfalls in serum free thyroxine measurements in infants with and without congenital hypothyroidism. *Horm Res* 1999;51 (suppl 2):17.

57. Francois M, Bonfils P, Leger J, et al. Role of congenital hypothyroidism in hearing loss in children. *J Pediatr* 1994;124:444.

58. Rovet J, Walker W, Bliss B, et al. Long-term sequelae of hearing impairment in congenital hypothyroidism. *J Pediatr* 1996;128:776.

59. Simoneau-Roy J, Marti S, Deal C, et al. Cognition and behavior at school entry in children with congenital hypothyroidism treated early with high-dose levothyroxine. *J Pediatr* 2004;144:747.

60. Haddow JE, Palomaki GE, Allan WC, et al. Maternal thyroid deficiency during pregnancy and subsequent neuropsychological development of the child. *N Engl J Med* 1999;341:549.

61. Lavado-Autric R, Auso E, Garcia-Velasco JV, et al. Early maternal hypothyroxinemia alters histogenesis and cerebral cortex cytoarchitecture of the progeny. *J Clin Invest* 2003;111:1073.

75C HYPOTHYROIDISM IN INFANTS, CHILDREN, AND ADOLESCENTS: ACQUIRED HYPOTHYROIDISM

GUY VAN VLIET

The unique feature of hypothyroidism in infants, children, or adolescents is that, if diagnosis is delayed, the condition may have a profound impact on skeletal growth and maturation, pubertal development, and adult height. When it occurs before birth, hypothyroidism may retard skeletal maturation, but it does not result in stunted intrauterine growth. However, starting immediately after birth (1), and until epiphyseal fusion, longitudinal bone growth is exquisitely sensitive to thyroid hormone deficiency. Thus, slowing of linear growth is the most sensitive clinical indicator of hypothyroidism in children. On the other hand, hypothyroidism in children 3 years of age or older does not have the same dramatic potential consequence of irreversible brain damage as when it is present at birth or soon thereafter. However, the initiation of treatment of severe hypothyroidism acquired during childhood and adolescence may transiently decrease learning ability and alter behavior, sometimes dramatically.

EPIDEMIOLOGY AND CAUSES OF ACQUIRED HYPOTHYROIDISM IN CHILDREN

The causes of acquired hypothyroidism in children and adolescents are shown in Table 75C.1. In addition to these disorders, in some infants with congenital hypothyroidism the onset of symptoms and signs of hypothyroidism may be delayed, and affected children may therefore present as

TABLE 75C.1.   CAUSES OF ACQUIRED HYPOTHYROIDISM IN CHILDREN AND ADOLESCENTS

Primary hypothyroidism
  Hashimoto's thyroiditis (goitrous and atrophic forms)
  Irradiation of the thyroid
    External irradiation for head and neck tumors
    Radioactive iodine treatment for hyperthyroidism
  Thyroidectomy
  Drug-induced (interferon-α, lithium, iodine-containing drugs)
  Consumptive (liver or skin hemangiomas)
  Iodine deficiency
Central hypothyroidism
  Tumors or infiltrative diseases of the hypothalamo-pituitary area
  Part of evolving hypopituitarism associated with:
    Developmental defects (e.g., pituitary stalk interruption)
    Pituitary transcription factor mutations

if they have acquired hypothyroidism. This is most common in children with inborn errors of thyroid hormone biosynthesis (see Chapter 48), but the mechanism of the delayed expression of the gene defect is unknown (2). On the other hand, children with central hypothyroidism caused by mutations in the β-subunit of thyrotropin (TSH) are missed by TSH-based neonatal screening programs and may only be recognized later.

Although the prevalence of congenital hypothyroidism is well known and varies little from country to country, there are relatively few studies of the prevalence of acquired hypothyroidism in children. In a recent study of 103,500 people aged 0 to 22 years in Scotland, 140 patients (0.14%) had received prescriptions for thyroxine (T_4) on a regular basis (2a). The male to female ratio was 1:2.8. A review of these patients' charts revealed that 75% had acquired hypothyroidism. The vast majority had primary hypothyroidism and evidence of autoimmune thyroid disease, 3.5% had type 1 diabetes mellitus, 2% had juvenile rheumatoid arthritis, and 1.5% had Down's syndrome. Geographic variations in the prevalence of hypothyroidism caused by autoimmune thyroid disease suggest that iodine deficiency may be protective (3). Hashimoto's thyroiditis is a common diagnosis in pediatric endocrine clinics in iodine-replete North America, but is much rarer in European countries such as Belgium, in which iodine intake is marginal.

Much less common than hypothyroidism due to autoimmune thyroid disease is radiation-induced hypothyroidism. This may occur as a result of external radiation therapy for tumors of the head and neck, or after radioiodine therapy for thyrotoxicosis (see Chapter 76) (4). Hypothyroidism after thyroidectomy is rare in children, because few children undergo thyroid surgery. Hypothyroidism due to drugs is also rare. Interferon-α, lithium,

and iodine-containing drugs can cause hypothyroidism in children, as in adults, primarily in children with preexisting chronic autoimmune thyroiditis.

An exceptional cause of hypothyroidism is consumptive hypothyroidism, resulting from the overexpression of type 3 deiodinase (see Chapter 7) by large liver or cutaneous hemangiomas (5). Although some of these infants have hypothyroidism at birth (6), most presented in the first few months of life, when hemangiomas are typically at their maximal size. One young adult with this syndrome has also been reported (7). Importantly, severe primary hypothyroidism requiring a high dose of T_4 was the presenting manifestation of multiple hepatic hemangiomas in one child, suggesting that a search for these tumors should be undertaken in any child with unexplained primary hypothyroidism who requires a high dose of T_4 (8).

Lastly, iodine deficiency remains an important cause of hypothyroidism worldwide (see section on iodine deficiency in Chapter 11 and Chapter 49). Although acquired hypothyroidism due to iodine deficiency is rare in North America and other countries where iodized salt is available, it can occur in children whose diets are severely restricted in salt and iodine-containing foods (9).

Acquired central hypothyroidism is typically associated with other pituitary hormone deficiencies. It is rarely the first or presenting manifestation of hypothalamic or pituitary disease, including tumors and infiltrative diseases such as histiocytosis, or of developmental defects with delayed expression.

CLINICAL PRESENTATION

The symptoms and signs of acquired hypothyroidism in children and adolescents depend on its severity and duration. Some patients present with a relatively short history of fatigue, constipation, dry skin, and cold intolerance, without a change in their growth pattern and without retardation of bone maturation, reflecting a sudden onset of hypothyroidism. However, in the vast majority of patients, assessment of growth reveals long-standing hypothyroidism. Typically, there is a rather abrupt deceleration in height gain at some time in the more or less distant past, whereas weight gain is relatively preserved. Thus, the patients present with short stature and relative weight excess, but they are seldom obese (Fig. 75C.1). The effect of hypothyroidism on bone maturation is even more pronounced than its effect on linear growth, so that the bone age is often younger than the height age (i.e., the age at which the child's height corresponds to the 50th percentile). Tooth eruption is also delayed. Other skeletal effects of hypothyroidism in children include stippling of the epiphyses and a slipped capital femoral epiphysis (see Chapter 62) (10).

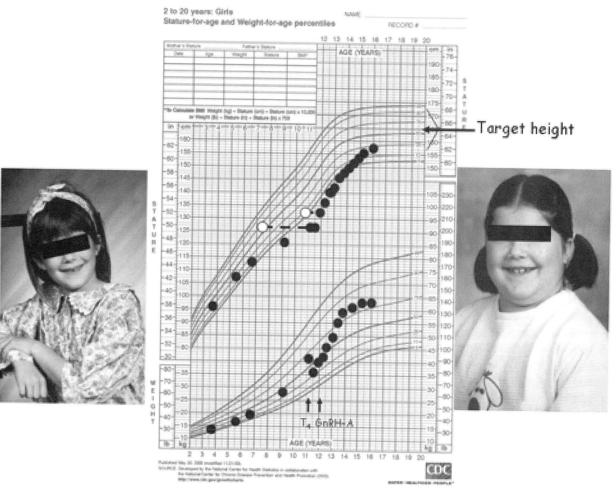

FIGURE 75C.1. Stature and weight curves of a girl with long-standing severe primary hypothyroidism caused by Hashimoto's thyroiditis. Her height and weight increased normally until she was about 7 years old (left picture), when height gain started to decrease while weight gain accelerated. At age 11.25 years, she had no fatigue, constipation, or cold intolerance, but her facial appearance had changed (right picture). Physical examination at that time revealed facial puffiness, very dry skin, and a small goiter. Her serum TSH concentration was 695 mU/L, her serum free thyroxine (T_4) concentration was 0.2 ng/dL (2.6 pM), and her serum titer of antithyroid peroxidase antibodies was 1:1,600. Bone age was 7.5 years (*open circle on left*). During the first months of T_4 therapy (*left vertical arrow*), she lost weight. This was followed by catch-up growth, progressive breast development, and rapid progression of bone maturation [bone age 11 years at chronological age 12 years (*open circle on right*)]. Despite treatment with a long-acting gonadotropin-releasing hormone agonist (GnRH-A) from age 12 to age 16 years to slow maturation (*right vertical arrow*), her adult height is below her target height (*right horizontal arrow*).

Because long-standing hypothyroidism retards bone maturation, it is often assumed that it invariably retards pubertal development. However, pubertal development may occur at a normal age. In some children, the effect of sex steroids on bone maturation seems to override that of hypothyroidism, resulting in an adult height below genetic potential. Rare children with severe primary hypothyroidism have sexual precocity (11): this appears to result from activation of follicle-stimulating hormone receptors by very high serum TSH concentrations. Accordingly, affected boys have testicular enlargement without excess testosterone secretion (12,13), and affected girls have functional ovarian cysts with vaginal bleeding, either with no other signs of puberty (14) or with breast development and galactorrhea but no pubic hair (11).

Hypothyroidism acquired after 3 years of age (the critical period during which it has an irreversible effect on brain development) does not typically affect school performance and progression. If the hypothyroidism is severe and of long duration, the child may require more time to accomplish the assigned tasks, but will rarely be held back academically. In fact, more often, school performance deteriorates after treatment is started.

Aside from its effects on growth, maturation, and puberty, the symptoms and signs of acquired hypothyroidism in children and adolescents are similar to those in adults (see Chapters 46, and 52 to 64). Thus, a constellation of increasing fatigue, constipation, cold intolerance, and puffiness of the face should alert the clinician to the possibility of hypothyroidism. Hypothyroidism has also been reported in otherwise asymptomatic children with hypercholesterolemia, and serum TSH should be measured in children with any type of hyperlipidemia (15).

In children with any symptoms and signs of hypothyroidism, the size of the thyroid should be determined. The World Health Organization definition that a goiter is present when the thyroid lobes are larger than the distal phalanx of the thumb of the child may seem rather crude, but is useful in children given their greatly varying size (16). In iodine-sufficient areas, the most common cause of goiter associated with hypothyroidism is Hashimoto's thyroiditis, in which case both lobes of the thyroid are usually moderately enlarged, firm, and irregular ("pebbly"). Nodules greater than 1 cm in diameter are rare, but a "Delphian node" is a frequent finding (a lymph node sometimes as small as a grain of rice that can be palpated above the isthmus, close to the midline). A family history of autoimmune thyroid disease is often elicited. Although a goiter is usually present at the time of diagnosis of Hashimoto's thyroiditis, the gland will usually gradually atrophy later. Thyroid atrophy may be present at diagnosis at any age, but this appears to be more common in infants (17).

Imaging of the pituitary is often performed when growth decelerates. It is important to remember that children and adolescents, as well as adults, with long-standing primary hypothyroidism can have pituitary enlargement, caused by hypertrophy and hyperplasia of the thyrotrophs (see Chapter 3). The enlargement may mimic that of a pituitary tumor, but is reversed by T_4 therapy (18). Thus, neuroradiologic studies should not be ordered in children with growth deceleration before serum TSH is measured. The shrinking of an enlarged pituitary may be responsible for the rare occurrence of transient growth hormone deficiency during the first years of T_4 therapy in children with hypothyroidism (19).

DIAGNOSTIC EVALUATION

Primary Hypothyroidism

A clinical suspicion of hypothyroidism should always be confirmed by measurements of serum TSH and free T_4. On the other hand, the serendipitous discovery of a high serum TSH concentration in a normally growing child or adolescent without any symptoms and signs of hypothyroidism should be verified before embarking on long-term treatment, because transient hypothyroidism may occur in autoimmune thyroiditis. If a diagnosis of primary hypothyroidism is confirmed, the next step is to determine its etiology. In infants, a radionuclide scan should be done to rule out a congenital cause that may have been missed on neonatal screening or if the onset of hypothyroidism was delayed. As stated above, most infants with congenital hypothyroidism in whom the onset of symptoms is delayed have some type of thyroid dyshormonogenesis (2,20), but one boy with normal blood-spot TSH and T_4 values at neonatal screening who had severe hypothyroidism due to ectopic thyroid tissue documented by radionuclide imaging at age 3 years has been reported (21). Intense radionuclide uptake by a normal-sized or enlarged thyroid in an infant with acquired hypothyroidism may suggest the presence of consumptive hypothyroidism (8).

In older infants, children, and adolescents, serum antithyroid peroxidase antibodies should be measured. A high concentration confirms the diagnosis of chronic autoimmune thyroiditis, whether the patient has a goiter (Hashimoto's thyroiditis, goitrous autoimmune thyroiditis) or not (atrophic autoimmune thyroiditis). On radionuclide imaging studies, the size of the thyroid may vary from small to large, and the heterogeneous pattern of uptake often seen in adults, which probably results from areas of fibrosis, is rarely seen in children (22). On ultrasonography, heterogeneous echogenicity is usually present (see Chapter 16) (23). In fact, neither scintigraphy nor ultrasonography is necessary to establish the diagnosis of chronic autoimmune thyroiditis. Imaging should be restricted to those children with a palpable thyroid nodule.

The child's growth trajectory should be carefully reconstructed and analyzed. Even if previous growth data are unavailable, a radiograph of the left hand and wrist should be obtained if hypothyroidism is severe, because its duration can be estimated by the degree of retardation of bone maturation.

As mentioned above, chronic autoimmune thyroiditis is more prevalent in children with type 1 diabetes. It is also more prevalent in children with chromosomal disorders, principally aneuploidies [trisomy 21 (24) and Turner's syndrome (25); the evidence for an association with Klinefelter's syndrome is less clear (26)]. Hypothyroidism is seldom the presenting feature of the polyglandular autoimmune syndromes.

Central Hypothyroidism

Central hypothyroidism is much less common than primary hypothyroidism in children and adolescents, and it is harder to diagnose. The symptoms and signs of hypothyroidism are usually more subtle, although slow growth and delayed bone maturation remain the most common presenting problems (27). Once a diagnosis of central hypothyroidism has been documented by measurements of serum free T_4 (low) and TSH (low, normal, or only slightly high) (see Chapter 51), other pituitary functions should be evaluated and neuroradiologic studies, preferably magnetic resonance imaging, should be performed. Most patients with central hypothyroidism have other pituitary hormone deficiencies, especially growth hormone deficiency, and TSH deficiency is seldom the first deficiency to be identified.

Some children with growth hormone deficiency may develop central hypothyroidism when they are treated with growth hormone, and hypothyroidism is one reason for a poor therapeutic response to growth hormone. This central hypothyroidism is generally due to evolving hypothalamic or pituitary disease. It should be distinguished from the decrease in serum free T_4 concentrations that occurs consistently during the first few months of growth hormone treatment in both growth hormone–deficient (28) and –sufficient humans (29), and which appears to be due mainly to increased conversion of T_4 to T_3. On the other hand, an increase in hypothalamic somatostatin secretion during growth hormone treatment may induce a decrease in serum TSH concentrations and true central hypothyroidism (30). However, treatment of growth hormone–deficient children with T_4 may result in a greater acceleration of bone maturation than of linear growth (31), and should therefore not be undertaken lightly. Despite these diagnostic difficulties, children who have a suboptimal response to growth hormone therapy, coupled with symptoms and signs of hypothyroidism and unequivocally low serum free T_4 concentrations, should be treated with T_4. This occurs mainly in children with organic hypopituitarism (32).

Whether a thyrotropin-releasing hormone (TRH) stimulation test should be performed before treatment is controversial (33). In children and adolescents with central hypothyroidism, administration of TRH typically induces an ample and sustained serum TSH response, with a peak serum TSH concentration at 60 minutes or later. This response suggests that the pituitary thyrotrophs are not only present but also store rather than secrete TSH because of lack of stimulation from endogenous TRH (34). The TSH produced in these patients has low bioactivity (35). Imaging studies usually reveal an interrupted pituitary stalk, often associated with other developmental defects such as an ectopic posterior pituitary gland (36). This type of hypothyroidism is caused by a disconnection between the hypothalamic TRH neurons and the pituitary thyrotrophs.

In the rare cases of central hypothyroidism resulting from pituitary transcription factor mutations, the serum TSH response to TRH is blunted or absent, and the pituitary stalk is normal on imaging (37). Thus, aside from it being required in all patients with central hypothyroidism

to rule out space-occupying lesions or infiltrative processes of the hypothalamic–pituitary area, imaging clarifies the developmental defects underlying many of the other cases.

TREATMENT

As in adults, the treatment of choice for children and adolescents with either primary or central hypothyroidism is the daily oral administration of T_4. An anticipated full replacement dose may be prescribed from the outset in children and adolescents. A rapid return to the euthyroid state is occasionally accompanied by dramatic psychological changes; and a few adolescents have an acute (and transient) psychosis. However, such cases are exceptional, and some have occurred even after gradual dose escalation (38). Another rare side effect during the early phase of T_4 therapy in children is benign intracranial hypertension; this, too, can occur despite gradual dose escalation (39). Thus, parents should be warned that dramatic behavioral changes may occur after therapy is begun, and that the onset of severe headaches should lead to prompt fundoscopic examination.

A full daily replacement dose of T_4, expressed as µg/kg of body weight, is about 5 for children 1 to 5 years old, 4 for children 6 to 12 years old, and 3 for adolescents. These doses correspond to about 100 µg/m^2 of body surface area (40). The needed dose is usually lower in patients with central hypothyroidism. However, there is substantial variation in the effect of T_4 in different patients, so these estimates are only a rough guide for the dose likely to be needed for an individual patient. The dose appropriate for a patient with primary hypothyroidism should be adjusted so that the patient's serum TSH concentration is normal. Absorption may be better if T_4 is administered 30 minutes or more before meals, and it may be decreased by the simultaneous intake of iron and calcium supplements (41, 42).

After therapy is started, the appearance of children with severe long-standing hypothyroidism changes dramatically, and initially weight may be lost (Fig. 75C.1). Subsequently, catch-up growth in height with proportionate weight gain occurs. In prepubertal children with severe hypothyroidism, pubertal development and bone maturation should be monitored closely, because progression may be too rapid. When this occurs, administration of a gonadotropin-releasing hormone agonist to decrease sex steroid secretion and delay epiphyseal maturation may be considered, although the impact of combined T_4 and agonist therapy on adult height is uncertain (43). Diagnosis of hypothyroidism before it has had an important impact on growth—which can be achieved if linear growth in children is followed longitudinally—is obviously preferable.

Because equilibration is slow, serum TSH should not be measured less than 6 weeks after therapy is started or changed. Once the patient's serum TSH concentration is normal, growth, pubertal development, and serum TSH should be monitored yearly.

T$_4$ therapy in patients with central hypothyroidism should be monitored by measurements of serum free T$_4$. In those patients in whom serum TSH concentrations were normal before therapy, undetectable values suggest overtreatment, even if their serum free T$_4$ concentrations are in the normal range. This should be avoided because it may lead to accelerated bone maturation, and the dose should be the lowest possible for optimal growth and maturation.

PROGNOSIS

In peripubertal children with severe long-standing hypothyroidism, the prognosis regarding adult height should be guarded (44). On the other hand, hypothyroidism acquired after the critical period of brain development during infancy does not carry a risk for irreversible long-term effects on cognition. In most patients, and specifically those who have chronic autoimmune thyroiditis, hypothyroidism will likely be permanent. However, as in many other autoimmune diseases, there may be periods of remission. In particular, thyroid function may fluctuate, sometimes widely (45), and it may therefore be appropriate to withdraw T$_4$ for 6 to 8 weeks every several years or at the end of growth. This is not necessary in patients who have high serum TSH concentrations while taking T$_4$, or in those who had severe hypothyroidism with thyroid atrophy at the time of diagnosis.

Adolescent girls should be informed that they may need more T$_4$ if they take an estrogen-containing oral contraceptive, although currently used oral contraceptives have only a minimal influence on thyroid function in normal women (46). More important, they should be advised that the adequacy of treatment should be determined before and as soon as possible after they become pregnant, because most pregnant women with hypothyroidism need a higher dose of T$_4$ than when they are not pregnant (see Chapters 67 and 80). Among those with chronic autoimmune thyroiditis, serum TSH receptor–blocking antibodies may be present, but rarely in sufficient quantities to affect fetal thyroid function (47).

Other factors that may lead to the need for an increase in T$_4$ include treatment with phenytoin, carbamazepine, or rifampin. These drugs increase the clearance of T$_4$; unlike normal subjects, patients with hypothyroidism cannot increase T$_4$ secretion to compensate for the increase in clearance. Other substances, for example, iron and calcium, can reduce intestinal absorption of T$_4$, thereby necessitating an increase in T$_4$ dose (see Chapter 67).

REFERENCES

1. Leger J, Czernichow P. Congenital hypothyroidism: decreased growth velocity in the first weeks of life. *Biol Neonate* 1989;55:218.
2. de Zegher F, Vanderschueren-Lodeweyckx M, Heinrichs C, et al. Thyroid dyshormonogenesis: severe hypothyroidism after normal neonatal thyroid stimulating hormone screening. *Acta Paediatr* 1992;81:274.
2a. Hunter I, Greene SA, MacDonald TM, et al. Prevalence and aetiology of hypothyroidism in the young. *Arch Dis Child* 2000; 83;207.
3. Pearce EN, Farwell AP, Braverman LE. Thyroiditis. *N Engl J Med* 2003;348:2646.
4. Ward L, Huot C, Lambert R, et al. Outcome of pediatric Graves' disease after treatment with antithyroid medication and radioiodine. *Clin Invest Med* 1999;22:132.
5. Huang SA, Tu HM, Harney JW, et al. Severe hypothyroidism caused by type 3 iodothyronine deiodinase in infantile hemangiomas. *N Engl J Med* 2000;343:185.
6. Ayling RM, Davenport M, Hadzic N, et al. Hepatic hemangioendothelioma associated with production of humoral thyrotropin-like factor. *J Pediatr* 2001;138:932.
7. Huang SA, Fish SA, Dorfman DM, et al. A 21-year-old woman with consumptive hypothyroidism due to a vascular tumor expressing type 3 iodothyronine deiodinase. *J Clin Endocrinol Metab* 2002;87:4457.
8. Konrad D, Ellis G, Perlman K. Spontaneous regression of severe acquired infantile hypothyroidism associated with multiple liver hemangiomas. *Pediatrics* 2003;112:1424.
9. Pacaud D, Van Vliet G, Delvin E, et al. A third world endocrine disease in a 6-year-old North American boy. *J Clin Endocrinol Metab* 1995;80:2574.
10. Burrow SR, Alman B, Wright JG. Short stature as a screening test for endocrinopathy in slipped capital femoral epiphysis. *J Bone Joint Surg Br* 2001;83:263.
11. Van Wyk JJ, Grumbach MM. Syndrome of precocious menstruation and galactorrhea in juvenile hypothyroidism: an example of hormonal overlap in pituitary feedback. *J Pediatr* 1960;57:416.
12. Bruder JM, Samuels MH, Bremner WJ, et al. Hypothyroidism-induced macroorchidism: use of a gonadotropin-releasing hormone agonist to understand its mechanism and augment adult stature. *J Clin Endocrinol Metab* 1995;80:11.
13. Lado-Abeal J, Molinaro E, DeValk E, et al. The effect of short-term treatment with recombinant human thyroid-stimulating hormones on Leydig cell function in men. *Thyroid* 2003;13:649.
14. Gordon CM, Austin DJ, Radovick S, et al. Primary hypothyroidism presenting as severe vaginal bleeding in a prepubertal girl. *J Pediatr Adolesc Gynecol* 1997;10:35.
15. Lavin A, Nauss AH. Hypothyroidism in otherwise healthy hypercholesterolemic children. *Pediatrics* 1991;88:332.
16. Van Vliet G, Delange F. Goiter and thyroiditis. In: Bertrand J, Rappaport R, Sizonenko PC, eds. *Pediatric endocrinology: physiology, pathophysiology, and clinical aspects.* Baltimore: Williams & Wilkins, 1993:270.
17. Foley TP Jr, Abbassi V, Copeland KC, et al. Hypothyroidism caused by chronic autoimmune thyroiditis in very young infants. *N Engl J Med* 1994;330:466.
18. Papakonstantinou O, Bitsori M, Mamoulakis D, e al. MR imaging of pituitary hyperplasia in a child with growth arrest and primary hypothyroidism. *Eur Radiol* 2000;10:516.
19. Dahlem ST, Furlanetto RW, Moshang T Jr, et al. Transient growth hormone deficiency after treatment of primary hypothyroidism. *J Pediatr* 1987;111:256.

20. Vincent MA, Rodd C, Dussault JH, et al. Very low birth weight newborns do not need repeat screening for congenital hypothyroidism. *J Pediatr* 2002;140:311.

21. Rochiccioli P, Dutau G, Augier D. Thyroid ectopia, a cause of error in neonatal screening for hypothyroidism. *Arch Fr Pediatr* 1983;40:405.

22. Alos N, Huot C, Lambert R, et al. Thyroid scintigraphy in children and adolescents with Hashimoto disease. *J Pediatr* 1995;127:951.

23. Set PA, Oleszczuk-Raschke K, von Lengerke JH, et al. Sonographic features of Hashimoto thyroiditis in childhood. *Clin Radiol* 1996;51:167.

24. Noble SE, Leyland K, Findlay CA, et al. School based screening for hypothyroidism in Down's syndrome by dried blood spot TSH measurement. *Arch Dis Child* 2000;82:27.

25. Radetti G, Mazzanti L, Paganini C, et al. Frequency, clinical and laboratory features of thyroiditis in girls with Turner's syndrome. The Italian Study Group for Turner's Syndrome. *Acta Paediatr* 1995;84:909.

26. Kondo T. Klinefelter syndrome associated with juvenile hypothyroidism due to chronic thyroiditis. *Eur J Pediatr* 1993;152:540.

27. Collu R, Tang J, Castagne J, et al. A novel mechanism for isolated central hypothyroidism: inactivating mutations in the thyrotropin-releasing hormone receptor gene. *J Clin Endocrinol Metab* 1997;82:1561.

28. Jorgensen JO, Pedersen SA, Laurberg P, et al. Effects of growth hormone therapy on thyroid function of growth hormone-deficient adults with and without concomitant thyroxine-substituted central hypothyroidism. *J Clin Endocrinol Metab* 1989;69:1127.

29. Grunfeld C, Sherman BM, Cavalieri RR. The acute effects of human growth hormone administration on thyroid function in normal men. *J Clin Endocrinol Metab* 1988;67:1111.

30. Lippe BM, Van Herle AJ, Lafranchi SH, et al. Reversible hypothyroidism in growth hormone-deficient children treated with human growth hormone. *J Clin Endocrinol Metab* 1975;40:612.

31. Van den Brande JL, Van Wyk JJ, French FS, et al. Advancement of skeletal age of hypopituitary children treated with thyroid hormone plus cortisone. *J Pediatr* 1973;82:22.

32. Giavoli G, Porretti S, Ferrante E, et al. Recombinant hGH replacement therapy and the hypothalamus-pituitary-thyroid axis in children with GH deficiency: when should we be concerned about the occurrence of central hypothyroidism? *Clin Endocrinol (Oxf)* 2003;59:806.

33. Mehta A, Hindmarsh PC, Stanhope RG, et al. Is the thyrotropin-releasing hormone test necessary in the diagnosis of central hypothyroidism in children. *J Clin Endocrinol Metab* 2003;88:5696.

34. Suter SN, Kaplan SL, Aubert ML, et al. Plasma prolactin and thyrotropin and the response to thyrotropin-releasing factor in children with primary and hypothalamic hypothyroidism. *J Clin Endocrinol Metab* 1978;47:1015.

35. Beck-Peccoz P, Amr S, Menezes-Ferreira MM, et al. Decreased receptor binding of biologically inactive thyrotropin in central hypothyroidism. Effect of treatment with thyrotropin-releasing hormone. *N Engl J Med* 1985;312:1085.

36. Hamilton J, Blaser S, Daneman D. MR imaging in idiopathic growth hormone deficiency. *AJNR* 1998;19:1609.

37. Ward L, Chavez M, Huot C, et al. Severe congenital hypopituitarism with low prolactin levels and age-dependent anterior pituitary hypoplasia: a clue to a PIT-1 mutation. *J Pediatr* 1998;132:1036.

38. Rovet JF, Daneman D, Bailey JD. Psychologic and psychoeducational consequences of thyroxine therapy for juvenile acquired hypothyroidism. *J Pediatr* 1993;122:543.

39. Van Dop C, Conte FA, Koch TK, et al. Pseudotumor cerebri associated with initiation of levothyroxine therapy for juvenile hypothyroidism. *N Engl J Med* 1983;308:1076.

40. Guyda HJ. Treatment of congenital hypothyroidism. In: Dussault JH, Walker P, eds. *Congenital hypothyroidism*. New York: Marcel Dekker, 1983:385.

41. Sherman SI, Malecha SE. Absorption and malabsorption of levothyroxine sodium. *Am J Ther* 1995;2:814.

42. Schneyer CR. Calcium carbonate and reduction of levothyroxine efficacy. *JAMA* 1998;279:750.

43. Teng L, Bui H, Bachrach L, et al. Catch-up growth in severe juvenile hypothyroidism: treatment with a GnRH analog. *J Pediatr Endocrinol Metab* 2004;17:345.

44. Rivkees SA, Bode HH, Crawford JD. Long-term growth in juvenile acquired hypothyroidism: the failure to achieve normal adult stature. *N Engl J Med* 1988;318:599.

45. Maenpaa J, Raatikka M, Rasanen J, et al. Natural course of juvenile autoimmune thyroiditis. *J Pediatr* 1985;107:898.

46. Wiegratz I, Kutschera E, Lee JH, et al. Effect of four oral contraceptives on thyroid hormones, adrenal and blood pressure parameters. *Contraception* 2003;67:361.

47. Brown RS, Bellisario RL, Botero D, et al. Incidence of transient congenital hypothyroidism due to maternal thyrotropin receptor-blocking antibodies in over one million babies. *J Clin Endocrinol Metab* 1996;81:1147.

GRAVES' DISEASE IN THE NEONATAL PERIOD AND CHILDHOOD

STEPHEN H. LAFRANCHI
CHERYL E. HANNA

Thyrotoxicosis is less common in children and adolescents than in adults, and it is rare in neonates. In all three groups, the cause is nearly always Graves' disease, as in adults. Most aspects of thyrotoxicosis (and Graves' disease) in neonates, children, and adolescents are similar to those in adults, but a few are age specific. For example, in neonates, the thyrotoxicosis is transient, and it has effects on growth and development of the nervous system. In children, thyrotoxicosis has effects on growth, pubertal development, and the skeleton that do not occur in adults. Graves' ophthalmopathy is seldom as severe as in adults, and localized myxedema is extremely rare. Furthermore, the differential diagnosis of hyperthyroxinemia is different in childhood; thyrotoxicosis is the most frequent cause, rather than pregnancy and estrogen therapy, and generalized resistance to thyroid hormones and inherited abnormalities in thyroxine (T_4) transport proteins are relatively more common than in adults. With respect to treatment of Graves' thyrotoxicosis, there is more reluctance to undertake destructive therapy than in adults, although radioiodine therapy is gaining acceptance in adolescents.

NEONATAL THYROTOXICOSIS

Incidence

Neonatal thyrotoxicosis is rare, accounting for at most 1% of the cases of thyrotoxicosis in childhood, and is nearly always associated with maternal Graves' disease. Usually, the mother has a history of Graves' thyrotoxicosis; in many cases, the mother had thyrotoxicosis during the pregnancy, but sometimes she had received destructive antithyroid treatment before the pregnancy and was taking T_4 during it. A few mothers have had chronic autoimmune thyroiditis (Hashimoto's disease) rather than Graves' disease. Neonatal Graves' thyrotoxicosis occurs in fewer than 2% of infants born to mothers who had Graves' thyrotoxicosis during or before the pregnancy [1], although a few neonates with mild thyrotoxicosis may escape detection. The condition occurs with equal frequency in boys and girls.

Pathogenesis

Graves' thyrotoxicosis in neonates is caused by the transplacental passage of thyrotropin (TSH) receptor–stimulating antibodies (TSHR-SAbs) [2–6], meaning that the mother must be producing these antibodies late in gestation. The mothers of many affected neonates have thyrotoxicosis during that pregnancy, but that is not essential, as noted above. In those mothers who did have thyrotoxicosis during pregnancy, the clinical severity of their thyrotoxicosis is a poor predictor of neonatal thyroid status, but measurements of TSHR-SAbs in maternal serum are useful in this regard [2,7–11]. Thyrotoxicosis is likely only in infants of mothers who have high serum TSHR-SAb values, for example, greater than 500% of control values in assays based on inhibition by serum of binding of radiolabeled TSH to TSH receptors [10,11]. Assays of this type do not measure biologic activity, and the prediction of neonatal thyrotoxicosis is more accurate when TSHR-SAbs are measured by biologic assays [7,9] (see Chapter 15 and section Pathogenesis in Chapter 23).

Serum TSHR-SAbs should be measured in mid- or late pregnancy in pregnant women with Graves' thyrotoxicosis to identify at-risk neonates, and measurements in the neonates also may be useful in identifying those likely to develop thyrotoxicosis if it is not present then, as in neonates of mothers who are receiving an antithyroid drug [12]. The occurrence of thyrotoxicosis only in neonates whose mothers have high serum TSHR-SAb values indicates that transplacental passage of the antibodies is limited.

Transplacental passage of maternal TSHR-SAbs can cause fetal as well as neonatal thyrotoxicosis. Placental transport of TSHR-SAbs from maternal to fetal circulation increases from 5% to 8% of maternal levels at 15 weeks' gestation to approximately maternal levels by 30 weeks' gestation [13]. Fetuses with thyrotoxicosis have tachycardia, hyperactivity, and poor growth, skeletal and brain maturation may be accelerated, and fetal hydrops has been described. Intrauterine death may also occur, particularly if the mother has severe (and usually untreated) thyrotoxicosis [13]. How often fetal thyrotoxicosis occurs is not known, but in mothers treated with an antithyroid drug, it is probably uncommon (see Chapter 80).

Graves' thyrotoxicosis in neonates subsides spontaneously as the maternal TSHR-SAbs disappear from the infant's serum. The serum half-life of immunoglobulin G in neonates is about 14 days; depending on the serum TSHR-SAb concentrations at the time of delivery, the thyrotoxicosis disappears in 3 to 12 weeks.

A rarer form of neonatal thyrotoxicosis is not associated with maternal autoimmune thyroid disease and persists indefinitely (13–15). It is caused by germ line mutations in the transmembrane region of the TSH receptor that result in constitutive activation of the receptor (see Chapter 25). These mutations may be inherited as an autosomal-dominant trait or occur sporadically as new mutations (15–19). Not all affected patients are neonates; the thyrotoxicosis may first become evident during childhood or even later. Cases of neonatal thyrotoxicosis associated with McCune-Albright syndrome also have been reported (20); these are caused by somatic activating mutations in the α subunit of the guanine nucleotide-binding protein (G protein), which is a component of the adenylyl cyclase signal transduction pathway.

Clinical Manifestations

The birth weight of neonates with thyrotoxicosis is often low. Delivery may be premature, according to postconception estimates, although skeletal maturation may be accelerated as a result of thyrotoxicosis *in utero* (21). They may have microcephaly, enlargement of their cerebral ventricles (22), frontal bossing, or triangular facies. Hyperphagia is common, but weight gain is poor despite a high caloric intake. They are irritable and difficult to console. Fever and diarrhea may also occur. Most have prominent eyes and a small diffuse goiter; rarely, the goiter may be large enough to cause tracheal obstruction. Tachycardia and bounding pulses are almost invariably present, and cardiomegaly, congestive heart failure, cardiac arrhythmias, systemic and pulmonary hypertension, jaundice, hepatosplenomegaly, and thrombocytopenia also may occur. Premature infants with thyrotoxicosis have similar abnormalities (23).

The onset, severity, and duration of symptoms in neonates with Graves' thyrotoxicosis are variable. Some are thyrotoxic at birth, but those whose mothers were receiving an antithyroid drug at the time of delivery may not become thyrotoxic for several days, until the drug is metabolized. Rarely, antibodies that block TSH action as well as those that mimic TSH action are passed transplacentally to the fetus; in one case, the blocking antibodies prevented the effect of the stimulating antibodies for 4 to 6 weeks, thus delaying the onset of thyrotoxicosis (24).

Diagnosis and Treatment

The diagnosis of neonatal thyrotoxicosis should be confirmed by measurements of serum total and free T_4 and serum TSH (see Chapter 44). Indeed, cord blood for these measurements should be obtained in any infant delivered by a woman with a history of Graves' thyrotoxicosis. It is important to note that the ranges for serum total and free T_4 [and triiodothyronine (T_3)] are higher in normal neonates than in normal adults (see Chapter 74).

Treatment should be initiated promptly in neonates with obvious thyrotoxicosis without awaiting laboratory confirmation. Either methimazole (MMI), 0.5 to 1 mg/kg daily, or propylthiouracil (PTU), 5 to 10 mg/kg daily, should be administered orally every 8 to 12 hours to inhibit thyroid hormone synthesis. The response to an antithyroid drug may be erratic in extremely premature infants, and they require more careful monitoring than do infants of more mature gestational age (23). In severely ill infants, propranolol, 2 mg/kg daily, is helpful in slowing the pulse rate and reducing hyperactivity. Inorganic iodine also may be given to inhibit thyroid hormone synthesis and release, in the form of low doses of Lugol's solution or potassium iodide (see Chapter 45). A more experimental, but apparently effective, method for giving iodine has been to administer iopanoic acid, an iodinated cholecystographic agent, in a dose of 100 to 200 mg daily or 500 mg every third day; this iodine-rich agent inhibits thyroid secretion and extrathyroidal conversion of T_4 to T_3 (it is no longer aailable in the United States) (25–27). Neonates with severe clinical thyrotoxicosis are often given a glucocorticoid, which in high doses decreases extrathyroidal conversion of T_4 to T_3 and also may inhibit thyroid secretion. Digoxin may be necessary for treatment of heart failure.

The rare neonates with thyrotoxicosis resulting from a TSH-receptor mutation or McCune-Albright syndrome also should be treated with an antithyroid drug initially. Because their thyrotoxicosis is permanent, however, they should be treated with radioiodine or thyroidectomy later (16–19,28).

With respect to fetal thyrotoxicosis, it should be suspected in a fetus with a heart rate exceeding 160 beats/min after 22 weeks' gestation, hyperactivity, and poor growth. Fetal thyrotoxicosis may have deleterious skeletal and neurologic effects; therefore, treatment should be considered if it is severe. Thyrotoxic fetuses may be treated by giving the mother an antithyroid drug; the dose should be adjusted to maintain a fetal heart rate of about 140 beats/min (29). Treatment should be monitored clinically and by ultrasonography; an enlarging thyroid gland is evidence of overtreatment. Normal reference values for fetal thyroid gland size throughout gestation have been established (30). Fetal blood sampling by cordocentesis can be done for laboratory tests (31,32), but can result in complications including fetal loss (13). Maternal and fetal thyrotoxicosis discovered during labor has been effectively treated with labetalol (33).

Prognosis

In most neonates, improvement is rapid, and treatment can be withdrawn in several weeks or months, according to the results of clinical examination and measurements of serum T_4 and TSH. In the rare infants in whom thyrotoxicosis persists longer than 3 to 4 months, it more likely is due to a TSH receptor mutation or the McCune-Albright syndrome than Graves' disease.

The mortality rate secondary to prematurity, congestive heart failure, and airway obstruction was estimated to be as high as 25% in the past, but is considerably lower now. Long-term morbidity, which includes growth retardation, craniosynostosis, hyperactivity, and impairment of intellectual function, is common (14,22,34), and may occur even in neonates treated promptly and adequately, suggesting that fetal thyrotoxicosis permanently affects the developing skeleton and brain. In addition, central (pituitary) hypothyroidism, which may be secondary to prenatal exposure of the hypothalamus and pituitary to high serum thyroid hormone concentrations during a critical stage of development, has been reported to follow neonatal thyrotoxicosis (35,35a).

THYROTOXICOSIS IN CHILDHOOD

The vast majority of cases of thyrotoxicosis in children and adolescents are caused by Graves' disease, and the proportion caused by Graves' disease is higher than in adults. It may begin in infancy, but it is rare in children less than 5 years old (30,32,33). The incidence progressively increases throughout childhood, with a peak incidence in children 11 to 15 years of age (36–38). Childhood Graves' thyrotoxicosis is still uncommon, however, accounting for fewer than 5% of all cases. The prevalence in children approximates 0.02%. Girls are more commonly affected than boys, with a female:male ratio of 3:1 to 6:1 (36–39). The incidence of Graves' disease in children varies on a geographic or racial/ethnic basis. In Denmark, the incidence was 0.79/100,000/year between 1982 and 1988 (40). In Hong Kong Chinese children under 15 years of age, the incidence was 3.2/100,000/year for the time period 1989 to 1993, and it was 6.5/100,00/year in 1994 to 1998 (41); the increase in incidence rate for girls was statistically significant (41).

Most children with Graves' thyrotoxicosis have a family history of some type of autoimmune thyroid disease (38), and some have other autoimmune endocrine diseases, such as type 1 diabetes mellitus and Addison's disease (42). Nonendocrine autoimmune disorders, such as systemic lupus erythematosus, rheumatoid arthritis, myasthenia gravis, vitiligo, idiopathic thrombocytopenic purpura, and pernicious anemia, also have been described in these children (42). Human leukocyte antigen DR haplotypes differ in patients according to their age of onset (see Chapter 20)

(43). In addition, Graves' thyrotoxicosis is more common in children with Down syndrome than in normal children (24,42). Graves' disease may also be part of the clinical spectrum associated with the 22q11.2 deletion (DiGeorge's) syndrome (44).

Clinical Features

The main clinical features of thyrotoxicosis in children and adolescents are similar to those in adults (36–39) (Table 76.1). Excluding weight loss and atrial fibrillation, the common symptoms and signs of thyrotoxicosis are at least as frequent in children as in adults (45). Onset is often insidious, and many children have what they and their parents recall as just a few symptoms for several months or even years before the child is brought for care, even though at that time a history of many symptoms is often elicited. In children, emotional lability and hyperactivity are often attributed to behavioral or other factors, and a small goiter and prominent eyes may go unnoticed. Prepubertal children tend to have a longer duration of symptoms at presentation than pubertal children (46).

Nervousness, emotional lability, behavioral changes, and deteriorating school performance are the symptoms likely to bring the child to medical attention. These symptoms often are noted by a parent or teacher rather than by the child. Referral for evaluation of hyperactivity and possible attention deficit disorder is common. Emotional outbursts, difficulty sleeping, and mood swings may lead to referral to a child psychiatrist or counselor. Fatigue, weak-

TABLE 76.1. FREQUENCY OF SYMPTOMS AND SIGNS OF THYROTOXICOSIS IN CHILDREN AND ADOLESCENTS

	Percentage
Goiter	99
Tachycardia	83
Nervousness	80
Increased pulse pressure	77
Hypertension	71
Exophthalmos	66
Tremor	61
Increased appetite	60
Weight loss	54
Thyroid bruit	53
Increased perspiration	49
Hyperactivity	44
Heart murmur	43
Palpitations	34
Heat intolerance	33
Fatigue	16
Headache	15
Diarrhea	13

Data from references 36–39.

ness, and dyspnea may lead to a reduction in activity and cessation of athletic activities.

Diffuse goiter is present in virtually all children with thyrotoxicosis caused by Graves' disease. The degree of thyroid enlargement is variable, but typically is not great. Thus, thyroid enlargement is usually not the chief complaint, and children rarely have symptoms from the enlargement. The thyroid gland is nontender, smooth, and firm, and a thyroid bruit may be heard. Thyroid nodules may be present; in a recent study of 468 patients 12 to 75 years of age, 12.8% had nodules. In six patients (1.3%), the nodule was a thyroid cancer (47).

Some ophthalmopathy is common, but severe ophthalmopathy is rare. Most children have stare and wide palpebral fissures, which are signs of thyrotoxicosis. Ophthalmic symptoms and signs such as tearing and eyelid, periorbital, or conjunctival swelling occur in about 10% to 15% of children (48–51). In the largest series (72 girls and 11 boys), 12% had exophthalmos, and punctate corneal erosions were seen in 13% (51). Exophthalmos is rarely the presenting complaint (52). Eye pain, diplopia, and ophthalmoplegia are rare. The stare and wide palpebral fissures improve with treatment of thyrotoxicosis; ophthalmopathy may persist but rarely requires treatment (see section Ophthalmopathy in Chapter 23).

Cardiac findings include tachycardia, a widened pulse pressure, and hyperactive precordium. Occasional children complain of heart "racing" or pounding. Left ventricular reserve may decrease, accounting at least in part for exercise intolerance (53), but arrhythmias and congestive heart failure almost never occur.

Most children with thyrotoxicosis have an increased appetite. Although weight loss is not as common as in adults, the children do not gain weight normally, indicating that the increase in appetite is inadequate to meet their caloric needs. On the other hand, some children truly overeat and therefore gain an excessive amount of weight. Increased stool frequency occurs in a minority of children, but diarrhea is rare. Once antithyroid treatment is instituted, some children continue to eat excessively and then may become obese. A conscious effort should be made to decrease excessive caloric intake after therapy is initiated.

Acceleration of linear growth is common in children with thyrotoxicosis, and many have an increase in height percentiles on the growth chart. The acceleration in growth is accompanied by increased epiphyseal maturation and advancement in bone age. Thus, epiphyseal closure may occur earlier. There is no increase in adult height. Thyrotoxicosis may impair mineralization of bone (54). At the time of diagnosis, bone mineral density is decreased; in one series 42% of children had severe osteopenia (55). Effective therapy results in restoration of normal bone mass for age (55).

Most children with thyrotoxicosis have a fine tremor and brisk deep tendon reflexes. The seizure threshold may

decrease, and seizures are a rare presenting feature of thyrotoxicosis (56). In children under 3 years of age, thyrotoxicosis may cause language delay or more global developmental delay, which may or may not be reversible with treatment (57). Muscle weakness and fatigue are common but seldom severe. Periodic paralysis has been described in children (58), but it is probably even rarer than in adults.

Heat intolerance and excessive perspiration occur in more than 30% of children. The skin is often warm and moist, and occasionally it is flushed. Localized myxedema and thyroid acropachy almost never occur in children with Graves' disease.

Diagnosis

For children and adolescents who present with obvious symptoms and signs of thyrotoxicosis, diffuse goiter, and ophthalmopathy, there should be no confusion regarding the diagnosis of thyrotoxicosis or its cause. In such children, laboratory tests confirm the presence of thyrotoxicosis, gauge its biochemical severity, and establish a baseline for treatment.

In others, the diagnosis of thyrotoxicosis may not be so obvious. These patients include seemingly asymptomatic children with diffuse or painful goiter or a thyroid nodule, and children with only a few symptoms or signs of thyrotoxicosis, such as weight loss, weakness, or change in behavior. In these children, laboratory tests are indicated primarily to identify the presence of thyrotoxicosis. (In other children, the possibility of thyrotoxicosis is considered only after thyroid function tests are done for some other reason, such as hyperactivity.)

The most appropriate tests in either group are measurements of serum TSH and free T_4, with measurement of serum T_3 if the serum free T_4 value is normal (see Chapters 13 and Chapter 44). Nearly all children with thyrotoxicosis, like adults, have low serum TSH and high serum total and free T_4 and T_3 concentrations. If the serum TSH value is normal (or high), the possibility of resistance to thyroid hormone should be considered (59) (see Chapter 81), and a TSH-secreting pituitary adenoma must be sought (see Chapter 24).

More than 75% of children with Graves' thyrotoxicosis have high serum concentrations of antithyroid peroxidase and antithyroglobulin antibodies, but the concentrations are not usually as high as in children with chronic autoimmune thyroiditis (60). These antibodies need not be measured unless evidence is being sought against the presence of Graves' disease. Similarly, TSHR-SAbs are present in the serum of more than 90% of children with Graves' disease, whether measured by receptor assay or bioassay (61,62). These antibodies also need not be measured routinely for diagnostic purposes. Measurements after some period of antithyroid drug therapy may provide information about the persistence of Graves' disease and, therefore, the likelihood of recurrent thyrotoxicosis if the drug is discontinued. The presence of TSHR-SAbs then would indicate a high probability of recurrence (see Chapter 15 and Chapter 45) (62,63).

Measurements of radioiodine uptake and radionuclide imaging are seldom needed in children. An uptake test may be helpful in those who have few clinical manifestations of thyrotoxicosis and low serum TSH but normal serum T_4 and T_3 concentrations (i.e., subclinical thyrotoxicosis); a high-normal or high value indicates Graves' disease, and a low value indicates thyroiditis or exogenous thyroid hormone ingestion. Thyroid radionuclide imaging is indicated only when one or more thyroid nodules are palpated. Although the coexistence of papillary thyroid cancer is uncommon, there may an increased risk in adults with Graves' thyrotoxicosis [1.8% in one study (64)]; palpable nodules in children should be evaluated for carcinoma.

Among the causes of thyrotoxicosis in children other than Graves' disease, the most common is probably an autonomously functioning thyroid adenoma. Painless or silent thyroiditis is virtually unreported in children (65) (see Chapter 27); subacute thyroiditis, toxic multinodular goiter, and exogenous thyrotoxicosis are rare; and TSH-secreting pituitary adenomas are extremely rare in all age groups (see Chapter 24). A thyroid adenoma should be detectable by physical examination; virtually all adenomas causing thyrotoxicosis are at least 2 cm in diameter. Most occur as isolated tumors, some of which contain activating mutations of the TSH receptor (see Chapter 25). A toxic thyroid adenoma (or a diffuse or toxic multinodular goiter) may occur as part of the McCune-Albright syndrome (café-au-lait pigmentation, precocious puberty, and polyostotic fibrous dysplasia) (20). Autosomal-dominant or sporadic nonautoimmune thyrotoxicosis due to germ line mutations in the TSH receptor can occur in children as well as in neonates (16,17); these children have diffuse goiters but no ophthalmopathy, and they may have a family history of thyrotoxicosis but not ophthalmopathy or chronic autoimmune thyroiditis. Exogenous thyrotoxicosis can be iatrogenic, occurring when high doses of T_4 are given to children with thyroid carcinoma or to decrease the size of a goiter. It can be surreptitious, for example, an adolescent taking thyroid hormone to lose weight. It can also be accidental, such as when a child takes a handful of thyroid pills belonging to another family member. The dose must be large (e.g., 0.5 mg/kg of T_4 or more), and even then not all children become thyrotoxic (66,67).

Disorders that must be distinguished from thyrotoxicosis are the thyroid hormone resistance syndromes (68) (see Chapter 81), and those disorders associated with increased serum binding of T_4 and T_3. The former may be associated with clinical thyrotoxicosis if the resistance is limited to the pituitary gland. Increased serum binding of T_4 results in hyperthyroxinemia (high serum total T_4 concentrations) but not thyrotoxicosis (see Chapter 13).

Treatment

Children and adolescents with Graves' thyrotoxicosis, like adults, can be treated effectively with an antithyroid drug, radioiodine, and thyroidectomy (69) (see Chapter 45). Both the natural history of Graves' disease and the effects (and side effects) of the three types of treatment are similar in the three age groups. Therefore, in children and adolescents, like in adults, choices are made more on the basis of physician, patient, and parent preferences than any other consideration. These are all treatments for the thyroid hypersecretion that causes thyrotoxicosis, not treatments for Graves' disease, unless antithyroid drugs indeed have immunosuppressive actions, as has been suggested (see Chapter 45). Among the three treatments, there are some differences in the time needed to reduce thyroid hypersecretion to normal, the required degree of patient and family compliance with treatment and follow-up visits, and the short- and long-term likelihood of recurrent thyrotoxicosis and hypothyroidism.

In contrast to adults, in whom radioiodine therapy alone or a relatively short course of an antithyroid drug followed by radioiodine therapy if remission does not occur is probably the most common therapeutic approach (70), most children with Graves' thyrotoxicosis are treated with an antithyroid drug for a long time. There are several reasons for this choice. First, in time, many patients do have a remission of the Graves' disease, and therefore remain euthyroid, and with normally regulated thyroid secretion, for long periods if not indefinitely after treatment is discontinued. Second, physicians, patients, and parents worry that radioiodine therapy may yet prove to have some long-term side effects, despite current evidence to the contrary. Third, few children or their parents accept subtotal thyroidectomy, and it requires careful medical preparation and experienced anesthesiologists and surgeons to avoid operative morbidity. Thus, even though radioiodine therapy or thyroidectomy is considered preferable initial treatment at some centers, we prefer antithyroid drug treatment in the hope that a remission of the Graves' disease will occur; radioiodine is a reasonable second choice in older children if the patient cannot tolerate drug therapy or does not have a remission.

Antithyroid Drug Treatment

The antithyroid drugs MMI, carbimazole, and PTU inhibit thyroid hormone biosynthesis (71) (see Chapter 45). PTU also inhibits extrathyroidal conversion of T_4 to T_3. In adults, and presumably also in children, MMI (and carbimazole) has a longer serum half-life, about 4 to 6 hours, as compared with 1 to 2 hours for PTU, and its intrathyroidal actions are considerably more prolonged (72,73); therefore single daily doses are adequate in most patients. The recommended initial dose of MMI is 0.5 to 1.0 mg/kg daily, given once daily, and that of PTU is 5 to 10 mg/kg daily, given three times daily. Children who are older, with longer duration of symptoms, larger goiters, or higher serum T_4 and T_3 concentrations, should be given the higher doses. Once the patient becomes euthyroid, the dose and frequency (in patients taking PTU) can usually be decreased. Conversely, occasionally the dose needs to be increased because the initial dose was too small or the thyrotoxicosis worsens. MMI is preferable to PTU because single daily doses are effective in most patients, and fewer tablets per day are needed because the MMI tablets that are available (5 and 10 mg) contain relatively more drug than the PTU tablet that is available (50 mg).

Antithyroid drugs, although they inhibit thyroid hormone synthesis, do not inhibit the release of preformed, stored hormone. Therefore, there is a lag period between initiation of therapy and achievement of the euthyroid state. The length of this period is correlated with the size of the patient's goiter, varying from 3 weeks to 2 months. During this period, propranolol, 0.5 to 2 mg/kg daily in divided doses, or another β-adrenergic antagonist drug may be given to alleviate the symptoms of thyrotoxicosis (74,75).

The results of eight studies of antithyroid drug treatment in children with Graves' thyrotoxicosis are shown in Table 76.2 (36,38,76–81). Thyrotoxicosis was controlled initially in 87% to 100% of the patients; failure of initial control was more likely if the patient had a large goiter or more severe clinical or biochemical thyrotoxicosis, or was poorly compliant with therapy. For these children, an alternative form of therapy must be selected. Although poor compliance with an antithyroid drug may be an indication for radioiodine or surgical treatment, the need for compliance often simply changes from compliance with an antithyroid drug to compliance with T_4.

Once the patient is euthyroid, either of two treatment plans may be implemented. One is to reduce the dose of antithyroid drug so as to maintain euthyroidism; the other

is to continue the same dose and add T_4 to prevent hypothyroidism. The first approach requires good clinical judgment, particularly because treatment may lead to low-normal serum T_4 and high-normal T_3 concentrations (82). Assessment of clinical status and measurements of serum TSH should lead to the correct therapeutic decisions. Because prolonged thyrotoxicosis may result in persistent suppression of TSH secretion, serum TSH measurements cannot be relied on to indicate overtreatment for 6 to 8 weeks after a patient becomes euthyroid (83). The second approach requires not only that the patient take two medications, when one would suffice, but the presence of thyrotoxicosis also may lead to confusion about whether to increase the antithyroid drug or decrease the dose of T_4. In addition, patients taking higher doses of antithyroid drug may have a higher risk for drug side effects, and the administration of T_4 makes it more difficult to determine if a remission of Graves' disease has occurred. Thus, we prefer the first approach.

Antithyroid drug treatment is continued either for a fixed time interval or until the patient remains euthyroid for several months while receiving a low dose of the drug. Treatment then is stopped to determine whether a remission has occurred, as defined by persistent euthyroidism. In the eight studies listed in Table 76.2, 34% to 64% of children had a remission after mean treatment periods of 2 to 4 years. Patients treated for fixed periods, usually 1 to 2 years, are less likely to have a remission than those treated indefinitely. Prepubertal children seem to need more prolonged treatment; in a study of 89 children, the median time to remission was 8 years in prepubertal children, compared with 4 years in pubertal children (46). In a study of 63 children and adolescents in which remission was analyzed by survival analysis, 25% had a remission every 2 years, and the 5-year remission rate was 50% (79).

Recurrence of thyrotoxicosis after cessation of antithyroid drug therapy occurs in 3% to 62% of children (Table

TABLE 76.2. RESULTS OF ANTITHYROID DRUG TREATMENT OF CHILDREN AND ADOLESCENTS WITH GRAVES' THYROTOXICOSIS

Study Location Reference	No. of Patients	Patients Achieving Control Initially (%)	Duration of Therapy yr (mean)	Remission (%)[a]	Relapse (%)[b]
Philadelphia (38)	95	87	2–4 (3.2)	40	13
Baltimore (36)	104	100	1–9 (2.9)	61	10
Helsinki (80)	38	100	1.6–6 (3)	50	6
USC (76)	60	100[c]	1–7 (2.9)	34	22[c]
Detroit (78)	182	87	0.5–10 (2)	38	36
UCLA (79)	63	97	0.4–12.4 (4.3)	25% every 2 yr	3
Boston (77)	53	98	0.25–8.7 (2.5)	64	47
London (81)	72	100	0.5–7 (3.3)	38	62

[a]Percentage of patients remaining euthyroid for a defined period after discontinuation of antithyroid drug therapy. This posttherapy period ranged from 1 to 3 months to 1 or more years in the different studies.
[b]Percentage of patients who became thyrotoxic after remaining euthyroid for a defined (variable) period after discontinuation of antithyroid drug therapy.
[c]Estimated; results not reported directly.

76.2). This wide range reflects to some extent different treatment approaches and different definitions of recurrence. In general, the rate of recurrence of thyrotoxicosis is higher in patients in whom the duration of treatment was shorter. Recurrence of thyrotoxicosis within a few weeks or months after cessation of therapy suggests that the patient had not had a remission of Graves' disease, but simply cessation of drug action in a patient with continuing Graves' disease. In contrast, later recurrence suggests that the patient had a remission of Graves' disease, but the disease then recurred. Late recurrence is less common, for example, occurring in only 3% of the patients in one study who remained euthyroid for 1 year after cessation of therapy (79).

In a study from Japan, the rate of recurrence was much lower in adults treated with MMI and T_4, and then T_4 alone, than in those treated only with MMI (84). In several subsequent studies, however, some of which included children, remissions of Graves' disease were no more common in patients treated with an antithyroid drug and T_4 than in those treated with an antithyroid drug alone (85–87). No studies of the two regimens have been conducted primarily in children. For the practical reasons described earlier, we do not recommend combination antithyroid drug and T_4 therapy.

Several clinical and biochemical markers may help to predict whether a recurrence of thyrotoxicosis is likely to occur before antithyroid drug therapy is begun or when it is discontinued, but their sensitivity and specificity are limited. A lower body mass index at the time of diagnosis favored recurrence in one study (88). Goiter size when treatment is discontinued is the best clinical predictor; the smaller the gland, the less likely a recurrence will occur (89). The most helpful biochemical marker appears to be measurement of serum TSHR-SAbs when therapy is discontinued; in one report, all children who had recurrent thyrotoxicosis tested positive for TSHR-SAbs at that time, and 78% of the children who remained euthyroid tested negative (61). In another study, the predictive value of this measurement was much lower (90). In practice, treatment simply should be discontinued and the patient followed periodically.

From 5% to 32% of children given MMI or PTU have a side effect of the drug, usually within the first several months of treatment, and care should be taken to inform all children and their parents about these side effects (36,38,76–81) (Table 76.3). The most common minor side effects are urticarial or papular skin rashes and transient granulocytopenia [<2,000/mm^3 (<2×10^9/L)], which occur in 1% to 9% of children. Others are hair loss, nausea, headache, abnormal taste sensation, and arthralgia. These side effects are dose dependent (91). In patients with nonhematologic side effects, the drug should be discontinued for a few days and then treatment with the other drug initiated; patients with symptomatic skin rashes may benefit from antihistamine or glucocorticoid therapy for a few days. Granulocytopenia is usually transient and does not necessitate discontinuation of therapy, but when the granulocyte count falls below 1,000/mm^3 (1×10^9/L), discontinuing the drug may avert agranulocytosis (92). From 0.1% to 0.2% of children develop agranulocytosis [<250/mm^3 (<0.25×10^9/L)]; it usually is accompanied by pharyngitis, fever, and other systemic symptoms of infection. We recommend white blood cell counts before initiation of treatment and during treatment if any of the findings that have been mentioned occur. Other serious drug toxic effects include a lupuslike syndrome, with rash, arthritis, and glomerulonephritis, mostly caused by PTU, and hepatitis (see Chapter 45) (93). The occurrence of any of these serious side effects necessitates immediate discontinuation of the drug; the other drug should not be given, but rather radioiodine therapy or thyroidectomy should be planned. Women of childbearing age who are taking MMI should be warned that it has been associated with an embryopathy, including cutis aplasia (94,95).

TABLE 76.3.   COMPLICATIONS OF ANTITHYROID DRUG TREATMENT OF CHILDREN AND ADOLESCENTS WITH GRAVES' THYROTOXICOSIS

Study Location (Reference)	Poor Compliance (%)	Overall Toxicity (%)	Major Toxicity[a] (%)	Minor Toxicity		Hypothyroidism (%)
				Rash (%)	↓WBC (%)	
Philadelphia (33)	17	5	0	1	3	8
Baltimore (31)	16	14	6	8	1	NR
Helsinki (57)	5	5	0	1.5	1.5	0
USC (61)	7	32	14	7.5	9	6
Detroit (63)	9	17	6	8	3	5
UCLA (64)	2	NR	2	NR	NR	NR
Boston (62)	13	11	4	7	2	11
London (81)	NR	5	3	3	0	0

[a]Agranulocytosis, lupus-like syndrome (e.g., rash, arthritis, glomerulonephritis), or hepatitis.
WBC, white blood cells; NR, not reported.

Radioiodine Therapy

Radioiodine (^{131}I) therapy has proved to be an effective therapy for children and adolescents with thyrotoxicosis due to Graves' disease. It is the preferred treatment in some centers, and in most others it is recommended for any patient who has a serious side effect or tires of antithyroid drug therapy. The dose, which is given orally, usually is calculated to deliver 50 to 200 μCi (1.85–7.4 MBq) of radioiodine per gram of thyroid tissue, estimated by physical examination or imaging, according to the following formula (96):

$$\frac{\text{Estimated thyroid weight (g)} \times 50 \text{ to } 200 \text{ μCi } ^{131}\text{I}}{\text{Fractional 24-hour uptake of } ^{131}\text{I}}$$

Younger children with smaller goiters usually are given lower doses, and those with larger goiters, higher doses. It is better to give more rather than less because the likelihood of persistent thyrotoxicosis, with need for retreatment, is lower. For example, among a group of children given 200 μCi (7.4 MBq) of ^{131}I/g of thyroid, 83% became euthyroid (78). In contrast, 54% of those given 50 μCi (1.85 MBq) of ^{131}I/g of thyroid had persistent thyrotoxicosis (97). Higher doses also may be associated with a lower risk for thyroid tumors (98). Pretreatment with an antithyroid drug is not necessary, but if used the drug should be discontinued 7 days before treatment to prevent interference with the uptake of radioiodine. Because the effects of a dose of radioiodine are not complete for several months or longer, adjunctive treatment with a β-adrenergic antagonist, as previously described, is recommended for patients with many symptoms. An antithyroid drug may also be given for a short time. The advantages of radioiodine treatment are its ease of administration, the lack of need for an antithyroid drug, and the high rate of permanent amelioration of thyrotoxicosis.

The major consequence of radioiodine therapy is hypothyroidism. It occurs in 20% to 40% of children in the first year after treatment and 2% to 3% per year thereafter, so most children eventually become hypothyroid (99). To ensure that thyrotoxicosis does not recur (and to reduce the risk for thyroid tumors), some pediatric endocrinologists believe that the dose should always be sufficient to result in hypothyroidism. In this regard, a recent study reported that doses of 110 μCi (4.1 MBq) of ^{131}I/g, 220 μCi (8.1 MBq) of ^{131}I/g, and 330 μCi (12.2 MBq) of ^{131}I/g resulted in hypothyroidism in 50%, 70%, and 95% of children with Graves' thyrotoxicosis, respectively (100). In another study in children given fixed doses of radioiodine (13.8–15.6 mCi [511–577 MBq]), all became hypothyroid on average 77 days after treatment (range 28–194 days) (101).

The main reservations about radioiodine therapy in children have centered around possible thyroid or other tumors and genetic damage. In a national collaborative study of 322 patients who received radioiodine therapy before age 20 years, the incidence of benign thyroid adenomas increased from an expected 0.6% to 1.9% (102). This risk appeared to be higher in patients given lower doses of radioiodine. In the same study, thyroid carcinomas were no more common in radioiodine-treated patients than those treated with an antithyroid drug or thyroidectomy. With respect to tumor formation, the thyroid glands of infants and young children are more susceptible to the effects of external radiation, and the same probably applies to radioiodine (see section Pathogenesis in Chapter 70) (103). In several long-term studies, mostly of adults, no evidence for an increased risk for leukemia or other cancers was found, with the possible exception of stomach cancer (relative risk 1.3) and breast cancer (relative risk 1.9) (104–107). Thyroid storm after radioiodine therapy has been reported in a single child; this child had earlier been treated with an antithyroid drug (108).

Another potential adverse effect of radioiodine therapy is the development or worsening of ophthalmopathy. In prospective studies in adults, ophthalmopathy was more likely to appear or worsen after treatment with radioiodine than during antithyroid drug therapy or after thyroidectomy (see Chapter 45) (109,110). In a retrospective study of children treated with radioiodine, eye signs improved in 90%, did not change in 8%, and worsened in 3% (99); much of the improvement was probably due to improvement in stare and lid retraction rather than infiltrative eye signs. In a recent study of eight children 4 to 14 years of age, none had deterioration of eye disease after radioiodine therapy (111).

Studies of offspring of children and adolescents previously treated with radioiodine revealed a 3% incidence of congenital anomalies, similar to that found in the general population (99). Karyotype studies revealed no increase in chromosomal aberrations of the type found after exposure to ionizing radiation (97). Furthermore, there are no reports of impaired fertility or an increase in miscarriage rate or fetal loss among girls treated with radioiodine, although continued surveillance is warranted.

In summary, there is little evidence of an increase in thyroid tumors or nonthyroid problems in more than 1,000 children treated with radioiodine for Graves' thyrotoxicosis with follow-up for up to 40 years. Given the increased sensitivity of the thyroid gland of young children to the effects of radiation, however, Rivkees et al. hypothesized in their review that the risk for thyroid cancer may be slightly increased; for this reason, most pediatric endocrinologists prefer not to treat children until they are 10 years of age or older (98). Surveillance should continue.

Thyroidectomy

Thyroidectomy is the most rapidly effective treatment for thyrotoxicosis. With appropriate preoperative preparation, the risks are similar to those of other major surgical procedures. It may be the best treatment for patients with markedly enlarged thyroid glands or those with severe ophthalmopathy who do not have a remission during antithyroid drug therapy (112).

To minimize surgical risks, the patient should be euthyroid, or nearly so, at the time of surgery. This is usually accomplished by administration of an antithyroid drug for several weeks and then addition of inorganic iodide for 7 to 14 days; the latter has an antithyroid action and also may reduce thyroid blood flow (see Chapter 45). Alternatively, patients may be prepared for surgery by administration of a β-adrenergic antagonist and inorganic iodine.

The operation of choice is near-total thyroidectomy; when less than 4 g of thyroid tissue remains, the likelihood of recurrent thyrotoxicosis is small (113,114). The likelihood of recurrence is even smaller after total thyroidectomy, but the morbidity rate is considerably higher. In a recent review of nine series, one death occurred in 555 children who underwent thyroidectomy for Graves' thyrotoxicosis (115). Subsequently, 42% became hypothyroid, 2% had hypoparathyroidism, and 1.2% had vocal cord paralysis. Bleeding, which may require tracheostomy, occurred in 0.25% and keloid formation in 1.7%. This summary covered the experience of many years. Because thyroidectomy is rarely done for Graves' thyrotoxicosis now, complications may well be more common.

OUTCOME OF CHILDHOOD GRAVES' DISEASE

Although there are potential complications unique to antithyroid drug, radioiodine, or surgical treatment of Graves' thyrotoxicosis, all may result in hypothyroidism or persistent thyrotoxicosis. In children treated with an antithyroid drug with follow-up of 8 to 22 years, about 10% eventually developed hypothyroidism caused by chronic autoimmune thyroiditis, either with destruction of the thyroid or production of antibodies that block the binding of TSH to its receptors (36,38,76–81,116) (Table 76.3). As noted earlier, hypothyroidism is common in children treated with radioiodine or subtotal thyroidectomy. On the other hand, persistent or recurrent thyrotoxicosis is fairly common in patients treated with an antithyroid drug. Therefore, whichever treatment is chosen, the child or adolescent requires lifelong follow-up.

REFERENCES

1. Ramsay I, Kaur S, Krassas G. Thyrotoxicosis in pregnancy: results of treatment by antithyroid drugs combined with T4. *Clin Endocrinol (Oxf)* 1983;18:73.
2. Dirmikis SM, Munro DS. Placental transmission of thyroid-stimulating immunoglobulins. *BMJ* 1975;2:665.
3. McKenzie JM. Neonatal Graves' disease. *J Clin Endocrinol Metab* 1964;24:660.
4. McKenzie JM, Zakarija M. Fetal and neonatal hyperthyroidism and hypothyroidism due to maternal TSH receptor antibodies. *Thyroid* 1992;2:155.
5. Smallridge RC, Wartofsky L, Chopra IJ, et al. Neonatal thyrotoxicosis: alterations in serum concentrations of LATS-protector, T_4, T_3, reverse T_3, and 3, 38 T2. *J Pediatr* 1978;93:118.
6. Sunshine P, Kusumoto H, Kriss JP. Survival time of circulating long-acting thyroid stimulator in neonatal thyrotoxicosis: implications for diagnosis and therapy of the disorder. *Pediatrics* 1965;36:869.
7. Matsura N, Konishi J, Fujieda K, et al. TSH-receptor antibodies in mothers with Graves' disease and outcome in their offspring. *Lancet* 1988;1:14.
8. Munro DS, Dirmikis SM, Humphries H, et al. The role of thyroid stimulating immunoglobulins of Graves' disease in neonatal thyrotoxicosis. *Br J Obstet Gynaecol* 1978;85:837.
9. Tamaki H, Amino N, Aozasa M, et al. Universal predictive criteria for neonatal overt thyrotoxicosis requiring treatment. *Am J Perinatal* 1988;5:152.
10. Zakarija M, McKenzie JM. Pregnancy-associated changes in the thyroid-stimulating antibody of Graves' disease and the relationship to neonatal hyperthyroidism. *J Clin Endocrinol Metab* 1983;57:1036.
11. Peleg D, Cada S, Peleg A, et al. The relationship between maternal serum thyroid-stimulating immunoglobulin and fetal and neonatal thyrotoxicosis. *Obstet Gynecol* 2002;99:1040.
12. Skuza KA, Sills IN, Stene M, et al. Prediction of neonatal hyperthyroidism in infants born to mothers with Graves' disease. *J Pediatr* 1996;128:264.
13. Zimmerman D. Fetal and neonatal hyperthyroidism. *Thyroid* 1999;9:727.
14. Hollingsworth DR, Mabry CC. Congenital Graves' disease: four familial cases with long-term follow-up and perspective. *Am J Dis Child* 1976;130:148.
15. Polak M. Hyperthyroidism in early infancy: pathogenesis, clinical features and diagnosis with a focus on neonatal hyperthyroidism. *Thyroid* 1998;8:1171.
16. Duprez L, Parma J, van Sande J, et al. Germline mutations in the thyrotropin receptor gene cause non-autoimmune autosomal dominant hyperthyroidism. *Nat Genet* 1994;7:396.
17. Schwab KO, Gerlich M, Broecker M, et al. Constitutively active germline mutation of the thyrotropin receptor gene as a cause of congenital hyperthyroidism. *J Pediatr* 1997;131:899.
18. Kopp P, van Sande J, Parma J, et al. Congenital hyperthyroidism caused by a mutation in the thyrotropin-receptor gene. *N Engl J Med* 1995;332:150.
19. de Roux N, Polak M, Couet J, et al. A neomutation of the thyroid-stimulating hormone receptor in a severe neonatal hyperthyroidism. *J Clin Endocrinol Metab* 1996;81:2023.
20. Mastorakos G, Mitsiades NS, Doufas AG, et al. Hyperthyroidism in McCune-Albright syndrome with a review of thyroid abnormalities sixty years after the first report. *Thyroid* 1997;7:433.
21. Farrehi C. Accelerated maturity in fetal thyrotoxicosis. *Clin Pediatr* 1968;7:134.
22. Kopelman AE. Delayed cerebral development in twins with congenital hyperthyroidism. *Am J Dis Child* 1983;137:842.
23. Smith C, Thomsett M, Choong C, et al. Congenital thyrotoxicosis in premature infants. *Clin Endocrinol (Oxf)* 2001;54:371.
24. Zakarija M, McKenzie JM, Hoffman WH. Prediction and therapy of intrauterine and late-onset neonatal hyperthyroidism. *J Clin Endocrinol Metab* 1986;62:368.
25. Joshi R, Kulin HE. Treatment of neonatal Graves' disease with sodium ipodate. *Clin Pediatr* 1993;32:181.

26. Karpman BA, Rapoport B, Filetti S, et al. Treatment of neonatal hyperthyroidism due to Graves' disease with sodium ipodate. *J Clin Endocrinol Metab* 1987;64:119.

27. Transue D, Chan J, Kaplan M. Management of neonatal Graves' disease with iopanoic acid. *J Pediatr* 1992;121:472.

28. Holzapfel H-P, Wonerow P, von Petrykowski W, et al. Sporadic congenital hyperthyroidism due to a spontaneous germline mutation in the thyrotropin receptor gene. *J Clin Endocrinol Metab* 1997;82:3879.

29. Cove DH, Johnston P. Fetal hyperthyroidism: experience of treatment in four siblings. *Lancet* 1985;1:430.

30. Radaelli T, Cetin I, Zamperini P, et al. Intrauterine growth of normal thyroid. *Gynecol Endocrinol* 2002;16:427.

31. Wenstrom KD, Weiner CP, Williamson RA, et al. Prenatal diagnosis of fetal hyperthyroidism using funipuncture. *Obstet Gynecol* 1990;76:513.

32. Nachum Z, Rakover Y, Weimer E, et al. Grave's disease in pregnancy: prospective evaluation of a selective invasive treatment protocol. *Am J Obstet Gynecol* 2003;189:159.

33. Bowman ML, Bergmann M, Smith JF. Intrapartum labetalol for the treatment of maternal and fetal thyrotoxicosis. *Thyroid* 1998;8:795.

34. Daneman D, Howard NJ. Neonatal thyrotoxicosis: intellectual impairment and craniosynostosis in later years. *J Pediatr* 1980;97:257.

35. Mandel SH, Hanna CE, LaFranchi SH. Diminished thyroid-stimulating hormone secretion associated with neonatal thyrotoxicosis. *J Pediatr* 1986;109:662.

35a. Kempers MJ, van Tijn DA, van Trostenburg AS, et al. Central congenital hypothyroidism due to gestational hyperthyroidism: detection where prevention failed. *J Clin Endocrinol Metab* 2003;88:5851.

36. Barnes H, Blizzard RM. Antithyroid drug therapy for toxic diffuse goiter (Graves' disease): thirty years experience in children and adolescents. *J Pediatr* 1977;91:313.

37. Saxena KM, Crawford JD, Talbot NB. Childhood thyrotoxicosis: a long-term perspective. *BMJ* 1964;2:1153.

38. Vaidya VA, Bongiovanni AM, Parks JS, et al. Twenty-two years experience in the medical management of juvenile thyrotoxicosis. *Pediatrics* 1974;54:565.

39. Kogut MD, Kaplan SA, Collip PJ, et al. Treatment of hyperthyroidism in children. *N Engl J Med* 1965;272:217.

40. Lavard L, Ranlov I, Perrild H, et al. Incidence of juvenile thyrotoxicosis in Denmark. 1982–88. A nationwide study. *Eur J Endocrinol* 1994;130:565.

41. Wong GWK, Cheng PS. Increasing incidence of childhood Graves' disease in Hong Kong: a follow-up study. *Clin Endocrinol (Oxf)* 2001;54:547.

42. Friedman JM, Fialkow PJ. The genetics of Graves' disease. *Clin Endocrinol Metab* 1978;7:47.

43. Chen Q-Y, Huang W, She J-X, et al. HLA-DRB1*08, DRB1*03/DRB3*0101, and DRB3*0202 are susceptibility genes for Graves' disease in North American Caucasians, whereas DRB1*07 is protective. *J Clin Endocrinol Metab* 1999;84:3181.

44. Kawame H, Adachi M, Tachibana K, et al. Graves' disease in patients with 22q11.2 deletion. *J Pediatr* 2001;139:892.

45. Nordyke RA, Gilbert FI, Harada ASM. Graves' disease: influence of age on clinical findings. *Arch Intern Med* 1988;148:626.

46. Shulman D, Muhar I, Jorgensen V, et al. Autoimmune hyperthyroidism in prepubertal children and adolescents: comparison of clinical and biochemical features at diagnosis and responses to medical therapy. *Thyroid* 1997;7:755.

47. Carnell NE, Valente WA. Thyroid nodules in Graves' disease: classification, characterization, and response to treatment. *Thyroid* 1998;8:647.

48. Young LA. Dysthyroid ophthalmopathy in children. *J Pediatr Ophthalmol Strabismus* 1979;16:105.

49. Uretsky SH, Kennerdell JS, Gutai JP. Graves' ophthalmopathy in childhood and adolescence. *Arch Ophthalmol* 1980;98:1963.

50. Gruters A. Ocular manifestations in children and adolescents with thyrotoxicosis. *Exp Clin Endocrinol Diabetes* 1999;107 (suppl 5):172.

51. Chan W, Wong GWK, Fan DSP, et al. Ophthalmopathy in childhood Graves' disease. *Br J Ophthalmol* 2002;86:740

52. Gorman CA. Temporal relationship between the onset of Graves' ophthalmopathy and the diagnosis of thyrotoxicosis. *Mayo Clin Proc* 1983;58:515.

53. Cavallo A, Casta A, Fawcett HD, et al. Is there a thyrotoxic cardiomyopathy in children? *J Pediatr* 1985;107:531.

54. Vestergaard P, Mosekilde L. Hyperthyroidism, bone mineral, and fracture risk-a meta-analysis. *Thyroid* 2003;13:585.

55. Lucidarme N, Ruiz JC, Czernichow P, et al. Reduced bone mineral density at diagnosis and bone mineral recovery during treatment in children with Graves' disease. *J Pediatr* 2000; 137:56.

56. Radetti G, Dordi B, Mengarda G, et al. Thyrotoxicosis presenting with seizures and coma in two children. *Am J Dis Child* 1993;147:925.

57. Segni M, Leonardi E, Mazzoncini B, et al. Special features of Graves' disease in early childhood. *Thyroid* 1999;9:871.

58. Drash PW, Money J. Motor impairment and hyperthyroidism in children: report of two cases. *Dev Med Child Neurol* 1966;8:741.

59. Caldwell G, Gow SM, Sweeting VM, et al. Value and limitations of a highly sensitive immunoradiometric assay for thyrotropin in the study of thyrotropin function. *Clin Chem* 1987;33:303.

60. Lavard L, Perrild H, Jacobsen BB, et al. Prevalence of thyroid peroxidase, thyroglobulin and thyrotropin receptor antibodies in a long-term follow-up of juvenile Graves' disease. *Autoimmunity* 2000;32:167.

61. Foley TP Jr, White C, New A. Juvenile Graves' disease: usefulness and limitations of thyrotropin receptor antibody determinations. *J Pediatr* 1987;110:378.

62. Botero D, Brown RS. Bioassay of the thyrotropin receptor antibodies with Chinese hamster ovary cells transfected with recombinant human thyrotropin receptor: clinical utility in children and adolescents with Graves' disease. *J Pediatr* 1998;132:612.

63. McKenzie JM, Zakarija M. The clinical use of thyrotropin receptor antibody measurements. *J Clin Endocrinol Metab* 1989; 69:1093.

64. Stocker DJ, Foster SS, Solomon BL, et al. Thyroid cancer yield in patients with Graves' disease selected for surgery on the basis of cold scintiscan defects. *Thyroid* 2002;12:305.

65. Fisher DA. The thyroid. In: Kaplan SA, ed. *Clinical pediatric endocrinology,* 2nd ed. Philadelphia: WB Saunders, 1990:110.

66. Litovitz TL, White JD. Levothyroxine ingestions in children: an analysis of 78 cases. *Am J Emerg Med* 1985;3:297.

67. Lewander WJ, Lacouture PG, Silva JE, et al. Acute thyroxine ingestion in pediatric patients. *Pediatrics* 1989;84:262.

68. Gharib H, Klee GG. Familial euthyroid hyperthyroxinemia secondary to pituitary and peripheral resistance to thyroid hormones. *Mayo Clin Proc* 1985;60:9.

69. Franklyn JA. The management of hyperthyroidism. *N Engl J Med* 1994;330:1731.

70. Wartofsky L, Glinoer D, Solomon B, et al. Differences and similarities in the diagnosis and treatment of Graves' disease in Europe, Japan, and the United States. *Thyroid* 1991;1:129.

71. Cooper DS. Antithyroid drugs in the management of patients with Graves' disease: an evidence-based approach to therapeutic controversies. *J Clin Endocrinol Metab* 2003;88:3474.

72. Shiroozu A, Okamura K, Ikenoue H, et al. Treatment of hyperthyroidism with a small single daily dose of methimazole. *J Clin Endocrinol Metab* 1986;63:125.

73. Okuno A, Yano K, Inyaku F, et al. Pharmacokinetics of methimazole in children and adolescents with Graves' disease. Studies on plasma and intrathyroidal concentrations. *Acta Endocrinol* 1987;115:112.

74. Codaccioni JL, Orgiazzi J, Blanc P, et al. Lasting remissions in patients treated for Graves' hyperthyroidism with propranolol alone: a pattern of spontaneous evolution of the disease. *J Clin Endocrinol Metab* 1988;67:656.

75. Feely J, Peden N. Use of β-adrenoceptor blocking drugs in hyperthyroidism. *Drugs* 1984;27:425.

76. Buckingham BA, Costin G, Roe TF, et al. Hyperthyroidism in children: a reevaluation of treatment. *Am J Dis Child* 1981; 135:112.

77. Gorton C, Sadeghi-Nejad A, Senior B. Remission in children with hyperthyroidism treated with propylthiouracil: long-term results. *Am J Dis Child* 1987;141:1084.

78. Hamburger JI. Management of hyperthyroidism in children and adolescents. *J Clin Endocrinol Metab* 1985;60:1019.

79. Lippe BM, Landau EM, Kaplan SA. Hyperthyroidism in children treated with long term medical therapy: twenty-five percent remission every two years. *J Clin Endocrinol Metab* 1987; 64:1241.

80. Maenpaa J, Kuusi A. Childhood hyperthyroidism. Results of treatment. *Acta Paediatr Scand* 1980;69:137.

81. Raza J, Hindmarsh PC, Brook CGD. Thyrotoxicosis in children: thirty years experience. *Acta Paediatr* 1999;88:937.

82. Chen JJS, Ladenson PW. Discordant hypothyroxinemia and hypertriiodothyroninemia in treated patients with hyperthyroid Graves' disease. *J Clin Endocrinol Metab* 1986;63:102.

83. Sills IN, Horlick MNB, Rapaport R. Inappropriate suppression of thyrotropin during medical treatment of Graves' disease in childhood. *J Pediatr* 1992;121:206.

84. Hashizume K, Ichikawa K, Sakurai A, et al. Administration of thyroxine in treated Graves' disease: effects on the level of antibodies to thyroid-stimulating hormone receptors and on the risk of recurrence of hyperthyroidism. *N Engl J Med* 1991; 324:947.

85. McIver B, Rae P, Beckett G. Lack of effect of thyroxine in patients with Graves' hyperthyroidism who are treated with an antithyroid drug. *N Engl J Med* 1996;334:220.

86. Rittmaster RS, Abbott EC, Douglas R, et al. Effect of methimazole, with or without L-thyroxine, on remission rates in Graves' disease. *J Clin Endocrinol Metab* 1998;83:814.

87. Hoermann R, Quadbeck B, Roggenbuck U, et al. Relapse of Graves' disease after successful ocutome of antithyroid drug therapy: results of a prospective randomized study on the use of levothyroxine. *Thyroid* 2002;12:1119.

88. Glaser N, Styne D. Predictors of early remission of hyperthyroidism in children. *J Clin Endocrinol Metab* 1997;82:1719.

89. Siok-Hoon T, Bee-Wah L, Hock-Boon W, et al. Relapse markers in childhood thyrotoxicosis. *Clin Pediatr* 1987;26: 136.

90. Ikenoue H, Okamura K, Kuroda T, et al. Prediction of relapse in drug-treated Graves' disease using thyroid stimulation indices. *Acta Endocrinol* 1991;125:643.

91. Reinwein D, Benker G, Lazarus JH, et al, and the European Multicenter Study Group on Antithyroid Drug Treatment. A prospective randomized trial of antithyroid drug dose in Graves' disease therapy. *J Clin Endocrinol Metab* 1993;76:1516.

92. Tajiri J, Joguchi S, Murakami T, et al. Antithyroid drug-induced agranulocytosis: the usefulness of routine white blood cell count monitoring. *Arch Intern Med* 1990;150:621.

93. Werner MC, Romaldini JH, Bromberg N, et al. Adverse effects related to thionamide drugs and their dosage regimen. *Am J Med Sci* 1989;297:216.

94. Clementi M, Di Giannantonio E, Pelo E, et al. Methimazole embryopathy: delineation of the phenotype. *Am J Med Genet* 1999;83:43.

95. Martin-Denavit T, Edery P, Plauchu H, et al. Ectodermal abnormalities associated with methimazole intrauterine exposure. *Am J Med Genet* 2000;94:338.

96. Levy WJ, Schumacher P, Gupta M. Treatment of childhood Graves' disease: a review with emphasis on radioiodine treatment. *Cleve Clin J Med* 1988;55:373.

97. Rapoport B, Caplan R, DeGroot LJ. Low-dose sodium iodide I 131 therapy in Graves' disease. *JAMA* 1973;244:1610.

98. Rivkees SA, Sklar C, Freemark M. The management of Graves' disease in children, with special emphasis on radioiodine treatment. *J Clin Endocrinol Metab* 1998;83:3767.

99. Safa AM, Schumacher OP, Rodriguez-Antunez A. Long-term follow-up results in children and adolescents treated with radioactive iodine for hyperthyroidism. *N Engl J Med* 1975;292: 167.

100. Rivkees SA, Cornelius EA. Influence of Iodine-131 dose on the outcome of hyperthyroidism in children. *Pediatrics* 2003;111: 745.

101. Nebesio TD, Siddiqui AR, Pescovitz OH, et al. Time course to hypothyroidism after fixed-dose radioablation therapy of Graves' disease in children. *J Pediatr* 2002 141:99.

102. Dobyns BM, Sheline GE, Workman JB, et al. Malignant and benign neoplasms of the thyroid in patients treated for hyperthyroidism: a report of the cooperative thyrotoxicosis therapy follow-up study. *J Clin Endocrinol Metab* 1974;38:976.

103. Brill AB, Becker DV. The safety of ^{131}I treatment of hyperthyroidism. In: Van Middlesworth L, Givins JR, eds. *The thyroid: a practical clinical treatise*. Chicago: Year Book Medical, 1986:347.

104. Hall P, Boice JD Jr, Berg G, et al. Leukaemia incidence after iodine-131 exposure. *Lancet* 1992;340:1.

105. Holm L-E, Hall P, Wiklund K, et al. Cancer risk after iodine-131 therapy for hyperthyroidism. *J Natl Cancer Inst* 1991;83:1072.

106. Goldman MB, Maloof F, Monson RR, et al. Radioactive iodine therapy and breast cancer. *Am J Epidemiol* 1988;127:969.

107. Ron E, Doody MM, Becker DV, et al. Cancer mortality following treatment for adult hyperthyroidism. *JAMA* 1998;280:347.

108. Kadmon PM, Noto RB, Boney CM, et al. Thyroid storm in a child following radioactive iodine (RAI) therapy: a consequence of RAI versus withdrawal of antithyroid medication. *J Clin Endocrinol Metab* 2001;86:1865.

109. Tallstedt L, Lundell G, Torring O, et al. Occurrence of ophthalmopathy after treatment for Graves' hyperthyroidism. *N Engl J Med* 1992;326:1733.

110. Bartelena L, Marcocci C, Bagozzi F, et al. Relation between therapy for hyperthyroidism and the course of Graves' ophthalmopathy. *N Engl J Med* 1998;338:73.

111. Cheetham TD, Wraight P, Hughes IA, et al. Radioiodine treatment of Graves' disease in young people. *Horm Res* 1998;49:258.

112. Bergman P, Auldist AW, Cameron F. Review of outcome of management of Graves' disease in children and adolescents. *J Paediatr Child Health* 2001;37:176.

113. Andrassy RJ, Buckingham BA, Weitzman JJ. Thyroidectomy for hyperthyroidism in children. *J Pediatr Surg* 1980;15:501.

114. Hayles AB, Chaves-Carballo E, McConahey WM. The treatment of hyperthyroidism (Graves' disease) in children. *Mayo Clin Proc* 1967;42:218.

115. Zimmerman D, Lteif AN. Thyrotoxicosis in children. *Endocrinol Metab Clin North Am* 1998;27:109.

116. Tamai H, Kasagi K, Takaichi Y, et al. Development of spontaneous hypothyroidism in patients with Graves' disease treated with antithyroid drugs: clinical, immunological, and histological findings in 26 patients. *J Clin Endocrinol Metab* 1989;69:49.

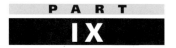

PART

IX

SPECIAL TOPICS
IN THYROIDOLOGY

MORBIDITY AND MORTALITY IN THYROID DYSFUNCTION AND ITS TREATMENT

JAYNE A. FRANKLYN
MICHAEL D. GAMMAGE

Overt thyroid dysfunction, defined as abnormal serum thyrotropin (TSH) and free thyroxine (T_4) concentrations, is common, and subclinical thyroid dysfunction (abnormal serum TSH but normal serum free T_4 concentrations) is even more common (see Chapter 19). For example, among 25,863 subjects attending a state-wide health fair in Colorado, the prevalence of overt hypothyroidism was 0.4% and that of overt thyrotoxicosis was 0.1%, and the respective prevalence rates for subclinical hypothyroidism and subclinical thyrotoxicosis were 9.0% and 2.1%, respectively (1). These abnormalities are more common in women, and the rates increase with age.

High serum TSH concentrations are found almost entirely in people with thyroid diseases, but low serum TSH concentrations have multiple causes. They include not only thyroid disease, and treatment for thyroid disease, but also nonthyroidal illness and treatment with drugs such as glucocorticoids and dopamine (see Chapter 13). Also, patients with hypothyroidism are often overtreated with T_4 or other thyroid hormone preparations (see Chapter 67) (1,2), and patients with thyrotoxicosis may have low serum TSH concentrations for prolonged periods despite restoration of normal serum T_4 and triiodothyronine (T_3) concentrations (see Chapter 45).

Most patients with overt thyroid dysfunction have some symptoms and signs (see Chapters 22 and 46), and before the advent of effective therapy they often died, typically from cardiovascular disease. In contrast, most patients with subclinical thyroid dysfunction do not have any more symptoms than do normal subjects (3). Nonetheless, subclinical thyroid dysfunction may be associated with an increase in morbidity and mortality. Cardiovascular disease remains the most important consequence of thyroid dysfunction, particularly thyrotoxicosis, and its treatment today. Other features of thyrotoxicosis, such as osteoporosis, may also result in substantial long-term morbidity. Finally, both thyroid dysfunction and its treatment have been implicated in the development of cancer, most attention focusing on the potential carcinogenic effect of radioiodine (iodine 131) therapy in patients with thyrotoxicosis.

CARDIOVASCULAR MORBIDITY AND MORTALITY IN THYROTOXICOSIS

Overt Thyrotoxicosis

Most patients with thyrotoxicosis have some abnormalities in cardiovascular function (see Chapter 31). Among them, the one most likely to be associated with adverse clinical events is atrial fibrillation. It occurs in approximately 5% to 15% of patients with overt thyrotoxicosis, especially older patients with ischemic heart disease or hypertension. For example, among 462 patients with thyrotoxicosis, 33% of those with coexisting ischemic heart disease and 41% of those with coexisting hypertension had atrial fibrillation (4). Effective treatment of thyrotoxicosis is associated with restoration of sinus rhythm in some, but not all, patients. In those with new-onset atrial fibrillation, spontaneous reversion to sinus rhythm may occur in up to 50%, and it typically does so within a few months after restoration of euthyroidism (5). Reversion to sinus rhythm is, however, much less likely in those with underlying heart disease and those in whom atrial fibrillation antedated thyrotoxicosis (4–6).

The main hazard of atrial fibrillation is arterial embolization, especially to the cerebral circulation. Few studies have investigated the rate of arterial embolism in patients with thyrotoxicosis and atrial fibrillation. In one study of 142 patients with thyrotoxicosis, 12 of the 30 patients with atrial fibrillation (40%) had an embolic event, as compared with none of the 112 patients who had a sinus rhythm (7). In another study of 610 patients with thyrotoxicosis, 12 of the 91 patients (13%) who had atrial fibrillation had an embolic event, as compared with 15 of the 519 patients (3%) who did not have atrial fibrillation (8). After adjustment for age, the presence of atrial fibrillation was not a risk factor for cerebrovascular events. However, during the first year after diagnosis of thyrotoxicosis, the frequency of cerebrovascular events among all 610 patients was higher than that expected in the general population. Taken together, the existing data suggest that the frequency of embolism, especially cerebral embolism occurring early in the course of thyrotoxicosis (9), is increased in patients with thyrotoxicosis and atrial fibrillation.

In addition to the association between atrial fibrillation and embolic complications in thyrotoxicosis described above, several studies have examined the relationship between overt thyrotoxicosis and other cardiovascular disease end points, including mortality. A follow-up study of 1,762 patients with thyrotoxicosis treated in the United States from 1946 to 1964 (80% of whom were treated with radioiodine) revealed, during a mean follow-up period of 17 years, an increase in mortality from all causes (standardized mortality ratio 1.3, 95% confidence interval 1.2–1.4), and an increase in mortality from diseases of the circulatory system (standardized mortality ratio 1.4, 95% confidence interval 1.3–1.6) (10). A larger study of 10,552 Swedish patients with overt thyrotoxicosis treated with radioiodine and followed for an average of 15 years revealed a similar increase in mortality from cardiovascular diseases (standardized mortality ratio 1.65, 95% confidence interval 1.59–1.71) (11). Lastly, among 7,209 patients with overt thyrotoxicosis treated with radioiodine between 1950 and 1989 in the United Kingdom, 3,611 had died by 1996, whereas the expected number of deaths was 3,196 (*p* < 0.001) (12) (Table 77.1). There were significant increases in risk of death for all categories of heart disease (rheumatic heart disease, hypertensive disease, ischemic heart disease; 240 excess deaths), and for cerebrovascular disease (159 excess deaths). The excess in mortality due to cardiovascular and cerebrovascular diseases was most marked in the first year after radioiodine therapy, and was associated with higher doses of radioiodine. There was excess mortality in all age groups; cardiovascular disease mortality was most

marked in those over 50 years of age when treated. The excess mortality in this cohort [and the Swedish cohort described above (11)] may have resulted from adverse effects of thyrotoxicosis, radioiodine therapy per se, or radioiodine-induced hypothyroidism or its treatment with T_4. In the U.K. study, the relationship between death and time after treatment, as well as the relationship between death and dose of radioiodine (an indirect marker of the severity of thyrotoxicosis), suggest that thyrotoxicosis itself was the major cause of the excess mortality. This is probably mediated through the effects of thyrotoxicosis on cardiac rate, rhythm, and function, as well as exacerbation of any underlying heart disease.

Subclinical Thyrotoxicosis

Atrial fibrillation has also been associated with subclinical thyrotoxicosis (see Chapter 79) (13–15). In the largest prospective study of this association, which involved 2,007 subjects 60 years of age or older followed for up to 10 years, the cumulative risk for atrial fibrillation was nearly three times higher (28%) in those subjects with a serum TSH concentration ≤ 1 mU/L at baseline than in those with normal serum TSH concentrations (>0.4–5.0 mU/L) (11%) (relative risk 3.1, 95% confidence interval 1.7–5.5; *p* < 0.001) (14) (Fig. 77.1). The incidence of atrial fibrillation in the subjects with slightly low serum TSH concentrations (>0.1–0.4 mU/L) and those with serum TSH concentrations greater than 5.0 mU/L was similar to that in the subjects with normal serum TSH concentrations (16% and 15%, respectively, vs. 11%). In a retrospective study of

TABLE 77.1. OBSERVED AND EXPECTED NUMBERS OF DEATHS AND STANDARDIZED MORTALITY RATIOS FOR CAUSES OF DEATH FOR WHICH THE RISK WAS ALTERED IN A COHORT OF 7,209 PATIENTS TREATED WITH RADIOIODINE FOR THYROTOXICOSIS

Cause of Death	ICD-9 Codes*	No. of Deaths Observed	No. of Deaths Expected	SMR (95% CI)	P Value
Endocrine and metabolic disease	240–279	159	51	3.1 (2.6–3.6)	<0.001
Disease of the circulatory system	390–459	1955	1577	1.2 (1.2–1.3)	<0.001
All cardiovascular diseases		1258	1018	1.2 (1.2–1.3)	<0.001
Rheumatic heart disease		67	21	3.2 (2.5–4.2)	<0.001
Hypertensive disease		59	28	2.1 (1.6–2.7)	<0.001
Ischemic heart disease		867	812	1.1 (1.0–1.1)	0.03
Diseases of pulmonary circulation and other heart disease		265	157	1.8 (1.5–1.9)	<0.001
Cerebrovascular disease		605	446	1.4 (1.2–1.5)	<0.001
Other diseases of the circulatory system		92	112	0.8 (0.7–1.0)	0.03
Injuries and poisoning	800–999	100	61	1.6 (1.3–2.0)	<0.001
Fractures		50	26	1.9 (1.4–2.6)	<0.001
All causes		3611	3186	1.1 (1.1–1.2)	<0.001

*ICD-9 denotes the ninth revision of the *International Classification of Diseases* (16); SMR, standardized mortality ratio; and CI, confidence interval. From Franklyn JA, Maisonneuve P, Sheppard MC, et al. Mortality after the treatment of hyperthyroidism with radioactive iodine. *N Engl J Med* 1998;338:712, with permission.

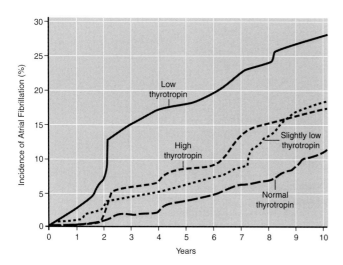

FIGURE 77.1. Cumulative risk of atrial fibrillation in subjects over 60 years of age followed for 10 years and divided according to serum thyrotropin concentration at baseline. (Adapted from Sawin CT, Geller A, Wolf PA, et al. Low serum thyrotropin concentrations as a risk factor for atrial fibrillation in older persons. *N Engl J Med* 1994;331:1249, with permission.)

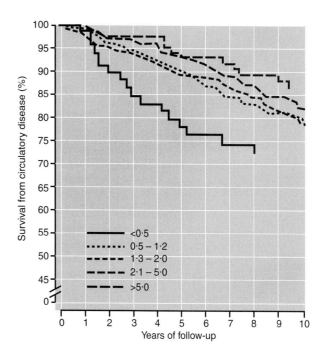

FIGURE 77.2. Kaplan-Meier survival plot of cardiovascular deaths in a cohort of 1,191 general practice patients over 60 years of age, subdivided according to their serum thyrotropin concentrations at baseline, followed for 10 years. (Adapted from Parle JV, Maisonneuve P, Sheppard MC, et al. Prediction of all-cause and cardiovascular mortality in elderly people from one low serum thyrotropin result: a 10-year cohort study. *Lancet* 2001;358:861, with permission.)

23,638 in- and outpatients in whom serum TSH was measured, 2% of those with normal serum TSH concentrations had atrial fibrillation, as compared with 14% of those with overt thyrotoxicosis, and 13% of those with subclinical thyrotoxicosis (15).

Subclinical thyrotoxicosis may also be associated with alterations in cardiac contractility and heart rate similar to but less marked than occur in overt thyrotoxicosis (see Chapter 31) (16,17). There is little evidence that these changes are associated with clinically important changes in cardiac function (3). In a study of hospital admission rates due to ischemic heart disease, there was an increase in risk for admission among patients taking T_4, as compared with those not taking T_4, but among those taking T_4 there was no difference between those with normal and those with low serum TSH concentrations (18). These results argue against an adverse effect of subclinical thyrotoxicosis secondary to ingestion of T_4 (exogenous subclinical thyrotoxicosis).

The risk for all-cause and cardiovascular disease mortality in relation to serum TSH concentration at baseline was studied in a cohort of 1,191 patients 60 years of age or older in the United Kingdom who were followed for 10 years (19,20). Causes of death for those who died during follow-up were compared with age-, sex-, and year-specific data for England and Wales. The all-cause standardized mortality rate for patients with subclinical thyrotoxicosis at year 2 was 2.1 (95% confidence interval 1.0–4.5), and the values for years 3, 4, and 5 were similar. This increase in all-cause mortality was almost completely accounted for by deaths caused by cardiovascular diseases (Fig. 77.2). The causes of the low serum TSH concentrations in this cohort were not determined, although about one third had a goi-

ter on physical examination, and serum free T_4 concentrations were higher in the patients with low serum TSH concentrations than in those with normal serum TSH concentrations, suggesting mild thyroid hormone excess as a general cause of TSH suppression. The absence of excess deaths from other common causes such as cancer or respiratory disease in the patients with low serum TSH concentrations suggests that the association of cardiovascular disease mortality with low serum TSH concentrations is not a nonspecific effect of nonthyroidal illnesses on TSH secretion. These results, along with the increased risk for atrial fibrillation cited above, support the view that antithyroid treatment should be considered in patients with persistent subclinical thyrotoxicosis, although evidence that intervention lowers the risk for atrial fibrillation or any other outcome is lacking (3).

CARDIOVASCULAR MORBIDITY AND MORTALITY IN HYPOTHYROIDISM

Overt Hypothyroidism

Severe overt hypothyroidism can lead to fatal myxedema coma (see Chapter 65) (21). Overt hypothyroidism has been reported to be associated with cardiovascular disease, although the evidence for an association is largely confined to older literature reporting findings from relatively small numbers of patients (22,23). Such an association is plausible, however, given the hypercholesterolemia, hyperhomocysteinemia, and diastolic hypertension found in patients with overt hypothyroidism (see Chapter 53).

Subclinical Hypothyroidism

The possibility of an association between subclinical hypothyroidism and cardiovascular disease has also been raised. Serum total and low-density lipoprotein cholesterol concentrations may be slightly high in these patients (see Chapter 78), but the concentrations do not decline consistently during T_4 therapy (24). There was an association between serum TSH concentrations and diastolic blood pressure in a study of 57 women with subclinical hypothyroidism and 34 normal women (25). Despite these potential mechanisms for increased cardiovascular risk, the prevalence of angina, myocardial infarction, peripheral arterial disease, and cerebrovascular disease among 3,678 subjects enrolled in the Cardiovascular Health Study was similar in those subjects with subclinical hypothyroidism and those with normal serum TSH concentrations (26). With respect to mortality, there was no increase in all-cause mortality or mortality from ischemic heart disease in subjects with subclinical hypothyroidism in the Whickham cohort followed for up to 20 years (27). These results are in agreement with the results of the 10-year follow-up study of a cohort of 1,191 patients described earlier, in that there was no increase in either all-cause or cardiovascular disease mortality in the patients who had subclinical hypothyroidism at baseline (20).

An association between subclinical hypothyroidism and ischemic heart disease was found in two small studies (28,29), and in a study of elderly subjects in a nursing home 32 of 56 subjects with subclinical hypothyroidism (58%) had coronary artery disease, as compared with 37 of 231 euthyroid subjects (16%) (30). The prevalence of peripheral arterial disease also was increased in these nursing home subjects (31). A study of 1,149 women 55 years of age and older in the Netherlands revealed an association between subclinical hypothyroidism and aortic calcification (odds ratio 1.9) and myocardial infarction (odds ratio 2.3) (32). There was no association with incident myocardial infarction.

FRACTURES AND THYROTOXICOSIS

Overt Thyrotoxicosis

Thyrotoxicosis results in net loss of bone and hence reduction in bone mineral density (see Chapter 40), but the evidence that patients with thyrotoxicosis have an increase in fracture is conflicting.

A large prospective study followed 9,516 white women over 65 years of age for an average of 4.1 years for incident

fractures of the femur. There was a 1.8-fold increase in risk for fracture among those women with a history of thyrotoxicosis (95% confidence interval 1.2–2.6) (33). Similarly, there was an increase in mortality from hip fracture among 7,209 patients with thyrotoxicosis treated with radioiodine (standardized mortality ratio 2.9, 95% confidence interval 2.0–3.9) (12). In contrast, there was no association between a history of thyrotoxicosis and fractures of the ankle and foot in a prospective study of over 9,000 postmenopausal women (34). A case control study of the occurrence of fracture before and after diagnosis of thyrotoxicosis found an approximate twofold increased incidence of fracture (of all sites) around the time of diagnosis, with return of the fracture rate to that in the control subjects thereafter (35). A smaller follow-up study of 630 patients who underwent thyroidectomy (only 85 of whom had thyrotoxicosis) revealed no association with fracture of the femur (36).

Subclinical Thyrotoxicosis

Like overt thyrotoxicosis, subclinical thyrotoxicosis (especially that associated with T_4 therapy) has been implicated in the development of osteoporosis (see Chapter 40). Most of the studies of subclinical thyrotoxicosis and bone disease have been conducted in patients receiving T_4, not patients with endogenous subclinical thyrotoxicosis.

Early studies reported significant reductions in bone mass in patients treated with T_4 for prolonged periods of time (37,38). However, several later studies failed to demonstrate any detrimental effect of T_4 therapy on bone, even in those taking sufficient T_4 to cause subclinical thyrotoxicosis (39,40). Two meta-analyses of the many studies of this topic suggested that T_4 therapy was associated with osteopenia in postmenopausal women (41,42), although these analyses are complicated by the heterogeneity of the women who were studied, particularly with respect to their history of thyrotoxicosis and extent of T_4 therapy. Bone density does increase when patients with subclinical thyrotoxicosis are treated with an antithyroid drug (43).

With respect to fracture, a study of 1,100 patients taking T_4 found no significant difference in fracture rate, as compared with the general population (18). In the prospective study of 9,516 white women over 65 years of age described above (33), there was an increased risk for incident fracture of the femur in women taking thyroid hormone (relative risk 1.6, 95% confidence interval 1.1–2.3), but this was no longer significant when adjusted for a history of thyrotoxicosis (present in 36% of those taking T_4). A prospective cohort study of 686 women over 65 years of age followed for a mean of 3.7 years revealed that women with baseline serum TSH concentrations < 0.1 mU/L had a threefold increased risk for hip fracture and fourfold increased risk for vertebral fracture, as compared with women with normal serum TSH concentrations (after adjusting for other factors including age, previous thyrotoxicosis, and estrogen therapy) (44). Among 23,183 patients (88% women) in the United Kingdom for whom T_4 had been prescribed, the occurrence of fracture of the femur was not higher than in 92,732 matched control patients (45). Prescription of T_4 was not an independent predictor of femoral fracture among the women (adjusted odds ratio 1.0, 95% confidence interval 0.9–1.2), but it was among men (adjusted odds ratio 1.7, 95% confidence interval 1.1–2.6).

Overall, the data regarding osteoporosis and thyroid status support an adverse effect of overt thyrotoxicosis on bone density and fracture risk, and the effect may be sustained despite successful antithyroid therapy. Subclinical thyrotoxicosis has little effect on bone density or fracture risk, except perhaps in patients with low serum TSH concentrations (some of whom may in fact have had overt thyrotoxicosis) and postmenopausal women.

CANCER RISK AND THYROID DYSFUNCTION AND ITS TREATMENT

Several studies have addressed the question of whether thyroid diseases are themselves associated with increased risk for thyroid and other cancers. In a retrospective study of 7,338 women followed on average for more than 15 years, there was a small but significant increase in total cancer deaths in those with nodular goiter, thyroid adenoma, thyrotoxicosis, and Hashimoto's thyroiditis, as compared with the general population, but women in the cohort who did not have thyroid disease also were more likely to die of cancer (46). The risk for cancer was not increased in a cohort of 57,326 patients discharged from a Danish hospital with a diagnosis of thyrotoxicosis, hypothyroidism, or goiter, but there was an increase in thyroid cancer, as well as cancer at some other sites, in all three groups of thyroid disease patients (47). These results may reflect true disease associations, associations between cancer risk and autoimmune disease (as the major underlying cause of thyroid dysfunction), or associations between cancer risk and thyroid hormone or antithyroid therapy.

Several studies have addressed a possible link between risk for breast cancer and thyroid disorders. Several found no association between either thyroid disorders or their treatment and breast cancer risk (48,49), although another study suggested there was a modest association (50). A recent case-control study involving 4,575 women with invasive breast cancer and 4,682 control women revealed that a history of any thyroid disorder was not associated with breast cancer risk (odds ratio 11.2, 95% confidence interval 0.9–1.2) (51). Only parous women with a diagnosis of thyroid cancer had increased risk. The results of similar case-control studies examining risk for other cancers, for example, ovarian cancer, were negative (52).

The introduction of radioiodine therapy for thyrotoxicosis in the 1940s was accompanied by questions concerning its long-term safety, especially in terms of cancer risk (53). These concerns, if anything, increased after recognition that irradiation of the head and neck caused thyroid cancer, whether from x-irradiation or exposure to the products of atomic bomb testing or nuclear power plant accidents (see section Pathogenesis in Chapter 70) (54,55).

Several studies of cancer risk in patients treated with radioiodine for thyrotoxicosis have been reported, with conflicting results. A study of a large cohort of patients in Sweden found no excess risk for leukemia or solid tumors in those exposed to ^{131}I, given either for diagnosis or treatment of thyrotoxicosis or thyroid cancer (56). Overall cancer incidence was increased (standardized incidence ratio 1.06, 95% confidence interval 1.01–1.11), and analysis of a subgroup of 10-year survivors revealed significantly increased risks for cancers of the stomach, kidney, and brain. Furthermore, the risk for stomach cancer has been reported to increase with time and with increasing dose of ^{131}I (57,58). However, a study comparing cancer risk in patients with thyrotoxicosis treated with ^{131}I or thyroidectomy revealed no differences in cancer incidence or mortality at these or other sites (59). In another study the incidence of cancer and mortality was determined in a cohort of 7,417 patients treated with ^{131}I for thyrotoxicosis (60). During 72,073 person-years of follow-up, 634 cancers were diagnosed, as compared with an expected number of 761 (standardized incidence ratio 0.83, 95% confidence interval 0.77–0.90). The risk for cancer mortality was also reduced in the cohort (observed cancer deaths 448; expected 499; standardized mortality ratio 0.90, 95% confidence interval 0.82–0.98). There were significant decreases in the incidence of cancers of the pancreas, bronchus and trachea, bladder, and lymphatic and hematopoietic systems, and mortality from cancers at each of these sites was also reduced. However, there was a small but statistically significant increase in incidence and mortality for cancer of the small bowel and thyroid, although the absolute risk for occurrence or death from these cancers was small.

Because the thyroid is the major site of radiation exposure after radioiodine treatment, attention has focused on risk for thyroid cancer. Patients given ^{131}I for diagnostic imaging have not had an increase in thyroid cancer (61). An analysis of 35,593 patients with thyrotoxicosis treated at 26 centers in the United States and United Kingdom between 1946 and 184, 65% of whom were treated with ^{131}I, did reveal an increase in thyroid cancer mortality (62). The cancer risk was increased in patients treated with ^{131}I and those treated with an antithyroid drug. In the cohort of 7,417 patients mentioned above (60), there was a small but statistically significant increase in incidence and mortality for thyroid cancer (standardized mortality ratio 2.8, 95% confidence interval 1.2–6.7), although the absolute risk for development or death from thyroid cancer was small.

Overall, these findings are reassuring in terms of the overall safety of ^{131}I treatment and cancer risk. The evidence does suggest an increased relative risk for thyroid cancer in patients with thyrotoxicosis treated with ^{131}I, although the absolute risk is small. If there is indeed an increase in risk, it may be caused by the underlying thyroid disease rather than ^{131}I therapy per se.

REFERENCES

1. Canaris GJ, Manowitz NR, Mayor G, et al. The Colorado thyroid disease prevalence study. *Arch Intern Med* 2000;160:526.
2. Parle JV, Franklyn JA, Cross KW, et al. Thyroxine prescription in the community: serum thyroid stimulating hormone level assays as an indicator of undertreatment or overtreatment. *Br J Gen Pract* 1993;43:107.
3. Surks MI, Ortiz E, Daniels GH, et al. Subclinical thyroid disease. Scientific review and guidelines for diagnosis and management. *JAMA* 2004;291:228.
4. Sandler G, Wilson GM. The nature and prognosis of heart disease in thyrotoxicosis. A review of 150 patients treated with 131 I. *QJM* 1959;28:347.
5. Nakazawa HK, Sakurai K, Hamada N, et al. Management of atrial fibrillation in the post-thyrotoxic state. *Am J Med* 1982;72:903.
6. Nordyke RA, Gilbert FI Jr, Harada AS. Graves' disease. Influence of age on clinical findings. *Arch Intern Med* 1988;148:626.
7. Bar-Sela S, Ehrenfeld M, Eliakim M. Arterial embolism in thyrotoxicosis with atrial fibrillation. *Arch Intern Med* 1981;141:1191.
8. Petersen P, Hansen JM. Stroke in thyrotoxicosis with atrial fibrillation. *Stroke* 1988;19:15.
9. Presti CF, Hart RG. Thyrotoxicosis, atrial fibrillation, and embolism, revisited. *Am Heart J* 1989;117:976.
10. Goldman MB, Maloof F, Monson RR, et al. Radioactive iodine therapy and breast cancer. A follow-up study of hyperthyroid women. *Am J Epidemiol* 1988;127:969.
11. Hall P, Lundell G, Holm LE. Mortality in patients treated for hyperthyroidism with iodine-131. *Acta Endocrinol (Copenh)* 1993;128:230.
12. Franklyn JA, Maisonneuve P, Sheppard MC, et al. Mortality after the treatment of hyperthyroidism with radioactive iodine. *N Engl J Med* 1998;338:712.
13. Tenerz A, Forberg R, Jansson R. Is a more active attitude warranted in patients with subclinical thyrotoxicosis? *J Intern Med* 1990;228:229.
14. Sawin CT, Geller A, Wolf PA, et al. Low serum thyrotropin concentrations as a risk factor for atrial fibrillation in older persons. *N Engl J Med* 1994;331:1249.
15. Auer J, Scheibner P, Mische T, et al. Subclinical hyperthyroidism as a risk factor for atrial fibrillation. *Am Heart J* 2001;142:838.
16. Biondi B, Fazio S, Carella C, et al. Control of adrenergic overactivity by beta-blockade improves the quality of life in patients receiving long term suppressive therapy with levothyroxine. *J Clin Endocrinol Metab* 1994;78:1028.
17. Biondi B, Palmieri EA, Fazio S, et al. Endogenous subclinical hyperthyroidism affects quality of life and cardiac morphology and function in young and middle-aged patients. *J Clin Endocrinol Metab* 2000;85:4701.
18. Leese GP, Jung RT, Guthrie C, et al. Morbidity in patients on L-thyroxine: a comparison of those with a normal TSH to those with a suppressed TSH. *Clin Endocrinol (Oxf)* 1992;37:500.
19. Parle JV, Franklyn JA, Cross KW, et al. Prevalence and follow-up of abnormal thyrotrophin (TSH) concentrations in the el-

derly in the United Kingdom. *Clin Endocrinol (Oxf)* 1991;34:77.
20. Parle JV, Maisonneuve P, Sheppard MC, et al. Prediction of all-cause and cardiovascular mortality in elderly people from one low serum thyrotropin result: a 10-year cohort study. *Lancet* 2001;358:861.
21. Yamamoto T, Fukuyama J, Fujiyoshi A. Factors associated with mortality of myxedema coma: report of eight cases and literature survey. *Thyroid* 1999;9:1167.
22. Steinberg AD. Myxedema and coronary artery disease—a comparative autopsy study. *Ann Intern Med* 1968;68:338.
23. VanHaelst L, Neve P, Chailly P, et al. Coronary-artery disease in hypothyroidism. Observations in clinical myxoedema. *Lancet* 1967;2:800.
24. Danese M,D, Ladenson PW, Meinert CL, et al. Effect of thyroxine therapy on serum lipoproteins in patients with mild thyroid failure: a quantitative review of the literature. *J Clin Endocrinol Metab* 2000;85:2993.
25. Luboshitzky R, Aviv A, Herer P, et al. Risk factors for cardiovascular disease in women with subclinical hypothyroidism. *Thyroid* 2002;12:421.
26. Cappola AR, Ladenson PW. Hypothyroidism and atherosclerosis. *J Clin Endocrinol Metab* 2003;88:2438.
27. Vanderpump MP, Tunbridge WM, French JM, et al. The development of ischemic heart disease in relation to autoimmune thyroid disease in a 20-year follow-up study of an English community. *Thyroid* 1996;6:155.
28. Dean JW, Fowler PB. Exaggerated responsiveness to thyrotrophin releasing hormone: a risk factor in women with coronary artery disease. *BMJ (Clin Res Ed)* 1985;290:1555.
29. Tieche M, Lupi GA, Gutzwiller F, et al. Borderline low thyroid function and thyroid autoimmunity. Risk factors for coronary heart disease? *Br Heart J* 1981;46:202.
30. Mya MM, Aronow WS. Subclinical hypothyroidism is associated with coronary artery disease in older persons. *J Gerontol A Biol Sci Med Sci* 2002;57:M658.
31. Mya MM, Aronow WS. Increased prevalence of peripheral arterial disease in older men and women with subclinical hypothyroidism. *J Gerontol A Biol Sci Med Sci* 2003;58:68.
32. Hak AE, Pols HA, Visser TJ, et al. Subclinical hypothyroidism is an independent risk factor for atherosclerosis and myocardial infarction in elderly women: the Rotterdam Study. *Ann Intern Med* 2000;132:270.
33. Cummings SR, Nevitt MC, Browner WS, et al. Risk factors for hip fracture in white women. Study of Osteoporotic Fractures Research Group. *N Engl J Med* 1995;332:767.
34. Seeley DG, Kelsey J, Jergas M, et al. Predictors of ankle and foot fractures in older women. The Study of Osteoporotic Fractures Research Group. *J Bone Miner Res* 1996;11:1347.
35. Vestergaard P, Mosekilde L. Fractures in patients with hyperthyroidism and hypothyroidism: a nationwide follow-up study in 16,249 patients. *Thyroid* 2002;12:411.
36. Melton LJ III, Ardila E, Crowson CS, et al. Fractures following thyroidectomy in women: a population-based cohort study. *Bone* 2000;27:695.
37. Paul TL, Kerrigan J, Kelly AM, et al. Long-term L-thyroxine therapy is associated with decreased hip bone density in premenopausal women. *JAMA* 1988;259:3137.
38. Ross DS, Neer RM, Ridgway EC, et al. Subclinical hyperthyroidism and reduced bone density as a possible result of prolonged suppression of the pituitary-thyroid axis with L-thyroxine. *Am J Med* 1987;82:1167.
39. Franklyn JA, Betteridge J, Daykin J, et al. Long-term thyroxine treatment and bone mineral density. *Lancet* 1992;340:9.
40. Hanna FW, Pettit RJ, Ammari F, et al. Effect of replacement doses of thyroxine on bone mineral density. *Clin Endocrinol (Oxf)* 1998;48:229.

41. Faber J, Galloe AM. Changes in bone mass during prolonged subclinical hyperthyroidism due to L-thyroxine treatment: a meta-analysis. *Eur J Endocrinol* 1994;130:350.

42. Uzzan B, Campos J, Cucherat M, et al. Effects on bone mass of long term treatment with thyroid hormones: a meta-analysis. *J Clin Endocrinol Metab* 1996;81:4278.

43. Mudde AH, Houben AJ, Nieuwenhuijzen Kruseman AC. Bone metabolism during anti-thyroid drug treatment of endogenous subclinical hyperthyroidism. *Clin Endocrinol (Oxf)* 1994;41:421.

44. Bauer DC, Ettinger B, Nevitt MC, et al. Risk for fracture in women with low serum levels of thyroid-stimulating hormone. *Ann Intern Med* 2001;134:561.

45. Sheppard MC, Holder R, Franklyn JA. Levothyroxine treatment and occurrence of fracture of the hip. *Arch Intern Med* 2002; 162:338.

46. Goldman MB, Monson RR, Maloof F. Cancer mortality in women with thyroid disease. *Cancer Res* 1990;50:2283.

47. Mellemgaard A, From G, Jorgensen T, et al. Cancer risk in individuals with benign thyroid disorders. *Thyroid* 1998;8:751.

48. Kalache A, Vessey MP, McPherson K. Thyroid disease and breast cancer: findings in a large case-control study. *Br J Surg* 1982;69: 4345.

49. Weiss HA, Brinton LA, Potischman NA, et al. Breast cancer risk in young women and history of selected medical conditions. *Int J Epidemiol* 1999;28:816.

50. Moseson M, Koenig KL, Shore RE, et al. The influence of medical conditions associated with hormones on the risk of breast cancer. *Int J Epidemiol* 1993;22:1000.

51. Simon MS, Tang MT, Bernstein L, et al. Do thyroid disorders increase the risk of breast cancer? *Cancer Epidemiol Biomarkers Prev* 2002;11:1574.

52. Parazzini F, Moroni S, La Vecchia C, et al. Ovarian cancer risk and history of selected medical conditions linked with female hormones. *Eur J Cancer* 1997;33:1634.

53. Baxter MA, Stewart PM, Daykin J, et al. Radioiodine therapy for hyperthyroidism in young patients—perception of risk and use. *QJM* 1993;86:495.

54. Gilbert ES, Tarone R, Bouville A, et al. Thyroid cancer rates and ^{131}I doses from Nevada atmospheric nuclear bomb tests. *J Natl Cancer Inst* 1998;90:1654.

55. Moysich KB, Menezes RJ, Michalek AM. Chernobyl-related ionising radiation exposure and cancer risk: an epidemiological review. *Lancet Oncol* 2002;3:269.

56. Hall P, Boice JD Jr, Berg G, et al. Leukaemia incidence after iodine-131 exposure. *Lancet* 1992;340:1.

57. Holm LE, Hall P, Wiklund K, et al. Cancer risk after iodine-131 therapy for hyperthyroidism. *J Natl Cancer Inst* 1991;83: 1072.

58. Hall P, Berg G, Bjelkengren G, et al. Cancer mortality after iodine-131 therapy for hyperthyroidism. *Int J Cancer* 1992;50: 886.

59. Hoffman DA, McConahey WM, Diamond EL, et al. Mortality in women treated for hyperthyroidism. *Am J Epidemiol* 1982; 115:243.

60. Franklyn JA, Maisonneuve P, Sheppard M, et al. Cancer incidence and mortality after radioiodine treatment for hyperthyroidism: a population-based cohort study. *Lancet* 1999;353: 2111.

61. Dickman PW, Holm LE, Lundell G, et al. Thyroid cancer risk after thyroid examination with ^{131}I: a population-based cohort study in Sweden. *Int J Cancer* 2003;106:580.

62. Ron E, Doody MM, Becker DV, et al. Cancer mortality following treatment for adult hyperthyroidism. Cooperative Thyrotoxicosis Therapy Follow-up Study Group. *JAMA* 1998;280: 347.

SUBCLINICAL HYPOTHYROIDISM

DOUGLAS S. ROSS

The term "subclinical hypothyroidism" was first introduced in the early 1970s coincident with the introduction of serum thyrotropin (TSH) measurements. This term eventually replaced other terms, such as "preclinical myxedema," "compensated euthyroidism," "preclinical hypothyroidism," and "decreased thyroid reserve." Subclinical hypothyroidism is defined biochemically as a high serum TSH concentration and normal serum free thyroxine (T_4) and triiodothyronine (T_3) concentrations. Some investigators, especially those studying the neuropsychiatric aspects of hypothyroidism, also consider patients who have normal basal serum TSH concentrations and supranormal serum TSH responses to thyrotropin-releasing hormone (TRH) to have hypothyroidism. Table 78.1 defines the several grades of hypothyroidism that have been suggested (1,2). By definition, patients with subclinical hypothyroidism cannot be identified on the basis of symptoms and signs (3).

ETIOLOGY

The causes of subclinical hypothyroidism are the same as the causes of overt hypothyroidism (see Chapter 46) and are listed in Table 78.2. Most patients have chronic autoimmune thyroiditis, as defined by high serum concentrations of antithyroid peroxidase (anti-TPO) antibodies. In a Michigan outpatient practice, 54% of patients with subclinical hypothyroidism had chronic autoimmune thyroiditis (4), and in a community survey in Whickham, England, 67% of women and 40% of men with high serum TSH concentrations also had high serum antibody values (5). Destructive therapy for thyrotoxicosis caused by Graves' disease is another major cause of subclinical hypothyroidism, accounting for 39% of the cases in the Michigan study (4). Among clinically euthyroid patients who have received radioiodine therapy for Graves' thyrotoxicosis, the majority have high serum TSH concentrations (6,7), and, in one survey, 65% of clinically euthyroid patients treated surgically for Graves' thyrotoxicosis had high serum TSH concentrations (8). Several drugs may cause subclinical (or overt) hypothyroidism, including lithium carbonate, iodine, iodine-containing drugs such as amiodarone, and iodine-containing radiographic contrast agents. Smoking may exacerbate subclinical hypothy-roidism and its metabolic consequences (9). External radiation therapy to the neck also may cause subclinical hypothyroidism. Another important cause of subclinical hypothyroidism is inadequate thyroid hormone therapy for overt hypothyroidism. In a community-based study (in Framingham, Massachusetts), 37% of older patients taking a thyroid hormone preparation for hypothyroidism had high serum TSH concentrations (10). Inadequate thyroid therapy may have been intentional in some patients because of coexisting heart disease, but more often it is caused by poor patient compliance or inadequate monitoring of therapy.

DIFFERENTIAL DIAGNOSIS

Several causes of high serum TSH concentrations do not properly fit the definition of subclinical hypothyroidism (Table 78.2). One is during recovery from nonthyroidal illness, during which time serum TSH concentrations may be transiently high for a week or occasionally longer. Studies of subclinical hypothyroidism based on serum TSH measurements in hospitalized patients may be invalid because of failure to recognize this cause of high serum TSH values. An occasional serum TSH determination may exceed the normal reference range because of a robust pulse of TSH secretion, especially at night, or because of assay variability.

Therefore, slightly high serum TSH concentrations should be confirmed before the diagnosis of subclinical hypothyroidism is accepted. Artifactual increases in serum TSH values may be caused by heterophile antibodies, for example, in patients treated with monoclonal mouse antibody preparations, which interfere with TSH measurement, although this technical problem has been corrected by most manufacturers of TSH assay materials. Serum TSH concentrations also may be high in patients with adrenal insufficiency and occasionally during treatment with metoclopramide or domperidone. Rare causes of slightly high serum TSH concentrations are TSH-secreting pituitary adenomas and resistance to thyroid hormone; patients with the former have thyrotoxicosis, whereas those with the latter are euthyroid or possibly thyrotoxic.

TABLE 78.1. GRADES OF HYPOTHYROIDISM

Grade	Symptoms and Signs	Serum T$_4$	Serum T$_3$	Serum TSH	Serum TSH Response to TRH
Overt	Obvious	Low	Usually low	Very high	Supranormal
Mild	Minimal	Low	Normal	Moderately high	Supranormal
Subclinical	None or few	Normal	Normal	Slightly high	Supranormal
Presubclinical	None	Normal	Normal	Normal	Supranormal

T$_3$, triiodothyronine; T$_4$, thyroxine; TRH, thyrotropin-releasing hormone; TSH, thyrotropin.

EPIDEMIOLOGY

Several population-based studies have defined the prevalence of subclinical hypothyroidism. In England (the Whickham Survey), the prevalence of serum TSH concentrations higher than 6 mU/L in the absence of overt hypothyroidism was 7.5% in women and 2.8% in men (5) (see Chapter 19). An age-dependent increase in serum TSH concentrations was found in women only when those with high serum antithyroid antibody concentrations were included in the analysis. In women over 75 years of age, the prevalence of subclinical hypothyroidism was 17.4%. In the United States, the National Health and Examination Survey (NHANES III) found a 4.3% prevalence of subclinical hypothyroidism (11); in blacks the prevalence was only 1.6%. In Detroit, the prevalence of high serum TSH concentrations was 8.5% in women and 4.4% in men over age 55 years (12). The higher prevalence of subclinical hypothyroidism in older people was confirmed by data from the Framingham Study, in which the prevalence of minor elevations in serum TSH concentrations in people over 60 years of age was 8.2% in men and 16.9% in women (13), and by a Dutch study in which the prevalence of subclini-

cal hypothyroidism in a group of women (mean age 55 years) was 4%; the rate was 7.3% in the same women 10 years later (14). The prevalence of subclinical hypothyroidism may be lower in elderly women; in an English study, the prevalence was 13.7% in women 60 to 69 years of age and 6.2% in women over 80 years of age (15).

Subclinical hypothyroidism is more prevalent in areas of higher, as compared with lower, but not deficient, iodine intake. Among nursing home residents with a mean age of 80 years and similar prevalence of high serum anti-TPO antibody concentrations, the prevalence of subclinical hypothyroidism was 4.2% in relatively iodine-deficient northern Hungary; 10.4% in Slovakia, where iodinated salt prophylaxis had been mandated for 40 years; and 23.9% in eastern Hungary, where iodine intake is high (16).

Subclinical hypothyroidism is more prevalent in patients with Down syndrome (17), type 1 diabetes mellitus (18), and probably other autoimmune diseases. In a survey of pregnant women in the United States, 2% had subclinical hypothyroidism, 58% of whom had high anti-TPO antibody concentrations (19).

TABLE 78.2. COMMON CAUSES OF SUBCLINICAL HYPOTHYROIDISM

Subclinical hypothyroidism
  Chronic autoimmune (Hashimoto's) thyroiditis
  Radioiodine or surgical treatment of Graves' thyrotoxicosis
  Inadequate thyroid hormone replacement therapy for overt hypothyroidism
  Lithium carbonate therapy
  Iodine and iodine-containing drugs and contrast agents
  External radiotherapy to the neck
Serum TSH elevations not associated with subclinical hypothyroidism
  Nonthyroidal illness
  Pulsatile TSH secretion, nocturnal surge in TSH secretion
  Assay variability
  Heterophile antibodies
  Metoclopropamide, domperidone
  TSH-secreting pituitary adenomas
  Thyroid hormone resistance syndromes

TSH, thyrotropin.

NATURAL HISTORY

In a follow-up study of persons from the original Whickham Survey (20), women who had high serum TSH and antithyroid antibody concentrations developed overt hypothyroidism at a rate of 4.3% yearly over 20 years, whereas women who had only high serum TSH concentrations or only high antibody concentrations developed overt hypothyroidism at annual rates of 2.6% and 2.1%, respectively. In a Swiss study of women with known thyroid disease followed prospectively for 9 years, overt hypothyroidism developed in 0%, 43%, and 77% of women with serum TSH concentrations of 4 to 6 mU/L, greater than 6 to 12 mU/L, and greater than 12 mU/L, respectively, and was 2.5-fold more likely in those with high serum anti-TPO antibody concentrations (21). In a New Mexico study of asymptomatic ambulatory subjects over 60 years of age with subclinical hypothyroidism (22), one third developed overt hypothyroidism during 4 years of follow-up; among them were all those whose initial serum TSH concentrations were higher than 20 mU/L and 80% of those whose serum anti-TPO antibody titers were 1:1600 or higher, but none with lower titers. In an English study of persons with subclinical hypothyroidism followed for 1 year, 18% developed overt hypothyroidism, 6% had normal serum TSH concentrations, and 77% had persistent subclinical hypothyroidism (15).

The underlying cause of subclinical hypothyroidism also may predict progression to overt hypothyroidism. In one study, 53% of patients with subclinical hypothyroidism followed for 8 years had overt hypothyroidism, and 47% continued to have subclinical hypothyroidism (23). The former group included all patients with autoimmune thyroid disease, prior radioiodine therapy, high-dose external radiotherapy, and long-term lithium therapy, whereas the latter group included patients who had thyroid or neck surgery for indications other than thyrotoxicosis or external neck radiotherapy during childhood.

BIOLOGIC IMPORTANCE

The fundamental clinical question regarding patients with subclinical hypothyroidism is whether they require treatment with thyroid hormone. Based on the natural history of subclinical hypothyroidism alone, one can argue that treatment should be started to prevent the development of overt hypothyroidism. Additionally, goiter, if present, decreases in size in some patients (24). This section summarizes several randomized trials of thyroid hormone therapy and other studies that compared various measures of tissue thyroid hormone action in patients with subclinical hypothyroidism with those in euthyroid subjects (Table 78.3).

RANDOMIZED TRIALS

The first randomized trial of T_4 therapy in 33 patients with subclinical hypothyroidism included patients with serum TSH values as high as 55 mU/L (25). It was a 1-year study, the T_4 dose was adjusted to normalize serum TSH concentrations, and symptoms were assessed based on a standardized hypothyroidism diagnostic index (26). The T_4-treated patients had no change in weight, basal metabolic rate, serum cholesterol or triglyceride concentrations, ratio of preejection period to left ventricular ejection time ratio (PEP:LVET ratio), or QKd (the interval from the Q wave on the electrocardiogram to the pulse arrival time at the brachial artery). A subgroup of patients with high PEP:LVET ratios had normal values during therapy. The major finding of this study was that half the patients with subclinical hypothyroidism had fewer symptoms during treatment.

A second randomized trial was a 1-year double-blind crossover study of 20 women with subclinical hypothyroidism (serum TSH values as high as 16 mU/L) (27). All patients received 0.15 mg of T_4 daily. Because this is an above-average replacement dose, some patients probably had subclinical thyrotoxicosis during treatment, as reflected by a shortening of systolic time intervals to subnormal values (see Chapter 79). During the 6-month T_4 therapy period, serum procollagen II peptide concentrations increased; but heart rate, serum cholesterol, creatine kinase, or sex hormone–binding globulin concentrations, body mass, blood pressure, or hemoglobin concentration did not change. Psychometric test scores and hypothyroid symptoms improved during T_4 administration, and many patients correctly distinguished the T_4 treatment period from the placebo period. Thus, the major findings in this study were improved results of psychometric testing and fewer hypothyroid symptoms when the patients were receiving T_4.

A third randomized trial was a 10-month double-blind placebo-controlled study of 37 patients with serum TSH values as high as 32 mU/L (28). The T_4-treated patients had a significant improvement in psychometric test scores related to memory, but no improvement in scores of several other cognitive function tests or in health-related quality of life, as assessed by several standardized questionnaires, including one used in the first trial.

In a fourth 48-month trial of 66 patients with serum TSH values as high as 50 mU/L (mean 12.8 mU/L), T_4 therapy resulted in improvement in symptom scores and lower serum total and low-density lipoprotein (LDL) cholesterol concentrations, but had no effect on serum high-density lipoprotein (HDL) cholesterol, triglyceride, apoprotein A1, or lipoprotein(a) concentrations (29).

A fifth randomized trial of 40 patients who had serum TSH concentrations between 5 and 10 mU/L revealed no improvement in symptom scores, body mass index, energy expenditure, or serum lipid concentrations (30). In a randomized trial in 49 patients with serum TSH values between 3.6 and 15 mU/L in which only serum lipids were measured, serum concentrations of total and LDL cholesterol decreased, whereas those of HDL cholesterol, apoprotein A1 or B, or lipoprotein(a) did not change (31). A randomized trial using Doppler echocardiography and videodensitometric analysis found that T_4 therapy normalized the low cyclic variation index and reduced the PEP:LVET ratio and isovolumetric relaxation time (32). Finally, neither T_4 nor placebo given for 48 weeks altered serum homocysteine and C-reactive protein concentrations in 63 women with subclinical hypothyroidism (33).

In summary, in patients with subclinical hypothyroidism, T_4 therapy resulted in improvement in psychometric test scores in both studies in which the tests were conducted, improvement of hypothyroid symptoms in three of five studies, improvement in serum lipid levels in

TABLE 78.3. SUBCLINICAL HYPOTHYROIDISM: BIOLOGIC EFFECTS

	Cross-sectional Studies			Clinical Trials	
	Increased	Decreased	Unchanged	Improved	Unchanged
Serum lipid and apoprotein concentrations					
Total cholesterol	31,34–38		14,39–46	29,31,38,42[a],48, 54[b],55[b],56[a],57[a]	24,25,27,28,36, 43,45,49–53
Low-density lipoprotein cholesterol	31,34,36,38		41,42,44–47	29,31,42[a],48,52, 54[b],56[a],57[a]	24,28,30,36,45, 50,53
High-density lipoprotein cholesterol		37,39,43	31,41,42,44–46	43	24,28,29–31,43, 45,48–50,52,53
Apoprotein A1	37,44		13,41,43,45	43	29,31,38,43,45, 48,50,52
Apoprotein B	31,36–38		14,43–45	38,52	29,31,36,38,43, 45,48,50,52
Apoprotein A2			43		43
Lipoprotein lipase activity					50
Lipoprotein(a)	36,37,58		31,45	38,58	29,31,36,38,48, 58
Cardiac function					
Systolic time intervals	32		44,60,62	25[a],27[c],51[c,d],61[f],62[c]	
Isovolumetric relaxation time	63,64			63	
Myocardial contractility				49,66	
Heart rate			32		27,32,49
Blood pressure	46		32	67	27,61
Cardiac output				67[g]	
Systemic vascular resistence				67[g]	
Other measurements					
Depression/psychiatric features	68–71				
Hypothyroid/somatic complaints	71			25,27,29,71	28,30
Psychometric test scores		71		27,28,71,72	
Achilles tendon reflex time	44,62			62[c]	
Amplitude of the stapedial reflex		55		55	
Intraocular pressure	79			79	
Basal metabolic rate					25
Body mass or weight			31,32,46		25,27,30,32,50
Nerve conduction velocity			75		49
Brainstem auditory evoked potentials			75		
Serum myoglobulin	44				
Increase in serum lactate with exercise	77				
Response to TRH					
Serum α-subunit	40,44[e]				
Serum prolactin	44		73	25	
Serum insulin and glucagon					50
Serum sex hormone–binding globulin, and corticosteroid-binding globulin					27
Serum creatine kinase			44		27
Serum ionized calcium		78		78	
Serum homocysteine			33,46,81		33,81
Serum C-reactive protein	33				33
Bone density					28,82

[a]Values improved in a subgroup of patients with abnormal baseline values.
[b]Meta-analysis.
[c]Some patients may have received excess doses of thyroid hormone.
[d]Some patients may have had mild hypothyroidism.
[e]Values abnormal only in postmenopausal women.
[f]During exercise only.
[g]Upright posture only.
TRH, thyrotropin-releasing hormone.

two of six studies, and improvement in cardiac function in one study.

SERUM LIPID AND APOPROTEIN CONCENTRATIONS

The serum total cholesterol concentrations in patients with subclinical hypothyroidism were high in six studies (31, 34–38) but not different from those in normal subjects in most other studies (1,14,39–46) (Table 78.3). In a survey of 25,862 people, the 1,799 subjects who had serum TSH concentrations of 5.1 to 10 mU/L had a mean serum cholesterol concentration of 223 mg/dL (5.8 mM), as compared with 216 mg/dL (5.6 mM) in the 22,842 subjects with normal serum TSH concentrations (35). Serum cholesterol concentrations decreased in response to T_4 therapy in three studies (31,38,47,48), but not in many other studies (24–28,36,43,45,49–53). In two meta-analyses of the treatment studies, serum total cholesterol concentrations decreased by 9 to 15 mg/dL (0.2–0.4 mM) during T_4 therapy (54,55).

Patients with subclinical hypothyroidism had high serum LDL cholesterol concentrations in six studies (31,34,36–38) and normal concentrations in six studies (41,42,44–47). The values were reduced by T_4 therapy in five studies (29,31,38,48,52) but not in seven others (24, 28,30,36,35,50,53). In a meta-analysis, T_4 therapy reduced serum LDL cholesterol concentrations by 11 mg/dL (0.3 mM) (54). T_4 therapy is more likely to lower serum total and LDL cholesterol concentrations in patients who have high values and in those with higher serum TSH concentrations (37,45,56,57).

Patients with subclinical hypothyroidism had lower serum HDL cholesterol concentrations than normal subjects in three studies (37,39,43), but the values were similar in six studies (31,41,42,44–46). Among the studies of the effect of T_4 therapy on serum HDL cholesterol in patients with subclinical hypothyroidism (24,28,29–31, 43,45, 48–50,52,53), the concentrations increased in only one (43).

Serum apoprotein A1 concentrations were high in two studies (37,44) and were not different from normal subjects in four studies (14,31,43,45); there was a decrease during T_4 therapy in only one (43) of eight studies (29,31,38,43,45,48,50,52). Serum apoprotein B concentrations were high in four studies (31,36–38) and did not differ from normal subjects in four studies (14,43–45); during T_4 therapy, the concentrations decreased in two (38,52) of nine studies (29,31,36,38,43,45,48,50,52). Lastly, serum lipoprotein(a) concentrations were high in three (36,37,58) of five studies (31,36,37,45,58), and they decreased during T_4 therapy in two (38,58) of six studies (29,31,36,38,48,58).

In a study of 1,149 Dutch women (mean age 69 years), aortic atherosclerosis and a history of myocardial infarction were increased in patients with subclinical hypothyroidism independent of other risk factors (59).

In summary, despite variable findings in multiple studies, subclinical hypothyroidism is likely associated with a small increase in serum total and LDL cholesterol concentrations that improve slightly with treatment. A response to treatment is more likely in patients with higher serum TSH concentrations (e.g., >10 mU/L), or those with initially higher serum lipid concentrations.

CARDIAC FUNCTION

Patients with subclinical hypothyroidism had no differences in the duration of electromechanical systole (Q-A2), LVET, or PEP:LVET ratio, as compared with normal subjects (60). In another study, resting PEP, LVET, and QKd values decreased during T_4 therapy (51); however, 25% of the patients had baseline serum TSH concentrations above 40 mU/L, and 20% were overtreated. There was no change in the PEP:LVET ratio or QKd in patients with subclinical hypothyroidism who received T_4 therapy in one of the randomized trials discussed previously (25), but in another group of patients an initially high PEP:LVET ratio became normal during T_4 therapy. In another study of T_4 therapy, resting PEP did not change, but there was a decrease in PEP during exercise and in left ventricular diastolic dimensions at rest (61). Two of these trials are flawed because of possible overtreatment. In one trial, patients treated with 20 μg T_3 twice daily had shorter systolic time intervals, but so, too, did normal subjects receiving the same regimen (62). In the randomized trial discussed previously in which all the patients received 0.15 mg of T_4 daily, the mean values for Q-A2, PEP, and the PEP:LVET ratio all decreased, but some patients had subclinical thyrotoxicosis (27).

Isovolumetric relaxation time was increased in two studies (63,64) and improved with T_4 therapy in one study (63). The ratio of velocity of blood flow across the mitral valve during early and late diastole was lower in patients with subclinical hypothyroidism, as compared with normal subjects, and became normal during T_4 therapy (63). The time to peak ventricular filling rate was high and became normal with treatment (65). In other studies of T_4 therapy, there was no change in left ventricular ejection fraction at rest or with moderate exercise, but it was higher during maximal exercise, and there also was an increase in the slope of the ratio of systolic blood pressure to end-systolic volume at maximal exercise (but not at rest), indicating improved myocardial contractility (49,66). Among 16 women with subclinical hypothyroidism (mean serum TSH 17.1 mU/L) who were treated with T_4 (mean serum TSH 2.2 mU/L), cardiac output increased by 14% and systemic vascular resistance (upright) decreased by 14% (67). Diastolic blood pressure was high in one study (46) and declined with treatment in another study (67).

Thus, some patients with subclinical hypothyroidism have subtle abnormalities in systolic time intervals, diastolic function, and myocardial contractility that may improve during treatment.

NEUROPSYCHIATRIC FEATURES

Reports of an increased prevalence of subclinical hypothyroidism in patients with depression or bipolar affective disorders need careful assessment because of frequently inadequate control groups, coincident lithium therapy, and the inclusion of patients with normal serum TSH values whose thyroid abnormality is limited to either an increased response of serum TSH after TRH administration or high serum antithyroid antibody concentrations (2). Nonetheless, several studies suggest an association of subclinical hypothyroidism with neuropsychiatric abnormalities. In one study of hospitalized patients, the prevalence of hypothyroidism was 14.8% in those with neurotic depression and 2.3% in those with senile and multiinfarct dementia, as compared with 1.9% in those with no psychiatric disorder (68). Patients with depression and subclinical hypothyroidism had a higher prevalence of associated panic disorder and a poorer response to antidepressant drug therapy than depressed euthyroid patients (69). Randomly selected women with subclinical hypothyroidism who had formal psychiatric assessment before assessment of thyroid function had a higher lifetime frequency of depression than euthyroid women (70). Women found to have subclinical hypothyroidism after presenting to a clinic for assessment of goiter had increased rates of free-flowing anxiety, somatic complaints, depressive features, and hysteria, as compared with euthyroid women with goiter, and these abnormalities improved during treatment with T_4 (71). Psychometric test scores in this (71) and one other study (72) were also abnormal and improved with therapy, confirming the results of two randomized trials of T_4 therapy discussed above (27,28).

OTHER MEASUREMENTS

Patients with subclinical hypothyroidism have a normal thyroidal response to TSH stimulation and no abnormality in volume of the sella turcica (40). They may have supranormal increases in the serum concentrations of glycoprotein hormone α subunit and TSH-β subunit in response to TRH administration (40). The serum prolactin response to TRH administration was increased in one study (34) and normal in another study (73).

The Achilles tendon reflex time is prolonged (44,62), and treatment with T_3 restores it to normal (62). The amplitude of the stapedial reflex is low and returns to normal with T_4 therapy (74). Brainstem auditory evoked potentials are normal (75). A peripheral neuropathy is suggested by prolonged latency in distal motor nerves during electrophysiologic testing (76); however, nerve conduction velocity is normal (75) and does not change during T_4 therapy (49). Serum myoglobin concentrations may be high (44), and excess lactate is released during exercise (77). More frequent neuromuscular symptoms, reduced serum ionized calcium, and repetitive discharges on surface electromyography were found in 33 patients; T_4 therapy reversed all these changes (78). Intraocular pressure may be high but decreases during T_4 therapy (79). Endothelium-dependent vasodilatation is impaired (80). Serum homocysteine concentrations are normal (33,46,81) and do not change during T_4 therapy (33,81). Serum C-reactive protein concentrations were slightly high in one study of 63 patients but did not decrease during T_4 therapy (33). Bone density was not reduced in patients with subclinical hypothyroidism after 14 months of T_4 therapy (82). Subclinical hypothyroidism is not more prevalent among women with premenstrual syndrome (74). Subclinical hypothyroidism during pregnancy may be a risk factor for poor developmental outcome in offspring (see Chapter 80) (83).

CONCLUSION

Subclinical hypothyroidism is common, especially among older women. Treatment may be indicated to prevent progression to overt hypothyroidism; this seems most appropriate for patients who have serum TSH concentrations greater than 10 mU/L and high serum anti-TPO antibody concentrations. The major immediate benefit of treatment is an improvement in symptoms and memory in some patients, a small decrease in serum total and LDL cholesterol concentrations, and possible increases in cardiac systolic and diastolic function. However, patients with subclinical hypothyroidism who have symptoms suggestive of hypothyroidism should be advised that treatment may not ameliorate those symptoms. Treatment may also be indicated to reduce thyroid enlargement.

The benefit of treatment is much less certain in patients with serum TSH concentrations less than 10 mU/L. However, pregnant women with any increase in serum TSH concentration should be treated.

Arguments against treatment include the limited clinical benefit, based on the results of the therapeutic trials described above, the relatively low rate of progression, the cost of therapy and the cost of monitoring therapy, and the lifelong commitment to daily medication in patients who have few if any symptoms. Rarely, therapy may exacerbate angina pectoris or a cardiac arrhythmia (84). If treatment is given, careful monitoring to avoid the adverse effects of subclinical thyrotoxicosis is mandatory.

REFERENCES

1. Evered DC, Ormston BJ, Smith PA, et al. Grades of hypothyroidism. *BMJ* 1973;1:657.
2. Haggerty JJ Jr, Golden RN, Garbutt JC, et al. Subclinical hypothyroidism: a review of neuropsychiatric aspects. *Int J Psych Med* 1990;20:193.
3. Bemben DA, Hamm RM, Morgan L, et al. Thyroid disease in the elderly. 2. Predictability of subclinical hypothyroidism. *J Fam Pract* 1994;38:583.
4. Hamburger JI, Meier DA, Szpunar WE. Factitious elevation of thyrotropin in euthyroid patients. *N Engl J Med* 1985;313:267.
5. Tunbridge WMG, Evered DC, Hall R, et al. The spectrum of thyroid disease in a community: the Whickham Survey. *Clin Endocrinol (Oxf)* 1977;7:481.
6. Tunbridge WMG, Harsoulis P, Goolden AWG. Thyroid function in patients treated with radioactive iodine for thyrotoxicosis. *BMJ* 1974;3:89.
7. Toft AD, Irvine WJ, Hunter WM, et al. Plasma TSH and serum T$_4$ levels in long-term follow-up of patients treated with ^{131}I for thyrotoxicosis. *BMJ* 1974;3:152.
8. Evered D, Young ET, Tunbridge WMG, et al. Thyroid function after subtotal thyroidectomy for hyperthyroidism. *BMJ* 1975;1:25.
9. Muller B, Zulewski H, Huber P, et al. Impaired action of thyroid hormone associated with smoking in women with hypothyroidism. *N Engl J Med* 1995;333:964.
10. Sawin CT, Geller A, Hershman JM, et al. The aging thyroid: the use of thyroid hormone in older persons. *JAMA* 1989;261:2653.
11. Hollowell JG, Staehling NW, Flanders WD, et al. Serum TSH, T$_4$, and thyroid antibodies in the United States population (1988 to 1994): National Health and Nutrition Examination Survey (NHANES III). *J Clin Endocrinol Metab* 2002;87:489.
12. Bagchi N, Brown TR, Parish RF. Thyroid dysfunction in adults over age 55 years: a study in an urban US community. *Arch Intern Med* 1990;150:785.
13. Sawin CT, Chopra D, Azizi F, et al. The aging thyroid. Increased prevalence of elevated serum thyrotropin levels in the elderly. *JAMA* 1979;242:247.
14. Geul KW, van Sluisveld ILL, Grobbee DE, et al. The importance of thyroid microsomal antibodies in the development of elevated serum TSH in middle-aged women: associations with serum lipids. *Clin Endocrinol (Oxf)* 1993;39:275.
15. Parle JV, Franklyn JA, Cross KW, et al. Prevalence and follow-up of abnormal thyrotrophin (TSH) concentrations in the elderly in the United Kingdom. *Clin Endocrinol (Oxf)* 1991;34:77.
16. Szabolcs I, Podoba J, Feldkamp J, et al. Comparative screening for thyroid disorders in old age in areas of iodine deficiency, long-term iodine prophylaxis and abundant iodine intake. *Clin Endocrinol (Oxf)* 1997;47:87.
17. Rubello D, Pozzan GB, Casara D, et al. Natural course of subclinical hypothyroidism in Down's syndrome: prospective study results and therapeutic considerations. *J Endocrinol Invest* 1995;18:35.
18. Gray RS, Borsey DQ, Seth J, et al. Prevalence of subclinical thyroid failure in insulin-dependent diabetes. *J Clin Endocrinol Metab* 1980;50:1034.
19. Klein RZ, Haddow JE, Faix JD, et al. Prevalence of thyroid deficiency in pregnant women. *Clin Endocrinol (Oxf)* 1991;35:41.
20. Vanderpump MJP, Tunbridge WMG, French JM, et al. The incidence of thyroid disorders in the community: a twenty-year follow-up of the Whickham Survey. *Clin Endocrinol (Oxf)* 1995;43:55.
21. Huber G, Staub JJ, Meier C, et al. Prospective study of the spontaneous course of subclinical hypothyroidism: prognostic value of thyrotropin, thyroid reserve, and thyroid antibodies. *J Clin Endocrinol Metab* 2002;87:3221.
22. Rosenthal MJ, Hunt WC, Garry PJ, et al. Thyroid failure in the elderly: microsomal antibodies as discriminant for therapy. *JAMA* 1987;258:209.
23. Kabadi UM. "Subclinical hypothyroidism": natural course of the syndrome during a prolonged follow-up study. *Arch Intern Med* 1993;153:957.
24. Romaldini JH, Biancalana MM, Figueiredo DI, et al. Effect of L-thyroxine administration on antithyroid antibody levels, lipid profile, and thyroid volume in patients with Hashimoto's thyroiditis. *Thyroid* 1996;6:183.
25. Cooper DS, Halpern R, Wood LC, et al. L-thyroxine therapy in subclinical hypothyroidism: a double-blind, placebo-controlled trial. *Ann Intern Med* 1984;101:18.
26. Billewicz WZ, Chapman RS, Crooks J, et al. Statistical methods applied to the diagnosis of hypothyroidism. *QJM* 1969;38:255.
27. Nystrom E, Caidahl K, Fager G, et al. A double-blind cross-over 12-month study of L-thyroxine treatment of women with "subclinical" hypothyroidism. *Clin Endocrinol (Oxf)* 1988;29:63.
28. Jaeschke R, Guyatt G, Gerstein H, et al. Does treatment with L-thyroxine influence health status in middle-aged and older adults with subclinical hypothyroidism? *J Gen Intern Med* 1996;11:744.
29. Meier C, Staub JJ, Roth CB, et al. TSH-controlled L-thyroxine therapy reduces cholesterol levels and clinical symptoms in subclinical hypothyroidism: a double blind, placebo-controlled trial (Basel Thyroid Study). *J Clin Endocrinol Metab* 2001;86:4860.
30. Kong WM, Sheikh MH, Lumb PJ, et al. A 6-month randomized trial of thyroxine treatment in women with mild subclinical hypothyroidism. *Am J Med* 2002;112:348.
31. Caraccio N, Ferrannini E, Monzani F. Lipoprotein profile in subclinical hypothyroidism: response to levothyroxine replacement, a randomized placebo-controlled study. *J Clin Endocrinol Metab* 2002;87:1533.
32. Monzani F, Di Bello V, Caraccio N, et al. Effect of levothyroxine on cardiac function and structure in subclinical hypothyroidism: a double blind, placebo controlled study. *J Clin Endocrinol Metab* 2001;86:1110.
33. Christ-Crain M, Meier C, Guglielmetti M, et al. Elevated C-reactive protein and homocysteine values: cardiovascular risk factors in hypothyroidism? A cross-sectional and a double-blind, placebo-controlled trial. *Atherosclerosis* 2003;166:379.
34. Kanaya AM, Harris F, Volpato S, et al. Association between thyroid dysfunction and total cholesterol level in an older biracial population: the health, aging and body composition study. *Arch Intern Med* 2002;162:773.
35. Canaris GJ, Manowitz NR, Mayor G, et al. The Colorado thyroid disease prevalence study. *Arch Intern Med* 2000;160:526.
36. Efstathiadou E, Bitsis S, Milionis HJ, et al. Lipid profile in subclinical hypothyroidism: is L-thyroxine substitution beneficial? *Eur J Endocrinol* 2001;145:705.
37. Kung AWC, Pang RWC, Janus ED. Elevated serum lipoprotein(a) in subclinical hypothyroidism. *Clin Endocrinol (Oxf)* 1995;43:445.
38. Yildirimkaya M, Ozata M, Yilmaz K, et al. Lipoprotein(a) concentration in subclinical hypothyroidism before and after levothyroxine therapy. *Endocr J* 1996;46:731.

39. Althaus BU, Staub JJ, Ryff-de Leche A, et al. LDL/HDL-changes in subclinical hypothyroidism: possible risk factors for coronary artery disease. *Clin Endocrinol (Oxf)* 1988;28:157.

40. Bigos ST, Ridgway EC, Kourides IA, et al. Spectrum of pituitary alterations with mild and severe thyroid impairment. *J Clin Endocrinol Metab* 1978;46:317.

41. Parle JV, Franklyn JA, Cross KW, et al. Circulating lipids and minor abnormalities of thyroid function. *Clin Endocrinol (Oxf)* 1992;37:411.

42. Bogner U, Arntz H-R, Peters H, et al. Subclinical hypothyroidism and hyperlipoproteinaemia: indiscriminate L-thyroxine treatment not justified. *Acta Endocrinol* 1993;128:202.

43. Caron PH, Calazel C, Parra HJ, et al. Decreased HDL cholesterol in subclinical hypothyroidism: the effect of L-thyroxine therapy. *Clin Endocrinol (Copenh)* 1990;33:519.

44. Staub J-J, Althaus BU, Engler H, et al. Spectrum of subclinical and overt hypothyroidism: effect on thyrotropin, prolactin, and thyroid reserve, and metabolic impact on peripheral target tissues. *Am J Med* 1992;92:631.

45. Tzotzas T, Krassas GE, Konstantinidis T, et al. Changes in lipoprotein (a) levels in overt and subclinical hypothyroidism before and during treatment. *Thyroid* 2000;10:803.

46. Luboshitzky R, Aviv A, Herer P, et al. Risk factors for cardiovascular disease in women with subclinical hypothyroidism. *Thyroid* 2002;12:421.

47. Vierhapper H, Nardi A, Grosser P, et al Low-density lipoprotein cholesterol in subclinical hypothyroidism. *Thyroid* 2000;10:981.

48. Arem R, Escalante DA, Arem N, et al. Effect of L-thyroxine therapy on lipoprotein fractions in overt and subclinical hypothyroidism, with special reference to lipoprotein(a). *Metabolism* 1995;44:1559.

49. Bell GM, Todd WTA, Forfar JC, et al. End-organ responses to thyroxine therapy in subclinical hypothyroidism. *Clin Endocrinol (Oxf)* 1985;22:83.

50. Lithell H, Boberg J, Hellsing K, et al. Serum lipoprotein and apolipoprotein concentrations and tissue lipoprotein-lipase activity in overt and subclinical hypothyroidism: the effect of substitution therapy. *Eur J Clin Invest* 1981;11:3.

51. Ridgway EC, Cooper DS, Walker H, et al. Peripheral responses to thyroid hormone before and after L-thyroxine therapy in patients with subclinical hypothyroidism. *J Clin Endocrinol Metab* 1981;53:1238.

52. Arem R, Patsch W. Lipoprotein and apolipoprotein levels in subclinical hypothyroidism: effect of levothyroxine therapy. *Arch Intern Med* 1990;150:2097.

53. Franklyn JA, Daykin J, Betteridge J, et al. Thyroxine replacement therapy and circulating lipid concentrations. *Clin Endocrinol (Oxf)* 1993;38:453.

54. Danese M, Ladenson P, Meinert C, et al. Effect of thyroxine therapy on serum lipoproteins in patients with mild thyroid failure: a quantitative review of the literature. *J Clin Endocrinol Metab* 2000;85:2993.

55. Tanis BC, Westendorp RGJ, Smelt AHM. Effect of thyroid substitution on hypercholesterolaemia in patients with subclinical hypothyroidism: a reanalysis of intervention studies. *Clin Endocrinol (Oxf)* 1996;44:643.

56. Diekman T, Lansberg PJ, Kastelein JJ, et al. Prevalence and correction of hypothyroidism in a large cohort of patients referred for dyslipidemia. *Arch Intern Med* 1995;155:1490.

57. Michalopoulou G, Alevizaki M, Piperingos G, et al. High serum cholesterol levels in persons with "high-normal" TSH levels: should one extend the definition of subclinical hypothyroidism? *Eur J Endocrinol* 1998;138:141.

58. Milionis HJ, Efstathiadou Z, Tselepis AD, et al. Lipoprotein (a) levels and apolipoprotein (a) isoform size in patients with subclinical hypothyroidism: effect of treatment with levothyroxine. *Thyroid* 2003;13:365.

59. Hak AE, Pols HA, Visser TJ, et al. Subclinical hypothyroidism is an independent risk factor for atherosclerosis and myocardial infarction in elderly women: the Rotterdam Study. *Ann Intern Med* 2000;132:270.

60. Bough EW, Crowley WF, Ridgway EC, et al. Myocardial function in hypothyroidism: relation to disease severity and response to treatment. *Arch Intern Med* 1978;138:1476.

61. Arem R, Rokey R, Kiefe C, et al. Cardiac systolic and diastolic function at rest and exercise in subclinical hypothyroidism: effect of thyroid hormone therapy. *Thyroid* 1996;6:397.

62. Ooi TC, Whitlock RML, Frengley PA, et al. Systolic time intervals and ankle reflex time in patients with minimal serum TSH elevation: response to triiodothyronine therapy. *Clin Endocrinol (Oxf)* 1980;13:621.

63. Biondi B, Fazio S, Palmieri EA, et al. Left ventricular diastolic dysfunction in patients with subclinical hypothyroidism. *J Clin Endocrinol Metab* 1999;84:2064.

64. Vitale G, Galderisi M, Lupoli GA, et al. Left ventricular myocardial impairment in subclinical hypothyroidism assessed by a new ultrasound tool: pulsed tissue Doppler. *J Clin Endocrinol Metab* 2002;87:4350.

65. Brenta G, Mutti LA, Schnitman M, et al. Assessment of left ventricular diastolic function by radionuclide ventriculography at rest and exercise in subclinical hypothyroidism, and its response to L-thyroxine therapy. *Am J Cardiol* 2003;91:1327.

66. Forfar JC, Wathen CG, Todd WTA, et al. Left ventricular performance in subclinical hypothyroidism. *QJM* 1985;57:857.

67. Faber J, Peterson L, Wiinberg N, et al. Hemodynamic changes after levothyroxine treatment in subclinical hypothyroidism. *Thyroid* 2002;12:319.

68. Tappy L, Randin JP, Schwed P, et al. Prevalence of thyroid disorders in psychogeriatric inpatients: a possible relationship of hypothyroidism with neurotic depression but not with dementia. *J Am Geriatr Soc* 1987;35:526.

69. Joffe RT, Levitt AJ. Major depression and subclinical (grade 2) hypothyroidism. *Psychoneuroendocrinology* 1992;17:215.

70. Haggerty JJ, Stern RA, Mason GA, et al. Subclinical hypothyroidism: a modifiable risk factor for depression? *Am J Psychiatry* 1993;150:508.

71. Monzani F, Del Guerra P, Caraccio N, et al. Subclinical hypothyroidism: neurobehavioral features and beneficial effect of L-thyroxine treatment. *Clin Invest* 1993;71:367.

72. Baldini IM, Vita A, Mauri MC, et al. Psychopathological and cognitive features in subclinical hypothyroidism. *Prog Neuropsychopharmacol Biol Psychiatry* 1997;21:925.

73. Casper RF, Patel-Christopher A, Powell AM. Thyrotropin and prolactin responses to thyrotropin-releasing hormone in premenstrual syndrome. *J Clin Endocrinol Metab* 1989;68:608.

74. Goulis DG, Tsimpiris N, Delaroudis S, et al. Stapedial reflex: a biological index found to be abnormal in clinical and subclinical hypothyroidism. *Thyroid* 1998;8:583.

75. Ozata M, Ozkardes A, Corakci A, et al. Subclinical hypothyroidism does not lead to alterations either in peripheral nerves or in brainstem auditory evoked potentials (BAEPs). *Thyroid* 1995;5:201.

76. Misiunas A, Niepomniszce H, Ravera B, et al. Peripheral neuropathy in subclinical hypothyroidism. *Thyroid* 1995;5:283.

77. Monzani F, Caraccio N, Siciliano G, et al. Clinical and biochemical features of muscle dysfunction in subclinical hypothyroidism. *J Clin Endocrinol Metab* 1997;82:3315.

78. Monzani F, Caraccio N, Del Guerra P, et al. Neuromuscular symptoms and dysfunction in subclinical hypothyroid patients:

beneficial effect of L-T$_4$ replacement therapy. *Clin Endocrinol (Oxf)* 1999;51:237.

79. Centanni M, Cesareo R, Verallo O, et al. Reversible increase of intraocular pressure in subclinical hypothyroid patients. *Eur J Endocrinol* 1997;136:595.

80. Taddei S, Caraccio N, Virdis A, et al. Impaired endothelium-dependent vasodilatation in subclinical hypothyroidism: beneficial effect of levothyroxine therapy. *J Clin Endocrinol Metab* 2003; 88:3731.

81. Deicher R, Vierhapper H. Homocysteine: a risk factor for cardiovascular disease in subclinical hypothyroidism? *Thyroid* 2002;12:733.

82. Ross DS. Bone density is not reduced during the short-term administration of levothyroxine to postmenopausal women with subclinical hypothyroidism: a randomized, prospective study. *Am J Med* 1993;95:385.

83. Haddow JE, Palomaki GE, Allan WC, et al. Maternal thyroid deficiency during pregnancy and subsequent neuropsychological development of the child. *N Engl J Med* 1999;341:549.

84. Chu JW, Crapo LM. The treatment of subclinical hypothyroidism is seldom necessary. *J Clin Endocrinol Metab* 2001;86: 4591.

SUBCLINICAL THYROTOXICOSIS

DOUGLAS S. ROSS

The introduction of serum thyrotropin (TSH) measurements into clinical practice during the early 1970s provided the necessary tool for defining subclinical hypothyroidism, although it took several years for our present understanding and an accepted definition of this entity to evolve (see Chapter 78). Similarly, the introduction in the 1980s of sensitive immunometric TSH assays allowed detection of subnormal serum TSH values in patients with no symptoms or signs of thyrotoxicosis. Subclinical thyrotoxicosis is best defined as a low serum TSH concentration and normal serum free thyroxine (T_4) and triiodothyronine (T_3) concentrations associated with few or no symptoms or signs of thyrotoxicosis. Patients with low serum TSH concentrations who have high serum free thyroid hormone concentrations are defined as having overt thyrotoxicosis. Before the introduction of sensitive assays for serum TSH, subclinical thyrotoxicosis could be demonstrated by the finding of blunted responses of serum TSH after administration of thyrotropin-releasing hormone (TRH). Now, however, TRH testing is not necessary because serum TSH responses to TRH are usually proportional to basal serum TSH concentrations. The studies reviewed in this chapter document the biologic importance of subclinical thyrotoxicosis; however, no consensus has been reached regarding the indications for treatment.

ETIOLOGY

The major causes of subclinical thyrotoxicosis are similar to those of overt thyrotoxicosis (Table 79.1). Conceptually, there are two groups of patients: those who have subclinical thyrotoxicosis caused by exogenous thyroid hormone therapy and those in whom it is caused by slight endogenous overproduction of T_4 and T_3.

Exogenous Subclinical Thyrotoxicosis

As many as 10 million people in the United States, and perhaps as many as 200 million people worldwide, are taking thyroid hormone and are therefore at risk for subclinical thyrotoxicosis because of either overzealous replacement therapy or intentional suppressive therapy. When sensitive methods for measuring serum TSH first became available, an estimated 40% to 50% of patients taking T_4 replacement therapy had subnormal serum TSH concentrations (1), but the proportion has diminished as a result of the use of these assays to monitor therapy and recognition of the potential dangers of overreplacement. Patients with thyroid cancer, thyroid nodules, or multinodular or diffuse goiter who are treated with T_4 to suppress TSH secretion to below normal have subclinical (if not overt) thyrotoxicosis. In these patients, the benefits of TSH suppression are considered to exceed the potential risks of subclinical thyrotoxicosis.

Endogenous Subclinical Thyrotoxicosis

The most common causes of endogenous subclinical thyrotoxicosis include multinodular goiter, autonomously functioning thyroid adenomas, Graves' disease, and subacute lymphocytic and subacute granulomatous thyroiditis (2). In one study, 6 of 15 patients had "patchy or irregular" uptake on thyroid radionuclide imaging, suggesting multinodular goiter and the possibility of autonomous thyroid secretion (3). Low serum TSH concentrations also have been found in apparently healthy people who had no evidence of thyroid disease.

The prevalence of autonomously functioning adenomas and multinodular goiter varies considerably from one region of the world to another. This variation is the result of differences in dietary iodine intake and perhaps also genetic differences. For example, in a U.S. study, the ratio of patients with thyrotoxicosis caused by an autonomously functioning adenoma to those with thyrotoxicosis caused by Graves' disease was 1:50 (4), whereas in Switzerland it was 1:2 (5); the ratios for subclinical thyrotoxicosis are probably similar. In Europe, 22% of patients with nontoxic multinodular goiter had blunted serum TSH responses to TRH consistent with subclinical thyrotoxicosis, and 28% had autonomous areas on thyroid radionuclide imaging (6). Subclinical thyrotoxicosis also occurs in patients with Graves' disease; they include patients who had overt thyrotoxicosis and are asymptomatic after radioiodine or surgical treatment, patients who remain asymptomatic (are in remission) after a course of antithyroid drug therapy, and

TABLE 79.1. COMMON CAUSES OF SUBCLINICAL THYROTOXICOSIS

Exogenous subclinical thyrotoxicosis
  Overzealous thyroid hormone replacement therapy
  Thyroid hormone suppressive therapy
Endogenous subclinical thyrotoxicosis
  Thyroid gland autonomy
    Autonomously functioning thyroid adenomas
    Multinodular goiter
  Graves' disease
    After radioiodine or surgical treatment
    During remission after antithyroid drug therapy
    Euthyroid (ophthalmic) Graves' disease
TSH suppression not associated with subclinical thyrotoxicosis
  Central hypothyroidism
  Severe nonthyroidal illness, glucocorticoid or dopamine
    therapy
  After treatment of thyrotoxicosis, before recovery of the
    pituitary–thyroid axis
  Interference of high serum human chorionic gonadotropin
    concentrations in immunometric assays for TSH
  Laboratory error

TSH, thyrotropin.

those with only ophthalmic manifestations of Graves' disease. For example, 64% of a group of Japanese patients with Graves' ophthalmopathy but no symptoms of thyrotoxicosis had subnormal serum TSH responses to TRH (7), and in another study 4% of patients with Graves' thyrotoxicosis in apparent remission were found to have subclinical thyrotoxicosis (by TRH testing) (8). It is likely that Graves' disease is the cause of subclinical thyrotoxicosis in some patients who have no history of thyroid disease and little or no thyroid enlargement (2). Patients with subacute lymphocytic thyroiditis (painless or silent thyroiditis and postpartum thyroiditis) may present with subclinical thyrotoxicosis (2), and it also occurs in patients with subacute granulomatous thyroiditis. The thyrotropic activity of high serum chorionic gonadotropin concentrations during early pregnancy also may cause a transient increase in serum free T_4 and T_3 concentrations within the normal range and low serum TSH concentrations (9).

Differential Diagnosis

There are other causes of low serum TSH concentrations, but many of the patients have abnormal serum T_4 and T_3 concentrations (Table 79.1). Patients with pituitary or hypothalamic disease who have hypothyroidism may have low serum TSH concentrations, and the concentrations are often low in patients with severe nonthyroidal illness, especially those receiving glucocorticoid or dopamine therapy (10). Low serum TSH concentrations may be associated with low or normal serum T_4 and T_3 concentrations shortly after treatment or spontaneous resolution of overt thyrotoxicosis because of persistent suppression of TSH secretion.

EPIDEMIOLOGY AND NATURAL HISTORY

In the United States, among 13,344 people with no known thyroid disease in the National Health and Nutrition Examination Survey (NHANES III), 0.7% had subclinical thyrotoxicosis (11). In a Swedish community-based study of 2000 people attending a medical clinic, 3.3% had low serum TSH concentrations without overt thyrotoxicosis (12); only 9% of the subjects with subclinical thyrotoxicosis had thyroid abnormalities (e.g., multinodular goiter, thyroiditis), and 40% had a normal serum TSH concentration on recall a few weeks later. In a U.S. study of 968 subjects over 55 years of age, 0.7% had endogenous subclinical thyrotoxicosis (13). In another U.S. study, 46 of 2411 subjects (1.9%) over 60 years of age had subclinical thyrotoxicosis, with serum TSH values less than 0.1 mU/L (14); during a 4-year follow-up period, only two developed overt thyrotoxicosis, and serum TSH concentrations became normal in most of the remainder. In a similar study from England, 6.3% of women and 5.5% of men had low serum TSH concentrations (< 0.5 mU/L); a year later, the serum TSH values were normal in 60% of these subjects, and only one (1.5%) had overt thyrotoxicosis (15). In Sweden, 1.8% of 886 subjects 85 years of age or older had subclinical thyrotoxicosis (16). Thus, the prevalence of subclinical thyrotoxicosis in the community has varied from 0.7% to 6.0%, depending on the criteria used and the age of the population. More than half of these subjects, especially those with slightly low serum TSH values, had normal values when retested during follow-up, and few developed thyrotoxicosis (see Chapter 19).

Although no long-term studies of the natural history of subclinical thyrotoxicosis have been reported, data are available regarding the natural history of autonomously functioning thyroid adenomas. In a U.S. study, 8.8% of initially euthyroid patients with these tumors developed overt thyrotoxicosis during a 6-year follow-up period (4); in a European study, 18% of patients developed overt thyrotoxicosis during a 7-year follow-up period (17).

BIOLOGIC IMPORTANCE

Although suppression of TSH secretion defines subclinical thyrotoxicosis, the increases in serum free thyroid hormone concentrations that cause the suppression may also cause symptoms suggestive of thyrotoxicosis and may have effects on other tissues similar to but less marked than those of overt thyrotoxicosis. Both the pituitary and the systemic effects of the increases are considered here.

PHYSIOLOGY OF SUPPRESSION OF TSH SECRETION

The negative feedback relationship between serum TSH and free T_4 (and T_3) concentrations is log-linear. Therefore, very small increases in endogenous thyroid hormone production, or only slightly excessive doses of the exogenous thyroid hormone, decrease serum TSH concentrations to below the normal range (18) (see Regulation of Thyrotropin Secretion, Chapter 10D). Groups of patients with low serum TSH concentrations who receive slightly excessive doses of T_4 have serum T_4 and T_3 concentrations greater than the mean values for normal subjects but within the respective normal ranges. Presently, most clinicians accept serum TSH measurements as the most sensitive indicator of thyroid hormone status (in the absence of pituitary or hypothalamic disease). Several findings, however, raise the question of whether this is always the case. In laboratory animals, intrapituitary deiodination of T_4 to T_3, a reaction that is catalyzed primarily by type 2 T_4-5'-deiodinase (see Chapter 7), contributes more of the T_3 bound to the T_3 nuclear receptors, and serum T_3 contributes less, compared with most other organs (19). Hence, the extent of T_3-induced inhibition, or lack thereof, of TSH secretion, may vary somewhat independently of the serum T_3 concentration. In addition, the concentrations of the different isoforms of the T_3 nuclear receptor are different in the pituitary and peripheral organs (see Chapter 8), and these concentrations are altered discordantly in states of thyroid hormone excess or deficiency (20). Some euthyroid elderly patients with low serum T_4 and normal serum TSH concentrations appear to have a decreased set point for T_4- and T_3-mediated feedback inhibition of TSH secretion (21). Finally, some patients with hypothyroidism feel better subjectively when they are given a slightly higher dose of T_4 than that needed to normalize their TSH secretion (18).

BONE AND MINERAL METABOLISM

Thyroid hormone has a direct resorptive effect on bone, and overt thyrotoxicosis is associated with increased bone resorption and, to a lesser extent, increased bone formation and an increase in fracture rate (22) (Table 79.2). Cortical bone is affected more than trabecular bone. In two studies patients with nodular goiter and subclinical thyrotoxicosis had lower bone density than comparable normal subjects (23,24), although in one study significant reductions in bone density occurred only in sites rich in cortical bone in postmenopausal women (24), and in a study of 15 premenopausal women bone density was not reduced (25). In two nonrandomized trials, postmenopausal women with nodular goiter and subclinical thyrotoxicosis treated with an antithyroid drug (26) or radioiodine (27) had higher

bone density after 2 years than similar women who were not treated. Serum concentrations of osteocalcin, a marker of bone formation, are high in patients with subclinical thyrotoxicosis and are inversely correlated with serum TSH concentrations (28).

Whether T_4 therapy in doses that result in subclinical thyrotoxicosis causes low bone density is controversial. Bone density may be low in premenopausal women receiving suppressive or overzealous replacement doses, but women receiving lower but still suppressive or slightly excessive replacement doses have normal bone density (22, 29). As in endogenous subclinical thyrotoxicosis, bone density more often is reduced at sites rich in cortical bone (e.g., wrist and hip) than sites rich in trabecular bone (e.g., lumbar spine), and postmenopausal women are more likely to be affected than premenopausal women (22). A meta-analysis concluded that low bone density occurs only in postmenopausal women (30). The adverse effect of T_4 on bone density is associated with doses in excess of 1.6 µg/kg (31). Estrogen therapy appears to protect against T_4-induced bone loss in postmenopausal women (31). In a study of postmenopausal women taking T_4 who had subclinical thyrotoxicosis, bone density increased when the T_4 dose was reduced and serum TSH concentrations increased to normal (32).

Other measures of bone turnover, in addition to serum osteocalcin, are abnormal in patients who have subclinical thyrotoxicosis. Urinary excretion of bone collagen–derived pyridinoline cross-links and hydroxyproline (33,34) and serum concentrations of carboxyl-terminal-1-telopeptide, markers of bone resorption, are increased (35). In women with thyroid cancer receiving T_4 suppression therapy, serum C-terminal telopeptide and osteocalcin concentrations and urinary excretion of N-terminal telopeptide of type I collagen were high in those who were postmenopausal, but not those who were premenopausal (36). Among patients with Graves' thyrotoxicosis treated with an antithyroid drug who had normal serum T_4 and T_3 concentrations, those who had persistently low serum TSH concentrations had higher serum alkaline phosphatase concentrations and urinary excretion of pyridinoline cross-links as compared with those who had normal serum TSH concentrations (37). Serum osteocalcin and TSH concentrations are also inversely correlated in patients with exogenous subclinical thyrotoxicosis (38).

Data regarding the risk for fracture in patients with subclinical thyrotoxicosis are still preliminary. In one study of women over 65 years of age, the overall fracture rate was 0.9% in those with normal serum TSH values, and it was 2.5% in those with low values; this difference was not statistically significant (39). An interview-based study did not find an increased fracture risk in women taking T_4 (40). In a third study, the risk for hip fracture was increased 1.6 times in women taking thyroid hormone; serum TSH val-

TABLE 79.2. BIOLOGIC EFFECTS OF SUBCLINICAL THYROTOXICOSIS

Measurements Reported to Be Abnormal	Change	References
Skeletal effects		
Bone density	↓	23,30,31
Biochemical markers of bone mineral metabolism		
Serum osteocalcin	↑	28,38
Urinary excretion of bone collagen–derived pyridinoline cross-links	↑	33
Urinary excretion of hydroxyproline	↑	34
Serum carboxyl-terminal-1-telopeptide	↑	35
Cardiac effects	↑	48,49
Heart rate	↑	49
Premature atrial contractions	↑	43–45
Risk of atrial fibrillation	↑	49
Cardiac contractility		
Systolic time intervals		
Preejection period divided by LV ejection time	↓	51,52
Isovolumetric contraction time	↓	49,50
Isovolumetric relaxation time	↑	56
Left ventricular mass index, intraventricular septal, and posterior wall thickness	↑	49,56
Left ventricular diastolic filling	↓	54
Exercise tolerance and maximal oxygen uptake	↓	56
Mortality from circulatory disease	↑	59
Other effects		
Serum total and low-density lipoprotein cholesterol	↓	60
Erythrocyte ouabain-binding capacity	↓	61
Serum alanine aminotransferase, glutathione S-transferase, and γ-glutamyl transferase	↑	62
Serum creatine kinase	↓	62
Ratios of urinary sodium excretion and urine flow during the day to those in the night[a]	↓	48
Serum sex hormone–binding globulin	↑	28,30
Time asleep at night	↓	64
Hyperthyroid symptoms (Short Form 36 Health Survey)	↑	65
Mood (using multidimensional scale for state of well-being)	↑	64
Dementia	↑	66

[a]Urine sodium excretion and flow rate are increased at night in patients with overt thyrotoxicosis.

ues were not reported (41). Finally, in a study of postmenopausal women with serum TSH concentrations of 0.1 mU/L or lower, there was an increased risk for both hip and vertebral fracture; however, serum T_4 was not measured, so the proportion of patients with overt thyrotoxicosis is unknown (42).

CARDIAC FUNCTION

The risk for atrial fibrillation is increased in patients with subclinical thyrotoxicosis (Table 79.2). In a community-based study of 2007 subjects 60 years of age or older followed for 10 years, the cumulative incidence of atrial fibrillation was 28% among those with serum TSH concentrations of 0.1 mU/L or less, 16% among those with serum TSH concentrations greater than 0.1 to 0.4 mU/L, and 11% among those with normal serum TSH concentra-

tions (43); the relative risk for atrial fibrillation was three-fold higher in the group with the lowest serum TSH concentrations. In a study of hospitalized patients, 13% of 613 patients with subclinical thyrotoxicosis, 14% of 725 patients with overt thyrotoxicosis, and 2% of 22,300 euthyroid patients had atrial fibrillation (44). In a study of 80 patients, the prevalence of atrial fibrillation was two times higher in those with subclinical thyrotoxicosis, as compared with matched control patients with normal serum TSH concentrations (45), and during a 2-year follow-up period, 9% of the patients with subclinical thyrotoxicosis developed atrial fibrillation, as compared with none of the control group.

Patients presenting with atrial fibrillation may prove to have subclinical thyrotoxicosis. Of 126 consecutive patients presenting to a hospital with atrial fibrillation, 2 had overt thyrotoxicosis, and 13 (10%) had subclinical thyrotoxicosis (46). The arrhythmia may remit with antithyroid therapy (47). Subclinical thyrotoxicosis is also associated with an increase in heart rate and an increase in atrial premature beats (48,49).

Both cardiac contractility and left ventricular hypertrophy may be increased in patients with exogenous subclinical thyrotoxicosis. Echocardiography reveals higher values for the percentage of fractional shortening and the rate-adjusted mean velocity of shortening, and a reduction in the isovolumetric contraction time (the time between mitral value closure and aortic value opening) (49,50). Systolic time intervals, measured as the ratio of the preejection period to the left ventricular ejection time (PEP:LVET ratio), also are reduced in patients with subclinical thyrotoxicosis (51,52). Left ventricular mass index, the thickness of the intraventricular septum, and left ventricular posterior wall thickness are all increased in patients with subclinical thyrotoxicosis (49). The increase in left ventricular mass index is proportional to the duration of subclinical thyrotoxicosis (49), and it is prevented by β-adrenergic blocking drugs (53). Impaired left ventricular diastolic filling, which is associated with reduced exercise capacity, is found in some patients with subclinical thyrotoxicosis and also is prevented by β-adrenergic blocking drugs (54). These results suggest that subclinical thyrotoxicosis could aggravate angina pectoris or congestive heart failure, although there are no data that address these possibilities. These measurements of cardiac function have not been abnormal in all studies (55), and most of the studies in which abnormalities were found were conducted in patients who had serum TSH concentrations well below 0.1 mU/L. In one study (56), significant abnormalities in left ventricular mass index, end-diastolic dimension, exercise tolerance, and maximal oxygen uptake at peak exercise became normal after the dose of T_4 was reduced and serum TSH concentrations increased to approximately 0.1 mU/L.

In two small studies in patients with endogenous subclinical thyrotoxicosis, cardiac function improved after antithyroid treatment (57,58). In one study, 10 patients treated with methimazole had a lower heart rate, fewer atrial premature beats, and a reduction of left ventricular mass index, interventricular septum thickness, and left ventricular posterior wall thickness when their serum TSH concentrations increased to normal (57). In the other study, six patients treated with radioiodine had a decrease in heart rate and cardiac output and an increase in systemic vascular resistance when their serum TSH concentrations returned to normal (58).

Subclinical thyrotoxicosis may be associated with increased mortality. In a population-based study of 1191 subjects 60 years of age or older who were not taking T_4, 10-year mortality was increased among those with low serum TSH concentrations, primarily due to a twofold increase in the standardized mortality ratio from cardiovascular diseases (59) (see Chapter 77). Thyroid hormone therapy was associated with an increased risk for ischemic heart disease in patients under 65 years of age, but this did not

correlate with their serum TSH concentrations (39). This observation may reflect undertreatment or poor compliance with thyroid hormone therapy, because subclinical hypothyroidism is associated with high serum lipid concentrations (see Chapter 78), whereas patients with subclinical thyrotoxicosis tend to have low serum lipid concentrations (60).

OTHER MEASUREMENTS

Other clinical, biochemical, and physiologic measurements that are often abnormal in patients with overt thyrotoxicosis may be abnormal in patients with subclinical thyrotoxicosis. The numbers of sodium pump sites on erythrocytes, estimated by measuring ouabain-binding capacity, were reduced by 15% in patients with exogenous subclinical thyrotoxicosis (61). Serum alanine aminotransferase, glutathione S-transferase, and γ-glutamyl transferase values may be high (62). Serum creatine kinase concentrations may be low (62). The ratios of urinary sodium excretion and urine flow during the day to those during the night are decreased (48). Serum sex hormone–binding globulin concentrations may be high in patients with either endogenous or exogenous subclinical thyrotoxicosis (28,63). Patients with subclinical thyrotoxicosis sleep less than normal subjects and have a better mood (64). In the standardized Short Form 36 Health Survey, patients with exogenous subclinical thyrotoxicosis had more symptoms consistent with thyroid hormone excess (65). Finally, in a population-based study of 1843 elderly Dutch subjects, subclinical thyrotoxicosis was associated with a threefold increased risk for dementia (66).

PREVENTION AND TREATMENT

Both low bone density and an increased risk for atrial fibrillation may result in substantial morbidity in older patients with subclinical thyrotoxicosis. These and other adverse effects of exogenous subclinical thyrotoxicosis can and should be avoided or minimized by careful titration of thyroid hormone therapy using serum TSH measurements. Patients who are receiving T_4 replacement therapy should have the dose adjusted to maintain a normal serum TSH concentration. Subclinical thyrotoxicosis cannot be avoided in patients treated with T_4 to decrease goiter size, prevent recurrent goiter, or prevent recurrence or minimize growth of thyroid carcinoma. The efficacy of suppressive therapy of goiter or thyroid nodules is controversial (see Chapter 73) (67), and data that support specific goals for serum TSH concentrations are contradictory. In one study of patients with a nodular goiter, the nodules were more likely to regress if serum TSH concentrations were reduced to less than 0.1 mU/L (68), while in another study the response to T_4 was similar in patients whose serum TSH concentrations were reduced to 0.4 to 0.6 mU/L and those whose concentrations were reduced to less than 0.01 mU/L (69). Many thyroidologists suggest giving sufficient T_4 to lower serum TSH concentrations to slightly low values in patients with benign thyroid diseases and to lower values (e.g., <0.05 mU/L) only in patients with thyroid cancer who have recurrent local or metastatic disease.

Few data are available to guide clinical decisions regarding the treatment of patients with endogenous subclinical thyrotoxicosis. However, the studies reviewed previously demonstrate that antithyroid drug or radioiodine therapy increases bone density in postmenopausal women with subclinical thyrotoxicosis (26,27), and it improves several measures of cardiac function in most patients with subclinical thyrotoxicosis (57,58). These results suggest that cardiac status and skeletal integrity should be carefully assessed, and the possible coexistence of other risk factors for cardiac disease and osteoporosis should be determined in patients with subclinical thyrotoxicosis. Treatment should be seriously considered in those patients considered at risk, especially those whose serum TSH concentrations are very low (e.g., <0.1 mU/L).

REFERENCES

1. Ross DS, Ardisson LJ, Meskell MJ. Measurement of thyrotropin in clinical and subclinical thyrotoxicosis using a new chemiluminescent assay. *J Clin Endocrinol Metab* 1989;69:684.
2. Charkes ND. The many causes of subclinical thyrotoxicosis. *Thyroid* 1996;6:391.
3. Stott DJ, McLellan AR, Finlayson J, et al. Elderly patients with suppressed serum TSH but normal free thyroid hormone levels usually have mild thyroid overactivity and are at increased risk of developing overt thyrotoxicosis. *QJM* 1991;78:77.
4. Hamburger JI. Evolution of toxicity in solitary nontoxic autonomously functioning thyroid nodules. *J Clin Endocrinol Metab* 1980;50:1089.
5. Horst W, Rosler H, Schneider C, et al. Three hundred six cases of toxic adenoma. *J Nucl Med* 1967;8:515.
6. Rieu M, Bekka S, Sambor B, et al. Prevalence of subclinical thyrotoxicosis and relationship between thyroid hormonal status and thyroid ultrasonographic parameters in patients with nontoxic nodular goitre. *Clin Endocrinol (Oxf)* 1993;39:67.
7. Kasagi K, Hatabu H, Tokuda Y, et al. Studies on thyrotropin receptor antibodies in patients with euthyroid Graves' disease. *Clin Endocrinol (Oxf)* 1988;29:357.
8. Murakami M, Koizumi Y, Aizawa T, et al. Studies of thyroid function and immune parameters in patients with hyperthyroid Graves' disease in remission. *J Clin Endocrinol Metab* 1988; 66:103.
9. Glinoer D, De Nayer P, Bourdoux P, et al. Regulation of maternal thyroid during pregnancy. *J Clin Endocrinol Metab* 1990; 71:276.
10. Spencer C, Eigen A, Shen D, et al. Specificity of sensitive assays of thyrotropin (TSH) used to screen for thyroid disease in hospitalized patients. *Clin Chem* 1987;33:1391.
11. Hollowell JG, Staehling NW, Flanders WD, et al. Serum TSH, T4, and thyroid antibodies in the United States population (1988 to 1994): National Health and Nutrition Examination Survey (NHANES III). *J Clin Endocrinol Metab* 2002;87:489.
12. Eggertsen R, Petersen K, Lundberg P-A, et al. Screening for thyroid disease in a primary care unit with a thyroid stimulating hormone assay with a low detection limit. *BMJ* 1988;297:1586.
13. Bagchi N, Brown TR, Parish RF. Thyroid dysfunction in adults over age 55 years: a study in an urban U.S. community. *Arch Intern Med* 1990;150:785.
14. Sawin CT, Geller A, Kaplan MM, et al. Low serum thyrotropin (thyroid stimulating hormone) in older patients without thyrotoxicosis. *Arch Intern Med* 1991;151:165.
15. Parle JV, Franklyn JA, Cross KW, et al. Prevalence and follow-up of abnormal thyrotropin (TSH) concentrations in the elderly in the United Kingdom. *Clin Endocrinol (Oxf)* 1991;34:77.
16. Sundbeck G, Jagenburg R, Johansson P-M, et al. Clinical significance of low serum thyrotropin concentration by chemiluminometric assay in 85-year-old women and men. *Arch Intern Med* 1991;151:549.
17. Sandrock D, Olbricht T, Emrich D, et al. Long-term follow-up in patients with autonomous thyroid adenoma. *Acta Endocrinol* 1993;128:51.
18. Carr D, McLeod DT, Parry G, et al. Fine adjustment of thyroxine replacement dosage: comparison of the thyrotropin releasing hormone test using a sensitive thyrotrophin assay with measurement of free thyroid hormones and clinical assessment. *Clin Endocrinol (Oxf)* 1988;28:325.
19. Silva JE, Larsen PR. Contributions of plasma triiodothyronine and local thyroxine monodeiodination to triiodothyronine to nuclear triiodothyronine receptor saturation in pituitary, liver, and kidney of hypothyroid rats. *J Clin Invest* 1978;61:1247.
20. Hodin RA, Lazar MA, Chin WW. Differential and tissue-specific regulation of the multiple rat c-erbA messenger RNA species by thyroid hormone. *J Clin Invest* 1990;85:101.
21. Lewis GF, Alessi CA, Imperial JG, et al. Low serum free thyroxine index in ambulatory elderly is due to a resetting of the threshold of thyrotropin feedback suppression. *J Clin Endocrinol Metab* 1991;73:843.
22. Ross DS. Thyrotoxicosis, thyroid hormone therapy, and bone. *Thyroid* 1994;4:319.
23. Mudde AH, Reijnders FJL, Nieuwenhuijzen Kruseman AC. Peripheral bone density in women with untreated multinodular goitre. *Clin Endocrinol (Oxf)* 1992;37:35.
24. Foldes J, Tarjan G, Szathmari M, et al. Bone mineral density in patients with endogenous subclinical thyrotoxicosis: is this thyroid status a risk factor for osteoporosis? *Clin Endocrinol (Oxf)* 1993;39:521.
25. Gurlek A, Gedik O. Effect of endogenous subclinical hyperthyroidism on bone metabolism and bone mineral density in premenopausal women. *Thyroid* 1999;9:539.
26. Mudde AH, Houben AJHM, Nieuwenhuijzen Kruseman AC. Bone metabolism during anti-thyroid drug treatment of endogenous subclinical thyrotoxicosis. *Clin Endocrinol (Oxf)* 1994; 41:421.
27. Faber J, Jensen IW, Petersen L, et al. Normalization of serum thyrotrophin by means of radioiodine treatment in subclinical thyrotoxicosis: effect on bone loss in postmenopausal women. *Clin Endocrinol (Oxf)* 1998;48:285.
28. Faber J, Perrild H, Johansen JS. Bone Gla protein and sex hormone-binding globulin in nontoxic goiter: parameters for metabolic status at the tissue level. *J Clin Endocrinol Metab* 1990; 70:49.
29. Baldini M, Gallazzi M, Orsati A, et al. Treatment of benign nodular goiter with mildly suppressive doses of L-thyroxine: effects on bone mineral density and on nodule size. *J Intern Med* 2002;251:407.
30. Faber J, Galloe AM. Changes in bone mass during prolonged subclinical thyrotoxicosis due to L-thyroxine treatment: a meta-analysis. *Eur J Endocrinol* 1994;130:350.

31. Schneider DL, Barrett-Connor EL, Morton DJ. Thyroid hormone use and bone mineral density in elderly women: effects of estrogen. *JAMA* 1994;271:1245.

32. Guo CY, Weetman AP, Eastell R. Longitudinal changes of bone mineral density and bone turnover in postmenopausal women on thyroxine. *Clin Endocrinol (Oxf)* 1997;46:301.

33. Harvey RD, McHardy KC, Reid IW, et al. Measurement of bone collagen degradation in thyrotoxicosis and during thyroxine replacement therapy using pyridinium cross-links as specific urinary markers. *J Clin Endocrinol Metab* 1991;72:1189.

34. Krakauer JC, Kleerekoper M. Borderline-low serum thyrotropin level is correlated with increased fasting urinary hydroxyproline excretion. *Arch Intern Med* 1992;152:360.

35. Loviselli A, Mastinu R, Rizzolo E, et al. Circulating telopeptide type I is a peripheral marker of thyroid hormone action in thyrotoxicosis and during levothyroxine suppressive therapy. *Thyroid* 1997;7:561.

36. Mikosch M, Obermayer-Pietsch B, Jost R, et al. Bone metabolism in patients with differentiated thyroid carcinoma receiving suppressive levothyroxine treatment. *Thyroid* 2003;13:347.

37. Kumeda Y, Inaba M, Tahara H, et al. Persistent increase in bone turnover in Graves' patients with subclinical thyrotoxicosis. *J Clin Endocrinol Metab* 2000;85:4157.

38. Ross DS, Ardisson LJ, Nussbaum SR, et al. Serum osteocalcin in patients taking L-thyroxine who have subclinical thyrotoxicosis. *J Clin Endocrinol Metab* 1991;72:507.

39. Leese GP, Jung RT, Guthrie C, et al. Morbidity in patients on L-thyroxine: a comparison of those with a normal TSH to those with a suppressed TSH. *Clin Endocrinol (Oxf)* 1992;37:500.

40. Solomon BL, Wartofsky L, Burman KD. Prevalence of fractures in postmenopausal women with thyroid disease. *Thyroid* 1993; 3:17.

41. Cummings SR, Nevitt MC, Browner WS, et al. Risk factors for hip fracture in white women. *N Engl J Med* 1995;332:767.

42. Bauer DC, Ettinger B, Nevitt MC, et al. Risk for fracture in women with low serum levels of thyroid-stimulating hormone. *Ann Intern Med* 2001;134:501.

43. Sawin CT, Geller A, Wolf PA, et al. Low serum thyrotropin concentrations as a risk factor for atrial fibrillation in older persons. *N Engl J Med* 1994;331:1249.

44. Auer J, Scheibner P, Mische T, et al. Subclinical thyrotoxicosis as a risk factor for atrial fibrillation. *Am Heart J* 2001;142:838.

45. Tenerz A, Forberg R, Jansson R. Is a more active attitude warranted in patients with subclinical thyrotoxicosis? *J Intern Med* 1990;228:229.

46. Monreal M, Lafoz E, Foz M, et al. Occult thyrotoxicosis in patients with atrial fibrillation and an acute arterial embolism. *Angiology* 1988;39:981.

47. Forfar JC, Feek CM, Miller HC, et al. Atrial fibrillation and isolated suppression of the pituitary–thyroid axis: response to specific antithyroid therapy. *Int J Cardiol* 1981;1:43.

48. Bell GM, Sawers JSA, Forfar JC, et al. The effect of minor increments in plasma thyroxine on heart rate and urinary sodium excretion. *Clin Endocrinol (Oxf)* 1983;18:511.

49. Biondi B, Fazio S, Carella C, et al. Cardiac effects of long term thyrotropin-suppressive therapy with levothyroxine. *J Clin Endocrinol Metab* 1993;77:334.

50. Tseng KH, Walfish PG, Persaud JA, et al. Concurrent aortic and mitral valve echocardiography permits measurement of systolic time intervals as an index of peripheral tissue thyroid functional status. *J Clin Endocrinol Metab* 1989;69:633.

51. Jennings PE, O'Malley BP, Griffin KE, et al. Relevance of increased serum thyroxine concentrations associated with normal serum triiodothyronine values in hypothyroid patients receiving

thyroxine: a case for "tissue thyrotoxicosis." *BMJ* 1984;289: 1645.

52. Banovac K, Papic M, Bilsker MS, et al. Evidence of thyrotoxicosis in apparently euthyroid patients treated with levothyroxine. *Arch Intern Med* 1989;149:809.

53. Biondi B, Fazio S, Cardella C, et al. Control of adrenergic overactivity by b-blockade improves the quality of life in patients receiving long term suppressive therapy with levothyroxine. *J Clin Endocrinol Metab* 1994;78:1028.

54. Biondi B, Fazio S, Cuocolo A, et al. Impaired cardiac reserve and exercise capacity in patients receiving long term thyrotropin suppressive therapy with levothyroxine. *J Clin Endocrinol Metab* 1996;81:4224.

55. Shapiro LE, Sievert R, Ong L, et al. Minimal cardiac effects in asymptomatic athyreotic patients chronically treated with thyrotropin-suppressive doses of L-thyroxine. *J Clin Endocrinol Metab* 1997;82:2592.

56. Mercuro G, Panzuto MG, Bina A, et al. Cardiac function, physical exercise capacity, and quality of life during long-term thyrotropin-suppressive therapy with levothyroxine: effect of individual dose tailoring. *J Clin Endocrinol Metab* 2000;85:159.

57. Sgarbi JA, Villaca FG, Carbeline B, et al. The effects of early antithyroid therapy for endogenous subclinical thyrotoxicosis in clinical and heart abnormalities. *J Clin Endocrinol Metab* 2003; 88:1672.

58. Faber J, Wiinberg N, Schifter S, et al. Haemodynamic changes following treatment of subclinical and overt thyrotoxicosis. *Eur J Endocrinol* 2001;145:391.

59. Parle JV, Maisonneuve P, Sheppard MC, et al. Prediction of all-cause and cardiovascular mortality in elderly people from one low serum thyrotropin result: a 10-year cohort study. *Lancet* 2001;358:861.

60. Franklyn JA, Daykin J, Betteridge J, et al. Thyroxine replacement therapy and circulating lipid concentrations. *Clin Endocrinol (Oxf)* 1993;38:453.

61. Wilcox AH, Levin GE. Erythrocyte ouabain binding in patients receiving thyroxine. *Clin Endocrinol (Oxf)* 1987;27:205.

62. Gow SM, Caldwell G, Toft AD, et al. Relationship between pituitary and other target organ responsiveness in hypothyroid patients receiving thyroxine replacement. *J Clin Endocrinol Metab* 1987;64:364.

63. Bartalena L, Martino E, Pacchiarotti A, et al. Factors affecting suppression of endogenous thyrotropin secretion by thyroxine treatment: retrospective analysis in athyreotic and goitrous patients. *J Clin Endocrinol Metab* 1987;64:849.

64. Schlote B, Schaaf L, Schmidt R, et al. Mental and physical state in subclinical thyrotoxicosis: investigations in a normal working population. *Biol Psychiatry* 1992;32:48.

65. Biondi B, Palmieri EA, Fazio S, et al. Endogenous subclinical thyrotoxicosis affects quality of life and cardiac morphology and function in young and middle-aged patients. *J Clin Endocrinol Metab* 2000;85:4701.

66. Kalmijn S, Mehta KM, Pols HA, et al. Subclinical thyrotoxicosis and the risk of dementia: the Rotterdam study. *Clin Endocrinol (Oxf)* 2000;53:733.

67. Ross DS. Thyroid hormone suppressive therapy of sporadic nontoxic goiter. *Thyroid* 1992;2:263.

68. Papini E, Petrucci L, Guglielmi R, et al. Long term changes in nodular goiter: a 5 year prospective randomized trial of levothyroxine suppressive therapy for benign cold thyroid nodules. *J Clin Endocrinol Metab* 1998;83:780.

69. Kroc M, Ersoz, HO, Akpinar I, et al. Effect of low- and high-dose levothyroxine on thyroid nodule volume: a crossover placebo-controlled trial. *Clin Endocrinol (Oxf)* 2002;57:621.

THYROID DISEASE DURING PREGNANCY

DANIEL GLINOER

REGULATION OF THYROID FUNCTION IN NORMAL PREGNANCY

Thyroidal Economy in Normal Pregnancy

Numerous hormonal changes and metabolic demands occur during pregnancy, resulting in profound and complex effects on thyroid function. Because thyroid diseases are common in women during the childbearing period, it is important to envisage both the expected changes in thyroid function tests taking place during a normal pregnancy and how pregnancy may affect the presentation and course of preexisting diseases such as thyroiditis, hypothyroidism, and Graves' disease. Over the past decade, new information regarding the relationship between pregnancy and the thyroid has permitted a major clarification of the complex interactions that take place between gestational processes and regulation of the thyroid system, both in normal individuals and in patients with thyroid disorders. Because the expecting mother is the "natural vector" allowing a future child to be born, a better understanding of the complexities in maternal-fetal interrelationships is primordial to ensure the best possible health status of both the mother and progeny. Normal changes in thyroid function are discussed in both iodine-sufficient and iodine-deficient women. In addition, those aspects of the diagnosis and treatment that must be kept in mind in the management of pregnant patients with thyroid disease are emphasized.

Early in pregnancy, renal blood flow and glomerular filtration increase, leading to an increase in iodide clearance from the plasma, and resulting in a decreased plasma iodide and an increased requirement for iodide in the diet (1,2). In pregnant women with iodine sufficiency, there is little impact of the obligatory increase in renal iodine losses, because the intrathyroidal iodine stores are plentiful at the time of conception and they remain unaltered throughout gestation (3). In pregnant women with iodine restriction, even though urinary iodine concentrations (UICs) may transiently show an early increase, there is, thereafter, a steady decrease in UIC from the first to third trimesters of gestation, hence revealing the underlying tendency toward iodine deficiency associated with the pregnant state (4).

Human chorionic gonadotropin (hCG) is a peptide hormone composed of two subunits termed the α and β chains. Whereas the α subunit is identical to that of thyrotropin (TSH), the β chains differ between both molecules and confer ligand specificity. The partial structural homology between hCG and TSH explains why hCG may act as a thyrotropic hormone, by overlap of their natural functions ("spillover" mechanism). Current evidence has clearly established that hCG is a direct thyroid stimulator and perhaps even a thyroid growth promotor (5–8). During normal pregnancy, the stimulatory effect of hCG on the thyroid induces a small and transient increase in free thyroxine (T_4) near the end of the first trimester and in turn a partial TSH suppression (9–11). The thyrotropic role of hCG during normal pregnancy is illustrated in Figure 80.1, depicting the inverse relationship between serum hCG and TSH concentrations. At the end of the first trimester, there is a mirror image between serum TSH (nadir) and hCG (peak) levels. In one fifth of otherwise euthyroid pregnant women at this time of gestation, serum TSH may even be transiently lowered below the normal range. The figure also shows the direct relationship between circulating free T_4 and hCG concentrations at the time of peak hCG values. The parallelism between peak hCG levels, the increases in free T_4 and triiodothyronine (T_3), and the TSH suppression provide compelling arguments for the thyrotropic role of hCG during normal pregnancy. An interesting study of desialylated and deglycosylated hCG, in a serum-free culture system using human thyroid follicles, showed that removal of sialic acid or carbohydrate residues from native hCG transformed such hCG variants into thyroid-stimulating superagonists (12). Further evidence supporting a pathophysiologic role of hCG in stimulating the human thyroid gland was found in studies of patients with hydatidiform mole and choriocarcinoma (13). In these conditions, clinical and biochemical manifestations of thyrotoxicosis often occur and, as expected, the abnormal stimulation of the thyroid is rapidly relieved after appropriate surgical treatment.

The increased plasma concentration of thyroxine-binding globulin (TBG), together with the increased plasma volume, results in a severalfold increase in the total thyroxine pool during pregnancy. Although the changes in TBG are most dramatic during the first trimester, the increase in plasma volume continues until delivery. Thus, if

conducted three decades ago: the
excretion was 145 µg/L, compared
the previous period (32). Thus, eve
dine intake levels in the United St
appear to be comfortably above th
mum, this survey showed that perh
the women in childbearing age, ar
during a pregnancy, had iodine ex
range of moderate ID, namely belo
the same lines, a recent study showe
efforts to implement the mandatory
Switzerland for many years, mild II
Berne area (34). Another considerati
iodine deprivation during pregnancy
locally, because mild to moderate II
are not immediately recognized as ioe
stance, a study in the southwest of Fra
75% of pregnant women in the area
levels below 100 µg/L (35). A third (
notion that the iodine intake may
within a given country: this occurs p
with mild to moderate ID, because of
in the natural iodine content of food
illustrated by a Danish study: pregn
iodine supplements had a median iodi
62 µg/g creatine in Copenhagen, con
µg/g creatine in East Jutland; further
differences were not alleviated in pregn
receive iodine supplements in the sam

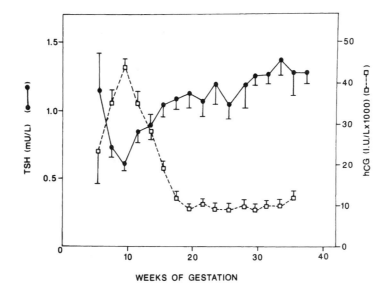

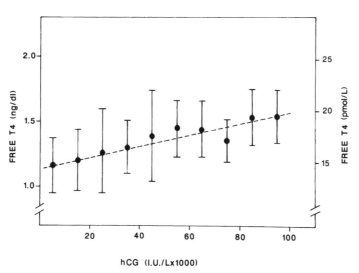

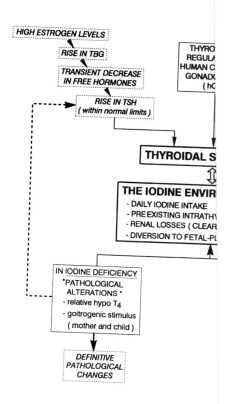

FIGURE 80.1. TOP: Serum thyrotropin (TSH) and human chorionic gonadotropin (hCG) as a function of gestational age in a large group of healthy pregnant women. Between 8 and 14 weeks' gestation, the changes in hCG and TSH levels are mirror images of each other, and there is a significant negative correlation between the individual TSH and hCG levels ($p<0.001$). **Bottom:** Scattergram of free thyroxine (T_4) levels in relation to hCG concentrations in the first half of gestation. When peak hCG values are plotted for 10,000 IU/L increments in circulating hCG, the graph shows the direct relationship with progressively increasing free T_4 levels in healthy pregnancies. (Reproduced from Glinoer D, De Nayer P, Bourdoux P, et al. Regulation of maternal thyroid function during pregnancy. *J Clin Endocrinol Metab* 1990;71:276–287, with permission.)

the free T_4 concentration is to remain unaltered, the T_4 production rate must increase (or its degradation rate decrease) to allow the additional T_4 to accumulate (2,10,14). In a situation where the T_4 input is constant, it would be predicted that there is an iterative increment in T_4 as TBG increases as a result of the reduced availability of T_4 to degradative enzymes. The evidence that levothyroxine requirements are markedly enhanced during pregnancy in hypothyroid women clearly indicates that not only is T_4 degradation decreased during early pregnancy but also that increased T_4 production must occur throughout gestation.

The placenta contains high concentrations of D3, the type 3 iodothyronine deiodinase (15–17). Inner ring deiodination of T_4 catalyzed by this enzyme is the source of high concentrations of reverse T_3 present in amniotic fluid.

The enzyme may function to reduce T_3 and T_4 concentrations in fetal circulation, although fetal tissue T_3 levels can reach adult levels as the result of D2's local action. D3 also may indirectly provide a source of iodide for the fetus through iodothyronine deiodination. Despite the presence of placental D3, transplacental passage of maternal T_4 occurs, and fetal serum T_4 levels are about one third of normal (18). Thyroxine is also detectable in amniotic fluid before the onset of fetal thyroid function (19). Thus, the placental barrier to maternal iodothyronines, even as late as the third trimester of gestation, appears not to be impermeable to the passage of maternal thyroid hormones. Although quantitatively small, such hormone concentrations may qualitatively represent an extremely important source of thyroid hormones to ensure the adequate development of the feto-maternal unit (20–23).

The only direct measureme
rates in pregnancy were obtaine
and the T_4 turnover rates were
nificantly from those of nonpre
more recent work, however, com
suggest that T_4 production rates
pregnancy. Evidence supporting
from analyses of the repercussior
roxine treatment in patients witl
In women with primary hypoth
ing stable doses of levothyroxine,
crease in serum TSH during ge
compensatory increase in levoth
euthyroidism (25,26). These resu
increase in T_4 requirements, beg
and persisting until the time of d
view of maternal thyroid functic
now widely accepted that there is
T_4 production during gestation (2

Thyroid Function Param
in Normal Pregnancy

Thyroxine-Binding Globulin

The increase in total serum T_4 ar
pregnancy is due to an increase in :
appears early; TBG concentratio
weeks' gestation. The cause of
serum TBG may be multifactorial.
increase in serum TBG synthesis ir
patocytes from rhesus monkeys pri
There is also an increase in the frac
lylated, and therefore more negativ
TBG in the sera of pregnant or e
uals. Because this increase in siali
inhibits the uptake of the protein
hepatocytes, the more heavily si
pregnant sera have a longer plasma
addition to stimulatory effects of es
sis, a major contribution to the inc
tion during pregnancy is the reduce
highly sialylated forms of the prote
two- to threefold increases in ser
creases in both serum transthyretin (
also commonly found in pregnancy

Total and Free T_4 and T_3

The increase in TBG during gestatio
total serum thyroid hormones. To
mone concentration, a thyroid ho
(THBR), free T_4 index, or direct
must be obtained. Because the redu
tion of T_3 is approximately equal to tl

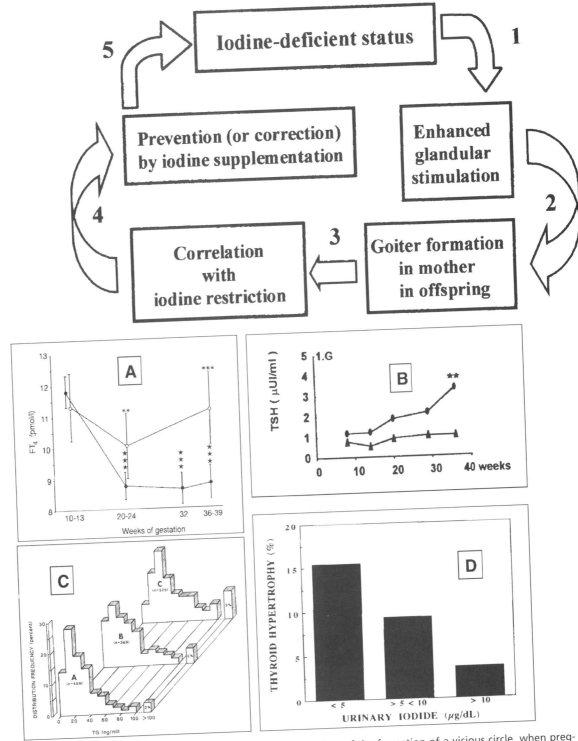

FIGURE 80.3. TOP: Schematic representation of the formation of a vicious circle, when pregnancy takes place in conditions with iodine deficiency. **A:** The progressive lowering in free thyroxine (T_4) concentrations in Sudanese pregnant women with iodine deficiency (●), compared with unaltered serum free T_4 in pregnancies in Sweden with an adequate iodine nutrition status (○). **B:** The increase in serum thyrotropin (TSH) (*circles*) in Sicilian pregnancies from an area with iodine deficiency, compared with unaltered TSH levels in Sicilian pregnant women from an area with iodine sufficiency (*triangles*). **C:** The progressive increase in serum thyroglobulin (*TG*) levels during pregnancy in Belgian pregnant women without iodine supplementation, in first trimester (*A*), at the end of second trimester (*B*), and immediately after parturition (*C*). **D:** The inverse correlation between glandular hypertrophy (%) and the severity of iodine restriction (based on urinary iodine concentration) in pregnant women in the southwest of France. [Modified from Glinoer D. Feto-maternal repercussions of iodine deficiency during pregnancy. *Ann Endocrinol (Paris)* 2003;64:37–44, with permission.]

are (a) relative hypothyroxinemia, with serum free T_4 frequently found near the lower limit of normality; (b) changes in serum TSH (usually remaining within the normal range), with a frequent doubling of initial TSH values near term; (c) changes in thyroglobulin (Tg) concentrations, with a progressive increase as gestation progresses; and (d) urinary iodine concentrations. Examples of the

successive steps in the formation of a vicious circle are given in the different graphs shown on Figure 80.3. Figure 80.3A shows the progressive lowering in free T_4 in pregnant women with ID in Sudan, compared with unaltered free T_4 concentrations in pregnant women in Sweden (39). Figure 80.3B illustrates changes in serum TSH in pregnant women from one area with ID in Sicily, compared with io-

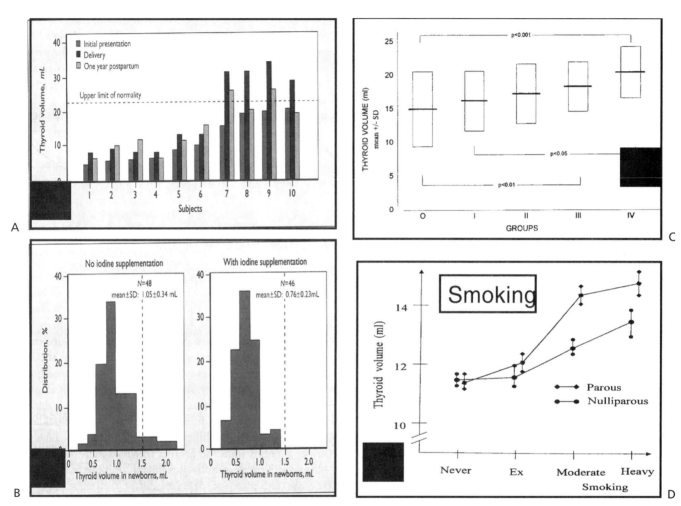

FIGURE 80.4. A: Thyroid volume (TV) determined by echography in 10 selected pregnant women at initial presentation in first trimester (*left set of bars*), at delivery (*middle set of bars*), and 12 months postpartum (*right set of bars*). The dotted line represents the upper limit of TV normality (i.e., 22 mL). (Reproduced from Glinoer D, Lemone M, Bourdoux P, et al. Partial reversibility during late postpartum of thyroid abnormalities associated with pregnancy. *J Clin Endocrinol Metab* 1992;74:453–457, with permission.) **B:** Distribution frequencies of TVs in neonates born to mothers without (on the left) and with (on the right) iodine supplementation received during pregnancy. Iodine supplementation allowed for a marked 38% average reduction in mean TV and for the complete prevention of neonatal thyroid hyperplasia. The upper limit of normal TV in newborns is indicated by the vertical dotted lines (at 1.5 mL). (Reproduced from Glinoer D, De Nayer P, Delange F, et al. A randomized trial for the treatment of mild iodine deficiency during pregnancy: maternal and neonatal effects. *J Clin Endocrinol Metab* 1995;80: 258–269, with permission.) **C:** Progressive changes in TV between group 0 (nulliparous) and group IV (Group I, one pregnancy; group II, two pregnancies; group III, three pregnancies; group IV, four or more pregnancies) in a retrospective study of the changes in TV in relation to parity in Italy (Naples). (Reproduced from Rotondi M, Caccavale C, Di Serio C, et al. Successful outcome of pregnancy in a thyroidectomized-parathyroidectomized young woman affected by severe hypothyroidism. *Thyroid* 1999;9:1037–1040, with permission.) **D:** The effect of parity and smoking on thyroid size in women in Denmark. (Reproduced from Knudsen N, Bülow I, Laurberg P, et al. Parity is associated with increased thyroid volume solely among smokers in an area with moderate to mild iodine deficiency. *Eur J Endocrinol* 2002;146:39–43, with permission.)

mild thyroid insufficiency, and give such patients the potential benefit of levothyroxine treatment (66). To date, only one such prospective trial has been reported, with promising results. In this study, women with TAI and recurrent early miscarriages were given levothyroxine treatment, both before and during pregnancy, and the researchers reported a significant reduction in the rate of miscarriages: 81% of the women who received thyroid hormone had live births, compared with only 55% in those given immunoglobulin injections (67). Obviously, conclusions must be considered with caution and balanced with the small number of patients investigated and the fact that there was no strict randomization. Despite these limitations, the study constitutes the first therapeutic intervention trial showing an effect of thyroid hormone administration in women who were habitual aborters. If delayed conception plays a role to decrease fertility in women with TAI, this would also constitute a strong argument for systematically screening infertile women for thyroid underfunction, particularly when seeking medical advice before *in vitro* fertilization procedures. Finally, women with TAI could be advised to plan for pregnancy at a younger age, although this type of medical advice is more easily written than practically applicable.

Effects of Pregnancy on Thyroid Function in Women with Thyroid Autoimmunity

When systematically screened in the early stages of pregnancy, 5% to 10% of women have thyroid autoantibodies with normal thyroid function. Despite the expected decrease in the titers of thyroid antibodies during gestation, the parameters of thyroid function show a gradual deterioration toward subclinical hypothyroidism in a significant fraction of women with TAI. Already in the first trimester, serum TSH, albeit normal, is shifted to slightly higher values, compared with antibody-negative pregnant controls. Thus, women with TAI usually are able to maintain normal thyroid function during early gestation, as a result of sustained thyrotropic stimulation. Thereafter, a marked reduction in free T_4 values is often observed with the progression of gestation, and at delivery, almost one half of women with TAI have free T_4 values in the hypothyroid range, hence confirming their reduced functional thyroid reserve (68). At the individual level, it is possible to predict the risk for progression to subclinical hypothyroidism, based on serum TSH levels and thyroid peroxidase (TPO) antibody titers: when serum TSH is greater than 2.0 mU/L and/or TPO antibody titers are greater than 1250 U/mL before 20 weeks' gestation, these markers reveal the propensity to develop hypothyroidism before the end of pregnancy (69). These observations provide clinicians with simple tools to help identify those women who carry the highest risk during early gestation. As a consequence, thy-

roid function can be more closely monitored and preventive levothyroxine treatment administered to avoid potentially deleterious effects of hypothyroxinemia on both maternal and fetal outcome.

PRIMARY HYPOTHYROIDISM

The most common cause of primary hypothyroidism in women in reproductive age is chronic autoimmune thyroiditis. This occurs in both the goitrous and atrophic forms of the disease. One percent to 2% of pregnant women are already receiving levothyroxine therapy for hypothyroidism (70,71). Population-based studies have evaluated the prevalence of elevated serum TSH concentrations in the early part of gestation in women without apparent hypothyroidism: 2% to 2.5% of apparently healthy unselected pregnant women were found to have elevated TSH levels (68,72).

Effect of Hypothyroidism on Pregnancy Outcome

Until recently, hypothyroidism has been considered to be relatively rare during pregnancy, presumably because of the increased infertility and miscarriage rates associated with hypothyroidism (73). Nowadays, however, this view has changed. Several studies have shown that when hypothyroid women become pregnant and maintain the pregnancy, they carry an increased risk for both maternal obstetric and fetal complications. These complications are more frequent and more severe in pregnant women with overt hypothyroidism, when compared with subclinical hypothyroidism. The older data concerning obstetric repercussions refer to a period when the diagnosis of hypothyroidism was not always made before conception, when levothyroxine was given during late gestation only, when thyroid function was not adequately monitored, and finally when the adaptation of levothyroxine doses was not systematically implemented (71,74). Such studies also frequently mention the association of hypothyroidism with other conditions (hypertension or diabetes) that may also have increased the overall obstetric risks (75). There are relatively few reports on the outcome of pregnancy in untreated hypothyroid pregnant women, but available information indicates that levothyroxine therapy greatly improves, but does not entirely suppress, the frequency of obstetric complications (76–78). Recently it was shown that when hypothyroid patients were not rendered euthyroid, pregnancy either ended in spontaneous abortion (in >60% of the cases) or led to an increased prevalence of preterm deliveries. Conversely, in hypothyroid women with adequate treatment, the frequency of abortions was minimal and pregnancies were in general carried to term without complications (79).

TPO antibodies are undetectable, free T$_4$ and hCG c$\ldots$
centrations should be determined. The second branch
the algorithm allows for the diagnosis of nonautoimmu
hCG-induced thyrotoxicosis (GTT), corresponding to
proximately 20 to 30 cases per year given a similar hosp
setting. In women with a history of Graves' disease (pre
or past, active or considered cured), TSHR antibody t
and free T$_4$ concentrations should be determined w
women have a history of Graves' disease before concep
In women with both active disease or "metabolically" c
Graves' disease, but in whom high titers of Graves' IgG
found, TSHR antibody titers should be monitored
later stage during gestation, preferably near the end c
second trimester. This strategy allows for the diagno
maternal immunity related to Graves' disease and f
potential suspicion of fetal thyrotoxicosis, thus indi
the need for a careful monitoring of fetal developme
nally, all cases with thyrotoxicosis of autoimmune
diagnosed during pregnancy require a close monito
thyroid antibody titers (both TPO antibodies and
antibodies) and thyroid function during the first yea
partum because of the significant risk for developin
partum thyroiditis or postpartum exacerbation of
toxicosis.

NODULAR THYROID DISEASE

Risk for Thyroid Cancer

A thyroid nodule or a dominant nodule within
nodular gland may be recognized for the first tim
pregnancy (151,152). Evaluation of a nodul
pregnancy relies on the use of ultrasound and fi
aspiration biopsy (FNAB). FNAB is indicated ir
nant women with a nodule larger than 1 cm, or
during gestation, or when it is associated witl
cervical lymph nodes. If FNAB is highly sug
malignancy, thyroid surgery should be perfor
though the patient is pregnant, although surg
safely deferred until after delivery (153). If FN
show a possible follicular neoplasm or is mi
cious, surgery is usually deferred until after the
and breast-feeding periods (154–156). There
evidence that the natural history of any fo
roid cancer is significantly modified by pregr
159). The outcome of thyroid cancer diagn
pregnancy was reevaluated recently in a study
dian follow-up period of 14 years (160). Th
showed that differentiated thyroid cancer p
pregnancy generally has an excellent prognos
disease is discovered early in pregnancy, surg
considered in the second trimester. Radioiod
phies and treatment can safely be deferred u
livery. Treatment, however, should not be
than a year.

Diagnosis
Hypothyr$\ldots$

The diagnosis
nancy can be r
and free T$_4$ (or
total serum T$_4$
n*M*) in the preg
normal. The si
similar to those
may be difficul
such as the fatig
nancy.

Because thyr$\ldots$
young female s
often remain un
proposing to sys
ing pregnancy. A
eral scheme is sh
thyroid antibodi
Based on recent
perhaps occur ir
serum TSH eleva
a free T$_4$ determi
vated or free T$_4$ is
the presence (or a
should be considϵ
underfunction an
pregnancy. Conce
antibodies, medic
serum TSH levels
below 2 mU/L, m
low titers of thyroi
not warranted, and
end of the secono

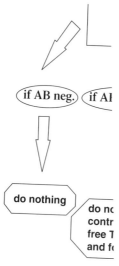

if AB neg.   if Al$\ldots$

do nothing

do nc
contr
free T
and fϵ

Therapeutic Considerations

In the newly diagnosed hypothyroid pregnant patient, a
full replacement dose of levothyroxine should be instituted immediately, assuming there are no abnormalities
in cardiac function. To normalize the extrathyroidal thyroxine pool more rapidly, therapy may be initiated by
giving for 2 to 3 days a dose that is two to three times the
estimated final replacement daily dose; this will allow for
a more rapid return to a euthyroid state. Several studies
have confirmed that levothyroxine requirements in most
women with preexisting hypothyroidism must be increased by approximately 50% on average during pregnancy (25,26,69). Adjustment of levothyroxine doses
should be implemented early in pregnancy, preferably in
the first trimester. If the pregnancy is planned, the patient should have thyroid function tests soon after the
missed menstrual period. If serum TSH is not increased
at that time, tests should be repeated (at 8–12 and 20
weeks) because an increase in hormone requirements may
not become apparent until later during gestation (80,
81). The magnitude of the increment depends in part on
the cause of hypothyroidism. Women without residual
thyroid tissue (after radioiodine ablation for thyrotoxicosis or surgery for thyroid cancer) require a larger increment in levothyroxine, whereas women with with some
residual functional thyroid tissue (Hashimoto's disease)
require a smaller increment (26) (Table 80.2). The need
to adapt levothyroxine doses is highly variable among
hypothyroid patients; therefore, treatment monitoring
should be tailored individually (69,82,83). Finally, women
with subclinical hypothyroidism who are already taking
small levothyroxine doses before pregnancy may not require a change systematically during gestation (although
they frequently do) if their functional reserve remains adequate.

Fetal and Neonatal Consequences
of Maternal Thyroid Underfunction

In general, infants born to hypothyroid mothers appear
healthy and without evidence of thyroid dysfunction, provided that there was no severe iodine deficiency *in utero*.
Clearly, maternal hypothyroidism during pregnancy raises a
serious concern about long-lasting psychoneurologic consequences for the progeny, due to the risk for insufficient placental transfer of maternal thyroid hormones to the developing fetus during the first half of gestation. Because the fetal
thyroid gland becomes operational only after midgestation,
thyroid hormones transferred transplacentally from mother
to fetus are important, both before and after the onset of
fetal thyroid function. Development of the fetal brain (with
neuronal multiplication, migration, and architectural organization) during the second trimester corresponds to a phase
during which the supply of thyroid hormones to the growing fetus is almost exclusively of maternal origin. During
later phases of fetal brain development (with glial cell multiplication, migration, and myelinization), from the third trimester onward, the supply of thyroid hormones to the fetus
is essentially of fetal origin. Therefore, whereas severe maternal hypothyroidism during the second trimester will result
in irreversible neurologic deficits, maternal hypothyroxinemia occurring at later stages will result in less severe, and also
partially reversible, fetal brain damage (18,19,21–23,84,85).

In disease, three sets of clinical disorders ought to be
considered and are schematically illustrated in Figure 80.5.
For infants with a defect of thyroid gland ontogeny leading
to congenital hypothyroidism, the participation of maternal hormones to the fetal circulating thyroxine environment is unaffected and the risk for brain damage results exclusively from insufficient fetal hormone production. In
contrast, when the maternal thyroid is deficient (i.e., in
women with TAI), it is both the severity and temporal oc-

TABLE 80.2.   DAILY THYROXINE DOSE REQUIRED FOR MAINTAINING NORMAL SERUM THYROTROPIN CONCENTRATION DURING PREGNANCY IN PATIENTS WITH PRIMARY HYPOTHYROIDISM[a]

	Patients with Hashimoto's Disease (*n* = 15)		Patients with Thyroid Ablation (*n* = 18)	
	Before	During	Before	During
T$_4$ dose (µg/day)	111 ± 25	139 ± 52	114 ± 33	166 ± 64[a]
T$_4$ dose (µg/kg/day)	1.7 ± 0.6	1.9 ± 0.9	1.8 ± 0.5	2.3 ± 0.8[a]
Serum TSH (mU/L)	2.0 ± 1.8	1.8 ± 1.1	1.5 ± 1.3	1.9 ± 1.1

[a]*p* <0.01.
T$_4$, thyroxine.
Adapted from Kaplan MM. Monitoring thyroxine treatment during pregnancy. *Thyroid* 1992;2:147–152, with permission.

based on molecular mimicry between hormone
and their receptors (96). An interesting, but unr
question is whether the thyroid gland is a "pas
stander" (or a victim) of an abnormal thyrotro
activity in GTT, or whether the gland itself, via
degrees of sensitivity of the TSH receptor (TSHR
role in its responsiveness to the effects of hCC
only one clinical example has been reported wi
stantially increased sensitivity of the TSHR to st
by hCG, due to a single mutation (K183R) in
cellular domain of the TSHR (143). The muta
was more sensitive than the wild-type recepto
thus accounting for recurrent hyperthyroidisr
nancy in the presence of normal hCG levels. T
raises the possibility that some women who de
may have an abnormality at the level of the th
ular cell. In elaborate studies of the structure
relationship of the TSHR, the group of Gil
performed site-directed mutagenesis, substit
183 in the ectodomain of the TSHR by a vari
acids expressing different physicochemica
(144,145). They obtained unexpected rest
TSHR mutants displayed a widening of the
toward hCG stimulation. Modeling of the m
tors indicated that the increased gain in sen
have resulted from the release of a near
residue (in position E157) from a salt bridg
K183.

Gestational transient thyrotoxicosis is o
with morning sickness, increased vomiting, a
gravidarum, a severe condition requiring hos
definitive treatment (134,146–148). There i
tion between the intensity of emesis and th

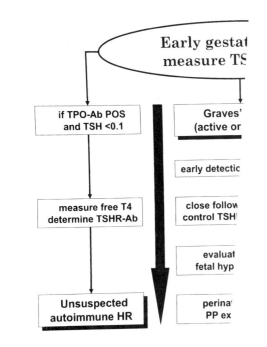

Early gestat
measure TS

if TPO-Ab POS
and TSH <0.1

Graves'
(active or

early detectic

measure free T4
determine TSHR-Ab

close follow
control TSH

evaluat
fetal hyp

Unsuspected
autoimmune HR

perina
PP ex

currence of r
resulting conse
nally, in iodin
roid functions
ity of iodine de
for fetal neurol
of an importar
logical develop
of age, born to
ficiency during
tors recruited c
serum TSH at
logical testing c
trols) showed t
and had a mean
points below tha
analyzed in the
were left untrea
and the average
the controls. In

125. Lamberg BA, Ikonen E, Osterlund K, et al. Antithyroid drug treatment of maternal hyperthyroidism during lactation. *Clin Endocrinol* 1984;21:81–87.
126. Mandel SJ, Cooper DS. The use of antithyroid drugs in pregnancy and lactation. *J Clin Endocrinol Metab* 2001;86:2354–2359.
127. Amino N, Mori H, Iwatani Y, et al. High prevalence of transient post-partum thyrotoxicosis and hypothyroidism. *N Engl J Med* 1982;306:849–852.
128. Amino N, Tada H, Hidaka Y. Autoimmune thyroid disease and pregnancy. *J Endocrinol Invest* 1996;19:59–70.
129. Browne-Martin K, Emerson CH. Postpartum thyroid dysfunction. *Clin Obstet Gynecol* 1997;40:90–101.
130. Tada H, Hidaka Y, Tsuruta E, et al. Prevalence of postpartum onset of disease within patients with Graves' disease of childbearing age. *Endocr J* 1994;41:325–327.
131. Momotani N, Noh J, Ishikawa N, et al. Relationship between silent thyroiditis and recurrent Graves' disease in the postpartum period. *J Clin Endocrinol Metab* 1994;79:285–289.
132. Hidaka Y, Tamaki H, Iwatani Y, et al. Prediction of post-partum Graves' thyrotoxicosis by measurements of thyroid stimulating antibody in early pregnancy. *Clin Endocrinol* 1994;41:15–20.
133. Yoshida S, Takamatsu J, Kuma K, et al. Thyroid-stimulating antibodies and thyroid stimulation-blocking antibodies during the pregnancy and postpartum period: a case report. *Thyroid* 1992;2:27–30.
134. Goodwin TM, Montoro M, Mestman JH. Transient hyperthyroidism and hyperemesis gravidarum: clinical aspects. *Am J Obstet Gynecol* 1992;167:648–652.
135. Kimura M, Amino M, Tamaki H, et al. Gestational thyrotoxicosis and hyperemesis gravidarum: possible role of hCG with higher stimulating activity. *Clin Endocrinol* 1993;38:345–350.
136. Tsuruta E, Tada H, Tamaki H, et al. Pathogenic role of asialo human chorionic gonadotropin in gestational thyrotoxicosis. *J Clin Endocrinol Metab* 1995;80:350–355.
137. Ramsey PS, Ramin KD. 24-year-old pregnant woman with nausea and vomiting. *Mayo Clin Proc* 2000;75:1317–1320.
138. Tanaka S, Yamada H, Kato EH, et al. Gestational transient hyperthyroxinaemia (GTH): screening for thyroid function in 23163 pregnant women using dried blood spots. *Clin Endocrinol* 1998;49:325–329.
139. Yeo CP, Hsu Chin Khoo D, Hsi Ko Eng P, Tan HK et al. Prevalence of gestational thyrotoxicosis in Asian women evaluated in the 8th to 14th weeks of pregnancy: correlations with total and free beta human chorionic gonadotrophin. *Clin Endocrinol* 2001;55:391–398.
140. Grün JP, Meuris S, De Nayer P, et al. The thyrotropic role of human chorionic gonadotropin (hCG) in the early stages of twin (versus single) pregnancy. *Clin Endocrinol* 1997;46:719–725.
141. Vassart G, Dumont JE. The thyrotropin receptor and the regulation of thyrocyte function and growth. *Endocr Rev* 1992;13:596–611.
141a. Ginsberg J, Levanczuk RZ, Honore LH. Hyperplacentosis: a novel cause of hyperthyroidism. *Thyroid* 2001;11:393–396.
142. Kosugi S, Mori T. TSH receptor and LH receptor. *Endocr J* 1995;42:587–606.

143. Rodien P, Brémont C, Sanson M-L, et al. Familial gestational hyperthyroidism caused by a mutant thyrotropin receptor hypersensitive to human chorionic gonadotropin. *N Engl J Med* 1998;339:1823–1826.
144. Smits G, Govaerts C, Nubourgh I, et al. Lysine 183 and glutamic acid 157 of the TSH receptor: two interacting residues with a key role in determining specificity toward TSH and human CG. *Mol Endocrinol* 2002;16:722–735.
145. Rodien P. Un récepteur de la TSH hypersensible à l'hCG responsable d'une hyperthyroïdie gestationelle récidivante et familiale. *Reprod Hum Horm* 2001;14:655–660.
146. Goodwin TM, Hershman JM. Hyperthyroidism due to inappropriate production of human chorionic gonadotropin. *Clin Obstet Gynecol* 1997;40:32–44.
147. Bober SA, McGill AC, Tunbridge WMG. Thyroid function in hyperemesis gravidarum. *Acta Endocrinol (Copenh)* 1986;111:404–410.
148. Lao TT, Chin KH, Chang AMZ. The outcome of hyperemetic pregnancies complicated by transient hyperthyroidism. *Aust N Z J Obstet Gynaecol* 1987;27:99–101.
149. Wilson R, McKillop JH, McLean M, et al. Thyroid function tests are rarely abnormal in patients with severe hyperemesis gravidarum. *Clin Endocrinol (Oxf)* 1992;37:331–334.
150. Tan JY, Loh KC, Yeo GS, et al. Transient hyperthyroidism of hyperemesis gravidarum. *Br J Obstet Gynaecol* 2002;109:683–688.
151. Rosen IB, Walfish PG. Pregnancy as a predisposing factor in thyroid neoplasia. *Arch Surg* 1986;121:1287–1290.
152. Hamburger JI. Thyroid nodules in pregnancy. *Thyroid* 1992;2:165–168.
153. Moosa M, Mazzaferri EL. Outcome of differentiated thyroid cancer diagnosed in pregnant women. *J Clin Endocrinol Metab* 1997;82:2862–2866.
154. Tan GH, Gharib H, Goellner JR, et al. Management of thyroid nodules in pregnancy. *Arch Intern Med* 1996;156:2317–2320.
155. Glinoer D. Nodule et cancer thyroïdiens chez la femme enceinte. *Ann Endocrinol (Paris)* 1997;58:263–267.
156. Marley EF, Oertel YC. Fine-needle aspiration of thyroid lesions in fifty seven pregnant and postpartum women. *Diagn Cytopathol* 1997;16:122–125.
157. Hod M, Sharony R, Friedman S, et al. Pregnancy and thyroid carcinoma: a review of incidence, course, and prognosis. *Obstet Gynecol Surv* 1989;44:774–779.
158. Asteris GT, DeGroot LJ. Thyroid cancer: relationship to radiation exposure and pregnancy. *J Reprod Med* 1976;4:1287–1291.
159. Mc Clellan DR, Francis GL. Thyroid cancer in children, pregnant women, and patients with Graves' disease. *Endocrinol Metab Clin North Am* 1996;25:27–48.
160. Vini L, Hyer S, Pratt B, et al. Management of differentiated thyroid cancer diagnosed during pregnancy. *Eur J Endocrinol* 1999;140:404–406.
161. Struve C, Haupt S, Ohlen S. Influence of frequency of previous pregnancies on the prevalence of thyroid nodules in women without clinical evidence of thyroid disease. *Thyroid* 1993;3:7–9.
162. Kung AW, Chau MT, Lao TT, et al. The effect of pregnancy on thyroid nodule formation. *J Clin Endocrinol Metab* 2002;87:1010–1014.

RESISTANCE TO THYROID HORMONE

SAMUEL REFETOFF

Functional Domains

CpG
dinucleotic

Mutations Associated with RTH

●■▲ mu
○□△▽◇

FIGU
thyro
main:
with
tion)
tom:
tion c
in the
relate
muta:
ticall)
acids
ing tc
ditior
phipa
(23); :
(Mod
lar ge

in 4 others, producing
amino acids in the TF
cleotide substitutions p
tion and a premature
trinucleotide deletions
acid, while insertion of

Resistance to thyroid hormone (RTH) is a syndrome of reduced responsiveness of target tissues to thyroid hormone (TH). More than 1,000 cases have been described that appear to fit this definition. In practice, such patients are identified by their persistent elevation of circulating free thyroxine (FT_4) and free triiodothyronine (FT_3) levels in association with nonsuppressed serum thyrotropin (TSH), and in the absence of intercurrent illness, drugs, or alterations of TH transport serum proteins. More importantly, higher doses of exogenous TH are required to produce the expected suppressive effect on the secretion of pituitary TSH and on the metabolic responses in peripheral tissues.

Although the apparent resistance to TH may vary in severity, it is always partial. The variability in clinical manifestations may be due to the severity of the hormonal resistance, the effectiveness of compensatory mechanisms, the presence of modulating genetic factors, and the effects of prior therapy. The magnitude of the hormonal resistance is, in turn, dependent on the nature of the underlying genetic defect. The latter is usually, but not always, a mutation in the TH receptor (TR) β gene (1,2).

Despite a variable clinical presentation, the common features characteristic of the RTH syndrome are (a) elevated serum levels of free T_4 and T_3, (b) normal or slightly increased TSH level that responds to TRH, (c) absence of the usual symptoms and metabolic consequences of TH excess, and (d) goiter.

CLINICAL CLASSIFICATION

The diagnosis is based on the clinical findings and standard laboratory tests and, when possible, confirmed by genetic studies. Before TR gene defects were recognized, the proposed subclassification of RTH was based on symptoms, signs, and laboratory parameters of tissue responses to TH (3). Not withstanding the assessment of TSH feedback regulation by TH, the measurements of most other responses to the hormone are insensitive and relatively nonspecific. For this reason, all tissues other than the pituitary have been grouped together under the term *peripheral tissues*, on which the impact of TH was roughly assessed by a combination of clinical observation and laboratory tests.

The majority of patients appeared to be eumetabolic and maintained a near normal serum TSH concentration. They were classified as having generalized resistance to TH (GRTH). In such individuals, the defect seemed to be compensated by the high levels of TH. In contrast, patients with equally high levels of TH and nonsuppressed TSH that appeared to be hypermetabolic, because they were restless or had sinus tachycardia, were classified as having selective pituitary resistance to TH (PRTH). Finally, the occurrence of isolated peripheral tissue resistance to TH (PTRTH) was reported in a single patient studied in detail (4). In this individual with partial thyroid gland ablation, although serum TSH was suppressed with physiologic doses of liothironine ($L-T_3$), supraphysiologic doses of this hormone failed to produce symptoms and signs of thyrotoxicosis or to increase oxygen consumption and pulse rate. No mutation in the TRβ gene of this patient was found (5) and no similar cases have been reported. More common in clinical practice is the apparent tolerance of some individuals to the ingestion of supraphysiologic doses of TH.

The earliest suggestion that PRTH may not constitute an entity distinct from GRTH can be found in a study by Beck-Peccoz et al. (6). In a group of 15 patients with PRTH, these investigators found that the serum level of the peripheral tissue marker of TH action, sex hormone–binding globulin (SHBG), was not increased as it should have been if the hormonal resistance were confined to the pituitary and hypothalamus. In a recent comprehensive study involving 312 patients with GRTH and 72 patients with PRTH, it was conclusively shown that the response of SHBG and other peripheral tissue markers of TH action were equally attenuated in GRTH and PRTH (7). The frequency of symptoms and signs were also similar in patients under both classifications. More importantly, identical mutations were found in individuals classified as having GRTH and PRTH, many of whom belonged to the same family (8). It was therefore concluded that these two forms of RTH are the product of the subjective nature of symptoms and poor specificity of signs (see later section on the Molecular Basis of the Defect). Thus, it is uncertain whether PRTH exists as a true TH resistance entity, except in association with TSH-producing pituitary adenomas (9,10).

INCIDENCE

The precise inc
tine neonatal scr
nation of TSH
(11). A limited
concentration
40,000 live birt
1,000, of which
tail (1).

Although mo
in women, RTH
both genders. T
graphic distribu
Africans, and As
ferent ethnic gro

Familial occu
approximately
those families in
jects have been s
is 21.3%. This i
the frequency of
The reports of a

Inheritance i
clearly recessive
in a family with
duced a homoz

TABLE 81.1.

Type

Substitution—sin
Substitution—din

Deletion—single
Deletion—trinucl

Deletion—all cod
Insertion—single
Insertion—trinucl
Duplication—seve
Mutations at CpG

De novo mutation
Total

in CpGs
No TRβ gene mut

---

[a]Not included are s
[b]Families with TRβ
[c]Not applicable.
[d]Total number of f

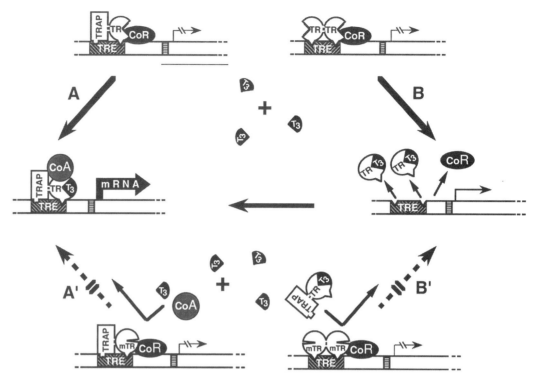

FIGURE 81.2. Mechanism of the dominant expression of RTH. In the absence of triiodothyro-nine (T_3), occupancy of TRE by TR heterodimers (TR-TRAP) or dimers (TR-TR) suppresses transacti-vation through association with a corepressor (CoR). **A:** T_3-activated transcription mediated by TR-TRAP heterodimers involves the release of the CoR and association with coactivators (*CoA*) as well as **(B)** the removal of TR dimers from TRE releases their silencing effect and liberates TREs for the binding of active TR-TRAP heterodimers. The dominant negative effect of a mutant TR (*mTR*), which does not bind T_3, can be explained by the inhibitory effect of mTR-containing dimers and heterodimers that occupy TRE. Thus, T_3 is unable to activate the mTR-TRAP het-erodimer (A′) or release TREs from the inactive mTR homodimers (B′). (Modified from Refetoff S, Weiss RE, Usala SJ. The syndromes of resistance to thyroid hormone. *Endocr Rev* 1993;14:348–399, with permission.)

ent. Indeed, more severe RTH and interference with the function of the WT-TRβ, despite mild impairment of T_3 binding or no binding defect at all, has been also observed (88). Two such mTRβs, R243Q and R243W, located in the hinge region of the receptor, have no significant im-pairment of T_3 binding when tested in solution, yet both clinically and *in vitro* manifested relatively severe RTH and impairment of transactivation function, respectively. The demonstration of normal nuclear translocation but re-duced ability of T_3 to dissociate homodimers formed on TRE suggested that these mutant TRβs have reduced af-finity for T_3 only after they bound to DNA (88). This has been confirmed by measurement of T_3 binding after com-plexing to TRE (89). Another mTRβ, L454V located in the AF2 domain (Fig. 81.1) and with near normal T_3 bind-ing, exhibited altered transcriptional function and RTH because of attenuated interaction with the CoA (74). Fi-nally, some mTRβs, such as R383H, exhibit a delay in CoR release despite minimal reduction of T_3 binding (90).

In general the relative degree of impaired function among various mTRβs is similar whether tested using TRE-controlled reporter genes that are negatively or posi-tively regulated by T_3. Exceptions to this rule are the mTRβs R383H and R429Q, which show greater impair-ment of transactivation on negatively than positively regu-lated promoters (87,90,91). The reason for this discrep-ancy is a matter of conjecture. Given the fact that R429Q binds T_3 normally, it is possible that T_3 binding to these mTRβs is allosterically modulated by the different TREs and cofactors (92,93).

MOLECULAR BASIS OF THE VARIABLE PHENOTYPE OF RESISTANCE TO THYROID HORMONE

The extremes of the RTH phenotype have a clear molecu-lar basis. Subjects heterozygous for a TRβ gene deletion are normal because the expression of a single TRβ allele is suf-ficient for normal function. RTH manifests in homozy-gotes completely lacking the TRβ gene and in heterozygotes that express an mTRβ with a dominant negative effect. The most severe form of RTH, with extremely high TH levels and signs of both hypothyroidism and thyrotoxicosis, occur in a homozygous individual expressing only mutant TRs (29,67). The severe hypothyroidism manifesting in bone and brain of this subject can be explained by the silencing effect of a double-dose mTR and its strong interference with the function of TRα (94), a situation that does not occur in homozygous subjects with TRβ deletion. In contrast, the manifestation of thyrotoxicosis in other tissues, such as the heart, may be explained by the effect that high TH levels have on tissues that normally express predominantly TRα1 (95,96) (see later section on Animal Models of Resistance to Thyroid Hormone). It is for the same reason that tachycardia is a relatively common finding in RTH (97).

Various mechanisms can be postulated to explain the tissue differences in TH resistance within the same subject and among individuals. The distribution of receptor isoforms varies from tissue to tissue (46,98,99). This likely accounts for greater hormonal resistance of the liver as compared with the heart. Differences in the degree of resistance among individuals harboring the same mTRβ could be explained by the relative level of mutant and WT-RT expression. Such differences have been found in one study (100) but not in another (64).

Although in a subset of mTRβs a correlation was found between their functional impairment and the degree of thyrotroph hyposensitivity to TH, it is surprising that this correlation was not maintained with regard to the hormonal resistance of peripheral tissues (87). Subjects with the same mutations, even belonging to the same family, showed different degrees of RTH. A most striking example is that of family G.H., in which the mTRβ R316H did not cosegregate with the RTH phenotype in all family members (101). This variability of clinical and laboratory findings was not observed in affected members of two other families with the same mutation (7,102). A study in a large family with the mTRβ R320H suggests that genetic variability of factors other than TR may modulate the phenotype of RTH (103).

RESISTANCE TO THYROID HORMONE WITHOUT THYROID HORMONE RECEPTOR GENE MUTATIONS

The molecular basis of non-TR-RTH remains unknown. Since the first demonstration of non-TR-linked RTH (2), 29 subjects belonging to 23 different families have been identified (39,104,105). The phenotype is indistinguishable from that in subjects harboring TRβ gene mutations (see later section on Differential Diagnosis). Distinct features are an increased female:male ratio of 2.5:1 and the high prevalence of sporadic cases. Of the 21 families in whom both parents, all siblings, and progeny were examined, the occurrence of RTH in another family member was documented in only 4. In those instances, and as in the case of TRβ-linked RTH, the inheritance pattern is dominant. Although it has been postulated that non-TR-RTH is likely caused by a defect in one of the cofactors involved in the mediation of TH action, proof supporting this contention is lacking. Indeed a search for abnormalities in several corepressors, coactivators, coregulators, and a TH membrane transporter yielded negative results (106,107).

ANIMAL MODELS OF RESISTANCE TO THYROID HORMONE

TRβ Gene Manipulations

Understanding of TH action *in vivo,* particularly the mechanisms underlying abnormalities observed in patients with RTH, has been bolstered by observations made in genetically manipulated mice. Three types of genetic manipulations have been applied: (a) transgenic mice that overexpress a receptor; (b) deletion of the receptor (knockout or KO mice); and (c) introduction of mutations in the receptor (knock-in or KI mice). The latter two types of gene manipulation, species differences notwithstanding, have yielded true models of the recessively and dominantly inherited forms of RTH, respectively (108).

The features of RTH found in patients homozygous for TRβ deletion also manifest in the TRβ-deficient mouse (109–111) (Table 81.2). Special features, such as sensorineural deafness and monochromatic vision, are characteristic and shared by mice (112,113) and humans (27,62). This indicates that the lack of TRβ per se, rather than deletion of other genetic material, is responsible for the deaf mutism and color blindness in affected members of the family (28). The mouse model allowed for investigations in greater depth into the mechanisms responsible for the development of these abnormalities. Thus, TRβ1 deficiency retards the expression of fast-activating potassium conductance in inner hair cells of the cochlea that transforms the immature cells from spiking pacemaker to high-frequency signal transmitters (114). TRβ2 interacts with transcription factors involved in photoreceptor development to provide timed and spatial order for cone differentiation, resulting in the selective loss off M-opsin (113). The downregulation of hypothalamic TRH is also TRβ2 specific (115). Mice deficient in TRβ have an increased heart rate that can be decreased to the level of the WT mouse by reduction on the TH level (111). This finding, together with the lower heart rate in mice selectively deficient in TRα1 (116), indicates that TH-dependent changes in heart rate are mediated through TRα, and explains the tachycardia observed in some patients with RTH. TRβ is also required for the T_3-mediated regulation of hepatic cholesterol metabolism, which cannot be compensated by TRα1 (117).

TABLE 81.2. TESTS OF THYROID FUNCTION IN MICE AND HUMANS WITH RESISTANCE TO THYROID HORMONE CAUSED BY TRβ GENE MUTATIONS

Genotype		T_4		T_3		TSH	
		μg/dL	%WT	ng/dL	%WT	μU/mL	%WT
WT	Mouse	3.8 ± 0.7	—	84 ± 11	—	25 ± 20	—
	Human	7.8 ± 0.9	—	119 ± 32	—	3.1 ± 2.2	—
Hetorozygous KO	Mouse	4.3 ± 0.7	113	98 ± 14	117	19 ± 21	76
	Human	7.6 ± 1.5	97	102 ± 11	86	3.5 ± 2.5	113
Homozygous KO	Mouse	7.8 ± 2.0	205	142 ± 43	169	136 ± 116	544
	Human	15.6 ± 4.5	203	209 ± 21	176	5.5 ± 2.6	177
WT	Mouse	3.0 ± 0.8	—	147 ± 46	—	58 ± 41	—
	Human	8.0 ± 0.7	—	115 ± 30	—	2.1 ± 1.0	—
Heterozygous KI	Mouse	6.3 ± 1.2	210	283 ± 83	193	129 ± 140	230
	Human	18.3 ± 4.6	230	286 ± 87	250	3.5 ± 3.4	170
Homozygous KI	Mouse	36 ± 14	1210	1,257 ± 507	855	19,485 ± 6,520	34,790
	Human	54	680	850	740	840	40,000

KI, knock-in; KO, knockout; WT, wild-type; T_3, triiodothyronine; T_4, thyroxine; TSH, thyrotropin.

The combined deletion of TRα1 and α2 produces no important alterations in TH or TSH concentrations in serum (51). However, expression of the carboxyl-terminal fragment of the TRα, due to the presence of a natural promoter and a transcription start site in intron 5, produces in the context of deficient intact TRα severe neonatal hypothyroidism that is lethal but can be rescued by short-term treatment with TH (118). The complete lack of TRs, both α and β, is compatible with life (51,52). This contrasts with the complete lack of TH, which in the athyreotic Pax8-deficient mouse results in death prior to weaning, unless rescued by TH treatment (119). The survival of combined TR-deficient mice is not due to expression of a yet unidentified TR but to the absence of the noxious effect of aporeceptors. Indeed, removal of the TRα gene rescues Pax8 KO mice from death (120). The combined TRβ- and TRα-deficient mice have serum TSH levels that are 500-fold higher than those of WT mice and T_4 concentrations 12-fold above the average normal mean (51). Thus, in this instance, the presence of an aporeceptor does not seem to be required for the up-regulation of TSH.

The first, partial model of the dominantly inherited RTH used somatic gene transfer of a mutant TRβ1, G345R, by means of a recombinant adenovirus (121). The liver of these mice was resistant to TH, as demonstrated by the reduced responsiveness of TH controlled genes to the administration of L-T_3. Overexpression of the WT TRβ increased the severity of hypothyroidism in the TH-deprived mouse, confirming that the unliganded TR has a constitutive effect *in vivo* as *in vitro*. Similarly, the response to TH is enhanced in animals that overexpress the WT TR. Transgenic mice have also been developed that express mTRβ1 genes (122). True mouse models of dominantly inherited RTH were recently generated by targeted muta-

tions in the TRβ gene (123,124). Mutations were modeled on those formerly identified in humans with RTH [frameshift resulting in 16 carboxyl-terminal nonsense amino acids (PV mouse) and T337Δ]. As in humans, the phenotype manifested in the heterozygous KI animals, and many of the abnormalities observed in humans were reproduced in these mice (Table 81.2).

Recent work has shown that NcoA (SRC-1) deficient mice have RTH manifesting with elevated T_4, T_3, and TSH concentrations (125). A more mild form of RTH was identified in mice deficient in RXRγ (126). Animals show reduced sensitivity to T_3 in terms of TSH down-regulation but not metabolic rate. These data indicate that abnormalities in cofactors can produce RTH.

The Phenotype of TRα Gene Mutation in the Mouse

The question of why mutations in the TRα gene have not been identified in humans was partially answered by the study of mice with targeted gene manipulations. As stated in the preceding section, TRα gene deletions, total or only α1, failed to produce an RTH phenotype. Similarly, mice with targeted TRα gene mutations failed to manifest the phenotype of RTH. Human mutations known to occur in the TRβ gene were targeted in homologous regions of the TRα gene of the mouse. These were the PV frameshift mutation in the carboxyl-terminus of TRα1 (35), TRα1 R348C [equivalent to TRβ R438C (36)] and P398H [equivalent to TRβ P453H (37)]. The resulting phenotypes were variable but did not exhibit RTH. In the heterozygous state, the former two show severe retardation in postnatal development and growth, while the latter has an increase in body fat and insulin resistance. Decreased heart rate and cold-induced thermogenesis, as well as reduced fertility, were also observed. The TRαPV KI mice exhibited severe reduction in brain glucose utilization and synaptic density (127,128). All three TRα KIs were lethal in the homozygous state, recapitulating the noxious effect of unliganded TRα1.

PATHOGENESIS

The reduced sensitivity to TH in subjects with RTH is shared to a variable extent by all tissues. The hyposensitivity of the pituitary thyrotrophs results in nonsuppressed serum TSH, which in turn increases the synthesis and secretion of TH. The persistence of TSH secretion in the face of high levels of free TH contrasts with the low TSH levels in the more common forms of TH hypersecretion that are TSH independent. This apparent paradoxic dissociation between TH and TSH is responsible for the wide use of the term "inappropriate secretion of TSH" to designate the syndrome. However, TSH hypersecretion is not at all inappropriate, given the fact that the response to TH is reduced. It is compensatory and appropriate for the level of TH action mediated through a defective TR. As a consequence, most patients are eumetabolic, although the compensation is variable among affected individuals and tissues in the same individual. However, the level of tissue responses do not correlate with the level of TH, probably owing to a discordance between the hormonal effect on the pituitary and other body tissues. Thyroid gland enlargement occurs with chronic, though minimal, TSH hypersecretion due to increased biologic potency of this glycoprotein through increased sialylation (129). Administration of supraphysiologic doses of TH are required to suppress TSH secretion without induction of thyrotoxic changes in peripheral tissues.

When sought, TSH-binding antibodies could not be detected (130,131). Thyroid-stimulating antibodies, which are responsible for the thyroid gland hyperactivity in Graves' disease, have been conspicuously absent in patients with RTH. Another potential thyroid stimulator, human chorionic gonadotropin, is also not involved (132,133).

The selectivity of the resistance to TH has been convincingly demonstrated. When tested at the pituitary level, both thyrotrophs and lactotrophs were less sensitive only to TH. Thyrotrophs responded normally to the suppressive effects of the dopaminergic drugs L-dopa and bromocriptine (131,134) as well as to glucocorticoids (131,135,136). Studies conducted in cultured fibroblasts confirm the *in vivo* findings of selective resistance to TH. The responsiveness to dexamethasone, measured in terms of glycosaminoglycan (137) and fibronectin synthesis (138), was preserved in the presence of T_3 insensitivity (Fig. 81.3).

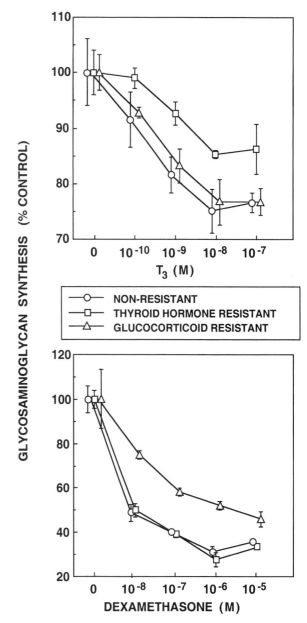

FIGURE 81.3. The inhibitory effect of triiodothyronine (T_3) and dexamethasone on glycosaminoglycan synthesis in fibroblasts from subjects with TH and glucocorticoid resistance compared with that in fibroblasts from a normal (nonresistant) subject. Note that fibroblasts from the patient with RTH had an attenuated response to T_3 but not to dexamethasone, while those from the patient with glucocorticoid resistance showed an attenuated response to dexamethasone only. (Modified from Refetoff S, Weiss RE, Usala SJ. The syndromes of resistance to thyroid hormone. *Endocr Rev* 1993;14:348–399, with permission.)

Several of the clinical features encountered in some patients with RTH may be the manifestation of selective tissue deprivation of TH during early stages of development. These clinical features include retarded bone age, stunted growth, mental retardation or learning disability, emotional disturbances, attention deficit/hyperactivity disorder

(ADHD), hearing defects, and nystagmus (1). A variety of associated somatic abnormalities appear to be unrelated pathogenically and may be the result of involvement of other genes such as in major deletions of DNA sequences (28). However, no gross chromosomal abnormalities have been detected on karyotyping (27,139).

PATHOLOGY

Little can be said about the pathologic findings in tissues other than the thyroid gland because of unavailability of autopsy data from patients with RTH. Electron microscopic examination of striated muscle obtained by biopsy from one patient revealed mitochondrial swelling, also known to be encountered in thyrotoxicosis (27). This is compatible with the predominant expression of TRα in muscle (140), resulting in a low level of expression of the mutant TRβ and unobstructed action of the excessive amount of circulating TH available to this tissue. Light microscopy of skin fibroblasts stained with toluidine blue showed moderate to intense metachromasia (141) as described in myxedema and is probably a manifestation of a decreased TH action in this tissue. However, in contrast to patients with myxedema due to TH deficiency, treatment with the hormone failed to induce a disappearance of the metachromasia in fibroblasts from patients with RTH.

Thyroid tissue, obtained by biopsy or at surgery, revealed various degrees of hyperplasia of the follicular epithelium (130,131,142,143). The follicles may vary in size, from small to large. Some specimens have been described as "adenomatous goiters," others as "colloid goiters," and

still others as normal thyroid tissue. Occasional lymphocytic infiltration, a finding not related to the syndrome, is due to the fortuitous coexistence of thyroiditis (144).

CLINICAL FEATURES

Characteristic of the RTH syndrome is the paucity of specific clinical manifestations. When present, manifestations are variable from one patient to another. Investigation leading to the diagnosis has been undertaken because of the presence of goiter, hyperactive behavior or learning disabilities, developmental delay, and sinus tachycardia (Fig. 81.4). The finding of elevated serum TH levels in association with nonsuppressed TSH is usually responsible for the pursuit of further studies leading to the diagnosis.

The majority of untreated subjects maintain a normal metabolic state at the expense of high levels of TH. The degree of this compensation of tissue hyposensitivity to the hormone is, however, variable among individuals as well as in different tissues. As a consequence, clinical and laboratory evidence of TH deficiency and excess often coexist. For example, RTH can present with a mild to moderate growth retardation, delayed bone maturation, and learning disabilities suggestive of hypothyroidism, along with hyperactivity and tachycardia, compatible with thyrotoxicosis. The more common clinical features and their frequency are given in Table 81.3. Frank symptoms of hypothyroidism are more common in those individuals who, because of erroneous diagnosis, have received treatment to normalize their circulating TH levels. In such patients, symptoms of fatigue, somnolence, depression, weight gain,

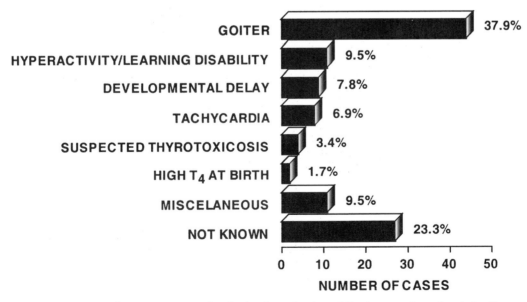

FIGURE 81.4. The reasons prompting further investigation of the key member of each family with resistance to thyroid hormone.

TABLE 81.3. CLINICAL FEATURES

Findings	Frequency (%)
Thyroid gland	
Goiter	66–95
Heart	
Tachycardia	33–75
Nervous system	
Emotional disturbances	60
Hyperkinetic behavior	33–68
Attention deficit hyperactivity disorder	40–60
Learning disability	30
Mental retardation (IQ <70)	4–16
Hearing loss (sensorineural)	10–22
Growth and development	
Short stature (<5%)	18–25
Delayed bone age >2 SD	29–47
Low body mass index (in children)	33
Recurrent ear and throat infections	55

Data derived from references 1, 7, and 145.

and bradycardia were noted. In children, inappropriate treatment has aggravated the delay in growth and development (1).

On physical examination, goiter is by far the most common abnormality. It has been reported in 66% to 95% of cases. In some patients without clinically obvious thyroid gland enlargement, goiter could be detected by ultrasonography, was absent due to prior surgery, or was present in other affected members of the family. Gland enlargement is usually diffuse; nodular changes and gross asymmetry are found in recurrent goiters after surgery.

Sinus tachycardia is also common, with some studies reporting frequency as high as 80% (7). Palpitations often bring the patient to the physician, and the finding of tachycardia is the most common reason for the erroneous diagnosis of autoimmune thyrotoxicosis or the suspicion of PRTH.

Careful evaluation of subjects with RTH has shown that about half have some degree of learning disability with or without ADHD (1,146). One fourth have intellectual quotients (IQs) of less than 85, but frank mental retardation (IQ <60) has been found only in 3% of cases. Impaired mental function was found to be associated with impaired or delayed growth (<5th percentile) in 20% of subjects, although growth retardation alone is rare (4%) (1). Despite the high prevalence of ADHD in patients with RTH, the occurrence of RTH in children with ADHD must be rare, none having been detected in 330 such children studied (147,148). Current data do not support a genetic linkage of RTH with ADHD. Rather, the higher prevalence of low IQ scores may confer a higher likelihood for subjects with RTH to exhibit ADHD symptoms (102).

A variety of physical defects that cannot be explained on the basis of TH deprivation or excess have been recorded.

These include major or minor somatic defects, such as winged scapulae, vertebral anomalies, pigeon breast, prominent pectoralis, birdlike facies, scaphocephaly, craniosynostosis, short fourth metacarpals, as well as Besnier's prurigo, congenital ichthyosis, and bull's eye type macular atrophy (1). No particular defect appears to be prevalent in RTH. A distinct body habitus and deaf-mutism occurred in all three affected members of a single family with TRβ gene deletion (27).

COURSE OF THE DISEASE

The course of the disease is as variable as is its presentation. Some subjects have normal growth and development, and lead a normal life at the expense of high TH levels and a small goiter. Others have variable degrees of mental and growth retardation. Symptoms of hyperactivity tend to improve with age, but this is not characteristic of RTH since it has been also observed in subjects with ADHD only.

Goiter has recurred in every patient who underwent thyroid surgery. As a consequence, some subjects have been submitted to several consecutive thyroidectomies or treatments with radioiodide (143,149–151).

Only in one patient is RTH believed to have contributed to his demise. This child, homozygous for a dominantly inherited TRβ mutation and a resting heart rate of 190 beats/minute (29), died from cardiogenic shock complicating staphyloccocal pneumonia (B.B. Bercu, personal communication).

LABORATORY FINDINGS

Thyroid Hormone and Its Metabolites in Serum

In the untreated patient, elevation in the concentration of serum free T_4 is a sine qua non requirement for the diagnosis of RTH. It is accompanied by high serum levels of T_3. Serum TBG and TTR concentrations are normal. The resin T_3 uptake is usually high, as is the case in patients with thyrotoxicosis.

Serum T_4 and T_3 values vary from just above to several-fold the upper limit of normal. Although the levels may vary in the course of time in the same patient (7), the degree of T_4 and T_3 elevation is usually congruent, resulting in a normal T_3:T_4 ratio (1). This is in contrast to the disproportionate increase in serum T_3 concentration relative to that of T_4, characteristic of autoimmune thyrotoxicosis (152). This observation has led some investigators to consider the possibility of reduced extrathyroidal conversion of T_4 to T_3 in patients with RTH (143).

Reverse T_3 concentration is also high in patients with RTH, as is that of another product of T_4 degradation, 3,3′-T_2 (130). Serum thyroglobulin concentration also tends to be high, and the degree of its elevation reflects the level of TSH-induced thyroid gland hyperactivity.

Thyrotropin and Other Thyroid Stimulators

A characteristic, if not pathognomonic, feature of the syndrome is the presence of TSH in serum and preservation of its response to TRH despite an elevated TH level (153). In most cases, the basal serum TSH concentration is normal and the circadian rhythm is unaltered (154,155). TSH values above 10 mU/L occur in subjects that have received treatment aimed at reducing their high level of TH. The TSH response to TRH is either normal or exaggerated.

Thyrotropin has increased biologic activity (129,156), and the concentration of its free α subunit is not disproportionately high. Except for the rare occurrence of coincidental autoimmune thyroiditis (157), serum is free of thyroid-stimulating immunoglobulins as well as antibodies against thyroglobulin and thyroid peroxidases.

Thyroid Gland Activity and Integrity of Hormone Synthesis

The fractional uptake of radioiodide by the thyroid gland is high, as is the absolute amount of accumulated iodide. The latter is normally organified, since no discharge of trapped iodide has been observed following the administration of perchlorate (27,149,158). No abnormal iodide-containing compounds have been detected in the circulation (27,141).

Turnover of Thyroid Hormone

In vivo turnover kinetics of T_4 showed a normal or slightly increased volume of distribution and fractional disappearance rate of the hormone. However, because of the high concentration of T_4 in serum, the extrathyroidal pool and absolute daily production of T_4 are increased, up to twofold the upper limit of normal, and that of T_3 is increased by about two- to fourfold (133,141,149,159,160). However, the extrathyroidal conversion of T_4 to T_3 is normal (160).

In Vivo Effects of Thyroid Hormone

The impact of TH on peripheral tissues has been assessed *in vivo* by a variety of tests. By and large, results have been normal and, given the high serum levels of TH, suggest a reduced biologic response to the hormone (1,7). The metabolic status has been evaluated by measurements of the basal metabolic rate (BMR), serum cholesterol, carotene, triglycerides, creatine kinase, alkaline phosphatase, angiotensin-converting enzyme, SHBG, ferritin, and osteocalcin, all of which usually have been within the normal range. Urinary excretion of magnesium, hydroxyproline,

creatine, creatinine, carnitine, and cyclic adenosine monophosphate (cAMP), all found to be elevated in thyrotoxicosis, have been normal or low, suggesting normal or slightly reduced TH effect. With the exception of an increased resting pulse rate in about half of the patients with RTH, the cardiac function is only minimally altered. Two-dimensional and Doppler echocardiography showed mild hyperthyroid effect on cardiac systolic and diastolic function of the myocardium, whereas other parameters, such as ejection and shortening fractions of the left ventricle, systolic diameter, and left ventricle wall thickness, were normal (97). The Achilles tendon reflex relaxation time has also been normal or slightly prolonged. The PRL response to TRH was not blunted as it is in patients with thyrotoxicosis. In fact, the PRL hyperresponsiveness in some patients with RTH may be due to the functional TH deprivation at the level of the lactotrophs (153).

Other Endocrine Tests

Evaluation of endocrine function by a variety of tests has failed to reveal significant defects other than those related to the thyroid. The following laboratory analyses have been conducted in patients with RTH and were found to be within the normal range: serum levels of cortisol and its diurnal rhythm; testosterone, estrogens, and progesterone; gonadotropins and their response to gonadotropin-releasing hormone; adrenocorticotropic hormone; insulin; prolactin and its response to TRH, L-dopa and glucocorticoids; growth hormone and its response to insulin hypoglycemia, arginine, and pyrogen; as well as the urinary excretion of 17-hydroxycorticoids, 17-ketosteroids, vanillylmandelic acid, adrenaline, and noradrenaline. Radiologic and magnetic resonance examinations of the pituitary gland and sella turcica have shown no anatomic abnormalities.

Bone Age

Radiologic evidence of delayed bone maturation has been observed in one half of patients with RTH diagnosed during infancy or childhood (1). However, the majority achieve normal adult stature. It is unclear whether the presence, in some cases, of stippled epiphyses is also the consequence of reduced TH action.

IN VITRO TESTS OF THYROID HORMONE ACTION

The normal stimulatory effect of T_3 on the degradation rate of low-density lipoproteins was reduced in cultured skin fibroblasts obtained from three affected members of one family (151). Similarly, T_3 and T_4, but not dexamethasone, failed to produce the normal inhibitory effect on the synthesis of glycosaminoglycans in fibroblasts from four of six patients with RTH (137) (Fig. 87.3). In contrast, T_3 normally stimulated glucose consumption by cultured fibroblasts from a patient with RTH (136,161). *In vitro* demonstration of TH resistance has been most consistent by measurement of the normal inhibitory effect of T_3 on the synthesis of fibronectin and its mRNA in skin fibroblasts maintained in culture. Of 12 patients with RTH who were studied, 11 showed either an attenuated or paradoxic response (138).

Responses to the Administration of Thyroid Hormone

Because reduced responsiveness to TH is central in the pathogenesis of the syndrome, patients have been given TH in order to observe their responses and thereby establish the presence of hyposensitivity to the hormone. Unfortunately, data generated have been discrepant, not only because of differences in the relative degree of resistance to TH among patients, but also because of lack of uniformity in the manner the hormone trials have been performed. These include differences in hormonal preparations, dosages, duration of treatment, and the type of observations and measurements performed, not to mention the conspicuous lack of adequate control studies.

Administration of TH ultimately suppresses TSH secretion, resulting in a decrease and eventually the abolition of the TSH response to TRH. The amount of TH necessary to produce such an effect has been variable, as has been the relative effectiveness of L-T_3 as compared with L-T_4. Such observations have led to earlier speculations that some patients may have an abnormality in conversion of T_4 to T_3 (142,143). The decreased TSH secretion during the administration of supraphysiologic doses of TH is accompanied by a reduction in the thyroidal radioiodide uptake and, when exogenous T_3 is given, a reduction in the pretreatment level of serum T_4 (132,133, 143,149,151).

Various responses of peripheral tissues to the administration of TH have been quantitated. Most notable are measurements of the BMR, pulse rate, reflex relaxation time, serum cholesterol, lipids, enzymes, osteocalcin and SHBG, and urinary excretion of hydroxyproline, creatine, and carnitine. Either no significant changes were observed, or they were much reduced relative to the amount of TH given (1).

Of great importance are observations on the catabolic effect of exogenous TH. In some subjects with RTH, L-T_4 given in doses of up to 1,000 µg/day, and L-T_3 up to 400 µg/day, failed to produce weight loss without a change in calorie intake, nor did they induce a negative nitrogen balance (131,132,141). In contrast, administration of these large doses of TH over a prolonged period of time was apparently anabolic, as evidenced by a dramatic increase in growth rate and accelerated bone maturation (11,131).

Effects of Other Drugs

As expected, administration of the TH analogue 3,5,3′-triiodo-L-thyroacetic acid (TRIAC) to patients with RTH produced attenuated responses (141,155,162).

Administration of glucocorticoids promptly reduced the TSH response to TRH and the serum T_4 concentration (131,132,135,142,159).

Administration of L-dopa and bromocriptine produced a prompt suppression of TSH secretion, as well as a diminution of the thyroidal radioiodide uptake and serum T_3 level (131,134,142). Domperidone, a dopamine antagonist, caused an increase in the serum TSH level when given to patients with RTH (155). These observations indicate that, in this syndrome, the normal inhibitory effect of dopamine on TSH is intact.

The response to antithyroid drugs has shown some variability. Methimazole and propylthiouracil, in doses usually effective in reducing the high serum TH level of hyperthyroidism of autoimmune etiology, had no effect in two patients (141). However, in other cases of RTH, antithyroid drugs induced some decrease in the circulating level of TH, producing a reciprocal change in the TSH concentration (32,139,158,163). Administration of 100 mg of iodine daily had a similar effect in one patient (133), but 4 mg potassium iodide per day produced no changes in another (141).

Observations on the effect of other drugs such as diazepam and chlorpromazine are limited. With one exception (141), propranolol and atenolol caused a significant reduction in heart rate.

DIFFERENTIAL DIAGNOSIS

Because the clinical presentation of RTH is variable, detection requires a high degree of suspicion. The differential diagnosis includes all possible causes of hyperthyroxinemia. The sequence of diagnostic procedures listed in Table 81.4 is suggested.

The presence of elevated serum T_4 concentration with nonsuppressed TSH needs to be confirmed by repeated testing. The possibility of an inherited or acquired increase in serum TBG must be excluded by direct measurement and by estimation of the circulating free T_4 level. The presence of a high serum T_3 level must also be documented because reduced conversion of T_4 to T_3 by peripheral tissues may occasionally give rise to the elevation of total and free T_4 but not T_3 levels. This may occur transiently in a variety of nonthyroidal illnesses or during the administration of some drugs (see Chapter 11). A familial form of hyperthyroxinemia, presumably due to a defective T_4 monodeiodination, has been also described (164). The inherited abnormality of T_4 binding to an albumin presents with high serum T_4 but normal T_3 concentration (see Chapters 6 and

TABLE 81.4. SUGGESTED SEQUENCE OF DIAGNOSTIC PROCEDURES IN SUSPECTED RESISTANCE TO THYROID HORMONE

1. Usual presentation: high serum levels of free T_4 and T_3 with nonsuppressed TSH.
2. Confirm the elevated serum levels of free thyroid hormone (T_4 and T_3) and exclude TH transport defects.
3. Obtain tests of thyroid function in first-degree relatives: parents, siblings, and children.
4. In the absence of similar TH test abnormalities in other family members, exclude the presence of a pituitary adenoma by measurement of α subunit in serum.
5. Demonstrate a blunted TSH suppression and metabolic response to the administration of supraphysiologic doses of TH (see L-T_3 suppression protocol, Fig. 87.5).
6. Perform linkage analysis and demonstrate a TH receptor gene defect.

T_3, triiodothyronine; T_4, thyroxine; TH, thyroid hormone; TSH, thyrotropin.

13). A rare cause of elevated serum T_4 and T_3 level is the endogenous production of antibodies directed against these hormones, which can be excluded by direct testing

Most useful is the measurement of the serum TSH. Under most circumstances, patients with high concentrations of circulating free TH have virtually undetectable serum TSH levels, which characteristically fail to increase in response to TRH. This is true even when the magnitude of TH excess is minimal and therefore subclinical both on physical examination or by other laboratory tests (see Chapters 13 and 79). The combination of elevated serum levels of TH and nonsuppressed TSH narrows the differential diagnosis to RTH and autonomous hypersecretion of TSH associated with pituitary tumors. The latter should be suspected when other members of the family, particularly the parents of the patient, fail to exhibit thyroid test abnormalities. Rarely, endogenous antibodies to TSH or some of the test components can give rise to false increases in serum TSH values.

In addition to symptoms and signs of thyrotoxicosis, some patients with TSH-producing (thyrotroph) pituitary adenomas may present with acromegaly due to the concomitant hypersecretion of growth hormone by the tumor. Galactorrhea and amenorrhea in association with hyperprolactinemia have also been reported (see Chapter 24). The tumors may be demonstrated by computed tomography or by magnetic resonance imaging of the pituitary. A typical finding in patients with TSH-producing pituitary adenomas is a disproportionate abundance in serum of free α subunit of TSH relative to whole TSH (165). Moreover, with rare exceptions (166), serum TSH fails to increase above the basal level in response to TRH or to decrease during the administration of TH. Ectopic production of TSH has not been unequivocally demonstrated (see Chapter 26). It is uncertain that endogenous TRH hypersecretion could maintain high TSH levels and induce hyperthyroidism.

Because the etiology of PRTH is not distinct from that of RTH, failure to demonstrate an anatomic defect in the pituitary gland by imaging does not exclude the presence of a small adenoma or thyrotroph hyperplasia. Furthermore, absence of conspicuous signs and symptoms of hypermetabolism are not sufficient to rule out thyrotoxicosis. The occurrence of an apparent selective hyposensitivity to T_4, but not T_3, has been reported in one family (167). Initially attributed to a putative defect in type II 5′-deiodinase, it was recently shown that affected family members had the TRβ R320L mutation (D. Gross, P.R. Larsen, and W.W. Chin, personal communication).

Proving the existence of peripheral tissue resistance to TH is not simple. Lack of clinical symptoms and signs of hypermetabolism are not sufficient to establish the diagnosis of RTH, and no single test objectively proves the existence of eumetabolism. Because resistance to the hormone is variable in different tissues, no single test measuring a particular response to TH is diagnostic. Furthermore, results of most tests that measure the effect of TH on peripheral tissues show considerable overlap among thyrotoxic, euthyroid, and hypothyroid subjects. The value of these tests is enhanced if measurements are obtained before and following the administration of supraphysiologic doses of TH.

Although the demonstration of TRβ gene mutation is sufficient to establish the diagnosis of RTH, *in vivo* demonstration of tissue resistance to TH is required when RTH is not associated with a TR gene mutation (2). A standardized diagnostic protocol, using short-term administration of incremental doses of L-T_3 and outlined in Fig. 81.5, is recommended. It is designed to assess several parameters of central and peripheral tissue effects of TH in the basal state and in comparison with those elicited following the administration of L-T_3. The three doses given in sequence are a replacement dose of 50 µg/day and two supraphysiologic doses of 100 and 200 µg/day. The hormone is administered in a split dose every 12 hours, and each incremental dose is given for the period of 3 days. Doses are adjusted in children and in adults of unusual size to achieve the same level of serum T_3. L-T_3, rather than L-T_4, is used because of its direct effect on tissues, bypassing potential defects of T_4 transport and metabolism, which may also produce attenuated responses. In addition, the more rapid onset and shorter duration of T_3 action reduces the period required to complete the evaluation and shortens the duration of symptoms that may arise in individuals with normal responses to the hormone. Responses to each incremental dose of L-T_3 are expressed as increments and decrements or as a percentage of the value measured at baseline. The results of such a study are shown in Figs. 81.6 and 81.7.

Failure to differentiate RTH from ordinary thyrotoxicosis has resulted in the inappropriate treatment of nearly one third of patients. The diagnosis requires awareness of the

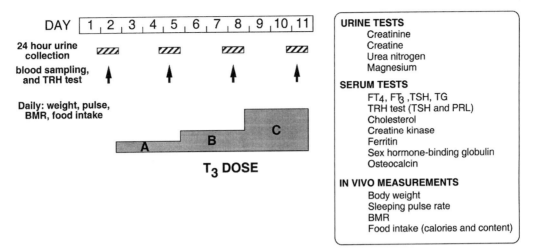

FIGURE 81.5. Schematic representation of a protocol for the assessment of the sensitivity to thyroid hormone using incremental doses of liothyronine (L-T$_3$). (Adapted from Refetoff S, Weiss RE, Usala SJ. The syndromes of resistance to thyroid hormone. *Endocr Rev* 1993;14: 348–399, with permission.)

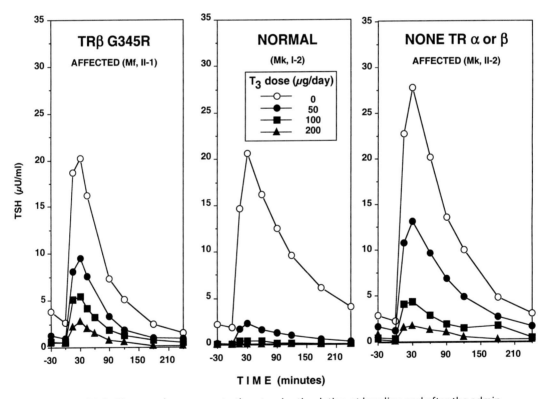

FIGURE 81.6. Thyrotroph responses to thyrotropin stimulation at baseline and after the administration of graded doses of liothyronine (L-T$_3$). The hormone was given in three incremental doses, each for 3 days as depicted in Fig. 81.5. Results are shown for patients with resistance to thyroid hormone (RTH) in the presence (left) or absence (right) of a TRβ gene mutation, together with the unaffected mother of the patient with non-TR-RTH (center).

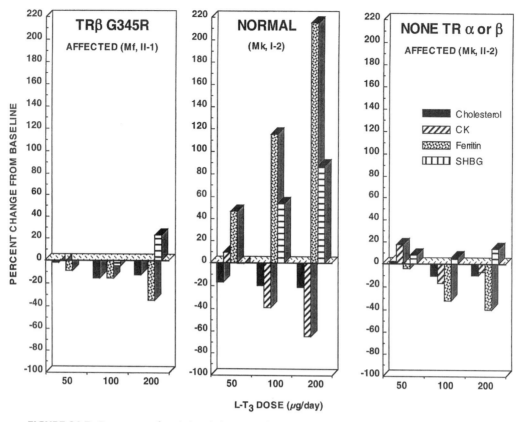

FIGURE 81.7. Responses of peripheral tissues to the administration of liothyronine (L-T$_3$) in the presence or absence of mutations in the TRβ gene. The hormone was given as described in Fig. 81.6. Note the stimulation of ferritin and sex hormone binding globulin (*SHBG*) and the suppression of cholesterol and creatine kinase (*CK*) in the normal subject. Responses in affected subjects, with or without a TRβ gene mutation, were blunted or paradoxic.

possible presence of RTH, usually suspected when high levels of circulating TH are not accompanied by a suppressed TSH.

TREATMENT

Although no specific treatment is available to fully and specifically correct the defect, the ability to identify specific mutations in the TRs provides a means for prenatal diagnosis and appropriate family counseling. This is particularly important in families whose affected members show evidence of growth or mental retardation. Fortunately, in most cases of RTH, the partial tissue resistance to TH appears to be adequately compensated for by an increase in the endogenous supply of TH. Thus, treatment need not be given to such patients. This is not the case in patients with limited thyroidal reserve due to prior ablative therapy. In these patients, the serum TSH level can be used as a guideline for hormone dosage.

Not infrequently, some peripheral tissues in patients with RTH appear to be relatively more resistant than the pituitary. Thus, compensation for the defect at the level of

peripheral tissues is incomplete. In such instances, judicious administration of supraphysiologic doses of the hormone is indicated. Because the dose varies greatly among cases, it should be individually determined by assessing tissue responses. In childhood, particular attention must be directed to growth, bone maturation, and mental development. It is suggested that TH be given in incremental doses and that the BMR, nitrogen balance, and serum SHBG be monitored at each dose, and bone age and growth on a longer term. Development of a catabolic state is an indication of overtreatment.

The exact criteria for treatment of RTH in infancy have not been established. This is often an issue when the diagnosis is made at birth or in early infancy. In infants with elevated serum TSH levels, subclinical hypothyroidism may be more harmful than treatment with TH. Indications for treatment may include a TSH level above the upper limit of normal, retarded bone development and failure to thrive. The outcome of affected older members of the family who did not receive treatment may serve as a guideline. Longer follow-up and psychological testing of infants who have been given treatment will determine the efficacy of early intervention.

A recent survey has shown an increased miscarriage rate and low birth weight of normal infants born to mothers with RTH (168). It is unclear at this time whether intervention during early gestation is appropriate. However, mothers with RTH should be followed carefully during pregnancy and not allowed to have low serum TSH values. The wisdom of *in utero* treatment is questionable (169, 170).

Patients with more severe thyrotroph resistance and symptoms of thyrotoxicosis may require therapy. Symptomatic treatment with an adrenergic β-blocking agent, preferably atenolol, usually suffices. Treatment with antithyroid drugs or thyroid gland ablation increase TSH secretion and may result in thyrotroph hyperplasia. Development of true pituitary tumors, even after long periods of thyrotroph overactivity, is extremely rare (171).

It has been shown recently that treatment with supraphysiologic doses of L-T_3, given as a single dose every other day, is successful in reducing goiter size with remarkable cosmetic benefits and without causing side effects (172). This appears to be the treatment of choice considering that postoperative recurrence of goiter is the rule. The L-T_3 dose must be adjusted in increments until TSH and TG are suppressed and reduction of goiter size is observed.

Patients with presumed isolated peripheral tissue resistance to TH present a most difficult therapeutic dilemma. The problem is, in reality, diagnostic rather than therapeutic. Many, if not most, patients falling into this category are habitual TH users. Gradual reduction of the TH dose and psychotherapy is recommended.

ACKNOWLEDGMENTS

This work was supported in part by U.S. Public Health Grants DK15070 and RR00055.

REFERENCES

1. Refetoff S, Weiss RE, Usala SJ. The syndromes of resistance to thyroid hormone. *Endocr Rev* 1993;14:348–399.
2. Weiss RE, Hayashi Y, Nagaya T, et al. Dominant inheritance of resistance to thyroid hormone not linked to defects in the thyroid hormone receptors α or β genes may be due to a defective co-factor. *J Clin Endocrinol Metab* 1996;81:4196–4203.
3. Weintraub BD, Gershengorn MC, Kourides IA, et al. Inappropriate secretion of thyroid stimulating hormone. *Ann Intern Med* 1981;95:339–351.
4. Kaplan MM, Swartz SL, Larsen PR. Partial peripheral resistance to thyroid hormone. *Am J Med* 1981;70:1115–1121.
5. Usala SJ. Molecular diagnosis and characterization of thyroid hormone resistance syndromes. *Thyroid* 1991;1:361–367.
6. Beck-Peccoz P, Roncoroni R, Mariotti S, et al. Sex hormone-binding globulin measurement in patients with inappropriate secretion of thyrotropin (IST): evidence against selective pituitary thyroid hormone resistance in nonneoplastic IST. *J Clin Endocrinol Metab* 1990;71:19–25.
7. Beck-Peccoz P, Chatterjee VKK. The variable clinical phenotype in thyroid hormone resistance syndrome. *Thyroid* 1994;4:225–232.
8. Adams M, Matthews C, Collingwood TN, et al. Genetic analysis of 29 kindreds with generalized and pituitary resistance to thyroid hormone: identification of thirteen novel mutations in the thyroid hormone receptor β gene. *J Clin Invest* 1994;94:506–515.
9. Ando S, Sarlis NJ, Krishan J, et al. Aberrant alternative splicing of thyroid hormone receptor in a TSH-secreting pituitary tumor is a mechanism for hormone resistance. *Mol Endocrinol* 2001;15:1529–1538.
10. Ando S, Sarlis NJ, Oldfield EH, et al. Somatic mutation of TR-beta can cause a defect in negative regulation of TSH in a TSH-secreting pituitary tumor. *J Clin Endocrinol Metab* 2001;86:5572–5576.
11. Weiss RE, Balzano S, Scherberg NH, et al. Neonatal detection of generalized resistance to thyroid hormone. *JAMA* 1990;264:2245–2250.
12. LaFranchi SH, Snyder DB, Sesser DE, et al. Follow-up of newborns with elevated screening T_4 concentrations. *J Pediatr* 2003;143:296–301.
13. Feng W, Ribeiro RCJ, Wagner RL, et al. Hormone-dependent coactivator binding to a hydrophobic cleft on nuclear receptors. *Science* 1998;280:1747–1749.
14. Chen JD, Evans RM. A transcriptional co-repressor that interacts with nuclear hormone receptors. *Nature* 1995;377:454–457.
15. Hörlein AJ, Näär AM, Heinzel T, et al. Ligand-independent repression by the thyroid hormone receptor mediated by a nuclear receptor co-repressor. *Nature* 1995;377:397–404.
16. Busch K, Martin B, Baniahmad A, et al. At least three subdomains of v-erbA are involved in its silencing function. *Mol Endocrinol* 1997;11:379–389.
17. Forman BM, Samuels HH. Interactions among a subfamily of nuclear hormone receptors: the regulatory zipper model. *Mol Endocrinol* 1990;4:1293–1301.
18. O'Donnell AL, Koenig RJ. Mutational analysis identifies a new functional domain of the thyroid hormone receptor. *Mol Endocrinol* 1990;4:715–720.
19. Kurokawa R, Yu VC, Naar A, et al. Differential orientations of the DNA-binding domain and carboxy-terminal dimerization interface regulate binding site selection by nuclear receptor heterodimers. *Genes Dev* 1993;7:1423–1435.
20. Au-Fliegner M, Helmer E, Casanova J, et al. The conserved ninth C-terminal heptad in thyroid hormone and retinoic acid receptors mediates diverse responses by affecting heterodimer but not homodimer formation. *Mol Cell Endocrinol* 1993;13:5725–5737.
21. Beck-Peccoz P, Chatterjee VKK, Chin WW, et al. Nomenclature of thyroid hormone receptor β-gene mutations in resistance to thyroid hormone: consensus statement from the first workshop on thyroid hormone resistance, July 10–11, 1993, Cambridge, United Kingdom. *J Clin Endocrinol Metab* 1993; 78:990–993.
22. Tone Y, Collingwood TN, Adams M, et al. Functional analysis of a transactivation domain in the thyroid hormone β receptor. *J Biol Chem* 1994;269:31157–31161.
23. Baniahmad A, Leng X, Burris TP, et al. The T_4 activation domain of the thyroid hormone receptor is required for release of a putative corepressor(s) necessary for transcriptional silencing. *Mol Cell Biol* 1995;15:76–86.
24. Hamy F, Helbecque NJ, Henichart P. Comparison between synthetic nuclear localisation signal peptides from the steroid thyroid hormone receptor superfamily. *Biochem Biophys Res Commun* 1992;183:289–293.
25. Wurtz J-M, Bourguet W, Renaud J-P, et al. A canonical structure for the ligand-binding domain of the nuclear receptors. *Nat Struct Biol* 1966;3:87–94.

26. Refetoff S, Weiss RE. Resistance to thyroid hormone. In: Thakker TV, ed. *Molecular genetics of endocrine disorders.* London: Chapman & Hill, 1997:85–122.

27. Refetoff S, DeWind LT, DeGroot LJ. Familial syndrome combining deaf-mutism, stippled epiphyses, goiter, and abnormally high PBI: possible target organ refractoriness to thyroid hormone. *J Clin Endocrinol Metab* 1967;27:279–294.

28. Takeda K, Sakurai A, DeGroot LJ, et al. Recessive inheritance of thyroid hormone resistance caused by complete deletion of the protein-coding region of the thyroid hormone receptor-β gene. *J Clin Endocrinol Metab* 1992;74:49–55.

29. Ono S, Schwartz ID, Mueller OT, et al. Homozygosity for a "dominant negative" thyroid hormone receptor gene responsible for generalized resistance to thyroid hormone. *J Clin Endocrinol Metab* 1991;73:990–994.

30. Frank-Raue K, Höppner W, Boll HU, et al. Severe form of thyroid hormone resistance in a homozygous mutation in the thyroid hormone receptor β gene [Abstract]. *Exp Clin Endocrinol Diabetes* 1998;106(suppl 1):16.

31. Usala SJ, Bale AE, Gesundheit N, et al. Tight linkage between the syndrome of generalized thyroid hormone resistance and the human c-erbAβ gene. *Mol Endocrinol* 1988;2:1217–1220.

32. Sakurai A, Takeda K, Ain K, et al. Generalized resistance to thyroid hormone associated with a mutation in the ligand-binding domain of the human thyroid hormone receptor β.. *Proc Natl Acad Sci U S A* 1989;86:8977–8981.

33. Usala SJ, Tennyson GE, Bale AE, et al. A base mutation of the c-erbAβ thyroid hormone receptor in a kindred with generalized thyroid hormone resistance. Molecular heterogeneity in two other kindreds. *J Clin Invest* 1990;85:93–100.

34. Weiss RE, Weinberg M, Refetoff S. Identical mutations in unrelated families with generalized resistance to thyroid hormone occur in cytosine-guanine-rich areas of the thyroid hormone receptor beta gene: analysis of 15 families. *J Clin Invest* 1993; 91:2408–2415.

35. Kaneshige M, Suzuki H, Kaneshige K, et al. A targeted dominant negative mutation of the thyroid hormone alpha 1 receptor causes increased mortality, infertility, and dwarfism in mice. *Proc Natl Acad Sci U S A* 2001;98:15095–15100.

36. Tinnikov A, Nordstrom K, Thoren P, et al. Retardation of postnatal development caused by a negatively acting thyroid hormone alpha1. *EMBO J* 2002;21:5079–5087.

37. Liu YY, Schultz JJ, Brent GA. A thyroid hormone receptor alpha gene mutation (P398H) Is associated with visceral adiposity and impaired catecholamine-stimulated lipolysis in mice. *J Biol Chem* 2003;278:38913–38920.

38. McCabe CJ, Gittoes NJ, Sheppard MC, et al. Thyroid receptor α1 and α2 mutations in nonfunctioning pituitary tumors. *J Clin Endocrinol Metab* 1999;84:649–653.

39. Sadow P, Reutrakul S, Weiss RE, et al. Resistance to thyroid hormone in the absence of mutations in the thyroid hormone receptor genes. *Curr Opin Endocrinol Diabetes* 2000;7:253–259.

40. Mitsuhashi T, Tennyson GE, Nikodem VM. Alternative splicing generates messages encoding rat c-erbA proteins that do not bind thyroid hormones. *Proc Natl Acad Sci U S A* 1988;85:5804–5805.

41. Macchia PE, Takeuchi Y, Kawai T, et al. Increased sensitivity to thyroid hormone in mice with complete deficiency of thyroid hormone receptor alpha. *Proc Natl Acad Sci U S A* 2001;98:349–354.

42. Chassande O, Fraichard A, Gauthier K, et al. Identification of transcripts initiated from an internal promoter in the c-erb-Aα locus that encode inhibitors of retinoic acid receptor-α and triiodothyronine receptor activities. *Mol Endocrinol* 1997;11:1278–1290.

43. Williams GR. Cloning and characterization of two novel thyroid hormone receptor beta isoforms. *Mol Cell Biol* 2000; 20:8329–8342.

44. Gauthir K, Plateroti M, Harvey CB, et al. Genetic analysis reveals different functions for the products of the thyroid hormone receptor alpha locus. *Mol Cell Biol* 2001;21:4748–4760.

45. Casas F, Rochard P, Rodier A, et al. A variant form of the nuclear triiodothyronine receptor c-ErbAalpha1 plays a direct role in regulation of mitochondrial RNA synthesis. *Mol Cell Biol* 1999;19:7913–7924.

46. Hodin RA, Lazar MA, Chin WW. Differential and tissue-specific regulation of the multiple rat c-erbA messenger RNA species by thyroid hormone. *J Clin Invest* 1990;85:101–105.

47. Macchia E, Nakai A, Janiga A, et al. Characterization of site-specific polyclonal antibodies to c-erbA peptides recognizing human thyroid hormone receptors α1, α2, and β and native 3,5,3'-triiodothyronine receptor, and study of tissue distribution of the antigen. *Endocrinology* 1990;126:3232–3239.

48. Strait KA, Schwartz HL, Perez-Castillo A, et al. Relationship of c-erbA mRNA content to tissue triiodothyronine nuclear binding capacity and function in developing and adult rats. *J Biol Chem* 1990;265:10514–10521.

49. Mannavola D, Moeller LC, Beck-Peccoz P, et al. A novel splice variant involving the 5' untranslated region of the thyroid hormone receptor β1 (TRβ1). *J Endocrinol Invest* 2004;27:318–322.

50. Frankton S, Harvey CB, Gleason LM, et al. Multiple mRNA variants regulate cell-specific expression of human thyroid hormone receptor β1. *Mol Endocrinol* 2004;18:1631–1642.

51. Gauthier K, Chassande O, Plateroti M, et al. Different functions for the thyroid hormone receptors TRα and TRβ in the control of thyroid hormone production and post-natal development. *EMBO J* 1999;18:623–631.

52. Göthe S, Wang Z, Ng L, et al. Mice devoid of all known thyroid hormone receptors are viable but exhibit disorders of the pituitary-thyroid axis, growth, and bone maturation. *Genes Dev* 1999;13:1329–1341.

53. Escriva H, Safi R, Hänni C, et al. Ligand binding was acquired during evolution evolution of nuclear receptors. *Proc Natl Acad Sci U S A* 1997;94:6803–6808.

54. Forman BM, Casanova J, Raaka BM, et al. Half-site spacing and orientation determines whether thyroid hormone and retinoic acid receptors and related factors bind to DNA response elements as monomers, homodimers, or heterodimers. *Mol Endocrinol* 1992;6:429–442.

55. Glass CK. Differential recognition of target genes by nuclear receptor monomers, dimers and heterodimers. *Endocr Rev* 1994; 15:391–407.

56. Brent GA, Dunn MK, Harney JW, et al. Thyroid hormone aporeceptor represses T3-inducible promoters and blocks activity of the retinoic acid receptor. *New Biologist* 1989;1:329–336.

57. Koenig RJ. Thyroid hormone receptor coactivators and corepressors. *Thyroid* 1998;8:703–713.

58. Pazin MJ, Kadonaga JT. What's up and down with histone deacetylation and transcription? *Cell* 1997;89:325–328.

59. Yen PM, Darling DS, Carter RL, et al. Triiodothyronine (T3) decreases binding to DNA by T3-receptor homodimers but not receptor-auxiliary protein heterodimers. *J Biol Chem* 1992;267:3565–3568.

60. Glass CK, Rose DW, Rosenfeld MG. Nuclear receptor coactivators. *Curr Opin Cell Biol* 1997;9:222–232.

61. Fondell JD, Guermah M, Malik S, et al. Thyroid hormone receptor-associated proteins and general positive cofactors mediate thyroid hormone receptor function in the absence of the TATA box-binding protein-associated factors of TFIID. *Proc Natl Acad Sci U S A* 1999;96:1959–1964.

62. Newell FW, Diddie KR. Typische Monochromasie, angeborene Taubheit und Resistenz gegenüber der intrazellulären Wikung des Thyroideahormons. *Klin Mbl Augenheilk* 1977;171:731–734.

63. Jones I, Srinivas M, Ng L, et al. The thyroid hormone receptor beta gene: structure and functions in the brain and sensory systems. *Thyroid* 2003;13:1057–1068.

64. Hayashi Y, Janssen OE, Weiss RE, et al. The relative expression of mutant and normal thyroid hormone receptor genes in patients with generalized resistance to thyroid hormone determined by estimation of their specific messenger ribonucleic acid products. *J Clin Endocrinol Metab* 1993;76:64–69.

65. Sakurai A, Miyamoto T, Refetoff S, et al. Dominant negative transcriptional regulation by a mutant thyroid hormone receptor β in a family with generalized resistance to thyroid hormone. *Mol Endocrinol* 1990;4:1988–1994.

66. Chatterjee VKK, Nagaya T, Madison LD, et al. Thyroid hormone resistance syndrome. Inhibition of normal receptor function by mutant thyroid hormone receptors. *J Clin Invest* 1991;87:1977–1984.

67. Usala SJ, Menke JB, Watson TL, et al. A homozygous deletion in the c-erbAβ thyroid hormone receptor gene in a patient with generalized thyroid hormone resistance: isolation and characterization of the mutant receptor. *Mol Endocrinol* 1991;5:327–335.

68. Yen PM, Sugawara A, Refetoff S, Chin WW. New insights on the mechanism(s) of the dominant negative effect of mutant thyroid hormone receptor in generalized resistance to thyroid hormone. *J Clin Invest* 1992;90:1825–1831.

69. Piedrafita FJ, Ortiz MA, Pfahl M. Thyroid hormone receptor-β mutants, associated with generalized resistance to thyroid hormone show defects in their ligand-sensitive repression function. *Mol Endocrinol* 1995;9:1533–1548.

70. Hao E, Menke JB, Smith AM, et al. Divergent dimerization properties of mutant β1 thyroid hormone receptors are associated with different dominant negative activities. *Mol Endocrinol* 1994;8:841–851.

71. Nagaya T, Jameson JL. Thyroid hormone receptor dimerization is required for the dominant negative inhibition by mutations that cause thyroid hormone resistance. *J Biol Chem* 1993;268:15766–15771.

72. Yoh SM, Chatterjee VKK, Privalsky ML. Thyroid hormone resistance syndrome manifests as an aberrant interaction between mutant T₃ receptor and transcriptional corepressor. *Mol Endocrinol* 1997;11:470–480.

73. Tagami T, Gu W-X, Peairs PT, et al. A novel natural mutation in the thyroid hormone receptor defines a dual functional domain that exchanges nuclear receptor corepressors and coactivators. *Mol Endocrinol* 1998;12:1888–1902.

74. Collingwood TN, Rajanayagam O, Adams M, et al. A natural transactivation mutation in the thyroid hormone β receptor: impaired interaction with putative transcriptional mediators. *Proc Natl Acad Sci U S A* 1997;94:248–253.

75. Liu Y, Takeshita A, Misiti S, et al. Lack of coactivator interaction can be a mechanism for dominant negative activity by mutant thyroid hormone receptors. *Endocrinology* 1998;139: 4197–4204.

76. Collingwood TN, Wagner R, Matthews CH, et al. A role for helix 3 of the TRβ ligand-binding domain in coactivator recruitment identified by characterization of a third cluster of mutations in resistance to thyroid hormone. *EMBO J* 1998;16: 4760–4770.

77. Nagaya T, Madison LD, Jameson JL. Thyroid hormone receptor mutants that cause resistance to thyroid hormone. Evidence for receptor competition for DNA sequences in target genes. *J Biol Chem* 1992;267:13014–13019.

78. Nagaya T, Fujieda N, Seo H. Requirement of corepressor binding of thyroid hormone receptor mutants for dominant negative inhibition. *Biochem Biophys Res Commun* 1998;247:620–623.

79. Hayashi Y, Sunthornthepvarakul T, Refetoff S. Mutations of CpG dinucleotides located in the triiodothyronine (T₃)-binding domain of the thyroid hormone receptor (TR) β gene that appears to be devoid of natural mutations may not be detected because they are unlikely to produce the clinical phenotype of resistance to thyroid hormone. *J Clin Invest* 1994;94:607–615.

80. Rastinejad F, Perlmann T, Evans F, et al. Structural determinants of nuclear receptor assembly on DNA direct repeats. *Nature* 1995;375:203–211.

81. Wagner RL, Apriletti JW, McGrath ME, et al. A structural role for hormone in the thyroid hormone receptor. *Nature* 1995; 138:690–697.

82. Wagner RL, Huber BR, Shiau AK, et al. Hormone selectivity in thyroid hormone receptors. *Mol Endocrinol* 2001;15:398–410.

83. Marimuthu A, Feng W, Tagami T, et al. TR surfaces and conformations required to bind nuclear receptor corepressor. *Mol Endocrinol* 2002;16:271–286.

84. Huber BR, Desclozeaux M, West BL, et al. Thyroid hormone receptor-beta mutations conferring hormone resistance and reduced corepressor release exhibit decreased stability in the N-terminal ligand-binding domain. *Mol Endocrinol* 2003;17: 107–116.

85. Meier CA, Dickstein BM, Ashizawa K, et al. Variable transcriptional activity and ligand binding of mutant β1 3,5,3′-triiodothyronine receptors from four families with generalized resistance to thyroid hormone. *Mol Endocrinol* 1992;6:248–258.

86. Nagaya T, Eberhardt NL, Jameson JL. Thyroid hormone resistance syndrome: correlation of dominant negative activity and location of mutations. *J Clin Endocrinol Metab* 1993;77:982–990.

87. Hayashi Y, Weiss RE, Sarne DH, et al. Do clinical manifestations of resistance to thyroid hormone correlate with the functional alteration of the corresponding mutant thyroid hormone-β receptors? *J Clin Endocrinol Metab* 1995;80:3246–3256.

88. Yagi H, Pohlenz J, Hayashi Y, et al. Resistance to thyroid hormone caused by two mutant thyroid hormone receptor β, R243Q and R243W, with marked impairment of function that cannot be explained by altered *in-vitro* 3,5,3′-triiodothyronine binding affinity. *J Clin Endocrinol Metab* 1997;82:1608–1614.

89. Safer JD, Cohen RN, Hollenberg AN, et al. Defective release of corepressor by hinge mutants of the thyroid hormone receptor found in patients with resistance to thyroid hormone. *J Biol Chem* 1998;273:30175–30182.

90. Clifton-Bligh RJ, de Zegher F, Wagner RL, et al. A novel mutation (R383H) in resistance to thyroid hormone syndrome predominantly impairs corepressor release and negative transcriptional regulation. *Mol Endocrinol* 1998;12:609–621.

91. Flynn TR, Hollenberg AN, Cohen O, et al. A novel C-terminal domain in the thyroid hormone receptor selectively mediates thyroid hormone inhibition. *J Biol Chem* 1994;629:32713–32716.

92. Kurokawa R, DiRenzo J, Boehm M, et al. Regulation of retinoid signaling by receptor polarity and allosteric control of ligand binding. *Nature (Lond)* 1994;371:528–531.

93. Zamir I, Zhang J, Lazar MA. Stoichiometric and steric principles governing repression by nuclear hormone receptors. *Genes Dev* 1997;11:835–846.

94. Duncan Bassett JH, Williams GR. The molecular actions of thyroid hormone in bone. *Trends Endocrinol Metab* 2003;14:356–364.

95. Johansson C, Göthe S, Forrest D, et al. Cardiovascular phenotype and temperature controlin mice lacking thyroid hormone receptor β or both α1 and β. *Am J Physiol* 1999;276:H2006–H2012.

96. Gloss B, Trost SU, Bluhm WF, et al. Cardiac ion channel expression and contractile function in mice with deletion of thyroid hormone receptor alpha or ss. *Endocrinology* 2001;142:544–550.

97. Kahaly GJ, Matthews CH, Mohr-Kahaly S, et al. Cardiac involvement in thyroid hormone resistance. *J Clin Endocrinol Metab* 2002;87:204–122.

98. Lazar MA. Thyroid hormone receptors: multiple forms, multiple possibilities. *Endocr Rev* 1993;14:184–193.

99. Falcone M, Miyamoto T, Fierro-Renoy F, et al. Antipeptide polyclonal antibodies specifically recognize each human thyroid hormone receptor isoform. *Endocrinology* 1992;131:2419–2429.

100. Mixson AJ, Hauser P, Tennyson G, et al. Differential expression of mutant and normal beta T$_3$ receptor alleles in kindreds with generalized resistance to thyroid hormone. *J Clin Invest* 1993;91:2296–2300.

101. Geffner ME, Su F, Ross NS, et al. An arginine to histidine mutation in codon 311 of the C-erbAβ gene results in a mutant thyroid hormone receptor that does not mediate a dominant negative phenotype. *J Clin Invest* 1993;91:538–546.

102. Weiss RE, Stein MA, Duck SC, et al. Low intelligence but not attention deficit hyperactivity disorder is associated with resistance to thyroid hormone caused by mutation R316H in the thyroid hormone receptor β gene. *J Clin Endocrinol Metab* 1994;78:1525–1528.

103. Weiss RE, Marcocci C, Bruno-Bossio G, et al. Multiple genetic factors in the heterogeneity of thyroid hormone resistance. *J Clin Endocrinol Metab* 1993;76:257–259.

104. Vlaeminck-Guillem V, Margotat A, Torresani J, et al. Resistance to thyroid hormone in a family with no TRβ gene anomaly: pathogenic hypotheses. *Ann Endocrinol (Paris)* 2000;61:194–199.

105. Parikh S, Ando S, Schneider A, et al. Resistance to thyroid hormone in a patient without thyroid hormone receptor mutations. *Thyroid* 2002;12:81–86.

106. Pohlenz J, Weiss RE, Macchia PE, et al. Five new families with resistance to thyroid hormone not caused by mutations in the thyroid hormone receptor β gene. *J Clin Endocrinol Metab* 1999;84:3919–3928.

107. Reutrakul S, Sadow PM, Pannain S, et al. Search for abnormalities of nuclear corepressors, coactivators and a coregulator in families with resistance to thyroid hormone without thyroid hormone receptor β or α genes mutations. *J Clin Endocrinol Metab* 2000;85:3609–3617.

108. Flamant F, Samarut J. Thyroid hormone receptors: lessons from knockout and knock-in mutant mice. *Trends Endocrinol Metab* 2003;14:85–90.

109. Forrest D, Hanebuth E, Smeyne RJ, et al. Recessive resistance to thyroid hormone in mice lacking thyroid hormone receptor β: evidence for tissue-specific modulation of receptor function. *EMBO J* 1996;15:3006–3015.

110. Weiss RE, Forrest D, Pohlenz J, et al. Thyrotropin regulation by thyroid hormone in thyroid hormone receptor β-deficient mice. *Endocrinology* 1997;138:3624–3629.

111. Weiss RE, Murata Y, Cua K, et al. Thyroid hormone action on liver, heart and energy expenditure in thyroid hormone receptor β deficient mice. (Erratum 2000;141:4767). *Endocrinology* 1998;139:4945–4952.

112. Forrest D, Erway LC, Ng L, et al. Thyroid hormone receptor β is essential for development of auditory function. *Nat Genet* 1996;13:354–357.

113. Ng L, Hurley JB, Dierks B, et al. A thyroid hormone receptor that is required for the development of green cone photoreceptors. *Nat Genet* 2001;27:94–98.

114. Rüsch A, Erway LC, Oliver D, et al. Thyroid hormone receptor β-dependent expression of a potassium conductance in inner hair cells at the onset of hearing. *Proc Natl Acad Sci U S A* 1998;95:15758–15762.

115. Abel ED, Boers ME, Pazos-Moura C, et al. Divergent roles for thyroid hormone receptor beta isoforms in the endocrine axis and auditory system. *J Clin Invest* 1999;104:291–300.

116. Wikström L, Johansson C, Salto C, et al. Abnormal heart rate and body temperature in mice lacking thyroid hormone receptor α1. *EMBO J* 1998;17:455–461.

117. Gullberg H, Rudling M, Salto C, et al. Requirement for thyroid hormone receptor Beta in t(3) regulation of cholesterol metabolism in mice. *Mol Endocrinol* 2002;16:1767–1777.

118. Fraichard A, Chassande O, Plateroti M, et al. The T$_3$Rα gene encoding a thyroid hormone receptor is essential for post-natal development and thyroid hormone production. *EMBO J* 1997;16:4412–4420.

119. Mansouri A, Chawdhury K, Gruss P. Follicular cells of the thyroid gland require Pax8 gene function. *Nat Genet* 1998;19:87–90.

120. Flamant F, Poguet AL, Plateroti M, et al. Congenital hypothyroid Pax8(−/−) mutant mice can be rescued by inactivating the TRalpha gene. *Mol Endocrinol* 2002;16:24–32.

121. Hayashi Y, Mangoura D, Refetoff S. A mouse model of resistance to thyroid hormone produced by somatic gene transfer of a mutant thyroid hormone receptor. *Mol Endocrinol* 1996;10:100–106.

122. Wong R, Vasilyev VV, Ting Y-T, et al. Transgenic mice bearing a human mutant thyroid hormone β1 receptor manifest thyroid function anomalies, weight reduction, and hyperactivity. *Mol Med* 1997;3:303–314.

123. Kaneshige M, Kaneshige K, Zhu X-g, et al. Mice with a targeted mutation in the thyroid hormone β receptor gene exhibit impaired growth and resistance to thyroid hormone. *Proc Natl Acad Sci U S A* 2000;97:13209–13214.

124. Hashimoto K, Curty FH, Borges PP, et al. An unliganded thyroid hormone receptor causes severe neurological dysfunction. *Proc Natl Acad Sci U S A* 2001;98:3998–4003.

125. Weiss RE, Xu J, Ning G, et al. Mice deficient in the steroid receptor coactivator-1 (SRC-1) are resistant to thyroid hormone. *EMBO J* 1999;18:1900–1904.

126. Brown NS, Smart A, Sharma V, et al. Thyroid hormone resistance and increased metabolic rate in the RXR-γ-deficient mouse. *J Clin Invest* 2000;106:73–79.

127. Itoh Y, Esaki T, Kaneshige M, et al. Brain glucose utilization in mice with a targeted mutation in the thyroid hormone alpha or beta receptor gene. *Proc Natl Acad Sci U S A* 2001;98:9913–9918.

128. Esaki T, Suzuki H, Cook M, et al. Functional activation of cerebral metabolism in mice with mutated thyroid hormone nuclear receptors. *Endocrinology* 2003;144:4117–4122.

129. Persani L, Borgato S, Romoli R, et al. Changes in the degree of sialylation of carbohydrate chain modify the biological properties of circulating thyrotropin isoforms in various physiological and pathological states. *J Clin Endocrinol Metab* 1998;83:2486–2492.

130. Lamberg B-A, Liewendahl K. Thyroid hormone resistance. *Ann Clin Res* 1980;12:243–253.

131. Refetoff S, Salazar A, Smith TJ, et al. The consequences of inappropriate treatment because of failure to recognize the syndrome of pituitary and peripheral tissue resistance to thyroid hormone. *Metabolism* 1983;32:822–834.

132. Bode HH, Danon M, Weintraub BD, et al. Partial target organ resistance to thyroid hormone. *J Clin Invest* 1973;52:776–782.

133. Tamagna EI, Carlson HE, Hershman JM, et al. Pituitary and peripheral resistance to thyroid hormone. *Clin Endocrinol* 1979;10:431–441.

134. Bajorunas DR, Rosner W, Kourides IA. Use of bromocriptine in a patient with generalized resistance to thyroid hormone. *J Clin Endocrinol Metab* 1984;58:731–735.

135. Refetoff S, DeGroot LJ, Barsano CP. Defective thyroid hormone feedback regulation in the syndrome of peripheral resistance to thyroid hormone. *J Clin Endocrinol Metab* 1980;51:41–45.

136. Kaplowitz PB, D'Ercole AJ, Utiger RD. Peripheral resistance to thyroid hormone in an infant. *J Clin Endocrinol Metab* 1981; 53:958–963.

137. Murata Y, Refetoff S, Horwitz AL, et al. Hormonal regulation of glycosaminoglycan accumulation in fibroblasts from patients with resistance to thyroid hormone. *J Clin Endocrinol Metab* 1983;57:1233–1239.

138. Ceccarelli P, Refetoff S, Murata Y. Resistance to thyroid hormone diagnosed by the reduced response of fibroblasts to the triiodothyronine induced suppression of fibronectin synthesis. *J Clin Endocrinol Metab* 1987;65:242–246.

139. Mäenpää J, Liewendahl K. Peripheral insensitivity to thyroid hormones in a euthyroid girl with goitre. *Arch Dis Child* 1980; 55:207–212.

140. White P, Burton KA, Fowden AL, et al. Developmental expression analysis of thyroid hormone receptor isoforms reveals new insights into their essential functions in cardiac and skeletal muscles. *FASEB J* 2001;15:1367–1376.

141. Refetoff S, DeGroot LJ, Benard B, et al. Studies of a sibship with apparent hereditary resistance to the intracellular action of thyroid hormone. *Metabolism* 1972;21:723–756.

142. Cooper DS, Ladenson PW, Nisula BC, et al. Familial thyroid hormone resistance. *Metabolism* 1982;31:504–509.

143. Vandalem JL, Pirens G, Hennen G. Familial inappropriate TSH secretion: evidence suggesting a dissociated pituitary resistance to T$_3$ and T$_4$. *J Endocrinol Invest* 1981;4:413–422.

144. Lamberg BA, Sandström R, Rosengård S, et al. Sporadic and familial partial peripheral resistance to thyroid hormone. In: Harland WA, Orr JS, eds. *Thyroid hormone metabolism*. London: Academic, 1975:139–161.

145. Brucker-Davis F, Skarulis MC, Grace MB, et al. Genetic and clinical features of 42 kindreds with resistance to thyroid hormone. The National Institutes of Health prospective study. *Ann Intern Med* 1995;123:573–583.

146. Hauser P, Zametkin AJ, Martinez P, et al. Attention deficit-hyperactivity disorder in people with generalized resistance to thyroid hormone. *N Engl J Med* 1993;328:997–1001.

147. Weiss RE, Stein MA, Trommer B, et al. Attention-deficit hyperactivity disorder and thyroid function. *J Pediatr* 1993;123: 539–545.

148. Elia J, Gulotta C, Rose SR, et al. Thyroid function and attention-deficit hyperactivity disorder. *J Am Acad Child Adolesc Psychiatry* 1994;33:169–172.

149. Lamberg BA. Congenital euthyroid goitre and partial peripheral resistance to thyroid hormones. *Lancet* 1973;1:854–857.

150. Bantle JP, Seeling S, Mariash CN, et al. Resistance to thyroid hormones: a disorder frequently confused with Graves' disease. *Arch Intern Med* 1982;142:1867–1871.

151. Chait A, Kanter R, Green W, et al. Defective thyroid hormone action in fibroblasts cultured from subjects with the syndrome of resistance to thyroid hormones. *J Clin Endocrinol Metab* 1982;54:767–772.

152. Schimmel M, Utiger R. Thyroidal and peripheral production of thyroid hormones: review of recent findings and their clinical implications. *Ann Intern Med* 1977;87:760–768.

153. Sarne DH, Sobieszczyk S, Ain KB, et al. Serum thyrotropin and prolactin in the syndrome of generalized resistance to thyroid hormone: responses to thyrotropin-releasing hormone stimulation and triiodothyronine suppression. *J Clin Endocrinol Metab* 1990;70:1305–1311.

154. Kasai Y, Aritaki S, Utsunomiya M, et al. Twin sisters with Refetoff's Syndrome. *J Jpn Pediatr Assoc* 1983;87:1203–1212.

155. Hughes IA, Ichikawa K, DeGroot LJ, et al. Non-adenomatous inappropriate TSH hypersecretion and euthyroidism requires no treatment. *Clin Endocrinol* 1987;27:475–483.

156. Persani L, Asteria C, Tonacchera M, et al. Evidence for secretion of thyrotropin with enhanced bioactivity in syndromes of thyroid hormone resistance. *J Clin Endocrinol Metab* 1994;78: 1034–1039.

157. Lamberg BA, Rosengård S, Liwendahl K, et al. Familial partial peripheral resistance to thyroid hormones. *Acta Endocrinol* 1978;87:303–312.

158. David L, Blanc JF, Chatelain P, et al. Goitre congénital avec résistance péripherique partielle aux hormones thyroïdiennes. Ou syndrome de pseudo-hyperthyroïdie. *Pediatrie* 1979;34:443–449.

159. Gómez-Sáez JM, Fernández Castañer M, Navarro MA, et al. Resistencia parcial a las hormonas tiroideas con bocio y eutiroidismo. *Med Clin* 1981;76:412–416.

160. Gheri RG, Bianchi R, Mariani G, et al. A new case of familial partial generalized resistance to thyroid hormone: study of 3,5,3'-triiodothyronine (T$_3$) binding to lymphocyte and skin fibroblast nuclei and *in vivo* conversion of thyroxine to T$_3$. *J Clin Endocrinol Metab* 1984;58:563–569.

161. Refetoff S, Matalon R, Bigazzi M. Metabolism of L-thyroxine (T$_4$) and L-triiodothyronine (T$_3$) by human fibroblasts in tissue culture: evidence for cellular binding proteins and conversion of T$_4$ to T$_3$. *Endocrinology* 1972;91:934–947.

162. Kunitake JM, Hartman N, Henson LC, et al. 3,5,3'-triiodothyroacetic acid therapy for thyroid hormone resistance. *J Clin Endocrinol Metab* 1989;69:461–466.

163. Magner JA, Petrick P, Menezes-Ferreira MM, et al. Familial generalized resistance to thyroid hormones: report of three kindreds and correlation of patterns of affected tissues with the binding of [^{125}I] triiodothyronine to fibroblast nuclei. *J Endocrinol Invest* 1986;9:459–470.

164. Maxon HR, Burman KD, Premachandra BN, et al. Familial elevation of total and free thyroxine in healthy, euthyroid subjects without detectable binding protein abnormalities. *Acta Endocrinol* 1982;100:224–230.

165. Beck-Peccoz P, Persani L, Faglia G. Glycoprotein hormone α-subunit in pituitary adenomas. *Trends Endocrinol Metab* 1992; 3:41–45.

166. Mornex R, Tommasi M, Cure M, et al. Hyperthyroidie associée à un hypopituitarisme au cours de l'evolution d'une tumeur hypophysaire secretant T.S.H. *Ann Endocrinol (Paris)* 1972;33: 390–396.

167. Rösler A, Litvin Y, Hage C, et al. Familial hyperthyroidism due to inappropriate thyrotropin secretion successfully treated with triiodothyronine. *J Clin Endocrinol Metab* 1982;54:76–82.

168. Anselmo J, Cao D, Karrison T, et al. Fetal loss associated with excess thyroid hormone exposure. *JAMA* 2004;292:691–695.

169. Asteria C, Rajanayagam O, Collingwood TN, et al. Prenatal diagnosis of thyroid hormone resistance. *J Clin Endocrinol Metab* 1999;84:405–410.

170. Weiss RE, Refetoff S. Treatment of resistance to thyroid hormone—primum non nocere. *J Clin Endocrinol Metab* 1999; 84:401–404.

171. Safer JD, Colan SD, Fraser LM, et al. A pituitary tumor in a patient with thyroid hormone resistance: a diagnostic dilemma. *Thyroid* 2001;11:281–291.

172. Anselmo J, Refetoff S. Regression of a large goiter in a patient with resistance to thyroid hormone by every other day treatment with triiodothyronine. *Thyroid* 2004;14:71–74.

INDEX